Pathology

Pathology

Edited by

Emanuel Rubin, M.D.

Gonzalo E. Aponte Professor and Chairman
Department of Pathology
Jefferson Medical College
Thomas Jefferson University
Philadelphia, Pennsylvania

John L. Farber, M.D.

Professor of Pathology
Jefferson Medical College
Thomas Jefferson University
Philadelphia, Pennsylvania

With 40 contributors

Illustrations by
Dimitri Karetnikov

J. B. Lippincott Company
Philadelphia
London   Mexico City   New York
St. Louis   São Paulo   Sydney

To our parents:
Jacob and Sophie Rubin,
Lionel and Freda Farber

and our wives:
Linda Anne and Susan

Acquisitions Editor: Lisa Biello
Developmental Editor: Richard Winters
Manuscript Editor: Patrick O'Kane
Indexer: Julia Schwager
Design Coordinator: Michelle Gerdes
Interior Designer: Bill Boehm
Cover Design: Anthony Frizano
Production Supervisor: Carol Florence
Production Coordinator: Charlene Catlett Squibb
Compositor: Ruttle, Shaw, and Wetherill
Printer/Binder: R.R. Donnelley & Sons Co.

3 5 6 4 2

Library of Congress Cataloging in Publication Data

Pathology/edited by Emanuel Rubin, John L. Farber;
40 contributors. p. cm.
  Includes bibliographies and index.
  ISBN 0-397-50698-8
  1. Pathology.   I. Rubin, Emanuel.   II. Farber, John L.
  [DNLM: 1. Pathology. QZ 4 P29854]
RB25.P38 1988
616.07—dc19
DNLM/DLC
for Library of Congress   87-36647
                                               CIP

The authors and publisher have exerted every effort to ensure
that drug selection and dosage set forth in this text are in accord
with current recommendations and practice at the time of
publication. However, in view of ongoing research, changes in
government regulations, and the constant flow of information
relating to drug therapy and drug reactions, the reader is urged
to check the package insert for each drug for any change in
indications and dosage and for added warnings and precautions.
This is particularly important when the recommended agent is a
new or infrequently employed drug.

Contributors

Vernon W. Armbrustmacher
Col. USAF, MC
Deputy Director, Armed Forces
  Institute of Pathology
Washington, DC

Károly Balogh, M.D.
Associate Professor of Pathology
Harvard Medical School;
Pathologist, New England
  Deaconess Hospital
Boston, Massachusetts

Sue A. Bartow, M.D.
Associate Professor of Pathology
University of New Mexico School
  of Medicine;
Director of Surgical Pathology
University of New Mexico
  Hospital
Albuquerque, New Mexico

Earl P. Benditt, M.D.
Professor of Pathology Emeritus
University of Washington
School of Medicine
Seattle, Washington

Hugh Bonner, M.D.
Adjunct Associate Professor of
  Pathology and Pathology in
  Medicine
University of Pennsylvania
  School of Medicine
Philadelphia, Pennsylvania;
Pathologist, Chester County
  Hospital
West Chester, Pennsylvania

Thomas W. Bouldin, M.D.
Associate Professor of Pathology
University of North Carolina
  School of Medicine
Chapel Hill, North Carolina

Stephen W. Chensue, M.D.
Assistant Professor of Pathology
The University of Michigan
  Medical School
Ann Arbor, Michigan

Wallace H. Clark, Jr., M.D.
Professor of Dermatology and
  Pathology
University of Pennsylvania
  School of Medicine
Philadelphia, Pennsylvania

Daniel H. Connor, M.D., C.M.
Chairman, Department of
  Infectious and Parasitic Disease
  Pathology
Armed Forces Institute of
  Pathology
Washington, DC

John E. Craighead, M.D.
Professor and Chairman,
  Department of Pathology
University of Vermont College of
  Medicine;
Director of Laboratories, Medical
  Center Hospital of Vermont
Burlington, Vermont

Ivan Damjanov, M.D., Ph.D.
Professor of Pathology
Jefferson Medical College
Thomas Jefferson University
Philadelphia, Pennsylvania

Maire Duggan, M.B., M.R.C.
  Path., F.R.C.P.(C)
Assistant Professor of Pathology
University of Calgary;
Staff Pathologist
Foothills Hospital
Calgary, Alberta, Canada

Joseph C. Fantone, M.D.
Associate Professor of Pathology
The University of Michigan
  Medical School
Ann Arbor, Michigan

John L. Farber, M.D.
Professor of Pathology
Jefferson Medical College
Thomas Jefferson University
Philadelphia, Pennsylvania

Cecilia M. Fenoglio-Preiser,
  M.D.
Professor of Pathology
University of New Mexico School
  of Medicine;
Chief of Laboratory Services
Veterans Administration Medical
  Center
Albuquerque, New Mexico

Dean W. Gibson, Ph.D.
Research Microbiologist
Department of Infectious and
  Parasitic Disease Pathology
Armed Forces Institute of
  Pathology
Washington, DC

Victor E. Gould, M.D.
Professor of Pathology
Rush Medical College;
Senior Attending Pathologist
Rush-Presbyterian-St. Luke's
  Medical Center
Chicago, Illinois

Donald B. Hackel, M.D.
Professor of Pathology
Duke University Medical School
Durham, North Carolina

Robert B. Jennings, M.D.
James B. Duke Professor and
  Chairman, Department of
  Pathology
Duke University Medical School
Durham, North Carolina

Kent J. Johnson, M.D.
Professor of Pathology
The University of Michigan
  Medical School
Ann Arbor, Michigan

Robert Kisilevsky, M.D., Ph.D.,
  F.R.C.P.(C)
Professor and Head of Pathology
Queen's University;
Pathologist-in-Chief
Kingston General Hospital
Kingston, Ontario, Canada

Gordon K. Klintworth, M.D.,
  Ph.D.
Professor of Pathology
and Joseph A.C. Wadsworth
  Research Professor of
  Ophthalmology
Duke University Medical School
Durham, North Carolina

Steven L. Kunkel, Ph.D.
Associate Professor of Pathology
The University of Michigan
  Medical School
Ann Arbor, Michigan

Robert J. Kurman, M.D.
Professor of Pathology and
  Obstetrics and Gynecology
Georgetown University School of
  Medicine
Washington, DC

Antonio Martinez-Hernandez,
  M.D.
Professor of Pathology
Jefferson Medical College
Thomas Jefferson University
Philadelphia, Pennsylvania

Wolfgang J. Mergner, M.D.,
  Ph.D.
Professor of Pathology
University of Maryland School of
  Medicine
Baltimore, Maryland

Roberta R. Miller, M.D.,
  F.R.C.P.(C)
Clinical Assistant Professor of
  Pathology
University of British Columbia;
Associate Pathologist
Vancouver General Hospital
Vancouver, British Columbia
Canada

Robert O. Petersen, M.D., Ph.D.
Staff Pathologist
Fox Chase Medical Center;
Jeanes Hospital;
American Oncologic Hospital
Philadelphia, Pennsylvania

Stanley J. Robboy, M.D.
Professor and Chairman,
  Department of Pathology
New Jersey Medical School
University of Medicine and
  Dentistry of New Jersey
Newark, New Jersey

Emanuel Rubin, M.D.
Gonzalo E. Aponte Professor and
  Chairman, Department of
  Pathology
Jefferson Medical College
Thomas Jefferson University
Philadelphia, Pennsylvania

Dante G. Scarpelli, M.D., Ph.D.
Professor and Chairman,
  Department of Pathology
Northwestern University Medical
  School
Chicago, Illinois

Alan L. Schiller, M.D.
Professor of Pathology
New York University School of
  Medicine
New York, New York;
Chief of Ancel U. Blaustein M.D.
  Department of Pathology and
  Laboratory Medicine
Booth Memorial Medical Center
Flushing, New York;
Consultant in Pathology
Massachusetts General Hospital
  and Harvard Medical School
Boston, Massachusetts

Stephen M. Schwartz, M.D.,
  Ph.D.
Professor of Pathology
University of Washington
  School of Medicine
Seattle, Washington

Sheldon C. Sommers, M.D.
Clinical Professor of Pathology
Columbia University College of
  Physicians and Surgeons;
Consultant in Pathology
Lenox Hill Hospital
New York, New York

Benjamin H. Spargo, M.D.
Professor of Pathology
University of Chicago
Chicago, Illinois

James R. Taylor, M.D.
Clinical Assistant Professor
University of Oklahoma
Tulsa Medical College;
Pathologist, St. Francis Hospital
Tulsa, Oklahoma

W. M. Thurlbeck, M.B., F.R.C.P.(C)
Professor of Pathology
University of British Columbia;
Pathologist, B.C. Children's Hospital;
Consultant Pathologist
University of British Columbia
Health Sciences Centre and Shaughenessy Hospital
Vancouver, British Columbia
Canada

Benjamin F. Trump, M.D.
Professor and Chairman, Department of Pathology
University of Maryland School of Medicine
Baltimore, Maryland

F. Stephen Vogel, M.D.
Professor of Pathology
Duke University Medical School
Durham, North Carolina

Peter A. Ward, M.D.
Professor and Chairman, Department of Pathology
The University of Michigan Medical School
Ann Arbor, Michigan

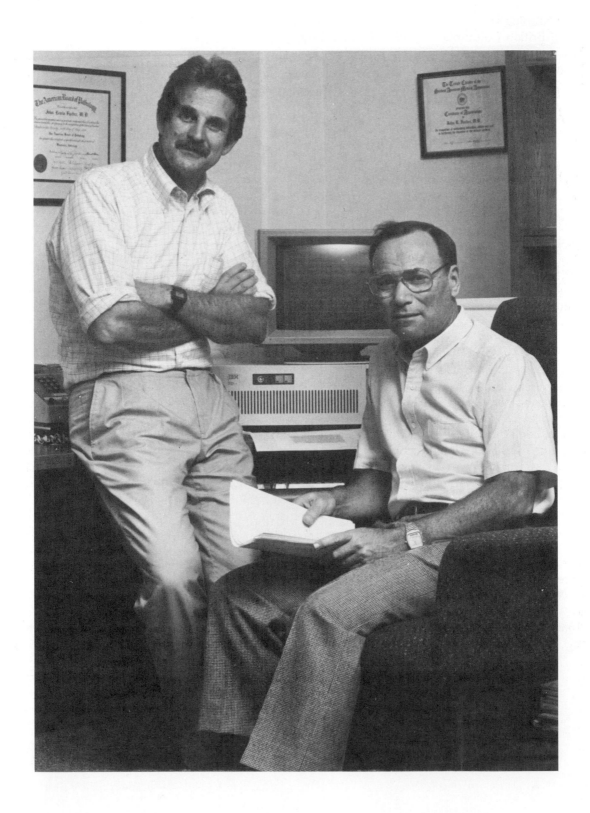

Preface

Pathology has been defined as the medical science that deals with all aspects of disease, but with special reference to the essential nature, the causes, and the development of abnormal conditions. In this sense, literacy in pathology is the bedrock of practice and research for the student of medical science. This book provides such a foundation by presenting classical general pathology and systemic pathologic anatomy in the context of modern biology.

To aid the reader in understanding and retaining complex and detailed information, we have devoted much space to graphic representations of the pathogenesis of disease, the complications of various disorders, and sequences of pathologic alterations. Because graphic images take advantage of pattern recognition, one of the most fundamental characteristics of the human brain, they powerfully communicate abstract and complex material, as any lecturer who has presented a graph will attest. At the same time, we have been guided by Einstein's admonition that "everything should be made as simple as possible, but not simpler." Whereas photomicrographs invariably include some distracting details and artifacts, graphics concentrate only on the essential features. They provide a direct route to the important principles—a "road map" to the basic concepts of pathology. Furthermore, graphics avoid semantic ambiguities and serve as effective summaries of the material presented in the text.

Every photograph included in this work had to pass two tests. It had to illustrate an important morphologic entity by supplementing its description in the text as well as serving as an example of a disease process. We further required that each photograph be sufficiently representative, technically precise, and devoid of artifact as to be clearly interpretable independent of its description in the text.

The scope of contemporary pathology can only be encompassed in a work such as this one through the participation of recognized authorities who are also experienced teachers. Yet we realized that a consistent literary style—beyond that usually found in multi-authored works—coupled with a constant graphic approach was essential for a coherent presentation. This goal required an unusually close working collaboration between the editors, the contributors, and the artist, Dimitri Karetnikov.

In the preparation of this book, we were mindful of the unparalleled advances in biology that have occurred over the past half century. The towering achievements in the study of ultrastructure, biochemistry, immunology, and molecular genetics have had a profound effect on current thinking about the pathogenesis of disease. At the same time, we remained dedicated to Virchow's original concept that ". . . the cell is really the ultimate morphological element in which there is any manifestation of life, and . . . we must not transfer the seat of real action to any point beyond the cell." The marriage of classical morphologic descriptions of disease and contemporary scientific concepts in this book serves to join traditional pathology with the modern revolution in biology.

Emanuel Rubin
John L. Farber

Contents

1 Cell Injury 2
Emanuel Rubin and John L. Farber

2 Inflammation 34
Joseph C. Fantone and Peter A. Ward

3 Repair, Regeneration, and
Fibrosis 66
Antonio Martinez-Hernandez

4 Immunopathology 96
Kent J. Johnson, Steven W. Chensue,
Steven L. Kunkel, and Peter A. Ward

5 Neoplasia 140
Emanuel Rubin and John L. Farber

6 Developmental and Genetic
Diseases 196
Ivan Damjanov

7 Hemodynamic Disorders 250
Wolfgang J. Mergner and
Benjamin F. Trump

8 Environmental and Nutritional
Pathology 274
Emanuel Rubin and John L. Farber

9 Infectious and Parasitic
Diseases 326
Daniel H. Connor and Dean W. Gibson

10 Blood Vessels 452
Earl P. Benditt and Stephen M. Schwartz

11 The Heart 496
Donald B. Hackel and Robert B. Jennings

12 The Respiratory System 542
William M. Thurlbeck and
Roberta R. Miller

13 The Gastrointestinal Tract
628
Emanuel Rubin and John L. Farber

14 The Liver and Biliary Tract
722
Emanuel Rubin and John L. Farber

15 The Pancreas 808
Dante G. Scarpelli

16 The Kidney 832
Benjamin H. Spargo and James R. Taylor

17   *The Urinary Tract and Male Reproductive System*   890
Robert O. Petersen

18   *The Female Reproductive System*   942
Stanley J. Robboy, Maire Duggan, and Robert J. Kurman

19   *The Breast*   990
Sue A. Bartow and Cecilia M. Fenoglio-Preiser

20   *The Blood and the Lymphoid Organs*   1014
Hugh Bonner

21   *The Endocrine System*   1118
Victor E. Gould and Sheldon C. Sommers

22   *Diabetes*   1164
John E. Craighead

23   *Amyloidosis*   1178
Robert Kisilevsky

24   *The Skin*   1194
Wallace H. Clark, Jr.

25   *The Head and Neck*   1260
Károly Balogh

26   *Bones and Joints*   1304
Alan L. Schiller

27   *Skeletal Muscle*   1394
Vernon W. Armbrustmacher

28   *The Nervous System*   1416
F. Stephen Vogel and Thomas W. Bouldin

29   *The Eye*   1500
Gordon K. Klintworth

Acknowledgments   1533

Index   1535

Pathology

1

Cell Injury

Emanuel Rubin and John L. Farber

Cellular Patterns of Response to Stress

Reversible Cell Injury

Morphologic Reactions to Persistent Stress

Irreversible Cell Injury

Calcification

Hyaline

Cellular Aging

Figure 1-1. Interior of an idealized cell.

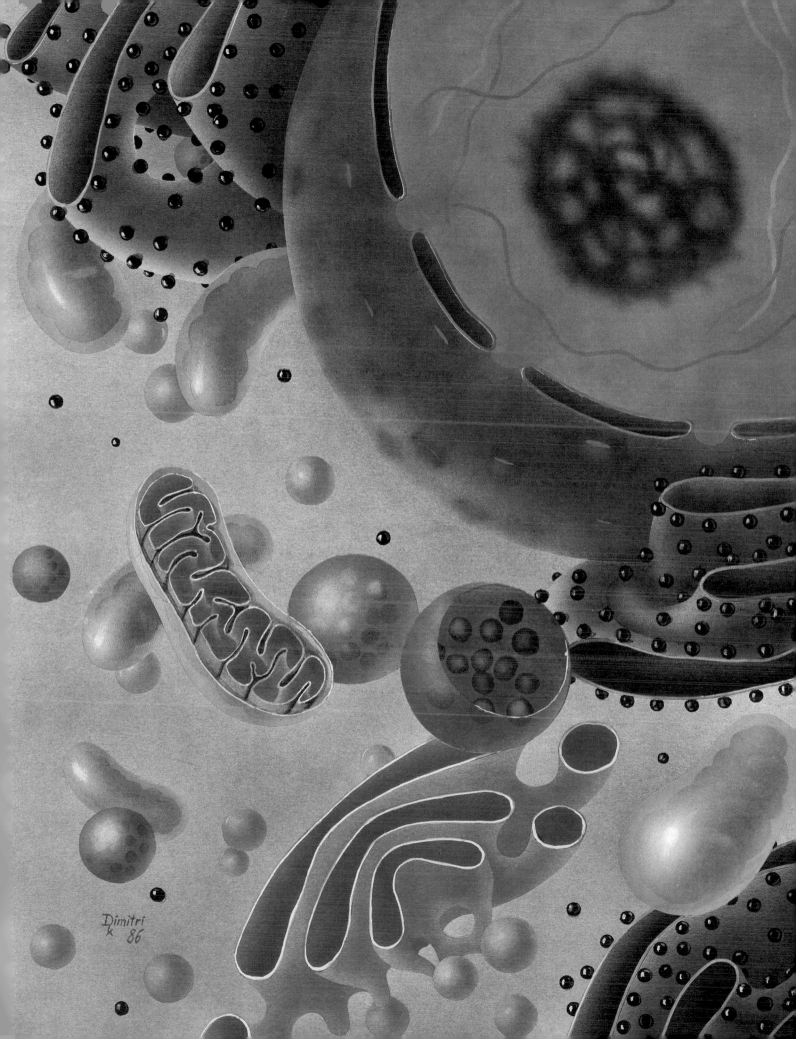

Pathology in its simplest sense is the study of structural and functional abnormalities that are expressed as diseases of organs and systems. Classical theories of disease attributed all disorders to systemic imbalances or to noxious effects of humors on specific organs. In the 19th century, Rudolf Virchow, often referred to as the father of modern pathology, broke sharply with such traditional concepts by proposing that the basis of all disease is injury to the smallest living unit of the body, namely the cell. More than a century later, clinical and experimental pathology remain rooted in Virchow's cellular pathology.

To appreciate the mechanisms of injury to the cell, it is useful to consider its global needs in a philosophical sense. In the reaction against mystical or vitalistic theories of biology, teleology—the study of design or purpose in nature—was discredited as a means of scientific investigation. Nevertheless, although facts can only be established by observations, teleologic thinking can be important in framing questions. As an analogy, without an understanding of the goals of chess and prior knowledge that a particular computer is programmed to play it, no analysis of the machine would be likely to uncover its method of operation. Moreover, it would be futile to search for the sources of defects in the specific program or overall operating system while lacking an appreciation of the goals of the device. In this sense, it is helpful to understand the problems with which the cell is confronted and the strategies that have evolved to cope with them.

If one accepts the premise that a living cell must maintain an organization capable of producing energy, then the most pressing need for a free living cell, whether prokaryotic or eukaryotic, is to establish a structural and functional barrier between its internal milieu and a hostile environment. The plasma membrane serves this purpose in three ways: it maintains a constant internal ionic composition against very large chemical gradients between the interior and exterior compartments; it selectively admits some molecules while excluding or extruding others; and it provides a structural envelope to contain the informational, synthetic, and catabolic constituents of the cell. At the same time, in order to survive, the cell must be able to adapt to adverse environmental conditions, such as changes in temperature, solute concentrations, or oxygen supply, the presence of noxious agents, and so on. The evolution of multicellular organisms eased the hazardous lot of individual cells by establishing a controlled extracellular environment in which temperature, oxygenation, ionic content, and nutrient supply are relatively constant. It also permitted the luxury of differentiation of cells for such widely divergent functions as nutrient storage (liver cell glycogen and adipocytes), communication (neurons), contractile activity (heart muscle), synthesis of proteins or peptides for export (liver, pancreas, and endocrine cells), absorption (intestine), and defense against foreign invaders (polymorphonuclear leukocytes, lymphocytes, and macrophages).

Cells encounter many stresses as a result of changes in their internal and external environments. The patterns of response to this stress constitute the cellular bases of disease. If an injury exceeds the adaptive capacity of the cell, it dies. A cell exposed to persistent sublethal injury has a limited repertoire of responses, the expression of which we interpret as evidence of cell injury. In general, the mammalian cell adapts to injury by conserving its resources; it decreases or ceases its differentiated functions and reverts to its ancestral, unicellular character, which is concerned with functions exclusively dedicated to its own survival. In this perspective, **pathology is the study of cell injury and the expression of a preexisting capacity to adapt to such injury, on the part of either injured or intact cells.** Such an orientation leaves little room for the concept of parallel—normal and pathologic—biologies.

Cellular Patterns of Response to Stress

All cells have efficient mechanisms to deal with shifts in environmental conditions. Thus, ion channels open or close, harmful chemicals are detoxified, metabolic stores such as fat or glycogen may be mobilized, and catabolic processes lead to the segregation of internal particulate materials. It is when environmental changes exceed the capacity of the cell to maintain normal homeostasis that we recognize acute cell injury. If the stress is removed in time, or if the cell is able to withstand the assault, cell injury is reversible, and complete structural and functional integrity is restored. For example, this is the situation when circulation to the heart is interrupted for less than one-half hour. The cell can also be exposed to persistent, sublethal stress, as in mechanical irritation of the skin or exposure of the bronchial mucosa to tobacco smoke. In such instances the cell has time to adapt to reversible injury in a number of ways, each of which has its morphologic counterpart.

On the other hand, if the stress is severe, irreversible injury leads to death of the cell. The precise moment when reversible gives way to irreversible injury, the "point of no return," cannot at present be identified. **The morphologic pattern of cell death occasioned by disparate exogenous environmental stresses is coagulative necrosis.** This type of necrosis is common to almost all forms of cell death and precedes the other forms described below.

Reversible Cell Injury

Hydropic Swelling

Acute cell injury may result from such disparate causes as chemical and biologic toxins, viral or bacterial infections, ischemia, excessive heat or cold, and so on. Regardless of the cause, reversibly injured cells are often enlarged. The greater volume reflects an increased water content and is known as **hydropic swelling, a condition characterized by a large, pale cytoplasm and a normally located nucleus** (Fig. 1-2). The number of organelles is unchanged, although they appear dispersed in a larger volume. The term "cloudy swelling" refers to the gross appearance of injured tissue, but is archaic.

Hydropic swelling results from impairment of cellular volume regulation, a process which controls ionic concentrations in the cytoplasm. This regulation, particularly for sodium, operates at three levels: the plasma membrane itself, the plasma membrane sodium pump, and the supply of ATP. The plasma membrane imposes a barrier to the flow of sodium down a concentration gradient into the cell and prevents a similar efflux of potassium from the cell. The barrier to sodium is imperfect, and the relative leakiness to that ion permits the passive entry of sodium into the cell. To compensate for this intrusion, the energy-dependent plasma membrane sodium pump (Na^+, K^+-ATPase), which is fueled by adenosine triphosphate (ATP), extrudes sodium. Injurious agents may interfere with this membrane-regulated process by increasing the permeability of the plasma membrane to sodium, thereby exceeding the capacity of the pump to extrude sodium; by damaging the pump directly; or by interfering with the synthesis of ATP, thus depriving the pump of its fuel. In any event, the accumulation of sodium in the cell leads to a water increase to maintain isosmotic conditions, and the cell swells.

Ultrastructural Changes

Changes in the ultrastructure of intracellular organelles occur in reversibly injured cells.

Endoplasmic Reticulum With swelling of the cell, the cisternae of the endoplasmic reticulum become

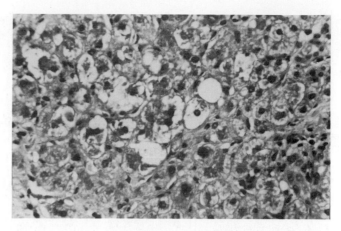

Figure 1-2. Hydropic swelling of liver cells in alcoholic liver injury. The hepatocytes in the center show central nuclei and cytoplasm distended (ballooned) by excess fluid.

dilated, presumably because of shifts in ions and water (Fig. 1-3). Independently, membrane-bound polysomes may undergo disaggregation and detach from the surface of the rough endoplasmic reticulum (Fig. 1-4).

Mitochondria In some forms of injury, particularly ischemia, mitochondria swell (Fig. 1-5). This enlargement is probably caused by the dissipation of the energy gradient and consequent impairment of mitochondrial volume control. Amorphous densities rich in phospholipid may appear, but these effects are fully reversible upon recovery.

Plasma Membrane Blebs of the plasma membrane—that is, focal extrusions of the cytoplasm—are occasionally noted. These can be pinched off and released while the cell remains viable.

Nucleolus In the nucleus, reversible injury is reflected principally in changes in the nucleolus, characterized by the separation of fibrillar and granular components, or a diminution in the latter, leaving naked fibrillar cores.

It is important to recognize that after withdrawal of an acute stress that has led to reversible cell injury, by definition, the cell returns to its normal state.

Morphologic Reactions to Persistent Stress

Persistent stress is often described as leading to chronic cell injury. Yet few if any of the morphologic changes at the cellular level reflect the type of chronic

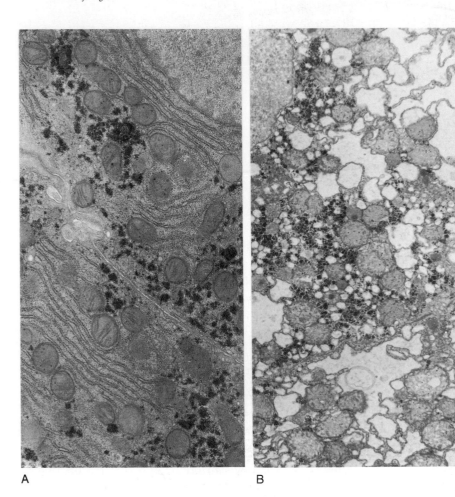

A   B

Figure 1-3. Ultrastructure of hydropic swelling of a liver cell. (*A*) Two apposed normal hepatocytes with tightly organized, parallel arrays of rough endoplasmic reticulum. (*B*) Swollen hepatocyte in which the cisternae of the endoplasmic reticulum are dilated by excess fluid.

damage seen in chronically injured organs. Similar responses to insults at the cellular level can produce different gross appearances in injured organs. For example, chronic ischemia of the brain leads to permanent injury and shrinkage of that organ. Chronic liver injury produces irreversible damage in the form of a diffuse scarring, called cirrhosis. In general, **permanent organ injury** is associated with the **death of individual cells.** By contrast, the cellular response to **persistent sublethal injury,** whether chemical or physical, reflects **adaptation of the cell** to a hostile environment. Again, these changes are, for the most part, reversible upon discontinuation of the stress. In response to persistent stress, a cell dies or adapts. Cells experiencing persistent stress manifest few if any of the characteristic alterations described for acute cell injury. It is thus our view that **at the cellular level** it is more appropriate to speak of **chronic adaptation** than of **chronic injury** (Fig. 1-6). The major adaptive responses are **atrophy, hypertrophy, metaplasia, dysplasia,** and **intracellular storage.** According to some theories, certain forms of neoplasia may also result from adaptive responses.

Atrophy

Atrophy is a decrease in the size and function of a cell. It is often seen in areas of vascular insufficiency or chronic inflammation and may result from disuse of skeletal muscle. Atrophy may be thought of as an adaptive response to stress in which the cell shrinks in volume and shuts down its differentiated functions, thus reducing its need for energy to a minimum. Upon restoration of normal conditions, atrophic cells are fully capable of resuming their differentiated functions; size increases to normal, and specialized functions, such as protein synthesis or contractile force, return to their original levels. Atrophy occurs under a variety of conditions outlined below.

Reduced Functional Demand

The most common form of atrophy follows reduced functional demand. For example, after immobilization of a limb in a cast as treatment for a bone fracture, or after prolonged bed rest, muscle cells atrophy

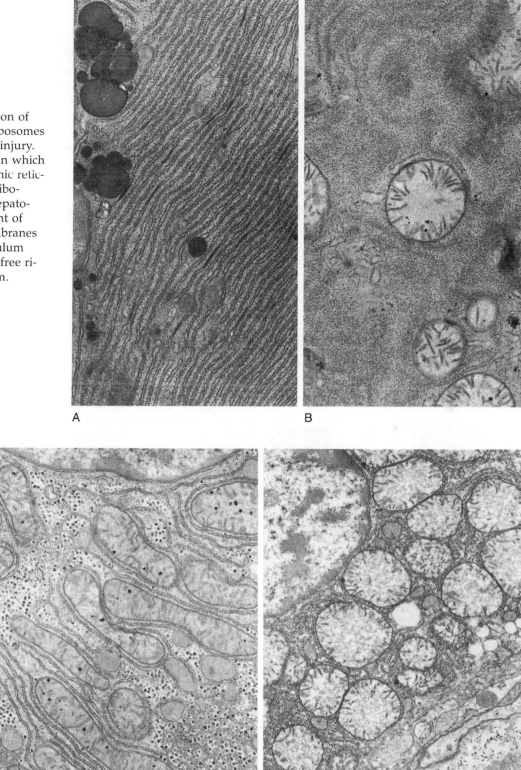

Figure 1-4. Disaggregation of membrane-bound polyribosomes in acute, reversible liver injury. (*A*) Normal hepatocyte, in which the profiles of endoplasmic reticulum are studded with ribosomes. (*B*) An injured hepatocyte, showing detachment of ribosomes from the membranes of the endoplasmic reticulum and the accumulation of free ribosomes in the cytoplasm.

A

B

A

B

Figure 1-5. Mitochondrial swelling in acute ischemic cell injury. (*A*) Normal mitochondria are elongated and display prominent cristae, which traverse the mitochondrial matrix. (*B*) Mitochondria from an ischemic cell are swollen and round, and exhibit a decreased matrix density. The cristae are less prominent than in the normal organelle.

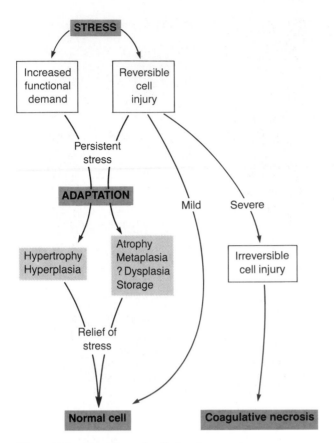

Figure 1-6. Reaction of cells to stress.

and muscular strength is reduced. With resumption of normal activity, normal size and function are restored.

Inadequate Supply of Oxygen

Interference with blood supply to tissues is known as ischemia. Total ischemia, with cessation of oxygen perfusion of tissues, results in cell death. However, partial ischemia occurs after incomplete occlusion of a blood vessel or in areas of inadequate collateral circulation following a complete vascular occlusion. This results in a chronically reduced oxygen supply, a condition often compatible with cell viability. Under such circumstances, cell atrophy is common. It is frequently seen around the inadequately perfused margins of ischemic necrosis (infarcts) in the heart, brain, and kidneys following vascular occlusion in these organs.

Insufficient Nutrients

Starvation or inadequate nutrition associated with chronic disease leads to cell atrophy, particularly in skeletal muscle. From a teleologic point of view, it is striking that reduction in mass is particularly prominent in cells that are not vital to survival of the organism. One cannot dismiss the possibility that a portion of the cell atrophy caused by partial ischemia reflects a lack of nutrients.

Interruption of Trophic Signals

The functions of many cells depend on signals transmitted by chemical mediators. Examples include the endocrine system and neuromuscular transmission. The demands placed on the cell by the actions of hormones or, in the case of skeletal muscle, by synaptic transmission, can be eliminated by removing the source of the signal. This can be accomplished through, for example, ablation of an endocrine gland or denervation. If the anterior pituitary is surgically resected, the loss of thyroid-stimulating hormone (TSH), adrenocorticotropic hormone (ACTH), and follicle-stimulating hormone (FSH) results in atrophy of the thyroid, adrenal cortex, and ovaries, respectively. Atrophy secondary to endocrine insufficiency is not restricted to pathologic conditions—witness the atrophy of the endometrium caused by decreased estrogen levels following menopause. Moreover, even cancer cells can be induced to undergo atrophy, to some extent, by hormonal deprivation. Androgen-dependent cancer of the prostate partially regresses after castration. The growth of certain types of thyroid cancer is halted by inhibiting pituitary TSH secretion with thyroxin. Neurologic conditions resulting in denervation of muscle, and thus in loss of the neuromuscular transmission necessary for muscle tone, cause atrophy of the affected muscles. The wasting caused by poliomyelitis or traumatic paraplegia falls into this category.

Persistent Cell Injury

Persistent cell injury is most commonly caused by chronic inflammation associated with prolonged viral or bacterial infections. Chronic inflammation may be seen in a variety of other circumstances, including immunologic and granulomatous disorders (see Chapter 4). Whether cell injury results from the inciting agent, the inflammatory process itself, or both, is not always clear. In any event, cells in areas of chronic inflammation are often atrophic. Persistent toxic injury, as exemplified by the action of cigarette smoke on the bronchial mucosa, can also cause atrophy. Even physical injury, such as prolonged pressure in inappropriate locations, produces atrophy. Heart failure leads to increased pressure in sinusoids of the liver because the heart cannot efficiently pump the venous return from that organ. Accordingly, the cells exposed to the greatest pressure—those in the center of the liver lobule—become atrophic.

Aging

As discussed below, cell aging is a process independent of disease. One of the hallmarks of aging, particularly in non-replicating cells such as those of the brain and heart, is cell atrophy. The size of all the parenchymal organs of the body decreases with age. The size of the brain is invariably decreased, while in the very old the size of the heart may be so diminished that the term "senile atrophy" has been used.

Hypertrophy

Hypertrophy is an increase in the size of a cell accompanied by an augmented functional capacity. Unlike hydropic swelling, the hypertrophied cell does not contain excess water or electrolytes. Hypertrophy is a response to trophic signals or increased functional demands and is commonly a normal process. **Physiologic hypertrophy** occurs during maturation under the influence of a **variety of hormones.** Sex hormones at puberty lead to hypertrophy of the juvenile sex organs and organs associated with secondary sex characteristics. The lactating woman, under the influence of prolactin and estrogen, exhibits hypertrophy, as well as hyperplasia, of breast tissue.

Although hypertrophy results from certain normal hormonal signals, it is also a response to abnormal levels of hormones. Exogenous anabolic steroids are taken by athletes precisely for their capacity to induce muscle hypertrophy. Endogenous overproduction of TSH by the pituitary is responsible for the thyroid enlargement (goiter) seen with nutritional iodine deficiency. In the absence of sufficient iodine, thyroid hormone is not produced. Consequently there is no feedback inhibition of TSH secretion, and the unopposed TSH, acting as a trophic hormone, induces hypertrophy of thyroid follicular cells. Increased hormone levels can also result from abnormal hormone production by tumors. For example, secretion of ACTH by pituitary tumors results in hypertrophy of the adrenal cortex.

Hypertrophy caused by an **increased functional demand** is exemplified by increased muscle size and strength following repeated exercise. In an analogous fashion, one places an **exogenous** metabolic demand on the liver cell by administering drugs that must be detoxified by the mixed-function oxidase system. Cytochrome P_{450} and other enzymes of this drug-metabolizing system reside in the smooth endoplasmic reticulum. The liver cell responds to the metabolic

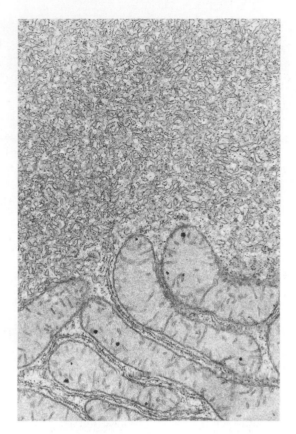

Figure 1-7. Proliferation of smooth endoplasmic reticulum in a liver cell in response to phenobarbital administration.

demand of detoxification by increasing the amount of smooth endoplasmic reticulum, with consequent hypertrophy of the cell (Fig. 1-7). Hypolipidemic drugs cause proliferation of peroxisomes with accompanying liver cell hypertrophy (Fig. 1-8).

Increased demand occurs under pathologic conditions as well. The heart may be called upon to increase its contractile force because of mechanical interference with the aortic outflow, or because of systemic hypertension, a condition requiring the heart to eject blood under higher pressure (Fig. 1-9). As in exercise-induced hypertrophy of skeletal muscle, the myocardial cells enlarge, and the heart may double in weight. Increased demand also results from the loss of functional mass. If one kidney is surgically removed or rendered inoperative because of vascular occlusion, the contralateral kidney hypertrophies to accommodate the increased demand.

It should be emphasized that although the stimulus for hypertrophy may assume various forms, the process must involve complex signals that eventuate in gene expression. Moreover, increased demand may itself lead to hormonal changes, which in turn may interact with other signals.

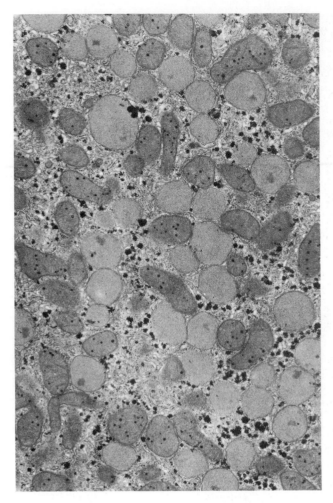

Figure 1-8. Increased number of peroxisomes (*lighter bodies*) in a liver cell exposed to a hypolipidemic drug.

Hyperplasia

While an organ may respond to hormonal signals or increased demands by increasing the size of individual cells, it can also augment function by increasing **the number of cells,** a process known as **hyperplasia.** Hypertrophy and hyperplasia are not mutually exclusive and are often seen concurrently. **Hormonal signals** can induce a physiologic hyperplastic effect. For example, the normal increase in estrogen levels at puberty and during the early phase of the menstrual cycle leads to an increased number of both endometrial and uterine stromal cells. A similar hyperplastic response commonly is produced by the administration of exogenous estrogen in postmenopausal women. Estrogens also produce hyperplasia in men. Gynecomastia, an enlargement of the male breast characterized by hyperplasia and hypertrophy of breast ducts, occurs after the treatment of prostatic carcinoma with exogenous estrogens. Similarly, gynecomastia is seen in patients with chronic liver disease, a malady in which circulating estrogen levels are raised because of diminished hepatic inactivation. Hormones produced by tumors can also lead to hyperplasia. For example, secretion of erythropoietin by cancer of the kidney leads to an increase in the number of red blood cell precursors in the bone marrow.

Hyperplasia, like hypertrophy, may also follow **increased physiologic demand**. Residence at high altitude, where the oxygen content of the air is relatively low, leads to compensatory hyperplasia of red blood cell precursors in the bone marrow and an increased number of circulating red blood cells (secondary polycythemia). The decrease in the amount of oxygen carried in each red blood cell is balanced by an increase in the number of cells. Upon return to sea level, the number of red blood cells promptly falls to normal. Similarly, chronic blood loss, as in abnormal uterine bleeding, causes hyperplasia of erythrocytic elements. The immune system's response to many antigens—a vital mechanism for protection from foreign invaders—constitutes another example of demand-induced hyperplasia. Morphologically, lymphocyte hyperplasia is conspicuous in chronic inflammation caused by conditions such as bacterial infection or transplant rejection. An increased demand for parathyroid hormone results in hyperplasia of the parathyroid glands, a sequence seen in some cases of chronic renal disease. In such cases, decreased calcium absorption from the small intestine results in mobilization of calcium from the bones to maintain appropriate blood calcium levels. This demand is mediated by parathyroid hormone, and the gland responds with an increase in the number of cells.

Persistent cell injury may lead to hyperplasia. Whether such hyperplasia should be viewed as a compensatory response to decreased function or simply as a manifestation of mitotic signals generated by injury is a philosophical question. The point is that, especially in the skin and the lining epithelium of some viscera, chronic inflammation or chronic exposure to physical or chemical injury results in a hyperplastic response. For instance, pressure from ill-fitting shoes causes hyperplasia of the skin of the foot, so-called corns or calluses. It is not too fanciful to consider the primary function of the skin as protection of underlying structures. In this perspective such hyperplasia, with resultant thickening of the skin, serves to enhance functional capacity. Chronic inflammation of the bladder (chronic cystitis) commonly causes hyperplasia of the bladder epithelium, a condition easily viewed grossly by endoscopy as whitish plaques of the bladder lining. Abnormal hyperplasia can itself be harmful—witness the unpleas-

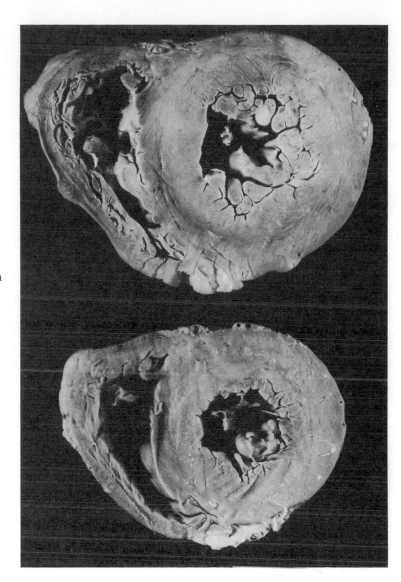

Figure 1-9. Myocardial hypertrophy. Cross section of the heart of a patient with longstanding hypertension (*top*), contrasted with a normal heart (*bottom*). The hypertensive left ventricle is uniformly thickened because of muscular hypertrophy.

ant consequences of psoriasis, a malady of unknown etiology characterized by conspicuous hyperplasia of the skin (Fig. 1-10).

Metaplasia

Metaplasia is the replacement of one differentiated cell type by another, the most common sequence being the replacement of a glandular epithelium by a squamous one. It is almost invariably a response to persistent injury and can be thought of as an adaptive mechanism. Columnar or cuboidal lining cells committed to differentiated functions, such as mucus production, assume a simpler form providing more protection against a pernicious chemical action or the effects of chronic inflammation. Prolonged exposure

of the bronchi to tobacco smoke leads to squamous metaplasia of the bronchial epithelium. A comparable response, associated with chronic infection, is seen in the endocervix (Fig. 1-11).

Metaplasia is not restricted to squamous differentiation; it may consist of replacement of one glandular epithelium by another. In chronic gastritis, a disorder of the stomach characterized by chronic inflammation, atrophic gastric glands are replaced by cells resembling those of the small intestine. The adaptive value of this condition, known as intestinal metaplasia, is not apparent. One also sees metaplasia of transitional epithelium to glandular epithelium in chronic inflammation of the bladder (cystitis glandularis).

It should be emphasized that metaplasia is not necessarily a harmless process, even though this response may be thought of as adaptive. Squamous

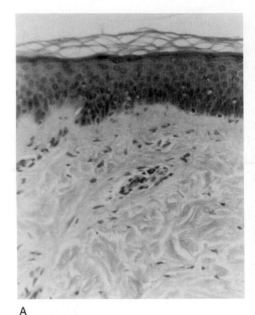

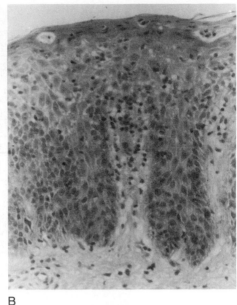

A   B

Figure 1-10. Epidermal hyperplasia. (*A*) Normal epidermis. (*B*) Epidermal hyperplasia in psoriasis, shown at the same magnification as in *A*. The epidermis is thickened, owing to an increase in the number of squamous cells.

metaplasia can impair bronchial function and predispose an individual to recurrent pneumonia. Furthermore, neoplastic transformation may occur in metaplastic epithelium; cancers of the lung, cervix, stomach, and bladder have their origins in such areas. It is unlikely that the metaplastic epithelium itself is responsible for cancer formation. More probably, the noxious stimuli leading to metaplasia are also carcinogenic to metaplastic cells.

Metaplasia is fully reversible. If the stimulus is removed—for example, when one stops smoking—the metaplastic epithelium returns to normal.

Dysplasia

The cells comprising an epithelium normally exhibit regularity of size, shape, and nucleus. Moreover, they are arranged in a regular fashion, as in the progression from plump basal cells to flat superficial cells in a squamous epithelium. **When we speak of dysplasia, we mean that this monotonous appearance is disturbed by variations in the size and shape of the cells; by enlargement, irregularity, and hyperchromatism of the nuclei; and by disorderly arrangement of the cells within the epithelium.** Dysplasia occurs most commonly in hyperplastic squamous epithelium, as seen in epidermal actinic keratosis (caused by sunlight), and in areas of squamous metaplasia, such as in the bronchus or the cervix. It is not, however, exclusive to squamous epithelium. Ulcerative colitis, an inflammatory disease of the large intestine, often is complicated by dysplastic changes in the mucosal cells.

Like metaplasia, dysplasia reflects the persistence of injurious influences and will customarily regress upon, for example, cessation of smoking or cure of chronic cervicitis. However, dysplasia shares many cytologic features with cancer, and the line between the two may be very fine indeed. For example, a common diagnostic problem for the pathologist is the distinction between severe dysplasia and early cancer of the cervix. It is established that dysplasia is a preneoplastic lesion, in the sense that it is a necessary stage in the multi-step cellular evolution to cancer. Severe dysplasia, therefore, is considered an indication for aggressive preventive therapy to cure the underlying cause, eliminate the noxious agent, or surgically remove the offending tissue.

Dysplasia as a process is not easy to reconcile with adaptation. Yet in a teleologic sense, it can be included in this category. The dysplastic cell is less differentiated than its hyperplastic or metaplastic neighbors and is likely more resistant to injury. Although not autonomous in its growth, its replication is clearly not as well regulated as that of the hyperplastic or metaplastic cell. Thus, in terms of its own survival, the dysplastic cell has found ways to cope with a dangerous environment. Such adaptation could be considered beneficial. It not only enhances the survival of the individual cell but also protects the integrity of the tissue. It would not do to have a gaping hole in the bronchus because the epithelial cells were destroyed by cigarette smoke. Unfortunately, the system is not so finely tuned that adaptation stops with dysplasia, and it can overshoot its adaptive mark. The ultimate adaptation is transformation to a cancer cell—a return to the conditions of

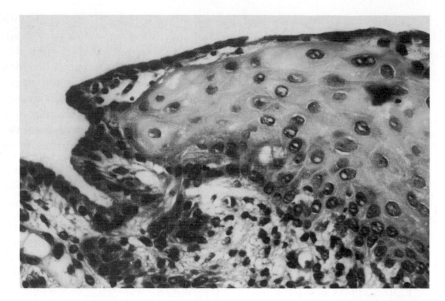

Figure 1-11. Squamous metaplasia. A section of endocervix shows the normal columnar epithelium on the left and metaplastic squamous epithelium on the right.

the free living cell—free of endogenous growth restraints and free to wander, perhaps to a more hospitable environment. Here the needs of the cell clash with those of the organism, since no case can be made for the advantage to the individual of metastatic cancer. Yet cancer has little if any evolutionary impact, since most cancers occur well after the reproductive period.

Intracellular Storage

Intracellular storage is a necessary function of the tissues of multicellular organisms. Bacteria and other unicellular organisms continuously ingest nutrients. By contrast, man is freed from the necessity of continuous eating. He can eat periodically and can survive a prolonged fast because he can store nutrients in specialized cells for later use—fat in adipocytes and glycogen in the liver, heart, and muscle. Yet excess storage of nutrients is not beneficial. Overeating leads to the storage of excess calories as fat—that is, to obesity. Hereditary defects in glycogen metabolism cause excess storage of glycogen, an effect resulting in malfunctions of the organs in which it is normally stored.

Storage is also the mechanism by which certain cells normally deal with substances that cannot be eliminated by intracellular digestion. For example, people living in urban environments commonly inhale carbon particles in the form of soot derived from the burning of fossil fuels. These carbon particles cannot be metabolized or dissolved and would accumulate indefinitely in the alveoli if they were not engulfed by long-lived macrophages. Macrophages containing stored carbon pigment accumulate around respiratory bronchioles, beneath the pleura, and in hilar lymph nodes, an appearance labeled "anthracosis." Anthracosis has no apparent deleterious effect on the macrophage, nor does it lead to any significant loss of pulmonary function. Coal miners may inhale very large quantities of particulate carbon and develop a particularly severe form of anthracosis, so-called **black lung**.

These examples illustrate the important point that **the normal storage functions of specialized cells are exaggerated under a variety of circumstances encountered in human disease.** This can lead to excess intracellular accumulation and storage of a number of substances, such as lipids, pigments, and dusts. In general, the storage of such substances represents a quantitative rather than a qualitative change from the normal. For instance, liver cells always contain some triglycerides because free fatty acids released from adipose tissue are taken up by the liver, where they are either oxidized or converted to triglycerides. Most of the newly synthesized triglycerides are secreted as lipoproteins by the liver. When the delivery of free fatty acids to the liver is increased, as in diabetes, or when the intrahepatic metabolism of lipids is disturbed, as in alcoholism, triglycerides accumulate in the liver cell. Fatty liver is identified morphologically by the presence of lipid globules in the cytoplasm. Other organs, including the heart and the kidney, also store fat. It is important to recognize that fat storage is always reversible, and there is no evidence that the presence of excess fat in the cytoplasm interferes in any way with the function of the cell.

About 25% of the body's total iron content is in an intracellular storage pool composed of the iron-storage proteins, ferritin and hemosiderin. The liver and bone marrow are particularly rich in ferritin, although it is present in virtually all cells. Hemosiderin is a partially denatured form of ferritin that easily aggregates and is recognized microscopically as yellow-brown granules in the cytoplasm. Normally, hemosiderin is found mainly in the spleen, bone marrow, and Kupffer's cells of the liver.

Total body iron may be increased by enhanced intestinal iron absorption, as in an anemia other than that produced by iron deficiency itself, or by parenteral administration of iron-containing red blood cells in a transfusion. In either case, the excess iron is stored intracellularly as both ferritin and hemosiderin. Increasing the body's total iron content results in a progressive accumulation of hemosiderin, a condition labeled "hemosiderosis." In this condition, iron is present not only in the organs in which it is normally found, but also throughout the body, in such places as the skin, pancreas, heart, kidneys, and endocrine organs. The intracellular accumulation of iron in hemosiderosis does not injure the cells. However, there are a number of situations in which the increase in total body iron is extreme; we then speak of **hemochromatosis,** a disorder in which iron deposition is so severe that it damages vital organs—the heart, liver, and pancreas. Severe iron overload of this kind can result from maladies that augment iron absorption, such as chronic liver disease or a hereditary abnormality in iron absorption, or from multiple blood transfusions such as those required in treating hemophilia or certain hereditary anemias.

Excessive iron storage in some organs is also associated with an increased risk of cancer. The pulmonary siderosis encountered among certain metal polishers is accompanied by an increased risk of lung cancer. Hemochromatosis of the liver leads to a higher incidence of liver cancer. The storage of other metals also presents dangers. In Wilson's disease, a hereditary disorder of copper metabolism, storage of excess copper in the liver and brain leads to severe chronic disease of those organs.

Irreversible Cell Injury

If the acute stress to which a cell must react is too great, the resulting changes in structure and function lead to the death of the cell. Among the more common causes of cell death are viruses, reduction in blood supply (ischemia), and physical agents such as ionizing radiation, extreme temperatures, or toxic chemicals. Cell death is almost invariably accompanied by a number of morphologic changes recognizable by the naked eye and by light microscopy, and labeled **coagulative necrosis.** In a few specific circumstances, cell death can be dissociated from coagulative necrosis—for example, in the killing of a cell in tissue culture or by fixation of a biopsy specimen. **It should be emphasized, however, that when a tissue is examined for morphologic evidence of irreversible injury, coagulative necrosis is the criterion by which cell death is identified.** This is not to deny that there is a definable point prior to the appearance of coagulative necrosis when cell injury is irreversible—the point of no return. If such a point exists, however, it cannot be appreciated in any morphologic alteration of the injured cell.

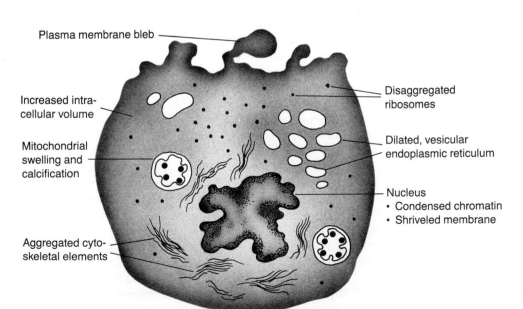

Plasma membrane bleb

Increased intra-cellular volume

Mitochondrial swelling and calcification

Aggregated cyto-skeletal elements

Disaggregated ribosomes

Dilated, vesicular endoplasmic reticulum

Nucleus
• Condensed chromatin
• Shriveled membrane

Figure 1-12. Ultrastructural features of coagulative necrosis.

The Morphology of Necrosis

Coagulative necrosis includes changes in both the cytoplasm and the nucleus (Figs. 1-12 and 1-13). When stained with the usual combination of hematoxylin and eosin, the cytoplasm is more eosinophilic than usual, owing both to a loss of basophilia and to an increased affinity of the cytoplasmic proteins for eosin. The nucleus displays an initial clumping of the chromatin followed by a redistribution along the nuclear membrane. The nucleus then becomes smaller and stains deeply basophilic as chromatin clumping continues. This process is called **pyknosis.** The pyknotic nucleus may break up into many smaller fragments scattered about the cytoplasm, an appearance termed **karyorrhexis.** Alternatively, the pyknotic nucleus may be extruded from the cell, or it may manifest progressive loss of chromatin staining. We then use the term **karyolysis.** The coagulative necrosis of single cells, as occurs with the formation of acidophilic bodies in viral hepatitis, has been called by some "apoptosis."

There are a few instances in which the specific circumstances responsible for cell killing modify the morphologic manifestations of the resulting coagulative necrosis. These changes result in a number of historically well-recognized types of necrosis. With coagulative necrosis, the dead cells persist *in situ* long enough to be identified. In most cases, the necrotic tissue is eventually removed by an inflammatory reaction. When there are particularly large areas of coagulative necrosis, as with the occlusion of a coronary artery and the death (infarction) of a large area of the myocardium, the central region may be inaccessible to the inflammatory process. The necrotic tissue will then persist in place, sometimes for years. In the usual case, regenerative or repair mechanisms accomplish the active removal of necrotic tissue. However, there are two circumstances in which the rate of dissolution of the necrotic cells is considerably faster than the rate of repair. The polymorphonuclear leukocytes of the acute inflammatory reaction are endowed with potent hydrolases capable of completely digesting dead cells. A sharply localized collection of these acute inflammatory cells, generally in response to a bacterial infection, produces the rapid death and dissolution of tissue, so-called **liquefactive necrosis.** The result is often an **abscess** (Fig. 1-14). Coagulative necrosis of the brain as a result of cerebral artery occlusion is frequently followed by rapid dissolution—liquefactive necrosis—of the dead tissue by a mechanism that cannot be attributed to the action of an acute inflammatory response. It is not clear why coagulative necrosis in the brain, and not elsewhere, is followed by the dissolution of the necrotic cells, but the phenomenon may be related to the presence

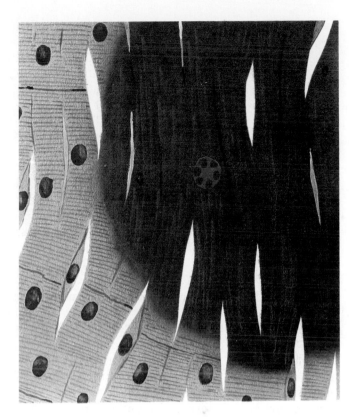

Figure 1-13. Acute myocardial infarction. Obstruction of a coronary artery leads to coagulative necrosis of the myocardium in the ischemic area. The deeply eosinophilic necrotic cells have lost their nuclei and cross striations.

of more abundant lysosomal enzymes or different hydrolases specific to the cells of the central nervous system. The liquefactive necrosis of large areas of the central nervous system can result in the formation of an actual cavity or cyst that will persist for the life of the individual.

Fat necrosis specifically affects adipose tissue and most commonly results from pancreatitis or trauma (Fig. 1-15). The unique feature determining this type of necrosis is the presence of triglycerides in adipose tissue. The process is begun when digestive enzymes, normally found only in the pancreatic duct and small intestine, are released from injured pancreatic acinar cells and ducts into the extracellular spaces. Upon extracellular activation, these enzymes digest the pancreas itself, as well as the surrounding tissues, including adipose cells. Phospholipases and proteases attack the plasma membrane of the fat cells, releasing their stored triglycerides. Pancreatic lipase then hydrolyzes the triglycerides, a process that produces free fatty acids. The fatty acids are precipitated as calcium soaps, which accumulate microscopically as amorphous, basophilic deposits at the periphery of the irregular islands of necrotic adipocytes. On

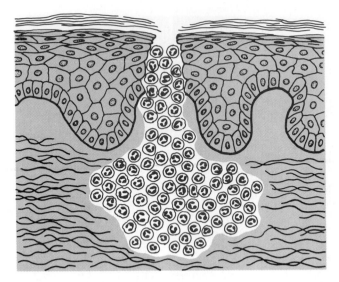

Figure 1-14. Liquefactive necrosis in the epidermis and dermis in an abscess of the skin. The abscess cavity is filled with polymorphonuclear leukocytes.

gross examination, fat necrosis appears as an irregular, chalky white area embedded in otherwise normal adipose tissue. In the case of traumatic fat necrosis, we presume that triglycerides and lipases are released from the injured adipocytes.

Caseous necrosis is characteristic of tuberculosis (Fig. 1-16). The lesions of tuberculosis are the tuberculous granulomas, or tubercles. In the center of such a granuloma, the accumulated mononuclear cells mediating the chronic inflammatory reaction to the offending mycobacteria are killed. In caseous necrosis, unlike coagulative necrosis, the necrotic cells do not retain their cellular outlines. They do not, however, disappear by lysis, as in liquefactive necrosis. Rather, the dead cells persist indefinitely as amorphous, coarsely granular, eosinophilic debris. Grossly, this debris appears greyish-white and is soft and friable. It resembles clumpy cheese, hence the name **caseous** necrosis. This distinctive type of necrosis is generally attributed to the toxic effects of the unusual cell wall of the mycobacterium, which contains complex waxes (peptidoglycolipids) that exert potent biologic effects.

Finally, there is an alteration of blood vessels known as **fibrinoid necrosis** (Fig. 1-17). In this case, the proximity of the blood allows insudation and accumulation of plasma proteins that cause the injured vessels to stain intensely eosinophilic, hence the name fibrinoid necrosis. This term is something of a misnomer, however, because the eosinophilia of the accumulated plasma proteins obscures the underlying alterations in the blood vessel, making it difficult, if not impossible, to determine whether there truly is necrosis of the vascular wall.

The Pathogenesis of Coagulative Necrosis

The morphologic changes constituting coagulative necrosis of cells are not specific for a particular insult. The morphologic manifestation of cell death—coagulative necrosis—is the same regardless of whether the cells have been killed by a virus, by ionizing radiation, or by an interruption in blood supply.

Living cells exist in striking disequilibrium with their external environment. The plasma membrane is the barrier separating the intracellular and extracellular environments. By both passive and active mechanisms, the plasma membrane maintains the numerous concentration gradients that characterize the difference between the intracellular and extracellular milieu. With cell death, these gradients are dissipated. The largest gradient in all living cells is that of calcium. The concentration of calcium ions in extracellular fluids is in the millimolar range ($10^{-3}\,M$). By contrast, the concentration in the cytosol is some 10,000-fold lower, on the order of $10^{-7}\,M$. This large concentration gradient is maintained by both the passive impermeability of the plasma membrane to calcium ions and by the active extrusion of calcium from the cell. It is not surprising, therefore, that coagulative necrosis is accompanied by the accumulation of calcium ions in the dead cells (Fig. 1-18). Calcium ions are biologically very active, and their accumulation in dead or dying cells may actually contribute to the morphologic transformations that characterize coagulative necrosis. The influx and accumulation of calcium ions, and the resultant morphologic changes of coagulative necrosis, can account for the common morphology of cell death. The sequence of events leading to coagulative necrosis may then be described

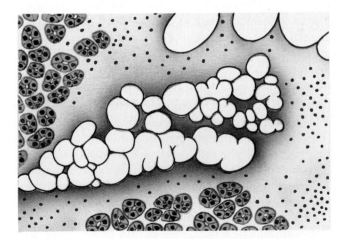

Figure 1-15. Fat necrosis in acute pancreatitis. The release and activation of lipolytic pancreatic enzymes results in the necrosis of surrounding adipose tissue. The hydrolysis of the triglycerides releases free fatty acids, which precipitate as calcium soaps in the necrotic debris.

as (1) irreversible injury and cell death; (2) loss of the plasma membrane's ability to maintain a gradient of calcium ions; (3) an influx and accumulation of calcium ions in the cell; and (4) the morphologic appearance of coagulative necrosis. Under such a scheme, coagulative necrosis occurs after the point of no return—that is, after irreversible injury and "death" of the cell.

Alternatively, cell injury may lead to potentially reversible plasma membrane damage. As a result of this damage, however, the large gradient of calcium ions can no longer be maintained. Excess calcium ions then accumulate in the injured cells and **cause** coagulative necrosis. This second scheme has two specific implications. First, it does not define a stage of cell death distinct from coagulative necrosis. Second, it envisions the accumulation of calcium ions as the point at which potentially reversible cell injury becomes irreversible. There is some experimental data to support such a hypothesis. Agents that block calcium fluxes across biologic membranes have been shown to prevent the coagulative necrosis that usually follows reperfusion of liver cells otherwise irreversibly injured by ischemia. Such experiments are difficult to interpret, however, because we cannot specifically implicate the inhibition of calcium accumulation as the mechanism by which the drug prevents coagulative necrosis. Any alternative action of the drug that results in cyto-protection would similarly prevent the accompanying accumulation of calcium.

The above discussion is summarized by emphasizing that, whatever the role of calcium, **the disruption of the permeability barrier of the plasma membrane seems to be a critical event in lethal cell injury. Loss of the plasma membrane's barrier function results in an equilibration of the concentration gradients that characterize living cells.** As these gradients are dissipated, the cells are transformed into necrotic debris. Necrotic cells accumulate calcium ions. It is also possible that an alteration in intracellular calcium homeostasis is a specific functional consequence of plasma membrane damage. The resultant increase in intracellular calcium possibly determines the loss of reversibility and may mediate the coagulative necrosis of the cells.

Ischemic Cell Injury

The interruption of blood flow—ischemia—is probably the most important cause of coagulative necrosis in human disease. The complications of atherosclerosis, for example, are generally the result of ischemic cell injury in the brain, heart, small intestine, kidneys, and lower extremities. Highly differentiated cells, such as the proximal tubular cells of

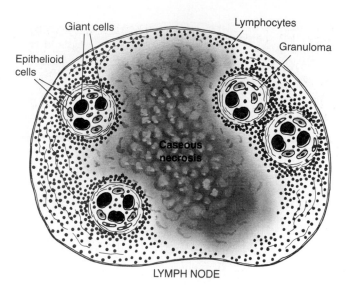

Figure 1-16. Caseous necrosis in a tuberculous lymph node, showing the typical amorphous, granular, eosinophilic, necrotic center surrounded by granulomatous inflammation.

the kidney, cardiac myocytes, and the neurons of the central nervous system, depend on aerobic respiration to produce ATP for the performance of their specialized functions. When ischemia limits the supply of oxygen and ATP is depleted, these cells rapidly manifest many changes in structure and function.

The effects of ischemic injury are all reversible if the duration of ischemia is short. For example, changes in myocardial contractility, membrane potential, metabolism, and ultrastructure are short-lived if the circulation is rapidly restored. However, when ischemia persists, the affected cells become irreversibly injured—that is, the cells continue to deteriorate and become necrotic despite reperfusion with arterial blood. By definition, all metabolic alterations associated with **reversible** ischemic cell injury are either quantitatively or qualitatively insufficient to produce irreversible injury. With longer periods of ischemia, some biochemical alteration develops that causes **irreversible** injury.

Two phenomena illustrate the difference between irreversibly and reversibly injured ischemic cells. An inability to reverse mitochondrial dysfunction upon reperfusion or reoxygenation correlates with a similar inability to reverse the cell injury in general. This finding was originally interpreted as indicating that ischemic cell death is a **consequence** of irreversible mitochondrial injury, particularly since mitochondria develop a series of structural and functional abnormalities with ischemia. However, recent studies have shown that the environment to which reperfusion exposes irreversibly injured cells does not allow mi-

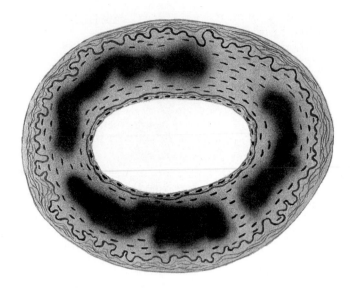

Figure 1-17.   Fibrinoid necrosis in a medium-sized artery. The muscular media contains sharply demarcated, homogeneous, deeply eosinophilic areas of necrosis.

tochondria to recover from injury that would otherwise be reversible. In particular, it has been shown that during reperfusion of irreversibly injured cells a large influx of Ca^{2+} ions occurs. An excess of Ca^{2+} ions is known to induce loss of mitochondrial function, and it may be that the inability to reverse mitochondrial dysfunction reflects the flooding of the cells with Ca^{2+}, rather than being a consequence of the mitochondrial abnormalities themselves.

A disturbance in membrane function in general, and in the plasma membrane in particular, is the second characteristic of the loss of reversibility in ischemic injury. Some have therefore maintained that defective cell membrane function is the primary event in the genesis of irreversible cell injury in ischemia. Indeed, the results of morphologic, functional, and biochemical studies clearly suggest that defects in cell membranes are an early feature of irreversible ischemic cell injury. Yet a definitive understanding of the mechanism underlying membrane damage in irreversible ischemic injury remains elusive. There are, however, potential candidates for this mechanism.

Activated Oxygen

A popular theory postulates a role for partially reduced—and thereby activated—oxygen species in the genesis of membrane damage in irreversible ischemia. The general problem of how activated oxygen species may injure cells is discussed later in this chapter; here, we consider the mechanisms by which activated oxygen is formed in ischemia and the evidence that it injures ischemic cells.

It might seem paradoxical that oxygen species cause cell injury when that injury is attributed to an insufficient oxygen supply. This apparent dilemma is resolved with the realization that toxic oxygen species are generated not during the period of ischemia itself but rather on restoration of blood flow, or reperfusion—hence the term **reperfusion injury.**

A hypothetical scheme holds that some metabolic event occurs during the period of ischemia that results in an overproduction of toxic oxygen species on restoration of the oxygen supply. In particular, xanthine dehydrogenase may be converted by proteolysis into a xanthine oxidase. On return of the oxygen supply, the abundant purines derived from the catabolism of ATP allow oxygen species to be overproduced. This model is supported by the fact that allopurinol, an inhibitor of xanthine oxidase, has the ability to protect cells from reperfusion injury. Antioxidants such as superoxide dismutase, a scavenger of superoxide anions, have the ability to reduce the extent of cell injury, which also supports the hypothesis that activated oxygen damages ischemic cells during reperfusion. Recently it has been suggested that polymorphonuclear leukocytes entering areas of ischemic injury during reperfusion are also a source of toxic oxygen species.

The specific role that reperfusion injury plays in the genesis of irreversible ischemic injury in human disease remains to be defined. Experimental analysis of this phenomenon has progressed rapidly, however, because one can readily control the length of the ischemic insult. We can put reperfusion injury in perspective by emphasizing that there are three different degrees of cell injury, depending on the duration of the ischemia. With short periods of ischemia, reperfusion (and, therefore, the resupply of oxygen) completely restores the structural and functional integrity of the cell. Cell injury in this case is completely reversible. With longer periods of ischemia, reperfusion is not associated with restoration of cell structure and function, but rather with deterioration and death of the cells. As we have seen, this seemingly paradoxical response to reoxygenation is a consequence of the formation of reduced oxygen species upon reperfusion, and it is these activated oxygen species that injure the cells. It is important to emphasize that, in this case, lethal cell injury occurs during the period of reperfusion. The third form of cell injury is characterized by the development of lethal cell injury during the period of ischemia itself; reperfusion is not a factor. A longer period of ischemia is needed to produce this third type of cell injury. In this case, cell damage is not dependent on the formation of activated oxygen species. When cells are reperfused after periods of ischemia that produce this third type of injury, there is an explosive accumulation of sodium and calcium ions in the cells. This accumulation is a result of plasma membrane damage that developed during the period of ischemia—not during reperfusion. How can we account for this membrane damage?

Altered Phospholipid Metabolism

Liver ischemia produces an accelerated phospholipid degradation and accompanying membrane dysfunction. Hepatic microsomal membranes prepared from ischemic livers exhibit, in addition to a variety of other dysfunctions, a 25- to 50-fold increase in their passive permeability to calcium. Microsomes and plasma membranes display aggregations of intramembranous particles, a finding suggestive of phase separations in the lipid bilayer. More recent studies have documented domains of differing fluidity in ischemic microsomal membranes. Interfaces between lipid domains of differing phase or fluidity are thought to be sites of increased permeability. Similar interfaces in the plasma membranes may be the molecular basis of the increased permeability that is evident on reperfusion. Disordered phospholipid metabolism is possibly the critical alteration producing irreversible cell injury, at least in liver ischemia. Fig-

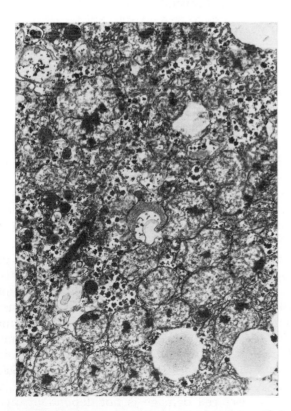

Figure 1-18. Calcium deposits in mitochondria with ischemic necrosis.

ure 1-19 reconstructs events that may produce coagulative necrosis in liver ischemia.

Are disturbances in phospholipid metabolism the basis for irreversible cell injury in myocardial ischemia? Phospholipid degradation is accelerated in myocardial ischemia, but the time frame of net phospholipid loss does not necessarily correlate with the more rapid disruption of the plasma membrane in myocardial cells. On the other hand, the release of arachidonic acid that occurs early in myocardial ischemia may reflect changes in plasma membrane structure that alter membrane permeability, thereby contributing to lethal injury. There is no evidence, however, that the released arachidonate originates from the phospholipids of the plasma membrane.

Cytoskeletal Alterations

The ultrastructural appearance of a disrupted plasma membrane in myocardial cells irreversibly injured by ischemia suggests alternative explanations of plasma membrane damage. Fragmentation of the plasma membrane in ischemic myocardial cells is associated with subsarcolemmic blebs that separate the membrane from underlying myofibrils. These fluid-containing blebs are not present in reversibly injured myocytes. Experimentally, plasma membrane fragmentation identical to that observed in lethal ischemic injury is seen when depletion of high-energy phosphates is combined with cell swelling. With prolonged periods of energy depletion, the plasma membrane becomes injured through an undefined mechanism. This injury then causes the membrane to rupture when the cell swells during ischemia and reperfusion.

The effect of ischemia on the cytoskeleton is another possible mechanism by which plasma membrane structure and function are altered. Microfilaments and intermediate filaments both interact with cell membranes, and several different types of cytoskeleton-membrane interactions have recently been described. Components of the cytoskeleton are observed in cardiac muscle at Z-lines, and intermediate filaments are probably attached to integral proteins of the plasma membrane. The subsarcolemmic blebs seen in ischemic or anoxic myocytes extend over many Z-lines, an appearance indicating loss of their attachments to the plasma membrane. It is possible that cytoskeletal interactions with the plasma membrane are impaired by the high levels of calcium-activated proteases, occasioned by the rise in cytosolic free calcium in cellular anoxia.

Calcium

Calcium ions are sequestered within mitochondria by the energy of the electrochemical gradient (negative

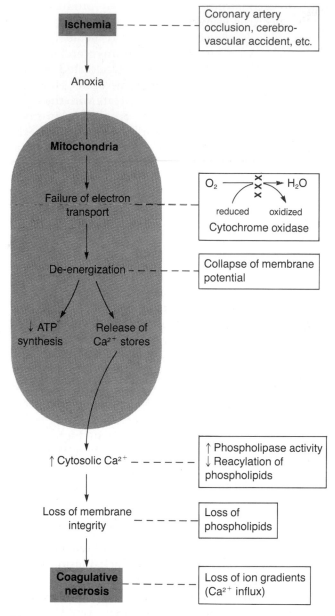

Figure 1-19. Possible sequence of events in the pathogenesis of irreversible cell injury with anoxia-ischemia.

inside) across the inner membrane. Cellular anoxia prevents electron transport, resulting in dissipation of the mitochondrial membrane potential. As a consequence, the sequestered stores of calcium are released from the mitochondria into the cytosol. Cultured cells, however, are relatively resistant to injury if they are depleted of calcium before being made anoxic. This resistance to injury occurs despite collapse of the mitochondrial membrane potential and depletion of ATP. How do changes in intracellular calcium homeostasis in anoxic cells influence the genesis of plasma membrane damage? An elevated cytosolic calcium ion concentration might activate

membrane-associated phospholipases, leading to accelerated phospholipid degradation. Alternatively, an elevated cytosolic calcium ion concentration might activate calcium-dependent proteases.

Cell Injury Caused By Oxygen Radicals

Oxygen has a major metabolic role as the terminal acceptor for mitochondrial electron transport. Cytochrome oxidase catalyzes the four-electron reduction of O_2 to water. The resultant energy is harnessed as an electrochemical potential across the mitochondrial inner membrane.

There are three partially reduced species that are intermediate between O_2 and H_2O, representing transfers of varying numbers of electrons. They are O_2^-, superoxide (one electron); H_2O_2, hydrogen peroxide (two electrons); and $OH\cdot$, the hydroxyl radical (three electrons). These partially reduced oxygen species are not produced by cytochrome oxidase, but are derived from other enzymatic and nonenzymatic reactions (Fig. 1-20).

Superoxide

Components of the mitochondrial electron transport chain may be directly auto-oxidized by O_2 to yield superoxide anions (O_2^-). Superoxide anions are also produced by enzymes such as xanthine oxidase and cytochrome P_{450}. Phagocytosis by polymorphonuclear leukocytes and macrophages is accompanied by increased oxygen consumption, which largely represents the formation of O_2^- by an oxidase in the plasma membrane. O_2^- anions produced in the cytosol or mitochondria are catabolized by superoxide dismutase (SOD). One molecule of H_2O_2 and one molecule of O_2 are formed from two molecules of O_2^-. Hydrogen peroxide is also produced directly by a number of oxidases in cytoplasmic peroxisomes (see Fig. 1-20).

Hydrogen Peroxide

Most cells have efficient mechanisms for removing H_2O_2. Two different enzymes reduce H_2O_2 to water: catalase within the peroxisomes and glutathione peroxidase in both the cytosol and the mitochondria (see Fig. 1-20). Glutathione peroxidase uses reduced glutathione (GSH) as a cofactor, producing two molecules of oxidized glutathione (GSSG) for every molecule of H_2O_2 reduced to water. GSSG is re-reduced to GSH by glutathione reductase with reduced nicotinamide adenine dinucleotide phosphate (NADPH) as the cofactor.

Hydroxyl Radical

Hydroxyl radicals are known to be formed in biological systems in only two ways: by the radiolysis of

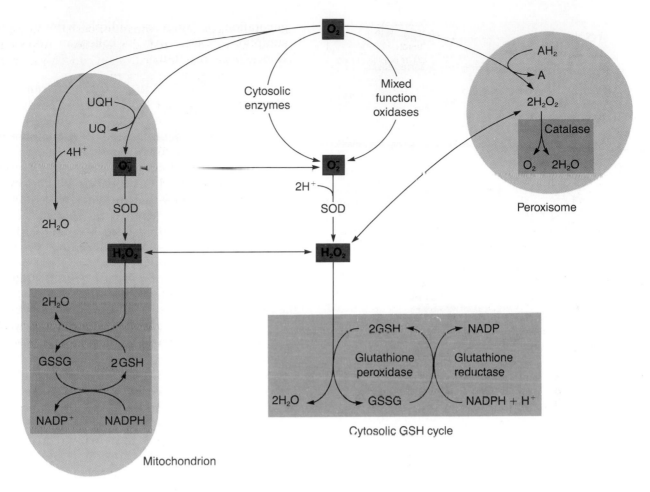

Figure 1-20. Cellular metabolism of oxygen and the accompanying antioxidant defense mechanisms.

water or by the reaction of hydrogen peroxide with ferrous iron (the Fenton reaction).

Activated Oxygen and Disease

Partially reduced oxygen species have been identified as the likely cause of cell injury in an increasing number of diseases (Fig. 1-21). We referred earlier to reperfusion injury when discussing the mechanism of cell injury in ischemia. The inflammatory process, whether acute or chronic, can cause considerable tissue destruction. Partially reduced oxygen species produced by phagocytic cells are important mediators of cell injury in such circumstances. Damage to cells resulting from oxygen radicals formed by inflammatory cells has been implicated in diseases of the joints and of many organs, including the kidney, lungs, and heart. The toxicity of many chemicals may reflect the formation of toxic oxygen species. The killing of cells by ionizing radiation is most likely the result of the direct formation of hydroxyl radicals from the radiolysis of water. There is also recent evidence of

a role for oxygen species in chemical carcinogenesis, during either initiation or promotion.

Cells also may be injured when oxygen is present at concentrations greater than normal. In the past, this occurred largely in those therapeutic circumstances in which oxygen was given to patients at concentrations greater than the normal 20% of inspired air. The lungs of adults and the eyes of premature newborns were the major targets of such oxygen toxicity.

The Role of Iron

How do oxygen species actually produce membrane damage that can result in irreversible cell injury? Although there is little question that partially reduced oxygen species in general can be toxic, there is continuing controversy over the particular role of any one of them. Recent evidence concerning a role for iron in cell injury caused by oxygen species has shed some light on this problem.

All respiring cells require iron; it is used, for ex-

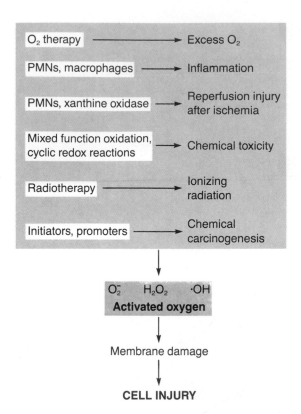

Figure 1-21. The role of activated oxygen species in human disease.

ample, to form cytochromes for electron transport in the mitochondria. Cells obtain iron from the plasma as ferric iron bound to transferrin. Transferrin binds to specific receptors on the cell surface and is delivered to the cytoplasm within an endosome, where an acidic environment releases free ferric iron. Free iron first is used for the synthesis of hemoproteins and then is stored as ferritin; it is subsequently returned to newly synthesized or recycled transferrin and is then secreted by the cell. Cellular iron stores may be mobilized by the autophagocytosis of ferritin. Following fusion of the autophagosome with lysosome, the acid proteases activated by the low pH release free ferric iron. Figure 1-22 summarizes these events, emphasizing the presence of a **pool of free ferric iron formed as a result of both the uptake and the release of iron from cells.**

It is this pool of free ferric iron that seems to be required for partially reduced oxygen species to injure cells. Free ferric iron can be reduced by superoxide anions to ferrous iron. Hydrogen peroxide, formed either directly or (more commonly) by the dismutation of superoxide anions, then reacts with the ferrous iron by the Fenton reaction to produce hydroxyl radicals. This sequence, starting with superoxide anions and ferric iron and leading to the

generation of hydroxyl radicals without the consumption of ferric iron, is called an iron-catalyzed Haber-Weiss reaction.

Hydroxyl Radicals and Lipid Peroxidation

The hydroxyl radical ($OH\cdot$) is an extremely reactive species, and there are several mechanisms by which it might damage membranes. The best known relates to $OH\cdot$ as an initiator of lipid peroxidation (Fig. 1-23). The hydroxyl radical removes a hydrogen atom from the unsaturated fatty acids of membrane phospholipids, a process that forms a free lipid radical. The lipid radical, in turn, reacts with molecular oxygen and forms a lipid peroxide radical. Like the hydroxyl radical, this peroxide radical can function as an initiator, removing another hydrogen atom from a second unsaturated fatty acid. A lipid peroxide and a new lipid radical result, and a chain reaction is initiated.

Lipid peroxides are unstable and break down into smaller molecules (hydroxyaldehydes) that either remain attached to the glycerol backbone of the phospholipid or are released into the cytosol. The destruction of the unsaturated fatty acids of phospholipids results in a loss of membrane integrity. Antioxidants, such as vitamin E, prevent the injury that usually follows exposure of cells to partially reduced oxygen species. This protection is attributed to the inhibition of lipid peroxidation by antioxidants.

Hydroxyl radicals may damage membranes in ways other than lipid peroxidation. Hydroxyl radicals may cause cross-linking of membrane proteins through the formation of disulfide (S—S) bonds. The resulting aggregation of membrane proteins may form ion channels or may otherwise disrupt membrane structure and function. The SH groups of membrane proteins can also be modified by the formation of mixed disulfides in a reaction with GSH, a process dependent on the hydroxyl radical. This modification of membrane proteins has recently been suggested as an alternative to lipid peroxidation as a mechanism by which oxygen species produce irreversible cell injury. Figure 1-24 summarizes the mechanisms of cell injury by activated oxygen species.

How Ionizing Radiation Kills Cells

The discussion of activated oxygen species can be extended to include the mechanism by which ionizing radiation injures cells. The adjective "ionizing" in reference to electromagnetic radiation connotes an ability to effect the radiolysis of water, thus directly forming hydroxyl radicals. These hydroxyl radicals then produce membrane injury by the mechanisms already discussed.

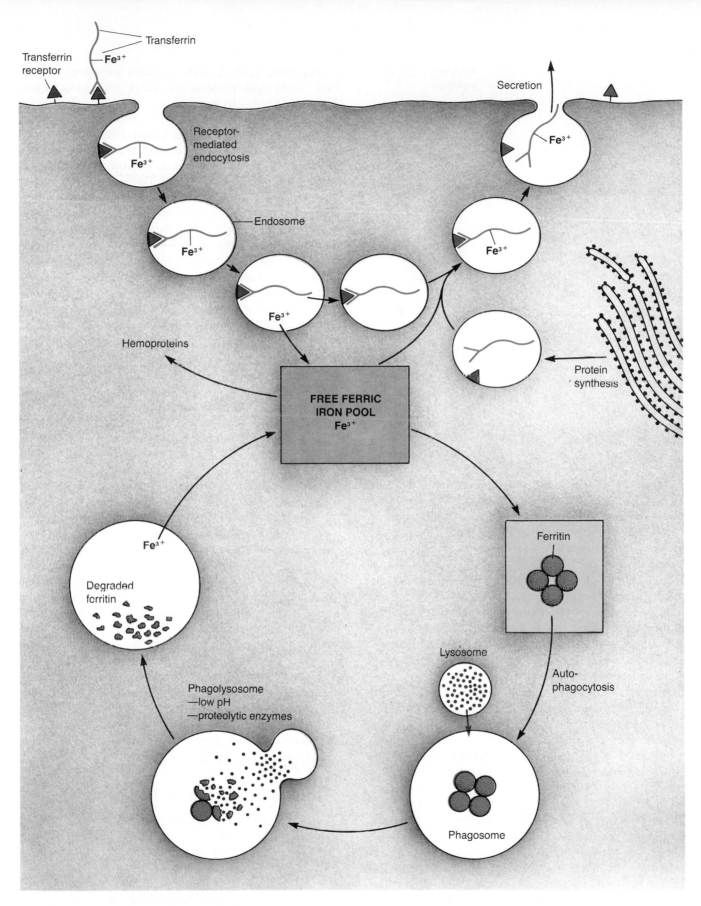

Figure 1-22. Cellular metabolism of iron.

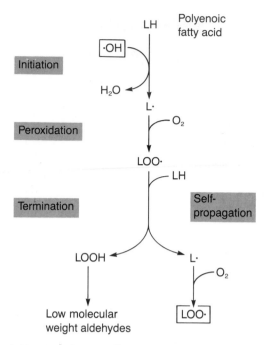

Figure 1-23. Lipid peroxidation initiated by the hydroxyl radical.

Hydroxyl radicals can also interact with DNA. An important functional consequence of such damage is the inhibition of DNA replication. For a nonproliferating cell, such as a hepatocyte or a neuron, the inability to replicate DNA is of little consequence. For a proliferating cell, however, the inability to replicate DNA represents a catastrophic loss of function. Experimental data suggest that once a proliferating cell is prevented from replicating, a mechanism is set in motion that leads to its demise. This mechanism may involve synthesis of new proteins, since it has been shown that an inhibition of protein synthesis prevents cell loss. An induction of cell death on inhibition of cell replication would clearly serve to rid the body of those cells that had lost their prime function. However, further confirmation of this sequence is needed.

Figure 1-25 summarizes the mechanisms of cell killing by ionizing radiation.

How Viruses Kill Cells

Viruses kill cells in two distinct ways. The infection of a cell by a **directly cytopathic virus** leads to lethal injury without the participation of the host immune system. **Indirectly cytopathic viruses**, on the other hand, require the participation of the immune system.

The polio virus is typical of the group of viruses that is directly cytopathic. It consists of a single strand of RNA surrounded by a protein capsule. After binding to specific receptors on the surface of the target cell, the virus is internalized by endocytosis. The endosome fuses with a cellular lysosome to form a phagolysosome, after which the protein capsule is removed by proteolysis. The viral genome is released into the cytosol and is recognized by the protein synthetic apparatus as just another messenger RNA molecule. As a result, the viral genome is translated by the host cell into capsular proteins and a specific RNA polymerase. The polymerase, in turn, leads to replication of the viral genome. Virally coded proteins insert into the host cell plasma membrane and form a pore, or channel, that disrupts the permeability barrier, allowing equilibration of ionic gradients. Potassium ions leave, and sodium and calcium ions enter. The cell is dead.

The hepatitis B virus is an example of an indirectly cytopathic virus. This agent consists of a double-stranded DNA genome enclosed in a protein capsule. Like the polio virus, the hepatitis B virus binds to specific receptors on the target cell surface, is internalized, and has its capsule removed by acidic proteases after the phagosome fuses with a lysosome. Unlike the polio virus, however, the viral DNA genome cannot be directly translated by the protein synthetic machinery. It must first be transcribed into viral messenger RNA before it can be translated into viral proteins. The transcription of the viral DNA genome is accomplished in the nucleus by the host cell's DNA-dependent RNA polymerase. The resulting viral RNAs are transported to the cytoplasm, where they are translated into proteins. The viral proteins include a DNA polymerase that replicates the viral genome and the capsular proteins. Progeny viruses are assembled and released from the host cell without lethal cell injury. Yet all is not well. It is thought that the process of viral assembly or release

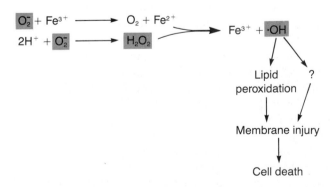

Figure 1-24. Possible mechanisms of cell injury by activated oxygen species.

exposes viral proteins on the external surface of the plasma membrane. These proteins are recognized by the immune system as non-self, or foreign, antigens. A cellular and humoral immune response develops in reaction to the viral proteins on the surface of the infected host cells. **It is this immune response that seems to be responsible for the lethal injury of the virus-infected cell.** T cells recognizing the viral antigens release a protein that interacts with the target cell plasma membrane. Disruption of the membrane's functional integrity and cell death proceed in a manner similar to that seen with the directly cytopathic viruses.

Figure 1-26 summarizes the mechanisms of cell killing by directly and indirectly cytopathic viruses.

How Chemicals Kill Cells

There are innumerable chemicals that can damage almost any cell in the body. The science of toxicology attempts to define the mechanisms that determine both the target cell specificity and the mechanism of action of such chemicals. Toxic chemicals are divided into two general classes: those that interact directly with cellular constituents without requiring metabolic activation, and those that are themselves not toxic but are metabolized to yield an ultimate toxin that interacts with the target cell. This target cell need not be the same cell that metabolizes the toxin.

Toxic Liver Necrosis

Studies of a few compounds that produce liver cell necrosis in rodents have enhanced our understanding of how chemicals injure cells. These studies have focused principally on those compounds that are converted to toxic metabolites.

Carbon tetrachloride, acetaminophen, and bromobenzene are well-studied hepatotoxins. Each is metabolized by the mixed function oxidase system of the endoplasmic reticulum, and each causes liver cell necrosis. How does this metabolic process relate to damage of the plasma membrane that results in irreversible injury? Each of the three hepatotoxins is metabolized in a somewhat different manner, and it is possible to relate the subsequent evolution of lethal cell injury to the specific features of this metabolism.

The active site of cytochrome P_{450} contains ferric iron. During substrate binding, NADPH-cytochrome P_{450} reductase transfers a single electron to the cytochrome P_{450}-substrate complex, thereby reducing ferric to ferrous iron. Molecular oxygen then binds to the cytochrome P_{450}-substrate complex in much the same way as it reacts with the ferrous iron of hemoglobin. O_2 is reduced to superoxide (O_2^-) by the transfer of an electron from the ferrous iron, thus

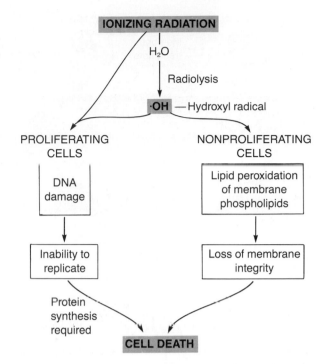

Figure 1-25. Possible mechanisms of cell injury by ionizing radiation.

initiating the reductive activation of oxygen. A second electron is added to form a peroxyl radical. The oxygen-oxygen bond is broken in such a manner that the two electrons are given to one of the oxygen atoms, thus reducing it to water. The remaining activated oxygen atom bound to the cytochrome-substrate complex is highly reactive. Through a mechanism still poorly understood, the substrate is oxidized by reaction with this activated oxygen atom. The final products are native ferric cytochrome P_{450}, one molecule of oxidized substrate, and one molecule of water. The equation for the oxidation of a given substrate (RH) can then be summarized as follows:

$$RH + 2e^- + O_2 + 2H^+ \rightarrow ROH + H_2O$$

Carbon Tetrachloride The metabolism of carbon tetrachloride (CCl_4), a model compound for toxicologic studies, is a variation on the mechanism described above. Again, when most chemicals bind to the ferric cytochrome P_{450}, an electron is added to the complex. With CCl_4, however, the addition of an electron immediately results in the reductive cleavage of a carbon-chlorine bond rather than in the reduction of iron. The products are a chlorine atom and a highly reactive trichloromethyl free radical. Oxygen is not involved in the metabolic activation of CCl_4.

Thus, the toxicity of CCl_4 (Fig. 1-27) depends on its metabolism and relates to the formation of the tri-

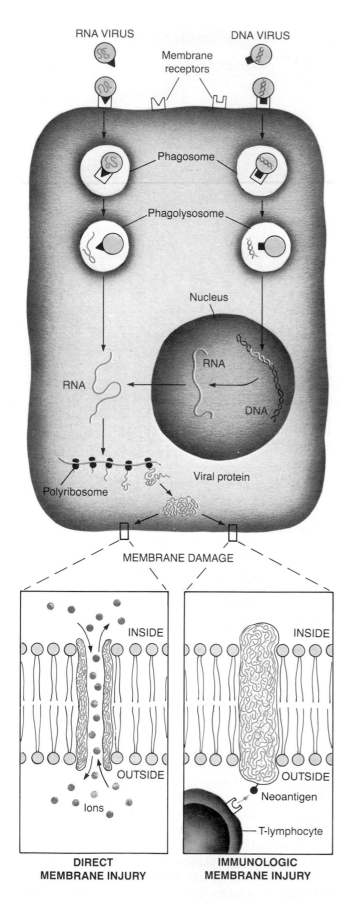

RNA VIRUS

DNA VIRUS

Membrane receptors

Phagosome

Phagolysosome

Nucleus

RNA

RNA

DNA

Polyribosome

Viral protein

MEMBRANE DAMAGE

INSIDE

OUTSIDE

Ions

DIRECT MEMBRANE INJURY

INSIDE

OUTSIDE

Neoantigen

T-lymphocyte

IMMUNOLOGIC MEMBRANE INJURY

chloromethyl free radical. Like the hydroxyl radical, the trichloromethyl radical is a potent initiator of lipid peroxidation. It abstracts a hydrogen atom from unsaturated fatty acids of the membrane phospholipids of the endoplasmic reticulum. Chloroform is produced and a lipid radical is formed. The reaction of the lipid radical with O_2 then initiates the peroxidative decomposition of the phospholipids of the endoplasmic reticulum. However, the liver cells do not die because of damage to the endoplasmic reticulum alone. Peroxidizing lipids release soluble products that can diffuse over significant distances and produce further membrane injury at other cellular loci, such as the plasma membrane. Figure 1-27 summarizes a possible sequence of events in the pathogenesis of liver cell necrosis from CCl_4.

Acetaminophen and Bromobenzene It has been suggested that the hepatotoxicity of the two model hepatotoxins, bromobenzene and the analgesic acetaminophen, might reflect covalent binding of electrophilic metabolites to critical cellular macromolecules. Bromobenzene is metabolized to a reactive, electrophilic epoxide, which can react with glutathione (GSH). If glutathione is depleted, the epoxide is free to react with cellular macromolecules. Acetaminophen is also metabolized to an electrophilic intermediate that can react with both GSH and cellular macromolecules. However, recent studies of the mechanisms by which bromobenzene and acetaminophen kill liver cells have suggested an alternative to the covalent binding of electrophilic metabolites. It has been possible to dissociate covalent binding from cell killing, and it is possible that liver necrosis is actually related to the toxicity of activated oxygen species. How are these species formed?

Acetaminophen is oxidized to the metabolite N-acetylimidoquinone without addition of oxygen. Like CCl_4, acetaminophen is metabolized by a modification of the normal cytochrome P_{450} cycle, in which a number of electron transfer reactions result in the formation of superoxide and hydrogen peroxide. The liver cells may then be lethally injured by these ac-

Figure 1-26. Mechanisms of cell killing by directly and indirectly cytopathic viruses. Membrane damage is the final common pathway by which both types of viruses produce cell death. The directly cytopathic viruses create a transmembrane channel by inserting their proteins into the plasmalemma, disrupting its function as a permeability barrier. The indirectly cytopathic viruses also insert into the plasma membrane and create a target for cytotoxic T-lymphocytes.

tivated oxygen species through mechanisms similar to those discussed above.

The metabolism of bromobenzene to produce an epoxide is a standard mixed function oxidation, without the kinds of modifications characterizing the metabolism of CCl_4 and acetaminophen. How then are the liver cells injured by activated oxygen species? There are two possible mechanisms. On the one hand, the mixed function oxidation of many substrates produces superoxide anions because the intermediate complex of cytochrome P_{450}, substrate, and reduced oxygen is inherently unstable; it may dissociate spontaneously to yield native cytochrome P_{450}, the original substrate, and superoxide. On the other hand, it is possible that as a result of GSH depletion from the reaction with the bromobenzene epoxide, the anti-oxidant defenses of the cells are so weakened that they become sensitive to endogenous activated oxygen species.

To summarize, the metabolism of hepatotoxic chemicals by mixed function oxidation leads to irreversible cell injury through mechanisms that may be unrelated, at least in part, to the covalent binding of reactive metabolites. What is emerging is a common theme of membrane damage as a result of the peroxidation of the constituent phospholipids. Lipid peroxidation is initiated by a metabolite of the original compound (as with CCl_4) or by activated oxygen species formed during the metabolism of the toxin (as with acetaminophen), the latter augmented by weakened anti-oxidant defenses.

Chemicals That Are Not Metabolized

Directly cytotoxic chemicals do not have to be metabolized to injure the target cell. Such compounds are inherently reactive and combine directly with cellular constituents. The class of directly cytotoxic chemicals includes many of the cancer chemotherapeutic agents and toxic heavy metals, such as mercury, lead, and iron. Because of the inherent reactivity of directly cytotoxic chemicals, many of the constituents of the target cell are damaged. This plethora of alterations has made it difficult to single out the critical interaction that leads to irreversible cell injury. We suspect that directly cytotoxic chemicals either interact directly with the plasma membrane or produce plasma membrane injury as a consequence of their interaction with other cellular constituents, such as glutathione.

Figure 1-28 reviews the various mechanisms we have discussed by which cellular membranes may be damaged in human disease. The functional consequence of these changes is usually coagulative necrosis.

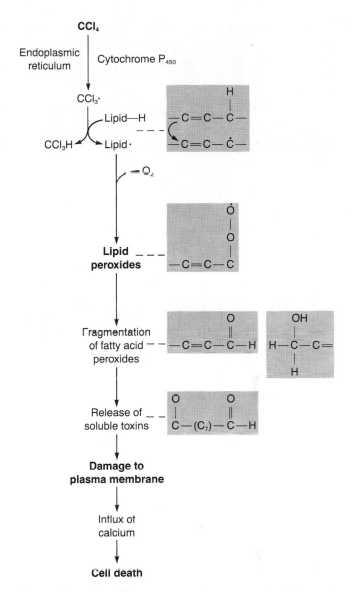

Figure 1-27. Possible sequence of events in the killing of liver cells by carbon tetrachloride.

Calcification

The deposition of mineral salts of calcium is, of course, a normal process in the formation of bone from cartilage. As we have learned, calcium entry into dead or dying cells is usual, owing to the inability of such cells to maintain a steep calcium gradient. This cellular calcification is not ordinarily visible except as inclusions within mitochondria (see Fig. 1-18).

Dystrophic calcification refers to the macroscopic deposition of calcium salts in injured tissues. This type of calcification does not simply reflect an accu-

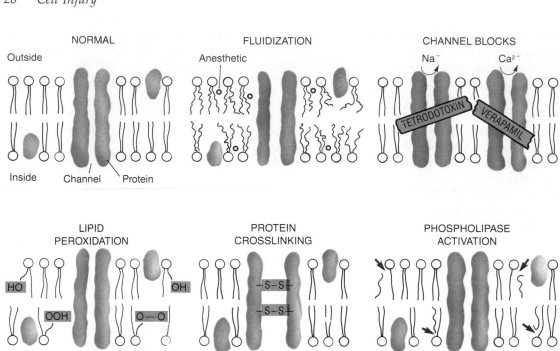

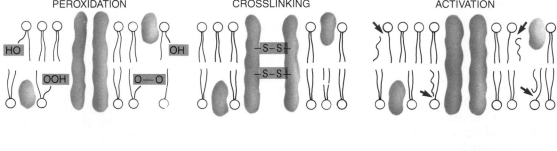

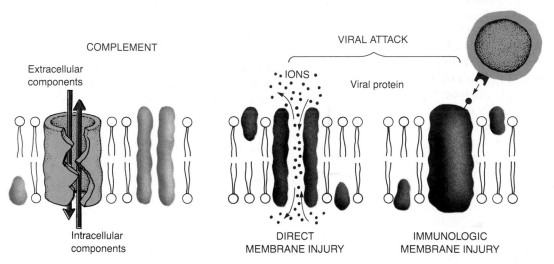

Figure 1-28.　Mechanisms of membrane damage in disease.

mulation of calcium derived from the bodies of dead cells, but rather represents an extracellular deposition of calcium from the circulation or interstitial fluid. Dystrophic calcification apparently requires the persistence of necrotic tissue; it is often visible to the naked eye, and ranges from gritty, sandlike grains to firm, rock-hard material. In many locations, such as in cases of tuberculous caseous necrosis in the lung or lymph nodes, calcification has no functional consequences. However, dystrophic calcification may also occur in crucial locations, such as in the mitral or aortic valves after rheumatic fever. In such instances, calcification leads to impeded blood flow because it produces inflexible valve leaflets and narrowed valve orifices (mitral and aortic stenosis). Dystrophic calcification in atherosclerotic coronary arteries contributes to narrowing of those vessels.

Dystrophic calcification also plays a role in diagnostic radiography. Mammography is based principally on the detection of calcifications in breast cancers; diagnosis of congenital toxoplasmosis, an infection involving the central nervous sytem, is suggested by the visualization of calcification in the infant brain.

Whereas dystrophic calcification has its origin in cell injury, **metastatic calcification** reflects deranged calcium metabolism, a change associated with an increased serum calcium concentration (hypercalcemia). In general, almost any disorder that increases the serum calcium level can lead to calcification in such inappropriate locations as the alveolar septa of the lung, renal tubules, and blood vessels. Calcification is seen in various disorders, including chronic renal failure, vitamin D intoxication, and hyperparathyroidism. In contrast to dystrophic calcification, the metastatic variety does not require pre-existing cell injury.

Another form of pathologic calcification is the formation of stones containing calcium carbonate in sites such as the gallbladder, renal pelvis, bladder, and pancreatic duct. Under certain circumstances, the mineral salts precipitate from solution and crystallize about foci of organic material. Those who have suffered the agony of gallbladder or renal colic will attest to the unpleasant consequences of this type of calcification.

Hyaline

The student will encounter the term **hyaline** in classical descriptions of diverse and unrelated lesions. Standard terminology includes hyaline arteriolosclerosis, alcoholic hyaline in the liver, hyaline membranes in the lung, and hyaline droplets in various cells. **The word hyaline simply refers to any material that exhibits a reddish, homogeneous appearance when routinely stained with hematoxylin and eosin.** The various lesions called hyaline actually have nothing in common. Alcoholic hyaline is composed of cytoskeletal filaments; the hyaline found in arterioles of the kidney is derived from basement membranes; and hyaline membranes consist of plasma proteins deposited in alveoli. The term is anachronistic and of questionable value, except as a handy morphologic descriptor.

Cellular Aging

Old age is a consequence of civilization; it is a condition rarely encountered in the animal kingdom or in primitive societies. From an evolutionary perspective, the aging process presents conceptual difficulties. Since animals in the wild do not attain their maximum longevity, how did aging evolve? On the other hand, if it is longevity that evolved, one might intuitively expect that a trait which is invariably lethal would be subject to evolutionary selective pressure. The consequences of aging arise after the reproductive period, and thus should not have an evolutionary impact.

Aging must be distinguished from mortality, on the one hand, and from disease on the other. Death is an accidental event; an aged individual who does not succumb to the most common cause of death will die from the second, third, or fourth most common cause. While the increased vulnerability to disease among the elderly is an interesting problem, disease itself is entirely distinct from aging.

Life Span

Millenia ago the psalmist sang of a natural life span of 70 years, which with vigor may extend to 80. On an evolutionary scale, biblical figures lived in our era of literate civilization. By contrast, it is estimated that the usual age at death of neolithic man was 20 to 25 years, and the average life span in many primitive cultures today is often barely 10 years more.

The difference between man in primitive and in civilized environments is analogous to that observed between animals in their natural habitat and those in a zoo (Fig. 1-29). For animals in the wild, after an initial high mortality during maturation, a progressive linear decline in survival is noted, ending at the maximum life span of the species. This steady decrease in the number of mature animals reflects not aging but random events, such as encounters with beasts of prey, accidental trauma, infections, starvation, and so on. On the other hand, survival in the

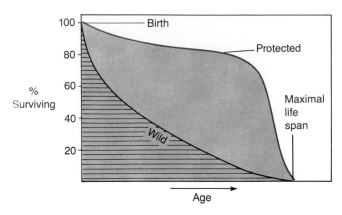

Figure 1-29. Life span of animals in their natural environment compared to a protected habitat. Note that both curves reach the same maximal life span.

protected environment of a zoo is characterized by slow attrition until senescence, at which time the steep decline in numbers is attributable to aging. Of interest is the fact that the maximum life span attained is not significantly altered by a protected environment. An analogous situation is seen in studies of human mortality (Fig. 1-30). Less than a century ago, the steep linear slope of mortality in the adult principally reflected random accidents and infections. With greater attention to safety and sanitation, the development of antibiotics and other specific drugs, safer blood transfusions, and improved diagnostic and therapeutic methods, mortality through the middle years has substantially decreased. Yet mortality

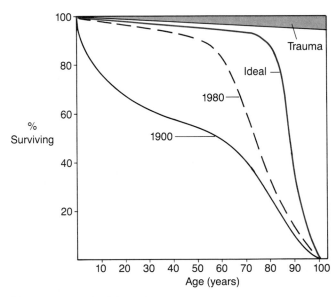

Figure 1-30. Ideal human life span contrasted with that seen in 1900 and 1980. Note again that the same maximal life span is reached in all cases.

during old age remains steep, and the maximum human life span has remained constant at about 110 years. What would happen if diseases associated with old age, such as coronary artery disease and cancer, were eliminated? Such triumphs might lead to an **ideal survival curve** (Fig. 1-30), but only a modest increase in average life expectancy. A long period of good health and low mortality would inevitably be followed by a precipitously increased mortality owing to aging itself; the life span would, for practical purposes, remain on the lower side of 100. Given the current mean life expectancy, which in women is approaching 80, the prevention or cure of the causes of premature death would have little impact on mean longevity.

Functional and Structural Changes

The insidious effects of aging can be detected in otherwise healthy individuals. The great leaps of imagination by theoretical physicists and mathematicians are almost exclusively the province of the young, and an athlete in his thirties may be referred to as "aged." Even in the absence of specific diseases or vascular abnormalities, beginning in the fourth decade of life there is a progressive decline in many physiologic functions (Fig. 1-31), including such easily measurable parameters as muscular strength, cardiac reserve, nerve conduction time, pulmonary vital capacity, glomerular filtration, and vascular elasticity. These functional deteriorations are accompanied by structural changes (Fig. 1-32). Lean body mass decreases and the proportion of fat rises. Constituents of the connective tissue matrix are progressively cross-linked. Lipofuscin ("wear and tear") pigment accumulates in the cytoplasm of organs such as the brain, heart, and liver.

The salient characteristic of aging is not so much a decrease in basal functional capacity as it is a reduced ability to adapt to environmental stress. Although the resting pulse is unchanged, the maximal increase with exercise is reduced with age, and the time required for return to a normal heart rate is prolonged. Similarly, the aged show an impaired adaptive response to ingested carbohydrates. Although the fasting blood sugar level in old age is normal compared to that of the young, it rises higher after a carbohydrate meal and declines more slowly.

The Cellular Basis of Aging

Although the biologic basis for aging is obscure, there is general agreement that its elucidation, as in all pathologic conditions, should be sought at the cel-

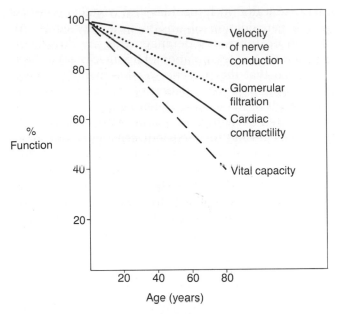

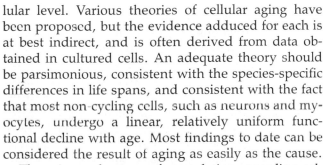

Figure 1-31. Decrease in human physiological capacities as a function of age.

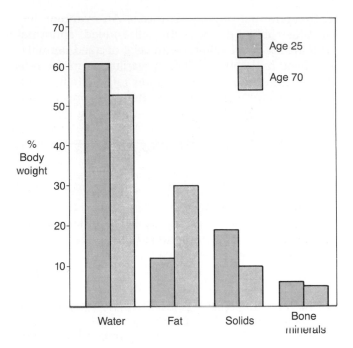

Figure 1-32. Structural changes with age in the human body.

lular level. Various theories of cellular aging have been proposed, but the evidence adduced for each is at best indirect, and is often derived from data obtained in cultured cells. An adequate theory should be parsimonious, consistent with the species-specific differences in life spans, and consistent with the fact that most non-cycling cells, such as neurons and myocytes, undergo a linear, relatively uniform functional decline with age. Most findings to date can be considered the result of aging as easily as the cause.

There is no shortage of speculation regarding cellular aging, but the fundamental information necessary for a coherent theory is lacking. In general, current theories propose that aging results either from **extrinsic** events that progressively damage cells or from **intrinsic** characteristics of the cell, such as genetic programming.

Random Event (Stochastic) Theories

According to stochastic theories, random environmental insults to the cells persist and, over time, accumulate to a lethal level. The most prominent example is the **somatic mutation theory,** which is based on the notion that background radiation produces random genetic damage in all cells. When enough genetic loci are altered, critical functions are impaired and the cell dies. The theory that background radiation is responsible for aging was in vogue during the height of research in radiation bi-

ology following World War II. It relies heavily on the observations that irradiation of experimental animals shortens life span. There is, however, no direct evidence linking the accelerated aging produced by radiation to normal aging. If the theory were true, one might expect a difference in aging between those living at high altitude, where background radiation is more intense, and those at sea level. No such difference has been reported. Inbred animals, which are homozygous at most genetic loci, should live longer than outbred animals because if one allele is damaged, the function of a homozygous gene is more likely to be maintained than that of a heterozygous one. It is well known, however, that outbred animals usually outlive inbred ones. Certain insects can be maintained in the haploid or diploid condition. As expected, the haploid variety is indeed more sensitive to radiation, owing to the lack of an allele. Yet, in the natural or unirradiated state, haploid and diploid insects have the same life spans. These observations are not consistent with a theory of somatic mutation.

Another theory is based on the mechanism of protein synthesis. Because the mechanism is not perfect, it may occasionally produce an erroneous copy of a protein. Such defective molecules are eventually replaced by normal catabolic processes. **The error theory of aging,** also based on random or stochastic events, holds that erroneous copies of protein molecules associated with the chromosomes may lead to genetic abnormalities, which in turn, result in persistently abnormal protein synthesis. An eventual "error catastrophe" destroys the cell. Indeed, abnormal proteins are more common in cells of aged animals, but these probably result from variations in the rate of post-translational modification rather than errors in protein synthesis. The error theory is conceptually elegant but devoid of adequate supporting data.

Developmental-Genetic Theories

The distinctive life spans of different species and the invariable senescence of certain cells and organs during embryogenesis suggest that aging is controlled by some intrinsic program, probably linked to the genetic apparatus. **Neuroendocrine** theories emphasize the role of the hypothalamic-pituitary system as the master timekeeper of the body. An age-related loss of function in the cells of this system leads to hormonal deficits, and thus to decreased systemic function. This theory has more credibility for higher vertebrates than for simple organisms that do not have highly developed neuroendocrine systems.

In an attempt to bridge the differences between stochastic theories and the perceived genetic basis of the maximum life span, the **theory of intrinsic mutagenesis** holds that the fidelity of genetic replication is different for each species. As a consequence, the genetic error rate is different for each species; thus, the life span varies. Although there is some evidence for a rough correlation between the levels of DNA repair mechanisms and species life spans, there are exceptions, and the theory remains controversial.

The functional capacity of the immune system—for example, T cell function—declines with age. Moreover, its fidelity appears to be impaired, as indicated by an age-related increase in autoimmune phenomena. These observations have led to an **immunologic theory of aging.** Interestingly, congeneic animals that differ only at the major histocompatibility locus exhibit different maximal life spans, an observation suggesting that this locus plays a role in longevity. The histocompatibility locus is involved not only with immune regulation but also with the regulation of superoxide dismutase and the mixed function oxidase system. Thus, supporters of this theory can claim a relation between the immune and lipid peroxidation theories of aging. On the other hand, the immune theory suffers from a lack of universality because it does not explain aging in simple animals lacking a well-developed immune system.

Lipid Peroxidation

Aging is accompanied by the deposition of lipofuscin pigment, principally in postmitotic cells of organs such as the brain, heart, and liver. This brown pig-

ment is located in lysosomes and contains products of the peroxidation of unsaturated fatty acids. Although no functional derangements are directly attributed to the accumulation of lipofuscin, it has been proposed that the presence of this pigment reflects continuing lipid peroxidation of cellular membranes as a result of inadequate defenses against the stress of activated oxygen. Presumably, an overload of rancid lipids results in persistent cell injury and, consequently, in aging. This theory is based to some extent on several observations: that the generation of activated oxygen species is directly related to body size; that metabolic rate is inversely related to body size (the larger the animal, the lower the metabolic rate); and that larger animals usually have longer life spans than smaller ones.

Some have speculated, therefore, that differences in species life spans reflect a species-specific endowment in the total number of calories that can be burned in a lifetime. Thus, animals that burn calories at a faster rate will use up their allotment in a shorter time. Experimentally, caloric restriction can increase life span by up to 50%. Moreover, superoxide dismutase activity in the livers of different primates has

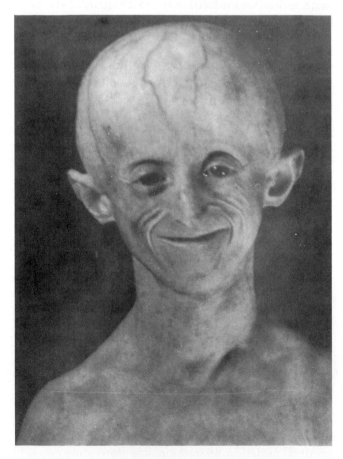

Figure 1-33. Progeria. A 14-year-old boy shows the signs of accelerated aging.

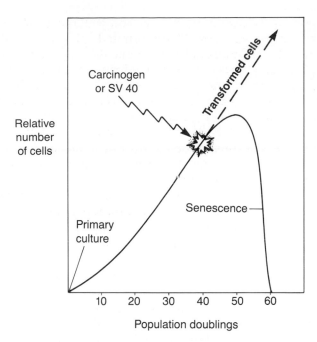

Figure 1-34. Number of cultured cells as a function of the number of population doublings. Note that after about 50 population doublings the cells no longer divide and the culture dies out. However, if the cells are transformed with a virus or a chemical, cellular senescence is not seen, and the cells continue to divide indefinitely.

been reported to be proportional to the maximal life span. In view of the experimental demonstration that lipid peroxidation may lead to cell death, and the likelihood that all varieties of cells can be so damaged, this theory has some credibility. However, phospholipid turnover in cell membranes is rapid, and no evidence is available for the accumulation of peroxides within the lipid bilayer of cell membranes *in vivo*. As with most theories of aging, the evidence for lipid peroxidation is circumstantial.

Aging as a Genetic Program

Every species has an appointed life span which, within limits, is immutable. Given an adequate environment, life span may be genetically determined. In humans, the modest correlation in longevity between related people and the excellent agreement among identical twins lend credence to this assumption. In addition, the entire process of aging, including features such as male pattern baldness, cataracts, and coronary artery disease, is compressed into a span of under 10 years in progeria (Fig. 1-33). Accelerated aging is also seen in other genetic diseases, such as Werner's and Down's syndromes.

Major support for the concept of a genetically programmed life span comes from studies of replicating cells in tissue culture. Unlike cancer cells, normal cells in tissue culture do not exhibit an unrestrained capacity to replicate. Cultured human fibroblasts undergo about 50 population doublings, after which they no longer divide and the culture dies out (Fig. 1-34). If the cells are transformed into cancer cells, by exposure to the SV 40 virus or a chemical carcinogen, they continue to replicate; in a sense, they become immortal. A rough correlation between the number of population doublings in fibroblasts and life span has been reported in several species. As an example, rat fibroblasts exhibit considerably fewer doublings than do human ones. Moreover, cells obtained from patients with precocious aging, such as those with progeria, also display a conspicuously reduced number of population doublings *in vitro*

There is no demonstrable age-related change *in vivo* in the replicative capacity of rapidly cycling cells, such as epithelial cells of the intestine. Therefore, one is left with the apparent paradox that replicating cells in culture have a limited life span but aging *in vivo* seems principally to affect the functional capacity of postmitotic cells. In other words, people do not age because the cells of the intestinal tract fail to replicate. However, if one considers that the **function** of cells *in vitro* is to proliferate, then they indeed display a major failure in functional capacity. Thus, cells in culture do represent a model for the study of aging.

SUGGESTED READING

BOOKS

Perez-Tamayo R: Mechanisms of Disease. An Introduction to Pathology, 2nd ed. Chicago, Year Book Medical Publishers, 1985

Hallowell B, Gutteridge JMC: Free Radicals in Biology and Medicine. Oxford, Clarendon Press, 1985

Poli G, Cheeseman KH, Dianzani MU (eds): Free Radicals in Liver Injury. Oxford, IRL Press, 1985

REVIEW ARTICLES

Farber JL: Biology of disease: Membrane injury and calcium homeostasis in the pathogenesis of coagulative necrosis. Lab Invest 47:114, 1982

Farber JL: Xenobiotics, drug metabolism, and liver injury. In Farber E, Phillips MJ, Kaufman N (eds): Pathogenesis of Liver Diseases. Baltimore, Williams & Wilkins, 1987

Fantone JC, Ward PA: Polymorphonuclear leukocyte–mediated cell and tissue injury: Oxygen metabolites and their relations to human disease. Hum Pathol 16:973, 1985

Cristafalo VJ: The biology of aging: An overview. In Horan MJ, Steinberg GM, Dunbar JB, et al (eds): Blood Pressure Regulation and Aging. New York, Biomedical Information Corp, 1986

2

Inflammation

Joseph C. Fantone and Peter A. Ward

Vascular Permeability

Sources of Vasoactive Mediators

Complement System

Phospholipid Metabolism and Arachidonic Acid Metabolites

Cellular Recruitment

Inflammatory Cell Activation

Modulation of Inflammatory Cell Function

Mechanisms of Injury Produced by Polymorphonuclear Leukocytes

Cell Adherence and Tissue Injury

Chronic Inflammation

Granulomatous Inflammation

Systemic Manifestations of Inflammation

Figure 2-1. Participants in acute and chronic inflammatory reactions.

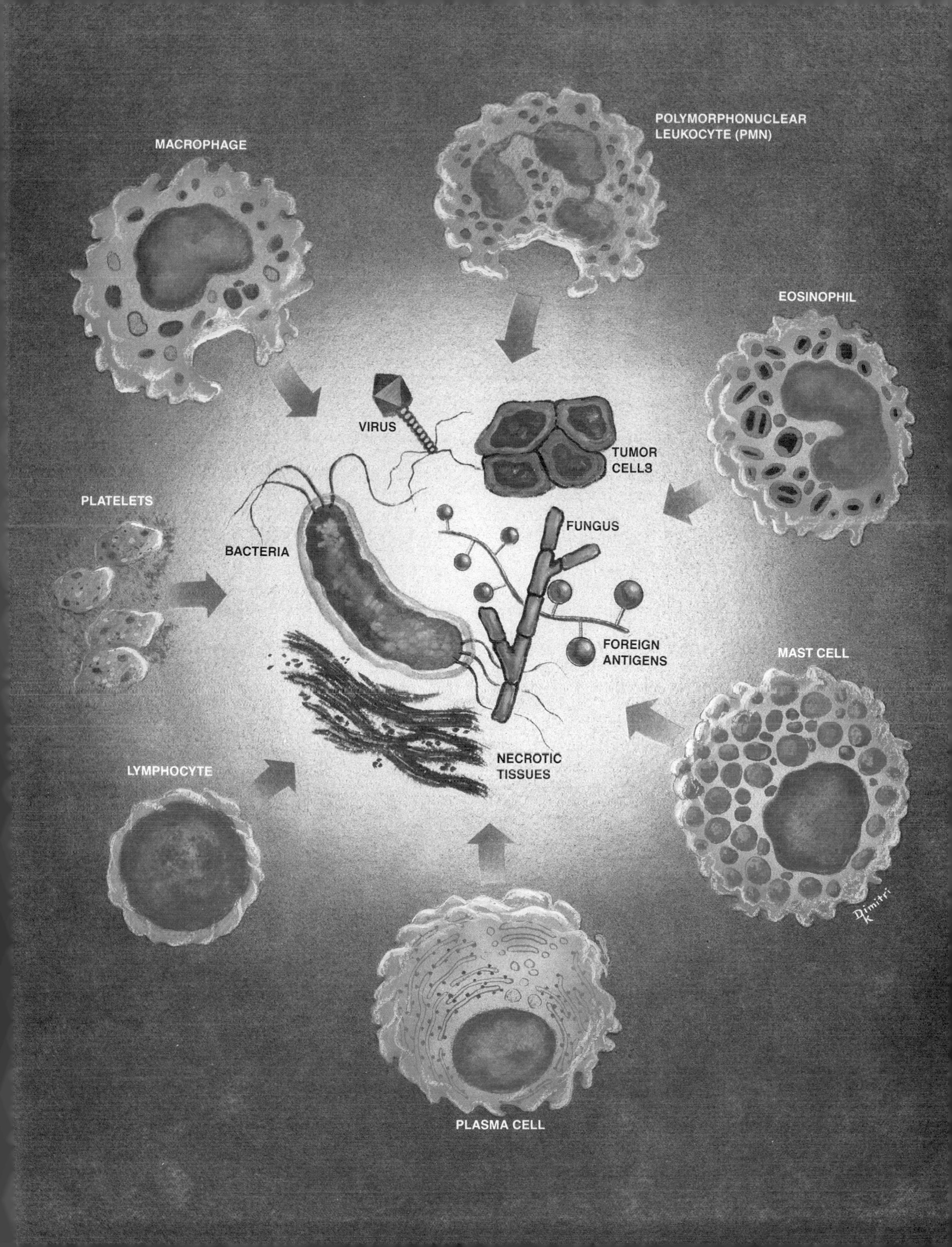

MACROPHAGE

POLYMORPHONUCLEAR
LEUKOCYTE (PMN)

EOSINOPHIL

PLATELETS

VIRUS

TUMOR
CELLS

FUNGUS

BACTERIA

FOREIGN
ANTIGENS

MAST CELL

LYMPHOCYTE

NECROTIC
TISSUES

PLASMA CELL

Inflammation is a reaction of the microcirculation characterized by movement of fluid and white blood cells from the blood into extravascular tissues. This is frequently an expression of the host's attempt to localize and eliminate metabolically altered cells, foreign particles, microorganisms, or antigens. The clinical signs of inflammation were described in Classical times; the Greeks and Romans noted the association of redness (rubor), heat (calor), swelling (tumor), and pain (dolor) with acute injury to tissues. These are the clinical signs with which we are most familiar and with which we associate response to injury.

Under normal conditions the inflammatory response eliminates the pathogenic insult and removes injured tissue components. This process accomplishes either regeneration of the normal tissue architecture and return of physiologic function or the formation of scar tissue to replace what cannot be repaired. Further extension of injury or the effects of the inflammatory response itself may lead to loss of function of the organ or tissue. The mechanisms responsible for the localization and clearance of foreign substances and injured tissues are initiated by the recognition that injury to tissues has occurred. This is followed by an amplification phase of the inflammatory response, in which both soluble mediators and cellular inflammatory systems are activated. After generation of inflammatory agents and elimination of the foreign agent, inflammatory responses are terminated by specific inhibitors of the mediators. Under certain conditions the ability to clear injured tissue and foreign agents is impaired, or the regulatory mechanisms of the inflammatory response are altered. In these circumstances inflammation is harmful to the host and leads to excessive tissue destruction and injury. In other instances, an immune response to residual microbial products or to altered tissue components also triggers a persistent inflammatory reaction.

Initiation of the inflammatory response following tissue injury occurs within the microvasculature at the level of the capillary and postcapillary venule. Within this vascular network are the major components of the inflammatory response, including plasma, platelets, red blood cells, and circulating white blood cells (Figs. 2-1 and 2-2). Normally these components are confined within the intravascular compartment by a continuous layer of endothelium that is connected by tight junctions and separated from the tissue by a limiting basement membrane. Following injury to a tissue, changes occur in the structure of the vascular wall, leading to a loss of endothelial cell integrity, leakage of fluid and plasma components from the intravascular compartment, and emigration of both red and white blood cells from the intraluminal space into the extravascular tissue.

Specific inflammatory mediators produced at the sites of injury (Fig. 2-3) regulate the response of the vasculature to injury. Among these mediators are vasoactive molecules that act directly on the vasculature to increase vascular permeability. In addition, chemotactic factors are generated that recruit white blood cells from the vascular compartment into the injured tissue. Once present in tissues, recruited white blood cells secrete additional inflammatory mediators that either enhance or inhibit the inflammatory response.

Historically, inflammation has been referred to as either **acute or chronic inflammation,** depending on the persistence of the injury, its clinical symptomatology, and the nature of the inflammatory response. **The hallmarks of acute inflammation include accumulation of fluid and plasma components in the affected tissue, intravascular stimulation of platelets, and the presence of polymorphonuclear leukocytes** (Fig. 2-4). **By contrast, the characteristic cell components of chronic inflammation are macrophages, lymphocytes, and plasma cells** (Fig. 2-5).

Activation of the inflammatory response results in one of three distinct outcomes. Under ideal conditions the source of the tissue injury is eliminated, the inflammatory response resolves, and normal tissue architecture and physiologic function are restored. In some cases, however, the nature of the acute inflammatory reaction is such that the area is walled off by the collection of inflammatory cells, a process that results in destruction of the tissue by products of the polymorphonuclear leukocytes (also known as neutrophils). This is the mechanism by which an **abscess** is formed. Alternatively, if the tissue is irreversibly injured despite elimination of the initial pathologic insult, the affected tissue's normal architecture is often replaced by scar. The third possibility is that the inflammatory cells may fail to eliminate the pathologic insult, in which case the inflammatory reaction persists. The area of chronic inflammation often expands, leading to fibrosis and scar formation.

Vascular Permeability

Alterations in the anatomy and function of the microvasculature are among the earliest responses to tissue injury (Fig. 2-6). An early vascular response to mild injury of the skin involves a transient vasoconstriction of arterioles at the site of injury. This

vasoconstriction is mediated by both neurogenic and chemical mediator systems, and usually resolves within seconds to minutes. **Vasodilation** of precapillary arterioles follows, with an increase in blood flow to the tissue. **This vasodilation is caused by the release of specific mediators and is responsible, in part, for the redness and warmth at sites of tissue injury.**

In conjunction with the vasodilation and increased blood flow, alterations in the permeability of the endothelial cell barrier result in increased leakage of fluid from the intravascular compartment into extravascular spaces. If not effectively cleared by lymphatics, fluid accumulates in the extravascular space. A net increase in extravascular fluid is called **edema**; its clinical manifestation is swelling. The loss of fluid from the intravascular compartment as blood passes through the capillary venules leads to local stasis and plugging of dilated small vessels with red blood cells. These changes are reversible following mild injury, and within several minutes to hours the extravascular fluid is cleared through lymphatics. The endothelial injury is reversed and the normal structure of the microcirculation is reestablished.

The pathologic changes described above are characteristic of the classic "triple response" first described by Sir Thomas Lewis. In the original experiments, a dull red line developed at the site of mild trauma to the skin, followed by the development of a red halo (flare) and associated swelling (wheal). Lewis postulated the presence of a vasoactive mediator that causes vasodilatation and increased vascular permeability at the site of injury.

Injury to the vasculature is a dynamic event and frequently involves sequential physiologic and pathologic changes. **Vasoactive mediators**, originating from both plasma and cellular sources, are generated at sites of tissue injury by a variety of mechanisms (Fig. 2-7). These mediators bind to specific receptors on vascular endothelial and smooth muscle cells, causing vasoconstriction or vasodilatation. Vasoconstriction of arterioles decreases blood flow to a tissue; arteriolar vasodilatation increases blood flow and can exacerbate fluid leakage into the tissue. In contrast, vasoconstriction of venules increases the hydrostatic pressure in the capillary bed, potentiating edema formation. Vasodilatation of venules decreases capillary hydrostatic pressure and inhibits the movement of fluid into the extravascular spaces. Therefore, when the role of a particular vasoactive mediator in the development of inflammatory response is being examined, the effects of this mediator on specific tissues and components of the vasculature must be identified.

Binding of vasoactive mediators to endothelial cells results in a complex series of biochemical events causing endothelial cell contraction and gap formation. This break in the endothelial barrier leads to an extravasation (leakage) of intravascular fluids into the extravascular space. **The postcapillary venule is the primary site at which the vasoactive mediators induce endothelial changes.** Endothelial retraction and gap formation is a reversible process. Local injection of classic vasoactive mediators into the skin results in an acute change in vascular permeability that peaks between 15 and 20 minutes after injection. Vascular integrity is restored within an hour. In contrast, direct injury to the endothelium, such as that caused by burns or caustic chemicals, may result in irreversible damage. In such cases the endothelium is separated from the basement membrane, an effect that leads to cell blebbing, that is, the appearance of blisters or bubbles between the endothelium and the basement membrane, and areas of denuded basement membrane. Mild, direct injury to the endothelium may result in a biphasic response: an early change in permeability occurs 15 to 30 minutes after the injury, followed by a second increase in vascular permeability after 3 to 5 hours. When damage is severe the exudation of intravascular fluid into the extravascular compartment increases progressively, reaching a peak between 3 and 4 hours after injury.

Accumulation of fluid within the extravascular compartment and interstitial tissues is referred to as **edema;** excess fluid in the cavities of the body is labeled an **effusion.** Edema fluid with a low protein content (specific gravity of <1.0) is called a **transudate.** Edema fluid with a high protein concentration (specific gravity >1.0) is termed an **exudate;** it is frequently characterized by a high lipid content and cellular debris. Exudates are observed early in acute inflammatory reactions and are produced by mild injuries, such as sunburn or traumatic blisters. When exudates or effusions occur in tissues in the absence of a prominent cellular response, they are termed **serous.** A serous fluid usually has a yellow, strawlike color, but when red blood cells are present the fluid has a red tinge and is referred to as **serosanguineous.** Under conditions that activate the coagulation system, large amounts of fibrin may be deposited in tissues, a process that results in a **fibrinous** exudate. An inflammatory exudate or effusion that contains prominent cellular components is described as **purulent. Purulent exudates and effusions are frequently identified with pathologic conditions such as pyogenic bacterial infections, in which the predominant cell type is the polymorphonuclear leukocyte.**

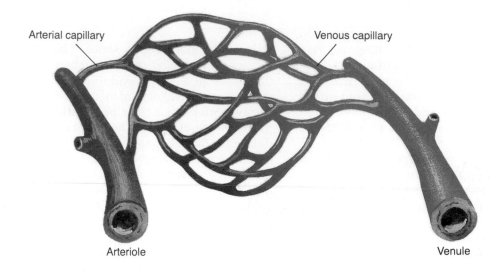

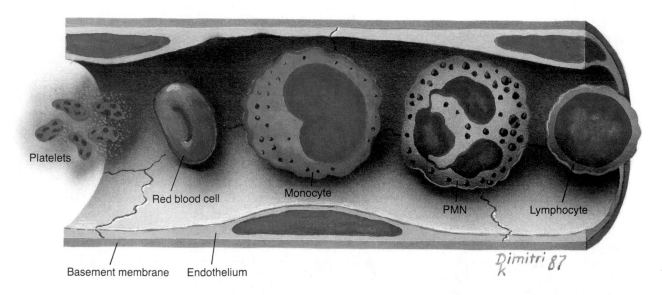

Figure 2-2. The microcirculation and cellular components of the blood.

Sources of Vasoactive Mediators

The primary sources of vasoactive mediators are cells and plasma. Important cellular sources of vasoactive mediators are circulating platelets, tissue mast cells, and basophils.

Platelets

The platelet plays a primary role in normal homeostasis and in the initiation and regulation of clot formation. It is also an important source of inflammatory mediators, including potent vasoactive substances and growth factors that modulate mesenchymal cell proliferation (Fig. 2-8). The platelet is a cell approximately 2 μm in diameter, lacking a nucleus but containing at least three distinct kinds of granules: dense granules rich in serotonin, histamine, Ca^{2+}, and adenosine diphosphate (ADP); α-granules containing fibrinogen, coagulation proteins, platelet-derived growth factor (PDGF), and other peptides and proteins; and lysosomes containing acid hydrolases.

When platelets come in contact with fibrillar collagen (following vascular injury that exposes the interstitial matrix proteins) or thrombin (following

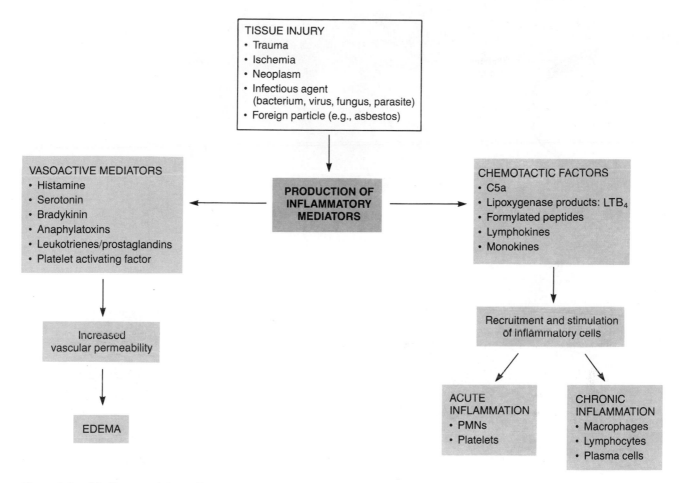

Figure 2-3. Mediators of the inflammatory response.

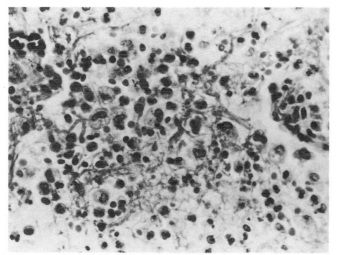

Figure 2-4. Acute inflammation. Interstitial edema and numerous polymorphonuclear leukocytes are present.

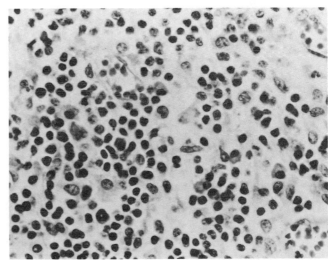

Figure 2-5. Chronic inflammation. Macrophages, lymphocytes and plasma cells predominate.

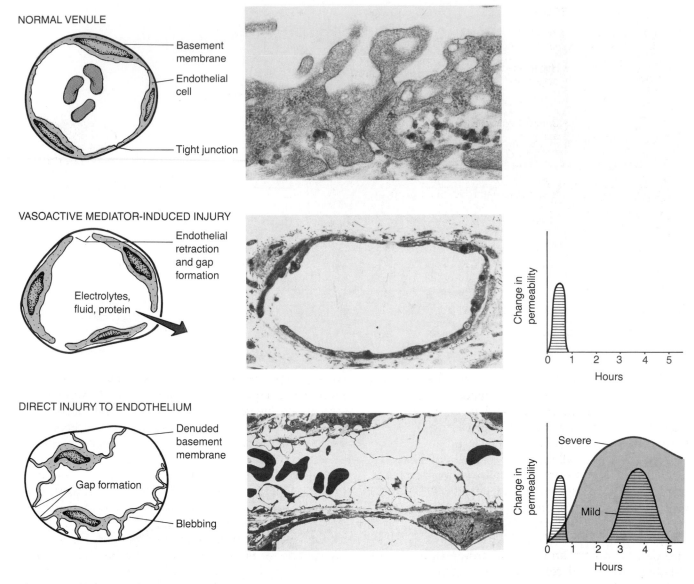

NORMAL VENULE

Basement membrane

Endothelial cell

Tight junction

VASOACTIVE MEDIATOR-INDUCED INJURY

Endothelial retraction and gap formation

Electrolytes, fluid, protein

DIRECT INJURY TO ENDOTHELIUM

Denuded basement membrane

Gap formation

Blebbing

Figure 2-6. Response of the microvasculature to injury. The wall of the normal venule is sealed by tight junctions between adjacent endothelial cells. During mild injury, the endothelial cells separate and permit the passage of the fluid constituents of the blood. With severe direct injury, the endothelial cells form blebs and separate from the underlying basement membrane. Areas of denuded basement membrane allow a prolonged escape of fluid elements from the microvasculature.

activation of the coagulation system), platelet adherence, aggregation, and degranulation may occur. Degranulation is associated with the release of **serotonin (5-hydroxytryptamine) and histamine,** mediators that directly induce changes in vascular permeability. In addition, the arachidonic acid metabolite **thromboxane A_2** is produced. Thromboxane A_2 not only plays a key role in the second wave of platelet aggregation, but also possesses smooth muscle constrictive properties.

Mast Cells and Basophils

The mast cell and basophil are additional cellular sources of vasoactive mediators. When antigen binds to IgE immunoglobulin and cross-links these molecules on basophil and mast cell surfaces, secretory release of these mediators from electron-dense cytoplasmic granules into extracellular tissues occurs (Fig. 2-9). These granules contain histamine, acid mucopolysaccharides (including heparin), and chemotactic

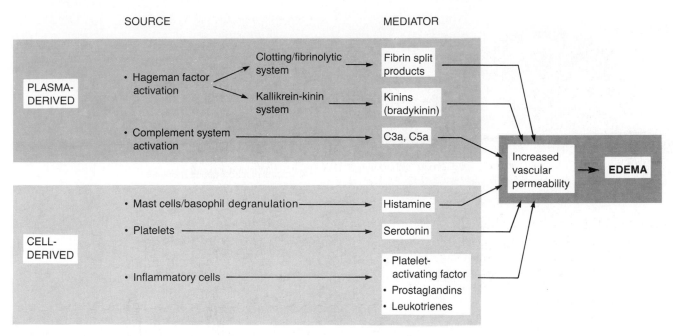

SOURCE   MEDIATOR

Figure 2-7. Vasoactive mediators of increased vascular permeability.

mediators for neutrophils and eosinophils. Because of their ability to secrete specific mediators following stimulation, both mast cells and basophils play an important role in the regulation of vascular permeability and bronchial smooth muscle tone, especially in many forms of allergic hypersensitivity reactions (see Chapter 4). Histamine is released from the electron-dense granules when IgE-sensitized cells are stimulated with antigen or the anaphylatoxins derived from the third and fifth components of the complement system (C3a and C5a). When injected into skin, both histamine and serotonin induce reversible endothelial cell contraction, gap formation, and edema.

The most important effects of histamine and serotonin occur early in the evolution of inflammatory reactions. The action of histamine on the vasculature is a result of its binding to specific H_1 receptors in the vascular wall, an effect that can be inhibited pharmacologically by H_1-receptor antagonists. Degranulation of mast cells and basophils may also be induced by physical agonists, such as cold and trauma, as well as by cationic proteins derived from platelets and neutrophil lysosomal granules.

Stimulation of mast cells and basophils also leads to the release of products of arachidonic acid metabolism, including the so-called **slow-reacting substances of anaphylaxis (SRS-As). The SRS-As consist**

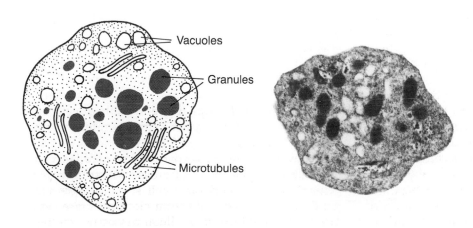

CHARACTERISTICS AND FUNCTIONS
• Thrombosis; promotes clot formation
• Regulates permeability
• Regulates proliferative response of mesenchymal cells

PRIMARY INFLAMMATORY MEDIATORS
• Dense granules
  –Serotonin
  –Ca^{2+}
  –ADP
• α-granules
  –Cationic proteins
  –Fibrinogen and coagulation proteins
  –Platelet-derived growth factor (PDGF)
• Lysosomes
  –Acid hydrolases
• Thromboxane A_2

Figure 2-8. Platelets: morphology and functions.

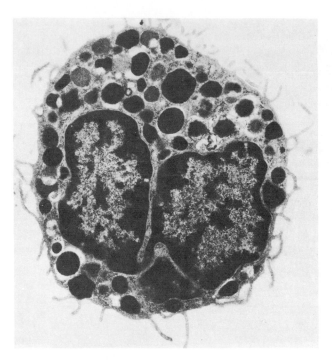

Mast Cell (Basophils)

CHARACTERISTICS AND FUNCTIONS
• Binds IgE molecules
• Contains electron-dense granules

PRIMARY INFLAMMATORY MEDIATORS
• Histamine
• Leukotrienes (LTC$_4$, LTD$_4$, LTE$_4$)
• Platelet activating factor
• Eosinophil chemotactic factors

Figure 2-9.   Mast cells: morphology and functions.

of leukotriene C$_4$ (LTC$_4$), leukotriene D$_4$ (LTD$_4$) and leukotriene E$_4$ (LTE$_4$). These lipoxygenase products of arachidonic acid metabolism induce smooth muscle contraction and increase vascular permeability in the skin. They produce their effects by binding to specific receptors on cell membranes and are important in delayed changes in vascular permeability at sites of inflammation.

Platelet Activating Factor

Stimulation of mast cells and leukocytes results in the generation of another class of vasoactive mediators, first characterized as a platelet activating factor (PAF), having the structure of an acetylated lysophospholipid. The biochemical structure of this compound varies with the species of origin. In the rabbit, PAF has been characterized as 1-0-hexadecyl/octyl-decyl-2-acetyl-sn-glycero-3-phosphocholine (AGEPC), a compound that has potent biologic effects at nanomolar concentrations. PAF induces platelet aggregation and degranulation at sites of tissue injury and enhances the release of serotonin and histamine, thereby causing changes in vascular permeability. In addition, it enhances arachidonic acid metabolism in neutrophils, an effect associated with increased motility, superoxide production, and degranulation of the polymorphonuclear leukocyte. PAF also has direct effects on the microvasculature, causing vasodilatation and enhancing vascular permeability at sites of tissue injury.

Hageman Factor (Factor XII)

Additional sources of vasoactive mediators are generated within plasma (Fig. 2-10). Activation of Hageman factor (clotting Factor XII) by exposure to negatively charged surfaces, such as basement membrane, proteolytic enzymes, bacterial lipopolysaccharides, and foreign materials (including urate crystals as occur in gout) results in the proteolytic activation of several additional plasma proteins. The list includes conversion of plasminogen to plasmin, conversion of prekallikrein to kallikrein, and activation of the alternative complement pathway.

Plasmin generated by activated Hageman factor induces fibrinolysis. The products of fibrin degradation augment vascular permeability in both the skin and the lung. In addition, plasmin cleaves components of the complement system in an action that generates biologically active products, including the anaphylatoxins C3a and C5a. C3a and C5a increase vascular permeability in the skin both directly and indirectly (e.g., by a mast cell–dependent mechanism).

Plasma kallikrein generated by activated Hageman factor cleaves high-molecular-weight kininogen, thus generating several vasoactive low-molecular-weight peptides, collectively referred to as **kinins** (Fig. 2-11). The best characterized of these vasoactive kinins is **bradykinin**. Bradykinin is a nanopeptide that, when injected into skin, elicits reversible changes of the endothelium that lead to edema. Many kinins are

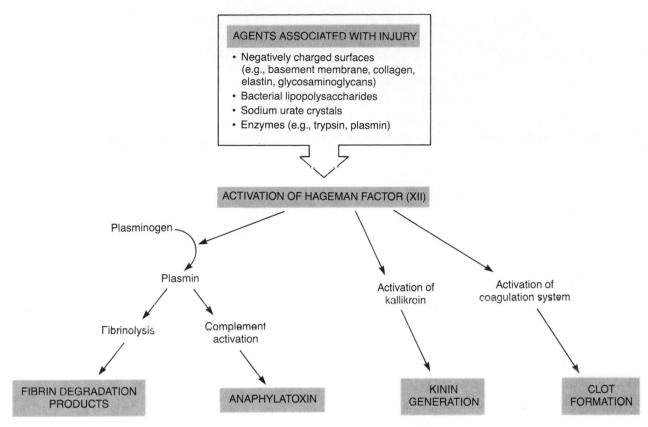

Figure 2-10. Hageman factor activation and inflammatory mediator production.

under the tight regulatory control of specific inactivating enzymes. For instance, two enzymes present in plasma, carboxypeptidase N (kininase I) and a dipeptidase referred to as angiotensin-converting enzyme (kininase II), selectively cleave the carboxy-terminal peptide and dipeptides of bradykinin, respectively. This renders the molecule biologically inactive.

The permeability changes induced by the vasoactive mediators are enhanced by the local production of vasodilative substances. In particular, the vasodilative prostaglandins (PGI$_2$, PGE$_2$, and PGD$_2$) increase edema formation when injected locally at sites of tissue injury. One proposed mechanism for the anti-inflammatory effects of aspirin, indomethacin, and other nonsteroidal anti-inflammatory drugs is their inhibition of prostaglandin production.

Complement System

The complement system consists of a group of 20 plasma proteins. In addition to being a source of vasoactive mediators, components of the complement system are an integral part of the immune system and play an important role in host defense against bacterial infection. Originally described as a biologic effect of serum responsible for the lysis of antibody-coated cells, it is now known that this activity is present in an inactive form in plasma. These proteins are sequentially activated by two independent pathways, termed "classical" and "alternative" (Fig. 2-12).

Classical Pathway

Activators of the classical pathway (Table 2-1) include antigen–antibody immune complexes and products of bacteria and viruses. The activation of the classical pathway involves recognition of the inflammatory agent by the first component of complement, C1. C1 consists of three separate proteins, C1q, C1r, and C1s. When IgM immunoglobulin or molecules of specific IgG subclasses are bound to soluble or fixed antigens on target cells or tissue substrates, alterations in the conformation of the Fc component initiate binding of C1q. This results in sequential enzymatic activation of C1r and C1s. Two additional components of the complement system, C4 and C2, serve as the substrate for the enzymatically active C1s. The action of C1s on C4 and C2 is responsible for the

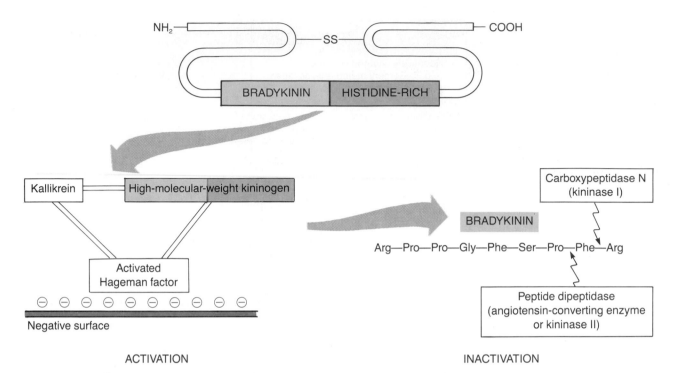

Figure 2-11.   The bradykinin precursor, kininogen, interacts with kallikrein and activated Hageman factor to form a trimolecular complex. Kallikrein releases bradykinin from kininogen. Bradykinin is, in turn, inactivated by kininases.

release of the first soluble anaphylatoxin, C4a, and the generation of the complex C4b2a. This complex, in turn, has proteolytic activity for the C3 molecule and has been defined as a C3 convertase. The C3 convertase cleaves C3, generating a second soluble anaphylatoxin molecule, C3a, and a residual product of C3 cleavage, C3b. The resulting multimolecular complex formed with C4b2a binds C5 and initiates hydrolysis of the C5 molecule, a process that generates a third complement-derived anaphylatoxin, C5a, and a residual component of C5 cleavage, C5b. The C5b molecule serves as a nucleus on target cell surface membranes for the sequential binding of C6, C7, and C8, and the polymerization of C9 molecules. This cascade leads to the formation of a macromolecular complex termed the **membrane attack complex.**

The assembly of the membrane attack complex on target cell surfaces occurs through hydrophobic interactions of the molecules. Morphologically, the injury by the membrane attack complex appears as a cylindrical hole in the cell membrane. As a consequence of its highly lipophilic nature, the membrane attack complex alters the phospholipid bilayer and membrane functions, which may ultimately result in the loss of cell membrane integrity, followed by cell lysis. Gram-negative bacteria are protected from the cytolytic action of the membrane attack complex by

a peptidylglycan layer. However, lysozyme, an enzyme present in the granules of phagocytic cells, is capable of cleaving the peptidylglycan layer. Once the bacteria are exposed to this enzyme, the membrane attack complex inserts into the cell membrane and lysis is initiated.

Alternative Pathway

Activation of the alternative pathway of the complement system is initiated through derivative products of infectious organisms and through foreign materials (Table 2-1) via a cascade-like interaction of specific plasma proteins. In the alternative pathway, unlike the classical pathway, C1, C4, and C2 are not involved. Activation of the alternative pathway occurs through the binding of C3 with two plasma proteins, factor B and factor D. This results in the formation of an enzymatically active derivative of factor B. The larger fragment, termed Bb, catalyzes the conversion of C3 to C3b and C3a. When C3b is bound to Bb, a C3 convertase is generated, thus greatly amplifying subsequent conversion of C3 and generating additional C3b and C3a. In addition, C5 convertase is formed, which in turn generates C5b (soluble C5a), and the membrane attack complex is subsequently

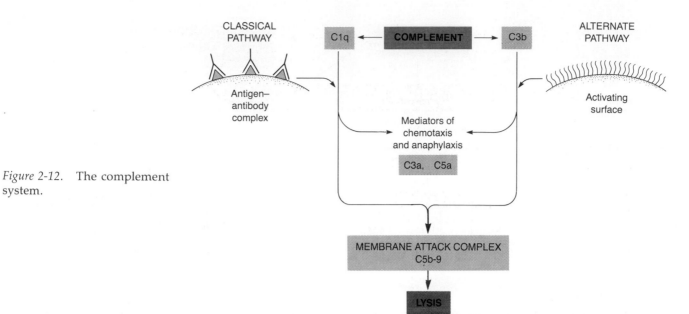

Figure 2-12. The complement system.

assembled. Thus, whether the alternative or the classical complement pathway is activated, the end result is the same: formation of a membrane attack complex capable of inducing cell lysis and generation of the biologically active anaphylatoxins C3a and C5a.

Anaphylatoxins

The anaphylatoxins C3a, C4a, and C5a are important products of complement activation via the classical pathway. Each of these molecules has been shown to have potent effects on smooth muscle and the vasculature, including enhancement of smooth muscle contraction and increasing vascular permeability (Fig. 2-13). Both C3a and C5a also induce mast cell and basophil degranulation, and the consequent release of histamine further potentiates the increase in vascular permeability. In addition to their effects on

vascular smooth muscle, the anaphylatoxins stimulate contraction of bronchial smooth muscle and cause airway narrowing. This effect is produced in two ways. The first is dependent on arachidonic acid metabolism in the lung; the second is mediated by the release of mast cell products.

C5a is also a potent chemotactic factor for neutrophils, monocytes, eosinophils, and basophils and induces low levels of neutrophil degranulation and superoxide anion production. Additional effects of C5a stimulation of neutrophils include enhancement of both the phagocytic response and, in response to a second stimulus, degranulation and superoxide anion production. This enhancement effect is referred to as "cell priming." C3a and C5a also modulate certain immune responses. Whereas C3a inhibits T-lymphocyte proliferation, C5a promotes immune reactions. These immune-regulatory properties of C3a and C5a are discussed in greater detail in Chapter 4.

Regulation of the Complement System

Activation of the complement system is regulated by three mechanisms. One mechanism involves the spontaneous decay of the individual enzymatically active complexes C4b2a, C3bBb, or cleavage products C3b and C4b. A second regulatory mechanism involves the proteolytic inactivation of specific components by inhibitors present in plasma, including factor I (an inhibitor of C3b and C4b) and serum carboxypeptidase N (SCPN). SCPN cleaves the carboxy-terminal arginine from the anaphylatoxins C4a,

Table 2-1 Activators of the Complement System

CLASSICAL	ALTERNATIVE
Immune complexes (IgM, IgG)	Zymosan (yeast cell wall)
Aggregated antibody	Cobra venom factor (CVF)
Proteases	Endotoxin (lipopolysaccharides)
Urate crystals	Polysaccharides
Polyanions (polynucleotides)	X-ray contrast media
	Dialysis membranes
	Parasites, fungi, and viruses

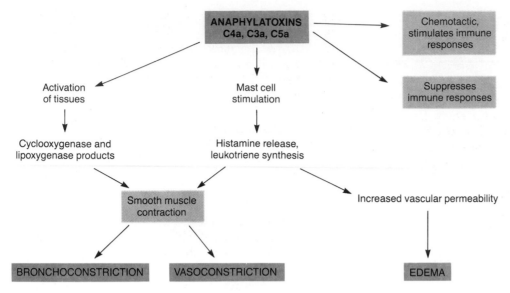

Figure 2-13. Biologic activity of the anaphylatoxins.

C3a, and C5a in a manner similar to that of brady-kinin. Cleavage of the single amino acid markedly decreases the biologic activity of each of these molecules. A third mechanism of regulation of the complement system relates to the binding of active components by specific proteins in the plasma. The C1 esterase inhibitor (C1INA) regulates the activation of the classical pathway by binding C1r and C1s, forming an irreversibly inactive complex. Additional binding proteins present in plasma include factor H and C4b binding protein. These proteins form complexes with C3b and C4b, respectively, and enhance their susceptibility to proteolytic cleavage by factor I.

The complement system plays an important role in many forms of immunologic tissue injury (Chapter 4). In addition, it is an important host defense mechanism against bacterial infection. Bacterial activation of the complement system may occur either by direct activation of the alternative pathway or as an outcome of antibody binding to the surface of the bacterium and activation of the classical pathway. Once the complement system is activated, bacteriolysis may follow, either by means of the assembled membrane attack complex or by enhanced bacterial clearance following opsonization. Bacterial **opsonization** is the process by which a specific molecule (e.g., IgG or C3b) binds to the surface of the bacterium. The process enhances phagocytosis by enabling receptors on the phagocytic cell membrane (e.g., the Fc or the C3b receptor) to recognize and bind to the opsonized bacterium. Viruses, parasites, and transformed cells also activate the complement system by similar mechanisms, resulting in their inactivation or death.

The importance of an intact and appropriately regulated complement system as a component of host defense is exemplified in individuals who have deficiencies of either specific complement components or regulatory proteins. **Deficiencies of complement components may be either acquired or congenital.** The most common congenital defect is a C2 deficiency, which is inherited as an autosomal codominant trait with a gene frequency of approximately 1%. Acquired deficiencies of early complement components may occur in patients with certain autoimmune diseases, especially those associated with circulating immune complexes. These include certain forms of membranous glomerulonephritis and systemic lupus erythematosus. Patients with congenital deficiencies in the early components of the complement system have recurrent symptoms resembling those of systemic lupus erythematosus. Patients with deficiencies of the middle (C3, C5) and terminal (C6, C7, or C8) complement components are particularly susceptible to pyogenic bacterial and neisserial infections, respectively—a circumstance that indicates the importance of individual components of the complement system in host surveillance against bacterial infection. Congenital defects have been reported in regulatory proteins of the complement system, including deficiencies of C1INA and SCPN. Deficiency of C1INA is associated with the syndrome of hereditary angioedema. The syndrome is characterized by episodic, painless, nonpitting edema of soft tissues, particularly the subepithelial areas, gastrointestinal tract, and upper respiratory areas. It may become life threatening if the larynx is affected.

Phospholipid Metabolism and Arachidonic Acid Metabolites

Among the mediators generated by inflammatory cells and injured tissues, certain derivatives of phospholipids and fatty acids are important. Depending on the specific inflammatory cell and the nature of the stimulus, activated cells generate arachidonic acid by one of two pathways (Fig. 2-14). The first pathway involves stimulus-induced activation of phospholipase A_2, which enhances the hydrolysis of arachidonic acid from the glycerol backbone of membrane phospholipids. In particular, phosphatidylcholine is an important substrate of phospholipase A_2 and is thus the major source of arachidonic acid in inflammatory cells. The second mechanism by which arachidonic acid is generated is the metabolism of phosphatidylinositol by phospholipase C to diacylglycerol and inositol phosphates. Diacylglycerol lipase then cleaves arachidonic acid from diacylglycerol. Once generated, arachidonic acid, a polyunsaturated (20:4) fatty acid, is metabolized via two pathways: cyclo-oxygenation, with the subsequent production of prostaglandins and thromboxanes; and lipoxygenation, to form monohydroxyeicosatetranoic and dihydroxycicosatetranoic acids (HETEs and diHETEs) and leukotrienes.

Specific cyclo-oxygenase enzymes in inflammatory cells generate endoperoxide derivatives of arachidonic acid, including prostaglandin G_2 (PGG$_2$) and prostaglandin H_2 (PGH$_2$). These endoperoxides are unstable and, depending on the specific inflammatory cell or tissue, are metabolized to more stable prostaglandins, including PGI$_2$ (also known as prostacyclin), PGF$_{2\alpha}$, PGE$_2$, PGD$_2$ and thromboxane A$_2$ (TxA$_2$). The primary cyclo-oxygenase metabolite in platelets is thromboxane A$_2$; endothelial cells secrete principally PGI$_2$. Macrophages, depending on their state of activation, produce any or all of these derivative products.

PGI$_2$ and PGE$_2$, owing to their vasodilatory effects, enhance vascular permeability at sites of inflammation; thromboxane A$_2$ is a potent vasoconstrictor and plays an important role in the mediation of the "second wave" of platelet aggregation. PGI$_2$ and PGE$_2$ bind to specific receptors on inflammatory cells, thereby activating adenylate cyclase and increasing intracellular cyclic adenosine monophosphate (cAMP) levels, thereby inhibiting their functional responses to other inflammatory stimuli.

A second pathway by which arachidonic acid is metabolized in inflammatory cells and tissues is lipoxygenation and the formation of hydroperoxyeicosatetranoic acid compounds (HPETEs). Hydroperoxy- compounds may be metabolized to hydroxyeicosatetranoic acids (HETEs) or to leukotriene A$_4$, which contains three conjugated double bonds and serves as a precursor for other leukotriene molecules. In the neutrophil and in certain macrophage populations, leukotriene A$_4$ is metabolized to leukotriene B$_4$, a compound with potent chemotactic activity for neutrophils, monocytes, and macrophages. In other cell types, especially mast cells, basophils, and macrophages, the addition of glutathione to leukotriene A$_4$ results in the formation of leukotriene C$_4$. Leukotrienes D$_4$ and E$_4$ are formed following sequential removal of the amino acids glycine and glutamine, respectively. LTC$_4$, LTD$_4$, and LTE$_4$ are collectively known as **slow-reacting substances of anaphylaxis (SRS-As)**. They stimulate the contraction of smooth muscle and enhance vascular permeability. The generation of leukotriene B$_4$ at sites of tissue injury plays an important role in the recruitment of polymorphonuclear leukocytes, while the production of leukotrienes C$_4$, D$_4$, and E$_4$ is responsible for the development of much of the clinical symptomatology associated with allergic-type reactions.

The importance of arachidonic acid metabolites in mediating many of the effects of the inflammatory response is demonstrated by the ability of inhibitors of the involved enzymes to attenuate both the pathologic changes and clinical symptomatology (Table 2-2). Corticosteroids are widely used to inhibit the tissue destruction associated with many inflammatory diseases, including allergic responses, rheumatoid arthritis, and systemic lupus erythematosus. Corticosteroids induce the synthesis of an inhibitor

Table 2-2 Biologic Activity of Arachidonic Acid Metabolites

METABOLITE	BIOLOGIC ACTIVITY
PGE$_2$, PGD$_2$	Induce vasodilation, bronchodilation Inhibit inflammatory cell function
PGI$_2$	Induces vasodilation, bronchodilation Inhibits inflammatory cell function
PGF$_{2\alpha}$	Induces vasodilation, bronchoconstriction
TxA$_2$	Induces vasoconstriction, bronchoconstriction Enhances inflammatory cell functions (esp. platelets)
LTB$_4$	Chemotactic for phagocytic cells Stimulates phagocytic cell adherence Enhances microvascular permeability
LTC$_4$, LTD$_4$, LTE$_4$	Induce smooth-muscle contraction Constrict pulmonary airways Increase microvascular permeability

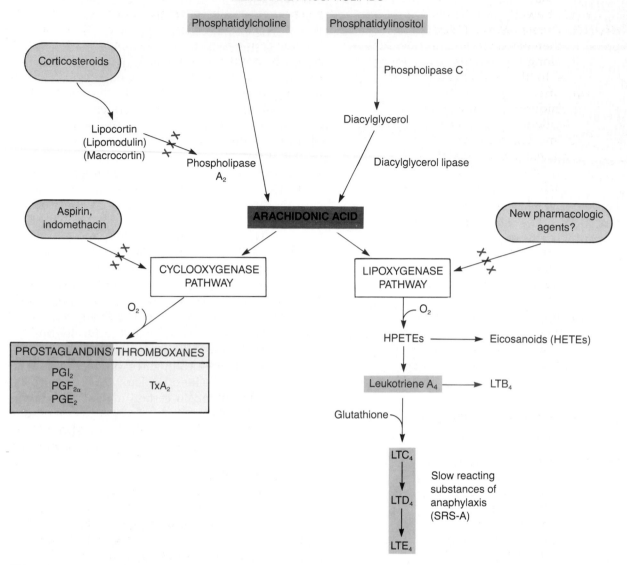

Figure 2-14. Arachidonic acid metabolism.

of phospholipase A_2 and block the release of arachidonic acid in inflammatory cells. Originally described as two proteins, lipomodulin and macrocortin, this regulatory inhibitor is now known to be a single protein, referred to as **lipocortin.**

A second class of anti-inflammatory agents that is widely used in the treatment of inflammatory diseases comprises the nonsteroidal anti-inflammatory drugs. These compounds—including aspirin, indomethacin, ibuprofen, and piroxicam—inhibit cyclooxygenase, and thus the synthesis of prostaglandins and thromboxanes. A third class of compounds that block specific lipoxygenase activities in inflammatory cells is currently being developed.

Cellular Recruitment

The second phase of the acute inflammatory response involves the accumulation of leukocytes— especially polymorphonuclear leukocytes (PMNs)— at sites of tissue injury (Fig. 2-15). During the first 24 hours (and sometimes even in the first few hours) after initiation of injury, many polymorphonuclear leukocytes accumulate. The sequence of events leading to this accumulation at inflammatory sites is initiated by locally generated soluble chemical mediators. These mediators, collectively referred to as **chemotactic factors,** are generated in high concentrations at sites of tissue injury, with a progressively decreasing gradient away from the injured tissue.

The physiologic responses of circulating leukocytes exposed to chemotactic factors include margination of the cells along the vascular wall, adherence of the leukocytes to the endothelium or vascular basement membrane, emigration through the vascular wall, and unidirectional migration toward increasing concentrations of the chemotactic agent (**chemotaxis**). The most important chemotactic factors for polymorphonuclear leukocytes are C5a derived from complement, low-molecular-weight N-formylated peptides (such as N-formyl-methionyl-leucyl-phenylalanine) derived from bacteria and mitochondria, and specific products of lipid metabolism, including leukotriene B_4.

Chemotactic factors for other cell types, including monocytes, lymphocytes, basophils, and eosinophils, are also produced at sites of tissue injury. Low-molecular-weight secretory products of lymphocytes (referred to as lymphokines) are chemotactic, as are secretions of monocytes and tissue macrophages (monokines). Proteases from neutrophils and macrophages also cleave C5 to generate C5a or C5a-related peptides.

Inflammatory Cell Activation

The polymorphonuclear leukocyte, mast cell, mononuclear phagocytic cells and platelet are important cellular components of the inflammatory reaction. Once stimulated, these cells release inflammatory mediators that cause tissue injury.

The polymorphonuclear leukocyte is activated in response to phagocytic stimuli or by binding of chemotactic mediators or antibody–antigen complex to specific receptors on its cell membrane. Neutrophil receptors react with the Fc portion of IgG and IgM molecules; with complement system components C5a, C3b, and C3bi; with arachidonic acid metabolites (e.g., leukotriene B_4); and with formylated low-molecular-weight chemotactic peptides.

Mast cells, platelets, and mononuclear phagocytic cells are also activated in a receptor-specific manner. **The process by which diverse stimuli lead to the functional responses of inflammatory cells (e.g., degranulation or aggregation) is referred to as "stimulus–response coupling."** Common pathways associated with inflammatory cell activation are stimulus-induced increases in phospholipid metabolism of cell membranes, raised intracellular calcium levels, and augmented protein kinase activity within the cell (Fig. 2-16).

The binding of a chemotactic factor to a specific receptor on the cell membrane results in the formation of a ligand–receptor complex (Fig. 2-17). A guanine-nucleotide regulatory protein couples the ligand–receptor complex to a specific phosphodiesterase in the inflammatory cell membrane, a process that activates the esterase. In the neutrophil this phosphodiesterase activity is phospholipase C. Stimulus-induced activation of phospholipase C enhances phosphoinositide turnover and the formation of two potent metabolites, diacylglycerol and inositol trisphosphate. Inositol trisphosphate releases calcium from intracellular stores. The release of intracellular calcium in conjunction with an influx of calcium ions from the extracellular environment contributes to an increase in free intracellular calcium—a critical event for the activation of most inflammatory cells. The increase in free intracellular calcium may have many effects, including the potentiation of phospholipase A_2 activity and the activation of multiple protein kinases that phosphorylate a variety of proteins. In addition, calmodulin (a high-affinity calcium-binding protein) is important in the activation of inflammatory cells. The mobilization of intracellular calcium is also closely linked to the activation of cytoskeletal elements. Assembly of the microtubular system and activation of actin–myosin complexes are crucial for the secretion of cytoplasmic granules and for chemotaxis of neutrophils and other inflammatory cells.

A second product of phospholipase C activity, diacylglycerol, mediates additional responses within the cell. Diacylglycerol activates protein kinase C, a cytosolic enzyme that associates with the cell membrane following cell stimulation. Protein kinase C phosphorylates several substrate proteins within the cell, including cytoskeletal elements, and alters their functional properties.

As described above, phospholipase A_2 is also activated by stimulation of inflammatory cells. This calcium-activated phospholipase releases arachidonic acid from membrane phospholipids; its subsequent metabolism to biologically active compounds is important in both inflammatory cell activation and the development of the inflammatory response.

Phospholipase A_2 activity is regulated by lipocortin (see Fig. 2-14). The dephosphorylated form of lipocortin inhibits phospholipase A_2 activity and the release of arachidonic acid. Thus, the phosphorylation of lipocortin during inflammatory cell activation frees phospholipase A_2 activity from inhibition, resulting in an increased release of arachidonic acid. The induction of elevated levels of dephosphorylated lipocortin within inflammatory cells has been postulated

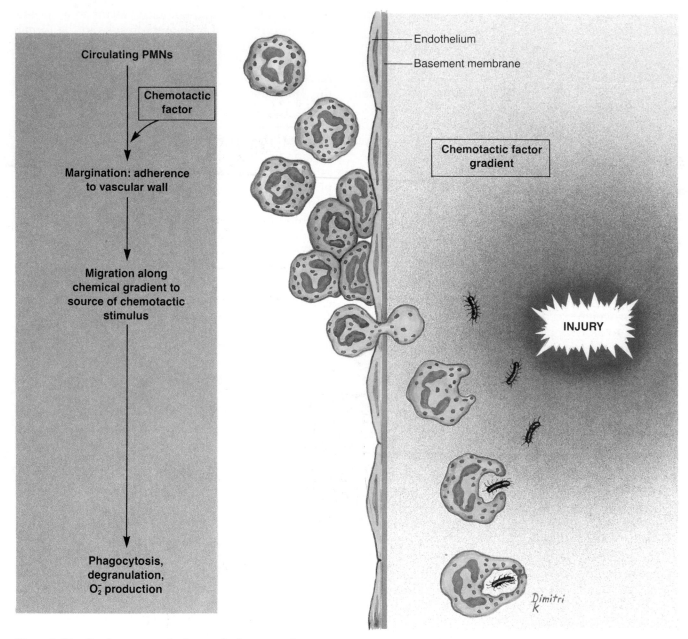

Figure 2-15. Leukocyte exudation and phagocytosis.

as a mechanism for the anti-inflammatory effects of corticosteroids.

The activation of methyltransferases following inflammatory cell stimulation also affects the phospholipid components of inflammatory cell membranes. Two methyltransferases that catalyze the methylation of phosphatidylethanolamine to phosphatidylcholine have been identified in the mast cell and basophil. The generation of phosphatidylcholine via transmethylation reactions is thought to be important for antigen-induced degranulation of mast cells and basophils.

An understanding of inflammatory cell stimulation will provide the basis for new strategies for therapeutic modulation of inflammation in human disease. For instance, specific lipoxygenase or phospholipase inhibitors could be developed to inhibit the early activation processes of inflammatory cells, thus suppressing the tissue injury associated with certain diseases.

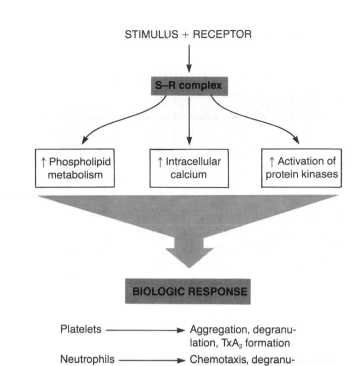

Figure 2-16. Mechanisms of inflammatory cell activation.

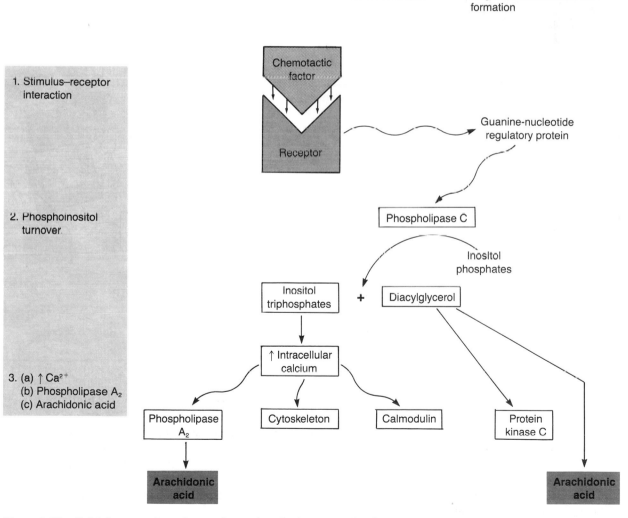

Figure 2-17. Initial events in polymorphonuclear leukocyte activation.

REVIEW ARTICLES

Fantone JC, Ward PA: Role of oxygen derived free radicals and metabolites in leukocyte-dependent inflammatory reactions. Am J Pathol 107:397-418, 1982

Elsbach P, Weiss J: Oxygen-dependent and oxygen-independent mechanisms of microbial activity of neutrophils. Immunol Letters, 11:159-163, 1985

Cochrane CG: Mechanisms coupling stimulation and function in leukocytes. (Minisymposium). Fed Proc 43:2729-2763, 1984

Synderman R, Pike MC: Chemoattractant receptors on phagocytic cells. Ann Rev Immunol 2:257-281, 1984

Becker EL: Leukocyte stimulation: Receptor, membrane, and metabolic events. (Minisymposium). Fed Proc 45:2148-2161, 1985

Berridge MJ: Inositol trisphosphate and diacylglycerol as second messengers. Biochem J 220:345-360, 1984

O'Flaherty JT: Lipid mediators of inflammation and allergy. Lab Invest 47:314-329, 1982

Samuelson B: Leukotrienes: Mediators of immediate hypersensitivity reactions and inflammation. Science 220:568-575, 1983

Goetzl EJ, Payan DG, Goldman DW: Immunopathogenetic roles of leukotrienes in human diseases. J Clin Immunol 4:79-84, 1984

Marcus AJ: The eicosanoids in biology and medicine. J Lipid Res 25:1511-1516, 1984

Weiss SJ, LoBulgio AF: Biology of disease: Phagocyte-generated oxygen metabolites and cellular injury. Lab Invest 47:5-18, 1982

Fantone JC, Ward PA: Polymorphonuclear leukocyte-mediated cell and tissue injury. Human Pathol 16:973-978, 1985

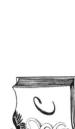

MC/VISA
PHONE ORDERS
Tel: 800-288-9777
Tel: (617) 262-5162
Fax: (617) 266-4458

Brown & Connolly
Medical Bookstore
1315 Boylston Street
Boston, Massachusetts 02215

3

Repair, Regeneration, and Fibrosis

Antonio Martinez-Hernandez

The Extracellular Matrix

The Repair Reaction

Wound Healing

Healing in Specific Tissues

Figure 3-1. Collagen synthesis, secretion, and assembly. The initial steps of collagen synthesis, namely translation by membrane-bound ribosomes and passage of the nascent chains into the rough endoplasmic reticulum (RER), follow pathways common to all proteins. In the cisternae of the RER the prepeptide sequences are removed, proline and lysine residues become hydroxylated, the propeptides are glycosylated, individual α chains associate by disulfide bonds, and triple helixes are formed. After all these post-translational modifications take place, individual procollagen molecules are secreted to the extracellular space. In the case of type I collagen, at least, the propeptides must be cleaved before fiber assembly can occur. The current theory is that partially confined spaces formed by invaginations of the cell membrane are the sites of extracellular processing and fiber assembly. Several collagen molecules associate in a quarter-staggered manner to form collagen fibrils, and fibrils associate to form collagen fibers with the characteristic cross-banding. In turn, collagen fibers associate to form bundles recognizable by light microscopy.

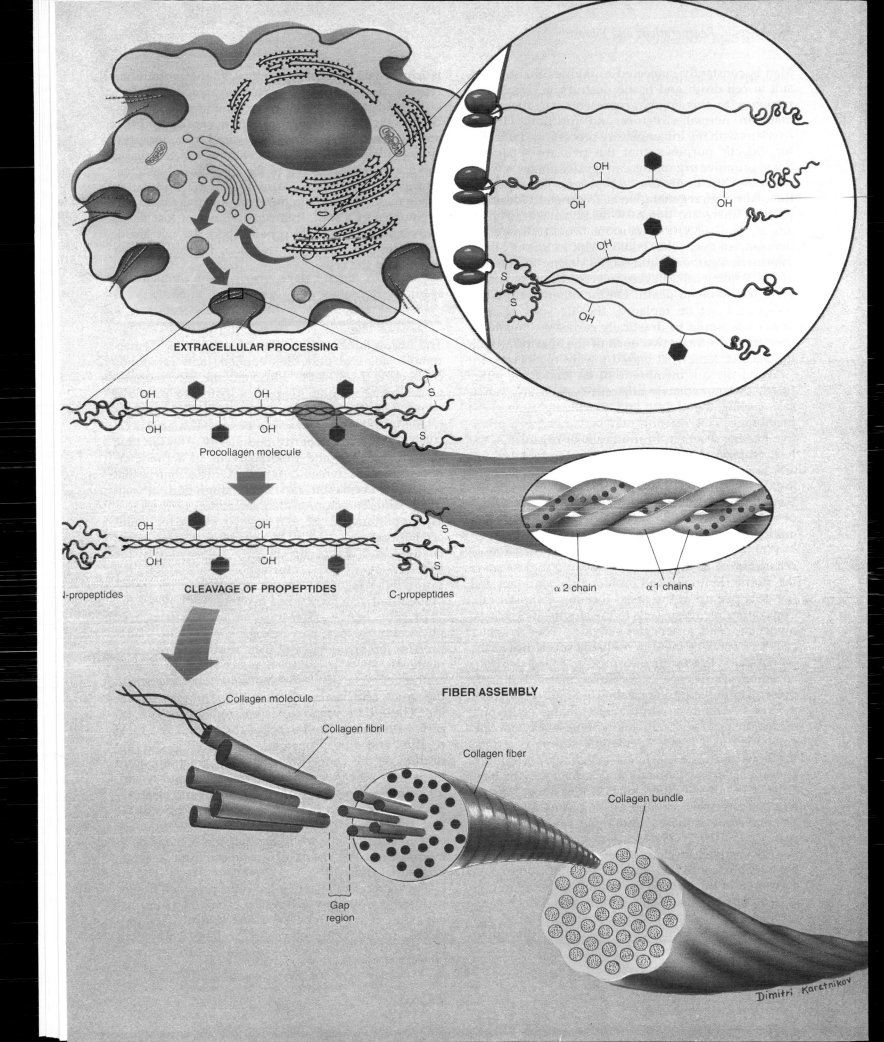

EXTRACELLULAR PROCESSING

OH   OH   S

OH   OH   S

Procollagen molecule

OH   OH   S

OH   OH   S

N-propeptides   **CLEAVAGE OF PROPEPTIDES**   C-propeptides

α 2 chain   α 1 chains

Collagen molecule

Collagen fibril

FIBER ASSEMBLY

Collagen fiber

Collagen bundle

Gap region

Dimitri Karetnikov

4

Immunopathology

Kent J. Johnson, Stephen W. Chensue,
Steven L. Kunkel, and Peter A. Ward

Cellular Components of the
Immune Response

Immunologically Mediated
Tissue Injury

Immune Reactions to
Transplanted Organs and
Tissues

Assessment of Immune
Status

Immunodeficiency Diseases

Autoimmunity

Figure 4-1. Demonstration by immunofluorescence of an extensive deposition of IgG in a renal glomerulus from a patient with systemic lupus erythematosus.

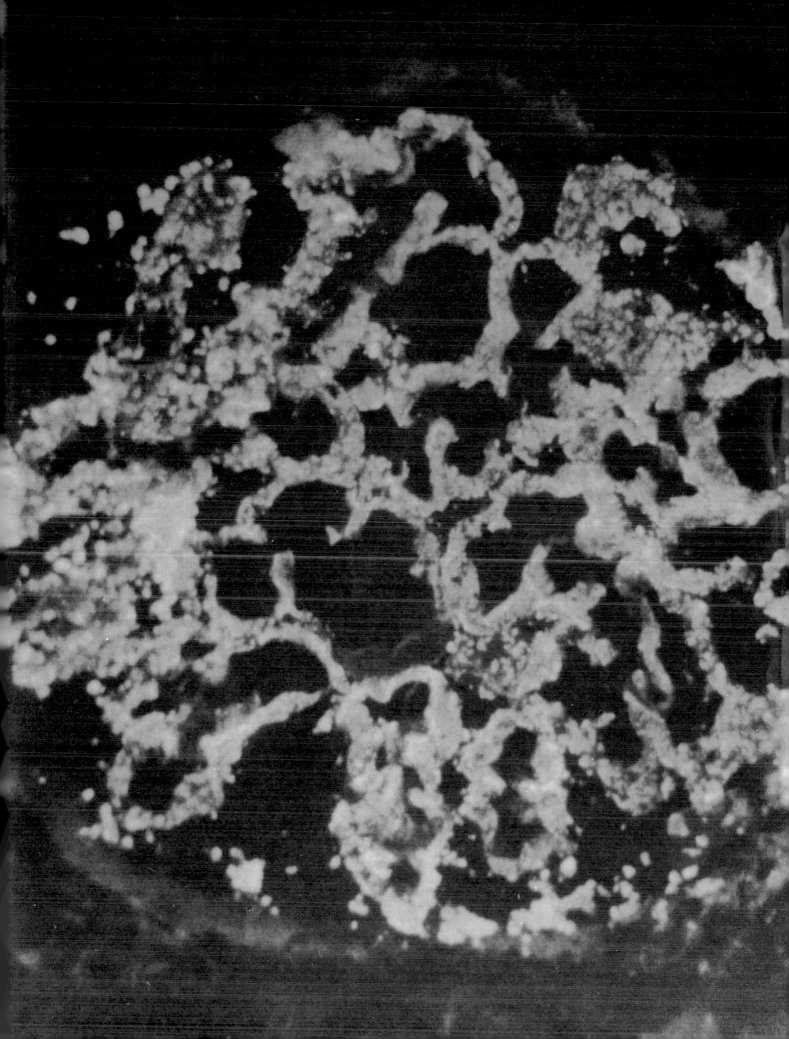

Cellular Components of the Immune Response

The immune system comprises an exquisitely complex network of cellular and humoral elements that promote defense against a vast spectrum of microbial agents, ranging from viruses to multicellular parasites. Many of the cellular and humoral components of this system have been described in Chapter 2. Here, we extend the discussion of the cells that orchestrate immune responses and describe the immunopathologic manifestations of exaggerated or dysfunctional immune responses.

Lymphocytes

Lymphocytes, because they have the capacity to recognize and react with specific foreign molecules, are primary directors of antigen-specific immune responses. The traditional model of lymphocyte development was that all follow one of two major pathways of development (Fig. 4-2). All lymphocytes originate from primitive yolk sac stem cell precursors that, depending on subsequent migration and molecular signals, become either T cells or B cells. In addition, however, a third class of lymphocytes lacking the defining characteristics of T and B cells has been recognized. The ontogeny of these "null" cells is unclear. The natural killer cells, which are described later, belong in this category. T- and B-lymphocytes are defined on the basis of several functional and phenotypic characteristics acquired during their ontogeny.

T Cells

Figure 4-3 summarizes T cell ontogeny in the thymus. The stem cell precursors interact with thymic epithelium, which provides the molecular signals that cause sequential expression of genes conferring the specific functional and phenotypic characteristics of T cells. A spectrum of functionally related T cell membrane antigens has been defined with monoclonal antibody reagents, thus enabling the maturational stage of the T cell to be identified. **T cells at different stages of maturation are characterized by the surface markers that they express.**

T cell development begins with proliferation of antigen-specific clones in the cortical regions of thymic lobes. The early, or least mature, cortical thymocytes comprise about 10% of the lymphocytes and express membrane antigens designated T9, T10, and T11. The T11 antigen is essentially a universal T cell marker and persists throughout subsequent maturation. Antibodies to T11 interfere with the characteristic ability of human T cells to bind sheep erythrocytes, an effect that suggests an association of the T11 antigen with the sheep erythrocyte receptor. T9 and T10 antigens are markers of activation—that is, they are associated with proliferating or metabolically stimulated T cells. The T9 antigen is the receptor for transferrin and provides a means to acquire iron during active metabolic states. Late cortical thymocytes comprise 80% of the thymic population and express new antigens, designated T1, T4, T6, and T8. They lose the early T9 antigen. Whereas the T1 antigen persists on all T cells, the T6 antigen is transient and is lost by the time thymocytes migrate to medullary areas. In these areas, the T4 and T8 antigens are distributed among two separate cell populations, which display helper and suppressor/cytotoxic functions, respectively. The medullary T cells also acquire the T3 membrane marker, which is associated with the antigen receptor and persists for the life of the cell. The expression of antigen-specific receptors does not require the presence of antigen, but seems to be the result of programmed gene expression and modification. The final stage of development occurs with the migration of T cells to blood and the lymphatic system, where the T10 antigen is lost. **In the blood and peripheral lymphoid organs, T4+ cells comprise 65% and T8+ cells 35% of all T cells.**

T cells recognize specific antigens—usually proteins or haptens bound to proteins—and respond as directed by endogenous maturational factors and exogenous molecular signals. Experimental studies suggest that T4+ and T8+ cells are, in fact, subsets of T cells that have varied effector or regulatory functions. **Effector functions include secretion of proinflammatory mediators and cytotoxic responses to cells containing foreign or altered membrane antigens. Regulatory functions include augmentation or suppression of immune responses, usually by secretion of specific helper or suppressor molecules.** One such helper molecule is **interleukin-2 (IL-2)**, which promotes the growth of activated T cells. **In general, T4+ cells perform helper functions and secrete proinflammatory lymphokines. By contrast, T8+ cells generally perform suppressor and cytotoxic functions.** Clearly, however, there is overlap, since T8+ cells secrete lymphokines and T4+ cells induce suppressor activity. A summary of some of the important T cell lymphokines and their effects is provided in Table 4-1.

An interesting aspect of T cell antigen recognition is the requirement for antigens to be presented in the context of self-histocompatibility membrane proteins.

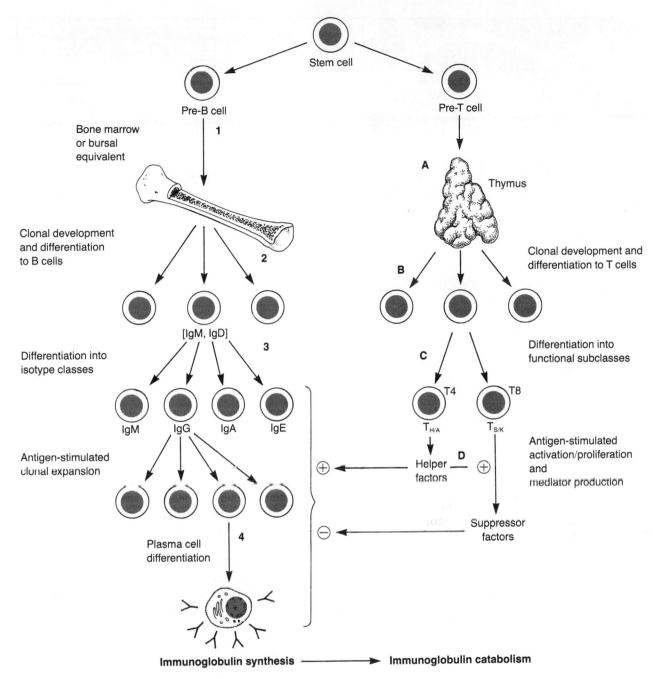

Stem cell

Pre-B cell

Pre-T cell

Bone marrow
or bursal
equivalent

1

A

Thymus

Clonal development
and differentiation
to B cells

2

Clonal development and
differentiation to T cells

B

[IgM, IgD]

3

Differentiation into
isotype classes

C

Differentiation into
functional subclasses

IgM   IgG   IgA   IgE

T4   T8

$T_{H/A}$ $T_{S/K}$

Antigen-stimulated
clonal expansion

⊕   Helper
factors   **D**   ⊕

Antigen-stimulated
activation/proliferation
and
mediator production

⊖   Suppressor
factors

Plasma cell
differentiation

4

Immunoglobulin synthesis ⟶ **Immunoglobulin catabolism**

Figure 4-2. Major maturational stages of lymphocytes.

In other words, T cells have a membrane receptor complex that, for a maximal immune response, must interact not only with foreign but also with self-histocompatibility molecular structures. Thus, accessory cells that bear appropriate histocompatibility antigens, such as macrophages, B cells, or biologically and chemically altered self-membrane proteins, must present antigen to T cells. The relevant histocompatibility antigens are derived from genes in the **major** **histocompatibility complex** (MHC). This region codes for class I and class II membrane proteins, a subject that will be discussed in greater detail below. In general, T8+ cells recognize antigen and class I molecules, whereas T4+ cells recognize antigen and class II molecules. It should be noted that histoincompatible foreign class I and II antigens are themselves potent immunogens and are recognized by host T cells.

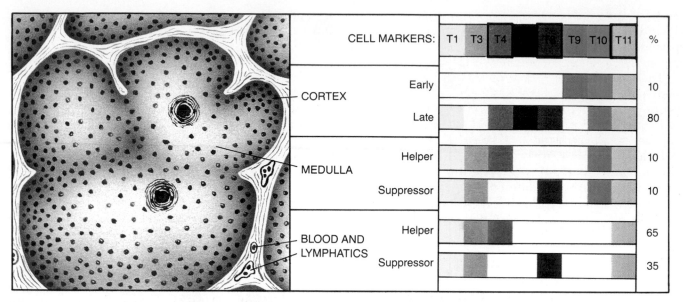

Figure 4-3. Membrane marker changes during thymic T cell maturation.

B Cells

B cells are defined as lymphocytes that bear membrane immunoglobulin and under appropriate conditions differentiate into antibody-secreting cells. As illustrated in Figure 4-2, following development in the embryonic yolk sac, precursor B cells migrate to the fetal liver and later to the bone marrow. The signal for B cell differentiation is provided at some point during the migration, but the source and nature of this signal are unclear. In birds this signal is provided by a specialized hindgut organ called the bursa of Fabricius.

Pre-B cells contain cytoplasmic heavy-chain μ immunoglobulins, but no light-chain or surface immunoglobulins. However, membrane receptors for complement fragment C3b and HLA class II proteins are present. In the fetal liver and bone marrow, pre-B cells multiply and diversify into a vast number of clones. Immature B cells are recognized by the appearance of surface monomeric IgM. With subsequent maturation involving gene rearrangements, B cells acquire surface IgD. Other membrane markers are also acquired—for example, receptors for IgG-Fc component, complement fragment C3d, and Epstein-Barr virus.

The next stage of B cell development involves further gene rearrangements, a process that results in **isotype switching.** In other words, in the absence of antigenic stimulation, a proportion of the B cell clones proceed to express other heavy-chain isotypes: IgG (γ_1, γ_2, γ_3), IgA (α_1 or α_2), or IgE (ϵ). In the presence of antigen, T cells produce differentiation factors that either stimulate B cell isotype switching or induce the proliferation of particular committed isotype populations.

Mature B cells are primarily in a resting state, awaiting activation by foreign antigen. Activation involves cross-linking of membrane immunoglobulin receptors by antigens presented on accessory cells. This initial stimulus leads to proliferation and clonal expansion, which can be amplified by macrophage-

Table 4-1 T Cell Products and Their Biologic Activity

LYMPHOKINE	TARGET CELL AND ACTION
B cell growth factor (BCGF)	Stimulates proliferation and differentiation of B cells
B cell differentiation factor (BCDF)	Causes differentiation of terminal plasma cells
Colony stimulating factor (CSF)	Stimulates differentiation of monocytes from bone marrow stem cells
Fibroblast activating factor (FAF)	Promotes proliferation of fibroblasts
Gamma-interferon (γIF)	Activates macrophages and promotes cytotoxic functions
Interleukin-2 (IL-2)	Stimulates proliferation of activated T cells
Interleukin-3 (IL-3)	Stimulates differentiation of bone marrow stem cells
Leukocyte inhibition factor (LIF)	Inhibits random migration of neutrophils
Lymphotoxin (LT)	Kills target tumor or virus-infected cells
Migration inhibition factor (MIF)	Inhibits random migration of macrophages

and T cell–derived factors, such as interleukin-1 (IL-1) and B cell growth factor. If no further signal is provided, the proliferating B cells return to the resting state and enter the **memory cell** pool.

The final stage of B cell differentiation into antibody-synthesizing plasma cells generally requires exposure to additional T cell products—for instance, B cell differentiation factors. This is the case for responses to most protein antigens. However, some polyvalent agents directly induce B cell proliferation and antibody synthesis, bypassing the requirements for B cell growth and differentiation factors. Such agents are called polyclonal B cell activators because they do not interact with antigen-binding sites and hence are not antigen-specific. Examples of these antigens are bacterial products (lipopolysaccharide, protein A) and certain viruses (Epstein-Barr virus, cytomegalovirus).

It is noteworthy that the spectrum of immunoglobulins produced during immune responses changes with age. Neonates tend to produce predominantly IgM; in contrast, older children and adults show rapid shifts toward IgG synthesis following antigenic challenge. Thus, B cell responses continue to be modified during early childhood.

In addition to antibodies, B cells also produce lymphokines that modulate immune responses.

Natural Killer Cells

One population of lymphocytes has the capacity to recognize directly and kill various tumor and virus-infected cells *in vitro*. These large lymphocytes with cytoplasmic granules cannot be precisely classified as T, B, or myelomonocytic cells. Thus, they represent a subset of so-called **null** cells and are termed **natural killer (NK) cells.** These cells possibly have several receptors for various target cell membrane structures.

Natural killer cells are affected by several molecular mediators. For example, interleukin-2 supports their growth, and interferons promote their killing activity. By contrast, prostaglandin E_2 is highly suppressive of NK cell activity.

NK cells also seem to have Fc receptors and thus kill target cells by an antibody-dependent mechanism. This null cell function was previously attributed to a population of K (killer) cells.

Mononuclear Phagocytes

***Mononuclear phagocyte* is a general term applied to populations of phagocytic cells found in virtually all organs and connective tissues. Among these cells are macrophages, monocytes, Kupffer's cells of the liver, and the so-called histiocytes.** These cells are identified by their nonsegmented nuclei, relatively abundant cytoplasm, and phagocytic function. Recent evidence suggests that there may be subpopulations of macrophages with different functional and phenotypic characteristics. Precursor cells (monoblasts and promonocytes) arise in the bone marrow, enter the circulation as monocytes, and then migrate to tissues, where they take up residence as "tissue" macrophages—that is, histiocytes. In the lung, liver, and spleen, large numbers of macrophages populate sinuses and capillaries to form an effective filtering system that removes effete cells and foreign particulate material from the blood. This system was formerly known as **the reticuloendothelial system** but is also termed the **mononuclear phagocytic system.** In addition to this housekeeping role, macrophages play a critical role in the induction of immune responses, as well as in the maintenance and resolution of inflammatory reactions.

Macrophages are important accessory cells by virtue of their expression of class II histocompatibility antigens. They actively ingest and process antigens for presentation to T cells in conjunction with class II antigens. The subsequent T cell responses are further amplified by macrophage-derived monokines. One of the best-characterized of these is interleukin-1 (previously known as T cell growth factor), which promotes the expression of interleukin-2 receptor by T cells, thereby augmenting interleukin-2–driven T cell proliferation. **Interleukin-1 also has a broad spectrum of effects on other tissues and, in general, prepares the body to combat infection—for example, it induces fever and promotes catabolic metabolism.**

Macrophages are dominant participants in subacute and chronic inflammatory reactions. During inflammation, increased numbers of monocytes are recruited from the bone marrow. Under chemotactic influences they migrate to sites of inflammation and mature into macrophages. Both recruited and local tissue macrophages participate and proliferate at these foci. Table 4-2 summarizes some of the many secretory products of macrophages that can play a role at sites of inflammation. Among these are proteins, lipids, nucleotides, and reactive oxygen metabolites. Functionally, these molecules are digestive, opsonic, cytotoxic, growth promoting, or growth inhibiting. Thus, macrophages are ideal cells both to effect and to direct inflammatory events, locally and systemically.

The functional activity of macrophages and the spectrum of molecules that they produce are regulated by external factors, such as T cell–derived lymphokines. Macrophages exposed to such factors become "activated"; that is, they acquire a greater capacity to release oxygen metabolites and kill tumor cells and intracellular microbes. Yet they show de-

---

Table 4-2 Major Macrophage Products

Proteins

Enzymes:
    Neutral proteinases (e.g., plasminogen activator elastase, collagenases)
    Lysozyme
    Arginase
    Lipoprotein lipase
    Angiotensin-converting enzyme
    Acid hydrolases
Plasma proteins:
    Coagulation proteins
    Complement components
    α_2-Macroglobulin
    Fibronectin
Monokines:
    Interleukin-1
    Tumor necrosis factor
    Interferon alpha
    Angiogenesis factor

Reactive Oxygen Species

    Superoxide anion
    Hydrogen peroxide
    Oxygen radicals

Bioactive Lipids

    Prostaglandin E_2
    Prostacyclin I_2
    Thromboxane B_2
    Leukotriene B_4, C_4, D_4, E_4
    Hydroxyeicosatetraenoic acids

Nucleotides

    Thymidine, uracil
    cAMP
    Uric acid

---

creased production of other molecules, such as interleukin-1 and prostaglandins. If the agent inciting an inflammatory process is poorly digestible, a granulomatous reaction may ensue. Under such conditions, macrophages show additional maturation and become so-called epithelioid cells and multinucleated giant cells. Epithelioid cells are macrophages with abundant eosinophilic cytoplasm that appear to be predominantly secretory. Giant cells may be fused macrophages or macrophages that have undergone mitosis without cytoplasmic division. Both epithelioid and giant cells probably function to sequester and digest foreign material.

Human Major Histocompatibility Complex (HLA Complex)

The discovery that the sera of multiparous women and multiply-transfused patients contain antibodies against blood leukocytes initiated the definition of an intricate system of membrane proteins known as **major histocompatibility complex** (MHC) antigens or **human leukocyte antigens** (HLA). These proteins, which are highly polymorphous within the human population, are **the main target antigens during rejection of transplanted organs.** We now know that such antigens allow for self-recognition during cell–cell interactions, especially in immune responses.

The HLA gene complex is located on the short arm of chromosome 6 (Fig. 4-4). Three major classes of molecules, designated I, II, and III, are coded for. The class III antigens represent certain complement components and are not histocompatibility antigens.

The class I antigens were the first MHC antigens to be defined, using the sera of multiparous women, and were found to be coded for by genes in the A, B, and C regions. These loci code for molecules of similar structure and are expressed in virtually all tissues. The molecule consists of two chains, a 44,000-dalton polymorphic transmembrane glycoprotein and a 12,000-dalton nonpolymorphic molecule called β_2-microglobulin. The latter is a superficial membrane protein in noncovalent association with the larger chain and is coded for by a gene on chromosome 15. The heavy chain contains the polymorphic antigenic determinants defining the many alleles that occupy the three class I loci. The alleles are expressed co-dominantly. Thus, tissues bear antigens for both parents. **Class I antigens are recognized by cytotoxic T cells during graft rejection or during killing of virus-infected cells.**

Class II molecules are coded for by genes in the D region; at least three major loci are defined: DP (formerly SB), DQ (formerly DC, MB, DS), and DR. These antigens are defined by specific antisera and mixed leukocyte reactions to be discussed below. These loci also code for molecules of similar structure and **are expressed primarily on macrophages and B cells.** Class II antigens are also referred to as Ia antigens because they are analogous to the mouse MHC genes that are associated with the immune response. Class II molecules consist of two noncovalently linked glycoprotein chains. The α-chain is 34,000 daltons and has a single disulfide bond. The β-chain is 29,000 daltons and has two disulfide bonds. Both are transmembrane proteins. As with class I antigens, alleles are expressed co-dominantly. **Class II molecules are important for interactions between immune cells, particularly in antigen presentation to T cells.**

Table 4-3 summarizes the methods used to define class I and II antigens for tissue typing prior to organ transplantations. **Class I antigens are serologically defined.** Briefly, a battery of defined antisera directed against various antigens are tested against the patient's white cells. Known antigens are named and

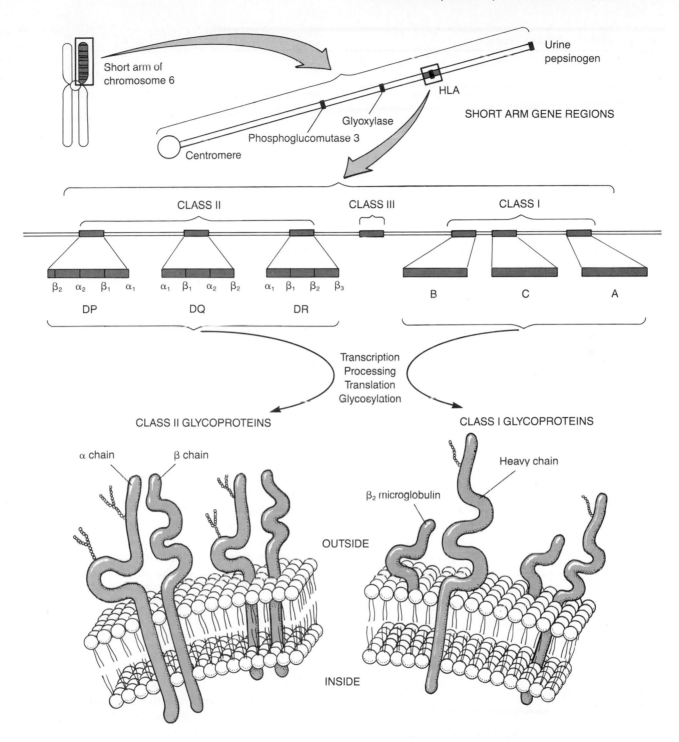

Figure 4-4. The genes of the human major histocompatibility complex (MHC) and their protein products.

Table 4-3 Methods of Tissue Typing

METHOD	ANTIGENS DETECTED	PRINCIPLE
Microcytotoxicity assay	Class I and some class II	Defined antibodies directed against specific HLA antigens are mixed with patient's cells in presence of complement. Cells bearing the specific antigens are lysed.
One-way mixed leukocyte	Class II (DQ, DR)	Mitomycin treated, HLA-defined typing cells are mixed with patient's cells. The patient's cells will not proliferate in response to cells with compatible antigens.
Primed lymphocyte typing assay	Class II (DP)	Defined typing cells "primed" to react with antigens are mixed with patient's cells treated with mitomycin. The primed cells will proliferate in response to cells bearing the specific antigens.

numbered according to the loci of origin—for example A1, A2, A3, B4, B6, C1, C2, and so on. **Tissue typing reveals two antigens for each locus, except when there is homozygosity at a locus.**

Class II DQ and DR antigens are defined serologically and by mixed lymphocyte reaction; that is, they are **lymphocyte-defined.** The mixed lymphocyte reaction is a sensitive method that uses a battery of mitomycin-treated, homozygous, typing cells that are mixed with cells of unknown HLA type. The unknown cells proliferate in response to incompatible typing cells, but do not respond to compatible cells. The unknown cells are assigned the DQ or DR type of the compatible cells. Class II DP antigens are defined by the primed lymphocyte typing assay. This assay uses a battery of cells that are presensitized to particular DP antigens. These cells are mixed with mitomycin-treated unknown cells. The typing cells proliferate in response to their target antigen. If a response is obtained, the unknown cells are assumed to bear the target DP antigen.

Immunologically Mediated Tissue Injury

Although the immune response is a protective mechanism to combat invasion by foreign organisms, it is apparent that immune responses often lead to tissue damage. Many inflammatory diseases are based on immune mechanisms. A wide variety of foreign substances (dust, pollen, bacteria, viruses, etc.) are capable of acting as antigens and provoking a protective immune response. In certain situations the protective effects of the immune response give way to deleterious events that may produce temporary discomfort or substantial injury to the host. For example, in the process of phagocytizing and destroying bacteria, phagocytic cells (neutrophils and macrophages) often cause injury to the surrounding tissue. **An immune response that results in tissue injury is broadly referred to as a "hypersensitivity" reaction and is associated with a group of diseases categorized as immune or immunologically mediated disorders.** In these conditions the immune response to a foreign or self-antigen causes injury. Immune- or hypersensitivity-mediated diseases are common; among them are asthma, hay fever, hepatitis, glomerulonephritis, and arthritis.

The most useful classification of hypersensitivity reactions is that of Gell and Coombs (Table 4-4), which lists these reactions according to the type of immune mechanism involved. **Types I to III hypersensitivity reactions all require the formation of a specific antibody against an exogenous or endogenous antigen. However, the class of antibody formed varies, and the antibody class is a critical determinant in the mechanism by which tissue injury occurs.** For example, in type I, or immediate-type, hypersensitivity reactions, IgE antibody is formed and binds to receptors on mast cells and basophils. In the presence of antigen reactive with the IgE, products are released from these cells—a sequence that results in the development of the characteristic symptoms of diseases such as asthma or anaphylaxis. In type II hypersensitivity reactions, IgG or IgM antibody is formed against an antigen, usually on a cell surface or (less commonly) a component of extracellular matrix, such as basement membrane. This antigen-antibody coupling causes complement activation, which in turn is responsible for causing lysis (cytotoxicity) of the cell or damage to the extracellular matrix.

In type III hypersensitivity reactions, the antibody responsible for tissue injury is also IgM or IgG, but here the mechanism of tissue injury differs. The antigen is usually not fixed to the cell surface, but circulates in the vascular compartment and is eventually deposited in tissues. In those sites complement activation leads to recruitment of leukocytes, which are responsible for the subsequent tissue injury.

Type IV (cell-mediated or delayed-hypersensitivity) reactions do not require the formation of an antibody. Rather, there is antigenic activation of T-lymphocytes, usually with the help of macrophages. The products of either activated lymphocytes or macrophages lead to subsequent tissue injury.

Although the Gell and Coombs classification is useful in classifying immunologically mediated tissue injury, it is important to remember that it is oversimplified. Many immunologic diseases are mediated by more than one type of hypersensitivity reaction. Perhaps the best example is hypersensitivity pneumonitis, a condition in which lung injury results from hypersensitivity to an inhaled extrinsic mold antigen. Types I, III, and IV hypersensitivity reactions are all involved in events leading to this disease. Although this may be an extreme example, it is clear that more than one type of immune mechanism may be involved in many immunologic diseases of humans. With this in mind we will briefly describe the immunologic mechanisms involved in the various hypersensitivity reactions.

Type I Hypersensitivity (Immediate Type or Anaphylaxis)

Immediate-type hypersensitivity or anaphylaxis is manifested by a localized or generalized reaction that occurs immediately (within minutes) after exposure to an antigen to which the individual has previously become sensitized. The reactions depend on the site of antigen exposure. For example, when the reactions involve the skin, the characteristic local reaction is swelling and edema **(hives).** Another common example of the localized manifestations of immediate hypersensitivity is hayfever, which involves the upper respiratory tract and conjunctiva, causing sneezing and conjunctivitis. In its generalized, most severe form, the immediate hypersensitivity reaction is associated with bronchial constriction, airway obstruction, and circulatory collapse, as seen in the **anaphylactic syndrome.** Fortunately, severe anaphylaxis reactions are rare, even though immediate-type hypersensitivity reactions, particularly of the localized variety, are common (millions of people every year have allergic rhinitis).

The mechanism involved in all immediate hypersensitivity reactions is related to the formation of IgE antibody. **IgE antibodies are formed by a T cell–dependent mechanism and bind avidly to Fc receptors on mast cells and basophils.** This avid and specific binding accounts for the term "cytotropic" antibody. An individual, once exposed to a specific allergen that has resulted in formation of IgE, is "sensitized," in the sense that subsequent responses to the allergen induce the immediate hypersensitivity reaction. Unlike the situation in which immune responses involve other classes of antibody (IgG and IgM), once an individual forms IgE antibody, reexposure to antigen often results in production of additional IgE antibody rather than "class switching." For example, IgM antibody responses after subsequent exposure to the same antigen result in production of IgG antibody. It should also be stressed that IgE bound to receptors on mast cells and basophils persists for long periods of time (weeks), a

Table 4-4 Classification of Hypersensitivity Reactions

TYPE	IMMUNOLOGIC MECHANISM	EXAMPLES
Type I (anaphylactic type): Immediate hypersensitivity	IgE antibody mediated—mast cell activation and degranulation	"Hayfever," asthma, anaphylaxis
Type II (cytotoxic type): Cytotoxic antibodies	Cytotoxic (IgG, IgM) antibodies formed against cell surface antigens. Complement is usually involved.	Autoimmune hemolytic anemias, antibody-dependent cellular cytotoxicity (ADCC), Goodpasture's disease
Type III (immune complex type): Immune complex disease	Antibodies (IgG, IgM, IgA) formed against exogenous or endogenous antigens. Complement and leukocytes (neutrophils, macrophages) are often involved.	Autoimmune diseases (SLE, rheumatoid arthritis), most types of glomerulonephritis
Type IV (cell-mediated type): Delayed type hypersensitivity	Mononuclear cells (T lymphocytes, macrophages) with interleukin and lymphokine production	Granulomatous diseases (tuberculosis, sarcoidosis)

feature unique to IgE. **The reaction of antigen with IgE coupled to the surface receptor activates mast cells and basophils, an event that releases the potent inflammatory mediators that are responsible for the development of the hypersensitivity reactions.** As shown in Figure 4-5 the antigen (allergen) binds to IgE antibody via its Fab sites. A binding or bridging of the antigen to more than one IgE antibody molecule, attached to receptors on mast cells and basophils, activates the cells. Cells can also be activated by agents other than antibodies. As shown in Figure 4-5, the complement anaphylatoxin peptides, C3a and C5a, directly stimulate mast cells by a different receptor-mediated process to cause release of granule constituents or the rapid synthesis and release of other mediators. Other compounds, including mellitin (from bee venom) and drugs (morphine, for example), also directly activate mast cells and cause release of granule constituents.

No matter how the mast cell activation sequence is initiated, calcium influx into the cell cytoplasm is required. The rise in cytosolic free calcium is associated with increases in cyclic AMP, the activation of several metabolic pathways within the cell, and the subsequent secretion of two main groups of products. Potent preformed mediators are rapidly released from granules. Because they are preformed and stored in granules, these mediators exert immediate biologic effects following their release. Of the granule constituents listed in Figure 4-5, histamine is perhaps the most important. **Histamine causes rapid contraction of airway smooth muscles as well as an increase in vascular permeability. These effects account for the classic early manifestations of immediate hypersensitivity: bronchospasm, vascular congestion, and edema.** Other preformed products released from mast cell granules are heparin, proteolytic enzymes, and at least two chemotactic factors: a neutrophil chemotactic factor and an eosinophil chemotactic factor, the latter being responsible for the accumulation of eosinophils so characteristic of immediate hypersensitivity.

When the mast cell is activated, the synthesis of potent inflammatory mediators is also initiated. Foremost among these mediators are the various products of the arachidonic acid pathway that are formed following the activation of phospholipase. Products derived from the activities of cyclooxygenase (PGD_2, PGE_2, PGF_2^α, thromboxane) and lipoxygenase (LTB_4, C_4, D_4, E_4) are formed. These arachidonate products, which are also generated by a variety of other cells, induce effects such as smooth muscle contraction, vasodilation, and edema. Of particular interest is the finding that leukotrienes C_4, D_4, and E_4 are the slow reacting substances of anaphylaxis (SRS-A), sub-stances that are important in the delayed bronchoconstriction phase of anaphylaxis. Leukotriene B_4, a potent chemotactic factor for neutrophils, macrophages, and eosinophils, is formed during anaphylaxis and may be involved in attracting inflammatory cells into tissues.

Another inflammatory mediator synthesized by the mast cell is platelet activating factor (PAF), a lipid derived from phospholipids (see Chapter 2). As the name implies, platelet activating factor is a potent agonist of platelet aggregation and the release of vasoactive amines from platelets. It has a broad range of biologic activity and is able to stimulate all types of phagocytic cells.

In summary, the Type I (immediate) hypersensitivity reaction is characterized by a specific cytotropic antibody that binds to receptors on basophils and mast cells and reacts with a specific antigen. This results in the activation of mast cells and basophils and the release of preformed (granule) products as well as the synthesis of mediators that cause the classic manifestations of immediate hypersensitivity.

Type II Hypersensitivity (Cytotoxic Type)

Type II hypersensitivity reactions are also caused by an antigen-antibody reaction but, as the name implies, the antibodies formed are often cytotoxic and are directed against antigens on cell surfaces or in connective tissues. IgG and IgM are the classes of antibody usually involved in these reactions. The most important characteristic of these antibodies is their ability to activate the complement system via Fc receptors. There are several antibody-dependent mechanisms of cytotoxicity.

The classical model of antibody-mediated cytotoxicity of red blood cells is illustrated in Figure 4-6. IgM or IgG antibody binds to an antigen on the surface of the erythrocyte membrane. As discussed in Chapter 2, this antibody binding induces activation of the complement system via the classical pathway through interaction with C1q. Once activated, complement leads to the destruction of the target cell by two distinct mechanisms. Complement products directly lyse the target cells, as shown in Figure 4-6, by the formation of a complex of C5b-9 complement components. This complex is referred to as the "membrane attack complex" because of its ability to form "holes" or ionic channels in the cell membrane, thus inducing lysis of the cell. This type of cell lysis in human diseases is exemplified in certain types of autoimmune hemolytic anemias caused by the for-

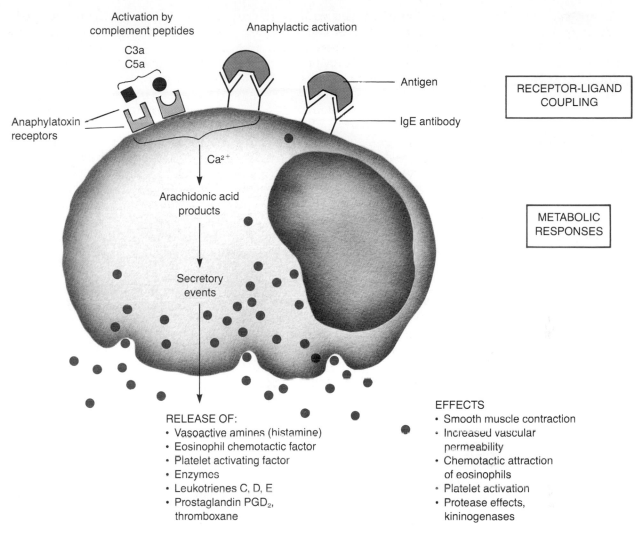

Figure 4-5. Type I hypersensitivity. Activation of the mast cell and the potent inflammatory mediators released or synthesized by the cell.

mation of cold reactive antibodies against erythrocyte blood group antigens. In transfusion reactions, in which hemolysis occurs as a result of a major blood group incompatibility, there is a potent activation of complement and red blood cell destruction, because the isoantibodies (anti A and anti B) of humans are of the IgM class.

Complement also indirectly enhances the destruction of a target cell by opsonization. As shown in Figure 4-7, this involves complement interaction on the target cell surface, with the formation of C3b. Many phagocytic cells, including neutrophils and macrophages, contain receptors for C3b on the cell membrane. Thus, **C3b bridges the target cell and the effector (phagocytic) cell, enhancing phagocytosis and intracellular destruction of the complement-** **coated cell.** Certain types of autoimmune hemolytic anemias and some drug reactions are mediated by this type of complement-associated opsonization.

In the two examples of type II hypersensitivity (cytotoxicity) already discussed, complement activation is required for the destruction of the target cell. There is another type of antibody-mediated cytotoxicity that does not require participation of the complement system. **This type of cytotoxicity is referred to as antibody-dependent, cell-mediated cytotoxicity (ADCC) and involves the destruction of antibody-coated cells by leukocytes that attack the antibody-coated target cells via Fc receptors.** Effector cells involved in these types of reactions are phagocytic cells, as well as a type of lymphocyte referred to as a null or K cell. The mechanism by which the target

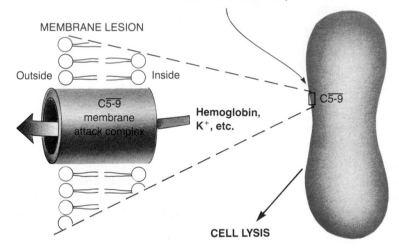

B antigen

Anti-B antibody (IgM)

ABO INCOMPATIBILITY

Immune complex formation

Activation of complement

C$\overline{5}$-$\overline{9}$ membrane attack complex

Type B
RBC

MEMBRANE LESION

Outside   Inside

C$\overline{5}$-9
membrane
attack complex

**Hemoglobin,
K$^+$, etc.**

C$\overline{5}$-$\overline{9}$

CELL LYSIS

Figure 4-6.   Type II hypersensitivity. Antibody- and complement-mediated red cell lysis due to complement activation and the formation of the C5-9 membrane attack complex (MAC).

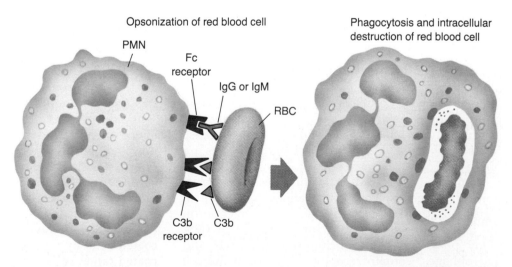

Opsonization of red blood cell

Phagocytosis and intracellular destruction of red blood cell

PMN

Fc
receptor

IgG or IgM

RBC

C3b
receptor

C3b

Figure 4-7.   Type II hypersensitivity. Antibody- and complement-dependent opsonization.

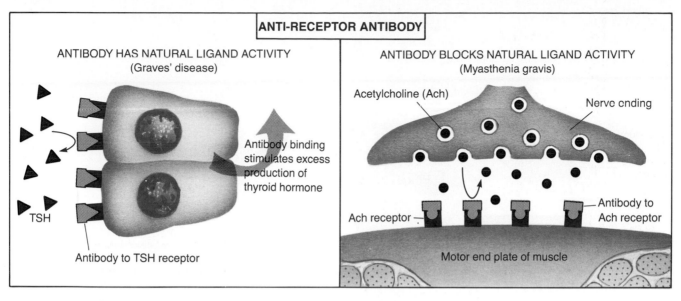

Figure 4-8.   Type II hypersensitivity. Noncytotoxic antireceptor antibody in Graves' disease and myasthenia gravis.

cell is destroyed in these reactions is not clear. It appears that these effector cells synthesize homologues of terminal complement proteins, and these homologues may be related to the cytotoxic events. Antibody-dependent, cell-mediated cytotoxicity may be involved in the pathogenesis of some autoimmune diseases, such as autoimmune thyroiditis.

In some type II reactions, antibody binding to a specific target cell receptor does not lead to death of the cell, but rather to physiological changes in the target cells. As shown in Figure 4-8, the autoimmune diseases myasthenia gravis and thyroiditis (Graves' disease) feature autoantibodies against cell receptors for hormones such as TSH and acetylcholine, respectively. In thyroiditis the autoantibody against the receptor (referred to as "long-acting thyroid stimulator") simulates the effect of TSH, thereby stimulating thyroid acinar cells. By contrast, in myasthenia gravis the autoantibody competes for the acetylcholine receptor in the neuromuscular end plate and inhibits synaptic transmission. Autoantibodies have also been described for receptors for insulin, prolactin, and growth hormone.

Finally, some type II hypersensitivity reactions occur as a result of the formation of antibody against a connective tissue component. Classic examples are Goodpasture's syndrome and the bullous skin diseases pemphigus and pemphigoid. In these diseases there is evidence of a circulating antibody against a fixed connective tissue antigen. The antibody binds to the antigen in the tissues and evokes a local in-

flammatory response. In the case of Goodpasture's disease (Fig. 4-9), an autoantibody binds to an antigen, or antigens, in pulmonary and glomerular basement membranes. Complement activation occurs locally, and injury develops because of recruitment of neutrophils into the site, although direct complement damage to the basement membrane via formation of the membrane attack complex may also be involved.

In summary, type II hypersensitivity reactions are generally directly or indirectly cytotoxic and involve the formation of antibodies against antigens on cell surfaces or in connective tissues. Complement is required for many of these cytotoxic events. Lysis is mediated directly by complement or indirectly by opsonization or the chemotactic attraction of phagocytic cells. Complement-independent reactions, such as antibody-dependent, cell-mediated cytotoxicity also fall into this category. Many human diseases, including the autoimmune hemolytic anemias, Goodpasture's syndrome, pemphigus and pemphigoid, Graves' disease, and myasthenia gravis are mediated by type II hypersensitivity reactions.

Type III Hypersensitivity: Immune Complex Diseases

Type III hypersensitivity reactions involve tissue injury mediated by immune complexes. IgM, IgG, or IgA is formed against a circulating antigen or one derived from tissues. Primarily on the basis of the

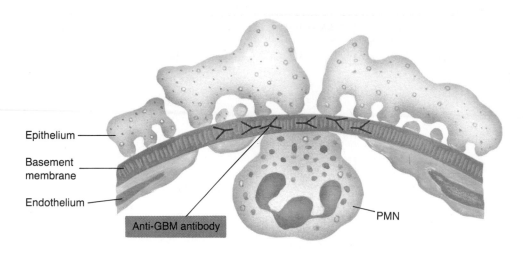

Epithelium

Basement membrane

Endothelium

Anti-GBM antibody

PMN

Figure 4-9. Type II hypersensitivity. Antibody against glomerular basement membrane antigens in Goodpasture's disease.

physiochemical characteristics of the immune complexes, such as size, charge, and so on, antigen-antibody complexes formed in the circulation are deposited in tissues, including the renal glomerulus, skin capillary venules, choroid plexus, lung, and synovium. Once deposited in tissues, immune complexes call forth an inflammatory response by activating complement, thereby leading to chemotactic recruitment of neutrophils or macrophages to the site. These cells are then activated and release their tissue-damaging substances, such as proteases and oxygen radicals.

Immune complexes have been implicated in the pathogenesis of many human diseases. The most compelling case is one in which the demonstration of immune complexes in the injured tissue correlates with the development of the injury. A convincing example of this is the lesions of periarteritis nodosa, in which medium-size arteries contain immune complexes of IgG and the hepatitis virus antigen (HbsAg) in the vessel wall. In many diseases immune complexes are detected in plasma without concomitant evidence of tissue injury. The physiochemical properties of these circulating complexes differ from those of complexes deposited in tissues, the presence of which is correlated with tissue injury. In some cases vasopermeability factors may play a key role in the localization of circulating immune complexes. In this regard, there is evidence that immune complex deposition in the renal glomerulus is facilitated by interaction of antigen with IgE-coated basophils. This binding results in the release of histamine and a local increase in permeability, thus permitting complexes to pass beyond the endothelial barrier. This is an example of a type I reaction that affects the outcome of a type III reaction. It is not known whether this IgE mechanism is involved in the deposition of circulating immune complexes in human tissues. The diseases that seem to be most clearly attributable to immune complexes are autoimmune diseases of connective tissue, such as systemic lupus erythematosus and rheumatoid arthritis, some types of vasculitis, and most varieties of glomerulonephritis.

Several experimental models of immune complex injury allow a precise definition of the mediation of this type of injury. Foremost among these models is acute serum sickness in the rabbit. Serum sickness is an acute, self-limited disease that occurs 6 to 8 days after the injection of a foreign protein (bovine albumin) and is characterized by fever, arthralgias, vasculitis, and an acute glomerulonephritis. As shown in Figure 4-10, the levels of exogenously injected antigen in the circulation remain constant until about day 6, at which time they fall rapidly. At the same time, immune complexes (containing IgM or IgG and the antigen) appear in the circulation. Simultaneously, some of these circulating immune complexes begin to deposit in tissues such as the renal glomeruli and blood vessels. As shown in Figure 4-10, tissue deposition of these immune complexes is enhanced by their interaction with the complement system, a process that renders the complexes more soluble. The interaction with complement also generates C3a and C5a, which increase vascular permeability by the mechanisms described above.

Once immune complexes are deposited in tissues, they induce an inflammatory response. The mediation of this response revolves around the local acti-

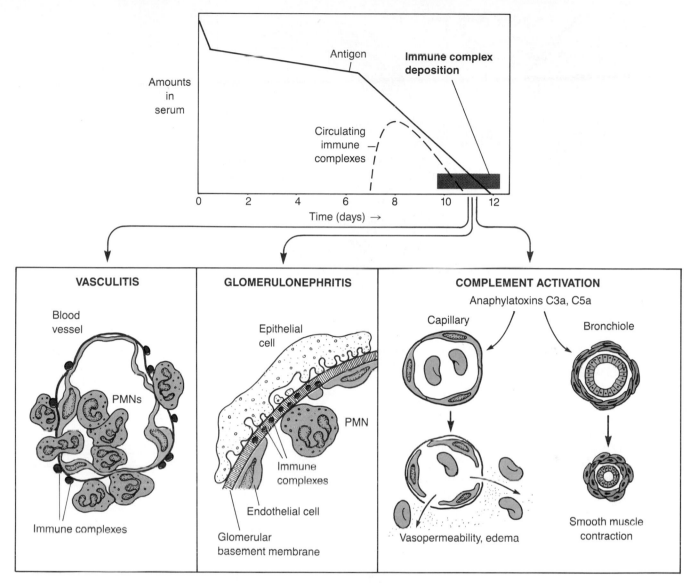

Figure 4-10. Type III hypersensitivity. In the serum sickness model of immune complex tissue injury, antibody forms against a circulating antigen and immune complexes form in the circulation. These complexes deposit in tissues such as blood vessels and glomeruli and, augmented by complement activation, induce tissue injury.

vation of the complement system by the complexes and the resulting formation of C5a, which functions as a chemoattractant for the accumulation of neutrophils. Once neutrophils arrive they are activated, usually through contact with and ingestion of immune complexes. In the process they release many inflammatory mediators, such as proteases, oxygen radicals, and arachidonic acid products, which collectively produce tissue injury. The serum-sickness–induced injury, such as that seen in the renal glomerulus, mimics the histologic appearance of many types of human glomerulonephritis.

An example of a localized injury induced by immune complexes is an experimental vasculitis model, the Arthus reaction (Fig. 4-11). This reaction is classically induced in the dermal blood vessels by the local injection of an antigen to which the animal has been previously sensitized (i.e., against which it has circulating antibody). The circulating antibody and locally injected antigen diffuse toward each other and form immune complex deposits in the walls of small blood vessels. The ensuing vascular injury is mediated by complement activation followed by recruitment and stimulation of neutrophils, which release

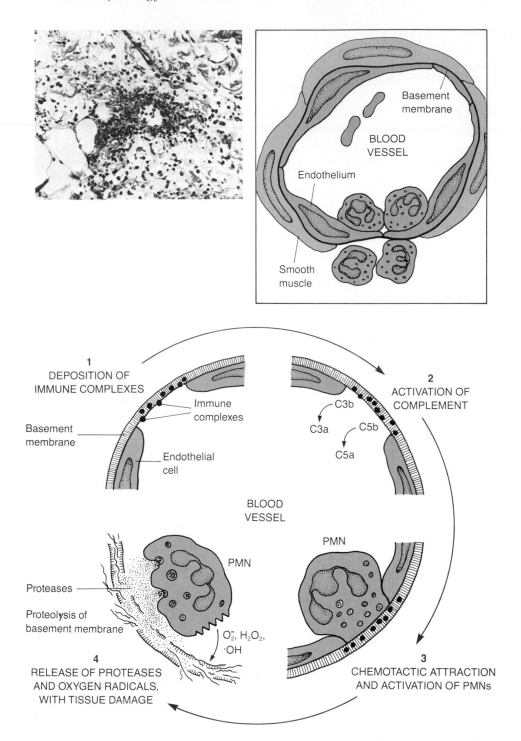

Figure 4-11.   Type III hypersensitivity. Localized immune-complex–induced vasculitis in the Arthus reaction is depicted. The formation of immune complexes in the vessel wall leads to localized complement activation and the recruitment of neutrophils, as shown in the photomicrograph. The neutrophils induce injury to the vessel wall with edema, hemorrhage, and fibrin deposition.

their tissue-damaging factors. Because the injury is caused by recruited neutrophils and their products, several (2–6) hours are required for evidence of tissue injury, in marked contrast to type I hypersensitivity reactions. Histologically, the affected vessels show large numbers of neutrophils and evidence of damage to the vessel, with edema and hemorrhage into the surrounding tissue (Fig. 4-11). In addition, the presence of fibrin creates the classic appearance of an immune-complex–induced vasculitis referred to as **fibrinoid necrosis.** This experimental model of localized vasculitis is the prototype for many types of vasculitis seen in man—for example, the various types of cutaneous vasculitides seen in drug reactions.

In summary, type III hypersensitivity reactions represent the classic example of immune complex-mediated injury in which antigen-antibody complexes, which are usually not organ-specific, are formed in the circulation and mainly directly in the tissues. Once deposited in the tissues, these complexes induce an inflammatory response by activating the complement system, consequently attracting neutrophils and macrophages. Activation of these cells by the immune complexes, with the release of potent inflammatory mediators, is directly responsible for the injury. Many human diseases, including anti-immune diseases such as systemic lupus erythematosus, as well as most types of glomerulonephritis, appear to be mediated by type III hypersensitivity reactions.

Type IV Hypersensitivity: Cell-Mediated Immunity

Cell-mediated hypersensitivity is defined as an antigen-elicited cellular immune reaction that results in tissue damage and does not require the participation of antibodies. These reactions often occur along with superimposed antibody reactions, which makes it difficult to define them under natural circumstances. Studies with several experimental models suggest that the type of tissue response largely depends on the nature of the inciting agent.

Delayed-Type Hypersensitivity

Classically, delayed-type hypersensitivity is defined as a tissue reaction, primarily involving lymphocytes and mononuclear phagocytes, that occurs in response to the subcutaneous injection of a soluble protein antigen and reaches greatest intensity 24 to 48 hours after injection. A naturally occurring example of this reaction is the contact sensitivity response to poison ivy. Although the chemical ligands in poison ivy are not proteins, they can bind covalently to cell membrane proteins and can therefore be recognized by antigen-specific lymphocytes.

Figure 4-12 summarizes the main stages of the delayed-type hypersensitivity reaction. In the initial phase, foreign protein antigens or chemical ligands interact with accessory cells bearing class II, HLA-D molecules. Soluble protein antigens are actively processed by macrophages and then presented in conjunction with HLA-D molecules. Small reactive chemical ligands interact directly with membrane proteins and thereby alter their structure. The foreign antigens are then recognized by antigen-specific T cells. The latter are called T effector or delayed hypersensitivity cells, and usually have the T4 phenotype. These cells become activated and begin synthesis of a spectrum of lymphokines (see Table 4-1). The lymphokines recruit and activate lymphocytes, monocytes, fibrocytes, and other inflammatory cells. If the antigenic stimulus is eliminated, the reaction spontaneously resolves after 48 hours, with only a scar remaining, as the result of fibroblast activity. If the stimulus persists, the response evolves into a granulomatous reaction in an attempt to sequester the inciting agent.

T Cell-Mediated Cytotoxicity

Another mechanism by which T cells effect tissue damage is the direct cytolysis of target cells. This immune mechanism is important for the destruction and elimination of cells infected by viruses and, possibly, tumor cells that express neoantigens. Cytotoxic T cells also play an important role in graft or transplant rejection.

Figure 4-13 summarizes the events in T cell–mediated cytotoxicity. In contrast with the delayed hypersensitivity reaction, the cytotoxic or killer T cell must interact with both the target and the class I major histocompatibility complex (MHC) antigens, HLA-A, B, or C. In the case of virus-infected and tumor cells, self-MHC antigens are recognized in addition to the viral antigens or tumor neoantigens. In graft rejection, foreign MHC antigens are potent activators of killer cells. T-killer cells bear the T8 phenotype marker. Once activated by the antigenic stimulus, the proliferation of these cells is promoted by helper or amplifier cells. This amplification is mediated by soluble growth factors such as interleukin-1. An expanded population of antigen-specific killer

(Text continues on p. 116)

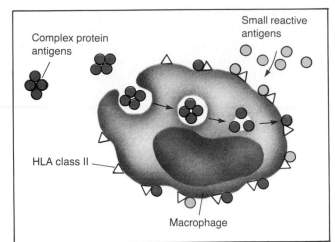

ANTIGEN PROCESSING
AND PRESENTATION
• Complex protein
  antigens are ingested
  by macrophages, pro-
  cessed, and then
  presented on the
  surface in association
  with class II HLA
  molecules
• Small reactive antigens
  may bind directly to
  class II molecules

Figure 4-12.   Delayed-type hypersensitivity reaction.
(*Panel 1*) Complex antigens are
phagocytosed and "processed" by
macrophages, then presented in
the membrane complexes with
class II (Ia) antigens. Chemically
reactive ligands then may bind directly to macrophage membrane
proteins.
(*Panel 2*) Antigen-specific T cells
recognize the membrane protein–
antigen complexes and receive
growth promoting signals (monokines), such as interleukin-1,
from macrophages. T cells then
become activated and begin synthesis and secretion of molecular
mediators (lymphokines).
(*Panel 3*) The generated lymphokines, as well as monokines, recruit additional inflammatory cells,
predominantly mononuclear cells.

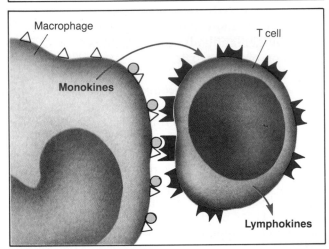

ANTIGEN RECOGNITION
AND T CELL ACTIVATION
• Antigen-specific T cells
  recognize antigen plus
  class II molecules
• T cells are stimulated
  to synthesize and re-
  lease lymphokines;
  macrophage-derived
  monokines promote this
  activation

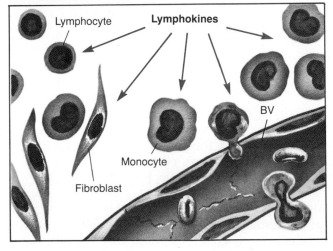

AMPLIFICATION AND
RECRUITMENT
• Lymphokines produce
  numerous effects,
  including recruitment
  of additional inflam-
  matory cells and
  activation of macro-
  phages and fibroblasts

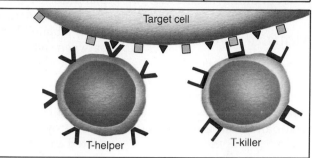

TARGET CELLS		
Viral	HLA	Tumor

TARGET ANTIGENS
- Virally-coded membrane antigen
- Foreign or modified histocompatibility antigen
- Tumor-specific membrane antigens

Target cell

T-helper   T-killer

RECOGNITION OF ANTIGEN BY T CELLS
- T-helper cells recognize antigen plus class II molecules
- T-cytotoxic/killer cells recognize antigen plus class I molecules

Figure 4-13. T cell-mediated cytotoxicity.

(*Panel 1*) Potential target cells of T cells include virally-infected cells, histoincompatible cells (e.g., transplanted organ), and tumor cells expressing neoantigens.

(*Panel 2*) T cells recognize foreign antigens and class I histocompatibility antigens.

(*Panel 3*) T cells become activated and begin to proliferate. T-helper cells release lymphokines that amplify proliferation.

(*Panel 4*) T-killer cell binds to target cell and delivers a signal resulting in disruption of the sodium-potassium pump. The target cell is then lysed.

T_K

T_H

IL-2

IL-2

T_K cytotoxic or killer cells

Helper lymphokines

T_H helper/amplifier cells

ACTIVATION AND AMPLIFICATION
- T-helper cells activate and proliferate, releasing helper molecules (e.g., IL-2)
- T-cytotoxic/killer cells proliferate in response to helper molecules

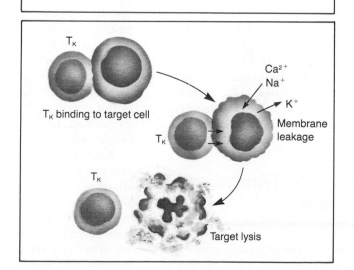

T_K

T_K binding to target cell

Ca^{2+}
Na^+
K^+

T_K

Membrane leakage

T_K

Target lysis

TARGET CELL KILLING
- T-cytotoxic/killer cells bind to target cell
- Killing signals released and target cell loses membrane integrity
- Target cell undergoes lysis

cells is thus generated for attacking target cells. The actual killing event requires energy-dependent binding of the killer to the target cell. The killer cell next delivers a molecular signal that disrupts the membrane permeability of the target, causing an influx of sodium, calcium, and water, and ultimate lysis. Once the cytotoxic signal is delivered, the subsequent lytic events are energy-independent and irreversible.

Natural Killer Cell-Mediated Cytotoxicity

The defining characteristics of natural killer (NK) cells have been described, but the extent to which such cells participate in tissue-damaging immune reactions is unclear. Mounting evidence indicates that they have both important effector and immunoregulatory functions.

Figure 4-14 summarizes the events of target-cell killing by NK cells. Unlike T-killer cells, NK cells recognize a variety of target cells. Thus, they bear receptors that recognize either several different antigenic structures or similar antigens on different target cells. The target antigens are membrane glycoproteins that are expressed by certain virus-infected or tumor cells. In a series of events similar to that described for killer T cells, NK cells bind to the target cell via their membrane receptors and then deliver a molecular signal that results in lysis. NK cells also have membrane Fc receptors. Thus, they acquire antibodies that allow for binding and killing of target cells by an antibody-directed mechanism—that is, antibody-dependent cell-mediated cytotoxicity.

In summary, the type IV hypersensitivity reaction, unlike the other types of hypersensitivity reactions, is not an antibody-mediated response. Rather, antigens are processed by macrophages and presented to antigen-specific T-lymphocytes. These lymphocytes become activated and release a variety of mediators toward lymphokines, which recruit and activate lymphocytes, macrophages, and fibroblasts. The resulting injury is caused by the T-lymphocytes themselves, the macrophages, or both. The granulomatous inflammation of diseases such as sarcoidosis or tuberculosis is an important example of type IV granulomatous reactions in human disease.

Immune Reactions to Transplanted Organs and Tissues

The introduction of organ transplantation has initiated intense investigation into the immune mechanisms that cause rejection. **These efforts have re-vealed the role of histocompatibility antigens as critical immunogenic molecules stimulating rejection episodes.**

It is clear that optimal survival of a graft requires that the recipient and donor be as closely matched as possible with regard to histocompatibility antigens. This is especially so in the case of renal transplantation. Thus, HLA matching is a crucial step in organ transplantation. In practice, an exact match is rarely obtained, except in the case of transplantation between monozygotic twins. As a result, vigilant monitoring of the status of the graft and immunosuppressive therapy are required after transplantation. When rejection does occur, any number or combination of the immune responses may be engaged to destroy the graft. This variety of responses is reflected in differing clinical and histologic manifestations of rejection.

Host Versus Graft

The histopathologic features of graft rejection are well demonstrated in rejected renal allografts. Three major types of rejection, based on the time of onset of the rejection episode and corresponding histologic features, have been described. These three types—hyperacute, acute, and chronic rejection—are illustrated in Figure 4-15.

Hyperacute rejection occurs within the first days after transplantation and is manifested clinically as a sudden cessation of urine output accompanied by fever and pain in the area of the graft site. This reaction necessitates prompt surgical removal of the kidney. **The histologic features of hyperacute rejection within the transplanted kidney are vascular congestion, fibrin-platelet thrombi within capillaries, neutrophilic vasculitis with fibrinoid necrosis, prominent interstitial edema, and neutrophilic infiltrates. This rapid form of rejection is mediated by preformed antibodies and complement activation products, including chemotactic and other inflammatory mediators.** Fortunately, this form of rejection is not common if appropriate antibody screening is performed, using recipient lymphocytes as the target cell for the antibody assay.

Acute rejection characteristically occurs in the first few weeks or months after transplantation. Clinically, there is sudden onset of azotemia and oliguria that may be associated with fever and graft tenderness. A needle biopsy is often performed to differentiate between a rejection episode and acute tubular necrosis or toxicity from immunosuppressive agents. **The microscopic findings of acute graft rejection include interstitial infiltrates of lymphocytes and macro-**

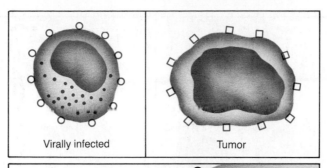

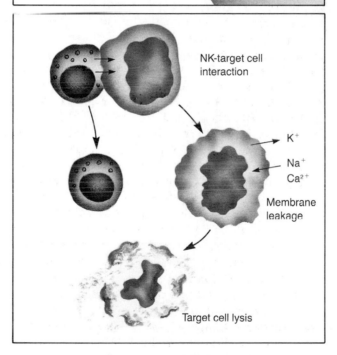

TARGET CELLS
- Virally-infected cells
- Tumor cells

RECOGNITION
- The natural killer (NK) cell binds to target via undefined receptor (possibly involving transferrin receptor)

TARGET CELL KILLING
- NK cell releases signals that commit target to lysis
- Target membrane integrity is lost, NK cell is detached
- Target undergoes lysis

Figure 4-14. Natural killer cell-mediated cytotoxicity.
(*Panel 1*) Potential targets of natural killer cells include virally infected cells and tumor cells.
(*Panel 2*) Recognition of antigen. Natural killer cells bear receptors for a variety of membrane glycoproteins, allowing for cell–cell binding.
(*Panel 3*) Following binding, the NK cell delivers the killer signal. The target cell sodium-potassium pump is disrupted, and the target cell is lysed.

phages, with associated edema. In addition, there is lymphocytic tubulitis and tubular necrosis. The most severe form also shows vascular damage, manifested as an arteritis, with thrombosis and fibrinoid necrosis. Vascular involvement is an ominous sign because it usually means the rejection episode will be refractory to therapy. Acute cellular rejection likely involves both cell-mediated and humoral mecha-

nisms of tissue damage. If detected in its early stages, acute rejection can be reversed with immunosuppressive therapy.

Chronic rejection occurs several months to years after transplantation. Clinically, the patient develops progressive azotemia, oliguria, hypertension, and weight gain. If indeed there is chronic rejection, a biopsy specimen will show the characteristic histo-

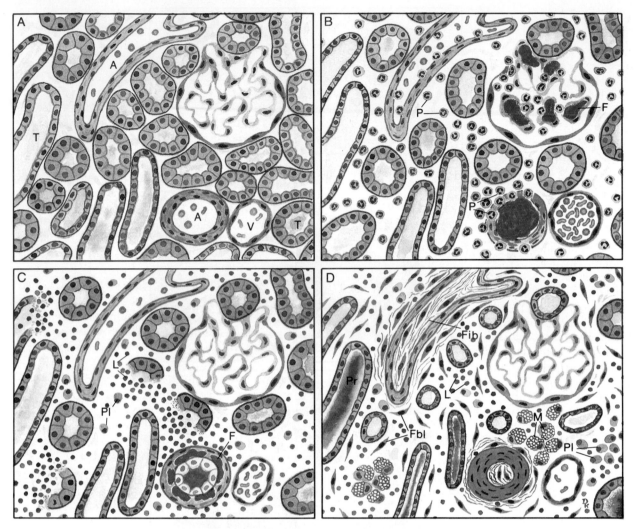

Figure 4-15. Histologic features of major forms of renal transplant rejection. (*A*) Normal kidney. (*B*) Hyperacute rejection occurs in minutes to hours and is characterized by interstitial edema, infiltrates of polymorphonuclear leukocytes, intravascular fibrin-platelet thrombi, and fibrinoid necrosis of arterioles. (*C*) Acute cellular rejection occurs in the first weeks to months and is characterized by interstitial edema, infiltrates of mononuclear cells, tubular damage, and vasculitis associated with thrombosis and fibrinoid necrosis. (*D*) Chronic rejection occurs months to years after transplantation and is characterized by arterial and arteriolar sclerosis, tubular atrophy, interstitial fibrosis, and glomerular capillary wall thickening. *P*, polymorphonuclear leukocyte; *F*, fibrin; *T*, tubule; *A*, artery; *V*, vein; *Fbl*, fibroblast; *Pl*, plasma cell; *L*, lymphocyte; *M*, macrophage; *Fib*, fibrous tissue.

logic picture. **The dominant features of chronic rejection are arterial and arteriolar intimal thickening, causing stenosis or obstruction. This is associated with thick glomerular capillary walls, tubular atrophy, and interstitial fibrosis.** The interstitium often has scattered mononuclear infiltrates and tubules containing proteinaceous casts. Chronic rejection may be the end result of repeated episodes of cellular rejection, either clinical or subclinical in presentation.

This advanced state of damage is not responsive to therapy.

It should be noted that the histologic features described above may overlap and vary in degree, such that a distinct picture may not be apparent on renal biopsy. Moreover, immunosuppressive drugs, such as cyclosporin, have complicated the histologic diagnosis by modifying immune responses as well as by having direct toxic effects on renal tubular cells.

Graft Versus Host

The above discussion describes rejection of an organ grafted to a recipient with an intact immune system. In recent years, bone marrow transplantation to bone marrow–depleted or immunodeficient patients has resulted in the complication of **graft-versus-host** (GVH) disease. Immunocompetent lymphocytes in the grafted marrow attempt to reject the host tissues. GVH also occurs when severely immunodeficient patients are transfused with blood products containing HLA-incompatible lymphocytes.

Clinically, graft-versus-host disease manifests as skin rash, diarrhea, abdominal cramps, anemia, and liver dysfunction. Histologically, the skin and gut show mononuclear cell infiltrates and epithelial cell necrosis. The liver shows periportal inflammation, damaged bile ducts, and liver cell injury. A chronic form of graft-versus-host disease is characterized by dermal sclerosis, sicca syndrome (dry eyes and dry mouth secondary to chronic inflammation of the lacrimal and salivary glands), and immunodeficiency. Treatment of graft-versus-host disease usually involves immunosuppressive therapy.

Assessment of Immune Status

Immunodeficiency is usually suspected in an infant or adult with chronic, recurrent, or unusual infections. The specific type of immunodeficiency is suggested by the kinds of infections developed and other clinical features. However, diagnosis and confirmation usually require laboratory studies. A number of laboratory methods are used to assess the various components of immunity—that is, antibody-mediated immunity (B cells), cell-mediated immunity (T cells), phagocytosis, and complement.

Immunoglobulin levels are crudely measured by **serum protein electrophoresis.** In this technique, serum proteins are separated electrophoretically, stained, and then quantitated by densitometry. Figure 4-16A shows the characteristic patterns of both a normal and a hypogammaglobulinemic individual, and their corresponding densitometric tracings. The immunoglobulins comprise the gammaglobulin fraction, which migrates cathodically and is significantly reduced in hypogammaglobulinemic patients.

Immunoglobulins (Ig) are more precisely measured by quantitation of individual Ig subclasses. Various methods are used (radial immunodiffusion, nephelometry, radioimmunoassay), but all employ antibodies directed against the different heavy-chain isotypes. Quantitation allows the detection of selective deficiencies of Ig subclasses and provides a measure of total available Ig. A number of conditions have been described in which there is a specific deficiency of IgA, IgM, or IgG.

Serologic methods for evaluating antibody-dependent immunity measure levels of circulating antibodies to specific antigens to which a person has been introduced through vaccination or environmental exposure (tetanus, diphtheria, typhoid, rubella, and major blood groups). These methods uncover more subtle deficiencies that may be present even when levels of immunoglobulin are normal.

Cell-mediated immunity is also evaluated by a number of techniques. Since most blood lymphocytes are T cells, the total lymphocyte count is a crude indication of cell-mediated immunity. Functional screening of delayed hypersensitivity is done through intradermal injection of antigens to which most of the population should be sensitive (*Candida albicans*, tetanus toxoid, streptokinase, streptodornase). A normal response is notable swelling, redness, and induration (>5 mm) at the skin injection site.

More sophisticated methods assess T-lymphocyte function *in vitro*. Figure 4-16B diagrams a commonly employed assay in which lymphoid cells are isolated from a blood sample and then incubated with a polyclonal T cell mitogen (phytohemagglutinin), a common microbial antigen (*Candida*, streptokinase, etc.), or histoincompatible cells. Normal T cells proliferate in response to such stimuli. A poor or absent response suggests a qualitative, quantitative, or regulatory lymphocyte defect.

Both antibody-mediated and cell-mediated immunity are evaluated by quantitation of peripheral blood T- and B-lymphocyte populations. For example, T cells are measured by their ability to bind sheep erythrocytes spontaneously and form rosettes *in vitro*. B cells are easily identified with fluorochrome-labeled rabbit or goat antibodies directed against human immunoglobulins. These antibodies bind to B cells, which are identified by fluorescence microscopy.

Recently, the development of laser technology and monoclonal antibodies with specificities for lymphocyte subpopulations has enabled more detailed analyses of lymphoid cells by the method of **flow cytometry.** The principles of this method are outlined in Figure 4-17. Briefly, lymphocyte preparations are stained with a fluorochrome-labeled monoclonal antibody specific for the target population—for instance, T4, T8, and so on. The cells are then passed individually through a narrow beam of laser light of

(Text continues on p. 122)

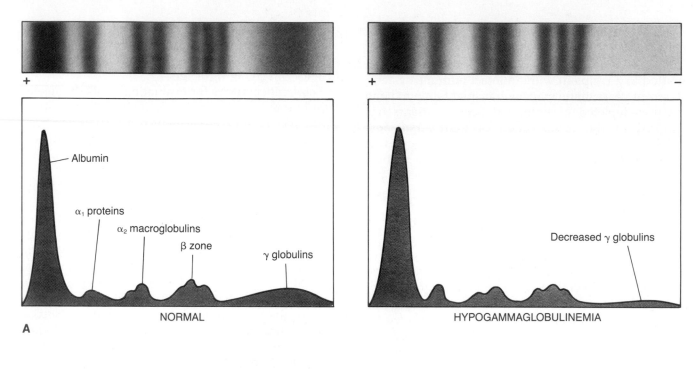

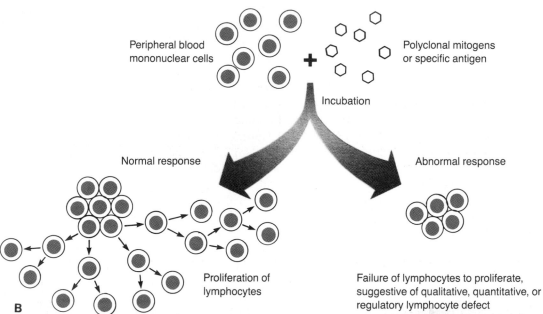

Figure 4-16. (*A*) Normal and hypogammaglobulinemic serum protein electrophoresis (SPEP). The SPEP provides a relatively rapid means to evaluate the major protein components of serum. (*B*) T cell mitogenic or blastogenic response assay. This assay tests the capacity of peripheral blood T cells to respond to mitogenic or antigenic stimuli.

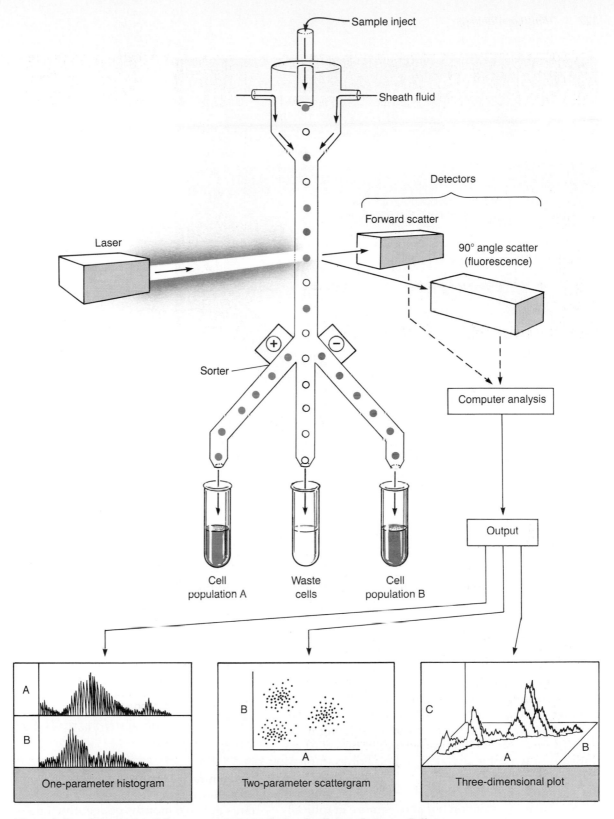

Figure 4-17. Schematic of flow cytometric analysis of cell populations. Cells treated with population-specific antibodies labeled with fluorochromes are passed individually through an incident beam of laser light. The diffracted and fluorescent light is monitored by forward scatter and 90° angle fluorescent light detectors. The monitored light is subjected to computer analysis. Cells with specific markers can be sorted and collected using electroplates.

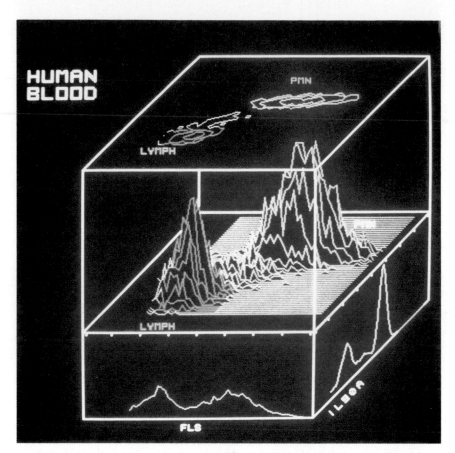

Figure 4-18.   Flow cytometric analysis of peripheral blood white cells presented as a three-dimensional plot.

appropriate wavelength. Diffracted light is analyzed by a forward light scatter detector. Various blood cell types, lymphocytes, neutrophils, monocytes, and so on, are recognized by their characteristic forward light scatter pattern. A second detector positioned at 90° to the incident beam monitors cells for fluorescent intensity. The information from both detectors is subjected to computer analysis and is expressed in various ways. The simplest plot is the one-parameter histogram, which is a graph of cell numbers versus fluorescence intensity. The generated plot shows the number of cells that stain with a particular marker, either A or B, and the distribution of staining intensity. The two-parameter scatter plot shows the relationship of two phenotypic markers. For example, it displays populations staining with only A, only B, or with both A and B. The three-dimensional plot provides similar information but shows more graphically the number of cells in various populations. In Figure 4-18 is a plot of light scatter analysis showing the major white cell populations in blood. A further advantage of flow cytometry is its capacity to sort and enrich particular cell populations for further investigational purposes.

Immunodeficiency Diseases

Immunodeficiency disorders are classified into antibody (B cell), cellular (T cell), and combined T and B cell deficiencies. In many cases functional defects are localized to particular points in the ontogeny of the immune system. The defects are congenital or acquired and their precise etiologies are often unclear.

Deficiencies of Antibody (B Cell) Immunity

Congenital (Bruton's) X-linked infantile hypogammaglobulinemia is generally observed in male infants at 5 to 6 months of age, the time when maternal antibody levels begin to decline. The infant usually presents with recurrent pyogenic infections, severe hypogammaglobulinemia, and an absence of mature peripheral blood B cells. Pre-B cells, however, can be detected. Thus, there is a defect early in the maturation of B cells, at the point at which pre-B cells receive the maturation signal from the bursal equivalent (see Fig. 4-2, step 2). A flow cytometry profile of a patient with Bruton's agammaglobulinemia is shown in Figure 4-19. Note that the levels of mature B cells are severely decreased, whereas pre-B cells are still detectable by the HLA-D/DR marker.

Another congenital form of hypogammaglobulinemia is known as **transient hypogammaglobulinemia of infancy.** The condition is characterized by prolonged hypogammaglobulinemia after maternal antibodies have reached a nadir. Some affected infants develop recurrent infections and require therapy, but all eventually produce immunoglobulins. Such infants have mature B cells that are temporarily unable to produce antibodies. The defect is thought to be at the level of the helper T cell signal.

An interesting congenital immunodeficiency exhibits low levels of IgG and IgA, but normal to elevated levels of IgM. The defect appears to be at the level of the "switch" to other heavy-chain isotopes (see Fig. 4-2, step 3); in this condition, B cells, although capable of producing IgM, secrete inadequate levels of other isotypes.

Common variable immunodeficiency is a severe hypogammaglobulinemia (IgG) that is manifested years to decades after birth. The mean age of onset is 31 years. These patients present with recurrent, severe pyogenic infections, especially pneumonia, as well as diarrhea, often due to *Giardia lamblia*. Different maturational and regulatory defects of the immune system result in the same clinical presentation, recognized as common variable immunodeficiency. Thus, this disorder probably represents several diseases rather than one.

The most common immunodeficiency syndrome, selective IgA deficiency, occurs in one of every 700 persons. Individuals with IgA deficiency are asymptomatic or present with severe respiratory or gastrointestinal infections. There is also a strong predilection for allergies and collagen vascular diseases. These individuals generally have normal numbers of IgA-bearing B cells. Therefore, their defect seems to be an inability to synthesize and secrete IgA (see Fig. 4-2, step 4). Similar selective deficiencies have been described for the IgG subclasses and IgM, but are quite rare.

Deficiencies of Cell-Mediated (T Cell) Immunity

DiGeorge syndrome is one of the severest forms of deficient T cell immunity. The disease usually presents in an infant with congenital heart defects and severe hypocalcemia (due to hypoparathyroidism) and is recognized shortly after birth. Infants who survive the neonatal period are subject to recurrent or chronic viral, bacterial, fungal, and protozoal infections. **The condition is caused by defective embryologic development of the third and fourth pharyngeal pouches, which become the thymus and parathyroid glands.** In the absence of a thymus, T cell maturation is interrupted at the pre-T cell stage (see Fig. 4-2, stage A). The disease can be corrected by transplanting thymic tissue.

Some patients have a **partial DiGeorge syndrome,** in which a small remnant of thymus is present. With time, these individuals recover T cell function without treatment. Figure 4-19 shows a flow cytometric profile of such a patient. Before thymic function has fully recovered, a large proportion of peripheral T cells still express the T10 marker, having not quite reached maturity.

Chronic mucocutaneous candidiasis, another congenital defect in T cell function, is characterized by susceptibility to candidal infections. The condition is associated with an endocrinopathy (hypoparathyroidism, Addison's disease, diabetes mellitus). Although most T cell functions are intact, there is a defective response to *Candida* antigens. The precise cause of the defect is unknown, but it could occur at any of several points during T cell development. Among the possibilities are failure to develop T cell clones that are specific for *Candida* antigens (see Fig. 4-2, stage B) and failure to proliferate and produce inflammatory mediators in response to *Candida* antigens (see Fig. 4-2, stage D).

Combined T and B Cell Deficiencies

Severe combined immunodeficiency disease is characterized by recurrent viral, bacterial, fungal, and protozoal infections with onset at about 6 months of age. The disease occurs in X-linked and autosomal recessive (Swiss type) forms. Both forms are associated with a virtually complete absence of T cells and severe hypogammaglobulinemia. Many of these infants have severely reduced lymphoid tissue and an immature thymus that lacks lymphocytes. In some patients, the undefined defect or defects manifest very early in the developing immune system. Specifically, lymphocytes fail to develop beyond the pre-B and pre-T cell level (see Fig. 4-2, stages 1 and A). In other patients, mature lymphocytes are present but fail to function, possibly because of a lack of helper cell activity.

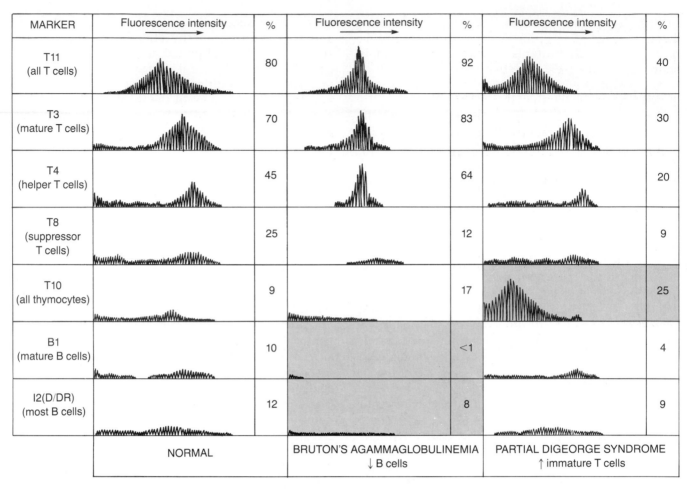

MARKER	Fluorescence intensity	%	Fluorescence intensity	%	Fluorescence intensity	%
T11 (all T cells)		80		92		40
T3 (mature T cells)		70		83		30
T4 (helper T cells)		45		64		20
T8 (suppressor T cells)		25		12		9
T10 (all thymocytes)		9		17		25
B1 (mature B cells)		10		<1		4
I2(D/DR) (most B cells)		12		8		9
	NORMAL		BRUTON'S AGAMMAGLOBULINEMIA ↓ B cells		PARTIAL DIGEORGE SYNDROME ↑ immature T cells	

Figure 4-19. Flow cytometric profiles in immunodeficiency states. Bruton's agammaglobulinemia—marked reduction in the number of circulating mature B cells (B1 marker); some immature B cells present (D/DR marker). Partial DiGeorge's syndrome—marked decrease in the number of mature T cells (T3, T4, T8 markers); increased numbers of immature T cells present (T11 marker). Acquired immunodeficiency syndrome (AIDS)—decreased numbers of helper T cells (T4 marker); normal, increased, or decreased numbers of suppressor T cells (T8 marker). B cell leukemia—increased B cells; decreased T cells.

In about half of patients with the autosomal recessive form of combined immunodeficiency, production of adenosine deaminase is defective. This enzyme takes part in the catabolism of purine nucleotides, specifically converting adenosine to inosine or deoxyadenosine to deoxyinosine. If it is defective or absent, deoxyadenosine and deoxy-ATP accumulate. Deoxy-ATP then inhibits ribonucleotide reductase, causing depletion of deoxyribonucleoside triphosphates and defective lymphocyte function. The clinical manifestations of adenosine deaminase deficiency range from mild to severe dysfunctions of T and B cells. Another enzyme involved in purine metabolism, nucleoside phosphorylase, is also deficient in some persons with immune defects. With this deficiency, however, unlike adenosine deaminase deficiency, B cell function is preserved.

There are a number of other congenital immunodeficiency diseases of varying degrees of severity. In most of these diseases a precise etiology has not been established.

Acquired Immunodeficiency

Immunodeficiency states can be secondary to a large number of conditions, including infections (viral, bacterial, and fungal), malnutrition, autoimmune diseases (systemic lupus erythematosus, rheumatoid arthritis), nephrotic syndrome, uremia, sarcoidosis,

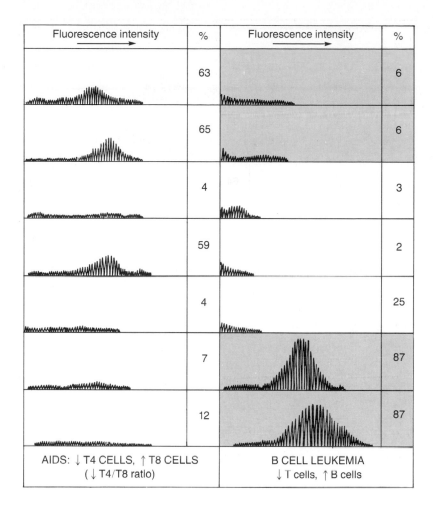

Fluorescence intensity	%	Fluorescence intensity	%
	63		6
	65		6
	4		3
	59		2
	4		25
	7		87
	12		87
AIDS: ↓ T4 CELLS, ↑ T8 CELLS (↓ T4/T8 ratio)		B CELL LEUKEMIA ↓ T cells, ↑ B cells	

cancer (lymphoid and nonlymphoid), and treatment with immunosuppressive agents (radiation, steroids, chemotherapy, cyclosporin A, etc.). The widespread use of immunosuppressive agents is today the main cause of immunodeficiency and the resulting increased risk for opportunistic infection.

The **acquired immunodeficiency syndrome (AIDS)** has become recognized as a fatal and increasingly prevalent disease. AIDS exhibits a spectrum of clinical manifestations, including an asymptomatic state with only laboratory evidence of immunodeficiency; a prodromal state manifested by fever, weight loss, and lymphadenopathy; and the classic picture of opportunistic infections and Kaposi's sarcoma. Table 4-5 summarizes the current classification of AIDS,

issued by the Centers for Disease Control in 1986. Figure 4-20 summarizes a few of the common conditions associated with the classic form of AIDS. Herpesvirus and candidal fungal infections involve the skin and mucosal surfaces. The protozoan *Pneumocystis carinii* is a rare cause of pneumonia in the general population but is common in AIDS patients. Opportunistic organisms, such as *Giardia*, and cryptosporidia, cause gastrointestinal infections. It should be emphasized that many other infectious agents, such as atypical mycobacteria (especially *M. avium-intracellulare*), *M. tuberculosis*, cytomegalovirus and toxoplasma, are seen in AIDS. Kaposi's sarcoma, a multicentric vascular neoplasm, develops in about one-third of AIDS patients, and the incidence of lym-

Table 4-5 Classification of HIV Infections

GROUP	TYPE	DESCRIPTION
Group I	Acute infection	Mononucleosis-like syndrome with associated sero-conversion for HIV antibody.
Group II	Asymptomatic infection	No signs or symptoms of HIV. There may or may not be laboratory evidence of disease.
Group III	Persistent generalized lymphadenopathy	Lymphadenopathy ($\geq$1 cm) at two or more extrainguinal sites persisting for more than 3 months in the absence of a condition other than HIV infection to explain the findings. There may or may not be laboratory evidence of disease.
Group IV	Other disease	*Subgroup A.* Constitutional disease, fever (>1 month), weight loss (>10% of baseline), or diarrhea (>1 month), in the absence of a condition other than HIV infection to explain the findings.
		Subgroup B. Neurologic disease such as dementia, myelopathy, or peripheral neuropathy in the absence of a condition other than HIV infection to explain the findings.
		Subgroup C. Diagnosis of an infectious disease associated with HIV infection or at least moderately indicative of a defect in cell-mediated immunity.

Category C-1. Disease due to at least one of the following:

Pneumocystis carinii	Cytomegalovirus
Toxoplasma	Cryptosporidia
Strongyloides (extraintestinal)	Isosporidia
Cryptococcus	*Candida* (esophageal, pulmonary or bronchial)
Atypical mycobacteria (*avium* complex or *kansasii*)	*Candida* (chronic mucocutaneous)
	Histoplasma
Progressive multifocal leukoencephalopathy	Herpes simplex (disseminated)

Category C-2. Disease due to one of the following:

Oral hairy leukoplakia	Multidermatomal herpes zoster
Nocardia	*Salmonella* bacteremia (recurrent)
Tuberculosis	
Oral candidiasis	

Subgroup D. Secondary cancers known to be associated with HIV infection; Kaposi's sarcoma, non-Hodgkin's lymphoma, or primary lymphoma of the brain

Subgroup E. Clinical conditions not defined above that may be due to HIV infection or indicative of defective cell-mediated immunity. Also included are patients with signs and symptoms that may be due to HIV or other clinical illness.

phoma and other neoplasms is also increased. Epidemiologically, in the United States AIDS has been largely restricted to homosexual men, intravenous drug abusers, hemophiliacs and other recipients of blood products, and Haitians. In Africa heterosexual transmission appears to be common, and as AIDS increases in prevalence in the United States, the disease is affecting a wider population.

Immunologically, AIDS patients show defects in both T cell and B cell function: delayed-type hypersensitivity is impaired, T cell cytotoxicity is reduced, and responses to mitogens and histocompatibility antigens are stunted. There is usually an increase in total plasma gammaglobulin level, but this is due to a nonspecific polyclonal activation of B cells. In fact, AIDS patients fail to mount specific antibody responses to immunizing antigens.

The major laboratory features of AIDS are lymphopenia and the loss of circulating T4 (helper/amplifier) lymphocytes. The numbers of T8 (suppressor/

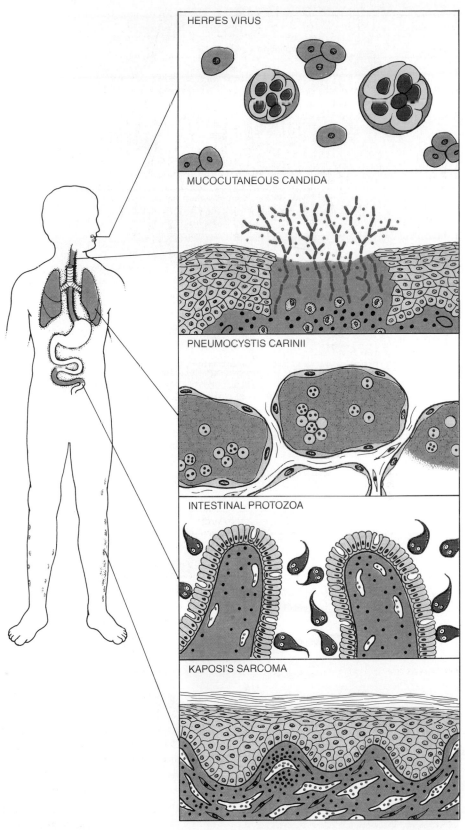

HERPES VIRUS

MUCOCUTANEOUS CANDIDA

PNEUMOCYSTIS CARINII

INTESTINAL PROTOZOA

KAPOSI'S SARCOMA

Figure 4-20. Diseases and opportunistic infections of acquired immunodeficiency syndrome.

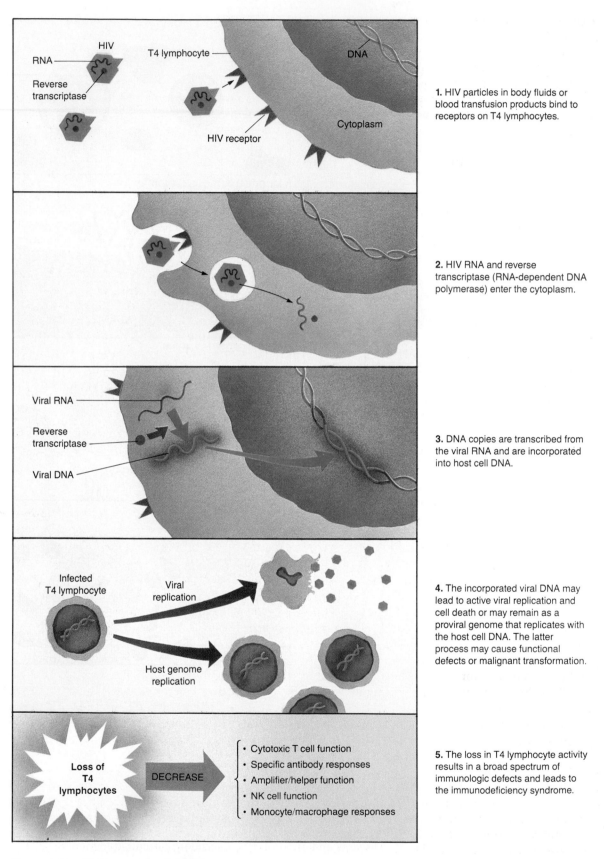

RNA

HIV

Reverse transcriptase

T4 lymphocyte

DNA

HIV receptor

Cytoplasm

1. HIV particles in body fluids or blood transfusion products bind to receptors on T4 lymphocytes.

2. HIV RNA and reverse transcriptase (RNA-dependent DNA polymerase) enter the cytoplasm.

Viral RNA

Reverse transcriptase

Viral DNA

3. DNA copies are transcribed from the viral RNA and are incorporated into host cell DNA.

Infected T4 lymphocyte

Viral replication

Host genome replication

4. The incorporated viral DNA may lead to active viral replication and cell death or may remain as a proviral genome that replicates with the host cell DNA. The latter process may cause functional defects or malignant transformation.

Loss of T4 lymphocytes

DECREASE

- Cytotoxic T cell function
- Specific antibody responses
- Amplifier/helper function
- NK cell function
- Monocyte/macrophage responses

5. The loss in T4 lymphocyte activity results in a broad spectrum of immunologic defects and leads to the immunodeficiency syndrome.

Figure 4-21.   Pathogenesis of AIDS.

cytotoxic) cells can be elevated, normal, or decreased. The **T4/T8 ratio**, which is about 2/1 in normal individuals, can be completely inverted (0.5) in AIDS patients. Figure 4-19 shows a flow cytometric profile of an AIDS patient. Other conditions, such as acute viral infections, can also cause inversions of the T4/T8 ratio, but these are usually not associated with a net loss of T4 cells.

The etiologic agent of AIDS is now known to be a retrovirus originally called HTLV-III (human T cell leukemia/lymphoma virus). Subsequently, an international conference of AIDS investigators renamed the virus as human immunodeficiency virus (HIV). This RNA virus is one of a family of human T cell viruses that cause leukemias and lymphomas. HIV specifically infects and kills the T4 subpopulation of T-lymphocytes (Fig. 4-21). However, it should be noted that HIV has also been recovered from monocytes and macrophages. The broad immunosuppressive action of the disease reflects the importance of T4 cells in amplifying immune responses.

Currently, research efforts are directed at vaccine development and methods of early detection and diagnosis. The only practical serologic test detects serum antibodies against HIV. This test indicates prior exposure to the virus but does not detect active infection. Moreover, HIV variants may complicate diagnostic efforts. Therefore, better screening and diagnostic tests will need to be developed.

Autoimmunity

Autoimmunity implies that an immune response has been generated against self-antigens (autoantigens). Central to the concept of autoimmunity is the breakdown in the ability of the immune system to differentiate between self- and nonself-antigens. Autoimmunity was classically interpreted as an abnormal immune response that invariably caused disease. However, it is now clear that autoimmune responses are common and are necessary for regulation of the immune system. The development of anti-idiotypic antibodies, which serve as important regulatory proteins for the immune response, is by definition an autoimmune response. Therefore, the **regulated production of autoantibodies is a normal event.** When the normal regulatory mechanisms are in some way deflected, the uncontrolled production of autoantibodies, or the appearance of abnormal cell–cell recognition, produces disease. The mere presence of autoantibodies is not sufficient for a designation of autoimmune disease. It is necessary to demonstrate a cause and effect relationship in which the autoim-

mune reaction (whether cellular or humoral) is directly related to the disease process. At present only a few diseases, such as lupus erythematosus and thyroiditis, fit this criterion.

An abnormal autoimmune response to self-antigens implies that there is a loss of immune tolerance. The term "tolerance" traditionally denotes a condition in which there is no measurable immune response to specific (usually self-) antigens. The reasons for this loss of tolerance in autoimmune diseases are not understood. Experimental studies suggest that normal tolerance to self-antigens is an active process requiring contact between self-components and immune cells. In the fetus, tolerance is readily established to antigens that in the adult cause vigorous immune responses. Induction of tolerance to an antigen is partly related to the dose of antigen to which cells of the intact organism are exposed. In contrast to the classical theory of Burnet, who postulated that tolerance is caused by "clonal deletion" of antigen-reactive T cells, there is extensive evidence that induction of tolerance is an active immune response that can be produced in a variety of ways. **Tolerance is best looked on as a diversion of the immune system to an active state of nonreactivity: that is, the immune response is blocked by inhibitory products.** Both T and B cells are rendered tolerant—T-helper cells after exposure to low doses of the antigen and B cells after large doses.

The most popular theories explaining the loss of tolerance in autoimmune disease are listed in Table 4-6. The simplest hypothesis states that an immune reaction develops to self-antigen not normally present in the circulation. The tissue antigens are usually bound in tissues and are not exposed or released until some type of tissue injury occurs. At that time these antigens are released into the circulation, and an immune response develops. Examples of this type of response are antibody formation against spermatozoa, lens tissue, and myelin. Whether these autoantibodies are capable of directly inducing injury is another matter. In the case of antisperm antibodies, outside of a localized orchitis there is no evidence that they induce generalized injury. **Thus, although autoantibodies form against such "sequestered antigens," there is little evidence that they are pathogenic.**

Another theory holds that autoimmune reactions develop as a result of abnormalities in the T cell system. Most immune responses require T cell participation to cause antigen-specific B cell activation. Alterations in the number or functional activities of T-helper or T-suppressor cells would be expected to influence the ability of the host to mount an immune

Table 4-6 Postulated Mechanisms by which Autoimmunity Develops

MECHANISM	EXAMPLES
Release of sequestered antigens	Antibodies to spermatozoa, lens tissue, myelin
Abnormal T cell function:	
Diminished suppressor-cell function	Systemic lupus erythematosus and other autoimmune diseases
Enhanced helper-cell function	Drug-induced hemolytic anemias
Polyclonal B cell activation	Systemic lupus erythematosus, other autoimmune diseases; Epstein-Barr virus–induced anti-DNA antibody

response. In fact, defects in T cells have been described in many autoimmune diseases. Most of the interest has centered on T-suppressor cells. For example, there are reports of defective suppressor cell activity in human and experimental systemic lupus erythematosus. Lymphocytotropic antibodies have also been described in patients with the disease. Abnormalities in suppressor cell function characterize other autoimmune diseases, including primary biliary cirrhosis, thyroiditis, multiple sclerosis, myasthenia gravis, rheumatoid arthritis, and scleroderma. However, the critical question is whether these alterations in suppressor cell function are the primary cause of these diseases or merely a secondary response. **Most evidence suggests that numerical decreases in suppressor cells are not directly the cause of autoimmune diseases.** Defects in suppressor cell function have also been described in individuals with no evidence of autoimmune disease.

There has also been interest in abnormalities in T-helper cell function in autoimmune disease. T-helper cells are defined by their role in antigen-specific B cell activation. It is believed that these cells maintain the tolerance induced by low doses of antigen. Experimentally it is possible to "break" this type of tolerance by altering the antigen in such a way that the T-helper cell is activated and triggers the B cell. Examples are antigen modification by partial degradation and antigen complexing to a carrier (protein). In some rheumatic diseases, autoantibodies to partially degraded connective tissue proteins, such as collagen or elastin, are demonstrated, and in some drug-induced hemolytic anemias the binding of the drug to the red cell membrane induces the hemolytic reaction.

A second mechanism by which the T-helper cell tolerance is overcome involves antibodies that are formed against foreign antigens but crossreact with self-antigens. Here the T-helper cell functions correctly and does not induce autoantibody formation. Rather, the efferent limb of the immune response is abnormal. An example is rheumatic heart disease, in which antibody formed against streptococcal bacterial antigens crossreacts with antigens from cardiac muscle (a process known as "biologic mimicry").

Finally, another postulated mechanism to explain the loss of tolerance involves polyclonal B cell activation, in which B-lymphocytes are directly activated by complex substances that contain many antigenic sites (such as bacterial cell walls and viruses). This type of B cell activation is independent of T cells. Therefore, it could lead to the loss of the normal T cell surveillance mechanism. **There is some evidence that polyclonal B cell activation may be involved in the formation of autoantibodies.** The development of rheumatoid factor and anti-DNA and other autoantibodies after bacterial, viral, or parasitic infections has been described. This mechanism may be involved in diseases such as rheumatoid arthritis and lupus erythematosus.

Mediation of Tissue Injury in Autoimmune Diseases

Traditionally, autoimmune diseases have been considered to be prototypes of immune complex disease—the immune complexes forming in either the circulation or the tissues. Thus, types II and III hypersensitivity reactions are implicated as the cause of tissue injury in most types of autoimmune diseases. Although it is probably true that these types of hypersensitivity reactions explain most of the autoimmune tissue injury, the story is actually more complicated. In some types of autoimmune diseases, T cells sensitized to self-antigens (such as thyroglobulin) may directly cause tissue injury, but it is not clear to what extent.

Examples of autoimmune diseases presumably mediated by type II hypersensitivity reactions are listed in Table 4-7. In these diseases an antibody is formed against either a cell surface antigen or connective tissue. As mentioned above, local complement activation by the antibody, with either direct complement-mediated lysis or opsonization for phagocytic cells, causes most of the injury. Another mechanism of tissue injury is antibody-directed cellular cytotoxicity. However, not all autoantibodies cause injury by cytotoxic reactions. In the antireceptor antibody diseases, such as Graves' disease or myasthenia gravis, the autoantibody binds to the receptor but has no toxic effect itself. Anti-insulin receptor antibodies have also been described in dis-

Table 4-7 Types of Hypersensitivity Reactions Involved in Autoimmune Disease

REACTION TYPE	DISEASE
Type II	Autoimmune hemolytic anemias, neutropenias, lymphopenias, thrombocytopenias
	Goodpasture's disease
	Antireceptor antibody diseases
	Myasthenia gravis
	Graves' disease
	Anti-insulin antibody
	Bullous skin diseases
	Pemphigus
	Pemphigoid
Type III	Systemic lupus erythematosus
	Rheumatoid arthritis
	Sjögren's disease
	Scleroderma
	Polymyositis–dermatomyositis

eases such as acanthosis nigricans and ataxia telangiectasia.

Type III hypersensitivity reactions explain tissue injury in some types of autoimmune diseases. As shown in Table 4-7, the prototypical disease of this kind is systemic lupus erythematosus, in which DNA–anti-DNA complexes formed in the circulation are deposited in tissues and induce various diseases, such as vasculitis, glomerulonephritis, and arthritis. Other examples are rheumatoid arthritis, scleroderma, polymyositis-dermatomyositis, and Sjögren's disease. All of these diseases are characterized by circulating immune complexes and deposition in tissue; they are classified under the general heading of "collagen-vascular" diseases. **Because the pathogenesis of these maladies largely involves circulating immune complexes, the clinical manifestations are systemic, and many organs and systems are involved. By contrast, the Type II–mediated autoimmune reactions, for the most part, are organ-specific.**

In the following sections we will briefly describe those systemic diseases for which there is good evidence of an autoimmune etiology.

Systemic Lupus Erythematosus

Systemic lupus erythematosus (SLE) is a chronic multisystem, inflammatory disease that may involve almost any organ but characteristically affects the kidneys, joints, serosal membranes, and skin (Table 4-8). It is the prototype of a systemic autoimmune disease in which autoantibodies are formed against a variety of self-antigens, including plasma proteins (complement components and clotting factors), cell surface antigens (lymphocytes, neutrophils, platelets, erythrocytes), and intracellular cytoplasmic and nuclear components (microfilaments, microtubules, lysosomes, ribosomes, DNA, RNA, histone).

The most important autoantibodies are those against nuclear antigens—in particular, antibody to double-stranded DNA and to the SM antigen, a soluble nuclear antigen. A high titer of these two autoantibodies (called antinuclear antibodies) is pathognomonic of SLE. These antinuclear antibodies are usually not directly cytotoxic by themselves. Antigen-antibody complexes form in the circulation and deposit in tissues, creating the characteristic injury of vasculitis, synovitis, and glomerulonephritis. It is for this reason that SLE is considered the prototype of type III hypersensitivity reactions. Occasionally in this disease, some directly cytotoxic antibodies are present—particularly antibodies formed against cell surface antigens of leukocytes and erythrocytes.

Etiology

The etiology of SLE is unknown. The characteristic feature of the disease—the presence of numerous autoantibodies, particularly antinuclear antibodies—suggests that there is a breakdown in the normal immune surveillance mechanisms, a defect that leads to a loss of the normal self-tolerance mechanisms.

There appear to be many factors that predispose to the development of SLE. In the past there was widespread interest in C-type virus particles in experimental models of the disease in mice. Recent evidence suggests that the virus is not necessary for the development of the disease in mice. In humans there is little evidence that viruses initiate SLE, although there is still interest in the possible role of the Epstein-Barr virus. This agent induces polyclonal B cell activation, a characteristic of the disease.

There is a clear female predisposition for SLE, women accounting for 90% of cases between ages 12 and 40. For unknown reasons, this female-to-male predominance is true for all autoimmune diseases. Sex hormones may in part be the explanation. In mouse models of lupus, estrogens accelerate progression of the disease, whereas androgens have a retarding effect. Estrogens have been described experimentally as increasing the likelihood of overcoming tolerance.

There also appears to be some genetic predisposition to lupus, and a higher incidence is described in families and monozygotic twins. The incidence of lupus (and the other autoimmune diseases) is higher among those exhibiting certain HLA and DR antigens of the major histocompatibility complex (MHC)—in the case of lupus, DR2 and DR3. These genes perform

Table 4-8 Primary Organ System Involvement in Systemic Lupus Erythematosus

ORGAN SYSTEM	PERCENTAGE	CHARACTERISTIC PATHOLOGY
Joints	90	Nonerosive synovitis with neutrophils and mono-nuclear cells
Kidney	75	Immune complex glomerulonephritis, interstitial nephritis
Serosal membranes	35	Pluritis, pericarditis peritonitis secondary to immune complex depostition
Heart	45–50	Pericarditis, myocarditis, endocarditis

two unlinked functions, namely participation in immunoregulation and the effector limb of the immune response. Thus, the HLA B8 haplotype, which is often found in association with autoimmune diseases, is also associated with the DR antigens in certain immunoregulatory abnormalities, including abnormal lymphocyte responses to antigens, decreased numbers of circulating suppressor cells, and increased numbers of B cells in the blood. Among the effector functions associated with these HLA haplotypes is a decrease in C3b receptors on cells that clear circulating immune complexes. Further evidence to support a critical role for the D/DR region in the pathogenesis of SLE comes from the observation that inherited deficiencies of certain complement components, particularly C2 and C4, are associated with an increased incidence of the disease. The genes that code for these early complement components are within the HLA region, close to the D/DR site. **Thus, many genetic factors seem to predispose to SLE, including defects in both immunoregulation and immune effector mechanisms.**

Immunologic Abnormalities

As noted earlier, **autoantibody production to nuclear antigens is characteristic of SLE.** This autoantibody production is linked to B cell hyperreactivity, the major effector mechanism of this disease. B cell hyperreactivity is genetically determined (DR locus) and, being polyclonal, is independent of T cells. B cells from patients with lupus show greatly increased spontaneous proliferation and antibody formation, and the antibodies formed are not exclusively against self-antigens. Therefore, this B cell hyperreactivity cannot be explained by the activation of T cell–dependent monoclonal antibody to self-antigens. Various abnormalities in T cells, particularly decreased levels of suppressor T cells, have also been described, most completely in the mouse models. However, in man no consistent defect in suppressor cells has been found. Thus, any abnormalities in T cells noted in lupus appear to be a function of the disease rather than the cause.

Pathogenesis

The evidence for the hypothesis that SLE is caused by a type III hypersensitivity reaction is as follows: During the active disease stages of lupus it is often possible to measure the levels of circulating immune complexes that contain nuclear antigens. Secondly, in lupus-induced tissue injury—for example, vasculitis or glomerulonephritis—immune complexes are identified in injured tissues by immunofluorescence. Finally, immune complexes extracted from the tissues contain nuclear antigens. Thus, there is good evidence that the bulk of the injury seen in lupus is due to immune complexes formed against self, particularly against DNA. Type II hypersensitivity reactions may also have a role in lupus, since cytotoxic antibodies against leukocytes, erythrocytes, and platelets have been described.

Because circulating immune complexes deposit in almost all tissues, virtually every organ in the body can be involved. Skin involvement is common and is manifested by an erythematous rash in sun-exposed sites, a "butterfly" malar rash being the most characteristic. Microscopically, the skin exhibits a perivascular lymphoid infiltrate and liquefactive degeneration of the basal cells. The organs with the most serious involvement by SLE are shown in Figure 4-22 and Table 4-8. **Joint involvement is the most common manifestation of SLE; over 90% of patients have polyarthralgias.** Although an inflammatory synovitis occurs, unlike rheumatoid arthritis there is usually no injury to the joint itself.

Although most of this multisystem involvement in SLE can be traced to the deposition of circulating preformed immune complexes in the tissues, recent evidence suggests that under certain conditions the formation of immune complexes occurs *in situ*—that is, in the tissues rather than in the circulation. Perhaps the best example of this *in situ* formation of immune complexes in SLE is seen with membranous lupus glomerulonephritis. As described below, this type of glomerulonephritis is generally associated with subepithelial immune deposits in the glomeruli, with no evidence of circulating immune complexes.

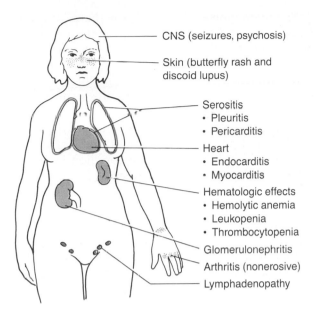

CNS (seizures, psychosis)

Skin (butterfly rash and discoid lupus)

Serositis
• Pleuritis
• Pericarditis

Heart
• Endocarditis
• Myocarditis

Hematologic effects
• Hemolytic anemia
• Leukopenia
• Thrombocytopenia

Glomerulonephritis

Arthritis (nonerosive)

Lymphadenopathy

Figure 4-22. Complications of systemic lupus erythematosus.

Experimentally, it appears that these subepithelial deposits are formed *in situ*, which explains the absence of circulating immune complexes. Therefore, while the deposition of preformed circulating immune complexes in tissues may be responsible for the bulk of the tissue injury in SLE and other immune complex diseases, *in situ* formation of immune complexes in the tissues also appears to be important.

Renal involvement, in particular glomerulonephritis, is very common and as **many as 75% of patients with SLE have evidence of renal disease at autopsy.**

Four main histologic types of glomerulonephritis can be distinguished, as defined in the World Health Organization classification of lupus nephritis. The mildest form of renal involvement is **mesangeal lupus nephritis.** In this disorder immune complexes and complement deposit almost exclusively in the mesangeal regions of the glomeruli, but there are only slight increases in mesangeal cells and mesangeal matrix (Fig. 4-23). These patients have only mild renal dysfunction, characterized by mild proteinuria and hematuria. The prognosis is excellent.

The next category is **focal proliferative lupus nephritis.** Some glomeruli, but not all (focal), show increased cellularity (Fig. 4-24), characterized both by a proliferation of resident glomerular endothelial and mesangeal cells and by infiltrating neutrophils and monocytes. Necrosis and fibrin deposition are also often present. Immunofluorescence studies and electron microscopy demonstrate deposition of immunoglobulin and complement, primarily in the mesangeal regions of the glomeruli. The prognosis of patients with this form of lupus nephritis is mixed. Some remain with only mild disease, whereas others progress to renal failure.

The third type, **diffuse proliferative lupus nephritis,** is the most serious. It occurs in as many as 50% of lupus patients with renal involvement and is associated with conspicuous increases in glomerular cellularity, fibrin deposition, and necrosis (Fig. 4-25). Epithelial crescents are also commonly seen. By immunofluorescence and electron microscopy widespread deposition of immune complexes is seen throughout the glomeruli, primarily in the mesan-

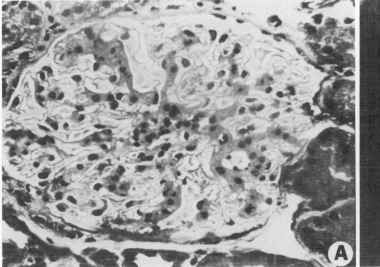
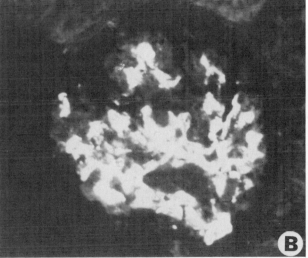

Figure 4-23. Mesangeal form of lupus nephritis. (*A*) Histologically there is a slight increase in mesangeal matrix and cellularity. (*B*) Immunofluorescence studies reveal immunoglobulin and complement deposition in the mesangium.

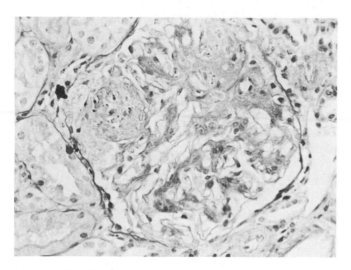

Figure 4-24. Focal proliferative lupus nephritis. Note the segmental necrosis in the glomerulus.

gium and underneath the glomerular basement membrane (subendothelial). Many patients with this form of lupus nephritis progress to renal failure.

The final type of lupus nephritis is **membranous lupus nephritis,** which is associated with massive proteinuria. Membranous lupus nephritis resembles other forms of membranous glomerulonephritis. There is no hypercellularity, but instead diffusely thickened glomerular capillary loops caused by the deposition of immunoglobulin and complement on the epithelial surface of the glomerular basement membrane (subepithelial). This pattern of lupus involvement is usually not associated with renal failure.

Although glomerulonephritis is the most common renal manifestation of SLE, occasionally an interstitial nephritis or (rarely) a vasculitis is associated with the disease. In many of these cases, immunoglobulins and complement are present in the interstitium and blood vessels of the kidney. Involvement of serous membranes is common in SLE. More than a third of patients have a pleuritis and a pleural effusion. Pericarditis and peritonitis occur less frequently.

Cardiac involvement is also common in SLE, but congestive heart failure is rare and is usually associated with a myocarditis. All layers of the heart may be involved, with pericarditis being the most common finding. Endocarditis is usually not clinically significant and is characterized by small vegetations along the lines of closure of the valve leaflets. These small nonbacterial vegetations constitute **Libman-Sacks endocarditis,** and they should be differentiated from the larger, more bulky vegetations of bacterial endocarditis.

Other organ involvement occurs less frequently and is often due to a vasculitis, which is also characteristic of lupus. Thus, splenic involvement is characterized by thickening and concentric fibrosis of the penicilliary arteries—the so-called onion-skin pattern. **Involvement of the central nervous system is a life-threatening complication of lupus. Its nature is not well understood, but vasculitis, hemorrhage and infarction of the brain may be seen.**

In summary, the primary abnormality in systemic lupus erythematosus is polyclonal B cell hyperactivity, which is associated with a loss of normal self-tolerance and autoantibody formation to a variety of

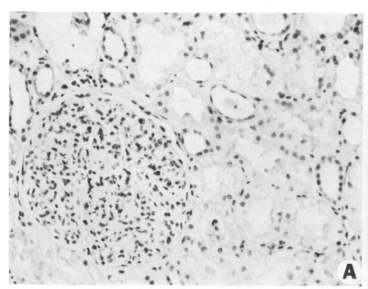
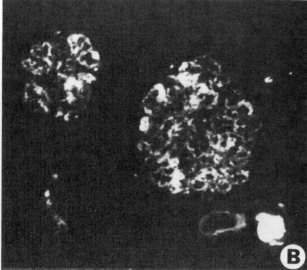

Figure 4-25. Diffuse proliferative lupus nephritis. (*A*) Marked diffuse cellularity increase in the glomerulus. (*B*) Immunofluorescence showing intense immunoglobulin and complement deposition in mesangial and capillary wall locations.

self-antigens, the most important of which is against DNA (Fig. 4-26). The reason for this B cell hyperactivity is not clear, but it is not associated with consistent T cell abnormalities. The systemic injury seen in lupus is caused by the deposition of these autoantibodies in tissues, which triggers acute inflammation.

Sjögren's Disease

Sjögren's disease is an autoimmune disorder characterized by keratoconjunctivitis sicca (dry eyes) and xerostomia (dry mouth) in the absence of other connective tissue diseases. This definition is used to separate primary Sjögren's disease from secondary types that are occasionally associated with other disorders of connective tissue, such as SLE or rheumatoid arthritis.

The main target in Sjögren's disease is the major and minor salivary glands, but the primary type is also frequently associated with involvement of other organs, including the thyroid gland, the lung, and the kidney.

Primary Sjögren's disease is the second common connective tissue disorder, after lupus. Like most autoimmune diseases, it occurs primarily in women (30-65 years). There are strong associations between primary Sjögren's disease and certain HLA types, notably HLA-DW3, DR3, DW2, and MT2, a B cell alloantigen. Familial clustering occurs, and in these families there is also a high incidence of other autoimmune diseases.

Immunologic Abnormalities

Production of autoantibodies, particularly antinuclear antibodies, occur in patients with Sjögren's disease. These autoantibodies may be directed against DNA, histones, or nonhistone proteins in the nucleus. **Autoantibodies to the soluble nuclear nonhistone proteins characterize primary Sjögren's disease, particularly the antigens SS-A and SS-B. However, autoantibodies to DNA or histones are rare. The presence of these antibodies suggests secondary Sjögren's disease due to lupus.** Rheumatoid factor is also commonly present in saliva, tears, and the circulation. Organ-specific autoantibodies, such as those directed against salivary gland antigens, are rare.

Pathogenesis

The etiology of Sjögren's disease is unknown, and the autoantibody production appears to be caused by a polyclonal B cell proliferation. This proliferation is

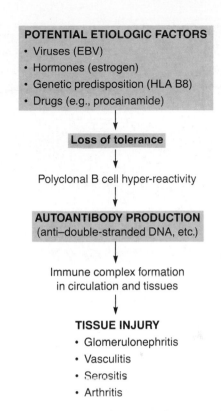

POTENTIAL ETIOLOGIC FACTORS
- Viruses (EBV)
- Hormones (estrogen)
- Genetic predisposition (HLA B8)
- Drugs (e.g., procainamide)

↓

Loss of tolerance

↓

Polyclonal B cell hyper-reactivity

↓

AUTOANTIBODY PRODUCTION
(anti–double-stranded DNA, etc.)

↓

Immune complex formation
in circulation and tissues

↓

TISSUE INJURY
- Glomerulonephritis
- Vasculitis
- Serositis
- Arthritis

Figure 4-26. Pathogenesis of systemic lupus erythematosus.

possibly triggered by the Epstein-Barr virus or cytomegalovirus. These viruses are commonly present in salivary glands, and the autoantibody directed against the SS-B antigen selectively binds to EBV RNA of the Epstein-Barr virus. Infection with this virus is associated with the development of nasopharyngeal carcinoma. An intense lymphocytic infiltrate, which resembles that seen in Sjögren's disease, occurs with this neoplasm. However, direct proof to incriminate the Epstein-Barr virus is lacking.

Pathology

Sjögren's disease is characterized by an intense lymphocytic infiltrate of the major and minor salivary glands (Fig. 4-27). Minor salivary glands are the usual biopsy sites, and focal lymphocytic infiltrates are initially observed in a periductal location. The majority of gland lobules, especially the centers of the lobules, are affected. Well defined germinal centers are rare. The lymphoid infiltrates destroy acini and ducts, and the latter often become dilated and filled with cellular debris. The stroma of the gland is preserved, an appearance that helps to differentiate this disorder from a lymphoma. The lymphocytic infiltrates in the glands are predominantly T cells; lesser numbers of B cells are present.

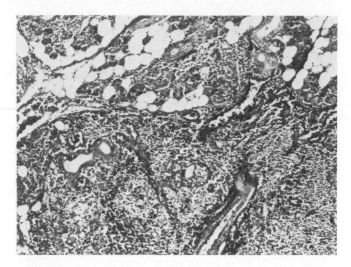

Figure 4-27. Sjögren's disease involving a major salivary gland. Focal intense lymphoid infiltrates are destroying the gland acini but sparing the ducts.

Involvement of extraglandular sites is also common in Sjögren's disease. Pulmonary involvement occurs in most patients, and bronchial glands atrophy following lymphoid infiltration. This causes thick tenacious secretions, focal atelectasis, recurrent infections, and bronchiectasis.

The disease also affects the gastrointestinal tract, and many patients have difficulty in swallowing (dysphagia). The submucosal glands of the esophagus are infiltrated by lymphocytes. In addition, atrophic gastritis occurs secondary to lymphoid infiltrates of the gastric mucosa. Liver involvement is present in 5% to 10% of patients and is associated with cholangitis and nodular lymphoid infiltrates. Interstitial nephritis and thyroid involvement are occasionally seen.

Progressive Systemic Sclerosis (Scleroderma)

Progressive systemic sclerosis, or scleroderma, is an autoimmune disease of connective tissue characterized by excessive collagen deposition in the skin and in internal organs.

The disease occurs primarily in women, but familial incidence is not a feature. There is also no association between HLA haplotypes and scleroderma. Nevertheless, almost all (96%) of patients with scleroderma have chromosomal abnormalities, such as chromatid breaks, translocations, and deletions. These abnormalities appear to be acquired rather than transmitted and are associated with a "serum breaking factor." The significance of these chromosomal abnormalities is unclear.

Immunologic Abnormalities

Patients with scleroderma exhibit abnormalities of the humoral and cellular immune systems. The number of circulating B-lymphocytes is normal, but there is evidence of hyperactivity, as manifested by hypergammaglobulinemia and cryoglobulinemia. Antinuclear antibodies are commonly present, but are usually in a lower titer than in lupus. However, **some types of antinuclear antibodies—for example, nucleolar autoantibody—are highly specific for scleroderma. Even more specific for scleroderma are antibodies to ScL-70, a nonhistone nuclear protein, and anticentromere antibodies.** Anticentromere antibodies are also present in the milder CREST variant of scleroderma, a form that is characterized by calcinosis (C), Raynaud's phenomenon (R), esophageal dysfunction (E), sclerodactyly (S), and telangiectasia (T). There is usually no severe systemic involvement in the CREST variant. There is no correlation between the titer of antinuclear antibodies and the severity of the disease process. Rheumatoid factor is also commonly present, and autoantibodies are occasionally directed against other tissues, such as smooth muscle, thyroid gland, and salivary glands. Antibodies against types I and IV collagen have also been described, and may be relevant to the pathogenesis of this disease.

Cellular immune derangements in progressive systemic sclerosis include a decrease in the number of circulating T cells, a decrease in T-helper cells, and an increase in T-suppressor cells. Although functional lymphocyte studies are inconclusive, lymphocytes from patients with this disease are sensitized to skin extracts or collagen, to which they respond by proliferating and by producing lymphokines, which may cause chemotaxis and enhanced collagen synthesis by fibroblasts.

Pathogenesis

Progressive systemic sclerosis is characterized by excessive collagen deposition in many tissues. This fibrosis may be due to an abnormality in the function of fibroblasts. Fibroblasts from patients with this disorder show spontaneously increased collagen synthesis in tissue culture. The reason for this increase is unknown, but it may relate to lymphokine production by T cells sensitized to collagen.

Pathology

The skin in scleroderma displays early edema and then induration, the latter characterized by the following:

- A striking increase in collagen fibers in the reticular dermis
- Thinning of the epidermis with loss of rete pegs
- Atrophy of dermal appendages
- Hyalinization and obliteration of arterioles
- Variable mononuclear infiltrates, consisting primarily of T cells

This stage of induration may progress to atrophy or revert to normal.

Similar histologic alterations occur in the synovium, lungs, gastrointestinal tract, heart, and kidneys. Alterations of the arteries, arterioles, and capillaries are typical of—and in some cases may be the first effect of—the disease. There is initial subintimal edema with fibrin deposition, followed by thickening and fibrosis of the vessel and reduplication or fraying of the internal elastic lamina (Fig. 4-28). Involved vessels are usually severely restricted in terms of blood flow, and may actually be thrombosed.

The most significant systemic involvement occurs in the kidneys, lungs, and heart. The kidneys, which are involved in more than half of the patients, show marked vascular changes, often with focal hemorrhage and cortical infarcts. Among the most severely affected vessels are the interlobular arteries and afferent arterioles. Early fibromucosal thickening of the subintima causes luminal narrowing, which is followed by fibrosis (Fig. 4-28). "Fibrinoid" necrosis is commonly seen in afferent arterioles. The glomerular alterations are nonspecific, and focal changes range from necrosis extending from the afferent arterioles to fibrosis. There is diffuse deposition of immunoglobulin, complement, and fibrin in affected vessels

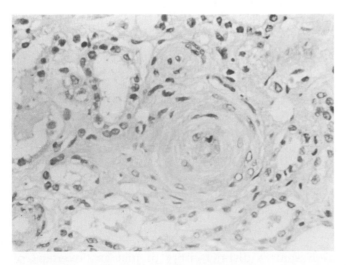

Figure 4-28. Scleroderma with characteristic renal vascular involvement. The interlobular artery shows a marked intimal thickening with virtual obliteration of the lumen.

early in the disease, probably because of increased vascular permeability.

In the lungs the primary abnormality is diffuse interstitial fibrosis. The lungs may progress to end-stage fibrosis, eventuating in a "honeycomb" lung.

Primary myocardial necrosis is seen with progressive systemic sclerosis, but does not reflect obstruction of the coronary arteries and ischemic necrosis. It is, rather, a primary event. In a quarter of patients the myocardial fibrosis is extensive, involving 10% or more of the myocardium.

Finally, progressive systemic sclerosis can involve any portion of the GI tract. Most commonly, esophageal dysfunction is the most significant gastrointestinal complication. Atrophy of the smooth muscle and fibrous replacement are seen in the lower esophagus.

Polymyositis/Dermatomyositis

Polymyositis/dermatomyositis is a multisystem autoimmune disease primarily involving skin and muscle. It occurs in both children and adults, and there is an increased frequency of HLA-B8 and DR3 in the childhood form of the disease. Women are affected twice as frequently as men.

Immunologic Abnormalities

Defects in both cellular and humoral mechanisms occur in these patients. Various autoantibodies against muscle are commonly present, and almost all patients (90%) have antibodies against myosin. Antibodies to myoglobin are also common. Various antinuclear and anti-DNA autoantibodies are found, including antibodies to ribonucleoprotein (RNP). Anti-RNP, present in high titer in patients with mixed connective tissue disease, is seen in some patients with polymyositis/dermatomyositis. Antibodies directed against the extractable nuclear antigens PM-1 and JO-1 are the most specific. Cell-mediated immune derangements have been described. Both the activity and the absolute numbers of T-suppressor cells have been described as either normal or elevated.

Pathogenesis

In polymyositis/dermatomyositis, as in all of the systemic autoimmune diseases, the causative agent is not known. The mechanisms directly responsible for the injury are also obscure, but both humoral and cell-mediated mechanisms of injury have been implicated. Many patients have circulating immune complexes, and it has been postulated that these complexes deposit in blood vessels of the muscle and induce vascular and muscle necrosis. Deposition of immunoglobulin and complement is often found in blood vessels.

There is also evidence that cell-mediated immune mechanisms are involved. A prominent lymphoid infiltrate in affected muscles contains a predominance of activated T cells as well as NK cells. *In vitro*, these lymphocytes have been shown to display sensitization to muscle antigens and cytotoxicity to muscle fibers. Antibody-dependent cellular cytotoxicity has also been postulated.

Pathology

The diagnosis of polymyositis rests not only on the histologic appearance of the involved muscles but also on the location of the involved muscles, on electromyographic alterations, and on elevated activities of muscle enzymes in the blood, the MM isoenzyme of including creatine phosphokinase (CPK) and aldolase. The disease typically involves proximal muscle groups of the upper and lower extremities, and is symmetrical. Skin involvement may or may not be present. Histologically, the skeletal muscle shows evidence of necrosis, regeneration, and a mononuclear inflammatory infiltrate. In chronic cases dense fibrous tissue replaces muscle fibers.

Skin involvement occurs in about 40% of patients and is manifested by an erythematous rash on the face resembling that seen in SLE. However, the rash is also present elsewhere; if it involves the eyelids (heliotropic rash), it is considered specific for dermatomyositis. The skin changes, as in SLE, involve a perivascular lymphoid infiltrate and liquefactive degeneration of the basal epithelial cells. Immunofluorescence studies of skin are helpful to differentiate these two entities. In SLE, granular immunoglobulin and complement deposition at the dermal-epidermal junction, which occurs in uninvolved and involved skin, is virtually pathognomonic. By contrast, dermatomyositis is not associated with the deposition of immune components at the dermal-epidermal junction. Other organ systems are involved, including joints, kidneys, lungs, and gastrointestinal tract. In the childhood form of the disease, a vasculitis may also be present. Many patients with polymyositis/dermatomyositis, particularly adult men, are also at increased risk for developing cancers. Renal involvement was initially thought to be rare, but newer reports suggest that a small percentage of patients (5%–10%) do have immune complex renal disease. Dermatomyositis usually responds to treatment with ad-

renocortical steroids, and the prognosis is generally considered good. Some patients, however, develop classic scleroderma, and others have significant pulmonary and brain involvement.

Mixed Connective Tissue Disease

Mixed connective tissue disease (MCTD) was first described as a separate entity in 1972. The disease combines features of SLE (skin rash, Raynaud's phenomenon, arthritis, arthralgias), scleroderma (swollen hands, esophageal hypomotility, pulmonary interstitial disease), and polymyositis (inflammatory myositis). Some patients also develop symptoms suggestive of rheumatoid arthritis. Patients with this disease have been reported to respond well to corticosteroid therapy, although newer studies have challenged this assertion.

The relative incidence of mixed connective tissue disease is unknown. Between 80% and 90% of patients are female, and most are adults (mean age 37 years).

Patients with this disorder often have hypergammaglobulinemia and a positive rheumatoid factor. Antinuclear antibodies are present, but, unlike SLE, are usually not against double-stranded DNA. The most distinctive antinuclear antibody is directed against an extractable nuclear antigen. Specifically, these patients have high titers of antibody to ribonucleoprotein in the absence of other extractable nuclear antigens, including PM-1 and JO-1. Anti-ribonucleoprotein antibodies are also occasionally seen in SLE, but usually in lower titer than is seen in mixed connective tissue disease.

The etiology and pathogenesis of this malady are unknown. The cause of the formation and maintenance of high titers of anti-ribonucleoprotein antibody is unclear. There is no direct evidence that these antibodies induce the characteristic involvement of the various organ systems. There is also controversy over whether mixed connective tissue disease is a separate disease entity or represents a heterogeneous collection of patients with SLE, scleroderma, or polymyositis, who do not present initially with the classic manifestations of these diseases. For example, some cases in which the original diagnosis was mixed connective tissue disease evolve into typical scleroderma. Also, some patients do develop evidence of renal disease, a finding that is suggestive of SLE. Therefore, whether mixed connective tissue disease represents a distinct entity or just an "overlap" of symptoms from patients with other types of collagen vascular diseases remains an open question.

SUGGESTED READING

BOOKS

Roitt I, Brosoff J, Male D: Immunology. St. Louis, CV Mosby, 1985

REVIEW ARTICLES

Alarcon-Segawa D: Mixed connective tissue disease: A disorder of immune regulation. Semin Arthritis Rheum 13 (suppl):114-120, 1983

Bril H, Benner R: Graft-vs-host reactions: Mechanisms and contemporary theories. CRC Crit Rev Clin Lab Sci 22:43-95, 1985

Fauci AS: Immunoregulation in autoimmunity. J Allergy Clin Immunol 66:5-17, 1980

Fox RI, Howell FV, Bone RC, et al: Primary Sjögren syndrome: Clinical and immunopathologic features. Semin Arthritis Rheum 14:77-105, 1984

Harry P: Immunobiology of transplant rejection. Ann Clin Res 13:172-198, 1981

Haynes DC, Gershwin ME: The immunopathology of progressive systemic sclerosis (PSS). Semin Arthritis Rheum 1112:331-351, 1982

Herberman RB, Ortaldo JR: Natural killer cells: Their role in defense against disease. Science 214:24, 1981

Hill HR: Immunodeficiency diseases. Prog Clin Pathol 8:205-238, 1981

Jimenez SA: Cellular immune dysfunction and the pathogenesis of scleroderma. Semin Arthritis Rheum (suppl) 13(1):104-113, 1983

Klein J, Fiquerca F, Nagy AZ: Genetics of the major histocompatibility complex: The final act. Annu Rev Immunol 1:119-142, 1983

Lane HC, Fauci AS: Immunologic abnormalities in the acquired immunodeficiency syndrome. Annu Rev Immunol 3:477-500, 1985

Mastaglia FL, Oyeda VJ: Inflammatory myopathies, part 2. Ann Neurol 17:317-323, 1985

Miller KB, Schwartz RS: Autoimmunity and suppressor T-lymphocytes. Ann Intern Med 27:281-313, 1982

Pachman LM, Friedman JM, Maryjowski-Sweeney ML, et al: Immunogenetic studies of juvenile dermatomyositis. III. Study of antibody to organ-specific and nuclear antigens. Arthritis Rheum 28:151-157, 1985

Reveille JD, Wilson RW, Provost TT, et al: Primary Sjögren's disease and other autoimmune diseases in families: Prevalence and immunogenetic studies in six kindreds. Ann Intern Med 101:748-756, 1984

Shoenfeld Y, Schwartz RS: Immunologic and genetic factors in autoimmune disease. N Engl J Med 311:1019-1029, 1984

Smith HR, Steinberg AD: Autoimmunity: A perspective. Annu Rev Immunol 1:75-210, 1983

Theofilopoulos AN, Dixon FJ: Autoimmune diseases: Immunopathology and etiopathogenesis. Am J Pathol 108:321-365, 1982

ORIGINAL ARTICLES

Habets WJ: Antibodies against distinct nuclear matrix proteins are characteristic for mixed connective tissue disease. Clin Exp Immunol 54:265-276, 1984

Postlethwaite AE, Kang AH: Pathogenesis of progressive systemic sclerosis. J Lab Clin Med 103:506-510, 1984

5

Neoplasia

Emanuel Rubin and John L. Farber

Benign versus Malignant
Tumors

Classification of Neoplasms

Histologic Diagnosis of
Malignancy

Invasion and Metastasis

Grading and Staging of
Cancers

The Biochemistry of the
Cancer Cell

The Growth of Cancers

The Causes of Cancer

Tumor Immunology

The Remote Effects of Cancer
on the Host

Heredity and Cancer

The Epidemiology of Cancer

Figure 5-1. Cancer epidemiology. The influence of environmental factors on the incidence of cancer is illustrated by the results of several classic epidemiologic studies of migrant populations. Offspring of Japanese migrants to Hawaii exhibited a decreased incidence of stomach cancer, an increased incidence of cancers of the breast, colon, and prostate, and an increased incidence of Hodgkin's disease. The incidence of nasopharyngeal carcinoma decreased in the offspring of migrants to the United States from China. Eastern Europeans who migrated to the United States showed an increased incidence of carcinoma of the breast, colon, and prostate. Finally, the incidence of Burkitt's lymphoma changed in Africans who migrated from the central highlands to coastal lowlands or to the United States.

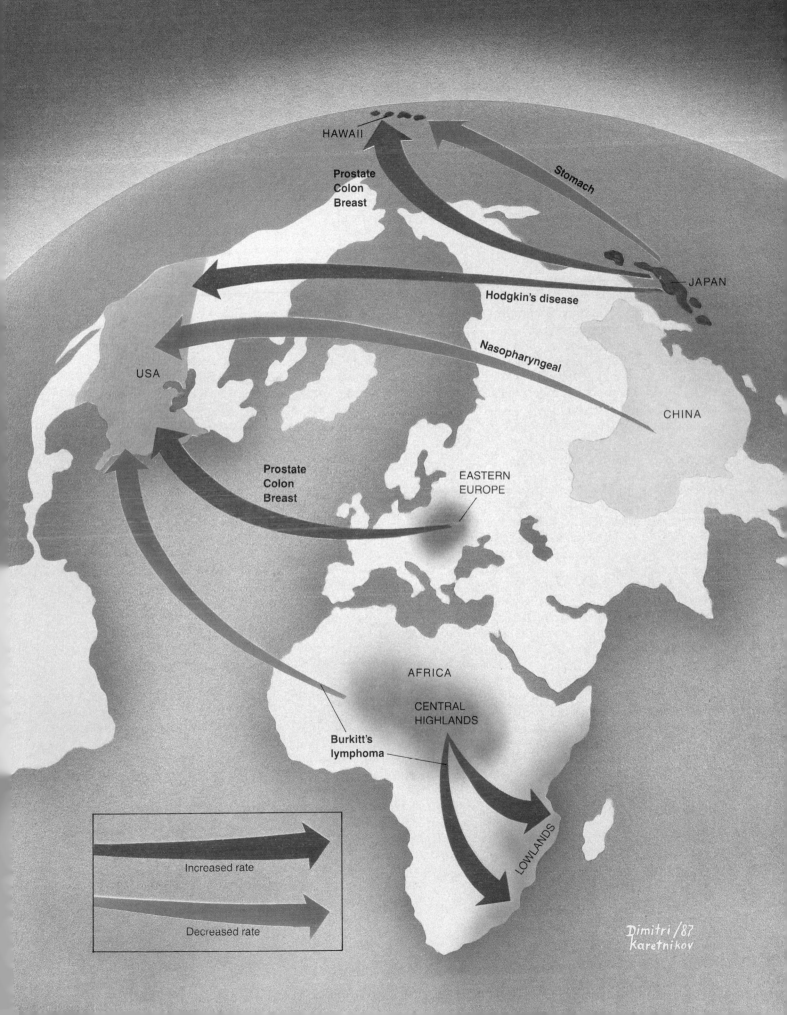

HAWAII

**Prostate
Colon
Breast**

Stomach

USA

Hodgkin's disease

Nasopharyngeal

CHINA

JAPAN

**Prostate
Colon
Breast**

EASTERN
EUROPE

AFRICA

CENTRAL
HIGHLANDS

**Burkitt's
lymphoma**

LOWLANDS

Increased rate

Decreased rate

*Dimitri /87
Karetnikov*

Cancer is an uncontrolled proliferation of cells that express varying degrees of fidelity to their precursors. The structural resemblance of the cancer cell to its putative cell of origin enables specific diagnoses as to the source and potential behavior of the neoplasm. Although the causes of most cancers are not identified, and the mechanisms of carcinogenesis remain obscure, considerable data on the biologic attributes of neoplasia are available. A wide variety of human and experimental data suggests that the neoplastic process entails not only cellular proliferation but also a modification of the differentiation of the involved cell types. Thus, in a sense cancer may be viewed as a burlesque of normal development.

Cancer is not a new disease. Evidence of bone tumors has been found in prehistoric remains, and the disease is mentioned in ancient writings from India, Egypt, Babylonia, and Greece. Hippocrates is actually reported to have distinguished benign from malignant growths. He also introduced the term *karkinos*, from which our term "carcinoma" is derived. In particular, Hippocrates described cancer of the breast, and Paul of Aegina in the seventh century A.D. commented on its frequency. This is especially relevant to the contemporary epidemiology of breast cancer.

The incidence of neoplastic disease increases with age, and the greater longevity of modern times necessarily enlarges the population at risk. Hence, for this reason alone, the overall incidence of cancers is increasing. People of previous generations, on average, did not live long enough to develop many cancers that are peculiar to middle and old age, such as cancer of the prostate, colon, pancreas, and kidney. Despite assertions that contemporary society is or will be subject to an "epidemic" of cancer, the numbers and nature of age-specific cancers have not changed dramatically during the last five decades. The notable exception is cancer of the lung, a disease clearly caused by smoking.

A neoplasm is an abnormal mass of cells that exhibits uncontrolled proliferation and that persists after cessation of the stimulus that produced it. **In general, neoplasms are irreversible, and their growth is, for the most part, autonomous.** Several observations are important at this point: First, neoplasms are derived from cells that normally maintain a proliferative capacity. Thus, mature neurons and cardiac myocytes do not give rise to tumors. Second, a tumor may express varying degrees of differentiation, from relatively mature structures that mimic normal tissues to a collection of cells so primitive that the cell of origin cannot be identified. Third, the stimulus responsible for the uncontrolled proliferation may not be identifiable; in fact, it is not known for most human neoplasms.

Benign versus Malignant Tumors

Benign tumors remain as localized overgrowths in the area in which they arise. **By definition, benign tumors do not penetrate (invade) adjacent tissue borders, nor do they spread (metastasize) to distant sites.** As a rule, benign tumors are more differentiated than malignant ones—that is, they more closely resemble their tissue of origin. **By contrast, malignant tumors, or cancers, have the added property of invading contiguous tissues and metastasizing to distant sites, where subpopulations of malignant cells take up residence, grow anew, and again invade.**

In common usage the terms "benign" and "malignant" refer to the overall biologic behavior of a tumor rather than to its morphologic characteristics. As a general rule, malignant tumors kill and benign ones do not. However, so-called benign tumors in critical locations can be deadly. For example, a benign intracranial tumor of the meninges (meningioma) can kill by exerting pressure on the brain. A minute benign tumor of the ependymal cells of the third ventricle (ependymoma) can block the circulation of cerebrospinal fluid, and the resulting hydrocephalus is lethal. A benign mesenchymal tumor of the left atrium (myxoma) may kill suddenly by blocking the orifice of the mitral valve. In certain locations the erosion or necrosis of a benign tumor of smooth muscle can lead to serious hemorrhage—witness the peptic ulceration of a gastric leiomyoma. On rare occasions a functioning, benign endocrine adenoma can be life-threatening, as in the case of the sudden hypoglycemia associated with an insulinoma of the pancreas or the hypertensive crisis produced by a pheochromocytoma of the adrenal medulla. Conversely, certain types of malignant tumors are so indolent that many are curable by surgical resection. In this category are a considerable proportion of cancers of the breast and some malignant tumors of connective tissue, such as fibrosarcoma.

There are a number of tumors that pose a nosologic dilemma because they do not fit all the criteria for either benign or malignant neoplasms. The best-known example is basal cell carcinoma of the skin, which is histologically malignant (i.e., it invades aggressively) but does not metastasize to distant sites. Similarly, the local growth of mixed tumors of the salivary glands, which are classified as benign, may be so aggressive that they defy surgical cure.

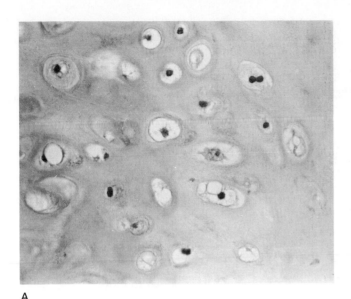
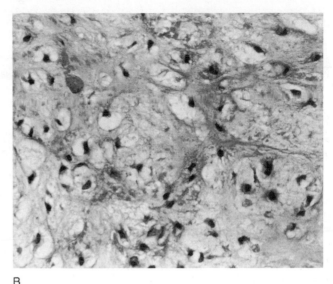

A   B

Figure 5-2.   Benign chondroma. *(A)* Normal hyaline cartilage. *(B)* A benign chondroma closely resembles normal cartilage.

Classification of Neoplasms

In any language the classification of objects and concepts is pragmatic, and useful only insofar as its general acceptance permits effective communication. Similarly, the nosology of tumors reflects historical concepts, technical jargon, location, origin, descriptive modifiers, and predictors of biologic behavior. Although it is unrealistic to expect the language of tumor classification to be rigidly logical or consistent, it still serves as a reasonably unambiguous mode of communication.

The primary descriptor of any tumor, benign or malignant, is its cell or tissue of origin. The classification of benign tumors is the basis for the names of their malignant variants. **Benign tumors are identified by the suffix "oma," which is preceded by reference to the cell or tissue of origin.** For instance, a benign tumor that resembles chondrocytes is termed a "chondroma" (Fig. 5-2). If the tumor resembles the precursor of the chondrocyte, it is labeled a "chondroblastoma". When a chondroma is located entirely within the bone, it is designated an "enchondroma". Tumors of epithelial origin are given a variety of names based on what is thought to be their outstanding characteristic. Thus, a benign tumor of the squamous epithelium may be called simply an "epithelioma" or, when branched and exophytic, may be termed a "papilloma". Benign tumors arising from glandular epithelium, such as in the colon or

the endocrine glands, are termed "adenomas". Accordingly, we refer to a thyroid adenoma (Fig. 5-3) or an islet cell adenoma. In some instances the predominating feature is the gross appearance, in which case we speak, for example, of an "adenomatous polyp" of the colon or the endometrium. Benign tumors that arise from germ cells and contain derivatives of different germ layers are labeled "teratomas". These occur principally in the gonads and occasionally in the mediastinum and may contain a variety of structures, such as skin, neurons and glial cells, thyroid, intestinal epithelium, and cartilage. Localized, disordered differentiation during embryonic development results in a "hamartoma", a disorganized caricature of normal tissue components (Fig. 5-4). Such tumors, which are not strictly neoplasms, contain varying combinations of cartilage, ducts or bronchi, connective tissue, blood vessels, and lymphoid tissue. Ectopic islands of normal tissue, termed "choristoma", may also be mistaken for true neoplasms. These small lesions are represented by pancreatic tissue in the wall of the stomach or intestine, adrenal rests under the renal capsule, and nodules of splenic tissue in the peritoneal cavity. Certain benign growths, recognized clinically as tumors, are not truly neoplastic but rather represent overgrowth of normal tissue elements. Examples are vocal cord polyps, skin tags, and hyperplastic polyps of the colon.

In general, the malignant counterparts of benign tumors usually carry the same name, except that the

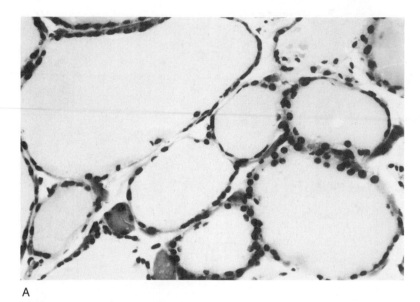

A

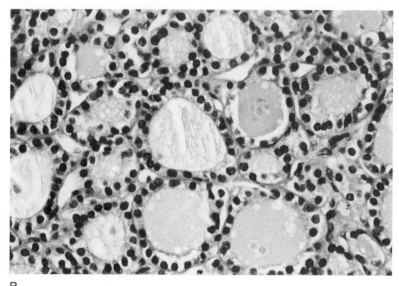

B

Figure 5-3.   Benign thyroid adenoma. *(A)* Normal thyroid. *(B)* The follicles of a thyroid adenoma are similar to those of the normal thyroid tissue. Both types of follicles (shown here at the same magnification) are lined by regular epithelial cells and contain colloid.

suffix **carcinoma** is applied to epithelial cancers and **sarcoma** to those of mesenchymal origin. For instance, a malignant tumor of the stomach is a *gastric adenocarcinoma* or *adenocarcinoma of the stomach*. *Squamous cell carcinoma* is an invasive tumor of the skin (Fig. 5-5) or the metaplastic squamous epithelium of the bronchus or endocervix, and *transitional cell carcinoma* is a malignant neoplasm of the bladder. By contrast, we speak of *chondrosarcoma* (Fig. 5-6) or *fibrosarcoma*. Sometimes the name of the tumor suggests the tissue type of origin, as in *osteogenic sarcoma* or *bronchogenic carcinoma*. Some tumors display neoplastic elements of different cell types but are not germ cell tumors. For example, fibroadenoma of the breast, composed of epithelial and stromal elements,

is benign, whereas, as the name implies, *adenosquamous carcinoma* of the uterus or the lung is malignant. A rare malignant tumor that contains intermingled carcinomatous and sarcomatous elements is known as *carcinosarcoma*.

The persistence of certain historical terms adds a note of confusion. *Hepatoma* of the liver, *melanoma* of the skin, *seminoma* of the testis, and the lymphoproliferative tumor, *lymphoma,* are all highly malignant. On the other hand, basal cell carcinoma is labeled by many as *basal cell epithelioma* to emphasize its localized nature. **Tumors of the hematopoietic system** are a special case in which the relationship to the blood is indicated by the **suffix "emia."** Thus *leukemia* refers to a malignant proliferation of white blood cells.

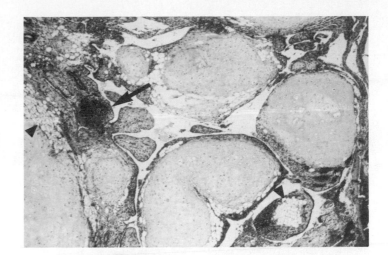

Figure 5-4. Hamartoma of the lung. The tumor contains islands of cartilage and clefts lined by a cuboidal epithelium. A lymphoid follicle *(arrow)* and foci of fat cells *(arrowheads)* are evident.

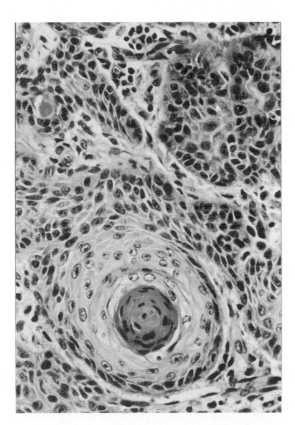

Figure 5-5. Squamous cell carcinoma of the skin. The tumor is composed of islands of neoplastic squamous cells. In the lower portion of the field, well-differentiated keratinized tumor cells have degenerated to form a concentric mass of keratin and pyknotic nuclei, termed an epithelial "pearl."

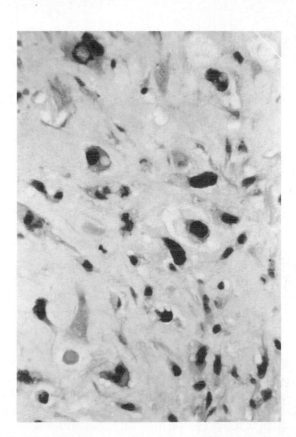

Figure 5-6. Chondrosarcoma of bone. The tumor is composed of malignant chondrocytes, which have bizarre shapes and irregular, hyperchromatic nuclei, embedded in a cartilaginous matrix. Compare with Figure 5-2.

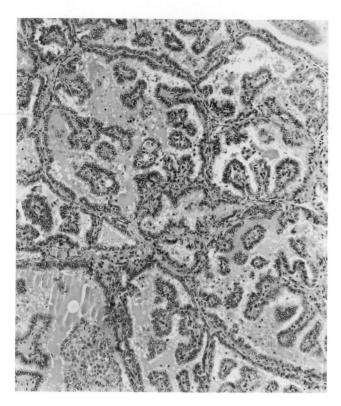

Figure 5-7. Papillary adenocarcinoma of the thyroid. The tumor exhibits numerous fronds, lined by malignant thyroid epithelium, which project into distended colloid-containing follicles.

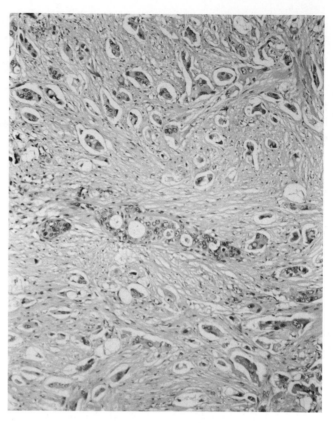

Figure 5-8. Scirrhous adenocarcinoma of the breast. Nests of cancer cells are embedded in a dense fibrous stroma.

Secondary descriptors (again, with some inconsistencies) refer to a tumor's morphologic and functional characteristics. For example, the term *papillary* refers to a frondlike structure (Fig. 5-7). *Medullary* signifies a soft, cellular tumor with little connective stroma, while *scirrhous* or *desmoplastic* implies a dense fibrous stoma (Fig. 5-8). *Colloid* carcinomas secrete abundant mucus in which float islands of tumor cells. *Comedocarcinoma* is an intraductal neoplasm in which necrotic material can be expressed from the ducts. Certain visible secretions of the tumor cells lend their characteristics to the classification—for example, production of mucin or serous fluid. A further designation describes the gross appearance of a cystic mass. From all these considerations we derive such common terms as *papillary serous cystadenocarcinoma* of the ovary, *comedocarcinoma* of the breast, *adenoid cystic carcinoma* of the salivary glands, *polypoid adenocarcinoma* of the stomach, and *medullary carcinoma* of the thyroid. Finally, tumors in which the histogenesis is poorly understood are often given an eponym—as in, for example, Hodgkin's disease, Ewing's sarcoma of bone, or Brenner tumor of the ovary.

Histologic Diagnosis of Malignancy

The distinction between benign and malignant tumors is, from a practical point of view, the most important diagnostic challenge faced by the pathologist. In most cases, the differentiation poses few problems, and in a few, careful study is required before an accurate diagnosis is secure. However, there remain tumors that defy the diagnostic skills and experience of any pathologist; in these cases correct diagnosis must await clinical outcome. In effect, the criteria used to assess the true biologic nature of any tumor are based not on scientific principles, but rather on a historical correlation of histologic and cytologic patterns with clinical outcomes. It must be recognized that established criteria vary by organ and tumor type, and although general criteria are recognized, they must be used with caution in specific cases. For instance, a reactive proliferation of connective cells termed *nodular fasciitis* (Fig. 5-9) has a more alarming histologic appearance than many fibrosarcomas, and misdiagnosis can lead to unnec-

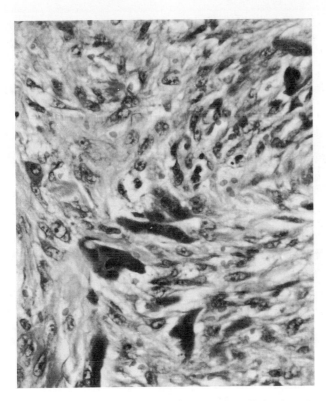

Figure 5-9. Nodular fasciitis. This highly cellular reactive lesion contains atypical and bizarre fibroblasts, which may be mistaken for a fibrosarcoma.

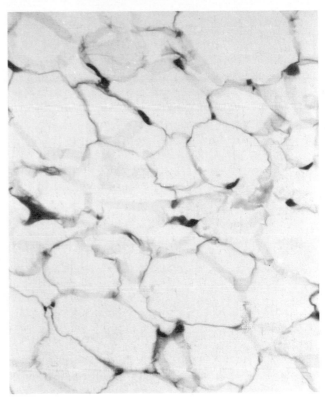

Figure 5-10. Lipoma. This nodular tumor of adipocytes is grossly and microscopically indistinguishable from normal fat.

essary surgery. Conversely, many well-differentiated endocrine adenocarcinomas are histologically indistinguishable from benign adenomas.

Benign tumors in general resemble their parent tissues, both histologically and cytologically. For example, lipomas, despite their often lobulated gross appearance, seem to be composed of normal adipocytes (Fig. 5-10). Fibromas are composed of mature fibroblasts and a collagenous stroma. Chondromas exhibit chondrocytes dispersed in a cartilaginous matrix. Thyroid adenomas form acini and produce thyroglobulin. The gross structure of a benign tumor may depart from the normal and assume papillary or polypoid configurations, as in papillomas of the bladder and skin and adenomatous polyps of the colon. However, **the lining epithelium of a benign tumor resembles that of the normal tissue.** Although many benign tumors are circumscribed by a connective tissue capsule, many equally benign neoplasms are not encapsulated. In the latter category are such benign tumors as papillomas and polyps of the visceral organs, hepatic adenomas, many endocrine adenomas, and hemangiomas. **It bears repetition that the defi-**

nition of a benign tumor resides above all in an inability to invade adjacent tissue and to metastasize.

Malignant tumors depart from the parent tissue morphologically and functionally, although an accurate diagnosis of their origin depends not only on the location but also on a histologic and cytologic resemblance to a normal tissue. The lack of differentiated features in a cancer cell is referred to as **anaplasia** or **cellular atypia,** and in general the degree of anaplasia correlates with the aggressiveness of the tumor. Cytologic evidence of anaplasia includes variation in the size and shape of cells and cell nuclei *(pleomorphism),* enlarged and hyperchromatic nuclei with coarsely clumped chromatin and prominent nucleoli, atypical mitoses, and bizarre cells, including tumor giant cells (Fig. 5-11). Abundant mitoses are characteristic of many malignant tumors, but are not a necessary criterion. However, in some cases—for example, leiomyosarcomas—the diagnosis of malignancy is based on the finding of even a few mitoses. Malignancy is proved by the demonstration of invasion, particularly of blood vessels and lymphatics. In some circum-

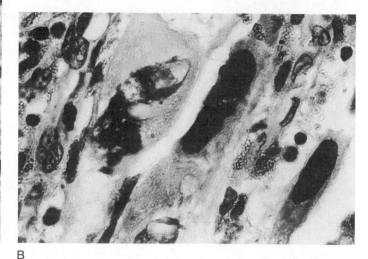

A

B

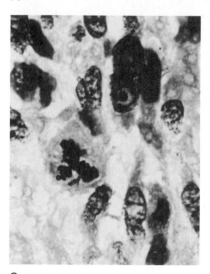

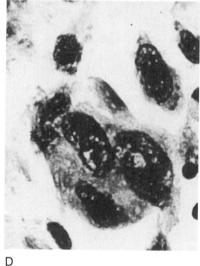

C

D

Figure 5-11. Anaplastic features of malignant tumors. *(A)* The cells of this anaplastic carcinoma are highly pleomorphic (i.e., they vary in size and shape). The nuclei are hyperchromatic and are large relative to the cytoplasm. *(B)* These extremely pleomorphic cancer cells show bizarre shapes and deeply hyperchromatic nuclei. *(C)* A malignant cell in metaphase exhibits an abnormal tripolar mitotic figure. *(D)* A multinucleated tumor giant cell.

stances, such as squamous carcinoma of the cervix or carcinoma arising in an adenomatous polyp, the diagnosis of malignant transformation is made on the basis of local invasion. It is intuitively obvious that the presence of metastases identifies a tumor as malignant, but occasionally it reveals the true nature of a tumor previously considered benign. In metastatic disease that was not preceded by a clinically diagnosed primary tumor, the site of origin is often not readily apparent from the morphologic characteristics of the tumor. In such cases electron microscopic examination and the demonstration of a specific tumor marker may establish the correct diagnosis.

Electron Microscopy of Tumors

The study of the ultrastructure of malignant tumors has failed to enhance our understanding of the *pathogenesis* of cancer. It is clear that in general the organization of the cytoplasm becomes simpler with increasing anaplasia. Thus, anaplastic tumors from highly differentiated tissues often do not show the rich cytoplasmic complexity of the parent tissue, in terms of organelles and specialized cytoplasmic components. However, **there are no specific determinants of malignancy or even of neoplasia itself that can be detected by electron microscopy.** On the other hand, electron microscopy has proved of significant value in the diagnosis of poorly differentiated cancers, whose classification is difficult by routine light microscopy. For example, it is often difficult to decide by light microscopy whether a poorly differentiated tumor is a carcinoma, a sarcoma, or a lymphoma. However, by electron microscopy, carcinomas often exhibit desmosomes and specialized junctional complexes, structures that are not typical of mesenchymal tumors and are absent in lymphomas.

Characteristically, the microvilli of carcinomas are short and blunt and are associated with a terminal web. By contrast, the microvilli of lymphoid and mesenchymal tumors do not show a terminal web. Cells of ectodermal origin often have many cilia, in contrast to the solitary cilia occasionally found in other cell types. The presence of bundles of tonofilaments is highly suggestive of an epithelial tumor, whereas slender microfilaments are more common in mesenchymal tumors. A metastatic tumor can often be correctly identified by visualizing cytoplasmic granules and identifying their nature. For example, the presence of melanosomes signifies a melanoma, whereas small, membrane-bound granules with a dense core are features of endocrine neoplasms (Fig. 5-12). Another example of a diagnostically useful granule is the characteristic crystal-containing granule of an insulinoma derived from the pancreatic islets.

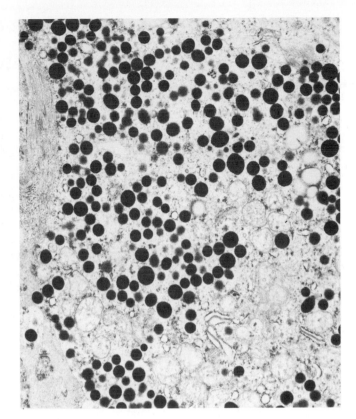

Figure 5-12. Metastatic cancer of the adrenal medulla (pheochromocytoma). The neuroendocrine origin of this poorly differentiated tumor was identified by the presence of characteristic cytoplasmic secretory granules.

Tumor Markers

The ultimate tumor marker would be one that allows the distinction between benign and malignant cells, but unfortunately no such marker is in sight. Nevertheless, markers do exist that are often useful in identifying the cell of origin of a metastatic or poorly differentiated primary tumor. Among these diagnostically useful markers are such diverse substances as immunoglobulins, fetal proteins, enzymes, hormones, and cytoskeletal and junctional proteins.

Metastatic tumors may be so undifferentiated microscopically as to preclude even the distinction between an epithelial and a mesenchymal origin. Tumor markers rely on the preservation of characteristics of the progenitor cell or the synthesis of specialized proteins by the neoplastic cell to make this distinction. For example, they can be used to determine the presence of neuroendocrine features in apparently undifferentiated small cell carcinomas. One of the markers used in this determination is **neuron specific enolase** (NSE), a glycolytic enzyme of normal neurons and neuroendocrine cells that is also produced by their transformed counterparts. A family of neurosecretory granule matrix proteins termed **chromogranins** and an integral membrane glycoprotein called **synaptophysin** also are markers for neuroendocrine cells. A third, readily available, group of markers enabling the specific diagnosis of functioning neuroendocrine tumors consists of antibodies against serotonin and a broad spectrum of neuropeptide hormones (e.g., ACTH, bombesin, calcitonin, gastrin, insulin, and somatostatin).

Intermediate filaments also serve as immunomarkers. These filaments tend to be cell type specific, and that relative specificity is retained after neoplastic transformation. Thus, antibodies to intermediate filaments allow a reliable discrimination among poorly differentiated epithelial, mesenchymal, and neural neoplasms.

Intermediate filaments fall within five distinct classes:

Cytokeratins, a multigene family of proteins comprising at least 19 distinct polypeptides, are characteristic of epithelial cells and carcinomas.
Vimentin is found in mesenchymal cells and sarcomas.

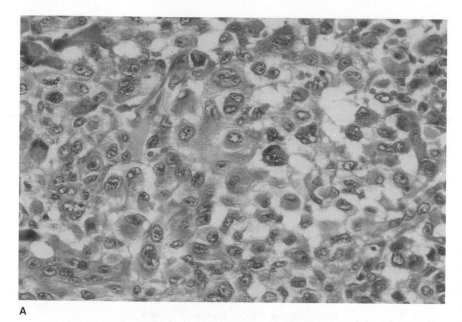

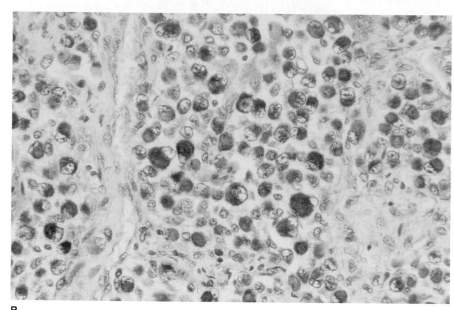

Figure 5-13. Tumor markers in the identification of undifferentiated neoplasms. *(A)* A metastatic undifferentiated malignant melanoma stained with hematoxylin and eosin does not exhibit melanin pigment by light microscopy. *(B)* An immunoperoxidase stain of the same tumor shows numerous cells positive for S-100 protein, a commonly used marker for cells of melanocytic origin.

Desmin is found in smooth muscle and striated muscle cells and neoplasms.

Glial filament protein, also known as glial fibrillary acidic protein (GFAP), is typical of glial cells and gliomas.

Neurofilament proteins are apparent in neurons and paraganglia cells and in neurogenic neoplasms.

Insoluble proteins of high molecular weight associated with desmosomal junctions are termed **desmoplakins.** Following the application of desmoplakin antibodies to tissue sections, single desmosomes can readily be seen. In most instances desmosomes are associated with cytokeratin polypeptides and are, therefore, markers of epithelial differentiation. However, desmoplakins are also found in association with desmin in cardiac muscle cells and occasional muscle sarcomas, and in association with vimentin in arachnoidal cells and meningiomas. These and other exceptions must be considered when intermediate filaments and desmoplakin antibodies are used in the differential diagnosis of tumors. Other diagnostically significant, though not pathognomonic, tumor markers are S-100 protein, an excellent marker for melanomas (Fig. 5-13); Factor VIII–related antigen, a good marker for endothelial cells; alpha-fetoprotein, which exists in hepatocellular carcinomas and yolk sac carcinomas; thyroglobulin, which may help in identifying thyroid carcinomas; prostatic acid phosphatase and prostate-specific antigen, which are useful for the differentiation between prostatic carcinomas and carcinomas of other sites; and human chorionic gonadotropin, which marks trophoblastic tumors. Carcinoembryonic antigen (CEA), although neither site-nor tumor-specific, is nevertheless a useful marker for gastrointestinal and related cancers.

Invasion and Metastasis

The two properties that are unique to cancer cells are the capacity to invade locally and the capacity to metastasize to distant sites. It is these properties that are responsible for the vast majority of deaths from cancer; the primary tumor itself is generally amenable to surgical extirpation.

Patterns of Spread

Direct Extension

Malignant tumors characteristically grow within the tissue of origin, where they enlarge and infiltrate normal structures. They may also extend directly beyond the confines of that organ to involve adjacent tissues. In some cases the growth of the cancer may be so extensive that replacement of the normal tissue results in functional insufficiency of the organ. Such a situation is not uncommon in primary cancer of the liver. Tumors of the brain, such as astrocytomas, infiltrate the brain until they compromise vital regions. The direct extension of malignant tumors within an organ may also be life-threatening because of their location. A common example is the intestinal obstruction produced by cancer of the colon (Fig. 5-14).

The invasive growth pattern of malignant tumors often leads to their direct extension outside the tissue of origin, in which case the tumor may secondarily impair the function of an adjacent organ. Squamous carcinoma of the cervix often grows beyond the genital tract to produce vesicovaginal fistulas and obstruction of the ureters. Neglected cases of breast cancer are often complicated by extensive ulceration of the skin. Even small tumors can produce severe consequences when they invade vital structures. A small cancer of the lung can cause a bronchopleural fistula when it penetrates the bronchus, or exsan-

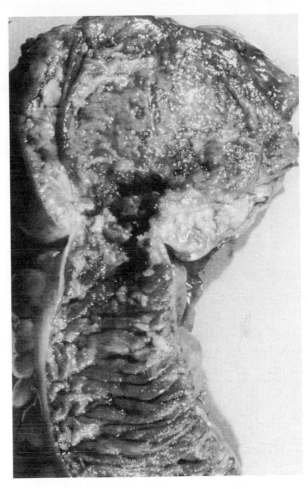

Figure 5-14. Adenocarcinoma of the colon with intestinal obstruction. The lumen of the colon at the site of the cancer is narrowed. The colon proximal to the obstruction is dilated.

guinating hemorrhage when it erodes a blood vessel. The agonizing pain of pancreatic carcinoma results from direct extension of the tumor to the celiac nerve plexus. Tumor cells that reach serous cavities—for example, those of the peritoneum or pleura—spread easily by direct extension or can be carried by the fluid to new locations on the serous membranes. The most common example is the seeding of the peritoneal cavity by certain types of ovarian cancer (Fig. 5-15). Although malignant brain tumors do not customarily metastasize extracranially, cells that reach the cerebrospinal fluid may be transported to other sites within the central nervous system.

Metastatic Spread

The invasive properties of malignant tumors bring them into contact with blood and lymphatic vessels. **In the same way that they can invade parenchymal**

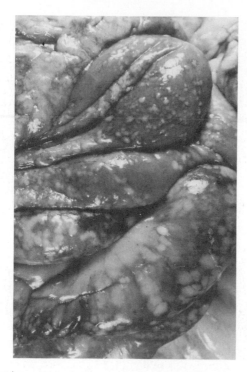

Figure 5-15. Peritoneal carcinomatosis. Loops of small intestine show peritoneal seeding by metastatic carcinoma, which appears as small whitish plaques on the serosal surface.

vessels, either to endothelial cells or to naked basement membranes, although the mechanisms remain a matter of speculation. This sequence of events explains why the liver and the lung are so frequently the sites of metastases. Because abdominal tumors seed the portal system, they lead to hepatic metastases, while other tumors penetrate systemic veins that eventually drain into the vena cava and hence to the lungs. In this respect it should be noted that some tumor cells released into the venous system survive passage through the microcirculation and are thereby transported to more distant organs. For instance, tumor cells may traverse the liver and produce pulmonary metastases, and neoplastic cells may also survive passage through the pulmonary microcirculation to reach the brain and other organs via arterial dissemination. Neoplastic cells arrested in the microcirculation are thought to penetrate the vessel walls at the site of metastasis by the same mechanisms with which the primary tumor invades.

tissue, neoplastic cells also can penetrate vascular and lymphatic channels. For metastases to appear, after the invasion of lymphatics or blood vessels the neoplastic cells must be released from the primary tumor, be transported through the circulation, lodge in the microcirculation of an organ, penetrate the vessel in the reverse direction, and grow autonomously in this new location. In general, metastases resemble the primary tumor histologically, although they are occasionally so anaplastic that their cell of origin is obscure.

Hematogenous Metastases

Cancer cells commonly invade capillaries and venules, whereas the thicker-walled arterioles and arteries are relatively resistant. The appearance of malignant cells in the blood should not be construed as synonymous with metastasis, because most of these cells are destroyed in the circulation. Nevertheless, it is likely that the probability of viable metastases correlates directly with the number of malignant cells released into the circulation. Before they can form viable metastases, circulating tumor cells must lodge in the vascular bed of the metastatic site (Fig. 5-16). Here they presumably attach to the walls of blood

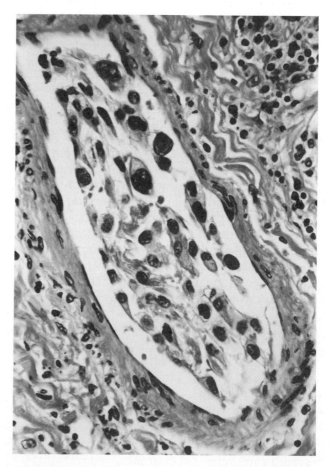

Figure 5-16. Hematogenous spread of cancer. Malignant cells fill a small pulmonary artery.

Lymphatic Metastases

A historical dogma of metastatic spread held that epithelial tumors (carcinomas) preferentially metastasize through lymphatic channels whereas mesenchymal neoplasms (sarcomas) are distributed hematogenously. This distinction is no longer considered valid, because of clinical observations of metastatic patterns and the demonstration of numerous connections between the lymphatic and vascular systems. Tumors arising in tissues that have a rich lymphatic network—for instance, the breast—often metastasize by this route, although the particular properties of specific neoplasms may play a role in the route of spread.

Basement membranes envelop only the large lymphatic channels; they are lacking in the lymphatic capillaries. Thus, there is reason to believe that invasive tumor cells may penetrate lymphatic channels more readily than blood vessels. Once in the lymphatic vessels, the cells are carried to the regional draining lymph nodes, where they initially lodge in the marginal sinus and then extend throughout the node. Lymph nodes bearing metastatic deposits may be enlarged to many times their normal size, often exceeding the diameter of the primary lesion. The cut surface of the lymph node usually resembles that of the primary tumor in color and consistency and may also exhibit the necrosis and hemorrhage commonly seen in primary cancers (Fig. 5-17).

The regional lymphatic pattern of metastatic spread is most prominently exemplified by cancer of the breast. In breast cancer the initial metastases are almost always lymphatic, and these regional lymphatic metastases have considerable prognostic significance. Cancers that arise in the lateral aspect of the breast characteristically spread to the lymph nodes of the axilla, whereas those arising in the medial portion drain to the internal mammary lymph nodes in the thorax.

Lymphatic metastases are occasionally found in lymph nodes distant from the site of the primary tumor; these are termed **"skip"** metastases. For example, abdominal cancers may initially be signaled by the appearance of an enlarged supraclavicular node, the so-called sentinel node. A graphic example of the relationship of lymphatic anatomy to the spread of malignant tumors is afforded by cancers of the testis. Rather than metastasizing to the regional nodes, as do other tumors of the male external genitalia, testicular cancers typically involve the abdominal peri-aortic nodes. The explanation lies in the descent of the testis from an intra-abdominal site to the scrotum, during which it is accompanied by its own lymphatic supply.

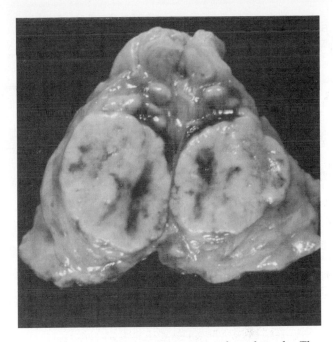

Figure 5-17. Metastatic carcinoma in a lymph node. The bisected node, embedded in fat tissue, is enlarged and indurated by metastatic carcinoma of the colon. Necrosis and hemorrhage are seen as dark, irregular areas.

It is of clinical importance to realize that lymph nodes that drain a tumor may be enlarged not only by the presence of metastases but also by **reactive hyperplasia,** which is presumably a response to the released antigens and cell debris from necrotic tumor cells. As is discussed below, viable tumor cells also shed membrane antigens, which may stimulate the proliferation of sensitized lymphocytes. Thus, the clinical presence of an enlarged lymph node is not necessarily synonymous with a metastasis. Conversely, the absence of tumor cells in a resected lymph node does not guarantee that there is no underlying cancer.

Biology of Invasion and Metastasis

It is intuitively clear that for invasion to occur, tumor cells must escape the confines of the basement membrane of their tissue of origin, traverse the extracellular matrix of the surrounding normal tissues, and penetrate the basement membranes of blood vessels. Invasive cancers, unlike their benign counterparts, do not generally produce basement membranes.

The penetration of the basement membrane of the host tissue and the invasion of the surrounding ex-

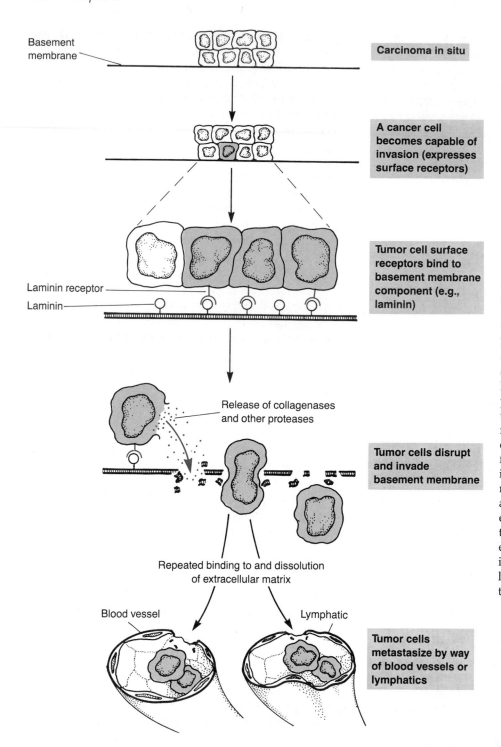

Basement membrane

Carcinoma in situ

A cancer cell becomes capable of invasion (expresses surface receptors)

Laminin receptor
Laminin

Tumor cell surface receptors bind to basement membrane component (e.g., laminin)

Release of collagenases and other proteases

Tumor cells disrupt and invade basement membrane

Repeated binding to and dissolution of extracellular matrix

Blood vessel   Lymphatic

Tumor cells metastasize by way of blood vessels or lymphatics

Figure 5-18. Mechanisms of tumor invasion. The mechanism by which a malignant tumor initially penetrates a confining basement membrane and then invades the surrounding extracellular environment is thought to involve three steps. The tumor must first acquire the ability to bind to a component of the basement membrane. This is depicted as the acquisition of receptors that bind to laminin, one component of the basement membrane. As a consequence of the binding to laminin, collagenases and other proteases are released from the tumor cells, and the basement membrane is lysed. The cancer cell then moves through the defect in the basement membrane into the extracellular environment. By repeatedly binding to and lysing components of the extracellular matrix, the invading tumor penetrates farther into the extracellular environment. The invasion of blood vessels and lymphatics occurs by essentially the same mechanisms.

tracellular environment is thought to involve three steps (Fig. 5-18): binding of the tumor cell to a matrix component; enzymatic lysis of this structure; and movement through the resulting defect. The initial binding may involve such tissue matrix components as fibronectin, laminin, proteoglycans, and collagen, which may be lysed by certain proteases and collagenases found in tumor cells. An attractive hypothesis holds that binding occurs by way of specific laminin receptors on the tumor cell membrane. The specific binding of human breast carcinoma cells to surface laminin is fifty times greater than that of normal breast tissue or benign lesions. In addition, malignant cells exhibit greater collagenase production, including a type IV collagenase (active against the collagen of basement membranes), than do normal cells. It is postulated that the enhanced attachment of tumor cells to connective tissue matrix components permits collagenases and other proteases to lyse the basement membrane and other connective tissue elements, after which the ameboid movement of the tumor exploits the resulting fault.

Although it appears that malignant tumors have the capacity to destroy connective tissue, they also frequently stimulate fibrosis, a process termed *desmoplasia*. In some tumors the desmoplastic response, rather than the accumulation of tumor cells, accounts for the clinical appearance of the cancer. In this category is the hard lump of infiltrating carcinoma of the breast and the "leather bottle stomach" of gastric carcinoma. The mechanisms underlying the desmoplastic response are not understood, and even the nature of the fibrogenic cell is debated. Recent studies have suggested that the myofibroblast may be involved, but the subject requires further research.

The anatomy of the vascular system and the vascularity of specific organs unquestionably influence the pattern of metastatic spread, but it is also true that certain tumors seem to prefer some organs over others, presumably because of interactions between tumor cells and the host organ. It is noteworthy that despite their size and abundant blood flow, neither the spleen nor skeletal muscle are common sites of metastases.

The need for a hospitable host environment has been elegantly demonstrated experimentally. Grafts of various organs were transplanted into the skeletal muscle of inbred mice, after which the animals were injected with mouse tumor cells. Metastases appeared only in grafts from organs that normally are the locale of secondary tumors. The mechanism underlying such preferential "homing" of neoplastic cells to specific organs is not well understood, but there is experimental evidence to suggest that the surface properties of the cells are involved.

As will be discussed below, **cancer is generally monoclonal—that is, the tumor is derived from the transformation of a single cell.** This circumstance might lead to the expectation that the progeny of the originally transformed cell are all alike. This assumption is not true. **Tumors are composed of heterogeneous cell populations.** This fact has important implications for the metastatic potential of tumors. A tumor must surmount a variety of hurdles before becoming established as a metastasis. When neoplastic cells are injected into an animal, as few as one in a thousand survives to establish a metastasis. Mechanical factors and host defenses undoubtedly play an important role in this reduction, but the question remains whether the survivors are selected randomly or are endowed with specific properties not inherent in the other elements of the primary neoplastic population.

It has long been known that by transplanting successive generations of metastatic cells from one animal to another it is possible to produce cells that have a far greater metastatic potential than the original tumor cells. In vitro, certain properties of neoplastic cells correlate with metastatic potential, including resistance to immunologic attack, the ability to invade other tissues, the capacity to digest type IV collagen, and detachment from a monolayer culture. Cells selected for such properties in vitro show enhanced metastatic potential in vivo.

An important demonstration of tumor heterogeneity has come from experiments in which a variety of epithelial and mesenchymal tumors were cloned in vitro and each clone was individually injected into a host animal. If the tumor cells were originally homogeneous, then a comparable number of metastases would be expected in each animal. In fact, however, the clones, which had not been treated or selected in any manner, displayed widely varying metastatic activity. **This heterogeneity of the primary tumor suggests that the survival of malignant cells in the form of metastases is not due to a random process, but rather is a manifestation of the selective growth of subpopulations of cells that are endowed with the properties necessary for survival and growth in potentially inhospitable places.** This concept of tumor heterogeneity extends beyond metastatic potential to include the expression of hormone receptors and, of great importance, sensitivity to chemotherapeutic agents.

The Grading and Staging of Cancers

In an attempt to predict the clinical behavior of a malignant tumor and to establish criteria for therapy, many cancers are classified according to a cytologic and histologic grading scheme or by staging protocols that describe the extent of spread. **Cytologic/histologic grading, which is necessarily subjective and at best semiquantitative, is based on the degree of anaplasia and on the number of proliferating cells.** The degree of anaplasia is determined from the shape and regularity of the cells, and the presence of distinct differentiated features, such as functioning glandlike structures in adenocarcinomas or epithelial pearls in squamous carcinomas. Evidence of rapid or abnormal growth is provided by large numbers of mitoses, the presence of atypical mitoses, nuclear pleomorphism, and tumor giant cells. Most grading schemes classify tumors into three or four grades of increasing degrees of malignancy (Fig. 5-19). Cytologic grading must not be confused with the classification of tumor variants, which is particularly important in the assessment of hematologic cancers, such as Hodgkin's disease and the non-Hodgkin's lymphomas. The general correlation between the cytologic grade and the biologic behavior of a neoplasm is not invariable: There are many examples of tumors of low cytologic grades with substantial malignant properties.

The choice of surgical approach or the selection of treatment modalities is influenced more by the stage of a cancer than by its cytologic grade. Moreover, most statistical data related to cancer survival are based on the stage rather than the cytologic grade of the tumor. Clinical staging according to the extent of spread of the tumor is independent of cytologic grading. **The significant criteria used for staging vary with different organs. Commonly used criteria include tumor size; the extent of local growth, whether within or without the organ; the presence of lymph node metastases; and the presence of distant metastases.** These criteria have been codified in the inter-

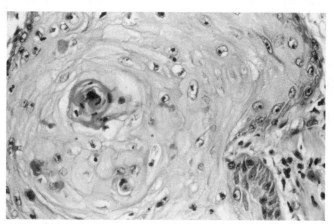

A

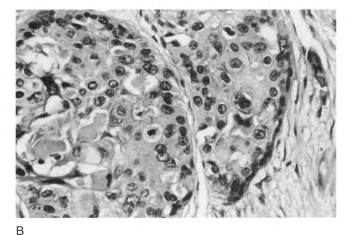

B

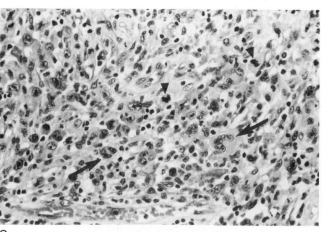

C

Figure 5-19. Cytologic grading of squamous cell carcinoma of the lung. *(A)* Well-differentiated (grade 1) squamous cell carcinoma. The tumor cells bear a strong resemblance to normal squamous cells and are synthesizing keratin, as evidenced by the epithelial pearl. *(B)* Moderately differentiated (grade 2) squamous cell carcinoma. The tumor cells are more pleomorphic and are less similar to squamous cells than those in *A*. Individual cells still produce keratin. *(C)* Poorly differentiated (grade 3) squamous cell carcinoma. The malignant cells are no longer identifiable as of squamous origin. Tumor giant cells *(arrows)* and atypical mitoses *(arrowhead)* are present.

national **TNM cancer staging system,** in which T refers to the size of the primary tumor, N to the number and distribution of lymph node metastases, and M to the presence and extent of distant metastases.

In some cases the distinction between benign and malignant tumors is based solely on size, as in the case of renal carcinoma. On the basis of clinical experience, tumors below 2 cm in diameter are considered benign adenomas, whereas those of larger size are labeled carcinomas. The choice of surgical therapy is often influenced by size alone. For example, a primary breast cancer smaller than 2 cm in diameter can be treated with local excision and radiation therapy, whereas larger masses necessitate mastectomy. Local extension, too, can be used to estimate prognosis, as in the Dukes classification of colorectal cancer. Penetration of the tumor into the muscularis and serosa is associated with a poorer prognosis than that of a more superficial tumor. Clearly, the presence of lymph node metastases mandates more aggressive treatment than their absence, whereas the presence of distant metastases is generally a contraindication to surgical intervention other than for palliation. In some cases, however, a primary tumor may be resected even when distant metastases are present in order to "debulk" the tumor before chemotherapy is begun.

The Biochemistry of the Cancer Cell

Despite more than a half-century of intensive investigation of the biochemical basis of neoplasia, no alterations unique to cancer cells or crucial to carcinogenesis have emerged. Among the earliest studies the most prominent were those of Warburg, who proposed that the biochemical basis of neoplasia was the dependence of tumor cells on anaerobic glycolysis rather than aerobic respiration. According to Warburg's theory the neoplastic stimulus is an irreversible injury to respiration, followed by a compensatory increase in fermentation and the production of a neoplastic cell. However, although it is true that most cancers do display high glycolytic rates, many display normal rates. An increase in glycolysis seems, therefore, to be a characteristic of only some tumors and to be an effect rather than a cause of neoplastic transformation. Later investigations found an association between neoplasia and numerous enzyme deficits, lowered protein levels, the appearance of unusual isozymes, and the production of fetal proteins. However, detailed studies of tumors with varying degrees of differentiation have clearly shown that this phenotypic heterogeneity of cancer cells simply reflects the variable degree of differentiation. **The search for a common qualitative biochemical defect to explain neoplasia has to date been unsuccessful.**

The Growth of Cancers

Cell Cycle Kinetics

Historically, cancer was considered to result from a totally unregulated growth of cells, and a logical corollary was that neoplastic cells proliferate at a faster rate than normal ones. When tritiated thymidine became available, accurate measurements of growth kinetics were made possible. The observation that the cell cycle time of intestinal cells was shorter than that of very rapidly growing tumors cast doubt on the validity of these basic assumptions. The fact that **tumor cells do not necessarily proliferate at a faster rate than their normal counterparts** is now well established and suggests that tumor growth depends on other factors, such as the proportion of cycling cells (growth fraction) and the rate of cell death. In normal proliferating tissues, such as the intestine and the bone marrow, an exquisite balance between cell renewal and cell death is strictly maintained. By contrast, **the major determinant of tumor growth is clearly the fact that more cells are produced than die in a given time.**

The growth of a tumor may be expressed in terms of the doubling time—that is, the time taken for the number of cells in the mass to double. Importantly, it has been shown in experimental and human tumors that the doubling time is not necessarily correlated with the growth fraction. Since the duration of mitosis in cancer cells is often prolonged, the number of mitoses in a histologic section can be misleading as an indicator of overall growth. For example, a doubling in mitotic time will result in twice as many visible mitoses without any real increase in the rate of growth. In most cases the theoretical tumor doubling time, calculated from the growth fraction and the cell cycle time, bears little relation to the actual clinical situation. For example, if a tumor weighing 1 g (often the smallest size clinically detectable) produces about two new cells per 1000 cells in each mitotic cycle the theoretical net increase would be a staggering 10^6 cells per hour, a figure totally at variance with the experience with most solid tumors. **Because of this difference between the theoretical and observed growth of tumors, it has been estimated that in human skin tumors as many as 97% of proliferated**

cells die spontaneously. The causes of tumor cell death are not precisely defined, but probably include such factors as inherent genetic programs (programmed cell death); inadequate blood supply with consequent ischemia; a paucity of nutrients; and vulnerability to specific and nonspecific host defenses.

Growth Factors and Neoplasia

The recent discovery of polypeptide growth factors (PGFs) has led to an enormous research effort aimed at defining their roles in the regulation of normal growth and the preservation of viability of many cell types. PGFs have been implicated in the regulation of embryogenesis, growth and development, selective cell survival, hematopoiesis, tissue repair, immune responses, atherosclerosis, and neoplastic growth. The molecular structures of a number of PGFs—for example epidermal growth factor (EGF), interleukin-2 (T-cell growth factor), nerve growth factor (NGF), and platelet-derived growth factor (PDGF)—have been determined. Numerous other growth factors have been partially characterized, while a number of naturally occurring substances, such as insulin, prolactin, thrombin, and transferrin, have been identified as growth regulators. It must be admitted that despite many studies in vitro, the mechanism of action for any PGF remains to be defined. Although processes and events associated with the binding of PGFs to their respective cell surface receptors have been amply described, the basic signals that trigger the cellular responses have not been definitively elucidated.

For a substance to qualify as a PGF, its production, transportation, and interaction with target cells must occur in a fashion consistent with a normal or regulated physiologic process. PGFs have the following characteristics: most of the structure consists of polypeptide material; binding at the cell surface initiates the cellular response; the response is initiated exclusively by the formation of a specific PGF-receptor complex; a specific hypertrophic or hyperplastic response is produced by the PGF-receptor complex; the PGF-receptor complex is internalized by receptor-mediated endocytosis.

A direct link between PGFs and events involved in the initiation or expression of the neoplastic state remains to be proved, but several important facts suggest that a relationship indeed exists.

1. In some instances PGFs related to epidermal growth factor and derived from both normal and neoplastic cells have the capacity to transform normal cells in vitro.

2. PGDF is virtually identical to a major sequence found in the product of a viral oncogene. A viral oncogene is a genetic locus of an RNA-transforming virus (retrovirus) whose activity is responsible for the initiation and maintenance of neoplastic transformation. The oncogenes of retroviruses are, in turn, close copies of cellular genes, known as proto-oncogenes or cellular oncogenes. In this context it is intriguing that PDGF is also involved in the normal proliferative responses of wound healing and repair—processes that have classically been thought to have certain analogies with neoplasia.

3. The receptors for PDGF, EGF, and insulin possess tyrosine-specific kinase (phosphorylating) activity. The product of the Rous sarcoma viral oncogene displays similar activity.

4. EGF enhances the synthesis of a viral gene product (poly(A^+)RNA, known as VL 30) that has been linked to the growth response of normal and transformed cells.

5. Certain chemicals (phorbol esters) that promote the development of skin tumors in vivo can regulate the affinity and number of EGF receptors.

6. A PGF coded for by an oncogene can, in turn, induce the expression of a second oncogene, an observation that is consistent with the multistep nature of carcinogenesis.

7. Small molecules, such as retinoids, that under certain circumstances prevent the development of cancer, modulate the expression of oncogenes or PGFs.

Most of our knowledge about the cellular responses to growth factors has been derived from studies of cultured cells, particularly mouse fibroblasts. When the culture medium used to incubate these cells is depleted of essential nutrients, including exogenous growth factors, the cells cease proliferating and leave the cell cycle by passing from the G_1 to the G_0 phase. This arrest of growth is reversible, and the cells can be reactivated by rescue with defined growth factors. By contrast, when virally transformed cells are subjected to starvation, they remain in the cell cycle but die within a few days. Cells transformed by chemical carcinogens behave differently. Although they are similar to cultured fibroblasts in ceasing to grow, they do not leave the cell cycle, but rather are arrested in G_1. Whereas normal cells require the addition of specific growth factors to reenter the cell cycle, chemically transformed cells can be rescued simply with nutrients such as amino acids and carbohydrates. **These studies demonstrate that transformed cells are less dependent on exoge-**

nous growth factors than normal cells. Since some of the oncogenes of neoplastic cells seem to code for products that are related to PGFs or their receptors, **cancer cells may not submit to the normal control by exogenous growth factors.**

Although our knowledge of the mechanism by which growth factors act is far from complete, a framework is beginning to emerge from the study of early mitogenic signals. When PDGF and other growth factors bind to their specific high-affinity receptors, they stimulate a complex sequence of early events:

Ion fluxes: PDGF and other growth factors produce an immediate entry of sodium into the cell by a sodium/hydrogen exchange mechanism, thereby causing alkalinization of the cytoplasm. Since a mitogenic response depends on intracellular pH and K^+ concentrations remaining above critical levels, these ionic events may be important. In addition to these changes in the fluxes of monovalent ions, PDGF causes a rapid release of calcium from intracellular stores into the cytosol. The mobilization of calcium reflects the activation of the phosphoinositide pathway, in which binding of the PDGF leads to the hydrolysis of phosphatidylinositol and the release of inositol trisphosphate (IP_3). IP_3 is a second messenger that stimulates the release of calcium from intracellular stores, probably the endoplasmic reticulum. This pathway is shown graphically in Chapter 2.

Activation of protein kinase C: In addition to IP_3 the other product derived from the hydrolysis of phosphatidylinositol is the lipid moiety of the phospholipid—namely, diacylglycerol (DAG). DAG activates protein kinase C, an enzyme that phosphorylates many proteins and that may be important in the production of a mitogenic response. Activation of this enzyme may also contribute to the alkalinization of the cytoplasm, since it increases the activity of the sodium/hydrogen antiport system. Protein kinase C appears to participate in a feedback system inhibiting the binding of growth factors to their receptors.

Increase in cyclic AMP levels: A sustained increase in the cytoplasmic concentration of cyclic AMP (cAMP) is now recognized as a mitogenic signal. PDGF raises cAMP levels by an indirect mechanism. Arachidonate derived from DAG is converted to various prostaglandins, including prostaglandin E, which binds to its own receptor and stimulates cAMP synthesis.

Expression of cellular oncogenes: PDGF and other growth factors rapidly induce the expression of the cellular oncogenes *c-fos* and *c-myc*, an effect that is probably mediated by the cytoplasmic events described above. Since these oncogenes encode nuclear proteins, their expression may play a role in the transduction of the mitotic stimulus to the nucleus.

While the relationship of the various effects listed above to mitogenesis remains hypothetical, a set of recent predictive experiments provides compelling evidence that such a relationship does indeed exist. Any agent that binds to a specific membrane receptor and produces all of the early events identified with PDGF should be a mitogen. This prediction has been validated for bombesin and related peptides, including gastrin-releasing peptide and the neuromedins. Furthermore, if there is a relationship between the early events provoked by PDGF and bombesin and mitogenesis, then agents that induce some but not all of these events in isolation should induce mitogenesis when added in combinations that totally reconstitute all the early events. This prediction has also been confirmed. Agents (e.g., phorbol ester) that evoke all the events except the increase in cAMP, stimulate DNA synthesis when added in combination with agents (e.g., cholera toxin) that raise cAMP levels but do not activate protein kinase C.

The Causes of Cancer

The morphologic appearance and biologic behavior of established cancers are well known. The underlying mechanisms of carcinogenesis, however, and the molecular description of the neoplastic state remain mysterious. Although we know of many agents that can cause cancer in man and experimental animals, we are ignorant of the proportion of human cancers that may be attributed to them. In some instances, it is clear that the majority of the cancers relate to a specific agent. For instance, most cancers of the lung are unquestionably examples of chemical carcinogenesis by tobacco smoke. On the other hand, although both high-dose radiation and an aromatic hydrocarbon, benzene, are known to cause leukemia, we do not know whether radiation- or chemical-induced leukemias comprise more than a small proportion of all granulocytic leukemias. Notwithstanding correlations with age, hormonal status, diet, genetic factors, and environmental agents, the etiology of many of the most common cancers, such as those of the breast, colon, and prostate, remains obscure. Despite the enormous gaps in our knowledge, an appreciation of carcinogenesis associated with chemicals, viruses, and physical agents is important, because the mechanisms of these processes may also underlie the induction of the majority of cancers, which are of unknown etiology.

Chemical Carcinogenesis

A brief historical overview of chemical carcinogenesis is not only of inherent interest, but also points the way to the details that require amplification. The entire field of chemical carcinogenesis originated some two centuries ago in descriptions of an occupational disease. This was not the first recognition of an occupation-related cancer (a peculiar predisposition of nuns to breast cancer was appreciated even earlier), but to the English physician Sir Percival Pott goes the credit for relating cancer of the scrotum in chimney sweeps to a specific chemical exposure, namely soot. Interestingly, the great German pathologist Rudolf Virchow attributed these scrotal tumors to irritation rather than to chemicals, even though at about the same time the high incidence of skin cancer in some German workers had been ascribed to an exposure to coal tar, whose ingredients were known to be remarkably similar to soot. Almost a century elapsed between those observations and the realization that other products of the combustion of organic materials are responsible for a man-made epidemic of cancer: cancer of the lung in cigarette smokers.

The experimental production of cancer by chemicals dates to 1915, when Japanese investigators produced skin cancers in rabbits with coal tar. Since that time, the list of organic and inorganic carcinogens has grown exponentially. Yet a curious paradox existed for many years. Many compounds known to be potent carcinogens are relatively inert in terms of chemical reactivity. The solution to this riddle became apparent in the early 1960s, when it was shown that **most, although not all, chemical carcinogens require metabolic activation before they can react with cell constitutents.** On the basis of those observations and the close correlation between mutagenicity and carcinogenicity, an in vitro test for screening potential chemical carcinogens—the Ames test—was developed a decade later. The experimental study of the actions of carcinogenic chemicals also led to the realization that **cancer is the result of a multistep process.** Initially, it was found that a single application of a carcinogen to the skin of a mouse is not, by itself, sufficient to produce cancer (Fig. 5-20). However, when a proliferative stimulus is then applied locally, in the form of a second, noncarcinogenic, irritating chemical—for example, a phorbol ester—tumors appear. The first effect is irreversible but not detectable by current methods, and is termed **initiation.** The action of the second, noncarcinogenic chemical is called **promotion.** This concept of a two-stage carcinogenic process has been expanded to a multistep process by numerous further experiments, principally centered on the liver.

Chemical Carcinogens and Their Metabolism

Chemicals cause cancer either directly or, more often, after metabolic activation. The direct-acting carcinogens are inherently sufficiently reactive to bind covalently to cellular macromolecules. In addition to a number of organic compounds, such as nitrogen mustard, bis(chloromethyl)ether and benzyl chloride, certain metals (discussed below) are included in this category. The great majority of organic carcinogens, however, require conversion to an ultimate, more reactive compound. This conversion is enzymatic and, for the most part, is effected by the cellular systems involved in drug metabolism and detoxification. Many cells in the body, particularly liver cells, possess enzyme systems that are capable of converting procarcinogens to their active forms. Yet each carcinogen has its own spectrum of target tissues, often limited to a single organ. The basis for organ specificity in chemical carcinogenesis is not well understood, but there is experimental evidence to suggest that other factors are required for initiation in certain tissues, such as the suspected role of cystitis in bladder cancer.

Figure 5-20. The concept of initiation and promotion. *(A)* The single application of an initiator to the skin of a mouse produces initiated cells, but no papillomas form. *(B)* Likewise, the application of a promotor alone to the skin produces no papillomas. *(C)* If the promoter is applied to the skin before the application of the initiator, no papillomas form, although initiated cells are present. *(D)* When the skin is first exposed to the initiator, the subsequent application of the promoter results in papillomas. If the promoter is withdrawn, the papillomas regress, leaving initiated cells in their place. When the promoter is applied to mouse skin bearing papillomas, invasive squamous cell carcinomas are produced.

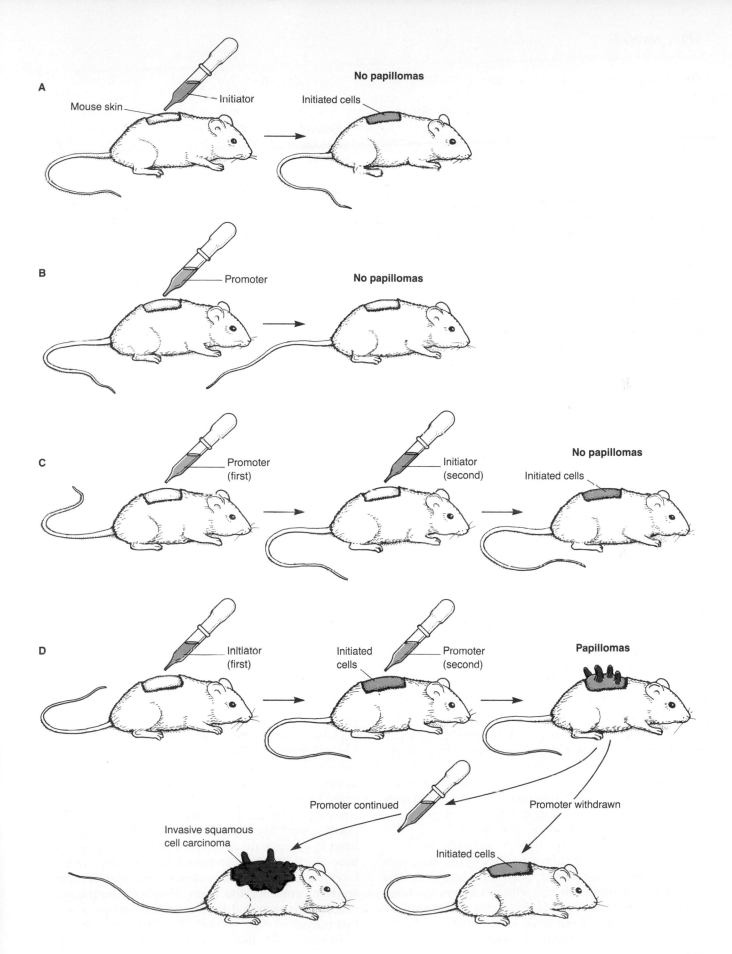

161

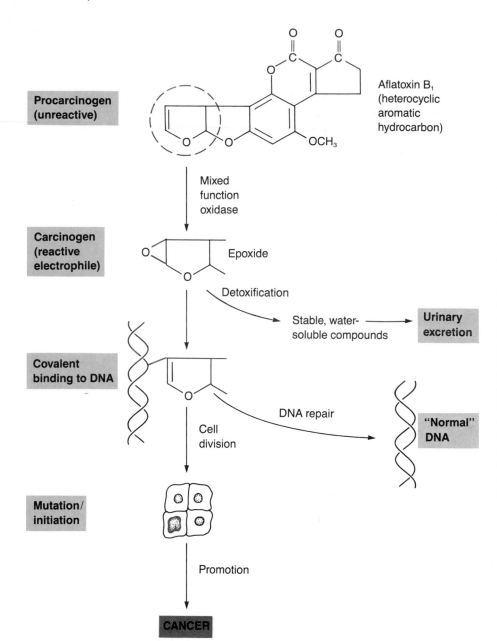

Procarcinogen (unreactive)

Aflatoxin B$_1$ (heterocyclic aromatic hydrocarbon)

Mixed function oxidase

Carcinogen (reactive electrophile)

O — Epoxide

Detoxification

Stable, water-soluble compounds → **Urinary excretion**

Covalent binding to DNA

DNA repair → **"Normal" DNA**

Cell division

Mutation/ initiation

Promotion

CANCER

Figure 5-21. Metabolic activation of aflatoxin B$_1$. The unreactive procarcinogen aflatoxin B$_1$ is metabolized by the mixed function oxidase of the hepatic endoplasmic reticulum to yield an epoxide. This electrophilic metabolite can be detoxified by conjugation with GSH and excreted in the urine. Alternatively, the epoxide of aflatoxin B$_1$ can covalently bind to liver cell macromolecules, and in particular can bind to DNA. The resulting DNA damage can be repaired, a process that restores the integrity of the DNA. If the hepatocyte divides before DNA repair is complete, initiated liver cells result. With the appropriate regimen, these initiated hepatocytes can be promoted to a hepatocellular carcinoma.

The **polycyclic aromatic hydrocarbons,** originally derived from coal tar, are among the most extensively studied carcinogens. In this class are such model compounds as benzo(a)pyrene, 3-methylcholanthrene, and dibenzanthracene. These compounds have a broad range of target organs and generally produce cancers at the site of application. The specific type of cancer produced varies with the route of administration and includes tumors of the skin, soft tissues, and breast. Since polycyclic hydrocarbons have been identified in cigarette smoke, it has been suggested that they may be involved in the production of carcinoma of the lung.

Polycyclic hydrocarbons are metabolized by cyto-

chrome P$_{450}$–dependent mixed function oxidases to electrophilic epoxides, which in turn react with proteins and nucleic acids. The formation of the epoxide depends on the presence of an unsaturated carbon–carbon bond. For example, **vinyl chloride,** the simple two-carbon molecule from which the widely used plastic polyvinyl chloride is synthesized, is metabolized to an epoxide, which is why it has carcinogenic properties. Workers exposed to the vinyl chloride monomer in the ambient atmosphere later developed angiosarcomas of the liver. However, better safety precautions have led to the virtual disappearance of this tumor.

In contrast to the polycyclic hydrocarbons, which

are for the most part formed either by the combustion of organic material or synthetically, a heterocyclic hydrocarbon, **aflatoxin B₁**, is a natural product of the fungus *Aspergillus flavus*. Like the polycyclic aromatic hydrocarbons, aflatoxin B₁ is metabolized to an epoxide, which is either detoxified or binds covalently to DNA (Fig. 5-21). Aflatoxin B₁ is among the most potent liver carcinogens recognized, producing tumors in fish, birds, rodents, and primates. Since *Aspergillus* species are ubiquitous, contamination of vegetable foods, particularly peanuts and grains exposed to the warm moist conditions that favor the growth of this mold, may result in the formation of significant amounts of aflatoxin B₁. It has been suggested that aflatoxin-rich foods may contribute to the high incidence of cancer of the liver in parts of Africa and Asia. This suggestion, however, must be viewed with caution, since hepatitis B is also endemic in these areas and has been incriminated as a cause of primary hepatocellular carcinoma.

Aromatic amines and **azo dyes,** in contrast to the polycyclic aromatic hydrocarbons, are not ordinarily carcinogenic at the point of application but commonly produce bladder and liver tumors, respectively, when fed to experimental animals. Both aromatic amines and azo dyes are primarily metabolized in the liver. The activation reaction undergone by aromatic amines is N-hydroxylation to form the hydroxylamino derivatives, which are then detoxified by conjugation with glucuronic acid. In the bladder, hydrolysis of the glucuronide releases the reactive hydroxylamine. **Occupational exposure to aromatic amines in the form of aniline dyes has resulted in bladder cancer.** Aminoazo dyes are also known to be carcinogenic. At one time butter yellow (dimethylaminoazobenzene) was used to color margarine or pale winter butter to simulate the richness of summer butter, and maraschino cherries were tinted with scarlet red, a structural component of which is o-aminoazotoluene. However, there are no documented cases of cancer in humans from these agents.

Carcinogenic **nitrosamines** are a subject of considerable study because it is suspected that they may play a role in human gastrointestinal neoplasms and possibly other cancers. The simplest nitrosamine, dimethylnitrosamine, produces kidney and liver tumors in rodents. Nitrosamines are also potent carcinogens in primates, although unambiguous evidence of cancer induction in humans is lacking. However, the extremely high incidence of esophageal carcinoma in the Hunan province of China (100 times higher than in other areas) has been correlated with the high nitrosamine content of the diet. There is concern that nitrosamines may also be implicated in other gastrointestinal cancers because nitrites, commonly added to preserve processed meats and other foods, may react with other dietary components to form nitrosamines. Nitrosamines are activated by hydroxylation, followed by formation of a reactive alkyl carbonium ion. A carbonium ion is also formed in the liver by the metabolism of carcinogenic **pyrrolizidine alkaloids,** which are important constituents of medicinal bush and herbal teas in undeveloped countries.

A number of metals or metal compounds can induce cancer, but the mechanisms by which they do so are unknown. Divalent metal cations, such as Ni^{2+}, Pb^{2+}, Cd^{2+}, Co^{2+}, and Be^{2+}, are electrophilic and can, therefore, react with macromolecules. In addition, metal ions react with guanine and phosphate groups of DNA. A metal ion such as Ni^{2+}, can depolymerize polynucleotides. Some metals can bind to the purine and pyrimidine bases through covalent bonds or pi electrons of the bases. These reactions all occur in vitro, but the extent to which they occur in vivo is not known. Most metal-induced cancers occur in an occupational setting, and the subject is, therefore, discussed in more detail in Chapter 8, which deals with environmental pathology.

Factors Influencing Chemical Carcinogenesis

Chemical carcinogenesis in experimental animals is influenced by a variety of factors, including species and strain, age and sex of the animal, hormonal status, diet, and the presence or absence of inducers of drug-metabolizing systems and tumor promoters. A similar role for such factors in humans has been postulated on the basis of epidemiologic studies. In the context of chemical carcinogenesis, it is appropriate to focus on the effects of modifiers of the metabolism of carcinogens.

The activity of the **mixed function oxidases** is genetically determined, and a correlation has been observed between the levels of these enzymes in various strains of mice and their sensitivity to chemical carcinogens. The levels of drug-metabolizing enzymes in newborn animals are very low and take some time to reach adult levels. Therefore, the greater sensitivity of young animals to induction of some tumors seems paradoxical. By way of example, polycyclic hydrocarbons, which do not produce liver tumors in adult rodents, are carcinogenic for young animals. However, this inconsistency can be readily accounted for by the higher proliferative activity of tissues in young animals.

The effects of **sex and hormonal status** are important determinants of susceptibility to chemical carcinogens but are highly variable and in many instances not readily predictable. In most experimental species, male animals are more susceptible to the aromatic amine liver carcinogens than are females. By contrast, female mice are more sensitive to the carcinogenic effects of aminoazotoluene and diethylnitrosamine. Moreover, in some instances, when a carcinogen is administered to a sexually immature animal, there still is a sex-linked incidence of cancer in organs that are not primarily endocrine responsive, such as the liver.

The **composition of the diet** can affect the level of drug-metabolizing enzymes. A low-protein diet, which reduces the hepatic activity of mixed function oxidases, is associated with a decreased sensitivity to hepatocarcinogens. In the case of dimethylnitrosamine, the decreased incidence of liver tumors is accompanied by an increase in that of kidney tumors, an observation that emphasizes the fact that the metabolism of carcinogens may be regulated differently in different tissues. Much attention has recently been focused on an alleged association between fat in the diet and the incidence of breast and colon cancers. Although it has been clearly shown experimentally that a diet high in fat increases susceptibility to chemically produced breast cancer, the number of confounding factors in epidemiologic studies suggests caution in extrapolating these data to humans. Dietary fiber has also been suggested as an influence on the occurrence of colorectal cancer. In this case a plausible explanation lies in the effect of fiber on increasing the motility of the gut and thereby hastening the elimination of potentially harmful chemicals in the fecal stream. However, despite the recommendations of health officials and the claims of manufacturers of certain foods, there is no clinical or epidemiologic evidence that the introduction of more fiber into the Western diet reduces the risk of colorectal cancer.

As already noted, most chemical carcinogens require metabolic activation. It follows that agents that enhance the activation of procarcinogens to ultimate carcinogens should lead to greater carcinogenicity, whereas those that augment the detoxification pathways should reduce the incidence of cancer. In general this is the case. Since man is exposed to many chemicals that may modify the metabolism of xenobiotics, in the diet, drinking water, and the workplace, such an interaction is potentially significant.

Chemical Carcinogens as Mutagens

Associations between exposure to a specific chemical and human cancers have historically been established on the basis of epidemiologic studies. These studies have numerous inherent disadvantages, including uncertainties in estimated doses, variability of the population, long and variable latency, and dependence on clinical and public health records of questionable accuracy. Moreover, a negative result—that is, a lack of association between the chemical and cancer—often does not necessarily exclude a weak carcinogenic effect. As an alternative to epidemiologic studies, investigators turned to the use of studies involving animals—indeed, such studies are legally required before the introduction of a new drug. Yet the logarithmic increase in the number of chemicals synthesized every year makes even this method prohibitively cumbersome and expensive. The search for rapid, reproducible, and reliable screening assays for potential carcinogenic activity has centered on the relationship between carcinogenicity and mutagenicity.

A mutagen is an agent that can permanently alter the genetic constitution of a cell. The most widely used screening test, **the Ames test,** utilizes the appearance of mutants in a culture of bacteria of the *Salmonella* species (Fig. 5-22). About 90% of known carcinogens are mutagenic in this system. Moreover, most, but not all, mutagens are carcinogenic. (This close correlation between carcinogenicity and mutagenicity presumably reflects the fact that both damage DNA.) Thus, while not infallible, the in vitro mutagenicity assay has proved to be a valuable tool in screening for the carcinogenic potential of chemicals.

Chemical Carcinogenesis as a Multistep Process

We have previously mentioned that experimentally chemical carcinogenesis is a multistep process, the details of which have been best defined in the rodent liver. The carcinogenic process in the liver from the administration of the carcinogen to the appearance of a hepatocellular carcinoma has been dissected into at least seven steps (Fig. 5-23):

1. **Biochemical lesion.** Most hepatocarcinogens react with DNA as the initial event. If this damage is not repaired, such an interaction may result in mutations, chromosomal translocations, inactivation of regulatory genes, or more subtle changes. Since the repair of the DNA damage is complete in 4 days, the biochemical change is shortlived.
2. **Fixation of the biochemical lesion by cell proliferation.** Most chemical carcinogens do not produce tumors in the normal adult liver even though they damage DNA. If initiation is to

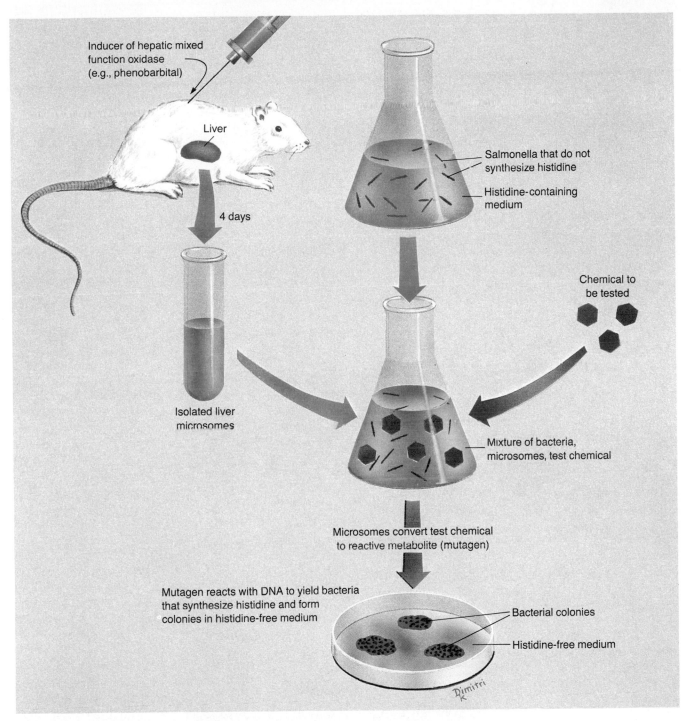

Figure 5-22. The Ames test. The Ames test is a method for screening chemicals for possible carcinogenicity. It is based on the strong correlation between mutagenicity and carcinogenicity, and determines the ability of the test chemical to induce mutations in a strain of *Salmonella* bacteria. A male rat is injected with an inducer of hepatic mixed function oxidase activity, such as phenobarbital. Several days later, microsomes are prepared from the liver. The test chemical and the microsomes are then incubated with the bacteria, which cannot synthesize histidine and which require histidine supplementation for growth. The bacteria are subsequently cultured on a histidine-free medium, which does not support growth. Mutants that do not require histidine are recognized by colony formation.

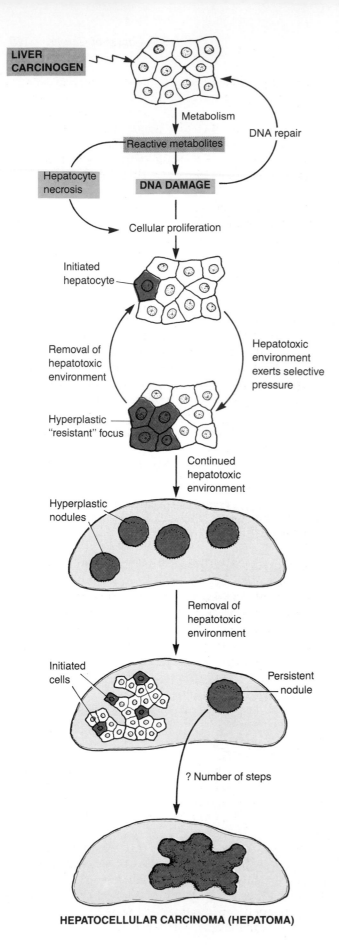

Figure 5-23. Hepatocarcinogenesis in the rat.

occur there must be cell proliferation before DNA repair is completed. Such proliferation can be induced by partial hepatectomy; by toxic necrosis, produced by either the carcinogen itself or another nonspecific agent; or by the physiologic growth of the newborn animal.

3. **Microscopic foci of altered cells.** During the process of promotion, initiated cells grow to form microscopic foci of phenotypically altered cells.

4. **Hepatocyte nodules.** Nodules are defined as macroscopically visible focal proliferations of altered hepatocytes that compress the surrounding liver. They may measure up to 1 cm in diameter in the rat liver. On removal of the promoting stimulus, the vast majority of nodules (95–98%) eventually remodel to the appearance of normal liver as their cells return to a more differentiated state. However, the preneoplastic process is evidenced by the persistence of a small minority of nodules (2–5%). These persistent nodules exhibit autonomous cell proliferation and are the precursors of the eventual hepatocellular carcinoma.

5. **Cell proliferation and cell death in the persistent nodules.** The persistent nodules at first display synchronous cell proliferation, which may be ten times faster than that of the surrounding normal liver. This growth is almost always balanced by an accelerated cell death, and the nodules, therefore, enlarge only slowly.

6. **Defective control of the cell cycle.** Eventually, a small subset of hepatocytes in the persistent nodules acquire a new property: namely, the capacity to continue cycling indefinitely, without the usual arrest after one or two cell divisions. For the first time these cells will form nodules, and eventually hepatocellular carcinomas, on transplantation to the spleen.

7. **Progression to hepatocellular carcinoma.** This step probably consists of a number of separate and distinct events, but the nature of these is obscure. It is clear that progression to cancer is subject to delay by dietary and hormonal influences. By 9 to 12 months after initiation, unequivocal hepatocellular carcinomas are seen.

From these observations, one can abstract four hypothetical stages of chemical carcinogenesis. The first stage, **initiation,** is followed by a stage of **promotion,** which is characterized by an excess of cell proliferation over cell death. During this second stage the altered cells do not exhibit autonomous growth, but remain dependent on the continued presence of the promoting stimulus. In the third stage, growth is autonomous, and **progression** to cancer is independent of the carcinogen or the promoter. When the cells acquire the capacity to invade and metastasize, the tumor is labeled **"cancer."**

While the process of initiation is most consistent with a mutational event, the mechanism of promotion is more controversial. In some cases, the selective stimulation of initiated cells may account for their differential growth. In other circumstances, initiated cells seem to be more resistant than normal cells to the toxic effects of the promoter and have, therefore, a selective growth advantage. The latter possibility is analogous to the emergence of antibiotic-resistant bacteria or to the development of resistance to chemotherapeutic agents by cancer cells. The autonomous growth that characterizes progression may be related to the growth properties previously described for cancer cells. In any event, the multistep pattern of chemical carcinogenesis in rat liver seems to be analogous to the multistep development of cancer in the squamous epithelium of the skin and the metaplastic epithelium of the endocervix and bronchus, the glandular cells of the colon, pancreas, and breast, and the transitional epithelium of the urinary bladder.

Physical Carcinogenesis

The physical agents of carcinogenesis discussed here are ultraviolet light, asbestos, and foreign bodies. Because of the significant implications for public health stemming from the diagnostic and therapeutic use of x-rays and radioisotopes in medicine, and because of the widespread concern about the safety of nuclear reactors and the dangers of atomic war, radiation carcinogenesis is discussed in Chapter 8, which is concerned with environmental pathology.

Ultraviolet Radiation

Among fair-skinned people a glowing tan is commonly considered the mark of a successful holiday. However, this overt manifestation of the alleged healthful effects of the sun conceals underlying tissue damage. The harmful effects of solar radiation were recognized by ladies of a bygone era, who shielded themselves from the sun with parasols in order to maintain a "roses and milk" complexion and to prevent wrinkles. The current fad for a tanned complexion has been accompanied by an increase in the incidence of the major skin cancers.

Ultraviolet (UV) radiation is the short wavelength portion of the electromagnetic spectrum adjacent to the violet region of visible light. The earth is shielded from much of the UV radiation from the sun by the ozone layer. Unfortunately, there is reason to believe that this layer is being depleted by industrial gases, and the long-term consequences are possibly unpleasant. The first evidence of cell damage produced by UV radiation dates to a century ago, when it was reported that this form of energy rendered bacteria inactive. Subsequently it was found that the effectiveness of energy of different wavelengths in killing bacteria paralleled the absorption spectrum of nucleic acids. **The effects of UV radiation on cells include enzyme inactivation, inhibition of cell division, mutagenesis, cell death, and cancer.** It appears that only certain portions of the UV spectrum are associated with tissue damage, and a carcinogenic effect is noted at wavelengths between 290 and 320 nm.

Appreciation of the carcinogenic effect of UV radiation in humans is based principally on clinical and epidemiologic observations. **Cancers attributed to sun exposure—namely basal cell carcinoma, squamous carcinoma, and melanoma—occur predominantly in whites;** the skin of the darker races is presumably protected by the increased concentration of melanin pigment, which absorbs UV radiation. In fair-skinned people the areas exposed to the sun are most prone to develop skin cancer. Moreover, there is a direct correlation between total exposure to sunlight and incidence of skin cancer.

It now appears that the most important biochemical effect of UV radiation is the formation of **pyrimidine dimers in DNA,** although other photoproducts may also play a role. Pyrimidine dimers may form between thymine and thymine, between thymine and cytosine, or between cytosine pairs alone. Dimer formation leads to a cyclobutane ring, which distorts the phosphodiester backbone of the double helix in the region of each dimer. The central role of pyrimidine dimers in the tissue injury caused by UV radiation is demonstrated by the fact that restoring these dimers to their original monomeric state by photoreactivation protects against UV-induced damage. Enzyme-catalyzed photoreactivation is a well-documented form of DNA repair, present in most nonmammalian cells. (Mammals depend on other complex DNA repair mechanisms.) The enzyme binds specifically to UV-damaged DNA, where it uses the energy of visible light to convert the dimer to two monomers. The induction of thyroid neoplasms by UV light is inhibited by visible light in species that contain the photoreactivating enzyme. In addition, in vitro transformation of cultured cells parallels the production of pyrimidine dimers by UV radiation of different wavelengths.

The importance of DNA repair in protecting against the harmful effects of UV radiation is exemplified by the autosomal recessive disease **xeroderma pigmentosum.** In this rare disease a sensitivity to sunlight is accompanied by a high incidence of skin cancers, including basal cell carcinoma, squamous cell carcinoma, and melanoma. Both the neoplastic and non-neoplastic disorders of the skin in this disease are attributed to an impairment in the excision of UV-damaged DNA.

Asbestos

Pulmonary asbestosis and asbestosis-associated neoplasms are discussed in Chapter 12, which deals with diseases of the lungs. Here we will review possible mechanisms of carcinogenesis attributed to asbestos. In this context, it is not conclusively established whether the cancers related to asbestos exposure should be considered as chemically or physically induced.

Asbestos, a material widely used in construction, insulation, and manufacturing, is a family of related fibrous silicates, which are classed as "serpentines" or "amphiboles." Serpentines, of which chrysotile is the only example of commercial importance, occur as flexible fibers, whereas the amphiboles, represented principally by crocidolite and amosite, are firm narrow rods.

Asbestos fibers are inhaled during mining, manufacturing, and the installation of asbestos insulation, in the vicinity of asbestos plants, from contaminated air in buildings undergoing repair or demolition, or from the clothing of asbestos workers. The deposition of asbestos fibers in the lung relates more to their diameter than to their length. The thick fibers lodge in the upper respiratory tract, but thin ones are deposited in the terminal airways and alveoli. Asbestos fibers can be coated with complexes of iron and protein and are then visualized particularly well with iron stains, which reveal so-called **ferruginous bodies (asbestos bodies).** However, most asbestos fibers remain uncoated and are, therefore, not visible by light microscopy.

The characteristic tumor associated with asbestos exposure is malignant mesothelioma of the pleural and peritoneal cavities. This cancer, which is exceedingly rare in the general population, has been reported to occur in 2% to 3% (in some studies even more) of heavily exposed workers. The latent period—that is, the interval between exposure and the appearance of a tumor—is usually about 20 years, but may be twice that figure. Fibrotic pleural lesions are often found in those exposed to asbestos but are not related to the development of malignant mesothelioma. It is reasonable to surmise that mesotheliomas of both the pleura and the peritoneum reflect the close contact of these membranes with asbestos fibers transported to them by lymphatic channels.

The pathogenesis of asbestos-associated mesotheliomas is obscure. In rats the dimensions of the fiber, rather than its chemical composition, were reported to be crucial. Long, thin fibers deposited in the pleural space produced tumors, while short, thick fibers did not. This finding is compatible with the clinical observation that the long, thin crocidolite fibers are associated with a considerably greater risk of mesothelioma than the shorter and thicker amosite fibers or the flexible chrysotile fibers. However, the distinction between these fibers in the causation of human disease should not be taken as absolute, particularly since mixtures of these fibers are characteristically found in human lungs. It has been speculated that mesothelioma related to asbestos exposure may be a human counterpart of the foreign-body sarcomas produced in rodents and described below.

An association between cancer of the lung and asbestos exposure is clearly established in smokers. A small increase in the prevalence of lung cancer has been found in nonsmokers exposed to asbestos, but the data base of the studies was small, and the subject would benefit from further investigation. An increased incidence of cancer of the larynx has also been reported among asbestos workers who smoke. Claims that exposure to asbestos increases the risk of gastrointestinal cancer have not withstood statistical analysis of the collected data.

Foreign Body Carcinogenesis

A number of different sarcomas have been induced in rodents by the implantation of inert materials, such as plastic and metal films, various fibers (including fiberglass), plastic sponges, glass spheres, and dextran polymers. The chemical nature of these implants does not seem to be the critical feature, since disks made of pure carbon also produce sarcomas. Rather, the size, smoothness, and durability of the implanted surface are important. This form of cancer is highly species-specific. For example, rats and mice are highly susceptible to foreign-body carcinogenesis but guinea pigs are resistant. Humans are certainly highly resistant, as evidenced by the lack of cancers following the implantation of prostheses constructed of plastics and metals. A few reports of cancer developing in the vicinity of foreign bodies in humans

probably reflect scar formation, which in some organs seems to be associated with an increased incidence of cancers. As an aside, it should be pointed out that despite numerous contrary claims in lawsuits, there is no evidence that a single traumatic injury can lead to any form of cancer.

A special case of possible foreign-body carcinogenesis are the tumors associated with certain parasitic infestations. Carcinoma of the bladder in persons harboring *Schistosoma haematobium* in that organ has long been recognized. Carcinoma of the bile ducts occasionally follows infection with the liver fluke *Clonorchis sinensis*, which takes up residence in the biliary passages. It is not clear whether the development of cancer reflects the foreign-body reaction itself or the release of carcinogens from the parasites.

Viral Carcinogenesis

The role of viruses in the spontaneous appearance and experimental induction of cancer in animals is thoroughly established. Yet, despite strong epidemiologic associations between viruses and a number of human cancers, no virus has yet been unequivocally shown to cause human cancer. The strongest association between viruses and cancer in humans are the RNA retrovirus HTLV I and T cell leukemia/lymphoma; the human papillomavirus (DNA) and squamous carcinoma of the cervix; and the hepatitis B virus (DNA) and primary hepatocellular carcinoma.

Historical Overview of Oncogenic Viruses in Animals

Chicken leukemias and **lymphomas** were at one time not uncommon and appeared in epidemic form. The transmissibility of avian erythroblastosis by cell-free extracts from diseased chickens was recognized shortly after the turn of the century, but the successful transfer of chicken lymphomatosis by cell extracts was not accomplished until 1941. Ten years later a vaccine against chicken lymphomatosis, the first anticancer vaccine, successfully eradicated this economic hazard from poultry flocks. It should be noted that the horizontal spread of chicken lymphomatosis from one animal to another is similar to that of many classic infectious viral diseases, such as influenza or the common cold. Moreover, the avian leukosis virus (RNA) is also transmitted vertically from parent to offspring via the egg.

The **Rous sarcoma virus** (RNA) was originally derived in 1910 from a cell-free extract of a breast sarcoma in a chicken. When injected into young chickens, sarcomas developed at the site of injection and metastasized to many other organs.

The **Shope papilloma virus** (DNA) was isolated from warty growths in wild cottontail rabbits in the early 1930s. The virus-induced tumor grows slowly in wild rabbits but rapidly when passed to a domestic rabbit. Furthermore, extracts from the tumors of the domestic animals failed to produce tumors in other rabbits, wild or domestic. This masking of the virus in the domestic rabbit will be explained below.

It has long been known that certain strains of mice have a high incidence of mammary tumors, whereas other strains have virtually none. Although the susceptibility to mammary cancer clearly seemed to be hereditary, it does not follow Mendelian laws. When the mother is from a tumor-susceptible strain, the daughters are susceptible. On the other hand, when the father is from a susceptible strain and the mother from a resistant strain, the daughters of the cross do not develop mammary tumors. Bittner in 1936 discovered that the factor that promotes mammary cancer is in the mother's milk, rather than in her genes. He showed that, if the offspring are delivered by caesarean section and suckled by dams from a tumor-free strain, the daughters do not develop cancer. Conversely, when young newborn mice from a tumor-free strain are suckled by dams of a susceptible strain, they develop mammary cancer. However, it is important to point out that the **Bittner milk factor** only produces tumors in certain strains, an observation that demonstrates the importance of hereditary factors. Moreover, if the offspring are castrated, no mammary tumors develop. It is, therefore, clear that the Bittner virus (RNA) induces mammary carcinoma only in the proper genetic and hormonal environment. Furthermore, age also plays an important role. Exposure to the virus at birth invariably leads to mammary carcinoma under the appropriate conditions, but exposure later in life is accompanied by far fewer tumors.

The **polyoma virus** (DNA), discovered in the 1950s, produces an astonishing variety of carcinomas and sarcomas in mice, rats, rabbits, and hamsters, the last being especially sensitive. The virus is exceedingly difficult to isolate from tumor-bearing animals but is easily passed in tissue culture, where it also transforms a wide range of cells. The explanation for this seeming paradox lies in the strong antigenicity of the virus, which elicits high titers of polyoma-specific antibodies.

In the succeeding 20 years many new oncogenic DNA viruses were found to produce solid tumors and lymphoproliferative disorders in a variety of species, including frogs, birds, rodents, and monkeys.

Another important oncogenic DNA virus, the **SV-40 virus (simian virus),** was isolated from monkey cells and shown to be a potent transforming agent in vitro.

During this same period many new oncogenic RNA viruses were also found to produce similar neoplasms in comparably diverse species. These include the Gross, Friend, Maloney, Kirsten, and Rauscher leukemia viruses. In 1970 the discovery of reverse transcriptase revolutionized the study of oncogenic RNA viruses and led to their being renamed **retroviruses.**

DNA Viruses

Papillomaviruses

As noted above, a viral etiology of human cancers has yet to be proved conclusively, but the evidence that human papillomaviruses (HPV) can induce cancer in man is highly suggestive. The similarity between the human diseases associated with HPV and those produced in animals is striking, and if any human cancers are definitely shown to be caused by viruses, HPV is a likely candidate for first honors. Animal papillomaviruses manifest a pronounced tropism for epithelial tissues, unlike other tumor viruses, which are associated principally with sarcomas and hematopoietic neoplasms. In animals papillomaviruses produce benign papillomas of squamous epithelia (for example, the skin and esophagus), adenomas of the glandular epithelium of the intestine, and papillomas in the bladder. A significant proportion of these benign animal tumors progress to frank malignancy. A similar situation is seen in humans. As in animals, HPV definitely causes benign lesions of squamous epithelium, including warts, laryngeal papillomas, and condylomata accuminata (genital warts) of the vulva, penis, and perianal region. Occasionally condylomata accuminata and laryngeal papillomas undergo malignant transformation to squamous cell carcinoma. Although warts of the skin invariably remain benign, in a rare hereditary disease termed "epidermodysplasia verruciformis" HPV produces flat warts that commonly progress to squamous carcinoma. It is noteworthy that all of these malignant transformations of benign squamous lesions in animals and humans exemplify the multistep nature of cancer development, proceeding through dysplasia and carcinoma in situ to frank invasion.

It is of great interest that **HPV has now been associated with the development of cervical intraepithelial neoplasia and invasive squamous carcinoma.** HPV-induced lesions in the uterine cervix are clinically equivalent to cervical intraepithelial neoplasia—that is, they can progress to carcinoma in situ. Progression to malignancy apparently depends on the demonstrated integration of the HPV DNA into the host cell DNA. Animal experiments suggest that genetic factors may also play a permissive role. Despite the persuasive circumstantial evidence presented, many questions must be answered before HPV can be unequivocally accepted as the cause of human cervical cancer.

Polyomaviruses

The prototype of all the polyomaviruses, the **polyoma virus** itself, produces tumors in a wide variety of organs in newborn mice or hamsters. **SV-40,** another important virus of this group, produces tumors only in the baby hamster, including lymphocytic leukemia, lymphoma, and osteogenic sarcoma. Two widespread human viruses, BK and JC viruses, are closely related to SV-40 and are responsible for a fatal demyelinating disease, **progressive multifocal leukoencephalopathy (PML).** Monkeys, which are the natural host of SV-40, show a similar disease, and SV-40, rather than JCV, has been isolated from two human cases of PML. The human viruses BK and JC also transform cultured cells and produce tumors in a number of animals, although no human tumors have been attributed to them.

Transformation by polyoma viruses has been a widely studied model for in vitro viral tumorigenesis (Figure 5-24). Cells are transformed if they do not permit replication of the virus or if they are infected with inactivated viral particles. This observation is explained by the fact that before transformation can occur, viral DNA must be integrated into the DNA of the host cell. In such a location the viral genome is not replicated independently of the host genome, as it is in a productive, lytic infection. Rather, the viral genome is expressed as a cellular gene. Only that portion of the viral genome that encodes for tumor antigens is expressed. These proteins initiate and maintain the transformed state, but their specific functions are unknown. It appears that the T antigen in some way stimulates the synthesis of DNA by the host cell and is responsible for sustaining transformation properties. The T antigen also serves as a transplantation antigen that stimulates the host immune response. The t antigen is also necessary for conserving the transformed phenotype, presumably by complementing the functions of the T antigen.

Interestingly, cells transformed with the polyoma virus also express a plasma membrane antigen, the so-called middle t antigen, that displays **tyrosine kinase activity,** as do the receptors for a number of growth factors and the product of the Rous sarcoma viral oncogene. Such an enzyme activity may provide

a link between the tumorigenic effects of DNA and RNA viruses.

Herpesviruses

Many herpesviruses produce lymphomas in animals or transform cells in vitro. In humans three herpesviruses—the Epstein-Barr virus (EBV), herpes simplex virus type 2, and cytomegalovirus—have been strongly associated with certain cancers.

EBV is so widely disseminated that 80% of adults in the world have antibodies to it. This virus infects B lymphocytes in humans and other primates, a situation similar to the tropism of other herpesviruses of nonhuman primates. Of all cells only B lymphocytes possess receptors for EBV, the virus that transforms these cells into lymphoblasts with an indefinite lifespan. In a small proportion of primary infections with EBV, this lymphoblastoid transformation is manifested as **infectious mononucleosis.** However, in Africa, principally in children, and in sporadic cases elsewhere, EBV has been closely associated with **Burkitt's lymphoma,** a B cell neoplasm in which the neoplastic lymphocytes contain EBV in DNA and manifest EBV-related antigens. A similar correlation, though perhaps not as persuasive, is reported with **nasopharyngeal carcinoma.** It remains to be proved whether the association of EBV with these tumors is causal.

A putative association between infection with herpes simplex type 2, the agent of genital herpes, and cervical cancer was claimed on the basis of the demonstration that women with genital herpes have a high incidence of cervical carcinoma, and that women with cervical carcinoma have a higher incidence of antibodies to the virus. However, a causal relationship between herpes simplex type 2 and cervical cancer has been seriously questioned. Since it is well established that the virus is transmitted venereally, it is possible that both the infection and the tumor are related to sexual activity.

Infection with cytomegalovirus is widespread, but under ordinary circumstances it causes no disease. However, when cell-mediated immunity is deficient, as in the fetus and newborn and in patients with AIDS, symptomatic infections of many organs occur. Recently it has been suggested that cytomegalovirus, a transforming agent in vitro, may cause Kaposi's sarcoma, the most common tumor complicating AIDS.

Hepatitis B virus (HBV)

Hepatitis B virus, a partially double-stranded DNA virus, infects only humans, although separate,

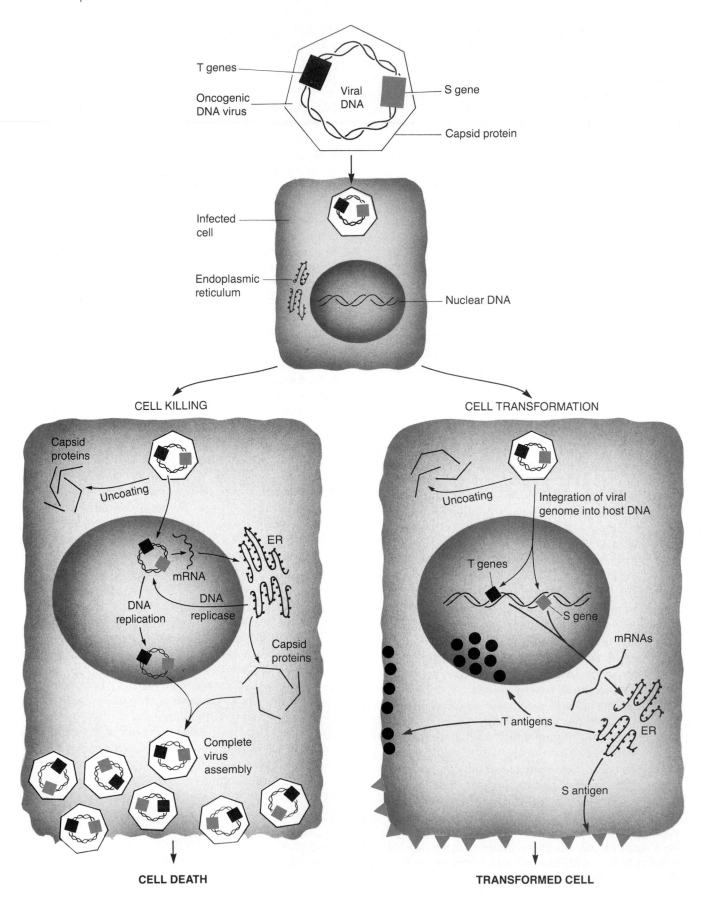

closely related viruses infect woodchucks, ground squirrels, and domestic ducks. Epidemiologic studies have clearly established an association between chronic infection with HBV and the development of primary hepatocellular carcinoma. Animals chronically infected with related hepatitis viruses also exhibit a high incidence of primary hepatocellular carcinoma. The demonstration that the HBV genome is integrated into host liver cell DNA suggests that this virus should now be considered a putative oncogenic virus. Study of the mechanism by which HBV may induce neoplasms has been hampered by the failure of this agent to grow in tissue culture or to transform cells in vitro.

Poxviruses and Adenoviruses

The poxviruses and adenoviruses, members of the group of DNA-containing viruses, are oncogenic in animals but have not been associated with any human tumors.

RNA Viruses (Retroviruses) and the Genetic Basis of Cancer

The discovery of DNA as the basis of heredity was entirely consistent with the transforming capability of DNA-containing viruses. It was argued that the induction of the permanent, heritable characteristics of the transformed cell reflects the incorporation of the viral DNA into the cellular genome. However, the transforming properties of RNA-containing viruses posed a dilemma, since the central dogma of molecular biology held that information flowed in a unidirectional manner, from DNA to RNA to protein. How then, could the genetic information encoded in RNA be communicated to subsequent generations of stable lines of transformed cells? In the mid-1960s a revolutionary hypothesis was put forward to the effect that the genome of RNA-containing oncogenic viruses is transcribed into DNA by a reversal of the usual direction of information flow. This hypothesis implied that the DNA segment derived from viral RNA, after integration into the host genome, functions as a gene and that messenger RNA is, in turn,

transcribed from it. Moreover, the theory implied that the messenger RNA transcribed from the integrated segment of DNA becomes the genome of nascent viral progeny. This hypothesis was validated by the demonstration of **reverse transcriptase** in 1970. This discovery opened a new era of research into the molecular biology of cancer.

While DNA viruses have been closely associated with the development of a number of epithelial, mesenchymal, and hematopoietic cancers, the RNA viruses to date have been implicated in only one human cancer, the rare T cell leukemia/lymphoma seen in Japan and the Caribbean region. Yet despite this apparently slight clinical impact, experimental studies of these viruses have added considerably to our understanding of the molecular biology of cancer.

Study of the tumorigenic properties of retroviruses led directly to deeper insights into the genetic basis of neoplasia. The belief that cancer has a genetic basis, embodied in the concept of "cancer genes," has been prevalent for most of this century and is rooted in the recognition of four factors: hereditary predisposition, the presence of chromosomal abnormalities in neoplastic cells, a correlation between impaired DNA repair and the occurrence of cancer, and the close association between carcinogenesis and mutagenesis. More recently, research on retroviruses has pointed to the existence of cellular genes, termed **proto-oncogenes,** which, in another form—namely, as **oncogenes**—may play a central role in neoplasia.

Retroviral Oncogenes

Infection by a retrovirus introduces new genetic material into the host cell. The viral RNA is transcribed into DNA by reverse transcriptase, and this DNA is then integrated into the host's chromosomal DNA. In this position there are two general mechanisms by which the viral DNA can influence the transformation of the cell (Figure 5-25). In one, cellular genes undergo abnormal regulation by the viral genome. This process has been named **insertional mutagenesis.** In the second, genetic recombination causes cellular genes to be implanted within the viral genome, in which case the cellular gene may become a viral oncogene. The process by which retroviral oncogenes

Figure 5-24. The cellular consequences of infection with a DNA tumor virus. Cells are either killed or transformed, depending on whether or not the viral DNA is integrated into the host genome. Viral replication directed by unintegrated viral DNA results in cell death. By contrast, integration of the viral genome into the host DNA results in the cellular expression of viral antigens, presumably associated with the process of transformation.

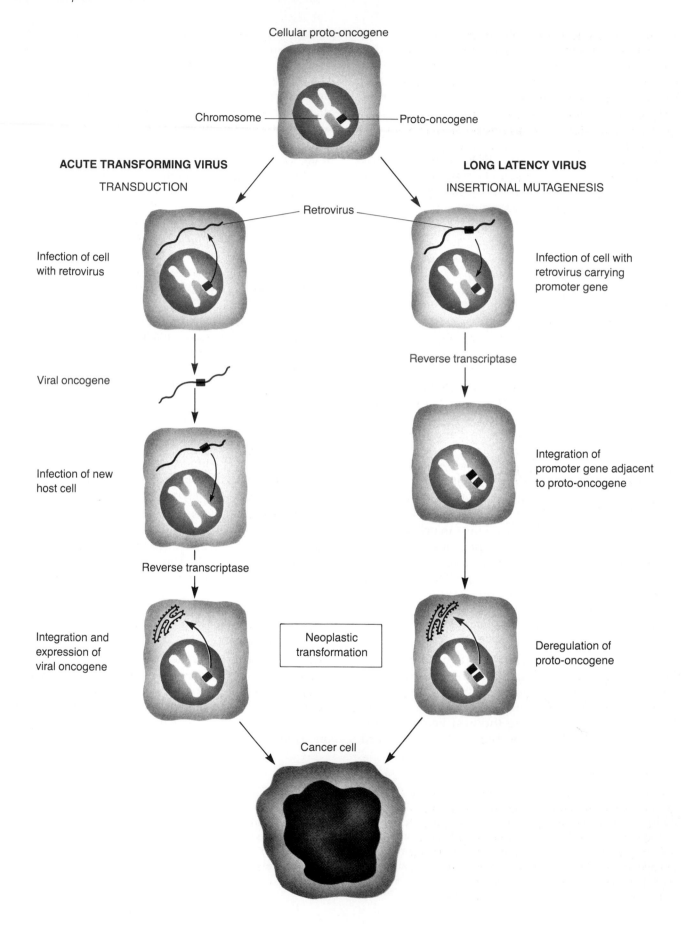

Cellular proto-oncogene

Chromosome — Proto-oncogene

ACUTE TRANSFORMING VIRUS

TRANSDUCTION

LONG LATENCY VIRUS

INSERTIONAL MUTAGENESIS

Retrovirus

Infection of cell with retrovirus

Infection of cell with retrovirus carrying promoter gene

Viral oncogene

Reverse transcriptase

Infection of new host cell

Integration of promoter gene adjacent to proto-oncogene

Reverse transcriptase

Integration and expression of viral oncogene

Neoplastic transformation

Deregulation of proto-oncogene

Cancer cell

are formed from such cellular proto-oncogenes is termed **transduction.** To date, close to two dozen retroviral oncogenes have been recognized, each of which encodes a protein whose biochemical action is amenable to study. In almost half of these viral oncogenes, corresponding cellular proto-oncogenes have been implicated in carcinogenesis. Despite the large number of viral and cellular oncogenes identified, only four biochemical mechanisms by which they may act have been recognized. These are protein phosphorylation of tyrosine or serine and threonine; metabolic regulation by proteins that bind GTP, in a manner resembling the normal B or N proteins; control of gene expression by influence on the biogenesis of mRNA; and participation in the replication of DNA. Many of these biochemical mechanisms relate, in turn, to the actions of polypeptide growth factors (Figure 5-26).

The question arises, what are the properties of the transduced oncogenes of retroviruses—presumably formed from apparently innocuous cellular genes—that cause them to be tumorigenic? The answer is twofold. In the first place, the expression of the transduced oncogenes is stimulated by signals from the viral genome in a manner not coordinated with the ordinary metabolism of the cell. Second, during the recombinations that lead from a proto-oncogene to a viral oncogene, the transduced genes often undergo mutations, such as point mutations, deletions, and genetic substitutions. Such mutations have been shown in some cases to increase the activities of the gene products, particularly tyrosine kinases. In other words, **transformation may induce sustained high levels of otherwise normal biochemical activities.**

It is not necessary for a retrovirus to possess an oncogene in order for it to cause cancer. In some virally induced tumors, a cellular proto-oncogene—for example, *c-myc* or *c-ras*—is activated by the insertion of retroviral sequences adjacent to it, a process that results in the ungoverned expression of the previously regulated or silent gene. The integrated viral DNA may function as a powerful promotor itself or it may activate a host promotor.

Chromosomal Alterations and Cancer

Studies of viral oncogenesis have also provided a better understanding of the mechanisms by which altered chromosomes in cancer cells may directly relate to the neoplastic phenotype. It is now well recognized that specific alterations in particular chromosomes are associated with certain types of tumors or with neoplasia in general. The study of these nonrandom karyotypic changes, particularly the **reciprocal chromosome translocations** in Burkitt's lymphoma and chronic myelogenous leukemia, has shed further light on the potential role of cellular proto-oncogenes in neoplasia. Most cases of Burkitt's lymphoma exhibit a reciprocal translocation involving chromosomes 8 and 14. The human *c-myc* gene on chromosome 8 has been mapped to the break point on that chromosome in Burkitt's lymphoma, and the immunoglobulin genes on chromosome 14 have also been traced to the break point. The translocation of the *c-myc* gene to the region adjacent to the immunoglobulin genes on chromosome 14 presumably leads to the deregulation of the expression of the *c-myc* oncogene (Fig. 5-27). The *c-myc* gene product is a nuclear protein whose normal function is believed to involve the growth regulation of lymphocytes and other cells. Thus, theoretically, deregulation of this gene in Burkitt's lymphoma could provide an unremitting growth stimulus to the cell. It is significant that other B-cell lymphomas and leukemias, which are far more common than Burkitt's lymphoma in most parts of the world, also display characteristic chromosomal translocations involving the terminal portion of chromosome 14, the site of the immunoglobulin genes, although it is likely that other translocations and gene rearrangements also play a role in the pathogenesis of B-cell neoplasms.

The first and still the best-known example of an acquired chromosomal anomaly in a human cancer is the **Philadelphia chromosome, found in most cases of chronic myelogenous leukemia.** The anomaly has now been identified as a translocation of the

Figure 5-25. Mechanisms of tumorigenesis by RNA retroviruses. Acute transforming RNA viruses contain a viral oncogene formed by transduction of a cellular proto-oncogene. Infection of a cell by such a virus results in the integration and expression of the viral oncogene, presumably leading to neoplastic transformation. By contrast, long-latency RNA-transforming viruses do not contain a viral oncogene, but rather a promoter gene. The integration of this promoter gene deregulates the expression of a cellular proto-oncogene (a process called insertional mutagenesis), again presumably leading to neoplastic transformation.

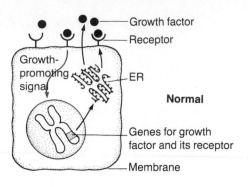

Growth factor

Receptor

Growth-promoting signal

ER

Normal

Genes for growth factor and its receptor

Membrane

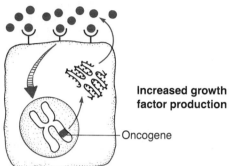

Increased growth factor production

Oncogene

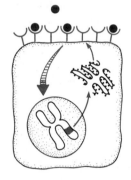

Increased number of receptors

Figure 5-26. Possible interactions between oncogenes and growth factors. Oncogenes may code directly for growth factors, alter the number or affinity of growth factor receptors, or change the sensitivity of the cell to growth factors.

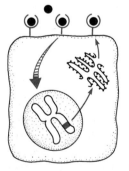

Increased affinity of receptors

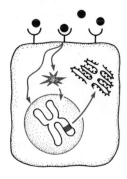

Increased sensitivity of cell (cytoplasm or nucleus) to signal

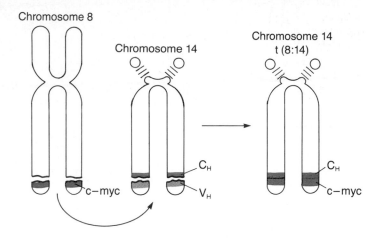

Figure 5-27. Chromosomal translocation in Burkitt's lymphoma. During interphase, the cellular *myc* gene (*c-myc*) on chromosome 8 is translocated to chromosome 14 adjacent to the gene coding for the constant region of an immunoglobulin heavy chain (C$_H$). A reciprocal translocation of the gene coding for the variable region of the heavy chain (V$_H$) from chromosome 14 to chromosome 8 occurs. During metaphase the altered chromosomes are duplicated, a process that results in both chromatids of each chromosome bearing the translocated genes. The expression of *c-myc* is enhanced by its new association with the actively transcribed immunoglobulin genes.

c-abl cellular proto-oncogene from its site on chromosome 9 to a critical region of chromosome 22. Unlike the situation in Burkitt's lymphoma, in which the *c-myc* gene product is unchanged in structure, the translocation producing the Philadelphia chromosome leads to a transcript that codes for an abnormal protein that has a much greater tyrosine kinase activity than the normal *c-abl* gene product. In other words, **the translocation produces a mutation that affects the biochemical function (a qualitative change) rather than the level of expression (a quantitative change) of a gene product.**

Reciprocal translocations are not the only form of chromosomal alterations that may be involved in carcinogenesis. Other nonrandom karyotypic abnormalities are trisomies, which represent the gain of a whole chromosome, and monosomies, which reflect a loss. For instance, trisomy 8 is common in acute leukemia and trisomy 12 in chronic B-cell leukemia. Extra copies of chromosome 7 have been noted in many melanomas and are consistently associated with the expression on the tumor cells of the receptor for epidermal growth factor. **A nonrandom loss of a whole chromosome or chromosomal segment is common in many leukemias.**

Gene deletion has been most extensively studied in children who harbor a hereditary predisposition to develop retinoblastoma, an otherwise rare ocular neoplasm. The disease is inherited as an autosomal recessive trait. These children typically show deletion of a segment of both copies of chromosome 13. Although the missing gene product has not been identified, some suspect it be an inhibitor of a normal process, possibly involving growth regulation.

Another type of genetic aberration that has been associated with changes in the function of oncogenes is gene dosage, represented by the term **gene ampli-**fication. This may take the form of many chromosomal copies of either the same gene or labile alternative forms. In some instances these changes have been shown to involve cellular or proto-oncogenes. Interestingly, it has been shown in cases of neuroblastoma that multiple copies of the *c-myc* gene are associated with the more aggressive stages of the tumor. Furthermore, amplification of a gene in the *erb* oncogene family to more than double the normal activity was a significant predictor of overall survival and time to relapse in patients with carcinoma of the breast. These observations on genetic alterations in cancer permit us to speculate that chromosome translocation may be an early event in the development of tumors, but that gene amplification is more important in the progression of the disease.

Gene Transfer as a Method of Cell Transformation

The DNA extracted from a malignant tumor has the ability to transform cells in culture, a process known as **transfection** (Fig. 5-28). Such transforming activity has been demonstrated in the DNA of 20% of a wide variety of primary human tumors and their cell lines. It is significant that the transforming oncogenes that have been identified by this technique of gene transfer are somatic mutants of normal proto-oncogenes restricted to tumor tissue. For example, the point mutations in the *c-ras* genes of human bladder, colon, and lung carcinomas encode proteins that bind to GTP but are not regulated by its hydrolysis. By contrast, the protein derived from the *neu* oncogene in a human cancer is a cell surface receptor that possesses tyrosine kinase activity and exhibits an extracellular domain resembling that of the epidermal

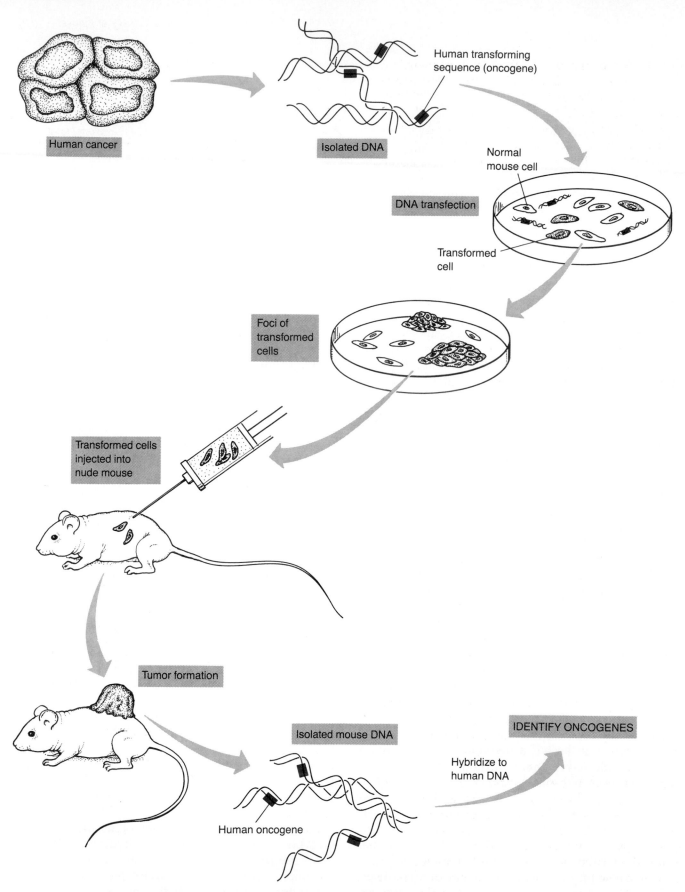

Human cancer

Isolated DNA

Human transforming
sequence (oncogene)

DNA transfection

Normal
mouse cell

Transformed
cell

Foci of
transformed
cells

Transformed cells
injected into
nude mouse

Tumor formation

Isolated mouse DNA

IDENTIFY ONCOGENES

Hybridize to
human DNA

Human oncogene

Figure 5-28. Identification of human oncogenes by DNA transfection. DNA from
a human cancer transforms cultured mouse cells. When injected into a nude
mouse, the transformed cells form tumors. DNA from the nude mouse tumor
contains the human oncogene, which is identified by hybridization with human DNA.

growth factor receptor. Although it is unclear why such a receptor should be oncogenic, the change in the configuration of the protein may be similar to that produced by the binding of a physiologic ligand, in which case unrestrained transduction of a growth signal might be maintained. Of great interest is the demonstration that antibodies against the products of the *c-ras* and *c-neu* oncogenes suppressed the neoplastic phenotype of cells carrying transforming alleles of these genes.

The Clonal Origin of Cancer

Studies of human and experimental tumors have provided strong evidence that most cancers arise from a single transformed cell. This theory has been most thoroughly examined in connection with proliferative disorders of the hematopoietic system. The most common piece of clinical evidence in its favor is the production of a single immunoglobulin unique to that patient by the neoplastic plasma cells of multiple myeloma. Indeed, such a "monoclonal spike" in the serum electrophoresis in a patient with suspected myeloma is regarded as conclusive evidence of the disease. Similarly, cell surface markers have also been used to establish a monoclonal origin for many other hematopoietic malignant disorders.

One of the most important observations in regard to the monoclonal origin of cancer was derived from the study of glucose-6-phosphate dehydrogenase in women who were heterozygous for its two isozymes, A and B (Fig. 5-29). These isozymes are encoded in genes located on the X chromosome, but only one of these genes is expressed in any given cell. Thus, whereas the genotypes of all cells are the same, their phenotypes vary with regard to the expression of isozyme A or B. An examination of benign uterine smooth muscle tumors (leiomyomas or "fibroids") revealed that all the cells in an individual tumor expressed only A or B, indicating that those cells were all derived from a single progenitor cell.

Despite their monoclonal origin, tumors often express considerable genetic instability as they progress. Neoplastic cells seem to be more susceptible than normal ones to chromosomal breakage, nondisjunction, sister chromatid exchange, and other alterations. There is reason to believe that this genetic instability may be related to the progress of cancer to more malignant phenotypes and perhaps even to the acquisition of invasive properties. **Although cancer may be caused by many agents, chemical, physical, and viral, they may all have a final common pathway, namely, damage to DNA.** The circumstantial evidence, while still not conclusive, incriminates cel-

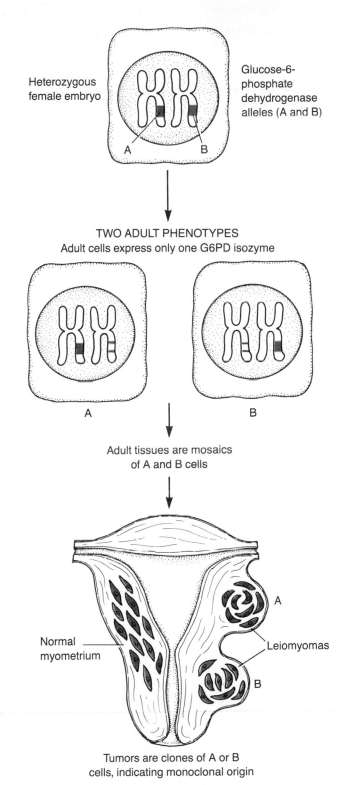

Figure 5-29. Monoclonal origin of human tumors.

lular proto-oncogenes as an important target of this damage.

Cancer As Altered Differentiation

The view that cancer represents aberrant cell differentiation is widely held. The altered phenotype of malignant cells has classically been interpreted as a "reversion" of the cell to a more primitive ancestral state. Such widely used terms as **"dedifferentiation"** and **"oncofetal gene expression"** attest to the prevailing view that malignant cells result from an alteration in a normal program of cellular differentiation. An alternative theory holds that cancer cells result from a maturation arrest in the sequence of development to a terminally differentiated cell—that is, human cancers are derived from normal stem cells. In many tumors **most of the neoplastic cells are outside the cell cycle and, thus, do not contribute to the malignancy of the tumor.** For example, as previously noted, fewer than 3% of the cells in a squamous carcinoma maintain the malignant potential of the tumor, and most differentiate and die spontaneously. **When such terminally differentiated tumor cells are transplanted into appropriate hosts, they do not grow, whereas their undifferentiated counterparts from the same tumor form typical squamous carcinomas.** Such observations raise the interesting possibility that the initial step in the development of some cancers is a **failure of the stem cell to differentiate normally.**

Evidence to support the concept of cancer as a failure of differentiation has come from the study of experimental, malignant germ cell tumors (teratocarcinomas). A single embryonal carcinoma cell, the stem cell of a teratocarcinoma, when transplanted into a mouse, gives rise to a tumor that contains cells derived from all three germ layers. Clearly, the progeny of the original transplanted tumor cell differentiate into more mature cells, which express recognizable phenotypes of more fully differentiated tissues. When these differentiated tissues of the teratocarcinoma are separated from the malignant embryonal cells and transplanted into compatible hosts, they not only survive, but function with no detriment to the host. These cells are clearly benign, and the dogma that "once a cancer cell, always a cancer cell" does not hold in this case.

A further refinement of this approach involves the transplantation of a single teratocarcinoma stem cell from one mouse into an early mouse embryo. At term, the entirely normal pup is a mosaic composed of cells derived from both the embryo proper and the teratocarcinoma. The progeny of the malignant cell, under the influence of normal epigenetic developmental controls, has differentiated into mature tissue elements. Thus, at least in the experimental situation, the altered expression of genetic information inherent in the definition of a cancer may be redirected into modes of expression that are normal for that particular cell.

Clinical analogies to the experimental situation do exist. The best known is illustrated by the rare spontaneous conversion of a malignant neuroblastoma to its better-differentiated, benign counterpart, the ganglioneuroma.

The most comprehensive systematic analysis of human neoplasia from the perspective of developmental biology has come from the study of leukemias and lymphomas. During normal B- and T-lymphocyte maturation, there are well-documented sequential changes of membrane antigens and rearrangements of immunoglobulin and T-cell receptor genes. In acute lymphoblastic leukemia of childhood, the neoplastic cells exhibit only partial assembly of the cell surface receptor molecules that characterize mature lymphocytes. In other words, the leukemic cell phenotype bears a strong resemblance to lymphocytes that appear transiently during the developmental sequence of the normal lymphocyte. Thus, the leukemic cells appear to be "frozen" in the act of receptor gene assembly and expression. Acute myeloid leukemia is similar to acute lymphoblastic leukemia in that the malignant cells express phenotypes of transient, immature myeloid populations. Likewise, studies of chronic lymphocytic leukemias and lymphomas have revealed that these malignant disorders represent clonal expansions of mature lymphocyte populations corresponding to subsets found in normal lymphoid tissue.

In normal hematopoietic maturation, differentiation is tightly coupled to proliferation—that is, terminally differentiated cells are continually lost, to be replaced by newly proliferated and differentiated cells. By contrast, the data reviewed above suggest that **certain leukemias and lymphomas are not truly proliferative disorders, but rather reflect an uncoupling of differentiation from proliferation, with the resulting accumulation of cells that have not attained terminal differentiation.** According to this theory, leukemia and lymphoma may represent the stabilization of a phenotype that is also expressed, though only transiently, in developing normal cells. It has been said that the cell phenotypes in a leukemia or lymphoma can be compared to the phenotype of the ostrich, which is thought to be "primitive and conserved rather than degenerate."

The view that certain cancers may reflect impaired differentiation has led to a search for maturation-enhancing drugs. The prototype of such an agent is a vitamin A derivative, the retinoid 13-cis-retinoic acid. The interest in the retinoids derives from experiments showing that administration of excess vitamin A or its derivatives inhibited chemically induced carcinogenesis in the skin, lung, bladder, colon, and mammary gland. However, as yet, there have not been adequate trials to assess the possible role of retinoids in the prevention or treatment of human cancer.

Conclusions

It is clear that many agents are capable of causing cancer and that no single known mechanism is sufficient to account for all the phenomena observed in neoplastic cells. The observations and theories discussed above are not mutually exclusive, and cancer may eventually be understood as a term that encompasses a variety of diseases, each with its distinct etiology and pathogenesis.

Tumor Immunology

It has long been recognized that malignant tumors elicit a chronic inflammatory response that is unrelated to necrosis or infection of the tumor. This observation led early investigators to postulate a host immune reaction to the neoplastic cells, but a refined understanding awaited the development of modern immunology. The inflammatory reaction is correlated with a better prognosis in some tumors, such as medullary carcinoma of the breast and seminoma, but in general no clear correlation exists. Although the infiltrate is composed principally of T cells and macrophages, suggesting a cell-mediated immune response, in most cases the antigens to which the cells respond have not been identified. Despite the paucity of direct evidence, it is clear from animal experiments that immune defenses against malignant tumors exist and may be important in humans.

To invoke a role for an immune defense against cancer, it is necessary to postulate that tumor cells express antigens that are different from normal cells and that are recognized as foreign by the host. Such a condition has been indirectly demonstrated in experiments with inbred mice (Fig. 5-30). When cells from a chemically or virally induced tumor are transplanted into a syngeneic mouse, the cells form a tumor. When cells from this tumor are passed into a second mouse, they again form a tumor. On the other hand, if the first transplanted tumor is removed before it metastasizes (i.e., the mouse is cured of its tumor), re-injection of the tumor cells back into the cured mouse will not produce a tumor. **The transplanted tumor is rejected because of immunity acquired as a result of the first tumor transplant.** Moreover, irradiated tumor cells or preparations of tumor cell membranes, when injected experimentally, augment resistance to tumor growth.

An important observation is that tumors induced by the same chemical in different mice are antigenically distinct, whereas those induced by the same virus express the same virally determined antigen. Accordingly, mice sensitized to one chemically induced tumor accept a second such tumor, whereas mice that have received a virus-induced tumor reject another similar tumor. These experiments provide compelling evidence that immunologic mechanisms can play a role in host defenses against tumors. However, the fact that tumor antigens can be demonstrated experimentally does not mean that they exist in all human cancers. Even if they do, their antigenicity and the strength of the immune response to them are not known.

Mechanisms of Immunologic Cytotoxicity

The specific rejection of transplanted tumors is mediated by T cells, as evidenced by the demonstration that lymphocytes from tumor-bearing hosts can transfer tumor immunity when injected into normal animals. Moreover, the transferred immunity is eliminated by the administration of antibodies directed against T cell antigens. The mechanisms of T-cell-mediated immunologic cell killing have been discussed in Chapter 4.

Another set of lymphocytes, the **natural killer (NK) cells,** have tumoricidal activity that is not dependent on prior sensitization. NK cells are identical with the large granular lymphocytes. Although tumors vary in their sensitivity to NK cells, these lymphocytes are generally more effective in killing tumor cells than untransformed cells. A different population of naturally occurring lymphocytes, **natural cytotoxic (NC) cells,** exerts a tumoricidal effect on some target cells that are resistant to NK cells. These lymphoid cells are clearly different from NK cells in their response to stimulation by interleukin-2 and in their resistance to corticosteroids. Proliferation of a third group of cells, the **lymphokine-activated killer (LAK) cells,** is also stimulated by interleukin-2, an effect that has been reported to hold some promise for cancer treatment.

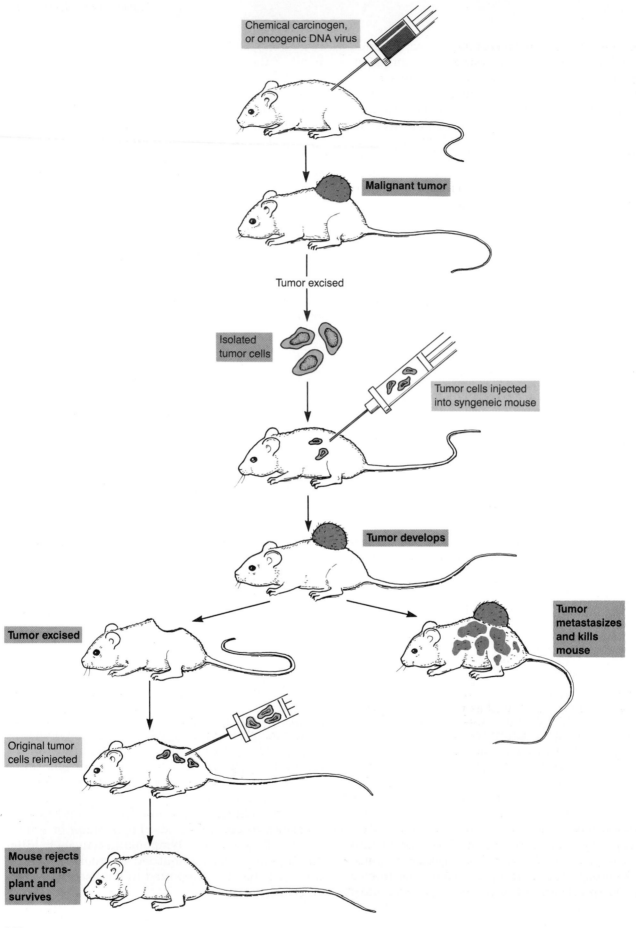

Chemical carcinogen, or oncogenic DNA virus

Malignant tumor

Tumor excised

Isolated tumor cells

Tumor cells injected into syngeneic mouse

Tumor develops

Tumor excised

Tumor metastasizes and kills mouse

Original tumor cells reinjected

Mouse rejects tumor transplant and survives

Macrophages are capable of killing tumor cells nonspecifically. Of the many lymphokines that stimulate macrophages, the most potent appears to be gamma interferon. Potential mediators of macrophage-mediated cytotoxicity are lysosomal enzymes, proteases, activated oxygen, and a cytotoxic protein resembling T cell "lymphotoxin." However, the role of macrophages in the immune control of malignant tumors is far from clear, since under some circumstances in vitro factors derived from macrophages can stimulate the proliferation of tumor cells and inhibit T-cell–mediated immunity.

Although tumor-associated antigens are capable of eliciting a humoral antibody response, these immunoglobulins by themselves are not capable of killing tumor cells. However, as discussed in Chapter 4, such antibodies can participate in antibody-dependent cell-mediated cytotoxicity and complement-dependent cell killing. Briefly, the antibody simultaneously binds to the tumor antigen and the Fc receptor of the effector cell, thereby bringing the effector cell into direct contact with its target. Depending on the conditions, the effectors may be lymphocyte killer cells, macrophages, or neutrophils. Alternatively, binding of an antibody to a tumor-associated antigen may trigger the complement cascade and lead to lysis of the malignant cell.

The mechanisms underlying immunologic cytotoxicity are summarized in Figure 5-31.

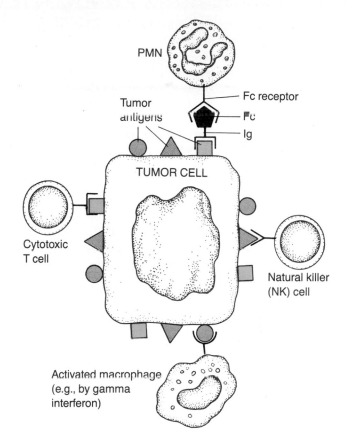

Figure 5-31. Mechanisms of immunologic tumor cytotoxicity.

Evasion of Immunologic Cytotoxicity

In view of the fact that cancer is alive and well despite the presence of potent immunologic defenses, it is necessary to postulate mechanisms by which tumors can evade immune destruction. It is intuitively clear that a lack of expressed antigens or a weak immunologic response to them will permit unhampered growth of the neoplasm. Certainly, **tumor-specific antigens have not been found as yet in the majority of human tumors,** and substantial variations in immunologic response, presumably of genetic origin, have been demonstrated in many clinical situations. Even when present, tumor antigens are not uniformly expressed in a given population of neoplastic cells. Since a few tumor cells lack the antigen, they will not be subject to immune attack and, therefore, will be selected for survival. Thus, in theory a tumor may initially be relatively vulnerable to immunologic defenses but may develop resistance in much the same way as bacteria develop resistance to antibiotics.

Tumor cells may also escape detection by the immune system by modulating their expression of surface membrane antigens. In the presence of antibodies against specific tumor antigen, this determinant may disappear from the cell surface, only to reappear after removal of the antibody. Although this modulation does not apply for all antigens, it remains a

Figure 5-30. Immunogenicity of tumors. Cancer cells injected into a syngeneic mouse form tumors, which metastasize and kill the animal. Excision of the tumor before it has metastasized allows the rejection of a second tumor implant, presumably as a consequence of immunity acquired from exposure to the original tumor.

possible mechanism by which tumor cells can escape from immunologic control.

Tumor cells may release antigens to the blood as secretory proteins (e.g., alpha-feto-protein) or as membrane vesicles. These antigens can then combine with circulating antibodies to form circulating immune complexes. Indeed, such complexes have been found in the blood of patients with a variety of tumors, although it has proved more difficult to identify the antigen in the circulating complexes. Moreover, the occurrence of membranous glomerulonephritis in patients with a number of epithelial neoplasms is attributed to the deposition in the kidney of immune complexes derived from antibodies that are specific for tumor plasma membrane antigens (e.g., carcinoembryonic antigen). Formation of circulating complexes might be expected to reduce the antibody titer in the blood and thus weaken antibody-dependent tumor cell killing. In addition, circulating immune complexes inhibit the effector cells involved in antibody-dependent cell killing.

When an antigen is injected intravenously, it bypasses the antigen-processing system of the lymph nodes and preferentially induces the proliferation of suppressor T cells. By contrast, the same antigen injected subcutaneously induces cell-mediated immunity. Since tumor cells release antigens directly into the circulation, it is possible that in addition to stimulating antibody production they may also stimulate the production of suppressor cells, thereby inhibiting the cell-mediated immune response. Cell-mediated immunity may also be inhibited by an alternative mechanism in which some epitopes of tumor-associated antigens trigger the proliferation of suppressor T cells directly.

Several nonspecific mechanisms have been invoked as inhibitors of the immune response to cancer. It is known that under some circumstances activated macrophages inhibit the proliferation of T cells, an activity possibly mediated by prostaglandins. In addition, a number of polypeptides secreted by tumors have been shown to inhibit proliferation of lymphocytes and chemotaxis. A third mechanism may stem from acute-phase reactants, which are secreted as a nonspecific reaction to injury, principally by the liver, and exert immunosuppressive effects.

Immune Surveillance

Considering the enormous number of chemical, viral, and physical agents that have been identified as potential carcinogens, it seems remarkable that the incidence of cancer is not far greater than current statistics indicate. Although it may be argued that exposure to these factors is random and that cancer develops only in those who are particularly susceptible, an equally attractive hypothesis holds that incipient neoplasms appear in the population at large with considerable frequency but are immediately recognized and eliminated. Shortly after the promlugation of the clonal selection theory of immune reactivity, it was postulated that cell-mediated immune responses recognize and expunge mutant clones with neoplastic potential.

This theory of **immune surveillance** has been supported by a number of experimental and clinical observations. The strongest evidence for immune surveillance by T cells comes from the observation that there is an increase in tumor induction by oncogenic DNA viruses in T-cell–deficient mice. (This increase is evident both in naturally deficient mice and in mice made deficient by thymectomy or treatment with thymus-specific antibodies.) About 10% of patients with a genetic T-cell deficiency develop cancer, principally of the lymphoproliferative variety. The occurrence of cancers in the immunosuppressed patients with AIDS also supports the immune surveillance concept. Immunosuppression to prevent transplant rejection has also been followed by a higher incidence of certain cancers.

It has been pointed out that the evidence for immune surveillance—that is, for a common mechanism for the elimination of all incipient neoplasms—is indirect, and wanting in many respects. Although a strong case can indeed be made in the case of highly antigenic oncogenic DNA-viruses, the theory appears weak with respect to other mechanisms of carcinogenesis. Nude mice, which are genetically deficient in T cells, do not exhibit an increased incidence of spontaneous tumors and are not more susceptible to tumor induction by RNA viruses or carcinogenic chemicals. In this regard, it is interesting to note that the tumors associated with AIDS—Kaposi's sarcoma and Burkitt's lymphoma—are suspected to result from infection with oncogenic DNA viruses, namely cytomegalovirus and Epstein-Barr virus, respectively. The theory of immune surveillance has now been revised to suggest that T cells are less important for surveillance than other effector cells, such as NK and NC cells and activated macrophages.

The Remote Effects of Cancer on the Host

The symptoms of cancer are, for the most part, referable to the local effects of either the primary tumor or its metastases. However, in a minority of patients, cancer produces remote effects that are not attributable to tumor invasion or to metastasis, and that are collectively termed **paraneoplastic syndromes.** Although such effects are rarely lethal, in some cases they dominate the clinical course. It is important to recognize these syndromes for several reasons. First, the signs and symptoms of the paraneoplastic syndrome may be the first clinical manifestation of a malignant tumor. When they are recognized, the cancer may be detected early enough to permit a cure. Second, the syndromes may be mistaken for those produced by advanced metastatic disease and may, therefore, lead to inappropriate therapy. Third, when the paraneoplastic syndrome itself is disabling, treatment directed toward alleviating those symptoms may have important palliative effects. Finally certain tumor products that result in paraneoplastic syndromes provide a means of monitoring recurrence of the cancer in patients who have had surgical resections or are undergoing chemotherapy or radiotherapy.

Fever

It is not uncommon for cancer patients to present initially with fever of unknown origin that cannot be explained by an infectious disease. Fever attributed to cancer correlates with tumor growth, disappears after treatment, and reappears on recurrence. The cancers in which this most commonly occurs are Hodgkin's disease, renal cell carcinoma, and osteogenic sarcoma, although many other tumors occasionally are complicated by fever. Tumor cells can themselves produce pyrogens, but the mechanism underlying tumor associated fever has not been elucidated.

Anorexia and Weight Loss

A paraneoplastic syndrome of anorexia, weight loss, and cachexia is very common in patients with cancer, often appearing before its malignant cause becomes apparent. Although cancer patients often have a decreased caloric intake because of anorexia and abnormalities of taste, restricted food intake does not explain the profound wasting so common among them; in fact, the mechanisms responsible are poorly understood. It is known, however, that unlike starvation, which is associated with a lowered metabolic rate, cancer is often accompanied by an elevated metabolic rate. Also of note is the recent discovery that **tumor necrosis factor,** a macrophage-derived substance that mediates tumor cell necrosis, is identical with **cachectin,** a similarly derived factor, which has profound catabolic effects at the cellular level. It is intriguing to speculate that the host reaction to the tumor may also be responsible for the wasting of cancer patients.

Endocrine Syndromes

Malignant tumors may produce a number of peptide hormones whose secretion is not under normal regulatory control. Most of these hormones are normally present in the brain or gastrointestinal tract, or in normal endocrine organs. Their inappropriate secretion can cause a variety of effects, as discussed below.

Cushing's Syndrome

Ectopic secretion of ACTH by a tumor leads to features of Cushing's syndrome, including hypokalemia, hyperglycemia, hypertension, and muscle weakness. The other prominent features of this syndrome, such as obesity, buffalo hump, and a moon facies, are less common. ACTH production is most commonly seen with cancers of the lung, particularly small cell (oat cell) carcinoma. It also complicates carcinoid tumors, thymomas and neuroendocrine tumors, such as pheochromocytomas, neuroblastomas, and medullary carcinomas of the thyroid.

Inappropriate Anti-Diuresis

The inappropriate production of arginine vasopressin (anti-diuretic hormone) causes sodium and water retention to such an extent that it is manifested as water intoxication, resulting in altered mental status, seizures, coma, and sometimes death. The tumors that most often produce this syndrome are small cell carcinomas of the lung, but it is also reported with carcinomas of the prostate, gastrointestinal tract, and pancreas, thymomas, lymphomas, and Hodgkin's disease.

Hypercalcemia

Hypercalcemia, a paraneoplastic complication that afflicts 10% of all cancer patients, is usually caused by metastatic disease of bone. However, in about one tenth of cases it occurs in the absence of bony metastases. In the latter situation, the tumor may produce parathormone, prostaglandins, osteoclast activating factor, and possibly other osteolytic agents. Hypercalcemia from bony involvement is most common with cancer of the breast and multiple myeloma; in the absence of metastases lung cancer is the usual culprit.

Hypocalcemia

Cancer-induced hypocalcemia is actually more common than hypercalcemia and complicates osteoblastic metastases from cancers of the lung, breast, and prostate. The cause of hypocalcemia is not known, but a role for tumor-secreted calcitonin has been postulated.

Hypophosphatemic Osteomalacia

Certain benign mesenchymal tumors are complicated by a vitamin D–resistant osteomalacia, characterized by phosphaturia and low serum phosphate and normal serum calcium levels. This syndrome is usually associated with neoplasms such as giant cell tumors of bone and large hemangiomas. The cause is obscure but may involve a vitamin D antagonist, abnormal metabolism of vitamin D, or a direct effect on the renal tubule to inhibit reabsorption of phosphate.

Gonadotropic Syndromes

Gonadotropins may be secreted by germ cell tumors, gestational trophoblastic tumors (choriocarcinoma, hydatidiform mole) and pituitary tumors. Less commonly, gonadotropin secretion is observed with hepatoblastomas in children and cancers of the lung, colon, breast, and pancreas in adults. High gonadotropin levels lead to precocious puberty in children, gynecomastia in men, and oligomenorrhea in premenopausal women.

Hyperthyroidism

A "hypermetabolic state" in cancer patients is not unusual, and frank hyperthyroidism is occasionally reported. This disorder may be caused by inappropriate secretion of the thyroid-stimulating hormone (TSH) or by very high levels of human chorionic gonadotropin (hCG) associated with choriocarcinoma.

Hypoglycemia

The best-understood cause of hypoglycemia associated with tumors is excessive insulin production by islet cell tumors of the pancreas. Other tumors, especially large mesotheliomas and fibrosarcomas, and primary hepatocellular carcinoma, are associated with hypoglycemia. The cause of hypoglycemia in nonendocrine tumors is not established, but the most likely candidate is production of somatomedins, a family of peptides normally produced by the liver under regulation by growth hormone.

Neurologic Syndromes

Neurologic disorders are common in cancer patients, usually resulting from metastases or from endocrine or electrolyte disturbances. Vascular, hemorrhagic, and infectious conditions affecting the nervous system are also common. However, there remains a small group of cancer patients who suffer from a variety of neurologic complaints without any demonstrable cause. Such disorders are thought to reflect remote effects of cancer on the nervous system. Cerebral complications may present as dementia, subacute cerebellar degeneration, or limbic encephalitis. In the spinal cord, a subacute motor neuropathy characterized by slowly developing lower motor neuron weakness without sensory changes is so strongly associated with cancer that an intensive search for an occult neoplasm, often a lymphoma, should be made in patients who present with these symptoms. In addition, a form of amyotrophic lateral sclerosis is well described among cancer patients, and conversely, many patients with this disease are found to have cancer. A rapidly ascending motor and sensory paralysis to the throacic level, with severe destruction of gray and white matter, has been described.

The peripheral nerves are also the site of paraneoplastic effects. A sensory-motor peripheral neuropathy, characterized by distal weakness and wasting and sensory loss, is common in cancer patients, and when not associated with an overt neoplasm suggests the possibility of an occult tumor. Interestingly, the removal of the primary tumor usually does not reverse the neuropathy. Autonomic and gastrointestinal neuropathies, manifested as orthostatic hypotension, neurogenic bladder, and intestinal pseudoobstruction, are associated with small cell carcinoma of the lung.

Paraneoplastic effects are also seen in the muscle and neuromuscular junction. Patients with dermatomyositis or polymyositis have an incidence of cancer five to seven time higher than the general population. The association is most striking in affected men over the age of 50 years, in whom more than 70% have a cancer. In most cases the muscle disorder and cancer present within a year of each other. An uncommon myasthenic (Eton-Lambert) syndrome is strongly associated with small cell carcinoma of the lung. Although the symptoms superficially resemble those of true myasthenia gravis, muscle strength improves with exercise and there is a poor response to an anti-cholinesterase (Tensilon). The association of true myasthenia gravis with thymoma is well recognized, although a wide variety of other tumors have on occasion been linked to this disorder of the neuromuscular junction.

Hematologic Syndromes

The most common hematologic complications of neoplastic disease result either from direct infiltration of the marrow or from treatment. However, hematologic paraneoplastic syndromes, which antedate the modern era of chemotherapy and radiotherapy, are well described. Cancer-associated erythrocytosis is a complication of some tumors, particularly renal cell carcinoma, primary hepatocellular carcinoma, and cerebellar hemangioblastoma. Interestingly, benign kidney disease, such as cystic disease or hydronephrosis, and uterine myomas can lead to erythrocytosis. Elevated erythropoietin levels are found in the tumor and in the serum in about half of the patients with erythrocytosis. The diagnosis of erythrocytosis is made when there is an increased red blood cell mass.

One of the most common findings in patients with cancer is anemia, but the mechanism for this disorder is not clear. The anemia is usually normocytic and normochromic, although iron deficiency anemia is common in cancers that bleed into the gastrointestinal tract, such as colorectal cancers. Pure red cell aplasia, often associated with thymomas, and megaloblastic anemia are sometimes encountered. Autoimmune hemolytic anemia may be associated with B-cell neoplasms and with solid tumors, particularly in the elderly. In fact, autoimmune hemolytic anemia in an older person suggests the possibility of an underlying neoplasm. Microangiopathic hemolytic anemia is occasionally seen, often in association with disseminated intravascular coagulation and thrombotic thrombocytopenic purpura.

The peripheral granulocyte count in patients with many nonhematologic cancers may be raised to over 20,000/μl, a finding that may lead to an erroneous diagnosis of leukemia. The mechanism underlying this paraneoplastic effect is not understood. Eosinophilia is occasionally noted, particularly in Hodgkin's disease, where it may occur in one-fifth of cases. Between 30% and 40% of cancer patients exhibit a thrombocytosis, with platelet counts above 400,000/μl. The platelet count usually returns to normal with successful treatment of the malignant disease. Thrombocytopenia, similar to that of idiopathic thrombocytopenic purpura, is seen in rare instances. However, an immune mechanism has not been demonstrated.

The Hypercoagulable State

The association between cancer and **thrombophlebitis** was noted more than a century ago. Since then other abnormalities resulting from a hypercoagulable state—for example **disseminated intravascular coagulation** and **nonbacterial thrombotic endocarditis**—have been recognized. The cancers most commonly associated with thrombophlebitis are carcinoma of the lung, pancreas, and gastrointestinal tract, but tumors of the breast, ovary, prostate, and other organs may also lead to this complication. The cause of this hypercoagulable state is debated.

Disseminated intravascular coagulation in association with cancer may come to attention because of the chronic occurrence of thrombotic phenomena or an acute hemorrhagic diathesis, or as a coagulation disorder detected by laboratory tests alone. This complication is most commonly found with acute promyelocytic leukemias and adenocarcinomas. Nonbacterial thrombotic endocarditis—the presence of noninfected verrucous deposits of fibrin and platelets adherent to the left-sided heart valves—occurs with or without disseminated intravascular coagulation. Although the effects on the heart are not of clinical importance, emboli to the brain present a great danger. Paraneoplastic endocarditis may develop early in the course of a cancer and signal its presence long before the tumor would otherwise become symptomatic. This cardiac complication is most common with solid tumors, but may occasionally be seen with leukemias and lymphomas.

Gastrointestinal Syndromes

About half of cancer patients develop histologic abnormalities of the small intestine, and some of these are associated with **malabsorption** of a variety of dietary components. The classic tumor associated with malabsorption is lymphoma of the small intestine. However, such changes can occur even with tumors that do not directly involve the bowel. In a few cases the very common finding of **hypoalbuminemia,** usually a result of paraneoplastic depression of albumin synthesis by the liver, is attributable to a **protein-losing enteropathy.** In this paraneoplastic disorder, there is an exudative loss of proteins into the bowel lumen, sometimes as a result of mucosal inflammation and occasionally without recognizable morphologic abnormalities.

Renal Syndromes

It is well known that patients with cancer develop the **nephrotic syndrome** as a consequence of **renal vein thrombosis** or amyloidosis. In addition, however, the nephrotic syndrome may represent a paraneoplastic complication in the form of lipoid nephrosis (glomerular epithelial cell disease) or a glomerulonephritis produced by the deposition of immune complexes. Although the antigens in glomerulonephritis of this kind are not generally identified, tumor-specific antibodies and carcinoembryonic antigen-antibody complexes have been eluted from the kidneys in a few cases.

Cutaneous Syndromes

Pigmented lesions and keratoses are well-recognized paraneoplastic effects. **Acanthosis nigricans,** a cutaneous disorder marked by hyperkeratosis and pigmentation of the axilla, neck, flexures, and anogenital region is of particular interest. **More than half of patients with acanthosis nigricans have cancer.** Development of the disease may precede, accompany, or follow the detection of the cancer. Over 90% of the cases occur in association with gastrointestinal carcinomas, tumors of the stomach accounting for half to two-thirds. Regression of the skin lesions after removal of the cancer has been recorded in a few cases. In rare instances the sudden development or rapid increase in the size of **seborrheic keratoses** heralds the presence of a malignant tumor. Certain lymphomas and Hodgkin's disease are complicated by an **exfoliative dermatitis** without any cutaneous involvement by tumor. An unusual skin disorder, **erythema gyratum repans,** which presents with scaling and itching, is seen almost exclusively in cancer patients.

Amyloidosis

About 15% of cases of **amyloidosis** occur in association with cancers, particularly with multiple myeloma and renal cell carcinoma but also with other solid tumors and lymphomas. The presence of amyloidosis implies a poor prognosis; in myeloma patients with the disorder the median survival is 14 months or less.

Heredity and Cancer

The etiology of cancer, as of most diseases, is intertwined with both hereditary and environmental factors. As an example, although smoking is unques-
tionably an environmental cause of cancer, only a minority of smokers develop any of the cancers associated with it. A parallel can be drawn with the effects of radiation. Although the incidence of leukemia was considerably increased in the Japanese survivors of the atom bomb explosions, only a small proportion of these individuals developed leukemia or any other cancer. In both of these examples, "constitutional" or hereditary factors presumably influence the development of cancer. In as genetically diverse a population as man, it is unlikely that many cancers have either a purely environmental or an unequivocally hereditary etiology. In all probability they constitute a continuum in which both these components contribute to a greater or lesser extent. Compounding this uncertainty is our ignorance of most of the environmental and hereditary factors that may be involved. Against this background we shall discuss those malignant disorders in which we know that genetic determinants are crucial because they are inherited according to Mendelian laws.

The hereditary tumors can be arbitrarily divided into three categories: malignant tumors inherited as such—for example, retinoblastoma, Wilms' tumor, and many endocrine tumors; benign inherited tumors that remain benign or have a malignant potential, as in familial polyposis of the colon; and inherited syndromes associated with a high risk of malignant tumors, such as Bloom's syndrome and ataxia-telangiectasia. Most of these are discussed in detail in the chapters dealing with specific organs, and selected examples are given in Table 5-1. In most cases the underlying genetic defect responsible for the tumor development is totally unknown, but in a few cases there are hints as to the underlying abnormality. Patients with Bloom's syndrome, ataxia-telangiectasia, and Fanconi's anemia display defects in DNA repair. Adenomatous polyps are the precursor of most colorectal adenocarcinomas, and it is not surprising that familial polyposis of the colon is associated with a high incidence of intestinal cancer. Similarly, von Recklinghausen's disease (neurofibromatosis) is complicated by malignant schwannomas and neurogenic sarcomas, and hereditary multiple trichoepitheliomas convert to basal and squamous cell carcinomas.

Some disorders that are difficult to classify, called **phakomatoses,** have both developmental and neoplastic features. The tumors associated with these syndromes mostly involve the nervous system.

Although only a small proportion of all cancers show a Mendelian pattern of inheritance, certain cancers show an undeniable tendency to run in families. It is estimated that for many tumors other members of the family of an affected individual have a twofold

Table 5-1. Inherited Neoplasia Syndromes

DISEASE	ASSOCIATED NEOPLASMS	INHERITANCE*
Chromosomal Instability Syndromes		
Bloom's syndrome	Leukemia, gastrointestinal cancer	R
Fanconi's anemia	Leukemia, squamous cell carcinoma, hepatoma	R
Werner's syndrome	Sarcomas	R
Hereditary Skin Diseases		
Nevi	Malignant melanoma	D
Giant hairy nevi	Malignant melanoma	D
Xeroderma pigmentosum	Skin cancers	R
Multiple trichoepitheliomas	Basal and squamous cell carcinomas	D
Epidermodysplasia verruciformis	Basal cell carcinoma, Bowen's disease, squamous carcinoma	R
Familial atypical nevi	Malignant melanoma	D
Nevoid basal carcinoma syndrome	Basal cell carcinoma, medulloblastoma, ovarian carcinoma	D
Tylosis	Esophageal cancer	D
Endocrine System		
Multiple endocrine neoplasia syndromes	Adenomas of endocrine glands	D
Nervous System		
Retinoblastoma	Retinoblastoma	D
Neuroblastoma	Neuroblastoma	R
Phacomatoses		
Neurofibromatosis (von Recklinghausen's disease)	Fibrosarcoma, schwannoma, meningioma, optic glioma	D
Tuberous sclerosis	Glial tumors, rhabdomyoma of heart, amgiomyolipoma of kidney	D
von Hippel-Lindau syndrome	Cerebellar hemangioblastoma, retinal angioma, other hemangiomas	D and R
Sturge-Weber syndrome	Multiple angiomas	D
Gastrointestinal System		
Familial polyposis coli	Intestinal polyps and carcinomas	D
Gardener's syndrome	Intestinal polyps and cancers, osteomas, fibromas	D
Peutz-Jegher's syndrome	Intestinal polyps and cancers	D
Vascular Syndromes		
Osler-Weber-Rendu syndrome	Angiomas	D
Multiple angiolipomas	Angiolipomas	D
Ataxia-telangiectasia	Lymphoma, leukemia, gastric cancer, brain tumors	R
Urogenital System		
Gonadal dysgenesis	Gonadoblastoma, dysgerminoma	R
Wilms' tumor		R and D
Immunologic Syndromes		
Agammaglobulinemia (Swiss type)	Lymphoma, leukemia	R
X-linked agammaglobulinemia	Lymphoma, leukemia	XR
DiGeorge syndrome	Squamous carcinoma of upper respiratory tract	D
Wiscott-Aldrich syndrome	Lymphoma	XR
Severe combined immunodeficiency	Lymphoma, leukemia, sarcoma	XR
Family Cancer Syndrome	Carcinomas of colon, breast, endometrium, lung	D

*D, autosomal dominant; R, autosomal recessive; XR, X-linked recessive to threefold increase in risk of developing the same cancer. This predisposition is particularly marked for cancer of the breast and colon. The interplay of heredity and environment is exemplified by the case of lung cancer. Smokers who are closely related to a person with lung cancer have a higher risk of developing lung cancer themselves than smokers without this familial background.

The Epidemiology of Cancer

The causes of cancer in humans are clearly not accessible at the present time, but there is ample reason to believe that, at least in some cases, chemical, viral, physical, and genetic factors are involved. This is not to deny the possibility that other agents or mechanisms, as yet unknown, may also be important in the pathogenesis of many human cancers. Experimental studies require exposure of animals to specific agents, and obviously this approach cannot be used for the study of human neoplasia. In attempts to identify the etiologies of human cancers, epidemiologic studies have been used. Such studies, which correlate the occurrence of cancers in defined human populations residing in specified geographic locations with genetic and environmental factors have yielded important clues. In the following discussion we will not deal with occupational epidemiology or exposure to specific agents, such as tobacco smoke or alcohol, since these are treated in Chapter 8.

The mere compilation of raw epidemiologic data is of little use unless they are subjected to careful analysis. In evaluating the relevance of epidemiologic observations to cancer causation, the following criteria are germane:

Strength of the association
Consistency under different circumstances
Specificity
Temporality (i.e., the cause must precede the effect)
Biologic gradient (i.e., there is a dose-response relationship)
Plausibility
Coherence (i.e., a cause-and-effect relationship does not violate basic biologic principles)
Analogy to other known associations.

It is not mandatory that a valid epidemiologic study satisfy all these criteria, nor does adherence to them guarantee that the hypothesis derived from the data is necessarily true. However, as a guideline they remain useful.

The major epidemiologic studies have been concerned with the incidence of and mortality from cancers in different populations, in defined populations at different times, in specified geographic areas, and in migrants from one locale to another. We will here discuss only a few representative examples.

The Incidence of Cancer in the United States

Cancer accounts for one fifth of the total mortality in the United States, and is the second leading cause of death after cardiovascular diseases and stroke. For most cancers death rates in the United States have largely remained flat over the last 50 years, with some notable exceptions (Figure 5-32). The death rate from cancer of the lung among men has risen dramatically from 1930, when it was an uncommon tumor, to the present, when it is by far the most common cause of death from cancer in men. As discussed in Chapter 8, the entire epidemic of lung cancer deaths is attributable to smoking. Among women, smoking did not become fashionable until World War II. Considering the time lag needed between starting to smoke and the development of cancer of the lung, it is not surprising that the increased death rate from cancer of the lung in women did not become significant until after 1965. By 1983 the death rate from lung cancer in women exceeded that for breast cancer in nine states, and it is now, as in men, the most common fatal cancer. By contrast, for reasons difficult to fathom, cancer of the stomach, which in 1930 was by far the most common cancer in men, and was only slightly less common than breast cancer in women, has shown a remarkable and sustained decline in frequency. Similarly, there has been an unexplained decline in the death rate from cancer of the uterus, although better screening, diagnostic, and therapeutic methods may account for some of this reduction. The ranking of the incidence of tumors in men and women in the United States is shown in Table 5-2.

Individual cancers have their own age-related profiles, but for most, increased age is associated with an increased incidence. The most striking example of the dependency on age is carcinoma of the prostate, in which the incidence increases 30-fold between age 50 and 85 years. Certain neoplastic diseases, such as acute lymphoblastic leukemia in children and testicular cancer in young adults, show different age-related peaks of incidence (Fig. 5-33).

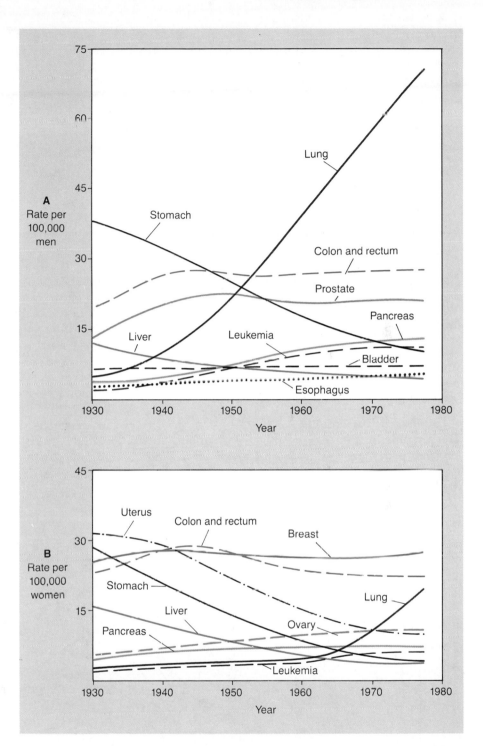

Figure 5-32. Cancer death rates in the United States over the last 50 years. *(A)* In men a striking increase in the incidence of cancer of the lung is attributable to smoking, whereas the sharp decline in stomach cancer is unexplained. *(B)* Increased smoking among women has led to a corresponding increase in cancer of the lung. The unexplained decrease in cancer of the stomach has been paralleled by a similar reduction in cancer of the uterus.

Table 5-2 Most Common Tumor Types in Men and Women

MEN		WOMEN	
TYPE	%	TYPE	%
Lung	20	Breast	27
Prostate	20	Colon and rectum	16
Colon and rectum	14	Lung	11
Urinery	10	Uterus	10
Leukemia and lymphoma	8	Leukemia and Lymphoma	7
Oral	4	Ovary	4
Skin	3	Urinery	4
Pancreas	3	Pancreas	3
All others	18	Skin	3
		Oral	2
		All others	13

Geographic and Ethnic Differences in Cancer Incidence

Nasopharyngeal Cancer

Nasopharyngeal cancer is rare in most of the world except for certain regions of China, Hong Kong, and Singapore. This type of cancer has been associated with infection by the Epstein-Barr virus.

Esophageal Carcinoma

The range in incidence of esophageal carcinoma varies from extremely low in Mormon women in Utah to a value some 300 times higher in the female population of Northern Iran. Particularly high rates of esophageal cancer are noted in a so-called Asian esophageal cancer belt, which includes the great landmass stretching from European Russia to Eastern China. Interestingly, throughout this belt, as the incidence rises the proportional excess in males decreases, and in some of the areas of highest incidence there is even a female excess. The disease is also more common in certain regions of black Africa and among blacks in the United States. The causes of esophageal cancer are obscure, but it is known that it disproportionately affects the poor in many areas of the world, and the combination of high alcohol consumption and smoking is associated with a particularly high risk.

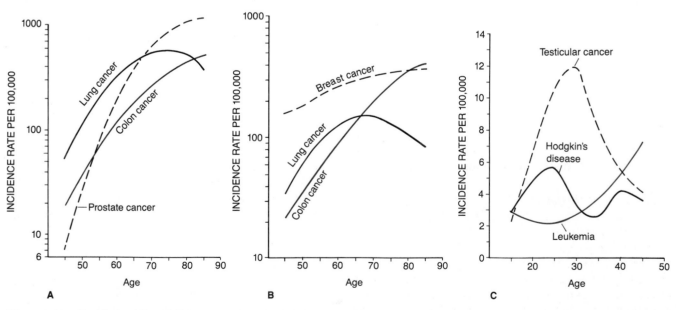

Figure 5-33. Incidence of specific cancers as a function of age. *(A)* Men. *(B)* Women. *(C)* Testicular cancer in men and Hodgkin's disease and leukemia in both sexes. The incidence of these cancers in *C* peaks at younger ages than do those in *A* and *B*.

Stomach Cancer

The highest incidence of stomach cancer is seen in Japan, where the disease is almost ten times as frequent as it is among American whites. A high incidence has also been observed in Latin American countries, particularly Chile. Stomach cancer is also common in Iceland and Eastern Europe.

Colorectal Cancer

The highest incidence of colorectal cancer is found in the United States, where it is three or four times more common than in Japan, India, Africa, and Latin America. It has been theorized that the high fiber content of the diet in low-risk areas and the high fat content in the United States are related to this difference.

Liver Cancer

There is a strong correlation between the incidence of primary hepatocellular carcinoma and the prevalence of hepatitis B infection. Endemic regions for both diseases include large parts of sub-Saharan Africa and most of the Orient, Indonesia, and the Philippines. It must be remembered, too, that levels of aflatoxin B_1 are high in the staple diets of many of the high-risk areas.

Skin Cancers, Including Melanoma

As previously noted the rates for skin cancers vary with skin color and exposure to the sun. Thus, particularly high rates have been reported in Northern Australia, where the population is principally of Celtic origin and sun exposure is intense. Increased rates of skin cancer have also been noted among the white population of the American Southwest. The lowest rates are found among people with pigmented skin, for example Japanese, Chinese, and Indians. The rates for African blacks, despite their heavily pigmented skin, are occasionally higher than those for orientals, because of the higher incidence of melanomas of the soles and palms in this groups.

Carcinoma of the Breast

Breast cancer, the most common female cancer in many parts of Europe and North America, shows considerable geographic variation. The rates in African and Asian populations are only a fifth to a sixth of those prevailing in Europe and the United States. Epidemiologic studies have contributed little to our understanding of the etiology of breast cancer. Although hormonal factors are clearly involved, except for a good correlation with age at first pregnancy, few confirmed correlations have surfaced.

Cancer of the Cervix

Striking differences in the incidence of squamous carcinoma of the cervix exist between ethnic groups and different socioeconomic levels. For instance, the very low rate in Ashkenazi Jews of Israel contrasts with a 25 times greater rate in the Hispanic population of Texas. In general, groups of low socioeconomic status have a higher incidence of cervical cancer than the more prosperous and better educated. This cancer is also directly correlated with early sexual activity and multiparity and is rare among women who are not sexually active, such as nuns. It is also uncommon among women whose husbands are circumcised. An association with human papillomaviruses has been demonstrated, and cervical cancer may eventually be classed as a venereal disease.

Choriocarcinoma

Choriocarcinoma, an uncommon cancer of trophoblastic differentiation, is found principally in women following a pregnancy, although it can present as a testicular tumor. The rates of this disease are particularly high in the rim of Asia (Singapore, Hong Kong, Japan, and the Philippines).

Prostatic Cancer

Very low incidences are reported for oriental populations, particularly Japanese, whereas the highest rates described are in American blacks, in whom the disease occurs some 25 times more often. The incidence in American and European whites is intermediate.

Testicular Cancer

An unusual aspect of testicular cancer is its universal rarity among black populations. Interestingly, while the rate in American blacks is only about one-fourth that in whites, it is still considerably higher than the rate among African blacks.

Cancer of the Penis

This squamous carcinoma is virtually nonexistent among circumcised men of any race, but is common in many parts of Africa and Asia. Interestingly, in the highlands of New Guinea, where both circumcision and washing are rarely practiced, this tumor is also rare, a finding that is contrary to expectation.

Cancer of the Urinary Bladder

The rates for transitional cell carcinoma of the bladder are fairly uniform. Squamous carcinoma of the bladder, however, is a special case. Ordinarily far rarer than transitional cell carcinoma, it has a high incidence in areas where schistosomal infestation of the bladder (bilharziasis) is endemic.

Burkitt's Lymphoma

Burkitt's lymphoma, a disease of children, was first described in Uganda, where it accounts for half of all childhood tumors. Since then a high frequency has been observed in other African countries, particularly in hot, humid lowlands. It has been noted that these are areas where malaria is also endemic. High rates have been recorded in other tropical areas, such as Malaysia and New Guinea, but European and American cases are encountered only sporadically. In view of the association between Burkitt's lymphoma and infection with the Epstein-Barr virus, it has been postulated that very early exposure to this virus, combined with chronic antigenic stimulation such as occurs in malaria, may lead to the development of malignant lymphoma.

Multiple Myeloma

This malignant tumor of plasma cells is uncommon among American whites but displays a three to four times higher incidence in American and South African blacks.

Chronic Lymphocytic Leukemia

Chronic lymphocytic leukemia is common among elderly people in Europe and North America, but is considerably less common in Japan.

Studies of Migrant Populations

Although planned experiments on the etiology of human cancer are hardly feasible, certain populations have unwittingly performed such experiments by migrating from one environment to another. Initially at least, the genetic characteristics of such people remained the same, but the new environment differed in climate, diet, infectious agents, occupations, and so on. Consequently, **epidemiologic studies of migrant populations (see Fig. 5-1) have provided many intriguing clues to the factors that may influence the pathogenesis of cancer.** The United States, which has been the destination of one of the greatest population movements of all time, is the source of most of the important data in this field.

Cancer of the Stomach

A study of Japanese residents of Hawaii found that migrants from Japanese regions with the highest risk of stomach cancer continued to exhibit an excess risk in Hawaii. By contrast, their offspring who were born in Hawaii had the same incidence of this cancer as American whites. Although dietary factors, such as pickled vegetables and salted fish, have been postulated to account for the higher incidence in Japan and the lower incidence in Hawaii, no firm evidence has been adduced to support this contention. More recently it has been shown in Japan that the population in regions at high risk for stomach cancer also display a high prevalence of chronic atrophic gastritis with intestinal metaplasia, lesions that are considered precursors of gastric cancer. Interestingly, when individuals from these regions move to low-risk areas, they carry the high prevalence of intestinal metaplasia with them. Thus, the environmental factors associated with stomach cancer may not be directly carcinogenic but rather may be related to atrophic gastritis and intestinal metaplasia.

Colorectal, Breast, Endometrial, Ovarian, and Prostatic Cancer

Migrant studies of the incidence of colorectal cancer show opposite trends to those of stomach cancer. Migrants from low-risk areas in Europe and Japan exhibit an increased risk of colorectal cancer in the United States. Moreover, their offspring continue at higher risk and reach the incidence levels of the general American population. This rule for colorectal cancer also obtains for cancers of the breast, endometrium, ovary, and prostate.

Cancer of the Liver

As previously noted, primary hepatocellular carcinoma is common in Asia and Africa, where it has been associated with hepatitis B. In American blacks and orientals, however, the neoplasm is no more common than in American whites, a situation that presumably reflects the low prevalence of hepatitis B in the United States.

Burkitt's Lymphoma

Emigrants to lowland areas from highland regions in Central Africa, where Burkitt's lymphoma is rare, develop tumors at an older age than do those born in endemic areas. This presumably reflects a later age of exposure to the Epstein-Barr virus or a more potent stimulation of the antigenic response by malaria. Moreover, the incidence of Burkitt's lymphoma is higher among emigrants to high-risk areas than among the same group who stay in the low-risk areas, and, indeed, higher than among adults who were born in the high-risk area. It is probable that many adults in the high-risk areas who have escaped Burkitt's lymphoma in their youth are immune to the disease.

Hodgkin's Disease

In general, in poorly developed countries the childhood form of Hodgkin's disease is the one seen most often. In the developed Western countries, by contrast, the disease is most common among young adults. Such a pattern is characteristic of certain viral infections, although there is no evidence for an infectious etiology of Hodgkin's disease. An exception to this generalization is noted in Japan, a developed country where young adult disease is distinctly uncommon. Further evidence for an environmental influence is the increased incidence of Hodgkin's disease in Americans of Japanese descent compared to that in Japan.

SUGGESTED READING

Books
DeVita VT, Jr, Hellman S, Rosenberg SA: Cancer: Principles and Practice of Oncology, 2nd ed. Philadelphia, JB Lippincott, 1985

Pitot HC: Fundamentals of Oncology, 3rd ed. New York, Marcel Dekker, 1986

Review Articles
Baserga R: The cell cycle. New Engl J Med 304; 453, 1981
Bishop JM: Cellular oncogenes and retroviruses. Annu Rev Biochem 52:301, 1983
Bishop JM: The molecular basis of cancer. Science 235:305, 1987
Farber E, Sarma DSR: Hepatocarcinogenesis: A dynamic cellular perspective. Lab Invest 56:4, 1987
Greaves MF: Differentiation-linked leukemogenesis in lymphocytes. Science 234:697, 1986
Nowell PC, Croce CM: Chromosomes, genes, and cancer. Am J Pathol 125:8, 1986
Pierce GB: Neoplasms, differentiations and mutations. 77:103, 1974
Duesberg PH: Activated proto-onc genes: Sufficient or necessary for cancer? Science 228:669, 1985

Original Articles
Slamon DJ, Clark GM, Wong SG, et al: Human breast cancer: Correlation of relapse and survival with amplification of the HER-2/neu oncogene, Science 235:177, 1987

6

Developmental and Genetic Diseases

Ivan Damjanov

Magnitude of the Problem

Principles of Teratology

Errors of Morphogenesis

Chromosomal Abnormalities

Single-Gene Abnormalities

Multifactorial Inheritance

Prenatal Diagnosis of Genetic Disorders

Diseases of Infancy and Childhood

Figure 6-1. Squash preparation of human chromosomes stained by the Giemsa banding technique. The X chromosome is enlarged and depicted schematically.

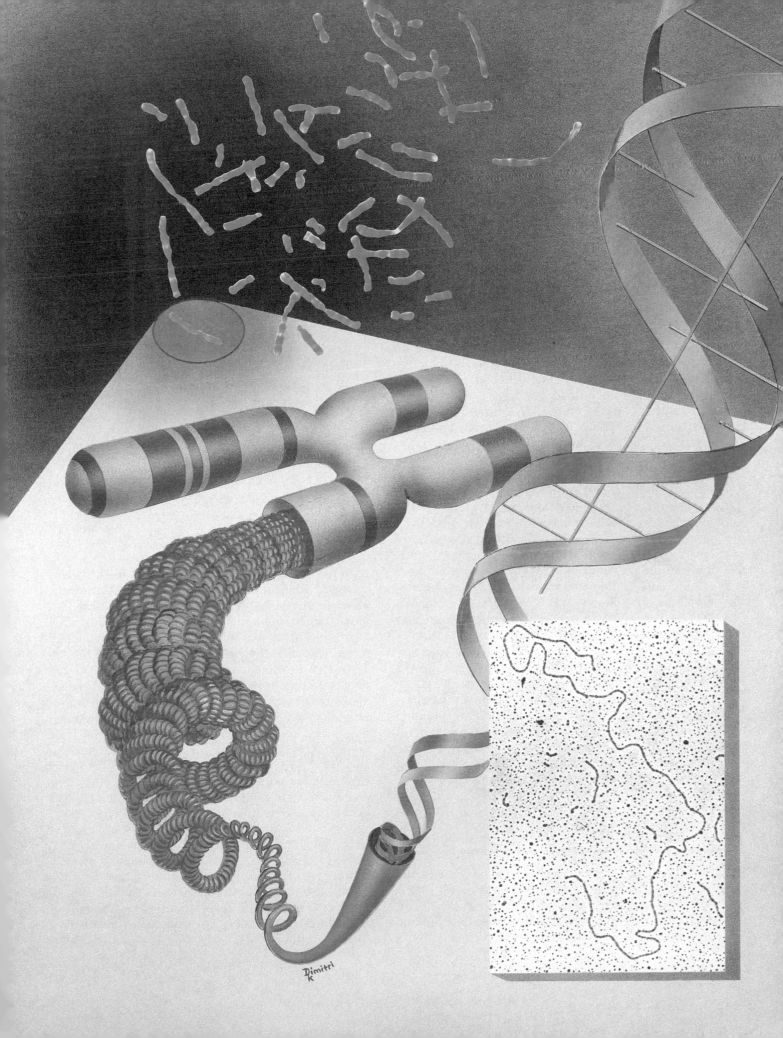

It has been known since biblical times that certain disorders are inherited or related to disturbances in intrauterine development. The earliest sanitary codices contain guidelines on how to choose a healthy spouse, how to conceive healthy children, and what to do or not do during pregnancy. Nevertheless, most of our present scientific knowledge about developmental and genetic disorders has been gathered only within the last three decades, and the exponential growth of molecular genetics promises that the coming years will witness even more progress in this area, appropriately called **prenatal medicine.**

Disorders that can be traced to prenatal stages of human development form a heterogeneous group that is best considered as a broad spectrum. At one end of the spectrum are diseases caused by adverse exogenous influences. At the other end are the disorders that are genetically determined and are not related to environmental factors. Between these two extremes are numerous pathologic conditions that are genetically predetermined but have a pathogenesis that depends largely on the interaction between the developing organism, the maternal body, and other external influences.

For didactic purposes it is customary to classify the origins of developmental and genetic disorders as **errors of morphogenesis, cytogenetic (chromosomal) abnormalities, single-gene defects, or multifactorial (polygenic) inheritance.** For the sake of completeness, we also include fetopathies due to **adverse transplacental influences** during intrauterine life, **fetal deformities and injuries** caused by mechanical intrauterine and intrapartal trauma, and **diseases of infancy and childhood.** It is important to remember that such classifications are artificial and arbitrary and that many categories overlap. Thus, many errors of morphogenesis are caused by a faulty gene, and several chromosomal abnormalities occur in families—a finding that suggests the existence of a heritable disease. It is even more important to maintain perspective and realize that some conditions now assigned to one category will eventually be reclassified in another because of the discovery of a subtle chromosomal abnormality or an abnormal gene activity that underlies the pathogenesis of faulty morphogenesis.

Magnitude of the Problem

Each year, about a quarter of a million babies are born in the United States with a birth defect that is either evident at the time of birth or initially latent, only to become clinically manifest later in childhood or in adult life. Several surveys from different coun-

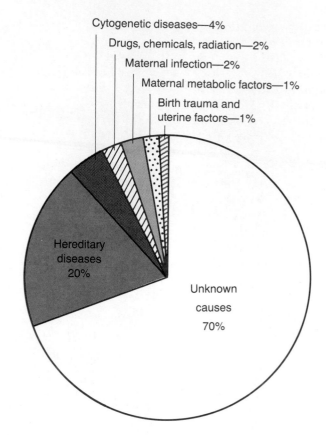

Figure 6-2. Causes of birth defects in man. Most birth defects have unknown causes.

tries have shown that, worldwide, at least 1 in 50 newborn infants has a major congenital anomaly, about 1 in 100 has a single-gene abnormality, and about 1 in 200 has a major chromosomal abnormality.

In more than two-thirds of all birth defects diagnosed clinically, the cause is not determined (Fig. 6-2). In a minority of cases the defect can be related to uterine factors (<1%), maternal factors, such as metabolic imbalance (1–2%), maternal infections during pregnancy (2–3%), or other adverse environmental influences, such as exposure to drugs, chemicals, or radiation (1–3%). Genetic diseases account for the remaining 15% to 20% of disorders. In 3% to 5% of children born with a congenital anomaly, cytogenetic analysis reveals an abnormal karyotype (i.e., a structural or numerical chromosomal abnormality).

Although chromosomal abnormalities account for only a small fraction of birth defects in newborn infants, cytogenetic analysis of fetuses spontaneously aborted in early pregnancy indicates that approximately two-thirds show chromosomal abnormalities. The incidence of specific numerical chromosomal abnormalities in the abortuses is several times higher than in term infants, indicating that **most inborn**

chromosomal defects are lethal. The conceptus dies in early pregnancy, and only a small number of children with cytogenetic abnormalities are born alive.

In highly developed Western countries, developmental and genetic birth defects account for approximately half of the total mortality in infancy and childhood. This contrasts with the situation in less developed countries, where 95% of infant mortality is attributable to environmental causes, such as poor sanitation and nutrition. In these countries, improved economic conditions should reduce infant mortality. In contrast, genetic counseling, early prenatal diagnosis, identification of high-risk pregnancies, and avoidance of possible exogenous teratogens are at the present time the only practical approaches that can reduce the mortality due to birth defects in the more developed countries.

Principles of Teratology

The discipline concerned with the study of developmental anomalies is called **teratology** (Greek *teraton,* "monster"). Chemical, physical, and biological agents that cause developmental anomalies are known as **teratogens.** There are very few agents of proven teratogenicity in humans, but many drugs and chemicals are teratogenic in animals and should, therefore, be considered as potentially teratogenic for humans.

A morphologic defect or abnormality of an organ, part of an organ, or anatomical region that results from perturbed or abnormal morphogenesis is called a **malformation.** Exposure to a known teratogen may, but does not invariably, result in a malformation. These and similar observations have led to the formulation of the following five general principles of teratology.

Susceptibility varies with the individual. The genotypes of the conceptus and the mother are the primary determinants of susceptibility to teratogens. Some strains of inbred mice are susceptible to particular exogenous stimuli to which other strains are resistant. This principle is the one most likely operative in humans. A good example is the fetal alcohol syndrome, which affects only some children born to alcoholic mothers, whereas others do not bear the stigmata of this disorder.

Susceptibility is specific for each developmental stage. The timing of exposure to a teratogen is of paramount importance. Most agents are teratogenic only during critical stages of development (Fig. 6-3). For example, maternal rubella infection causes abnormalities in the fetus only during the first 3 months of pregnancy.

Pharmacologic or biologic mechanisms are specific for each teratogen. The teratogenicity of each chemical depends, to a large extent, on the mechanisms of its action. Teratogenic drugs inhibit the activity of crucial enzymes or receptors, interfere with the formation of the mitotic spindle, or block energy sources, and thus inhibit metabolic steps critical for normal morphogenesis. Many drugs and viruses affect specific tissues ("neurotropism", "cardiotropism") and thus damage some developing organs more than others.

Response is related to dose. Teratogens act in a dose-dependent manner, a higher dose being more toxic than a smaller one. Theoretically this means that for each teratogen one can determine a "safe" dose, which should have no consequences. In practice, however, because of the multivariant determinants of teratogenesis, all established teratogens should be avoided during human pregnancy; an absolutely safe dose cannot be predicted for each individual.

The outcome of teratogenic influences is death, growth retardation, malformation, or functional impairment. The outcome depends on the interaction between the teratogenic influences, the maternal organism, and the fetal placental unit.

The search for human teratogens requires (1) a systematic approach based on population surveys, (2) prospective and retrospective studies to establish the cause of single malformations, or (3) the investigation of a reported adverse effect of drugs or other chemicals. The list of proven teratogens includes most cytotoxic drugs, alcohol, some antiepileptic drugs, heavy metals, and thalidomide, among others. On the other side of the spectrum are the drugs and chemicals that have been declared as safe for use during pregnancy, primarily on the basis of a negative outcome of teratogenic studies in laboratory animals. However, there is species specificity for every drug, and the fact that a drug is not teratogenic for mice and rabbits is not necessarily evidence that it is innocuous for humans. In fact, the best known drug-related teratogenic incident—complex malformations related to the ingestion of the hypnotic drug **thalidomide**—occurred after the drug was found to be nonteratogenic in mice and rats. Subsequently, long after the drug was found to be teratogenic in man, its teratogenicity was also demonstrated in rabbits and monkeys.

Errors of Morphogenesis

Normal intrauterine and postnatal development depend on sequential activation and repression of genes inherited from the parents and transmitted at con-

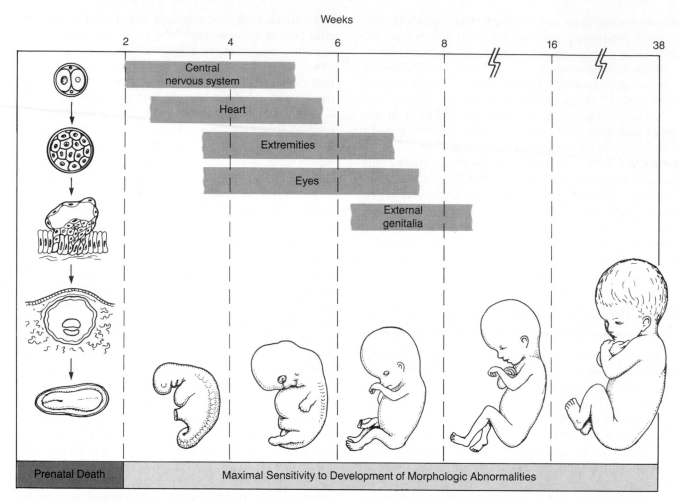

Figure 6-3. Critical stages of human development in utero. Exposure to adverse influences in the preimplantation and early postimplantation stages of development leads to death. Periods of maximal sensitivity to teratogens (*red bars*) vary for various organ systems, but overall are limited to the first 8 weeks of pregnancy.

ception. Although the fertilized ovum (zygote) has all the genes found in the adult organism, most of these genes are inactive. As the zygote enters cleavage stages of development, individual genes or sets of genes are activated in a stage-specific manner. Initially, activation involves only genes essential for cellular replication and growth, cell-to-cell interaction, and the regulation of important morphogenetic movements. **Abnormally activated or structurally abnormal genes in the zygote and early embryonic cells result in early death.**

Early descendants of the zygote (i.e., the blastomeres that form the two-cell and four-cell embryos) are developmentally equipotent, and each could give rise to most tissues found in the adult organism or even form the entire organism. Separation of blastomeres at this stage results in identical twins or

quadruplets. Since the blastomeres are equipotent and interchangeable, loss of a single blastomere at this stage of development may pass without any serious consequences. On the other hand, since the blastomeres are identical, if one blastomere contains a set of lethal genes it is likely that other blastomeres contain the same genes. Their activation, thus, invariably leads to the death of the conceptus. Furthermore, if the conceptus is exposed to untoward exogenous influences, the noxious agent exerts the same effect on all blastomeres and also causes death. Thus, adverse environmental influences on preimplantation stage embryos exert an **all or nothing** effect; either the the conceptus dies or development proceeds uninterrupted, since the interchangeable blastomeres replace the loss. As a rule, exogenous toxins acting on preimplantation stage embryos do not produce errors of morphogenesis and do not result in malformations (see Fig. 6-3). **The most common consequence of toxic exposure at the preimplantation stage is embryonic death, which often passes unnoticed or is perceived as heavy, albeit somewhat "delayed," menstrual bleeding.**

Malformations resulting from nonlethal injuries during preimplantation stages of embryogenesis are rare, since few embryos survive injury at early stages of development. Injury during the first 8 to 10 days after fertilization usually results in an incomplete separation of blastomeres, an effect that leads to the formation of **double monsters.** Symmetrical double monsters represent incompletely separated twins ("Siamese twins") joined at various anatomical sites, such as the head (craniopagus), thorax (thoracopagus) or rump (ischiopagus). Asymmetrical double monsters have one well-developed and one rudimentary or hypoplastic twin. The rudimentary twin is always abnormal, and is either externally attached to or internally included in the body of the better-developed sibling *(fetus in fetu).* Some of the congenital teratomas, especially those in the sacrococcygeal area, are actually asymmetrical monsters.

Most complex developmental abnormalities affecting several organ systems are due to injuries inflicted during embryogenesis, from the time of implantation of the blastocyst through early organogenesis. In addition to rapid cell division, this period is characterized by differentiation of cells and formation of so-called **developmental fields,** in which cells interact one with another and determine each other's developmental fate. Induction and formation of developmentally programmed structures leads to irreversible differentiation of groups of cells. Complex morphogenetic movements form **organ primordia** ("anlage"), and organs are then interconnected in functionally active systems. This is the most susceptible period for teratogenesis, and many major developmental abnormalities are probably due to faulty gene activity or the deleterious effects of exogenous toxins on the embryo at this stage of development (see Fig. 6-3).

Disorganized or disrupted morphogenesis may have minor or major consequences at the level of cells and tissues, organs or organ systems, and anatomical regions. Representative examples given here reflect the disturbance of some specific morphogenetic processes.

Agenesis is the complete absence of an organ primordium. It may manifest as complete absence of an organ, as in unilateral or bilateral agenesis of kidneys; as the absence of part of an organ, as in agenesis of the corpus callosum of the brain; or as the absence of tissue or cells within an organ, as in the absence of testicular germ cells in congenital infertility ("Sertoli cell only" syndrome).

Aplasia is absence of the organ coupled with persistence of the organ anlage or a rudiment that never developed completely. Thus, aplasia of the lung refers to a condition in which the main bronchus ends blindly in nondescript tissue composed of rudimentary ducts and connective tissue.

Hypoplasia refers to reduced size due to the incomplete development of all or part of an organ. Examples are microphthalmia (small eyes), micrognathia (small jaw), and microcephaly (small brain and head).

Dysraphic anomalies are defects caused by failure to fuse. Spina bifida is an anomaly in which the spinal canal has not closed completely and the overlaying bone and skin have not fused, thus leaving a midline defect.

Involution failures are defects due to the persistence of embryonic or fetal structures that should involute at certain stages of development. A persistent thyroglossal duct is the result of incomplete involution of the tract that connects the base of the tongue with the developing thyroid.

Division failures are defects caused by incomplete cleavage, when that process depends on the involution and programmed death of cells. Fingers and toes are formed at the distal end of the limb bud through programmed death of cells between the primordia that contain the cartilage. If these cells do not die in a predetermined manner, the fingers will be conjoined or incompletely separated ("syndactyly").

Atresia refers to defects caused by incomplete formation of a lumen. Many hollow organs originate as strands and cords of cells, the centers of which are programmed to die, thus forming a central cavity or lumen. Atresia of the esophagus is characterized by partial occlusion of the lumen, which was not fully established in embryogenesis.

Dysplasia is a defect caused by abnormal organization of cells into tissues, a situation that results in abnormal histogenesis. (*Dysplasia* has a different meaning here from that used in characterizing the precancerous lesion epithelial dysplasia [see Chapter 1].) Tuberous sclerosis is a striking example of dysplasia, being characterized by abnormal development of the brain, which contains aggregates of normally developed cells arranged into grossly visible "tubers."

Ectopia or heterotopia is an anomaly in which an organ is outside its normal anatomical site. Thus, ectopic heart is located outside the thorax. Heterotopic parathyroid glands can be located within the

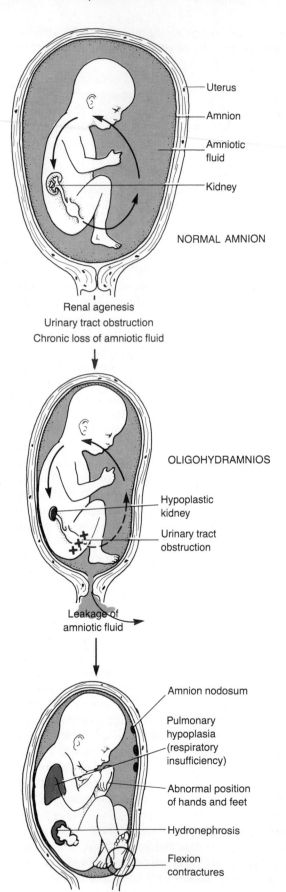

Renal agenesis
Urinary tract obstruction
Chronic loss of amniotic fluid

NORMAL AMNION

— Uterus

— Amnion

— Amniotic fluid

— Kidney

OLIGOHYDRAMNIOS

Hypoplastic kidney

Urinary tract obstruction

Leakage of amniotic fluid

Amnion nodosum

Pulmonary hypoplasia (respiratory insufficiency)

Abnormal position of hands and feet

Hydronephrosis

Flexion contractures

thymus in the anterior mediastinum. **Dystopia** is the term used to denote the retention of an organ in a site at which it is usually located during development. For example, the kidneys are initially located in the pelvis, and move thereafter into a more cranial lumbar position. Dystopic kidneys are those that remain in the pelvis. Dystopic testes are retained in the inguinal canal, not having completed their descent into the scrotum.

Developmental anomalies due to interference with morphogenesis are often multiple. This is either because the noxious agent affects several organs that are simultaneously in the critical stages of development (the so-called **polytopic effect)** or because a single localized **(monotopic)** anomaly causes a cascade of pathogenetic events. Multiple anomalies that form a pattern that can be related to a single anomaly or pathogenetic mechanism are called **developmental sequence, anomalad,** or **complex anomalies.** In a developmental sequence anomaly, different distinct causes lead to the same functional and anatomical consequences through a common pathogenetic pathway. This is best illustrated in Potter's complex (Fig. 6-4). The typical features of Potter's complex—pulmonary hypoplasia, external signs of intrauterine fetal compression, and morphologic changes of the amnion—are all related to **oligohydramnios.** Oligohydramnios (i.e., a severely reduced amount of amniotic fluid) is due either to inadequate production of fetal urine or to leakage of fluid from the amniotic sac. The fetus enclosed in an amniotic sac devoid of fluid develops several distinctive anomalies involving the face, skeleton, and extremities. Although this complex has several causes, the end results in each case are similar.

Multiple anomalies that are pathogenetically related form a **developmental syndrome.** The term "syndrome" implies a single cause for anomalies in anatomically distant organs that have been damaged

Figure 6-4. Potter's complex. The normal fetus swallows amniotic fluid and, in turn, excretes urine, thereby maintaining a normal volume of amniotic fluid. In the face of urinary tract disease, such as renal agenesis or urinary tract obstruction, or leakage of amniotic fluid, the volume of amniotic fluid decreases, a situation termed oligohydramnios. Oligohydramnios results in a number of congenital abnormalities, termed Potter's complex, which includes pulmonary hypoplasia and contractures of the limbs. The amnion has a nodular appearance. In cases of urinary tract obstruction, congenital hydronephrosis is also seen, although this abnormality is not considered part of Potter's complex.

by the same polytopic effect during a critical developmental period. Many of the developmental syndromes are related to chromosomal abnormalities or single-gene defects. The nonrandom occurrence of multiple anomalies not due to the polytopic field defect (sequence or syndrome) is called **developmental association or syntropy.** This term refers to multiple anomalies that are associated statistically but do not necessarily share the same pathogenetic mechanisms. Many of the anomalies that now seem unrelated may one day prove to have the same pathogenesis and be due to the same cause. However, until such associations are proved, it is important to note that not all multiple congenital defects are interrelated. In practical terms the birth of a child with multiple anomalies does not prove that the mother was exposed to an exogenous teratogen or that all the diverse anomalies are caused by the same genetic defect. The recognition of specific syndromes, and their distinction from random associations, is essential for the estimation of the risk of recurrence of similar anomalies in subsequent children in the same family.

After the third month of pregnancy, exposure of the human fetus to teratogenic influences rarely results in major errors of morphogenesis. However, subcellular, histologic, and, especially, functional consequences are still found in children exposed to exogenous teratogens during the fetal stages of development—that is, the second and third trimesters of pregnancy. Although organs have already been formed by the end of the third month of pregnancy, most still undergo restructuring, maturation, and functional adaptation to the changing internal milieu and to the ever-increasing metabolic requirements associated with preparation for extrauterine life. Functional maturation proceeds at different rates in different organs. For example, the central nervous system does not attain functional maturity until several years after birth, and is, thus, susceptible to adverse exogenous influences not only during pregnancy but for some time after birth.

Most anatomical defects caused by adverse influences in the fetal stage of pregnancy fall into the category of **deformations,** defined as abnormalities of form, shape, or position of a part of the body caused by mechanical forces. These forces may be external—for instance, amniotic bands in the uterus—or intrinsic, as in fetal hypomobility due to a central nervous system injury. Thus, a deformity known as equinovarus foot can be due to the compression of the extremities by the uterine wall in oligohydramnios or to spinal cord abnormalities that lead to defective innervation and movement of the foot.

Clinically Important Malformations

The causes of most errors of morphogenesis remain undetermined. As an illustration of the difficulty encountered in searching for the cause of congenital malformations we shall discuss the **anencephaly-spina bifida** complex, a major error of morphogenesis of unknown origin. Some important **drug-induced** errors of morphogenesis and defects caused by **infectious agents** will be analyzed to emphasize that these pathogenetic agents can be identified, and therefore avoided.

Anencephaly and Spina Bifida

Anencephaly is a dysraphic defect of neural tube closure. During development the neural plate invaginates and is transformed by posterior fusion into a neural tube (Fig. 6-5). Overlying mesenchyma then molds the skull and the vertebral arches posterior to the spinal cord. If the neural tube does not fuse, the overlying bony structures may not fuse either. If the skin and subcutaneous tissue do not form, a huge defect remains, exposing the malformed neural tissue directly to the exterior. Anencephalic fetuses thus lack the calvarium and the soft tissues of the cranium. The brain is incompletely formed and, owing to its unprotected position, is further damaged mechanically by the uterine wall. In most instances, the base of the skull contains only fragments of the neuropil, some ependymal tissue and residues of the meninges. The defective closure may involve only the calvarium and the brain (acrania) or may extend into the spinal cord and vertebral column (craniorachischisis). **Spina bifida,** the incomplete closure of the spinal cord canal and vertebral column, is usually localized to the lumbar region and represents the mildest dysraphic anomaly of the central nervous system. The etiology and pathogenesis of the anencephaly/spina bifida complex remain unclear. It has been estimated that craniorachischisis is caused by an injury between the 17th and 23rd day of pregnancy. **Acrania** is thought to result from an injury between the 23rd and 26th day, and spina bifida from an insult between the 25th and 30th day of pregnancy. These periods reflect the timetable for the sequential closure of the neural tube.

Anencephaly is a typical multifactorial birth defect. In the United States the frequency of anencephaly is about 1 in 1000 live births. However, there is worldwide geographic variation in the incidence of this anomaly. The highest incidence, up to 5 to 6 per 1000 live births, has been reported in Ireland and Wales. Interestingly, parts of the United States populated by

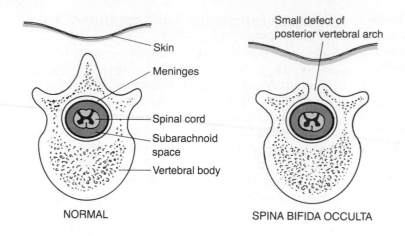

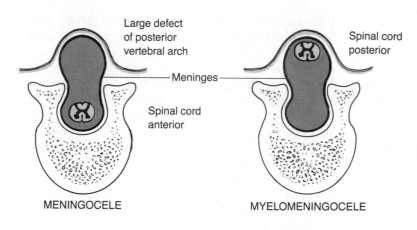

Figure 6-5. Dysraphic defects of the neural tube. Incomplete fusion of the neural tube and overlying bone, soft tissues, or skin leads to several defects, varying from mild anomalies, such as spina bifida, to severe anomalies, such as anencephaly.

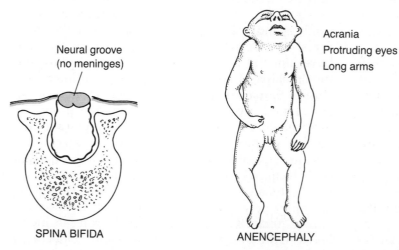

Irish immigrants show the highest incidence of anencephaly in North America, although the rate is lower (2-3 per 1000 live births) than in Ireland. The incidence of anencephaly is low in blacks, a fact that suggests racial predisposing factors.

Epidemiologic data from Ireland indicating that a higher incidence of anencephaly coincided with a severe potato blight led to theories linking the anencephaly to toxins produced by the potato blight fungus, or to antifungal substances produced by the infested potato. However, this theory was not experimentally proven, and the search for other exogenous teratogens was also unproductive. The high incidence of anencephaly in Iran was linked to a lack of zinc in the soil and water. This theory received support from experiments in which experimental animals fed a zinc-deficient diet produced anencephalic pups. Anencephaly can also be produced experimentally by hypervitaminosis A, specific antibodies, and many metabolic inhibitors given during the period of organogenesis. However, none of these teratogenic regimens is epidemiologically related to anencephaly in man. Further, the disorder affects female fetuses twice as often as male ones, and it occurs with higher incidence in certain families. It has been calculated that there is a 5% chance of recurrence in the same marriage; if two offspring are affected the risk rises to 20% to 25% for each subsequent pregnancy. Thus, genetic factors also play a role.

Children born with anencephaly are shortlived; most, in fact, are stillborn. Spina bifida, with or without myelomeningocele, is compatible with life, and the degree of neurologic impairment depends on the extent of the lesion. There are no known preventive measures.

Thalidomide-Induced Malformations

Limb-reduction deformities, involving one or up to all four extremities, are rare congenital defects of unknown origin that affect 1 in 5000 live babies. These defects have been known for ages: a Goya depiction of a typical example is in the Louvre Museum in Paris. In the 1960s a sudden increase in the incidence of limb-reduction deformities in Germany and England was epidemiologically linked to maternal intake of a sedative during the early stages of pregnancy. Known under the generic name of thalidomide, but marketed under several proprietary names, this derivative of glutamic acid is teratogenic between the 28th and 50th day of pregnancy. Many of the children born to mothers exposed to thalidomide presented with skeletal deformities and pleomorphic defects in other organs, most commonly the

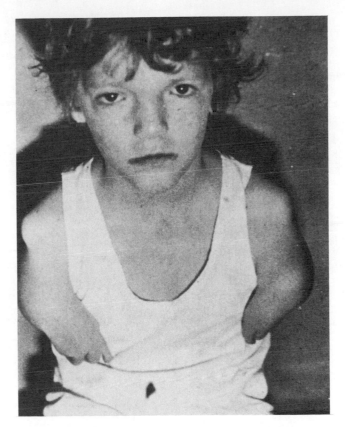

Figure 6-6. Thalidomide-induced deformity of the arms. This defect is called phocomelia because the extremities resemble the flippers of a seal (Gr. *phoke* seal).

ears (**microtia** and **anotia**) and the heart. Typically, the arms of the affected children were short and malformed (Fig. 6-6) and resembled the flippers of the seal (**phocomelia**). Sometimes limbs were completely missing (**amelia**). The central nervous system was not involved, and the children had normal intelligence. After it was recognized that the defects were causally linked to thalidomide, the drug was banned from the market, but not before an estimated 3000 malformed children were born.

Fetal Hydantoin Syndrome

Approximately 10% of children born to epileptic mothers treated during pregnancy with antiepileptic drugs such as hydantoin show characteristic facial features, hypoplasia of nails and digits, and various congenital heart defects. Since this syndrome occurs only two to three times more often in treated epileptics than in nontreated ones, it is uncertain whether the defects are entirely due to the adverse effects of the drug. Both the genetic factors that in some instances play a pathogenic role in epilepsy and the

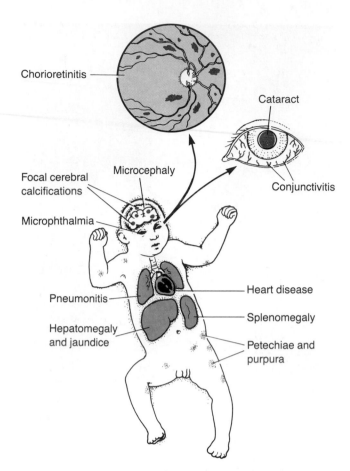

Figure 6-7. TORCH complex. Children infected in utero with toxoplasma, rubella, cytomegalovirus, or herpes simplex virus show remarkably similar symptoms.

unfavorable influence of seizures during pregnancy may also contribute to the development of this poorly understood syndrome. Since epilepsy is often exacerbated during pregnancy, pregnant women should be informed of the risk. In most instances it is not practical to discontinue drug treatment during pregnancy because the risk of injury to the mother from seizures outweighs the danger to the fetus.

Fetal Alcohol Syndrome

Although the association between alcohol intake and malformations has only recently been recognized, **ethyl alcohol is today one of the best known human teratogens.** It has been estimated that the fetal alcohol syndrome occurs in one of every 600 to 1000 liveborn children in the United States. Alcohol consumption during pregnancy increases the rate of miscarriages and stillbirths. Perinatal mortality is also augmented. The syndrome is both dose-dependent and under the influence of genetic factors. Approximately 30% to

50% of all children born to chronic alcoholic women who consume more than 125 grams of ethanol per day are born with the fetal alcohol syndrome, but even as little as 28 to 36 grams of pure ethanol (about 3 ounces of 86-proof whiskey) per day may adversely affect the conceptus.

Most children suffering from the fetal alcohol syndrome exhibit growth retardation, microcephaly, and mild-to-moderate mental retardation. Typical facial features include short palpebral fissures, epicanthal folds, ptosis, a short nose, a hypoplastic philtrum, and a thinned vermilion border of the upper lip. Commonly, the children have a short, upturned nose and a hypoplastic maxilla. Other malformations involve the extremities, kidneys, and heart. The fetal alcohol syndrome is easily prevented by abstaining from or, at the very least, drastically curtailing alcohol intake, especially during the first trimester of pregnancy. Since alcohol may potentiate the damaging effects of other drugs, and vice versa, the combined intake of alcohol and other drugs should be strictly avoided during pregnancy.

TORCH Complex

Neonatologists dealing with infants who were damaged *in utero* or perinatally by infectious agents noticed that the same complex of symptoms is produced by different microorganisms. **Toxoplasma, rubella, cytomegalovirus, and herpes simplex virus** were found to be the most frequent causes of this syndrome, and their initials were used to form the acronym **TORCH.** In this term the only unaccounted letter, namely "O", stands for all **O**thers. The term was coined to alert pediatricians to the fact that the infections in fetus and newborn by TORCH agents are usually indistinguishable from each other, and that testing for one of the four major TORCH agents should include testing for the other three and for some possible "others" as well (Fig. 6-7).

Infections with TORCH agents occur in 1% to 5% of all liveborn children in this country. It has been estimated that intrauterine toxoplasma infection occurs at a rate of 0.1% of all pregnancies, rubella and herpes simplex occur at a rate of 0.05%, and cytomegalovirus, at up to 2%. Intrapartum infection with herpes and cytomegalovirus, which are common veneral diseases, usually doubles or triples the total number of infected neonates. The exact figures for the prevalence of TORCH agents in neonates are unknown because most infants have no symptoms. Infection in the mother is also clinically inapparent in most instances. However, retrospective studies on mothers whose infants had clinically apparent symptoms disclosed that less than 1% of mothers who displayed antibodies to cytomegalovirus had symptoms of the disease. Less than 10% of mothers whose infants were infected with toxoplasma had an infectious mononucleosis-like disease or rash. Twenty percent of mothers whose babies suffered from herpes infection had signs of genital herpes infection, whereas about half of mothers of infants with rubella had exhibited a rash and fever. Rubella in mothers is obviously diagnosed much more easily than other causes of the TORCH complex.

All microorganisms of the TORCH complex cross the placenta and infect the conceptus, even before the placenta is functional. Toxoplasma is usually transmitted from a recently infected mother who experienced her primary infection while pregnant. Chronic infection is not unduly hazardous for the fetus, although women with chronic toxoplasmosis have a high rate of spontaneous abortions. This suggests that the full-blown syndrome is not seen in the offspring because the infected embryo is aborted early in pregnancy. Cytomegalovirus and herpes simplex virus infections are transmitted to the fetus from chronic carrier mothers; activation of the virus presumably facilitates its transmission to the infant. Herpes-related blisters in the vagina or the vulva are a major source of perinatal herpes infection. Cytomegalovirus infection of the genitalia is usually inapparent, but as many as 20% of asymptomatic women have the virus in the cells of the cervix and vagina.

Rubella virus harms the fetus only during acute infection, and only if the acute infection occurs during the first 20 weeks of pregnancy. Infection within the first 10 weeks is more dangerous than infection during the period from 10 to 20 weeks of gestation. Transplacental transmission of the virus to the fetus rarely occurs after the 20th week of pregnancy; infections in late pregnancy usually do not produce malformations. Active immunity to the rubella virus, due to a previous infection or active immunization, usually provides protection. However, pregnant women should avoid rubella patients with active rubella infection, since there is always a possibility that a mutant virus might reinfect even an immunized person, cross the placenta in late pregnancy, and damage the fetus at any time.

Clinical and pathologic findings in the symptomatic fetus and newborn infected with TORCH agents vary, and only a minority present with a multisystemic disease and the full-blown syndrome (Table 6-1).

Congenital rubella is a prototype of the entire syndrome. In the classic form the syndrome includes ocular defects, cardiac defects, and sensorineural deafness. Most infants also have thrombocytopenia,

Table 6-1 Pathologic Findings in the Fetus and Newborn Infected with TORCH Agents

General	Prematurity, intrauterine retardation
Central Nervous System	Encephalitis Microcephaly Hydrocephaly Intracranial calcifications Psychomotor retardation
Ear	Inner ear damage with hearing loss
Eye	Chorioretinitis (TCH) Pigmented retina (R) Keratoconjunctivitis (H) Cataracts (RH) Glaucoma (R) Visual impairment (TRCH)
Liver	Hepatomegaly Liver calcifications (R) Jaundice
Hematopoietic System	Hemolytic and other anemias Thrombocytopenia Splenomegaly
Skin and Mucosae	Vesicular or ulcerative lesions (H) Petechiae and ecchymoses
Cardiopulmonary System	Pneumonitis Myocarditis Congenital heart disease
Skeleton	Various bone lesions

T, toxoplasma; R, rubella; C, cytomegalovirus; H, herpes virus

hepatosplenomegaly, and lesions of the central nervous system. Toxoplasmosis is usually dominated by chorioretinitis and calcifications in the brain. Hepatosplenomegaly, thrombocytopenia, and brain lesions characterize congenital cytomegalovirus infection. Herpes simplex infection presents with brain or hepatosplenic involvement, and the diagnosis is facilitated by the presence of mucocutaneous vesicles.

Toxoplasma gondii is an intracellular parasite. The tachyzoites are seen in acute lesions as sickle-shaped organisms, measuring up to 6 μm. Bradyzoites, which are encapsulated in larger cysts, are more easily visualized. Rubella virus has no specific morphologic manifestations with the light microscope. By contrast, cytomegalovirus forms large intranuclear and cytoplasmic basophilic inclusions that are easily recognized by light microscopy (Fig. 6-8). Cells infected with the herpes simplex virus show a ground-glass appearance of the nuclear chromatin. The virions are identified either by electron microscopy or immunohistochemically with monospecific antibodies.

The most serious pathologic changes in TORCH-

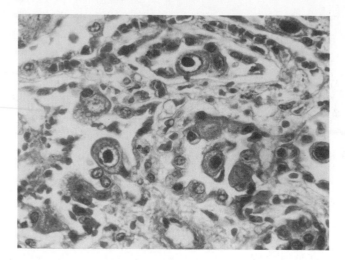

Figure 6-8. Cytomegalovirus inclusions of epithelial cells lining the alveoli of the lung. Note the enlargement of the cells harboring the virus.

infected children are found in the brain. Acute encephalitis is associated with foci of necrosis, which are initially surrounded by inflammatory cells. In later stages the lesions become calcified and are visible radiologically, most prominently in congenital toxoplasmosis. Microcephaly and hydrocephalus are frequently evident on gross examination. Abnormally shaped gyri and sulci (microgyria, oligogyria), defects of cerebral matter (porencephaly), missing olfactory bulbs, and other major brain defects are also identified by radiologic imaging. Severe brain damage is the cause of psychomotor retardation, neurologic defects, lethargy, and seizures.

Ocular symptoms are prominent in the TORCH complex. Rubella embryopathy, found in more than 70% of all affected children, typically presents with unilateral or bilateral **cataracts** and **microphthalmos.** Cataracts are not apparent at birth, although the clouding of the lens usually becomes noticeable within the first few weeks. Other ocular abnormalities include **glaucoma, choroidoretinitis,** and **coloboma** of the retina. Choroidoretinitis is also very common in congenital toxoplasmosis. The condition is mostly bilateral and presents with typical funduscopic changes, in the form of gray, yellow, or white mottled areas, surrounded peripherally by a pigmented rim. Similar retinal changes dominate congenital cytomegalovirus infection. **Keratoconjunctivitis** is the most common ocular lesion in children afflicted with herpes simplex. **Cardiac defects** occur in many children with the TORCH complex, but are most typical of congenital rubella. The commonest lesions are patent ductus arteriosus and various septal defects. Stenosis of the pulmonary artery and complex cardiac anomalies are also found.

Clinical recognition of the TORCH complex should be followed by serologic and microbiologic tests to establish the exact diagnosis. The diagnosis of toxoplasmosis is established by an indirect immunofluorescence test based on the demonstration of IgM antibodies that bind to the organism. IgM antibodies to *Toxoplasma* in a titer of 1:16 or higher are diagnostic of the disease in infants. Rubella infection is detected serologically, mostly by hemagglutination or complement fixation techniques. Rubella virus is isolated from the oropharynx of infected children up to several years after infection. Virus is also found in the cells of affected organs, in the fluid of the anterior chamber of the eye, and in the cerebrospinal fluid. Viral culture is the method of choice for the diagnosis of cytomegalovirus infection. This virus is isolated from urine, cerebrospinal fluid, saliva, and directly from affected tissues. Cytomegalovirus induces typical cytopathic effects on human cells grown in culture. The diagnosis of congenital herpes infection is best confirmed by direct isolation of the virus from mucocutaneous vesicles, the oropharynx or clinically affected tissues. The herpes virus grows rapidly *in vitro* and produces a typical cytopathic effect on human cells in culture. The infection may be caused by both type I and type II virus. The serotype of the causative agent is of no practical significance.

TORCH complex infections are major causes of morbidity among newborn children in the United States. Severe lesions inflicted by these organisms are mostly irreparable, and prevention is the only alternative. Best results in preventing rubella embryopathy have been achieved by active immunization of women prior to pregnancy. The prevention of congenital toxoplasmosis is based on avoidance of cats and other sources of acute infection in pregnancy, such as raw meat. Some apparently asymptomatic women with chronic toxoplasma infection may also transmit the organism to their offspring. No techniques for the prevention of cytomegalovirus have been devised. Transplacental infection with herpes also cannot be prevented. Intrapartum infection of the infant by cytomegalovirus and herpes simplex virus is circumvented by elective cesarean section, which is indicated if florid genital lesions are present at the time of delivery.

Congenital Syphilis

Infection with *Treponema pallidum* is transmitted to fetuses *in utero* by mothers who acquire syphilis during pregnancy. There is a possibility that the fetus will be infected if the mother became infected in the 2 years preceding the pregnancy and was not treated adequately, but the actual risk cannot be accurately assessed. It has been estimated that congenital syphilis affects 1 in 2000 liveborn children in the United States.

T. pallidum invades the fetus at any point during pregnancy. Early infections most likely induce abortions, and the grossly visible signs of congenital syphilis appear only in fetuses infected after the 16th week of pregnancy. The spirochetes grow in all fetal tissues and the clinical presentation is thus characterized by protean manifestations. Destruction of tissues is caused by direct invasion by spirochetes, treponemal vasculitis, and gumma formation. Fetal lesions are, thus, due in part to direct tissue invasion by the spirochete and in part to the host's response to infection. The placenta is also infected, and its function may be impaired.

Children born with congenital syphilis are initially normal or show symptoms clinically indistinguishable from the TORCH complex. Many are asymptomatic, only to develop the typical stigmata of tardive syphilis several years later. Skin lesions include **macules, papules,** and **vesicular and annular skin eruptions**. Palmar and plantar sloughing of the epithelium, and circumoral and circumanal **rhagades,** with oozing, may be the only signs of intrauterine infection. Involvement of the nasopharynx presents as a serosanguineous nasal discharge **(sniffles)**. Anemia, hepatosplenomegaly, jaundice, and signs of mild meningeal irritation are common. Osteochondritis involves the long bones, and occasionally the small bones of the extremities. Pneumonitis **(pneumonia alba)** is found only in severe congenital syphilis (Fig. 6-9). All these lesions contain spirochetes. The tissues are infiltrated with lymphocytes and plasma cells, and show inflammatory changes of small arteries and arterioles and fully developed gummas. Late symptoms of congenital syphilis become apparent many years after birth. Most of them reflect slowly evolving tissue destruction and repair of subclinical lesions, and are also due to the immune response of the body.

Prominent among the symptoms of tardive syphilis is the **Hutchinson's triad,** considered for many years to be the hallmark of the disease. It includes interstitial **keratitis,** sensorineural **deafness,** and **deformed teeth**. Dental lesions typically involve permanent teeth. Notched edges of the anterior teeth, which are usually narrower at the apical than the basal side, produces a typical change known as **Hutchinson's teeth**. Deformed molars, known as **mulberry molars,** are another sign of deranged dentition and impaired enamel formation. Other symptoms of tardive syphilis are predominantly found in the skeleton; they include **saddle deformity** of the nose, perforation of the hard palate, and **saber deformity** of the shin. Perforation of the palate and saddle deformity of the nose are caused by the destruction of the facial bones by gummas. Disturbed

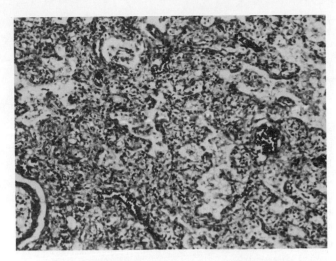

Figure 6-9. Syphilitic pneumonia in a newborn child. The spaces are collapsed and the alveolar walls have lost their normal outlines. The alveolar septa are infiltrated with mononuclear cells, and the alveolar spaces are airless. Because of the impaired blood flow through such a lung, the organ appears pale on gross examination and lacks the crepitance of the normal lungs (pneumonia alba).

ossification and chronic periostitis lead to the "sabre deformity" of the shin, which can be traced to anterior bowing of the tibia and thinning of cortical bone in one area in conjunction with excessive formation of subperiosteal bone in other parts. Heart disease is not a feature of congenital syphilis. Symptoms of brain involvement are protean.

The diagnosis of congenital syphilis is suggested by clinical findings and a history of maternal infection. Serologic confirmation of syphilitic infection may be difficult in the newborn because the transplacental transfer of maternal IgG gives false-positive results. If the infant presents with skin lesions, the diagnosis is established by demonstrating *T. pallidum* in swabs from tissue. In children born to syphilitic mothers who do not present with clinically detectable disease, one should perform monthly quantitative reagin tests in an attempt to detect the infant's own immune response to *T. pallidum*. If positive serologic test results reflect the transfer of maternal antibodies, the titer in the infant's serum slowly decreases over 2 to 3 months. Intrauterine infection with syphilis causes the titers of reaginic antibodies to remain high or even increase. Penicillin is still the drug of choice for both intrauterine and postnatal syphilis. If penicillin is given during intrauterine life or during the first 2 years of postnatal life, the prognosis is excellent, and most symptoms of early and tardive congenital syphilis will be prevented.

Chromosomal Abnormalities

During cell division, the nuclear material condenses to form distinct threadlike particles, the **chromosomes.** Every nucleated somatic cell in the human body contains 46 chromosomes: 44 autosomes and 2 sex chromosomes. Chromosomes are readily prepared for light microscopic examination and are routinely analyzed in many clinical situations. The discipline concerned with the study of chromosomes and chromosomal abnormalities is called **cytogenetics.** We shall discuss chromosomal or cytogenetic disorders that fall into two major categories: structural chromosomal abnormalities and numerical chromosomal disorders.

Normal Chromosomes

Chromosomes are distinct nuclear organelles composed of nucleic acids and proteins. The morphologic appearance of human chromosomes in metaphase has been studied in detail. The classification system now in use is the International System for Human Cytogenetic Nomenclature (ISCN).

Cytogenetic analysis can be performed on any spontaneously dividing cell. However, in most instances the analysis is performed on circulating lymphocytes, which are readily available in peripheral blood and are easily stimulated to undergo mitosis. Mitotic cells are treated with colchicine to arrest them in metaphase, after which they are spread on glass slides to disperse the chromosomes. The chromosomes are stained with standard hematologic stains and by more sophisticated techniques that enable more precise identification of chromosomes on the basis of distinct bands. Using hematologic stains such as Giemsa, the chromosomes are classified according to their **length** and the positioning of the constriction, or **centromere.** The centromere is the point at which the two identical double helices of the chromosomal DNA, called sister **chromatids,** attach to each other. The location of the centromere is used to classify the chromosomes as **metacentric, submetacentric,** or **acrocentric.** In metacentric chromosomes (numbers 1, 3, 19, and 20) the centromere is exactly in the middle. In submetacentric chromosomes the centromere divides the chromosomes into a short arm (p—from French *petit*), and a long arm (q—next letter in the alphabet). Acrocentric chromosomes (numbers 13, 14, 15, 21, 22, and Y) have very short arms or stalks and satellites attached to an eccentrically located centromere. Chromosomes of many animal species have terminally located centromeres, but these **telocentric** chromosomes are not found in man.

Hematologic stains provide sufficient data to classify chromosomes into seven groups, conventionally labeled with letters from A to G. Thus, group A contains two large metacentric and a large submetacentric chromosome, group B contains two distinct large submetacentric chromosomes, group C contains 6 submetacentric chromosomes, and so forth. In order to identify each chromosome individually, additional techniques are applied. These **banding** techniques delineate specific bands of different staining intensity on each chromosome. **The pattern of bands is unique to each chromosome and makes possible the pairing of two homologous chromosomes, the recognition of each chromosome, and the identification of defects on each segment of a chromosome.**

Chromosome bands are traditionally labeled with letters denoting the technique used to produce them. **G bands** refer to Giemsa stained preparations, and **Q bands** to fluorescent bands in preparations stained with quinacrine. Although produced by different techniques, Q bands correspond to G bands. On the other hand, **R bands** are produced by controlled denaturation and represent the reverse image of G and Q bands. **C banding** is the technique of choice for the staining of centromeres and other portions of chromosomes containing so-called constitutive heterochromatin. By contrast, facultative heterochromatin forms the inactive X chromosome of the Barr body. **NOR (nucleolar organizer region) staining** is useful for visualization of secondary constrictions (stalks) of chromosomes with satellites, and **T banding** is useful for staining of the terminal ends of chromosomes.

Structural Abnormalities

Structurally abnormal chromosomes arise during cell division (Fig. 6-10). In dividing somatic cells, these abnormalities usually either are of no consequence or lead to lethal traits that cause extinction of the abnormal cell clone. It has become evident that some structural chromosomal abnormalities are pathogenetically related to some forms of cancer. However, most of these **somatic cell mutations** are limited to a few cell lines and have little effect on fetal development. **Much more important from the embryological point of view are the structural chromosomal abnormalities that originate during gametogenesis, because these are transmitted to all somatic cells and result in hereditary transmissible traits.**

During meiosis homologous chromosomes pair to form bivalents. Their chromatids are broken, and crossing of portions of chromatids normally occurs. Exchange of fragmented chromatids during the first

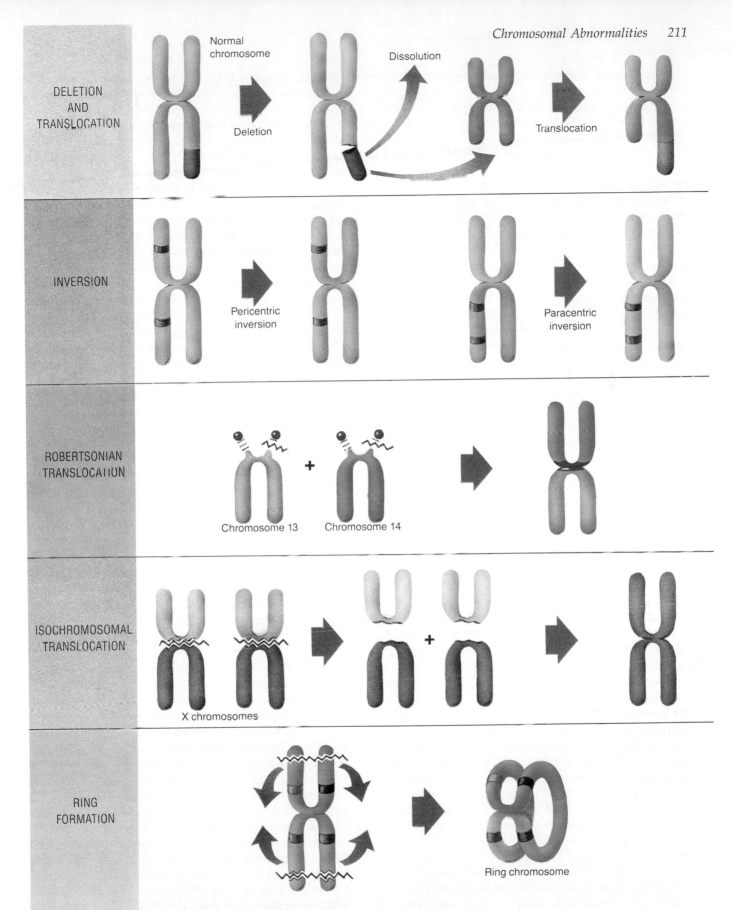

Figure 6-10. Structural abnormalities of human chromosomes. Such abnormalities evolve during either mitosis or meiosis.

meiotic division also occurs between nonhomologous chromosomes, a process that results in **translocation.** In **reciprocal translocation** acentric segments of chromatid from one chromosome are exchanged for a similar segment from a heterologous chromosome. Reciprocal translocations are not detected in routine chromosome preparations and are apparent only after banding with special techniques.

Robertsonian translocations, or centric fusion, involve the centromere and can be recognized in routine chromosomal preparations. In such cases two acrocentric chromosomes, broken near the centromere, exchange two arms and form a new, large, metacentric chromosome and a small fragment. This fragment is devoid of a centromere and is usually lost during subsequent divisions. If there is no loss of genetic material, this translocation is called **balanced.** Individuals with such abnormalities are usually normal, but may suffer from infertility. When fertile, they have a higher than normal risk of giving birth to malformed children. Apparently, the translocation that was "balanced" in the cells of a parent may become "unbalanced" when it is transmitted in the haploid gamete and is paired with a new set of genes from the other parent.

The overall risk for the development of cancer because of translocations in germ cells is only now being assessed. Nevertheless, it is already evident that certain forms of translocation in somatic cell lineages are associated with an increased risk of tumor formation. The best examples are the translocations between chromosomes 8 and 14 and between 22 and 9 in malignant lymphomas and leukemias. The Robertsonian translocation of chromosome 21 plays a role in hereditary Down's syndrome.

Meiotic disturbances, or single breaks of chromatids in somatic cells, induced by physical, chemical, and biological agents cause formation of acentric fragments that are not incorporated into any of the 46 chromosomes and may be lost in subsequent cell divisions. This loss of genetic material is called **deletion** and involves either the terminal or the intercalary (middle) portion of a chromosome. The shortening of the chromosome because of a deletion may be apparent in routinely stained chromosome preparation. Banding techniques are applied to determine whether the arm of the chromosome is shortened because of a deletion of the terminal portion or because of a double break in the more central portions, an event that leads to intercalary deletion and subsequent fusion of adjoining residual fragments.

Deletion can be associated with either normal or abnormal development. The best example is the "cri du chat" syndrome, which is associated with the deletion of part of the short arm of chromosome 5. Deletion is pathogenetically related to several cancers in man, including some hereditary forms of cancer. For example, **retinoblastomas** are associated with the deletion of the long arm of chromosome 13. **Wilms' tumor aniridia syndrome** is associated with deletion of the short arm of chromosome 11.

The break of a chromosome at two points, followed by **inversion** of the intermediate segment and reunion, results in the formation of chromosomes with a rearranged distribution of genes in the restructured chromatid. Inversions are called **pericentric** or **paracentric,** depending on whether the rotation occurs around the centromere or only on the acentric portion of the arm. Homologous chromosomes with inverted segments do not undergo regular pairing during meiosis. They do not exchange segments of chromatids as readily as normal chromosomes, because of interference with meiotic pairing. Although this has little consequence for the affected individual, it may be important from the evolutionary point of view, since certain genes are transmitted in groups as units. This may lead to clustering of certain hereditary features.

Ring chromosomes are formed by a break involving both telomeric ends of a chromosome, followed by deletion of the broken acentric fragment and end-to-end fusion of the remaining portion. The consequences depend primarily on the amount of genetic material lost because of the break. The abnormally shaped chromosome may impede normal meiotic division, but in most instances this chromosomal abnormality is of no consequence.

Isochromosomes are formed by the faulty division of the centromere. Normally, centromere division occurs in a plane parallel to the long axis of the chromosome, leading to the formation of two identical hemichromosomes. If the centromere divides transversely to the long axis, pairs of isochromosomes are formed, one corresponding to the short arms attached to the upper portion of the centromere and the other to the long arms attached to the lower segment. The most important clinical condition involving isochromosomes is **Turner's syndrome**, in which approximately 15% of those affected have an isochromosome of the X chromosome. Thus, a woman with a normal X chromosome and an isochromosome composed of long arms of the X chromosome is monosomic for all the genes located on the missing short arm (i.e., the other isochromosome, which is lost during the meiotic division). She is trisomic for the genes located on the long arm. The absence of the genes from the short arm accounts for the abnormal development in these individuals.

Table 6-2 Numerical Chromosomal Aberrations

EUPLOIDY	ANEUPLOIDY
Haploid (n) = 23	Hypodiploid 2n − 1, − 2 etc.
Diploid (2n) = 46	(monosomy)
Triploid (3n) = 69	Hyperdiploid 2n + 1, + 2,
	etc. (trisomy)
Tetraploid (4n) = 92	
Polyploid	

Numerical Aberrations

Every mammalian species has a characteristic number of chromosomes corresponding to two **haploid** sets of homologous chromosomes. In man each haploid set includes 23 chromosomes; the **diploid** number is, therefore, 46. Any multiple of the haploid number is termed **euploid,** whereas karyotypes that are not exact multiples of the haploid number are called **aneuploid.** Children born with a triploid or tetraploid chromosome number are thus also euploid, although these cases obviously represent serious numerical aberrations that are incompatible with life. Karyotypes that contain multiples of the haploid number are labeled **polyploid** (Table 6-2).

Numerical chromosomal abnormalities arise primarily from **nondisjunction. Nondisjunction is a failure of paired chromosomes or chromatids to separate and move to opposite poles of the mitotic spindle at anaphase.** Nondisjunction occurs during mitosis or meiosis. It leads to aneuploidy if only one pair of chromosomes is involved and to polyploidy if the entire set fails to divide and all the chromosomes are segregated in a single daughter cell. In somatic cells aneuploidy due to nondisjunction results in one daughter cell exhibiting **trisomy** and the other **monosomy** for the affected chromosome pair (2n + 1 or 2n − 1). Aneuploid germ cells have two copies of the same chromosome or lack the affected chromosome entirely (n + 1 or n − 1).

A special form of nondisjunction involves single pairs of chromosomes and is called **anaphase lag.** In this process, one chromosome or a chromatid fails to synapse with its pair at the same time as the other chromosomes. It lags behind the others on the nuclear spindle and is, thus, not incorporated into the nucleus of the daughter cell in telophase. As the result of the lag in anaphase, one daughter cell is euploid and the other is monosomic for the missing chromosome.

The causes of chromosomal aberrations are obscure. Putative exogenous factors, such as radiation, viruses, and chemicals, affect the mitotic spindle or DNA synthesis and produce mitotic and meiotic disturbances in experimental animals. However, the role of these factors in the production of human chromosomal abnormalities remains conjectural. Immune factors have been invoked, in view of the correlation between autoantibodies and chromosomal anomalies in families with autoimmune thyroid disorders. The familial occurrence of meiotic failure and chromosomal anomalies provides some evidence for the existence of human genes that predispose to faulty cell division. However, these explanations are hypothetical, and there are only two phenomena known to be of importance in aberrations of human development: (1) **Disturbances of meiotic division are more common in individuals with structurally abnormal chromosomes.** This is probably related to the fact that structurally abnormal chromosomes do not pair or segregate as readily as normal chromosomes, and therefore nondisjunction occurs more frequently. (2) **Children born to older women show chromosomal aberrations more frequently than those born to younger mothers.** Maternal age obviously plays an important role, but there is no precise explanation for the higher incidence of nondisjunction in older women.

Abnormal ova or spermatozoa resulting from nondisjunction transmit the genetic defect through all cell lineages derived from the division of the zygote. In most instances the genetic imbalance has a lethal effect on the developing conceptus and leads to early death of the embryo or spontaneous abortion in the early stages of pregnancy. Most major chromosomal abnormalities are, thus, incompatible with life.

Autosomal aneuploidies associated with the loss of genetic material (monosomies) generally do not even reach the terminal stages of pregnancy. **Monosomy** of sex chromosomes, on the other hand, is compatible with life, but only if the conserved chromosome is an X. Female fetuses with only one X chromosome (45,X) are also less viable than their normal counterparts and about 90% are lost in pregnancy. The karyotype 45,Y absolutely precludes normal embryonic development and invariably results in early abortion.

Autosomal trisomies—that is, aneuploidies with an additional chromosome—are associated with several developmental abnormalities. Many fetuses with trisomy are viable throughout the pregnancy, and some are even liveborn. Liveborn infants with autosomal trisomy die soon after birth, except for those with trisomy 21. These infants express the stigmata

Table 6-3 Approximate Incidence of Chromosomal Aberrations in Newborn Infants

TYPE OF ABERRATION	INCIDENCE
Autosomal	
Trisomies	
Trisomy 13	1/20,000
Trisomy 18	1/8,000
Trisomy 21	1/800
Other	1/50,000
Translocations	
Balanced	1/500
Unbalanced	1/2000
Sex Chromosome	
Monosomy X (45,X) and X deletion variants	1/3000
Trisomies	
47,XXY	1/1000
47,XXX	1/1000
47,XYY	1/1000
Total	1/500

of **Down's syndrome,** and can survive for years. Sex chromosome trisomies may result in abnormal development but are not lethal.

Mitotic nondisjunction may involve embryonic cells during early stages of development and result in chromosomal aberrations. These are transmitted selectively through some cell lineages but not through others. The condition in which the body contains two or more karyotypically different cell lines is called **mosaicism.** Like all chromosomal abnormalities related to nondisjunction, mosaicism may involve autosomes or sex chromosomes. The phenotype of a mosaic individual depends on the chromosome involved and the extent of mosaicism. Autosomal mosaicism is rare, most likely because this condition is usually lethal. On the other hand mosaicism involving sex chromosomes is common and is found in patients with gonadal dysgenesis who present with Turner's or Klinefelter's syndromes.

Nomenclature of Chromosomal Aberrations

Structural and numerical chromosomal abnormalities are classified according to an international convention that includes the number of chromosomes, the number of the affected chromosomes, and the nature and exact location of the defect. According to this system, 47,XX +21 denotes trisomy 21 in a female with Down's syndrome. The first number, indicating the total number of chromosomes, is followed by the

symbols for the two sex chromosomes. The plus sign denotes an additional chromosome 21. The designation 46,XX del (5) (qter p 13): denotes deletion of the terminal portion of the long arm of chromosome 5 seen in **cri du chat syndrome.** The colon at the end indicates where the break occurred and that the segment distal to band 13 of the chromosome 5 has been deleted.

Clinically Important Syndromes

Estimates are that 5 to 7 per 1000 liveborn infants have a structural or numerical chromosomal aberration. The most common aberrations are balanced translocations, which are usually not associated with obvious clinical symptoms. Clinically, the most important cytogenetic disorder is trisomy 21 (Down's syndrome). The approximate incidence of various chromosomal aberrations in newborn infants is presented in Table 6-3.

Trisomy 21 (Down's Syndrome)

Trisomy 21 is one of the commonest clinically recognized chromosomal disorders and also the single most common cause of mental retardation. Liveborn infants represent only a fraction of all conceptuses with this chromosomal defect. Two-thirds are aborted spontaneously or die *in utero.* Life expectancy is also reduced: 30% die within the first year of life, 50% succumb before the age of 5 years and only 8% survive beyond 40 years. Recent advances in the therapy of infections, operations for congenital heart defects, and chemotherapy for leukemia—the leading causes of death in patients with Down's syndrome—are rapidly changing these statistics.

Most patients with Down's syndrome (92-95%) have trisomy 21, approximately 2% are mosaics, and 5% have translocation of an extra chromosome 21 to another acrocentric chromosome. **The extra chromosome in classical trisomy is the result of nondisjunction during meiosis in one of the parents. The incidence of trisomy 21 correlates strongly with maternal age.** The risk of giving birth to abnormal children rises with age, which suggests that **nondisjunction during oogenesis is the underlying cause of this chromosomal anomaly,** at least in older mothers. The influence of advanced paternal age has not been definitely established. The risk of giving birth to a trisomic child is constant at about 0.9 per 1000 liveborns for women in their mid- to late thirties. The risk then dramatically increases, to reach an incidence of 1 in

30 pregnancies at age 44 years (Fig. 6-11). The fact that a few children with Down's syndrome are mosaics indicates that the trisomy found in one of the somatic cell lines is due to **mitotic nondisjunction in early stages of embryogenesis.** By contrast, nondisjunction during mitosis is not related to maternal age. The risk for this form of Down's syndrome is equal in women of all ages.

The risk of recurrence of Down's syndrome in subsequent children born to the same mother is approximately 1% irrespective of maternal age, unless the syndrome is associated with translocation of chromosome 21. Translocation of an extra chromosome 21 to another acrocentric chromosome, most frequently chromosome 14 or 21, is associated with a normal number of chromosomes, and it may be balanced and asymptomatic. However if the translocated chromosome is transmitted to the offspring, the infant may carry a karyotype designated as 46,XX, − 14, + t (14q;21q) or 46,XY, − 21, + t (21q;21q). These karyotypes are clinically manifested as Down's syndrome. Parents of children born with this translocation-related form of Down's syndrome should, therefore, be karyotyped to determine whether the translocation in the child was transmitted from one of the parents or occurred de novo. Some asymptomatic parents may be mosaic for the translocation. Fortunately the translocation t(21;21) is only exceptionally found in a balanced form, and asymptomatic carriers are rare. More commonly chromosome 21 is translocated to one of the D chromosomes (13, 14, 15). Balanced translocation in the mother carries a 16% risk of a child being born with Down's syndrome; in the father, it carries about a 5% risk. This actual risk and the sex differences in transmission differ from the theoretical calculations and cannot be fully explained. Irrespective of the risk, in clinical practice it is customary to perform cytogenetic studies in each subsequent pregnancy following the birth of an infant with Down's syndrome.

The diagnosis of Down's syndrome is usually made at the time of birth and is confirmed by chromosomal analysis. The infant is hypotonic and displays the typical craniofacial features (Fig. 6-12). These include a flat facial profile, a low-bridged nose, reduced interpupillary distance, oblique palpebral fissures, and epicanthal folds on the eyes, imparting an Oriental appearance. The iris may be speckled (Brushfield spots). The mouth is often open and the tongue is enlarged, protruding, coarsely furrowed, and without a central fissure. The hands are broad and short and exhibit a transverse simian crease. The middle phalanx of the fifth finger is hypoplastic, a

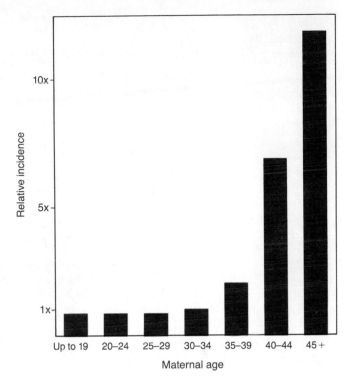

Figure 6-11. Incidence of Down's syndrome as a function of maternal age. A dramatic rise in the incidence of this chromosomal anomaly is seen in mothers over 35 years of age.

feature resulting in clinodactaly (inward curvature). The imprint of the palms and fingers leaves a characteristic dermatoglyphic pattern. The feet and toes show equivalent abnormalities. Other skeletal defects include those of the rib cage, pelvis, and long bones, which are shorter than average. Congenital heart defects are common. Malformations of other organ systems occur at an increased rate but are not standard features of this syndrome. **Mental retardation is usually severe, and the intelligence quotient (IQ) is, in most instances, lower than 50.**

Down's syndrome is associated with an increased incidence of acute lymphoblastic and myeloblastic leukemia. Neuropathologic changes indistinguishable from those in Alzheimer's disease occur in adults who survive into their 40s and 50s.

Sex Chromosome Trisomies

Trisomies of sex chromosomes (Fig. 6-13) are considerably more common than those involving autosomes. The reasons are not obvious, but it appears that additional sex chromosomes produce less genetic imbalance than extra autosomes and do not disturb

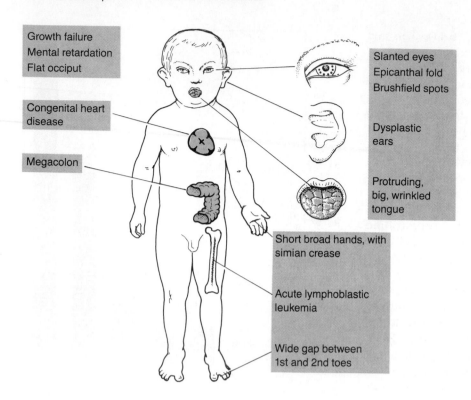

Growth failure
Mental retardation
Flat occiput

Congenital heart disease

Megacolon

Slanted eyes
Epicanthal fold
Brushfield spots

Dysplastic ears

Protruding, big, wrinkled tongue

Short broad hands, with simian crease

Acute lymphoblastic leukemia

Wide gap between 1st and 2nd toes

Figure 6-12.   Clinical features of Down's syndrome.

Gametes	SPERM	X		Y		XY		0	
OVUM									
X		XX Normal ♀		XY Normal ♂		XXY Klinefelter ♂		XO Turner ♀	
XX		XXX Triple X ♀		XXY Klinefelter ♂		XXXY Klinefelter ♂		XXO Normal ♀	
XXX		XXXX 48, XXXX ♀		XXXY Klinefelter ♂		XXXXY 49, XXXXY ♂		XXXO Triple X ♀	
0		OX Turner ♀		OY LETHAL		OXY LETHAL		OO LETHAL	

X chromatin (Barr body)
Y chromatin

Figure 6-13.   Pathogenesis of sex chromosome aberrations. Nondisjunction in either the male or female gamete is the principal cause of these numerical chromosomal abnormalities.

critical stages of development. Sex chromosome abnormalities that do cause severe disturbances of development probably result in early abortion.

Individuals born with an extra Y chromosome (47,XYY) are phenotypically male, and although very tall, do not exhibit any symptoms. Thus, a dose effect of double or multiple Y chromosomes is not readily detectable. Multiplicity of X chromosomes over the normal XX or XY complement is often accompanied by mental retardation, which roughly correlates with the number of extra X chromosomes. This is especially true in males, who also show some degree of feminization. Females with three X chromosomes are usually normal, whereas those with four or five are mentally retarded. The reasons for the adverse effects of extra X chromosomes are not obvious, since all the X chromosomes but one are inactivated and attached to the nuclear membrane as heteropyknotic chromatin, or **Barr body.** Although the inactivation of the extra X chromosomes occurs during early embryogenesis, it is apparently not early enough to be without an effect on the developing nervous system and gonads. It is also possible that the inactivation of an extra X chromosome does not occur simultaneously in all cell lineages. Since multiple X chromosomes produce more mental retardation than a single additional one, perhaps inactivation of multiple X chromosomes takes longer than that of the normal complement.

Clinically, the most important sex chromosome trisomy presents as **Klinefelter's syndrome,** or testicular dysgenesis (Fig. 6-14). The syndrome is related to the presence of one or more X chromosomes in excess of the normal male XY complement. Approximately 80% of those affected have a 47,XXY karyotype. The remainder are mosaics or have more than two X chromosomes. The additional chromosome affects the development of gonads and influences the development of intelligence. Abnormalities of sexual development and intelligence are usually not apparent until later in childhood. The testicles are small, and at puberty the body does not assume the typical male characteristics and proportions. Individuals with Klinefelter's syndrome are tall, with long arms and legs, and have a small penis. Feminization is typified by a female pattern of pubic hair, gynecomastia, and a high-pitched voice. All these changes are related to hypogonadism and inadequate Leydig cells. Low levels of testosterone in serum and urine are associated with elevated serum levels of follicle-stimulating hormone (FSH), indicating that the pituitary is normal but that the testicular hormone-producing cells do not respond to the stimulus. Testicular biopsy reveals prominent interstitial fibrosis

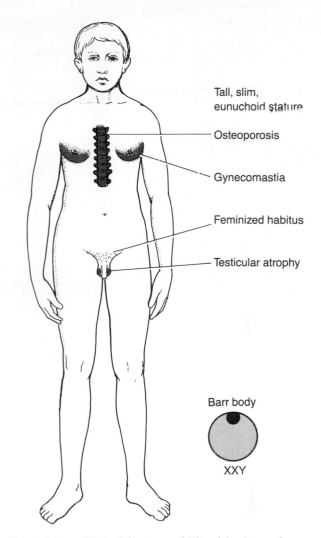

Tall, slim, eunuchoid stature

Osteoporosis

Gynecomastia

Feminized habitus

Testicular atrophy

Barr body

XXY

Figure 6-14. Clinical features of Klinefelter's syndrome.

replacing normal Leydig cells and surrounding atrophic tubules. A low sperm count or aspermatogenesis is reflected in infertility. Exogenous testosterone given at time of puberty or thereafter induces the development of secondary male characteristics, but does not remedy infertility or improve intelligence.

Monosomy X

The X chromosome is essential for the viability of the fetus, and those missing both X chromosomes or having the 45,Y karyotype die *in utero*. Almost all fetuses with the 45,X karyotype are spontaneously aborted. About one-tenth of spontaneously aborted fetuses have a 45,X karyotype.

Infants born with the 45,X karyotype display the clinical features of **Turner's syndrome** (Fig. 6-15). In

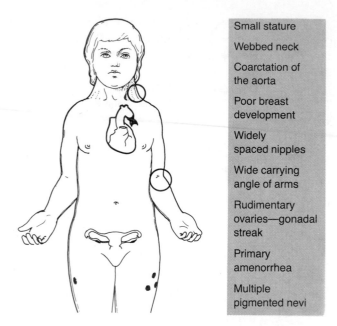

Small stature

Webbed neck

Coarctation of
the aorta

Poor breast
development

Widely
spaced nipples

Wide carrying
angle of arms

Rudimentary
ovaries—gonadal
streak

Primary
amenorrhea

Multiple
pigmented nevi

Figure 6-15.   Clinical features of Turner's syndrome.

80% of these cases, the single X chromosome is of maternal origin, indicating that the **missing X was most commonly lost in paternal meiosis.** Stigmata of Turner's syndrome are also found in individuals with 45,X/46,XX mosaicism, those missing a portion of one X chromosome, and those with one normal chromosome and an isochromosome or ring chromosome X. Approximately half of patients with Turner's syndrome have classic monosomy X, whereas the others have variant forms—namely, mosaicism and abnormal X chromosomes. **Structurally abnormal chromosomes are often of paternal origin, and this anomaly may be causally related to advanced age of the father.** The diagnosis of Turner's syndrome is suggested at the time of birth by lymphedema of the extremities and the neck but is easier to make later in life. The only constant and typical features of the syndrome are the streak gonads and growth retardation.

During intrauterine life the ovaries are initially normal. Fetal ovaries contain primordial follicles, which degenerate at a rapid rate and, in most children with Turner's syndrome, completely disappear from the gonads by the time of puberty. The gonads, devoid of oocytes, transform into fibrous streaks, but the fallopian tubes, uterus, and vagina develop normally. Menarche does not occur, and sterility is the rule. Estrogen production is low, and serum gonadotropin levels are elevated. Secondary sexual characteristics remain infantile but may be artificially induced to develop with exogenous estrogens.

Other somatic features of Turner's syndrome are highly variable, depending on the nature of the chromosomal defect. Common features are a short, broad neck with low hairline, web neck (**"pterygium coli"**), shield chest with widely spaced nipples, cubitus valgus, short metatarsal and metacarpal bones, numerous pigmented nevi, lymphedema of hands and feet, hypoplasia of nails, miscellaneous renal malformations, coarctation of the aorta, ventricular septal defect, and craniofacial peculiarities, such as epicanthal folds, abnormal teeth, and a high arched palate. In most instances intelligence is normal. For unknown reasons the incidence of autoimmune thyroiditis and hypothyroidism is increased. A substantial number of patients with Turner's syndrome develop essential hypertension, but life expectancy is normal.

Single-Gene Abnormalities

Single genes that **encode identifiable traits, segregate sharply within families, and transmit according to the classic laws of inheritance outlined by Gregor Mendel are called "mendelian."** Each mendelian trait is specified by two variants of the same gene, called **alleles,** which are located on the same locus of two homologous chromosomes. Genes are classified as **autosomal** if located on autosomes, as **sex-linked** if located on the X and Y chromosomes. Genes that are expressed only when they present in identical form on both chromosomes (i.e., when the individual is homozygous for that pair of genes) are called **recessive.** Genes that require only one copy—that is, genes that are expressed in homozygous and heterozygous form—are called **dominant.** A variant of dominance in which both alleles in a heterozygous gene pair are fully expressed is called **codominance**—an example is provided by the AB blood group genes. Mendelian traits are classified as autosomal dominant or recessive and sex-linked dominant or recessive. Sex-linked dominant traits are rare and of little practical significance.

The Biochemical Basis of Single-Gene Abnormalities

Mendelian traits can be identified only by a study of pedigree and transmission patterns through generations; they cannot be recognized by chromosomal analysis. Gene linkage analysis and somatic cell genetics have enabled the assignment of specific mendelian genes to individual chromosomes. Gene mapping of chromosomes has linked certain genetic defects with specific structural chromosomal defects and thus formed a bridge between mendelian genetics and cytogenetics.

The genetic message is encoded in sequences of DNA. The **codon,** the basic genetic unit, consists of a triplet of DNA bases. A **gene** contains codons transcribed in series. Through messenger RNA, the sequence of DNA is translated into a sequence of amino acids that forms the final product of the gene, the polypeptide chain. Although slightly modified by recent advances, the concept that one gene codes for one polypeptide chain is the basic tenet of modern genetics.

A series of genes codes for a series of enzymes of a specific metabolic pathway, which catalyzes the conversion of substrate A through several intermediate metabolites (B and C) to the final product, D.

A	$\rightarrow$	B $\rightarrow$ C	$\rightarrow$	D
initial substrate		intermediary metabolites		end product

A single-gene defect can have several possible consequences:

- **Failure to complete a metabolic pathway.** In this situation the end product is not formed because an enzyme that is essential for the completion of a metabolic sequence is missing.

$$A \rightarrow B \rightarrow C \rightarrow (D)$$

An example is albinism due to tyrosinase deficiency. Tyrosinase catalyzes the formation of dihydroxyphenylalanine (DOPA), an intermediary metabolite in the metabolic pathway leading to the synthesis of melanin from tyrosine. In the absence of this enzyme, melanin is not formed, and the affected individual is devoid of pigment ("albino") in all organs that normally contain it, primarily the eyes and skin.

- **Accumulation of unmetabolized substrate.** In these circumstances the enzyme that converts the initial substrate into the first intermediary metabolite is missing. Absence of the enzyme results in an excessive accumulation of the initial substrate. Intermediary metabolites and the final end product are usually formed through other metabolic pathways, but in reduced amounts.

$$A (\uparrow) \xrightarrow[x]{x} B (\downarrow) C (\downarrow) D (\downarrow)$$

A typical example of this sequence of events is glycogenosis caused by a deficiency of glucose-6-phosphatase. This enzyme is essential for normal utilization of glycogen, and without it unmetabolized glycogen accumulates in the cells. Defective mobilization of glycogen leads to low blood glucose levels, which in turn produce other metabolic disturbances in a number of organs.

- **Storage of an intermediary metabolite.** In this situation an intermediary metabolite, which is readily processed into the final product and is normally present only in minute amounts, accumulates in large quantities. The subsequent intermediary metabolites and the end product may be reduced in amount.

$$A \rightarrow B (\uparrow) C (\downarrow) D (\downarrow)$$

Lysosomal storage diseases are typical examples of this metabolic derangement. An enzyme deficiency causes intermediary metabolites to accumulate in the lysosomes in various conditions, such as Tay-Sachs disease, Niemann-Pick disease, and other gangliosidoses, mucopolysaccharidoses, and lipid storage diseases.

- **Activation of an alternate metabolic pathway.** In this sequence of events, an enzyme deficiency leads to the accumulation of intermediary metabolites, which are then channeled into an alternate pathway. Metabolites normally formed in minute amounts are produced excessively and accumulate in the body.

$$\begin{aligned} A \rightarrow B &\rightarrow C (\downarrow) D (\downarrow) \\ &\rightarrow X \, Y \, Z \end{aligned}$$

This type of genetic disorder is exemplified by phenylalanine hydroxylase deficiency, the major cause of phenylketonuria. The deficiency of this enzyme, which catalyzes the conversion of phenylalanine to tyrosine, results in both the accumulation of toxic phenylketones and a deficiency in the normal end products of tyrosine metabolism, a pathway essential for the functioning of many cell systems.

- **Formation of abnormal end product.** In this situation an altered genetic code perturbs the synthesis of a structural protein that will form the normal equivalent.

$$A \rightarrow B \rightarrow C \rightarrow d$$

AUTOSOMAL DOMINANT

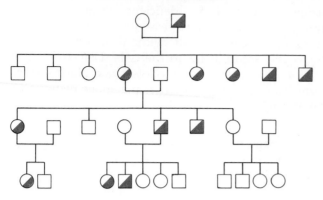

■, ● Heterozygote with disease

Figure 6-16. Autosomal dominant inheritance. Only symptomatic individuals transmit the trait to the next generation, and heterozygotes are symptomatic. Both males and females are affected.

In sickle cell anemia, one such defect, the sequencing of amino acids is normal, except that valine is substituted for glutamine at the sixth position of the beta chain of hemoglobin.

Autosomal Dominant Disorders

The salient features of autosomal dominant traits are the following:

- The gene is located on an autosome.
- The gene produces its effects in both the homozygous and heterozygous states.
- The trait transmitted by the gene appears in every generation, unless it has a low penetrance or its expression has been modified by additional mutations.
- Unaffected members of the family do not transmit the trait to their offspring.
- Affected individuals are usually heterozygous for the trait and transmit it to only one half of their offspring.
- Males and females are equally affected.

Figure 6-16 illustrates the pattern of inheritance of autosomal dominant traits. **More than a thousand human diseases are inherited as autosomal dominant traits, but most of them are rare.** Examples of such diseases are systemic disorders of connective tissue (the Marfan syndrome), skeletal abnormalities (achondroplastic dwarfism), developmental disturbances of the kidneys (polycystic kidneys), maladies of the brain (tuberous sclerosis, Huntington's chorea), hemoglobinopathies (sickle cell anemia, thalassemia), impaired metabolism of cholesterol (familial hypercholesterolemia) and even familial tumors, such as polyposis coli and neurofibromatosis.

Clinically Important Autosomal Dominant Disorders

Heritable Diseases of Connective Tissue

The numerous genetic disorders of collagen are heterogeneous and, in many instances, difficult to classify (Fig. 6-17). This discussion will be limited to three of the most common and best studied entities: the Marfan syndrome, Ehler-Danlos syndrome, and osteogenesis imperfecta. Even in these well-delineated disorders, the clinical symptomatology often overlaps. For instance, some patients exhibit the joint dislocations typical of the Ehlers-Danlos syndrome while other members of the same family suffer from the multiple fractures characteristic of osteogenesis imperfecta. Yet other individuals in the family, with the same genetic defect, may be totally without symptoms. It is clear, therefore, that the current classifications, which are based on clinical criteria, will eventually be replaced by references to specific gene defects, in a manner analogous to the hemoglobinopathies.

The gross structure of connective tissue varies in different organs. For instance, collagen fibrils in tendons are arranged as thick, parallel bundles of fibers. By contrast, the connective tissue of the skin contains randomly oriented collagen fibrils. The collagen fibrils of bone form a complex network around the haversian canals that is reinforced by calcium in the form of hydroxyapatite. In addition, differences in the extracellular matrix proteins of various tissues also reflect the presence of specific gene products. An example is the aorta, a blood vessel that contains a great deal of elastin and an associated microfibrillar protein, as well as a unique mixture of several types of collagen. The strength of collagen resides not only in its intrinsic molecular structure, but also in its crosslinking by covalent bonds between adjacent chains.

Type I collagen is synthesized from two structural genes, and a mutation in either is expressed in all tissues that contain type I collagen. Other types of collagen may also be involved in heritable diseases. For instance, Ehlers-Danlos syndrome, type IV, is caused by mutations in the genes for type III procollagen. The disease is expressed in tissues that are rich in type III collagen—namely, the skin, aorta, and

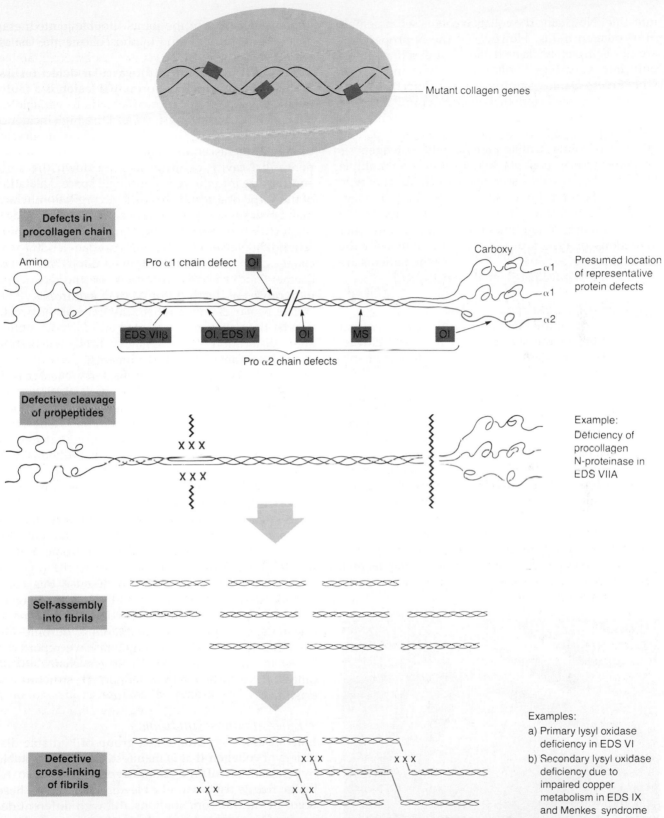

Figure 6-17. Synthesis of type 1 collagen fibers. Collagen genes are initially translated into procollagen chains. The amino and carboxy terminal propeptides are cleaved and the resulting collagen molecules self-assemble into fibrils, which cross-link for stability. Defects in procollagen, propeptide cleavage, or cross-linking lead to disorders of collagen metabolism.

intestine. Normally, the collagen chains self-assemble into collagen fibrils. However, if the N-propeptides are not completely cleaved, the chains self-assemble only into very thin fibrils. Thus, some individuals with Ehlers-Danlos syndrome have defective genes for type I procollagen that do not permit efficient cleavage of the N-propeptides; they are, therefore, afflicted principally by dislocations of the hips and other large joints. Unlike patients with osteogenesis imperfecta, these patients do not suffer from multiple fractures, because the assembly of thick fibrils of type I collagen is not as important for the structural integrity of bone as it is for the ligaments of the joints. On the other hand, certain mutations that result in other alterations of type I procollagen interfere with the mineralization of bone, in which case the patients are considered to have osteogenesis imperfecta.

The Marfan Syndrome

The hallmarks of the Marfan syndrome are structural abnormalities of the skeletal system, the cardiovascular system, and the eye. The skeletal derangements are characterized by dolichomorphism (Gr. *dolichos* long).

The patients are usually (but not invariably) tall, and the lower body segment (pubis-to-sole) is longer than the upper body. A slender habitus, which reflects a paucity of subcutaneous fat, is complemented by long, thin extremities and fingers, the latter accounting for the term "arachnodactyly" (spider fingers) (Fig. 6-18). Overall, the affected individuals resemble figures in a painting by El Greco.

Disorders of the ribs are conspicuous and produce pectus excavatum (concave sternum) and pectus carinatum (pigeon breast). The tendons, ligaments, and joint capsules are weak, a condition that leads to

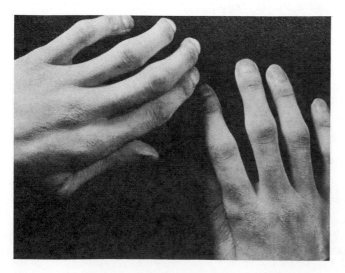

Figure 6-18. Arachnodactyly of Marfan's syndrome.

hyperextensibility of the joints (double-jointedness), dislocations, hernias, and kyphoscoliosis, the last often severe.

The most important cardiovascular defect resides in the aorta, in which the principal lesion is a faulty media. Weakness of the media leads to variable dilatation of the ascending aorta and to a high incidence of dissecting aneurysms. The dissecting aneurysm, usually of the ascending aorta, may rupture into the pericardial cavity or make its way down the aorta and rupture into the retroperitoneal space. Dilatation of the aortic ring results in aortic regurgitation, which may be so severe as to produce angina pectoris and congestive heart failure. The mitral valve may exhibit redundant valve leaflets and chordae tendineae—changes that result in the so-called floppy valve syndrome. Cardiovascular disorders are the most common causes of death in the Marfan syndrome.

The ocular changes reflect the generalized weakness in the structure of collagen and include subluxation (dislocation) of the lens, cataracts (opacification of the lens), and retinal detachments.

Microscopic examination of the aorta reveals a conspicuous fragmentation and loss of elastic fibers, accompanied by an increase in metachromatic mucopolysaccharide. Focally, the defect in the elastic tissue results in discrete pools of amorphous metachromatic material, reminiscent of that seen in Erdheims's idiopathic cystic medial necrosis of the aorta. Smooth muscle cells are enlarged and lose their orderly circumferential arrangement.

The molecular defect in the Marfan syndrome has not been unequivocally identified. Experimental lathyrism, an analogue of the Marfan syndrome, is produced by feeding beta-aminoproprionitrile (derived from sweet clover) to animals. Because this compound interferes with the cross-linking of collagen, it has been postulated that such a defect plays a major role in the pathogenesis of the Marfan syndrome. On the other hand, some investigators have reported a defect in one of the type II collagen chains, while others have proposed an abnormal structure of elastin.

Ehlers-Danlos Syndrome

Ehlers-Danlos syndrome is a group of heritable disorders of collagen that is manifested by a remarkable hyperelasticity of the skin, hypermobility of the joints, fragile tissues, and a bleeding diathesis. These occur in various combinations and with different degrees of severity. The most prominent physical feature of the syndrome is the cutaneous disorder, and patients typically are able to stretch the skin many centimeters. The skin is also unusually fragile, and trivial injuries can lead to serious wounds. Sutures do not hold well and dehiscence of surgical incisions is common. The hypermobility of the joints allows unusual flexion and extension, a circumstance that accounts for the "human pretzel" and other contortionists in the freak shows of an earlier age. The eyes may exhibit blue sclerae (as in osteogenesis imperfecta) and assorted disorders, such as ectopia lentis, a microcornea, retinal detachment, and glaucoma. The internal organs are friable, and spontaneous intestinal perforation, dissecting aortic aneurysm, and hemorrhage in a number of organs have been described. Excessive bleeding during surgery, after trauma or a tooth extraction, or after vigorous brushing of the teeth is a well-known characteristic.

A number of variants (at least eight) of the Ehler-Danlos syndrome have been catalogued according to the predominating clinical features, but all show a **genetic defect in the formation of procollagen.** Some variants show an autosomal dominant pattern of inheritance, whereas others are autosomal recessive. One X-linked recessive form has been described.

Osteogenesis Imperfecta

Osteogenesis imperfecta, or brittle bone disease, is a group of diseases principally inherited in an autosomal dominant pattern, although there are rare cases that are autosomal recessive. A detailed pathologic description is found in the chapter on bone pathology (Chapter 26). **The basic defect is the synthesis of an abnormal type 1 procollagen,** which is manifested mainly as a deficiency in the formation of the bone matrix; in this respect the disorder may be thought of as a hereditary form of osteoporosis. The most striking clinical feature of the disorder is the tendency to sustain multiple bone fractures with even minor trauma.

The disease is divided into two clinical forms— **osteogenesis imperfecta congenita** and **osteogenesis imperfecta tarda.** The congenital variety is fatal *in utero* or shortly after birth owing to the numerous fractures occasioned by normal movements. The skull is thin and soft, and the extremities are short and resemble those of achondroplasia.

The clinical expression of the tarda variety of osteogenesis imperfecta is highly variable, and bone fractures range from severe to minimal. In a severe case trivial trauma can result in fracture of almost any bone: the patient is often said to be as fragile as a china doll. The bones are more radiolucent than normal and have a radiologic appearance resembling that of osteoporosis. As in the Marfan and Ehlers-Danlos syndromes, the joints are hypermobile. The eyes exhibit the classic hallmark of the disease; namely, **blue sclerae.** This appearance reflects a defect in the col-

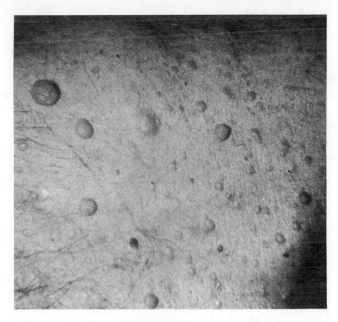

Figure 6-19. Multiple pedunculated neurofibromas on the skin of a patient with neurofibromatosis.

lagen of the sclerae that causes them to be more translucent. Many other ocular disorders have also been described. The skin tends to be thin and, like the sclerae, translucent.

Deafness is not uncommon, owing to defects or fractures in the bones of the middle ear, which lead to otosclerosis. The teeth tend to be opalescent and display a bluish tint, which comes from the blood. Often the teeth have no pulp canal, and dental drilling causes no pain. The dental abnormality is thought to reside in the dentine. Cardiovascular changes like those in the Marfan syndrome have been described occasionally.

Among the collagen abnormalities that have been identified in various types of osteogenesis imperfecta are amino acid substitutions, short peptide deletions, total deficiencies of protein chains, and strangely migrating protein chains.

Neurofibromatosis (von Recklinghausen's Disease)

Neurofibromatosis is one of the most common autosomal disorders. It has been estimated that in the United States there are three million people with some features of this syndrome. At least 50% of cases represent new mutations. In the classic form, neurofibromatosis presents with a triad consisting of **multiple nerve tumors** (Fig. 6-19) (neurofibromas and neurilemmomas); **pigmented skin macules** called "café au lait spots"; and **pigmented nodules of the iris** (Lisch nodules).

Abnormalities of other organ systems are common. About one-third of patients have skeletal lesions, such as scoliosis of the spine, multiple intraosseous and subperiosteal cysts, and various degenerative changes of the joints. Affected individuals are at high risk for developing various tumors—most commonly pheochromocytoma, meningioma, Wilm's tumor, and medullary carcinoma of the thyroid. Pheochromocytomas are found in 1% of patients with this syndrome. Neurofibromatosis associated with pheochromocytoma and medullary carcinoma of the thyroid form the typical clinical triad of the hereditary multiple endocrine neoplasia (MEN) syndrome.

Achondroplastic Dwarfism

Achrondroplastic dwarfs have short limbs and a large head, with a bulging forehead and a deeply indented bridge of the nose. The abnormal gene affects the proliferation of cartilage cells and causes impaired epiphyseal bone growth (see Chapter 26). The condition is more severe in homozygotes, who usually die in early infancy.

Familial Hypercholesterolemia

Familial hypercholesterolemia is one of the most common autosomal dominant disorders and affects at least one in 500 adults in the United States. This topic is treated in greater detail in Chapter 10. Briefly, the genetic defect involves the low density lipoprotein (LDL) receptor on the cell surface, which is crucial for the regulation of the level of LDL and cholesterol in plasma and of cholesterol metabolism in the cells. In familial hypercholesterolemia a deficiency of LDL receptors prevents entry of LDL-cholesterol into the cell, and endogenous cholesterol synthesis is, therefore, not regulated. Overproduction and maldistribution of cholesterol at the cellular level and in various compartments of the body leads to severe complications, primarily affecting the cardiovascular system. In heterozygotes suffering from familial hypercholesterolemia, the number of cell surface receptors for LDL is reduced to a variable extent; in homozygotes they may be lacking entirely. Cholesterol-LDL complexes are still removed from the blood, but only through a less efficient, receptor-independent mechanism. Heterozygotes have a twofold to threefold elevation of plasma cholesterol, whereas in homozygotes the cholesterol levels are five to six times higher than normal. **Patients with hypercholesterolemia develop atherosclerosis at an accelerated rate and suffer at an early age from myocardial infarc-**tion, cerebrovascular accidents, and occlusive peripheral vascular disease.

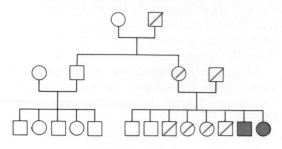

AUTOSOMAL RECESSIVE

■, ● Homozygote with disease

▨, ⊘ Heterozygote without disease (silent carrier)

Figure 6-20. Autosomal recessive inheritance. Symptoms of the disease appear only in homozygotes, male or female. Heterozygotes are asymptomatic carriers.

Autosomal Recessive Disorders

Essentially all clinically identified inborn errors of metabolism and storage diseases, and many of the hereditary traits that have only marginal significance for the practice of medicine, exhibit an autosomal recessive pattern of inheritance. The characteristics of this pattern are as follows:

- The gene is located on an autosome. The effects of the gene are obvious only in the homozygous state.
- Both parents are usually heterozygous for the trait and are clinically unaffected.
- Symptoms appear in one-quarter of the offspring.
- One-half of all siblings are heterozygous for the trait and are thus asymptomatic.
- Males and females are equally affected.

Figure 6-20 illustrates the pattern of autosomal recessive inheritance. The pathogenesis of these disorders follows the principle of "one gene, one enzyme," and the deficient enzyme has been identified in many conditions. Among these are lysosomal storage diseases (glycogenoses, lipidoses, mucopolysaccharidoses), deficiencies of synthetic enzymes (agammaglobulinemia, albinism), transport enzymes (cystinuria), and many others. However, the basic defect in some major autosomal recessive disorders—cystic fibrosis, for instance—has not been identified.

Clinically Important Autosomal Recessive Diseases

Cystic Fibrosis

Cystic fibrosis is the most common clinically important autosomal recessive disorder in Caucasian children, having an incidence of 1 in 2500 newborn white children. More than 95% of cases have been recorded in whites. The disease is found only exceptionally in blacks and almost never in Orientals. Since the condition is autosomal recessive, the afflicted children are obviously homozygous for the trait. According to the Hardy-Weinberg law of human population genetics, the frequency of dominant (d) and recessive (r) genes is calculated from the known incidence of the disease in homozygotes, according to the formula $d^2 + 2dr + r^2 = 100\%$. Since the incidence of cystic fibrosis is 1/2500, or 0.0004, the frequency of the recessive gene (r) is the square root of this number—0.02, or 2%. The dominant gene thus has a frequency of 98% and the $2dr$ frequency of heterozygotes is 0.04 (4%), or 1 in 25 individuals. Recombinant DNA technology has enabled the identification in fetal tissue of restriction fragment length polymorphisms (RFLPs) within the human *mer* gene that predict inheritance of cystic fibrosis.

Cystic fibrosis is a systemic disease that affects essentially all exocrine glands of the body and results in abnormal sweat electrolyte content and hyperviscous secretions in the pancreas, biliary tract, and bronchial tree. The original name, cystic fibrosis of the pancreas, denotes foremost the typical changes in that organ. The ducts are cystically dilated, and fibrosis replaces pancreatic acini destroyed by stagnant pancreatic enzymes. Viscous mucus, which accounts for the synonymous term **"mucoviscidosis"** causes comparable changes in salivary and other mucus-secreting glands, and in organs containing mucus-secreting cells, such as the bronchi, biliary tree, epididymis, and intestine. (Fig. 6-21)

The basic defect in cystic fibrosis is not known. Many theories have been proposed to explain the increased viscosity of the mucus and the biochemical changes found in the sweat, but no unifying concept has emerged. A deficiency in transmembrane transport seems likely. Most of the research has concentrated on the biochemical analysis of the mucus and the role of hormones, minerals, and transport proteins that regulate various cellular secretory mechanisms. Electrolyte disturbances are detectable in the sweat of affected individuals and serve as a test for early diagnosis. **The sodium and chloride content of sweat is two to three times normal, and levels of 60 mEq/liter are diagnostic.** Pilocarpine iontophoresis facilitates the collection of sweat and is the basic test for diagnosis of cystic fibrosis, with an accuracy of over 95%.

Clinically the condition presents even *in utero*. Viscous contents of the gut (**meconium**) cause obstruction, which is associated with forceful peristaltic movements. This blockage results in ileus or peritonitis, owing to the extravasation of intestinal contents (**meconium peritonitis**). In infancy and early childhood, nutritional deficiency is the major clinical problem. Because the pancreatic ducts are obstructed, digestive enzymes do not reach the intestine. Consequently, the patient shows the typical symptoms of malabsorption, such as lipid intolerance, bulky fatty stools (**steatorrhea**), and deficiencies of the fat-soluble vitamins (A,D,K). Obstruction of the biliary tree is another contributory cause of malabsorption.

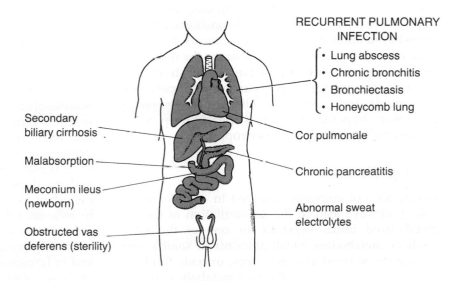

Figure 6-21. Clinical features of cystic fibrosis.

RECURRENT PULMONARY INFECTION
- Lung abscess
- Chronic bronchitis
- Bronchiectasis
- Honeycomb lung

Secondary biliary cirrhosis

Malabsorption

Meconium ileus (newborn)

Obstructed vas deferens (sterility)

Cor pulmonale

Chronic pancreatitis

Abnormal sweat electrolytes

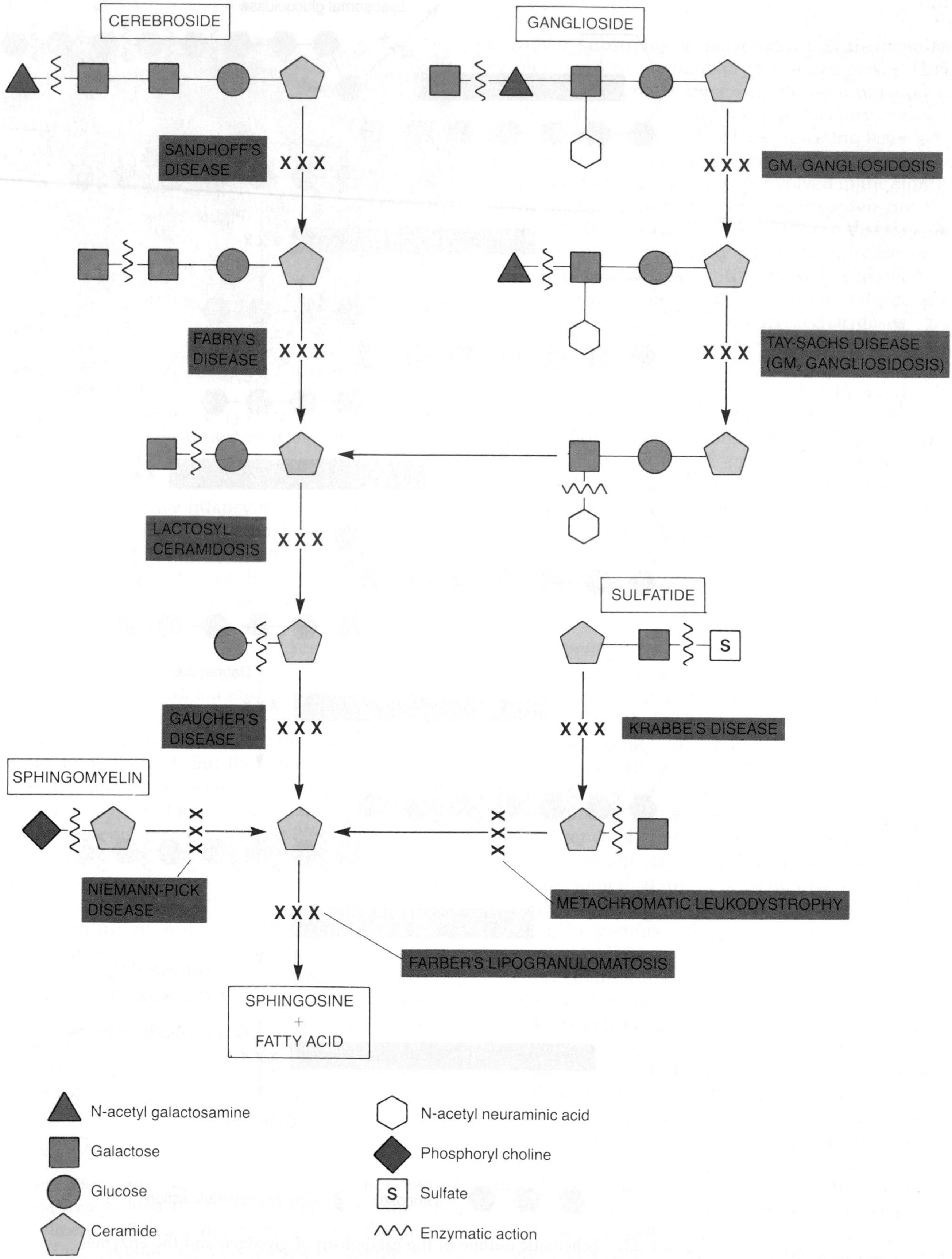

Figure 6-24.   Disturbances of lipid metabolism in various sphingolipidoses.

zymatic deficiency. For instance, acid maltase is a lysosomal hydrolase, and its deficiency disease is, thus, characterized by storage of glycogen in lysosomes.

Sphingolipidoses

The sphingolipidoses are the most important group of disorders involving disturbances of lipid metabolism. Sphingolipids consist of a basic structural unit, ceramide, composed of a long-chain base, sphingosine, linked by an amide bond to a long-chain fatty acid. Two forms of sphingolipids, called cerebrosides and gangliosides, are formed from this basic unit through the addition of various oligosaccharide chains attached to the first carbon of the sphingosine. Sphingolipidoses are inborn errors of metabolism that are characterized by deficiencies of lysosomal enzymes responsible for cleaving various moieties from cerebrosides and gangliosides in the catabolic pathway that ends in sphingosine and fatty acids (Fig. 6-24). Cerebrosides, gangliosides, and various degradation products accumulate in lysosomes, which contain whorls of concentrically layered membranes. The specific enzyme deficiency is determined biochemically in cultured cells from a skin biopsy, blood, or amniotic fluid.

The brain is commonly affected in Fabry's disease and variants of the Niemann-Pick disease. The salient features of Tay-Sachs disease and Gaucher's disease will be discussed.

Tay-Sachs disease was described in the 1880s as "familial amaurotic idiocy," a term designating mental deterioration and blindness as the major clinical findings. Initially, affected children appear normal, but in early infancy the disease evolves rapidly, and most children succumb by the age of 3 years. The basic defect is a deficiency of hexosaminidase A, with a compensatory increase in hexosaminidase B. **GM_2 ganglioside accumulates in the lysosomes of all organs, but it most dramatically affects the neurons and retinal cells.** Owing to the pallor of the lipid-laden retinal cells, the normal red color of the choroid of the macula appears more prominent and is labeled the **cherry-red spot.** The lipid-laden neurons appear enlarged and vacuolated in histologic sections. Electron microscopy reveals lipid accumulation in lysosomes, which appear filled with whorls of lipid-rich membranes ("myelin figures") (Fig. 6-25). Because of the progressive loss of neurons, the brain exhibits narrow gyri, although excessive accumulation of ganglioside may even result in enlargement of the brain. The degenerative changes in the brain interrupt normal development, motor and mental functions rapidly deteriorate, and death is inevitable within 2 to 3

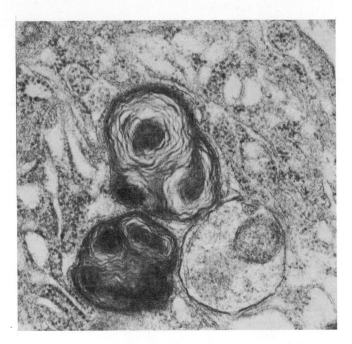

Figure 6-25. Tay-Sachs disease. The cytoplasm of the nerve cell contains lysosomes filled with whorled membranes.

years after the onset of symptoms.

Tay-Sachs, an autosomal recessive disorder, primarily afflicts Ashkenazi Jews. Approximately 1 in 30 Ashkenazi Jews is a carrier of the defective gene. Heterozygous carriers are detected with appropriate biochemical tests, and the affected fetus can be identified by amniocentesis or chorionic villus sampling.

Gaucher's disease reflects a deficiency of glucocerebrosidase, the lysosomal enzyme that cleaves glucose from the ceramide backbone. This enzyme degrades glycolipids formed continuously from turnover of lipid-rich cell membranes. For example, it is involved in the degradation of glycolipids liberated from the membranes of senescent red blood cells taken up by the reticuloendothelial cells in the liver and spleen. Since the brain contains more lipid than most other tissues, and since the reticuloendothelial cells of the spleen and liver are the major degradation sites for the senescent erythrocytes, it is understandable that deficiency of glucocerebrosidase primarily affects those organs.

There are three forms of Gaucher's disease. In the most common form—type I or **adult Gaucher's disease**, found primarily in Ashkenazi Jews—the disease presents with hepatosplenomegaly, but without any neurologic symptoms. The adult form does not pose any serious symptoms and does not shorten the life span. In the type II form, also called **infantile Gaucher's disease**, both the brain and the reticuloendoth-

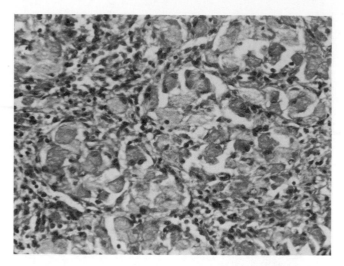

Figure 6-26. The spleen in Gaucher's disease. Typical Gaucher's cells have foamy cytoplasm and eccentrically located nuclei.

elial system are involved. The disease, which shows no predilection for Jews, begins in early infancy, and death occurs early. The third form of the disorder is termed **juvenile Gaucher's disease**. There is no ethnic predominance, and the clinical presentation is intermediate between the adult and infantile forms. Patients with type I disease have reduced levels of glucocerebrosidase, patients suffering from type II disease have no measurable enzyme activity, and type III patients are somewhere in between. Although all three forms of Gaucher's disease involve the same enzyme, the differences in enzyme activity indicate that the disorders may be caused by different mutations.

Gaucher's cells—reticuloendothelial cells filled with glucocerebroside—have a characteristic microscopic appearance. They are large and display abundant, vacuolated, lipid-laden cytoplasm. (Fig. 6-26). The cytoplasm is rich in carbohydrates, as evidenced by strong staining with the PAS technique. By electron microscopy, the storage material is found within the lysosomes and appears as parallel layers of twisted membranes.

Mucopolysaccharidoses

Mucopolysaccharides are high-molecular-weight polymers composed of hexosamines and hexuronic acid. Complexed with protein to form proteoglycans, they are integral components of the extracellular matrix. Connective tissue cells synthesize the mucopolysaccharides and are also involved in their degradation.

Mucopolysaccharidoses are inborn errors of metabolism involving the lysosomal enzymes engaged in the degradation of mucopolysaccharides (Fig. 6-27). Fibroblasts and other connective tissue cells that produce mucopolysaccharides excrete most of the synthesized material. However, a small fraction remains in the cytoplasm and is degraded by lysosomal enzymes, such as alpha-L-iduronidase or beta-glucosaminidase. A lack of one of these enzymes results in the **accumulation of mucopolysaccharides in the lysosomes,** primarily in connective tissue cells but also in other cells, most notably neurons. Although there are several distinct clinical entities having different underlying enzyme deficiencies, in all cases the storage material consists of one or more of the four mucopolysaccharides: heparan sulfate, dermatan sulfate, keratan sulfate, and chondroitin sulfate.

The clinical presentation of each disease has its own peculiarities, but most mucopolysaccharidoses also have certain common features, including skeletal deformities, aortic and cardiac valvular lesions, and corneal clouding. Mental retardation is invariably present in all mucopolysaccharidoses. Many of the patients are dwarfs and show coarse facial features and hepatosplenomegaly, a picture resembling the gargoyle figures from Gothic cathedrals. Hence, the term "gargoylism" applied to patients with the prototype of this group of disorders, namely **Hurler's syndrome**. Most patients with mucopolysaccharidoses have a shortened life span. Cardiovascular changes, due to deposits of mucopolysaccharides in the coronary arteries and valves and the aorta are major causes of morbidity and mortality. Except for Hunter's syndrome, which is X linked recessive, all are autosomal recessive traits. Excessive amounts of mucopolysaccharides in the blood, urine, and amniotic fluid serve as the basis for diagnosis. This is confirmed by analyzing the cells (skin or amniotic fluid) for specific enzyme deficiencies.

Inborn Errors of Amino Acid Metabolism

Many enzyme deficiencies involve the metabolism of amino acids. Some present serious clinical problems, whereas others are of lesser importance. Only a short discussion of the closely related metabolic pathways of phenylalanine and tyrosine will be presented.

Phenylalanine is an essential amino acid derived from dietary protein. Tyrosine is also obtained principally from food, but it is also formed by the action of phenylalanine hydroxylase. Through an intermediary product, tyrosine serves as a starting point for the synthesis of melanin, epinephrine, and thyroid hormones. The degradation pathway of tyrosine begins through its conversion into homogentisic acid and ends in formation of CO_2 and H_2O. Phenylalanine that does not enter into the tyrosine pathway is converted into phenylpyruvic acid, which in turn gives rise to phenylketones that are excreted in the urine. Enzyme deficiencies that interrupt these metabolic pathways produce distinct chemical syndromes, known as phenylketonuria (PKU), tyrosinosis, ochronosis, alkaptonuria, hypothyroidism and albinism (Fig. 6-28).

Phenylketonuria

In phenylketonuria **a deficiency of phenylalanine hydroxylase** prevents the conversion of phenylalanine into tyrosine, and all the dietary phenylalanine is shunted into the formation of phenylketones. Early in childhood, neurological dysfunction, typified by hyperirritability, tremor, and hypertonicity, gives rise to slowly progressive mental deterioration. An excess of phenylacetic acid accounts for a peculiar "mousey" odor. The phenylketones also competitively inhibit the enzyme that mediates the conversion of tyrosine to melanin. The children are, therefore, fair-haired and have hypopigmented skin. Elevated levels of serum phenylalanine and urinary phenylketones can be detected biochemically in newborn infants, but not prenatally: The fetus is generously supplied with maternally produced phenylalanine and does not use the phenylketone-producing pathway.

If an affected child is placed on a phenylalanine-deficient diet early in life, mental retardation can be prevented. In fact, children placed on an appropriate diet at not later than 3 months of age achieve normal intelligence. The diet must be continued for at least 6 to 8 years. The degree of mental deficiency correlates with the delay in instituting the diet. A phenylalanine-deficient diet is of no help after 1 year of age.

Albinism

Albinism is a common inborn error of metabolism that is related to several defects in the synthesis of melanin. Melanin synthesis starts with the initial conversion of tyrosine to 3,4-dihydroxyphenylalanine (DOPA), which is then converted to melanin. Both steps are catalyzed by tyrosinase, and a deficiency of this enzyme results in deficient melanin synthesis, or albinism. The skin and eyes of those affected are devoid of pigment. It should be noted that tyrosinase deficiency accounts for only some forms of albinism. The enzymatic defect in the other group, called **ty-**

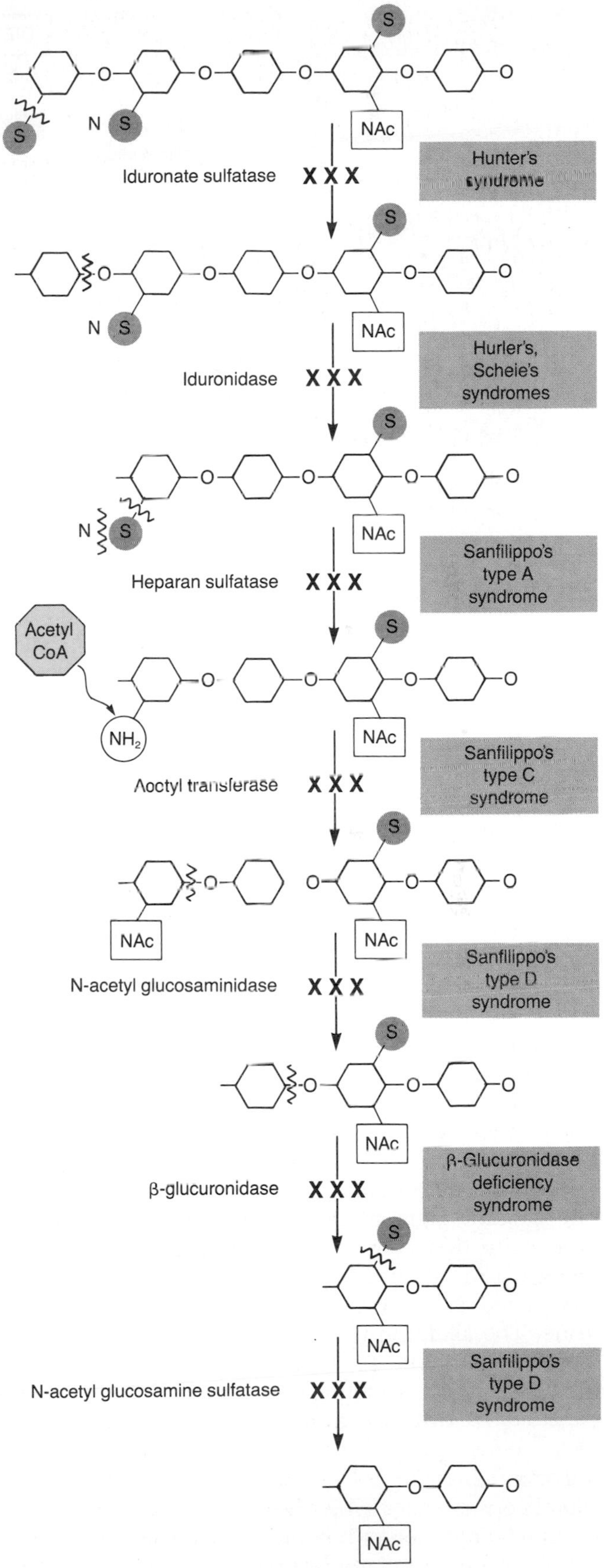

Figure 6-27. Metabolic disturbances in various mucopolysaccharidoses.

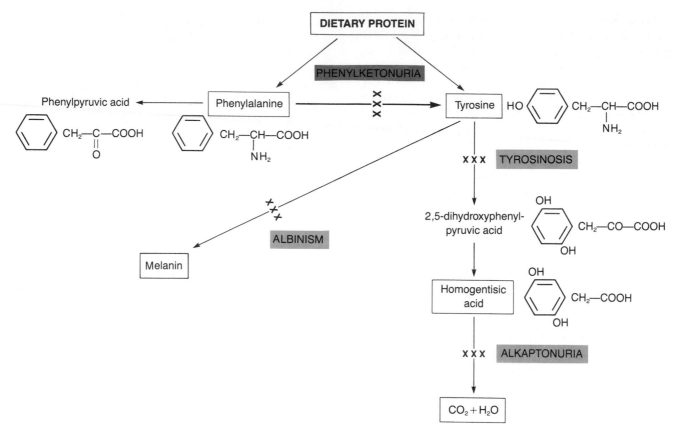

Figure 6-28. Disturbances of phenylalanine and tyrosine metabolism causing albinism, tyrosinosis, and alkaptonuria.

rosinase-positive albinism, has not been fully identified.

Ochronosis (Alkaptonuria)

Oxidative degradation of tyrosine leads to formation of homogentisic acid, which is further degraded to water and CO_2. **Ochronosis or alkaptonuria is caused by a deficiency of homogentisic acid oxidase,** which blocks further degradation of homogentisic acid. The acid undergoes spontaneous conversion into a black pigment called **alkapton**, which accumulates in the body. Alkapton formed from homogentisic acid excreted in the urine turns black and is recognized as dark spots on diapers soaked with urine. The alkapton formed from homogentisic acid deposited in connective tissue and cartilage causes dark discoloration of the ear lobes and sclera, and degenerative arthropathy.

Tyrosinemia

Inborn errors that involve the enzymes responsible for the degradation of tyrosine (i.e., errors that cause tyrosine to accumulate) are rare. The only common disorder is neonatal tyrosinemia. At least 30% of pre-

mature and 10% of term infants develop neonatal tyrosinemia. Other than a high level of tyrosine in the blood, this transitory condition has no clinical significance. The disorder reflects the slow activation of p-hydroxyphenylpyruvic acid oxidase (p-HPPA), an enzyme that is present in inadequate amounts before birth.

A genetic deficiency of p-HPPA causes the rare condition called **hereditary tyrosinemia**, a disease that presents in an acute and chronic form. The acute form presents 2 to 3 months after birth and manifests as an enlarged liver and hepatic insufficiency. The chronic form is seen in late infancy and early childhood and is manifested primarily as a renal absorptive defect, which leads to aminoaciduria, rickets, and complex metabolic disturbances. Serum levels of tyrosine greater than 3 mg/dl are always found. Both acute and chronic forms are invariably lethal.

Sex-Linked Disorders

The term sex-linked inheritance primarily denotes conditions that are recessive and caused by genes located on the X chromosome. Recessive mutations involving genes on the X chromosome are not expressed in females, because the homologous X chromosome contains the dominant allele. If the same recessive gene is present in the male, however, there is no hindrance to its expression, since the Y chromosome does not have a homologous allele. X-linked recessive genes may be expressed in females, but only in individuals homozygous for the trait.

Certain recessive X-linked traits are partially expressed in females. This fact is best explained in light of Lyons' hypothesis, which states that one of the two X chromosomes in the cells is inactivated. Since this inactivation (**Barr body** formation or heteropyknosis) occurs at random in various cell clones, it follows that a woman with one recessive and one dominant allele on the X chromosomes will at random inactivate one or the other. Some cells thus express the dominant and others the recessive gene. This is illustrated by glucose-6-phosphate dehydrogenase (G6PD) deficiency, an X-linked trait that predisposes to hemolysis of blood exposed to various chemicals. For the sake of simplicity, one could designate the enzyme activity in a normal man as 100 and that in an afflicted recessive man as 10. Recessive women, being mosaics, have red blood cells with either the active or inactive X chromosome. In this instance glucose-6-phosphate dehydrogenase activity is intermediate between 10 and 100, depending on the number of clones with inactivated X chromosomes.

The pattern of X-linked recessive inheritance is illustrated in Figure 6-29. The principles of this form of inheritance are as follows:

- The gene is located on the X chromosome.
- The recessive traits are fully expressed in heterozygous males and rarely in homozygous females.
- Partial expression may occur in heterozygous females, a phenomenon that reflects the random inactivation of one X chromosome.
- A trait is usually transmitted by asymptomatic females.

- Each son of a heterozygous female carrier has a 1 in 2 chance of being affected.
- Unaffected males do not transmit the gene.
- Affected males do not transmit the trait to their sons, but only to daughters. These daughters then become asymptomatic carriers. Rarely, if they inherit the second recessive allele from a carrier mother, daughters homozygous for the trait may present with symptoms.

There are close to 100 identified genes on the X chromosomes. Important clinical conditions inherited as X-linked recessive traits include hemophilia A and B, red-green color blindness, Duchenne's muscular dystrophy, glucose-6-phosphate dehydrogenase deficiency, diabetes insipidus, and some congenital immunodeficiency syndromes, such as Bruton's agammaglobulinemia, the Wiskott-Aldrich syndrome, and the Lesch-Nyhan syndrome.

Clinically Important Disorders

Hemophilia

Hemophilia is an inborn bleeding disorder that occurs in two forms, known as hemophilia A (classic hemophilia), and hemophilia B (Christmas disease). Factor VIII:C is missing in hemophilia A and Factor IX in hemophilia B. Since the gene for Factor VIII:C is very large and occupies about 0.1% of the entire X chromosome, it is understandable that point mutations or deletions occur more often in this region than in the smaller region that codes for factor IX. Accordingly, hemophilia A occurs six times more often (1:5000 males) than hemophilia B (1:30,000 males). The mutation or deletion rate for the locus that codes for factor VIII:C is high, as evidenced from the fact that one in four patients presents without any family history. The complexity of the factor VIII:C gene accounts, in part, for the variable symptoms of the disease, which may present in a spectrum from a

X-LINKED RECESSIVE

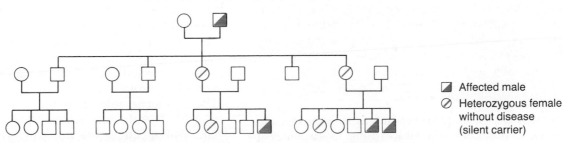

Figure 6-29. X-linked recessive inheritance. Only males are affected; females are asymptomatic carriers. Asymptomatic males of the kindred do not transmit the trait.

mild to a severe bleeding disorder. About 20% of patients have subclinical disease and have no bleeding problems at all. Another 25% have considerable disturbances of coagulation, and the remaining half of all patients suffer from severe, debilitating coagulopathy. These patients have factor VIII:C levels that are less than 5% of normal. The situation is made even more complicated by the fact that 6% of patients treated by transfusions (usually those with lowest levels of factor VIII:C) develop autoantibodies called factor VIII:C inhibitors. Hemophilia B presents invariably as a severe bleeding disorder.

Muscular Dystrophy

Duchenne's muscular dystrophy is the most important of the three clinically distinct forms of muscle disease transmitted as X-linked recessive traits. The disease is rare, affecting one to four males per 100,000. "Spontaneous" mutations involve the relevant genetic region at a rate estimated to be one per million, and the number of affected individuals has been increasing.

The trait is transmitted by the mother, but the disease affects only boys. Symptoms appear in early childhood, and by school age most patients are incapacitated. The muscle wasting first involves the pelvic and femoral muscles, but the disease progressively spreads to the extremities and finally paralyzes the truncal muscles. Most affected individuals are confined to a wheelchair by puberty and do not survive beyond 20 years. All of them also have reduced intelligence. Histologically, the dystrophic muscles show degeneration and necrosis, and compensatory

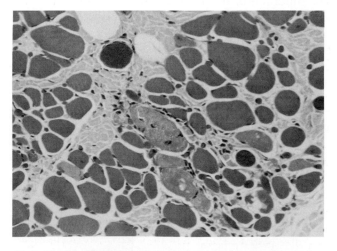

Figure 6-30. Dystrophic skeletal muscle in Duchenne's muscular dystrophy. Note the variation in size and shape of muscle cells and the intrafascicular fibrosis.

hypertrophy of the remaining fibers (Fig. 6-30). Connective tissue ultimately replaces the wasted muscle fibers. Replacement of muscle cells with fat cells accounts for the weakness of bulging calf muscles, a prominent clinical finding appropriately designated as "pseudohypertrophy." Loss of muscle fibers is accompanied by elevation of serum **creatine phosphokinase** (CPK) levels. Female carriers do not have symptoms but may have elevated levels of CPK.

Multifactorial Inheritance

Most human traits are inherited neither as dominant nor as recessive mendelian characteristics, but in a more complex manner known as **multifactorial inheritance.** This type of inheritance is determined by a combination of many genetic and nongenetic factors, each of which exerts a minor, but nevertheless distinct, effect. The contribution of each gene cannot be measured in exact units. Neither is it possible to predict whether their interaction will be additive or substractive. Furthermore, disorders stemming from multifactorial inheritance cannot easily be recognized as mendelian traits by analyzing family pedigrees. Still, the concept of multifactorial inheritance has been tested and proved in both experimental animals and man.

Multifactorial inheritance is best studied by population genetics or by the analysis of concordance in twins and families affected by rare diseases. Most of the quantifiable traits—for example, height or intelligence—have a distribution in the general population that corresponds to the gaussian (bell-shaped) curve. These traits are examples of **continuous multifactorial** characteristics that exhibit a range of values, with a continuous gradation between two extremes. Arterial hypertension and diabetes mellitus are diseases that belong to this category.

The so-called **discontinuous multifactorial traits,** less common but pathogenetically more important, account for a considerable number of **congenital malformations and common adult diseases (Table 6-4).** Discontinuous multifactorial traits produce clinical effects only if the ratio of underactive (mutant) and normally active genes reaches a critical threshold. The predisposition to develop clinical signs of such a trait is graphically represented as a gaussian curve, but the affected individuals represent only that fraction of the total number above a critical threshold. The incidence rate in the population reflects this threshold, and is determined by the number of mutant genes. Thus, the offspring of parents with a more severe defect (which is presumably produced

Table 6-4 Multifactorial Traits

CONTINUOUS		DISCONTINUOUS	
TRAITS	DISEASES	CONGENITAL MALFORMATIONS	DISEASES
Height	Hypertension	Cleft lip and pal-	Manic-depressive psychosis
Intelligence	Diabetes	ate	Schizophrenia
Blood pressure		Pyloric stenosis	Rheumatoid arthritis
Skin color		Anencephaly	
Metabolic		Congenital heart	
parameters		disease	

by more mutant genes) have a greater chance of expressing the defect than those born to less affected individuals. Moreover, the close relatives of an affected person have more mutant genes than the population at large and have a greater chance of exhibiting signs of the trait. For first-degree relatives this chance is in the range of 2% to 7%. The concordance of discontinuous multifactorial traits in identical twins is not complete and usually varies from 20% to 40%, suggesting that environmental factors are crucial determinants for the regulation of expression.

The following characteristics of multifactorial inheritance are useful in determining whether a condition is a multifactorial or a single-gene trait.

- The expression of symptoms is proportional to the number of mutant genes. The chances of expressing the same number of mutant genes are highest in identical twins, who express the trait concordantly about one-third of the time.
- Environmental factors influence the expression of the trait. Thus, concordance of the expression is seen in fewer than half of monozygotic twin pairs. As a rule, if the concordance rate for a particular trait in monozygotic twins is double that in dizygotic twins, the trait is not inherited as a mendelian dominant. If the concordance is more than four times higher, mendelian recessive inheritance can be excluded and the trait is most likely inherited as multifactorial.
- Relatives of those affected have an increased risk of disease. For all first-degree relatives, parents, siblings and children, the risk is the same (2–7%). The risk is considerably lower for second-degree relatives.
- The probability of the trait's being expressed in later offspring is influenced by whether or not it was expressed in earlier offspring. If one or more children are born with a multifactorial defect, the overall chances for recurrence rise from 2–7% to 9%. This contrasts with mendelian traits, in

which the probability of occurrence is independent of the number of affected siblings.
- The more severe the defect the higher are the chances that it will be transmitted to offspring or recur in subsequent pregnancies. Individuals with more severe defects have presumably more mutant or inactive genes, and their offspring thus have a greater chance of inheriting some of the abnormal genes than offspring of a less affected individual.

Clinically Important Disorders

Cleft Lip and Cleft Palate

At about the 35th day of pregnancy, the frontal prominence fuses with the maxillary process to form the upper lip. **Many processes of upper lip formation are easily disturbed, thereby leading to malformations.** Any disturbance of morphogenesis of the facial structures may interfere with the proper fusion of the fetal rudiments and lead to cleft lip, with or without cleft palate (Fig. 6-31). This anomaly may be part of a systemic malformation syndrome due to various well-known teratogens (rubella, anticonvulsants) and is often encountered in children with chromosomal abnormalities. The incidence of cleft lip is 1 in 1000 in white and 0.4 in 1000 in black American children. In addition to this racial difference, 60% to 80% of affected individuals are male. The clinical consequences vary from a minor cosmetic defect to a serious anatomical anomaly that impairs normal speech and feeding.

Cleft lip and palate are an excellent paradigm to illustrate the principles of multifactorial inheritance. If one child is born with cleft lip, the chances are 4% that the second child will also exhibit the defect. If the first two children have the defect, the risk increases to 9% for the third child. The severity of the defect also influences the risk.

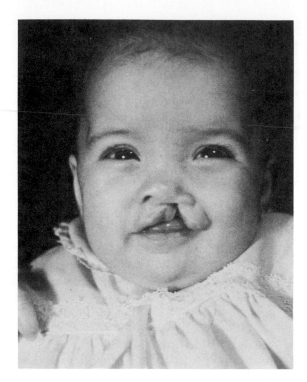

Figure 6-31. Cleft lip and palate.

Since the anomaly occurs less frequently in females than in males, one could speculate that the threshold for the number of mutant genes is higher in females. If this is true, the offspring of affected females should be at higher risk than those of similar males. Indeed, sons of women with cleft lip and palate have a four times higher risk of expressing the defect than sons of affected males.

Prenatal Diagnosis of Genetic Disorders

Amniocentesis and chorionic villus biopsy are the most important diagnostic methods for the diagnosis of developmental and genetic disorders (Fig. 6-32). Both procedures are safe, reliable, and easily performed. The indications for chorionic villi biopsy or amniocentesis in pregnant women are as follows:

- **Age 35 years old and over.** The risk of having a child with Down's syndrome is about 1 in 300 for the 40-year-old woman, compared to 1 in 1200 at age 25. This risk rises even higher with advanced maternal age.
- **Previous chromosomal abnormality.** The risk of recurrence of Down's syndrome in a succeeding child of a woman who has already borne an infant with trisomy 21 (Down's syndrome) is about 1%. There are no data to predict the risk for recurrence of other autosomal trisomies and sex chromosome abnormalities.
- **Translocation carrier.** Estimates of risks to the offspring of translocation carriers vary from 3% to 15% for D/G translocation carriers to 100% for 21/21 translocation carriers. The risks of hereditary diseases to children of carriers of uncommon translocations are unknown.
- **History of familial inborn errors of metabolism.** The recessive inborn errors of metabolism have a risk of 25% for each child. Prenatal diagnosis should be considered in all of these disorders for which a definitive biochemical diagnosis can be made.
- **Identified heterozygotes.** Carrier detection programs, such as the Tay-Sachs Disease Prevention Program, detect couples in which both spouses are carriers of the same recessive gene. Each pregnancy to such couples has a 25% risk of an affected child, and prenatal diagnosis should routinely be made.
- **Family history of X-linked disorders.** Fetal sex determination, using amniotic cells, should be offered to women known to be carriers for X-linked disorders. The diagnosis of some of these conditions can be corroborated biochemically by amniotic fluid analysis.
- **Occurrence of neural tube anomalies in a previous pregnancy.** The recurrence risk for a neural tube disorder, when a couple has had such a child, is 15%. First-degree relatives of affected persons may have a high enough risk themselves to warrant alpha-fetoprotein determination in amniotic fluid.

Diseases of Infancy and Childhood

The period from birth to puberty has been traditionally subdivided into several stages: neonatal age, spanning the first 4 weeks; infancy (first year); early childhood (1–4 years); and late childhood (5-14 years). Although growth is continuous, each of these periods has its own distinct anatomical, physiologic, and immunologic characteristics, which determine the nature and form of various pathologic processes. Morbidity and mortality rates in the neonatal period differ considerably from those in infancy and childhood.

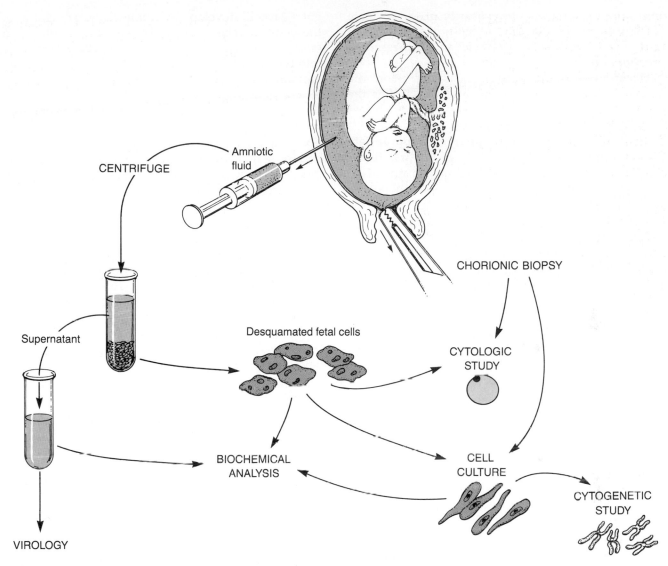

Figure 6-32. Principles of prenatal diagnosis. It is possible to sample the amniotic fluid or the chorionic villi for cytogenetic and biochemical tests.

In the neonatal period, which is a continuation of intrauterine life, the major health problems are directly related to developmental pathology, as influenced by inherited traits in the fetus, maternal influences, and environmental factors acting through the mother and the placenta. Genetic and developmental factors have been discussed; here we will deal only with maternal influences operating in late pregnancy. Infants and children are not simply "small adults," and they may be afflicted by many systemic and organ-specific diseases unique to their particular age group. Most of these conditions will be discussed in the chapters dealing with specific organ pathology.

Disorders Related to Maturity of the Neonate

Normal human pregnancy lasts 40 ± 2 weeks, and most babies born at term weigh 3300 ± 600 g. The duration of pregnancy and the weight of the newborn are good estimates of neonatal maturity, but certain babies may reach maturity even before the 38th week of pregnancy, and at least 10% of term babies weigh less than 2500 g. The term **prematurity,** indiscriminately applied to all neonates weighing less than 2500 g or born before term, is still clinically useful, although body weight and duration of pregnancy are only rough estimates. **The maturity of the neonate is the sum of the maturity of its organs, which in turn may be precisely evaluated and expressed in functional terms.**

In contrast to birth at term, deliveries before the 38th week are called **preterm,** and those after the 42nd week **post term.** Term babies who weigh less than 2500 g are called **small for gestational age** (SGA), while other newborns are labeled **appropriate for gestational age** (AGA) and **large for gestational age** (LGA) infants. Preterm babies may also be SGA, and a combination of these two factors doubles the risk of neonatal death and adversely affects life expectancy. Below a gestational age of 34 weeks, the weight of the baby does not influence the prognosis, and the overall morbidity and mortality depend almost exclusively on the duration of pregnancy—the shorter the pregnancy the greater the risk.

The causes of intrauterine growth retardation that result in an SGA birth belong to several classes: fetal factors, maternal factors, and defined environmental influences. In one-third of SGA infants the cause of intrauterine growth retardation cannot be determined. **Placental insufficiency,** an imprecise term, has been invoked to explain some idiopathic cases.

When intrauterine growth retardation exists in the presence of an adequate nutritional supply and in the absence of adverse environmental or maternal metabolic conditions, it is usually due to fetal abnormalities. These include various genetic metabolic disorders, chromosomal anomalies, and developmental malformations. **Identifiable exogenous causes include infections, smoking, alcohol, and drug abuse.** Inadequate maternal nutrition may be a significant contributory factor, but no clearcut relationship between SGA and nutritional factors has been established. Maternal diabetes and renal and cardiac disease all predispose to intrauterine growth retardation. SGA babies usually reach normal size by late infancy or early childhood. Identifiable fetal abnormalities, low gestational age, and serious postnatal complications adversely affect the neural development of SGA babies, which is the most serious consequence of this condition.

The maturity of the neonate can be defined in anatomical and physiologic terms. The maturing organs differ morphologically from those in term babies, although complete morphologic and physiologic maturity of many organs is not achieved until later in life.

The **maturity of the lungs** is of paramount importance for normal postnatal life. The fetal lungs develop as branching tubes that originate from the foregut. Alveoli develop as terminal outpouching of these tubes. The fetal alveoli are thick-walled and only in late pregnancy do the lining cells differentiate into type I and II pneumocytes. Fetal alveoli are only partially expanded and are filled with amniotic fluid. At the time of birth the amniotic fluid pours out of the lungs and air expands most of the respiratory spaces. Sluggish respiratory movements do not suffice to evacuate the amniotic fluid from the lungs, and those neonates who die at this point have incompletely expanded lungs. On histologic examination the alveolar ducts, bronchioles, and larger bronchi contain squames, lanugo hair, and protein-rich amniotic fluid (Fig. 6-33). Some alveoli contain the same material, whereas most of the others appear collapsed; that is, they display **atelectasis.** This residual amniotic fluid is often called **amniotic fluid aspiration,** although this "aspiration" reflects only the inability of the fetus to expel all the fluid from the lungs.

Alveoli expanded through the first inspiration collapse again unless they are kept open by the elastic tension generated by the connective tissue in the septa and by the cell surface tension generated by surfactant. **Pulmonary surfactant** is a complex mixture of several major phospholipids produced by type II alveolar pneumocytes. In the adult lung 75% of the surfactant consists of phosphatidylcholine (lecithin), 10% is phosphatidylglycerol, and the remainder consists of several other minor components, including 1.5% sphingomyelin. In the adult lung lecithin is of the surface-active dipalmitic phosphatidylcholine

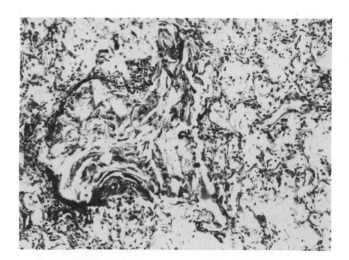

Figure 6-33. Incompletely expanded fetal lung with retention of amniotic fluid. Amniotic fluid contains desquamated fetal skin and lanugo hair. Such squames are readily recognizable in the fetal airspaces.

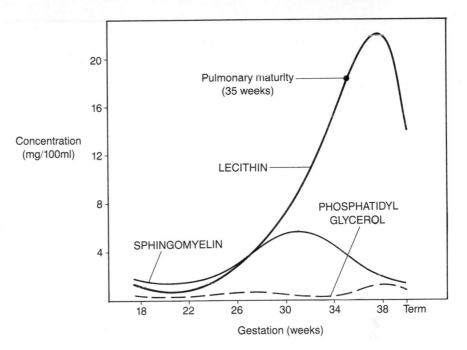

Figure 6-34. Changes in the amniotic fluid composition during pregnancy. The onset of pulmonary maturity is enhanced by a surge of lecithin and a concomitant decrease of sphingomyelin. Phosphatidyl glycerol is a good marker of fetal lung maturity, but it appears late (i.e., 35 weeks) and is thus of limited practical value in earlier stages of pregnancy.

type; in the fetal lung, however, the less active alpha palmitic, beta myristic lecithin predominates. Furthermore, phosphatidylglycerol is not present in the lungs before 36 weeks of pregnancy. Before the 35th week of pregnancy the immature fetal lungs secrete surfactant that differs from adult surfactant in several respects: (1) it contains a higher proportion of sphingomyelin; (2) instead of the surface-active dipalmitic lecithin, it contains alpha palmitic, beta myristic lecithin; and (3) it does not contain phosphatidylglycerol. Fetal pulmonary surfactant is released into the amniotic fluid, which can be sampled in pregnancy to determine fetal lung maturity (Fig. 6-34). Most often, a lecithin:sphingomyelin ratio above 2:1 indicates that the fetus will survive without developing the respiratory distress syndrome. The appearance of phosphatidylglycerol is the best available biochemical proof of fetal lung maturity. This compound is not present in fetal lungs before the 35th week and is, therefore, of little practical significance before that time.

The **liver** of premature infants has the basic structure of the adult organ, and the only obvious sign of immaturity is the residual foci of extramedullary hematopoiesis. The functional immaturity of hepatocytes cannot be assessed morphologically, but it presents in many forms. **The most obvious evidence of hepatic immaturity is the inability of the liver to conjugate and excrete bilirubin—a failure that leads to jaundice.** Jaundice (**icterus neonatorum**), due in part to the rapid destruction of fetal erythrocytes and

in part to a deficiency of glucuronyl transferase, appears often in neonates. It is more pronounced in premature babies and usually lasts longer in these infants than in those born at term. Other liver functions are also not fully operational, but the deficiencies are easily overcome with adequate medical support.

The **brain** of an immature neonate differs significantly from that of an adult. Although these differences are easily identified morphologically, the immaturity of the brain rarely presents clinical problems. The fetal **kidneys** and **adrenals,** although also different from the adult organs, are usually mature enough to sustain extrauterine life, even in extremely premature babies.

A clinical assessment of neonatal maturity is usually performed at 1 minute and 5 minutes after delivery, and the vital signs are scored according to the criteria recommended by Virginia Apgar (Table 6-5). The Apgar score has considerable prognostic value and is widely used in the evaluation of newborn infants.

Respiratory Distress Syndrome of the Newborn

The respiratory distress syndrome is one of the major clinical problems affecting premature babies. Although the exact pathogenesis of the syndrome has not been fully elucidated, the evidence indicates that

Table 6-5 Apgar Score

SIGN	0	1	2
Heart rate	Not detectable	Below 100/min	Over 100/min
Respiratory effort	None	Slow, irregular	Good, crying
Muscle tone	Poor	Some flexion of extremities	Active motion
Response to catheter in nostril	No response	Grimace	Cough or sneeze
Color	Blue, pale	Body pink, extremities blue	Completely pink

Sixty seconds after the completion of birth the five objective signs above are evaluated and each is given a score of 0, 1, or 2. A maximum score of 10 is assigned to infants in the best possible condition.

it is related to or caused by immaturity of the lung and inadequate release or storage of surfactant by type II pneumocytes.

At term the fetal lungs are anatomically mature and functionally prepared to adapt for the transition from an intrauterine to an extrauterine environment. The alveoli are fully formed by the 25th week, and by the 31st week the type II pneumocytes already produce adequate amounts of surfactant, which still differs from that of the term newborn. The bronchial and pulmonary circulations are characterized *in utero* by **high pressure** and **low flow**. This situation leads to a high pulmonary resistance, which exceeds the systemic resistance. Most of the blood circulates through the placenta, and only 5% to 10% perfuses the lungs.

Neuromuscular control of respiration is effectively established long before birth. External compression of the thorax during passage through the vaginal canal ejects some of the amniotic fluid from the lungs and also leads to subsequent recoil of the chest wall. These actions facilitate the first active inspiratory movement and the entry of air into the lungs, which inflates the alveoli. The amniotic fluid is exhaled and resorbed, leaving the alveoli coated with surfactant. This sequence of events decreases the external compression of the capillaries in the alveolar walls, and the pulmonary blood flow suddenly rises. Increased alveolar oxygen tension further expands the precapillary vascular space through dilatation of arteries and arterioles. Decreased vascular pressure in the entire pulmonary circulation, accompanied by an enormous influx of blood from the right ventricle, further facil-

itates the absorption of the alveolar fluid and results in augmented lymph flow and increased flow of oxygenated blood into the left atrium. These events, followed in early infancy by the closure of the ductus arteriosus, lead to the transformation of the **fetal high-resistance, low-flow** pulmonary circulation into the **adult low-resistance, high-flow** circulation.

Disturbances in lung maturation and in the various transitions from fetal to adult pulmonary circulation, mechanical factors, and disturbances in the neural control of respiration all cause respiratory distress in the newborn. Among the identifiable causes are incidents affecting the respiratory center in the central nervous system. For example, oversedation of the mother during the delivery may affect the fetal brain. Traumatic brain injury of the fetus at birth, with bleeding into or ischemic necrosis of the respiratory centers, prevents normal respiration. Asphyxia may be due to mechanical factors, birth trauma, or umbilical cord strangulation. Metabolic disorders in the mother—for instance, diabetes mellitus—may impair respiration. Blockage of the air passages due to particulate matter, blood clots, or aspirated meconium from the amniotic fluid can also cause respiratory distress. However, more common than all other forms of respiratory distress is the **idiopathic syndrome,** presumed to be due to functional and anatomical immaturity of fetal lungs.

The **idiopathic respiratory distress syndrome of neonates** is usually a disease of preterm AGA babies. Most infants appear normal and have a good Apgar score. However, some were born in protracted labor, showed intrapartum asphyxia, and needed resusci-

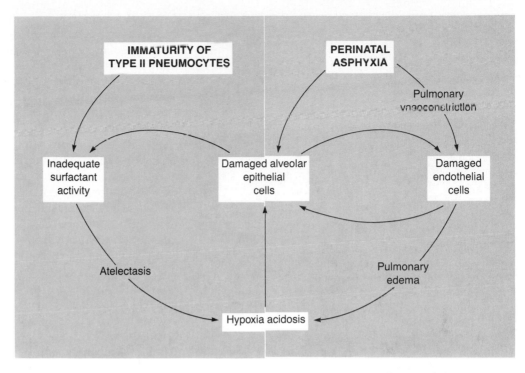

Figure 6-35. Pathogenesis of the idiopathic respiratory distress syndrome of the neonate. Immaturity of the lungs and perinatal asphyxia are the major pathogenetic factors.

tation. Typically, increased respiratory effort is the first symptom and is easily recognizable 30 to 60 minutes after birth. The infants show forceful intercostal retraction and use accessory neck muscles. A loud expiratory grunt is produced by the forceful passage of air through the partially closed glottis. Partial closure of the glottis represents a Valsalva maneuver to maintain the positive end-respiratory pressure and keep the alveoli open. However, as the compliance of the lungs diminishes, this maneuver becomes less efficient and the baby cannot compensate for the respiratory insufficiency by closing the glottis.

To meet the demand for oxygen, the respiratory center increases the number of respirations to more than 100 per minute, and the accessory thoracic respiratory muscles are used to maintain the terminal airways open by forcing the expansion of lungs through negative intrathoracic pressure. A characteristic seesaw respiration reflects the diminished compliance of the lungs, which forces the protrusion of the diaphragm into the abdominal cavity and, thus, the bulging of the abdomen with each inspiration. Finally, the sternum and the anterior portion of the ribs collapse under the negative intrathoracic pressure.

The skin is pale because of peripheral vasoconstriction, but the internal organs are congested with unoxygenated blood. Edema, most prominent on the face, palms, and soles, becomes generalized (anasarca). The chest radiograph shows a characteristic "ground glass" granularity, with prominent bronchi extending into the pulmonary periphery. In terminal stages the fluid-filled alveoli contribute to the complete "whiteout" of the chest. The infant becomes progressively obtunded and flaccid and experiences long periods of apnea interspersed with periods of irregular breathing. Many infants are saved by intensive care and assisted ventilation, but the mortality is still high. Type II pneumocytes need 3 to 4 days to become fully functional. If the child survives these first few days, it often recovers. Recovery, unless there are major complications, is usually quite satisfactory. After protracted respiratory distress and prolonged treatment with a respirator, a few babies develop chronic pulmonary disease.

A basic defect causing the idiopathic respiratory distress syndrome in preterm babies is the immaturity of the lungs, particularly type II pneumocytes (Fig. 6-35). Qualitatively and quantitatively, fetal surfactant is less efficient than adult surfactant in lowering the alveolar surface tension and keeping the

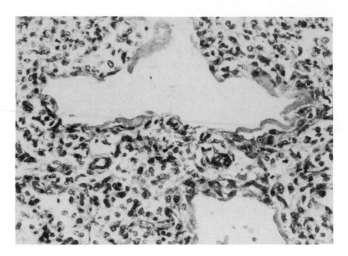

Figure 6-36. The lung in idiopathic respiratory distress syndrome of the neonate. The alveoli are atelectatic, and the dilated alveolar ducts are lined with fibrin-rich hyaline membranes.

alveoli open. Because lung compliance is low, the critical negative pressure needed to allow influx of air into the lungs cannot be attained. The collapse of alveoli (atelectasis) not adequately coated with surfactant reduces the pulmonary surface, allowing exchange of gases only through the walls of alveolar ducts and terminal bronchioles—structures that are not suitable for that purpose. Anoxia and hypercapnia cause acidosis, leading to peripheral vasodilation and pulmonary vasoconstriction. This situation, in turn, leads to the reestablishment of a partial fetal circulatory pattern. Right-to-left shunting of unoxygenated blood through the ductus arteriosus and foramen ovale further contributes to hypoperfusion of the lungs, jeopardizing the respiratory oxygen supply even more. Hypoxia adversely affects pulmonary cells, and necrosis of endothelial, alveolar, and bronchial cells takes place. Vascular disruption causes transudation of plasma into the alveolar spaces and layering of fibrin ("hyaline membranes") along the surface of alveolar ducts and respiratory bronchioles partially denuded of their normal cell lining. This in turn further impedes the passage of oxygen from the alveolar spaces across the respiratory surface into the pulmonary vasculature. Moreover, extravasation of blood into the respiratory passages, combined with the collapse of the alveoli, further contributes to the consolidation of the lungs. In terminal stages air is found only in bronchi and dilated bronchioles, and the rest of the lung is consolidated and airless.

On histologic examination the lungs have a characteristic appearance. The alveoli are collapsed and the alveolar ducts and respiratory bronchioli are dilated. Within these spaces cellular debris, proteinaceous edema fluid, and some red blood cells accumulate. The lining of the dilated alveolar ducts is covered with fibrin-rich hyaline membranes. The walls of the collapsed alveoli are thick, the capillaries are congested, and the lymphatics are filled with proteinaceous material (Fig. 6-36).

The outcome of the idiopathic respiratory distress syndrome of the neonate depends on the severity of the disease, the gestational age of the infant at birth, and the presence of complications or aggravating conditions. The overall mortality is still about 30%, and in infants born before 30 weeks of pregnancy it is over 50%. Aggravating factors, such as maternal diabetes, anoxia during delivery, or extensive blood loss, also adversely influence the outcome. Rapid development of profound respiratory insufficiency unresponsive to standard treatment is a bad omen and is associated with high mortality. Mild cases can be salvaged with oxygen alone, whereas more serious distress requires intensive care to correct acidosis, sustain the failing circulation, and assist the respiration.

Major complications of the idiopathic respiratory distress syndrome of the neonate are **intraventricular cerebral hemorrhage**, persistence of the **patent ductus arteriosus** and **necrotizing enterocolitis**. These pathologic changes are consequences of anoxia, hypercapnia, and acidosis.

The **periventricular germinal matrix** in the brain is especially susceptible to injury in neonates with respiratory distress. Dilated, thin-walled veins in this area rupture easily, leading to extravasation of blood into the brain and destruction of nerve cells . Bleeding often extends into the ventricles and causes **hematocephalus** (Fig. 6-37). Factors invoked to explain the pathogenesis of this injury include the lack of connective support of the germinal matrix blood vessels, impaired vascular autoregulation, hypoxia leading to venous sludging, thrombosis, and direct injury to periventricular capillaries, and increased fibrinolytic activity in the fetal brain that allows the formation of large hematomas. None of these theories provides a full explanation for the occurrence of this complication.

The clinical diagnosis may be suspected on the basis of an acute onset of hypotension, acidosis, flaccidity, hypoventilation, and a sudden drop in he-

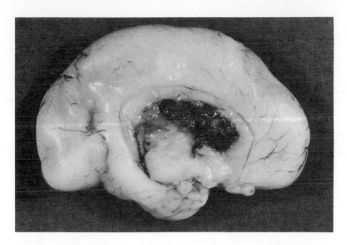

Figure 6-37. Hemorrhage into the periventricular matrix in a premature infant suffering from the idiopathic respiratory distress syndrome of the neonate. The hemorrhage has penetrated into the lateral ventricle and caused hematocephalus.

matocrit in an otherwise stable infant. The mortality of intracerebral and intraventricular hemorrhage exceeds 50%. However, this serious complication is not invariably lethal, and many children recover without significant neurologic deficits. Posthemorrhagic hydrocephalus is found in 20% of survivors.

Persistence of the ductus arteriosus is a serious consequence of the respiratory distress syndrome that is due to the partial preservation of the fetal circulation. Blood is shunted from right to left through the foramen ovale and the ductus, thus bypassing the lungs. In many neonates who survive the syndrome, the ductus remains patent. Circulatory recovery reverses the shunt and forces blood from the arterial side into the pulmonary circulation. Pulmonary congestion and right sided heart failure may ensue and are clinically apparent in almost one-third of all infants recovering from the respiratory distress syndrome.

Necrotizing enterocolitis, a less common but serious complication, is the most common acquired gastrointestinal emergency in neonates. The pathogenesis of this condition is not fully understood. It has been suggested that the lesion is initiated by anoxic necrosis of intestinal mucosal cells, leading to ulceration, perforation, and finally peritonitis. Bacterial infection is always evident but is thought to be superimposed on the initial injury caused by anoxia. Necrotizing enterocolitis occurs in neonates who have been fed formula fluids. It is thought that various components or the hypertonicity of the formulas may potentiate the effects of ischemia and facilitate bacterial overgrowth. Penetrating ulcers are usually localized to the ileum and cecum.

Bronchopulmonary dysplasia is a late complication of the respiratory distress syndrome that usually occurs in infants who weigh less than 1500 g and were maintained on a respirator for more than 6 days. Radiographically the lungs show focal emphysema and atelectasis. Exudative inflammation in the alveoli leads to the formation of granulation tissue, which progresses to fibrosis. In the final stages the lungs show focal fibrosis and bullous emphysema. Pulmonary hypertension and eventually cor pulmonale develop. In order to prevent bronchopulmonary dysplasia, respirator treatment should be as short as possible, and attempts to close the patent ductus arteriosus should be made. Despite precautions, bronchopulmonary dysplasia will develop in some infants.

Erythroblastosis Fetalis and Neonatal Hemolytic Anemia

Erythroblastosis fetalis is defined as hemolytic disease in the fetus or newborn caused by transplacental passage of maternal antibodies directed against paternally inherited antigens on fetal red blood cells. Since the fetal red blood cells, like other cells, express both maternally and paternally inherited gene products, paternal gene products could, theoretically, be recognized by the maternal immune system as foreign. However, the placenta and the fetal membranes provide a barrier that prevents immunization of the mother by paternal antigens. **Maternal-fetal blood group incompatibility may, nevertheless, result in hemolytic anemia in the fetus**.

In order to understand maternal-fetal blood group incompatibility, it is helpful to compare the Rh and ABO systems. The **Rh blood group system** consists of a group of some 25 components, of which only the alleles cde/CDE are strong antigens. In practice, Rh serotyping is limited to the strongest of these three antigens, namely d/D—*D* denoting the Rh-positive and *d* the Rh-negative individuals. Rh-negative persons comprise approximately 15% of the Euro-American Caucasian population, and 5% of Afro-American blacks. Japanese, Chinese, and North American Indian populations contain essentially no Rh-negative individuals.

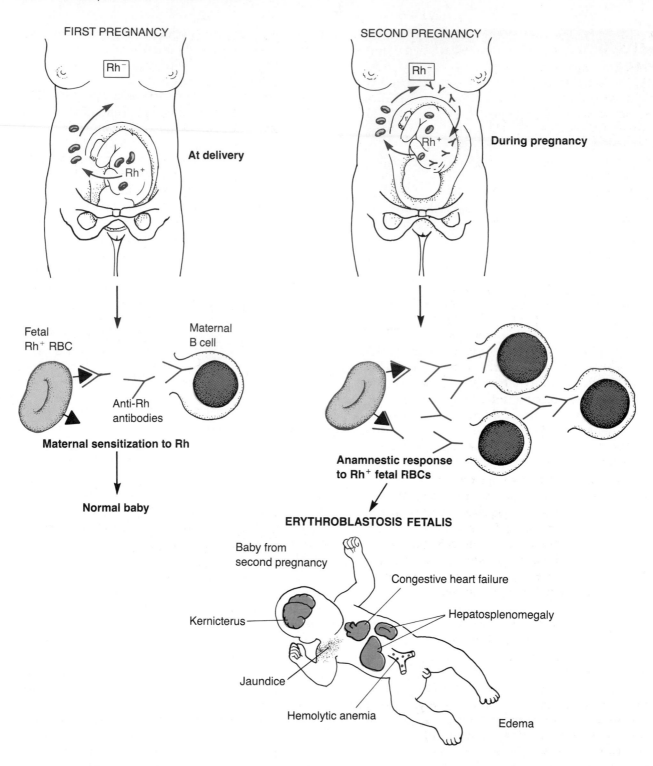

FIRST PREGNANCY

Rh⁻

At delivery

SECOND PREGNANCY

Rh⁻

During pregnancy

Rh⁺

Rh⁺

Fetal
Rh⁺ RBC

Maternal
B cell

Anti-Rh
antibodies

Maternal sensitization to Rh

**Anamnestic response
to Rh⁺ fetal RBCs**

Normal baby

ERYTHROBLASTOSIS FETALIS

Baby from
second pregnancy

Congestive heart failure

Kernicterus

Hepatosplenomegaly

Jaundice

Hemolytic anemia

Edema

Figure 6-38. Pathogenesis of erythroblastosis fetalis due to maternal-fetal Rh incompatibility. Immunization of the Rh-negative mother with Rh-positive erythrocytes in the first pregnancy leads to the formation of anti-Rh antibodies of the IgG type. These antibodies cross the placenta and damage the Rh-positive fetus in subsequent pregnancies.

In contrast to the naturally occurring antibodies against the major ABO blood group antigens, antibodies to Rh antigens are found only in Rh-negative people who are immunized with Rh-positive blood. Typical antibodies to ABO are of the IgM class, and only some persons of type O have natural IgG anti-A or anti-B. Whereas the initial immunization with Rh-positive cells produces a surge of IgM antibodies, the second exposure leads to the production of IgG antibodies. This is of particular importance in pregnancy, since **only IgG crosses the placenta.**

A characteristic sequence leading to Rh-related erythroblastosis fetalis starts with immunization of an Rh-negative mother with blood of an Rh-positive infant, who has inherited the D antigen from an Rh-positive father (Fig. 6-38). Immunization usually occurs at the time of delivery, owing to the passage of fetal blood into maternal uterine veins. Immunization can also occur during the late stages of pregnancy because of **transplacental transfusions,** but since only minute amounts of fetal blood cross the placenta, this is rarely the case. Other forms of immunization include spontaneous or induced abortion, with entry of Rh-positive fetal blood into the mother, and transfusion of Rh-positive blood into an Rh-negative person. As already stated, this initial exposure to Rh-positive blood leads to IgM antibody formation, which is of little clinical significance. A surge of IgG antibodies after the second exposure to Rh-positive blood—usually a second pregnancy with an Rh-positive fetus—hemolyzes the fetal red blood cells.

An Rh-positive fetus in an isoimmunized Rh-negative mother develops normally through the first two trimesters. As the transplacental transport of immunoglobulins becomes more efficient in the third trimester, and as the paternal antigens become fully expressed on fetal red blood cells, immune hemolysis increases. Fetal injury presents in three clinical forms of graded severity. The most severe is **hydrops fetalis** (Fig. 6-39). Less severe is **icterus gravis**, and the mildest form is **congenital anemia of the newborn.** Because of the destruction of red blood cells, generalized anoxia develops, affecting most prominently the heart, liver, and brain. Hypoxic liver cells produce less serum proteins, an effect that decreases the oncotic pressure of the plasma. Together with the inefficient pumping of blood by the anoxic heart, this leads to generalized edema, or hydrops fetalis.

Hemolyzed red blood cells release hemoglobin, which is degraded to bilirubin. In the fetus or neonate, an oversupply of bilirubin, combined with functional immaturity of the liver and anoxia of liver cells, leads to jaundice. Unconjugated bilirubin is normally

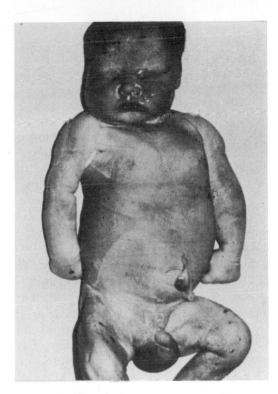

Figure 6-39. Hydrops fetalis. The stillborn infant shows anasarca and desquamation of the skin due to intrauterine death and maceration of the skin by the amniotic fluid.

bound to albumin in the serum. Since dysfunction of the liver cells leads to hypoalbuminemia, much of the bilirubin is not complexed to albumin and crosses the blood-brain barrier, to be deposited in the brain substance. Unconjugated bilirubin is toxic to the brain and causes edema and yellowish discoloration, most prominently in the basal ganglia. Jaundice of basal nuclei is known by the German term **kernicterus** (Kern = nucleus).

On external examination the fetus affected by the severe form of erythroblastosis fetalis *in utero* is born edematous and pale, the pallor being due to anemia. Jaundice—that is, yellowish discoloration of the sclerae and skin—is mild, because the excess bilirubin is cleared through the placenta. Hepatosplenomegaly is prominent. The most prominent histologic findings are in the liver and the placenta. The liver shows prominent extramedullary hematopoiesis. The placental villi are extremely edematous. Their loose connective tissue contains prominent lipid-laden placental macrophages (**Hofbauer cells**), and the fetal blood vessels are packed with nucleated red blood cells. The surface of the chorionic villi is covered with cytotrophoblastic cells, even in the late stages of pregnancy, when the trophoblast normally consists predominantly of syncytiotrophoblastic cells and contains only scattered cytotrophoblastic cells. The pathologic changes in milder forms of the disease are not diagnostic, are usually transient, and do not have serious consequences. Kernicterus may result in mild to severe neurologic deficits.

The clinical diagnosis of erythroblastosis, which is suspected on the basis of the maternal-fetal blood group incompatibility, is corroborated by laboratory tests that indicate immune hemolysis. A direct Coombs' test performed on fetal red blood cells demonstrates the presence of hemolytic immunoglobulins on the surface of the cells; this result is the most important evidence that the hemolysis in the neonate is immunologically mediated. Serologic tests are used to determine whether the hemolysis is due to antibodies directed to Rh antigens or to the ABO blood group antigens.

Since 15% of white women are Rh-negative, and since they have an 85% chance of marrying an Rh-positive man, 13% of all marriages are theoretically at risk for maternal-fetal Rh-incompatibility. The actual risk for the fetus is, however, much smaller. First, isoimmunization of the mother occurs only if the fetus is Rh-positive. Thus, if the father is heterozygous D/d, the fetus has only a 1 in 2 chance of inheriting the Rh-positivity. Second, the risk for isoimmunization of the mother is directly proportional to the amount of fetal blood that reaches the mother during pregnancy or at birth. If the amount of fetal blood does not exceed 0.1 ml—and this is the case in most instances—the chances for isoimmunization are slim. Third, if there is an ABO blood group incompatibility between the mother and the fetus, even if more than 0.1 ml fetal blood enters into maternal circulation, most fetal cells carrying the foreign antigens will be coated with the natural maternal antibody and eliminated before immunization of the mother can take place.

With appropriate medical care erythroblastosis fetalis can be almost completely prevented. **Rh immunoprophylaxis is based on the administration of anti-D immunoglobulin to all Rh-negative women within 72 hours after delivery of an Rh-positive infant.** This treatment interdicts isoimmunization of 98% of all Rh-negative women and efficiently prevents erythroblastosis fetalis. Unfortunately 2% of Rh-negative women become sensitized during pregnancy or in the immediate postpartum period, and are not helped by this prophylactic procedure. Exchange transfusions and intensive care of affected neonates saves most infants from even these high-risk pregnancies.

Because of the efficient immunoprophylaxis of erythroblastosis fetalis due to Rh incompatibility, hemolytic disease of the newborn caused by **ABO and other minor blood group antigens** has achieved relative prominence. Fortunately, hemolysis of fetal red blood cells in these cases is usually much milder than with Rh incompatibility. One might expect a considerable number of pregnancies to exhibit maternal-fetal incompatibility of the ABO system, but only 10% of these children show mild hemolysis, and only 1 in 200 presents with symptoms that require treatment. Usually the hemolytic disease occurs in group O mothers carrying an A, B, or AB fetus. Infants with the A_1 blood group, antigen for which is usually strongly expressed on fetal red blood cells, are at highest risk. Some blood group O mothers have peculiar natural IgG antibodies to AB antigens. Since these antibodies are not elicited by previous sensitization in pregnancy, the first infant may also be affected.

The reasons for the infrequent occurrence of hemolytic disease due to ABO maternal-fetal incompatibility are several. Natural antibodies to AB are IgM and do not cross the placenta. Even if IgG antibodies reach the fetus, hemolysis is weak because the fetal red blood cells do not strongly express the ABO antigens. Major blood group antigens are also expressed on fetal and placental blood vessels, which bind a significant amount of these antibodies and eliminate them from circulation. Finally, there are no efficient ways of predicting or preventing hemolytic disease of the newborn caused by ABO incompatibility. Since the disease is mild in most instances, it does not present a major public health problem.

Birth Injury

Natural birth lasts, in most instances, several hours and is associated with considerable stress on both the mother and the fetus. Injuries occur easily and although most of them are minor—for example caput **succedaneum** and **cephalhematoma**—a considerable number of mishaps contribute significantly to morbidity in infancy and disability later in life.

The **head, skeleton, liver,** and **peripheral nerves** are most frequently affected. Compression of the head during the passage through the birth canal or by forceps may cause a tear in the falx cerebri, tentorium cerebelli, or dural sinuses, with massive **subdural or epidural hematomas.** The fragile brain tissue is also easily bruised, especially in premature infants and term infants large for gestational age. Massive intracranial hemorrhage causes an acute onset of neurological symptoms and results in death. Birth injury of the brain can also have disturbing chronic consequences, including **cerebral palsy.**

Bones are easily **fractured** during birth, but many of these fractures are partial and heal easily, and they are generally subclinical. Due to the occipital positioning of the fetus in the uterine canal the humerus is more often broken than the leg bones. The clavicle is actually the most commonly fractured bone, but this fracture usually presents no clinical problems and passes unnoticed.

Birth trauma may affect nerves and result in subsequent paralysis. **Facial nerve injury** and **tearing of the brachial plexus** are the most common forms of injury, again reflecting the most common, head-first form of natural birth. Rupture of large abdominal organs, primarily liver and spleen, is a rare but potentially serious birth injury.

Sudden Infant Death Syndrome (SIDS)

The sudden infant death syndrome (SIDS), also known as "crib death," is a term given to "sudden and unexpected death of an infant who was either well or almost well prior to death, and whose death remains unexplained after the performance of an adequate autopsy." SIDS is one of the major causes of infant mortality, an estimated 10,000 cases occurring annually in the United States.

Typically, SIDS occurs in 2- to 4-month old infants, most of whom seem perfectly healthy or have only a minor respiratory illness. The infants usually die unexpectedly during the night. There are no satisfactory explanations for the occurrence of sudden death, and there are no reliable means to identify children at risk. Autopsy usually reveals minor signs of anoxia, but the findings are nonspecific and cannot be interpreted unequivocally. There exist children who experienced prolonged apnea but were saved and resuscitated by a watching parent. Such cases, which are considered to represent "near misses," suggest that some infants in this age group have labile cardiorespiratory centers that inadequately control cardiovascular function. However, it is uncertain whether central disturbances of respiration or heart function indeed represent the basic defect in all affected infants, or whether the condition has more than one cause and pathogenetic pathway.

Tumors of Infancy and Childhood

Although tumors of infancy and childhood do not account for more than 2% of all neoplasms, they are responsible for about 10% of all deaths in this age group. Some tumors are diagnosed at birth or in the immediate neonatal period and have obviously evolved *in utero.* In addition to these **developmental tumors,** others originate in **abnormally developed organs, organ primordia, and displaced organ rests,** an observation suggesting that somatic and neoplastic development represent two diametrically opposite aspects of ontogenesis.

Under normal circumstances the embryonic cells differentiate into specialized somatic descendants through a series of events that ultimately limits the capacity of the cells to proliferate and endows them with highly specialized functions. This progressive, but differential, gene repression and activation is called **differentiation.** If the embryonic cells do not reach the level of differentiation essential for the functional integrity of the organ, but rather continue to proliferate as undifferentiated or only partially differentiated stem cells, a tumor forms. Many embryonic tumors are composed of undifferentiated cells that do not differ from normal embryonic cells except that they proliferate without any obvious reason. Other tumors contain endogenous growth promoters, oncogenes, or point mutations, which make them aberrant and morphologically "malignant." It is important to realize that tumors of infancy and childhood often exhibit some basic features of normal embryonic or fetal cells and that under appropriate conditions these malignant cells can cease their proliferation and transform into nonproliferating, terminally differentiated descendants. Thus, a neonatal neuroblastoma may be "spontaneously" cured by differentiating into benign ganglioneuroma. The good prognosis of most saccrococcygeal teratomas is attributed to a "maturation" with age, the tumor changing from fetal to adult tissues. These examples demonstrate the ability of some tumors of infancy and childhood to revert from a malignant phenotype to a nonproliferating benign form in a process that resembles normal organ maturation.

Benign Tumors and Tumor-like Conditions

Most benign tumors encountered in infancy and childhood are actually developmental abnormalities and cannot be clearly separated from hamartomas and choristomas. **Hamartomas** represent an excessive

7

Hemodynamic Disorders

Wolfgang J. Mergner and Benjamin F. Trump

Circulatory Anatomy,
Physiology, and Regulation

Hemodynamic Disorders of
Perfusion

Disorders of Water and
Electrolytes

Embolism

Shock

Figure 7-1. Capillary system of the heart. The coronary arteries were washed with Ringer's solution and filled with a low-viscosity plastic. Subsequently the heart tissue was digested with concentrated KOH. The cast of the capillaries was then observed under low-magnification scanning electron microscopy. *C,* capillary; *A,* arteriole.

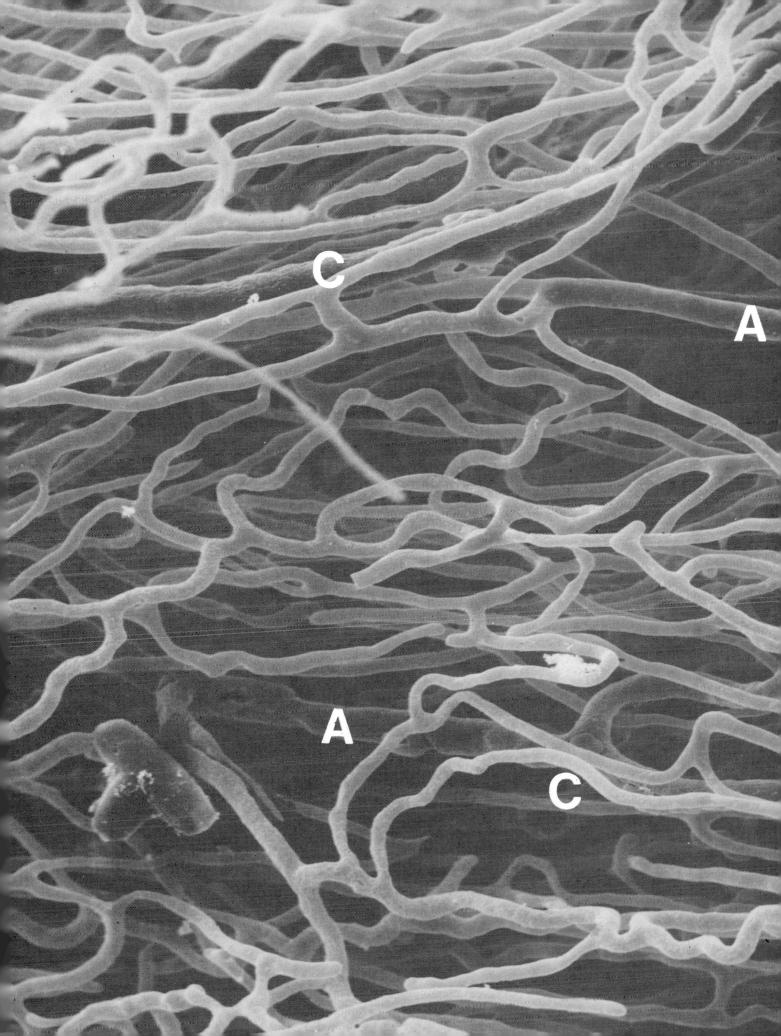

Circulatory Anatomy, Physiology, and Regulation

The metabolism of organs and cells depends on an intact circulation for the continuous delivery of oxygen, nutrients, hormones, electrolytes, and water, and for the removal of metabolic waste and carbon dioxide. **Delivery and elimination at the cellular level are controlled by exchanges among the intravascular space, interstitial space, cellular space, and lymphatic space.**

The **intravascular space** is the sum of the volumes of the lumina of capillaries, veins, and arteries. The tightness of the capillary barrier varies from organ to organ; the brain has a very tight barrier, called the "blood–brain barrier," while the liver has permeable sinuses with large gaps between the sinusoidal lining cells.

The **interstitial space** between the blood capillaries and the membranes of parenchymal and connective tissue cells is filled by collagen fibers and interstitial substances, including glycosaminoglycans. This interstitial gel prevents fluids from moving freely but does not limit their filtration and reabsorption along the capillaries. Moreover, it does not significantly interfere with the movement of molecules and metabolites. The pleural cavity, the pericardium, and the peritoneal cavity are extensions of the interstitial space.

The **cellular space** is the sum of the spaces within the confines of the plasma membranes of all cells. The plasma membrane controls access to the cellular space by the expenditure of energy.

The **lymphatic space** is surrounded by the lymphatic endothelial cells. The driving force for lymph is the difference in pressure between the interstitial space and the thoracic duct system. Increased production of interstitial fluid increases interstitial pressure and leads to an elevated lymphatic flow. Interstitial fluid production may increase if capillary permeability increases or if hydrostatic pressure in capillaries increases. It has been proposed that the large lymphatics produce a slightly negative pressure, owing to contractile elements in their wall. The average lymph flow is 2 to 4 liters/24 hr, or 2 ml/min.

Diffusion, Filtration, and Transport

The movement of solids, fluids, and gases across the barriers between compartments occurs by diffusion, filtration, and vesicular transport. The barrier between all compartments is modified by cells and cell membranes. In diffusing, lipid-soluble substances such as gases can utilize the entire endothelial capillary cell surface—a total of 6,000 square meters. This diffusion occurs at a rate of 55,000 ml/min in both directions. Oxygen, carbon dioxide, glucose, and other nutrients are exchanged in this way.

The movement of fluid between compartments is called **filtration** and occurs passively along pressure gradients—the hydrostatic pressure gradient and the osmotic pressure gradient. The **hydrostatic pressure** at the site of the arteriolar capillary is 32 mm Hg, while at mid-capillary it is 20 mm Hg. This hydrostatic pressure difference, together with a 5 mm Hg interstitial osmotic pressure, represents an **outward force** in the intravascular space. This outward force is balanced by an interstitial hydrostatic pressure of 3 mm Hg plus an osmotic pressure of 26 mm Hg in the intravascular space. The net pressure difference causes outward fluid filtration across the capillaries at a rate of 14 ml/min at the arterial end. Osmotic reabsorption produces an inward movement of 12 ml/min at the venous segment. Lymphatic flow drains the remaining 2 ml/min, so that in equilibrium there is no net fluid gain or loss.

The major function of filtration is the regulation of plasma volume. The anatomic site of filtration still has not been precisely identified; it is thought to be between endothelial cells, an area amounting to approximately 0.2% of the entire potential exchange area. The filtration fluid contains 0.2% protein, which, since it cannot normally reenter the circulation, must be cleared by the lymphatics. The protein content of lymphatics varies with the organ; lymph from the extremities, for example, contains 1% protein, while that from the liver contains 6%.

The Heart

The heart is a two-chambered pump, with the two vascular circuits placed in series. The amount of blood pumped by the right ventricle must, over time, equal the amount of blood pumped by the left ventricle. The hemodynamically important parameters are cardiac output, perfusion pressure, and resistance. The function of the heart determines the cardiac output and perfusion pressure. Cardiac output is the volume of blood pumped by each ventricle per minute, and represents the blood flow in the pulmonary and systemic circulations. Perfusion pressure (also called "driving pressure") is the difference in the dynamic pressure between two points along a tube or vessel. Blood flow to any segment of the circulation is ultimately dependent on the arterial driving pressure. However, each organ can autoregulate flow and thereby determine the amount of blood that it receives from the circulation. The sum of the factors that determine regional flow in each organ determines the total vascular resistance. The sum of all regional flows equals the venous return, which in turn determines the cardiac output.

The Aorta and Arteries

The aorta and major arteries are "conducting vessels" whose major functions are the transport of blood to the organs and the conversion of pulsatile flow into sustained regular flow. The latter function derives from the elastic properties of the aorta and the resistance produced by the arteriolar sphincters.

The Microcirculation

The velocity of the blood in the microcirculation (Fig. 7-1) is 1 mm/sec. The average length of a capillary is 1 mm. Blood from an arteriole enters the capillaries, which freely anastomose with each other either directly or through metarterioles. Entry into the capillary system is guarded by **precapillary sphincters,** except in the case of **thoroughfare channels** that bypass capillaries and are always open. Since not all capillaries are open at all times, blood flow can be increased by recruiting capillaries. The sum of the flow through the capillary bed, the thoroughfare channels, and the arteriovenous anastomoses determines the regional blood flow. The exact means by which an organ regulates blood flow according to its metabolic needs is still debated, but there is a link between oxygen demand and blood flow. In the heart, blood flow is adjusted on a second-to-second basis. Proposed as factors that mediate and link metabolic vasodilatation to cellular metabolism are adenosine, other nucleotides, certain prostaglandins, carbon dioxide, and pH.

Hemodynamic Disorders of Perfusion

Hemodynamic disorders are those diseases that disturb perfusion and result in organ and cellular injury. They include:

- Hemorrhage
- Hyperemia (active or passive)
- Heart failure (pump failure)
- Occlusion of blood vessels by thrombi or emboli
- Occlusion of blood vessels by atherosclerosis
- Abnormal permeability of the endothelial barrier
- Decreased blood or fluid supply in shock or dehydration
- Increased fluid loss from burns
- Abnormal drainage of lymphatics
- Abnormal distribution of blood in septic shock

Hemorrhage

Hemorrhage (i.e., bleeding) is a discharge of blood from the vascular compartment to the exterior of the body or into nonvascular body spaces. The most common and obvious cause is trauma—usually accidental, but often by the surgeon's scalpel. A blood vessel may be ruptured in ways other than laceration. For instance, severe atherosclerosis may so weaken the wall of the abdominal aorta that it balloons to form an aneurysm, which then bleeds into the retroperitoneal space. By the same token, an aneurysm may complicate a congenitally weak cerebral artery (berry aneurysm) and lead to cerebral (subarachnoid) hemorrhage. Certain infections—for example, pulmonary tuberculosis—erode blood vessels; a similar vascular injury is caused by invasive tumors.

Hemorrhage also results from damage at the level of the capillaries—for instance, the rupture of capillaries by blunt trauma. Increased venous pressure also causes extravasation of blood from capillaries in the lung. Vitamin C deficiency is associated with capillary fragility and bleeding, owing to a defect in the supporting structures. It is important to recognize that the capillary barrier by itself is not sufficient to contain the blood within the intravascular space. The minor trauma imposed on small vessels and capillaries by normal movement requires an intact coagulation system to prevent hemorrhage. Thus, a severe decrease in the number of platelets (thrombocytopenia) or a deficiency of a coagulation factor (e.g., factor VIII in hemophilia) is associated with spontaneous hemorrhages unrelated to any apparent trauma.

An individual may exsanguinate into an internal cavity, as in the case of gastrointestinal hemorrhage from a peptic ulcer (arterial hemorrhage) or esophageal varices (venous hemorrhage). In such cases large amounts of fresh blood fill the entire gastrointestinal tract. When a large amount of blood accumulates in soft tissue, we speak of a **hematoma.** Such a collection of blood can be merely painful, as in a muscle bruise, or fatal, if located in the brain.

Diffuse superficial hemorrhages in the skin are termed **purpura** or **ecchymoses.** Following a bruise or in association with a coagulation defect, an initially purple discoloration of the skin turns green and then yellow before resolving, a sequence that reflects the progressive oxidation of bilirubin released from the hemoglobin of degraded red blood cells. A good example of an ecchymosis is a "black eye."

A minute punctate hemorrhage, usually in the

skin or conjunctiva, is labeled a **petechia.** This lesion represents the rupture of a capillary or arteriole and is seen in conjunction with coagulopathies or vasculitis, the latter classically associated with bacterial endocarditis.

Hyperemia

Hyperemia, defined simply as an excess amount of blood in an organ, may be caused either by an increased supply of blood from the arterial system (active hyperemia) or by an impediment to the exit of blood through venous pathways (passive hyperemia or congestion).

Active Hyperemia

An augmented supply of blood to an organ is usually a physiological response to an increased functional demand, as in the case of the heart and skeletal muscle during exercise. Neurogenic and hormonal influences play a role in active hyperemia, seen particularly well at both extremes of the female reproductive span—namely, in the form of the blushing bride and the menopausal flush. Although these examples do not appear to promote any useful function, hyperemia of the skin in febrile states serves to dissipate heat. The increased blood supply is brought about by arteriolar dilatation and recruitment of inactive or latent capillaries. The most striking active hyperemia occurs in association with inflammation. Vasoactive materials released by inflammatory cells cause dilatation of blood vessels; in the skin this results in the classic "tumor, rubor, and calor" of inflammation. In pneumonia the alveolar capillaries are engorged with red blood cells as a hyperemic response to inflammation. Since inflammation can also damage endothelial cells and increase capillary permeability, the hyperemia of inflammation is often accompanied by edema and the local extravasation of red blood cells.

Passive Hyperemia (Congestion)

Any obstruction to the return of blood or its passage through the lungs to the heart results in a generalized increase in venous pressure, slower blood flow, and a consequent increase in the volume of blood in many organs, including the liver, spleen, and kidneys. In the past, heart failure from rheumatic mitral stenosis was a common cause of generalized venous congestion, but with the decline in the prevalence of rheumatic fever and the advent of surgical valve replacement, such cases are unusual. Congestive heart failure secondary to coronary artery disease and right-sided failure because of pulmonary disease are now more common causes. In **acute passive congestion** affected organs increase in size and assume a bluish color because of the presence of large amounts of deoxygenated blood.

The Lung

Chronic failure of the left ventricle constitutes an impediment to the exit of blood from the lungs and leads to **chronic passive congestion** of the lungs. As a result, the pressure in the alveolar capillaries is increased, and these vessels become engorged with blood. The increased pressure in the alveolar capillaries has four major consequences:

- Microhemorrhages release red blood cells into the alveolar spaces, where they are phagocytosed and degraded by alveolar macrophages. The released iron, in the form of hemosiderin, remains in the macrophages, which are then termed "heart failure cells."
- The increased hydrostatic pressure forces fluid from the blood into the alveolar spaces, resulting in pulmonary edema, a dangerous condition that interferes with gas exchange in the lung.
- The increased pressure, together with other poorly understood factors, stimulates fibrosis in the interstitial spaces of the lung. The presence of fibrosis and iron is viewed grossly as a firm, brown lung ("brown induration").
- The increased capillary pressure is transmitted to the pulmonary arterial system, a condition labeled pulmonary hypertension. This disorder leads to right-sided failure and consequent generalized venous congestion.

The Liver

The liver, with the hepatic veins emptying into the vena cava immediately inferior to the heart, is particularly vulnerable to chronic passive congestion. The central veins of the hepatic lobule become dilated. The increased venous pressure is transferred to the sinusoids, where it leads to dilatation of the sinusoids with blood and pressure atrophy of the centrilobular hepatocytes. Grossly, the cut surface of the liver exhibits dark foci of centrilobular congestion surrounded by paler zones of unaffected peripheral portions of the lobules. The result is a curious reticulated appearance, resembling a cross-section of a nutmeg, and is appropriately termed "nutmeg liver" (Fig. 7-2). Prolonged venous congestion of the liver eventually leads to thickening of the central veins and centrilobular fibrosis. Only in the most extreme cases of venous congestion (e.g., constrictive pericarditis or tricuspid stenosis) is the fibrosis sufficiently generalized and severe to justify the label "cardiac cirrhosis."

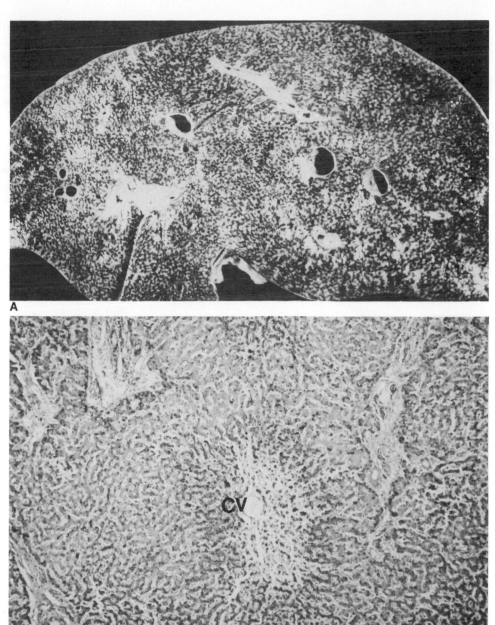

Figure 7-2. Passive congestion of the liver. (*A*) A gross photograph shows the pattern of chronic passive congestion, in which lighter-appearing tissue segments form an interlacing pattern with dark-staining centrilobular blood spaces. (*B*). In histologic sections of liver tissue from patients with chronic passive congestion, the central vein (*CV*) and central sinusoids appear distended. Adjacent liver cells may become atrophic because of hypoxia or compression. Chronic passive congestion of the liver may pass into central hemorrhagic necrosis, the distinguishing features of which are marked centrilobular dilatation and necrosis of adjacent hepatocytes.

The Spleen

Another organ that displays prominent congestive changes is the spleen. Increased pressure in the liver, whether from cardiac failure or from an intrahepatic obstruction to the flow of blood (e.g., cirrhosis), results in higher splenic vein pressure and congestion of the spleen. The organ becomes enlarged and tense, and the cut section oozes dark blood. In longstanding congestion diffuse fibrosis of the spleen is seen, together with iron-containing, fibrotic, and calcified foci of old hemorrhage (Gamna-Gandy bodies). Fibrocongestive splenomegaly may result in an organ that weighs 250 to 750 g, compared to a normal weight of 150 g. The enlarged spleen sometimes displays excessive functional activity—a condition termed hypersplenism—that leads to hematologic abnormalities.

Edema and Ascites

Venous congestion impedes the flow of blood in the capillaries, thus increasing hydrostatic pressure and promoting edema formation. The accumulation of edema fluid in heart failure is particularly noticeable in dependent tissues: the legs and feet in ambulatory patients and the back in bedridden individuals. Ascites, the accumulation of fluid in the peritoneal space, reflects (among other factors) the lack of tissue rigor, a condition in which there is no countervailing external pressure to oppose hydrostatic pressure.

Pathologic Conditions Altering Regional Perfusion

Vascular Stenosis

Vascular stenosis, a lesion that causes reduced blood flow, is most commonly a result of atherosclerotic lesions—for example, in the extramural coronary arteries. Maximal coronary flow in a single vessel begins to decline when 45% of the lumen is obstructed, although resting flow is not affected until 80 to 90% of the lumen is compromised. In individual patients, however, multiple lesions and their geometry make it difficult to use the diameter of the obstructed segment to predict the degree of reduction of coronary circulation. The geometry of the stenosis is important because it modifies the kinetic energy. Factors recognized as affecting flow in stenotic lesions are the entrance of a blood stream into a stenotic lesion, frictional loss of energy in the stenotic segment, and the turbulence at the exit. The parameters that ultimately determine the effect of a stenosis are resistance produced by the lesion and the pressure gradient across the lesion.

Vascular Spasm

Vascular spasm in the coronary circulation can produce clinically apparent ischemic attacks. Candidates for substances that can produce spasm are thromboxanes, platelet aggregates, and catecholamines. It has also been proposed that the atherosclerotic vascular wall has a lower response threshold to vasoactive agents. The presence of mast cells in the arterial media and adventitia has been linked to histamine- and serotonin-induced spasms.

Total Occlusion of Arterial Circulation

When an artery is suddenly occluded, ischemia occurs in the vascular bed it supplies (called the "area of risk"). The subsequent infarct, however, may not extend over the whole area served by the occluded vessel. The principal determinants of the size of the infarction relative to the area of risk are the extent to which perfusion has been occluded and the level of residual perfusion through the collateral circulation. The flow through collaterals is determined by the size and diameter of the collateral vascular bed and by the pressure gradient between the perfused and occluded vascular bed. The final size of the infarct is inversely related to the contribution of the collateral vascular bed. Recently, a leading role for leukocytes in advancing infarctions has been described.

Anemia and Polycythemia

Oxygen delivery to an organ is largely mediated by hemoglobin. Changes in **hemoglobin concentration** affect the oxygen-carrying capacity and viscosity of the blood. Factors that interfere with oxygen delivery can also alter vascular resistance. Severe **chronic anemia** causes an increase in cardiac output. The systolic pressure remains normal, but vasodilatation causes the diastolic pressure and peripheral vascular resistance to fall.

Polycythemia can cause a hemodynamic disorder that is also associated with systemic vascular effects. In patients with polycythemia vera, a disorder characterized by an increase in the number of red blood cells, the blood volume and cardiac output are increased, but the peripheral vascular resistance is normal. The increase in viscosity in this disease may become a critical factor in the presence of other diseases, such as infection or shock.

Pathology of Reduced Perfusion

Total occlusion of an artery produces an area of coagulative necrosis called an infarct. Partial occlusion—that is, stenosis—occasionally causes necrosis, but more commonly leads to a variety of degenerative cell changes. These changes include vacuolization of cells, atrophy, loss of muscle cell myofibrils, and interstitial fibrosis. Infarction of vital organs such as the heart, brain, and intestine may be life-threatening. If the individual survives, the infarct heals with a scar, which is the common occurrence in less vital organs.

Infarct Morphology

Morphologically, the necrotic tissue of an infarct swells, and the infarcted area often protrudes above the surface of the organ. As an infarct ages it undergoes fibrosis, reduces in size, and ultimately shrinks below the surface of the organ. A fresh infarct is pale because of the loss of red blood cells, an appearance reflected in the terms "white" or "pale" infarct (Fig. 7-3). Infarcts can also be red and hemorrhagic, particularly in the lung and the intestine. With time, the tissue surrounding an infarct forms granulation tissue rich in sprouting capillaries that bleed easily.

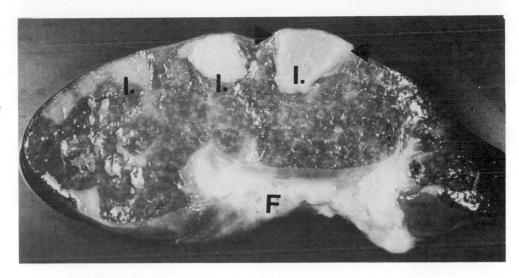

Figure 7-3. Spleen infarction. The gross photograph shows three wedge-shaped, pale infarcts of the spleen (*I*) bulging above the contour of the spleen and lifting the capsule. The pale region at the bottom (*F*) is hilar adipose tissue. Splenic infarcts are often encountered during autopsies and are often due to emboli that arise in the heart.

Therefore, the border of a healing infarct frequently is hemorrhagic. Table 7-1 summarizes the gross appearance and the usual outcome of the most frequent types of infarction. Figure 7-4 details the organs most commonly affected by infarction.

Myocardial Infarcts

Myocardial infarcts are divided into two classes: **transmural** and **subendocardial** infarcts. A transmural infarct results from complete occlusion of a major extramural coronary artery. A myocardial infarct is initially pale, but hemorrhage occurs with reflow into an injured vascular bed. Subendocardial infarction reflects prolonged ischemia caused by partially occluding stenotic lesions when the requirement for oxygen outstrips the supply.

Pulmonary Infarcts

Only about 10% of pulmonary emboli elicit clinical evidence of pulmonary infarction, usually after occlusion of a middle-sized pulmonary artery. **Infarction occurs if the circulation from the bronchial arteries inadequately compensates for the loss of supply from the pulmonary arteries.** Infarcts of the lung are pyramidal in shape with the base toward the pleural surface. Hemorrhage into the alveolar spaces of the necrotic lining tissue occurs within 48 hours.

Cerebral Infarcts

Infarction of the brain may be the result of local ischemia or of a generalized reduction in blood flow. A generalized reduction in blood flow resulting from systemic hypotension, as in shock, produces infarction in the border zones between the distributions of the major cerebral arteries. If prolonged, severe hy-

potension can cause widespread brain necrosis. The occlusion of a single vessel in the brain—for example, after an embolus has lodged—causes ischemia and necrosis in a well defined area. This type of cerebral infarct may be pale (nonhemorrhagic) or red (hemorrhagic), the latter being common with embolic occlusions. Infarcts in the areas supplied by small penetrating arteries are referred to as "lacunar infarcts." The occlusion of a large artery produces a wide area of necrosis that may ultimately resolve as a large fluid-filled cavity in the brain (Fig. 7-5).

Intestinal Infarcts

The earliest tissue changes in intestinal ischemia are necrosis of the tips of the villi in the small intestine and necrosis of the superficial mucosa in the large intestine. In either case more severe ischemia leads to hemorrhagic necrosis of the submucosa and muscularis, but not the serosa. Small mucosal infarcts heal in a few days, but more severe injury leads to

Table 7-1 Location, Appearance, and Lethality of Selected Infarcts

LOCATION	GROSS APPEARANCE	LETHALITY
Myocardial infarction	Pale	Frequently lethal
Pulmonary infarction	Hemorrhagic	Less commonly fatal
Cerebral infarction	Hemorrhagic or pale	Lethal only if massive
Intestinal infarction	Hemorrhagic	Frequently lethal
Renal infarction	Pale	Not lethal unless massive and bilateral

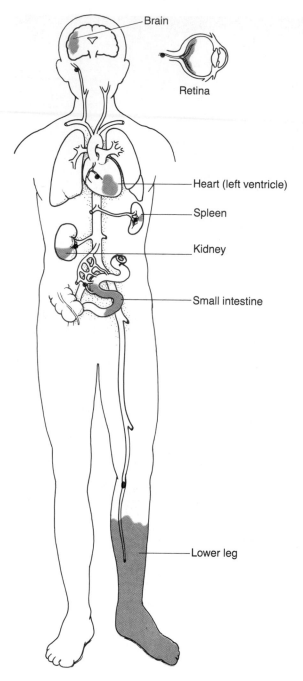

Figure 7-4. Common sites of systemic infarction from arterial emboli.

ulceration. These ulcers can eventually re-epithelialize. If the ulcers are large they are repaired by scar tissue, a process that may lead to strictures. Severe transmural necrosis may be associated with massive bleeding or perforation, complications that often result in irreversible shock, sepsis, and death.

Renal Infarcts

Renal infarcts are pyramidal in shape, with the base toward the capsule. These pale infarcts acquire a hemorrhagic border as granulation tissue develops. A gray rim in early infarcts is related to an exudate of polymorphonuclear leukocytes.

The methods for assessing the integrity of blood vessels on postmortem examination are detailed in Table 7-2.

Disorders of Water and Electrolytes

Effects and Causes of Edema

Mild degrees of **edema,** an excess of interstitial fluid, are not detectable clinically; tissue pressure remains negative. More severe derangements, however, appear as pitting edema over the extremities, as pleural or abdominal effusions, or as edema over soft connective tissue such as that of the orbit. Edema can be caused by an imbalance of the perfusion pressures or osmotic pressures that alters normal fluid transit. The mechanisms of edema formation are summarized in Table 7-3 and in Figure 7-6.

Severe edema alters perfusion by several mechanisms, among which are compression of the vascular bed and reduction in the circulating volume. For example, severe hypoalbuminemia occasionally precipitates acute prerenal failure because of low circulating volume. **Edema can be generalized or localized. Local edema** may be caused by local deep venous obstruction, by a thrombus, or by obstruction of lymphatic drainage by a tumor.

Generalized Edema and Salt Metabolism

The kidney maintains sodium homeostasis, thereby maintaining the intravascular volume and blood pressure. When the kidney senses a reduction in blood pressure it increases sodium retention, an effect that leads to water retention and, in turn, to expansion of the circulating intravascular volume. To understand the phenomenon one must differentiate between the "effective circulating volume" and the "total volume." It is the effective blood volume, sensed by baroreceptors in the kidney, that initiates the kidney's regulatory renin-angiotensin-aldosterone mechanisms. The total blood volume is determined primarily by the capacity of the vascular system. **In certain disease states—for example, congestive heart failure, ascites, and the nephrotic syndrome—the difference between the total blood volume and the effective blood volume initiates a counter-regulation that augments rather than decreases the trend to edema formation.** Thus, sodium retention in the interstitial space contributes to further edema formation. **Although the conditions re-**

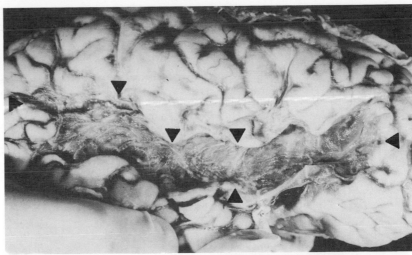

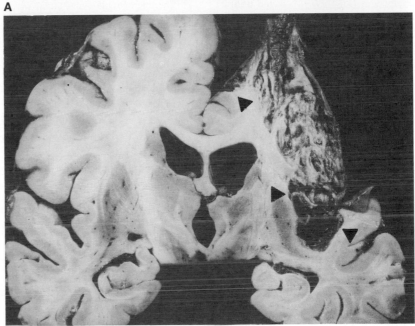

Figure 7-5. Cerebral infarction. (*A*) An old cystic infarction of the brain (*arrows*) is seen in the distribution of the middle cerebral artery. Cerebral infarctions are frequently pale, nonhemorrhagic infarctions. As seen here, healing of a cerebral infarct may lead to the generation of large cystic spaces. (*B*) A coronal cross section through the frontal lobe reveals a focal area of infarction. Note the destruction of the cortex.

sponsible for systemic edema differ, they share a deranged regulatory mechanism for sodium homeostasis.

Congestive Heart Failure

Congestive heart failure results from impaired cardiac emptying, which leads to a rise in ventricular end-diastolic pressure. Increased end-diastolic pressure is transmitted to the venous system as increased venous pressure. High venous pressure promotes exudation of fluid by decreased reabsorption, altered neurogenic precapillary resistance, hepatic congestion (which impairs renin clearance by the liver), and altered lymphatic drainage due to altered venous pressure relationships. The loss of water into the interstitial space, sensed as a contraction of the effective blood volume, activates salt-retaining mechanisms.

The clinical manifestations of congestive heart failure reflect either inadequate output or increased backward venous pressure. The major effects are, therefore, divided into "forward failure" and "backward failure." Failure to deliver blood as a result of insufficient cardiac output eventually can result in cardiogenic shock, manifested clinically as impaired perfusion. The lack of blood leads to hypotension, mental confusion, oliguria, and acidosis. Backward failure results in increased hydrostatic pressure in the

Table 7-2 Postmortem Examination of Blood Vessels

METHOD	PRINCIPLE	USE	COMMENT
Perfusion–Fixation	Following cleaning of vessels by saline solutions the fixative is infused under normal pressure.	Used to visualize true luminal narrowing; can be used for gross and histologic examination.	Limited to greater muscular arteries. Microvasculature is obscured by edema and rigor mortis.
Contrast Filling with Barium-Sulfate Latex	Cleaning as above; contrast material is infused under normal pressure into the vascular bed.	X-ray examination combined with gross and histologic examination.	Viscosity of the barium sulfate limits its use to greater arteries.
Silicon-Rubber Cast	Preparation as above; contrast material is injected until it hardens and flow ceases.	X-ray examination, histologic examination. The microcirculatory bed can be visualized if the tissue is made transparent by methylsalicylate.	Larger vessels and microcirculation can be seen.
Plastic Corrosion Cast	Preparation as above. Low-viscosity plastic is injected under normal pressure. Tissue is digested using KOH.	Preparation of casts of larger vessels and microcirculation.	Large vessels and capillaries can be seen grossly and by dissecting microscopy or by scanning electron microscopy.
Histochemistry	Enzyme, lipid, and immunohistochemistry is used to visualize lesions and vessels.	Tissue sections can be stained or vessels can be observed grossly and microscopically.	Capillaries, atherosclerotic plaques and sprouting vessels can be observed.

venous system, leading to pulmonary edema in left ventricular failure, systemic edema in right ventricular failure, and edema and cardiogenic shock in biventricular failure.

The heart is integrated into the regulation of the body fluid system by specific reflexes and by its endocrine functions. The most recent discovery is its secretion of **atrial natriuretic factor (ANF),** a powerful contributor to regulation of blood pressure, blood volume, and the excretion of water, sodium, and potassium. Thus, the heart maintains regulatory interactions with the blood vessels, kidneys, adrenal glands, and central nervous system. Atrial natriuretic factor is stored in granules within atrial cells, from which it is released on stretching of the atrial walls. The hormone interacts with the renin-angiotensin-aldosterone system and binds to specific receptors of target cells. One of these target cells is the renal tubular cell, where ANF regulates water, sodium, and potassium excretion. Another target cell is the

vascular smooth muscle cell, which it causes to relax. In the central nervous system the natriuretic factor acts on the center that controls blood pressure to inhibit production of vasopressin, an agent that constricts blood vessels. Though its effect on sodium homeostasis and peripheral vascular tone atrial natriuretic factor is important in the control of hypertension and congestive heart failure. Animals with longstanding heart failure exhibit both hypertrophy of endocrine-secreting atrial cells and depletion of endocrine granules, the latter suggesting secretory exhaustion. A deficiency of the hormone may contribute to the severe edema seen in congestive heart failure.

Pathology of Congestive Heart Failure

Congestive heart failure produces congestion in the dependent vascular system, organ enlargement, and serous effusions in the abdominal and chest cavities.

Table 7-3 Mechanisms of Edema Formation

Hydrostatic pressure	Increase in capillary transmural pressure caused by Severe arteriolar dilatation Increased venous pressure because of venous obstruction, left or right ventricular failure, or hypervolemia Increased gravitational pressure (postural).
Oncotic pressure	Decreased oncotic transmural pressure because of Plasma protein depletion Plasma protein dilution
Increased capillary permeability	Defective removal of interstitial fluid because of lymphatic obstruction.

As previously mentioned, visible edema is more severe in the dependent body regions: the legs in upright patients and the back in bedridden ones. The condition is called "pitting edema" because when the skin is depressed it does not immediately rebound, leaving a "pit."

Pathologically, the heart is enlarged and the chambers are dilated. Chronic passive congestion of the lungs, liver, and spleen associated with heart failure has been previously described.

Edema in Cirrhosis of the Liver

The events that lead to water and sodium accumulation in cirrhosis of the liver are complex. Scarring of the liver obstructs the portal flow and leads to **portal hypertension,** a condition that increases the hydrostatic pressure in the splanchnic circulation. Cirrhosis also augments **vasodilation** and opens arteriovenous bypasses. This situation is compounded by a **decreased synthesis of albumin** as a result of hepatic dysfunction. In combination these changes are sensed as a decrease in the effective blood volume and stimulate the **renin-angiotensin-aldosterone** mechanism. Elevated levels of these hormones are complicated by impairment of renin inactivation in the liver. A vicious cycle thus leads to chronic sodium retention. Furthermore, the increased **transudation of lymph from the liver capsule** adds to the accumulation of fluid in the peritoneal space.

Nephrotic Syndrome

The nephrotic syndrome is caused by a massive loss of protein to the urine, the magnitude of which exceeds the rate at which albumin is replaced by the liver. The resulting decline in the concentration of plasma proteins reduces the colloid-osmotic pressure in the venous circulation and diminishes the ability of the vascular system to reabsorb water from the extracellular space, producing edema. These events also decrease the total blood volume and effective blood volume. The decrease in effective blood volume stimulates the renin-angiotensin-aldosterone mechanism and leads to a further increase in sodium retention.

The edema in nephrotic syndrome shows a direct correlation with the plasma albumin concentration. The edema is generalized, but appears preferentially in soft connective tissues, the eyes, eyelids, and subcutaneous tissue. Ascites and pleural effusion also occur.

Edema in Special Organs

Cerebral Edema

Edema of the brain is extremely dangerous because the confined space of the cranium allows little expansion. Increased intracranial pressure compromises the blood supply and integrity of the brain. Cerebral edema is divided into three categories: vasogenic edema, cytotoxic edema, and interstitial or hydrocephalic edema.

Vasogenic edema is the result of increased vascular permeability, principally in the white matter. The usually tight endothelial junctions constituting the so-called blood-brain barrier are disrupted, resulting in an increase in the extracellular fluid volume by the addition of a plasma filtrate. Clinical disorders associated with cerebral vasogenic edema include trauma, tumors, encephalitis, abscesses, infarcts, hemorrhage, and toxic brain injury (e.g., lead poisoning).

Cytotoxic edema refers to cell swelling and occurs in response to cell injury, such as that produced by ischemia.

Interstitial or hydrocephalic edema results from decreased clearing of cerebrospinal fluid. In this condition the extracellular fluid volume is increased but the vascular permeability remains normal. Fluid accumulates in the cerebral ventricles and periventricular tissue, as seen in disorders such as hydrocephalus and purulent meningitis. In the latter case, the condition is referred to as "granulocytic edema."

At autopsy, a diffusely edematous brain is soft and heavy. The gyri are flattened and the sulci narrowed. Severe cerebral edema leads to herniation of the cerebellar tonsils.

Pulmonary Edema

Pulmonary edema refers to increased fluid in the interstitium of the lung or in the alveolar spaces.

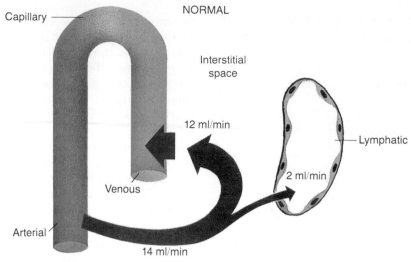

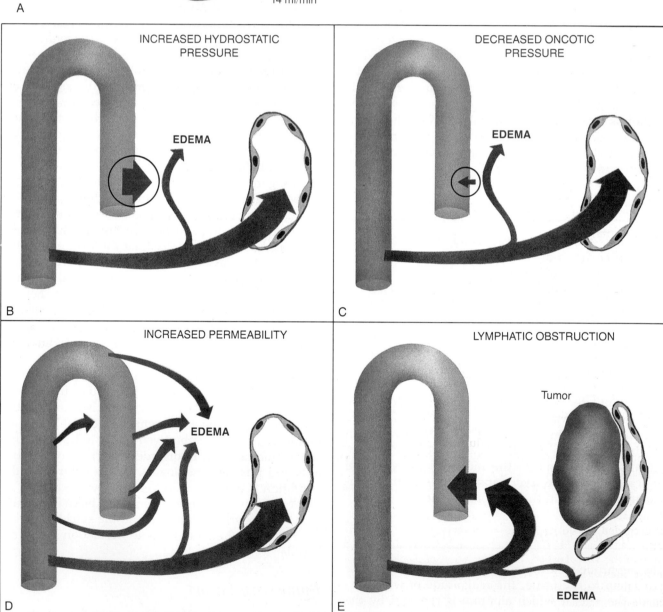

Pulmonary edema leads to decreased gas exchange in the lung, causing hypoxia and hypercapnia.

The lung is a loose tissue without much connective tissue support and, therefore, requires mechanisms to prevent the development of edema. Among these mechanisms are:

- Low hydrostatic pressure in the lung capillaries due to low right ventricular pressure.
- Effective draining of the interstitial space of the lung by lymphatics, which are under a slightly negative pressure and can accommodate up to 10 times the regular lymph flow.
- Tight cellular junctions between endothelial cells, controlling capillary permeability.
- Surfactant protection of the alveolar surface against the exudation of fluid into the alveolus.

If these protective mechanisms are perturbed, pulmonary alveolar edema results. Prolonged interstitial edema is also a strong stimulus for interstitial fibrosis in the lung. Clinical conditions that induce the formation of edema are **hemodynamic diseases** (including left heart failure, mitral valve stenosis or insufficiency, pulmonary veno-occlusive disease, head injury, and the physiologic effects of high altitude) or **changes in capillary permeability** (produced by irritant gases, aspiration of acidic material, near drowning, shock lung, fat embolism, viral infections, and uremia).

Pulmonary fluid accumulation may go unnoticed initially, but eventually dyspnea and coughing become prominent. If the edema is severe, large amounts of frothy sputum, often pink, are expectorated. Hypoxemia is manifested as cyanosis.

Pulmonary function is restricted in severe congestion and in interstitial pulmonary edema because the accumulation of fluid in the interstitial space causes reduced compliance—that is, a stiffening of the lung tissue. Thus, increased respiratory work is required to maintain ventilation. Since the alveolar walls are thickened, there is a greater barrier to the exchange of oxygen and carbon dioxide. The exchange of carbon dioxide is less affected than that of oxygen, a situation that results in hypoxia with near-normal carbon dioxide levels. As a result of capillary damage, which frequently accompanies vascular congestion, proteins and electrolytes drain into the interstitial space. Fluid accumulation in pulmonary alveoli (i.e., alveolar edema) further restricts the surface for pulmonary gas exchange.

In conditions of severe endothelial damage, a protein-rich fluid leaks into the alveoli. This fluid forms a foam when air is bubbled through it, leading to the frothy sputum seen in patients with pulmonary edema. Sections of the lung reveal severely congested alveolar capillaries and alveoli filled with a homogeneous, pink-staining fluid permeated by air bubbles. Cell debris, fibrin, and proteins may form films of proteinaceous material called "hyaline membranes."

Fluid Accumulation in Body Cavities

The body cavities, such as the pericardium and the pleural and peritoneal spaces, are extensions of the interstitial space. Fluid accumulates in them as an expression of generalized edema.

The Pleural Space

Fluid in the pleural space, also called **pleural effusion,** is a straw-colored transudate of low specific gravity that contains few cells (mainly exfoliated me-

Figure 7-6. The capillary system and mechanisms of edema formation. (*A*) **Normal:** The differential between the hydrostatic and oncotic pressure at the arterial end of the capillary system is responsible for the filtration into the interstitial space of approximately 14 ml of fluid per minute. This fluid is reabsorbed at the venous end at the rate of 12 ml/min. It is also drained through the lymphatic capillaries at a rate of 2 ml/min. Proteins are removed by the lymphatics from the interstitial space. (*B*) **Hydrostatic edema:** If the hydrostatic pressure at the venous end of the capillary system is elevated, reabsorption is decreased. As long as the lymphatics are able to drain the surplus fluid, no edema results. If their capacity is exceeded, however, edema fluid accumulates. (*C*) **Oncotic edema:** Edema fluid also accumulates if reabsorption is diminished by a decrease in the oncotic pressure of the vascular bed, owing to a loss of albumin. (*D*) **Inflammatory and traumatic edema:** Edema, either local or systemic, results if the vascular bed becomes leaky following injury to the endothelium. (*E*) **Lymphedema:** Lymphatic obstruction causes the accumulation of interstitial fluid because of insufficient reabsorption and deficient removal of proteins, the latter increasing the oncotic pressure of the fluid in the interstitial space.

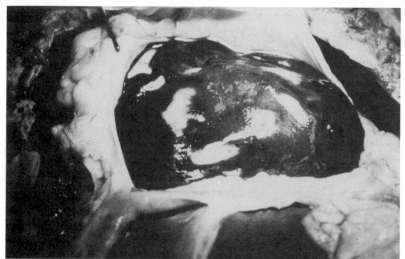

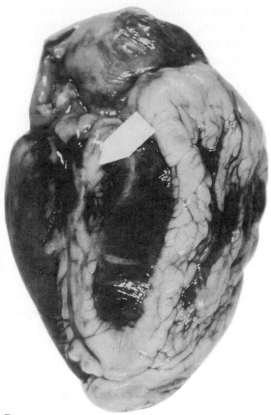

A

B

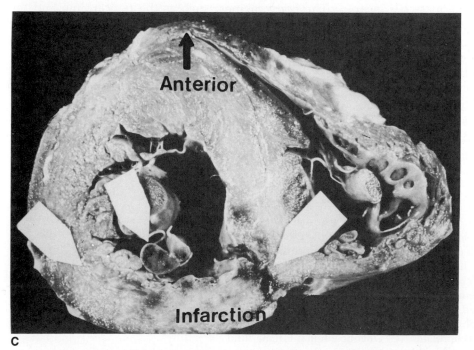

C

Figure 7-7. Pericardial tamponade. (*A*) The pericardium contains a large blood clot that was caused by bleeding through a perforation of the posterior wall of the left ventricle (*B*). (*C*) In this cross section through the right and left ventricles close to the level of the AV valves, the arrows delineate both the perforation (seen on the right as a dark channel crossing the posterior wall of the left ventricle) and the posterior wall infarct. Note that the perforation occurred at the border between normal and ischemic tissue. The blood distended the pericardium with pressure high enough to interfere with heart function.

sothelial cells). Fluid commonly accumulates as an expression of a generalized tendency to form edema in diseases such as the nephrotic syndrome, cirrhosis of the liver, and congestive heart failure. It may also accumulate in response to an inflammatory process or tumor in the lung or on the pleural surface.

The Pericardium

Fluid in the pericardium may accumulate slowly or quickly. A rapid accumulation is poorly tolerated because the distensibility of the pericardium is limited. Consequently, pericardial pressure rises rapidly, an effect—termed **tamponade**—that interferes with cardiac function (Fig. 7-7). If the fluid accumulates slowly, however, the pericardium expands without an increase in pericardial pressure. Although the upper tolerable limit may be 90 to 120 ml of fluid when a pericardial effusion forms quickly, a liter or more of fluid may be tolerated when the process is gradual.

The Peritoneum

Peritoneal effusion, also called **ascites,** causes distension of the abdomen. The main causes of ascites are cirrhosis of the liver, abdominal tumors, pancreatitis, cardiac failure, the nephrotic syndrome, and hepatic venous obstruction. The pathogenesis of ascites in cirrhosis of the liver was discussed earlier. Complications of ascites derive from increased abdominal pressure and include anorexia and vomiting, reflux esophagitis, dyspnea, ventral hernia, and leakage of fluid into the pleural space.

Fluid Loss and Overload

Excessive fluid loss (dehydration) and fluid overload are clinical situations with potentially grave consequences. Fluid imbalance causes hemodynamic disorders; alterations in the osmolality and quantity of the fluid in the intravascular, interstitial, and cellular spaces may affect perfusion or substrate, electrolyte, or fluid delivery.

Pathology of Dehydration

Dehydration refers to a condition in which there is inadequate fluid to fill the fluid compartments of the body. Such a condition results from inadequate fluid intake or from excessive fluid loss. Water loss may exceed intake in cases of vomiting, diarrhea, burns, excessive sweating, and diabetes insipidus. When excessive fluid loss occurs, fluid is recruited from the interstitial space to the plasma space. The fluids in the cell and within the interstitial and vascular compartments become more concentrated, particularly if there is a preferential loss of water, such as during inappropriate secretion of antidiuretic hormone. When patients suffer from burns, vomiting, excessive sweating, or diarrhea, they not only lose fluid but also suffer electrolyte disturbances. Only dryness of the skin and mucus membranes is noted initially, but as dehydration progresses the turgor of the skin is lost. If dehydration persists, oliguria occurs as compensation for the fluid loss. More severe degrees of fluid loss are accompanied by a shift of water from the intracellular to the extracellular space, a process that causes severe cell dysfunction, particularly in the brain. Shrinkage of brain tissue may result in the rupture of small vessels and subsequent bleeding. Systemic blood pressure falls with continuous dehydration, and declining perfusion may eventually lead to death.

Pathology of Overhydration

Excessive hydration occurs when fluid intake exceeds the compensatory capacity of the kidney to excrete a fluid overload. This is a rare situation unless renal injury limits the excretory function of the kidney, or unless the kidney is prevented from proper counter regulation (e.g., through excessive secretion of antidiuretic hormone).

Fluid excess also may be caused iatrogenically by administering excessive amounts of intravenous fluids. The most serious effect of this type of fluid overload is the induction of cerebral edema, which produces alterations in brain function, vomiting, disorientation, and convulsions.

Embolism

Embolism is the passage through the venous or arterial circulations of any material capable of lodging in a blood vessel and thereby obstructing the lumen. The usual embolus is a thromboembolus—that is, a blood clot formed in one location that detaches from the vessel wall and travels to a distant site.

Pulmonary Thromboembolism

For the clinician, pulmonary thromboembolism remains an important diagnostic and therapeutic challenge. Pulmonary thromboemboli are reported in as many as half of all autopsies. At autopsy, small peripheral emboli are often not detected, and only massive pulmonary emboli are recorded (Fig. 7-8). **The majority of emboli arise from the deep veins of the lower extremities; most of the fatal ones arise from**

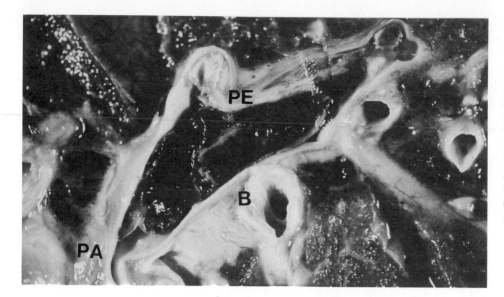

Figure 7-8. Pulmonary embolism. Pulmonary emboli (*PE*) can occlude the pulmonary artery (*PA*) or branches of the pulmonary artery. In this case a thromboembolus had occluded a branch of the main pulmonary artery of the right lobe close to the hilum of the lung. *B*, bronchus.

the ileofemoral veins (Fig. 7-9). Only half of patients with pulmonary thromboembolism have signs of thrombophlebitis. Some thromboemboli arise from the pelvic venous plexus and others from the right heart. The upper extremities are an extremely rare source of thromboemboli. Conditions that favor the development of pulmonary thromboembolism are:

- Stasis (heart failure, chronic venous insufficiency)
- Injury (trauma, surgery, parturition)
- Hormonal imbalance (oral contraceptive use)
- Advanced age
- Immobilization (orthopedic, paralysis, bed rest)
- Sickle cell disease

Clinical Features of Pulmonary Thromboembolism

Pulmonary Syndrome (Infarction)
The pulmonary syndrome clinically resembles pneumonia. Patients experience cough, stabbing pleuritic pain, shortness of breath, and occasional hemoptysis. Pleural effusion is common and often bloody. Pathologically, pyramidal segments of hemorrhagic infarction are seen at the periphery of the lung.

Circulatory Syndrome (Without Infarction)
The circulatory syndrome is characterized by dyspnea, cough, chest pain, and hypotension, with at-

tacks of shortness of breath. Embolism produces pulmonary hypertension by mechanical blockage of the arterial bed. Reflex vasoconstriction and bronchial constriction due to release of vasoactive substances may contribute to a reduction in the size of the functional pulmonary vascular bed. Whether a patient develops the pulmonary or the circulatory syndrome depends on the thromboembolic load and the availability of circulatory reserve of the bronchial arteries.

Massive Pulmonary Embolism
Massive pulmonary emboli typically cause sudden obstruction of blood flow through one or both of the major pulmonary arteries. The patient often goes into shock immediately—presumably because of certain neurologic reflexes—and may die within minutes. This catastrophe is characteristically precipitated when a patient who has been recuperating from surgery gets out of bed for the first time. Venous thrombi in the legs, formed because of stasis, are dislodged and travel to the lungs, resulting in **sudden death.**

Fate of Pulmonary Thromboemboli

Small pulmonary emboli may completely resolve, depending on the embolic load, the adequacy of the pulmonary vascular reserve, the state of the bronchial collateral circulation, and the activity of the thrombolytic process. The bronchial collateral circulation may be impaired in chronic pulmonary edema and

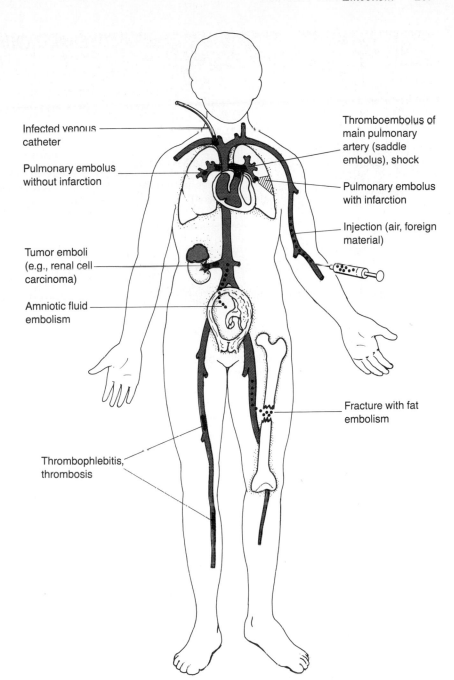

Figure 7-9.   Sources of venous emboli.

congestion, although the lung has an active thrombolytic system. Alternatively, thromboemboli may become organized and leave strings of fibrous tissue in the lumen of pulmonary arteries.

Paradoxical Embolism

Occasionally, emboli arising in the venous circulation may bypass the lungs by traveling through an incompletely closed foramen ovale, subsequently blocking flow in systemic arteries.

Emboli in Peripheral Arteries

The heart is the most common source of systemic emboli (Fig. 7-10), which usually arise from mural thrombi (Fig. 7-11) or diseased valves. Mural thrombi are seen in atrial fibrillation, mitral valve disease, myocardial infarction, left ventricular aneurysm, heart failure of any etiology, and cardiomyopathy, particularly the congestive type. Bacterial infection of diseased mitral or aortic valves **(bacterial endocarditis)** provides a source for septic emboli. Sterile

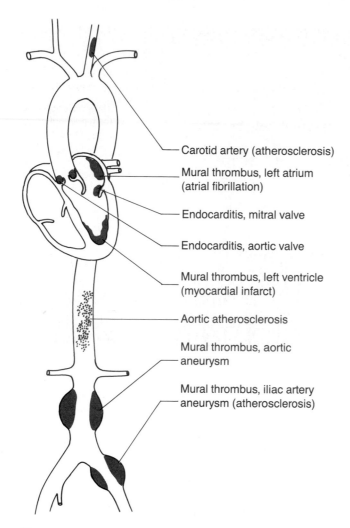

Carotid artery (atherosclerosis)

Mural thrombus, left atrium (atrial fibrillation)

Endocarditis, mitral valve

Endocarditis, aortic valve

Mural thrombus, left ventricle (myocardial infarct)

Aortic atherosclerosis

Mural thrombus, aortic aneurysm

Mural thrombus, iliac artery aneurysm (atherosclerosis)

Figure 7-10.   Sources of arterial emboli.

thrombi may form in the valves in certain debilitated states **(marantic endocarditis).** Emboli usually lodge at points where the vessel lumen narrows abruptly— for example, at bifurcations or in the area of an atherosclerotic plaque. The viability of the tissue supplied by the vessel depends on the availability of collateral circulation and on the fate of the embolus. The embolus may propagate locally and lead to a more severe obstruction, or it may fragment and dissolve. **Arterial emboli to the brain cause strokes. In the mesenteric circulation they cause infarction of the bowel,** a complication that presents as an acute abdomen and requires immediate surgery. **Embolism of an artery of the leg leads to sudden pain, absence of pulse, and a cold limb.** In some cases the limb must be amputated. **Renal artery embolism may infarct the entire kidney but more commonly results in small peripheral infarcts. Coronary artery embolism and resulting myocardial infarcts are reported, but are rare.** The more common sites of infarction are summarized in Figure 7-4.

Emboli Other Than Thromboemboli

Any material introduced into the lumen of an artery or vein may embolize and obstruct the circulation (see Fig. 7-9).

- **Air embolism.** Air may be introduced into the venous circulation through neck wounds, thoracocentesis, punctures of the great veins during invasive procedures, and hemodialysis.
- **Amniotic fluid embolism.** Amniotic fluid embolism is rare, but may be a catastrophic complication of childbirth. The pulmonary emboli are composed of the solid epithelial constituents contained in the amniotic fluid. Of greater importance is the initiation of a potentially fatal consumptive coagulopathy caused by the release of thromboplastic substances.
- **Fat embolism.** Severe trauma to fat-containing tissue, particularly the bone, can release fat emboli into damaged blood vessels. When these emboli lodge in the lung, pulmonary edema may result. Fatty acids released locally by lipases may act as a promoter of pulmonary edema. Fat emboli may also lodge in the brain, where they produce a change in consciousness.

Shock

Shock is a condition characterized by a reduction in tissue perfusion and oxygen delivery below the levels required to meet normal demands, and is ordinarily accompanied by a decreased arterial blood pressure. The term "shock" encompasses all the hemodynamic reactions that occur in response to such alterations of hemodynamic homeostasis.

Mechanisms and Types of Shock

Shock initiates compensatory mechanisms that, for a while, sustain the organism at borderline levels. If the compensatory mechanisms become exhausted, shock is said to enter an irreversible phase. **In the natural course of shock, a rapid circulatory collapse leads to impaired cellular metabolism and death.** Shock is not synonymous with low blood pressure, although hypotension is commonly a part of the shock syndrome. Hypotension is a late sign of shock and indicates failure of compensation. Blood flow is dependent on both perfusion pressure and vascular resistance. Peripheral flow can fall below critical levels, but extreme vasoconstriction can maintain central arterial blood pressure. This distinction between

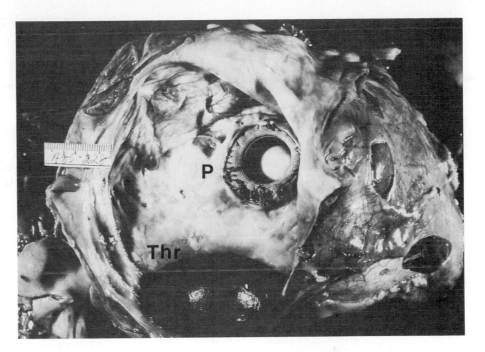

Figure 7-11. Mural thrombus, left atrium. The dilated left atrium contains a dark, almost round thrombus, which had been attached to the wall of the atrium. This mural thrombus had come free and had occluded the mitral valve prosthesis, killing the patient.

shock and hypotension is important clinically because the rapid restoration of **nutrient blood flow** is the primary goal in treating shock. When blood pressure alone is raised with vasopressive drugs, nutrient flow may actually be diminished.

Pathogenesis of Shock

Shock is a state in which the perfusion of body tissues is inadequate to meet normal metabolic demands. This decreased perfusion is generally the result of a decreased cardiac output, resulting either from the inability of the heart to pump the normal venous return or from a decreased volume of blood secondary to a decreased venous return. These two mechanisms, which lead to a decreased cardiac output, define the two major types of shock: **cardiogenic** and **hypovolemic** shock (Fig. 7-12). In cardiogenic shock due to myocardial infarction, myocarditis, or pericardial tamponade, a depressed systolic cardiac function (ejection fraction less than 20%) is responsible for the decreased cardiac output and, consequently, for the shock symptoms. In hypovolemic shock, however, a decreased blood volume is reflected in a reduced venous return to the heart, which in turn leads to a decreased cardiac output. A reduction in blood volume results from either **external** or **internal** fluid loss (Fig. 7-12). Hemorrhage, diarrhea, excessive urine formation, and perspiration are the major mechanisms of external fluid loss; internal fluid loss usually results from an increase in the permeability of the microvasculature caused by endotoxemia, burns, trauma, or anaphylaxis.

In the case of burn or trauma, direct damage to microcirculation is the mechanism by which vascular permeability is increased. Immunologic mechanisms, coupled to the activation of complement and the release of anaphylotoxins, increase vascular permeability in anaphylaxis.

Septic Shock

Septicemia with gram-negative organisms is the most common condition predisposing a patient to septic shock, but the mechanism for the increase in vascular permeability is not as straightforward. The entry of endotoxin into the blood stream triggers a series of reactions that involve leukocytes, platelets, complement, and a number of other blood factors. It is not clear whether endotoxin injures the endothelial cells directly or whether other mediators, such as polymorphonuclear leukocytes and complement, are necessary.

The lipopolysaccharide portion of bacterial endotoxins activates complement by two antibody-independent mechanisms. The lipid region of the lipopolysaccharide molecule (lipid-A) binds directly to C1 and initiates complement activation by the classical pathway. The polysaccharide portion of the molecule activates the alternative pathway by a mechanism that is independent of lipid-A. Complement activation generates potent chemotactic factors that cause leukocytes to marginate in the microcirculation, an event followed by degranulation and endothelial injury. The neutrophil has therefore been suggested as playing a central role in the pathogenesis of endotoxin-associated injury. Oxygen radicals and neutro-

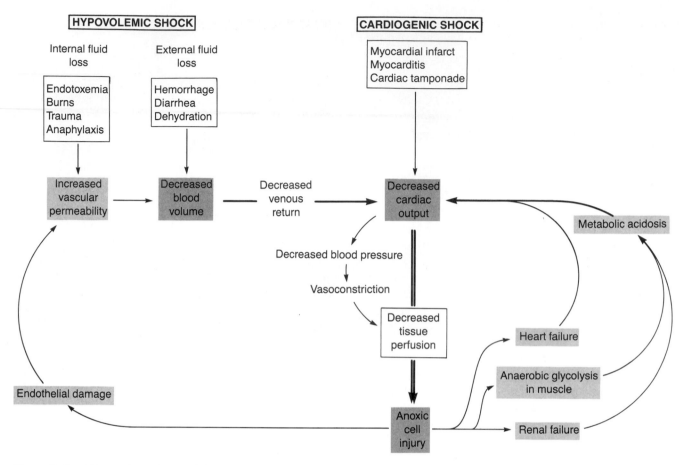

Figure 7-12. The pathogenesis of shock. This graph describes the integration of many factors in the progression of shock. Shock is initiated by one of two principal events: pump failure, or "cardiogenic shock"; and loss of circulatory volume, also called "hypovolemic shock." Hypovolemic shock follows **internal fluid loss**, such as that in endotoxemia, burns, trauma, or anaphylaxis, or from **external fluid loss** such as that caused by hemorrhage, diarrhea, and dehydration. The effect of both events is decreased cardiac output and decreased tissue perfusion. The resulting anoxic cell injury sets into motion several vicious cycles. Metabolic acidosis (renal failure, increased anaerobic glycolysis) and heart failure lead to a further decline in cardiac output. Endothelial damage increases vascular permeability and decreases effective blood volume, reducing venous return and decreasing cardiac output.

phil-derived proteases have, in turn, been implicated in neutrophil-mediated injury to the endothelium. Alternatively, it has been suggested that endotoxin injures endothelial cells directly, and that activated complement and neutrophils only exaggerate the injury by their interactions with the altered endothelium. At present, the many effects of endotoxin on coagulation and complement, platelets, polymorphonuclear leukocytes, endothelial cells, and macrophages/monocytes do not allow a simple explanation of the pathogenesis of microvascular injury that initiates septic shock.

In both hypovolemic and cardiogenic shock, a decreased cardiac output and resultant decreased tissue perfusion make up the essential pathogenetic mechanisms in the progression from reversible to irreversible shock. Anoxic injury is the common cellular consequence of the initial decrease in tissue perfusion (Fig. 7-12). A vicious cycle of decreasing tissue perfusion and further cell injury is perpetuated by two mechanisms: Injury to endothelial cells as a result of decreased tissue perfusion increases vascular permeability; in turn, the increased exudation of fluid from the circulation reduces blood volume, decreases venous return, and further decreases cardiac output, thus aggravating anoxic cell injury. Decreased perfusion of the kidneys and skeletal muscles results in metabolic acidosis, which in turn further decreases cardiac output and tissue perfusion; decreased perfusion of the heart injures the myocardial cells and decreases their ability to pump blood, further reducing cardiac output and tissue perfusion.

Vascular Compensatory Mechanisms in Shock

Feedback mechanisms maintain blood flow to the vital organs, the heart and the brain, shifting it away from the periphery, skeletal muscle, skin, splanchnic bed, adipose tissue, limbs, and some parenchymal organs. The compensatory mechanisms involve the sympathetic nervous system, the release of endogenous vasoconstrictors and hormonal substances, and local vasoregulation. The integrated regulatory response increases cardiac output by increasing the heart rate and myocardial contractility while constricting the arteries and arterioles.

The **increased sympathetic discharge** also increases adrenal catecholamine synthesis and the release of catecholamines by the adrenal medulla. The skeletal muscle, splanchnic bed, and skin arterioles respond to this increased sympathetic discharge, while the cardiac and cerebral arterioles are less reactive. In this manner the increased sympathetic tone affects volume regulation. The marked arteriolar vasoconstriction results in reduced capillary hydrostatic pressure and in less fluid shifted into the interstitium, thus permitting an osmotic fluid shift from the interstitium to the vascular system. The sympathetic-adrenal response can completely compensate for a blood loss of 10% of intravascular volume. With a greater volume deficit, cardiac output and blood pressure can no longer be properly maintained, and nutrient blood flow to tissue is reduced.

The **renin-angiotensin-aldosterone mechanism** also contributes to compensation. Renin converts the circulating angiotensinogen into angiotensin I, which subsequently is transformed to angiotensin II, the most potent endogenous vasoconstrictor. Angiotensin II also stimulates aldosterone secretion, which in turn stimulates sodium and water reabsorption, thus helping to maintain intravascular volume. A similar water-preserving action is provided by the pituitary antidiuretic hormone.

Vascular autoregulation preserves regional blood flow to vital organs, particularly the heart and the brain, by vasodilatation of the coronary and cerebral circulations in response to hypoxia and acidosis. The peripheral circulation of organs such as the skin and skeletal muscles, which are less sensitive to hypoxia, do not display such a tightly controlled autoregulation.

Pathology of Shock

Shock is associated with a number of specific changes in organs (Fig. 7-13), including acute tubular necrosis, acute respiratory distress syndrome, liver failure, depression of host defense mechanisms, and heart failure.

The Heart

Grossly, the heart shows petechial hemorrhages of the epicardium, particularly on the posterior aspect, and of the endocardium, especially the left outflow tract. Microscopically, there are necrotic foci in the myocardium, ranging from the loss of single fibers to large areas of necrosis. The affected fibers stain a deep red with eosin and the nuclei become pyknotic. Prominent contraction bands, although visible by light microscopy, are better seen by electron microscopy. Ultrastructurally, flattened areas of the intercalated disk are a sign of cell swelling, and invagination of adjacent cells is considered a catecholamine-induced lesion.

The Kidney

Acute renal failure has been divided into three phases: the **initiation phase,** from the onset of injury to the beginning of renal failure; the **maintenance phase,** from the onset of renal failure to a stable, reduced renal function; and the **recovery phase.** In survivors, the recovery phase begins about 10 days after an episode of severe systemic shock and lasts up to 8 weeks.

During acute renal failure the kidney is large, swollen, and congested, although the cortex may be pale. Cross section reveals blood pooling in the outer stripe of the medulla. Microscopically, fully developed acute tubular necrosis is manifested by dilatation of the proximal tubules and focal necrosis of cells. Frequently, pigmented casts in the tubular lumina indicate leakage of hemoglobin or myoglobin. Coarse, "ropy" casts are seen in the distal nephron and distal convoluted tubules. Interstitial edema is prominent in the cortex and mononuclear cells accumulate within the tubules and surrounding interstitium. Renal blood flow is restricted to one-third of normal following the acute ischemic phase, an effect that is even more severe in the outer cortex. The constriction of arterioles reduces the filtration pressure, thus reducing the amount of filtrate and contributing to oliguria. Interstitial edema occurs, possibly through a process termed "backflow." Excessive vasoconstriction is thought to be related to stimulation of the renin-angiotensin system.

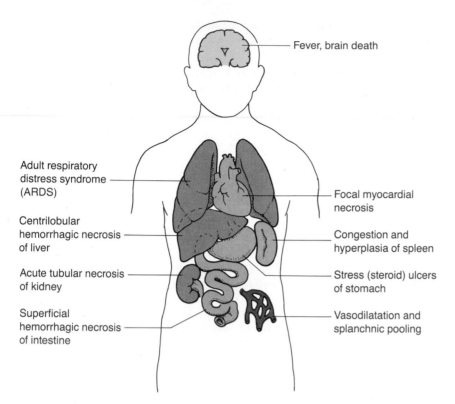

Figure 7-13.   Complications of shock.

The Lung

Following the onset of severe and prolonged shock, injury to the alveolar wall results in focal or generalized interstitial pneumonitis (shock lung). The sequence of changes is mediated by acute inflammatory cells and includes interstitial edema, necrosis of endothelial cells, microthrombi, and necrosis of the alveolar epithelium.

Grossly, the lung is firm and congested. Frothy fluid exudes from the cut surface. Interstitial edema is first seen around peribronchial connective tissue and lymphatics, subsequently filling the interalveolar connective tissue. In this initial period a large fluid volume drains into the pulmonary lymphatics. If removal of this fluid becomes insufficient, or if the balance of forces that keep the fluid in the interstitial space is disturbed, alveolar edema develops.

Edema of the lung is initiated by the loosening of intercellular junctions between the pulmonary capillary endothelial cells, a reaction that occurs at different speeds in different types of shock. It occurs within 2 to 3 minutes following endotoxemia and can be traced to the activation of complement and production of C5, a substance that is chemotactic for polymorphonuclear leukocytes. The significance of leukocyte trapping in the terminal vascular bed is not fully understood. Possibly the release of lysosomal enzymes or activated oxygen species from neutrophils mediates endothelial injury.

A reversible accumulation of platelets in the terminal vascular bed is characteristic of both hemorrhagic and endotoxin shock. Shock-induced lung injury leads to the appearance of hyaline membranes in the alveoli, which are frequently expelled into the alveolar ducts and terminal bronchioles. These lung changes may heal entirely, but in half of the patients the repair processes progress and cause a thickening of the alveolar wall. Type II pneumocytes proliferate and form a picket line of alveolar lining cells, interfering with gas exchange. Fibrous tissue proliferation also leads to organization of the alveolar exudate.

The Intestines

Injury to the gastrointestinal tract is one of the more serious consequences of shock, leading to **pancreatitis, duodenitis, and duodenal ulcer and rupture of the esophagus.** Insufficiency of the microcirculation has been thought to be the main cause of intestinal malfunction. The microvasculature shows thrombosis and increased fibrinolysis, processes that lead to interruption of the vessels and diffuse gastric hemorrhage. The high alpha adrenergic receptor activity in shock induces pronounced vasoconstriction and causes mucosal necrosis of varying degrees. The mucosal surface of the ascending colon is frequently the target of milder degrees of ischemia. Interruption of the barrier function of the intestine may be related to the development of septicemia. More severe necrotizing lesions are responsible for the deterioration in the final phase of shock.

The Liver

In patients who die in shock, the liver is heavy and enlarged and has a mottled cut surface that reflects marked centrilobular pooling of blood. The most prominent histologic lesion is centrilobular zonal necrosis, although it is not clear how important it is clinically. The cells in the center of the lobule are the most distant from the blood supply that comes from the portal tracts and are, therefore, presumably more vulnerable to circulatory disturbances.

Hypoxia of the liver leads to the development of cytoplasmic vacuoles, which represent dilated cisternae of the endoplasmic reticulum. An increase in intracellular fat is consistently noted in individuals who have survived shock for some time—2 to 24 hours, for example. Evidence of the disturbed microcirculation is best seen in the pooling of blood in the centrilobular region close to the central vein, although in severe cases the midzonal region is also involved. However, the liver shows little indication of fibrin deposits, platelet aggregates, or microthrombi. If the patient survives the shock for some time, large autophagic vacuoles develop. Kupffer cells are prominent and are packed with cellular debris.

The Exocrine Pancreas

The splanchnic vascular bed, which supplies the exocrine pancreas, is particularly affected by impaired circulation during shock. The resulting ischemic damage to the pancreas unleashes activated catalytic enzymes from exocrine pancreas and causes acute pancreatitis, a complication that further promotes shock.

Host Defenses

The alteration of the immunologic system and the host defenses in shock is not well defined, although clinically it is common that patients who survive the acute phase succumb to subsequent overwhelming infection. It may well be that several factors interact, namely ischemic colitis, tissue trauma, suppression of the immune system, and metabolic suppression of host defenses. Humoral immunity and phagocytic activity by leukocytes and mononuclear macrophages are both depressed, but the mechanisms of these effects are not clear.

The Brain

Brain lesions are rare. Occasionally, microscopic hemorrhages are seen, but patients who recover do not display neurologic deficits. In severe cases, particularly in individuals with cerebral atherosclerosis, hemorrhage and necrosis may appear in the overlapping region between the terminal distributions of major arteries, the so-called **watershed zone.**

The Adrenals

In severe shock the adrenal glands may exhibit conspicuous hemorrhage in the inner cortex. Frequently, this hemorrhage is only focal, but it can be massive and accompanied by hemorrhagic necrosis of the entire gland, as seen in the **Waterhouse-Friderichsen syndrome.**

SUGGESTED READING

Books

Badeer HS (ed): Cardiovascular Physiology. Basel, Karger, 1984

Cowley RA, Trump BF (eds): Pathophysiology of Shock, Anoxia, and Ischemia. Baltimore, Williams and Wilkins, 1982

Dole WP, O'Rourke PP: Hypotension and cardiogenic shock. In Stein JH (ed): Internal Medicine. Boston, Little, Brown & Co, 1983

Epstein M: Disorders of sodium balance. In Stein JH (ed): Internal Medicine. Boston, Little, Brown & Co, 1983

Fishman AP, Renkin EM: Pulmonary Edema. Bethesda, MD, American Physiological Society, 1979

McComb GJ, Davis RL: Choroid plexus, cerebrospinal fluid, hydrocephalus, cerebral edema, herniation. In Davis RL, Robertson DM (eds): Textbook of Neuropathology. Baltimore, Williams and Wilkins, 1985

McGovern VJ, Tiller DJ: Shock: A Clinicopathological Correlation. New York, Masson Publishing, 1980

Articles

DeBold AJ, Borenstein HB, Veress AT, et al: A rapid and potent natriuretic response to intravenous injection of atrial myocardial extracts in rats. Life Sci 28:89-94, 1981

Trump BF, Bejezesky IK: The role of calcium in cell injury and repair. Surv Synth Path Res 4:248-256, 1985

Trump BF, Laiho KU, Mergner WJ, Arstila AU: Studies on the subcellular pathophysiology of acute lethal cell injury. Beitr Path 152:243-271, 1974

8 Environmental and Nutritional Pathology

Emanuel Rubin and John L. Farber

Smoking

Alcoholism

Drug Abuse

Iatrogenic Drug Injury

Environmental Chemicals

Physical Agents

Nutritional Disorders

Figure 8-1. Diseases associated with cigarette smoking. The cancers whose incidences are known to be increased in cigarette smokers are shown on the left. The non-neoplastic diseases associated with cigarette smoking are shown on the right.

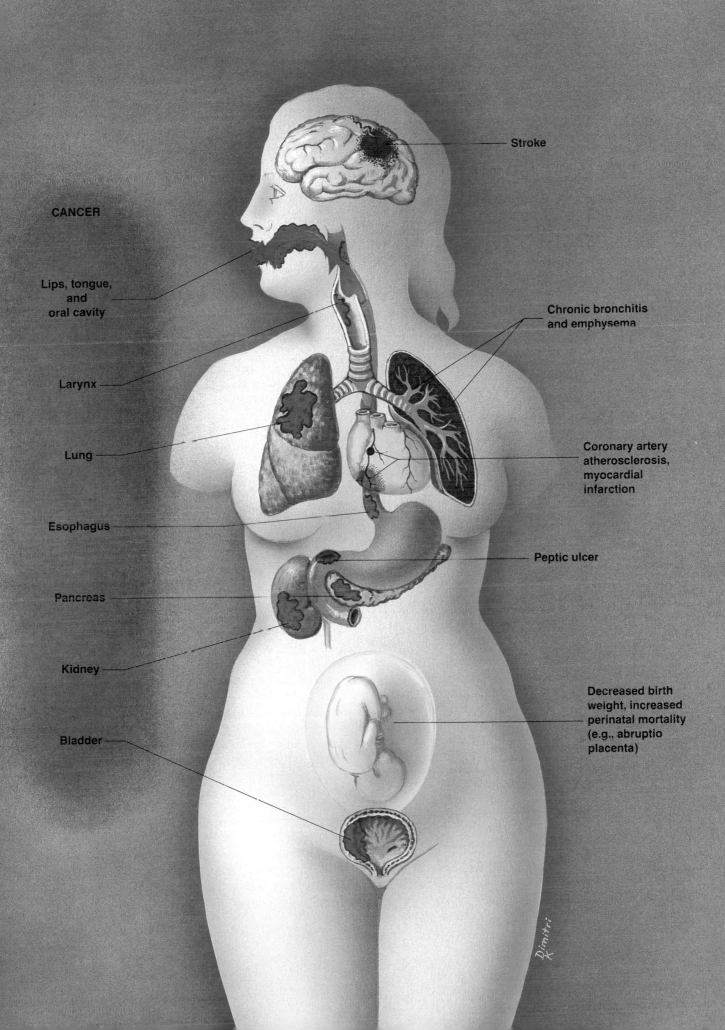

Stroke

CANCER

Lips, tongue, and oral cavity

Chronic bronchitis and emphysema

Larynx

Lung

Coronary artery atherosclerosis, myocardial infarction

Esophagus

Peptic ulcer

Pancreas

Kidney

Decreased birth weight, increased perinatal mortality (e.g., abruptio placenta)

Bladder

Dimitri

Environmental pathology, the field that deals with the diseases caused by exposure to harmful external agents and deficiencies of vital substances, in a sense encompasses all nutritional, infectious, chemical, and physical causes of illness. A half century ago a few physicians cultivated an interest in diseases that seemed to have strict geographical boundaries; as a result, a discipline called "geographic pathology" supplanted the more restricted "tropical medicine." Geographic pathology was concerned with diseases endemic to certain areas of the world, notably parasitic and infectious diseases that seemed unique to those locales. A minor component dealt with nutritional disease, and a separate discipline covered forensic medicine. With the discovery that chemical agents are mediators of a variety of tissue changes, and with the recognition that many of these causative agents are environmental contaminants, a component called "occupational disease" was added to the roster. Finally, disease due to contaminants in the broadest sense was included to constitute the field of "environmental pathology."

The mortality and morbidity from the voluntary intake of tobacco smoke, alcohol (ethanol, ethyl alcohol), and illicit psychoactive drugs dwarfs that from all other environmental hazards combined. For reasons that are difficult to fathom, the outrage directed against environmental pollution is curiously muted when the greatest of all environmental contaminants is discussed. Were tobacco or alcohol to be introduced at this time, it is inconceivable that either would be approved by the Food and Drug Administration. Because of ingrained cultural habits throughout the world, a simple prohibition of these substances is clearly not effective. The experiment with the legal prohibition of alcoholic beverages in the United States and the current inability to control the distribution and intake of illicit drugs attest to the difficulty of persuading people that exposure to culturally acceptable agents is indeed dangerous. With few exceptions, every type of physician is likely to have extensive experience with diseases related to the intake of these substances. Radiation, air pollution, and industrial exposures are relatively minor dangers compared to the problems that people willingly bring upon themselves.

Smoking

Smoking is the single largest preventable cause of death in the United States, with direct health costs to the economy of at least $25 billion a year. In 1979 there were 80,000 deaths from lung cancer and 22,000

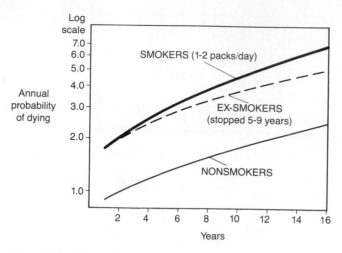

Figure 8-2. The risk of dying in smokers and nonsmokers. Note that the annual probability of an individual dying, indicated on the ordinate, is a log scale. Individuals who have smoked for 1 year have a twofold greater probability of dying than a nonsmoker, while those who have smoked for more than 15 years have more than a threefold greater probability of dying.

from other smoking-related neoplasms, 225,000 deaths from cardiovascular disease, and 19,000 deaths from chronic pulmonary disease. **About 350,000 deaths a year—one-sixth of the total mortality in the United States—occur prematurely because of smoking.** Life expectancy is shortened, and overall mortality is proportional to the duration of cigarette smoking (Fig. 8-2). For example, a person who smokes two packs of cigarettes a day at the age of 30 years will live an average of 8 years less than a nonsmoker. One of the less desirable fallouts from the feminist movement has been the assumption of the smoking habit by many women. As a result, the epidemic of smoking-related disease that assaulted men more than a generation ago has now reached the female population. Women whose smoking characteristics are similar to those of men exhibit mortality rates similar to men's. In fact, cancer of the lung, almost all of which is related to cigarette smoking, has now exceeded cancer of the breast as the most common malignant neoplasm in women in the United States. The excess mortality associated with cigarette smoking declines after cessation of the habit, and after 15 years of abstinence from cigarettes the mortality of ex-smokers is similar to that of those who have never smoked at all. Overall mortality among those who smoke only cigars or pipes is only slightly higher than that in the nonsmoking population.

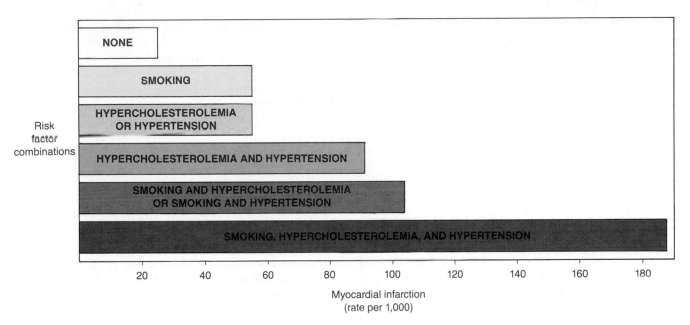

Figure 8-3. The risk of myocardial infarction in cigarette smokers. Smoking is an independent risk factor and increases the risk of a myocardial infarction to about the same extent as does hypertension or hypercholesterolemia alone. The effects of smoking are additive to those of these other two risk factors.

The major diseases responsible for the excess mortality seen in cigarette smokers are, in order of frequency, coronary heart disease, cancer of the lung, and chronic obstructive pulmonary disease (see Fig. 8-1). Smokers also suffer an increased incidence of cancer of the oral cavity, larynx, esophagus, pancreas, bladder, and kidney. The combination of smoking and alcohol abuse is particularly synergistic for cancer of the upper respiratory tract and the esophagus. In addition, smokers suffer excess mortality from atherosclerotic aortic aneurysms and peptic ulcer disease.

Cardiovascular Disease

Cigarette smoking is a major independent risk factor for myocardial infarction, and acts synergistically with other risk factors, such as high blood pressure and elevated blood cholesterol levels (Fig. 8-3). It not only serves to precipitate initial myocardial infarction, but also increases the risk for second heart attacks and diminishes survival after a heart attack among those who continue to smoke. Smoking also increases the incidence of sudden cardiac death, possibly by exacerbating regional ischemia, an effect that may promote electrical instability of the heart.

Cigarette smoking alone does not induce chronic hypertension and may even be associated with a mild chronic hypotensive effect. Thus, by itself, smoking is probably not associated with an increased incidence of strokes, since high blood pressure is the major risk factor for stroke. However, when hypertension is present, smoking acts synergistically to increase the risk not only of cardiac complications but of stroke as well. As will be discussed in the section on oral contraceptives, the combination of smoking and oral contraceptive use in women over 35 years of age greatly increases the risk of myocardial infarction. Similarly, the use of cigarettes by women who are on "the pill" significantly augments their risk of stroke.

Atherosclerosis of the coronary arteries and the aorta is more severe and extensive among cigarette smokers than among nonsmokers, and the effect is dose-related. As a consequence, cigarette smoking is a strong risk factor for atherosclerotic aortic aneurysms, the mortality ratio (death rate of smokers vs. nonsmokers) for this disorder being about 8 to 1. The incidence and severity of atherosclerotic peripheral vascular disease are remarkably increased by smoking.

In the earlier part of this century, a peculiar inflammatory and occlusive disease of the vasculature of the lower leg was described in a patient population consisting principally of Eastern European Jews, almost all of whom were heavy smokers. This disorder,

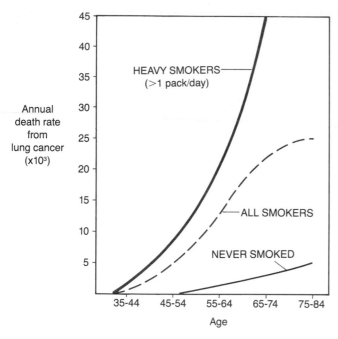

Figure 8-4. Death rate from lung cancer among smokers and nonsmokers. Non-smokers exhibit a small, linear rise in the death rate from lung cancer from the age of 50 onwards. By contrast, those who smoke more than 1 pack/day show an exponential rise in the annual death rate from lung cancer starting at about age 35. By age 70, heavy smokers have about a twentyfold greater death rate from lung cancer than nonsmokers.

termed **Buerger's disease,** was characterized by inflammation, fibrosis, and thrombosis of both the artery and its accompanying vein, leading to gangrene and amputation of the lower extremities. Although Buerger's disease is unquestionably related to smoking, it is rarely seen today.

Cancer

Cancer of the lung is today the single most common cancer in both men and women in the United States (Fig. 8-4). Its pathogenesis is discussed in detail in Chapter 12, which deals with lung disease. While the precise offenders in cigarette smoke have not been identified, it is clear that cigarette smoke is toxic to the bronchial mucosa. When cigarette smoke is passed through a filter it is separated into gas and particulate phases. Cigarette tar, the material that is deposited on the filter, contains more than 2000 compounds, many of which have been identified as carcinogens, tumor promoters, and ciliatoxic agents. Compounds with similar toxic properties are found in the gas phase, but they are fewer.

The initial change in the morphologic sequence leading to cancer of the lung is squamous metaplasia of the bronchial mucosa. As is often the case in a squamous mucosa—the cervix, for example—the metaplastic epithelium becomes dysplastic and eventually neoplastic. In time carcinoma in situ of the bronchial mucosa invades the basement membrane of the epithelium and metastasizes to regional nodes and distant sites. The risk of developing lung cancer is directly related to the number of cigarettes smoked (Fig. 8-5).

Cigarette smoking is also an important factor in the induction of lung cancer that is associated with certain occupational exposures. In general, it is difficult to separate damage due to smoking from that due to certain types of occupational exposures, but in some cases they appear to be additive. For instance, uranium miners have an increased rate of lung cancer, presumably because of the inhalation of radon daughters. However, the rate of lung cancer among smoking miners is considerably greater than that among non-miners with similar smoking habits.

Another example is the case of asbestos workers. It has been reported that asbestos workers who have never smoked exhibit a risk of contracting lung cancer three to five times greater than the general population not exposed to asbestos; these data, however, are based on small numbers of patients and require further study. In any event, whereas heavy smokers in the general population have a risk of lung cancer in excess of 20 times greater than nonsmokers, asbestos workers who smoke heavily have a risk that is more than 60 times that of nonsmokers. Thus, in this group, the risk is not simply additive, but seems to reflect a synergism. The subject is interesting from a legal point of view, since it is difficult to say whether asbestos exposure is particularly dangerous in smokers or smoking is more dangerous in asbestos workers; the relative contribution of each to the extraordinary incidence of cancer of the lung is debatable.

All forms of tobacco use—cigarette, cigar, and pipe smoking, as well as tobacco chewing—expose the oral cavity to the compounds found in raw tobacco or tobacco smoke. **Cancers of the lip, tongue, and buccal mucosa occur principally in tobacco users.** The precursor lesion—leukoplakia, a thickening and keratinization of the squamous mucosa—is followed by dysplasia and eventually neoplasia.

In the larynx the situation is similar. **Cancer of the larynx** accounts for about 1% of all cancer deaths in the United States. Among white male smokers the mortality ratio, compared to nonsmokers, varies from 6 to 13, and in some large studies all deaths from cancer of the larynx occurred in smokers.

The risk ratios for **cancer of the esophagus** in

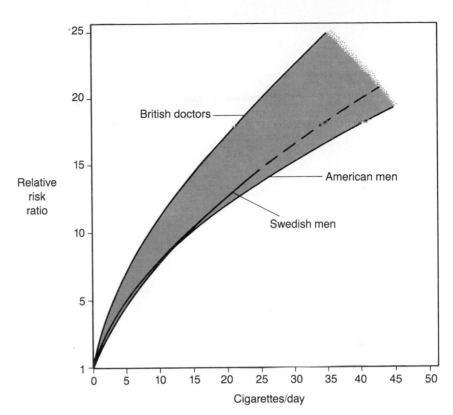

Figure 8-5. Dose-dependent relationship between cigarette smoking and the risk of lung cancer. Prospective studies of three different populations of smokers found a dependence of the risk of lung cancer on the number of cigarettes smoked per day. For example, there is about a threefold greater risk of developing lung cancer in those who smoke 15 cigarettes a day as opposed to those who smoke five. The dashed line is an extrapolation of the data for Swedish men who smoke from 25 to 50 cigarettes a day.

smokers in the United States and Great Britain is between 2 and 9. There is a pronounced synergism with excessive intake of alcohol.

Cigarette smokers are twice as likely to die from **cancer of the bladder** as nonsmokers, and 30% to 40% of all bladder cancers are attributable to smoking. As with most tobacco-related disorders, there is a clear dose–response relationship between the incidence of bladder cancer and the number of cigarettes smoked per day and the duration of cigarette smoking.

Retrospective studies of **primary adenocarcinoma of the kidney** have shown a 50% to a 100% increase in incidence among smokers. A modest increase in cancer of the renal pelvis has also been documented.

The steady increase in the incidence of **cancer of the pancreas** may, at least in part, be related to cigarette smoking. The risk ratio in male smokers for adenocarcinoma of the pancreas is 2 to 3, and a dose–response relationship exists (Fig. 8-6). In fact, men who smoke more than two packs a day have a five times greater risk than nonsmokers.

Non-neoplastic Diseases in Smokers

As discussed in Chapter 12, **it is now clear that smoking is the principal cause of chronic bronchitis and chronic obstructive lung disease** (Fig. 8-7). Not only

is this relationship established by pulmonary function studies and symptomatic histories, but cigarette smokers demonstrate more frequent abnormalities in macroscopic and microscopic lung sections at autopsy than do nonsmokers. Furthermore, there is a dose–response relationship between these changes and the intensity of smoking.

There is a 70% greater prevalence of peptic ulcer disease in male cigarette smokers than in nonsmok-

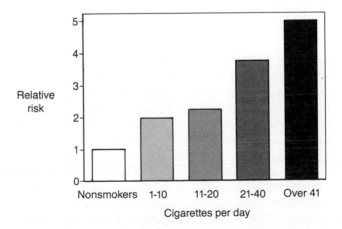

Figure 8-6. Dose-dependent relationship between smoking and the risk of pancreatic cancer. The relative risk of pancreatic cancer increases with the number of cigarettes smoked per day.

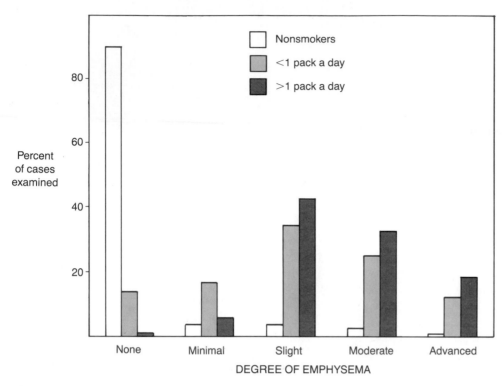

Figure 8-7. The association between cigarette smoking and pulmonary emphysema. Ninety percent of nonsmokers have no detectable emphysema at autopsy. In contrast, virtually all those who smoke more than one pack per day have morphologic evidence of emphysema at autopsy. Emphysema shows a slight dose dependence on the number of cigarettes smoked. Those who smoke less than one pack per day tend to have less severe emphysema, but 85% to 90% of such smokers have some emphysema at autopsy.

ers. The converse has also been shown: the proportion of smokers is higher among patients with peptic ulcer disease than among controls. Moreover, it now appears that smoking retards the healing of peptic ulcers of the stomach and duodenum.

Smoking and Women

Women share with men the numerous complications of smoking. In addition, it is now clear that women who smoke experience an **earlier menopause** than nonsmokers. Although the cause is not conclusively established, it may be related to the effects of tobacco on estrogen metabolism.

In the liver, estradiol is hydroxylated to estrone, which then enters one of two irreversible metabolic pathways (Fig. 8-8). In one, 16-hydroxylation leads to the production of estriol, a compound with potent estrogenic activity. In the other, which involves 2-hydroxylation, the end product is methoxyestrone, a compound that has no estrogenic activity. **In smoking women, the pathway leading to the inactive metabolite is stimulated and, as a result, circulating levels of the active estrogen, estriol, are reduced.** As well as earlier menopause, an increased incidence of postmenopausal **osteoporosis** in smoking women has been attributed to decreased estriol levels. In view of the alarming increase in smoking among teenage girls, it might be useful to make this information widely known.

The most dangerous effect of smoking that particularly affects women occurs in pregnancy. The dangers to the fetus are so varied that, in analogy to the fetal alcohol syndrome, the term "fetal tobacco syndrome" has been suggested. Babies born to women who smoke during pregnancy are, on average, 200 g lighter than babies born to comparable women who do not smoke. This decrease in birth weight is independent of other determinants of birth weight, since there is a downward shift of the entire set of weights of smokers' babies (Fig. 8-9). Thus,

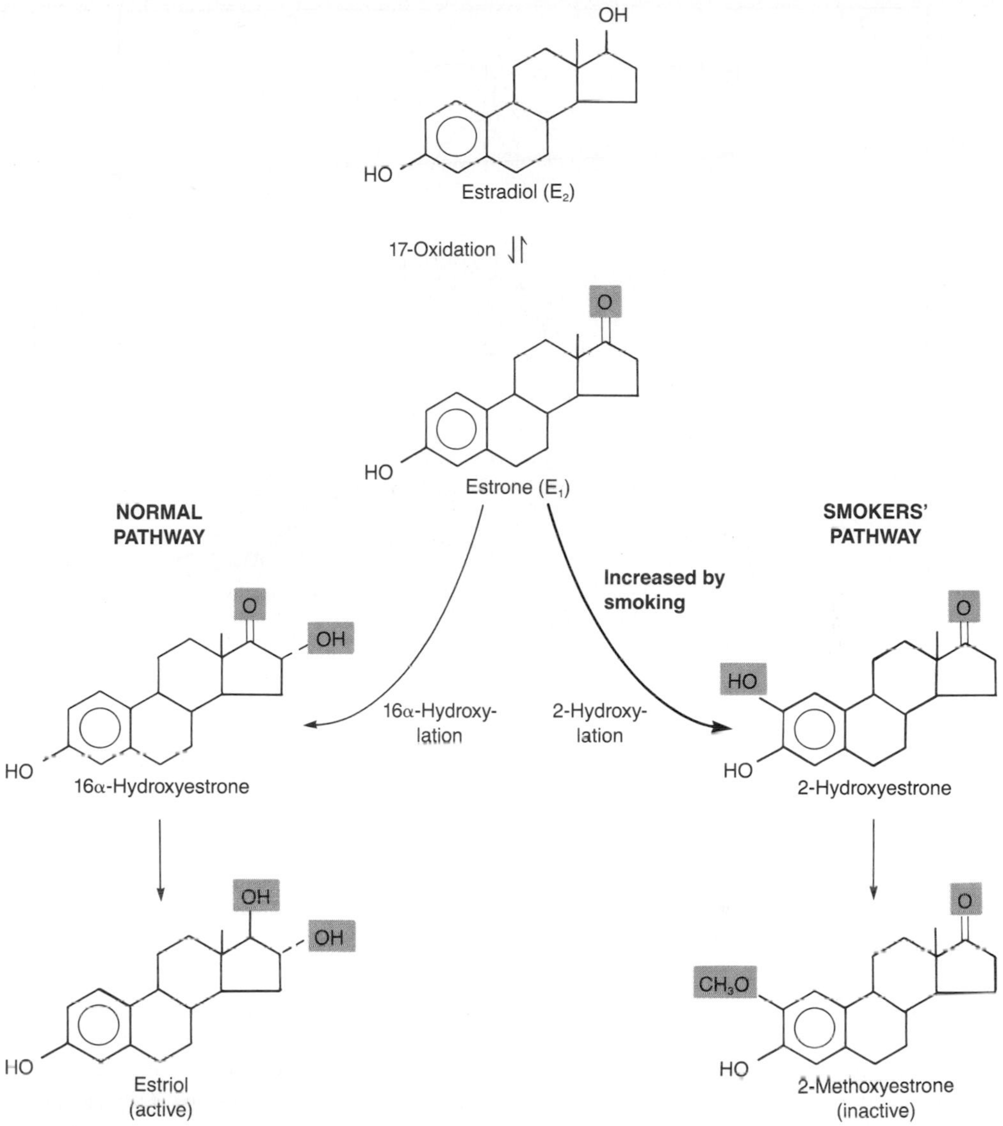

Figure 8-8. Effect of smoking on estrogen metabolism. Estradiol is converted in the liver to estrone, which is further catabolized by two different pathways. The major normal pathway, via 16-α-hydroxylation, leads to the production of estriol, a metabolite that retains estrogenic activity. In smokers, the activity of the pathway that involves 2-hydroxylation is increased. This results in the production of methoxyestrone, a derivative that lacks estrogenic activity.

this effect of smoking is not idiosyncratic, but reflects a direct retardation of fetal growth. These infants are not born preterm, but rather are small for gestational age at every stage of pregnancy. The prevalence of newborns weighing less than 2500 g is much greater among smoking mothers. Among light smokers there is a 50% increase in the number of newborns weighing less than 2500 g; among heavy smokers this figure is more than doubled. In fact, 20% to 40% of the incidence of low birth weight can be attributed to maternal cigarette smoking. Studies in India have shown that the use of chewing tobacco is also associated with low birth weight.

The noxious effect of smoking on the fetus is mirrored by its effect on the uteroplacental unit. Every major well-controlled study has shown perinatal mortality to be increased among the offspring of smokers, the increase ranging from 20% among the progeny of women who smoke less than a pack per day to almost 40% among the offspring of those who

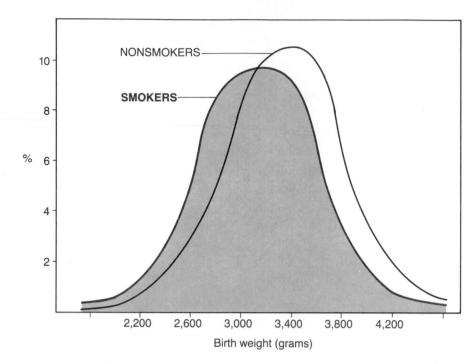

Figure 8-9. Effect of smoking on birth weight. Mothers who smoke give birth to smaller infants. In particular, the incidence of babies weighing less than 3,000 grams is very significantly increased by smoking.

smoke more than a pack per day. It is important to recognize that this excess mortality does not reflect specific abnormalities of the fetus, but rather problems related to the uteroplacental system. The incidences of **abruptio placentae, placenta previa, uterine bleeding and premature rupture of the membranes** are all increased (Fig. 8-10). These complications of smoking tend to occur at times when the fetus is not viable or is at great risk, namely from 20 weeks to 32 weeks of gestation.

There is substantial evidence that the injurious effects of maternal cigarette smoking are not limited to the fetus and the neonate but extend to the physical, cognitive, and emotional development of the children at older ages. Thus, in a number of studies the children of smoking mothers have exhibited measurable deficiencies in physical growth, intellectual maturation, and emotional development that are independent of other known predisposing factors. In the most comprehensive study to date, 17,000 children born during one week in Great Britain were studied at ages 7 and 11 years. The children of mothers who smoked 10 or more cigarettes a day during pregnancy were, on average, 1.0 cm shorter than children of nonsmoking mothers and were 3 to 5 months retarded in reading, mathematics, and general intellectual ability. Moreover, the deficits increased with the number of cigarettes smoked during pregnancy. These studies were carefully controlled

for associated social and biologic factors. A number of other studies have come to the same conclusions, and although the studies of performance on psychological tests have not shown statistically significant differences, the direction of differences is always in favor of the nonsmokers' child. Thus, it appears that the children of smoking women, on average, do not catch up with the fetal retardation induced by smoking. Although more data are needed, it is also possible that deficits in growth and development may occur in children of normal birth weight whose mothers were habituated to smoking.

Alcoholism

It is estimated that there are about 12 million alcoholics in the United States, or about one-tenth of the population at risk. The proportion may be even higher in other countries, particularly those in which wine is consumed in preference to water. Certain ethnic groups—for example, Native Americans and Eskimos—have notoriously high rates of alcoholism. By contrast, other groups, such as Chinese and Jews, experience little alcoholism. Although this addiction is more common in men, the number of female alcoholics has been rapidly increasing.

The definition of alcoholism is difficult and varies widely with different authors. In view of the large differences in individual susceptibility both to the acute intoxicating effects of alcohol and to the development of alcohol-related disease, it is difficult to derive a simple number for the consumption of ethanol above which a diagnosis of alcoholism can be made. It is sufficient that chronic alcoholism be defined as the regular intake of a quantity of alcohol that is enough to injure a person socially, psychologically, or physically. While there are no firm rules for most people, a daily consumption of more than 40 g alcohol should probably be discouraged. Intakes of 100 g or more a day may be dangerous (10 g alcohol = one ounce, or 30 ml, of 86° proof (43%) spirit).

The acute effects of alcohol on the brain need no elaboration, since they are familiar to most people, either through personal experience or through the observation of acute alcoholic intoxication. Although the mechanism of inebriation is not understood, alcohol, like other anesthetic agents, acts as a central nervous system depressant. However, it is such a weak anesthetic that it must be drunk by the glassful to exert any significant effect. Recent evidence suggests that it may act by opening the chloride channel of the neurons through an interaction with the receptor for gamma aminobutyric acid (GABA). In the normal person, characteristic behavioral changes can be detected at low alcohol concentrations (below 50 mg/dl). Levels above 100 mg/dl are usually associated with gross incoordination, and in most American jurisdictions are considered legal evidence of intoxication while driving a motor vehicle. Above 300 mg/dl most people become comatose, and at levels above 400 mg/dl death from respiratory failure is common. In man the LD_{50} is about 5 g alcohol per kg of body weight.

The situation is somewhat different in chronic alcoholics, who develop central nervous system tolerance to alcohol. Such individuals often easily tolerate blood alcohol levels of 100 to 200 mg/dl, and in fatal automobile accidents blood levels of 500–600 mg/dl

Figure 8-10. Effect of smoking on the incidence of abruptio placentae, placenta previa, and the premature rupture of amniotic membranes. In each the ordinate shows the probability of one of three complications of the third trimester of pregnancy. Note that it is a log scale. Smoking increases the probability of abruptio placentae and premature rupture of the amniotic membranes prior to 34 weeks of gestation, at which time the fetus is still premature. Smoking increases the risk of placenta previa up to 40 weeks of gestation.

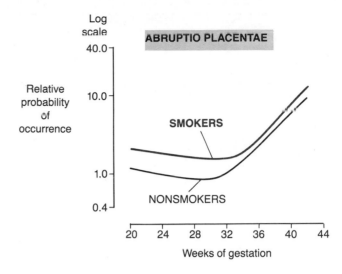

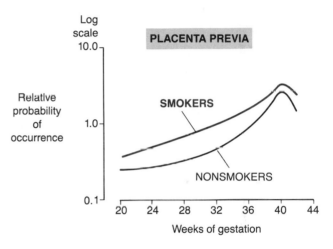

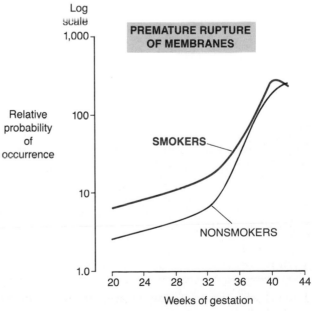

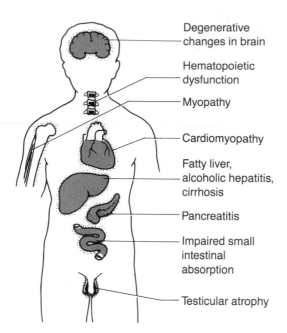

Degenerative changes in brain

Hematopoietic dysfunction

Myopathy

Cardiomyopathy

Fatty liver, alcoholic hepatitis, cirrhosis

Pancreatitis

Impaired small intestinal absorption

Testicular atrophy

Figure 8-11. Complications of chronic alcohol abuse.

or more have been found by medical examiners. The mechanism underlying tolerance has not been established for alcohol or any other drug. It has been shown that chronic alcohol intake leads to adaptive changes in neuronal membranes, but the subject requires further study.

Acute alcohol intoxication is hardly a benign condition. About half of all fatalities from motor vehicle accidents involve alcohol—about 25,000 deaths a year in the United States. Alcoholism is also a major contributor to fatal home accidents, death in fires, and suicide.

Many of the chronic diseases associated with alcoholism were, at one time, attributed to malnutrition, and it is true that some alcoholics suffer from nutritional deficiencies—for example, thiamine deficiency (Wernicke's encephalopathy) or folate deficiency (megaloblastic anemia). **However, most alcoholics have an adequate diet, and the great majority of alcohol-related disorders should be attributed to the toxic effects of alcohol.** The diseases associated with alcoholism are discussed in detail in chapters dealing with individual organs, and we shall restrict this discussion to the spectrum of disease (Fig. 8-11).

Liver

Liver disease associated with the excess consumption of alcoholic beverages has been recognized for several thousand years, having been implied in the Ayur

Veda, the ancient medical text of India. Almost 300 years ago the noted English clinician, Thomas Heberden, wrote about the increase in "scirrhous" livers in those who consume large quantities of "spirituous liquors." **Alcoholic liver disease, the most common medical complication of alcoholism, accounts for a majority of the cases of cirrhosis of the liver in the industrialized countries.** (In Asia and Africa, by contrast, most cirrhosis is due to infection with the hepatitis B virus.) The nature of the alcoholic beverage is largely irrelevant; consumed in excess, beer, wine, whiskey, hard cider, and so on all produce cirrhosis. Only the total daily dose of alcohol is relevant. Alcoholic liver disease is conventionally divided into three major phases: a reversible fatty liver, which has few functional consequences; alcoholic hepatitis, an inflammatory and necrotizing disease of the liver, which has a significant mortality; and cirrhosis, an irreversible scarring of the liver (Fig. 8-12). The last leads to liver failure or the consequences of portal hypertension, particularly gastrointestinal hemorrhage (Fig. 8-13).

Pancreas

The relationship of acute pancreatitis to alcoholism is unclear, but such episodes are seen with sufficient frequency to suggest that it is also a complication of alcoholism. **Chronic calcifying pancreatitis, on the other hand, is an unquestioned result of alcoholism,**

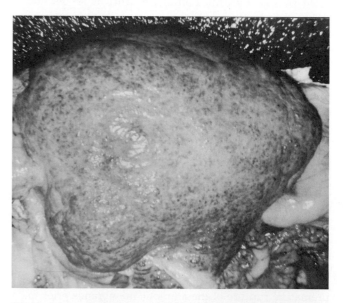

Figure 8-12. Cirrhosis of the liver in a chronic alcoholic. The liver is reduced in size and its surface displays innumerable small nodules of hepatocytes, separated by interconnecting bands of fibrous tissue.

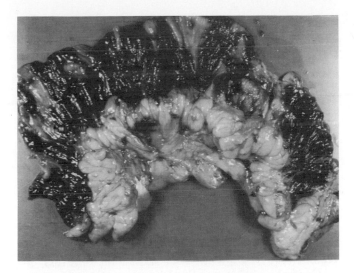

Figure 8-13. Gastrointestinal hemorrhage in a chronic alcoholic. Alcoholic cirrhosis caused portal hypertension, which in turn resulted in prominent submucosal esophageal varices. Rupture of such a varix led to massive upper gastrointestinal hemorrhage. The small intestine has been opened and contains fresh blood.

and is an important cause of incapacitating pain, pancreatic insufficiency, and pancreatic stones. Among men in the industrialized countries alcoholism may be the cause of the majority of cases of chronic pancreatitis.

Heart

Alcohol-related heart disease was recognized over a century ago in Germany, where it was referred to as the "beer-drinker's heart." This degenerative disease of the myocardium, termed **alcoholic cardiomyopathy,** leads to low-output congestive heart failure. Although the pathogenesis is obscure, it is widely accepted as a toxic effect of ethanol. This cardiomyopathy is clearly different from the heart disease associated with thiamine deficiency (beri-beri), a disorder characterized by high-output failure. Cardiac changes in alcoholics are far more common than are usually appreciated; up to 20% of confirmed alcoholics may show ultrastructural changes in the myocardium on endomyocardial biopsy. The alcoholic heart seems also to be more susceptible to arrhythmias, and the occurrence of abnormal cardiac rhythms after an alcoholic binge has been termed the "holiday heart." Many cases of sudden death in alcoholics are probably caused by sudden, fatal arrhythmias.

Skeletal Muscle

Muscle weakness is extremely common in alcoholics and is often attributed to general debility or nutritional deficiency. However, when carefully tested clinically, even well-nourished alcoholics usually show some weakness, particularly of the proximal muscles. A wide range of changes in skeletal muscle is seen in chronic alcoholics, varying from mild alterations in muscle fibers evident only by electron microscopy to a severe, debilitating chronic myopathy, with degeneration of muscle fibers and diffuse fibrosis. On rare occasions, **acute alcoholic rhabdomyolysis**—acute necrosis of muscle fibers and release of myoglobin to the circulation—is seen. This sudden event can be fatal, because of renal failure secondary to myoglobinuria.

Endocrine System

The principal endocrine effect of alcoholism in men is on the testes, which are reduced in size. Feminization of chronic alcoholics, together with loss of libido and potency, is common. The distribution of fat may change, giving the alcoholic male a female habitus. The breasts become enlarged (gynecomastia), body hair is lost, and a female distribution of pubic hair (escutcheon) develops. Some of these changes can be attributed to an impaired metabolism of estrogens due to chronic liver disease, but many of the changes—particularly atrophy of the testes—occur in the absence of any liver disease. Chronic alcoholism leads to lower levels of circulating testosterone because of a complex interference with the pituitary-gonadal axis, possibly complicated by an accelerated metabolism of testosterone by the liver. Alcohol has been shown to have a direct toxic effect on the testes; thus, sexual impairment in the male is one of the prices exacted by alcoholism.

Gastrointestinal Tract

Since the esophagus and stomach may be exposed to 10 molar ethanol, it is not surprising that a direct toxic effect on the mucosa of these organs is common. Injury to the mucosa of both organs is potentiated by the hypersecretion of gastric hydrochloric acid stimulated by ethanol. **Reflux esophagitis** may be particularly painful, and peptic ulcers are also more common in the alcoholic. Violent retching may lead to tears at the esophageal-gastric junction (**Mallory-Weiss syndrome**), sometimes so severe as to result in exsanguinating hemorrhage. The mucosal cells of the small intestine are also exposed to circulating alcohol, and a variety of absorptive abnormalities and ultrastructural changes have been demonstrated. Alcohol inhibits the active transport of amino acids, thiamine, and vitamin B_{12}.

Blood

Megaloblastic anemia secondary to a deficiency of folic acid is not uncommon in malnourished alcoholics. A nutritional deficiency of folic acid is the most important factor, but alcohol is itself considered a weak folic acid antagonist in man. Moreover, absorption of folate in the small intestine may be decreased in alcoholics. In addition, chronic ethanol intoxication leads directly to an **increase in red blood cell volume.** In the presence of alcoholic cirrhosis the spleen is often enlarged by portal hypertension; in such cases **hypersplenism** often causes **hemolytic anemia.** Acute transient **thrombocytopenia** is common after acute alcohol intoxication and may result in bleeding. Alcohol also interferes with the aggregation of platelets, thereby contributing to bleeding.

Immune System

Despite tantalizing clinical anecdotes and a substantial number of serious investigations, no consistent effect of alcohol on humoral or cell-mediated immunity has yet been conclusively established. Neither is there convincing evidence of an alcohol-related defect in neutrophils. Clinically, however, **alcoholics seem to be prone to many infections**—particularly pneumonias—with organisms that are unusual in the general population, such as *Haemophilus influenzae.*

Brain

A general cortical atrophy of the brain is common in alcoholics and may reflect a toxic effect of alcohol. By contrast, most of the characteristic brain diseases in alcoholics are probably a result of nutritional deficiency. **Wernicke's encephalopathy,** caused by thiamine deficiency, is characterized by mental confusion, ataxia, abnormal ocular motility, and polyneuropathy. The pathologic changes involve the diencephalon and brain stem. Lesions are always present in the mammillary bodies and are frequently present in the walls of the third ventricle and the periaqueductal gray matter. Necrosis of nerve cells and myelinated fibers, together with glial responses, are noted.

The retrograde amnesia and confabulatory symptoms of **Korsakoff's psychosis,** once thought to be pathognomonic of chronic alcoholism, have now been identified in a number of organic mental syndromes and are considered nonspecific. Alcoholic cerebellar degeneration is differentiated from other forms of acquired or familial cerebellar degeneration by the uniformity of its manifestations. Progressive unsteadiness of gait, ataxia, incoordination, and reduced deep tendon reflex activity are present. The cerebellar vermis displays varying degrees of shrinkage of the folia and widening of the sulci. At the microscopic level, the Purkinje cells are the neuronal elements primarily destroyed, but in advanced cases the molecular and granular cell layers are also affected.

Central pontine myelinolysis is another characteristic change in the brain of alcoholics, apparently caused by electrolyte imbalance—usually after electrolyte therapy, after an alcoholic binge, or during withdrawal. In this complication a progressive weakness of bulbar muscles causes dysphagia and dysarthria and may be rapidly succeeded by an inability to swallow. Quadriparesis and coma eventually terminate in respiratory paralysis. Microscopic examination reveals foci of demyelination in the pons. **Amblyopia** (impaired vision) is occasionally seen in alcoholics and may result from an alcohol-related decrease in tissue vitamin A, although other vitamin deficiencies may also be involved.

Alcoholism and Cancer

The incidence of cancer of the lung, upper respiratory tract, and esophagus is unquestionably greater in alcoholics than in the general population, but the precise relationship of cancer to alcohol consumption is confused by the fact that most alcoholics are also smokers.

Mechanism of Alcohol-Induced Tissue Injury

The mechanism by which alcohol injures any organ or tissue is not understood. In the liver, the change in the redox potential occasioned by the metabolism of ethanol has been proposed as a major factor. During the oxidation of ethanol to acetaldehyde, NAD is reduced to NADH, thereby greatly increasing the reducing power of the cell. However, although certain metabolic abnormalities may be attributed to this change in the NAD/NADH ratio, no tissue injury has been directly shown to be caused by it. Moreover, other organs that also exhibit alcohol-induced injury, such as the heart and the pancreas, do not metabolize ethanol to any appreciable extent. Another proposed factor in tissue injury is acetaldehyde, the highly toxic product of alcohol metabolism. In the liver, acetaldehyde is rapidly converted by aldehyde dehydrogenase to acetate, but measurable levels of acetaldehyde (usually <50 μM) can be found in the liver. However, circulating levels of acetaldehyde are extremely low, and it is difficult to attribute all of the changes associated with alcoholism to this metabolite.

An effect of ethanol common to all cells, regardless of their origin or location, is fluidization of cell membranes. Like all anesthetics, ethanol intercalates within the lipid bilayer and decreases the molecular order of the phospholipids (a process known as fluidization). As an adaptive response the composition of the membranes is changed, so that they become resistant to this fluidizing effect of ethanol. Such a mechanism may be important for central nervous system tolerance to alcohol, but its relationship to cell injury requires further study.

Drug Abuse

Drug abuse has been defined as "the use of any substance in a manner that deviates from the accepted medical, social, or legal patterns within a given society." For the most part, drug abuse involves agents that affect the higher functions of the brain and that are used to alter mood and perception. These chemicals include derivatives of opium (heroin, morphine), depressants (barbiturates, tranquilizers, alcohol), stimulants (cocaine, amphetamines), marijuana, psychedelic drugs (LSD), and inhalants (amyl nitrite, organic solvents such as those in glue). The use of psychotropic chemicals to produce euphoric states has a long history and a worldwide distribution. In addition to alcoholic beverages, examples are hashish in the Middle East, opium in the Far East, coca leaves in South America, and mescaline among Native Americans of the Southwest. However, the current epidemic of drug abuse in Western industrialized countries is of recent origin. A notable difference in the pattern of drug intake, namely the intravenous injection of illicit drugs, reflects the easy availability of syringes and hypodermic needles in industrialized societies. This change in the pattern of drug intake and the development of newer and more potent drugs have led to a profound change in the nature of the diseases related to drug abuse. The social and emotional consequences of drug abuse are beyond the scope of this chapter, but it should be noted that suicide, homicide, and accidents are responsible for one-quarter to one-half of deaths related to narcotic abuse.

The intravenous injection of excessive amounts of heroin and other "street drugs" accounts for more than one-half of all the deaths from drug abuse. Deaths from narcotic overdosage are not only caused by the pharmacologic effects of the drugs; they may be a result of cardiac arrhythmias, acute pulmonary edema, or otherwise unexplained hypoxia. The so-called narcotic lung represents a number of nonspecific, acute pulmonary complications related to respiratory depression, aspiration of gastric contents, and infection.

Apart from reactions related to the pharmacologic or physiological effects of substance abuse, the most common complications (15% of directly drug-related deaths) are caused by the introduction of infectious organisms by a parenteral route. The most common infections are local at the site of injection. Among these are cutaneous abscesses, cellulitis, and ulcers (Fig. 8-14). When these heal, "track marks" persist, and these areas may also exhibit hypo- or hyperpigmentation. Thrombophlebitis of the veins draining the sites of injection is common. Self-administration of street drugs is a major cause of tetanus, particularly when the injection is subcutaneous or intramuscular. The intravenous introduction of bacteria also leads to septic complications in many organs. Bacterial endocarditis, often involving *Staphylococcus aureus*, occurs on both sides of the heart (Fig. 8-15). Other complications of bacteremia are pulmonary, renal, and intracranial abscesses, meningitis, osteomyelitis, and mycotic aneurysms (Fig. 8-16).

Perhaps the most feared infectious complications today are of viral etiology. Addicts who exchange needles constitute one of the highest risk groups for AIDS and for viral hepatitis. Addicts also suffer from the complications of viral hepatitis, such as chronic active hepatitis, necrotizing angiitis, and glomerulonephritis. A focal glomerulosclerosis ("heroin nephropathy") has been described, characterized by the presence of immune complexes in the absence of a known antigen, and has been ascribed to an immune reaction to impurities contaminating illicit drugs. The prognosis in this form of glomerulonephritis is poor, and progression to uremia is common.

The intravenous injection of talc, a material used to dilute the pure drug, is associated with the appearance of foreign body granulomas in the lung. These may be severe enough to lead to interstitial pulmonary fibrosis. In some cases, talc-induced thrombosis of pulmonary vessels results in pulmonary hypertension or cor pulmonale.

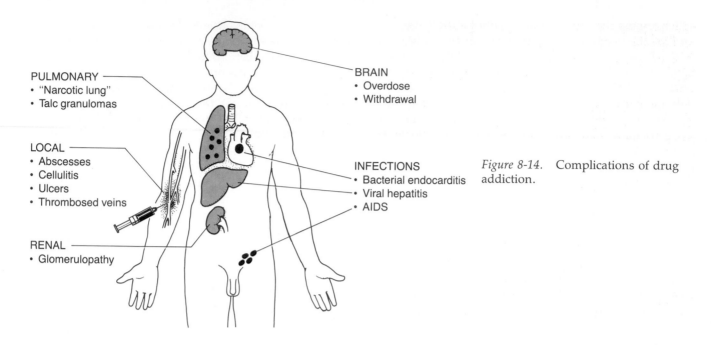

PULMONARY
• "Narcotic lung"
• Talc granulomas

BRAIN
• Overdose
• Withdrawal

LOCAL
• Abscesses
• Cellulitis
• Ulcers
• Thrombosed veins

INFECTIONS
• Bacterial endocarditis
• Viral hepatitis
• AIDS

RENAL
• Glomerulopathy

Figure 8-14.   Complications of drug addiction.

Drug addiction in pregnant women poses substantial risks for the fetus. Infants of drug-dependent mothers often exhibit a full-blown withdrawal syndrome. Moreover, the appearance of the drug withdrawal syndrome in the fetus during labor may result in excessive fetal movements and increased oxygen demand, a situation that increases the risk of intrapartum hypoxia and meconium aspiration. If labor occurs when maternal drug levels are high, often the infant is born with respiratory depression. Mothers who are addicted to drugs experience higher rates of toxemia of pregnancy and premature labor, although it is unclear to what extent smoking may also contribute to these events.

Iatrogenic Drug Injury

The basis of the scientific practice of medicine is rational drug therapy. Although few act as specifically and effectively as antibiotics, properly used drugs constitute the foundation of patient management. However, the administration of therapeutic agents exacts a price. Adverse reactions are surprisingly common, being found in 2% to 5% of patients hospitalized on medical services; of these reactions, 2% to 12% are fatal. The typical hospitalized patient is given about 10 different medications, and some receive five times as many. The risk of an adverse

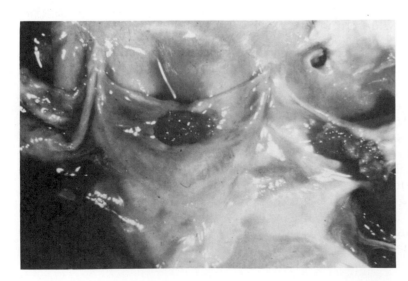

Figure 8-15.   Bacterial endocarditis in a drug addict. Two aortic valve cusps display adherent vegetations. A coronary artery ostium is visible in the upper right.

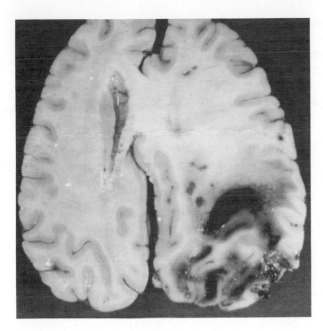

Figure 8-16. Brain abscess (lower right) in an intravenous drug abuser.

reaction increases proportionately with the number of different drugs; for example, the risk of injury is at least 40% when more than 15 drugs are administered. Because they are so ubiquitously prescribed, drugs represent a significant environmental hazard. Untoward effects of drugs result from overdose, an exaggerated physiologic response, a genetic predisposition, hypersensitivity mechanisms, interactions with other drugs, and other, unknown factors. It is beyond the scope of this chapter to describe in detail adverse reactions to individual drugs; the characteristic pathologic changes associated with these reactions are treated in chapters dealing with specific organs. Some general principles are discussed here.

An overdose implies an excessive pharmacologic effect of the drug. The intake of an inordinate amount of a drug can be a deliberate suicide attempt or can be accidental, as often happens in children or in those who are addicted to illicit drugs. The lethal physiological effect may be different from the desired effect at lower doses—for example, depression of the respiratory centers in barbiturate poisoning. A minor physiological effect may be dangerous in a susceptible person, as with lethal cardiac arrhythmias in some cocaine users. A dose considered safe for the general population may be excessive in someone who has a genetically slow metabolizing apparatus. Others may show an exaggerated reactivity (e.g., neurologic or cardiovascular) to the pharmacologic action of specific drugs. Drugs that have a wide therapeutic window—that is, a substantial distance between therapeutic and toxic levels—are less likely to produce these side effects than those with a steep dose–response curve. It is often not appreciated that drug reactions can produce a bewildering variety of disorders in virtually all organs. The following discussion deals with representative drug reactions, and is not meant to be all-inclusive.

Gastrointestinal Tract

Gastritis is a common reaction, particularly with aspirin and other nonsteroidal anti-inflammatory agents. This damage may progress to **hemorrhagic gastritis** severe enough to cause anemia and even exsanguination. **Peptic ulceration** is also seen with these agents, as well as with corticosteroids. **Jejunal ulceration** may be particularly troublesome with enteric-coated potassium supplements. **Pancreatitis,** another complication of treatment with corticosteroids, also occurs with thiazide diuretics. Certain broad-spectrum antibiotics lead to the overgrowth of intestinal bacteria and a severe **pseudomembranous enterocolitis. Gingival hyperplasia** is a characteristic side effect of chronic treatment with the anticonvulsant diphenylhydantoin.

Liver

The single most common cause of **jaundice** in the United States is probably drug toxicity. In most cases this jaundice is cholestatic—that is, the type resembling biliary obstruction. Representative drugs producing this condition are the phenothiazines, other tranquilizers, anabolic steroids, and oral contraceptives. Jaundice also accompanies the **hepatitis** produced by such drugs as halothane, isoniazid, and propylthiouracil. **Chronic hepatitis, fibrosis,** and **cirrhosis** may all result from drug reactions. Hepatic drug toxicity is discussed in detail in Chapter 14, which deals with diseases of the liver.

Nervous System

Cerebrovascular accidents complicate the use of anticoagulants and oral contraceptives. **Convulsive seizures** are occasionally produced by phenothiazines and certain other psychotropic agents. Extrapyramidal dysfunction, notably **tardive dyskinesia,** is a feared complication of chronic treatment with phenothiazines and other tranquilizing agents, particularly since it is often not reversible upon discontinuation of the medication. **Peripheral neuropathy** is one of the more common adverse reactions to drugs, as with the chemotherapeutic agent vincristine and the antimalarial chloroquine. A particularly distressing form of this complication is the **eighth nerve deafness** caused by streptomycin.

Skin

The cutaneous manifestations of drug reactions run the entire gamut of dermatologic disease, from **acne** to a fatal **exfoliative dermatitis.** Long-term corticosteroid treatment, leading to the development of Cushing's syndrome, is classically associated with acne. Among the most common drug reactions is **urticaria** ("hives"), a hypersensitivity response to agents such as penicillin, sulfonamides, and barbiturates. **Fixed drug eruptions** can be troublesome, and **alopecia** produced by chemotherapeutic agents may be embarrassing. **Erythema nodosum,** caused by such drugs as penicillin and sulfonamides, is unpleasant but reverses upon discontinuation of the offending drug. By contrast, a number of drugs, including penicillin, sulfonamides, hydantoins, and phenylbutazone, cause serious and occasionally life-threatening **exfoliative dermatitis, toxic epidermal necrolysis,** and the **Stevens-Johnson syndrome.**

Heart

The most common cardiac complications of drug therapy relate to the pharmacologic actions of the particular agents. **Arrhythmias** are associated with the administration of drugs as diverse as digitalis, propranolol, procainamide, and thyroxin. **Congestive heart failure** may be precipitated by drugs that increase blood volume (e.g., corticosteroids) or by intravenous fluid overload. A toxic, dose-related **cardiomyopathy** results from chemotherapy with doxorubicin (Adriamycin).

Metabolic Effects

Certain drugs, when used injudiciously, cause electrolyte imbalances, particularly **hyponatremia, hypokalemia, hyperkalemia,** and **metabolic acidosis.** Overdosage with vitamin D or treatment with thiazide diuretics can cause **hypercalcemia.** Acute episodes of **hepatic porphyria** are precipitated by barbiturates, hydantoins, and sulfonamides. Although alcohol is not considered a therapeutic agent, it is a potent stimulator of delta-aminolevulinic acid syn-

thetase, and therefore also precipitates acute hepatic porphyria. **Hyperuricemia** and associated **urate nephropathy** complicate the treatment of cancer with chemotherapeutic agents.

Blood

Aplastic anemia, often fatal, is associated with a variety of drugs on rare occasions, but is a notorious complication of chloramphenicol treatment. Depression of specific bone marrow precursors by antineoplastic agents, sulfonamides, and barbiturates causes **agranulocytosis** and **thrombocytopenia.** Immune **hemolytic anemia** complicates treatment with penicillin, quinidine, and the cephalosporins. In persons with a genetic deficiency of glucose-6-phosphate dehydrogenase, nitrofurans and sulfonamides cause a nonimmune hemolytic anemia. Folic acid antagonists, such as methotrexate and diphenylhydantoin, can induce a **megaloblastic anemia.**

Lungs

An important complication of treating cancer with certain chemotherapeutic agents, such as bleomycin, busulfan, cyclophosphamide, and methotrexate, is an acute **toxic alveolitis,** which can progress to **interstitial pulmonary fibrosis.** Similar reactions can follow the administration of other types of drugs, such as the antiarrhythmic agent amiodarone and the antibiotic nitrofurantoin (Fig. 8-17). **Asthma** is precipitated by nonsteroidal anti-inflammatory medications (aspirin, indomethacin) and the beta-adrenergic blocker propranolol. **Pulmonary infections** are a distressing complication of treatment with corticosteroids and other immunosuppressive drugs.

Kidney

Renal damage is a limiting factor in the use of a number of antibiotics, including such antibacterial drugs as gentamicin and kanamycin and the antifungal agent amphotericin B. These drugs produce **acute tubular necrosis** and, therefore, acute renal failure. A **nephrotic syndrome** results from the administration of some drugs (gold salts for rheumatoid arthritis, tolbutamide for diabetes, penicillamine for Wilson's disease, trimethadione for seizures). Analgesic abuse is associated with **chronic interstitial nephritis** and **papillary necrosis.**

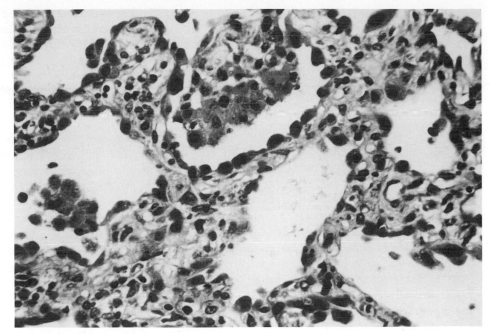

Figure 8-17. Diffuse interstitial pneumonitis in a patient treated with amiodarone for a cardiac arrhythmia. The alveolar walls are widened by edema and numerous inflammatory cells. The alveoli are lined by type II pneumocytes and contain desquamated epithelial cells.

Female Reproductive Tract

Oral Contraceptives

The most important contemporary drugs with important gynecologic effects are the oral contraceptives. These hormonal preparations, barely known a generation ago, are now the most commonly used method of contraception in industrialized countries. Almost all current formulations are combinations of synthetic estrogens and steroids with progesterone-like activity. The oral contraceptives act by either inhibiting the surge of gonadotropins in midcycle, thereby preventing ovulation, or inhibiting implantation by altering the phase of the endometrium. Most of the complications are produced by the estrogenic component, but some may be related to the progestin component or to a combination of the two (Fig. 8-18). The current preparations contain only one-fifth as much estrogen as earlier ones, and the incidence of side effects has progressively decreased as the amount of hormone in the proprietary oral contraceptives has been decreased.

Ethinyl estradiol, the synthetic estrogen in many oral contraceptives, augments the liver's synthesis of several globulins of the coagulation system, and may thereby cause a hypercoagulable state and thrombosis. An increased production of angiotensinogen may lead to an increase in the level of angiotensin II, thereby raising blood pressure. Estrogen's stimulation of tryptophan metabolism in the liver may lead to a decrease in the level of tryptophan in the blood; it may also lead to low levels of serotonin, the end product of tryptophan metabolism. Presumably this can produce depression and behavioral changes.

The progestational agents, or gestagens, are related structurally to androgenic steroids and therefore exert certain virilizing effects, including weight gain, acne, and amenorrhea. The weight gain is presumed to be an anabolic effect of the progestin component. The progestins decrease the number of estrogen receptors in the endometrium; endometrial growth is therefore decreased, leading to amenorrhea.

For reasons unknown oral contraceptives may induce an increased pigmentation of the malar eminences, called **chloasma,** which is accentuated by sunlight and persists for a long time after the contraceptives are discontinued. The incidence of **cholelithiasis** is increased twofold in women who have used oral contraceptives for 4 years or less, but decreases to lower than normal after that period of time (see Fig. 8-18). Thus, oral contraceptives accelerate the process of cholelithiasis but do not increase its overall incidence. The risk of deep vein **thrombophlebitis** is increased three to four times by oral contraceptive use, as is the risk of **thromboembolism.** The incidence of stroke is increased in women who use oral contraceptives, but the epidemiologic data are conflicting. It is probable that the increase is lim-

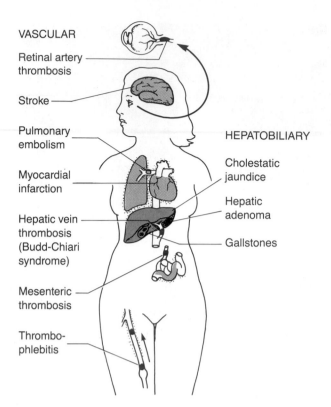

VASCULAR

Retinal artery thrombosis

Stroke

Pulmonary embolism

Myocardial infarction

Hepatic vein thrombosis (Budd-Chiari syndrome)

Mesenteric thrombosis

Thrombophlebitis

HEPATOBILIARY

Cholestatic jaundice

Hepatic adenoma

Gallstones

Figure 8-18.   Complications of oral contraceptives.

ited to women with preexisting hypertension and older women who smoke. The risk of **stroke** may be three times higher than normal, but the incidence is low—about 1 in 20,000 to 1 in 30,000 a year. Of particular concern is the fact that women over 35 who smoke or have another associated risk factor, such as hypertension or hypercholesterolemia, have an increased risk of developing **myocardial infarction** when using oral contraceptives. Nevertheless, the incidence of myocardial infarction is low—about one in 5,000 a year. For cardiovascular disease, although the relative-risk figure can be frightening, the absolute-risk figure in smoking women who use oral contraceptives and who do not have any other risk factors is negligible. The cause of myocardial infarction or stroke in users of oral contraceptives is usually arterial thrombosis, not atherosclerosis. A few women develop high blood pressure, but this reverses upon discontinuation of the oral contraceptives.

Benign liver adenomas occur with an estimated frequency of one in 30,000 to one in 50,000 a year in the general population. The incidence is higher in women who have used oral contraceptives for more than 5 years.

Despite earlier reports to the contrary, all of the

large prospective studies have shown that **the use of oral contraceptives does not increase the risk of any type of cancer.** Data that appeared to implicate oral contraceptives in an increased incidence of cervical cancer, breast cancer and melanoma are all plagued with confounding factors and have not been confirmed in other studies.

Absolute contraindications to oral contraceptive use are a past history of vascular disease (thromboembolism, thrombophlebitis, atherosclerosis, and stroke), a history of systemic vascular disease (lupus erythematosus, sickle cell disease), hypertension, diabetes mellitus with vascular disease and hyperlipidemia. Smoking in women over 35 is also an absolute contraindication. Patients who suffer from an estrogen-dependent tumor, such as cancer of the breast or endometrium, should probably not take oral contraceptives, although there are no data showing an ill effect. Pregnancy is a contraindication because of the masculinizing effect of the gestagens on the external genitalia of the female fetus. Patients with heart disease may develop congestive heart failure because of fluid retention. Women with active liver disease should not receive oral steroids because they are metabolized in the liver. Those over the age of 45 should not receive oral contraceptives except in unusual circumstances.

The use of oral contraceptives is also beneficial for some conditions. Protective effects have been shown against pelvic inflammatory disease, ovarian and endometrial carcinoma, and fibrocystic disease of the breast. Acne has been reported to be improved, and there is a decreased incidence of rheumatoid arthritis.

Other Drugs

The use of diethylstilbesterol by pregnant women is of historical interest. Although the women themselves suffered no appreciable untoward effects, years later their daughters developed **vaginal adenosis** and **adenocarcinoma.**

Drugs given to pregnant women may be potent teratogens, as exemplified by the epidemic of **congenital anomalies** following maternal ingestion of thalidomide. This subject is discussed in detail in Chapter 6, which deals with congenital disorders.

Musculoskeletal Effects

Myopathies and muscle weakness are well recognized as side effects of treatment with corticosteroids, chloroquine, and a number of other unrelated drugs. A serious complication of corticosteroid administration, and one that is not uncommon, is **osteoporosis.**

Long-term use of these steroids in children retards bone growth.

Immunologic Syndromes

Several hundred deaths occur every year in the United States because of severe **anaphylactic reactions to penicillin.** Individuals who become sensitized to a variety of other drugs can also exhibit anaphylactic reactions. Penicillin is the single most common cause of **serum sickness,** although other antibiotics and drugs, such as propylthiouracil and barbiturates, can also cause this syndrome. The same drugs, presumably acting by similar mechanisms, produce **vasculitis.**

A **lupus-like syndrome,** characterized by antinuclear antibodies, fever, muscle and joint pain, and (less commonly) rash and lymphadenopathy, results from the chronic administration of a number of drugs, including hydralazine, procainamide, penicillin, and hydantoins. Symptoms are generally reversible upon discontinuation of the medication.

Environmental Chemicals

Man's migrations and search for food placed him in localities where he was subject not only to attack by microorganisms and parasites, but also to injury by foreign chemicals and carcinogens. In addition, not all the foods with which early man experimented were nutritious, and some contained chemicals deleterious to his health. Not only did parasites grow upon his fresh foodstuffs, but his need to store food provided a further opportunity for contamination. The same situation that allowed for parasitism and saprophytic growth also provided a new set of biologically active molecules to which he was exposed. The introduction of man-made chemicals to increase food production, protect it from insects, and increase its "shelf life" has added 60 micrograms a day of man-made chemicals to the average human diet.

The environment through which man moved and the microenvironment he prepared for his own habitation harbored further dangers. The whale oil lamps of the Eskimos were so smoky that their lungs became distinctly black from carbon deposits. Endogenous material within water supplies—and even radioactivity in water—exposed man to hazards. (The word "hazard" should be considered here in context; not infrequently, areas became popular as "spas" because of these waters—for example, Baden-Baden, which became famous for the "curative" radioactivity of its natural elements.) A variety of parasitic organisms that enter the body through the skin lurked in the lakes and rivers in which he fished or traveled. Finally, man breathed air—initially clouded by dust, but more recently contaminated by his own industry. As the following quote from Maimonides shows, concerns about air pollution existed even in the 12th century.

> Comparing the air of cities to the air of deserts is like comparing waters that are befouled and turbid to waters that are fine and pure. In the city, because of the height of its buildings, the narrowness of its streets, and all that pours forth from its inhabitants, the air becomes stagnant, turbid, thick, misty, and foggy. If there is no choice in this matter, if we have grown up in the cities and become accustomed to them, we should endeavor at least to dwell out at the outskirts of the city. Wherever the air is altered ever so slightly you will find men develop dullness of understanding, failure of intelligence, and defects of memory.

Man inhales, bathes in, and eats a variety of chemical materials that are found as contaminants in foods and in the food chain, the water supply, and the general ecosystem in which he lives. In the last two decades man-made contamination and the effects of these chemicals have caused considerable alarm. However, predictions of widespread destruction of flora and fauna and an epidemic of human cancer have yet to materialize. In fact, recent attempts to quantitate the potency of environmental contaminants and to estimate past and present human exposure suggest that **naturally occurring chemicals pose a far greater hazard than man-made products,** and the former have been with us for millenia. Our natural environment is not without risk, and even oxygen can be harmful.

There are several important mechanisms that govern the effect of toxic agents, including the toxin's absorption, distribution, metabolism, and excretion. Absorption (whether through pulmonary, gastrointestinal, or dermal routes) depends in part on the chemical structure of the agent. For example, because of their solubility in lipids the insecticides chlordane and heptachlor are rapidly absorbed and stored in body fat. By contrast, the herbicide paraquat, because it is water soluble, is readily eliminated.

The effects of many chemicals are exerted by their metabolic products rather than by the parent compound. The capacity of the xenobiotic systems to modify these materials varies among tissues. Moreover, these detoxifying systems may produce different metabolites in different sites, which may vary in their capacity to produce disease. The cellular content of these enzyme systems varies with age, sex, hormonal and nutritional status, and previous drug intake.

The storage, distribution, and excretion of these materials control their concentrations in the organism at any given time. It follows that agents stored in adipose tissue exert a prolonged low-level effect, whereas the more water-soluble materials that are easily excreted by the kidney have a shorter duration of action.

It is worth pointing out that the fact that a toxic agent can be detected in the workplace does not mean that it necessarily produces disease. For example, carbon tetrachloride, a recognized species-dependent hepatotoxin, is used frequently in the machining of steel. Yet liver disease derived from this haloalkane is not an occupational hazard in the steel fabricating industry. Thus, although there is little question that chemicals can and do produce human disease, in many cases our information is far from conclusive.

Toxic vs. Hypersensitivity Responses

Many substances elicit disease in a variety of animal species in a dose-dependent manner, with a regular time delay and a predictable target-organ response. Furthermore, the morphologic changes in the injured tissues are constant and reproducible. By contrast, other agents show great variability in the production of disease, an irregular lag before any manifestation of injury, no dose-dependency, and a lack of reproducibility. It has been assumed that the predictable dose–response reactions reflect a direct action of the compound or its metabolite on a tissue—that is, a "toxic" effect. The second, unpredictable type of reaction is thought to reflect "hypersensitivity," or an immunologic response. Yet despite the wealth of information that has been accumulated about the mechanisms of cell injury, such a separation with respect to mechanisms of action has not been conclusively established. There are, clearly, immunologic responses, but the mechanisms by which delayed, irregular responses to toxic agents occur have yet to be explained.

Responses to Chemical Substances

Our current fund of information does not permit an easy cataloging of responses to the variety of man-made and natural products. For the purposes of this chapter we will discuss certain specific chemicals as

illustrations or because of the importance of the pathologic changes they induce.

Beginning with the industrial revolution there has been an exponential rise in the number of chemicals manufactured and a corresponding increase in the risk of human exposure. This potential problem has elicited widespread public concern, and has particularly attracted the attention of journalists and attorneys. In any consideration of this topic it is crucial to differentiate between the problems of acute poisoning and chronic toxicity. One must also distinguish industrial and accidental exposure from that which is likely to occur in the general environment. The lack of adequate quantitative data in humans and the obvious problem involved in obtaining such information have led to the extrapolation to humans of experimental data derived from animal studies. Such projections can be hazardous because of species differences in sensitivity, differing routes of administration, and use of unrealistically high concentrations of the test agent. Yet the doctrine is enshrined in American law that any agent that produces malignant tumors in any species, and at any dose, is unfit for human use. For example, large doses of the artificial sweeteners saccharin and the cyclamates were reported to be associated with the development of bladder tumors in experimental animals. As a result the cyclamates have been withdrawn from use and saccharin has been subjected to strong criticism. Yet there are no adequate epidemiologic data in humans that suggest a similar harmful effect among those who have regularly consumed these substances.

Except for certain hypersensitivity reactions in susceptible individuals, acute poisoning by environmental chemicals does not pose a threat to the general population. The concentrations necessary to cause acute functional disorders or structural damage are ordinarily encountered only in the workplace or as a consequence of uncommon accidents. The latter category includes the exposure to the largest amount of tetrachloro-dibenzo-dioxin (TCDD) ever to contaminate the environment, which followed an explosion in a chemical plant in Seveso, Italy, in 1976. This compound, a potent herbicide, is a byproduct of the synthesis of 2,4,5-trichlorphenoxyacetic acid (2,4,5-T), a defoliant used by the U.S. Army in Vietnam. As expected, some exposed individuals developed acute symptoms, although none died. It is noteworthy that more than a decade later, with the exception of chloracne, there have been no confirmed chronic effects in the people exposed at Seveso.

Similarly, although accidental mass poisonings with the pesticides endrin and parathion have led to as many as 100 deaths in a single event, no chronic sequelae among the survivors have been documented. Despite claims of an association between progressive chronic disease and exposure to pesticides, the small number of cases, coupled with the nonspecific nature of the complaints, does not permit such a conclusion. It should be stressed that the action of most environmental toxins is specific, and that a causal relationship to disease implies damage to a specific organ or organ system, with specific alterations of these tissues. As a corollary, multisystem involvement, particularly when the symptoms are vague, should be viewed with skepticism. The experimental literature dealing with the acute and chronic toxicity of industrial chemicals is voluminous and complicated, and often contradictory. It is for this reason that we shall largely restrict the following discussion to documented effects in man.

Volatile Organic Solvents and Vapors

Volatile organic solvents and vapors are widely used in industry to dissolve other compounds (degreasers) and as fuels. With few exceptions the exposures are industrial or accidental, and represent acute dangers rather than chronic toxicity. For the most part, exposure is by inhalation rather than by ingestion.

Chloroform ($CHCl_3$) and **carbon tetrachloride** (CCl_4) exert anesthetic effects on the central nervous system but are better known as hepatotoxins. With both, large doses lead to acute hepatic necrosis, fatty liver, and liver failure. Whereas chronic administration of carbon tetrachloride to rats invariably produces cirrhosis, such a situation does not obtain in man because each exposure to the toxin results in recognizable clinical liver injury. Unlike the rat, a person who suffers a bout of jaundice after exposure to carbon tetrachloride will not be permitted another episode of poisoning.

Trichloroethylene ($Cl_2C=CHCl$), a ubiquitous industrial solvent, in high concentrations depresses the central nervous system, but hepatotoxicity is minimal. There is no evidence for chronic sequelae in man following ordinary long-term industrial exposure.

Methanol (CH_3OH) was originally called "wood alcohol" because it was derived from the distillation of wood. Because the odor and taste of methanol are similar to those of ethanol, and because methanol does not carry the burden of a tax, it is used by impoverished chronic alcoholics as a substitute for ethanol or by unscrupulous merchants as an adulterant of alcoholic beverages. In methanol poisoning, inebriation similar to that produced by ethanol is succeeded by gastrointestinal symptoms, visual dysfunction, coma, and death. The major toxicity of methanol is thought to arise from its metabolism to formaldehyde, principally by alcohol dehydrogenase, followed by its oxidation to formic acid by aldehyde dehydrogenase. The most characteristic lesion of methanol toxicity is necrosis of retinal ganglion cells and subsequent degeneration of the optic nerve, a process presumably mediated by the metabolites of methanol oxidation. Interestingly, methanol-induced blindness occurs only in primates. It is not clear whether the metabolic acidosis seen in cases of methanol poisoning results from a direct effect of formate or from an inhibition of glucose oxidation.

Gasoline and **kerosene** are mixtures of aliphatic hydrocarbons and branched, unsaturated, and aromatic hydrocarbons. Despite prolonged exposure to gasoline, gas station attendants, auto mechanics, and so on do not manifest any evidence of toxicity. The increased use of kerosene as a home heating fuel has led to accidental poisoning of children.

Ethylene glycol ($HOCH_2CH_2OH$), commonly used as an antifreeze, has been ingested by chronic alcoholics as a substitute for ethanol for many years. Poisoning with this compound has recently come into prominence because it has been used to adulterate wines in Austria and Italy, owing to its sweet taste and solubility. Like methanol, ethylene glycol is much more toxic in man than in other animals. The major toxicity relates to acute tubular necrosis in the kidney. Oxalate crystals in the tubules and oxaluria are often noted.

Benzene (C_6H_6), the prototypic aromatic hydrocarbon, must be distinguished from benzine, a mixture of aliphatic hydrocarbons. Benzene is one of the most widely used chemicals in industrial processes, being employed as the starting point for innumerable syntheses, as a solvent, and as a constituent of fuels. Virtually all cases of acute and chronic benzene toxicity have occurred against the background of industrial exposure. Many instances have been reported in shoemakers and workers in shoe manufacturing, occupations which at one time were associated with heavy exposure to benzene-based glues. Acute benzene poisoning primarily affects the central nervous system, and death results from respiratory failure. However, it is the chronic effects of benzene exposure that have attracted the most attention. The bone marrow is the principal target in chronic benzene intoxication. Those who develop hematologic abnormalities characteristically exhibit **hypoplasia or aplasia of the bone marrow and pancytopenia.** Aplastic anemia usually is seen while the workers are still exposed to high concentrations of benzene. In a substantial proportion of cases of benzene-induced anemias, **acute myeloblastic leukemia** or erythroleukemia develops during continuing exposure to benzene or after a variable latent period following removal from the hazardous environment. Some cases of acute leukemia have occurred without a prior history of aplastic anemia. While instances of chronic myeloid and chronic lymphocytic leukemia have been reported, a cause-and-effect relationship with benzene exposure is less convincing than with cases of acute leukemia. There is no *a priori* reason to doubt a causal association, but the subject requires further careful epidemiologic studies before a definitive answer can be accepted. The closely related compound toluene, also widely used for its solvent properties, has not been incriminated as a cause of hematologic abnormalities.

Agricultural Chemicals

Pesticides, fungicides, herbicides, and organic fertilizers are crucial to the success of modern agriculture, and it is probable that without their use epidemic and endemic famine would again become commonplace. However, the realization that many of these chemicals persist in soil and water, thereby posing a potential long-term hazard, has caused substantial concern. The problem of acute poisoning with very large concentrations of any of these chemicals has already been alluded to, and it is clear that exposure to industrial concentrations or inadvertently contaminated food can cause severe acute illness. A particularly common acute poisoning occurs in children who ingest home gardening preparations. The symptoms of acute toxicity are often related to the mode of action of the toxin. For example, the organophosphate insecticides exert their effect by inhibiting acetylcholinesterase, and thus acute toxicity in humans is principally reflected in symptoms referable to the nervous system. If the acute incident is not fatal, in most cases there are no chronic sequelae. However, delayed neurotoxicity has been reported with a few compounds, the most notorious of which is triorthocresyl phosphate (TOCP). Acute poisoning with this compound leads to a peripheral neuropathy that progresses to motor weakness of limbs, which in some cases is only partially reversible. Contamination of illicit ginger liquor in the United States during the 1930s led to an epidemic of "ginger jake paralysis." In Morocco, the adulteration of cooking oil with lubricating oil containing TOCP produced an outbreak of a similar peripheral neuropathy.

The problem of widespread chronic human exposure to low levels of agricultural chemicals has profound health, economic, and legal implications. Because from a practical point of view these chemicals cannot be eliminated from our environment and because they produce a variety of diseases in experimental animals, it is appropriate to search for evidence of disease in humans. Potential effects that have elicited public concern include cancer, chronic degenerative diseases, congenital abnormalities, and a host of nonspecific complaints ranging from asthenia to impotence. A cause-and-effect relationship between the presence of agricultural chemicals in the environment and disease in humans can only be established by careful and well-controlled epidemiologic studies. The current state of our knowledge can be summarized with the simple recognition that although chronic toxicity and reproductive failure have been clearly established in predatory birds and fish, there are no reliable data to support a similar link in humans. Until such a connection has been validated, the burden of proof will remain on those who postulate a cause-and-effect relationship.

Aromatic Halogenated Hydrocarbons

The halogenated aromatic hydrocarbons that have received considerable attention recently include the polychlorinated biphenyls (PCBs), chlorophenols (pentachlorophenol, used as a wood preservative; hexachlorophene, used as an antibacterial agent in soaps), and the dioxin TCDD, a byproduct of the synthesis of herbicides and hexachlorophene, and therefore a contaminant of these preparations. TCDD has been mentioned above. The problem of the presence of PCBs in the environment resembles that of agricultural chemicals: Chronic animal toxicity is well documented, but a health hazard for humans remains to be established. The same situation obtains for hexachlorophene and pentachlorophenol.

Cyanide

Prussic acid (HCN) is the classic murderer's tool in detective fiction, where the smell of bitter almonds (*Amygdalus prunus*) betrays the crime. A more contemporary homicidal application of cyanide is its surreptitious addition to a number of commercially available medicinal capsules. Amygdalin, a glycoside found in the pits of several fruits (including apricots, peaches, and wild cherries) and in the seeds of almonds and hydrangeas, is a combination of glucose, benzaldehyde, and cyanide. While humans do not possess the beta-glucosidase needed to liberate the cyanide, intestinal flora are capable of effecting this release, thereby leading to cyanide intoxication. Amygdalin is, therefore, far more toxic when ingested than when injected intravenously. These considerations may appear esoteric, except for the fact that extracts of apricot pits are used in the formulation of fraudulent anticancer nostrums and have resulted in cases of cyanide poisoning.

Cyanide blocks cellular respiration, reversibly binding to mitochondrial cytochrome oxidase, the terminal acceptor in the electron transport chain, which is responsible for reducing molecular oxygen to water. The pathologic consequences are similar to those produced by any acute global anoxia.

Environmental dusts lead to pulmonary disease and are discussed in Chapter 12. **Environmental carcinogens** are dealt with in Chapter 5, which discusses neoplasia, and in the chapters that describe the pathology of individual organs.

Metals

Metals are an important group of environmental chemicals that have caused disease in humans from ancient times to the present. Although lead and mercury were known for centuries to cause disease, the industrial revolution was accompanied by a proliferation of occupational exposures to these and other toxic metals. In our own time, attention has increasingly turned to the ominous threat of the pollution of our environment by toxic metals.

Lead

Lead poisoning in the United States is mainly a pediatric problem related to pica, the habit of chewing on cribs, toys, furniture, and woodwork, and the eating of painted plaster and fallen paint flakes. Most dwellings built before 1940 were decorated with paint that contained lead, and children living in dilapidated, older residences that are heavily coated with flaking paint comprise the major group at risk for lead poisoning. In adults occupational exposure to lead occurs primarily among those engaged in the smelting of lead, a process that releases metal fumes and deposits lead oxide dust in the industrial environment. Lead oxide is a constituent of battery grids, and an occupational exposure to lead is a potential hazard in the manufacture and recycling of automobile batteries. Accidental poisonings occasionally occur from the use of pottery that has been improperly fired with a lead glaze, the renovation of an old residence heavily coated with lead paint, the consumption of "moonshine" whiskey made in lead stills, or the "sniffing" of lead-containing gasoline. It is still unresolved whether lead-containing automobile exhaust fumes contribute to clinically significant total body lead burdens, despite the clear lowering of mean blood levels in the United States since the introduction of unleaded gasoline.

Lead is absorbed either through the lungs or the gastrointestinal tract. Once in the blood, it rapidly equilibrates with the plasma and red cells. A portion of blood lead remains freely diffusible and enters either of two types of tissues. Bones, teeth, nails, and hair represent a tightly bound pool of lead that is not generally regarded as harmful. By contrast, the amount of lead in the brain, liver, kidneys and bone marrow is directly related to its toxic effects. With chronic exposure, 90% of the total body lead burden is in the bones. During metaphyseal bone formation in children, lead and calcium are deposited to produce the increased bone densities ("lead lines") seen radiographically at the metaphysis, thereby providing a simple method of detecting increased body stores of lead in children. Lead is excreted by the kidneys.

Lead toxicity is manifested in the dysfunction of three important organ systems: the nervous system, the kidneys, and the hematopoietic system (Fig. 8-19). **The central nervous system is the target of lead toxicity in children; adults usually present with manifestations of peripheral neuropathy.** Children with lead encephalopathy are typically irritable and ataxic. They may convulse or display altered states of consciousness, from drowsiness to frank coma. Children with blood lead levels above 80 μg Pb/ml but with concentrations lower than those in children with frank encephalopathy (120 μg Pb/ml), exhibit mild central nervous system symptoms such as clumsiness, irritability, and hyperactivity. In **lead encephalopathy,** the brain is edematous and displays flattened gyri and compressed ventricles. There may be herniation of the uncus and cerebellar tonsils. Microscopically, congestion, petechial hemorrhages, and foci of neuronal necrosis are seen. A diffuse astrocytic proliferation in both the gray and white matter may accompany these changes. Vascular lesions in the brain are particularly prominent, with dilatation and proliferation of capillaries. The most common manifestation of lead neurotoxicity in the adult is a **peripheral motor neuropathy,** typically affecting the radial and peroneal nerves and resulting in **wrist** and **foot drop,** respectively. Lead-induced neuropathy is probably also the basis of the paroxysms of gastrointestinal pain known as *lead colic.*

Lead intoxication also produces an **anemia** by disrupting heme synthesis in bone marrow erythroblasts through inhibition of delta-aminolevulinic acid dehyratase, the second enzyme in the de novo synthesis of heme, and through inhibition of ferrochelatase, the enzyme that catalyzes the incorporation of ferrous iron into the porphyrin ring. The resulting inability to produce heme adequately is expressed as a

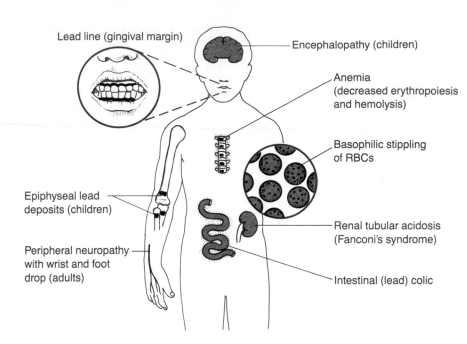

Lead line (gingival margin)

Encephalopathy (children)

Anemia (decreased erythropoiesis and hemolysis)

Basophilic stippling of RBCs

Epiphyseal lead deposits (children)

Peripheral neuropathy with wrist and foot drop (adults)

Renal tubular acidosis (Fanconi's syndrome)

Intestinal (lead) colic

Figure 8-19.   Complications of lead intoxication.

microcytic and hypochromic anemia resembling that seen in iron deficiency, where heme synthesis is also impaired. The anemia of lead intoxication is also characterized by prominent **basophilic stippling of the erythrocytes,** related to the clustering of ribosomes. The life span of the red blood cells is decreased; thus, the anemia of lead intoxication is due to both ineffective hematopoiesis and accelerated turnover.

Lead is toxic to the proximal tubular cells of the kidney. The resulting dysfunction is characterized by aminoaciduria, glycosuria and hyperphosphaturia (Fanconi's syndrome). Such functional alterations are accompanied by the formation of inclusion bodies in the nuclei of the proximal tubular cells. These inclusions are characteristic of **lead nephropathy** and are composed of a lead–protein complex containing more than 100 times as much lead as in the whole kidney.

Lead poisoning is treated with chelating agents such as calcium EDTA, either alone or in combination with dimercaptopropanol (BAL). Both the hematologic and renal manifestations of lead intoxication are usually reversible; the alterations in the central nervous system are generally irreversible.

Mercury

Mercury has been used since prehistoric times and has been known to be an occupation-related hazard at least since the Middle Ages. As the use of mercury has changed, so have the populations at risk. At first, mercurialism was mainly a disease of mercury miners. In the 16th and 17th centuries, mercury poison-

ing was an occupational disease among gilders of gold, silver, or copper, who used mercury in the process of preparing a surface to be decorated. Mercury was subsequently introduced into the manufacture of fur felt, and mercurialism became an occupational hazard of the hatting industry. The neurologic syndrome of tremor ("hatter's shakes") and mental symptoms ("mad as a hatter") was well known in the 19th century.

While mercury poisoning is still seen in some occupations, there has been increasing concern over the potential health hazards brought about by the contamination of many ecosystems following several well-known outbreaks of methylmercury poisoning. The most widely publicized episodes occurred in Japan, first in Minamata Bay in the 1950s and then in Niigata. In both cases local inhabitants developed severe, chronic organic mercury intoxication from the consumption of fish contaminated with mercury that had been discharged into the environment in the effluents from a fertilizer and a plastics factory. To date over a thousand cases of methylmercury poisoning have been reported from Japan. In the early 1970s, there was a more extensive outbreak of mercury poisoning in Iraq resulting from the consumption of bread made from cereal grains that had been treated with organic mercury fungicides. Six thousand people were affected, and 500 died.

In the last two decades it has become ominously clear that mercury released into the environment may be bioconcentrated and enter our food chain. Bacteria in the bottoms of bays and oceans can convert mercury compounds released from industrial wastes into highly neurotoxic organomercurials. These compounds are then transferred up the food chain and are eventually concentrated in the large carnivorous fish that make up a large part of the diet in many countries.

While inorganic mercury is not efficiently absorbed in the gastrointestinal tract, organic mercurial compounds are readily absorbed because of their lipid solubility. Both inorganic and organic mercury are preferentially concentrated in the kidney, and methylmercury also distributes to the brain. **Although the kidney is the principal target of the toxicity of inorganic mercury, the brain is damaged by organic mercurials.**

At one time mercuric chloride was widely used as an antiseptic, and acute mercuric chloride poisoning was much more common; the compound was ingested by accident or for suicidal purposes. Under such circumstances, **proximal tubular necrosis** was accompanied by oliguric renal failure. Mercurial diuretics were also widely prescribed in the past, and a chronic mercury nephrotoxicity was a not uncommon complication of their chronic use. Today, chronic mercurial nephrotoxicity is almost always a consequence of a chronic industrial exposure. Proteinuria is common with chronic mercurial nephrotoxicity, and there may be a nephrotic syndrome with more severe intoxication. Pathologically, there is a membranous glomerulonephritis with subepithelial electron-dense deposits, suggesting immune complex deposition.

Clinically the neurotoxicity of mercury, now known as **Minamata disease,** is manifested as a constriction of visual fields, paresthesias, ataxia, dysarthria, and hearing loss. Pathologically, there is cerebral and cerebellar atrophy. Microscopically the cerebellum exhibits atrophy of the granular layer, without loss of Purkinje cells, and spongy softenings in the visual cortex and other cortical regions.

Arsenic

The toxic properties of arsenic have been known for centuries. Arsenic-containing compounds are toxic to a broad spectrum of living systems and, therefore, have been widely used as insecticides, weed killers and wood preservatives. In the past the medicinal uses of arsenic ranged from the treatment of a variety of cancers to its use as a "tonic." In the United States the use of arsenicals in human medicine has declined, although they remain in common use in veterinary medicine and in agriculture. Arsenic compounds contaminate the soil and drinking water as a result of coal burning and the use of arsenical pesticides.

As with mercury, there is evidence for the bioaccumulation of arsenic along the food chain.

Acute arsenic poisoning is almost always the result of accidental or homicidal ingestion. Death is due to **central nervous system toxicity.** Chronic arsenic intoxication is characterized initially by such nonspecific symptoms as malaise and fatigue. Eventually gastrointestinal disturbances develop, along with changes in the skin and a peripheral neuropathy. The latter is characterized by paresthesias, motor palsies, and painful neuritis. Industrial and agricultural exposure to arsenic has been implicated, on epidemiologic grounds, in the etiology of **cancers of the skin and respiratory tract** in exposed populations. Arsenic in the drinking water has also been related to local increases in the incidence of skin cancer.

Cadmium

Cadmium is used in the manufacture of alloys, in the manufacture of alkali storage batteries, in electroplating of other metals (such as automobile parts and musical instruments), and as a pigment. Fumes of cadmium oxide are released in the course of welding steel parts previously plated with a cadmium anticorrosive.

Acute cadmium inhalation irritates the respiratory tract, with pulmonary edema the most dangerous result. The lungs and the kidneys are the principal target organs of chronic cadmium intoxication. Emphysema has been the major finding in the fatal cases of cadmium pneumonitis that have been studied. Proteinuria, which reflects tubular rather than glomerular damage, has been the most consistent finding in cadmium workers with renal damage.

Nickel

Nickel is a widely used metal in electronics, coins, steel alloys, batteries, and food processing. Dermatitis ("nickel itch"), the most frequent effect of exposure to nickel, may occur from direct contact with metals containing nickel, such as coins and costume jewelry. The dermatitis is a sensitization reaction; the body reacts to nickel-conjugated proteins formed following the penetration of the epidermis by nickel ions. Exposure to nickel, as to arsenic, increases the risk of development of specific types of cancer. Epidemiologic studies have demonstrated that workers who were occupationally exposed to nickel compounds have an increased incidence of **lung cancer** and **cancer of the nasal cavities.**

Iron

Iron deficiency anemia is a common disease, particularly in women. Oral iron preparations contain largely ferrous sulfate, the form absorbed by the gastrointestinal mucosa and then converted to the trivalent form. Acute poisoning from the accidental ingestion of ferrous sulfate tablets occurs chiefly in children, particularly those between the ages of 12 and 24 months. As little as 1 g to 2 g of ferrous sulfate may be lethal, but most fatal cases follow ingestion of 3 g to 10 g. Hemorrhagic gastritis and acute liver necrosis have been the most prominent findings at autopsy.

A chronic, excessive dietary intake of iron does not lead to abnormal iron accumulation in the body, except in the Bantus of South Africa, among whom it is common. These people have a high iron content in their diet. Although some of it is derived from iron cooking pots, the major source is the iron drums used for the preparation of fermented alcoholic beverages. The acidic pH of these brews readily solubilizes the iron, and their low alcohol content allows large volumes to be consumed. Whether or not this high dietary iron intake is solely responsible for the iron overload in these people is still debated. In any case, a large proportion of the excess iron is in the liver, and there is a correlation between the degree of siderosis and the presence of cirrhosis. There is also a high incidence of diabetes and heart disease in this "Bantu siderosis."

Miscellaneous Metals

In the 1960s an epidemic of an unusual cardiomyopathy, clinically characterized by fulminant congestive heart failure, appeared in drinkers of a particular brand of beer, first in the Canadian province of Quebec and subsequently in the United States and Europe. The heart disease was traced to an excessive intake of cobalt, which had been added to the beer to enhance foaming qualities. When the cobalt was removed from the beer, no further cases of heart disease were reported.

In 1972 a new syndrome, called "dialysis encephalopathy," was first reported in patients with uremia undergoing chronic renal dialysis. The subsequent finding of high concentrations of aluminum in the gray matter of the brains of patients who died led to the suggestion that the **encephalopathy** resulted from **aluminum intoxication.** Epidemiologic studies implicated the aluminum in the tap water used to prepare the dialysates, and the disease could be eliminated by removing aluminum from the water. Aluminum intoxication with encephalopathy and osteomalacia can occur in patients (generally children) with uremia who are not dialyzed, but who are given oral aluminum-containing phosphate-binding gels.

Physical Agents

Man is essentially a tropical animal who evolved at sea level in a warm climate with modest temperature fluctuations. Lacking natural thermal protection (fur or feathers) and the capacity to withstand significant ambient pressure changes, his body structure and physiology is adapted to this environment. However, unlike other fauna, man has succeeded in surviving in areas of habitation that are remarkably diverse, including arctic, alpine, and desert locations. These areas are inhospitable to most plants and animals, and natural selection has provided limited living companions in these zones. Man has outwitted slow, adapative evolutionary change by providing his own portable microenvironment for hostile surroundings. He fashions clothes instead of growing fur, and devises living quarters to maintain a reasonable temperature and shelter from the elements. The "prime" primate also has to provide for his nutritional base, and for the storage of food over long periods during long winters and drought. Initially, our ancestors were random feeders, depending on forage to find edibles with which to sustain their nutrition. From this beginning there developed several different societal types, primarily the food-gatherer and the hunter–gatherer. The geographical spread and growth in numbers of the human species followed, in part, the availability of food. As a direct result, historical diseases from which man suffered reflected exposures to areas containing diverse pathogens. In addition, many interactions with other members of his own species added physical and chemical threats to his existence. Man's capacity to eliminate members of his own species, with or without "purpose," is remarkable.

The recent homogenization of mankind as a result of the ease of travel and intermarriage has blurred many of the distinctions of genetic predisposition and geographic disease. The newer emphases in health research are related to societal development and activity (especially industrialism), and to the forces of nature.

Man's tolerance for or adaptation to a cold environment is particularly limited, as is his ability to adapt to pressure changes. Some means of regulating the thermal environment—for instance, clothing, shelter, and fire—are required to permit survival for long periods at temperatures much below 20°C (68°F). With this adaptation came the problems of smoke inhalation, burns, and insulation dusts (asbestos currently is considered the prime hazard in the latter category). Additionally, man developed at or near sea level, and is best adapted to an atmosphere with a pressure of 760 torr and containing roughly 20% oxygen. Reduction of the partial pressure of oxygen at high altitudes (over 3,000 meters) or increased atmospheric pressure (as in sea diving) produces disease.

Thermal-Regulatory Dysfunction

Body temperature is regulated by the thermal regulatory center of the hypothalamus, which modifies heat loss from the body, and by heat production, primarily from muscular activity. The hypothalamic center is sensitive to thermal, neural, and humoral stimulation. There is also evidence that it responds to changes in perfusing blood temperature of as little as half a degree Celsius. A lowering of skin temperature below 32.8°C causes a neural discharge of this center. A disturbance of thermal regulation characterized by temperature elevation (fever) is produced by a short polypeptide, interleukin-1, which is released from macrophages. There is also a diurnal variation in body temperature of about half a degree Celsius. Although this natural variation seems to be part of the biologic clock system, there is no good explanation for this temperature fluctuation.

Body heat is produced as a result of cellular metabolic activity and muscular work. It has been estimated that the skeletal muscle and skin contribute as much as 50% to overall heat production. Cold stress produces an increase in heat production of 50% to 100% by increasing muscle tone, a modification not associated with significant physical movement. Increased heat production beyond this level requires actual muscular contraction, often in the form of shivering, which can further increase the heat yield considerably.

Heat loss accounts for 50% of the heat produced; the remainder of the heat energy provides for the 37° ± 1°C body temperature. In large part, heat loss is regulated by the volume of blood that perfuses the superficial vascular arcades in the skin. Two major factors are involved in the dermal regulatory system: blood flow to the skin, and the use of that thermal energy to warm the portion of the skin surface that is wet with perspiration. Dilatation of these arcades to bring the blood nearer the skin surface facilitates the transfer of the heat, a process that underlies the flushed appearance during strenuous exercise or hot weather. The means for heat dissipation from the body are conduction, convection, and radiation of thermal energy, as well as the evaporation of sensible

and insensible perspiration from the surface of the skin. Under basal conditions, roughly 5% of the cardiac output goes to the skin, but when vasodilatation is called upon to increase heat loss this value may reach roughly half of the normal cardiac output. In the reverse process, environmental cold leads to vasoconstriction and a reduction in blood flow to the skin to as little as 30 ml/min, an effect seen as blanching.

Although the skin surface is the major avenue of heat loss, smaller quantities of heat energy are lost through the warming of inspired air and through sweating. The skin has abundant sweat glands whose orifices deposit perspiration on the surface. The evaporation of this fluid contributes to the loss of heat energy by extracting the heat of vaporization. At rest a person normally loses about a liter of insensible perspiration a day. During strenuous physical activity or in a hot environment, the production of sweat serves as an important additional source of cooling.

The dermis is also provided with a fatty layer that serves as an effective insulator—so effective, that aquatic mammals, which have a thick fatty layer, can flourish in waters that would literally freeze a human. Even man appears to use body fat as an adaptive device for cold climates. People living near and above the arctic circle frequently have thicker dermal fat layers than their southern counterparts.

Hypothermia

Hypothermia—a decrease in body temperature below 35°C—can result in systemic or focal injury, the latter exemplified by **trenchfoot** or **immersion foot.** In localized hypothermia of these types, actual tissue freezing does not occur. **Frostbite,** by contrast, involves the crystallization of tissue water. It should not be forgotten that the hospitalized patient, especially if sedated, is often placed in a thermal environment that is cooler than optimal and that can exert a stressful effect. Heat loss during a surgical procedure can be remarkable, and the administration of muscle relaxants further compromises the ability to generate heat.

Generalized Hypothermia
Most human studies of hypothermia have been based on observation of the effects of immersion in cold water. Interest in this area was stimulated in large part by the loss of soldiers, from time immemorial to our contemporary wars (the estimated life expectancy of fliers downed in the North Sea during World War

II was 5 minutes). Most data in humans were obtained from experiments carried out in German concentration camps in World War II. Unclothed, nonmedicated, partially starved prisoners were placed in vats of cold water, and a number of parameters recorded. The use of data obtained from these barbarous experiments is controversial. We believe that recording this information for the benefit of mankind serves as a memorial to the victims of the Third Reich.

Acute immersion at 4° to 10°C results in immediate increases in both ventilatory rate and respiratory tidal volume. The initial "gasp" response makes possible the aspiration of water, with resulting laryngospasm, asphyxia, and sudden death. The increased respiratory rate and depth of respiration result in decreased arterial carbon dioxide concentration and a secondary constriction of the cerebral vasculature. The reduction in central blood flow, coupled with the decreased core body temperature and lower temperature of the blood perfusing the brain, results in mental confusion. Muscle tetany makes swimming impossible. Furthermore, an increased vagal discharge leads to premature ventricular contractions, ventricular arrythymias, and even fibrillation.

In an attempt to increase heat production, the immersed body immediately responds by increasing muscle activity and oxygen consumption. However, there are limits to the sources of energy available for sustained warming. Within a half hour, heat loss exceeds heat production because of the combination of high direct conduction of heat from the whole skin surface and the altered muscle tone caused by decreased arterial carbon dioxide and exhaustion, and core temperature begins to fall. Peripheral vasoconstriction is another response to conserve heat. In addition, there is an increased sympathetic neural discharge, resulting in increased heart and basal metabolic rates and shivering. When the core temperature approaches 35°C, this activity may be three to six times above normal. Below this temperature a decline in respiratory rate, heart rate, and blood pressure ensues because of the decline in functional reserve.

With prolonged cooling, a "cold-induced" diuresis results in an increased blood viscosity. As a result, blood flow decreases and oxygen-hemoglobin association is less effective. Cardiac stroke volume decreases and peripheral vascular resistance increases as a direct result of both blood "sludging" and loss of plasma. The most important factor in causing death is cardiac arrhythmia or sudden arrest. These observations have been confirmed and extended in the last several decades, largely because the need to induce hypothermia in patients undergoing open-heart surgery. In fact, with careful pharmacologic control, prolonged periods of decreased body temperature can be achieved with no residual harm.

During prolonged hypothermia—for example, after an accident to a mountain climber—several of the consequences of decreased body temperature are related to altered cerebrovascular function. When the body core temperature reaches 32°C the individual becomes lethargic, apathetic, and withdrawn. A characteristic response is inappropriate behavior, including disrobing, even when cold. A further decline in temperature increases the lethargy to intermittent "stupor," and eventually coma. A core temperature below 28°C results in a weak pulse, feeble respiration, and unresponsive coma.

Although there are no specific morphologic changes in those who have succumbed to hypothermia, the skin exhibits red and purple discolorations, swelling of the ears and hands, and irregular vasoconstriction and vasodilatation. Areas of myocytolysis are seen within the heart. The lung may display pulmonary edema and intra-alveolar, intrabronchial, and interstitial hemorrhage.

Focal Thermal Alterations

As discussed previously, local reduction in tissue temperature, particularly in the skin, is associated with local vasoconstriction. Tissue water crystallizes if blood circulation is insufficient to counter persistent thermal loss. When freezing occurs slowly, ice crystals form within tissue cells and in the interstitial space. Concomitantly, electrolyte-rich gels are excluded. Injury to the cellular organelles reflects the drastic changes in ionic concentrations in the excluded volume. Denaturation of macromolecules follows, as well as physical disruption of cellular membranes by the ice. When freezing is rapid, a gel-like structure forms within the cell that lacks the crystalloids of water. This water-solid reduces the extent of mechanical and chemical injury. The most significant cellular damage apparently occurs on thawing, when mechanical disruption of membrane structures occurs. This may be the result of transformation of gel to crystal. The most biologically significant cell injury appears in the endothelial lining of the capillaries and venules, an effect that alters small vessel permeability, thereby initiating extravasation of plasma, formation of localized edema and blisters, and an inflammatory reaction. **Immersion foot (trenchfoot)** is caused by a prolonged reduction in tissue temperature to a point not low enough to freeze tissue. This cooling causes cellular disruption and vascular changes that resemble those observed during the healing phase of local tissue freezing. The target, again, seems to be the endothelial cell. Local thrombosis and changes caused by altered permeability are prominent. Vascular occlusion often leads to gangrene.

Hyperthermia

Tissue responses to hyperthermia are similar in some respects to those caused by freezing injuries. In both instances, injury to the vascular endothelium results in altered vascular permeability, edema, and blisters. The degree of injury is dependent on both the extent of temperature elevation and the rapidity with which it is reached. Clearly, increased temperature of any living system increases its metabolic rate. However, above a certain thermal limit, denaturation of enzymes and precipitation of other proteins occur. In addition, "melting" of the lipid bilayers of cell membranes takes place.

Systemic Hyperthermia

Elevation of body core temperature occurs because of increased heat production, decreased elimination of heat from the body (reflecting an aberrant response of the thermoregulatory center), or a disturbance of the thermal regulatory center itself. It can also occur because heat is being conducted into the body faster than the system can clear the additional "thermal load." During infectious processes and inflammatory responses, a circulating factor derived from macrophages apparently resets the body's "thermostat" to permit a higher body core temperature level. This small polypeptide, interleukin-1, may exert a direct effect or may have a prostaglandin intermediate. However, it may not be the sole thermal factor.

There is a finite level to which core temperature can rise, above which survival of the individual is no longer possible. A blood temperature higher than 42.5°C leads to profound functional disturbances, including general vasodilatation, inefficient cardiac function, and altered respiration. Isolated heart-lung preparations fail at about the same temperature, suggesting an inherent temperature limitation in the cardiovascular system and perhaps in the myocardial cells themselves. **In general, systemic temperature elevations above 41° to 42°C are not compatible with life.**

Systemic temperature elevations associated with infections are commonly designated "fever." There are few, if any, defined pathologic changes that are associated with fever alone. Physical findings include increased heart and respiratory rates, peripheral vasodilatation, and diaphoresis, all recognized mechanisms for thermoregulation. The central nervous system responds with irritability, restlessness, and, particularly in children, convulsions. The temperature at which convulsions occur differs for each individual, and may change during life. Nocturnal temperature elevations with "night sweats" are a feature of pulmonary granulomatous infection (especially tuberculosis) and are also seen in lymphoproliferative diseases. Prolonged temperature elevation can produce wasting, principally because of an increased metabolic rate. A peculiar thermal alteration that occurs during surgery in susceptible persons is designated **malignant hyperthermia.** The cause of this prolonged temperature elevation (over 40°C) is not known, but it may be a hypersensitivity response to anesthetic agents.

Localized Hyperthermia

Cutaneous burns are the most frequent form of localized hyperthermia. Both the elevated temperature and the rate of temperature change are important in determining the pattern of the tissue response. A temperature of 70°C or higher for several seconds causes necrosis of the entire dermal epithelium, whereas a temperature of 50°C may be sustained for 10 minutes or more without killing the cells.

Cutaneous burns have been separated into three categories of severity: first-, second- and third- degree burns (Fig. 8-20). A more contemporary classification refers to full thickness (third-degree) and partial thickness (first- and second-degree) burns. First-degree burns, such as a mild sunburn, are recognized by congestion and pain, but are not associated with necrosis. Mild endothelial injury produces vasodilatation, increased vascular permeability, and slight edema. Burns that cause necrosis of the epithelium but spare the dermis are termed second-degree burns. Clinically, these are recognized by blisters, in which the epithelium is separated from the dermis. Third-degree burns char both the epithelium and the underlying dermis. Histologically, the epidermis and the dermis are carbonized and the cellular structure is lost. The extent of anatomical change is related to the intensity of the thermal exposure and the rapidity of dissipation of heat energy. Flash burns resulting from atomic bomb explosions are associated with carbonization of the epithelial fragments, but show little evidence of deep thermal injury.

One of the most serious systemic disturbances caused by cutaneous burns arises from the fact that the denuded skin surfaces "weep" plasma. People with third-degree burns can lose about 0.3 ml body water per square centimeter of burned area a day. The resulting hemoconcentration and poor vascular

FIRST DEGREE

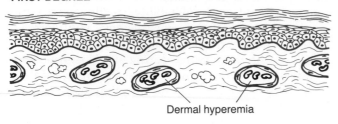

Dermal hyperemia

SECOND DEGREE

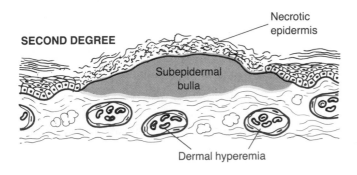

Necrotic epidermis

Subepidermal bulla

Dermal hyperemia

THIRD DEGREE

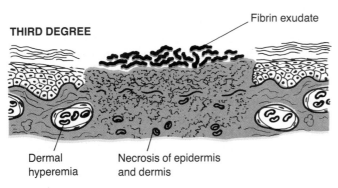

Fibrin exudate

Dermal hyperemia

Necrosis of epidermis and dermis

Figure 8-20. The pathology of cutaneous burns. A first-degree skin burn exhibits only dilatation of the dermal blood vessels. In a second-degree burn there is necrosis of the epidermis, and subepidermal edema collects under the necrotic epidermis to form a bulla. In a third-degree burn, both the epidermis and dermis are necrotic.

perfusion of the skin and other viscera complicate the recovery of these individuals.

The healing of cutaneous burns is related to the extent of the tissue destruction. First-degree burns, by definition, display little if any cell loss, and healing requires only repair or replacement of the injured endothelial cells. Second-degree burns also heal without a scar because the basal cells of the epidermis are not destroyed and serve as a source of regenerating cells for the epithelium. Third-degree burns, in

which there is destruction of the entire thickness of the epidermis, pose a separate set of problems. If the destruction spares the skin appendages, reepithelialization can arise from these foci. Initially, islands of proliferation at the orifices of these glands grow and coalesce to cover the surface. Saprophytic infection of the charred tissue is common, and poses another difficulty for healing. Deeper burns that destroy the skin appendages require new epidermis to be grafted to the debrided area to establish a functional covering. Burned skin that is not replaced by a graft heals with the formation of a dense scar. Since this connective tissue lacks the elasticity of normal skin, **contractures** which limit motion may be the eventual result.

Electrical Burns

Electrical injury produces damage through two modalities: first, through an electrical dysfunction of the cardiovascular conduction system and the nervous system, and second, through the conversion of electrical energy to heat energy when the current encounters the resistance of the tissues. **Because electrical energy has the potential to disrupt the electrical system within the heart, it frequently causes death through ventricular fibrillation.** The amount of current necessary to produce such a disruption depends in part on its pathway through the body and its ease in penetrating the skin. Someone who inadvertently touches a 120-volt line in a living room may suffer burns on the hand because of the electrical resistance of the skin that contacts the wire. The same person inadvertently touching the same line in a bathtub may have no cutaneous manifestations but be killed by disordered electrical activity in the heart. In the latter instance, the wet skin provides a low-resistance entry for the current, thereby permitting greater current flow to the entire body.

Electrical burns of the skin reflect the voltage, the area of electrical conductance, and the duration of current flow (Fig. 8-21). Very high voltage current chars the tissue and produces a third-degree burn. On the other hand, broad, moist surfaces exposed to the same flow exhibit less severe change. With very high voltage currents the force may be almost "explosive," in which case vaporization of tissue water produces extensive damage.

Altitude-Related Illnesses

The competition between man and other animals for food, the nature of the interactions in human society, and perhaps the lure of adventure itself causes subpopulations to seek out and live at different altitudes. Adaptive physiological responses, as well as disease,

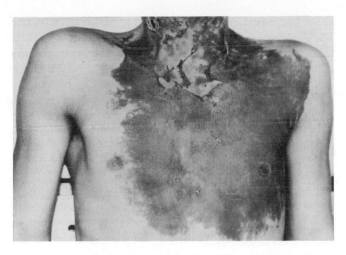

Figure 8-21. Electrical burns of the skin. The body of a young man killed by contact with a high voltage electrical line shows severe burns over the neck and chest.

are associated with both living and travel at high altitudes. From a physiological standpoint, altitudes are separated into three categories: below 2500 meters, 2500 to 4000 meters, and above 4000 meters. Altitudes of 2500 to 4000 meters are generally accessible in the United States, but altitude-related illness is rare under 2500 meters. Very high altitudes (above 4500 meters) are principally the domain of sportsmen. High altitude illness is rare, in large part, because of the acclimation of mountain climbers before extreme altitudes are achieved. However, there is an altitude limit beyond which human life cannot be sustained for prolonged periods. Communities in the Andes succeed at 4000 to 4300 meters. The indigenous people adapt to the decreased pressure and availability of oxygen by developing elevated hematocrits and large "barrel" chests with increased lung volume. Even those who live in this zone do not survive at elevations above 5500 to 6000 meters. Prolonged stays at this altitude result in weight loss, difficulty in sleeping, and lethargy, perhaps because of the redirection of cellular energy simply for survival. For example, of the oxygen obtained per inhalation at 6000 meters, 75% to 90% is utilized for the effort of inspiration alone.

The modifications induced by high altitude are related to a decreased atmospheric pressure and, therefore, to decreased oxygen availability. It has been suggested that the decreased oxygen tension and the limited ability of the lungs to extract oxygen at lower pressures produce the hypoxia that is probably the most important factor in causing high-altitude illness. The narrow reserve is illustrated by the observation that physical activity at these elevations leads to a decrease in the partial pressure of arterial oxygen, whereas comparable physical activity at sea level does not change oxygen saturation. At sea level, cardiac output limits exercise, whereas at high altitudes the diffusing capacity of the lung for oxygen seems to be the determinant. Acclimation to chronic hypoxia at high altitudes results in a reduced ventilatory drive. Acclimated individuals have an increased number of capillaries per unit of brain, muscle, and myocardium; increases in the amount of myoglobin within tissues; increased mitochondria per cell; and an increased hematocrit. An increase in erythrocyte levels of 2'3' diphosphoglycerate, which enhances oxygen delivery to tissues, occurs within hours, but the induction of polycythemia requires months. Some of the minor effects of high altitude are systemic edema, retinal hemorrhages, and flatus expulsion. The more serious nonfatal diseases are acute and chronic mountain sickness and high-altitude deterioration. Fatal disease can develop in the form of high-altitude pulmonary edema and high-altitude encephalopathy.

High-Altitude Systemic Edema

High-altitude systemic edema results from an asymptomatic modification of vascular permeability, particularly in the hands, face, and feet and most often occurs at elevations over 3000 meters. It is reflected only in weight gain; upon return to lower altitude, a diuresis causes the edema to disappear. This disorder is twice as common in women as in men. The cause of this peculiar condition is not known; an endothelial response to hypoxia provides only a partial explanation.

High-Altitude Retinal Hemorrhage

A critical analysis by funduscopic examination revealed that 30% to 60% of those sleeping above 5000 meters had retinal hemorrhage. The initial effect includes retinal vascular engorgement and tortuousness. Optic disc hyperemia is also noted, and multiple flame-shaped hemorrhages subsequently occur. These changes are reversible.

High-Altitude Flatus

Changes in external pressure and the production of intestinal gas provide for the expansion of the luminal contents of the intestine and increased flatus at altitudes above 3500 meters. No specific physical disease has been associated with these changes, although social problems have been encountered.

Acute Mountain Sickness

Acute mountain sickness is rare below 2500 meters, but is present to some degree in nearly everyone at 3000 to 3600 meters. The initial presentation includes headache, lassitude, anorexia, weakness, and difficulty in sleeping. The pathophysiological mechanism that underlies this disease is in part related to hypoxia and a shift in plasma fluid to the interstitial space. Adaptation through a modification of pulmonary function (increased respiratory rate) causes some amelioration of the disease. Descent to lower altitudes is certainly indicated. Chronic or subacute exacerbation of this disease also occurs, frequently at lower altitudes, and the symptoms may be severe. The basis of the disease is not known.

High-Altitude Deterioration

High-altitude deterioration, generally occurring at higher elevations (5500 meters or more), presents as a decrease in physical and mental performance. The combination of chronic hypoxia, inadequate fluid intake, and inadequate nutrition, together with decreased plasma volume and hemoconcentration, are aggravating factors.

High-Altitude Pulmonary Edema and Cerebral Edema

Serious high-altitude problems, including pulmonary edema and cerebral edema, can occur with a rapid ascent to heights over 2500 meters, particularly in susceptible individuals who poorly tolerate sleeping at higher altitudes. Tachycardia, right ventricular overload, and a marked reduction in arterial oxygen pressure, are seen, but there is no change in pH or carbon dioxide retention. A characteristic patchy pulmonary infiltrate is seen radiographically. Pulmonary hypertension due to increased resistance is common in patients with high-altitude pulmonary edema. Hypoxic vasoconstriction and intravascular thrombosis have been proposed as causes of pulmonary hypertension. Eventually, cardiac output is decreased and systemic blood pressure falls. The precapillary arterioles become dilated, increasing capillary bed pressure and inducing interstitial and alveolar edema. Autopsy findings include severe confluent pulmonary edema, proteinaceous alveolar exudates, and hyaline membrane formation. Capillary obstruction by thrombi has been noted. A dilated heart and enlarged pulmonary arteries are commonly found.

High-altitude encephalopathy is characterized by confusion, stupor, and coma. Autopsies have consistently revealed cerebral edema and vascular congestion. A proposed mechanism is severe cerebral hypoxia, with inhibition of the sodium pump and resultant intracellular edema.

Physical Injuries

The effect of mechanical trauma is related to the force transmitted to the tissue, the rate at which the transfer occurs, the surface area to which the force is transferred, and the area of the body that is injured. The disruption of the continuity of the tissue results in a wound. It should be remembered, however, that the transmission of the energy absorbed can produce alterations elsewhere in the body.

Force expended: The amount of energy released is related to the velocity and mass of the object that strikes the person, or to that of the person who collides with a stationary object. In addition to the lateral displacement, many objects that strike people—from bullets to car wheels—have rotational forces. Prolongation of the period of impact dissipates some of the energy, as when a boxer "rolls with a punch."

Transfer area: The area over which transfer of force occurs is particularly important. The intensity—that is, the force exerted per unit area—decreases with the increasing area. A protective helmet does not lessen the force of a blow or projectile, but diffuses it over a larger area.

Body area: The area of the body that is affected by physical trauma plays an important role. The compressibility of the tissue adjacent to the transmitted force in part determines its effect. A blow over a large muscle mass, such as the thigh or upper arm, is often less injurious than a direct blow to a poorly shielded bone, such as the anterior tibia. Furthermore, the distribution of the force is important. Blows over a hollow viscus can rupture the organ because of compression of the fluid or gas it contains; organs nestled beneath the skin, like the liver, can be easily ruptured. An impact directly over the heart can even disturb its electrical systems.

Contusions

A force with sufficient energy may disrupt capillaries and venules within an organ by physical means alone. If this occurs in the skin, a loss of blood into the tissue space occurs. The resultant altered coloration identifies a **contusion,** namely, a localized area of mechanical injury with focal hemorrhage. The change may be so limited that the only histologic change is hemorrhage in tissue spaces outside of the vascular compartment. The presence of a discrete blood pool within the tissue is termed a **hematoma.** Initially the deoxygenated blood renders the area blue to blue-black, as in the classic "black eye." Macrophages ingest the red blood cells and convert the hemoglobin to bilirubin, thus changing the color from blue to yellow. Both mobilization of the pigment by macrophages and further metabolism of bilirubin cause the yellow to fade to yellowish green and then to disappear.

Abrasions

A direct or tangential impact can crush or scrape the epithelial surface of the skin, producing a defect called an **abrasion.** The disruptive force may destroy some of the cells by crushing them, and thus may provide a portal of entry for microorganisms. There may be disruption of the epidermis itself, and there may also be vascular distortion of the cells within the dermis. The impact of the agent and its configuration are frequently seen in these wounds, and are of special interest to the forensic pathologist.

Lacerations

Should the force be greater, and should the tangential impact be stronger, the epithelium can split and tear, resulting in a **laceration.** Lacerations are usually the result of unidirectional displacement, but they may have crushed margins, in which case they are termed abraded lacerations.

Incisions

The deliberate opening of the skin by a cutting instrument, usually the surgeon's scalpel, is an **incision.** Incisions have particularly sharp edges and, importantly, spare no tissue to the depth of the wound. **Deep penetrating wounds** produced by high-velocity projectiles, such as bullets, are often deceptive because the energy of the missile as it passes through the body may be released at sites distant from the entrance itself. Bullets, because they rotate, produce a well-defined and usually round entrance wound. Once the projectile enters the flesh, however, it may fragment, tumble, or actually explode, resulting in a remarkable degree of tissue damage and a large, ragged exit wound. The interested student may refer to the reading list at the end of the chapter for further information in this area of forensic pathology.

Radiation

We can define radiation simply as the emission of energy by one body, its transmission through an intervening medium, and its absorption by another body. By this definition, radiation encompasses the entire electromagnetic spectrum and certain charged particles emitted by radioactive elements. However, since the latter also have wave characteristics, this distinction is to some extent arbitrary. Alpha particles, such as the radiation emitted by phosphorus-32, and the beta particles of elements such as tritium and carbon-14 are of immense use scientifically and diagnostically but pose few hazards for man. High-energy radiation, in the form of gamma or x-rays, is the mediator of most of the biologic effects discussed here.

Radiation can be employed in a benign or malignant manner. On the one hand, medical practice is inconceivable today without the use of diagnostic and therapeutic radioisotopes, clinical radiographs, and radiation therapy. On the other hand, nuclear explosions and accidental exposure to radiation in nuclear power plants have caused injury and death. Here, we focus on the pathologic consequences of radiation exposure.

Radiation is quantitated in a number of ways. The emission of radiant energy from a source is measured in **roentgens,** units that refer to the amount of ionization produced in air. The absorption of radiant energy—biologically, the more important parameter—is measured in terms of the **rad,** the unit that defines the ergs of energy absorbed by a tissue. A newer international unit is the **Gray,** which corresponds to 100 rads. Because low-energy particles produce more biologic damage than gamma or x-rays, the **rem** unit was introduced to describe the biologic effect produced by a rad of high-energy radiation. For the practical purposes of this discussion of radiation-induced pathology, the roentgen, rad, and rem are comparable. The details of radiation biology are the subject of a voluminous literature and the student may refer to this chapter's list of suggested reading.

At the cellular level, radiation essentially has two effects: a somatic effect, associated with acute cell killing, and its induction of genetic damage. Radiation-induced cell death, as discussed in Chapter 1, is attributed to the acute effects of the radiolysis of water. The production of activated oxygen species results in lipid peroxidation, membrane injury, and possibly an interaction with macromolecules of the cell. Genetic damage to the cell, whether caused by direct absorption of energy by DNA (the target theory) or caused indirectly by a reaction of DNA with oxygen radicals, is expressed either as mutation or as reproductive failure. Both mutation and reproductive failure may lead to delayed cell death, and the former is incriminated in the development of radiation-induced neoplasia.

The differential sensitivity of tissues to radiation has been recognized since the beginning of the century. For example, the intestine and the hematopoietic bone marrow are far more vulnerable to radiation than tissues such as bone and brain. These differences should not be construed as a reflection of variable sensitivity to acute cell killing (even though there may be slight differences in the acute, somatic response of cells to radiation based on anti-oxidant and other metabolic defenses). The important consideration is that the vulnerability of a tissue to radiation-induced damage depends on its proliferative rate, which in turn correlates with the natural life span of the constituent cells. Damage to the DNA of a long-lived, nonproliferating cell does not necessarily pose a threat to its function or viability because the reproductive and metabolic functions of the cell are distinct. By contrast, a short-lived, proliferating cell, such as an intestinal crypt cell or a hematopoietic precursor, must be rapidly replaced by division of the stem cells and the committed precursor. When radiation-induced DNA damage precludes mitosis of these cells, the mature elements are no longer replaced and the tissue can no longer function.

Before discussing the structural and functional injury produced by radiation, it is important to distinguish between whole-body irradiation and localized irradiation. Except for unusual circumstances, as in the massive irradiation that precedes bone marrow transplantation, significant levels of whole-body irradiation result only from industrial accidents or from the explosion of nuclear weapons. By contrast, localized irradiation is an inevitable byproduct of any diagnostic radiologic procedure, and it is the intended result of radiotherapy. Acute somatic cell death occurs only with extremely high doses of radiation, well in excess of 1000 rads. It is morphologically indistinguishable from the coagulative necrosis produced by other causes (see Chap. 1). Irreversible damage to the replicative capacity of cells requires far lower doses, possibly as little as 50 rads.

Whole-Body Irradiation

Fortunately, there have been few instances of human disease caused by whole-body irradiation, and most of our information has been derived from studies of Japanese atom bomb casualties. Further information may be forthcoming from study of the survivors of the much smaller sample of people exposed in the accident at the Chernobyl nuclear power plant in the USSR in 1986.

Since by definition the same dose of radiant energy is transmitted to all organs in whole-body irradiation, the development of the different acute radiation syndromes clearly reflects only the dissimilarities in vulnerability of the target tissues (Fig. 8-22). At a dose of approximately 300 rads, a syndrome characterized by **hematopoietic failure** develops within 2 weeks. Since all hematopoietic precursor elements are highly sensitive to radiant energy, a pancytopenia typically characterizes the hematopoietic whole-body irradiation syndrome. Following an initial depletion of circulating lymphocytes, a progressive decrease in formed elements of the blood eventually leads to bleeding, anemia, and infection. The last is often the cause of death. With more intense radiation, in the vicinity of 1000 rads, the principal cause of death is related to the **gastrointestinal system.** While gastrointestinal symptoms characterize the entire dose range of whole-body exposure, at higher levels severe destruction of the entire epithelium of the gastrointestinal tract occurs within 3 days, the time that corresponds to the normal life span of the villous and crypt cells. As a result the fluid homeostasis of the bowel is disrupted, and severe diarrhea and dehydration ensue. Moreover, the epithelial barrier to intestinal bacteria is breached, and bacteria invade and disseminate throughout the body. Shock and septicemia kill the victim.

With exposure to whole-body doses of 2000 rads and greater, central nervous system damage causes death within hours. In most cases, endothelial injury resulting in cerebral edema and loss of the integrity of the blood–brain barrier predominates, but with extreme doses radiation necrosis of neurons can be expected. Convulsions, coma, and death follow.

The effects of whole-body irradiation on the human fetus have been documented in studies of the survivors of the atom bomb explosions in Japan. Pregnant women exposed to doses of 25 rads or greater gave birth to infants with reduced head size, diminished overall growth, and mental retardation.* In studies of the clinical status of children who were exposed to therapeutic doses of radiation in utero, the most likely time for the production of growth retardation and microcephaly was between the third

---

* Intrauterine exposure to radiation at Nagasaki was significantly less teratogenic than at Hiroshima. This disparity has been attributed to a difference in the quality of the radiation in the two cities. The bomb dropped on Hiroshima produced far greater fast-neutron radiation (20% as opposed to 1% of the total energy released), which is lower in energy than comparable doses of gamma rays and, therefore, produces greater biologic damage.

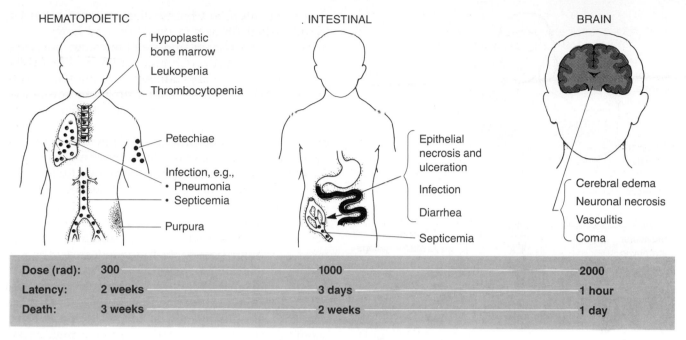

HEMATOPOIETIC

- Hypoplastic bone marrow
- Leukopenia
- Thrombocytopenia

- Petechiae

- Infection, e.g.,
  - Pneumonia
  - Septicemia

- Purpura

INTESTINAL

- Epithelial necrosis and ulceration
- Infection
- Diarrhea
- Septicemia

BRAIN

- Cerebral edema
- Neuronal necrosis
- Vasculitis
- Coma

Dose (rad):	300	1000	2000
Latency:	2 weeks	3 days	1 hour
Death:	3 weeks	2 weeks	1 day

Figure 8-22. Acute radiation syndromes. At a dose of approximately 300 rads of whole body radiation, a syndrome characterized by hematopoietic failure develops within 2 weeks. In the vicinity of 1,000 rads, a gastrointestinal syndrome with a latency of only 3 days is seen. With doses of whole body radiation of 2,000 rads or greater, disease of the central nervous system appears within 1 hour, and death ensues rapidly.

and twentieth week of gestation. Other effects of irradiation in utero include hydrocephaly, microphthalmia, chorioretinitis, blindness, spina bifida, cleft palate, club feet, and genital abnormalities. Data derived from experimental and human studies strongly support the conclusion that major congenital malformations are highly unlikely with doses of less than 20 rads after day 14 of pregnancy. This does not mean that lower doses cannot produce subtle effects, but these have not been documented. **To protect against such a possibility, the established maximum permissible dose to the fetus from exposure of the expectant mother is far below the known teratogenic dose.**

The potential genetic effects of radiation have been the source of considerable public alarm. Again, there is a dearth of evidence, and most of the data on which predictions of human genetic effects are based are derived from experimental data. **After long-term follow-up, even the survivors of Hiroshima and Nagasaki have failed to manifest evidence of genetic damage in the form of either congenital abnormalities or hereditary diseases in subsequent offspring or their descendants.** Animal experiments suggest that the risk of spontaneous mutations per rad is at most only 0.5% to 5% of the risk of spontaneous mutation, estimated to be 10% of live births. In other words, the experimental radiation exposure necessary to double the spontaneous mutation rate is 20 to 200 rads. **Thus, even with the most pessimistic estimates, the risk of genetic damage to future generations from radiation appears inconsequential.**

The finding that rodents exposed to whole-body irradiation have a shortened life span has led to the suggestion that radiation accelerates the aging process. A mortality study of the survivors of the atom bomb explosions in Japan has not disclosed any excess mortality not attributable to neoplasia. Nor is there any evidence of acceleration in disease among the survivors in any part of the age range. **Thus, the effects of ionizing radiation on mortality are specific and focal, and there is no reason to believe that premature aging in humans or radiation-induced carcinogenesis is due to a general acceleration of aging.**

Localized Radiation Injury Associated With Radiotherapy

In the course of radiotherapy for malignant neoplasms, some normal tissue is inevitably included in

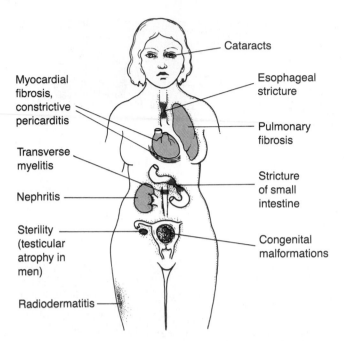

Figure 8-23.   The non-neoplastic complications of radiation exposure.

the radiation field. While almost any organ can be damaged by radiation, the clinically important tissues are the skin, lungs, heart, kidney, bladder, and intestine—organs that are difficult to shield (Fig. 8-23). Localized damage to the bone marrow is clearly of little functional consequence because of the immense reserve capacity of the hematopoietic system.

Persistent damage to radiation-exposed tissue can be attributed to two major factors: compromise of the vascular supply and a fibrotic repair reaction to acute necrosis and chronic ischemia. Radiation-induced tissue injury predominantly affects small arteries and arterioles. The endothelial cells are the most sensitive elements in the blood vessels and acutely exhibit swelling and necrosis. Chronically the walls become thickened by endothelial cell proliferation and subintimal deposition of collagen and other connective tissue elements (Fig. 8-24). Striking vacuolization of intimal cells, the so-called foam cell, is typical. Fragmentation of the internal elastic lamina, loss of smooth muscle cells and scarring in the media, and fibrosis of the adventitia are seen in the small arteries. The fibroblastic repair reaction is nonspecific but may be exaggerated, possibly owing to altered epithelial–mesenchymal interactions consequent on impaired regeneration. Bizarre fibroblasts with large, hyperchromatic nuclei are common and, again, probably reflect radiation-induced DNA damage.

Acute necrosis is represented by such disorders as **radiation pneumonitis, cystitis, dermatitis** and diar-

rhea from **enteritis.** Chronic disease is characterized by **interstitial fibrosis** in the heart and lungs, **strictures** in the esophagus and small intestine, and **constrictive pericarditis.** Chronic **radiation nephritis,** which simulates malignant nephrosclerosis, is primarily a vascular disease characterized by severe hypertension and progressive renal insufficiency.

Since radiotherapy inevitably traverses the skin it often leads to **radiodermatitis.** The initial damage is evidenced by dilatation of blood vessels, recognized as **erythema.** Necrosis of the skin may follow and linger as **indolent ulcers** that do not heal because the epithelium is unable to regenerate. A further consequence of this poor regenerative capacity is the difficulty faced by the surgeon, for whom the impairment of wound healing in irradiated areas poses a serious problem. **Poorly healed** or **dehisced wounds** or **persistent ulcers** often require full-thickness skin grafts. **Chronic radiodermatitis** results from the repair and revascularization of the skin, and is characterized by atrophy, hyperkeratosis, telangiectasia, and hyperpigmentation (Fig. 8-25).

Like other tissues that depend on continuous cell cycling, the **gonads,** both testes and ovaries, are exquisitely radiosensitive. The acute inhibition of mitosis in the testis results in necrosis of the germinal stem cells, the spermatogonia. The combination of radiation-induced vascular injury and direct damage to the germ cells leads to progressive atrophy of the seminiferous tubules, peritubular fibrosis, and loss of reproductive function. However, since the interstitial and Sertoli cells do not cycle rapidly, they are more resistant than the germ cells and so persist, thereby preserving the normal hormonal status. Comparable injury is seen in the irradiated ovary; the follicles become atretic, and the organ eventually becomes fibrous and atrophic. Should the eye lie in the path of the radiation beam, lenticular opacities—that is, **cataracts**— may result. The spinal cord is unavoidably irradiated during treatment of certain thoracic or abdominal tumors, and the vascular damage in the cord may bring about localized ischemia which can result in a **transverse myelitis** and paraplegia.

Radiation and Cancer

High doses of radiation cause cancer. The evidence is incontrovertible and comes both from animal experiments and from studies of the effects of occupational exposure, radiotherapy for non-neoplastic conditions, the diagnostic use of certain radioisotopes, and the atom bomb explosions (Fig. 8-26). In the early part of this century, scientists and radiologists tested their equipment by placing their hands in the path of the beam. As a result they developed basal and

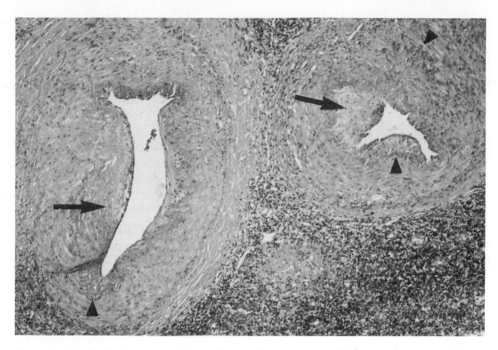

Figure 8-24.   Radiation vasculitis in tissue adjacent to a malignant tumor treated by radiotherapy. Intimal thickening *(arrows)* is conspicuous. Remnants of the original internal elastic lamina *(arrowheads)* are evident.

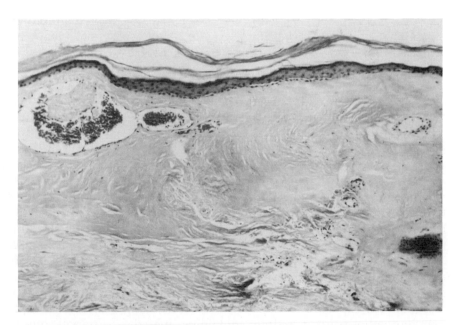

Figure 8-25.   Chronic radiodermatitis. The epidermis is atrophic. The dermis is densely fibrotic and contains dilated superficial blood vessels.

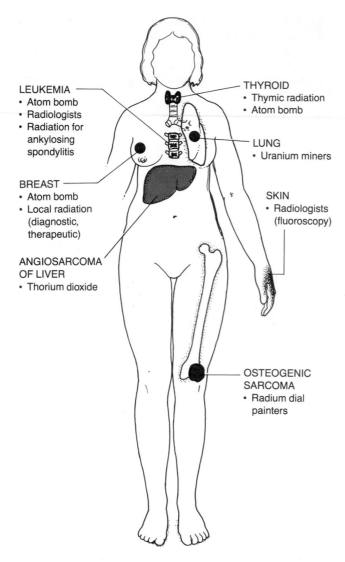

LEUKEMIA
• Atom bomb
• Radiologists
• Radiation for ankylosing spondylitis

BREAST
• Atom bomb
• Local radiation (diagnostic, therapeutic)

ANGIOSARCOMA OF LIVER
• Thorium dioxide

THYROID
• Thymic radiation
• Atom bomb

LUNG
• Uranium miners

SKIN
• Radiologists (fluoroscopy)

OSTEOGENIC SARCOMA
• Radium dial painters

Figure 8-26.   Radiation-induced cancers.

squamous cell carcinomas of the exposed skin. In addition, early instruments were not properly shielded, and the hazards associated with fluoroscopy were not appreciated. The radiologists of that era suffered an unusually high incidence of leukemia, a situation that has disappeared with the use of modern shielding and protective equipment. An unusual occupational exposure to radiation occurred among workers who painted radium-containing material onto watches to create luminous dials. These workers were in the habit of licking their paint brushes, which led to the ingestion of the radioactive element and its subsequent localization in their bones. As a consequence, these workers later experienced a high incidence of cancer of the bone and of the paranasal sinuses. Another example of the result of occupa-

tional exposure to a radioactive element is the high rate of lung cancer in uranium miners who inhaled radioactive dusts. Since most of these workers also smoke, it is difficult to distinguish the independent from the synergistic effects of radiation in the induction of their cancers, but the evidence favors a synergistic effect.

At one time, thymic irradiation of infants for a mysterious ailment known as "status thymico-lymphaticus" was popular. The infants showed no perceptible improvement in their overall health, but as adults they did develop cancer of the thyroid. Another example of iatrogenic cancer resulted in Great Britain from the widespread use of spinal irradiation as a treatment for ankylosing spondylitis. While a beneficial effect on the course of this disease was claimed, the penalty was the later development of aplastic anemia and myelogenous leukemia. Radiation delivered by long-lived radioactive isotopes used for diagnostic purposes was also not without danger. Thorium dioxide (Thorotrast), a material avidly ingested by phagocytic cells, was at one time used for radionuclide imaging. Its persistence in the liver resulted in the development of a number of tumors, particularly angiosarcomas.

The survivors of the atom bomb explosions suffered from a number of cancers. These people exhibited a more than tenfold increase in the incidence of leukemia, which reached its zenith from 5 to 10 years after exposure and subsequently declined to background rates.* Two-thirds were acute leukemia; the remainder were of the chronic myelogenous variety. Chronic lymphocytic leukemia, an uncommon disease in Japan, showed no increase in incidence. The risk of multiple myeloma increased fivefold and there was a small increment in the incidence of lymphoma. The risk of the development of solid tumors, although not as great as that for leukemia, was clearly increased for the breast, lung, thyroid, gastrointestinal tract, and urinary tract. The development of malignant tumors, including leukemia, showed a dose-response relationship.

Low-Level Radiation and Cancer   Few debates have engendered as much heat and as little light as that concerning the potential carcinogenic effect of low levels of radiation. All assumptions are based on extrapolations to zero of the risk of cancer at higher doses, or from epidemiologic studies to which valid exception may be taken. **The key question that needs**

* An increased incidence of leukemia was evident in those exposed to doses as low as 50 rads in Hiroshima, but required more than 100 rads in Nagasaki. As previously suggested, this difference in sensitivity may reflect the greater neutron component of the radiation in Hiroshima.

to be answered is whether there is a threshold dose of radiation below which there is no increase in incidence of cancer, or whether any exposure carries a significant risk.

The "no threshold hypothesis"—that is, the theory that postulates no safe dose—is based on a linear (proportional to dose) projection to zero. However, as is the case with many drugs, there is no *a priori* reason to accept such an assumption; an alternative analysis of the same data utilizes a quadratic (proportional to dose squared) dependence of risk on dose. With this analysis, the curve is steep at higher doses but is appreciably flattened at the lowest ones. A more sophisticated approach is the linear-quadratic analysis, in which the quadratic dependence gives way to a linear dependence at the lowest doses. At low doses the linear-quadratic model is intermediate between the highest level of risk of radiogenic cancer projected by the linear analysis and the lowest risk indicated by the quadratic projection. For instance, based on data from the Nagasaki survivors, the risk of leukemia from a 1-rad dose, expressed as excess cases per million per year, ranges from 2.5 for the linear model to 0.016 for the quadratic model—a 156-fold difference in risk. Comparable differences can be derived from other epidemiologic studies of cancer incidence. Human epidemiologic studies do not provide data precise enough to permit an accurate estimate of cancer risk from low-level radiation, except to suggest that it lies between 0 and some projected upper limit. However, experiments involving the effects of radiation on cells in culture and in other mammals suggest a dose relation that is less than linear for x- and gamma irradiation. Such a conclusion implies that the established permissible exposures to radiation (which are based on a linear relation) are highly conservative and may exaggerate the risks.

A discussion of the effects of low-level radiation must include consideration of naturally occurring background radiation—that is, the radiation derived from cosmic and terrestrial radiation and the inhalation and ingestion of natural and man-made radioactive isotopes. This background radiation is estimated at about 100 millirads per year. Since exposure to this radiation is universal, it is clearly impossible to determine directly whether this level of exposure contributes to the spontaneous incidence of cancer in man. However, using the linear hypothesis to estimate the risk from the low levels of background radiation, it has been estimated that the leukemia rate in 20- to 30-year-old women in the United States that can be attributed to this radiation is between 3 and 4 per million per year. The actual leukemia rate in this group is 18 per million per year; thus, background radiation can only account for about one-fifth. However, other attempts to estimate cancer incidence from the linear hypothesis have yielded conflicting conclusions. For example, a linear extension back from the observed cancer incidence and radiation exposure among uranium miners predicts a cancer rate that is four times higher than the rate actually observed in a population of nonsmokers. Cancer mortality has been recorded in two regions of China that have different levels of background radiation. In the low-background region, people were exposed to 72 millirads per year, while in the high-background region the exposure was almost three times greater. Despite this difference, no difference in cancer mortality existed. Moreover, pilots and cabin crews of commercial airlines, who are exposed to significantly higher doses of background radiation at high altitude, have not manifested any increased cancer incidence. These and other studies suggest that the contribution of background radiation to the occurrence of human cancer may not be as significant as many believe.

The arguments for a risk of radiogenic cancer from low-level radiation (between 1 and 10 rads) has been buttressed by a number of epidemiologic studies. It has been reported that children exposed to radioactive fallout from atmospheric testing of nuclear weapons had a higher incidence of leukemia than similar children not so exposed. However, close inspection of the data reveals that, oddly enough, this apparent increase is explained not by an increased incidence of leukemia relative to the general population, but rather by an unusually low leukemia rate in the controls. Interestingly, the incidence of other types of cancer was decreased in the high-fallout areas by a factor of two compared to immediately adjacent low-fallout areas, and this observed reduction is as significant statistically as the apparent increase in leukemia.

Another epidemiologic study of radiation associated with nuclear bomb tests involved military personnel engaged in exercises during and after the detonation of a nuclear device named "Smokey" in Nevada in 1957. An unusual feature of this study was the availability of film badges that measured the dose of external radiation. After a 20-year follow-up, seven cases of myelocytic leukemia were found, with a mean whole-body dose of 1 rad, compared to 1.8 cases expected from the spontaneous incidence of this disease. If these cases were induced by radiation, the risk can be calculated as 80 times greater than the risk established by all other major studies. Moreover, the unusually long latent period of 11 to 19 years for the occurrence of myelocytic leukemia is also at variance with the experience from the study of atom bomb survivors. Thus, the data from the "Smokey" episode should be interpreted with caution and with the recognition that other unrelated factors may have played a role. Equally compelling arguments can be raised against many other studies of the carcinogenic effect of low-level radiation, and there are also studies that failed to show such an effect. For example, analyses of cancer mortality among British radiologists, x-ray technicians trained during World War II, and women given radiotherapy for cervical cancer did not establish a higher risk of leukemia than the expected spontaneous rate.

In summary, the data currently available from radiation studies of cancer induction in animals, chromosomal damage in human cell cultures, malignant transformation of mammalian cells in vitro, and populations exposed to radiation show that the estimates of risk at low doses derived from a linear extrapolation from risk at high doses exaggerate the risk, perhaps by an order of magnitude. On the other hand, the data do not by any means show that the risk of radiogenic cancer from low-level radiation is zero. **When the data from atomic bomb survivors are subjected to a linear-quadratic analysis, the lifetime risk from 1 rad of whole-body x- or gamma irradiation is 1 excess cancer death per 10,000 persons.**

Microwave and Ultrasound Radiation

Microwaves, produced by ovens, radar, and diathermy, are electromagnetic waves that penetrate tissue but do not produce ionization. Unlike x- and gamma radiation, the absorption of microwave energy produces only heat. Thus, exposure to microwave radiation under ordinary circumstances is highly unlikely to produce any injury. Ultrasound, the vibrational waves in air above the audible range, produces mechanical compression but, again, no ionization. Highly focused and energetic ultrasound devices are used to disrupt tissue in vitro for chemical analysis and to clean various surfaces, including teeth. However, there is no reason to believe that diagnostic ultrasound or accidental exposure to any industrial device results in any measurable damage.

Nutritional Disorders

Obesity

Although obesity is the most common nutritional disorder in the industrialized countries, where it is far more common than all the nutritional deficiencies combined, a satisfactory definition is elusive. There is no single ratio of increased weight to height or body area at which an increased morbidity and mortality can be said to begin. Thus, as in the case of anemia or hypertension, arbitrary standards are employed. **If one defines obesity as beginning at 20% above the mean adiposity, then 20% of middle-aged American men and 40% of middle-aged American women are obese.** Although the prevalence of obesity declines in the elderly, it is possible that this reflects, in part, the increased mortality associated with obesity. Socioeconomic and cultural factors are important because they influence not only the type and amount of food, but the social acceptability of obesity as well. Genetic factors may also play a role in some ethnic and racial groups. For instance, blacks, particularly women, have a considerably higher prevalence of obesity than do whites in the United States. However, since there is a negative correlation, most pronounced in women, between socioeconomic status and obesity, it is not clear whether environmental or genetic factors are more important in this case.

Like the definition itself, the causes of obesity are not well delineated. **It is indisputable that obesity results from a chronic excess of caloric intake relative to the expenditure of energy.** However, the reasons for the inappropriate intake of food are not at all clear. The ability to store energy in the form of fat during plentiful times clearly confers an evolutionary advantage in an environment in which periods of food scarcity may occur. Presumably, evolution has been unable to anticipate the advances in societal organization and food production that have converted this evolutionary advantage into a leading cause of morbidity and mortality.

Although sharp distinctions cannot be made, there are two general types of obesity: that which begins in childhood and is lifelong, and that which begins in the adult. These are discussed in greater detail in Chapter 22, which deals with diabetes.

Lifelong obesity is associated with a larger than normal number of adipocytes, presumably a genetically determined phenomenon. By contrast, the obesity that begins in adult life develops against a background of larger—that is, hypertrophied—adipocytes, the number of which remains the same. These two types of obesity have been referred to as the hyperplastic and hypertrophic types, respectively. Both types reflect excess caloric intake, but they have different patterns of fat deposition. In adult-onset obesity fat is deposited principally on the trunk—that is, the hips and buttocks in women and the abdomen (pot belly) in men. In the type that begins in childhood, weight gain is distributed more peripherally, and is readily measured as an increase in the skin-fold thickness over the triceps muscle or in the subscapular area.

Despite numerous studies, it is not possible to attribute the common varieties of obesity to any specific metabolic or functional disturbance. In experimental animals, lesions of the hypothalamus have produced obesity, and it has been postulated that an "appetite center" has been damaged. This concept is supported by the occurrence of overeating and obesity in patients with tumors that impinge on the hypothalamus. However, it is now known that hypothalamic lesions directly influence lipogenesis and the secretion of insulin, and it is probable that obesity induced by hypothalamic lesions is secondary to these effects. Since the basal metabolic rate decreases progressively with age, it has been suggested that adult-onset obesity may simply reflect the maintenance of the usual food intake despite decreasing need. However, the decline in basal metabolic rate is not large enough to explain obesity. Lean body mass decreases with age, while the proportions of water and fat in the body increase. Thus, the basal metabolic rate per unit of lean body mass may actually not change, although the total caloric requirement seems to decrease. Under these circumstances, it is likely that the usual food intake becomes excessive in relation to the more sedentary life associated with aging in industrialized countries.

Numerous theories of obesity, invoking hormonal changes, alterations in enzymes associated with fat metabolism, and decreased thermogenesis, have been proposed, but none has been substantiated. The many hormonal and metabolic changes seen in obese persons appear to be results of the increased fat stores, rather than the cause of the obesity.

The most important consequence of obesity (Fig. 8-27) **is maturity-onset (Type II) diabetes, which is associated with normal or high levels of circulating insulin and peripheral resistance to insulin's action.** In the United States, more than 80% of Type II diabetes occurs in obese individuals. The precise mechanism is not understood, but in experimental animals it has been found that weight gain directly stimulates insulin secretion by the beta cells of the pancreas. Higher levels of circulating insulin decrease the number of insulin receptors on the surfaces of muscle and adipose cells—a form of negative feedback inhibition. This observation has led to the theory that this peripheral resistance to the action of insulin stimulates insulin production, leading to a further decrease in the number of receptors. Eventually the beta cell is unable to secrete enough insulin to overcome the peripheral resistance to its effect. In an analogy to

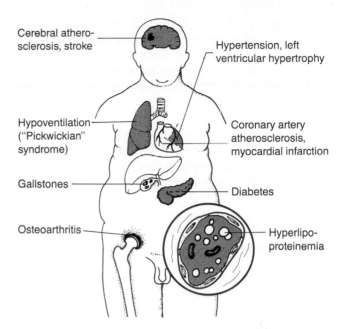

Figure 8-27. Complications of obesity.

the heart, the final result is "high output failure" of the beta cells of the pancreas. Weight reduction usually ameliorates the glucose intolerance of Type II diabetes, presumably owing to a decrease in the stimulus for insulin secretion by the pancreatic beta cells. This subject is more fully discussed in Chapter 22.

Obesity has also been linked to atherosclerosis and myocardial infarction. It is noteworthy that obesity is associated with all the major risk factors for myocardial infarction, including hypercholesterolemia, low levels of high-density lipoproteins (HDL), diabetes, and hypertension. The relationship of hypertension to obesity is not understood, but it may involve an increase in circulating blood volume and dietary salt intake. In addition to its deleterious effect on the heart, hypertension is also responsible for the greater incidence of stroke and vascular disease of the kidneys prevalent in obese individuals. Atherosclerosis seems to be linked to the disordered lipid metabolism associated with obesity. **Obesity and hypercholesterolemia are also linked to an increased incidence of gallstones, particularly in women.** Severe degrees of obesity result in the deposition of fat in the liver and minor functional changes, but these are generally of little clinical significance. For reasons that are not clear, blood uric acid levels are increased in obese individuals, as is the incidence of gout.

A number of complications can be traced simply to the physical effect of an increase in body weight and skin fold thickness. Osteoarthritis, or degenerative joint disease, is common in weight-bearing joints, such as those of the hip, knee, and spine. Excessive subcutaneous fat, particularly beneath the breasts and in the crural areas in women, often is responsible for an intertriginous dermatitis, owing to an accumulation of moisture and maceration of the epidermis. The moisture in the intertriginous areas may predispose to fungal infections of the skin. Hernias of the ventral abdominal wall and of the diaphragm are not uncommon. Because the fat deposits place greater pressure on the veins, and possibly because tissue turgor is decreased, varicose veins of the lower extremities are more common in obese persons, and the incidence of thrombophlebitis is increased correspondingly.

Obesity also poses a physical impediment to surgery, which is made more difficult technically. Because of the longer time needed for surgery, the risks of anesthesia, pulmonary complications, and infection are increased, and the overall surgical mortality for the obese is probably twice as great as that for persons of normal weight.

Obesity also has an important effect on the female reproductive system. **Oligomenorrhea and amenorrhea are common in premenopausal obese women.** Pregnant obese women have a higher incidence of toxemia of pregnancy. Postmenopausal obese women have higher rates of endometrial carcinoma and uterine fibroids. It has been postulated that the increased body fat provides a larger storage space for estrogens and that the conversion of adrenal androgens to compounds with estrogenic activity is increased. Such mechanisms might lead to greater hormonal stimulation of the endometrium and myometrium.

The treatment of obesity is difficult, especially in those who have been overweight since childhood. Despite the commercial success of innumerable fad diets that purport to enhance weight loss, there is no evidence that any particular form of caloric restriction is more effective than others. Simply put, any caloric intake that is less than energy expenditure will result in weight loss. Since some unusual diets (for example, protein hydrolysates) may actually pose health risks, such as cardiac arrhythmias, the most reasonable regimen for most people is a balanced diet containing less than 1000 calories a day. The use of diuretics to achieve weight loss borders on the fraudulent, and administration of thyroid hormone has a greater effect on lean body mass than on adipose tissue.

Protein-Calorie Malnutrition

Protein-calorie malnutrition is a direct result of inadequate dietary protein coupled with a deficient intake of the carbohydrates and lipids necessary to provide an adequate energy source. A secondary form of this condition arises when disease prevents absorption of nutrients from the intestine or provokes an increased nutritional demand. It should be recalled that a lack of carbohydrates and lipids results in the oxidation of endogenous protein, a complication that leads to wasting. These states are found not only in children and adults in endemic areas of restricted food supply, but also in as many as 25% of hospitalized adult patients, because of the increased nutritional needs associated with the underlying disease. The manifestations of protein-energy deficiency vary depending on the individual and his or her state of development. Infants and children are particularly susceptible because of their requirements for growth. There are two ends of the spectrum of protein-calorie malnutrition, reflecting the relative imbalance between the components of the diet. A deficiency of calories from all sources leads to **marasmus**, whereas a diet deficient in protein alone is associated with **kwashiorkor**. Actually, the classic manifestations of either of these conditions are uncommon when compared with the high prevalence of intermediate states of undernutrition. Moreover, both marasmus and kwashiorkor, as well as their intermediate states, are often complicated by deficiencies in vitamins and minerals.

Marasmus

Global starvation—that is, a deficiency of all elements of the diet—leads to marasmus. The condition is common throughout the nonindustrialized world, particularly when breast feeding is stopped and a child must subsist on a calorically inadequate diet. The pathologic changes are similar to those in starving adults, and consist of decreased body weight, diminished subcutaneous fat, a protuberant abdomen, muscle wasting, and a wrinkled face. In general, the child is a "shrunken old person." Wasting and increased lipofuscin pigment are seen in most visceral organs, especially the heart and the liver. No edema is present. The pulse, blood pressure, and temperature are low, and diarrhea is common. Because immune responses are impaired, the child suffers from numerous infections. An important consequence of marasmus is growth failure. If these children are not provided with an adequate diet during childhood, they will not reach their full potential stature as adults. The effects on ultimate intelligence are controversial.

Kwashiorkor

One of the most common diseases of infancy and childhood in the nonindustrialized world is **kwashiorkor** (Fig. 8-28), a syndrome that results from **a**

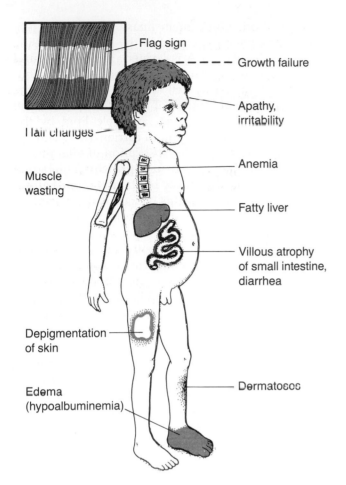

Flag sign

Growth failure

Apathy, irritability

Hair changes

Anemia

Muscle wasting

Fatty liver

Villous atrophy of small intestine, diarrhea

Depigmentation of skin

Edema (hypoalbuminemia)

Dermatoses

Figure 8-28. Complications of kwashiorkor.

generally life-threatening. The nonspecific effects on growth, pulse, temperature, and the immune system are similar to those in marasmus. It has been claimed that kwashiorkor not only impairs physical development, but also stunts later intellectual growth. However, the subject requires further study.

Microscopically, the liver in kwashiorkor is conspicuously fatty, and the accumulation of lipid within the cytoplasm of the hepatocyte displaces the nucleus to the periphery of the cell. The adequacy of dietary carbohydrate provides the lipid to the hepatocyte, but the inadequate protein stores do not permit the synthesis of enough apoprotein carrier to transport the lipid from the liver cell. The changes, with the possible exception of mental retardation, are fully reversible when sufficient protein is made available. In fact, the fatty liver reverts to normal after early childhood, even though the diet may remain deficient. In any event, the hepatic changes are not progressive and are not associated with the development of chronic liver disease. Earlier studies, which linked kwashiorkor in childhood to the development of hepatocellular carcinoma many years later, are questionable in light of the demonstrated association between infection with the hepatitis B virus and primary hepatocellular carcinoma in these geographic areas.

Vitamins

"Vitamin" is a general term for a number of unrelated organic catalysts that are not endogenously synthesized but are necessary for normal metabolic functions. **The body is therefore totally dependent on dietary sources for these crucial substances.** Critical to the definition of a vitamin is the demonstration that a lack of this compound results in a clearly definable disease. Thus, vitamins in one species are not necessarily vitamins in another. For example, whereas man is unable to synthesize ascorbic acid (vitamin C) and therefore requires dietary ascorbate to prevent scurvy, most lower animals are fully capable of producing their own ascorbic acid and do not require it as a vitamin. In contrast, the importance of the anti-oxidant vitamin E in rats is clear; however, its precise role in human nutrition has not been well elucidated, and a deficiency state is only poorly characterized. Another example is choline, a deficiency of which produces fatty liver and cirrhosis in rats. Thus, although not a vitamin, it may be considered an essential nutrient for that species. However, no lesions attributable to choline deficiency have been demonstrated in man. Vitamins A, D, and K are fat soluble, a property which allows for their storage in the liver, and which also accounts for their malab-

deficiency of protein in a diet relatively high in carbohydrates. As in the case of marasmus, the disorder commonly occurs after the baby is weaned, at which time a protein-poor diet, consisting principally of staple carbohydrates, replaces the mother's milk. Although there is generalized growth failure and muscle wasting, as in marasmus, the subcutaneous fat is normal, owing to an adequate caloric intake. Extreme apathy is a notable feature, in contrast to children with marasmus, who may be alert. Also in contrast to marasmus, severe edema, hepatomegaly, depigmentation of the skin, and dermatoses are usual. The "flaky paint" lesions of the skin, located on the face, extremities, and perineum, are dry and hyperkeratotic. The hair becomes a sandy or reddish color; a characteristic linear depigmentation of the hair ("flag sign") provides evidence of particularly severe periods of protein deficiency. The abdomen is distended because of flaccid abdominal muscles, hepatomegaly, and ascites. Along with generalized atrophy of the viscera, villous atrophy of the intestine may interfere with nutrient absorption, and diarrhea is common. Anemia is a usual feature, although not

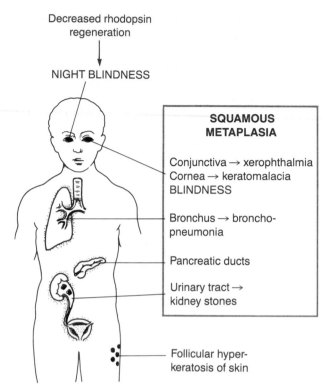

Decreased rhodopsin regeneration

↓

NIGHT BLINDNESS

SQUAMOUS METAPLASIA

Conjunctiva → xerophthalmia
Cornea → keratomalacia
BLINDNESS

Bronchus → broncho-pneumonia

Pancreatic ducts

Urinary tract → kidney stones

Follicular hyper-keratosis of skin

Figure 8-29.   Complications of vitamin A deficiency.

sorption in diseases that interfere with lipid absorption, such as pancreatic disease, biliary obstruction, and primary disease of the small bowel (sprue). Because the water-soluble vitamins—vitamin B complex and vitamin C—are not stored as efficiently as the fat-soluble vitamins, deficiency states occur more rapidly after deprivation of dietary sources.

Vitamin A Deficiency

Vitamin A, a fat-soluble substance, is important for the maintenance of a number of specialized epithelial linings, skeletal maturation, and the structure of the cell membranes. In addition, it is an important constituent of the photosensitive pigments in the retina. Vitamin A occurs naturally as retinoids or as a precursor, beta-carotene. The source of the precursor, carotene, is in plants, principally leafy, green vegetables. Fish livers are a particularly rich source of vitamin A itself. Both forms are absorbed from the intestinal mucosa, vitamin A as 80% to 90% of the available food load, and beta-carotene as only 40% to 50%. Beta-carotene is cleaved in the intestinal mucosa to the aldehyde and then reduced to retinoids. The retinoids are bound to palmitic acid, absorbed to chylomicrons, and transported by the lymph to the general circulation. Lipoprotein lipase releases the retinoid, after which it is stored in the liver, where 90% of the body's vitamin A is located. Retinol is bound to a retinol-binding protein, transported with albumin, and extracted by cell surfaces throughout the body. Usually, rapid transit of food through the small intestine, or modification of available lipid by the addition of nonabsorbable lipid carriers (for example, mineral oil), decreases the absorption of vitamin A.

The lack of vitamin A results principally in squamous metaplasia, especially in glandular epithelium (Fig. 8-29). One effect of this change is the formation of an epithelium whose structure is not adapted to functional needs. Stratified squamous epithelium keratinizes, and the keratin debris blocks sweat and tear glands. Squamous metaplasia is common in the trachea and the bronchi, and bronchopneumonia is a frequent cause of death. The lining epithelia of the renal pelvis, pancreatic ducts, uterus, and salivary glands are also commonly affected. Epithelial changes in the renal pelvis are occasionally associated with kidney stones. With further diminution of vitamin A stores, squamous metaplasia of the epithelial cells of the conjunctiva and tear ducts occurs, which leads to **xerophthalmia,** a dryness and wrinkling of the cornea. The cornea becomes softened **(keratomalacia)** and is vulnerable to ulceration and bacterial infection, complications which may lead to blindness. **Follicular hyperkeratosis,** a skin disorder that results from occluded sebaceous glands, is also a feature of this disease.

The earliest sign of vitamin A deficiency often is diminished vision in dim light. Vitamin A is a necessary component in the pigment of the retinal rods and is active in light transduction. Since the aldehyde of vitamin A, retinal, is constantly being degraded during the generation of the light signal, a continuous supply of vitamin A is necessary for night vision.

Large doses of vitamin A, usually from overenthusiastic administration of vitamin supplements to children, lead to lesions of vitamin A toxicity. (Early Arctic explorers were said to have experienced vitamin A toxicity because they ate polar bear livers, which are particularly rich in the vitamin.) An enlarged liver and spleen are common, and microscopically these organs show lipid-laden macrophages. In the liver, vitamin A is also present in hepatocytes, and prolonged vitamin A toxicity has been incriminated in the production of cirrhosis. Bone pain and neurologic symptoms such as hyperexcitability and headache may be the presenting symptoms. Discontinuation of excess vitamin A consumption reverses all or most of the lesions. Excessive carotene intake is benign and simply stains the skin yellow, an appearance that may be mistaken for jaundice.

Synthetic derivatives of retinoic acid are now increasingly used for their pharmacologic effect in alleviating severe acne. The dosage of these compounds, which display potent vitamin A activity, is limited by vitamin A toxicity. Retinoids are also effective in the treatment of certain experimental tumors, and may find a place in the treatment of human cancer.

Vitamin B Complex

Vitamins in the B group of water-soluble vitamins are numbered 1 through 12, but most are not distinct vitamins. The members of the complex currently recognized as true vitamins are vitamins B_1 (thiamine), B_2 (niacin, nicotinic acid), B_3 (riboflavin), B_6 (pyridoxine), and B_{12} (cyanocobalamin).

Thiamine Deficiency

With the exception of vitamin B_{12}, which is derived only from animal sources, the vitamins of the B complex, although chemically distinct, are found principally in leafy green vegetables, milk, and liver.

Thiamine was actually the active ingredient in the original description of vitamin B, which was defined as a water-soluble extract in rice polishings that cured beri-beri (clinical thiamine deficiency). This disease was classically seen in the Orient, where the staple food was polished rice that had been deprived of its thiamine content by processing. With increased awareness of the disease and improved nutrition in some areas, the disorder is less common now than in previous generations. In Western countries the disease occurs in alcoholics, neglected people with poor overall nutrition, and food faddists. **The cardinal symptoms of thiamine deficiency are polyneuropathy, edema, and cardiac failure** (Fig. 8-30). The deficiency syndrome is classically divided into **dry beri-beri,** with symptoms referable to the neuromuscular system, and **wet beri-beri,** in which the symptoms of cardiac failure predominate.

Patients with dry beri-beri present with paresthesias, depressed reflexes, and weakness and atrophy of the muscles of the extremities. Wet beri-beri is characterized by generalized edema, a reflection of severe congestive failure. The basic lesion is an uncontrolled, generalized vasodilatation and significant peripheral arteriovenous shunting. This combination leads to a compensatory increase in cardiac output, and eventually to a large dilated heart and congestive heart failure. In the absence of a documented metabolic disease (e.g., hyperthyroidism), high output failure and generalized edema are strongly suggestive of thiamine deficiency.

Thiamine deficiency in chronic alcoholics may be manifested by involvement of the brain in the form of **Wernicke's syndrome,** in which progressive **dementia, ataxia,** and **ophthalmoplegia** (paralysis of the extraocular muscles) are prominent. Korsakoff's syndrome, in which a thought disorder is conspicuous, at one time was attributed solely to thiamine deficiency, but it now appears to be a finding both in chronic alcoholics and in patients with other organic mental syndromes.

Pathologic examination of the nervous system in cases of thiamine deficiency has not defined a pathognomonic change in the peripheral nerves, since similar or identical changes can be seen in a variety of other diseases characterized by peripheral neuropathy. A characteristic alteration is degeneration of myelin sheaths, often beginning in the sciatic nerve and then involving other peripheral nerves, and sometimes the spinal cord itself. In the few advanced cases that have been studied, fragmentation of the

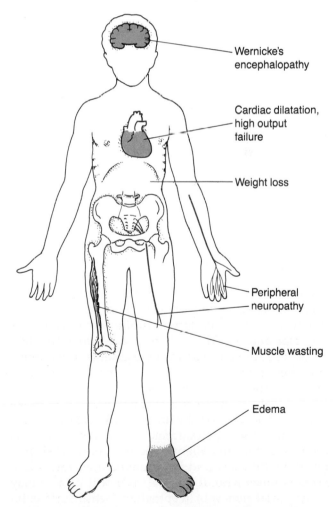

Figure 8-30. Complications of thiamine deficiency (beri-beri).

axons has been noted. In Wernicke's encephalopathy the most striking lesions are found in the mammillary bodies and surrounding areas that abut on the third ventricle. Indeed, atrophy of the mammillary bodies can be visualized in alcoholics by computerized tomography and magnetic resonance imaging. Microscopically, degeneration and loss of ganglion cells, rupture of small blood vessels, and ring hemorrhages are seen in the brain.

The changes in the heart are also nonspecific. Grossly, the heart is flabby, dilated, and increased in weight. The process may affect either the right or the left side of the heart, or both. The microscopic changes are nondescript, and include edema, inconsistent fiber hypertrophy, and occasional foci of fiber degeneration. At one time, all primary myocardial diseases in the alcoholic were considered to reflect thiamine deficiency, but it is now recognized that the large majority are unrelated to thiamine and are caused by a direct toxic effect of alcohol (alcoholic cardiomyopathy).

The most reliable diagnostic test for thiamine deficiency is an **immediate and dramatic response to parenteral thiamine.** Measurements of levels of thiamine in the blood and red blood cell transketolase activity are also useful. The biochemical basis of the symptoms in thiamine deficiency is not understood. As a result of the defect in the oxidative decarboxylation, pyruvate accumulates. However, experimental pyruvate administration does not produce the same lesions. Moreover, it is difficult to attribute the symptomatology to a generalized defect in energy metabolism.

Niacin Deficiency

Niacin refers to two chemically distinct compounds: nicotinic acid and nicotinamide. These biologically active components are derived from dietary niacin or are biosynthesized from available tryptophan. Niacin plays a major role in the formation of nicotinamide adenine dinucleotide (NAD) and its phosphate (NADP), compounds important in intermediary metabolism and a wide variety of oxidation-reduction reactions. Animal protein, as found in meat, eggs, and milk, is high in tryptophan, and is therefore a good source of endogenously synthesized niacin. Niacin itself is available in many types of grain. Like other deficiencies of the B vitamins, clinical niacin deficiency, called **pellagra,** is uncommon today; it is seen principally in patients who have been weakened by other diseases and in malnourished alcoholics. Food faddists who do not eat sufficient protein may suffer a deficiency of tryptophan, which in combination with a lack of exogenous niacin may result in mild pellagra. Malabsorption of tryptophan, as in Hartnup disease, or excessive utilization of tryptophan for the synthesis of serotonin in the carcinoid syndrome, may also lead to mild symptoms of pellagra. Pellagra is particularly prevalent in areas where maize is the staple food because the niacin in maize is chemically bound and thus poorly available. Maize is also a poor source of tryptophan. Deficiencies of pyridoxine and riboflavin increase the requirement for dietary niacin because both of these cofactors are required for the biosynthesis of niacin from tryptophan.

Pellagra (Italian, "rough skin") is characterized by the **three Ds of niacin deficiency: dermatitis, diarrhea, and dementia** (Fig. 8-31). Those areas exposed to light, such as the face and the hands, and those subjected to pressure, such as the knees and the elbows, exhibit a rough, scaly dermatitis. The involvement of the hands leads to so-called glove dermatitis. The lesions are discrete and show areas of pigmentation and of depigmentation. Microscopically, hyperkeratosis, vascularization, and chronic inflammation of the skin are characteristic. Subcutaneous fibrosis and scarring may be seen in late stages. Similar lesions are found in the mucous membranes of the mouth and vagina. In the mouth, inflammation and edema lead to a large, red tongue, which in the chronic stage is fissured and is likened to raw meat. A chronic, watery diarrhea is a typical feature of the disease, presumably caused by mucosal atrophy and ulceration in the entire gastrointestinal tract, particularly in the colon. The dementia, characterized by

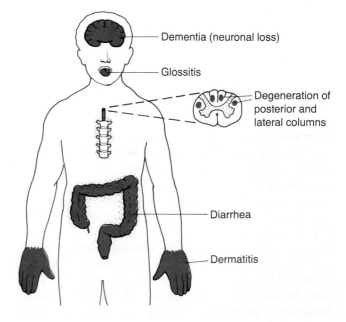

Figure 8-31.   Complications of niacin deficiency (pellagra).

aberrant ideation bordering on psychosis, is represented in the brain by degeneration of ganglion cells in the cortex. Myelin degeneration of tracts in the spinal cord resembles the subacute combined degeneration of vitamin B_{12} deficiency. Severe long-standing pellagra adds another D—death.

Riboflavin Deficiency

Riboflavin, a vitamin derived from many plant and animal sources, is important for the synthesis of flavin nucleotides, which play an important role in electron transport and other reactions in which the transfer of energy is crucial.

Riboflavin is converted within the body to flavin mononucleotides and dinucleotides. Riboflavin itself and flavin mononucleotides are absorbed from the proximal small bowel, whereas flavin adenine dinucleotide must be degraded to flavin mononucleotide prior to absorption. The conjugated and unconjugated forms circulate bound to serum proteins, but storage sites have not been clearly defined. Clinical symptoms of riboflavin deficiency are uncommon; they are usually seen only in debilitated patients with a variety of diseases and in poorly nourished alcoholics.

Deficiencies of thiamine, riboflavin, and niacin are unusual in the industrialized countries because bread and cereals are fortified with these vitamins. Occasionally a mild deficiency of riboflavin is seen during pregnancy and lactation or during the period of rapid growth of childhood and adolescence, when increased demands are combined with moderate nutritional deprivation.

Riboflavin deficiency is manifested principally by lesions of the facial skin and the corneal epithelium. **Cheilosis,** a term used for fissures in the skin at the angles of the mouth, is a characteristic feature (Fig. 8-32). These cracks in the skin may be painful and often become infected. Microscopically, hyperkeratosis and a mild mononuclear infiltrate of the skin are noted. **Seborrheic dermatitis,** an inflammation of the skin that exhibits a greasy, scaling appearance, typically involves the cheeks and the areas behind the ears. The tongue is smooth and a purplish (magenta) color owing to atrophy of the mucosa. The most troubling lesion may be an **interstitial keratitis of the cornea.** The conjunctivae are injected and severe photophobia is a problem. The cornea is initially vascularized by numerous sprouting capillaries. This process is followed by opacification of the cornea and eventual ulceration. The localization of the lesions in riboflavin deficiency is not explained by biochemistry.

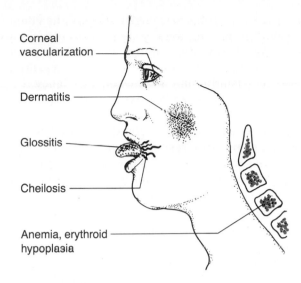

Figure 8-32. Complications of riboflavin deficiency.

Pyridoxine Deficiency

Vitamin B_6 activity is found in three related, naturally occurring compounds: pyridoxine, pyridoxal, and pyridoxamine. For the sake of convenience, they are all grouped under the heading pyridoxine. These compounds are widely distributed in vegetable and animal foods.

Pyridoxine is converted to pyridoxal phosphate, a coenzyme for many enzymes, including transaminases and carboxylases. Pyridoxine deficiency is rarely caused by an inadequate diet, although infants who have been fed a poorly prepared powdered formula in which the pyridoxine has been destroyed during preparation have suffered convulsions. A higher demand for the vitamin, such as may occur in pregnancy, may lead to a secondary deficiency state. Of particular concern is the deficiency of pyridoxine that follows prolonged medication with a number of drugs, particularly isoniazid, cycloserine, and penicillamine. A deficiency state is also occasionally seen in alcoholics.

There are no clinical manifestations of the disease that can be considered characteristic or pathognomonic. The usual dermatologic complications of other B vitamin deficiencies are seen with pyridoxine deficiency. **The primary expression of the disease is in the central nervous system, a feature consistent with the role of this vitamin in the formation of pyridoxal-dependent decarboxylase of the neurotransmitter gamma aminobutyric acid (GABA).** In infants and children, diarrhea, anemia, and seizures have occurred.

Conditions are encountered in which there is no clinical or biochemical evidence of pyridoxine deficiency, yet large (pharmacologic) doses of the vitamin are useful in treating the disorder. Such diseases are termed **pyridoxine-dependency syndromes,** and include anemia, convulsions, and homocystinuria caused by cystathionine synthetase deficiency. Pyridoxine-responsive anemia is hypochromic and microcytic, and therefore can be confused with iron deficiency anemia. Unlike iron-deficiency anemia, however, pyridoxine-responsive anemia is characterized by saturation of iron stores and an increased saturation of transferrin. Thus, administration of iron may simply make pyridoxine-responsive anemia worse. By definition, the anemia responds well to massive doses of pyridoxine.

Vitamin B₁₂ and Folic Acid Deficiencies

Deficiencies of vitamin B_{12} are almost always seen in cases of pernicious anemia and result from the lack of secretion of intrinsic factor in the stomach, which prevents absorption of the vitamin in the ileum. Since vitamin B_{12} is found in almost all animal protein, including meat, milk, and eggs, dietary deficiency is seen only in rare cases of extreme vegetarianism, and that only after many years of a restricted diet. Parasitization of the small intestine by the fish tapeworm, *Diphyllobothrium latum,* may lead to vitamin B_{12} deficiency because the parasite absorbs the vitamin.

Deficiency of folic acid, the trivial name for pteroylmonoglutamic acid, is commonly of dietary origin. Leafy vegetables, liver, kidney, and yeast are rich sources of folic acid. However, excessive cooking destroys much of the folic acid in foods. Dietary folic acid deficiency is usually accompanied by multiple vitamin deficiencies. Pregnancy increases the requirement for folic acid five- to tenfold. It has been estimated that **two-thirds of anemic pregnant women are folate deficient,** although this may be combined with iron deficiency. Folic acid is absorbed principally in the upper third of the small intestine, and therefore folate deficiency is common in certain diseases of malabsorption, notably nontropical and tropical sprue. The latter condition is responsive to treatment with folic acid.

Deficiencies of both vitamin B_{12} and folic acid are associated with **megaloblastic anemia.** In addition, pernicious anemia is complicated by a neurologic condition called **subacute combined degeneration of the spinal cord.** A comprehensive discussion of vitamin B_{12} and folic acid deficiencies is found in Chapter 20, which deals with hematologic disorders, and Chapter 28, which is devoted to neuropathology.

Vitamin C (Ascorbic Acid) Deficiency

Ascorbic acid is a powerful biologic reducing agent that is involved in numerous oxidation-reduction reactions and the transfer of protons. This vitamin is important in the synthesis of chondroitin sulfate and in the hydroxylation of proline to form the hydroxyproline of collagen. It serves many other important functions, such as preventing the oxidation of tetrahydrofolate and augmenting the absorption of iron from the gut. Without vitamin C the biosynthesis of certain neurotransmitters is impaired because of a reduction in the activity of dopamine-beta-hydroxylase. Wound healing and immune functions are also under the influence of ascorbic acid. The best dietary sources of vitamin C are citrus fruits, green vegetables, and tomatoes. Man and the guinea pig lack the ability to make ascorbic acid, an incapacity which can be explained only as an evolutionary quirk.

The clinical vitamin C deficiency state is termed **scurvy.** The first demonstration of the need for this vitamin was the remarkable effect of lime in preventing scurvy among 18th century British sailors. The distribution of limes in the British navy led to the term "limey" for the sailors. Scurvy is uncommon in the Western world, but is often seen in nonindustrialized countries in which other forms of malnutrition are prevalent. In the industrialized countries, scurvy is now a disease of people afflicted with chronic diseases who do not eat well, the neglected aged, and malnourished alcoholics. Elderly individuals who consume a "tea and toast" diet are particularly vulnerable to ascorbic acid deficiency because of an inadequate intake of the vitamin. The stress of cold, heat, fever, or trauma (accidental or surgical) leads to an increased requirement for vitamin C. Children who are fed only milk for the first year of life may develop scurvy, as do alcoholics. However, in alcoholics, vitamin C deficiency is not as common as a deficiency of the B vitamins.

The rate of catabolism of ascorbic acid is about 3% of the body pool a day, a value which is consistent with the fact that on a diet lacking in vitamin C the symptoms of scurvy take some months to develop.

In the early stages of vitamin C deficiency, nonspecific symptoms of weakness and lethargy are noted. **Most of the subsequent events are caused by the formation of abnormal collagen that lacks tensile strength** (Fig. 8-33). Within 1 to 3 months, subperiosteal hemorrhages lead to pain in the bones and joints. Petechial hemorrhages, ecchymoses, and purpura are common, particularly after mild trauma or at pressure points. Perifollicular hemorrhages in the skin are particularly typical of scurvy. In advanced

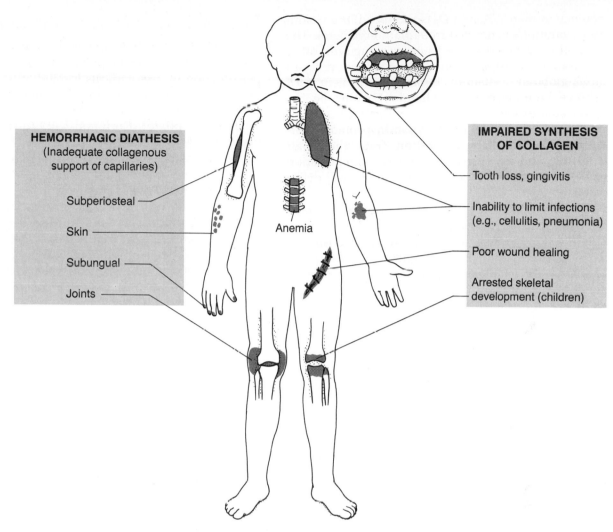

HEMORRHAGIC DIATHESIS
(Inadequate collagenous
support of capillaries)

Subperiosteal

Skin

Subungual

Joints

Anemia

IMPAIRED SYNTHESIS
OF COLLAGEN

Tooth loss, gingivitis

Inability to limit infections
(e.g., cellulitis, pneumonia)

Poor wound healing

Arrested skeletal
development (children)

Figure 8-33. Complications of vitamin C deficiency (scurvy).

cases, swollen, bleeding gums are a classic finding. Alveolar bone resorption results in loosening and loss of teeth. Wound healing is poor, and dehiscence of previously healed wounds occurs. Anemia may result from prolonged bleeding, impaired iron absorption, or an associated folic acid deficiency. In children, vitamin C deficiency leads to growth failure, and collagen-rich structures such as the teeth, bones, and blood vessels develop abnormally. The effects on developing bone are conspicuous and relate principally to impaired calcification. The effects of scurvy on bone are discussed in greater detail in Chapter 26, which deals with bone pathology. In addition to poor wound healing, scorbutic individuals have difficulty in walling off an infection to form an abscess, and infections therefore spread more easily. The diagnosis of scurvy is confirmed by finding low levels of ascorbic acid in the serum. Mild depression of ascorbate levels also occurs in other conditions, however, including cigarette smoking, tuberculosis, rheumatic fever, and many debilitating disorders. Some women who use oral contraceptives may have a mild decrease in serum vitamin C levels.

Widespread publicity has attended claims that very large doses of ascorbic acid are useful in the prevention of the common cold and in the treatment of metastatic cancer. There is little or no evidence to support either contention.

Vitamin D Deficiency

Vitamin D is a fat-soluble steroid hormone found in two forms: vitamin D_3 (cholecalciferol) and vitamin D_2 (ergocalciferol), both of which have equal biologic potency in man. Vitamin D₃ is produced in the skin, and vitamin D₂ is derived from plant ergosterol. The vitamin is absorbed in the jejunum along with other fats and is transported in the blood bound to an alpha-globulin, vitamin D–binding protein. **To achieve biologic potency, vitamin D must be hydroxylated to active metabolites in the liver and kidney. The active form of the vitamin promotes calcium and phosphate absorption from the small intestine,** and may directly influence mineralization of bone, although the latter effect is not well delineated.

Vitamin D deficiency results from insufficient vitamin D in the diet, insufficient production of vitamin D in the skin because of limited sunlight exposure as a result of occupation or dress, inadequate absorption of vitamin D from the diet (as in the fat malabsorption syndromes), or abnormal conversion of vitamin D to its bioactive metabolites. The last occurs in liver disease and chronic renal failure. **In children, vitamin D deficiency causes rickets; in adults, osteomalacia is seen.**

The bone lesions of vitamin D deficiency in children (rickets) have been recognized for centuries and were common in the Western industrialized world until recently. It was a disease that affected the urban poor to a much greater extent than their rural counterparts. A partial explanation for this difference lies in the greater exposure of rural residents to sunlight. The addition of vitamin D to milk and many processed foods, the administration of vitamin preparations to young children, and generally improved levels of nutrition have made rickets a curiosity in industrialized countries. A full discussion of the metabolism of vitamin D and its relationship to rickets and osteomalacia is found in Chapter 26.

The most common cause of excess vitamin D, or **hypervitaminosis D,** is the inordinate consumption of vitamin preparations. Abnormal conversion of vitamin D to biologically active metabolites is occasionally seen in granulomatous diseases such as sarcoidosis. In cases of calcium malabsorption, when the underlying disease is corrected the sensitivity of target tissues to vitamin D may be increased. The initial response to excess vitamin D is **hypercalcemia,** which leads to nonspecific symptoms such as weakness and headaches. The increased excretion of calcium by the kidneys results in **nephrolithiasis** or **nephrocalcinosis. Ectopic calcification** in other organs, such as blood vessels, the heart, and lungs, may be seen. Infants are particularly susceptible to excess vitamin D, and if the condition is not corrected they may develop premature arteriosclerosis, supravalvular aortic stenosis, and renal acidosis.

Vitamin E

Vitamin E is an antioxidant that, experimentally at least, protects membrane phospholipids against lipid peroxidation by free radicals formed by cellular metabolism. The activity of this fat-soluble vitamin is found in a number of dietary constituents, principally in alpha-tocopherol. Corn and soy beans are particularly rich in vitamin E. No specific carrier protein in the blood has been identified for vitamin E, nor is it stored in any specific organ. A dietary deficiency of vitamin E is rare, except among individuals receiving total parenteral nutrition. Low vitamin E levels have also been found in patients with disorders of fat absorption from the intestine. A clearly definable syndrome associated with vitamin E deficiency has not been identified in adults. Inconsistent reports of abnormalities of the posterior columns of the spinal cord, together with functional disturbances of gait, proprioception, and vibration have been recorded. Although the life span of the red blood cell may be shortened, clinical anemia is not attributable to vitamin E deficiency alone.

In premature infants, hemolytic anemia, thrombocytosis, and edema have been associated with a deficiency of vitamin E. Vitamin E has been claimed by food faddists and enterprising entrepreneurs to be an anti-aging vitamin and an enhancer of sexual potency. There is no objective evidence to support these claims. On the other hand, vitamin E therapy has been reported to improve hemolytic anemia in premature newborns, and may reduce the severity—but not the incidence—of retrolental fibroplasia. Vitamin E is reported to retard the development of cirrhosis in infants with congenital biliary atresia. A number of interesting experimental effects are produced by vitamin E, such as inhibition of (a) platelet aggregation, (b) the conversion of nitrites to nitrosamines, and (c) prostaglandin synthesis. Protection against toxins that exert their activity through the production of free radical oxygen species has also been shown. The applicability of these results to man requires further study.

Vitamin K

Vitamin K, a fat-soluble material, occurs in two forms: vitamin K₁, from plants, and vitamin K₂, which is principally synthesized by the normal intestinal bacteria. Green leafy vegetables are rich in vitamin K, and liver and dairy products contain smaller amounts. Dietary deficiency is very uncommon in the United States; most cases are associated with other disorders. However, inadequate dietary intake of vitamin K does occasionally occur in conjunction with chronic illness associated with anorexia.

Vitamin K deficiency is common in severe fat malabsorption, as seen in sprue and biliary tract obstruction. The destruction of intestinal flora by antibiotics may also result in vitamin K deficiency. Newborn infants frequently exhibit vitamin K deficiency because the vitamin is not transported well across the placenta, and the sterile gut of the newborn does not have bacteria to produce it. Vitamin K, which confers calcium-binding properties to certain proteins, is important for the activity of four clotting factors: prothrombin, factor VII, factor IX, and factor X. Deficiency of vitamin K can be serious, because it can lead to catastrophic bleeding. Parenteral vitamin K therapy is rapidly effective.

Minerals

The essential trace minerals are, for the most part, components of enzymes and cofactors necessary for metabolic functions. These include iron, copper, iodine, zinc, cobalt, selenium, manganese, nickel, chromium, tin, molybdenum, vanadium, silicon, and fluorine. Dietary deficiencies of these minerals are clinically important in the case of iron and iodine, and these are discussed in Chapters 20 and 21, which deal with blood diseases and endocrinologic pathology, respectively.

Chronic zinc deficiency has been reported in Iran and Egypt to result in hypogonadal dwarfism in boys. The children usually are those who eat clay, a substance that may bind zinc, but a deficiency in dietary protein is usually also present. An inherited disorder of zinc metabolism, acrodermatitis enterohepatica, which is a chronic form of pure zinc deficiency, is characterized by diarrhea, skin rash, hair loss, muscle wasting, and mental irritability. Similar symptoms are seen in acute zinc deficiency associated with total parenteral nutrition. Zinc deficiency is also seen in diseases that cause malabsorption, such as Crohn's disease, sprue, cirrhosis, and alcoholism.

Dietary copper deficiency is rare, but may occur in certain inherited disorders, malabsorption syndromes, and during total parenteral nutrition. The most common result is a microcytic anemia, although megaloblastic changes have also been described.

Manganese deficiency has been described and causes poor growth, skeletal abnormalities, reproductive impairment, ataxia, and convulsions. Industrial exposure to manganese causes symptoms closely related to those of Parkinsonism.

Conclusion

The dawn of life was marked by an incredibly hostile environment. The earth revolved on its axis more then 10^{12} times before a creature evolved who could consciously manipulate his environment. In the process, the 18-year average life span of Cro-Magnon man has risen for industrialized man to surpass the biblical three-score and ten. While this remarkable success should not lead us to complacency in our efforts to improve the quality and extent of life, it remains important to maintain a realistic perspective on the impact of civilization on the environment.

SUGGESTED READING

BOOKS

Alcohol, Drug Abuse, and Mental Health Administration: The Sixth Special Report to the US Congress on Alcohol and Health from the Secretary of Health and Human Services. Item no. 498-C-6. Rockville, MD, US Department of Health and Human Services, 1987

Committee on the Biological Effects of Ionizing Radiations (BEIR III): The Effects on Populations of Exposure to Low Levels of Ionizing Radiation. Washington, DC, National Academy of Sciences, 1980

Doull J, Klaassen CD, Amdur MO: Toxicology: The Basic Science of Poisons, 3rd ed. New York, Macmillan, 1986

Hall EJ: Radiobiology for the Radiologist, 3rd ed. Philadelphia, JB Lippincott, 1988

Office on Smoking and Health: The Health Consequences of Smoking: Cancer and Chronic Lung Disease in the Workplace. A Report of the Surgeon General. Item no. 85-50207. Rockville, MD, US Department of Health and Human Services, 1985

Rubin E (ed): Alcohol and the Cell. Ann. NY Acad Sci, vol 492, 1987

Strickland GT (ed): Nutritional Deficiencies and Heat-Associated Illnesses. In Hunter's Tropical Medicine, 6th ed. Philadelphia, WB Saunders, 1984

Tedeschi CG, Eckert WG, Tedeschi LG: Forensic Medicine: A Study in Trauma and Environmental Hazards. Philadelphia, WB Saunders, 1977

ARTICLES

Brent RL: The effects of ionizing radiation, microwaves, and ultrasound on the developing embryo: Clinical interpretations and applications of the data. Curr Probl Ped 14, 1984

Michenovicz JJ, Hershcopf RJ, Naganuma H, et al: Increased 2-hydroxylation of estradiol as a possible mechanism for the anti-estrogenic effect of cigarette smoking. N Engl J Med 315:1305, 1986

Webster EW: Garland Lecture. On the question of cancer induction by small x-ray doses. Am J Roentgenol 137:647, 1981

9 Infectious and Parasitic Diseases

Daniel H. Connor and Dean W. Gibson

Diseases Caused by Viruses

Diseases Caused by Mycoplasmas

Diseases Caused by Chlamydiae

Diseases Caused by Rickettsiae

Diseases Caused by Spirochetes

Diseases Caused by Bacteria

Diseases Caused by Filamentous Bacteria

Diseases Caused by the Mycobacteria

Diseases Caused by Protozoans

Diseases Caused by Fungi

Diseases Caused by Filarial Nematodes

Diseases Caused by Other Nematodes

Diseases Caused by Trematodes

Diseases Caused by Cestodes

Diseases Caused by Arthropods

Diseases Caused by Stinging Microorganisms (Marine Invertebrates)

Opportunistic Infections in the Acquired Immune Deficiency Syndrome (AIDS)

Figure 9-1. Epidemiology of yellow fever. The usual reservoir for the yellow fever virus is the tree-dwelling monkey. The virus is passed from monkey to monkey in the forest canopy by mosquitoes of the genus *Aedes*. Felling a tree brings mosquitoes down with the tree, increasing the chance of being bitten and inoculated with the virus.

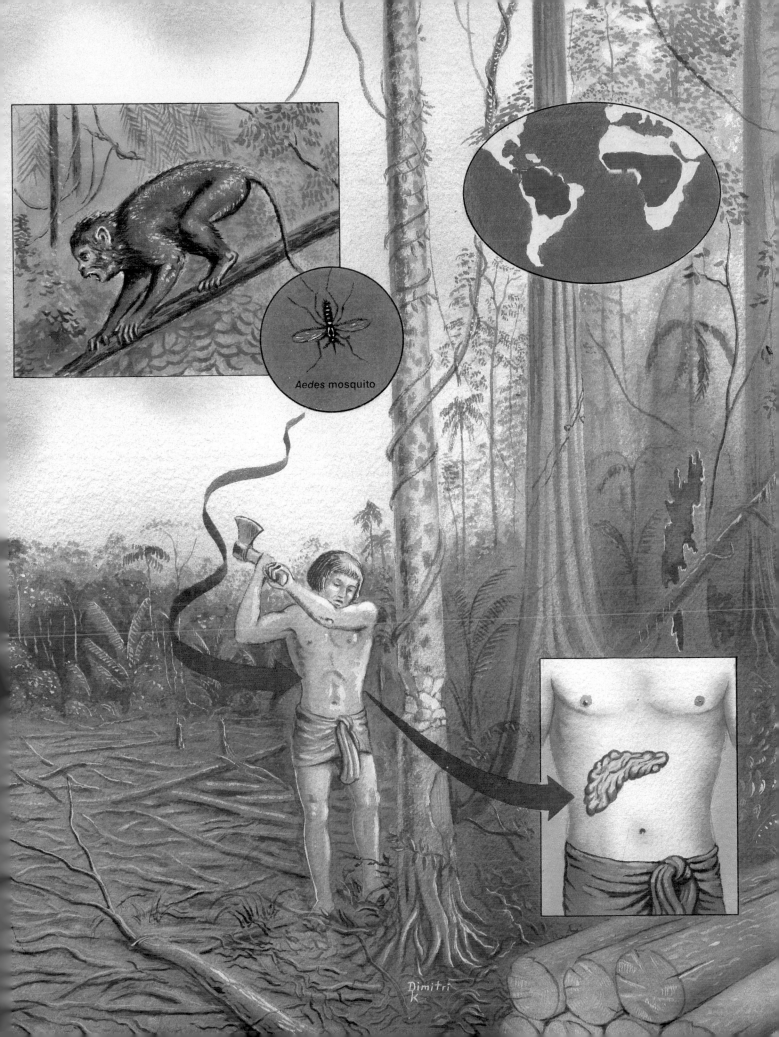

Aedes mosquito

Microorganisms are ubiquitous. They are in the soil, water, and atmosphere, and they cover our body surfaces. Some are distributed throughout the world, others have sharply limited geographical distributions. Genetic drift and mutation produce a steady stream of new variants, which constantly seek new niches to exploit. Many exploitable niches are in the tropical world, where poor sanitation, malnutrition, and crowding contribute to the propagation and transmission of organisms causing malaria, tuberculosis, schistosomiasis, filariasis, and leprosy. Other exploitable niches are debilitated patients in hospitals and persons with defective immune systems.

During the past century the pattern of infection in the developed world has changed dramatically. Tuberculosis, typhoid fever, cholera, smallpox, measles, pertussis, poliomyelitis, malaria, pneumococcal pneumonia, typhus, amebiasis, and syphilis no longer take their relentless toll. Vaccines have controlled or eliminated many diseases (e.g., smallpox, measles, pertussis, and poliomyelitis). Antibiotics have reduced or eliminated the threat of others (e.g., pneumococcal pneumonia). Insecticides have helped control malaria, schistosomiasis, and typhus. The purification of drinking water has lessened the threat of water-borne epidemics (e.g., amebiasis and hepatitis). In spite of these advances, infections still rank fourth as a cause of death in the United States, and the reasons are clear. New strains of microorganisms have emerged to exploit man's weaknesses. Microorganisms resistant to antimicrobial agents appear at regular intervals. Immunosuppressive therapy makes patients with malignant tumors and transplanted organs susceptible to opportunistic infections. Changes in cultural attitudes about sex have contributed to an epidemic of a heretofore unknown fatal disease—the acquired immunodeficiency syndrome (AIDS). Finally, there is the shift in attitudes about medical care. In recent decades medical treatment has become specific and effective, and this in turn has necessitated increasingly specific diagnosis. The trend over the last 50 years has been to bring increasing numbers of patients to the hospital, where the technology for specific diagnosis is concentrated. Although this practice has advantages, it also concentrates patients—many of whom are in weakened states—thus enabling opportunistic infections to flourish.

A focus on pathogenic microorganisms may obscure the fact that most microorganisms benefit us. Microorganisms, in fact, are essential for the "balance of nature" and for our survival. They generate oxygen and fix nitrogen, a process that enriches the soil, and they are the great biodegraders. They have a broad range of relationships with host-organisms, including symbiosis, commensalism, "true" parasitism, and saprophytism.

Symbiosis is defined as a cooperative association between two dissimilar organisms, beneficial to both and required for the survival of both (e.g., *E. coli* in the human intestinal tract).

Commensalism involves dissimilar organisms living together to the benefit of one (the commensal) without injury or benefit to the other. The arrangement is essential for the survival of the commensal organism but not for that of the host (e.g., *Demodex folliculorum* mites in human hair follicles).

True parasitism describes a state in which dissimilar organisms live together to the benefit of the parasite and the detriment of the host. The parasite needs the host for its own survival, so ideally the host survives also. Malaria, schistosomiasis, and other protozoal and helminthic infections involve parasites.

Saprophytism is the condition in which organisms live on dead tissue; for example, dermatophytes living in the surface layers of the skin.

We are thus surrounded and virtually covered by microorganisms. Many of them would invade our bodies were it not for our defenses, which include the following:

1. The integrity of the body surface—namely, the skin and mucous membranes, which constitute natural barriers to microorganisms.
2. The neutrophils, which mobilize in the inflammatory response.
3. The phagocytic cells of the monocyte-macrophage system.
4. The humoral and cellular immune systems.

When the body surfaces are breached or the immune mechanisms fail, organisms that are ordinarily benign invade the body and produce "opportunistic infections." Among the conditions that promote deficient immunity are:

Prematurity
Malnutrition
Congenital defects of immunity
Anatomical defects
Mental and physical stress
Diabetes
Transplantation of organs
Cancer and its treatments
Liver failure
Acquired immune deficiency syndrome

Almost a century ago, Robert Koch, a German microbiologist, formulated rules for establishing a causal connection between a microorganism and a disease. Koch's postulates state that in general (1) the cause of an infectious disease is present in all examples of that disease, (2) the causal organism is recovered in pure culture from lesions that characterize the disease, (3) on inoculation the organism produces similar lesions in animals, and (4) the organism is recovered again in pure culture from the lesions of the animals. Although limited when compared to modern techniques, Koch's postulates enable the microbiologist to recognize many pathogens and to screen out many microorganisms that contaminate lesions. Contrast these postulates with the pathologist's criteria for assigning causality to a microorganism (Table 9-1). First, the characteristic lesions of the disease are defined and contain the causal organism. Second, the causal organism is concentrated in the center of the lesion or has a symmetrical relationship to the lesion. Third, the number of infecting organisms increases while the lesion is active and expanding. Fourth, their numbers diminish and vanish as the lesion resolves.

The pathologist, by first identifying the cause of a disease, guides those attempting to culture the causal organism. For example, these criteria have enabled the identification of an acid-fast bacillus, *Mycobacterium leprae*, as the cause of leprosy. Yet attempts to culture *M. leprae* have been unsuccessful. Similarly, with cat scratch disease, we know by applying the pathologist's criteria that the cause is a gram-negative bacillus. Attempts at culture are now directed toward a bacillus, not toward a virus or chlamydia, as had been done previously. Clearly, the elucidation of the pathogenesis of infectious diseases requires the application of both Koch's postulates and the pathologist's criteria.

Diseases Caused by Viruses

Viral Hemorrhagic Fevers

Viral hemorrhagic fevers are a group of at least 13 distinct acute viral infections that cause varying degrees of hemorrhage and shock, and sometimes death. There are many similar viral hemorrhagic fevers in different parts of the world, often named for the area where they were first described. On the basis of differences in routes of transmission and other epidemiologic characteristics, the viral hemorrhagic fevers have been divided into four groups: mosquito-borne, tick-borne, zoonotic, and the Marburg and Ebola virus group, in which the route of transmission is unknown.

Table 9-1 Comparison of Microbiologist's Criteria (Koch's Postulates) and Pathologist's Criteria for Establishing a Microorganism as the Cause of a Disease or Lesion

Microbiologist's Criteria (Koch's Postulates)	Pathologist's Criteria
The causative organism	The causative organism
1. is in all patients with the disease	1. is in the lesion that characterizes the disease*
2. must be isolated from lesions in pure culture	2. is centered in, or has a symmetrical relationship to, the lesion
3. must reproduce the disease in susceptible animals	3. increases in number as the lesion expands
4. must be reisolated from lesions of experimentally infected animals	4. decreases in number and vanishes as the lesion resolves

* Many infectious organisms are also intracellular; they may invade somatic cells of the host, or they may be phagocytosed by neutrophils or by macrophages.

Mosquito-Borne Group (Aedes *Species as Vectors*)

Yellow Fever

Yellow fever is an acute viral hemorrhagic fever caused by a flavivirus of the family Togaviridae and characterized by jaundice and renal damage. It is primarily a zoonosis of simians that is transmitted by mosquitoes.

First described in the Caribbean, yellow fever is the oldest known viral hemorrhagic fever. The virus is restricted to certain regions of Africa and South America, including both jungle and urban settings, and is antigenically related to the flaviviruses that cause dengue and other hemorrhagic fevers.

The usual reservoir is tree-dwelling monkeys, the virus being passed among them in the forest canopy by mosquitoes. These monkeys are a good reservoir because the virus neither kills them nor makes them ill. Humans acquire jungle yellow fever by entering the forest and being bitten and inoculated by *Aedes* mosquitoes (Fig. 9-1). Felling trees increases the risk because mosquitoes are brought down with the tree. On returning to the village or city, the victim becomes the reservoir for epidemic yellow fever in the urban setting, where *Aedes aegyptii* is the vector.

In yellow fever there is usually a short incubation period (3–6 days), followed by sudden onset of high fever, chills, headache, and myalgia (lasting 3–4 days). A second stage consists of hepatic failure, renal failure, bleeding diathesis, leukopenia, and hypotension. Yellow fever tends to heal without sequelae, and mortality is less than 5%.

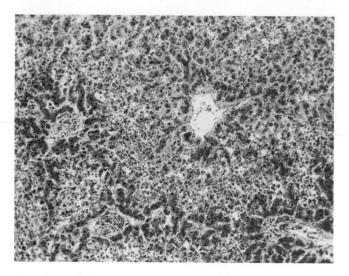

Figure 9-2. Yellow fever, showing midzonal necrosis in the liver. There is a rim of surviving parenchymal cells around the central veins and portal tracts.

The major pathologic changes are in the liver and kidney. The liver is bile-stained and has an accentuated lobular pattern caused by midzonal necrosis. Microscopically, there are three characteristic changes: **midzonal necrosis** (Fig. 9-2); **Councilman bodies**; and **microvesicular fat.** At first, there is focal coagulative necrosis of discrete liver cells and small clusters of cells. Necrotic areas coalesce to form broad patterns of midzonal necrosis. In later stages (e.g., beyond day 8), when the infection is fatal, the necrosis spreads to involve almost the entire lobule, but characteristically spares a single row of parenchymal cells around portal tracts. Councilman bodies are intensely eosinophilic oval bodies that represent necrotic parenchymal cells that have lost their nuclei and have been extruded from the liver cell plate. Councilman bodies are found free in the sinusoids or are phagocytosed by Kupffer's cells. Fat is a constant feature, and a diagnosis of yellow fever should not be made without it. Two less obvious features that help distinguish yellow fever from other kinds of necrotizing hepatitis are the preservation of the overall architecture of the liver, including the reticulin framework, and the lack of a significant inflammatory response in the parenchyma or the portal tracts (see Fig. 9-2). The microscopic differential diagnosis of the inflammatory and necrotizing changes in the liver includes viral hepatitis, dengue, and Weil's disease (leptospirosis).

The kidney exhibits coagulative necrosis of the proximal tubules, fat accumulation in the tubular epithelium, and hemorrhage. Changes in other organs include edema and petechial hemorrhages in the brain, degeneration of myofibrils and increased fat in the heart, follicular hyperplasia in the spleen and lymph nodes, and hemorrhages in the skin, gingiva, and gastrointestinal tract.

Dengue Fever

Uncomplicated dengue fever (breakbone fever), a disease of densely populated areas, is a benign, self-limited, febrile disease that affects muscles and joints. By contrast, dengue hemorrhagic fever, a severe and potentially fatal variant, is characterized by high fever, cutaneous and intestinal hemorrhage, thrombocytopenia, shock, and neurologic disturbances. First seen in an epidemic in the Philippines (1954), the variant spread during the 1950s and 1960s. It is a disease of children throughout Southeast Asia, Indonesia, and Pakistan, and there was an outbreak in Cuba in 1981. Transmission is highest during and after the rainy season, when mosquitoes are most numerous.

Chikungunya Hemorrhagic Fever

Chikungunya hemorrhagic fever is a rare variant of Chikungunya fever—the latter being characterized by fever, muscle and joint pains, myocarditis, hematemesis, melena, shock, and, rarely, death. Man is the only known vertebrate host. Chikungunya fever was first recognized in East Africa (1952) and occurs over an extensive area of subSaharan Africa, India, Southeast Asia, and the Philippines. An outbreak of the hemorrhagic variant occurred in Bangkok in 1962, and subsequently in India.

Rift Valley Fever

Rift Valley fever is an acute viral infection of sheep, cattle, and humans in which nonspecific, influenza-like symptoms (headache, fever, myalgia, etc.) are prominent. The disease was first described in Kenya, and there have been epizootics in southern and eastern Africa and in the Sudan and Egypt. Hemorrhagic complications resembling those of yellow fever develop in some patients and may be fatal.

Tick-Borne Group (Transmitted by the Bite of Infected Ticks)

Crimean Hemorrhagic Fever

Crimean hemorrhagic fever is distinguished by a diphasic high fever and hemorrhages in mucous membranes, lungs, and the genitourinary and gastrointestinal tracts. It is often accompanied by pneumonitis, pulmonary hemorrhages, and edema. Animal reservoirs are small wild mammals (especially rodents), domesticated animals (sheep, cattle, goats, and hares), and birds. It was originally reported among farm workers in Crimea, USSR (1944), and recurs annually in a wide belt across Africa, in the eastern Balkan States, and in the Soviet Central Asian republics bordering the shores of the Black and Caspian Seas.

Omsk Hemorrhagic Fever

Omsk hemorrhagic fever resembles Crimean fever and was first described in the Asiatic USSR (1947). Endemic to the forested steppe–lake region of western Siberia, its animal reservoir is principally rodents. Infections in humans come from the bites of infected ticks or from contact with muskrats killed by hunters, in which case the muskrats were bitten by ticks infected with the virus from small rodents.

Kyasanur Forest Disease

Kyasanur Forest disease, characterized by diphasic fever, hemorrhage, and nonspecific symptoms, was first identified in humans following an epizootic in monkeys in the Indian state of Mysore (1957). The reservoir is small rodents, but Rhesus and Langur monkeys and humans are infected, although they are not part of the natural chain.

The Zoonotic Group

Korean Hemorrhagic Fever

Hemorrhagic fever with renal syndrome (Korean hemorrhagic fever) occurs in rural communities exposed to saliva and urine of infected rodents. The illness was known to Russians in Vladivostok (1890), and similar diseases are found across the entire Eurasian land mass, from European and Asiatic Russia to Manchuria, Korea, and Japan. The disease became known to American medicine when it struck United Nations troops serving in Korea in 1951, hence the misnomer "Korean." Recovery is usual, but fatal cases do occur. In such cases, morphologic evidence of shock is present. There is a mononuclear cell infiltrate in the sinusoids of liver and spleen, and throughout the body damage to the capillaries is manifested by dilatation, engorgement, diapedesis of erythrocytes, and rupture. Recently, viral antigen has been found in endothelial cells.

Argentine Hemorrhagic Fever

Argentine hemorrhagic fever is a severe illness whose symptoms resemble those of "Korean" hemorrhagic fever. An epidemic developed in rural agricultural areas and villages northwest of Buenos Aires in 1958. The virus is found naturally in wild rodents and may be transmitted in food or contaminated airborne dust.

Bolivian Hemorrhagic Fever

Bolivian hemorrhagic fever is an acute febrile disease with hemorrhagic manifestations that are almost identical to those of Argentine hemorrhagic fever. The virus is similar to that which causes Argentine hemorrhagic fever, and its reservoir is also wild rodents. Bolivian hemorrhagic fever was first recognized in rural areas of northeastern Bolivia (1959), and there were two major epidemics in Bolivian villages during 1962-64.

Lassa Fever

Lassa fever is a serious, highly infectious, viral hemorrhagic disease characterized by high fever, prostration, generalized hemorrhages, abdominal pain, vomiting, diarrhea, severe pharyngitis, dyspnea, serous effusions, facial edema, and shock. It is fatal in almost half the cases. The Lassa virus emerged suddenly and may be a virulent mutant of the lymphocytic choriomeningitis virus. The Lassa virus appears to have a natural cycle of transmission in rodents and has been isolated repeatedly from a rat, *Mastomys natalensis*. Lassa fever was first recognized in herdsmen's villages in Nigeria in 1969 and also occurs in Liberia and Sierra Leone. The disease spreads from patients to uninfected persons in households and hospitals.

Marburg and Ebola Virus Group (Unknown Route)

Marburg Virus Disease

Marburg virus disease, a severe, distinctive hemorrhagic illness with a high rate of mortality, is heralded early by severe sore throat, a maculopapular rash, and a red exanthem on the hard and soft palate. Later, severe, generalized bleeding dominates the clinical course. The disease was first recognized in 1967 in Marburg, Germany, and in Yugoslavia among laboratory workers exposed to blood and tissues from African green monkeys imported from Uganda. There have been subsequent outbreaks in South Africa, Kenya, and Zimbabwe. The Marburg and Ebola viruses are interpreted as the first recognized viruses of a newly named family, the Filiviridae. Although the route of transmission is unproved, Marburg virus disease is probably transmitted in the blood of monkeys.

Ebola Virus Disease

Ebola virus disease is an acute hemorrhagic fever that closely resembles Marburg virus disease and also has a high mortality. The disease was first recognized in outbreaks in the Sudan and northern Zaire (1976).

Although the natural host and the route of transmission are uncertain, the Ebola virus appears to be spread mainly by close and prolonged contact with an infected person or by inoculation from contaminated syringes and needles.

Arthropod-Borne Viral Encephalitis (Arbovirus Encephalitis)

Arthropod-borne viruses (arboviruses) are a large, heterogeneous group of viruses transmitted between vertebrates by blood-sucking arthropod vectors, such as mosquitoes and ticks. Replication of the virus in vertebrates causes severe illness, but in the arthropod it is harmless. Most arbovirus infections are zoonoses among wild and domestic animals, especially birds and mammals. Man becomes accidentally infected if bitten by an infected arthropod. There are eight arboviruses that cause meningoencephalitis in man, and each of the arthropod-borne viral encephalitides is confined to a particular geographic area and a specific vector. In temperate zones, the climate affects the breeding of arthropods and the abundance of vertebrate hosts, thus resulting in seasonal variation in each disease. In tropical areas seasonal variation is less pronounced. The arthropod transmits the virus to a person from one of the reservoir animals but not from another person.

People of all ages are susceptible to these diseases. Clinical symptoms range from a mild grippe-like illness to fulminating and fatal encephalitis. The encephalitis usually begins abruptly, with fever, headache, disturbed consciousness and sometimes signs of meningitis, convulsions, or paralysis. The clinical course is usually short, not chronic as in some other viral infections. The diseases share many common features, but each type has a different course. For example, Eastern equine encephalitis is commonly a severe fulminant encephalitis that kills in a few days, whereas Venezuelan equine encephalitis is a mild disease.

The histologic findings in these encephalitides are usually confined to the central nervous system and are similar for all types. The lesions range from a mild meningitis with scattered lymphocytes to more severe inflammation of the gray matter, mainly around neurons, to prominent necrosis. Perivascular cuffing appears in the acute phase. In contrast to the other infections, Eastern equine encephalitis exhibits neutrophilic rather than lymphocytic inflammation and extensive meningitis, resembling a pyogenic infection. Vasculitis and thrombosis lead to numerous foci of necrosis, which extend into the white matter. Some of the necrotic foci resemble microabscesses.

Encephalitis Caused by Alphaviruses (Formerly "Group A" Arboviruses)

Eastern Equine Encephalitis

Eastern equine encephalitis (EEE) is encountered primarily in the eastern and north central United States and adjoining provinces of Canada. The reservoir is birds. Horses and humans have "dead-end" infections. Mosquitoes are vectors. Epizootics among horses usually precede epidemics in humans. EEE occurs primarily during summer in temperate zones.

Western Equine Encephalitis

Western equine encephalitis (WEE) is encountered primarily in the western and central United States and Canada (it is also found, less frequently, in Brazil); the reservoir is birds, but horses and humans have "dead-end" infections. Vectors are mosquitoes. WEE occurs primarily in May to September.

Venezuelan Equine Encephalitis

Venezuelan equine encephalitis (VEE) is encountered principally in Venezuela, Colombia, Central America, Mexico, and the southwestern United States. The reservoir is rodents, many other mammals, and birds. Horses and humans have "dead-end" infections. Vectors are mosquitoes. VEE occurs throughout the year.

Encephalitis Caused by Flaviviruses

St. Louis Encephalitis

St. Louis encephalitis (SLE) occurs throughout the United States (except New England), in Ontario, Canada, and less frequently in scattered areas in the Caribbean and Central and South America. **SLE is the most important arbovirus infection in North America.** The reservoir is birds; vectors are mosquitoes. SLE occurs during late summer and early fall.

Japanese B Encephalitis

Japanese B encephalitis (JBE) occurs in Japan, China, Korea, the Philippines, eastern and southeastern Asia, Siberia, India, and Nepal; the reservoir is birds and pigs, but humans have incidental "dead-end" infections; vectors are mosquitoes. JBE occurs during late summer and in epidemics of CNS disease throughout the orient.

Encephalitis Caused by a Bunyavirus

California Encephalitis

California encephalitis (CE) is encountered in California and the north-central United States. The reservoir is probably rodents such as squirrels, cotton rats, and rabbits; vectors are mosquitoes. CE occurs in summer.

Poliomyelitis

Poliomyelitis is an acute infection by polioviruses. Most infections are asymptomatic, but when the virus invades the central nervous system it destroys lower motor neurons, causing paralysis.

Sporadic infections may be seen at any time, but outbreaks occur mostly in summer. More recent epidemics have stricken adults as well as children. Polio was sporadic in earlier centuries, but became epidemic in the first decades of this century and subsequently pandemic, the incidence having peaked during the 1950s in many developed countries. Immunization has stopped its spread in the Western world, but polio remains a major public health problem in many developing countries where sewage is untreated.

Poliovirus is transmitted in drinking water contaminated with feces (Fig. 9-3). The virus replicates in the mucosa of the small intestine. Some virions pass from there into the feces, contaminating water and completing the cycle. Others enter the bloodstream (viremia) and extend to the spinal cord, where they infect and destroy the anterior horn cells, causing paralysis.

Smallpox (Variola)

Before its eradication, smallpox (variola) was an acute, highly contagious, exanthematous viral infection. The virus contains double-stranded DNA and produces a typical plaque, or "pock," when cultured on the chorioallantoic membrane of embryonated chicken eggs. Since Jenner's pioneering work in 1796, a similar virus—vaccinia, the causative agent of cowpox—has been used for "vaccination" to protect against smallpox.

Smallpox was evidently an ancient disease; a rash resembling smallpox was found in the mummified remains of the Egyptian Pharaoh Ramses V, who died in 1160 BC. The disease once had worldwide distribution in both urban and rural areas, afflicting persons of both genders and all ages, but particularly children.

In 1967, the World Health Organization began its uniquely successful campaign to eradicate smallpox. By then, smallpox had already been controlled in most developed countries but was still endemic in the less developed world. In 10 years the vaccination campaign eradicated the disease. The successful eradication of smallpox depended on several factors,

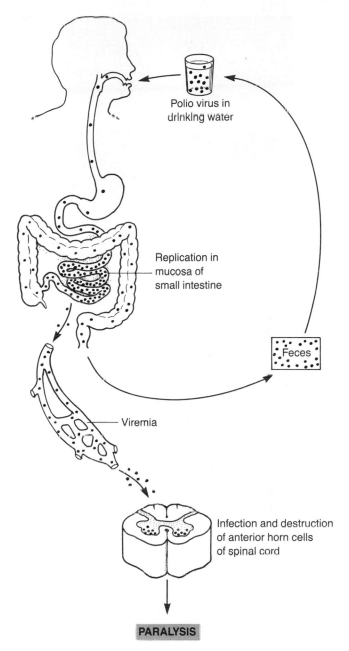

Figure 9-3. Poliovirus. Poliovirus is transmitted in drinking water contaminated with feces. Virions replicate in the mucosa of the small intestine, and some pass into the feces to contaminate water and complete the cycle. Others enter the circulation, invade the spinal cord, and destroy the anterior horn cells, causing paralysis of the lower motor neuron.

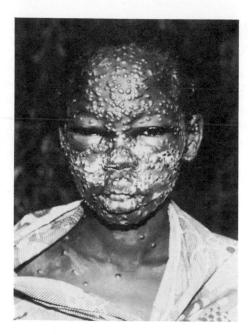

Figure 9-4.   Smallpox, eastern Zaire, 1968.

including the permanence of immunity following vaccination, the stability of the smallpox virus (in contrast to the genetic instability of influenza viruses and many others), and the lack of an animal reservoir for the virus.

Smallpox was transmitted in respiratory droplets and almost always involved face-to-face contact. The virus infected the oropharynx or nasopharynx, multiplied in lymphoid tissue of the upper respiratory tract for about 2 days, invaded the circulation for a 2-day period of viremia and then entered a 4- to 14-day "latent" period, when it was undetectable in the blood and was assumed to be multiplying in the reticuloendothelial system. After another 1- or 2-day period of viremia, there was a 2- to 4-day prodrome of nonspecific febrile symptoms.

The prodrome was followed by the characteristic eruption of smallpox, which evolved through several stages, beginning as macules, then progressing over a 1- to 2-week period through papules, vesicles, and pustules (Fig. 9-4). The pustules umbilicated within 2 weeks, and desiccated ("crust") to form scabs. The scabs, which contained the smallpox virus, usually sloughed from the skin, thereby creating fresh, pitted scars. Pitting or pockmarking was most common over facial areas that have numerous sebaceous glands. In the most severe form, black, "hemorrhagic smallpox", which was almost always fatal, there was bleeding into the vesicles and pustules. Histologic features of the earliest stage of the rash included

hyperemia, swelling of capillary endothelium, and perivascular infiltrates of lymphocytes and histiocytes in the upper dermis. Multiloculated vesicles developed by rupture of the membranes between degenerating epidermal cells. There was ballooning of cells in the lower levels of the stratum spinosum, and some degenerating cells fused into giant cells with two to four nuclei. Eosinophilic intracytoplasmic inclusion bodies **(Guarnieri's bodies)** were prominent in ballooned epithelial cells.

Secondary bacterial infections during the pustular stage led to complications such as keratitis, laryngitis, bronchitis, bronchopneumonia, encephalitis, osteomyelitis, and orchitis. Viral keratitis and secondary bacterial infections of the eyes were frequent complications. Many patients in Asia developed corneal ulcerations, and smallpox was usually the primary cause of blindness during epidemic periods. In pregnant women, the disease frequently caused abortion.

Herpesvirus Infections

Five herpesviruses infect man: varicella-zoster virus; herpes simplex virus, types 1 and 2; cytomegalovirus; and Epstein-Barr virus (EBV). Varicella-zoster virus causes chickenpox in nonimmune persons and shingles in those who have had chickenpox. Herpes simplex viruses 1 and 2 cause "fever blisters" and genital lesions, respectively. Cytomegalovirus is the agent of cytomegalic inclusion disease, and Epstein-Barr virus causes infectious mononucleosis. Each of these viruses may disseminate and kill patients with defective or suppressed immunity.

Herpesviruses are enveloped double-stranded DNA viruses with similar ultrastructural features. All have icosahedral symmetry and all are about the same size (approximately 200 nm across). They are among the largest viruses. They replicate in the cell nucleus, have an affinity for cells of ectodermal origin, produce vesicles or pocks, and produce latent infections. **A principal histologic feature is the formation of Cowdry type A intranuclear inclusions in epithelial and other cells of the host.** These acidophilic (red with eosin) inclusions have a diameter that exceeds half the diameter of the nucleus and are surrounded by a clear zone ("halo") of vacant nucleoplasm. Herpesvirus infections also cause the formation of syncytial giant cells by aggregation and fusion of infected epithelial cells. These giant cells may also contain intranuclear inclusions.

Varicella (Chickenpox)—Varicella-Zoster Virus

Varicella (chickenpox) is an acute vesicular exanthem caused by the varicella-zoster virus, an agent that has a worldwide distribution and for which humans are the only known host. Although all age groups are susceptible, in temperate zones chickenpox affects mostly children and in the tropics mostly young adults. The virus, which is spread through inhalation of droplets or by direct contact, is highly contagious from about 24 hours before the initial eruption to a week or more thereafter. Although infection with varicella-zoster virus establishes lifelong immunity and chickenpox does not recur, the latent viral genome may be activated years later to cause shingles.

Nonimmune persons (usually children) are susceptible to primary infection with varicella-zoster virus. Chickenpox begins as a "silent" infection of the nasopharynx, with local replication of varicella-zoster virus. After an incubation period of 10 to 23 days, the virus enters the bloodstream, causing viremia and a sudden onset of fever, malaise, and anorexia. In the circulation it seeds reticuloendothelial cells, an effect that leads to secondary waves of viremia. The virus then disseminates to skin and viscera, and within 24 to 48 hours a red maculopapular eruption develops, usually on the upper trunk and face. The papules rapidly become clear vesicles with an erythematous base. In the next 24 hours, the vesicles become cloudy, the eruption begins to itch, and scratching may rupture the vesicles. Separate crops appear for 3 to 6 days and spread peripherally. After the last crop, the scabs heal without scarring. Although vesicles of the skin are generally painless, painful lesions may develop on mucous membranes, such as the cornea and tympanic membrane. Complications include pneumonia, encephalitis, hepatitis, carditis, keratitis, orchitis, arthritis, hemorrhages, and acute encephalopathy with fat accumulation in the viscera (Reye's syndrome).

Histologically, the skin lesions initially show ballooning of epidermal cells. Later, unilocular vesicles containing proteinaceous fluid, degenerating cells, and syncytial giant cells are seen. Cowdry type A intranuclear inclusions are in epidermal cells, endothelial cells of superficial capillaries, reticuloendothelial cells, and fibroblasts. The affected organs in chicken pox exhibit spherical foci of coagulative necrosis. At the margin of these necrotic foci, surviving cells contain intranuclear inclusions, as shown in Figure 9-5.

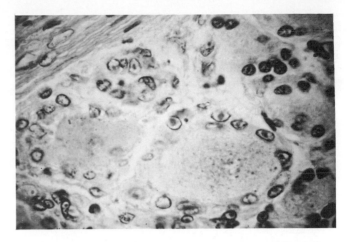

Figure 9-5. Section of cerebrum from a patient with necrotizing meningoencephalitis caused by varicella virus. Intranuclear inclusions in disseminated infections with herpesviruses (VZV, HSV-1, and HSV-2) are indistinguishable with routine stains. The inclusions are coalesced viral nucleoplasm typical of Cowdry type A inclusions. They are eosinophilic, more than half the diameter of the nucleus, and surrounded by a "halo."

Herpes Zoster (Shingles)—Varicella-Zoster Virus

Herpes zoster (shingles) is a recurrent, painful, erythematous vesicular eruption caused by the reactivation of latent varicella-zoster virus in an individual who had chickenpox years earlier. Adults with shingles may transmit the virus to children and cause chickenpox. During the latent phase, the virus resides in the dorsal root spinal ganglion or the cranial nerve ganglion (see Fig. 9-5). On reactivation, the virus spreads from the ganglia along sensory nerves to peripheral nerves of the sensory dermatomes. Attacks of shingles produce cutaneous lesions that resemble varicella. In shingles, however, the eruptions are limited to one or more sensory dermatomes, and the vesicles or bullae may be few. Shingles is painful, especially in older people, in contrast to the painless vesicles of children with chickenpox. Eventually the scales over the vesicles slough, and symptoms remit until another attack.

Herpes Simplex—Herpes Simplex Virus Type 1

Herpes simplex virus type 1 is responsible for a spectrum of vesicular and necrotizing lesions, principally on the skin, lips, and mucous membranes. Neonates

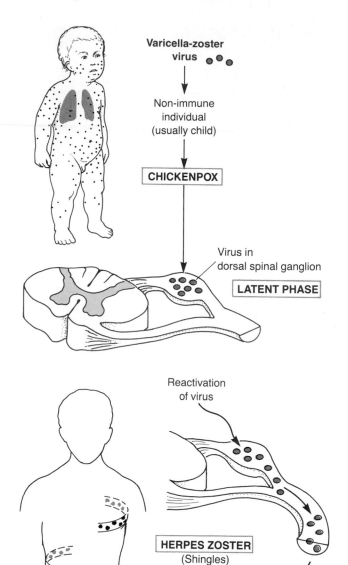

and immunodeficient patients may have disseminated infections, with involvement of many organs, including the liver, lung, and brain. Humans are the natural hosts for herpesvirus 1, but some animals are also susceptible. Transmission is usually by kissing, crowding, and direct contact, although fomites may also be infectious for a short time after contamination. The virus causes sporadic outbreaks in nurseries, schools, and hospitals. Primary lesions occur in those with no previous exposure and no antibodies. Recurrent lesions are common.

Those without debilitating disease or immunodeficiency, and infants older than 1 month, have a mild infection, lesions being localized to the oral cavity, lips, eyes, and skin. This includes gingivostomatitis—commonly known as a "fever blister" or "cold sore" (Fig. 9-7). Even in these "mild" forms, the lesions may be painful. On rare occasions, in patients of any age the virus may disseminate and kill. In addition to dissemination, complications include keratoconjunctivitis, meningoencephalitis, and aseptic spinal meningitis. Microscopically, the vesicular lesions and the foci of coagulation necrosis in parenchymatous organs are indistinguishable from those described for the varicella-zoster virus.

During acute gingivostomatitis or asymptomatic primary infection of the oropharynx, the virus invades nerve endings in mucous membranes of the mouth, ascends within axons, and establishes a latent infection in the trigeminal ganglion that persists for life. Various stimuli—e.g., fever, exposure to actinic light, respiratory infections, and stress—reactivate the latent virus. It then descends within the axon to peripheral nerve twigs, reinfects the lip or adjacent mucous membrane, and causes recurrent blisters.

Genital Herpes—Herpes Simplex Virus Type 2

Genital herpes, caused by herpes simplex virus type 2, is sexually transmitted and produces a spectrum of vesicular and necrotizing lesions on or about the genitalia (see Fig. 9-7). As with herpes simplex virus Type 1, primary lesions develop in those without previous exposure and without antibodies, and recurrent lesions are common. **Neonates are especially susceptible to disseminated herpes simplex virus Type 2.** Normal adults and infants older than 1 month have mild infections that present as vesicles on the mucous membranes of the genitalia and on the external genitalia. There may be large, solitary ulcers on the genitalia or lips, and swollen regional

Figure 9-6.   Varicella (chickenpox) and herpes zoster (shingles).

Varicella (chickenpox). Varicella-zoster virus (VZV) in droplets is inhaled by a nonimmune person (usually a child) and initially causes a "silent" infection of the nasopharynx. This progresses to viremia, seeding of reticuloendothelial cells, and dissemination of VZV to skin and viscera. The VZV resides in a dorsal spinal ganglion, where it remains dormant for many years.

Herpes zoster. Latent VZV is reactivated and spreads from ganglia along the sensory nerves to the peripheral nerves of sensory dermatomes.

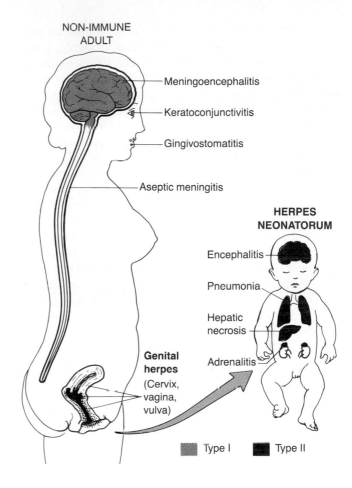

Figure 9-7. Herpesvirus infections.
Herpes simplex. Herpes simplex virus type 1 (HSV-1) infects a nonimmune adult, causing gingivostomatitis ("fever blister" or "cold sore"), keratoconjunctivitis, meningoencephalitis, and aseptic spinal meningitis.
Genital herpes. Herpes simplex virus type 2 (HSV-2) infects the genitalia of a nonimmune adult, involving the cervix, vagina, and vulva.
Herpes neonatorum. HSV-2 infects the fetus as it passes through the birth canal of an infected mother. The infant's lack of a mature immune system results in disseminated infection with HSV-2. The infection is often fatal, involving lung, liver, adrenal glands, and central nervous system.

lymph nodes. Microscopically, the vesicular lesions are indistinguishable from those of herpes simplex virus Type 1. Latent infections are established in a manner analogous to that for the Type 1 virus. During primary genital herpes (even when asymptomatic) the virus invades sensory nerve endings in the genital mucosa, ascends within axons, and establishes a latent infection in sensory neurons within the corresponding sacral ganglia. Months or years later, nonspecific stimuli, including menses and sexual intercourse, reactivate the virus, which descends within axons to the genital mucosa or skin and causes a recurrent genital herpetic lesion.

Cytomegalic Inclusion Disease— Cytomegalovirus

Cytomegalic inclusion disease, an infection with cytomegalovirus, may be congenital; perinatal; postnatal in infants after loss of maternal antibodies; "classic" in older adolescents and adults with "normal" immunity; or a disseminated, possibly lethal, opportunistic infection in immunodeficient persons, including those with lymphomas, leukemias, and AIDS. The general population has a high incidence of exposure to this virus, as indicated by seropositivity rates of 50% to 80% among adults. There is special concern for infection in pregnant women, because cytomegalovirus may be transmitted to the fetus or infant.

The modes of transmission are the following: (1) intrauterine, from the placenta and maternal circulation; (2) perinatal, as the fetus passes through the birth canal; (3) venereal, from semen or vaginal fluid; (4) mammary, from mother's milk; (5) respiratory, from inhalation of contaminated droplets; (6) transfusional, from latent virus in circulating leukocytes; and (7) transplantational, from grafts taken from donors with latent infections.

The target organs and severity vary with the mode of transmission. Infections *in utero* damage the brain, sometimes causing mental retardation or death of the fetus. Infants with congenital infections may be premature and exhibit anemia, thrombocytopenia, jaundice, purpura, hepatosplenomegaly (from extramedullary hematopoiesis), and interstitial pneumonitis. On the other hand, most congenital infections produce no clinically apparent lesions at birth. However, even asymptomatic congenital infections may enter the latent phase and be reactivated years later to cause more serious disease.

The most prominent feature of classic cytomegalic inclusion disease in neonates is the one for which it is named, **the cytomegalic inclusion.** Compared to epithelial cells without inclusions, those that contain inclusions are greatly enlarged. These inclusions, which are more characteristic than any of the other viral inclusions, are typically intranuclear, but may also be intracytoplasmic. The nucleus is enlarged and the chromatin marginated. The round nuclear inclusion is large, sharply outlined, and either amphophilic or eosinophilic. The cytoplasmic inclusions, when present, tend to be amphophilic and of variable shape.

Cytomegalic inclusions are seen in any organ, common sites being the salivary gland, lung, liver, kidney, intestine, pancreas, thyroid, adrenal gland, and brain. Inclusions may be observed in the urinary sediment. The small and large intestines may be ulcerated in addition to having cytomegalic inclusions. Lesions of the brain include focal acute inflammatory cell infiltrates, inclusions in endothelial cells of blood vessels and in subependymal and subpial tissue, calcifications about the ventricles, and damage to ganglion cells.

Postnatal infections during the first year of life develop after the loss of maternal antibodies, but they tend to be mild or asymptomatic. More severe cases present with hepatosplenomegaly and interstitial pneumonia. Infections are much less common in children 1 to 15 years of age, but occur with greater frequency in adolescents and adults who have "normal" immunity. In adult infections, cytomegalic inclusions are often limited to lung and intestine. Thus, pneumonia—sometimes prolonged—may be a prominent feature in adults but not in neonates. By contrast, brain involvement is rare in adults common in neonates.

Infectious Mononucleosis—Epstein-Barr Virus

Infectious mononucleosis, a benign, self-limited disease, results from infection with the Epstein-Barr virus. It is characterized by intense proliferation of lymphoid cells in the spleen, lymph nodes, and blood. Patients have "heterophile antibody" (agglutinin) in their serum. Epstein-Barr virus has the appearance of a herpesvirus, but it does not have significant serologic cross-reactivity with other viruses of the herpes group. Many people in western countries are asymptomatic carriers.

In most of the world, primary infection with Epstein-Barr virus is an asymptomatic childhood illness. On the other hand, infectious mononucleosis usually occurs in late adolescence in the upper socioeconomic classes—that is, among those who are unlikely to be exposed in childhood. The virus is commonly transmitted by kissing. In a seronegative person, the virus replicates within the salivary glands or pharyngeal epithelium and is shed into the saliva and respiratory secretions (Fig. 9-8). The virus then infects B-lymphocytes, which have receptors for the virus. Polyclonal activation of infected B cells leads to transformed B cells that activate two types of lymphocytes: T_K ("killer") lymphocytes, which kill B cells, and T_S ("suppressor") lymphocytes, which suppress polyclonal immunoglobulin production by B cells. **The activated T cells are the so-called atypical lymphocytes characteristic of infectious mononucleosis.**

The death of B cells causes immunologic responses that may be used to monitor the disease. Early IgM antibodies (heterophile antibodies) are followed by IgG antibodies to viral capsid antigen, virus-neutralizing antibodies, and antibodies to cell membranes of infected B cells. The heterophile antibody persists for only 3-6 months. After these immune responses "free" virus disappears from the blood, but the viral genome is "hidden" in a latent form being integrated into the DNA of virus-transformed B cells that remain in the circulation. This lifelong latent infection with Epstein-Barr virus is analogous to latent infections characteristic of the other herpes viruses.

The clinical features of infectious mononucleosis include **the triad of fever, sore throat and lymphadenopathy, atypical T_K ("killer") and B lymphocytes in the blood, and heterophile agglutinin in the serum.** In the blood there is an absolute increase in lymphocytes and monocytes, with more than 10% atypical lymphocytes. Splenomegaly is also a common feature. Chills, headache, rash, abdominal pain, arthralgia, anorexia, jaundice, and encephalitis are less common (Fig. 9-8). Ninety percent of patients have abnormal liver function, half have variable degrees of thrombocytopenia—some with petechiae—and 40% have hemolytic anemia caused by cold agglutinins.

The pathologic changes are prominent in the

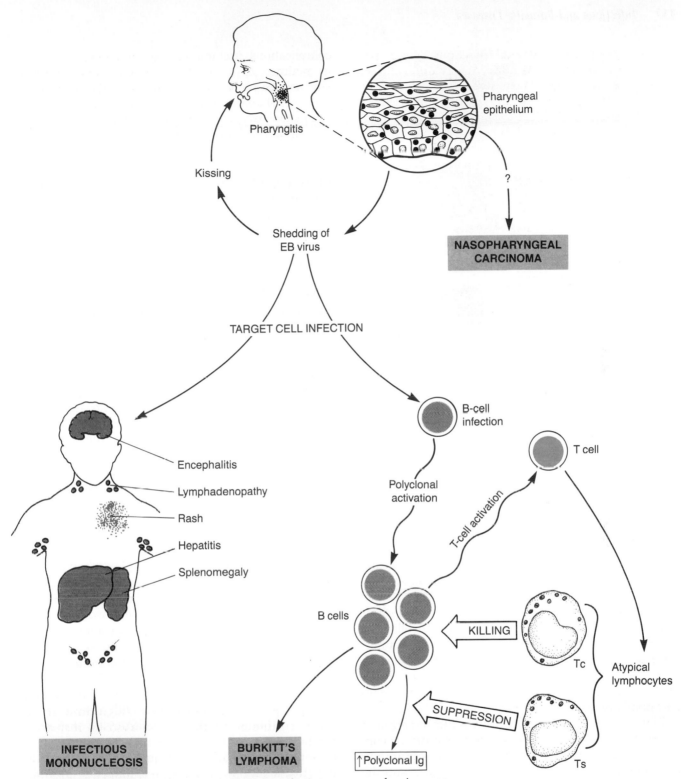

Figure 9-8. Role of Epstein-Barr virus (EBV) in infectious mononucleosis, nasopharyngeal carcinoma, and Burkitt's lymphoma. EBV invades and replicates within the salivary glands or pharyngeal epithelium, and is shed into the saliva and respiratory secretions. In some people, the virus transforms pharyngeal epithelial cells, leading to nasopharyngeal carcinoma. In people who are not immune from childhood exposure, EBV causes infectious mononucleosis. EBV infects B lymphocytes, which undergo polyclonal activation. These B cells stimulate the production of T_k and T_s lymphocytes in the blood of patients with infectious mononucleosis. Some infected B cells are transformed into immature malignant lymphocytes of Burkitt's lymphoma.

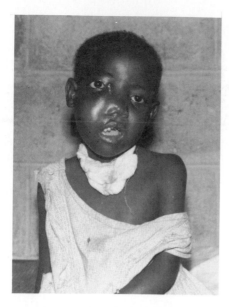

Figure 9-9. Burkitt's lymphoma involving the right maxilla and right mandible of a young African from eastern Zaire.

lymph nodes and spleen because of the underlying immunologic nature of the illness. In most patients the lymphadenopathy is symmetrical and most striking in the neck, and the nodes are movable, discrete, and tender. On gross examination they are soft and swollen, and the hyperemic (pink) cut surfaces occasionally display foci of necrosis. Microscopically, the general architecture is preserved. The germinal centers are large and have indistinct margins because of a proliferation of immunoblasts. They contain frequent mitoses and scattered nuclear debris, presumably from degenerated B cells. The nodes contain occasional large hyperchromatic cells with polylobated nuclei that resemble Reed-Sternberg cells. The immunoblastic hyperplasia and consequent architectural distortion, and the presence of atypical cells, may present diagnostic problems because of the morphologic similarity to Hodgkin's disease or non-Hodgkin's lymphoma.

The spleen is large and soft owing to hyperplasia of the red pulp and is susceptible to rupture. Many immunoblasts are present throughout the pulp and infiltrate the walls of vessels, the trabeculae, and the capsule. The edema and infiltration of the capsule probably account for the tendency to rupture. The liver is almost always involved, but the hepatitis is nonspecific. The sinusoids contain atypical lymphocytes, and there are mild lymphocytic infiltrates in the portal tracts.

Most patients recover completely, although convalescence may be protracted. Uncommon neurologic complications include diffuse or focal encephalitis (sometimes involving the cerebellum) and, occasionally, aseptic meningitis. In the rare fatal cases, meningoencephalitis is the most common cause of death.

Epstein-Barr virus was discovered during ultrastructural studies of endemic Burkitt's lymphoma in Africa. There is now strong evidence that the virus causes two cancers—endemic Burkitt's lymphoma in Africa (Fig. 9-9) and nasopharyngeal carcinoma, especially in the Orient.

Measles (Rubeola)

Measles (rubeola) is an acute, highly contagious, systemic infection of childhood caused by the measles (rubeola) virus. Humans are the only reservoir. Most commonly transmitted by inhalation, it may also be passed through the placenta. Unlike German measles (rubella), rubeola does not cause congenital abnormalities.

Infants up to about 6 months of age are protected by maternal antibodies, but thereafter are vulnerable. The highest incidence and mortality are in developing countries, where nutrition and hygiene tend to be poor. Epidemics of measles in the past have caused high mortality among Polynesians and Eskimos, the lack of prior exposure, racial susceptibility, and poor nutrition being possible factors. At one time the developed countries had epidemics, especially in winter and spring, but the measles vaccine has all but eliminated measles in much of the industrialized world.

The incubation period is 14 days (range 10-21 days). After contaminated droplets are inhaled, virions enter the lymphoid tissue of the tonsils, adenoids, and lymph nodes, cause leukopenia and hyperplasia of the reticuloendothelial system, and then enter the blood. The initial signs and symptoms of the prodrome are fever, conjunctivitis, prominent dry cough, coryza, and **"Koplik's spots,"** a hallmark. These spots on the buccal mucosa are red, irregular macules, 1 to 3 mm in diameter, with a central white speck. (Although these are characteristic of measles, similar spots are occasionally seen in other viral infections.) Other early symptoms include lymphadenopathy, splenomegaly, and respiratory symptoms.

The prodrome, which lasts 3 to 5 days, recedes with the appearance of the blotchy, erythematous rash of measles. The rash begins as pink macules behind the ears, quickly becomes maculopapular and rapidly spreads over the face and down the neck, trunk, and limbs. The macules often coalesce and become purple, with edema of the underlying skin, but the rash rarely becomes confluent. The nonproductive cough increases as the rash develops. The rash lasts a few days and then clears with epidermal scaling, while the fever and other symptoms rapidly abate. Rarely, patients develop a fulminating, hemorrhagic (black) measles that is often fatal.

Microscopically, the affected skin displays dilated epidermal vesicles, edema, and a nonspecific, moderate infiltrate of mononuclear cells and occasional neutrophils in the dermal capillary bed. Koplik spots contain giant cells and epithelial cells with intranuclear inclusions. Lymphoid tissue commonly shows follicular hyperplasia. The **"Warthin-Finkeldey" giant cells, which are pathognomonic for measles,** contain up to 100 nuclei (Fig. 9-10) and both intracytoplasmic and intranuclear inclusions. These cells are found in lymph nodes, other reticuloendothelial organs, and lymphoid tissues of the pharynx, bronchi, and gastrointestinal tract, including the appendix. Warthin-Finkeldey giant cells vanish when circulating antibodies appear.

Measles is usually benign in children with normal immunity, but can have serious or catastrophic complications in the malnourished, in the immunosuppressed, in neonates, and in the elderly. Complications and sequelae include otitis media, pneumonia (either measles virus or secondary bacterial pneumonia), measles encephalitis, subacute sclerosing panencephalitis, juvenile diabetes mellitus, and thrombocytopenic purpura.

German Measles (Rubella)

German measles, or rubella, is a mild, systemic illness of childhood caused by the rubella virus. Except for superficial similarity in the name, the rubella virus is not related to the measles (rubeola) virus. A worldwide disease, rubella is characterized by a measleslike rash, low-grade fever, and swollen posterior auricular and occipital lymph nodes.

Subclinical infections are common. The incubation period is 12 to 21 days, and the mild rash and other symptoms resolve within 3 days. Initially, swollen, nontender posterior auricular and occipital lymph nodes appear. A day or two later the nonpruritic rash begins on the face and rapidly spreads over the rest of the body, sparing the palms and soles.

The virus is very contagious and is shed from the nasopharynx. **The virus is also transmitted through the placenta, and rubella infections in pregnant women are a serious public health concern, because intrauterine infection causes spontaneous abortion, fetal death, and a variety of congenital abnormalities.** Infection during the first trimester is most serious. The principal congenital abnormalities are pat-

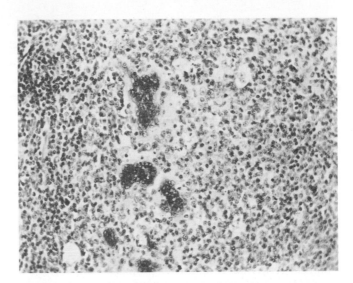

Figure 9-10. Lymph node from a patient with measles. Several Warthin-Finkeldey giant cells are seen in a germinal center.

ent ductus arteriosus, pulmonary and aortic stenosis, coarctation of the aorta, defects of the atrial or ventricular septum, ocular lesions (cataracts, glaucoma, and chorioretinitis), deafness, microcephaly, mental retardation, and retarded growth.

Mumps

Mumps is an acute but usually mild viral infection of childhood, characterized by swollen and inflamed salivary glands, most often the parotids. Less often the virus attacks the pancreas, ovaries, testes, and other organs. Mumps virus is a highly contagious paramyxovirus that is commonly transmitted in respiratory droplets. A vaccine made from attenuated live mumps virus has reduced the frequency. Most adults are immune. Nonimmune adults who acquire the infection may have a painful and debilitating illness.

The incubation period is 2 to 4 weeks, after which fever, headache, malaise, and swelling and inflammation of the salivary glands follow. Swelling and other acute symptoms usually subside within 2 weeks. Mumps is usually diagnosed clinically from swollen salivary glands and confirmed by finding rising titers to mumps virus in the serum of convalescent patients.

The histologic features of the swollen parotid glands include diffuse interstitial edema and an inflammatory infiltrate composed of histiocytes, lymphocytes, and plasma cells. This infiltrate may compress the acini and ducts, and the exudate may also spill into the epithelial layers.

Other organs may be affected whether the salivary glands are swollen or not. The most common complication is a painful orchitis with parenchymal hemorrhage. The tunica albuginea tightly contains the swollen testis, which may result in necrosis of seminiferous tubules, local hemorrhages, and microinfarctions sometimes leaving permanent fibrous scars. Mumps orchitis is usually unilateral and thus rarely causes male sterility. Infection of the pancreas leads to pancreatitis, characterized by necrosis of pancreatic and fat cells.

Viral Gastroenteritis

Gastroenteritis is a common illness that may be caused by a variety of bacteria and protozoa, but such pathogens have been absent from a large proportion of diarrheal stools, including those from about two-thirds of infants and young children hospitalized for diarrhea. Although it was long suspected that viruses might cause such "acute infectious nonbacterial gastroenteritis," attempts to propagate the causative viruses in conventional cell cultures were unsuccessful. Electron microscopic studies of gastrointestinal specimens and diarrheal stools have now identified two types of viral particles, **rotaviruses in infants and Norwalk-like viruses in adults,** that appear to cause most viral diarrheas. Enteric adenoviruses and other viruses may have minor etiologic roles.

Rotavirus Diarrhea

Rotaviruses contain double-stranded RNA, resemble a wheel, have icosahedral symmetry, and are "double-shelled" (with inner and outer capsids). Rotavirus particles have been found in the duodenal mucosa of children with acute gastroenteritis and in diarrheal stool specimens.

In developed countries rotavirus is the most common pathogen of childhood diarrhea. Rotavirus-induced diarrhea is an endemic problem throughout the world, the organisms being identified in half the children in developed countries and in almost half of those in developing countries. In temperate countries rotavirus diarrhea usually has a seasonal winter peak, but in tropical countries high rates are observed throughout the year. Nosocomial infections are common, and shedding of rotavirus has even been found in some (usually asymptomatic) newborns in communal obstetric nurseries within 3 or 4 days of birth. Antibodies to the rotavirus in colostrum and breast milk protect against infection. The highest incidence of symptomatic infection is in children aged 7 to 24 months. Most children have rotavirus antibodies by

the end of the third year, and nearly all infections in adults are subclinical.

Rotavirus is spread by fecal-oral transmission, typically by person-to-person contact or by contact with a contaminated object. Contaminated water may be an important mode of transmission in developing countries. After an incubation period of 2 to 3 days there is an abrupt onset of watery diarrhea, followed by dehydration and vomiting and, in a few days, by high fever. (The early vomiting and fever distinguish rotavirus diarrhea from diarrhea caused by enterotoxigenic *E. coli* or *Vibrio cholerae*.) The upper respiratory tract may also be affected. In developed countries, most children have a self-limited illness that lasts a few days. But coincidental infection with pathogenic enterobacteria may extend the duration, especially in developing countries. Moreover, in developing countries, severe life-threatening dehydration may be an important cause of mortality among children under 2 years of age.

Treatment of rotavirus diarrhea consists of prompt intravenous or oral rehydration. For prevention, "Jennerian" rotavirus vaccines are being developed, including strains of bovine rotavirus and rhesus rotavirus grown in conventional cell cultures. Animal studies have shown that resistance to rotavirus diarrhea depends primarily on local antibody to rotavirus in the lumen of the small intestine.

Diarrhea Caused by Norwalk-like Viruses

The prototype "Norwalk agent" was discovered in an outbreak of diarrhea and vomiting among elementary school students in Norwalk, Ohio. The virus has icosahedral symmetry, contains single-stranded RNA, and is now thought to be a calicivirus.

Norwalk-like viruses have been associated with gastroenteritis, primarily in adults and older children. Diarrhea and vomiting are of short duration, and dehydration is rare (as compared with rotavirus diarrhea). The outbreaks have occurred at all times of the year and have been associated with contaminated water and foods (oysters and clams), infected food-handlers, and person-to-person spread. Outbreaks have occurred in schools and college campuses, among families, in nursing homes, in communities with contaminated drinking or swimming water, and on cruise ships.

Rotavirus and Norwalk-like viruses multiply in epithelial cells lining villi of the small intestine, causing nonspecific inflammatory changes in the mucosa, including blunting of the villi, cytoplasmic vacuolization of epithelial cells, and a patchy, mononuclear, infiltrate of the lamina propria. The lysis of epithelial cells leaves the villi denuded and allows leakage of fluid and electrolytes into the lumen of the small intestine. Later there is contraction of denuded villi and transient replacement of mature, tall columnar epithelial cells by immature, cuboidal cells that migrate up from the crypts. Severe watery diarrhea and dehydration result from the decreased absorptive surface of the villi, decreases in the enzymatic activity of the brush border (including disaccharidases), and secretions by the immature crypt cells. Since the diet of young children is often based on milk, lactose malabsorption is of special concern. The diarrhea lasts only 1 to 3 days in most patients, and the intestinal mucosa is histologically normal within 3 to 4 weeks after onset of diarrhea. Histologic changes, however, persist in some children, especially among those less than 6 months old.

Diarrhea Caused by Enteric Adenoviruses and Other Viruses

Electron microscopic studies of diarrheal stools have revealed enteric adenoviruses in the stools of acutely ill patients but not in those of convalescent patients. Paired sera show seroconversion, indicating that adenoviruses cause a small but significant proportion of viral diarrheas. Enteric adenoviruses are morphologically indistinguishable from respiratory adenoviruses; both have icosahedral symmetry and contain double-stranded DNA. Adenovirus gastroenteritis occurs mainly in infants and young children, in small outbreaks, and primarily in developed countries. There is no striking seasonal variation, and dehydration is rare (as compared with rotavirus diarrhea).

Respiratory Viruses (Viral Pneumonias)

Respiratory disorders are caused by a wide variety of viruses, of different families, species, and serotypes. These include orthomyxoviruses (influenza A, B, and C), paramyxoviruses (respiratory syncytial virus), parainfluenza viruses, and measles virus, adenoviruses, herpesviruses (varicella-zoster virus), cytomegalovirus, and herpes simplex virus (HSV), picornaviruses (rhinoviruses, echoviruses, and coxsackieviruses), and human respiratory coronaviruses. Some of these—for example, rhinoviruses and coronaviruses—primarily cause upper respiratory infections. Many cause more serious lower respiratory infections, with variable degrees of bronchiolitis, inflammation of the pulmonary parenchyma (usually mononuclear and interstitial) and exudation of fluid into the alveoli. For simplicity the diseases are collectively termed "viral pneumonias." Most influenza viruses and adenoviruses are transmitted by inhalation of airborne droplets. Others are transmitted by direct contact with infected secretions. Some viruses reach the lung by hematogenous spread from other organs.

Viral pneumonias are common in children under 5 years of age, and are often complicated by superimposed bacterial pneumonias (*Staphylococcus aureus, Streptococcus pneumoniae, Haemophilus influenzae*). Viral pneumonias comprise a small minority of all pneumonias in healthy adults, but susceptibility is increased in debilitated people, women in the third trimester of pregnancy, and immunocompromised persons. In an exception to the general rule, the incidence of adenovirus pneumonia is high among presumably healthy military recruits. Uncomplicated viral pneumonias have a low mortality, and most deaths are caused by secondary bacterial infections.

Histopathologic changes seen in viral pneumonia include interstitial mononuclear cell infiltrates of the alveolar septa and peribronchial and septal connective tissues, squamous metaplasia of the bronchial epithelium, hyperplasia of type II pneumocytes, alveolar edema with or without mononuclear cell exudate, hyaline membranes lining the alveolar walls, and a mixture of other changes, such as hyperemia, atelectasis, and hemorrhage. These features are nonspecific and may be seen in many other nonbacterial pneumonias.

Orthomyxoviruses (Influenza)

Orthomyxoviruses (influenza A, B, and C viruses) are enveloped viruses that contain single-stranded RNA in a helical array of nucleoprotein. Inserted in the lipid envelope are two glycoproteins—the hemagglutinin (HA) and the neuraminidase (NA). **Influenza viruses have the unusual capability of changing the antigenic identities of their HA and NA polypeptides, thus creating numerous antigenic variants.** The hosts of different types of virus give their names to the disease, as in, for example, human, swine, and avian influenza.

Influenza viruses are highly contagious and afflict people of all ages. They are transmitted by aerosols generated by coughing and sneezing. Influenza A virus, the most common cause of viral pneumonia in adults, infects animals and man and produces pandemics. Influenza B virus is apparently restricted to man, causes epidemics, and is associated with Reye's syndrome in children and pneumonitis and croup in infants. Influenza C virus causes sporadic upper respiratory infections, but not epidemic influenza. Influenza has significant mortality and morbidity, and may have long-term sequelae. Patients with viral influenza during the third trimester of pregnancy, the aged, and persons with valvular heart disease or chronic bronchopulmonary disease all have increased susceptibility to bacterial superinfection. Superinfection usually occurs 1 to 5 days after the onset of the viral illness, while the patient appears to be getting well.

After an incubation period of 18 to 72 hours, the onset is characteristically abrupt, with fever, chills, generalized malaise, myalgias, and headache. As the fever and systemic symptoms subside, the respiratory symptoms become prominent. The histopathologic features include a necrotizing bronchitis and diffuse hemorrhagic necrotizing pneumonitis with pulmonary edema. Ciliated epithelial cells are destroyed and goblet cells and mucous glands disrupted. Bronchioles become thickened, distended, and infiltrated with mononuclear cells. There is often severe inflammatory edema, and a fluid exudate in the alveolar spaces has a hyaline appearance.

Paramyxoviruses

Paramyxoviruses (respiratory syncytial virus [RSV], parainfluenza viruses, and measles virus) are also spherical enveloped viruses that contain single-stranded RNA. They are transmitted by inhalation of droplets of aerosols.

Respiratory Syncytial Virus

The respiratory syncytial virus is the most common cause of viral pneumonia in children under 2 years of age and is a common cause of death in infants aged 1 to 6 months. This agent accounts for about one-third of hospital admissions for pneumonia and for up to 90% of those admitted for bronchiolitis. Susceptibility is also increased in elderly or immunocompromised patients. In temperate climates of the northern hemisphere, annual epidemics occur in midwinter (January–March). Histopathologic features include necrotizing bronchitis, bronchiolitis, and interstitial pneumonia. The infiltrate is purely mononuclear (predominantly lymphocytes). In many cases irregular intracytoplasmic inclusion bodies are seen in alveolar and bronchiolar epithelial cells, but intranuclear inclusions are not present.

Parainfluenza Viruses (Types 1–4b)

Type 3 parainfluenza is the most prevalent of the parainfluenzas, occurring endemically throughout the year. Infants are especially susceptible. Parainfluenza viruses are spread principally by direct contact or by large droplets (in contrast to the spread of influenza virus by inhalation of small droplets). Replication is restricted to the respiratory tract. The infection involves only the upper respiratory tract, except in some infants in whom the primary infection may also involve the larynx, trachea, and bron-

chioles. Histopathologic features include necrotizing bronchitis, bronchiolitis, and interstitial pneumonia.

Measles Virus (Rubeola) Pneumonia

Measles pneumonia occurs in up to half of patients with measles, usually within 5 days of development of the rash. There are rales and rhonchi on chest examination, and radiographs of the chest reveal interstitial pneumonia, commonly involving lower lobes. In immature or debilitated children, secondary bacterial infections are especially common. The histopathologic appearance, therefore, varies from pure interstitial (viral) pneumonia to lobar (bacterial) pneumonia. There are often pathognomonic multinucleated giant cells (Warthin-Finkeldey cells) (see Fig. 9-10), intranuclear and intracytoplasmic inclusions, and hyperplasia of distal bronchial cells. In immunocompromised patients measles pneumonia may occur without rash and is often fatal.

Adenovirus Pneumonia

Adenoviruses, nonenveloped icosahedral viruses that contain DNA, are isolated from the respiratory tract of man and other animals. Adenoviruses (subgroup B, types 4 and 7) are common causes of acute respiratory disease and adenovirus pneumonia in military recruits coming together for the first time for basic training. Adenoviruses (subgroup C) are also important causes of chronic pulmonary disease in infants and young children. Histopathologic features of adenovirus pneumonitis include necrotizing bronchitis and bronchiolitis, with necrosis and desquamation of the epithelium. Sloughed epithelial cells are subsequently mixed with mononuclear cells, mucus, and cell debris, so that the damaged bronchiole resembles a thrombosed blood vessel. There is interstitial pneumonia, with areas of consolidation showing extensive necrosis, hemorrhage, edema, and mononuclear inflammatory infiltrate. Two distinctive types of intranuclear inclusions—smudge cells and Cowdry type A intranuclear inclusions—are scattered throughout the lesions but primarily involve bronchiolar epithelial cells and alveolar lining cells.

Herpesvirus Pneumonias

Varicella pneumonia is rare in children, occurring mostly in adults or patients with depressed immunity. It may be a complication of pregnancy or of disseminated varicella infection following chemotherapy of leukemia or lymphoma. The pneumonia develops a few days after the onset of the vesicular rash. Varicella pneumonia is usually more severe than other forms of primary viral pneumonia and frequently involves both upper and lower lobes bilaterally. Throughout the lung there are nodular lesions that may coalesce and cause severe hypoxia. Frequently there is pleuritic pain, apparently caused by vesicular lesions on the pleura.

Cytomegalovirus pneumonia occurs in patients with impaired defenses—the debilitated, the elderly, and the immunosuppressed (especially those with leukemia or organ transplants). Characteristic cytomegalic intranuclear inclusions may be seen. Pneumonia is usually not a feature in infections of the newborn.

Herpes simplex pneumonia. Pneumonia is an infrequent complication in patients with depressed immunity who are infected with herpesvirus. Cowdry type A intranuclear inclusions are noted.

Picornavirus Pneumonias

Picornaviruses are animal viruses named for their small size and single-stranded RNA. Pneumonias may be a complication of some infections with three classes of picornavirus: rhinoviruses, echoviruses, and cosackieviruses.

Rhinoviruses, of which there are more than 100 species, are transmitted by direct contact with infected secretions, rather than by inhalation of aerosols. **These agents replicate in the epithelial cells of the nasal mucosa and are shed primarily from the nose. They are the most common cause of the "common cold."** In some patients with chronic bronchitis, rhinoviruses have been associated with abnormalities of pulmonary function.

Echoviruses and cosackieviruses are enteroviruses that infect man primarily through the ingestion of fecally contaminated material. After replicating in lymph nodes they may enter the bloodstream, replicate further in the reticuloendothelial system, and disseminate in the bloodstream, a process that infrequently results in respiratory disorders.

Human respiratory coronaviruses, which contain single-stranded RNA, are the second most common cause of the "common cold." They characteristically cause a profuse nasal discharge but have little or no effect on the lower respiratory tract.

Diseases Caused by Mycoplasmas

Mycoplasmas (formerly known as pleuropneumonia-like organisms [PPLO] or Eaton agents) are slowly growing polymorphous microorganisms, the pathogenicity of which is not well understood. They are larger than most viruses (300-800 nm across) but smaller than bacteria, and are the smallest free-living organisms. Unlike viruses, they replicate in cell-free media and divide by binary fission. Unlike bacteria, they lack a cell wall. Mycoplasmas morphologically resemble, but are not related to, transient cell-wall–defective variants of bacteria (the so-called L-forms). They are resistant to penicillins, cephalosporins, and other cell-wall active antimicrobials, but they are sensitive to antimicrobials that inhibit protein synthesis, such as tetracycline and erythromycin.

In special agar medium mycoplasmas form microscopic colonies of varying size (50-600 μm) that have a characteristic "fried egg" appearance, with an opaque central zone and a translucent peripheral zone. Mycoplasmas can also be grown in the yolk sac and in tissue cultures.

Mycoplasmas are widespread both geographically and ecologically, as saprophytes and as parasites of a broad range of animal and plants. They are heterogeneous and differ in DNA composition, nutritional requirements, antigenic composition, and host species specificity. They require lipids and lipid precursors for synthesis of their plasma membranes, and some require exogenous cholesterol for growth.

Mycoplasma Pneumonia

M. pneumoniae causes tracheobronchitis and "primary atypical pneumonias," most frequently in children and adolescents. Infections are worldwide and account for about 20% of all cases of pneumonia in some cities. Most infections occur in small groups of people who have frequent close contact, for example, families, college fraternities, military units, and closed institutions. The organism is spread by aerosol transmission from person to person over a period of several months, with an attack rate of greater than 50% within the group. The incubation period is 2 to 3 weeks, and the onset is insidious. Clinical features are an initial nonproductive cough followed by the production of watery or mucoid sputum, fever, rhinorrhea, chest pain, and generalized myalgia. The diagnosis is made by culturing *M. pneumoniae* in special cell-free media after inoculating specimens of sputum, throat swabs, pleural fluids, or tissues.

Infections commonly involve the oropharynx, trachea, bronchi, and lungs, usually causing unilateral pneumonia of the lower lobe. The radiographic appearance cannot be distinguished from that of other nonbacterial pneumonias. The infection is superficial, with the organisms attaching to ciliated epithelial cells. Electron microscopy reveals that the mycoplasma has a specialized tapered, filamentous tip with a rodlike core, which may attach the mycoplasma to the epithelial cell. *M. pneumoniae* does not produce endotoxin or exotoxin but does produce hydrogen peroxide and superoxide (O_2^-). Microscopically, there is a patchy interstitial pneumonia with swollen alveolar lining cells, bronchiolar walls thickened by congestion and edema, and an intraluminal exudate of neutrophils, epithelial cells, and proteinaceous debris. The initial infiltrate, predominantly a perivascular and peribronchial cuffing by lymphocytes, is followed by neutrophils and macrophages. The pulmonary changes are often complicated by bacterial superinfection. In rare instances other organs may be involved (central nervous system, pancreas, joints, skin, heart, and pericardium), probably as a result of hematogenous spread.

The diagnosis of infection with *M. pneumoniae* is made by detecting specific complement-fixing antibodies.

The symptoms and signs of mycoplasma pneumonia usually abate within 10 to 14 days, and recovery is hastened by treatment with broad-spectrum antibiotics. Patients continue to shed mycoplasmas for some time after therapy has been discontinued but usually recover without sequelae.

Diseases Caused by Chlamydiae

Chlamydiae are obligate intracellular gram-negative bacteria that have a unique two-stage cycle. The infectious "elementary body," representing the extracellular stage, is a 0.2- to 0.4-μm sphere that has a rigid cell envelope and is metabolically inactive. The intracellular second stage, the initial body, is larger—0.7 to 1.0 μm in diameter—and metabolically active, and multiplies by binary fission.

Chlamydial infections are widespread among birds and mammals, and perhaps 20% of the human population is infected. **Chlamydial diseases in humans include trachoma, inclusion conjunctivitis, psittacosis, lymphogranuloma venereum, infections of the urethra, cervix, and salpinx, and neonatal pneumonitis.** Chlamydial cervicitis and urethritis are the most common sexually transmitted diseases in North America.

Psittacosis (Parrot Fever, Ornithosis)

Psittacosis, a disease of birds that is transmissible to man, is an acute infection caused by *Chlamydia psittaci*. Once thought to infect only psittacine birds, *C. psittaci* is harbored by many other birds, including chickens, turkeys, pigeons, and sea gulls, and by many mammals. Man usually acquires the disease by contacting infected birds.

C. psittaci causes systemic disease in man, but pulmonary involvement is most prominent. The organisms are inhaled with dust-borne contaminated excreta or aerosolized droplets. The organisms are carried to the reticuloendothelial cells of the liver and spleen, proliferate, and disseminate to the lungs and other organs.

The disease ranges in severity from subclinical to fatal. After an incubation period of 7 to 21 days, an intense headache and fever herald the disease. A faint macular rash (Horder's spots), resembling the rose spots of typhoid fever, may be present. Pharyngitis, malaise, anorexia, and painful myalgias and arthralgias are common, as is hepatosplenomegaly. A persistent dry hacking cough, fine crepitant rales, and tachypnea are typical.

Psittacosis begins as an inflammatory process in the lung and progresses to consolidation, primarily lobular but occasionally lobar. It progresses through a sequence of congestion, edema, and red and gray hepatization. Histopathologically, fibrin, erythrocytes, and neutrophils appear early in the alveolar exudate. Later the alveoli contain large mononuclear cells and epithelial cells. Interstitial infiltration is not present in early stages, but as the disease progresses lymphocytes and monocytes invade the alveolar walls. Hyperplasia of alveolar type 2 pneumocytes is typical. In severe disease abscesses form in alveolar septa, and hemorrhage and fibrin may fill the alveoli. The hilar nodes show lymphadenitis and reticuloendothelial hyperplasia.

Elementary bodies in the alveolar lining cells appear as clusters of minute, intracytoplasmic, basophilic, coccobacillary inclusions 0.2 to 0.4 μm by 0.4 to 0.8 μm, up to 0.8 μm in greatest dimension. The organisms are dark blue with the Van Gieson and Giemsa stains and red against a blue background with the Gimenez or Machiavello stains. They are also demonstrated by direct immunofluorescence.

Dissemination is characterized by foci of necrosis in the liver and spleen and diffuse mononuclear cell infiltrates in the heart, kidneys, and brain. In the liver, swelling, vacuolization, and phagocytic activity of Kupffer's cells are prominent, and intracytoplasmic elementary bodies can be seen in the Kupffer cells. Focal necrosis in the spleen is accompanied by diffuse reticuloendothelial hyperplasia and desquamation of mononuclear cells into the splenic sinuses. Pericardial and myocardial inflammation have been described. The brain is rarely involved, but when it is, edema, congestion, and focal hemorrhage are present.

The clinical signs and symptoms are not diagnostic and routine laboratory findings are not specific; a history of exposure to birds may be the best clue.

Radiographs of the chest usually reveal a patchy lower lobe infiltrate, but findings vary. The diagnosis is made either by isolating *C. psittaci* from sputum, blood, or tissue specimens or by serologic tests.

The mortality rate in the pre-antibiotic era exceeded 20% but with antibiotic treatment is now only 1%. Immunity is incomplete and the carrier state may persist for years. Infection in birds is effectively controlled by adding tetracycline to their feed during quarantine.

Trachoma

Trachoma is a chronic progressive infection of the conjunctiva and cornea that may cause partial or total blindness. **Infection with *Chlamydia trachomatis*, subgroups A, B, Ba, and C, is the leading cause of preventable blindness in the world.** The disease is worldwide, associated with poverty, and most prevalent in dry or sandy regions. Only humans are naturally infected. Poor personal hygiene and inadequate public sanitation are common factors. Endemic regions have been reduced in size since World War II, but trachoma remains a major problem in parts of Africa, India, and the Middle East. In the United States, American Indians are most susceptible. Spread mostly by direct contact, trachoma is also transmitted by fomites, contaminated water, cosmetics, and probably flies. Subclinical infections are an important reservoir.

In endemic areas infection is acquired early in childhood, becomes chronic, and eventually progresses to blindness. An abrupt onset of palpebral and conjunctiva inflammation leads to lacrimation, purulent conjunctivitis, and photophobia. As chronic inflammation progresses over months and years, there is scarring of the upper tarsal plate and corneal keratitis, with the formation of a vascular pannus. Scarring, trichiasis, and entropion eventually interfere with normal ocular function. Secondary bacterial infections and corneal ulceration are common.

Histologic examination of the early lesions shows conjunctival hyperemia, degeneration of the epithelium, intracytoplasmic inclusions, epithelial hyperplasia, lymphocytic infiltrates, and the formation of small lymphoid follicles in the stroma. As the disease progresses, the reaction in the conjunctiva becomes more pronounced and deep glandlike crypts and papillary hypertrophy are seen. The cornea is eventually invaded by blood vessels and fibroblasts to form the pannus. Necrosis eventually occurs, especially in the lymphoid follicles, causing extensive conjunctival scarring. Resorption of lymphoid follicles at the limbus results in indentations called Herbert's pits.

The diagnosis of trachoma is based on characteristic clinical findings and the demonstration of organisms in smears or cultures. Scrapings of the superficial conjunctiva stained with Giemsa or by direct immunofluorescence may reveal diagnostic intracytoplasmic inclusions.

Trachoma responds to topical and systemic tetracycline, but endemic trachoma is difficult to treat because of repeated exposure. All members of a family or social group should be treated to prevent retransmission. Vaccines have been ineffective, and those administered systemically tend to exacerbate the disease. Improved hygiene and public sanitation are the most effective control measures.

Inclusion Conjunctivitis

Inclusion conjunctivitis is a self-limited suppurative conjunctivitis, acquired by newborns as they transit the birth canal. Adults are infected by direct contamination of the eye with genital secretions containing *C. trachomatis* (subgroups D–K), although there are reports of infection after swimming in unchlorinated pools.

In the newborn, inclusion conjunctivitis appears between the 2nd and 25th day of life, reaching a maximum intensity in 2 weeks, without pannus formation or scarring. Inclusion conjunctivitis in adults is less acute. After an incubation period of 4 to 12 days, patients present with unilateral or bilateral follicular conjunctivitis, with minimal suppuration, preauricular lymphadenopathy, and conjunctival lymphoid follicles. Symptoms include lacrimation, mild foreign body sensation, and lid fullness. Histologically, an exudate of neutrophils and monocytes develops in one or both eyes, with edema and congestion of the lids.

The diagnosis is made by isolating the organism in tissue culture or by identifying intracytoplasmic inclusions in smears stained by Giemsa or by direct immunofluorescent techniques. Tissue culture is more sensitive than microscopy, but smears are faster and may be advantageous when evaluating neonatal disease. Neonatal inclusion conjunctivitis must be differentiated from gonococcal conjunctivitis.

Lymphogranuloma Venereum

Lymphogranuloma venereum, a sexually transmitted disease of man caused by *C. trachomatis*, subgroups L_1, L_2, or L_3, is characterized by a transient primary cutaneous or mucosal lesion and regional lymphadenitis. Although the disease is present worldwide, the highest prevalence is in the tropics and subtropics: it accounts for up to 6% of sexually transmitted disease in Africa, Southeast Asia, and India. Lymphogranuloma venereum is diagnosed more frequently in men than in women, a situation that probably reflects underdiagnosis and asymptomatic disease in women. In North America and Europe, lymphogranuloma venereum is now primarily a disease of homosexual men.

After an incubation period of 4 to 21 days, a primary lesion develops at the site of infection. The painless, herpetiform lesion, varying in diameter from 1 to 6 mm, usually occurs on the penis, vagina, or cervix, but lips, tongue, and fingers are other primary sites. Before the primary lesion appears, *C. trachomatis* is carried in the lymphatics to regional lymph nodes. Here, after a latent period of 1 to 4 weeks, the nodes enlarge. Any group may be involved and enlargement may be unilateral or bilateral. Over the next few weeks, the nodes become tender and fluctuant, and frequently ulcerate and discharge pus. Lymphadenopathy and drainage may persist for several weeks or months. Involvement of the inguinal and femoral nodes may produce the "groove sign," in which the enlarged nodes are visibly separated by the inguinal ligament. Primary anorectal lymphogranuloma venereum, usually in homosexual men, causes severe proctocolitis, accompanied by tenesmus, diarrhea, bleeding, fever, and weight loss.

Patients with lymphogranuloma venereum usually present with lymphadenopathy, with or without systemic signs and symptoms, such as fever, chills, myalgias, arthralgias, headache, anorexia, and meningismus. Increased serum immunoglobulins, leukocytosis, an elevated erythrocyte sedimentation rate, and abnormal liver function are common. False-positive reagin tests for syphilis are a feature, but concurrent syphilis always must be considered.

Most infections resolve completely, with or without antimicrobial therapy, but there may be serious sequelae. Progressive ulceration of the penis, urethra, or scrotum, with fistulas and urethral stricture, develop in 5% of men with lymphogranuloma venereum. Chronic ulcers of the vulva (esthiomene) and smooth, pedunculated, perianal growths (lymphorrhoids) are occasional complications. Lymphatic obstruction develops in 10% to 20% of untreated patients and can cause genital elephantiasis in women. Rarely, the infection may disseminate to the lungs, kidneys, bones, joints, and brain system, in which case it may be fatal.

The primary cutaneous lesion is a superficial ulcer without specific features. **The lymph nodes contain characteristic multiple, coalescing abscesses, which have the appearance of granulomas.** There are neu-

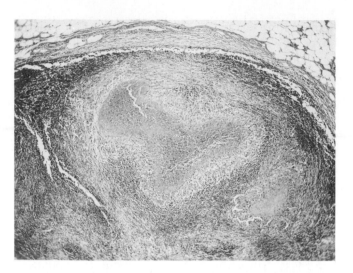

Figure 9-11.   Lymphogranuloma venereum. The necrotic central area of this lymph node is surrounded by a granulomatous zone with palisading epithelioid cells, macrophages, and occasional giant cells surrounded, in turn, by a wide zone of lymphocytes and plasma cells.

trophils and necrotic debris in the center, surrounded by a zone of palisaded epithelioid cells, macrophages, and occasional giant cells. In turn, this zone is surrounded by lymphocytes, plasma cells, and fibrous tissue (Fig. 9-11). Healing is by fibrosis with effacement of the normal architecture of the node. Lesions outside lymph nodes tend to be dominated by fibrous scarring. Granulomas in the nodes are identical to those of cat scratch disease but the bacilli of cat scratch disease, when present in the granulomas, are diagnostic.

The diagnosis of lymphogranuloma venereum is best made by isolating the appropriate subgroup of *C. trachomatis* in tissue culture, although cultures are positive in only 30% of patients. The diagnosis is most often made on clinical grounds and supported by serologic tests. The intradermal Frei test is insensitive and nonspecific and is no longer available in the United States.

Chlamydial Infections of the Genital Tract

Chlamydia trachomatis (D–K) causes urethritis, epididymitis, and proctitis in men and cervicitis, salpingitis, urethritis, and proctitis in women. **In adults, these infections are sexually transmitted; they have surpassed gonorrhea as the leading cause of sexually contracted disease in North America.** Recent studies implicate *C. trachomatis* in 20% of men with nongonococcal urethritis, and in a comparable proportion of men with gonococcal urethritis. *Chlamydia trachomatis* also causes epididymitis, usually in those under age 35, and may occasionally be responsible for chronic prostatitis. In women, *C. trachomatis* infection of the cervix is more common than gonorrhea. Thirty to sixty percent of women with gonorrhea have concurrent *C. trachomatis* infection, and this organism is now recognized as a cause of acute salpingitis.

The spectrum of disease parallels gonococcal disease. For instance, chlamydial urethritis in men typically causes dysuria and a scant mucoid discharge, and in women cervicitis causes a mucopurulent exudate in the cervical os, hypertrophic cervical erythema, and friable surface epithelium. The clinical presentation of acute chlamydial salpingitis—namely, pelvic pain and fever—resembles that of gonococcal salpingitis.

The diagnosis of chlamydial infections is best established by isolating the organism in tissue culture. Direct fluorescent staining of cervical or urethral smears with monoclonal reagents is diagnostic, but light microscopy seldom discloses chlamydial inclusions in smears from the genital tract. Serodiagnosis is also acceptable, particularly when there is a rising titer.

Diseases Caused by Rickettsiae

Epidemic Typhus (Louse-Borne Typhus) and Brill-Zinsser Disease

Epidemic typhus (louse-borne typhus) is caused by *Rickettsia prowazekii*. The disease is widely distributed in some regions of Africa, Asia, Europe, and the Western Hemisphere. Its devastating epidemics were associated with cold climates, poor sanitation, and crowding during natural disasters, famine, or war—as, for instance, the epidemics in Russia and eastern Europe during 1918-22. Epidemic typhus may kill 60% or more of the untreated aged, but kills only about 10% of untreated children.

R. prowazekii is a small gram-negative bacillus (rickettsia) that has a man–louse–man life cycle (Fig. 9-12). These rickettsiae infect and multiply in human endothelial cells. Infected endothelial cells detach and rupture, releasing organisms into the circulation (rickettsemia). A person is usually infectious for lice only during the febrile stage of the disease. A louse taking a blood meal becomes infected with rickettsiae, after which the organisms enter the epithelial cells of the midgut, multiply, and rupture the cells within 3 to 5 days. Large numbers of rickettsiae are

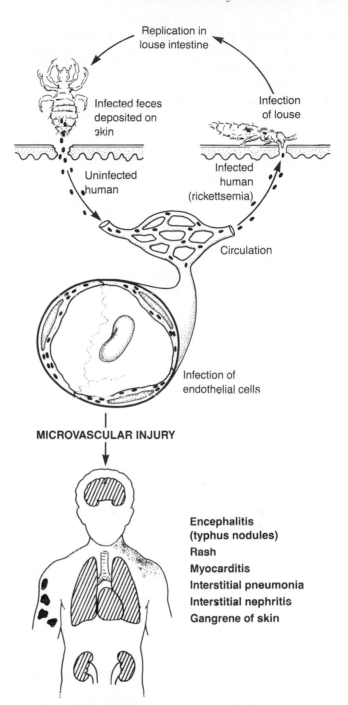

Figure 9-12. Epidemic typhus (louse-borne typhus). *R. prowazekii* has a man-louse-man life cycle. The organism multiplies in endothelial cells, which detach, rupture, and release organisms into the circulation (rickettsemia). A louse taking a blood meal becomes infected with rickettsiae, which enter the epithelial cells of its midgut, multiply, and rupture the cells, thereby releasing rickettsiae into the lumen of the louse intestine. Contaminated feces are deposited on the skin or clothing of a second host and penetrate an abrasion or are inhaled. The rickettsiae then enter endothelial cells, multiply, and rupture the cells, thus completing the cycle.

released into the lumen of the louse intestine. The louse deposits its contaminated feces on the skin or clothing of a second host, where the feces may remain infectious for more than 3 months. A person becomes infected when the contaminated louse feces penetrate an abrasion or scratch in the skin or when the person inhales airborne rickettsiae from clothing containing louse feces. After penetrating the skin or nasal mucous membrane, the rickettsiae enter the endothelial cells, multiply, and rupture the cells, thus completing the cycle.

An incubation period of 10 to 14 days is followed by the sudden onset of severe headaches, generalized aching, and high fever, which may continue 10 to 14 days before subsiding. About 4 to 6 days after the onset of symptoms, the patient develops a maculopapular rash on the back, chest, and abdomen. The rash is composed of 1-mm to 4-mm "spots," but in fatal cases commonly becomes confluent and purpuric. Mild rickettsial pneumonia is followed by a severe superimposed bacterial pneumonia. Although the brain, heart, and kidneys may be involved during the acute phase, patients who recover have no sequelae. Dying patients may exhibit encephalitis, myocarditis, interstitial rickettsial pneumonia, interstitial nephritis, and shock (see Fig. 9-12). Although rickettsiae do not produce local lesions on entering the skin or respiratory tract, they do cause a generalized vasculitis of minute blood vessels as they multiply within endothelial cells, and fibrin thrombi often form in capillaries, especially those of the brain, skin, and heart. Fibrin thrombi also occlude larger vessels, and cutaneous necrosis (gangrene of the skin) develops in a few patients.

At autopsy, there are few gross findings except for splenomegaly and occasional areas of necrosis. However, histologic sections commonly reveal collections of mononuclear cells in various organs; for example, the skin, brain, and heart. The mononuclear cell infiltrate includes mast cells, lymphocytes, plasma cells, and macrophages and are frequently arranged as **"typhus nodules"** around arterioles and capillaries. The Brown-Hopps tissue Gram stain (or the Giemsa stain) demonstrate the rickettsiae within endothelial cells. The rickettsiae divide by binary fission. When there are many rickettsiae in an endothelial cell, they are usually lined up in a "flotilla" pattern several columns wide, parallel to each other and to the longitudinal axis of the endothelial cell.

Brill-Zinsser disease is a recrudescence of a latent infection by *R. prowazekii* in people who have previously had epidemic typhus. In the past, the disease primarily affected older immigrants from Eastern Europe, especially those who had a weakened immune

system. Years after the initial infection, sporadic illness reappears, characterized by headache, fever and a macular rash. Histologic features are similar to but milder than those for the initial epidemic typhus. Lice fed with blood from these patients become infected with *R. prowazekii*. Epidemic typhus can be controlled by large-scale delousing of the population by, for example, steam sterilization of clothing or use of insecticides. Tetracycline antibiotics are the preferred treatment for rickettsial diseases.

Endemic (Murine) Typhus

Endemic or murine typhus is caused by *Rickettsia typhi*, a minute gram-negative bacillus. Humans become infected by interrupting the usual rat–flea–rat cycle of transmission. When the flea defecates on the surface of the skin, the feces contaminate the small wound made by the bite. The rickettsiae also contaminate clothes, become airborne and, when inhaled, cause pulmonary infection. Outbreaks are associated with an exploding population of rats, but sporadic infections continue in the southwestern United States. These are associated with rat-infested dwellings and with occupations that bring people into contact with rats, such as the handling and storage of grain.

Headache, myalgia, and fever begin 1 to 2 weeks after inoculation, and a macular rash is seen 3 to 5 days later. Obliterative thrombovasculitis and perivascular nodules of the skin resemble the effects of epidemic typhus. There is interstitial inflammation of the heart and testes and inflammation of meninges. The endothelial cells of the blood vessels contain bacteria.

Rocky Mountain Spotted Fever

Rocky mountain spotted fever is a severe, sometimes fatal systemic infection caused by *Rickettsia rickettsii* and transmitted by ticks. Ticks are the reservoir for *R. rickettsii* and pass the organism transovarially to their progeny. Rickettsiae in the salivary glands of the tick are inoculated while the tick is feeding. Attacks may be so mild that the patient remains ambulatory, or so severe that he dies.

Symptoms begin 2 to 14 days after the tick bite and include fever, headache, and myalgia. The rash, which appears 2 to 6 days after onset, begins on the wrists and ankles before extending rapidly over the body to include the palms and soles. The rash begins as pink macules, which become fixed, dark red or purple, and form petechiae and hemorrhages.

Cough, rash, nausea, vomiting, abdominal pain, stupor, meningismus, or ataxia are evidence of serious systemic spread. Those over 40 years of age and those with dark skins are at greater risk.

R. rickettsia is a minute gram-negative bacillus that invades blood vessels, especially the endothelial cells of the kidney, meninges, skin, and heart. The orientation of the bacilli in parallel rows and in an end-to-end pattern gives them the appearance of a "flotilla at anchor" facing the wind. In fatal infections the endothelial cells lift away from the vessel, leaving the internal elastic lamella bare. Thrombi form at these sites, platelet counts drop to below 100,000/ml, and disseminated intravascular coagulation is a terminal complication. Although rickettsiae are in blood vessels of all organs, they are most easily identified in the meninges and kidneys. Patients with longer clinical courses have a perivascular cuffing of lymphocytes, especially in the heart and brain. Degranulating mast cells are prominent near the vessels. There may be microinfarcts and ring hemorrhages around vessels of the brain. Biopsy of the skin for diagnosis should include the deep dermis because the rickettsiae are concentrated in the endothelial cells of vessels in this area.

Scrub Typhus

Scrub typhus (tsutsugamushi disease) is caused by *Rickettsia tsutsugamushi*. Infected mites pass the infection transovarially to their larvae, which crawl to the tips of vegetation and attach to passers-by rather than to the usual host, the rat. While feeding, the mite passes the rickettsia into the skin.

A multiloculated vesicle forms at the inoculation site and ulcerates, after which an eschar forms. As the eschar heals, there is a sudden onset of headache, malaise, anorexia, weakness, and fever, followed by pneumonia, a macular rash (on the trunk before the limbs), lymphadenopathy, hepatosplenomegaly, and conjunctivitis. Mild infections may exhibit only fever. Since multiple serotypes exist and cross-immunity is transient, recurrent infections are common. Severe infections are complicated by meningoencephalitis involving cranial nerves, focal myocarditis, pneumonia, and circulatory collapse. Mortality rates range up to 30%.

The rickettsiae grow in the endothelial cells and produce a vasculitis. There are "typhus nodules," but these are usually smaller than those of epidemic typhus. Necrosis of the skin and lymph nodes and a dense mononuclear infiltrate in the heart and lungs are seen in severe cases.

Q Fever

Q fever is caused by the rickettsia *Coxiella burnetii*, an organism that is worldwide and passes from the tick host to sheep or cattle. Humans become infected by drinking contaminated milk, breathing air contaminated by drying animal placentas or other products of birth, and by coming in contact with contaminated soil or wool. Laboratory workers and those handling meat, skin, milk, wool, and fertilizer are at risk. Aerosol droplets spread the infection from person to person.

Headache, fever, chills, myalgia, malaise, and anorexia begin 2 to 4 weeks after infection. Pulmonary symptoms include cough and discrete densities on radiographs of the chest. In chronic Q fever the liver is enlarged and tender. Two to 20 years after exposure, subacute endocarditis may develop and form vegetations.

Rickettsiae are seen as extracellular colonies in the vegetations on the valve. The characteristic lesion in both liver and lung is a granuloma rather than vasculitis. The granuloma in the liver is composed of focal collections of lymphocytes, plasma cells, and giant cells, and may have central necrosis. There is interstitial pneumonia resembling that of scrub typhus.

Diseases Caused by Spirochetes

Leptospirosis

Leptospirosis is caused by the spirochete *Leptospira interrogans*. The leptospires are 0.1 μm wide and 6 to 12 μm long, with 18 or more coils. Of over 170 varieties, serovar canicola is associated with dogs, serovar icterohemorrhagica with rodents, and serovar pomona with swine and cattle. Serovar icterohemorrhagica grows in the lumen of renal tubules in the rat and is shed in the urine for the life of the animal. The leptospires penetrate abraded skin or mucous membranes following contact with infected rats, contaminated water, or mud. Since warm, moist environments favor survival of the spirochetes, the incidence is greater in the tropics. Congenital infection causes fetal death.

Symptoms begin 4 to 19 days after inoculation. Ninety percent of infections have a mild, anicteric course with resolution of symptoms in about 1 week. However, those with severe infections have a sudden onset of fever, myalgia, headache, and nausea and vomiting in the leptospiremic stage. The symptoms abate after 4 to 9 days and leptospires cease to cir-

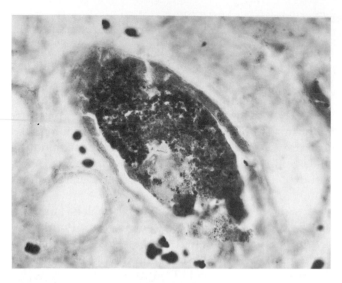

Figure 9-13. Leptospirosis, kidney. A distal tubule is obstructed by a bile-stained mass of hemoglobin and cellular debris. A leptospire is in the center of this mass.

culate. The second, or immune, stage known as **Weil's disease** follows after a latent period of 1 to 3 days in 10% of patients. Fever, headache (which signals the onset of meningismus), and the appearance of circulating IgM antibodies are characteristic. Severe myalgia, nausea, vomiting, abdominal pains, conjunctivitis, and hemorrhage into the conjunctiva are also features. Eventually, hepatic failure, renal failure, and shock may lead to death.

At autopsy there is bile staining of tissues, hemorrhages in many organs, and pulmonary edema. Microscopically, the liver shows dissociation of the liver cell plates, erythrophagocytosis of the Kupffer cells, necrosis of hepatocytes, neutrophils in sinusoids, and a mixed inflammatory cell infiltrate in portal tracts. In the kidney the tubular epithelium is swollen and necrotic. Spirochetes are numerous in the lumen of the tubules and particularly in bile-stained casts (Fig. 9-13).

In the first phase, culture of blood and cerebrospinal fluid is the most effective means of confirming the diagnosis. Leptospires grow from urine after the second week. Serologic tests are useful during the second phase. Antibiotics must be started within 4 days of onset. Large doses of penicillin and tetracyclines are useful.

Relapsing Fever

There are two main types of relapsing fever: epidemic (louse-borne), for which man is the reservoir, and endemic (tick-borne), for which rodents and other animals are the natural reservoir. Louse-borne relapsing fever is caused by the spirochete *Borrelia recurrentis*. Tick-borne relapsing fever is caused by several species, the most common being *B. turicatae*, *B. hermsii*, and *B. parkeri* in North America, *B. hispanica* in Spain, *B. persica* in Asia, and *B. duttonii* in Africa. Borrelias are 0.2 μm to 0.5 μm wide, 3 to 20 μm long, and they have three to ten coarse irregular coils.

The human body louse, *Pediculus humanus humanus* becomes infected with *B. recurrentis* when it feeds on an infected host. The borrelias cross the gut wall of the louse into the hemolymph, where they multiply. Here they remain unless the louse is crushed when feeding. If the louse is crushed, the borrelias escape and penetrate at the site of the bite or even through the intact skin. War, crowded migrant-worker camps, and heavy clothing during cold weather all favor mobilization of lice and the spread of relapsing fever. Furthermore, lice dislike the higher temperatures of the feverish victims and seek new hosts, another factor in the rapid spread of relapsing fever during epidemics.

In tick-borne relapsing fever, ticks are infected while biting rats and other animals. The borellias grow in the hemocoelom of the tick and invade other tissues including salivary glands. Man is infected by the saliva or coxal fluid of the tick. Ticks are much more durable than fleas and may harbor spirochetes for 12 to 15 years without a blood meal.

About 1 week after inoculation, fever, headache, myalgia, arthralgia, and lethargy begin suddenly. The liver and spleen enlarge, and there are petechiae of skin, conjunctival hemorrhages, and abdominal tenderness. In severe cases a rash, coma, meningitis, myocarditis, and liver failure may ensue. Three to nine days after onset the fever ends abruptly, only to begin again seven to ten days later. During the afebrile period the spirochetes disappear from the blood and change their antigenic coats. The symptoms are milder and the duration of illness is shorter for each relapse.

In fatal infections the spleen is enlarged and contains miliary microabscesses. Spirochetes form entangled masses around the necrotic centers. Lymphocytes and neutrophils infiltrate central and midzonal areas of the liver, where spirochetes lie free in the sinusoids. The pleura, peritoneum, brain, stomach, and intestines exhibit focal hemorrhage.

Wright's and Giemsa stained smears of blood, urine, and spinal fluid reveal spirochetes within or outside of leukocytes. Kelly's broth medium supports growth of borrelia. Specimens from patients injected into mice yield borrelia in the blood of the animal. Serologic tests for syphilis may also be positive. An-

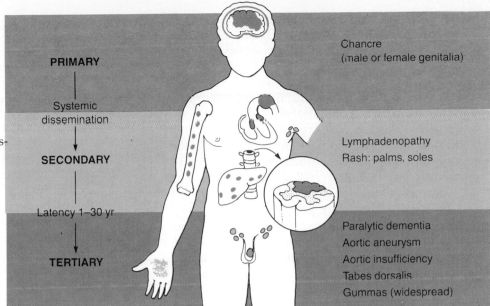

Figure 9-14. Clinical characteristics of the various stages of syphilis.

tibodies in the serum of convalescent patients agglutinize and immobilize spirochetes and fix complement.

Tetracycline and erythromycin are effective. Treatment can provoke a sudden drop of blood pressure, headache, myalgia, and sensation of cold. This reaction is thought to be related to the flooding of the blood by endotoxins when the spirochetes die, a process that activates fibrin and complement factors.

Syphilis (Lues)

Syphilis, a sexually transmitted disease of mankind caused by the spirochete *Treponema pallidum*, was first recognized in Europe in the 1490s, and has been related to the return of Christopher Columbus. Mass movements of peoples caused by war and urbanization contributed to its rapid spread. At that time, syphilis was an acute disease that caused destructive skin lesions and early death, but since then it has become milder, with a more protracted and insidious clinical course. **The disease is divided into three stages (Fig. 9-14): primary (the chancre), secondary (disseminated), and tertiary (with lesions of deep organs following a latent period of 2 to 20 years or more).** Congenital syphilis, acquired *in utero*, may have any of the secondary or tertiary lesions.

T. pallidum is a helical bacterium, 5 to 20 μm long and 0.1 to 0.2 μm wide, with 8 to 14 evenly distributed coils. The silver impregnation technique precip-

itates metallic silver on the wall of the spirochete, enlarging its outline and making it opaque, features that make it visible in tissue sections (Fig. 9-15). When smears from chancres or other syphilitic lesions are examined by darkfield microscopy, the spirochetes have the appearance of floating silver-white corkscrews on a black background, spinning on their long axes and flexing in the middle. Various direct and indirect immunofluorescent and immunoperoxidase staining procedures are also available for demonstrating spirochetes in tissue sections and smears.

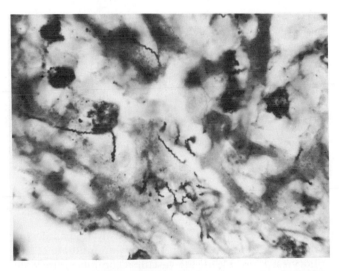

Figure 9-15. Syphilis, eye. Spirochetes of *Treponema pallidum* in the eye of a child with congenital syphilis.

Several serologic and immunofluorescent tests detect organisms or antigens, and the host's antibodies to them. One is the *Treponema pallidum* immobilization test, in which live spirochetes of *T. pallidum* are immobilized by antibody in the patient's serum. The standard method for demonstrating antibody in the serum is the indirect fluorescent treponemal antibody test, in which the antigen is lyophilized *T. pallidum*. To increase specificity, nonspecific antibodies in the patient's serum are first absorbed by nonpathogenic treponemes.

A nontreponemal antigen, cardiolipin from beef heart, is used for diagnostic screening and to assess treatment. Antigenically, it resembles a lipoid released by *T. pallidum* when it invades human tissues. The Veneral Disease Research Laboratory (VDRL) test and the rapid plasma reagin (RPR) test detect antibodies to cardiolipin. It is important to note that, although useful, these tests are not specific, because lipoidal antigen is released in patients with infectious mononucleosis, viral hepatitis, leprosy, and autoimmune diseases.

Spirochetes are very fragile and are killed by soap, antiseptics, drying, and cold. Person-to-person transmission requires direct contact between a rich source of spirochetes, for example the chancre, and mucous membranes or abraded skin of the genital organs, rectum, mouth, fingers, or nipples. Spirochetes enter the skin or mucous membrane, invade blood and lymph and disseminate almost immediately.

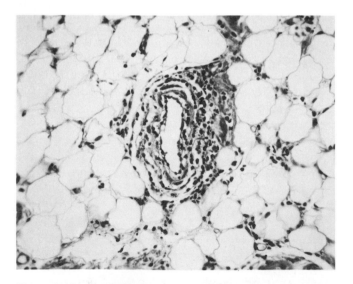

Figure 9-16. Syphilis. Luetic vasculitis in the panniculus. The wall of the vessel is expanded by an infiltrate of lymphocytes. If untreated, the vasculitis continues, the wall becomes fibrotic, and in the tertiary stage the lumen is reduced to a pinpoint opening.

Primary Syphilis

The chancre develops at the site of inoculation in 10 to 90 days (average 21 days). It begins as a small papule and may remain a papule. However, when the inoculum is large, the chancre develops into a shallow, painless ulcer with indurated margins. The base is covered by fibrin and cellular debris. Spirochetes may be anywhere in the chancre, but they concentrate in the walls of vessels and in the epidermis around the ulcer. Neutrophils migrate into the epithelium around the ulcer, drawn there by spirochetes. The upper dermis is congested and infiltrated with many lymphocytes and plasma cells; spirochetes shun the company of these inflammatory cells.

Chancres, as well as lesions of secondary, tertiary, and congenital syphilis, have a characteristic "luetic vasculitis," in which endothelial cells proliferate and swell, and the walls of the vessels become thickened by lymphocytes and fibrous tissue. Early in the vasculitis, lymphocytes are seen in the wall and there may be a cuff of plasma cells around the adventitia (Fig. 9-16). Gradually, the inflammatory cells diminish and fibrous tissue replaces the smooth muscle of the media. As the vasculitis continues the lumen narrows, and by the tertiary stage the lumen is reduced to a minute caliber. Spirochetes are visualized in the walls of the vessels in the primary and secondary stages, but not in the tertiary stage.

Regional lymph nodes draining the chancre are enlarged and firm, but painless. The chancre disappears in 3 to 12 weeks, and the patient is asymptomatic and immune to reinfection.

Secondary Syphilis

Secondary syphilis is characterized by dissemination and lesions in a variety of organs, most strikingly skin, mucous membranes, lymph nodes, stomach, and liver. At first there is a rash that appears 2 weeks to 6 months after the chancre heals. The rash is diffuse, macular, bilateral, and symmetrical and **often includes the palms and soles.** Next, the mucous membranes of the mouth and the moist genital surfaces display "mucous patches," which develop into shallow ulcers. There are a variety of secondary lesions, including condylomata lata (exudative plaques in the perineum, vulva, or scrotum); follicular syphilids (small papular lesions around hair follicles that cause loss of hair); and nummular syphilids (coinlike lesions involving the face and perineum). Condylomata lata are characterized by epithelial hyperplasia, acanthosis, infiltrates of plasma cells in the dermis, and a luetic vasculitis. These dermal and mucosal lesions teem with spirochetes.

Characteristic changes in lymph nodes include a thickened capsule, follicular hyperplasia, increased numbers of plasma cells, areas of fibro-histiocytic proliferation, clusters of histiocytes encroaching on the germinal centers, and luetic vasculitis. Focal abscesses and scattered granulomas containing giant cells are less common. Spirochetes abound in the walls of vessels, the areas of fibro-histiocytic proliferation, and abscesses.

In secondary syphilis of the stomach, a diffuse infiltrate of the wall by lymphocytes and plasma cells resembles lymphoma. Usually there are numerous spirochetes in the vessel walls and the loose connective tissue. In secondary syphilis of the liver, plasma cells, lymphocytes, and neutrophils infiltrate the portal tracts, in which there is a luetic vasculitis. The serum alkaline phosphatase activity is unusually high.

Infection of the meninges begins during the secondary stage and typically persists for life. There may also be optic neuritis during secondary syphilis. The cerebral spinal fluid is abnormal: the lymphocyte count is about 500 per mm^3 (pleocytosis), protein levels are increased, glucose levels are normal, and VDRL tests register positive. The serum likewise is VDRL-positive.

Latent Syphilis

When the lesions of secondary syphilis subside, there is a silent period of "well-being" that lasts for years or decades. However, during this latent period spirochetes continue to multiply, and the deep-seated lesions of tertiary syphilis gradually develop and expand. A few meningeal infections heal spontaneously, but most remain asymptomatic (latent) for years before some are reactivated during tertiary meningeal syphilis. The cerebral spinal fluid shows reduced pleocytosis (about 5 lymphocytes per mm^3), and both cerebral spinal fluid and serum are VDRL-positive. During this latent period, moreover, spirochetes may be passed in blood transfusions or across the placenta to the fetus.

Tertiary Syphilis

About 30% of untreated patients develop tertiary lesions. **Luetic aortitis,** a common tertiary lesion, is characterized by gradual weakening and stretching of the wall of the aorta to form an aneurysm. Grossly, the intima of the aorta appears rough and pitted; it has been described as having the appearance of tree bark (Fig. 9-17). This rough appearance is caused by degeneration of the media, and this in turn is caused by luetic vasculitis of the vasa vasorum. Over the

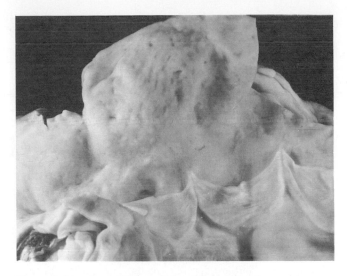

Figure 9-17. Syphilitic aortitis of the ascending aorta. The degeneration and destruction of the media makes the intima rough, "tree-barking".

years their lumens are gradually narrowed to the point of obliteration, causing ischemia of the wall of the aorta and degeneration of the media. The specialized arrangement of the aortic media, which includes a delicate and intimate weave of elastica, smooth muscle, and collagen, is gradually replaced by scar tissue. It is the specialized tissues of the media that give the aorta its strength and resiliency, and when these are replaced by scar, the aorta gradually stretches, becoming progressively thinner to the point of rupture, massive hemorrhage, and sudden death. **Damage to and scarring of the first part of the aorta commonly lead to stretching of the aortic ring, separation of the aortic cusps, and regurgitation through the aortic valve: so-called aortic insufficiency.** Luetic vasculitis of the coronary arteries may narrow or occlude the vessels and cause myocardial infarction.

Tertiary syphilis of the central nervous system (neurosyphilis) has many manifestations, which involve the meninges (with reactivation of the infection that began during secondary stage) and the arteries and parenchyma of the cerebral cortex. Meningovascular syphilis is characterized by an obliterative endarteritis of the meningeal vessels with subsequent arterial thrombosis and ischemic necrosis in the brain and spinal cord. Meningitis may also irritate the brain, causing grand mal or focal seizures, and may damage cranial nerves at the base of the brain.

Parenchymatous neurosyphilis is characterized by selective destruction of neurons, a process that leads to "general paresis of the insane." This syndrome

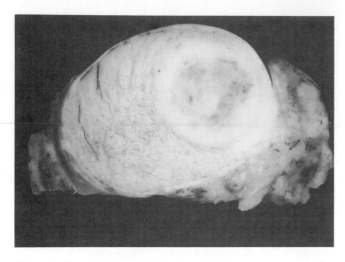

Figure 9-18. Tertiary syphilis, testis. The gumma in this testis is sharply circumscribed by a fibrogranulomatous wall. Only the center is necrotic.

starts with gradual loss of higher cognitive functions and progresses through various personality changes to dementia. Patients show impaired judgment, loss of memory, confusion, disorientation, grandiose but poorly developed delusions, hyperactive reflexes, and optic atrophy. **Inflammation of the dorsal roots causes secondary destruction of the dorsal columns (tabes dorsalis),** a disorder characterized by loss of the senses of joint position and vibration, wide-based gait, footslap, paresthesias of lower limbs, impotence, and episodes of intense referred pain (tabetic crisis). There may also be secondary, degenerative arthritis of one or more large joints (Charcot's joints). Sometimes there is simultaneous involvement of the parenchyma of both the spinal cord and the brain (taboparesis), usually preceded by generalized paresis.

The gumma, a characteristic lesion of tertiary syphilis, may form in any organ or tissue. This fibrotic and granulomatous lesion usually presents as an expanding tumor, commonly in the liver and testis (Fig. 9-18). In the liver, there may be a solitary gumma, several large gummas, or widespread small gummas that resemble cirrhosis. Gummas of the testis cause diffuse interstitial fibrosis and contraction of the testis into a round, hard mass. Microscopically, gummas are characterized by a central area of coagulative necrosis, surrounded by epithelioid cells, occasional giant cells, and a perimeter of fibrous tissue. The small vessels surrounding the gumma have thick walls and narrow lumens and resemble the vasa vasorum of luetic aortitis. Although infrequently seen, spirochetes are present in the necrotic centers of gummas.

Congenital Syphilis

Syphilis may be acquired *in utero*. The mother becomes infected within 5 years before the pregnancy. After about the fourth month of gestation, spirochetes in the maternal blood cross the placenta and invade the fetus. Infection may cause abortion or stillbirth or may remain inapparent for months or years. Infants also may be infected by contact with maternal lesions at the time of birth. **Patients with congenital syphilis have lesions of the skin, mucous membranes, bone, teeth, liver, lung, and central nervous system.** The rash may be of any type, including vesicular or bullous, and may be so severe that the epidermis sloughs. Target sites are anus, vulva, palms, soles, and mouth. The dermal vessels show luetic vasculitis, as already described, and the epidermis teems with spirochetes.

Spirochetes invade and grow in many fetal organs and tissues. Damage to bones and reconstruction by periosteum causes two characteristic lesions. The first is a depressed deformity of the bridge of the nose **(saddle nose),** and the second is anterior bowing of the tibias **(saber shins).** Infection of the enamel causes notched incisors **(Hutchinson's teeth).** In the liver, large areas of parenchymal cells are separated by loose fibrous connective tissue **(hepar lobatum).** Interstitial fibrosis and inflammatory cells in the lung **(pneumonia alba)** may prevent adequate pulmonary expansion and aeration. Spirochetes may infect the cornea, the optic nerve, and the eighth cranial nerve.

Penicillin arrests syphilis in all stages. Tetracycline is given to patients allergic to penicillin.

Bejel

Bejel is a syphilis-like disease transmitted by a nonvenereal route, such as from an infected baby to the breast of its mother, from mouth to mouth, or from utensils to mouth. Bejel is caused by a spirochete, *Treponema pallidum var. endemic*. Poor children who live in rural arid areas under unsanitary conditions are commonly affected.

Other than on the nursing breast, primary lesions are rare. Secondary lesions in the mouth are identical to the mucous lesions of venereal syphilis and may spread from the upper airway to the larynx. Lesions of perineum and bone and gummas of the breast occur, but cardiovascular and neurologic lesions and congenital transmission are rare. Spirochetes abound in the epidermis, neutrophils invade the skin, plasma cells are prominent in the dermis, and there is a syphilitic vasculitis.

Serologic tests for syphilis are positive, but the clinical presentation is different. Penicillin is an effective remedy.

Yaws

Yaws is a systemic treponematosis caused by *Treponema pertenue*, a spirochete that is morphologically and serologically indistinguishable from *T. pallidum*. Like syphilis, yaws has three stages and a period of latency, but it is nonvenereal and late lesions are limited to bone and skin. *T. pertenue* does not cause late lesions of the cardiovascular system, the central nervous system, or other deep organs. Children and adolescents living in deprived tropical regions are at risk. Transmission is by skin-to-skin contact and is facilitated by a break or abrasion.

Two to five weeks after inoculation, a single "mother yaw" appears at the site of inoculation, usually on an exposed part. It begins as a papule and becomes a "raspberry-like" papilloma, 2 to 5 cm across. The disseminated or secondary stage begins with the eruption of a similar, but smaller, raspberry-like lesion on other parts of the skin. Microscopically, the mother lesion and the disseminated lesions resemble each other. There is hyperkeratosis with a finely lobulated contour, papillary acanthosis, with elongation and pointing of the tips of the rete ridges, and an intense infiltrate of the epidermis by neutrophils. The epidermis dissolves at the apex of the papilloma, where neutrophils are concentrated, to form a shallow erosion of the surface. The dermal papillae are hyperemic and edematous. Plasma cells invade the upper dermis. Spirochetes are numerous in the dermal papillae, particularly in foci of neutrophils and in the superficial exudate. Unlike the causative organism of syphilis, *T. pertenue* does not invade, compromise, or destroy vessels. Painful papillomas on the soles lead the patient to walk on the sides of his feet like a crab, a condition called crab yaws. Shortly after inoculation the treponemes are borne by blood to bone, lymph nodes, and skin. Here they grow during a latent period of 5 or more years. This is followed by lesions of the late stage, which include gummas of the skin and periostitis, both of which are destructive. Periostitis of the tibia causes "saber shins" or "boomerang legs." Gummas of the skin are destructive in the face and upper airway.

Darkfield examinations of exudates, silver impregnation techniques on tissue sections, and all the serologic tests for syphilis are useful in the diagnosis of yaws. A single dose of long-acting penicillin is curative.

Pinta

Pinta, from the Spanish for blemish or painted, is a mild, systemic, nonvenereal treponemal infection caused by *Treponema carateum*. Pinta prevails in remote, arid inland regions and river valleys of the American tropics. Pinta, like syphilis, has been divided into three stages, but unlike syphilis all stages of pinta are limited to the skin, and lesions of the three stages tend to merge.

Transmission, usually after long intimate contact, is by skin-to-skin inoculation. Ten days later a small papule appears, most often on the leg. The papule grows and in 1 to 3 months may involve a 10-cm patch of skin. The lesion becomes flattened and displays irregular margins. The surface is scaly and pigmented, often appearing slate blue in dark-skinned patients. This lesion may persist for several years and on resolution leaves an area of hypopigmentation. In secondary pinta (5–18 months later) generalized pale-pink macules (pintids) concentrate on exposed surfaces. Later these lesions become depigmented and hyperkeratotic. There are numerous treponemes in the epidermis of the primary and secondary lesions, but not the late lesions. The lesions are characterized by acanthosis and hyperkeratosis of the epidermis, follicular plugging, elongation of rete ridges, intraepidermal microabscesses, and absence of pigment in the basal layer. The inflammatory infiltrate is diminished in the tertiary stage. Darkfield examination of exudate and serologic tests for syphilis are positive when the secondary lesions appear. A single dose of long-acting penicillin is curative.

Rat Bite Fever

Rat bite fever is a systemic infection that afflicts people in slums where rat control is lacking. There are two distinct organisms and hence two diseases. One of the agents is a spirochete, *Spirillum minor*, 0.15 μm wide and 2 to 5 μm long, with one to six spirals. Most of these infections are in Japan. The second cause is *Streptobacillum moniliformis*, a gram-negative bacillus, 0.1 to 0.7 μm wide and 1 to 5 μm long, which appears as clusters of organisms in tissue, forming long wavy chains or filaments.

Fever, chills, prostration, and myalgia begin 1 to 3 weeks after inoculation with the spirochetes at the site of the rodent bite. The site heals and then ulcerates. Lymphangitis, regional lymphadenitis, and generalized rash follow. Arthritis and endocarditis are less common. Febrile periods and remissions may alternate for years. The pathologic findings are unknown. *S. minor* is demonstrated in darkfield examination of specimens directly or after inoculation into an animal and examination of its blood. Penicillin is effective in *S. minor* infection.

Lyme Disease

Lyme disease, a tick-borne disease, is caused by *Borrelia burgdorferi*. Infection was first described in patients from Lyme, Connecticut, but was later recognized along the northeastern coast of the United States and in isolated foci in other regions of the United States and Europe. The peak season in the United States is summer and early fall. Ticks are infected while biting deer and mice.

Three days to four weeks after inoculation, a papule develops. A ringlike rash expands outward from the site of the bite and lasts from a month to a year. The majority of patients suffer from migratory polyarthritis, which may develop into chronic arthritis. Myocarditis and neurologic symptoms are seen in a minority of patients.

The papule shows acanthosis and necrosis of keratocytes in the epidermis. In the dermis and synovium, lymphocytes and histiocytes infiltrate neurovascular spaces. Spirochetes are found in vessel walls. The organisms are grown from blood, cerebrospinal fluid, and skin specimens. Penicillin V and tetracycline shorten the duration of the illness.

Diseases Caused by Bacteria

Anthrax

Anthrax, a rare zoonosis of man, is caused by *Bacillus anthracis*, a large, spore-forming, nonmotile, gram-positive bacillus. Goats, sheep, cattle, horses, pigs, and dogs are most susceptible. Spores form in the soil and dead animals, resisting heat, desiccation, and chemical disinfection for years. Man is infected when spores enter the body through breaks in skin, by inhalation, or by ingestion. Once in man, or another host, the spores germinate, yielding vegetative bacilli that produce potentially lethal toxins.

There are four forms of the disease—malignant pustule, septicemic, pneumonic, and gastrointestinal. The malignant pustule form is most common, accounting for 95% of infections. Those in contact with livestock, pastures, animal hides and carcasses, and other animal products are at greatest risk. Cutaneous lesions develop when bacilli or spores of *B. anthracis* enter traumatized skin. Several days later a small, red macule develops, which enlarges to form

a vesicle 0.5 to 1 cm across. Small satellite vesicles form around the primary lesions. Surrounding edema may be dramatic but is not constant. Vesicular fluid containing bloody, purulent exudate accumulates and gradually darkens to purple or black. In 2 to 4 days the vesicle ruptures, leaving a ragged, firm crater with a dark, leathery base. Reddened lymphatics reveal the path of drainage. Regional lymphadenitis portends a poor prognosis, because invasion of lymphatics precedes septicemia. In most patients, however, infection remains localized and subsides.

Pulmonary anthrax, sometimes called "wool sorters' disease," is a hazard of handling contaminated raw wool, and develops when spores of *B. anthracis* are inhaled. After an incubation period of 1 to 4 days there is an insidious onset of fever, malaise, and nonproductive cough. Several days later the patient experiences high fever, diaphoresis, prostration, dyspnea, tachycardia, and cyanosis. Pulmonary anthrax causes extensive serofibrinous exudate in large areas of the lung and sometimes consolidation of an entire lobe. The exudate contains many organisms but few neutrophils. There is a tendency for hemorrhagic necrosis of alveolar septa, and fibrin thrombi are seen in alveolar capillaries. The patient usually dies in the acute toxic stage.

Septicemia more commonly follows pulmonary anthrax than malignant pustule. In the former, bacilli are phagocytosed by alveolar macrophages and transported to the regional lymph nodes and then to the blood by way of the thoracic duct. Disseminated infection and localization in other organs follows. Disseminated intravascular coagulation complicates septicemia. In addition animal experiments have shown that a bacterial toxin causes a fatal depression of the respiratory center, which explains the fact that death can occur even when antibiotic therapy has cured the infection.

Anthrax of the gastrointestinal tract is rare and is probably acquired by eating contaminated meat. Ulceration of the stomach or bowel and invasion of regional lymphatics are the usual features. The hemorrhagic gastroenteritis of anthrax may cause obstruction or perforation, but death is commonly caused by electrolyte imbalance and hemoconcentration produced by fulminant diarrhea and massive ascites.

Salmonellosis (Gastroenteritis and Septicemia)

The genus *Salmonella* comprises a large, heterogeneous group of motile gram-negative bacilli that infect many animals and man. As a group, they are enteroinvasive and enteropathogenic and cause enteric fevers. Three species, associated with three distinct clinical entities, are identified; namely *S. enteritidis* (salmonella enteritis), *S. choleraesuis* (salmonella septicemia), and *S. typhi* (typhoid fever). *S. enteritidis* and *S. choleraesuis* are found in a wide range of animals, including reptiles, birds, and mammals. The only natural reservoir of *S. typhi* is man.

Gastroenteritis, caused by *S. enteritidis*, is an acute, self-limited infection of the small bowel, lasting 2 to 5 days. Symptoms include diarrhea, abdominal pain, and fever. Dehydration and electrolyte imbalance, probably caused by an enterotoxin similar to that of *E. coli*, can be a serious and even fatal complication in the very young and the very old. Organisms are isolated from stools for several weeks, but chronic infection is rare.

Septicemia, usually caused by *S. choleraesuis*, is characterized by prolonged fever and anemia. Focal suppurative lesions in many tissues and organs include osteomyelitis, pneumonia, pulmonary abscess, meningitis, and endocarditis. There are no gastrointestinal symptoms and the organisms are not cultured from the stools.

Typhoid Fever

Typhoid fever is an acute systemic illness caused by motile gram-negative bacilli of the genus *Salmonella* usually *S. typhi* or *S. enteritidis*. The organisms are gram-negative, flagellated, nonencapsulated, nonsporulating, facultative anaerobic bacilli, which have characteristic flagellar, somatic, and outer coat antigens. Typhoid fever, the most serious human salmonellosis, is characterized by prolonged fever, bacteremia, and multiplication of the organisms within mononuclear phagocytic cells of the liver, spleen, lymph nodes, and Peyer's patches.

Humans are the only natural reservoir for *S. typhi*, and typhoid fever therefore must be acquired from convalescing patients or from chronic carriers—especially older women with gallstones or biliary scarring, in whom *S. typhi* may colonize the gallbladder or biliary tree. Typhoid fever is spread primarily through ingestion of contaminated water and food (especially dairy products and shellfish), and much less commonly by direct finger-to-mouth contact with feces, urine, or other secretions. Although concentrations of *Salmonella typhi* in the water or food may be too low to cause infection, the organisms may proliferate sufficiently when environmental conditions are favorable to cause infection. Shellfish in contaminated water filter large volumes and concentrate the microbial content, a process that accumulates enormous doses of *S. typhi* in raw shellfish.

Urine from patients with pyelonephritis can be a significant source of *S. typhi*. Typhoid fever has become rare in countries with modern control of sewage and of water and milk supplies. Throughout history armies and refugees have been especially susceptible.

Untreated typhoid fever progresses through the following five stages: incubation (10-14 days); active invasion/bacteremia (1 week); fastigium (1 week); lysis (1 week); and convalescence (several weeks). Following ingestion, bacilli must first survive gastric acid. Thus, patients who ingest antacids, have had a gastrectomy, or have low gastric acidity for other reasons require fewer organisms for infection. Bacilli that survive gastric acidity attach preferentially to the tips of villi in the small intestine, invade the mucosa immediately, or multiply in the lumen for several days before penetrating the mucosa (Fig. 9-19). The bacilli then pass to the lymphoid follicles of the intestine and the draining mesenteric lymph nodes. Some organisms pass into the systemic circulation and are phagocytosed by reticuloendothelial cells of liver and spleen. Bacilli invade and proliferate further within the phagocytic cells of the intestinal lymphoid follicles, mesenteric lymph nodes, liver, and spleen. During this initial incubation period, therefore, the bacilli are primarily sequestered in the intracellular habitat of the intestinal and mesenteric lymphoid system.

Eventually, bacilli are released from the reticuloendothelial cells, pass through the thoracic duct, enter the bloodstream, and produce a primary transient bacteremia and clinical symptoms. During this active invasion/bacteremic phase, bacilli disseminate to and proliferate in many organs, but are most numerous in organs that possess significant phagocytic activity, namely the liver, spleen, and bone marrow. The Peyer's patches of the terminal ileum and the gallbladder are also hospitable sites. Bacilli invade the gallbladder from either blood or bile, after which they reappear in the intestine, are excreted in the stool, or reinvade the wall of the intestine.

Clinically, patients develop fever, diarrhea or constipation, vomiting, abdominal distention, myocarditis, splenomegaly, leukopenia, and mental changes. Infection of Peyer's patches leads to lymphoid hyperplasia, which can resolve without scarring or can progress to capillary thrombosis, with necrosis and ulceration. *S. typhi* in the blood during the second or third week of illness initiates prolonged bacteremia, often heralded by the transient appearances of "rose spots"—macular lesions on the limbs, lower abdomen, and chest that resemble petechial hemorrhages, but are actually foci of hyperemia (capillary atony). Microscopically, the macular lesions are edematous and infiltrated with histiocytes—an appearance that reveals that they are sites of bacterial localization and toxic injury.

The patient's temperature follows a characteristic pattern. It remains normal during the incubation period, undergoes daily stepwise elevations during active invasion, remains high during fastigium, falls slowly (with fluctuations) during lysis, and remains normal during convalescence. During the bacteremic phase, patients typically have a spiking afternoon fever that increases daily (up to 105°C) before stabilizing in the second or third week of illness. The high fever is often associated with prostration and delirium. Bacteria are seeded to other organs, including spleen, liver, kidneys, and gallbladder, and chronic cholecystitis may be established. Bacteria shed from the gallbladder reinfect the intestine, producing a tender abdomen and diarrheal disease, and they may also produce hepatosplenomegaly.

In the final phase, usually 3 to 5 weeks after onset, the patient is febrile and exhausted, but recovers if there are no complications. The most frequent and severe complication is intestinal perforation with peritonitis. Other problems are bleeding and thrombophlebitis, usually of the saphenous vein, cholecystitis, pneumonia, and focal abscesses in various organs and tissues. The mortality from these complications ranges from 2% to 10% without treatment. About 20% of untreated convalescent patients relapse.

The success of cultivation of *Salmonella* varies with stage and "tissue" (blood, urine, or stool). Cultures of blood may be positive during incubation and are usually positive during active invasion and fastigium; they are usually negative during lysis and convalescence. Cultures of urine and stool grow salmonella less frequently, but usually become positive toward the end of fastigium. Stool cultures remain positive until late convalescence. The Widal agglutination test, using H (flagellar) or O (somatic) antigens, becomes positive 10 or more days after onset, and titers continue to rise into convalescence.

The earliest pathologic changes are in the stages of bacterial attachment and penetration. Bacteria are firmly attached to intestinal epithelium with an accompanying degeneration of the brush borders. Later, as the salmonellae pass to lymphoid follicles of the intestine, there is diffuse enterocolitis and hypertrophy of Peyer's patches. This is followed by necrosis of intestinal and mesenteric lymphoid tissues, focal granulomas in the liver and spleen, and characteristic *mononuclear* inflammatory cells ("typhoid nodules") in many organs. Typhoid nodules are primarily aggregates of altered macrophages ("typhoid cells") that phagocytose bacteria, erythrocytes, and degenerated lymphocytes. These nodules also contain plasma cells and lymphocytes, but not typically neutrophils. The most common sites for typhoid nodules are the intestine, mesenteric lymph nodes, spleen, liver, and bone marrow. Less commonly, the kidney, testes, and parotid gland are affected.

Although the pathologic changes of typhoid fever may not correlate precisely with the clinical stages, certain patterns are characteristic. During the incubation stage there is a mild enteritis, mesenteric lymphadenitis, and hyperplasia of intestinal lymphoid tissue, primarily of Peyer's patches of the ileum and solitary lymphoid follicles of the cecum. The lymphoid hyperplasia may resolve or may progress to capillary thrombosis. Thrombosis causes the adjoining intestinal mucosa to enlarge during the phase of active invasion and then become necrotic. This pro-

---

Figure 9-19. Stages of typhoid fever.
Incubation (10–14 days). Water or food contaminated with *S. typhi* is ingested. Bacilli attach to the villi in the small intestine, invade the mucosa, and pass to the intestinal lymphoid follicles and draining mesenteric lymph nodes. The organisms proliferate further within mononuclear phagocytic cells of the lymphoid follicles, lymph nodes, liver, and spleen. Bacilli are sequestered intracellularly in the intestinal and mesenteric lymphatic system.
Active invasion/bacteremia (1 week). Organisms are released and produce a transient bacteremia. The intestinal mucosa becomes enlarged and necrotic, forming characteristic mucosal lesions. The intestinal lymphoid tissues become hyperplastic and contain "typhoid nodules"—aggregates of macrophages ("typhoid cells") that phagocytose bacteria, erythrocytes, and degenerated lymphocytes. Bacilli proliferate in several organs, reappear in the intestine, are excreted in stool, and may reinvade through the intestinal wall.
Fastigium (1 week). Dying bacilli release endotoxins that cause systemic toxemia.
Lysis (1 week). Necrotic intestinal mucosa sloughs, producing ulcers, which hemorrhage or perforate into the peritoneal cavity.

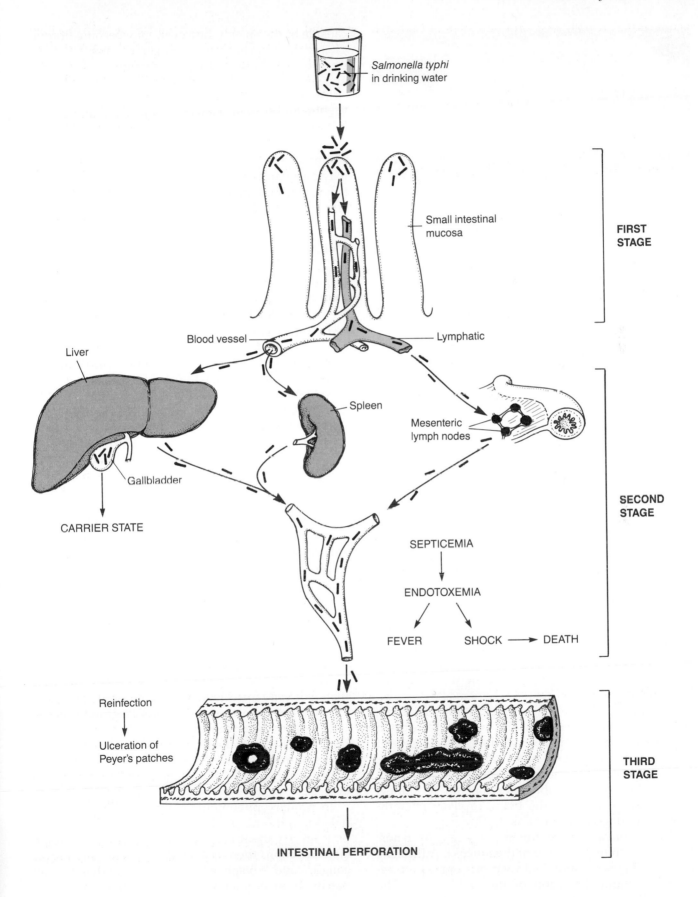

Salmonella typhi in drinking water

Small intestinal mucosa

FIRST STAGE

Blood vessel

Lymphatic

Liver

Spleen

Mesenteric lymph nodes

Gallbladder

CARRIER STATE

SECOND STAGE

SEPTICEMIA

ENDOTOXEMIA

FEVER

SHOCK ⟶ DEATH

Reinfection

Ulceration of Peyer's patches

THIRD STAGE

INTESTINAL PERFORATION

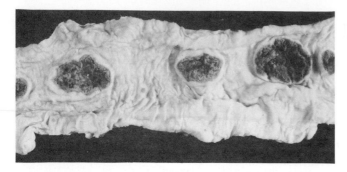

Figure 9-20. Ulcers of the terminal ileum in fatal typhoid fever. The ulcers have a longitudinal orientation because they are over hyperplastic and necrotic Peyer's patches.

cess gives rise to the characteristic lesions, which are elevated 0.1 to 0.4 cm above adjacent mucosa.

While bacilli continue to proliferate, dying bacilli release endotoxins that cause toxemia, beginning during invasion and becoming maximal in fastigium. The necrotic mucosa sloughs, usually during lysis, producing ulcers that conform to Peyer's patches and are concentrated along the antimesenteric border (Fig. 9-20). The ulcers may bleed or perforate, usually during lysis. Most perforations are near the ileocecal valve, measure less than 1 cm across, and lead to peritonitis. Interestingly, these areas become repopulated with lymphoid cells and heal without scarring.

During active invasion the mesenteric lymph nodes enlarge and develop typhoid nodules, focal hemorrhages, and necrosis, changes which resemble those in the intestinal lymphoid tissue. The spleen becomes large and hyperemic and microscopically shows typhoid nodules in the red pulp. The hyperplastic white pulp exhibits areas of focal necrosis. The enlarged liver displays sinusoids lined with swollen Kupffer's cells and histiocytes. Focal necrosis of liver cells is common. The lack of neutrophils in typhoid fever is conspicuous. The intestinal ulcers and focal areas of necrosis are bounded only by chronic inflammatory cells, and the patient is actually leukopenic.

Toxemia may cause other complications, including ileus; mild fatty liver; a flabby heart with dilated ventricles, vacuolization of cardiac myocytes, and cardiac arrhythmia that may cause sudden death; mild interstitial pneumonia; swelling and degeneration of the proximal tubular epithelium of kidney; "ring" hemorrhages in the brain; capillary microthrombi; and degeneration of skeletal muscles.

During convalescence, the intestine returns to normal, with minimal scarring of the mucosa. Adhesions are rare. Typhoid nodules in various organs are resorbed without distortion of the architecture. The

capsule of the spleen, however, may become fibrotic, giving the appearance of "sugar coating." Skeletal muscle regenerates and toxic changes of heart disappear.

The most widely used antibiotic for typhoid fever is chloramphenicol. However, this drug does not reduce the relapse rate, and convalescent excretors and chronic carriers are not cured. Moreover, some strains of *S. typhi* are resistant, and chloramphenicol may cause aplastic anemia. Other effective antibiotics (some without these disadvantages) are ampicillin, amoxicillin, and trimethoprim-sulfamethoxazole.

Plague

Plague is caused by *Yersinia pestis*, a plump, bipolar, staining coccobacillus. The Americas, Africa, and Asia are endemic areas. Wild rodents such as squirrels, chipmunks, mice, wood rats, and rabbits are reservoirs. Transmission from animal to animal is by fleas. Infected domestic animals bring the disease to humans by direct contact or flea bites.

Two to eight days after the flea bite, bubonic plague begins with chills, fever, nausea, vomiting, and rapid respiration and pulse. A painful lymph node (bubo) enlarges in the area drained by the bite. The architecture of the lymph node, including the capsule and perinodal fat, is obliterated by necrosis, hemorrhage, and finely granular material. This material comprises solid masses of gram-negative coccobacilli, the plague bacillus. Blood cultures are positive in 50% of patients. **Petechiae and ecchymoses lead to the "black death,"** 60 to 90% of those affected dying within 24 hours if untreated. Toxemia may kill even when antibiotics have arrested the growth of bacteria. The virulence of the plague bacillus partly reflects its resistance to phagocytosis and destruction. Furthermore, the bacillus elaborates an antigenic coat that, on the release of the organisms from phagocytic cells, enhances their resistance to further phagocytosis.

In primary systemic plague, the bacteria are inoculated directly into blood and do not produce a bubo. Patients die from the overwhelming growth of bacteria in the bloodstream. Fever, prostration, and meningitis occur suddenly, and death comes within 48 hours of onset. All vessels contain bacilli, and fibrin casts surround them in renal glomeruli and in dermal vessels.

In primary pneumonic plague, the bacilli are inhaled in airborne particles from carcasses of animals or from a patient's cough. Forty-eight to 60 hours after infection, there is a sudden onset of high fever, cough, and dyspnea. Radiographs demonstrate patchy bronchopneumonia or confluent consolidation. The sputum teems with bacilli. Respiratory insufficiency and shock from endotoxin and disseminated intravascular coagulation kill the patient in 1 to 2 days. Lobular pneumonia is characterized by necrotic alveolar walls, nodules of necrotic tissue and debris, intense hyperemia and hemorrhage, and myriad bacilli in the alveoli. Neutrophils are scant.

The diagnosis is made by blood culture and smears of aspirate from buboes, cerebrospinal fluid, sputum, and transtracheal aspirates. Tetracycline or streptomycin are effective if started early, and chloramphenicol is used in patients with meningitis.

Tularemia

Tularemia is an acute, febrile, granulomatous, zoonotic disease caused by *Francisella tularensis*. Rabbits and rodents are the most important reservoirs, but many other wild and domestic animals are infected. Humans become infected through broken skin or intact mucosa by handling infected animals and carcasses; by ingesting contaminated food and water; by inhaling bacteria; or by being bitten by infected insects, including ticks, deer flies, and mosquitoes. Human-to-human transmission has not been reported. The incidence of reported cases in the United States has decreased by a factor of ten in the last 50 years.

F. tularensis is a small (0.2 by 0.5 μm), aerobic, gram-negative bacillus that is not motile, encapsulated, or spore-forming. It does not grow on standard bacteriologic media, but will grow slowly on media enriched with cystine or cysteine. Two biovars of *F. tularensis* are identified. Type A is in the continental United States only, where it causes 90% of tularemia. It is highly virulent and is usually tick-borne and rabbit-associated. The mortality from untreated Type A tularemia ranges from 5% for ulceroglandular tularemia to 30% for the typhoidal and pneumonic forms. Type B is less virulent and has a worldwide distribution. It occurs in goats and may be transmitted to humans by mosquitos or ticks, or by water contaminated by infected rodents, such as beavers and muskrats. The mortality caused by Type B is less than 1%, even if the disease is left untreated.

Tularemia has four clinical presentations: ulceroglandular, oculoglandular, pneumonic, and typhoidal. Pneumonia may complicate any one of the types. The incubation period ranges from 1 to 20 days, depending on the dose and route of transmission, with a mean of 3 to 4 days. The duration of illness is 1 week to 3 months, but may be shortened by prompt treatment. The most common form of tularemia, **ulceroglandular,** begins as a tender erythematous pap-

ule at the site of inoculation, usually on a limb. This develops into a pustule, which ulcerates. The regional lymph nodes become large and tender, and may suppurate and drain through sinus tracts. In some patients an erythematous, maculopapular rash, thought to represent delayed hypersensitivity, may develop. The initial bacteremia is followed in a week by generalized lymphadenopathy and splenomegaly. Symptoms include fever, headache, myalgia, and occasionally prostration. Some patients develop meningitis, endocarditis, pericarditis, or osteomyelitis. The most serious infections are complicated by a secondary pneumonia and endotoxic shock, in which case the prognosis is grave. In **oculoglandular** tularemia the primary lesion is a papule in the conjunctiva, which becomes a pustule and ulcerates. This is accompanied by lymphadenopathy of the head and neck. Severe ulceration may penetrate the sclera entering the eye and infect the optic nerve, causing blindness. In **glandular tularemia** generalized lymphadenopathy is the first manifestation. A diagnosis of the **typhoidal form** is made when fever, hepatosplenomegaly, and toxemia, resembling salmonella sepsis, are the presenting features. Diagnostic antibody titers usually appear within 2 weeks of infection.

The initial skin lesion in tularemia is a pyogenic ulcer with purulent exudate. Later, disseminated lesions undergo central necrosis and are surrounded by a perimeter of granulomatous reaction resembling lesions of tuberculosis. The lymph nodes become large and firm from hyperemia and from large numbers of histiocytes in the subcapsular and peritrabecular sinusoids. Later they soften as areas of stellate necrosis and suppuration develop. By contrast, the enlarged spleen shows only congestion, nonspecific inflammatory cell infiltrates, and lymphoreticular hyperplasia. The lesions in the lung resemble those of primary tuberculosis (Fig. 9-21). On rare occasions bacilli may be identified in histocytes.

Haemophilus Influenzae *Infection*

Haemophilus influenzae is a gram-negative, pleomorphic, aerobic bacillus that is nonmotile and does not form spores. It is a strict parasite of humans, and causes pneumonia, meningitis, epiglottitis, pericarditis, bacteremia, cellulitis, pyarthrosis, and "pink eye"—an acute, purulent conjunctivitis. The presence or absence of a polysaccharide capsule determines the morphology of its colonies and its pathogenicity. Encapsulated bacteria secrete a capsular polymer that makes the colony appear umbilicated. Of six dissimilar antigens in the capsule, type b

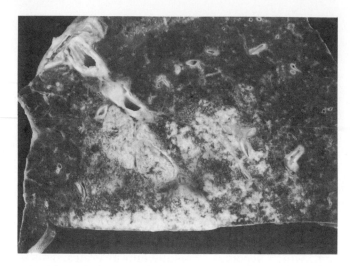

Figure 9-21. Fatal tularemia, lung. The white areas are firm, consolidated, and necrotic.

causes more than 90% of human infections and is **the most common cause of bacterial meningitis in the United States.** *H. influenzae* is recovered from 80% of healthy adults and is encountered worldwide. By 5 years of age, all children have *H. influenzae* in their nasopharynx, and 1 in 200 children will at some time have a systemic infection caused by type b. Some children who become infected before 18 months fail to develop adequate antibodies and may contract a second systemic infection with *H. influenzae*. Children under 2 years of age in day care centers or who are in families with an ill patient are at greater risk. These children should receive rifampin prophylaxis.

Meningitis caused by *H. influenzae* usually follows otitis, sinusitis, pneumonia, or impaired immunity. An early symptom is pain when the child sits up or is diapered. Upper respiratory symptoms, fever, vomiting, irritability, and lethargy accompany the meningitis, and 5% to 10% die within 48 hours. Neurologic deficits are permanent in one-third of those who survive. Bacteria, neutrophils, and fibrin form an exudate in the leptomeninges. The exudate extends from the basal portion of the subarachnoid space into the brain along the vessels. The typical gram-negative coccobacilli are in neutrophils in the exudate around the meningeal blood vessels.

Infection of lung by *H. influenzae* produces fever, cough, purulent sputum, dyspnea, and either bronchopneumonia or lobar pneumonia. The pneumonia usually complicates chronic lung disease and in half the patients follows a viral infection of the respiratory tract. The alveoli are filled with neutrophils, macrophages containing bacilli, and fibrin. The bronchial epithelium is necrotic and replaced by macrophages.

Bacilli are in macrophages and short and long filamentous bacilli are packed together in extracellular foci. Empyema may form and display a similar inflammatory reaction. Part of the pathogenicity of *H. influenzae* may be due to an extracellular toxin that arrests the action of cilia.

The onset of epiglottitis is sudden; fever, dysphagia, accumulation of oropharyngeal secretions, tachypnea, and retraction precede obstruction of airways. The epiglottis is swollen by edema, neutrophils, and macrophages. The infection may descend past the larynx into the trachea and bronchi, plugging the small airways with thick exudate.

Bacteremia may seed large weight-bearing joints, leading to pyarthrosis. There is fever, heat, erythema, swelling, pain on movement, and decreased movement. The diagnosis is made by culturing *H. influenzae* from the joint fluid.

Needle aspirates of exudates from empyema and lung, pericardium, joint, and blood or cerebral spinal fluid may be cultured for specific diagnosis. Chloramphenicol remains the drug of choice in meningitis. A polysaccharide vaccine for *H. influenzae* type b is under development.

Whooping Cough (Pertussis)

Whooping cough is caused by *Bordetella pertussis*, a nonmotile, gram-negative coccobacillus that forms a capsule in its virulent state. Humans provide the only reservoir. *B. pertussis* produces a heat-labile toxin, a heat-stable endotoxin, and a lymphocytosis-producing factor also called histamine-sensitizing factor. The heat-labile toxin is dermonecrotic in rabbits and paralyzes cilia in the lungs of mice, but its effect in man is unproved.

Pertussis is worldwide and passes from person to person in moist droplets containing *B. pertussis*. Nearly all susceptible contacts become infected. *B. pertussis* has a remarkable ability, probably enhanced by its pili, to attach to ciliated bronchial epithelium. Here the organisms proliferate, remain on the surface epithelium, and accumulate in great numbers. The bacteria stimulate the bronchial cells to produce a profuse, tenacious mucus that slows ciliary action and inhibits the bronchopulmonary toilet. Secondary bacterial infections and epithelial necrosis follow. A catarrhal stage begins 7 to 10 days after exposure and may last 1 to 2 weeks. There is low-grade fever, rhinorrhea, tearing, and conjunctivitis. During the catarrhal stage, when the patient is most infectious, *B. pertussis* proliferates, forms entangled masses mixed with the cilia, and elicits a neutrophilic exudate.

Cough progresses to severe paroxysms terminating in a gasping, strident, inspiratory effort. During inspiration, air is forcibly drawn through a narrow glottis, giving the characteristic "whoop." This paroxysmal stage begins 2 to 3 weeks after inoculation, lasts days to weeks, and is marked by as many as 50 paroxysms per day. The necrotic bronchial epithelium is covered by a thick mucopurulent exudate. The convalescent stage lasts weeks or (rarely) months.

The death rate is highest in infancy. Immunity is conferred by IgA antibody, which prevents bacterial attachment. Second attacks can occur but are caused by *B. parapertussis*, which may cause 20% of all whooping cough infections. Vaccination protects against *B. pertussis*, but not against *B. parapertussis*.

B. pertussis may be cultured from the posterior nasopharynx during the first 2 weeks. Smears from nasopharyngeal swabs can be tested with fluorescent-labeled antipertussis serum. A combination of culture and fluorescent-labeled smears gives the greatest diagnostic accuracy. Erythromycin is effective in the catarrhal stage and should be given to all contacts with positive nasopharyngeal smears. Antibiotics begun after the paroxysmal stage begins do not alter the clinical course.

Chancroid

Chancroid, the "third venereal disease", is an acute, sexually transmitted bacterial infection caused by *Haemophilus ducreyi*, a short gram-negative bacillus that appears in tissue as clusters of parallel bacilli and as chains—said to resemble schools of fish. The bacillus is highly infectious and invades on contact, through the skin or mucous membranes. Chancroid is most common in tropical and subtropical regions and especially in the Far East. It is more frequent in men than women and is associated with promiscuity and poor personal hygiene.

The lesions are located on the skin and mucous membranes of the genitalia. A papule develops 1 to 14 days after contact, becomes pustular, and ulcerates. The ulcers rarely exceed 2.0 cm in diameter, although large and mutilating ulcers have been described. Multiple ulcers are common, and in rare cases there are extragenital lesions of the tongue, lips, and fingers. Seven to 10 days after the appearance of the primary lesion, half of the patients develop unilateral, painful, suppurative, inguinal lymphadenitis (a bubo). The skin becomes inflamed, breaks down, and drains pus from the underlying node. At the time the bubo develops, the patient has systemic symptoms, including headache and fever.

Microscopically, the infected epithelium over the papule becomes acutely inflamed and necrotic, and sloughs. The typical ulcer has three zones, which overlap and merge. The superficial zone contains neutrophils, fibrin, erythrocytes, and debris. The broad middle zone comprises edematous, inflamed granulation tissue. Finally, a deep zone contains plasma cells and lymphocytes concentrated around vessels. The lymph nodes enlarge, become necrotic, and erupt through the skin. The diagnosis is made by identifying the bacillus in tissue sections or gram stained smears prepared from ulcers or aspirated buboes. *H. ducreyi* can be cultured on selective media, but with difficulty. Erythromycin is usually effective.

Legionellosis (Legionnaires' Disease)

Legionellosis is a severe, necrotizing pneumonia caused by a minute, gram-negative bacillus, *Legionella pneumophila*. About 6 months after an outbreak of a severe respiratory disease of unknown cause at the American Legion's state convention in Philadelphia in 1976, *L. pneumophila* was identified by workers at the Centers for Disease Control. Subsequently, retrospective serologic and immunofluorescent studies revealed antibodies in sera from previously unexplained epidemics. Of historical note is the first epidemic so recognized, in a meat packing plant in Minnesota in 1957. Legionnaires' disease occurs sporadically, as epidemics, and as nosocomial infections, especially in patients with compromised immunity. Those who abuse alcohol and smoke heavily are also at increased risk. Common source exposure is frequent. The organism has been recovered from soil, ponds, water systems, and air conditioning systems. Legionellosis has been recognized throughout the world, without a geographic pattern.

The disease presents as a rapidly progressive pneumonia, accompanied by fever, a nonproductive cough, and myalgias. The onset is abrupt, after an incubation period of 2 to 10 days. Within 2 days, most patients develop a persistent high fever and respiratory rales. Radiograms of the chest reveal unilateral, diffuse, patchy bronchopneumonia, progressing to widespread nodular consolidation, usually without cavitation. Toxic symptoms, hypoxia, and obtundation may be prominent, and death may follow in a few days. In those who survive, convalescence is prolonged. The antibiotic of choice is erythromycin.

The main changes in the lung include consolidation, necrosis, and acute congestion. Microscopically, the alveoli are packed with an exudate composed of histiocytes and fibrin (Fig. 9-22). The alveolar walls

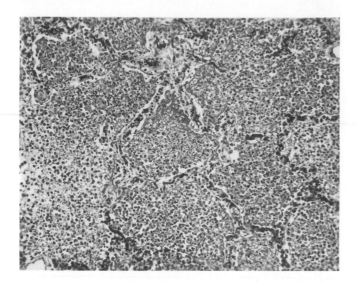

Figure 9-22. Fatal legionellosis, section of consolidated lung. The alveoli are packed with an exudate composed of histiocytes and fibrin.

become necrotic and are destroyed. Neutrophils accumulate as necrosis becomes more pronounced and eventually confluent. Many histiocytes show eccentric nuclei, pushed aside by cytoplasmic vacuoles containing *L. pneumophila*. Dissemination of *L. pneumophila* to the kidneys, spleen, bone marrow, and lymph nodes has been reported.

Isolation and identification of the bacilli is necessary for an unequivocal diagnosis, but isolation may be hazardous. The direct fluorescence antibody test for *L. pneumophila* can be performed on formalin-fixed, paraffin-embedded tissue and is thus valuable for confirming the diagnosis.

Cholera

Cholera is caused by the enterotoxin elaborated by *Vibrio cholerae*, a gram-negative bacillus (Fig. 9-23). The organism proliferates in the lumen of the small intestine and causes profuse watery diarrhea, rapid dehydration, and (if fluids are not restored) shock and death within 24 hours of the onset of symptoms. Enterotoxins of other vibrios (for instance *V. parahaemolyticus*) also cause diarrhea and mimic cholera, but symptoms are milder.

In the 19th century cholera was common in most parts of the world, but it periodically "disappears." There have been major pandemics; the seventh and most recent (1961–74) extended throughout Asia, the Middle East, southern Russia, the Mediterranean basin, and parts of Africa. Cholera persists in the delta of the Ganges river of India.

V. cholerae is a curved gram-negative bacillus with a polar flagellum that moves in a helical path, with a characteristic wobble. *V. cholerae* is destroyed by gastric acid. Successful colonization in the small intestine depends on (a) a reduction or dilution of gastric acid, (b) bacterial motility, pili, and production of enzymes (colicins, mucinase, neuraminidase), and (c) availability of binding sites for the organisms and the enterotoxin. Pathogenic strains adhere to cells of the intestinal mucosa.

Drinking water contaminated with *V. cholerae* and food prepared with contaminated water are infectious (Fig. 9-23). Those with a normal gastric acidity are much less susceptible than those with low levels of stomach acid as a result of a gastrectomy or other cause. Vibrios traverse the stomach, enter the small intestine and propagate. **They remain in the lumen and do not invade the intestinal mucosa.** They do, however, elaborate an enterotoxin, which contains A and B subunits. The B subunit binds the toxin to GM_1 ganglioside in the cell membrane at the brush border of the small intestine. The A subunit enters the cell and activates adenyl cyclase, thereby initiating a chain of reactions in the membrane (see Fig. 9-23). Symptoms begin when the massive secretion of water and sodium in the small intestine, a consequence of the activation of cyclic AMP, exceeds the resorptive capacity of the colon. The small intestine, however, is not damaged morphologically either by the vibrios or by the enterotoxin.

The loss of sodium and water causes severe diarrhea, called "ricewater stool." Fluid loss may exceed 1 liter per hour. Acute dehydration, hypovolemic shock, and metabolic acidosis follow quickly. The patient exhibits dry skin, sunken eyes, lethargy, cyanosis, a weak pulse, faint heart sounds, hemoconcentration, and elevation of serum proteins. The hematocrit may rise to 55–65 and the plasma specific gravity to 1.035–1.050. Patients are usually afebrile; in fact, body temperature may be subnormal. Treatment is prompt rehydration, and under such circumstances most patients survive. After the onset of diarrhea, urine production ceases, but renal function improves when fluid and electrolytes are replaced. Inadequate replacement, however, leads to prolonged renal failure, with acute damage of tubules and the vacuolar lesions of hypokalemia.

For many years, the intestinal changes in cholera could be studied only at autopsy. Degenerative changes in the intestinal epithelium, although observed repeatedly in victims of cholera, could not be distinguished from the autolysis that begins in the intestine at the moment of death. Specimens of the small intestine taken promptly after death have now

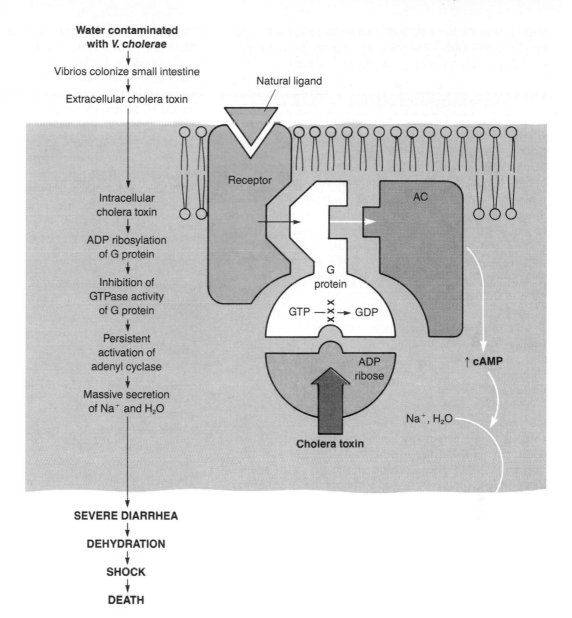

**Water contaminated
with *V. cholerae***
↓
Vibrios colonize small intestine
↓
Extracellular cholera toxin
↓
Intracellular
cholera toxin
↓
ADP ribosylation
of G protein
↓
Inhibition of
GTPase activity
of G protein
↓
Persistent
activation of
adenyl cyclase
↓
Massive secretion
of Na⁺ and H₂O

Natural ligand

Receptor

AC

G
protein

GTP —×××→ GDP

ADP
ribose

↑ **cAMP**

Na⁺, H₂O

Cholera toxin

SEVERE DIARRHEA
↓
DEHYDRATION
↓
SHOCK
↓
DEATH

Figure 9-23. Cholera. Infection comes from water contaminated with *Vibrio cholerae* or food prepared with contaminated water. The vibrios traverse the stomach, enter the small intestine, and propagate. Although they do not invade the intestinal mucosa, the vibrios elaborate a potent toxin that induces a massive outpouring of water and electrolytes, . Severe diarrhea ("ricewater stool") leads to dehydration and hypovolemic shock.

shown that cholera patients have an intact intestinal epithelium and, except for minor, nonspecific changes, a morphologically normal mucosa.

Vibrio parahemolyticus *Infection*

Vibrio parahemolyticus is a gram-negative bacillus that causes acute gastroenteritis. It is found in marine life and coastal waters around the world and causes outbreaks in summer; the gastroenteritis is associated with consumption of inadequately cooked or inadequately refrigerated seafood. Symptoms appear 12 to 24 hours after ingestion. The clinical course is short, usually lasting less than 1 week, and deaths have not been reported.

The usual clinical syndrome resembles salmonella enteritis, with explosive watery diarrhea, abdominal cramps, nausea, and vomiting. Occasionally *V. parahemolyticus* causes a shigella-like dysentery, characterized by abdominal pain, bloody mucoid stools, chills and fever. Serodiagnosis is not helpful, because *V. parahemolyticus* cross-reacts with other halophilic vibrios.

The pathogenic mechanisms are uncertain but studies suggest an enterotoxin antigenically related to shiga toxin. Adherence of the enterotoxin to the intestinal epithelium is required for pathogenicity. There is direct invasion of ilial mucosa in animal models, and this may explain the dysentery-like disease.

Shigellosis

Shigellosis is an acute bacterial dysentery caused by any of four species of shigellae, *S. dysenteriae, S. flexnerin, S. boydii*, and *S. sonnei*. Shigellae are among the most virulent enteropathogens. Disease is produced by the ingestion of as few as 10 to 100 organisms, and there are few asymptomatic carriers. *Shigella* enteritis ranges from mild diarrhea to incapacitating and life-threatening dysentery, the latter caused primarily by *S. dysenteriae* (the Shiga bacillus). This species caused the 1968 pandemic in Central and North America, in which mortality rates reached 20% to 50%. The enteric lesions, limited to the colon, are destructive, as evidenced by the bloody mucoid stools characteristic of shigellosis.

The shigellae are worldwide and are most important and conspicuous in tropical and developing countries, where they are a major cause of morbidity and mortality. Unlike the salmonellae, which also invade and colonize the intestinal mucosa, shigellae have no significant animal reservoir. Nor do shigellae survive well outside the stool, being transmitted mainly by direct fecal-oral contamination. Endemic shigellosis, therefore, tends to strike communities with poor standards of hygiene and sanitation. Shigellosis is also spread in closed communities, such as hospitals, barracks, and households. In developed countries, *S. flexneri* and *S. sonnei* are more common, and infection is sporadic.

Symptoms appear 2 to 5 days after the ingestion of bacteria. The dose of organisms and the status of host defenses influence the incubation period and severity. Milder infections are characterized by the onset of profuse diarrhea before other acute symptoms. Early onset of fever, diarrhea, abdominal pain, and tenesmus is more serious and may be life-threatening. Diffuse involvement of the colon is associated with high fever, shaking chills, toxemia, and shock. Appropriate antibiotic therapy is critical in shortening the illness, preventing relapse, and reducing transmission. The emergence of plasmid-mediated multiple drug resistance in shigellae requires that antibiotic sensitivity be determined for all isolates of shigellae.

The key to the pathogenicity of *Shigella* is its ability to invade and multiply in the epithelium and lamina propria of the terminal ileum and colon. The mucosa becomes edematous and hyperemic, and is covered by pus and mucus. The ulcerated mucosa becomes covered with a granular, dirty-yellow pseudomembrane, consisting of necrotic mucosa, neutrophils, fibrin, and erythrocytes. Sloughed pseudomembrane, together with blood-tinged mucus, comprise the characteristic dysenteric stool of shigellosis. The epithelium persists only in the depths of the crypts, and goblet cells contain no mucus in the acute stage. Epithelial regeneration is rapid and healing is complete in 2 weeks. Endotoxin probably adds to necrosis, but the role of enterotoxin produced by some species of *Shigella* in the pathogenesis of dysentery is uncertain. While clearly secondary to invasion, Shiga toxin probably contributes to the profuse diarrhea that precedes dysentery in some patients. This enterotoxin, which is related antigenically to the enterotoxin of enteropathogenic *E. coli*, activates membrane-associated adenyl cyclase. Thus, shiga toxin, like cholera toxin and *E. coli* enterotoxin, induces hypersecretion of fluid and electrolytes from the mucosa of the terminal ileum. Water and electrolyte balance must be maintained to prevent dehydration, prostration, and impaired mental status.

Escherichia coli *Infection*

Escherichia coli, a gram-negative bacillus that is part of the intestinal flora, is also an important opportunistic pathogen, causing diarrhea and dysentery, urinary tract infections, pneumonia, and neonatal meningitis.

E. coli causes at least three patterns of human enteric diseases: enterotoxigenic, enteroinvasive, and enteroadherent. Enterotoxigenic *E. coli* causes a diarrheal disease by elaborating two plasmid-mediated enterotoxins. The heat-labile toxin is antigenically, structurally, and functionally related to the cholera toxin, although the toxin of *E. coli* is less potent than that of cholera. The heat-labile toxin also binds to GM_1 ganglioside on the intestinal epithelial cells. As in cholera, the resulting activation of adenyl cyclase produces a hypersecretory diarrhea. The heat-stable toxin of *E. coli* is different from cholera toxin and apparently acts to impair sodium and chloride absorption and to reduce the motility of the small intestine through a mechanism dependent on cyclic GMP. Dehydration and electrolyte imbalance is a significant cause of morbidity and mortality when appropriate rehydration is lacking—a common combination among infants in less developed countries. Enterotoxigenic *E. coli* is also responsible for 50% of traveller's diarrhea.

The importance of enterotoxigenic *E. coli* in the United States is uncertain but an estimated 4% of childhood diarrhea in the United States is caused by this organism.

Enteroinvasive *E. coli* produces a dysentery-like disease resembling shigellosis, although it is less severe and requires a much larger infecting dose of organisms. Enteroinvasive *E. coli* invades the intestinal mucosa and causes local tissue destruction and sloughing of necrotic mucosa. Bloody mucoid stools contain neutrophils. The importance of enteroinvasive *E. coli* in the United States is also uncertain.

Enteroadhesive *E. coli* has only recently been associated with diarrheal diseases. Enteroadhesiveness is plasmid-dependent and is apparently mediated by pili, which bind tightly to receptors on the intestinal epithelial cells. The mechanism of diarrhea is unknown.

About 80% of all infections of the urinary tract in humans, ranging from mild cystitis to fatal pyelonephritis, are caused by *E. coli*. In addition, *E. coli* is the etiologic agent in many cases of nosocomial pneumonia, most often in elderly patients with underlying chronic disease. Aspirates of endogenous oral flora containing *E. coli* appear to be the cause of this bronchopneumonia, although in bacteremic patients pneumonia may result from seeding by septic emboli. Empyema is a common complication, especially in patients with disease lasting more than a week.

Only rarely does *E. coli* cause meningitis in adults, but it is a major cause of neonatal meningitis. Between 40% and 80% of infants with *E. coli* meningitis die, and the survivors frequently suffer from neurologic or developmental anomalies.

Yersiniosis

Yersiniosis is caused by *Yersinia enterocolitica* and *Y. pseudotuberculosis* (*Y. pestis* causes human plague and is described separately). *Y. enterocolitica* and *Y. pseudotuberculosis* are gram-negative, oval, coccoid or rod-shape bacteria. Both species are motile, facultative anaerobes found in the feces of wild and domestic animals, including rodents, sheep, cattle, dogs, cats, and horses. Birds such as turkeys, ducks, geese, pigeons, and canaries are common sources of *Y. pseudotuberculosis*. Both organisms have been isolated from drinking water and milk. *Y. enterocolitica* is more likely to be acquired from contaminated meat and *Y. pseudotuberculosis* from contact with infected animals.

Ingested *Y. enterocolitica* proliferates in the ileum, invades the mucosa, produces ulceration and necrosis of Peyer's patches, and migrates by way of the lymphatics to the mesenteric lymph nodes. Arthralgia, arthritis, and erythema nodosum are complications. Septicemia is an uncommon complication but kills about one-half of those affected. Fever, diarrhea—sometimes bloody—and abdominal pain begin 4 to 10 days after penetration of the mucosa. Abdominal pain in the right lower quadrant may lead to an incorrect diagnosis of appendicitis.

Ingested *Y. pseudotuberculosis* penetrates the ileal mucosa, localizes in ileocecal lymph nodes, and produces abscesses and granulomas in the lymph nodes, spleen, and liver. The granulomas may be centered in the lymphoid follicles. Diarrhea and abdominal pain with fever may lead to an erroneous diagnosis of appendicitis.

Streptomycin, gentamicin, tetracycline, and trimethoprim-sulfamethoxazole are the antibiotics of choice.

Campylobacter Enteritis

With reliable isolation and routine screening, *Campylobacter* species have emerged as the leading cause of acute bacterial enteritis. Formerly identified as vibrios, these flagellated, comma-shaped, gram-negative bacteria cause up to 11% of all infectious dysentery in U.S. hospitals, thus causing more enteritis than *Salmonella* species. *Campylobacter* enteritis is acquired by eating improperly cleaned and cooked food, usually poultry, contaminated by *C. jejuni*, an organism that colonizes poultry. In one study, *C. jejuni* was cultured from the body cavities of more than half of fresh and frozen chickens and turkeys in 10 major cities around the world.

C. jejuni, like *Salmonella*, are enteroinvasive and produce a spectrum of disease ranging from subclinical infection to severe dysentery. Illness appears 2 to 5 days after ingestion of contaminated food and lasts about 5 days. Symptoms include abdominal pain, diarrhea, nausea, vomiting, fever, and myalgia. Stools are malodorous and frequently bloody. Inflammation involves the gastrointestinal tract from jejunum to anus. Most patients have colonic crypt abscesses and ulcers resembling those in ulcerative colitis. Microscopically, the small bowel is edematous and hyperemic and is infiltrated with neutrophils, lymphocytes, and plasma cells. Comma-shaped organisms are seen in the intestinal mucosa and lamina propria. The disease is generally benign and self-limited.

Another species, *C. fetus*, is an infrequent but clinically important opportunistic pathogen that causes localized infections as well as sepsis. This organism is an economically important cause of septic abortion and infertility in sheep and cattle. It has been isolated from vaginal secretions of cows, from the prepuce and ejaculate of bulls, and from the placenta and tissues of abortuses. Cases of spontaneous abortion and infertility in humans may thus be caused by *C. fetus*, especially in populations exposed to livestock.

Melioidosis

Melioidosis is an uncommon infectious disease caused by *Pseudomonas pseudomallei*, a small gram-negative bacillus in the soil and surface water of Southeast Asia and other tropical areas. Synonyms include Rangoon beggar's disease and Whitmore's disease. Although melioidosis is endemic in Southeast Asia, there have been scattered infections of humans and animals in South and Central America, Africa, Turkey, Australia, and Guam. During the conflict in Vietnam, several hundred French, Vietnamese, and American servicemen acquired melioidosis. The organism flourishes in wet environments, such as rice paddies and marshes. The skin is the usual portal of entry, and organisms enter through preexisting lesions, including penetrating wounds and burns. Man may also be infected by inhaling contaminated dust or aerosolized droplets. The association of melioidosis with drug addiction implies transmission by contaminated needles and syringes.

The incubation period varies up to months and possibly years. The clinical course may be chronic, subacute or acute. The acute illness presents as a

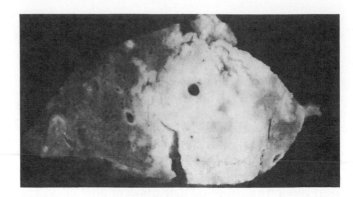

Figure 9-24.   Fatal melioidosis (*Pseudomonas pseudomallei*), lung. The lung is consolidated and necrotic.

pulmonary infection, with sudden onset, high fever, chills, malaise, myalgia, and a cough that may produce blood-stained mucopurulent sputum. The severity of pulmonary involvement varies from a mild tracheobronchitis to an overwhelming cavitary pneumonia (Fig. 9-24). Splenomegaly, hepatomegaly, and jaundice are sometimes present. The diarrhea may be as severe as in cholera. Fulminating septicemia, shock, coma, and death may develop in spite of antibiotic therapy.

Acute septicemic melioidosis causes discrete abscesses throughout the body. These occur most frequently in the lungs, liver, spleen, lymph nodes, and bone marrow, but any organ may be involved. Small, firm, and yellowish lesions are sharply delimited from surrounding normal tissue and are often bounded by a narrow hemorrhagic margin. The small foci may coalesce into larger abscesses.

Microscopically, the centers of the abscesses are necrotic and contain neutrophils in a fibrin mesh. A narrow necrotic rim containing histiocytes forms the boundary of the abscess. Necrosis is a prominent feature of even the very early lesions, a finding that probably reflects toxin production by *P. pseudomallei*. Large numbers of bacteria are seen in the abscesses, but seldom in the surrounding tissue.

Subacute melioidosis mimics tuberculosis and is characterized by fever, cough, and pneumonia. Melioidosis also occurs as a self-limited febrile disease lacking specific features. Some 20% of people living in endemic areas have antibodies against *P. pseudomallei*.

Chronic melioidosis is a localized, suppurative infection involving the lungs, skin, or bones. Clinically and radiologically it may resemble tuberculosis. Complications include osteomyelitis, psoas or subcutaneous abscesses, and lymphadenopathy. Chronic melioidosis may follow a mild acute illness, or it may lie dormant for months or years, only to appear suddenly—hence the colloquial appellation, "Vietnamese time bomb."

Chronic melioidosis is usually localized to a single organ, most often the lung. The lesions have a necrotic center surrounded by a granulomatous reaction and a perimeter of fibrous tissue. The central necrotic zone may be suppurative or caseous. In the lymph nodes stellate abscesses resemble lesions of lymphogranuloma venereum, cat scratch disease, and tularemia. Bacteria are seldom seen in chronic lesions, even though cultures may be positive.

The diagnosis is made by serologic tests or culture. The cultures must be handled carefully, since laboratory-acquired infection is possible. Tetracycline is the treatment of choice.

Glanders

Glanders is an infection of equine species and rarely of humans. It may be acute and severe or protracted and wasting. The cause is *Pseudomonas mallei*, a small, gram-negative, nonmotile bacillus.

Although uncommon, glanders remains endemic in South America, Asia, and Africa. In addition there have been rare infections of laboratory workers in the United States and Canada. The natural reservoir is equines, and transmission to humans is by contact through broken skin or by inhalation of contaminated aerosols. Glanders may also be transmitted from person to person.

The acute disease is characterized by a papule at the site of inoculation, followed by bacteremia with severe prostration, fever, vomiting, and generalized pain. The bacilli drain from the primary papule through lymphatics to regional lymph nodes and then to the bloodstream. Abscesses may form along the draining lymphatics, in the regional nodes and in many organs throughout the body, including the lung, liver, spleen, muscle, joints, and especially the subcutaneous tissues. The abscesses are composed of a central zone of neutrophils surrounded by a granulomatous perimeter. Patients with the chronic form of glanders show a low-grade fever, draining abscesses of skin, lymphadenopathy, and hepatosplenomegaly. The lesions begin as abscesses and evolve to granulomas, mimicking tuberculosis. In its acute form, glanders is almost always fatal, and in the chronic form mortality is more than 50%. Some success in treatment has been achieved with sulfonamides.

The lesions are not pathognomonic, and the di-

agnosis depends on the isolation of *P. mallei* or the detection of complement-fixing antibodies. Although *P. mallei* may be cultured from blood, sputum, or pus, its high potential for causing laboratory-acquired infection requires strict containment.

Brucellosis

Brucellosis, a zoonotic disease caused by several species of the genus *Brucella*, may present as an acute severe systemic disease or as a subacute or chronic malady. *Brucella* are small, nonmotile, nonsporulating, gram-negative coccobacilli, which may or may not be encapsulated. Four species infect humans, each from its own animal reservoir. *Brucella melitensis* infects sheep and goats; *Brucella abortus*, cattle; *Brucella suis*, swine; and *Brucella canis*, dogs. The disease is encountered worldwide and in all climates. Virtually every type of domestic animal and many wild ones are affected. The prevalence relates to occupational exposure, cultural or socioeconomic conditions resulting in close contact with animals, and consumption of contaminated milk or milk products. In the United States brucellosis is an occupational disease of farmers, employees of abattoirs, and veterinarians. In much of the world the most common cause of infection is unpasteurized dairy products. In the arctic and subarctic regions humans acquire brucellosis by eating raw bone marrow of infected reindeer. Infectious mastitis of cattle may persist for years after recovery from the acute infection and remain a reservoir of *Brucella*. Products of abortion may contain organisms and are infectious. Urine, manure, and vaginal discharges are also major sources of contamination.

The incubation period is 5 days to several months. The onset of symptoms may be abrupt or insidious. The three clinical types of brucellosis are acute malignant, recurrent, and chronic (intermittent). The presenting features of acute malignant brucellosis resemble those of influenza, and include the sudden onset of high fever, chills, prostration, and somatic aches and pains. Lymphadenopathy and a palpable spleen and liver are the only localized findings. Death may be sudden, within a few days of onset, or after a few weeks of delirium and coma. Recurrent brucellosis (**undulant fever**) is characterized by influenza-like signs and symptoms that recur in wavelike relapses. The cycles may persist for weeks, gradually decreasing in severity. Chronic (intermittent) brucellosis is caused primarily by *B. abortus*. The onset may be acute or there may be gradual increase in malaise, weakness, weight loss, and vague somatic aches and pains. Fever is usually mild, but weakness may be profound.

The most common complications of brucellosis involve the bones and joints and include spondylitis of the intervertebral area of the lumbar spine and localized suppuration in large joints. In addition, peripheral neuritis, meningitis, orchitis, suppurative endocarditis, and pulmonary lesions may develop.

Bacteria enter through skin abrasions, the conjunctiva, oropharynx, or lung and spread in the bloodstream to the liver, spleen, lymph nodes, and bone marrow, where they multiply in phagocytic cells. A generalized histiocytic hyperplasia ensues, with conspicuous noncaseating granulomas, causing lymphadenopathy and hepatosplenomegaly. Patients with chronic brucellosis may exhibit "coin" lesions in the lung resembling histoplasmomas or the lesions of tuberculosis. Acute bacterial endocarditis, myocardial abscesses, and focal suppurative lesions in the myocardium are occasionally encountered. The diagnosis must be confirmed by isolating the organism in culture or by serologic testing. Prolonged treatment with tetracycline and streptomycin is usually effective. Patients who recover from brucellosis are immune. Control of the disease depends on the elimination of brucellosis in animal reservoirs.

Listeriosis

Listeriosis is a systemic infection caused by *Listeria monocytogenes*, a small, motile, nonsporulating, hemolytic, gram-positive coccobacillus. On cultures the organism is easily confused with streptococci or corynebacteria. Listeriosis is usually sporadic but may also be epidemic. *L. monocytogenes* has been isolated worldwide from surface water, soil, vegetation, the feces of healthy people, from many species of domestic and wild mammals, and from several species of birds. In spite of this wide distribution, the spread of infection from animals to humans is rare. Most human infections are in urban rather than rural environments and occur during July and August, while the peak months of infections in animals are January through May. However, some infections have been traced to unpasteurized milk. *L. monocytogenes* grows at refrigerator temperatures, and outbreaks of listeriosis have been caused by contaminated cheeses and other dairy products.

Most infections fall into one or two groups. One, listeriosis of pregnancy, includes prenatal and postnatal infections. The other, listeriosis of the adult population, is characterized by meningoencephalitis and septicemia. Chronic alcoholics, patients with car-

cinoma, leukemia, or lymphomas, and those receiving immunosuppressive therapy are all susceptible.

Maternal infection early in pregnancy leads to abortion or prematurity. Infected live-born, premature infants show signs of infection within a few hours of birth. These include respiratory distress, pneumonia, hepatosplenomegaly, papular cutaneous and mucosal nodules, leukopenia, and thrombocytopenia. In neonatal listeriosis acquired during delivery, the onset is 3 days to 2 weeks after delivery.

Infections before birth involve many organs and tissues. The amniotic fluid, the placenta, and cord are all heavily infected. The cutaneous lesions are raised and necrotic with red margins. Abscesses are found in the liver, spleen, lymph nodes, adrenals, lungs, pleura, esophagus, posterior pharynx, and tonsils. Microscopically, the visceral lesions are foci of necrosis and suppuration that contain many bacteria. Older lesions contain histiocytes and occasionally epithelioid cells and lymphocytes, but not giant cells. Still older lesions have a fibrous wall. Neurologic sequelae are common, and the mortality is high even when therapy is prompt.

Meningitis is the most common form of listeriosis in adults, and resembles other bacterial meningitides. Microscopically, the leptomeninges are infiltrated with lymphocytes, plasma cells, macrophages, and neutrophils. The inflammation extends into the brain along the Virchow-Robin spaces.

Septicemic listeriosis in adults is most common in immunodeficient patients, and causes severe illness with high fever and prostration. Shock and disseminated intravascular coagulation may lead to an erroneous diagnosis of gram-negative sepsis. Listerial endocarditis resembles endocarditis caused by other bacteria. Septicemia may seed the brain with miliary abscesses and cause a suppurative leptomeningitis.

The diagnosis is made by isolating *L. monocytogenes* in culture or demonstrating the typical gram-positive bacilli in tissue sections. Prolonged treatment with antimicrobials is usually required, because patients tend to relapse if treatment is less than 3 weeks. Penicillin or ampicillin is the treatment of choice.

Clostridial Diseases

Clostridia are gram-positive, spore-forming bacilli that are obligate anaerobes. The vegetative bacilli are found in the gastrointestinal tract of herbivorous animals and man. Anaerobic conditions promote vegetative division, while aerobic conditions promote sporulation (Fig. 9-25). Spores pass in the animal feces, contaminate the soil and plants, and can survive unfavorable environmental conditions. Under anaerobic conditions the spores revert to vegetative cells, thus completing the cycle. During sporulation, the vegetative cells degenerate, and their plasmids produce a variety of specific toxins that cause widely different clostridial diseases, depending on the species. **Food poisoning and necrotizing enteritis ("pig bel") are caused by the enterotoxins of *Clostridium perfringens*, gas gangrene by the myotoxins of *C. perfringens*, *C. novyi*, *C. septicum*, and others, tetanus by the neurotoxin of *C. tetani*, and botulism by the neurotoxin of *C. botulinum*.**

Food Poisoning

C. perfringens has five serotypes (A–E), based on the combinations of antigens. Types A and C produce a toxin, alpha-enterotoxin, that causes food poisoning (see Fig. 9-25). *C. perfringens* is ubiquitous, and is the most widely disseminated of all pathogenic bacteria, typically being 10 to 100 times more numerous than *E. coli* in stool. Type A serotype is the only one commonly found in the colonic flora of animals and humans. It is also omnipresent in the environment, contaminating soil, water, and air samples, clothing, dust, and meat. Food poisoning from *C. perfringens* occurs throughout the world.

Most of the food poisoning is from contaminated beef, gravy, and other meat products. For example, a large piece of meat that is slowly cooling often has an internal temperature in the range of 43° to 47°C—optimal for the growth of *C. perfringens*. Heating the meat drives out enough air to make it anaerobic, a condition that is conducive to growth but not to sporulation. Thus the contaminated meat contains the vegetative clostridia, but little preformed enterotoxin. (This contrasts with the situation in botulism, in which preformed neurotoxin of *C. botulinum* is ingested.) When contaminated food is consumed, the ingested *C. perfringens* reach the intestine, where alpha-enterotoxin is produced during sporulation.

Symptoms may develop within 2 to 4 hours, but 8 to 12 hours is usual. Symptoms include cramping abdominal pain, sudden vomiting, and frequent episodes of watery diarrhea. The effect of the toxin appears to be greatest in the ileum. The patient usually recovers within 2 days.

Necrotizing Enteritis

C. perfringens Type C also produces beta-enterotoxin, which causes a necrotizing enteritis known as "pig bel." This necrotizing enteritis is seen in malnourished persons who have sudden dietary overindulg-ence, as was seen, for example, in impoverished children immediately after World War II. Necrotizing enteritis is endemic in the highlands of New Guinea, especially in children who have participated in pig feasts (whence the pidgin term, pig bel). Most adults have circulating antibodies and do not develop pig bel. Spit roasting of pig carcasses eaten at the feasts encourages the growth of *C. perfringens*. The normal diet of the children is vegetarian, more than 90% of calories being derived from sweet potatoes. The combination of inadequate protein consumption and the presence of a trypsin inhibitor in sweet potatoes renders the children deficient in intestinal proteases, to which beta-enterotoxin is very sensitive.

The usual incubation period is 48 hours after ingestion of contaminated meat. The presenting symptoms include severe abdominal pain and distention, vomiting, and passage of bloody or black stools. Patients with fulminating pig bel may die within 24 hours of onset. Other patients have mild pig bel that resembles gastroenteritis. Half of the patients require surgery.

Necrotizing enteritis is a segmental disease that may be restricted to a few centimeters or may involve the entire small intestine. Green, necrotic pseudomembranes are seen in segmental areas of necrosis and peritonitis. More advanced lesions may perforate the bowel wall. Histologic sections reveal infarction of the mucosa, with edema, hemorrhage, and suppurative infiltrate that extends transmurally. The pseudomembrane is composed of necrotic epithelium containing gram-positive bacilli.

Clostridial Myonecrosis (Gas Gangrene)

Gas gangrene is a rapidly progressive, life-threatening illness, in which necrosis of previously healthy skeletal muscle is caused by myotoxins elaborated by a few species of clostridia. *C. perfringens* Type A is the most common source of myotoxin (80–90% of cases), but myotoxin may also come from *C. novyi*, *C. septicum*, and rarely from three other species. The myonecrosis usually follows traumatic wounds or surgical procedures in which the site of the wound becomes contaminated with clostridia (see Fig. 9-25). However, only a small proportion of wounds contaminated with clostridia develop gas gangrene. Contributing factors include hypoxia from injury to blood vessels near the wound site, pressure dressings, tourniquets, local injection of vasoconstrictors, foreign bodies, damaged tissues from earlier injury, and concurrent microbial infections. Uterine gas gangrene most commonly follows "backroom" septic abortions, but may also occur postpartum.

Under anaerobic conditions clostridia grow rapidly and elaborate the myotoxin(s). Over twenty exotoxins have been identified from the species causing gas gangrene. Of these, the most important is alpha-toxin, produced by *C. perfringens* Type A (and four of the other five causative species). Alpha-toxin is a lecithinase that destroys cell membranes, thus altering capillary permeability and causing severe hemolysis.

The species responsible for gas gangrene are ubiquitous, and exposure is universal. In particular, *C. perfringens* Type A is in the colonic flora of animals and humans, and widely contaminates soil, water, dust, clothing, and meat. Clostridia are found on the skin, especially over the buttocks, thighs, and perineum. Thus, the incidence of gas gangrene depends more on wound management and asepsis during surgical procedures than on exposure to the clostridia. A critical factor in preventing gas gangrene is prompt and thorough debridement of traumatized tissue, in which the clostridia thrive. Commonly this involves excision of involved muscles, amputation of a limb, uterine curettage, or hysterectomy. Debridement is accompanied by antibiotic therapy, such as intravenous penicillin or chloramphenicol.

The incubation period is commonly 2 to 4 days after wounding, surgery, or abortion. Sudden, severe pain occurs at the site of injury, which is tender and edematous. The skin darkens because of hemorrhage and cutaneous necrosis. The lesion develops a thick, serosanguineous discharge that has a fragrant odor and may contain gas bubbles. Clinically, sweating, low-grade fever, and disproportionate tachycardia give way rapidly to hemolytic anemia, hypotension, and renal failure. In the terminal stages, coma, jaundice, and shock supervene. **Gas gangrene is characterized histologically by necrosis of muscle and overlying soft tissues, with little inflammatory cell reaction.**

Tetanus

Tetanus (lockjaw) is a severe, acute neurologic syndrome of humans and warm-blooded animals. It is caused by tetanus toxin (tetanospasmin), an extremely potent neurotoxic exotoxin elaborated by plasmids of *C. tetani*.

The vegetative cells of *C. tetani* inhabit the intestine of animals (especially horses and other herbivores) and man. The bacillus has terminal and spherical

---

Figure 9-25. Clostridial diseases. Clostridia in the vegetative form (bacilli) inhabit the gastrointestinal tract of humans and animals. Spores pass in the feces, contaminate soil and plant materials, and are ingested or enter sites of penetrating wounds. Under anaerobic conditions they revert to vegetative forms. Plasmids in the vegetative forms elaborate toxins that cause several clostridial diseases.
Food poisoning and necrotizing enteritis. Meat dishes left to cool at room temperature grow large numbers of clostridia (more than 10^6 organisms per gram). When contaminated meat is ingested, *C. perfringens* Types A and C produce alpha-enterotoxin in the small intestine during sporulation, causing abdominal pain and diarrhea. Type C also produces beta-enterotoxin.
Gas gangrene. Clostridia are widespread and may contaminate a traumatic wound or surgical operation. *C. perfringens* Type A elaborates a myotoxin (alpha-toxin), a lecithinase that destroys cell membranes, alters capillary permeability, and causes severe hemolysis following intravenous injection. The toxin causes necrosis of previously healthy skeletal muscle.
Tetanus. Spores of *C. tetani* are in soil, and enter the site of an accidental wound. Necrotic tissue at the wound site causes spores to revert to the vegetative form (bacilli). Autolysis of vegetative forms releases tetanus toxin. The toxin is transported in peripheral nerves and (retrograde) through axons to the anterior horn cells of the spinal cord. The toxin blocks synaptic inhibition, and the accumulation of acetylcholine in damaged synapses leads to rigidity and spasms of the skeletal musculature (tetany).
Botulism. Improperly canned food is contaminated by the vegetative form of *C. botulinum*, which proliferates under aerobic conditions and elaborates a neurotoxin. After the food is ingested, the neurotoxin is absorbed from the small intestine and eventually reaches the myoneural junction, where it inhibits the release of acetylcholine. The result is a symmetric descending paralysis of cranial nerves, trunk, and limbs, with eventual respiratory paralysis and death.

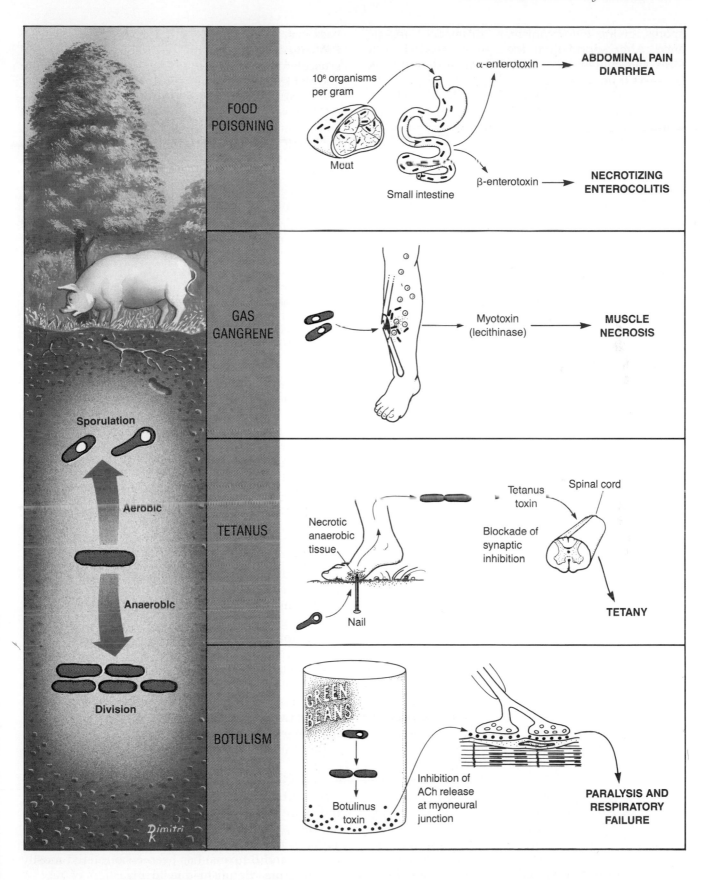

spores, giving the organism a "drumstick" appearance. After sporulation, the spores pass with the feces and contaminate the soil, where they survive for years if not exposed to sunlight. Spores enter the site of a traumatic, penetrating wound—for instance, from stepping on a nail (see Fig. 9-25) or a battle wound. Neonatal tetanus, a disease most prevalent in less developed countries, results when soil or dung contaminates the stump of the umbilical cord.

At the site of injury, necrotic tissue and suppuration contribute to the creation of an anaerobic environment, a condition that causes spores to revert to vegetative cells. Tetanus toxin, one of the most potent toxins known, is released from autolyzed vegetative cells and binds to ganglioside receptors on neuronal cell membranes, thereby causing discharge of local peripheral nerves and spasm of muscles. Although the clostridial infection remains localized, the neurotoxin then undergoes retrograde transport (via intra- and peri-axonal transport) through the ventral roots of peripheral nerves to the anterior horn cells of the spinal cord. The toxin there crosses the synapse and interacts with presynaptic terminals on motor neurons in the ventral horns, blocking release of inhibitory neurotransmitters. This causes uninhibited neural stimulation and sustained contraction of skeletal musculature (tetany) (see Fig. 9-25). Blockage of the inhibitory transmitters also induces acceleration of the heart rate, hypertension, and cardiovascular instability.

The incidence of tetanus varies in different areas of the world and is commonly high in warmer countries that are overcrowded and economically deprived. Contributing factors include soil conditions, the presence of herbivorous animals (especially equines and bovines), frequency of tetanus-prone wounds, care for such wounds, abortion practices, conditions during birth, and the immune status of the population. In some undeveloped countries, for example, lethal tetanus is associated with septic abortions. Unsanitary circumcisions provide another portal of entry for clostridial spores. Neonatal tetanus is associated with the custom of applying dung to umbilical stumps. In developed countries, tetanus is most frequently associated with drug addiction.

The clinical manifestations include generalized hypertonia (less frequently, localized hypertonia) of the skeletal musculature, accompanied by paroxysmal clonic muscular spasms. The incubation period is 1 to 3 weeks. An early symptom is difficulty in opening the jaw ("lockjaw" or trismus). As the disease progresses, increasing rigidity of the musculature leads to rigidity of the facial muscles ("risus sardonicus") and those of the neck, abdominal wall, back, lower limbs, and other sites. Rigidity of the muscles of the back may produce backward arching (opisthotonos). Prolonged spasms of the respiratory and laryngeal musculature lead to death. Tetanus immune globulin and penicillin are used in treatment.

The histologic changes are nonspecific. Tissue necrosis is seen at the site of the wound together with an inflammatory infiltrate and a mixed bacterial flora, including gram-positive bacilli that may suggest clostridia. Ganglion cells of the spinal cord and medulla may display swelling, nuclear alterations, and chromatolysis.

In cases of neonatal tetanus the initial symptom, after a 1-week incubation, is difficulty in sucking the breast. The subsequent progression is similar to that for adult tetanus. Muscle spasms are usually intense and frequent and convulsions occur. Spasms of the respiratory muscles result in apnea and death unless muscle-relaxing drugs are injected immediately.

Botulism

Botulism is a paralyzing illness that follows the ingestion of food containing the neurotoxins of *C. botulinum*. There have also been cases of "wound botulism," in which spores enter a penetrating wound with proliferation of clostridia and elaboration of neurotoxin in the tissue. Botulism is characterized by a symmetric descending paralysis of cranial nerves, limbs, and trunk.

The spores of *C. botulinum* are widely distributed in soil and animals, and contaminate many foods. The spores survive unfavorable conditions, and are especially resistant to drying and boiling. **In the United States the toxin is most commonly present in vegetables or other foods that have been improperly home-canned and stored without refrigeration, conditions that provide suitable anaerobic conditions for growth of the vegetative cells that elaborate the neurotoxins (A–G).** But botulism can also be contracted from home-cured ham and other meat that has been left unrefrigerated for several days and from raw, smoked, and fermented fish products. Infants may ingest spores in honey, establish an intestinal infection with *C. botulinum*, and develop botulism by absorbing neurotoxin from the gut.

Botulism occurs in all parts of the world, but the incidence varies with eating habits and with the control exercised over commercial food processing. The types of botulism also vary in prevalence. Types A and B are common in the United States and are associated with improperly home-canned vegetables, fruits, or prepared meats. Infant botulism (also from Types A and B toxins) has been encountered mostly in California. Botulism due to ingestion of raw or lightly smoked fish results from Type E neurotoxin, and commonly occurs in Japan, Scandinavia, the USSR, and the Great Lakes region of the United States.

After food containing neurotoxin is ingested, the toxin resists gastric digestion and is readily absorbed into the blood from the upper portions of the small intestine. Toxin in the circulation eventually reaches the cholinergic nerve endings at the myoneural junction. The toxin binds to membrane receptors (gangliosides) of the synaptic vesicles and inhibits release of acetylcholine, thus causing paralysis and respiratory failure (see Fig. 9-24).

The symptoms of botulism begin 12 to 36 hours after the ingestion of food containing toxin. Since the neurotoxin is preformed, there is no true "incubation" period for growth of organisms. The early clinical symptoms of nausea, vomiting, and diarrhea probably do not result from the neurotoxin. For "wound botulism," however, there is an incubation period of 4 to 14 days, during which the spores revert to the vegetative form, the bacterial infection becomes established, and the neurotoxin is produced. A specific antitoxin is available.

For both routes the neurotoxin leads to a symmetric, descending pattern of weakness or paralysis of the cranial nerves (especially nerve VI), limbs, and trunk. These symptoms may be accompanied by diplopia, dysarthria, dysphagia, and, in severe cases, respiratory paralysis. The last is clearly the most life-threatening aspect of botulism. Infant botulism may result in the sudden infant death syndrome.

The histologic changes are nonspecific and include hyperemia of the central nervous system and minute thromboses of small vessels, primarily in the brain and brain stem. Respiratory paralysis and vascular stasis produce hypoxic damage to vulnerable organs.

Diphtheria

Diphtheria is an acute disease that results from a localized infection and a systemic toxemia caused by exotoxin-producing strains of *Corynebacterium diphtheriae*. The name is derived from the Greek words *koryne* (club) and *diphtheria* (leather), the latter referring to the gray membrane at the site of infection. The membrane is most commonly in the pharynx, but the nasal fossae, tonsils, lower respiratory tract, gut, conjunctiva, umbilical stump, and skin are other sites. The exotoxin produces myocarditis and neuritis.

C. diphtheriae is a pleomorphic, nonmotile, gram-positive club-shaped bacillus. Its pathogenicity depends on the presence of a toxin-producing, lysogenic bacteriophage and a critical concentration of iron in the environment. **The exotoxin is one of the most toxic substances known, and a single molecule is sufficient to kill a cell.** It inactivates protein synthesis at the cellular level by modifying elongation factor 2, thus preventing elongation of the nascent protein chain at the ribosome.

Until an effective vaccine became available, diphtheria was a major cause of death in children. In the United States, the incidence is now less than 100 infections per year, which occur mainly in poor people living in crowded conditions. Infection of the pharynx is more common in children between 5 and 14 years of age, whereas cutaneous infections are more common in adults living in the tropics.

The infection spreads from person to person by infected droplets or exudates. Humans are the only significant reservoir and most people are asymptomatic carriers. An intradermal injection of diphtheria toxin (the Schick test) determines host susceptibility to the pathogenic strains of corynebacteria. The immune host neutralizes the antigen and there is no reaction.

Pharyngeal diphtheria is the most common presentation. After an incubation period of 1 to 7 days, during which the corynebacteria proliferate at the site of implantation, the patient experiences fever, sore throat, malaise, and sometimes nausea and vomiting. The gray-green membrane adheres to the underlying epithelium and leaves a bleeding surface when it is peeled away. The membrane may spread over the entire pharynx and in severe infections involves the larynx, trachea, and bronchi, thereby obstructing the airway. The term "bull neck" refers to the edema and cervical adenopathy that obscure the angle of the jaw, the contour of the anterior portion of the neck, and the clavicle. The ulcer of primary cutaneous diphtheria, which is usually located on the limbs, has a raised, firm border, and the base is covered by a membrane. Secondary cutaneous infections may develop at any site. **Absorption of the exotoxin in the nonimmune host causes cardiac enlargement, cardiac arrhythmias, and heart failure.** The exotoxin also causes neuritis, which may progress to paralysis.

Histologically, the membrane is composed of a coagulated fibrinopurulent exudate mixed with necrotic epithelial cells and masses of corynebacteria. The bacilli are concentrated deeply in the lesion beneath the necrotic epithelium. The adjacent soft tissues display vascular congestion, suppuration, and edema. The exotoxin produces diffuse myocarditis, with edema, focal and diffuse degeneration of myocardial fibers (Fig. 9-26), and increased fat within myocytes. The diphtheria exotoxin also causes demyelinization of nerves and interstitial nephritis with proteinuria. Those who survive have no residual effects.

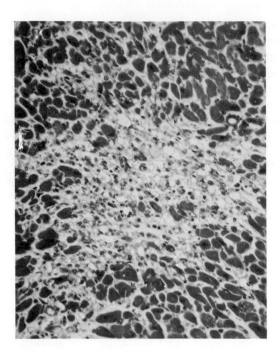

Figure 9-26. Diphtheria, heart, showing focal degeneration of myofibers.

Corynebacterium diphtheriae can be cultured on selective media. Smears of organisms reveal typical palisaded groups resembling Chinese characters. A clinical suspicion of diphtheria should prompt immediate treatment with antitoxin. Treatment with penicillin or erythromycin halts the proliferation of bacteria, but should not be given without antitoxin.

Rhinoscleroma

Rhinoscleroma is a chronic granulomatous disease of the nasal mucosa (less commonly, the nasopharynx, larynx, and trachea) caused by *Klebsiella rhinoscleromatis*, an encapsulated, nonsporulating, nonmotile gram-negative bacillus. Rhinoscleroma is prevalent in the USSR, Poland, and central Europe and is endemic in Mexico, Central America, and upper South America. Infections in the United States are rare.

Rhinoscleroma is a disease of young and middle-aged adults, slightly more common in women and without racial predisposition. The onset is slow and insidious, usually over many years, and the patient's general health is unaffected. At first, the symptoms are those of a common cold. An initial granularity of the nasal mucosa is replaced by reddish, waxy, granulomatous infiltrates and firm, nodular, intranasal masses. In fully developed rhinoscleroma hyperplastic changes of the alae and tip of the nose (the "Hebra nose") are severely disfiguring. Airway obstruction,

anosmia, and speech difficulties develop as the disease advances. Anesthesia of the soft palate and enlargement of the uvula suggest rhinoscleroma, but any part of the upper airway, the paranasal sinuses and orbit may be involved. Compressive destruction of bone and soft tissue mimics invasive tumors. Scar tissue persists after the disease runs its course.

Microscopically, the most conspicuous feature is the presence of histiocytic granulomas, with fibrosis and an abundant infiltrate of lymphocytes and plasma cells. The mucosal surfaces display variable changes, ranging from squamous metaplasia to extreme pseudoepitheliomatous hyperplasia. Large, vacuolated, "foamy" histiocytes, known as **Mikulicz cells**, are characteristic of rhinoscleroma and are most numerous in the nodular stage. *Klebsiella* organisms are seen within cells and in extracellular locations.

The diagnosis of rhinoscleroma is confirmed by isolating *Klebsiella rhinoscleromatis* in culture or by demonstrating the organism in tissue sections. Antibiotics of choice are streptomycin, tetracycline, and chloramphenicol. In some patients surgical intervention is necessary to relieve airway obstruction or to repair the facial features.

Friedlander's Bacillus (Klebsiella pneumoniae)

Klebsiella pneumoniae, known as Friedlander's bacillus, is a short, encapsulated, gram-negative bacillus that causes a necrotizing lobar pneumonia. This organism also causes 10% of all infections acquired in hospital, including pneumonia and infections of the urinary tract, biliary tract, and surgical wounds. Carriers are a special hazard among hospital personnel, especially when resistant strains of *K. pneumoniae* colonize their mouths, throats, and intestines. Predisposing factors are indwelling catheters and endotracheal tubes, old age, alcoholism, immunosupression, diabetes, congestive heart failure, obstructive pulmonary disease, and other debilitating conditions. Furthermore, secondary *Klebsiella* pneumonias may complicate influenza or other viral infections of the respiratory tract. **The combined mortality rate of primary and secondary *Klebsiella* pneumonias is about 50%,** because the necrotizing pneumonia is itself dangerous and because those stricken tend to be chronically ill or otherwise debilitated.

Clinically, the pneumonia has a sudden onset, characterized by fever, pleuritic pain, cough, and **thick mucoid sputum.** When infection is severe these symptoms progress to shortness of breath, cyanosis, and death in 2 to 3 days.

Pneumonia develops when the bacilli invade and multiply within the alveolar spaces. The pulmonary parenchyma becomes consolidated, and the mucoid exudate that fills the alveoli is dominated by macrophages, fibrin, and edema fluid. Neutrophils are inhibited by a neutral polysaccharide in the capsule of *K. pneumoniae*, and are not a significant part of the early exudate. Numerous encapsulated gram-negative bacilli appear free in the exudate and in alveolar macrophages. As the exudate accumulates the alveolar walls become compressed and then necrotic. Numerous small abscesses may coalesce and lead to cavitation.

The pneumonia, or other infections by *K. pneumoniae*, may be complicated by a fulminating, often fatal, septicemia, even without disseminated lesions in other tissues.

The diagnosis is by culture. Both an aminoglycoside and a cephalosporin are recommended for treatment.

Bartonellosis

Bartonellosis is an infection by *Bartonella bacilliformis*, a small, pleomorphic, multiflagellated, gram-negative coccobacillus, which is the only member of the genus *Bartonella* but is closely related to certain animal pathogens. The organisms parasitize erythrocytes *in vivo* and can be cultured in semisolid media or in embryonated eggs. In smears of blood and in tissue sections stained with Giemsa or Wright stain, the bacteria are reddish-violet. The organisms are small coccobacilli, occasionally curved, and may aggregate in chains of three or in "V" or "Y" forms.

The term bartonellosis encompasses two syndromes, both caused by *B. bacilliformis*—Oroya fever, the acute anemic phase; and verruga peruana, the chronic dermal phase. These present as a biphasic pattern, with the acute anemia first, followed some months later by the chronic dermal phase. Either phase may occur by itself.

Bartonellosis occurs only in Peru, Ecuador, and Colombia. The foci of endemic transmission are river valleys in the Andes at an elevation between 700 and 2,500 meters. The disease is transmitted by the sandflies *Phlebotomus verrucarum* and *Phlebotomus noguchi*. The vectors are sensitive to drying and cold, hence the absence of bartonellosis in coastal regions and at higher elevations. Humans provide the only reservoir and acquire bartonellosis at sunrise and sunset, when sandflies are most active. In endemic areas, 10% to 15% of the population have latent infections. Newcomers are susceptible, whereas the indigenous population is resistant, a difference explained by subclinical infection and immunity in the indigenous people.

The incubation period of the acute anemic stage is 3 weeks. The onset is abrupt, with fever, skeletal pains, and a severe hemolytic anemia that is often macrocytic. Lymphadenopathy and hepatosplenomegaly are usually present. Reticulocytosis, jaundice, and other changes of hemolytic anemia also occur. The anemia can be profound, and the blood erythrocyte count may fall in a few days from normal to less than 500,000/μl. Secondary septicemia caused by salmonellae is frequent and contributes to the high mortality of acute bartonellosis. About 40% of patients with untreated bartonellosis die in the anemic phase.

The dermal eruptive phase of bartonellosis sometimes coexists with the anemic phase, but they are usually separated by an asymptomatic interval of 3 to 6 months. Occasionally the eruptive form develops independently without prior evidence of bartonellosis. The eruption is usually miliary *(forma miliar)*, and many small hemangioma-like lesions of the dermis balloon outward and cause a studded appearance. Nodular lesions *(forma nodular)* are larger but fewer and may be more prominent on the extensor surfaces of the arms and legs. At times, a few large, deep-seated lesions, which tend to ulcerate, develop near joints and limit motion. The eruptive phase is often prolonged, but eventually heals spontaneously. The mortality in the eruptive phase is less than 5%.

Grossly, the acute phase causes changes characteristic of acute hemolytic anemia, with prominent pallor and jaundice. The bone marrow is hyperplastic. Lymphadenopathy, hepatomegaly, and splenomegaly are present, caused by the engorgement of the reticuloendothelial cells with bacteria, erythrocytes, and hemosiderin. Microscopically, the endothelial cells of the spleen are swollen with phagocytosed bacteria and debris. Thrombosis, with splenic infarcts and centrilobular hepatic necrosis, may be present.

The lesions of the dermal eruptive phase are nodular and sessile, usually with an epithelial collar and prominent capillary proliferation. Within the lesion are foci of large cells with prominent hyperchromatic nuclei and abundant, darkly staining cytoplasm. Although bacilli are present in the endothelial cells lining the vascular spaces, they are difficult to find. The lesions heal slowly by fibrosis. Clinically and microscopically these lesions must be distinguished from Kaposi's sarcoma and granuloma pyogenicum.

The diagnosis is made by demonstrating the bacilli in blood smears or tissue sections or by isolating the organism in cultures from blood or tissue. Serologic tests are not useful. Successful treatment of acute hemolytic bartonellosis has been reported with chloramphenicol, tetracycline, streptomycin, and penicillin, but bacteremia is not always eliminated by antimicrobial therapy. Antibiotic therapy of the dermal eruptions has been less successful.

Granuloma Inguinale

Granuloma inguinale is a sexually transmitted, chronic, superficial ulceration of the genitalia and inguinal and perianal regions caused by *Calymmatobacterium granulomatis*, a small, encapsulated, nonsporulating, nonmotile, gram-negative bacillus. It has been cultivated in the yolk sacs of embryonated chicken eggs and on media containing egg yolk. The disease has been produced in volunteers but not in laboratory animals, and there is no similar disease in animals.

Granuloma inguinale is rare in temperate climates, but common in the tropics and subtropics. New Guinea, central Australia, and India have the highest incidence. Individual susceptibility varies greatly, and the low level of infectivity has sparked controversy about sexual transmission. For instance, spouses of infected persons often remain uninfected despite repeated sexual contact. However, epidemiologic data favors sexual transmission. Most patients are 15 to 40 years of age, the period of greatest sexual activity. Because male homosexuals who take the passive role have only anal lesions, and because *C. granulomatis* has been isolated from feces, the organism is thought to inhabit the intestinal tract. It causes granuloma inguinale through autoinoculation, anal intercourse, or vaginal intercourse, when the vagina is colonized by enteric bacteria.

The incubation period varies from 1 week to 6 months, 2 to 4 weeks being the average. The initial lesion may be a papule, a subcutaneous nodule, or an ulcer. The lesion develops within several weeks into a raised, soft, painless, beefy-red, superficial ulcer. The exuberant granulation tissue resembles a fleshy mass herniating through the skin. In heterosexual men, early ulceration of the penoscrotal skin commonly extends to genitocrural and inguinal folds. In women ulcerations spread to the perineal and perianal skin. In homosexual men the lesions are perianal and anal.

Regional lymphadenopathy is not a feature. Occasionally, however, subcutaneous inflammation in the inguinal regions may be confused with the bubo of lymphogranuloma venereum.

Sometimes granuloma inguinale can infect the va-

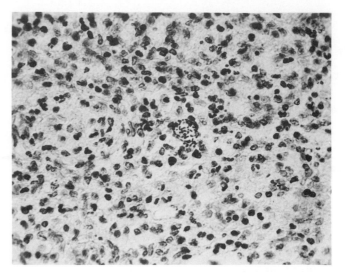

Figure 9-27. Granuloma inguinale, skin, showing *Calymmatobacterium granulomatis* (Donovan bodies), clustered in a large histiocyte. Intense silvering by the Warthin-Starry technique makes the organisms large, black, and easily seen.

gina and cervix and mimic carcinoma. Rarely, the infection disseminates to the pelvic organs, bone, and spleen following abortion or delivery. Extragenital lesions of the skin and mucous membranes of the oral cavity have been reported.

Untreated granuloma inguinale follows an indolent, relapsing course, often healing with an atrophic scar. Secondary fusospirochetal infection may cause ulceration, with mutilation or amputation of the genitalia. Massive cicatrization of the dermis and subcutis causes genital elephantiasis, probably by lymphatic obstruction. It is uncertain whether there is an association between granuloma inguinale and squamous cell carcinoma, because the diseases share common risk factors, such as poor hygiene, fusospirochetal flora, and a large number of sexual partners.

Microscopically, there is epithelial hyperplasia of the ulcer margin. The dermis and subcutis are infiltrated by numerous histiocytes and plasma cells and by fewer neutrophils and lymphocytes. The neutrophils in the ulcer bed are clustered into poorly defined microabscesses. Interspersed histiocytes contain many bacteria, which are called Donovan bodies (Fig. 9-27). The bacteria are difficult to see in routinely stained sections but are clearly revealed by silver impregnation. In older lesions, the inflammatory cell infiltrate is composed of lymphocytes and plasma cells, and the organisms are difficult to find.

The diagnosis of granuloma inguinale is suggested by the clinical appearance of the lesion and confirmed by the demonstration of *C. granulomatis* in smears of ulcer scrapings or in tissue sections. A combined regimen of trimethoprim and sulfamethoxazole is the treatment of choice.

Tropical Phagedenic Ulcer

Tropical phagedenic (rapidly spreading and sloughing) ulcer is a painful, necrotizing ulcer of the skin and subcutaneous tissues of the leg that afflicts young people living in tropical climates. Pathologic and bacteriologic studies implicate *Bacillus fusiformis* and *Treponema vincenti* as the cause. Malnutrition may predispose the patient to infection. The lesion usually starts on the skin at a point of trauma and develops rapidly. The surface sloughs to form an ulcer with raised borders and a cup-shaped crater (Fig. 9-28) that contains a gray, putrid exudate. The ulcer may be so deep that the underlying bone and tendons are exposed. The margin becomes fibrotic, but complete healing with re-epithelization may be delayed for years. In addition to secondary infection, tibial osteomyelitis and squamous cell carcinoma may be late complications. The carcinomas are well-differentiated, locally invasive, and destructive, but generally do not metastasize.

Sections through the ulcer reveal a coagulum of fibrin, containing degenerating cellular debris and masses of intermixed fusiform bacilli and spirochetes. The granulation tissue is infiltrated by leukocytes and supports the coagulum. The base of the ulcer contains a variety of inflammatory cells, including histiocytes, eosinophils, neutrophils, plasma cells, and lymphocytes. Occasional giant cells may also be present in deeper layers of scar tissue.

The diagnosis is made by the clinical presentation and the exclusion of other causes, such as Buruli ulcers and stasis ulcers. In some rural areas the ulcers are often treated with a wet compress of fresh papaya, which contains papain, a proteolytic enzyme that degrades the necrotic tissue. Penicillin, sulfonamides, tetracycline, and metronidazole have been effective. Reconstructive plastic surgery may be necessary to close the defect.

Noma

Noma, or cancrum oris, is a rapidly progressive necrosis of soft tissues and bones of the mouth and face, and, less commonly, other sites, such as chest, limbs, or genitalia. It afflicts malnourished children, many of whom are further debilitated by recent infections, for example, with measles, malaria, or kala-azar. Poor oral hygiene is an additional factor. A variety of bacteria may be recovered from these le-

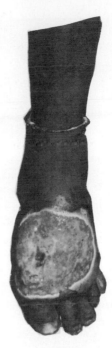

Figure 9-28. Tropical phagedenic ulcer (TPU), caused by infection with fuso-spirochetal organisms following penetrating trauma. TPUs are foul-smelling, painful, chronic, and an enormous public health problem in many parts of the third world.

sions, but *Treponema vincenti, Bacillus fusiformis, Bacteroides,* and *Corynebacterium* tend to dominate.

The ulceration is destructive and disfiguring, and usually unilateral (Fig. 9-29). The initial lesion is a small papule, often on the inner cheek opposite the molars or premolars. From this early lesion, large malodorous defects quickly develop. The lesions are painful and accompanied by variable systemic symptoms. Untreated, the patients often die.

Sections of the advanced lesions reveal coagulative necrosis of the epithelium, muscle, and adipose tissue. The surface of the exposed bone is often covered by a "fringe" or mixed bacterial growth. The diagnosis is based on the characteristic clinical appearance and the exclusion of other diseases, such as bacterial abscesses, actinomycosis, and maduromycosis. Systemic penicillin is the treatment of choice, together with cleansing of the lesion and a diet high in calories, protein, and vitamins. Reconstructive surgery may be required to repair extensive defects.

Staphylococcal Infections

Staphylococcal infections are caused by species of the genus *Staphylococcus.* These gram-positive cocci are ubiquitous, colonizing the skin and the anterior nasal vestibule of children and adults, and the umbilicus,

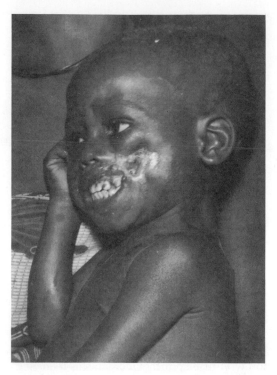

Figure 9-29. Noma (gangrenous stomatitis), a disease of malnourished children—frequently, children recovering from measles. There is massive destruction of the soft tissue and bones of mouth and cheek.

stool, and perineum of neonates. Three species are pathogenic in humans: *S. aureus, S. epidermidis,* and *S. saprophyticus.* About 20% to 40% of adults are nasal carriers of *S. aureus,* and many become carriers while in the hospital, perhaps because medical personnel are more frequent carriers than the general population. Large numbers of staphylococci are required for infection, and patients with more than 10^6 organisms per milliliter of nasal fluid tend to infect themselves and spread the staphylococci to others.

Most staphylococcal infections are caused by *S. aureus,* which grows especially well on skin and mucous membranes but can infect any part of the body. *S. aureus* causes a wide variety of suppurative diseases, including among others, **abscesses of the skin** (impetigo, boils, styes, carbuncles, breast abscesses, botryomycosis), **abscesses of bone** (osteomyelitis) and other deep organs, **infections of burns and surgical and other wounds, infections of the upper and lower respiratory tracts** (pharyngitis, bronchopneumonia, empyema), **purulent arthritis, septicemia, acute endocarditis,** and **meningitis.** *S. aureus* releases several exotoxins: enterotoxins (enteritis and food poisoning); exfoliative toxin (exfoliative skin disease);

and pyrogenic toxin (toxic shock syndrome). *S. epidermidis* causes only minor skin lesions, except in patients who have surgically inserted prostheses or are immunodeficient. *S. saprophyticus* is responsible for bladder infections.

S. aureus, named for its golden-yellow colonies on blood agar, produces coagulase (i.e., is "coagulase-positive"). *S. epidermidis* and *S. saprophyticus,* which form white colonies on blood agar (hence the former name *S. albus*), are coagulase-negative. Staphylococci are spherical and about 1 μm in diameter, a size that usually requires an oil immersion lens for identification in tissue sections. In liquid culture medium as well as in tissue, staphylococci grow in characteristic clusters, because they divide in successive perpendicular planes and daughter cells do not separate. These clusters distinguish staphylococci from streptococci, which grow in chains.

Many strains of staphylococci have developed resistance to penicillin and other antibiotics. Penicillin resistance is caused by plasmid-mediated production of penicillinase.

Infections of Skin

Impetigo is a skin infection that is caused by staphylococci (and by streptococci). Staphylococcal impetigo frequently afflicts school children who have a nasal discharge. Macular and pustular lesions begin around the nose and spread over the face, forming honey-yellow crusts, the hallmark of impetigo. These crusts are adherent to the surface of the skin, and removal leads to weeping skin lesions. Staphylococcal and streptococcal impetigo exhibit similar lesions, including folliculitis, pyoderma, wound infection, lymphatic spread, and sepsis. Staphylococcal impetigo leads to focal tissue necrosis and abscesses more frequently than does streptococcal impetigo.

Furuncles (boils) and styes. Boils are deep-seated infections with *S. aureus* in and around hair follicles, often in a nasal carrier. They occur only on hairy surfaces, such as the neck, thighs, and buttocks of men, and the axilla, pubic area, and eyelids of both sexes, the latter surfaces predisposed to boil formation by friction or maceration. The boil begins as a nodule at the base of the hair follicle, followed by a pimple that remains painful and red for a few days. A yellow apex forms, and the central core becomes necrotic and fluctuant. Rupture or incision of the boil relieves the pain. Several boils may occur in close proximity, and they often recur. Styes are boils that involve the sebaceus glands around the eyelid.

Carbuncles result from coalescing infections with

S. aureus around hair follicles and produce draining sinuses. Most carbuncles are on the neck, but they also occur on the limbs, trunk, face, and scalp. Necrosis spreads deeply into the skin, and some patients develop bacteremia, with a risk to life.

Breast abscesses usually arise within a few weeks after delivery, when staphylococci are transmitted from an infant with neonatal sepsis to the skin glands in the breasts of the nursing mother. The disease may be precipitated by the stasis of milk after weaning or a missed feeding.

Botryomycosis (a misnomer) is a chronic **bacterial** infection that may be caused by staphylococci (as well as by streptococci, *E. coli*, and other common bacteria). Botryomycosis presents as an indurated fibrotic mass with draining sinuses and grains in a purulent exudate and in tissue sections. Macroscopically, these grains cannot be distinguished from those of actinomycosis or a mycetoma. Microscopically, however, microcolonies of staphylococci in clusters within the grain are surrounded by an amorphous eosinophilic coating ("Splendore-Hoeppli phenomenon"). Botryomycosis resists antibiotic therapy, probably because the fibrosis and compactness of the grains prevents adequate levels of drug from reaching the bacteria. The lesion should be totally excised.

Abscesses of Bone (Osteomyelitis)

Acute staphylococcal osteomyelitis most commonly afflicts boys between 3 and 10 years of age, most of whom have a history of infection or trauma. The bones of the legs are involved in most patients. Many patients have an underlying bacteremia (*S. aureus*) with systemic symptoms. Osteomyelitis may become chronic if not properly treated.

Adults over 50 years of age are more frequently afflicted with osteomyelitis of the vertebra. The onset of localized back pain is usually abrupt, but may follow staphylococcal infection of the skin or urinary tract, prostatic surgery, infected abortion, puerperal infection, or a surgical procedure such as pinning a fracture.

Infections of Burns and Surgical Wounds

Burns and surgical wounds may become infected with *S. aureus* from the patient's own nasal carriage or from medical personnel. The appearance of visible pus in the wound depends on the interaction of bacteria, host factors, and foreign bodies. Neonates, the elderly, the malnourished, and the obese all have increased susceptibility.

Infections of the Upper and Lower Respiratory Tract (Pharyngitis, Bronchopneumonia, and Empyema)

Staphylococcal infections of the respiratory tract most commonly occur in infants less than 2 years of age, and especially in those under 2 months. They usually occur in winter, when viral respiratory diseases are prevalent. The child often has an underlying staphylococcal skin infection. Infection of the respiratory tract is mild at first, but suddenly worsens. Characteristic features include fever and spasms of dry coughing, followed by marked tachypnea with expiratory grunting, sternal retraction, cyanosis, progressive lethargy, and shock. There are ulcers of the upper airway and scattered foci of pneumonia. Other common complications are pleural effusion, empyema, and pneumothorax. Roentgenograms of the chest show patchy infiltrates, which progress rapidly. Gram-positive cocci are seen in aspirated tracheal or pleural fluid, which is often bloody. In adults, staphylococcal pneumonia may follow viral influenza, a disease that destroys the ciliated surface epithelium and leaves the bronchial surface vulnerable to secondary infections. Patients with chronic lung disease and chronic heart disease (especially rheumatic valve disease) are also at increased risk for staphylococcal pneumonia.

Acute and Chronic Bacterial Arthritis

S. aureus is the causative organism in half of all cases of septic arthritis. Most of those who have the disease are adults, 50 to 70 years old, and usually only a single joint is involved. Rheumatoid arthritis and steroid therapy are common predisposing conditions. The acute onset of staphylococcal arthritis is marked by severe, throbbing pain, often worse at night, which is accompanied by shaking chills and fever. Acute staphylococcal arthritis may be confused with an acute episode of rheumatoid arthritis.

Septicemia

Septicemia with *S. aureus* afflicts patients with lowered resistance who are in the hospital for other diseases or conditions. Some have underlying staphylococcal infections (for example, osteomyelitis or septic arthritis), some have had surgery (especially transurethral resection of the prostate), and some have infections from an indwelling intravenous catheter. Staphylococcal septicemia is associated with the common symptoms of bacteremia, such as shaking chills and fever. Miliary abscesses and staphylococcal endocarditis are serious complications.

Bacterial Endocarditis

Acute and subacute bacterial endocarditis are complications of septicemia caused by *S. aureus* (as well as by *S. epidermidis*). Endocarditis may develop spontaneously on normal valves or on valves damaged by rheumatic fever. It may also follow insertion of prosthetic valves or other intracardiac surgery. Those with intravenous heroin addiction also have an increased risk of endocarditis from infection with *S. aureus*. In addition to the symptoms of septicemia, a heart murmur is usual, with or without evidence of embolization to other organs.

Meningitis

Staphylococcal meningitis is a complication of surgical procedures on the central nervous system. Infections of shunts in the brain may be caused by *S. aureus* or *S. epidermidis*. Although staphylococcal meningitis is often not clinically evident, it may be found at autopsy in patients with septicemia or endocarditis.

Toxinoses

Staphylococcal **food poisoning** is caused by the ingestion of preformed staphylococcal enterotoxin in prepared food. This commonly involves food eaten in a restaurant (not industrially processed food), especially unrefrigerated meats, milk, or custard and other milk products. The food (**not** the patient's excreta) must be tested for staphylococci. Food that contains more than 10^8 staphylococci per gram contains enough enterotoxin to cause food poisoning. *S. aureus* has caused more than half of the food poisoning epidemics in which the causative agent has been identified. Thus, the incidence is much higher than that of epidemics caused by *Salmonella*, *Clostridia perfringens*, *Shigella*, or *Streptococcus*. At least six enterotoxins are produced by some of the coagulase-positive strains of *S. aureus*, and enterotoxins are also produced by a few coagulase-negative strains. Enterotoxins are resistant to heat and withstand cooking for 20 to 60 minutes. Usually, nausea and vomiting begin within a few hours of ingesting the toxin. In some cases, however, diarrhea and abdominal discomfort are the only symptoms. Patients with more severe food poisoning have bloody mucus in the vomitus and stools, as well as muscle cramps, head-

ache, and sweating. The acute phase commonly lasts 4 to 6 hours, and recovery is complete within 1 or 2 days.

Acute gastroenteritis is characterized by histologic changes in both stomach and small intestine. Within 2 hours of the introduction of enterotoxin, there is a neutrophilic exudate in the stomach. By 6 hours the gastric mucosal cells are depleted of mucus, and the mucosa is covered by a mucopurulent exudate. The inflammatory reaction in the stomach subsides within 24 hours. In the small intestine, by 4 hours there is focal degeneration of the epithelium of the villi, elongation of crypts, and infiltration of neutrophils in the lamina propria. After 12 hours regression begins, and by 48 to 72 hours the mucosa appears normal.

The exfoliative toxin of *S. aureus* causes the **"scalded skin syndrome,"** which afflicts neonates, infants, and young children, typically in the aftermath of conjunctivitis or minor staphylococcal infection. A painful, brick-red rash begins on the face, neck, axilla, and groin, and then becomes generalized. The rash leads to blisters or bullae, and the upper dermis is shed in large sheets.

Toxic Shock Syndrome (TSS)

The toxic shock syndrome is a sporadic, febrile illness that is characterized by fever, hypotension, and a desquamating rash. Some of the symptoms resemble those of scarlet fever, a malady caused by the erythrogenic toxin of *Streptococcus pyogenes*. The toxic shock syndrome may progress to renal and pulmonary failure and death. The disease afflicts young, menstruating women, in whom it is usually associated with some brands of tampons. The risk appears to be higher if tampons with high absorbency remain in place longer than usual. However, the syndrome may also afflict nonmenstruating women, men, and children, in association with staphylococcal empyema, septic abortions, fasciitis, osteomyelitis, and abscesses.

The toxic shock syndrome is thought to be caused by only some strains of *S. aureus*, namely those that grow well in the environment provided by the tampon. Some studies suggest that the DNA of a lysogenic bacteriophage in those strains may enable *S. aureus* to produce a specific toxin.

Histologic studies of the liver from patients with the toxic shock syndrome have shown acute cholangitis with little or no cholestasis. Acute cholangitis could account for the jaundice and hyperbilirubinemia reported in many patients with this condition. Circulating toxin is thought to damage the bile ducts, rather than bacterial infection *per se*.

Infections with S. epidermidis

As previously mentioned, *S. epidermidis,* an opportunistic pathogen, causes only minor skin lesions, except in patients undergoing surgery for insertion of prosthetic devices and patients with impaired immune systems. The organism is ubiquitous, and in healthy persons usually resides on the skin of the axilla, head, nose, and limbs. Infections with *S. epidermidis* are often associated with foreign bodies, such as prosthetic valves, shunts for cerebrospinal fluid, joint prostheses (especially replacements of the hip and femur), and vascular prostheses. Prosthetic valvular endocarditis, for example, may be caused by contaminated coronary suction lines during the insertion of prosthetic valves, with subsequent infection of repaired areas of the heart and prosthetic valve. Deep sternal wound infections may result, often in the first few weeks after the operation. *S. epidermidis* can be the direct cause (without foreign body) of bladder infections, endocarditis, and other infections. Strains of *S. epidermidis* are frequently resistant to penicillin and other antimicrobial agents, and infected protheses and grafted vessels often need to be replaced.

Infections with S. saprophyticus

S. saprophyticus resembles *S. epidermidis,* but biochemical assays and the pattern of drug resistance distinguish the two. For reasons unknown, *S. saprophyticus* causes bladder infections, primarily in young women. Strains of *S. saprophyticus* are sensitive to many antibiotics.

Streptococcal Infections

Streptococcal infections are caused by species of the genus *Streptococcus,* which includes *Streptococcus pyogenes* (group A), *S. agalactiae* (group B), *S. faecalis* (group D), *S. pneumoniae* (pneumococcus) and the viridans streptococci group. Although streptococci elicit suppurative inflammatory responses, there are several nonsuppurative complications that reflect immune responses and deposition of immune complexes. Streptococcal infections occur throughout the world, even where antibiotics are readily available. As in the case of many infections, problems with streptococci are greatest among underprivileged populations for whom penicillin and other antibiotics are not readily available.

Streptococci become nonvirulent on desiccation, and indirect spread rarely occurs. **To acquire infection, an individual must usually be inoculated with millions of streptococci, spread by close contact with a carrier or with someone who has an active infection.** But of those colonized with streptococci, few actually develop an overt infection. Whether or not infection by a streptococcus becomes clinically apparent, patients are at risk from the late, "nonsuppurative," immune complications; namely, rheumatic heart disease, acute glomerulonephritis, and erythema nodosum.

The streptococcus is gram-positive and is demonstrated in cultures, smears, and tissue sections. The organisms are spherical and very small (less than 2 μm diameter), and the oil immersion lens must be used in searching for them in tissue sections.

Cultural, biochemical, and immunologic studies have identified many groups and subtypes of streptococci:

Group A beta-hemolytic streptococci (for example *S. pyogenes*) cause nasopharyngeal and cutaneous lesions, different strains infecting these sites.

Group B streptococci produce infections of the newborn.

Group C, G, and other streptococci are responsible for respiratory infections

"Untypable" alpha (green) hemolytic streptococci (for instance *S. viridans*), are part of the flora of the mouth and cause about one-half of all bacterial endocarditis.

Group D streptococci (e.g., enterococci) are an important cause of infections of the urinary tract, endocarditis, postsurgical infections, septicemia, and other infections.

Pneumococci (*Streptococcus pneumoniae*) produce primary bacterial pneumonia, septicema, meningitis, and other infections.

Antigens and Exotoxins

The capsule of the streptococcus is a polysaccharide that contains hyaluronic acid. The cell wall contains antiphagocytic "M protein" (closely linked to virulence), and lipoteichoic acid, which is required for recognition of and adhesion to the host epithelial cell membranes. The structural backbone of the cell wall is a peptidoglycan that has pyrogenic properties and weak endotoxicity.

Group A streptococci produce several exotoxins, including erythrogenic toxins (pyrogenic exotoxins) and cytolytic toxins (streptolysins S and O). Erythrogenic toxins cause the rash of scarlet fever (not directly but by enhancing acquired hypersensitivity to diverse streptococcal products). Most, but not all, group A streptococci produce both streptolysin S and streptolysin O, which are not only "hemolysins" (lysing red blood cells), but also cytolytic: that is, they damage and lyse a broad spectrum of mammalian cells and cellular components. The surface hemolysis on blood agar plates is largely caused by streptolysin S, which also lyses bacterial protoplasts (L-forms) and probably destroys neutrophils after they ingest group A streptococci. This toxin influences T-lymphocytes to a much greater extent than B-lymphocytes and has antitumor activity. Because streptolysin S is not immunogenic, its effects may be unimpeded even after repeated streptococcal infections. By contrast, streptolysin O induces a persistently high antibody titer, an effect that provides a useful marker for the diagnosis and epidemiologic studies of group A streptococcal infections and the late nonsuppurative complications. Streptolysin O also has cardiotoxic properties, possibly playing a role in acute rheumatic fever and rheumatic heart disease.

Streptococcal infections and their nonsuppurative complications are outlined in Figure 9-30.

Primary Streptococcal Infections

Infections of the Upper Respiratory Tract
Infections of the upper respiratory tract are caused mainly by group A beta-hemolytic streptococci and present as pharyngitis, pneumonia, and pulmonary abscesses. The pharyngitis varies in intensity from mild lesions resembling the common cold, to more severe lesions that involve the epiglottis and the tonsillar crypts. These lesions commonly produce vasodilatation, spreading edema, and an exudate composed mostly of neutrophils, often mixed with macrophages. Streptococci may spread from the pharyngitis to the airways, especially if there is a peritonsillar or a retropharyngeal abscess.

Scarlet Fever
Scarlet fever, which results from an acute pharyngitis or tonsillitis caused by group A streptococci, is characterized by a rash produced by the erythrogenic toxin. The incubation period of 2 to 5 days is followed by chills and fever, fiery red pharyngeal mucosa, small crypt abscesses in enlarged tonsils, and a bright red tongue with edematous papillae ("raspberry tongue"). One to 3 days later there appears a diffuse, punctate, erythematous rash, most prominent over the trunk and inner aspects of the limbs and involving the face, except for a small area around the mouth ("circumoral pallor"). When the pharyngitis and rash subside, near the end of the first week, desquamation begins. Microscopically, an acute suppurative exudate on the pharynx and oropharynx contains streptococci. There is also an acute inflammatory reaction

in the lymph nodes. Hyperkeratosis of the reddened skin accounts for scaling during defervescence. The characteristic 1-week duration of scarlet fever is not appreciably shortened by antibiotic therapy, but suppurative complications, such as otitis media, sinusitis, and mastoiditis, are prevented. Scarlet fever is notorious for late nonsuppurative sequelae, which are also prevented by prompt treatment.

Erysipelas
Erysipelas, caused chiefly by beta-hemolytic group A streptococci, is the classic cutaneous streptococcal infection. It is common in warm climates, but is not often seen before the age of 20 years. Erysipelas is an erythematous swelling of the skin that usually begins on the face and spreads rapidly. The maplike area of brawny erythema has a sharp, well-demarcated, serpiginous border. A diffuse, edematous, acute inflammatory reaction in the dermis and epidermis extends into the subcutaneous tissues. The inflammatory infiltrate (mostly neutrophils) is most intense around vessels and adnexae of the skin. Cutaneous microabscesses and small foci of necrosis are not uncommon.

Impetigo
Impetigo, another infection of skin that may be caused by streptococci, has increasingly been reported as a cause of post-streptococcal complications in children. Streptococcal and staphylococcal impetigo have similar lesions, including folliculitis, pyoderma, wound infection, lymphatic spread, and sepsis. Streptococcal impetigo more often induces lymphangitis (red streaks along the draining lymphatics) than does staphylococcal impetigo, and less frequently causes focal tissue necrosis or abscesses.

Aphthous Ulcers
Recurrent aphthous ulcers of the lip (chancres) have been associated with and may be caused by *Streptococcus sanguis* in those who are susceptible.

Puerperal Sepsis
Puerperal sepsis, a result of infection by group A streptococci from the contaminated hands of attendants at delivery, was formerly common but, with the acceptance of the "germ theory" of disease and improved hygiene, is now rare in the developed countries. Group B streptococcus is an important neonatal pathogen, causing pneumonia, sepsis, and meningitis. Infants acquire the infection from their mothers during delivery, and mortality rates are high (50% or more) if the onset of infection is within 10 days of delivery.

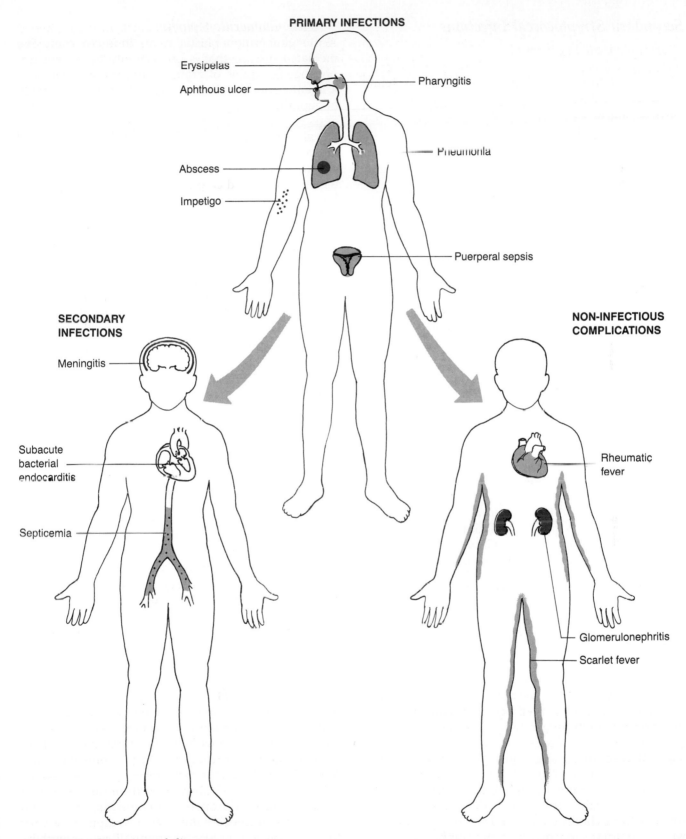

Figure 9-30. Streptococcal diseases.

Secondary Streptococcal Infections

Streptococcal Septicemia

Streptococcal septicemia with group A streptococci may spread from the nasopharynx to the systemic circulation and seed the lungs, meninges, or heart valves. Streptococcal septicemia can develop quickly, may be life-threatening, and is a particular hazard for splenectomized patients or those with abnormal splenic function.

Pneumococcal Pneumonia and Meningitis

Pneumococcal pneumonia and meningitis result from infection with *S. pneumoniae* (the pneumococcus), an organism that is responsible for 80% of all bacterial pneumonias. Pneumococci also spread from the nasopharynx through the systemic circulation and seed the meninges. Some patients develop meningitis from primary pneumococcal pneumonia. For example, in most parts of Africa, a meningitis is more commonly caused by the pneumococcus than by the meningococcus. The histologic features of pneumococcal meningitis resemble those described for meningococcal meningitis.

Bacterial Endocarditis

Bacterial endocarditis is a complication of streptococcal septicemia in which the organisms spread from a site of local infection through the circulation to colonize heart valves. The alpha-hemolytic streptococci are a leading cause of subacute bacterial endocarditis, whereas *Streptococcus pneumoniae* frequently produces acute bacterial endocarditis. Endocarditis caused by group A streptococci is rare. Group D streptococci (including enterococci) also cause endocarditis, but infection of the valves with group A streptococci is rare.

Nonsuppurative Complications

Rheumatic Fever

Rheumatic fever is an acute, recurrent, systemic inflammatory process that usually follows a pharyngeal infection by group A streptococci. Rheumatic fever probably results from a reaction between antibodies to streptococcal antigens and tissue antigens that takes place in many sites, but it is particularly dangerous in the heart. The disease is characterized by pancarditis, migratory polyarthritis of large joints, erythema marginatum of the skin, subcutaneous nodules, and chorea—the last a neurologic disorder with involuntary, purposeless movements. The clinical pathologic features of rheumatic fever and rheumatic heart disease are discussed in Chapter 11.

Acute Glomerulonephritis

Acute glomerulonephritis is an immune complex–mediated disease that is caused only by certain nephritogenic strains of group A streptococci. There is a latent period between the infection and the onset of nephritis during which the titer of antibodies (e.g., antistreptolysin-O) increases. Granular deposits in the glomeruli contain immunoglobulin and complement, a reflection of antigen–antibody complexes. The clinical and pathologic features of acute glomerulonephritis are discussed elsewhere.

Erythema Nodosum

Erythema nodosum is an inflammatory reaction of the subcutaneous adipose tissue (panniculitis) that is sometimes associated with infections, including those with group A streptococci. The connective tissue septa of the fat are widened by edema and an exudate of fibrin and neutrophils. Later the inflammatory infiltrate contains lymphocytes, histiocytes, giant cells, and occasional eosinophils.

Meningococcal Infections

The gram-negative, bean-shaped diplococcus *Neisseria meningitidis* causes a variety of clinical and pathologic manifestations, including pharyngitis, meningitis, and septicemia (Fig. 9-31). *N. meningitidis* may be cultured from the nasopharynx, blood, or cerebrospinal fluid. Meningococci are typed serologically by the protein antigens in their cell walls and the polysaccharide in their capsules. There are eight major serogroups, three of which (A, B, C) cause most infections. The exception is meningococcal pneumonia, produced by group Y.

Meningococci are ubiquitous and lead to meningitis throughout the world. Group A organisms cause major epidemics in a belt through the northern savanna of sub-Saharan Africa, from Gambia to Ethiopia. Groups B and C produce most endemic infections in Europe and the United States. In the African meningitis belt, the incidence is highest in children 5 to 14 years of age, but in developed countries it is highest in children under the age of 5 years. People with defective humoral immunity have an increased susceptibility. Those with anatomic defects that allow meningococci to spread from the nasopharynx into the cranium are also at risk.

Meningococci are transmitted from person to person by respiratory droplets. After exposure most people become carriers but develop no symptoms, except for an occasional mild pharyngitis. Less commonly, organisms invade the bloodstream to cause a fulminating meningococcemia, or to seed the meninges

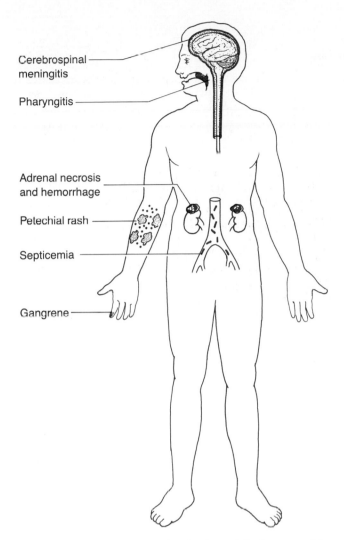

Cerebrospinal meningitis

Pharyngitis

Adrenal necrosis and hemorrhage

Petechial rash

Septicemia

Gangrene

Figure 9-31. Meningococcal infections. Meningococcal infections have a variety of clinical manifestations including pharyngitis, meningitis, septicemia, and associated complications.

and produce an acute suppurating meningitis. **Thus, the meningococcus is responsible for two distinct fatal lesions: septicemia (meningococcemia) and meningitis.**

Fever, tachycardia, and hypotension are early symptoms of acute meningococcemia. There is usually a leukocytosis, but critically ill patients may have leukopenia. Proliferating meningococci produce an endotoxin that causes circulatory collapse, a characteristic feature of meningococcemia. The toxemia is often sudden and kills the patient within a few hours. Thrombocytopenia and an increase in products of fibrin degradation, the features of disseminated intravascular coagulation, are usual. Fulminating meningococcemia is also the principal cause of the **Waterhouse-Friderichsen syndrome,** a complication seen mainly in children and characterized by purpura, circulatory collapse, and hemorrhage into the adrenal glands. Some patients who survive the early phase of meningococcemia develop late allergic complications, such as polyarthritis, cutaneous vasculitis, episcleritis, and pericarditis. Occasionally, severe vasculitis is associated with extensive cutaneous ulceration and sometimes even gangrene of the distal portions of limbs. At postmortem examination victims of acute meningococcemia have petechiae at multiple sites, hemorrhage into the adrenal medulla and other organs, encephalitis, and damage to small blood vessels.

Like meningococcemia, meningococcal meningitis develops suddenly and kills the patient quickly. Characteristically the patient suddenly experiences headache, stiff neck, and fever. A cardiac arrhythmia indicates myocardial damage. Typically there is a neutrophilic leukocytosis and the cerebrospinal fluid shows characteristic changes of acute pyogenic meningitis, including increased white blood cell levels (mainly neutrophils), high protein, and low glucose.

At autopsy the brain is covered with thick yellow-gray pus that extends inward along the Virchow-Robin (perivascular) spaces. Microscopically, the exudate is composed of fibrin and neutrophils, expands the subarachnoid space, and may also extend to the ventricles. Local production of endotoxins by meningococci in the meninges probably stimulates the formation of chemotactic complement components, which contribute to the meningeal exudate. Inflammatory cells may appear in the brain, indicating an encephalitis. Tissue Gram stains reveal meningococci in neutrophils and free in the exudate.

The diagnosis of meningococcal meningitis is established by culturing *N. meningitidis* or by detecting meningococcal antigen in the cerebrospinal fluid. Serum antibody levels are higher during convalescence than in the acute phase. For acute meningococcemia, the antibiotic of choice is penicillin given for at least 7 days, initially by intravenous infusion and subsequently by intramuscular injection. For meningococcal meningitis the antibiotic of choice is also penicillin, continued for 5 to 10 days.

Gonococcal Infections (Gonorrhea)

Gonorrhea is a sexually transmitted disease caused by various strains of the gram-negative diplococcus *Neisseria gonorrhoea* (Fig. 9-32). The infection is usually localized to the urogenital tract, most commonly the urethra of men and the endocervix of women. About one-half of infected women have no symptoms. In men, however, infection is usually symptomatic.

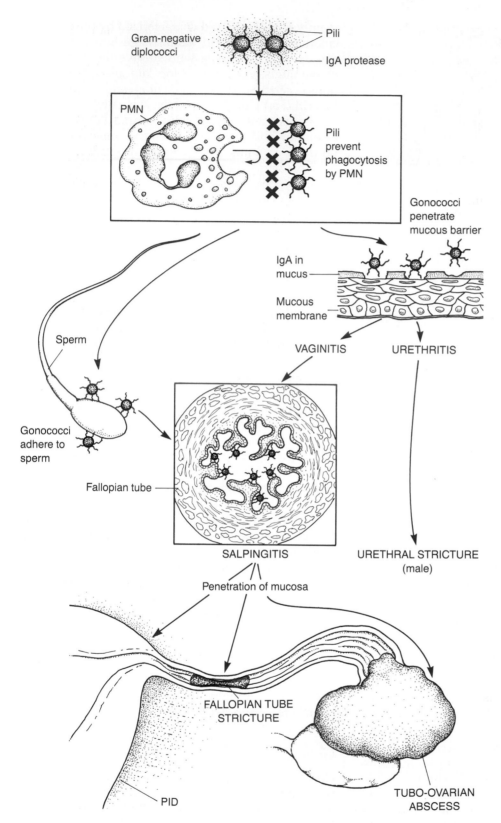

Figure 9-32. Pathogenesis of gonococcal infections. *Neisseria gonorrhoea* is a gram-negative diplococcus whose surface pili form a barrier against phagocytosis by neutrophils. The pili contain an IgA protease that digests IgA on the luminal surface of the mucous membranes of the urethra, endocervix, and fallopian tube, thus facilitating attachment of gonococci. Gonococci cause endocervicitis, vaginitis, and salpingitis. In men, gonococci attached to the mucous membrane of the urethra cause urethritis and, sometimes, urethral stricture. Gonococci may also attach to sperm heads and be carried into the fallopian tube. Penetration of the mucous membrane by gonococci leads to stricture of the fallopian tube, pelvic inflammatory disease (PID), or tubo-ovarian abscess.

Gonorrhea is a serious public health problem in most parts of the world, and is epidemic in many countries. It is especially common in the tropics, where the prevalence is high in prostitutes, who transmit it to migrant male workers.

Gonococci are readily seen in smears (urethral, endocervical, or conjunctival exudates) and cultures, and appear as bean-shaped pairs, with the flat sides apposed. The organisms are cultured from tampons, urethral swabs, urine, specimens from the endocervix, vagina, anus, and pharynx.

Gonorrhea begins as a surface infection of the mucous membranes; that is, a catarrh. The bacteria attach to and spread along the cells of the surface mucous membranes, after which they invade superficially and provoke acute inflammation. The mucous membranes of the urethra, endocervix, and salpinx are characteristic sites. The cell wall of *N. gonorrhoea* contains lipopolysaccharide, protein, and phospholipid. It lacks a true polysaccharide capsule, but projecting from the cell wall are hairlike extensions called pili. Within these pili is a protease that digests IgA on the surface of the mucous membrane, thus facilitating the attachment of gonococci to the columnar and transitional epithelium of the urogenital tract (see Fig. 9-32). "Smooth" strains with few pili are less virulent and less prone to cause urethritis or cervicitis.

After an incubation period of 3 to 5 days, men usually have purulent urethral discharge and dysuria. With prompt antibiotic treatment the infection is arrested and gonococci are confined to the mucosa of the anterior urethra. However, if treatment is not instituted promptly the organisms extend to the prostate, epididymis, and accessory glands, where they cause urethral stricture, epididymitis, orchitis, and sometimes male infertility. Urethral stricture may be associated with fistulas between the urethra and perineum ("watering can" perineum). Male homosexuals develop pharyngitis and proctitis.

The first manifestation of infection in women is usually endocervicitis, with vaginal discharge or bleeding. There may be urethritis, manifested by dysuria rather than by urethral discharge. In some women (usually during the first menses after exposure), the infection extends to the fallopian tubes, where it produces acute and chronic salpingitis and pelvic inflammatory disease (see Fig. 9-32). The fallopian tubes swell with pus, causing acute abdominal pain. Infertility occurs when inflammatory adhesions close the tubes at both ends, blocking the ascent of sperm and the descent of ova. Infected fallopian tubes ("pus tubes") have the shape of a retort flask (Fig. 9-33).

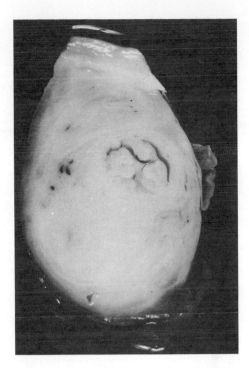

Figure 9-33. Gonorrhea, fallopian tube. Cross section of a "pus tube," showing thickening of the wall and a lumen swollen with pus.

From the fallopian tubes the infection may spread to the peritoneum, healing as fine adhesions ("violin string" adhesions) between the capsule of the liver and the parietal peritoneum. The vaginal discharge may infect the anal crypts, leading to mucopurulent anal discharge, rectal pruritus, and tenesmus. Chronic endometritis is a persistent complication of gonococcal infection and is usually a consequence of chronic gonococcal salpingitis. In such cases the endometrium contains many lymphocytes and plasma cells. Women (and to a lesser extent men) may also develop bacteremia, producing disseminated gonococcal infection, which in turn leads to monarthritis or polyarthritis.

Neonatal infections from infected amniotic fluid or an infected birth canal result in symptoms within a few days after birth. These infections involve the conjunctiva and constitute a major cause of blindness in much of Africa and Asia. Other sites of neonatal infection are the pharynx, respiratory tract, vagina, anus, leptomeninges, joints, and blood.

Uncomplicated gonococcal infections of the urethra and endocervix are treated with penicillin and other antibiotics. *N. gonorrhoea* is displaying increasing resistance to penicillin. Penicillinase-producing strains are especially common in Africa and Asia.

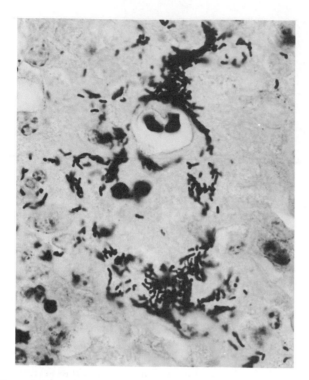

Figure 9-34. Cat scratch disease, lymph node. The wall of a small vessel is swollen and packed with the causal organism (unclassified and unnamed). The bacilli are gram-negative but difficult to see with tissue Gram stains; they are blackened by the Warthin-Starry silver-impregnation technique, however, making them more easily seen.

Cat Scratch Disease

Cat scratch disease is a usually self-limited infection by a gram-negative, bacterium that is as yet unnamed. The bacteria form filaments up to 10 μm or longer. It has not been cultured but is easily seen in tissue sections of the skin, lymph nodes, and conjunctiva, when stained by a silver impregnation technique. The reservoir is unknown, but infection begins when the organism is inoculated into the skin by the claws of cats and rarely by other animals, or by thorns or splinters. Sometimes the conjunctiva is contaminated by close contact with a cat, possibly by licking around the eye. Infections are more common in children (80%) than adults, and there may be clustering when a stray cat or kitten joins a family.

Most patients have a papule at the site of inoculation, but it may be small and overlooked. The papule, which begins 3 to 14 days after inoculation and may persist for 8 weeks, is followed by tenderness and enlargement of the regional lymph nodes. The nodes remain enlarged for 3 to 4 months and may drain through the skin. About one-half of the patients have other symptoms, including fever and malaise

and (rarely) splenomegaly, Parinaud's oculoglandular syndrome, rash, encephalitis (which typically has a sudden onset and sudden resolution), and erythema nodosum.

At the site of inoculation the bacteria multiply in the walls of small vessels and about collagen fibers, from which they move through draining lymphatics to regional lymph nodes, where they produce a pyogranulomatous lymphadenitis. In early lesions clusters of bacteria expand and obliterate the walls of small vessels (Fig. 9-34). The lesions in the skin and lymph nodes progress from abscesses to suppurating granulomas and finally to necrosis. Bacteria are abundant in early lesions and rare in late ones.

Without biopsy and the visualization of the characteristic bacteria, the diagnosis is supported when three criteria are met: contact with a cat, a cat scratch, or a primary lesion of the skin or conjunctiva; a positive skin test for cat scratch antigen; and negative results from laboratory studies for other causes of lymphadenopathy. No specific antibiotic has been accepted as beneficial.

Diseases Caused by Filamentous Bacteria

Actinomycosis

Actinomycosis is a chronic infection characterized by swelling, pain, and draining sinuses that discharge actinomycotic grains. A number of different anaerobic and microaerophilic bacteria cause actinomycosis. These are *Actinomyces israelii*, *A. naseslundii*, *A. viscosus*, *Arachnia propionica*, and *Bifidobacterium adolescentis*. The bacteria are long, gram-positive filaments 0.2 to 0.3 μm wide by at least 4.0 μm long. In tissue, actinomyces form round yellow grains, 100 to 300 μm across, which are cemented together by a mucosaccharide–protein matrix.

The actinomyces are saprophytes and may be part of the normal flora of the oral cavity, the intestine, and the vagina. A break in the epithelial surface and damage to the surrounding tissue allows the actinomycetes to invade and establish infection. Dental extractions, poor oral hygiene, abdominal surgery, appendicitis, and diverticulitis all predispose to actinomycosis. Pulmonary alveoli damaged by aspiration may also become infected by actinomycetes. Women with neglected intrauterine devices have increased actinomycotic flora of the vagina and cervix, and the attached IUD string becomes a nidus for actinomycotic growth. With continued neglect there

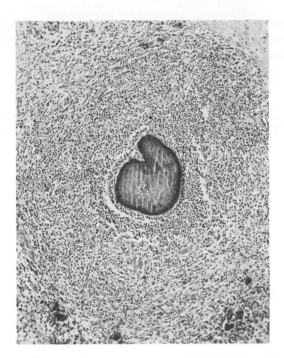

Figure 9-35. Actinomycosis, ovary. A typical grain lies within an abscess surrounded by a fibrogranulomatous reaction.

is a risk of uterine, tubal, or ovarian actinomycosis. Actinomycosis originating in a tooth socket or the tonsils is characterized by swelling of the face and neck, at first painless and fluctuant, but later painful. The infection spreads along tissue planes and by sinus tracts into bone and through the skin. In pulmonary infections sinus tracts may penetrate from lobe to lobe, through the pleura, and into ribs and vertebrae. Night sweats, weight loss, and cough are common and chest radiographs reveal abscesses, particularly at the lung bases. In the abdomen actinomycosis usually begins in the appendix or colon and extends to the abdominal wall, diaphragm, spine, liver, ovaries, kidney or urinary bladder.

Histopathologically, the grains stain deep purple with hematoxylin and are composed of packed actinomycetes in an eosinophilic matrix (Fig. 9-35). This matrix, also called Splendore-Hoeppli material, coats the actinomycetes projecting from the surface of the grain, giving the perimeter the appearance of radiating clubs. The grains lie in an abscess surrounded by a granulomatous reaction.

The key to diagnosis is the identification of the gram-positive filaments within the grain. Specimens taken for culture should include grains. Penicillin is given in high doses for 6 weeks and is followed by 6 to 12 months of tetracycline. Incision and drainage or surgical resection may also be necessary.

Nocardiosis

Nocardiosis is an infection of the lung that may spread to the brain and skin and, less commonly, to the thyroid, liver, or other organs. The causative organism is *Nocardia asteroides,* a gram-positive, aerobic, branching, filamentous bacillus that is weakly acid-fast and belongs to the order Actinomycetales. *Nocardia* species inhabit the soil and have worldwide distribution. Debility and immunosuppression predispose to infection. Invasion of the lung causes a bronchopneumonia, which may extend to become lobar. Fever, weight loss, night sweats, and cough are usual. Direct extension to the pleura, trachea, and heart and extension to the brain or skin through the circulation are recognized complications and carry a grave prognosis.

The gross appearance of the lung depends on the duration and extent of infection. The lesions may be focal or diffuse and usually have necrotic centers surrounded by a perimeter of organizing pneumonia. Microscopically, the necrotic centers are rich in fibrin and degenerating neutrophils. The nocardia infiltrate the pulmonary tissue freely and are most easily seen after silver impregnation. A modified acid-fast stain demonstrates weak and segmental staining (Fig. 9-36). For treatment, sulfadiazine and sulfisoxazole are the antibiotics of choice and are continued after recovery for 6 weeks to 12 months.

Two other pathogenic species of *Nocardia* that deserve mention are *N. brasiliensis* and *N. caviae.* Either of these may cause pulmonary nocardiosis resem-

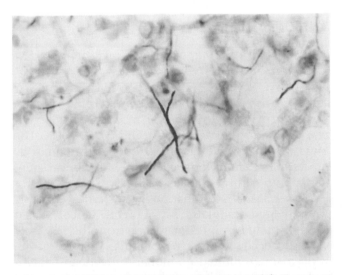

Figure 9-36. Nocardiosis, lung, showing acid-fast segments of *Nocardia asteroides* in a necrotic exudate in the lung.

bling that produced by *N. asteroides*, but more characteristically they are encountered in underdeveloped countries as a cause of mycetoma. They are inoculated into the skin and subcutaneous tissue at the time of penetrating trauma, grow slowly, and form nocardial grains. A pyogranulomatous reaction erupts through the skin to form draining sinuses. Nocardial mycetomas must be distinguished from the mycetomas caused by fungi and nonfilamentous bacteria.

Pitted Keratolysis

Pitted keratolysis is characterized by pits in the keratin layer of the soles and is caused by invasion of the stratum corneum by *Dermatophilus congolensis*, a gram-positive filamentous bacterium. The organism divides both longitudinally and transversely, giving an unmistakable appearance of reduplicating railroad tracks. Near the surface of the keratin short segments separate, and these resemble micrococci. The pits are multiple, painless, chronic, and most numerous over the heels and balls of the feet. In the tropics, where barefooted rural people are especially susceptible, they tend to recur during the rainy season. In temperate zones, those with hidrosis or other causes of chronically wet feet are also susceptible. The pits have sharp vertical walls and a punched-out appearance. Biopsy or culture confirms the diagnosis. The key to treatment is drying the soles and keeping them dry. A topical ointment containing formaldehyde has been successful.

Diseases Caused By the Mycobacteria

Tuberculosis

Tuberculosis is a chronic communicable disease caused by a variety of tubercle bacilli, especially *Mycobacterium tuberculosis hominis* and *M. t. bovis*. The lungs are the prime target, but any organ may be infected. The characteristic lesion is a spherical granuloma with central caseous necrosis.

M. t. hominis is ordinarily contracted by inhaling contaminated droplets. *M. t. bovis* is contracted through the gastrointestinal tract, from the raw milk of diseased cows. Most people, after exposure, develop a small, limited pulmonary infection. This infection is contained by an inflammatory reaction, and during its course the tuberculin skin test becomes positive. **Thus most tuberculous infections do not progress to clinical disease.**

Distributed throughout the world, tuberculosis is clearly one of the most important bacterial diseases of mankind. Although the risk of infection has been dramatically reduced in developed countries, it remains high for malnourished people in impoverished areas. In the United States, for example, the incidence is 12 per 100,000, and the mortality is one to two per 100,000. In some developing countries, the incidence reaches 450 per 100,000. The mortality data are usually poor, but the rates are certainly many times higher than in the United States. There are also racial and ethnic differences: Jews, other Caucasians, and Mongolians have greater natural resistance than Africans, Native Americans, and Eskimos. Age may also be a factor. In the United States, tuberculosis is highest among the elderly, possibly a reflection of infections acquired earlier in life before the decline in the prevalence of the disease.

Tubercle bacilli are slender, beaded nonmotile, acid-fast, and gram-positive bacilli, although their gram-positivity may be difficult to demonstrate. The cell wall is waxy and contains components that confer acid-fastness; that is, the retention of carbolfuchsin after rinsing with acid alcohol. **Tubercle bacilli are strict, obligate aerobes that proliferate within phagocytes.** They grow slowly in culture and require 3 or more weeks to develop colonies. The virulence of tubercle bacilli is associated with a tendency to aggregate and form filaments or cords in liquid media. The organisms resist heat and disinfectants but are killed quickly by ultraviolet light.

Delayed cell-mediated immunity to the tubercle bacillus is commonly measured by the Mantoux or Tine skin tests, which use as test antigen the "purified protein derivative" from media in which tubercle bacilli have grown. The skin test is positive if an area of induration at least 10 mm in diameter develops within 48 hours after the intradermal injection of the antigen. Patients usually develop this hypersensitivity 2 to 4 weeks after infection. Although a positive skin test indicates infection with tubercle bacilli, it is not necessarily associated with clinical disease. **Indeed, most people with positive skin tests have immune systems that have confined and limited the infection.** A positive skin test also develops after vaccination with bacille Calmette-Guérin (BCG). When BCG is used in an effort to control natural tuberculosis, the skin test is not reliable as an indicator of naturally acquired infection.

Once positive, the person remains so for life. Before the patient develops sensitivity, bacilli multiply unchecked and may move through lymphatics and bloodstream to distant sites. The cellular basis of the positive test is a granulomatous response, composed of epithelioid cells and giant cells. At first, when there is uncontrolled growth of bacilli, the reaction is histiocytic and necrotizing. But with time, the appearance of epithelioid cells signals the destruction of bacilli and the limitation of the infection. Hypersensitivity (resistance to infection) is associated with increased phagocytosis of bacilli, conversion of macrophages to epithelioid cells, the formation of giant cells, and the inhibition of intracellular replication of tubercle bacilli.

Primary Tuberculosis

Primary tuberculosis is an infection of persons who have not had prior contact with the tubercle bacillus. The bacilli usually enter the body by inhalation but can also enter through the gastrointestinal tract or by cutaneous or subcutaneous inoculation. Inhaled bacilli are commonly deposited in alveoli immediately beneath the pleura, usually in the lower part of the upper lobes or the upper part of the lower lobes. These areas receive the greatest volume of inspired air. The initial infection produces only slight abnormalities and may cause only slight malaise and mild fever. Since sensitized T cells are lacking, the tubercle bacilli multiply freely and enter the bloodstream and lymphatics. Cell-mediated immunity develops over a period of 3 to 6 weeks.

The primary infection characteristically produces a "Ghon complex"—that is, **a single lesion in the pulmonary parenchyma, usually subpleural, that is accompanied by a lesion of the hilar lymph nodes draining that part of the lung** (Fig. 9-37). The primary lesion, or Ghon focus, in the lung is typically a 1-cm, grayish, circumscribed nodule. It becomes granulomatous within a few days and by the second week has a soft, caseous, necrotic center. Tubercle bacilli drain through lymphatic channels to infect the hilar lymph nodes and form the second part of the Ghon complex.

In over 90% of normal adults the infection follows this self-limited course, because the cellular immune response is sufficient to control the multiplication of bacilli. Therefore, in both the lung and the lymph nodes the lesions of the Ghon complex heal, undergoing shrinkage, fibrous scarring, and calcification. Most of the organisms die, but a few remain viable for years. Later, if immune mechanisms wane or fail, the resting bacilli may break out and cause serious tuberculous infection.

Progressive primary tuberculosis is a rarer alternative course, in which the immune response fails to control multiplication of the tubercle bacilli (see Fig. 9-37). **Infection takes this course in less than 10% of normal adults, but it is common in children under 5 years of age.** In adults, progressive primary tuber-culosis most commonly occurs in patients with suppressed or defective immunity. The primary Ghon focus in the lung enlarges rapidly, erodes the bronchial tree, and spreads, a sequence that results in adjacent "satellite" lesions. This process is accompanied by caseous enlargement of the hilar lymph nodes, which may erode through the wall of a bronchus and discharge bacilli, thereby producing tuberculous pneumonia. Clinical manifestations are abrupt high fever (associated with progression to tuberculous pneumonia), pleurisy with effusion, and lymphadenitis. These highly active lesions may seed the bloodstream with tubercle bacilli and result in life-threatening dissemination of the bacilli.

Secondary Tuberculosis

Secondary (cavitary) tuberculosis usually results from reactivation of dormant, endogenous tubercle bacilli in a sensitized patient who has had previous contact with the tubercle bacillus (see Fig. 9-37). In some cases, the disease is caused by reinfection with exogenous bacilli. Secondary tuberculosis may develop any time after primary infection, even decades later. Reactivation typically begins in the apical or posterior segments of one or both upper lobes ("Simon's foci"), where the organisms were seeded during the primary infection. Radiographically, the lesions are spherical and cavitary—the so-called coin lesions. A fibrous capsule surrounds a caseous, acellular center, which contains numerous tubercle bacilli. From these cavitary nodules the organisms can spread through the lungs and be discharged into the air during bouts of coughing.

The symptoms of secondary tuberculosis begin with cough, which may be erroneously attributed to smoking or to a "cold." Low-grade fever develops, with general malaise, fatigue, anorexia, weight loss, and often night sweats. As the disease progresses, the cough worsens and the sputum may be streaked with blood. The rupture of a branch of the pulmonary artery in the wall of a cavity leads to massive hemoptysis and asphyxiation or exsanguination.

These pulmonary lesions of secondary tuberculosis are often complicated by a variety of secondary effects, including (1) scarring and calcification; (2) spread to other areas; (3) pleural fibrosis and adhesions, with associated pleurisy, sharp pleuritic pain, and shortness of breath; (4) rupture of a caseous lesion, which spills bacilli into the pleural cavity; (5) erosion into a bronchus, which seeds the mucosal lining of bronchioles, bronchi, and trachea; and (6) implantation of bacilli in the larynx, which causes laryngitis, hoarseness, and pain on swallowing. Lesions of secondary tuberculosis acquired through the

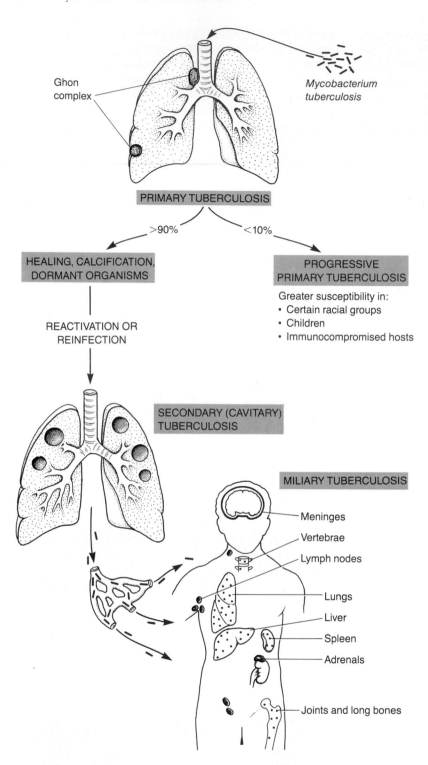

Ghon complex

Mycobacterium tuberculosis

PRIMARY TUBERCULOSIS

>90%   <10%

HEALING, CALCIFICATION, DORMANT ORGANISMS

PROGRESSIVE PRIMARY TUBERCULOSIS

Greater susceptibility in:
- Certain racial groups
- Children
- Immunocompromised hosts

REACTIVATION OR REINFECTION

SECONDARY (CAVITARY) TUBERCULOSIS

MILIARY TUBERCULOSIS

Meninges
Vertebrae
Lymph nodes
Lungs
Liver
Spleen
Adrenals
Joints and long bones

Figure 9-37.   Stages of tuberculosis. **Primary tuberculosis** (in a person lacking previous contact or immune responsiveness). Progressive primary tuberculosis develops in less than 10% of normal adults and more frequently in children and immunosuppressed patients. **Secondary (cavitary) tuberculosis** results from reactivation of dormant endogenous bacilli or reinfection with exogenous bacilli. **Miliary tuberculosis** is dissemination of tubercle bacilli to produce numerous, minute, yellow-white lesions (resembling millet seeds) in distant organs.

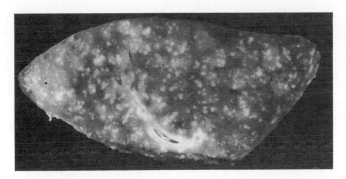

Figure 9-38. Miliary tuberculosis, lung. The tiny white foci are caseating granulomas.

gastrointestinal tract (usually with *M. t. bovis*) can lead to entrapment of bacilli in lymphoid patches of small and large bowel.

Miliary Tuberculosis

Miliary tuberculosis is the disseminated form of tuberculosis and is caused by seeding of the bacilli through lymphatics or blood vessels (see Fig. 9-37) **to produce minute, yellow-white lesions resembling millet seeds (hence "miliary").** The lung (Fig. 9-38), lymph nodes (Fig. 9-39), kidneys, adrenals, bone marrow, spleen, liver (Fig. 9-40), meninges, brain, eye grounds, and genitalia are all common sites of miliary lesions. Miliary tubercles rarely develop in the pancreas, thyroid, striated muscle, or heart. Regardless of the organs involved, all granulomas have similar features and follow the same progression, namely focal collections of histiocytes, followed by epithelioid cells, Langhans' giant cells, central caseation necrosis, and eventually fibrosis and mineralization.

Clinical suspicions of tuberculosis are confirmed by the microscopic demonstration of acid-fast bacilli within smears of sputum. The diagnosis is also confirmed by the demonstration, within tissue sections from affected organs, of bacilli that have a symmetric or consistent relationship to the lesions (Fig. 9-41). Bacilli are usually found in the caseous centers or in histiocytes or giant cells at the perimeter. Both *M. t. hominis* and *M. t. bovis* can be cultured from sputum or tissue specimens.

Tuberculosis is effectively treated with at least two bactericidal or bacteriostatic drugs: companion drugs are included to provide activity against bacilli that are resistant to the primary drug. To succeed, the chemotherapeutic regimen must eliminate extracellular bacilli in both solid and cavitary lesions, and intracellular bacilli in histiocytes or in giant cells. Among the drugs in use are isoniazid, rifampin, streptomycin, capreomycin and kanamycin, pyrazinamide, ethambutol, para-aminosalicylic acid (PAS), ethionamide, and thiacetazone. Isoniazid is the most valuable antituberculous drug, since it can be taken orally as well as parenterally and kills both extracellular and intracellular bacilli. Oral rifampin likewise kills both extracellular and intracellular bacilli and is especially important for eradicating "persisters" during the continuation phase.

Leprosy (Hansen's Disease)

Leprosy (Hansen's disease) is a chronic infection caused by *Mycobacterium leprae*. It affects the cooler parts of the body, especially the nasal mucosa, upper respiratory tract, peripheral nerves, testes, the skin of the ears, and the anterior segment of the eyes.

The World Health Organization estimates that worldwide over 15 million persons are infected, most in tropical countries (Fig. 9-42). **It is of historical interest that this was the first reported bacterial pathogen of mankind.** For centuries, leprosy was widespread in Europe and England. Indeed, in 1873 Hansen first saw the lepra bacillus in fresh mounts of

(Text continued on page 400.)

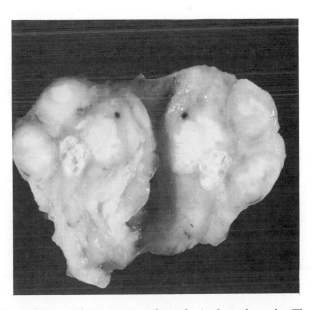

Figure 9-39. Fibrocaseous tuberculosis, lymph node. The substance of the lymph node is replaced by large granulomas with central areas of caseation, which have "stellate" patterns.

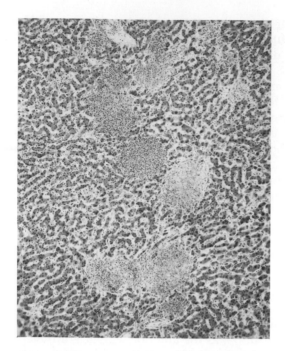

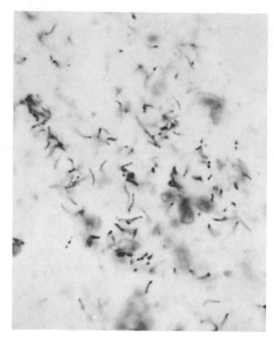

Figure 9-40. Miliary tuberculosis, liver. The lesions are anergic, lacking epithelioid cells, giant cells, and a perimeter of fibrous tissue.

Figure 9-41. Tuberculosis, lung. The bacilli are thin, curved, beaded, acid-fast, and concentrated in the necrotic centers of the granulomas.

Figure 9-42. (*A, top*) Lepromatous leprosy. There is diffuse involvement, including a leonine face, loss of eyebrows and eyelashes, and nodular distortions, especially on the face, ears, forearms, and hands—the exposed (cool) parts of the body. (*A, bottom*) The nodular skin lesion of advanced lepromatous leprosy. Swelling has flattened the epidermis (loss of Rete ridges). A characteristic "clear zone" of uninvolved dermis separates the epidermis from tumor-like accumulations of histiocytes, each containing numerous lepra bacilli (*Mycobacterium leprae*). (*B, top*) Tuberculoid leprosy on the cheek, showing a hypopigmented macule with a raised, infiltrated border. The central portion may be hypesthetic or anesthetic. (*B, bottom*) Macular skin lesion of tuberculoid leprosy. Skin from the raised "infiltrated" margin of the plaque contains discrete granulomas that extend to the basal layer of the epidermis (without a clear zone). The granulomas are composed of epithelioid cells and Langhan's giant cells, and are associated with lymphocytes and plasma cells. Lepra bacilli are rare. (C) Distribution of leprosy. Prevalence is greatest in tropical regions of Africa, Asia, and Latin America.

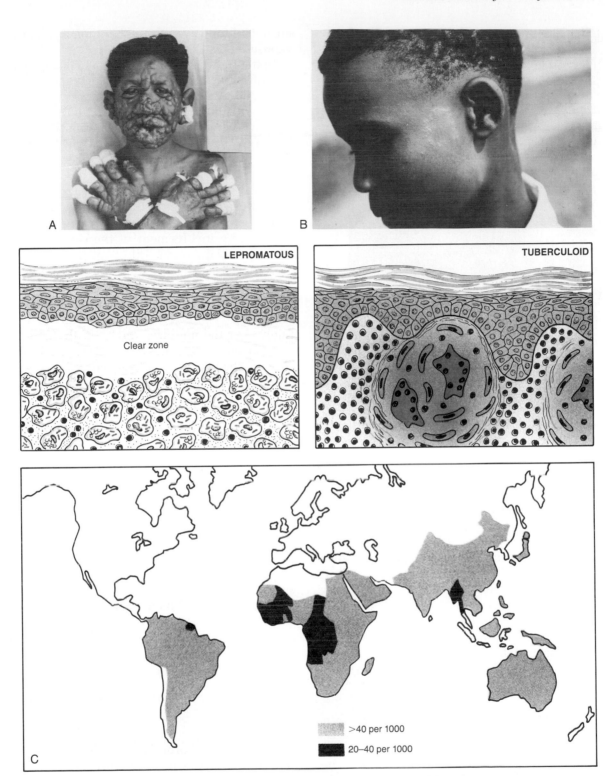

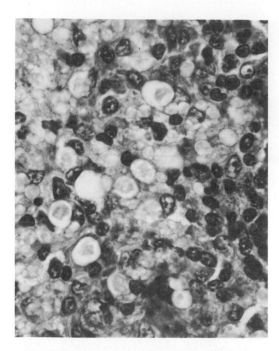

Figure 9-43. Lepromatous leprosy, skin, showing tumor-like mass of histiocytes. The faint masses within the vacuolated histiocytes are enormous numbers of acid-fast bacilli. The histiocytes show no tendency to inhibit proliferation of the lepra bacilli.

scrapings from a leproma of a Norwegian patient. A few patients still acquire leprosy in temperate regions, such as the United States and Europe, but most patients in temperate climates are immigrants who were infected elsewhere.

Lepra bacilli are slender, weakly acid-fast rods. To date, all attempts to culture the organism have failed or are unsubstantiated. Lepra bacilli multiply in experimental animals at sites with temperatures below that of the internal organs, such as the foot pads of mice, and the ear lobes of hamsters, rats, and other rodents. Naturally acquired leprosy has now been recognized in armadillos (Louisiana and Texas), in a chimpanzee trapped in Sierra Leone, and in a mangabey monkey captured in Nigeria. Lepra bacilli have been experimentally transmitted to armadillos, whose susceptibility is related, in part, to their low central body temperature (32–35°C).

Leprosy exhibits a bewildering variety of clinical and pathologic features. The lesions vary from the small, insignificant, and self-healing macules of tuberculoid leprosy to the diffuse, disfiguring, and sometimes fatal lesions of lepromatous leprosy. This extreme variation in the presentation of the disease is not fully understood, but is probably related to differences in immune reactivity. Ninety-five percent of all people have a natural protective immunity and

are not infected even through intimate and prolonged exposure.

In the susceptible 5% who may develop symptomatic infections, a broad immunologic spectrum ranges from anergy to hyperergy. **Anergic patients (i.e., those with little or no resistance) have lepromatous leprosy, whereas hyperergic patients (those with high resistance) develop tuberculoid leprosy.** "Borderline" leprosy is the term applied to the broad middle ground into which most patients fall.

Patients with lepromatous leprosy have nodular and diffuse infiltrates of the skin, eye, testes, nerves, and organs of the reticuloendothelial system. The most severe involvement of the skin is in exposed areas; the nodular distortions of the face are called "leonine facies" (see Fig. 9-42). The infiltrates are composed of tumor-like accumulations of histiocytes, each histiocyte containing enormous numbers of lepra bacilli (Fig. 9-43). The epidermis is stretched thinly over the nodules, and beneath it is a narrow, uninvolved "clear zone" of dermis. Rather than destroying the bacilli, the phagocytic cells appear to act as microincubators (see Fig. 9-43). Unchecked, these infiltrates expand slowly to distort and disfigure the face, ears, and upper airway and to destroy the eyes, eyebrows and eyelashes, nerves, and testes. Those who are untreated may die of asphyxiation from an obstructed airway or from secondary amyloidosis.

The other end of the spectrum is represented by patients with tuberculoid leprosy, a condition characterized by a single lesion or very few lesions of the skin. The hypopigmented macule, with a raised "infiltrated" border, may be hypesthetic or anesthetic. The lesion expands slowly over a period of months or years, and then gradually heals (see Fig. 9-42), although the hypesthesia or anesthesia remain. Microscopically, the tuberculoid lesion is a dermatitis characterized by discrete noncaseating granulomas in the dermis. The granulomas are composed of epithelioid cells and Langhan's giant cells and are associated with varying numbers of lymphocytes and plasma cells (see Fig. 9-42). Cutaneous nerves, including the small dermal nerve twigs, are eventually destroyed by the bacilli, which accounts for the sensory deficit.

Patients with borderline leprosy have an endless variety of features of both lepromatous and tuberculoid leprosy. The term "indeterminate" leprosy is used when the biopsy sample is taken from a lesion that is so early in the course of the disease that the cellular response does not reveal the type of leprosy. Thus, "indeterminate" lesions may heal spontaneously or progress to either lepromatous or tuberculoid forms.

The most commonly used drug, dapsone, rids the lepromatous patient of lepra bacilli in 4 to 5 years, but it must be continued indefinitely. Dapsone-resistant strains of *M. leprae* have developed, and multidrug regimens are now often used.

Buruli Ulcer (Mycobacterium ulcerans)

Buruli ulcers are indolent, necrotizing ulcers of the skin and panniculus. First described as a rare disease in Australia, these ulcers are now recognized as common in Uganda and Zaire and have been identified in other countries of West Africa, as well as in Southeast Asia and Central and South America. The name is derived from Buruli County in Uganda, where a cluster of patients was identified in the late 1950s. The reservoir and route of infection are unknown, but organisms are probably inoculated by minor penetrating trauma. The major endemic areas are sparsely populated river valleys and swampy lowlands.

Buruli ulcers are caused by *Mycobacterium ulcerans*, an acid-fast bacillus that grows slowly on routine mycobacteriological media at several degrees below body temperature. Most Buruli ulcers are on the limbs, frequently over joints. The bacilli proliferate in the skin and subcutaneous tissues and elaborate a cytotoxin that diffuses symmetrically and causes a contiguous necrosis of all structures in its path—namely, the epidermis, dermis, panniculus, deep fascia, nerves, vessels, and (rarely) underlying muscle and bone.

The lesion begins as a firm, painless, subcutaneus nodule that becomes papular and ulcerates. The perimeter of the ulcer is typically scalloped and often deeply undermined. At first the ulcers spread steadily, undermining the skin over large areas. After many months the perimeter stabilizes and healing begins, a process that requires many months. The eventual scar is broad and depressed and resembles a healed third-degree burn.

Microscopically, there is coagulation necrosis of the deep dermis and panniculus, with destruction of dermal collagen and all structures, including blood vessels, appendages, and nerves. Large extracellular clusters of acid-fast bacilli are concentrated in the necrotic exudate, in the ulcer bed, and in the necrotic adipose tissue of the undermined skin. Smears of necrotic tissue in the ulcer bed reveal the organisms.

Preulcerative infections may be cured by local wide excision. When excision is impractical, the most effective therapy is repeated debridement and grafting, combined with continuous heating of the area to 40°C, using a circulating water jacket. Rifampin is the chemotherapeutic agent of choice.

Atypical Mycobacterial Infections of Skin

The atypical mycobacteria were originally grouped only by their growth characteristics but are now individually classified (Table 9-2). "**Swimming pool granuloma**," the only common disease caused by a slow-growing atypical mycobacteria (*M. marinum*), is usually acquired in swimming pools. Those who keep tropical fish or who come into contact with coastal or brackish water are also at risk. Because of its cooler temperature requirement (30–32°C), infection by *M. marinum* is limited to the skin. The initial lesions are at sites of trauma, usually the hands, elbows, or knees. There may be satellite spread along draining lymphatics. Spontaneous cure within a few months is the rule, but untreated lesions may persist.

*Table 9-2 Runyon Classification of the Atypical Mycobacteria Causing Lesions of Skin in Man**

Group	Pigment Production In Culture	Growth Rate	Specifies Identified*
I	Photochromogens†	Slow	*Mycobacterium kansasii* *M. marinum*
II	Scrotochromogens‡	Slow	*M. scrofulaceum* *M. szulgai*
III	Nonphotochromogens§	Slow	*M. avium* *M. intracellular*
IV	Variable	Rapid	*M. fortuitum* *M. chelonei*

* Classification does not include *M. ulcerans*
† Pigment produced only on exposure to light
‡ Pigment produced in dark or light
§ Nonpigmented

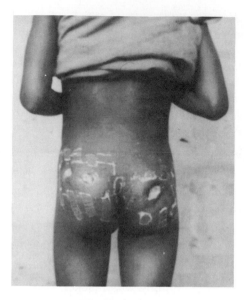

Figure 9-44. Cutaneous and subcutaneous infection caused by *Mycobacterium chelonei.* These are usually at the sites of injection. The reaction is both suppurative and granulomatous.

Typical early lesions are nodular and sometimes ulcerated. Initially the dermis displays lymphocytes, histiocytes, and neutrophils; later lesions show tuberculoid granulomas that contain foci of caseation necrosis. Few acid-fast bacilli exist in the tissue.

Among the fast-growing atypical mycobacteria, *M. fortuitum* and *M. chelonei* are ubiquitous saprophytes of soil and water and commonly cause "injection abscesses" or are introduced into the skin by trauma. Painless fluctuant abscesses appear at the site of inoculation, ulcerate, and gradually heal spontaneously (Fig. 9-44). In immunodeficient patients the organisms may disseminate. In contrast to the granulomatous reaction to other mycobacteria, neutrophilic infiltrates predominate, and there is prominent liquefactive necrosis. Acid-fast bacilli are concentrated in spherical vacuoles within the pus.

Diseases Caused by Protozoans

Chagas's Disease

Chagas's disease (American trypanosomiasis), a zoonotic infection by the protozoan *Trypanosoma cruzi*, causes acute, subacute, and chronic parasitemia, with dissemination to many organs, especially the heart, brain, esophagus, and colon. *T. cruzi* infects certain insects and mammals and is commonly transmitted to humans by species of reduviid bugs. American trypanosomiasis exists in every country of Central and South America, but is rarely seen in the United States, Mexico, and the Caribbean islands. Infection is promoted by contact between humans and infected bugs, usually in mud or thatched dwellings of the rural and suburban poor. The bugs hide in cracks of rickety houses and in vegetal roofing, come out at night, and feed on sleeping inhabitants.

Metacyclic trypomastigotes of *T. cruzi* are discharged in the feces of the reduviid bug while it takes its blood meal. Itching and scratching promotes contamination of the wound by the insect feces containing the trypomastigotes. These penetrate through the site of the bite or through other local abrasions, or they may penetrate the mucosa of eye or lips. Artificial transmission of *T. cruzi* has occurred through blood transfusion and laboratory accidents involving infected blood or cultures. Infection may be congenital from transplacental spread. Once in the body, trypomastigotes lose their flagella and undulating membranes, round up to become amastigotes, enter histiocytes, and there undergo repeated division by fission. The amastigotes also invade other sites, including myofibers (manifested in acute Chagasic myocarditis) and brain. Within the host cells, amastigotes differentiate into trypomastigotes, which break out and enter the bloodstream (Fig. 9-45). Ingested in a subsequent bite of a reduviid bug, trypomastigotes enter the alimentary tract of the insect, multiply, and differentiate into epimastigotes and metacyclic trypomastigotes. The metacyclic trypomastigotes congregate in the rectum of the bug and are discharged in the feces during another blood meal from a new host, thus completing the cycle.

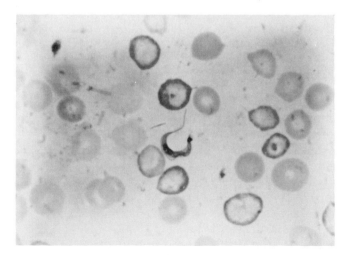

Figure 9-45. Chagas's disease (parasitemia), showing a trypanosome of *Trypanosoma cruzi* in a thin film of blood. It has a characteristic "C" shape, a flagellum, a nucleus, and a terminal kinetoplast.

Acute Chagas's Disease

In acute Chagas's disease, after an incubation period of about 1 to 2 weeks following inoculation with *T. cruzi*, a subcutaneous inflammatory nodule, the "chagoma", develops at the site. When trypomastigotes invade the conjunctiva there may be the characteristic "Romana's sign," consisting of unilateral conjunctivitis, palpebral and periorbital edema, and ipsilateral preauricular lymphadenopathy. Parasitemia (see Fig.9-45) appears 2 to 3 weeks after inoculation and is associated with fever, edema, lymphadenopathy, and hepatosplenomegaly. The dangerous complications are myocarditis (tachycardia, arrhythmia, cardiac failure) and encephalitis.

Grossly, the heart is enlarged and dilated with a pale, focally hemorrhagic myocardium. The liver, lungs, spleen, and intestine are congested, depending on the degree of cardiac failure. Microscopically, numerous parasites are seen in the heart, and amastigotes are evident within pseudocysts in myofibers (Fig. 9-46). There is extensive chronic inflammation, with lymphocytes, macrophages, and plasma cells. Phagocytosis of parasites is conspicuous. Myofibers are destroyed, and the heart shows interstitial edema, endocarditis, pericarditis, and inflammation and parasitization of the sinus node and atrioventricular node.

Congenital Chagas's Disease

In some pregnant women with parasitemia, infection of the placenta and fetus leads to spontaneous abortion. Some infants die of encephalitis within a few days or weeks. In the infrequent live births, acute necrotizing encephalitis and any of the lesions of acute Chagas's disease may be found.

Chronic Chagas's Disease

Chronic Chagas's disease is the most frequent and most serious consequence of infection by *T. cruzi* and afflicts several million people in Central and South America. The disease develops years or even decades after infection. In the heart the principal manifestations are cardiomegaly, electrocardiographic evidence of right and left bundle branch blocks, atrioventricular blocks, multifocal ventricular extrasystoles, and necrosis of the cardiac apex. The clinical course varies from sudden death (from arrhythmias) to slow but relentless loss of cardiac function and repeated episodes of cardiac failure, eventually leading to death. Emboli from mural thrombi in the ventricles and atria may produce cerebral and pulmonary infarcts. Some

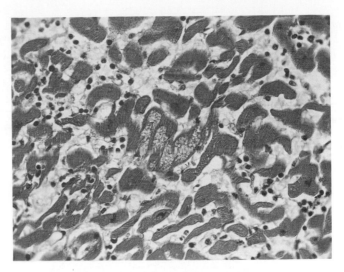

Figure 9-46. Chagas's disease, with myocarditis. The myofibers contain large numbers of amastigotes (leishmanial forms) of *T. cruzi*. There is edema and chronic inflammation.

patients in regions of Brazil, Chile, and Argentina (but not in Central America or other parts of South America) have massive dilatation of the esophagus (achalasia), or less often of the bronchi, ureters, duodenum, and stomach, owing to involvement of the myenteric plexus of these organs.

Chronic Chagas's disease characteristically causes chronic cardiomyopathy and in some geographic regions (Brazil and Chile) megaesophagus and megacolon. The cardiomyopathy is characterized by a dilated heart, prominent right ventricular outflow tract, and dilatation of the valve rings. The interventricular septum is often deviated to the right and may immobilize the adjacent tricuspid leaflet. Microscopically, the myocardium displays focal inflammatory infiltrates (lymphocytes and plasma), interstitial fibrosis, and hypertrophied myofibers. Parasites are difficult to find.

The early diagnosis of acute Chagas's disease is made by demonstration of *T. cruzi* in thick blood smears a few weeks before serologic and immunofluorescent tests become positive. The presence of IgM-specific antibodies is diagnostic of congenital infection. The diagnosis of chronic Chagas's disease depends on clinical findings, a positive complement fixation test and other serologic procedures, and demonstration of the parasite by culture or xenodiagnosis. Xenodiagnosis is established by the demonstration of epimastigotes of *T. cruzi* in the insect feces 10 days after a laboratory-reared, "clean" reduviid bug is allowed to bite the patient.

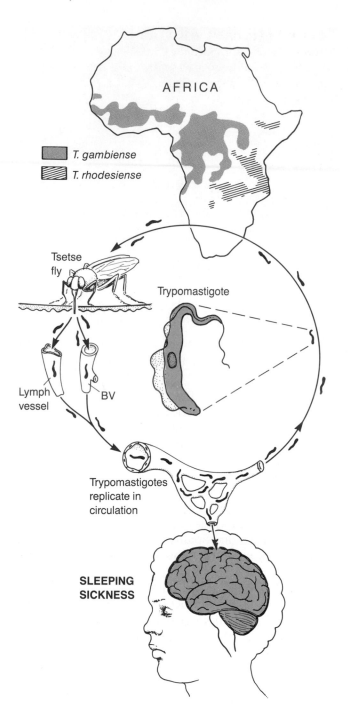

T. gambiense

T. rhodesiense

AFRICA

Tsetse fly

Trypomastigote

Lymph vessel

BV

Trypomastigotes replicate in circulation

SLEEPING SICKNESS

Figure 9-47. African trypanosomiasis (sleeping sickness). The distribution of Gambian and Rhodesian trypanosomiasis is related to the habitats of the vector tsetse flies (*Glossina* sp.). A tsetse fly bites an infected animal or human and ingests trypomastigotes, which multiply into infective, metacyclic trypomastigotes. During another fly bite, these are injected into lymphatic and blood vessels of a new host. A primary chancre develops at the site of the bite (Stage 1a). Trypomastigotes replicate further in the blood and lymph, causing a systemic infection (Stage 1b). Another fly ingests trypomastigotes to complete the cycle. In stage 2, invasion of the central nervous system by trypomastigotes leads to meningoencephalomyelitis and associated symptoms, including lethargy and daytime somnolence. Patients with Rhodesian trypanosomiasis may die within a few months.

Although no drugs are registered in the United States for chemoprophylaxis against Chagas's disease, nifurtimox (Lampit) and benzonidazole (Rochagan) are presently marketed in Latin America for specific treatment of *acute* human *T. cruzi* infections. The value of therapy in *chronic* infections is unclear. Both drugs usually abolish parasitemia in the acute phase, but prolonged follow-up may reveal lingering parasites by xenodiagnosis.

African Trypanosomiasis (Sleeping Sickness)

African trypanosomiasis (sleeping sickness) is a chronic infection with *Trypanosoma brucei gambiense* or an acute one with *T. b. rhodesiense*. These hemoflagellate protozoa are transmitted cyclically by several species of blood-sucking tsetse flies of the genus *Glossina*. The uneven distribution of African trypanosomiasis is related to the habitats of the tsetse flies (Fig. 9-47). In Gambian trypanosomiasis, *T. b. gambiense* is transmitted by tsetse flies of the riverine bush, mainly in focal areas of West and Central Africa. Man is the only important reservoir for *T. b. gambiense*, which causes a chronic infection often lasting more than a year. In Rhodesian trypanosomiasis, *T. b. rhodesiense* is transmitted by tsetse flies of the woodland savanna of East Africa. Antelope, other game animals and domestic cattle are natural reservoirs of *T. b. rhodesiense*. Incidental infection of man is an occupational hazard of game wardens, fisherman, and cattle herders. *T. b. rhodesiense* causes a disabling, acute, and fulminant infection in man, killing the patient in 3 to 6 months.

While biting an infected animal or man, the tsetse fly ingests trypomastigotes with the blood (see Fig. 9-47). These forms lose their coat of surface antigen, multiply in the midgut of the fly, migrate to the salivary gland, develop over a 3-week period through the epimastigote stage, and multiply in the fly's saliva as infective, metacyclic trypomastigotes. During another bite the metacyclic trypomastigotes are injected into the lymphatic and blood vessels of a new host. Trypomastigotes disseminate to the bone marrow and tissue fluids, and some eventually invade the central nervous system (see Fig. 9-47). After replicating by binary fission in blood, lymph, and spinal fluid, trypomastigotes are ingested in another fly bite, to complete the cycle.

The clinical manifestations of trypanosomiasis are divided into stage 1, primary chancre and systemic infection, excluding the brain; and stage 2, invasion of the brain.

Stage 1a (Primary Chancre)

After an incubation period of 5 to 15 days, the dermal inoculation site develops a primary trypanosomal chancre, a 3- to 4-cm papular swelling in the skin, topped by a central red spot, that subsides spontaneously within 3 weeks.

Stage 1b (Systemic Infection, Excluding the Brain)

Shortly after the appearance of the chancre (if any), and within 3 weeks after the bite, invasion of the bloodstream is marked by intermittent fever, which lasts up to a week and is often accompanied by splenomegaly and local and generalized lymphadenopathy. "Winterbottom's sign"—enlargement of the posterior cervical lymph nodes—is characteristic of Gambian trypanosomiasis. In both forms the evolving illness is marked by remittent, irregular fever, headache, joint pains, lethargy, anorexia, muscle wasting, and, in some patients, anemia. Myocarditis may be a complication, and is more common and severe in Rhodesian trypanosomiasis. Dysfunction of lungs, kidneys, liver, and endocrine system are frequently observed in both forms.

Stage 2 (Brain Invasion)

Differences between the forms of sleeping sickness are primarily a matter of time scale, especially in regard to invasion of the brain. Stage 2 (see Fig. 9-47) typically develops early (in weeks or months) in Rhodesian trypanosomiasis, or late (after months or years) in Gambian trypanosomiasis. Stage 2 is marked by apathy, irritability, changes in personality, lethargy, daytime somnolence, and sometimes coma. These symptoms are associated with a diffuse meningoencephalomyelitis and include tremors of the tongue and fingers; fasciculations of the muscles of the limbs, face, lips, and tongue; oscillatory movements of the arms, head, neck, and trunk; indistinct speech; and cerebellar ataxia, leading to problems in walking. Without treatment both forms are fatal.

The pathogenesis of African trypanosomiasis involves the formation of immune complexes by variant trypanosomal antigens and antibodies. The production of autoantibodies against antigenic components of red blood cells, brain, and heart is also a prominent feature. The trypanosome survives in the mammalian host by periodically altering its antigenic coat, which is composed of glycoproteins. These alterations take place in a genetically determined pattern, **not** by mutation. Thus, each new wave of circulating trypanosomastigotes includes immunologically distinct antigenic variants that are a step ahead of the immune response, providing a means of escaping host defenses.

Microscopic changes in the primary chancre have not been well described for human infections. In experimental infections, primary chancres show edema, proliferation of endothelial cells and fibroblasts, and trypanosomes. The trypanosomes move from the chancre to the general circulation either by direct invasion of dermal venules or by the lymphatic system.

The acute phase (stage 1b) is characterized by reactivity of lymphoid tissue. In later stages both cellular and humoral immunity are suppressed, with depletion of lymphocytes and plasma cells. IgM levels are strikingly increased (associated with various autoantibodies) and IgG levels moderately so. The reaction to various skin test antigens is reduced, and responses to viral and bacterial vaccines are diminished. Thrombocytopenia is common, with greater reductions in the platelet counts for *T. b. rhodesiense* than for *T. b. gambiense*.

In the acute stage the spleen and lymph nodes may be enlarged. Microscopic changes include foci of lymphocytic and histiocytic hyperplasia in spleen and lymph nodes, but trypanosomes are difficult to demonstrate in tissue sections.

Rhodesian trypanosomiasis and, less often, Gambian trypanosomiasis involve the heart. Microscopically, there is a pancarditis, with mononuclear cell infiltration (lymphocytes, plasma cells, and histiocytes) of the interstitium and the perivascular spaces of the endocardium, myocardium, and epicardium. Experimental studies in monkeys have revealed trypanosomes and inflammatory infiltrates in cardiac valves, the conducting system, cardiac lymph drainage, and apical aneurysms, a distribution suggesting partial obstruction of the cardiac lymph drainage.

In stage 2 trypanosomiasis, invasion of the brain, a meningoencephalomyelitis, is characterized by a perivascular infiltrate of lymphocytes, plasma cells, and histiocytes that thickens the leptomeninges and involves the Virchow-Robin spaces and, sometimes, the vessel walls. Two cytologic but inconstant abnormalities suggest African trypanosomiasis: lymphophagocytosis and morular (mulberry) cells of Mott. The latter are Russell bodies—that is, altered plasma cells containing clumped IgG. Gliosis of the brain, marked by proliferation of microglial rod cells and gemistocytic astrocytes, may be conspicuous.

Trypanosomes are rarely seen in tissue sections, and attempts to demonstrate them are an impractical approach to diagnosis. In the early stages a definitive diagnosis of African trypanosomiasis is made by demonstrating the organisms in aspirates from the chancre, in thick and thin blood films, in aspirates

from enlarged lymph nodes, and, later, in aspirates of bone marrow. Repeated examinations of the blood may be necessary because of cyclic fluctuations in parasitemia. In the late stage trypanosomes may be demonstrated in cerebrospinal fluid.

The key drugs used for therapy of African trypanosomiasis are pentamidine, for chemoprophylaxis; suramin, for the treatment of the early disease in which trypanosomes are found in the blood, lymph, and lymph nodes; and melarsoprol, for the later disease in which trypanosomes are located in the brain.

Leishmaniasis

Cutaneous and Mucocutaneous Leishmaniasis

Cutaneous and mucocutaneous leishmaniasis are caused by three species complexes, *Leishmania tropica*, *L. brasiliensis*, and *L. mexicana*. The amastigote stage, found in reticuloendothelial cells of the vertebrate host (including man), is round, 2 to 5 μm across, and has a thin cell membrane, a nucleus, and a rod-shaped kinetoplast. The amastigote is ingested from an infected host by blood-sucking sandflies (Fig. 9-48) (*Lutzomyia* in the New World, and *Phlebotomus* in the Old World). Within the digestive tract of the sandfly, amastigotes are transformed into promastigotes, each having a single flagellum. The promastigotes multiply in the gut of the sandfly and, in turn, are injected into the dermis of the next vertebrate host (animal or man). The promastigotes invade reticuloendothelial cells, transform into amastigotes, multiply, and invade other reticuloendothelial cells, thereby completing the cycle.

The diagnosis may be established by cultivating leishmania from lesions, or by a leishmanin skin test, which becomes positive within 3 months and remains positive for life.

Three species of the *L. tropica* complex are distinguished on ecological, biochemical, and serological grounds. The gerbil is the reservoir for *L. tropica major*, which causes cutaneous leishmaniasis ("tropical sore") in moist **rural** environments of the Middle East, Arabia, Russia, India, and sub-subSaharan Africa. Man and dogs are reservoirs for *L. tropica minor*, which causes cutaneous leishmaniasis in dry **urban** environments of the Middle East and the Mediterranean basin. The rock hyrax and tree hyrax (rabbit-like mammals) are reservoirs for *L. tropica aethiopica*, which causes diffuse (anergic) cutaneous leishmaniasis in people whose homesteads encroach on deforested mountain slopes of the Rift Valley in Ethiopia and Kenya. This variant is also caused by *L. mexicana*, which finds its reservoirs in rodents and marsupials of the Amazon basin, Venezuela, and, rarely, Mexico and Central America.

The primary lesion of cutaneous leishmaniasis is an itching papule, which expands over a period of weeks or months to form a shallow, indolent, slowly expanding ulcer. Histologically, at the site of inoculation the first reaction is an infiltrate of leishmania-containing histiocytes, which expand and proliferate to accommodate the increasing numbers of leishmania. This is followed by an infiltrate of neutrophils, necrosis, and sloughing of large numbers of organisms. Gradually the histiocytes lose their leishmania and become epithelioid cells, after which the reaction matures to a granuloma. During this transition increasing numbers of lymphocytes and plasma cells appear in the exudate. Satellite lesions develop along draining lymphatics. Healing usually begins at 3 to 6 months, but may take a year or longer.

Patients with diffuse cutaneous leishmaniasis are anergic, lacking **specific** cell-mediated immune responses to leishmania, although delayed hypersensitivity to tuberculin and other antigens appears to be normal. Diffuse cutaneous leishmaniasis begins as a single nodule, but adjacent satellite nodules slowly form, eventually involving much of the skin. Clinically and pathologically, these nodules resemble lepromatous leprosy so closely that some patients have been cared for in leprosaria. The nodule of anergic leismaniasis is caused by enormous numbers of histiocytes stuffed with leishmania.

Rodents and sloths are reservoirs for the *L. brasiliensis* complex, which causes mucocutaneous leishmaniasis in Central and South America. Mucocutaneous leishmaniasis is a late complication of cutaneous leishmaniasis. Years after the primary lesion has healed, an ulcer develops at a mucocutaneous junction, such as the larynx, nasal septum, anus, or vulva. These ulcers are destructive and disfiguring, and may kill the patient by obstructing the airway. Biopsies of mucocutaneous lesions reveal necrotizing granulomas, with many plasma cells and lymphocytes. Leishmania are rare.

Pentavalent antimonials, given intravenously or intramuscularly, are usually effective. Diffuse cutaneous leishmaniasis and mucocutaneous leishmaniasis are more resistant and may require a variety of antiprotozoan drugs. Amphotericin B has been successful in some patients.

Visceral Leishmaniasis (Kala-azar)

Visceral leishmaniasis (Kala-azar) (Fig. 9-49) is caused by the species complex *L. donovani*, which morphologically resembles the leishmania organisms previously described. Leishmania can be identified in

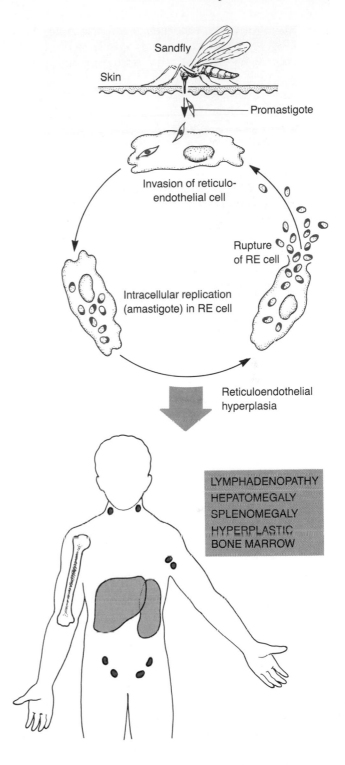

Figure 9-48. Leishmaniasis. Blood-sucking sandflies ingest amastigotes from an infected host. These are transformed in the sandfly gut into promastigotes, which multiply and are injected into the next vertebrate host. There they invade reticuloendothelial cells, revert to the amastigote form, and multiply, eventually rupturing the cell. They then invade other reticuloendothelial cells, thus completing the cycle.

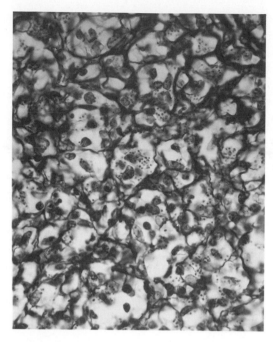

Figure 9-49. Visceral leishmaniasis, bone marrow. There are many leishmania in phagocytic cells.

smears or tissue specimens of the spleen, lymph nodes, liver, bone marrow, and skin, but splenic aspiration is the surest method of confirming the diagnosis.

The life cycle and insect vectors of *L. donovani* are the same as those described for the other *Leishmania* species.

Serologic tests for antibodies to leishmania are positive in 95% of cases, but the leishmanin skin test is uniformly negative in active visceral leishmaniasis. Some 90% of patients develop a positive skin test reaction within 6 weeks to a year after recovery.

The reservoirs of *L. donovani*, and the susceptible age groups, vary in different parts of the world. Man is the reservoir in India, foxes in Southern France, Central Italy, and some parts of South America. Jackals are the reservoir for sporadic cases in rural areas of the Middle East and central Asia. Dogs are reservoirs in the Mediterranean basin, China, and some parts of South America. The reservoirs in Africa are incompletely known but may include man, domestic dogs, rats, and other rodents.

Low-grade fever, malaise, and lassitude begin 10 days to 10 months after inoculation. The cardinal features of visceral leishmaniasis are fever, generalized lymphadenopathy, hepatosplenomegaly (see Fig. 9-48), pancytopenia, and cachexia. Fair skin turns dark ("kala-azar" is Hindi for "black fever"). Death is often caused by bacterial pneumonia, septicemia, tuberculosis, dysentery, and uncontrolled hemorrhage or by severe anemia with its sequelae. Some patients who survive kala-azar have dermal leishmaniasis that resembles advanced lepromatous leprosy.

Histologically, a granuloma develops at the site of inoculation, and amastigotes spread by the lymph to local lymph nodes and by the blood to the spleen, liver, and bone marrow. Histiocytic cells in the spleen proliferate, replace the parenchyma, and expand the organ. Many amastigotes accumulate in Kupffer cells of the liver and in phagocytic cells of bone marrow (see Fig. 9-49). The histiocytes are stuffed with amastigotes and resemble the foamy histiocytes of lepromatous leprosy. The heart, skin, and epididymis also contain numerous leishmania-containing histiocytes.

Treatment with pentavalent antimonials and meglumine antimoniate, administered intravenously or intramuscularly, is usually effective.

Malaria

Human malaria is an acute and chronic protozoal disease, caused by any one or a combination of four species of plasmodia, namely *Plasmodium falciparum*, *P. vivax*, *P. ovale* and *P. malariae*. *P. falciparum* is the most virulent of these and the only one that kills acutely. The other three species are "benign." Infections with *P. ovale* and *P. malariae* are now rare. The plasmodial parasites are transmitted by female mosquitoes of several species of the genus *Anopheles*, and hyperendemic breeding grounds for these mosquitoes are directly related to the prevalence of the disease.

The World Health Organization recognizes malaria as the world's major primary health problem, causing more morbidity and mortality than any other disease. Malaria has been eradicated in the United States, Canada, and Europe, but continues to be a scourge in tropical and subtropical areas, especially tropical Africa, parts of South and Central America, India, and Southeast Asia (Fig. 9-50). The rural poor, infants, children, the malnourished, pregnant women, and splenectomized individuals are all especially susceptible. All inhabitants of hyperendemic regions are presumed to harbor malarial parasites, even though they may have no clinical symptoms.

P. falciparum, the cause of malignant malaria, is distinguished from the other malarial parasites in four respects: it has no secondary exoerythrocytic stage, it parasitizes erythrocytes of any age, there may be several parasites in a single erythrocyte, and the parasitized erythrocyte is "sticky." This last feature leads to obstruction of small vessels by thrombi and is probably the most important factor in the virulence of *P. falciparum*.

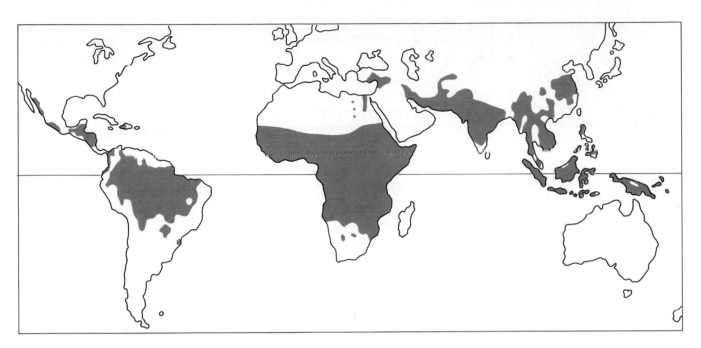

Figure 9-50.   The geographic distribution of malaria.

The plasmodia have a complex life cycle (Fig. 9-51). In the mosquito vector there is a single sexual multiplication, termed sporogony, which ends in the infective stage, the sporozoite being located in the salivary glands. The bite of a mosquito inoculates the sporozoites into the bloodstream of the vertebrate host, where asexual division (schizogony) takes place. Some sporozoites enter parenchymal cells of the liver and multiply asexually in exoerythrocytic schizogony, in which repeated nuclear division within the schizont stage eventually produce thousands of uninucleate merozoites. The merozoites penetrate erythrocytes and initiate the intraerythrocytic asexual cycle. The merozoites become trophozoites, which divide to form numerous schizonts. The schizonts, in turn, undergo nuclear division to form more merozoites. Merozoites released by the rupture of one erythrocyte reenter other red blood cells to begin a new cycle. The erythrocytic cycle of schizogony is repeated many times. Eventually subpopulations of merozoites differentiate into sexual forms, namely gametocytes, which include female macrogametocytes and male microgametocytes. A female anopheline mosquito feeding on an infected host ingests those gametocytes, which then undergo further development in the insect's stomach. The male microgamete and female macrogamete fuse to form the zygote. Sporogony involves several more stages and ends in infective sporozoites in the salivary glands, thus completing the cycle.

The cardinal clinical symptoms of malaria are cyclic paroxysms of high fever and chills, usually accompanied by varying degrees of anemia and splenomegaly. The major pathologic changes are a consequence of parasitization and destruction of erythrocytes (see Fig. 9-51). As succeeding populations of parasites mature within erythrocytes and destroy them, merozoites, malarial pigment, hemoglobin, and cellular debris are released into the bloodstream. Malarial pigment accumulates in phagocytic cells of the reticuloendothelial system, and hemoglobin is absorbed by renal tubular cells. Patients who have massive absorption of hemoglobin by the renal tubules may die with **hemoglobinuric nephrosis** ("blackwater fever") .

At autopsy, the spleen and liver in falciparum malaria are enlarged and all organs of the reticuloendothelial system are darkened ("slate gray") by malarial pigment. The gross lesions of the brain—congestion and petechiae—are limited to the white matter, a characteristic feature of cerebral malaria (Fig. 9-52). For reasons that are unclear, parasitized erythrocytes cling to endothelial cells. This "stickiness" has two practical implications. First, parasitized erythrocytes attached to endothelial cells do not circulate, so patients with severe falciparum malaria have few circulating parasites. Second, capillaries of deep organs, especially the brain, become obstructed, leading to hypoxia and death (Fig. 9-53). Phagocytosis of parasitized erythrocytes leads to reticuloendothelial hyperplasia and hepatosplenomegaly. Clusters of parasitized erythrocytes become bound in fibrin thrombi that obstruct small vessels and are

(Text continued on page 412.)

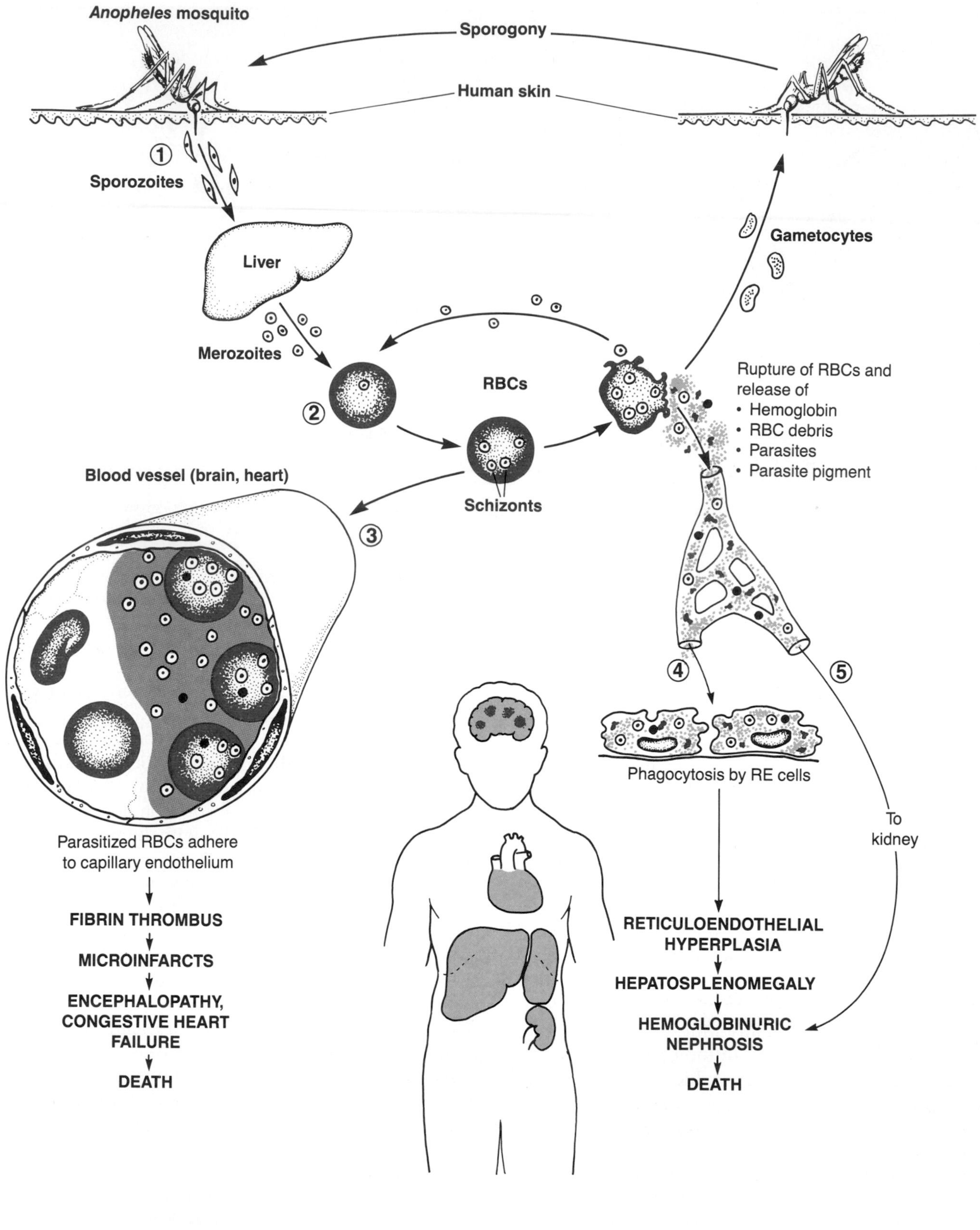

Anopheles mosquito

Sporogony

Human skin

① Sporozoites

Liver

Merozoites

②

RBCs

Schizonts

Gametocytes

Rupture of RBCs and release of
• Hemoglobin
• RBC debris
• Parasites
• Parasite pigment

Blood vessel (brain, heart)

③

Parasitized RBCs adhere
to capillary endothelium

↓

FIBRIN THROMBUS

↓

MICROINFARCTS

↓

**ENCEPHALOPATHY,
CONGESTIVE HEART
FAILURE**

↓

DEATH

④ ⑤

Phagocytosis by RE cells

To
kidney

**RETICULOENDOTHELIAL
HYPERPLASIA**

↓

HEPATOSPLENOMEGALY

↓

**HEMOGLOBINURIC
NEPHROSIS**

↓

DEATH

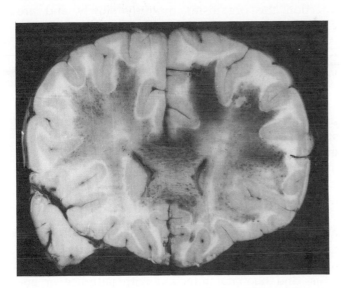

Figure 9-52.   Acute falciparum malaria of brain. There is severe, diffuse congestion of white matter with focal hemorrhages. This selective involvement of white matter is a characteristic feature of cerebral malaria.

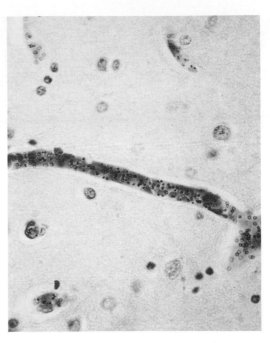

Figure 9-53.   Section of malarious brain showing a capillary packed with parasitized erythrocytes.

Figure 9-51.   Life cycle of malaria. An *Anopheles* mosquito bites an infected person, taking blood that contains micro- and macrogametocytes (sexual forms). In the mosquito, sexual multiplication ("sporogony") produces infective sporozoites in the salivary glands. *1.* During the mosquito bite, sporozoites are inoculated into the bloodstream of the vertebrate host. Some sporozoites leave the blood and enter the hepatocytes, where they multiply asexually (exoerythrocytic schizogony), and form thousands of uninucleated merozoites. *2.* Rupture of hepatocytes releases merozoites, which penetrate erythrocytes and become trophozoites, which then divide to form numerous schizonts (intraerythrocytic schizogony). Schizonts divide to form more merozoites, which are released on the rupture of erythrocytes and reenter other erythrocytes to begin a new cycle. After several cycles, subpopulations of merozoites develop into micro- and macrogametocytes, which are taken up by another mosquito to complete the cycle. *3.* Parasitized erythrocytes obstruct capillaries of the brain, heart, kidney, and other deep organs. Adherence of parasitized erythrocytes to capillary endothelial cells causes fibrin thrombi, which produce microinfarcts. These result in encephalopathy, congestive heart failure, pulmonary edema, and frequently death. Ruptured erythrocytes release hemoglobin, erythrocyte debris, and malarial pigment. *4.* Phagocytosis leads to reticuloendothelial hyperplasia and hepatosplenomegaly. *5.* Released hemoglobin produces hemoglobinuric nephrosis, which may be fatal.

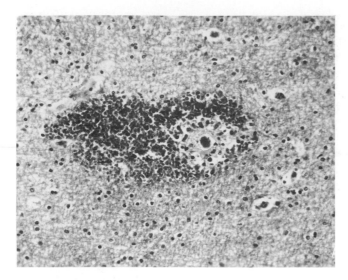

Figure 9-54.   Malarious brain with characteristic flame hemorrhage around the thrombosed capillary. The capillary contains parasitized erythrocytes in a fibrin thrombus.

associated with microhemorrhages and microinfarcts, if the patient lives long enough for these to develop (Fig. 9-54). Encephalopathy, congestive heart failure, pulmonary edema, and hemoglobinuric nephrosis with renal failure are all fatal complications.

The diagnosis of malaria is made by demonstrating plasmodia within erythrocytes, in thick or thin blood films, or in histologic sections. The demonstration of the different reproductive forms is important for determining the type of malaria. The chemoprophylaxis and treatment of active disease are complex.

Toxoplasmosis

Toxoplasmosis, infection by the protozoan *Toxoplasma gondii*, is worldwide and may be the most common infection of mankind. Most infections, however, are mild or asymptomatic, and clinical disease is uncommon. *T. gondii* infects a wide variety of mammals and birds as intermediate hosts. The final host is the cat, which ingests the cysts of bradyzoites in the tissues of an infected mouse or other intermediate host. Within the cat's intestinal epithelium, five multiplicative stages end with the shedding of oocysts, which sporulate in feces or soil and differentiate into two sporocysts. Oocysts are ingested by intermediate hosts such as birds, mice, or humans. The sporozoites within the oocysts develop in the intermediate host and form tachyzoites and bradyzoites to complete the life cycle.

T. gondii has two stages in tissue: tachyzoites and bradyzoites. Both are crescent-shaped and measure 2 μm × 6 μm. During acute infection tachyzoites

multiply rapidly to form "groups" within intracellular vacuoles of the parasitized host cells, a process that eventually destroys these cells. During chronic infection the organisms multiply slowly and are called bradyzoites. These bradyzoites store PAS-positive material, and hundreds of organisms are tightly packed in "cysts." The cysts originate in intracellular vacuoles, gradually enlarge beyond the usual size of the cell, and push the nucleus to the periphery.

Although infective forms enter through the gastrointestinal tract, there is no enteritis. Tachyzoites spread from the gut through the lymphatics to regional lymph nodes and through the blood to the liver, lungs, and other organs.

Toxoplasmosis manifests itself in several ways, including acute febrile disease, sometimes with pneumonia, myocarditis, and hepatitis; lymphadenopathy; acute or chronic encephalitis in an immunosuppressed host; chronic retinitis; asymptomatic maternal infection and transplacental infection of the fetus; and neonatal infection with jaundice or encephalitis.

In the acute disease the incubation period ranges from 7 to 17 days. The initial symptoms include headache, fever, myalgia, enlarged lymph nodes, and sometimes splenomegaly. Tachyzoites multiply in many tissues, destroy host cells, cause necrosis, and provoke inflammation. Hepatitis, myocarditis, and myositis have been documented (Fig. 9-55).

Toxoplasmic lymphadenitis most commonly involves the posterior cervical lymph nodes, although nodes at other sites may also be affected. Follicular

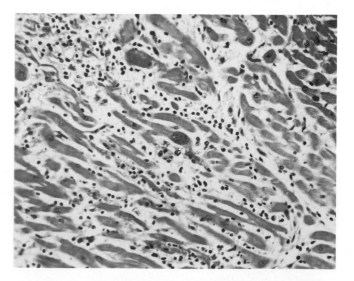

Figure 9-55.   Toxoplasmosis, heart. There is a cyst of bradyzoites *(Toxoplasma gondii)* within and expanding a myofiber with edema and inflammatory cells in adjacent tissue.

hyperplasia and characteristic small clusters of histiocytes are prominent throughout the parafollicular areas and, sometimes, within the follicles.

Patients with immunodeficiencies may have acute, recrudescent, necrotic lesions with huge numbers of tachyzoites, usually in only one organ, such as the brain, heart, or lung. Some immunosuppressed patients develop fatal toxoplasmic encephalitis (Fig. 9-56), in which case scattered areas of infarction are caused by vasculitis and thrombi.

In chronic toxoplasmosis, bradyzoites persist in tissue cysts and cause disease of many organs, especially striated muscle, brain, and retina. The retinal lesions, which may lead to blindness, are often recurrent and are usually the sequelae of congenital infection or exposure in childhood.

Asymptomatic maternal infections, although benign to the mother, are transmitted to the fetus in about a third of cases. The most important lesions in the neonate with congenital toxoplasmosis are in the brain. The lesions progress from small nodules containing tachyzoites through stages of vascular thrombosis, ependymal ulceration, and periventricular lesions with calcification, which may obstruct the aqueduct and kill the infant. Some newborns have hepatitis, with large areas of necrosis and giant cells, and others have adrenal necrosis.

The diagnosis is usually made by serologic tests. *T. gondii* can be isolated or tachyzoites or cysts of bradyzoites can be demonstrated in tissue sections or smears. The most effective treatment for toxoplasmosis consists of sulfadiazine and pyrimethamine.

Babesiosis (Piroplasmosis)

Babesiosis, an infection by protozoans of the genus *Babesia*, is transmitted by hard-bodied ticks. Although common in animals, babesiosis is rare in humans. The causative organisms, parasites resembling those of malaria, invade and destroy erythrocytes, but differ from malaria parasites in several important ways. They are transmitted by ticks, make no pigment, produce no sexual forms, and have no exerythrocytic stage. *Babesia* infect a variety of mammals including cattle, horses, and dogs. The parasites are ingested by ticks when they feed on infected mammals, multiply in the intestinal epithelium of the ticks, and spread through the insect bodies. The infective organisms are then transmitted in the saliva when the tick feeds again.

Babesiosis so far has been limited to Europe and North America. Infections in the United States have been concentrated in islands off the New England coast.

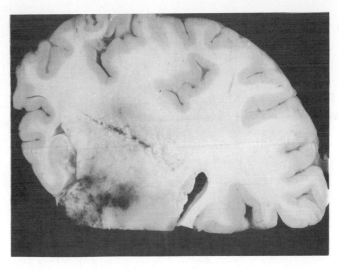

Figure 9-56. Toxoplasmosis, brain. There is a large area of necrosis with focal hemorrhage.

After inoculation by the tick, *Babesia* invade erythrocytes, where they appear as ameboid, round, rod-shaped or irregularly shaped organisms. They are 1 to 5 μm in diameter, and with the Giemsa stain have a blue cytoplasm and a mass of red chromatin.

Splenectomy and diabetes are predisposing factors. The incubation period varies from 2 to 6 weeks and is followed by sudden onset of chills and fever, sometimes with muscle aches and pains, prostration, jaundice, dark urine, diarrhea, and vomiting. The progressive invasion and destruction of red blood cells causes hemoglobinemia, hemoglobinuria, jaundice, and renal failure. The disease is usually self-limited, but uncontrolled infections can be fatal. Autopsies have found parasites in erythrocytes concentrated in congested capillaries of many organs, and especially in the hepatic sinusoids. The diagnosis is made by identifying *Babesia* in thin blood films. Parasitized erythrocytes may also be identified in tissue specimens.

Pneumocystosis

Pneumocystosis is an opportunistic infection of the lungs caused by the protozoan *Pneumocystis carinii*. Two stages, cyst and trophozoite, are both in the pulmonary alveoli. Cysts are 4 to 6 μm across and contain up to eight sporozoites. The trophozoite is 1.5 to 4 μm, thin-walled, round to crescent-shaped, mobile, and nucleated. The organism is worldwide, and since 75% of the population have acquired antibodies by 5 years of age, it is reasonable to assume that the organisms are inhaled regularly by all. In healthy people these organisms are killed by the pulmonary macrophages. When phagocytosis is defec-

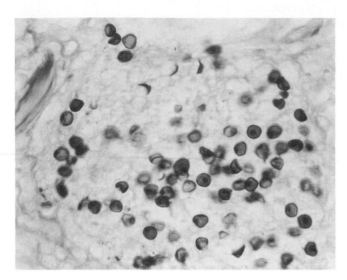

Figure 9-57. Pneumocystosis. The alveoli contain many cysts *(Pneumocystis carinii)*. The crescent-shaped organisms are collapsed and degenerated; others have a characteristic dark spot in their wall.

tive, however, organisms remain in the alveoli, proliferate, and eventually fill the alveoli with their carcasses. They do not invade the alveolar walls and provoke little inflammation. Pneumocystosis, therefore, although it may be fatal, is not an infection in the usual sense.

Pneumocystosis afflicts two distinct groups of patients. The first comprises premature and malnourished infants whose immune systems are not yet developed; the second comprises immunodeficient adults. **Pneumocystosis is now recognized as the most common infection of patients with the acquired immune deficiency syndrome (AIDS).**

The presenting symptom of pneumocystosis pneumonia is shortness of breath, with or without a nonproductive cough, that may progress to respiratory failure and death. Complications include pneumothorax, pneumomediastinum, and, in chronic cases, pulmonary fibrosis.

The lungs are consolidated and heavy, but not edematous. Microscopically, the alveoli contain a foamy eosinophilic, honeycombed material, which is composed of alveolar macrophages and cysts and trophozoites of *P. carinii*. There may be hyaline membranes and prominent type 2 alveolar lining cells. In newborns the alveolar septa are thickened by lymphoid cells and histiocytes. The prominence of plasma cells in the infantile disease led to the term "plasma cell pneumonia." This pneumocystic material may resolve when phagocytic function recovers, or it may return and lead eventually to diffuse interstitial pulmonary fibrosis. Rare, but well-docu-

mented, examples of disseminated pneumocystosis involving the eyes, liver, and spleen, have been reported.

The definitive diagnosis requires the identification of the organisms. *P. carinii* is easily seen in sections stained with Gomori's methenamine silver (Fig. 9-57). The organism can be demonstrated in open lung and transbronchial biopsy specimens, touch imprints of the lung, and smears of bronchial lavage or brushings. With silver impregnation the organisms have a thin, intensely silvered wall. Some organisms are wrinkled and collapsed. Thus, the organisms may be crescentic or folded. The organisms also stain with Giemsa, Gridley, and Gram-Weigert stains. Trimethoprim-sulfamethoxazole and pentamidine are effective and are used for both treatment and prophylaxis.

Amebiasis (Entamoeba histolytica)

Amebiasis refers to an infection by the ameba *Entamoeba histolytica*, the most important intestinal ameba of man (Fig. 9-58). *E. histolytica* is named for its lytic actions on tissue. Trophozoites invade and ulcerate the colonic mucosa, causing diarrhea, intermittent constipation, abdominal distention, and malodorous flatus. Complications include amebomas of the colon, stricture, amebic abscesses of the liver and lung, and cutaneous amebiasis.

Man is the principal reservoir. Amebiasis is worldwide but is more common and more severe in tropical and subtropical areas, where poor sanitation prevails. Amebiasis also tends to be severe, and even fatal, in some urban populations of both temperate and tropical areas (e.g., Durban, South Africa; Mexico City; and Medellín, Colombia).

E. histolytica has three distinct stages: the trophozoite (the ameboid form), the precyst, and the cyst. The trophozoites, 15 to 20 μm across, are found in the stools of patients with acute symptoms. They are spherical or oval, have a thin cell membrane, a single nucleus, condensed chromatin on the interior of the nuclear membrane, and a central karyosome. The PAS procedure stains the cytoplasm of the trophozoites and makes them stand out in tissue sections. Amebic cysts are found only in the stools, since they do not invade tissue. They are spherical, have thick walls, measure 5 to 25 μm across, and usually have four nuclei.

The cysts, found in contaminated water or food, are the infective stage (see Fig. 9-58). Ingested cysts pass through the stomach and excyst in the lower ileum. A metacystic ameba containing four nuclei divides to form four small metacystic trophozoites,

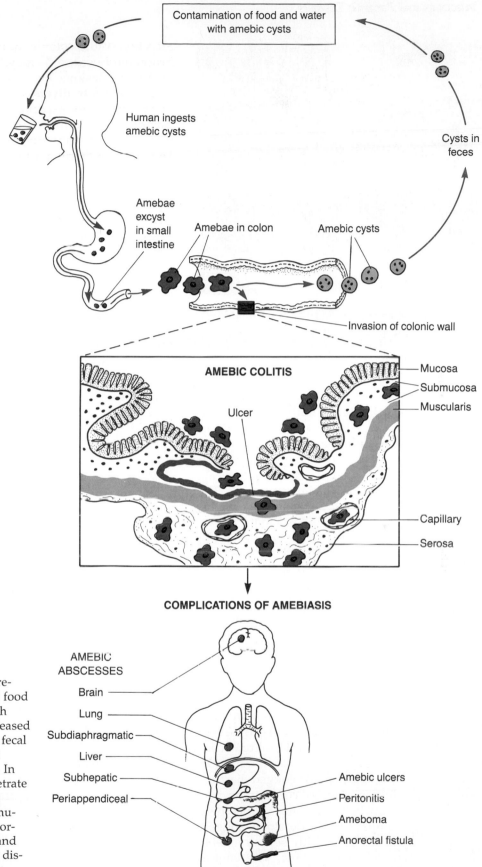

Contamination of food and water
with amebic cysts

Human ingests
amebic cysts

Cysts in
feces

Amebae
excyst
in small
intestine

Amebae in colon

Amebic cysts

Invasion of colonic wall

AMEBIC COLITIS

Ulcer

Mucosa
Submucosa
Muscularis

Capillary

Serosa

COMPLICATIONS OF AMEBIASIS

AMEBIC
ABSCESSES

Brain
Lung
Subdiaphragmatic
Liver
Subhepatic
Periappendiceal

Amebic ulcers
Peritonitis
Ameboma
Anorectal fistula

Fig. 9-58. Amebic colitis results from the ingestion of food or water contaminated with amebic cysts. Cysts are released into the feces, after which fecal contamination of food and water completes the cycle. In the colon the amebae penetrate the mucosa and produce a flask-shaped ulcer of the mucosa and submucosa. The organisms reach the serosa and invade capillaries, thereby disseminating throughout the body and producing local complications.

415

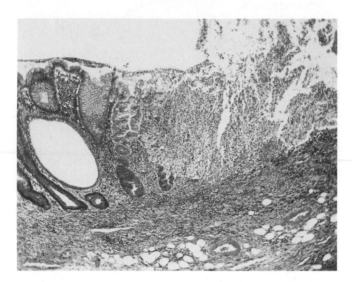

Fig 9-59. Amebiasis, colon. The mucosa is partly destroyed by invading trophozoites of *Entamoeba histolytica.* The advancing edge of the lytic action of the trophozoites is sharply delineated.

which then grow to full size. Trophozoites may colonize any portion of the large bowel, but the area of maximum disease is usually the cecum. Precyst and cysts form when bowel passage is slow. Precysts form a cyst wall and develop into a mature quadrinucleate cyst—the transmission state to the next host. The cysts contaminate water, food, or fingers, thus completing the cycle. Patients with symptomatic amebic colitis usually pass both cysts and trophozoites, but the trophozoites survive only briefly outside the body and are destroyed by gastric secretions.

Clinical responses vary, depending on the pathogenicity of the strain of *E. histolytica,* the intensity of the infection, the bacterial flora, and the site and extent of tissue damage. Only a small proportion of patients develop dysentery, perforation of the colon, liver abscess, or pleuropulmonary involvement.

The incubation period for acute amebic colitis is usually 8 to 10 days. Clinically, gradually increasing abdominal discomfort, tenderness, and cramps are accompanied by chills and fever. Nausea, severe vomiting, malodorous flatus, and intermittent constipation are typical features. Liquid stools (up to 25 a day) contain bloody mucus, and prolonged diarrhea may result in dehydration. Amebic colitis often persists for months or years; between acute attacks there may be recurring cramps; soft, loose stools suggest untreated parasitism. Patients with severe amebic colitis become emaciated and anemic. The clinical features may be bizarre and sometimes must be differentiated from those of appendicitis, cholecystitis, intestinal obstruction, diverticulitis, pneumonia, or lung abscess. In severe amebic colitis, massive destruction of the colonic mucosa, hemorrhage, perforation, and peritonitis may be fatal complications.

Amebic lesions begin as small foci of necrosis that progress to ulcers. Some remain small and discreet, but others expand. Undermining of the ulcer margin and confluence of one or more expanding ulcers lead to sloughing of the mucosa in broad, irregular geographic patterns. Typically the bed of the ulcer is gray and necrotic, being composed of fibrin and cellular debris. A sharp line divides the necrotic and viable mucosa, a feature that demonstrates the lytic action of the trophozoite (Fig. 9-59). The exudate raises the undermined mucosa, producing chronic amebic ulcers whose shape has been described as resembling a flask, a bottle neck, or a "sea anemone." Trophozoites are found on the surface of the ulcer, in the exudate, and in the crater. They are frequently also found in the submucosa, muscularis, serosa, and small veins of the submucosa. There is little inflammatory response in early ulcers. However, as the ulcer widens, there is an accumulation of neutrophils, lymphocytes, histiocytes, plasma cells and sometimes eosinophils.

An **ameboma** is an inflammatory thickening of the wall of the bowel that resembles carcinoma of the colon in location, symptoms, and gross and radiographic appearance. The ameboma tends to form a "napkin-ring" constriction. Histologic sections reveal granulation tissue, fibrosis, chronic inflammatory cells, and clusters of trophozoites, usually concentrated in the submucosa near small points of ulceration.

Intestinal perforation, most often in the cecum, is a feared complication. Slow leakage into the peritoneal cavity is more common than acute perforation and can cause peritonitis and intra-abdominal "abscesses." Patients may have single or multiple amebic liver "abscesses," which may be large enough to destroy an entire lobe. The so-called amebic abscess contains yellow or gray, opaque, amorphous liquid material that does not contain neutrophils. The wall contains abundant fibrin, and trophozoites are clustered in the fibrin at the junction of viable and necrotic tissue.

Liver abscesses may expand and perforate, thereby causing peritonitis. They may extend through the abdominal wall, where they erupt through the skin, or penetrate the diaphragm to involve the pleura and lung (see Fig. 9-58) and sometimes the pericardium. Involvement of the pericardium results in a pericardial effusion, amebic pericarditis, cardiac tamponade and cardiac failure.

Rarely, a liver abscess or even a lesion in the colon may spread amebae to the brain by a hematogenous route. Cerebral lesions, which localize in any part of the brain, begin as minute areas of softening and then expand to larger necrotic lesions containing yellowish-green material and hemorrhage.

Cutaneous amebiasis results from extension of rectal amebiasis (to the anus, perianal skin, and vulva), extension of an amebic liver abscess (to the skin of the abdominal wall or flank), or from anal intercourse (infecting the penile skin). Cutaneous lesions of the anus, perianal skin, and vulva are characterized by marked epithelial hyperplasia (with a cauliflower-like surface resembling carcinoma), punctuated by small circumscribed ulcers. Microscopically, there is papillary acanthosis of the epithelium and a chronic inflammatory response. Trophozoites are concentrated over points of ulceration, in adjacent epidermis, and in the superficial layers of the ulcer. Ulcers of the abdominal wall and penis, which may extend rapidly, are acutely tender and have a putrid odor and a gray-white necrotic base.

Demonstration of *E. histolytica* in stools or in tissue sections confirms the diagnosis. A variety of drugs is effective against amebiasis. The classic therapy for amebic colitis, emetine hydrochloride, has been largely replaced by metronidazole (Flagyl).

Amebic Meningoencephalitis (Naegleria fowleri).

Amebic meningoencephalitis, caused by *Naegleria fowleri*, is characterized by acute suppurative inflammation of the brain and meninges. *N. fowleri* is a nonparasitic, free-living soil ameba that causes rhinitis when introduced into the nasal cavity. The amebae may subsequently invade the olfactory nerves, migrate through the cribriform plate, and proliferate in the meninges and brain. The infections are fulminating and uniformly fatal.

The disease has been recognized in many parts of the world, including the United States, Europe, Australia, New Zealand, South America, and Africa. It has been diagnosed principally on histologic evidence, with only a few cases confirmed by cultures. Almost all patients give a history of swimming in freshwater lakes or pools shortly before the onset of symptoms.

In tissue sections, trophozoites of *Naegleria* measure from 8 to 15 μm across. The cytoplasm is not distinctive, but the nuclei are sharply outlined and deeply stained with hematoxylin. Some amebae have perinuclear vacuoles that tend to obscure the nuclear margin. Cysts of *Naegleria* have not been seen in tissue sections.

Clinically, acute and fulminating rhinitis and meningoencephalitis lead to death, usually within 1 to 2 weeks. Most victims have been in their teens or younger. The cerebrospinal fluid contains numerous neutrophils, blood, and amebae.

Grossly, the brain is swollen and soft, with vascular congestion and a thin purulent exudate on the meningeal surface, most prominent over the lateral and basal areas. There is massive destruction of the brain by amebae, which invade the brain along the Virchow-Robin spaces. Thrombosis and destruction of blood vessels are associated with extensive hemorrhage in the affected areas. The olfactory tract and bulbs are enveloped and destroyed, and there is an exudate between the bulb and the inferior surface of the temporal lobe.

Histologic sections show severe damage to the olfactory tract and bulb and invasion by amebae of nerve fibers in the passages through the cribriform plate. The exudate expands the subarachnoid space. Extensive proliferation of *Naegleria* in the brain often leads to formation of solid masses of amebae (amebomas).

Meningitis can extend the full length of the cord. The cerebellum is usually heavily involved, with amebae surrounding and damaging Purkinje cells. There may be large areas of necrosis in the gray matter of the cerebellum and cerebrum.

During life, diagnosis is made by finding organisms in the cerebral spinal fluid or in biopsy specimens. The fluid may be placed directly in the counting chamber, where motile amebae are seen.

Hartmannella-Acanthameba Group

Like the *Naegleria*, amebae of the Hartmannella-acanthameba group are free-living and cause acute suppurative meningoencephalitis. Unlike *Naegleria*, however, organisms of this group cause a chronic infection. Moreover, they are distinct from *N. fowleri* morphologically, immunologically, clinically, and epidemiologically. The Hartmannella-acanthameba organism causes meningoencephalitis much less frequently than *Naegleria*, and it has not been cultured from cerebral spinal fluid, brain, or meningeal exudate. Infections tend to develop in patients whose resistance has been lowered by disease or immunosuppression. The more virulent isolates have been called *H. culbersoni*; the less virulent are *H. rhysodes*.

Amebae of this group are 10 to 25 μm across. The nuclei are sharply outlined and have a dense nucleolus surrounded by a thin nuclear membrane, with a clear space between the two. The cytoplasm is indistinct.

Infections are associated with debilitating disease or trauma, and the clinical course is protracted. The gross lesions of the brain resemble those of infections with *Naegleria*, but are more focal. The Hartmannella-acanthameba organisms also cause large areas of necrosis in the cerebrum and cerebellum. Large trophozoites and characteristic cysts are present in the exudate. Thrombosed blood vessels are common.

These amebae are difficult to visualize in tissue sections. Antemortem diagnosis involves identifying the organism in the cerebrospinal fluid.

Balantidiasis (Balantidium coli)

Balantidiasis, infection by the protozoan *Balantidium coli*, is encountered worldwide, but infections are more common in tropical and subtropical regions. In temperate zones, high rates of infection may develop in institutions for the mentally retarded, in penitentiaries, and in any other environments with crowding and poor hygiene. *B. coli* infects many animals but pigs and rats are the most important reservoirs.

B. coli is a ciliated protozoan with two stages—cyst and trophozoites. In tissue sections, the trophozoites usually measure $25-45 \times 40-80$ μm. The trophozoites are oval, with a slightly pointed anterior end and a rounded posterior end. The thin cell membrane is ciliated. The foamy cytoplasm contains vacuoles, a large macronucleus, and a small micronucleus. Cysts are round or oval, 40 to 65 μm across, and have both a micro- and a macronucleus.

Trophozoites of *B. coli* live in the large intestine and are concentrated in the cecal and sigmoidorectal regions. They multiply by transverse binary fission and under some conditions transform into cysts that are passed in the stool. Humans become infected by ingesting cysts in water or food. After ingestion, the cyst wall dissolves and liberates trophozoites that invade the mucosa of the large intestine.

Most balantidial infections are asymptomatic or characterized by intermittent diarrhea or constipation. Severe infections may cause abdominal pain, colonic tenderness, fever, anorexia, and severe diarrhea. Other symptoms are headache, insomnia, nausea, vomiting, cachexia, pallor, weakness, anemia, dehydration, malaise, and distention. Stool specimens may be watery and contain blood, mucus, and pus.

Balantidia invade the bowel wall and cause ulcers that resemble amebic ulcers. The ulcers are flask-shaped with undermined edges and may involve the entire thickness of the intestine. The base of the ulcer is formed by a zone of coagulative necrosis that contains balantidial trophozoites. Beyond the necrotic bed the tissues are edematous and contain chronic inflammatory cells, mostly lymphocytes and plasma cells. Rarely, an ulcer may perforate the bowel wall.

Diagnosis is usually made by identifying trophozoites or cysts of *B. coli* in the stool or in a biopsy specimen taken through a sigmoidoscope, or by finding trophozoites in the ulcer at autopsy. Tetracycline or iodoquinol are treatments of choice.

Giardiasis (Giardia lamblia)

Giardiasis, an infection of the small intestine by the protozoan *Giardia lamblia*, has a worldwide distribution, with a prevalence that varies from 1% to more than 25%. The incidence is higher in warmer climates and in crowded, unsanitary environments. Children are about three times more susceptible than adults. Giardia are spread from person to person, or by water and food. This infestation may be epidemic, outbreaks having been noted in orphanages and institutions for the mentally retarded. Beavers are a reservoir and may contaminate streams.

Although the organism is a harmless commensal in most people, it can cause acute or chronic symptoms. Frequent or intermittent diarrhea is the most important clinical complaint. Chronic giardiasis may cause malabsorption, weight loss, and retarded growth in children.

G. lamblia has two stages, trophozoites and cysts. The trophozoites are flat, pear-shaped, binucleate organisms, with four pairs of flagella, and are most numerous in the duodenum and upper small intestine. A curved, disclike "sucker plate" on the ventral surface aids mucosal attachment. The ingested cysts, which contain two or four nuclei, revert spontaneously to trophozoites on reaching the intestine. The stools usually contain only cysts, but trophozoites may also be present in patients with diarrhea.

Biopsy of the small intestine reveals few to many trophozoites attached to the epithelial cells of the intestinal mucosa. The mucosa is essentially normal in many patients, but in others blunting and chronic inflammation of the villi are seen. Tissue invasion is rare, and the mechanism by which *G. lamblia* causes gastrointestinal dysfunction is unknown.

Giardiasis can be diagnosed from stool specimens, duodenal contents, or intestinal biopsy tissue. Motile trophozoites may be readily observed in fresh duodenal fluid. The organism is also seen in Giemsa-stained smears prepared from aspirated fluid or from a fragment of tissue or mucus contained within the biopsy capsule. Metronidazole, tinidazole, and quinacrine are effective drugs.

Isosporiasis (coccidiosis)

Isosporiasis is an acute or chronic diarrhea of humans and animals, caused by protozoa of the genus *Isospora*. The commonly encountered pathogen is *I. belli*.

Its oocysts are double-walled, refractile, ellipsoid structures.

Most coccidian infections are not serious and follow a benign course. Serious infections, however, begin with fever, diarrhea, and abdominal pain, soon followed by weight loss. Those affected usually recover spontaneously, but in some the disorder pursues a protracted and sometimes fatal course. Peripheral eosinophilia is common both in the initial illness and during relapse. Diarrhea is often complicated by steatorrhea and striking weight loss.

The histopathologic changes of isosporiasis are usually limited to the small intestine, although the colon may be involved in fatal infections. Characteristic changes include shortening and blunting of the villi, deepening of the crypts, and infiltration of the lamina propria with neutrophils, lymphocytes, plasma cells, and eosinophils. Intense parasitization may cause mucosal atrophy and consequent malabsorption. Sporozoites, schizonts, merozoites, and gametocytes may be seen in epithelial cells, and their identification confirms the diagnosis.

Since isospora invade and parasitize the mucosa of the small intestine, the diagnosis can be made by biopsy of small intestine, or by identifying oocysts in the feces or the contents of the small intestine. Combined therapy that includes sulfonamides is curative.

Sarcocystosis

Intestinal sarcocystosis is an infection by a coccidian parasite that has an obligatory two-host cycle. Humans are the final host and cattle and pigs are intermediate hosts. Although few human infections have been identified, the high incidence in beef and pork suggests that sarcocystosis may be common throughout the world.

Humans acquire sarcocystosis by ingesting bradyzoites from raw beef or pork. Bradyzoites invade the intestine and initiate the sexual phase by forming micro- and macrogametocytes. Following fertilization, a zygote develops by sporogeny to a cyst that contains two sporocysts, each with four elongated sporozoites. The oocyst ruptures, releasing infective sporocysts that pass in the feces. If the intermediate host ingests the sporocyst (cattle for *S. bovihominis*, pigs for *S. suihominis*), sporozoites are released and invade the intestinal mucosa, reaching endothelial cells, where they multiply by schizogony and produce many merozoites. These invade skeletal or cardiac muscle and multiply asexually into bradyzoites. These, in turn, form intramuscular cysts that become the vehicle of infection for man.

Sarcocystosis in man involves the intestine and, in rare instances, skeletal muscle. Following an incubation period of 3 to 6 hours after infected raw or undercooked beef is ingested, the affected person exhibits initial symptoms of nausea, abdominal pain, and diarrhea. Sporocysts then develop, and peak shedding, associated with diarrhea and abdominal pain, occurs 14 to 18 days later.

Cryptosporidiosis

Cryptosporidiosis, a well-known enteric infection of animals by a coccidian protozoan of the genus *Cryptosporidium*, is newly recognized in man, particularly patients with AIDS. It varies from a self-limited gastrointestinal infection to a potentially life-threatening infection in those with compromised immunity. Unlike toxoplasma and other coccidia, *Cryptosporidium* is an extracellular parasite. Transmission is presumed to be by the fecal-oral route and all stages of the organism are seen on the brush border of the intestinal epithelium of the host, including trophozoites, schizonts, merozoites, gametocytes, zygotes, and oocysts.

Many infections are asymptomatic. In patients with normal immune systems, gastrointestinal symptoms begin 4 to 12 days after exposure and resolve spontaneously within 2 weeks. Patients with AIDS and others with compromised immunity often have chronic and profuse watery diarrhea and malabsorption, which may be severe enough to kill the patient.

The infective oocysts invade the microvillous borders of the gut. The membrane of the host cell surrounds them, but they do not enter the cytoplasm. Infection is most common in the terminal ileum and cecum and may blunt and shorten the villi. Mild inflammatory changes, prominent Peyer's patches, and follicular hyperplasia of the draining lymph nodes are other features. In patients with defective immunity, the cryptosporidans have been found in the gallbladder, intrahepatic bile ducts, and appendix and throughout the gastrointestinal tract, from pharynx to rectum. No effective treatment is known.

Microsporidiosis

Microsporidans are parasitic protozoans that have spores containing characteristic spiral filaments, visible by electron microscopy. These obligate intracellular parasites infect all classes of animals, but humans are only rarely infected following ingestion of spores from either urine or insect excreta. When the spore approaches or touches a host cell—the intestinal epithelial cell, for example—the polar filament is discharged into the host cell and the sporoplasm

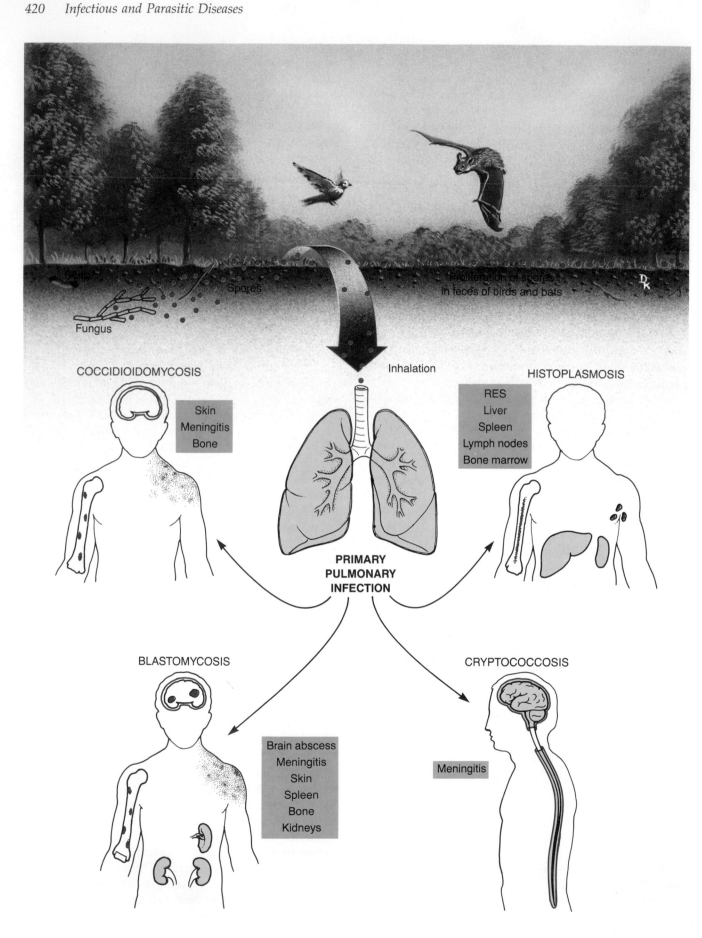

COCCIDIOIDOMYCOSIS

Skin
Meningitis
Bone

HISTOPLASMOSIS

RES
Liver
Spleen
Lymph nodes
Bone marrow

Inhalation

Spores

Fungus

Proliferation of spores
in feces of birds and bats

**PRIMARY
PULMONARY
INFECTION**

BLASTOMYCOSIS

Brain abscess
Meningitis
Skin
Spleen
Bone
Kidneys

CRYPTOCOCCOSIS

Meningitis

enters through the tubular polar filament. The organism reproduces by a series of divisions and accumulates as clusters in the host cells.

Microsporidans have caused encephalitis, enteritis, and keratitis. The diagnosis is made by identifying the spores in histologic sections or in body fluids. The most helpful diagnostic feature is the PAS-positive polar filament at the anterior end. Immunoassays are used to detect antibodies.

Diseases Caused by Fungi

Of more than 100,000 known fungi only a few invade and destroy human tissue. Of these, most are "opportunists"—that is, they infect only those with impaired immune mechanisms. Why are fungi, although abundant in nature, so poorly represented among the infectious agents of mankind? The reasons may be found in the hostile environment these organisms encounter in the human body. The elevated temperature arrests their growth, and cell-mediated immune mechanisms destroy them. Even the thermally dimorphic fungi (i.e., those that grow in living tissues as well as in soil) do not usually survive phagocytosis by neutrophils and histiocytes. Most invading fungi thus fail to establish infection, and most of those that do, infect only when cellular immunity fails. Although cell-mediated systems effectively protect against fungi, humoral antibodies play little or no role. Defective neutrophils, or the inhibition of the action of neutrophils or histiocytes, invites infection. Corticosteroid administration, other immunosuppressive therapy, and congenital or acquired T-cell deficiencies all predispose to mycotic infections.

Fungi and the diseases they cause are grouped according to anatomic location. The dermatophytes, for instance, colonize the epidermal surfaces and cause the superficial mycoses. *Phialophora* have lim-

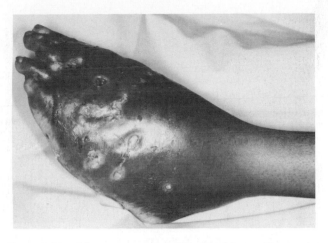

Figure 9-61. Mycetoma of foot. The foot is swollen, painful, and warm, and sinuses drain through the skin. Occasional grains are in the discharge. The foot was amputated.

ited virulence, but under the right circumstances they proliferate and cause a walled-off abscess in the panniculus. Some of the fungi that invade the deep organs are true pathogens, while others are opportunists. The inflammatory response to fungi spans the spectrum of inflammation, from virtually no response to fulminating septic thromboses with infarctions.

Mycetoma

Mycetomas are chronic, painful infections that cause swelling and deformity of a limb or other tissue and are characterized by draining sinuses that discharge bacterial or mycotic grains (Fig. 9-61). The grains are colonies of compact bacteria or fungi, cemented together by a mucopolysaccharide–protein matrix (Fig. 9-62). Sixty percent of the mycetomas are caused by

Figure 9-60. Pulmonary and disseminated fungal infection. Fungi grow in soil, air, and the feces of birds and bats, and produce spores, some of which are infectious. When inhaled, spores cause primary pulmonary infection. In a few patients the infection disseminates.
Histoplasmosis. Primary infection is in the lung. In susceptible patients, the fungus disseminates to target organs, namely the reticuloendothelial system, (liver, spleen, lymph nodes, and bone marrow), and the tongue, mucous membranes of mouth, and the adrenals.
Cryptococcosis. Primary infection of the lung disseminates to the meninges.
Blastomycosis. Primary infection of the lung disseminates widely. The principle targets are the brain, meninges, skin, spleen, bone and kidney.
Coccidioidomycosis. Primary infection of the lung may disseminate widely. The skin, meninges, and bone are common targets.

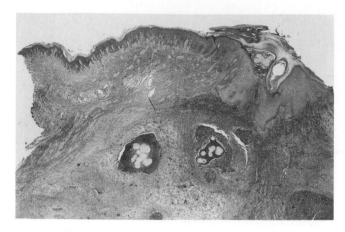

Figure 9-62.   Mycetoma, skin. There are mycotic grains in the dermis. These are clusters of fungi surrounded by an abscess with a granulomatous perimeter. The grains are erupting through the surface, and are in a tunnel in the keratin. The fungus is *Petriellidium boydii.*

actinomyces; these are discussed elsewhere. Forty percent are eumycetomas (i.e., mycetomas caused by true fungi). The fungi most commonly isolated are *Madurella mycetomatis, M. grisea, Leptosphaeria senegalensis, Petriellidium boydii, Aspergillus nidulans,* and *Acremonium,* and *Curvularia* species.

Eumycetomas are common in northern and tropical Africa, southern Asia, and the tropical Americas. The fungi are inoculated directly from soil into bare feet, from contaminated sacks carried on the shoulder, or into the hands from infected vegetation.

Sinus tracts, which discharge pus and grains, form several months after inoculation. The tracts tend to follow fascial planes in their lateral and deep spread through connective tissue, muscle, and bone. The sinus tracts contain purulent material, while the surrounding reaction is granulomatous. The treatment is radical excision, although meticulous microbiological studies of the causal organisms and specific therapy have been effective.

Aspergillosis

About 150 species of aspergillus are known, of which only three, *Aspergillus fumigatus, A. flavus-oryzae* and *A. niger* commonly infect man. These fungi are worldwide, ubiquitous, live in soil as saprophytes, and produce spores in great abundance. Because the spores are constantly inhaled, the lung is the most common site of infection, but any organ may be invaded, as well as virtually any orifice or surface, including the ear, nose, nasal sinuses, eye, skin, and intestine. Two lines of defense protect against infec-

tion. Alveolar macrophages kill inhaled spores and neutrophils kill growing hyphae. Corticosteroid therapy, which suppresses phagocytosis and promotes neutropenia is, thus, an obvious predisposing cause. Most patients, in fact, have one or more predisposing conditions, including diabetes, leukemia, lymphoma, or other malignant tumors, and treatment with cytotoxic agents, radiation, and broad-spectrum antibiotics.

Aspergillosis may be divided into three categories: aspergilloma, the fungus ball; acute aspergillosis, with or without dissemination; and allergic bronchopulmonary aspergillosis.

Aspergilloma   Almost all fungus balls (aspergillomas) are caused by *A. niger.* Airborne spores or mycelial fragments colonize a cavity or ectatic bronchus caused by prior tuberculosis, bronchiectasis, or histoplasmosis. Here the aspergilli grow in the moist, warm, dark, aerated, and protein-rich environment of the lung. The fungus ball is a layered compact mass of mycelium and cellular debris, in which the hyphae have a parallel or radial arrangement. Numerous fruiting heads are usually present. The cavity is lined by metaplastic squamous epithelium. Fungus balls are most often seen in the upper lobes and most commonly in the 4th, 5th, and 6th decades. The symptoms include cough, expectoration, hemoptysis, chest pain, wheezing, and night sweats. The treatment is surgical removal of the cavity and the fungus ball.

Acute Aspergillosis   Acute aspergillosis begins in the lung or intestine and spreads in the bloodstream to the brain, heart, kidney, and other organs. *A. fumigatus* is the most virulent of the aspergilli and the most common cause of acute and disseminated infection. Acute aspergillosis is characterized by an abundance of hyphae, which are arranged in a radial pattern and cause a purulent, necrotizing reaction. The hyphae are septate, 3 to 7 μm wide, and display dichotomous branching. They grow along tissue planes, invade vessels, and cause thrombi and septic infarction. Lesions in the brain are angiocentric and result from septic thrombosis of cerebral arteries and resultant septic infarction. Acute aspergillosis may start in a nasal sinus and spread to the face, orbit, or brain.

Primary Allergic Bronchopulmonary Aspergillosis   Patients with primary allergic bronchopulmonary aspergillosis are not infected. Rather, owing to sensitization to antigens of *Aspergillus* species, they have an exaggerated humoral response to inhaled spores. *A. fumigatus,* the prevailing saprophytic fungus in some environments, is the common offender. Inhalation of spores is followed by an attack of asthma, with productive cough, fever, malaise, and prostration. Some patients have transient pulmonary infiltrates and high levels of circulating eosinophils. The sputum is purulent and contains eosinophils and fungi. Although fungi are found in the sputum, infection plays no role. The patient recovers within 1 to 2 days.

Blastomycosis

Blastomycosis, a chronic infection caused by *Blastomyces dermatitidis*, affects the lungs and skin. Men with outdoor occupations in the Mississippi, Ohio, Missouri, and St. Lawrence River basins are most susceptible. The source and route of infection are unproved, but inhalation of conidia from the soil is most likely.

The primary infection is usually in the lung (see Fig. 9-60). It may resolve without residue, or it may disseminate to the skin, bone, urogenital organs, and, less commonly, the brain. Symptoms include mild to severe pleuritic pain, fever, productive cough, dyspnea, myalgia, and arthralgia. Amphotericin B is effective.

The pulmonary infection, which may be solitary or bilateral, results in consolidation and hilar lymphadenopathy. The reaction to the organism is mixed, having suppurative and granulomatous features. The infected areas contain numerous yeasts of *B. dermatitidis*, which are spherical and 8 to 14 µm across, with broad-based buds and multiple nuclei in the central body (Fig. 9-63). They may be found in epithelioid cells, histiocytes, or giant cells, or they may lie free in microabscesses. Although these lesions usually resolve by scarring, some patients develop progressive miliary lesions or focal consolidation with cavitation. Lesions in other organs exhibit the same mixed pyogranulomatous response. Skin lesions may show a pseudoepitheliomatous reaction that resembles squamous cell carcinoma.

Paracoccidioidomycosis

Paracoccidioidomycosis is a chronic infection caused by *Paracoccidioides brasiliensis*. The disorder is restricted to Central and South America, and Brazilians living in rural areas constitute the largest affected group. In most patients the primary infection is pulmonary and often inapparent. Although positive skin tests are equally distributed in men and women, the male to female ratio of patients with clinically significant infection is 9:1. Interestingly, *P. brasiliensis* has an estrogen-binding protein in the cytosol of the

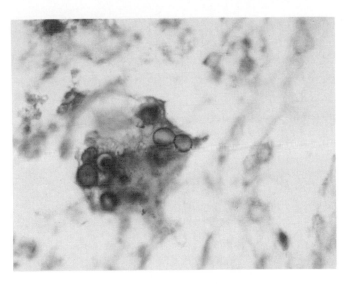

Figure 9-63. Blastomycosis, brain. The yeasts of *Blastomyces dermatitidis* have a doubly-contoured wall and nuclei in the central body. The buds have broad-based attachments.

yeast form, and estrogen inhibits transformation of the mycelium into a yeast, a combination that renders women more resistant. Paracoccidioidomycosis has three distinct presentations: pulmonary, either benign or progressive; mucocutaneous-lymphangitic; and disseminated.

Benign pulmonary infection is asymptomatic, and identification of past infection is based on the presence of residual calcifications in the lung and a reaction to paracoccidioidin skin tests. Progressive pulmonary infection simulates tuberculosis and other pulmonary mycoses and is characterized by productive cough, hemoptysis, weight loss, lethargy, and fever. Mucocutaneous infection produces indolent papules or vesicles, which ulcerate. Later, the lesions become proliferative and form vegetations. Regional lymphadenopathy is a characteristic feature. The infection rarely disseminates, but when it does, the liver, spleen, intestine, adrenals, and lymph nodes are target organs. Amphotericin B is effective.

P. brasiliensis produces a mixed purulent and granulomatous reaction, with necrosis in rapidly progressing lesions. Fibrosis dominates the chronic lesions. In tissue, *P. brasiliensis* is a large, round cell, 5 to 15 µm in diameter, that reproduces by budding. A diagnostic feature is the large yeast with small daughter cells budding from its surface (Fig. 9-64), which give an appearance that has been likened to a crown, a ship's wheel, or the radial engine of vintage aircraft. The organism can be recovered from sputum or pus.

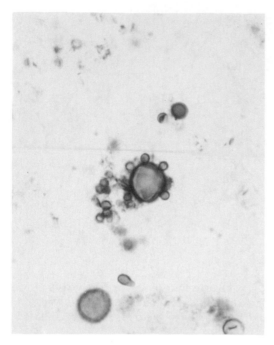

Figure 9-64. Paracoccidioidomycosis, lung, caused by *Paracoccidioides brasiliensis*. The parent cell has many external buds. Sometimes these are crowded, giving the appearance of a crown—a reliable diagnostic feature.

Candidiasis

Candidiasis is an opportunistic infection caused by *Candida albicans*, and occasionally by *C. tropicalis* and other species. **One of the most common fungal pathogens of mankind, Candida species are part of the normal flora of the skin and mucocutaneous areas, intestine, and vagina.** Infants are exposed to *Candida* at birth, after which the organisms colonize the intestinal tract and natural immunity develops. Disruption of the balance between the host and the organism leads to the expression of disease. A number of predisposing factors contribute to infections. Prolonged treatment with antibiotics, particularly with multiple antibiotic therapy, permits an overgrowth of *Candida* by eliminating and impairing the competing bacterial flora that holds *Candida* in check. The lack of a balanced flora predisposes newborns to thrush and diaper rash. During prolonged steroid administration, pregnancy, or endocrine disturbances *Candida* proliferate. In all these situations overgrowth of *Candida* usually resolves without treatment. With impaired immunity, however, superficial candidiasis may progress to mucocutaneous candidiasis and then to systemic infection.

Candida may involve the skin and mucosa or may invade deep organs. **Early in life, oral thrush is the commonest form of mucocutaneous candidiasis, and candidal vaginitis during pregnancy predisposes the neonate to infection.** In oral thrush, the lesions begin as a small focal areas of colonization of the mucosa that progress into confluent patches. Later, a creamy white pseudomembrane, composed of masses of fungi, covers the tongue, soft palate, and buccal mucosa. When detached, it leaves a reddened inflamed surface, which, in severe disease, may be ulcerated. Vaginal candidiasis is characterized by a thick yellow discharge and by patches of gray-white pseudomembranes on the mucosa. The lesions are pruritic and may extend to involve the vulva and perineum. Balanitis and balanoposthitis are less common and result from conjugal infection. Thrush or vaginitis are most intense when oral or vaginal pH is lowest. Oral contraceptives, diabetes, antibiotic therapy, polyendocrine disturbances, altered immunity, advanced neoplasia, and pregnancy are important contributing factors.

The most common forms of cutaneous candidiasis are paronychia and onychomycosis, particularly in people who frequently immerse their hands or feet in water. *Candida* also colonizes the intertriginous areas of the skin, axilla, groin, inframammary areas, intercrural and intergluteal folds, interdigital spaces, and umbilicus, especially in obese people or in tropical climates. It produces a pruritic eczematous reaction with an erythematous base, scalloped borders, and vesicles and pustules at the margins. In adult patients, drug-induced or secondary candidiasis develops in the form of cheilitis and anal pruritus. In patients, especially children, with a variety of genetic immune or endocrine defects, candidiasis is chronic and refractory to treatment, and develops into a generalized cutaneous disease with pronounced hyperkeratosis and granulomatous dermatitis.

Systemic candidiasis is rare and is usually a terminal event of an underlying disorder associated with an altered immune system. In addition to *C. albicans*, other candidal species are capable of producing invasive candidiasis. The organisms may enter through an ulcerative lesion of the skin or mucosa, or they may be introduced by iatrogenic means—for example, peritoneal dialysis, intravenous lines, urinary catheters. The urinary tract is most commonly involved and the incidence in women is four times greater than in men. Renal lesions may be blood borne or may arise from an ascending pyelonephritis. Candidal endocarditis is characterized by large vegetations on the valves and a high incidence of embolization to large arteries. In most patients with candidal endocarditis, the cause is not immunosuppression but unusual vulnerability. Drug addicts who use unsterilized needles for intravenous injections constitute such a group. Persons with pre-existing valvular disease who have had prolonged antibacterial therapy, indwelling catheters, or prolonged intravenous infusion (hyperalimentation) are at risk for endocarditis. This condition may also be seen after open heart surgery. One of the most serious complications of invasive candidiasis is septic emboli to the brain.

In mucocutaneous candidiasis masses of yeast cells and mycelia develop in the most superficial layers of the epithelium. The yeast cells are round, 3 to 4 μm in diameter, and exhibit septate hyphae or pseudohyphae. There is an acute diffuse inflammatory infiltrate and intraepithelial microabscesses. In chronic cutaneous candidiasis folliculitis, pseudoepitheliomatous hyperplasia and a granulomatous reaction are prominent. There is ulceration of the skin and mucous membranes, with focal invasion in the most severe presentations. The lesions of systemic candidiasis are extensive and polymorphous. In the kidney, yeast or pseudohyphae occupy the necrotic centers of multifocal microabscesses. Pulmonary lesions are focally hemorrhagic and necrotizing. Although primary pulmonary candidiasis is rare, secondary infections occur in patients with other primary lung diseases, such as tuberculosis or cancer. Cutaneous infection is treated topically, whereas amphotericin B is used for systemic candidiasis.

Because *Candida* is part of the flora, a positive culture does not represent proof of infection, especially if the culture is from materials passing through the mouth, vagina, or rectum. Isolation of the organism from the blood is significant. Although thrush in the newborn has a distinctive appearance and presents no diagnostic difficulty, in the adult the diagnosis depends on demonstrating the organism in smears or tissue sections. Serological tests for candidiasis are useful for monitoring therapy.

Coccidioidomycosis

Coccidioidomycosis, caused by the inhalation of arthrospores of *Coccidioides immitis*, is a chronic, necrotizing, mycotic infection that clinically and pathologically resembles tuberculosis. The inhaled arthrospore enlarges to become a spherule and then matures to a sporangium, which reaches 30 to 60 μm across. It gradually fills with endospores (sporangiospores), 1 to 5 μm across, which accumulate by endosporulation, a process unique among the pathogenic fungi (Fig. 9-65). The sporangia eventually rupture and release endospores, which then repeat the cycle.

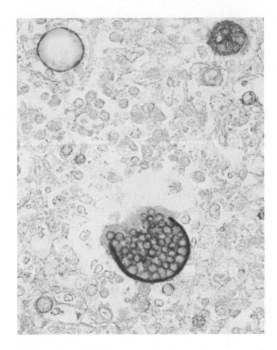

Figure 9-65. Coccidioidomycosis, lung. A ruptured sporangium of *Coccidioides immitis* is releasing endospores into the tissue.

Coccidioidomycosis is most prevalent in the western and southwestern United States and is particularly common in the San Joaquin Valley of California, where it is called "valley fever." Coccidioidomycosis also occurs in Mexico and parts of South America. The organism grows in the soil where rainfall is low and summer temperatures are high. In recent years better housing, with less exposure to dust, has reduced the size of the inoculum, reducing the risk of progressive infection and dissemination.

Approximately 60% of patients are unaware of their infections, and only skin sensitization to coccidioidin or spherulin (fungal antigens) discloses the existence of a past or present infection. Many symptomatic patients have reactive antibodies, and serologic tests are valuable in establishing the diagnosis.

Coccidioidomycosis is a disease of protean manifestations, which may vary from a subclinical respiratory infection to one that disseminates and is rapidly fatal. Practitioners in endemic areas who are most experienced in diagnosing coccidioidomycosis state that almost any complaint or syndrome may be a manifestation of coccidioidomycosis. It thus joins syphilis and typhoid fever as a "great imitator." The two most common types of coccidioidomycosis are primary pulmonary and disseminated.

Primary pulmonary coccidioidomycosis is an acute, self-limited infection. Although it may be mild or even asymptomatic, it provokes delayed hypersensitivity to the fungal antigens. The lesion is a solitary grayish focus of consolidation, 2 to 3 cm across, usually in the middle or lower lung fields. Occasionally, a more diffuse pneumonic consolidation or multiple scattered foci of consolidation appear. Hilar lymphadenopathy is usually absent. Symptomatic patients have fever, night sweats, pleuritic pain, dysphagia, cough, and shortness of breath.

Histologically, the primary pulmonary nodule is a caseating granuloma. Sproangia are free in the necrotic tissue or in epithelioid cells and giant cells of the granuloma. Endospores released within the granuloma provoke neutrophils, and these are sufficiently concentrated in some areas to form microabscesses. Diffuse suppuration indicates rapid proliferation of fungi. With time, the granulomas become scarred and calcified, thereby simulating tuberculosis.

Cavitation is the most frequent complication of pulmonary coccidioidomycosis. The cavity is usually solitary and may persist for years. In a few patients, progression or reactivation leads to destructive lesions in the lungs or, more seriously, to disseminated lesions throughout the body (see Fig. 9-60).

Primary involvement of the skin occasionally occurs, but skin involvement is more often a manifestation of progressive disease and hematogenous dissemination. Disseminated coccidioidomycosis occurs by hematogenous spread of sporangiospores from the lungs into the skin, bones, joints, adrenals, lymph nodes, spleen, liver, and meninges. At all of these sites the inflammatory response may be purely granulomatous, pyogenic, or mixed. Purulent lesions predominate in patients who lack a normal cell-mediated response. The gastrointestinal tract is spared, in contrast to tuberculosis, histoplasmosis, and paracoccidioidomycosis. The prognosis is poor in acute disseminated coccidioidomycosis, especially if there is meningitis. Even with amphotericin B therapy the course of the disease is marked by remissions and exacerbations.

Cryptococcosis

Cryptococcosis is a systemic mycosis with worldwide distribution caused by *Cryptococcus neoformans*. The most important lesions are in the lungs and meninges (see Fig. 9-60). Cryptococci are unique among pathogenic fungi in having a mucopolysaccharide capsule, which is essential for their pathogenicity. In routinely stained sections, the organisms appear as faintly stained basophilic yeasts that vary in size, 4 to 9 μm across, and have a clear mucinous capsule, 3 to 5 μm thick.

The main reservoir is pigeon droppings, which are alkaline and hyperosmolar. These conditions keep the cryptococci small, thus allowing them, on being inhaled, to penetrate to terminal bronchioles. Although inhaled cryptococci may infect the lung, ingested cryptococci are harmless. Clinically significant cryptococcosis is usually an opportunistic infection. For instance, patients with progressive cryptococcosis have abnormal cell-mediated immunity, and half of the patients with cryptococcal meninigitis have some lymphoid cancer.

People with normal immunity become infected, but the infection is silent and heals spontaneously. The lesion in these "normal" people, the primary pulmonary cryptococcoma, is a circumscribed nodule that has a necrotic center containing many cryptococci and a fibrous and granulomatous wall. These lesions do not calcify, so evidence of healed infection is not present on radiograms of the chest.

People with immunodeficiencies, on the other hand, develop progressive cryptococcal pulmonary infection, with cough, pleuritic pain, malaise, and fever. The lesions are frequently bilateral and localized in the lower lobes, but may involve an entire lobe or lobes and kill the patient quickly. Miliary granulomas, small abscesses, and large solid mucoid lesions are seen.

From the lung the cryptococci spread through the bloodstream to other organs, particularly the central nervous system, where the common presentation is meningitis. A gray mucinous exudate distends the subarachnoid space, especially at the base of the brain and over the cerebral convexities.

Untreated cryptococcal meningitis is uniformly fatal. Treatment with intravenous amphotericin B cures about 60% of patients, but many of these relapse. Untreated cryptococcal meningitis usually has a subacute or chronic course, with periods of spontaneous remission followed by recurrence and progressive deterioration over weeks to months. A few patients, however, have a fulminating meningoencephalitis that kills in a few days. The lesions in the brain are cystic, and are extensions from the meninges or from septic emboli. Solitary brain lesions may be confused with tumors. The diagnosis of cryptococcosis is sometimes evident only after brain surgery and biopsy of the lesion.

The inflammatory response may be inapparent in terminal cerebromeningeal infections because fungal cells with thick capsules grow in an unrestricted fashion through the tissue. Thus the lesions are mucinous, with large numbers of free organism and a minimal inflammatory cell response. On the other hand, poorly encapsulated ("dry") variants elicit a granulomatous reaction, with organisms mostly within giant cells. The early lesions tend to be mucinous, whereas older lesions become granulomatous. Disseminated cryptococcosis involves the skin, mucous membranes, bone, and deep organs. Lesions of skin present as papules or small abscesses. Mucocutaneous lesions are usually granulomatous.

The diagnosis is confirmed by cultivating *C. neoformans* and by identifying it in smears and tissue sections. In mucoid lesions, the diagnosis of cryptococcosis is made on routinely stained sections. Mucicarmine and alcian blue staining of the capsule aids in the identification of cryptococci. *C. neoformans* is harder to identify in granulomatous lesions because the mucinous capsule may not be apparent. The india ink preparation demonstrates cryptococci in spinal fluid, and the latex agglutination test detects capsular mucopolysaccharide in serum or spinal fluid. The infection is treated with amphotericin B.

Sporotrichosis

Sporotrichosis is a chronic infection of skin, subcutaneous tissues, and regional lymph nodes caused by *Sporothrix schenckii*, a ubiquitous fungus commonly found on decaying vegetation, on a wide variety of plants, and in the soil. Inoculation of the skin occurs by traumatic implantation from thorns or splinters, or by handling reeds, sphagnum moss, or grasses. Rose gardeners are at special risk. Dissemination is rare and may involve the bones and other organs. Primary infection of the lung is also recognized; it mimics tuberculosis and is prevalent among chronic alcoholics. Sporotrichosis is endemic in the Americas and South Africa.

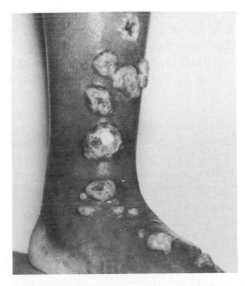

Figure 9-66. Sporotrichosis of leg, showing typical lymphocutaneous spread.

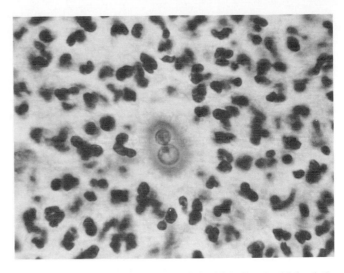

Figure 9-67. Sporotrichosis of skin. This "asteroid body" is composed of a pair of budding yeasts of *Sporothrix schenckii*, surrounded by a layer of Splendore Hoeppli substance, with radiating projections. The asteroid body is diagnostic of sporotrichosis.

About 75% of infections are on the arm, hands, or legs. The infection starts in a penetrating wound, usually of the hand or finger. After an incubation period of 3 weeks a firm, movable subcutaneous nodule develops at the site. Later, the nodule ulcerates, and satellite nodules and ulcers appear along the draining lymphatic vessels (Fig. 9-66).

The typical lesion is a granulomatous reaction, with central suppuration and fibrosis at the perimeter. In primary cutaneous lesions, rare yeasts are seen mainly in purulent exudate or within giant cells. The overlying epidermis is hyperkeratotic and acanthotic and may be ulcerated. The organism appears as round or elongated (cigar-shaped) cells. The yeasts are 2 to 3 μm in diameter and the "cigar" bodies, 1 to 2 μm thick and 4 to 5 μm long. Some of the yeasts are surrounded by an eosinophilic spiculated zone and are called asteroid bodies (Fig. 9-67). This material (Splendore-Hoeppli substance) is probably antigen-antibody complex on the surface of the yeast. A large variant of *S. schenckii* (var. *luriei*), 15-20 μm, grows on the timbers in the deep mines of South Africa and infects mine workers.

The diagnosis is most frequently established by culture, but serologic tests are also of value. Direct examination of pus is seldom helpful. Potassium iodide is the treatment of choice.

Histoplasmosis

Histoplasmosis is a worldwide systemic mycosis caused by *Histoplasma capsulatum*, a dimorphic fungus

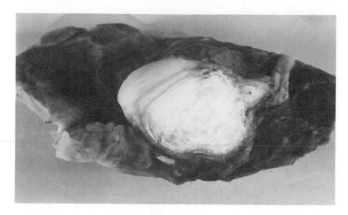

Figure 9-68. Histoplasmosis, lung, showing characteristic features of a histoplasmoma, a walled-off primary infection by *Histoplasma capsulatum*. It is subpleural, about 2 cm across, circumscribed and encapsulated, and has a laminated, mineralized interior. The diagnosis can be made by identifying the carcasses of yeasts in the central portion of the nodule. Most people resolve their primary infection as a subpleural nodule.

that grows in humans as a round or oval yeast, 2 to 4 μm in diameter. The reservoir for *H. capsulatum* is in bird droppings and in the soil. In the Americas, hyperendemic areas are in the eastern and central United States, western Mexico, Central America, the northern countries of South America, and Argentina. Starlings imported from Europe in 1890 became concentrated along the Ohio-Mississippi Valley and contributed to the establishment of this area as a major endemic focus. As a result, the population in this area displays a high prevalence of positive histoplasmin skin test results. In the tropics, bat nests, caves, and soil beneath trees are foci of exposure. In the soil *H. capsulatum* produces characteristic macroconidia, 8 to 16 μm in diameter, and microconidia, 2 to 5 μm in diameter. Because they are smaller, the microconidia usually reach the alveolar spaces, where they are transformed into yeasts. Inhalation of conidia causes a primary pulmonary infection, which in 95% of people is subclinical and transitory. The primary pulmonary infection is diagnosed by a positive histoplasmin skin test and radiologic findings of a spherical subpleural lesion, which may be calcified (Fig. 9-68).

Inhalation of a large number of conidia causes a more aggressive infection. The initial infection is followed by a transient fungemia. Symptoms develop in 8 to 15 days and include malaise, cough, and shortness of breath. Most patients abort their infection, leaving residual foci of calcification in the lungs and, sometimes, the spleen. Others develop chronic pulmonary histoplasmosis, which may be confused

with tuberculosis because the clinical and pathologic features are similar. Chronic cough, chest pain, fever, night sweats, malaise, and weight loss are all common to both histoplasmosis and tuberculosis. Radiographically, the lesions are segmental wedge-shaped shadows, usually in the apex. These may cavitate or heal with a fibrotic scar.

Infants, the elderly, and those with deficient immunity are all prone to disseminated histoplasmosis, a condition characterized by proliferation of the organism in phagocytic cells of the bone marrow, liver, and spleen (see Fig. 9-60). The patient suffers from generalized lymphadenopathy, hepatosplenomegaly, fever, anemia, weight loss, leukopenia, and thrombocytopenia. Lesions of the tongue, mouth, and adrenals are common. The yeast cell is round and has a central basophilic body surrounded by a clear zone or "halo," which in turn is encircled by a rigid cell wall, approximately 2 to 4 μm in diameter. In caseous lesions, where the yeasts are degenerating, silver impregnation is needed to identify the carcasses of the yeasts. Treatment is with amphotericin B.

Chromomycosis

Chromomycosis is a chronic infection of the skin caused by several species of brown fungi (*Phialophora* and *Cladosporium* species) that live as saprophytes in soil and decaying vegetable matter. Chromomycosis is most common in barefooted agricultural workers living in the tropics and subtropics. The fungus enters the skin by traumatic implantation, usually below the knee. The lesions begin as papules and, over the years, become verrucous, crusted, and sometimes ulcerated. The infection spreads by contiguous growth and by satellites along draining lymphatics. Eventually it may involve an entire limb.

Microscopically, there is marked epidermal thickening, caused by hyperkeratosis and epidermal hyperplasia. The dermis is edematous and contains an inflammatory cell exudate that is both suppurative and granulomatous. The fungi are brown, round, thick-walled, and about 8 μm across: They have been described as "copper pennies." The organisms are located in microabscesses, giant cells (Fig. 9-69), histiocytes, epithelioid cells and hyperplastic epithelium. Elongated rete ridges project into the dermis, where they surround some of the fungi, incorporate them into the epidermis, and carry them up with the maturating epidermal cells. The fungi are then extruded through the surface of the skin with the desquamating keratin. This process is called transepithelial elimination, and although it eliminates fungi from

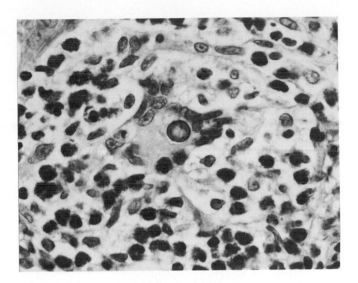

Figure 9-69. Chromomycosis of skin. the giant cell in the center contains a thick-walled, brown, sclerotic body; the fungus that causes chromomycosis.

the body it does not do it quickly enough to cure the infection.

The diagnosis of chromomycosis is made on the basis of a biopsy specimen in which the typical brown fungi are identified in the dermis and epidermis. In the early stages, chromomycosis can be cured by surgical excision, but in advanced infections, specific antifungal therapy is necessary.

Phaeomycotic Cyst

Phaeomycotic cyst is infection of the deep dermis and subcutaneous tissue by brown fungi—usually *Phialophora* species. These fungi are worldwide saprophytes, common in soil, decaying wood, and vegetation. They have low pathogenicity, and are inoculated with penetrating slivers and splinters, usually on the hands and feet. There are no systemic signs and symptoms, and regional lymph nodes are not involved. Altered immunity may predispose to infection.

The phaeomycotic cyst begins as a small firm, nontender lesion in the panniculus. It enlarges slowly, gradually softens, and finally becomes fluctuant. Histologically, the lesions progress from solid granulomas to stellate abscesses. The central cavity contains pus and is surrounded by a layer of granulomatous tissue. There is no ulceration and no sinus tracts. The fungi contain traces of brown pigment, are polymorphous, and are located in the pus and in the surrounding histiocytes and giant cells. The cysts "shell out" easily, and resection cures the lesion.

Zygomycosis

Several genera of Zygomycetes infect man, including *Rhizopus*, *Absidia*, *Mucor*, *Basidiobolus*, and *Entomophthora*. Zygomycetes have a characteristic appearance in tissue sections and usually can be distinguished from other pathogenic fungi. They are large (8–15 μm across), branch at right angles, have thin walls, and lack septa. In sections they appear as hollow tubes (lacking cross walls their liquid contents flow, leaving long empty segments) or as "twisted ribbons." The latter are collapsed hyphae, a consequence of their fragile walls.

Zygomycetes are the common bread molds and fruit spoilers. Therefore, isolates from body tissues and fluids must be interpreted with caution and identified as pathogens only when there is sufficient clinical and pathologic correlation.

Subcutaneous zygomycosis is limited to the tropics and is caused by *Basidiobolus haptosporus*. The fungus grows slowly in the panniculus, producing a gradually enlarging, hard, inflammatory mass, usually on the shoulder, trunk, buttock, or thigh. Characteristically, the mass has sharp edges and lifts easily away from the underlying fascia (Fig. 9-70). Microscopically, the fungi appear as tubular openings in the tissue, surrounded by a protein coagulum (Splendore-Hoeppli substance). The hyphae spread contiguously in the panniculus, but do not invade vessels.

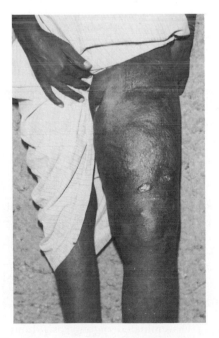

Figure 9-70. Subcutaneous zygomycosis (phycomycosis). The lesion is centered in the panniculus, is hard, has sharp edges, and lifts easily from the underlying fascia.

The inflammatory response is dominated by eosinophils, granulomas, and fibrous tissue. These lesions respond dramatically to orally administered potassium iodide.

Nasofacial zygomycosis, caused by *Entomophthora coronata*, resembles subcutaneous zygomycosis but involves the mucous membranes of the nose, paranasal sinuses, and subcutaneous tissues of the face. The infection progresses slowly, but relentlessly, to cause grotesque disfigurement. The appearance of the fungus in tissue and the reaction to it are identical to those of subcutaneous zygomycosis. Tragically, however, these infections do not respond to treatment with potassium iodide.

Rhinocerebral zygomycosis, caused by *Rhizopus, Absidia,* and *Mucor* species, is a rare, devastating infection of the nasal sinuses, eyes, and brain. **Most patients have diabetic acidosis or other predisposing factors which render the host susceptible to this usually harmless fruit mold.** The infection begins in the nasal turbinates and paranasal sinuses and quickly spreads into the eyes and brain. Frontal headache, blood-tinged nasal discharge, and fever are followed by orbital pain, a bulging eye, and fixed pupil. Of these features the bulging discolored eye is the most striking. The fungal hyphae grow into the arteries and cause a devastating, rapidly progressive, hemorrhagic and septic infarction. Extension into the brain leads to a fatal necrotizing, hemorrhagic encephalitis.

Cutaneous zygomycosis is rare, may be caused by a variety of genera, and is usually seen as a secondary infection of burns and other wounds. Because these infections tend to be chronic and difficult to treat,

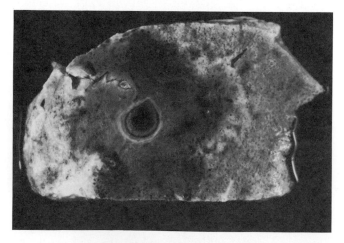

Figure 9-71. Disseminated zygomycosis, lung. The vessel in the center of the field is invaded by zygomycetes and is occluded by a septic thrombus. The surrounding tissue is infarcted and hemorrhagic.

they contribute to the delayed healing of burns and wounds.

Disseminated zygomycosis begins in the lung or gastrointestinal tract. In either site the infection may remain localized or may disseminate. Infections in the lung cause chest pain and bloody sputum (Fig. 9-71). With gastrointestinal infection, which is more common in malnourished children, the symptoms include abdominal pain, hematemesis, bloody stools, diarrhea, and in late stages, peritonitis from perforation of the intestine. Local spread takes place when fungi grow along tissue planes and invade the walls of arteries, a complication that leads to arteritis, septic thrombosis, hemorrhage, and infarction. Patients with diabetic acidosis or cancer and those receiving long-term steroid, antibiotic, or cytotoxic therapy are susceptible to infection. Amphotericin B is used in therapy.

Rhinosporidiosis

Rhinosporidiosis, a chronic mycosis caused by *Rhinosporidium seeberi*, is characterized by hyperplastic polypoid lesions of the nasal mucosa. Less frequently the infection involves the conjunctiva and mouth, and in rare instances it involves the skin and viscera. Infection is sporadic and has been related to contact with stagnant water or dust. The disease has been reported from all continents, but 90% of the 2000 reported cases have come from India and Sri Lanka. The mode of infection is unknown, but trauma may be a factor.

Patients seek attention when they feel a swelling or perceive a foreign body in a nostril, accompanied by itching, sneezing, mucous discharge, and mild bleeding. At first the nasal lesions are sessile, but they progress to large, pedunculated and distorted polypoid growths. Lesions high in the turbinates or nasal septum may protrude from the nares or into the nasopharynx, in which case they may lead to dysphagia and dyspnea. Most ocular infections involve the palpebral conjunctiva. Early lesions are asymptomatic but eventually cause excessive tearing, discharge, photophobia, redness, and secondary infection. Some conjunctival lesions have been misdiagnosed as hemangiomas. Lesions of the skin begin as papillomas, which become warty and exude myxomatous material.

The nasal polyps contain mature sporangia, which appear as minute white foci on the mucosal surface. Microscopically, granulation tissue contains plasma cells, lymphocytes, and focal collections of histiocytes and neutrophils. The overlying epithelium is usually

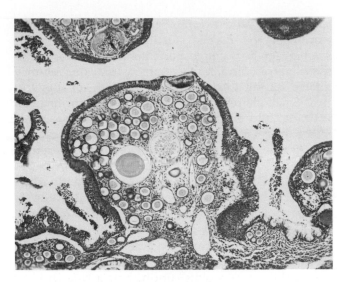

Figure 9-72. Rhinosporidiosis, nasal mucosa, through a polypoid lesion. The lesion contains many sporangia, one of which is about to rupture through the surface epithelium.

hyperplastic, with focal thinning and occasional ulceration. Fungi are numerous and appear as globular sporangia that range from 10 to 300 μm across, depending on their stage of maturation (Fig. 9-72). Young "trophic" forms, 10 to 100 μm across, have a central basophilic nucleus but lack spores. Mature sporangia have a chitinous wall up to 5 μm thick and contain spores in different stages of development. Spores are 8 to 10 μm across, and each contains 8 to 10 globular eosinophilic bodies. The largest sporangia are usually in a subepithelial location. Spores are released through a pore or by rupture of the wall at the site of a pore. Ruptured sporangia collapse and provoke a foreign body reaction. The released free spores incite a neutrophilic response in the tissue but are also passed in the nasal discharges. The spores in the tissue develop into small trophic forms, thus enlarging the lesion and perpetuating the infection.

Since *R. seeberi* cannot be routinely cultured, the diagnosis is confirmed by biopsy. Treatment is surgical excision. Recurrence is common and may require repeated excisions over a period of many years.

Superficial Fungi

Superficial fungi, which infect the hair, nails, and outer portions of the skin, are spread by direct person-to-person contact or by fomites. Dermatophytosis, the most important cutaneous mycosis, is caused by species of three genera, *Microsporum*, *Trichophyton*, and *Epidermophyton*. Tinea capitis is characterized by

patchy alopecia of the scalp, eyebrows, or eyelashes. Tinea barbae is acute folliculitis of the bearded area. Tinea corporis is an erythematous dermatitis with scaling urticarial papules. The fungi invade the stratum corneum and then the hair follicles. Certain species of *Trichophyton* invade the hair and form hyphae or arthrospores. Other species of *Trichophyton* and *Microsporum* form spores of varying size, hyphae, or arthrospores within (endothrix) and around (exothrix) the hair. Lymphocytes invade adjacent perivascular spaces in the corium, and rupture of hair follicles provokes a granulomatous reaction. In nonhairy skin, lymphocytes invade the perivascular spaces in response to the presence of the fungus in the epidermis. In hypersensitivity "id" reactions, *Trichophyton* infection of the skin of the feet provokes intraepidermal vesicles of the hand. In patients with deficient immunity, the superficial fungi may invade and disseminate to all organs of the body, and may kill the patient.

The diagnosis is made by direct microscopic examination of skin scrapings mounted in sodium hydroxide solution, by culture, or by demonstration of the fungus in tissue sections. The treatment consists of topical antifungal and keratolytic agents or oral griseofulvin.

Diseases Caused by Filarial Nematodes

Bancroftian and Malayan Filariasis

Bancroftian and Malayan filariasis are infections by *Wuchereria bancrofti* and *Brugia malayi*, respectively. The adult worms inhabit lymphatic vessels, most frequently those in the lymph nodes, testis, and epididymis. Both genera block lymphatic vessels, and they cause similar symptoms and lesions. The female worm discharges microfilariae that circulate in the blood.

The elephantiasis characteristic of filariasis was familiar to Hindi and Persian physicians as early as 600 B.C. Humans are the only definitive host of these worms. Insect vectors, which serve also as intermediate hosts, include at least 80 species of mosquitoes of the genera *Culex*, *Aedes*, *Anopheles*, and *Mansonia*. Bancroftian filariasis is endemic in large regions of Africa, coastal areas of Asia, western Pacific islands, and coastal areas and islands of the Caribbean basin.

Malayan filariasis is endemic in coastal areas of Asia and western Pacific islands.

Most of those infected remain asymptomatic throughout life. Those with symptoms show features of acute or chronic disease. Features of acute infection include fever, lymphangitis, lymphadenitis, orchitis, epididymitis, urticaria, eosinophilia, and microfilaremia. Chronic infection is characterized by enlarged lymph nodes, lymphedema, hydrocele, and elephantiasis. Elephantiasis afflicts only a small proportion of patients, and then only after years of infection. Filariasis also causes tropical eosinophilia (also known as Weingartner's syndrome, eosinophilic lung, and tropical pulmonary eosinophilia), which is characterized by cough, wheezing, eosinophilia, and diffuse pulmonary infiltrates.

The most significant pathologic changes are a consequence of adult worms living in the lymphatic vessels, especially in the lymph nodes, testis, epididymis, and spermatic cord. These lymphatic vessels become dilated and the endothelial lining is thickened. In the adjacent tissue a chronic inflammatory infiltrate, consisting of lymphocytes, histiocytes, plasma cells, and eosinophils, surrounds the worms. A granulomatous reaction may develop, and degenerating worms can provoke acute inflammation. The lumen of the lymphatic vessel eventually becomes obliterated. Microfilariae are seen within blood vessels and lymphatics, and degenerating microfilariae also provoke a chronic inflammatory reaction. Microfilariae that invade the walls of blood vessels may provoke a focal vasculitis and lead to thrombosis. The pulmonary lesions in tropical eosinophilia contain microfilariae surrounded by inflammation.

The diagnosis is usually made by identifying the microfilariae in blood, which should be obtained at night because of the periodicity of the microfilaremia. Microfilariae and adult worms are also identified in tissue sections. The drug of choice is diethylcarbamazine, which kills microfilariae and possibly adult worms.

Loiasis

Loiasis is infection by the filarial nematode, *Loa loa*, the African "eyeworm" or "loa" worm. It prevails in the rain forests of central and West Africa. Humans and baboons are definitive hosts and infection is transmitted by mango flies (*Chrysops* species). The adult *L. loa* migrates in the skin and occasionally crosses the eye beneath the conjunctiva, making the patient acutely aware of his infection. Gravid worms discharge microfilariae that circulate in the bloodstream during the day but reside in capillaries of the skin, lungs, and other organs at night.

Most infections are asymptomatic but persist for years. Some patients have pruritic, red, subcutaneous, "Calabar" swellings, which may be a reaction

to migrating adult worms or to microfilariae in capillaries of the dermis. Ocular symptoms include swelling of lids, congestion, itching, and pain. Female worms, and rarely male worms, may be extracted during their migration beneath the conjunctiva. Systemic reactions include fever, pain, itching, urticaria, and eosinophilia. Dead worms in or near major nerves may cause paresthesias and focal paralyses. Some patients have a regional lymphadenopathy, characterized by follicular atrophy, histiocytic hyperplasia, and eosinophilia. Treatment with microfilariacides may cause massive death of microfilariae and provoke fever, meningoencephalitis, nephritis, coma, and death.

Migrating worms cause no inflammation, but static worms are surrounded by plasma cells, lymphocytes, eosinophils, neutrophils, fibrin, and a foreign body giant cell reaction. At autopsy patients with acute generalized loiasis have obstructive fibrin thrombi, which contain degenerating, microfilariae, in small vessels of most organs. When the brain is involved, obstruction of vessels by filarial thrombi kills the patient through sudden and diffuse cerebral ischemia.

The diagnosis is made by identifying microfilariae in blood films taken during the day, by removal of adult worms from the conjunctiva or by identifying microfilariae or adult worms in biopsy specimens.

Onchocerciasis

Onchocerciasis, infection by the filarial nematode *Onchocerca volvulus*, is one of the world's major endemic diseases, afflicting an estimated 40 million people, of whom about 2 million are blind. Man is the only known definitive host. Onchocerciasis is transmitted by several species of blackflies of the genus *Simulium*, which breed in fast-flowing streams. There are endemic regions throughout tropical Africa and in focal areas of Central and South America.

The cardinal manifestations are subcutaneous nodules, dermatitis, sclerosing lymphadenitis, and eye disease. The adult worms live singly and as coiled entangled masses in the deep fascia and the subcutaneous tissues. The worms are detected clinically only when they become encapsulated by a fibrous scar, forming discrete onchocercal nodules (**onchocercomas**) in the deep dermis and subcutaneous tissues. Nodules form over bony prominences of the skull, scapula, rib, iliac crest, trochanter, sacrum, and knee. The adult worms are innocuous, but the gravid female worms produce millions of microfilariae, which migrate from the nodule into the skin, eyes, lymph nodes, and deep organs, thereby causing the corresponding onchocercal lesions. Onchocercal dermatitis presents a spectrum of clinical features, including itching, hypopigmented macules of the skin, and papular eruptions. Onchocercal lymphadenitis involves a progression of changes. The femoral and/ or inguinal lymph nodes become enlarged and then fibrotic. The consequent lymphatic obstruction leads to an overlying "hanging groin" (adenolymphocele) and genital elephantiasis. Ocular onchocerciasis results from the migration of microfilariae into all regions of the eye, from the cornea to the optic nerve head, and result in sclerosing keratitis, iridocyclitis, chorioretinitis, and optic atrophy.

Microscopically, the subcutaneous nodules contain coiled adult worms and have an outer fibrous layer and a central inflammatory exudate, which varies from suppurative to granulomatous. Arborization of capillaries around adult worms provides them with nutrition. The dermatitis begins when microfilariae degenerate in the dermis, an event that is accompanied by degranulation of eosinophils and deposition of eosinophil granule major basic protein on the cuticle. Onchocercal lymphadenitis is characterized initially by histiocytic hyperplasia and follicular atrophy, and later by fibrosis.

The diagnosis is made by identifying the microfilariae in tissue sections of skin, and the adult worms in the subcutaneous nodules. Another sensitive diagnostic test is the Mazzotti reaction to oral diethylcarbamazine (DEC), which kills microfilariae and produces allergic erythema and pruritus.

Nodulectomy removes adult worms in palpable nodules but misses deeper worms. Suramin kills adult worms, but has dangerous side effects. Oral DEC kills microfilariae (not adult worms), and remains the principal treatment, sometimes in combination with low, carefully controlled doses of suramin. A new drug, ivermectin, kills microfilariae, but with a lesser allergic reaction than DEC.

Mansonelliasis

Three species of *Mansonella* infect man: *M. perstans*, *M. ozzardi*, and *M. streptocerca*. *M. perstans* inhabits Africa and South America. *M. ozzardi* is restricted to areas of South America and the Caribbean, and *M. streptocerca* is found in portions of West and Central Africa. The symptoms caused by *M. perstans* and *M. ozzardi* are minor and nonspecific. Both worms live in the abdominal cavity, where they provoke little or no inflammation. The only sign of infection is usually circulating microfilariae. By contrast, the adult *M. streptocerca* lives in the dermis of the upper trunk, shoulders, and arms. The microfilariae are concentrated there, but have also been identified in lymph nodes. Infection by *M. streptocerca* causes itching and hypopigmented macules of upper trunk, shoulders, and arms. After treatment with diethylcarbamazine (a potent filariacide) microfilariae and adult worms degenerate in the dermis and cause diffuse and focal inflammation. The diagnosis is made by placing a skin snip in saline and watching the microfilariae emerge. The hypopigmented macules of streptocerciasis must be distinguished from macules of leprosy. Species of *Culicoides*, the biting midges, are intermediate hosts for all three species of *Mansonella*.

Dirofilariasis

Pulmonary Dirofilariasis

The filarial nematode *Dirofilaria immitis*, a common parasite of dogs and other mammals, is transmitted by mosquitoes. In humans the infective stage usually does not reach maturity, but is swept by the venous circulation into the lung, where it obstructs a pulmonary arteriole and causes a subpleural infarct, which resolves as a granuloma. Originally reported from Japan and Australia, pulmonary dirofilariasis is most common in the southern and eastern United States.

Most of these lesions are silent and are discovered as spherical, 1-cm to 3-cm, subpleural "coin lesions" during radiologic examination of the chest. Microscopically, a central area of coagulation necrosis is surrounded by a zone of granulomatous reaction. The coiled immature and degenerating *D. immitis* is located in an arteriole in the central zone of necrosis.

Subcutaneous Dirofilariasis

D. tenuis, a subcutaneous parasite of the raccoon, and *D. repens*, a subcutaneous parasite of dogs and cats in Europe, Africa, and Asia, cause subcutaneous dirofilariasis in humans. Each of these species is probably transmitted to humans by mosquitoes.

Before reaching maturity, the infective stage of the worm degenerates and provokes an abscess, usually surrounded by a granulomatous perimeter. The most common site is the subcutaneous tissue of the trunk, but the conjunctiva, eyelid, scrotum, and breast can also be affected. Clinically a subcutaneous tender nodule gradually enlarges for several weeks. Microscopically, a central abscess contains a single coiled worm. Older lesions are granulomatous. The diagnosis is made by identifying the worm in a biopsy specimen.

Diseases Caused by Other Nematodes

Dracunculiasis

Dracunculiasis, an infection with *Dracunculus medinensis*, the guinea worm, is transmitted in drinking water contaminated with the intermediate host, a microscopic crustacean of the genus *Cyclops*. It is common in Africa, the Middle East, and India.

The adult female *D. medinensis* lives in subcutaneous tissue. About a year after infection systemic symptoms of erythema and a pruritic urticarial rash appear. A few hours later a reddish papule, often around the ankles, appears and vesiculates. Beneath this sterile blister is the anterior end of the female. When the blister comes into contact with water it bursts, and the female worm partially emerges, spewing thousands of larvae into the water. These infect the intermediate host.

Because blisters often cause secondary infections (including tetanus), and because dead worms provoke an intense inflammatory response, dracunculiasis is a debilitating disease. Treatment is by manual removal of the worms or antihelminthic drugs.

Capillariasis

Capillariasis is an infection by *Capillaria philippinensis*, *C. hepatica*, or *C. aerophila*. *C. philippinensis* causes a malabsorption enteropathy that may be severe and even fatal. Infection with *C. hepatica* presents the clinical picture of acute or subacute hepatitis with hypereosinophilia. *C. aerophila* causes acute bronchitis, bronchiolitis, asthma, and cough.

The life cycle of *C. philippinensis* is not completely known, but infection is probably acquired by ingesting eggs or infective larvae in small fish. The organisms embed in the mucosa of the jejunum and interfere with absorption. Fatal infections are caused by extraordinarily heavy worm burdens. Larvae released from the female cause autoinfection.

In severe infections generalized abdominal pain, diarrhea, and pronounced borborygmi are followed by nausea and vomiting and intractable diarrhea, leading to severe malabsorption, cachexia, and death. The combination of muscular wasting and loss of body fat makes intestinal peristalsis visible and outlines muscles and tendons through the skin. The mortality ranges from 7% to 20%. At autopsy the small intestine is indurated, thickened, and distended with fluid. One liter of fluid may contain 200,000 adults and larvae. Adults, larvae and eggs of *C. philippinensis* are in the crypts and lamina propria of the duodenum, jejunum, and upper ileum. The diagnosis is made by identifying characteristic *C. philippinensis* eggs in the stool.

C. hepatica is a cosmopolitan parasite of mammals. Adult worms in the definitive host (the rat) deposit eggs in the liver. If this host is eaten by a cat or dog, the eggs pass with the animal feces. Eggs in the soil are eaten by humans and hatch in the small intestine. The larvae penetrate the intestinal wall and migrate to the liver, where they mature. *C. hepatica* in adults are the foci of intense granulomatous reactions. The diagnosis is made by identifying eggs or adult worms in the liver. Mebendazole is the drug of choice.

Trichinosis

Trichinosis, an infection by the nematode *Trichinella spiralis*, is cosmopolitan but is most common in eastern and central Europe, North America, and Central and South America. Although it prevails in areas where pork is eaten, many animals, including dogs, cats, rats, bears, foxes, and wolves, are reservoirs of infection. Humans become infected by eating undercooked or raw meat containing encysted larvae, mainly pork (Fig. 9-73). The cysts, located in striated muscle, are digested, liberating larvae that mature to adult worms that attach to the wall of the small intestine. Female worms there liberate larvae that invade the intestinal wall, enter the circulation, and penetrate striated muscle, where they encyst and remain viable for years.

The clinical features are highly variable, depending on the number of larvae ingested, and patients may be asymptomatic or die of a fulminating disease. In subclinical disease the only sign is eosinophilia. The invasion of muscle by the larvae is associated with muscle pain, swelling of the eyelids and facial edema, eosinophilia, and pronounced fever. Respiratory and neurologic manifestations may appear. Fatal cases are usually attributed to a severe myocarditis. During the chronic phase of the disease the symptoms gradually attenuate.

On invasion of the muscle the larvae cause inflammation and destruction of muscle fibers. A fibrous hyaline layer develops around a single coiled larva. Histiocytes and giant cells may surround the cyst, which eventually calcifies. The most frequently involved muscles are those of the limbs, diaphragm, tongue, jaw, larynx, ribs, and eye. Larvae in other organs, including the heart and brain, cause edema, necrosis, and focal infiltration of neutrophils, eosinophils, and lymphocytes, but they do not encyst.

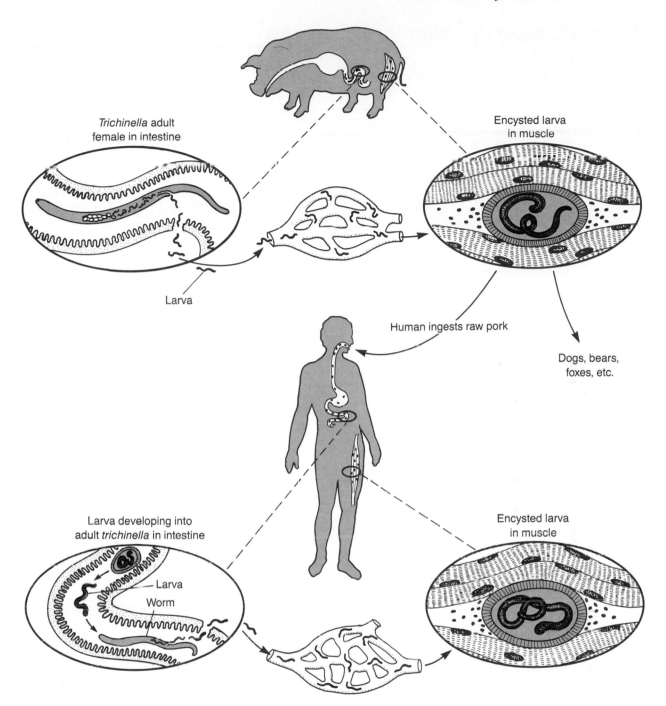

Figure 9-73. Trichinosis. After being ingested by the pig, cysts of *Trichinella* are digested in the gastrointestinal tract, liberating larvae that mature to adult worms. Female worms release larvae that penetrate the intestinal wall, enter the circulation, and lodge in striated muscle, where they encyst. When humans ingest inadequately cooked pork the cycle is repeated, resulting in the muscle disease characteristic of trichinosis.

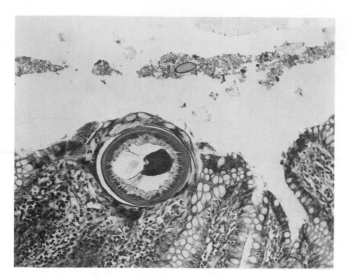

Figure 9-74.   Trichuriasis of the colon. The anterior "whip" end of *T. trichiura* is threaded into the mucosa, beneath the epithelium. A cross section of the worm is shown. There are inflammatory cells in the mucosa. The lumen contains an egg of *T. trichiura*.

The diagnosis is made by identifying larvae in muscle biopsies or by serologic tests. Antihelminthic drugs remove adult worms from the intestine.

Trichuriasis

Trichuriasis, an infection by the nematode *Trichuris trichiura* (the whipworm), is cosmopolitan but is more common and more severe in tropical and subtropical regions, where children are especially susceptible. Adult worms live in the cecum and upper colon, where they attach to the intestinal epithelium. Female worms discharge eggs that pass in the feces. Eggs embryonate in moist soil and become infective in about 3 weeks. Man is infected by ingesting eggs in contaminated soil, food, or drink. Eggs in the gut hatch larvae that grow and eventually mature into adult worms in the colon.

Most patients have light infections and are asymptomatic, but heavy infections cause abdominal pain, diarrhea, bloody stools, and anemia. *T. trichiura* may also obstruct the lumen of the appendix and cause acute appendicitis. Persistent diarrhea leads to weakness, dehydration, and emaciation. Edema of the face and hands, dyspnea, cardiac dilation, and convulsions have all been noted in fatal infections.

The adult worms thread their anterior (whip) end into the colonic mucosa just beneath the epithelium (Fig. 9-74), causing edema and inflammation.

The diagnosis is made by finding eggs in the stool or, occasionally, by identifying adult worms in paraffin sections of vermiform appendix or colon. Mebendazole is effective.

Ancylostomiasis

Ancylostomiasis is an infection of man by one of two hookworms, *Ancylostoma duodenale* or *Necator americanus*. Ancylostomiasis is encountered worldwide and causes serious public health problems across vast areas of the globe. In fact both *A. duodenale* ("Old World" hookworm) and *N. americanus* ("American" hookworm) prevail on most continents and have overlapping epidemiologic boundaries. In general, however, *A. duodenale* is rare in the Western Hemisphere, Australia, and Africa, where *N. americanus* is common. Likewise, *A. duodenale* is common around the Mediterranean, where there is no infection by *N. americanus*. Both species are common in Southeast Asia.

Tropical areas with poor sanitation are ideal for transmission. Warm, moist, sandy soil with adequate shade from direct sunlight favors survival of the soil-borne infective larvae. They may live for several months in soil either as infective filariform larvae or as free-living rhabdoid larvae and adults. On contact with human skin, filariform larvae penetrate the epidermis and enter the venous circulation. They are then swept through the right heart and into the pulmonary capillaries. Here they break through vessels into alveolar spaces, migrate to the epiglottis, are coughed up, and then swallowed. They molt in the duodenum, attach to the mucosal wall with toothlike buccal plates, clamp off a section of the villus, and ingest it (Fig. 9-75). Infection causes three main syndromes: a dermatitis when larvae penetrate the skin, a pneumonitis when larvae migrate through the lung, and severe iron deficiency anemia from loss of blood caused by the adult worms biting of bits of intestinal mucosa.

The diagnosis is confirmed by identifying eggs of *A. duodenale* or *N. americanus* in stool. Adult worms also pass with feces. The drug of choice is mebendazole.

Strongyloidiasis

Strongyloidiasis, an infection by the nematode *Strongyloides stercoralis*, is encountered worldwide but is most common in tropical climates. Epidemics may develop in institutions where personal hygiene is poor, such as hospitals for the mentally ill. *S. stercoralis* is a complex organism that has three life cycles. In one, parasitic parthenogenic females live in the human small intestine and lay eggs that hatch in the mucosal epithelium, releasing rhabdoid larvae. These larvae become infective within the intestine or on the perianal skin and invade human hosts directly (the

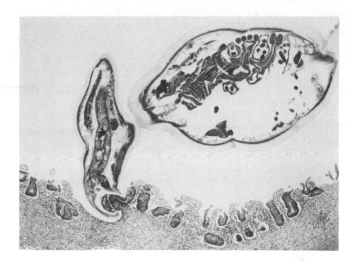

Figure 9-75. Ancylostomiasis of the ileum. Shown are two sections of a single adult worm, *Ancylostoma duodenale,* not connected in this plane of section. A plug of mucosa is in the buccal cavity of the hookworm.

autoinfection cycle). Alternatively, rhabdoid larvae pass in the feces, become infective larvae in the soil, and later penetrate human skin (the direct development cycle). In the third possible cycle (the indirect development cycle), rhabdoid larvae passed in the feces become free-living adults in the soil and eventually produce infective larvae. These infective larvae penetrate the skin, enter blood vessels, and pass to the lungs, where they invade alveolar spaces. They ascend the trachea, descend the esophagus, and mature to become parthenogenetic females in the small intestine.

Invading larvae cause transient dermatitis. Larvae migrating through the lungs may provoke cough, hemoptysis, and dyspnea, but most infections do not lead to pulmonary symptoms. Severe infection of the intestine is debilitating and causes vomiting, diarrhea, and constipation. This is often associated with the autoinfective cycle. In patients with suppressed immunity, infective larvae are more likely to penetrate the intestinal mucosa and invade the body. This "hyperinfection" strongyloidiasis may cause malabsorption and hypoproteinemia with anasarca, and may be severe enough to kill the patient. Obstruction from paralytic ileus and from thickening and immobility of the colon are characteristic of persistent hyperinfection.

Female worms and rhabdoid larvae living in jejunal crypts (Fig. 9-76) cause mild eosinophilia and chronic inflammation. By contrast, patients with hyperinfection may have ulceration, edema, congestion, fibrosis, and severe inflammation of the intestine. In such cases, filariform larvae invade both the small and large intestine and may travel to any organ.

Larvae in tissues may cause no reaction or may provoke microabscesses or granulomas.

The diagnosis is made by identifying larvae in the stool. Larvae may occasionally be in sputum, pleural effusions and urine. Chemotherapy is generally unsatisfactory, but thiabendazole may be useful.

Visceral Larva Migrans

Visceral larva migrans, also known as toxocariasis, is an infection of deep organs by helminthic larvae migrating in aberrant hosts. Toxocariasis is a sporadic disease, primarily of young children, that is often found in areas where there are overcrowded dwellings, dogs, and cats. *Toxocara* species are the most common cause of visceral larva migrans, but other parasites, such as *Ancylostoma, Strongyloides, Baylisascaris* (Nematoda), *Spirometra* (Crestoda), and *Alaria* (Trematoda), can also cause the disease.

The typical patient is a child with hypereosinophilia, pneumonitis, and hypergammaglobulinemia. Ocular visceral larva migrans is a distinct entity. The chief complaint is decreased vision in one or both eyes, and failure to treat ocular lesions may lead to retinal detachment. Generally, as with all forms of the disease, the infection is self-limited and symptoms disappear within a year. A presumptive diagnosis can be made serologically. Both diethylcarbamazine and thiabendazole are used to treat visceral larva migrans.

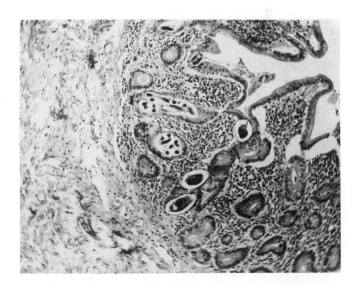

Figure 9-76. Strongyloidiasis, jejunum. The adult worms, larvae, and eggs of *Strongyloides stercoralis* are in the crypts of the glands. The mucosa is infiltrated with lymphocytes, plasma cells, and eosinophils. The patient had a massive infection, and presented with malabsorption syndrome.

Cutaneous Larva Migrans

Cutaneous larva migrans is caused by migration of larval nematodes through the epidermis. The migrating worms provoke severe inflammation, which appears as serpiginous urticarial trails (Fig. 9-77). The names applied to this condition are as varied as the organisms that cause it, and include creeping eruptions, sandworm, plumber's itch, duck hunter's itch, and epidermis linearis migrans. The common larval nematodes are *Strongyloides stercoralis, Ancylostoma brasiliensis, A. caninum, Uncinaria stenocephala, Bunostomum phlebotomum, Necator americanus, Strongyloides myopotami* and *Gnathostoma spinigerum.*

In a condition known as larva currens (creeping eruption), the agent is *Strongyloides stercoralis.* This disorder was first reported in prisoners of war held by the Japanese during World War II. Unlike cutaneous larva migrans, linear urticarial trails in the area of the anus are the only lesions.

Dogs and cats infected with hookworm are the major source of the disease. Outbreaks of cutaneous larva migrans occur at subtropical and tropical beaches. Plumbers who crawl under houses and animal caretakers are also frequently infected. The diagnosis is based on history and clinical appearance. Thiabendazole is the treatment of choice and is effective in either topical or oral preparations.

Angiostrongyliasis

Angiostrongyliasis is infection with *Angiostrongylus cantonensis* (cerebral) or *A. costaricensis* (abdominal). Both are parasites of rats that accidentally infect humans. In East Asia and the Western Hemisphere, rats are infected by eating infective larvae of *A. cantonensis* shed by snails. The larvae migrate to the gray matter of the brain, where they molt before ultimately lodging in a pulmonary artery. After maturation, the worms lay eggs in the lung that hatch in situ. Larvae are coughed up, swallowed, and passed in feces. The life cycle is completed when larvae infect snails, which in turn are eaten by humans. Migrating infective larvae or young adult worms die in and around blood vessels and arteries in the brain and provoke an eosinophilic meningoencephalitis, with a low mortality (less than 1%). The diagnosis is based on the demonstration of *A. cantonensis* in cerebrospinal fluid.

A. costaricensis, found exclusively in Central America, infects the mesenteric veins of rats near the cecum, where it deposits eggs. After hatching, larvae migrate to the fecal stream, pass with the feces, and infect snails or slugs. Infective larvae emerge from

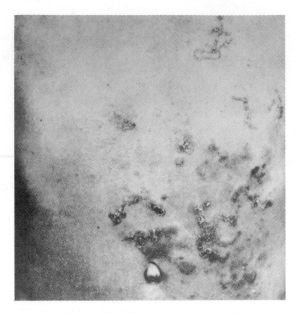

Figure 9-77. Cutaneous larva migrans. The "creeping eruptions" on the surface of the skin are tracks of migrating larvae of *Ancylostoma* species (sandworm).

the snails or slugs on the slime trail. Humans become infected by eating material contaminated with the slime trail. Worms reach maturity in the human host and produce viable progeny. Large nodules composed of scar tissue, eggs, and larvae cause lower right quadrant pain. Surgical excision of the nodules, together with the appendix, relieves the symptoms.

Enterobiasis

Enterobiasis, infection by the nematode *Enterobius vermicularis* (the pinworm), is encountered worldwide but is more frequent in temperate zones. A common helminthic infection in the United States, its prevalence is highest among children and tends to infect certain groups, especially people in institutions. Adult worms live in the lumen of the colon. After copulation gravid females migrate through the anus to deposit embryonated eggs on the perianal and perineal skin. These eggs are immediately infective and require no development in soil or an intermediate host. Humans become infected by ingesting the infective eggs from contaminated hands, clothing, food, and fomites. Ingested eggs hatch in the intestine, releasing larvae that develop into adult worms in the colon.

Some patients are asymptomatic, but most complain of anal pruritus. Scratching may cause perianal dermatitis, eczema, and secondary bacterial infections. Although a benign infection, adult worms may cause minute colonic ulcers and mild inflammation. Rare but serious complications arise when female worms migrate through the vagina, uterus, and fallopian tube, and reach the peritoneum and omentum. In these extraintestinal sites the worms die and provoke a granulomatous reaction.

The diagnosis is made by identifying eggs in the perianal area, using various swab techniques. Eggs are not usually found in feces. Antihelminthic drugs are effective.

Ascariasis

Ascariasis, infection by the large intestinal roundworm *Ascaris lumbricoides*, is cosmopolitan and probably **the most common helminthic infection.** Infection is more common in the tropics, in children, and in crowded rural communities with poor sanitation. Adult worms live in the small intestine, where gravid females discharge eggs that pass in the feces. Eggs develop in warm moist soil to become infective in 3 to 4 weeks. The eggs hatch when ingested, and the larvae penetrate the intestinal wall, enter the portal circulation, pass through the liver and heart, reach the lungs, and develop into third-stage larvae. The larvae migrate up the trachea and down the esophagus, reaching the small intestine, where they develop into adult worms. Humans acquire the infection by ingesting infective eggs in contaminated soil, food, or water.

Most patients have few or no symptoms. Infection with a few adult worms causes only vague abdominal pain, but heavy infections may cause vomiting, malnutrition, appendicitis, and sometimes intestinal obstruction (Fig. 9-78)

Adult worms in the small intestine usually cause no changes, but when worms migrate into the ampulla of Vater or the pancreatic or biliary ducts, they cause biliary obstruction, acute pancreatitis, suppurative cholangitis, and liver abscesses. Eggs deposited in the liver or other tissues produce necrosis, granulomatous inflammation, and fibrosis. *Ascaris* pneumonia, which is occasionally fatal, develops when larvae migrate within alveolar walls, air sacs, bronchioles, and bronchi. The exudate is composed of eosinophils, macrophages, and fibrin.

The diagnosis of ascariasis is made by identifying eggs in the feces. Occasionally, adult worms may pass with the stool or even emerge from nose or mouth. Ascaricidal drugs are effective.

Anisakiasis

Anisakiasis is infection by ascarid larvae of the genera *Anisakis, Phocanema, Terranova,* and *Contracaecum.* Aniskiasis is contracted when inadequately cooked fish containing these nematode larvae are eaten. Popular foods containing viable larvae are pickled herring in Scandinavian countries, sashimi in Japan, and cod, flounder, and tuna from the east coast of the United States. Nematodes causing anisakiasis have a marine mammal as the definitive host.

In humans the larvae penetrate the wall of the throat, stomach, intestine, or colon. Intestinal discomfort begins a few hours after eating the fish. Larvae are released from the muscle of the fish, penetrate the gastric or intestinal mucosa, or become attached in the throat without invasion of tissue. Infection is diagnosed after surgical intervention for intestinal obstruction or peritonitis, which is caused by necrotizing, eosinophilic, granulomatous inflammation. Worms in the throat or stomach are frequently vomited or coughed up, and a common clinical presentation is a wriggling sensation in the throat, with larvae appearing in the mouth of an alarmed patient.

Intestinal anisakiasis clinically resembles appendicitis, with right lower quadrant pain, nausea and vomiting. Continued migration to omentum or mes-

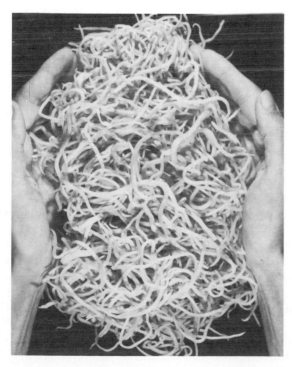

Figure 9-78. Ascariasis. This mass of over 800 worms *Ascaris lumbricoides* obstructed and infarcted the ileum of a 2-year-old girl in South Africa who died before she could be treated.

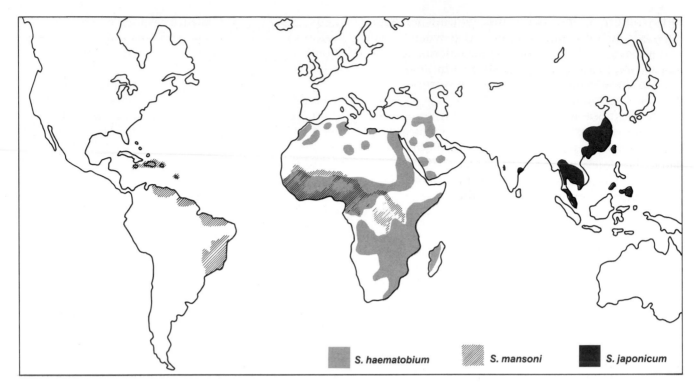

Figure 9-79. Distribution of schistosomiasis caused by *Schistosoma mansoni, S. haematobium,* and *S. japonicum.*

entery is common. Worms lodge in and thicken the gastric or bowel wall.

The identification of larvae provides the diagnosis. Infections of the small intestine, cecum, or colon are usually not diagnosed before exploratory laparotomy. Removal of worms relieves the symptoms.

Diseases Caused by Trematodes

Schistosomiasis

Schistosomiasis (bilharziasis) is a parasitic infection by flukes (trematodes) of three principal species, namely *Schistosoma haematobium, S. mansoni,* and *S. japonicum.* Since the intermediate hosts are freshwater snails, the geographic distribution of schistosomiasis depends on the presence of snails and opportunities for infection of both snail and humans. **Schistosomiasis is increasing in prevalence, affecting about 10% of the world's population and ranking second only to malaria as a cause of morbidity and mortality.** *S. haematobium* is found in large regions of tropical Africa and parts of Southwest Asia, *S. mansoni* in much of tropical Africa, parts of Southwest Asia, South America, and the Caribbean islands, and

S. japonicum in parts of Japan, China, the Philippines, India, and several countries in Southeast Asia (Fig. 9-79).

The schistosomes have complicated life cycles, alternating between asexual generations in the invertebrate host (snail) and sexual generations in the vertebrate host (Fig. 9-80). A schistosome egg hatches in fresh water, liberating a miracidium that penetrates a snail, where it develops through two stages of mother and daughter sporocyst to form the final larval stage, the cercaria. The cercaria escapes from the snail into fresh water and penetrates the skin of the human host, during which process it loses its forked tail and becomes a schistosomule. The shistosomule migrates through tissues, penetrates a blood vessel, and is carried to the lung and subsequently to the liver. In hepatic portal venules the schistosomules mature, forming pairs of male and female worms, with the female lying in the gynecophoral canal of the male worm. The "worm pairs" migrate to the small venules, where the female worm deposits immature eggs. *S. mansoni* and *S. japonicum* lay eggs in the intestine and *S. haematobium* in the urinary bladder. Embryos develop during the passage of eggs through the tissues, and the larvae are mature when the eggs pass through the wall of the intestine or the urinary bladder. The eggs hatch in fresh water and liberate miracidia, thus completing the cycle.

Penetration of the skin by cercariae may cause dermatitis. In acute schistosomiasis, symptoms begin 2 to 4 weeks after exposure to cercariae. The patient becomes febrile and frequently has a cough, asthma, hives, and dysentery, with a severe eosinophilia. If the patient survives, the acute phase tapers to an intermediate asymptomatic period. Months to years later, the clinical features of chronic schistosomiasis develop. The lesions of schistosomiasis vary in severity from insignificant to fatal, the latter occurring in only a small proportion of those infected. The chronic lesions reflect the sites of deposition of the eggs—namely, the bladder with *S. haematobium*, and the intestine and liver with *S. mansoni* and *S. japonicum*. **The basic lesion is a circumscribed granuloma around an egg, or a diffuse cellular infiltrate around it, mainly eosinophils and neutrophils.** In some granulomas an amorphous eosinophilic material (Splendore-Hoeppli substance) surrounds the eggs. Eggs of *S. haematobium* and *S. japonicum* often become calcified and surrounded by hyalinized scar tissue. Adult schistosomes provoke no inflammation while alive in the veins. Dead worms, however, dislodge and cause large focal lesions. For example, worms killed by schistosomicidal drugs may become entangled as "verminous emboli" and be swept from the portal veins to the liver or lungs, where they provoke intense reactions.

Intestinal schistosomiasis caused by *S. mansoni* and *S. japonicum* is associated with granulomas in the lamina propria and submucosa. In heavy infections by *S. mansoni* inflammatory polyps of the colon contain eggs. Eggs that fail to exit the body through the intestine are carried through the portal veins to the liver, where they provoke granulomas and fibrosis (Fig. 9-81). Gradually, broad tracts of portal scar tissue, so-called **pipestem fibrosis,** become obvious on gross examination of the liver (Fig. 9-82). Portal hypertension frequently complicates schistosomal pipestem fibrosis and leads to splenomegaly and other complications.

Urogenital schistosomiasis is caused by *S. haematobium*. Eggs are most numerous in the bladder, ureters, and seminal vesicles, but they may also reach the lungs, colon, and appendix. Numerous eggs in the urinary bladder and ureters lead to a granulomatous reaction, with evolution of polypoid patches. Eggs in the ureter can cause obstructive uropathy. **There is a high incidence of carcinoma of the bladder in patients with urogenital schistosomiasis.**

The diagnosis is made by finding characteristic schistosome eggs in the urine or feces, or in tissue sections. Chemotherapy is now highly effective.

Clonorchiasis

Humans acquire clonorchiasis—infection by *Clonorchis sinensis* (Chinese liver fluke)—by eating raw or undercooked fish. Adult worms are flat and transparent, live in the bile ducts, and pass eggs to the intestine and the feces. After ingestion by an appropriate snail, the egg hatches in a miracidium. Cercariae escape from the snail and seek out certain fish, which they penetrate and in which they encyst. When human hosts eat the fish the cercariae emerge in the duodenum, enter the common bile duct through the ampulla of Vater, and mature in the distal bile ducts to an adult fluke. The symptoms vary from mild to severe, depending on the number of flukes. An onset with chills and fever indicates bacterial infection from biliary obstruction. Patients with clonorchiasis may die from a variety of complications, including biliary obstruction, bacterial cholangitis, pancreatitis, and cholangiocarcinoma.

With massive infection the liver may be up to three times normal size. Dilated bile ducts are seen through the capsule, and the cut surface is punctuated with thick-walled, dilated bile ducts (Fig. 9-83). The flukes, sometimes in the thousands, can be expressed from the bile ducts. Microscopically, the epithelium lining the ducts is initially hyperplastic and then becomes metaplastic. The surrounding stroma is fibrotic. Secondary bacterial infection is common and associated with pus in the bile ducts. Eggs deposited in the hepatic parenchyma are surrounded by a fibrous and granulomatous reaction. Masses of eggs become lodged in the bile ducts and cause a cholangitis. The pancreatic ducts may also be invaded and become dilated, thickened, lined by metaplastic epithelium, and eventually surrounded by scar.

The diagnosis is made by identifying the eggs of *C. sinensis* in stools or in duodenal aspirates. Treatment is with praziquantel.

Cholangiocellular carcinoma, originating in either the intra- or extrahepatic bile ducts, is a complication of clonorchiasis. The similar liver fluke endemic in Thailand, *Opisthorchis viverrini*, also causes cholangiocellular carcinoma.

Paragonimiasis

Paragonimiasis is infection by the oriental lung fluke *Paragonimus westermani* or by one of several other species of *Paragonimus*. These are the only helminthic parasites of humans that, as adult worms, naturally infect the lungs. Paragonimiasis occurs in Asia, *(Text continued on page 444.)*

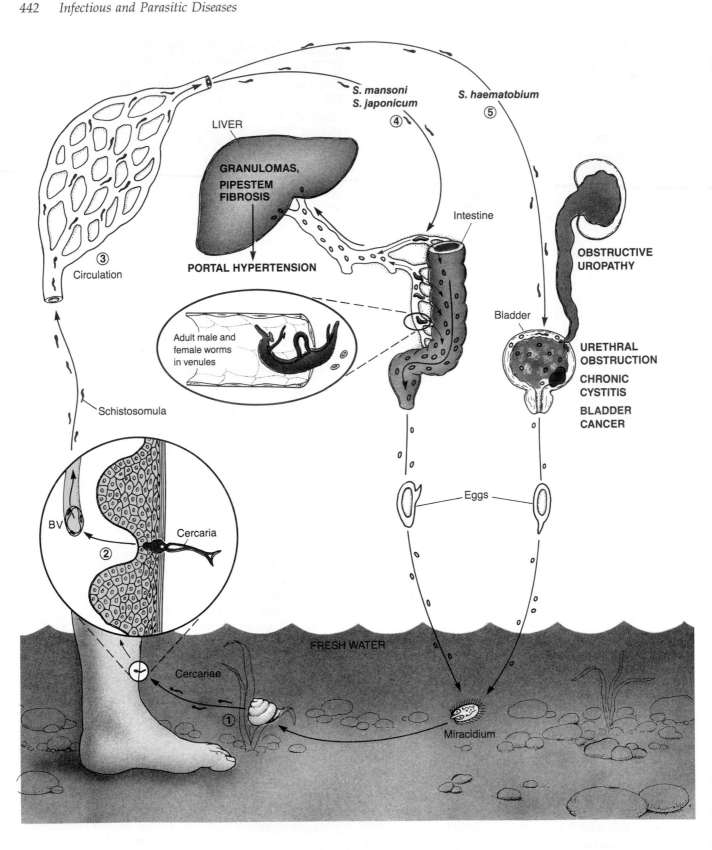

LIVER

GRANULOMAS, PIPESTEM FIBROSIS

PORTAL HYPERTENSION

③ Circulation

S. mansoni
S. japonicum

S. haematobium

④

⑤

Intestine

Adult male and female worms in venules

Bladder

OBSTRUCTIVE UROPATHY

URETHRAL OBSTRUCTION

CHRONIC CYSTITIS

BLADDER CANCER

Schistosomula

BV

Cercaria

②

Eggs

FRESH WATER

Cercariae

①

Miracidium

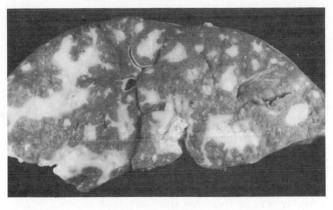

Figure 9-82. Schistosomiasis *(Schistosoma japonicum)* of liver, showing characteristic pipestem fibrosis.

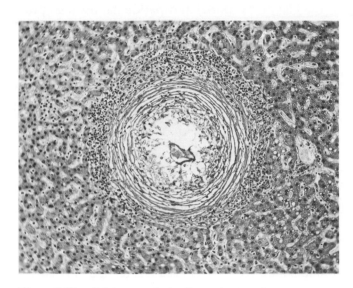

Figure 9-81. Schistosomiasis, liver. A granuloma in a portal tract of the liver surrounds a degenerating egg of *Schistosoma mansoni.*

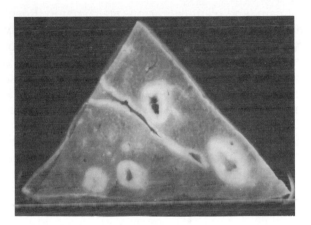

Figure 9-83. Clonorchiasis of liver. The bile ducts are greatly thickened and dilated because of the presence of adult flukes *(Clonorchis sinensis)* in the ducts.

Figure 9-80. Life cycle of *Schistosoma* and clinical features of schistosomiasis. The schistosome egg hatches in water, liberates a miracidium that penetrates a snail, and develops through two stages to sporocyst to form the final larval stage, the cercaria. (*l*) The cercaria escapes from the snail into water, "swims," and penetrates the skin of a human host. (2) The cercaria loses its forked tail to become a schistosomule, which migrates through tissues, penetrates a blood vessel, and (3) is carried to the lung and later to the liver. In hepatic portal venules the schistosomule becomes sexually mature and forms pairs, each with a male and a female worm, the female worm lying in the gynecophoral canal of the male worm. The organism causes lesions in the liver, including granulomas, portal ("pipestem") fibrosis, and portal hypertension. (4) The female worm deposits immature eggs in small venules of the intestine and rectum *(S. mansoni,* and *S. japonicum)* or (5) of the urinary bladder *(S. haematobium).* The bladder infestation leads to obstructive uropathy, ureteral obstruction, chronic cystitis, and bladder cancer. Embryos develop during passage of the eggs through tissues, and larvae are mature when eggs pass through the wall of the intestine or urinary bladder. Eggs hatch in water and liberate miracidia to complete the cycle.

Africa, and South America. Human hosts acquire the infection by eating raw infected crustaceans.

Paragonimus eggs are coughed up from the lungs, swallowed, and passed in the stool. Miracidia emerge in water and infect a molluscan intermediate host, after which a sporocyst and a generation of redia develop in the mollusc. Infective cercariae emerge and penetrate the gills of a crustacean. The larvae migrate to soft tissue and encyst. After a human host ingests the cyst a metacercaria emerges and penetrates the wall of the stomach, migrates to the diaphragm, bores through the pleura, and settles in the lung, where it matures into an adult worm, which survives for 20 years.

The clinical onset of pulmonary paragonimiasis is insidious, with a diagnostic triad of cough, hemoptysis, and eggs in sputa or stool. Night sweats, severe chest pain, and pleural effusions are common. Roentgenograms reveal transient diffuse pulmonary infiltrates. Although the adult worms cause pulmonary disease, the larvae occasionally produce lesions at ectopic sites, such as the brain, liver, gut, skeletal muscle, testes, and lymph nodes. The prognosis in pulmonary paragonimiasis is good, but ectopic lesions of brain are often fatal, even with aggressive treatment. The worms provoke leukocytic infiltrates and, later, fibrous encapsulation. Gravid female worms begin to lay eggs at about 70 days. Cavities that form around the eggs contain worms, eggs, and necrotic debris. When these cavities perforate into a bronchiole or bronchus, the eggs are coughed up or become lodged in the lung and provoke fibrosis.

Pulmonary paragonimiasis is frequently misdiagnosed as tuberculosis. Eggs in sputa or stools provide the definitive diagnosis. In pleural paragonimiasis, the pleura must be aspirated to obtain eggs. Praziquantel, the drug of choice, is effective against pulmonary paragonimiasis.

Fascioliasis

Fascioliasis is infection by *Fasciola hepatica*, the sheep liver fluke. Humans may acquire the infection wherever sheep are raised. The eggs, passed by the sheep in their feces, require 2 weeks in fresh water before a miracidium emerges. Miracidia infect a molluscan intermediate host (lymnaeid snails), after which infective cercariae emerge from the snail, and encyst on submerged vegetation. Humans become infected by eating vegetation, such as water cress, that is contaminated by the cysts. Metacercariae excyst in the duodenum, pass through the wall into the peritoneal cavity, penetrate the liver, and migrate through the hepatic parenchyma into the bile ducts. The larvae mature to adults and live in both the intrahepatic and extrahepatic bile ducts. Later, the adult flukes penetrate the wall of the bile ducts and wander back into liver parenchyma, where they feed on liver cells and deposit their eggs. The eggs lead to abscess formation, followed by a granuloma. The worms induce hyperplasia of the lining epithelium of the bile ducts, portal and periductal fibrosis, proliferation of bile ductules, and varying degrees of biliary obstruction. Eosinophilia, vomiting, and acute epigastric pain are features. Severe untreated infections may be fatal. Early diagnosis and aggressive treatment with praziquantel prevents irreparable damage to liver.

The diagnosis is made by recovering eggs from stools or from the biliary tract.

Fasciolopsiasis

Fasciolopsiasis, an infection by *Fasciolopsis buski*, the giant intestinal fluke, prevails throughout most of the Orient. Humans, the definitive hosts, acquire fasciolopsiasis by eating uncooked aquatic vegetables contaminated with the encysted cercariae of *F. buski*.

The worm is huge (3 × 7 cm) and attaches to the duodenal or jejunal wall. The point of attachment may ulcerate and become infected, causing pain that resembles that of a peptic ulcer. Acute symptoms may be caused by intestinal obstruction or by toxins released by large numbers of worms. The diagnosis is made by identifying the eggs of *F. buski*, which are similar to those of *F. hepatica*, in the stool. Treatment is with praziquantel.

Diseases Caused by Cestodes

Echinococcosis (Hydatid Disease)

Echinococcosis is a zoonotic infection caused by larval cestodes (tapeworms) of the genus *Echinococcus*. The most common offender is *E. granulosus* (cystic hydatid disease). Rarely, *E. multilocularis* (alveolar hydatid disease) and *E. vogeli* (polycystic hydatid disease) infect humans.

Figure 9-84 illustrates the life cycle of *E. granulosus*. The adult tapeworms are 2 to 6 mm long and live in the small intestine of a carnivorous host such as the wolf, fox, coyote, jackal, or dog. The tapeworm has a scolex with suckers and numerous hooklets for attachment to the intestinal mucosa. A short neck is followed by three segments or "proglottids" (one immature, one mature, and one gravid proglottid). The terminal, gravid proglottid breaks off and releases eggs, which are eliminated in the feces of the

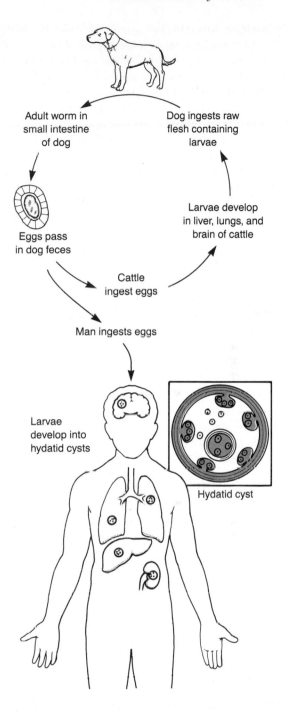

Figure 9-84. Life cycle of *Echinococcus granulosus* and cystic hydatid disease. The adult cestode lives in the small intestine of a dog (the definitive host). A gravid proglottid ruptures, releasing cestode eggs into the dog's feces. Cestode eggs are ingested by cattle or sheep (the intermediate hosts), hatch in the intestine, and release oncospheres that penetrate the wall of the gut, enter the bloodstream, disseminate to various deep organs, and grow to form hydatid cysts, containing brood capsules and scolices. When another dog ingests raw flesh from the cattle or sheep, the scolices are ingested and develop into mature worms in the dog's intestine to complete the cycle. A person who ingests cestode eggs in contaminated plant material becomes an accidental intermediate host. The larvae increase in size, but the parasite reaches a "dead-end" without developing into an adult tapeworm. Hydatid cysts in humans occur predominantly in the liver, but may also involve lung, kidney, brain, and other organs.

carnivore. Contaminated herbage is then eaten by herbivorous intermediate hosts, such as deer, moose, antelopes, sheep, cattle, and humans. Larvae released from the eggs penetrate the wall of the gut, enter the blood stream, and disseminate to deep organs, where they grow to form hydatid cysts containing brood capsules and scolices. When the flesh of the intermediate host, the herbivore, is eaten raw by a carnivore, the scolices develop into sexually mature worms in the intestine of the definitive host, thereby completing the cycle. Humans become infected by ingesting plant material contaminated by cestode eggs (see Fig. 9-84). Cystic hydatid disease (due to *E. granulosus*) is common in sheep- and cattle-raising areas of Australia, New Zealand, and East Africa, many Mediterranean and Middle Eastern countries, and several South American countries.

E. multilocularis causes alveolar hydatid disease in humans. The wild definitive host—the wolf, fox, and coyote—are predators of the intermediate hosts, the field mouse, mole, shrew, and lemming. Dogs and cats are domestic definitive hosts, and the domestic intermediate host is the house mouse. There have been rare cases of human infection by *E. multilocularis* in Germany, Switzerland, China, and the U.S.S.R.

Wild dogs are definitive hosts for *E. vogeli* and are predators of certain field rats. No domestic intermediate hosts other than humans have been reported. Nevertheless, humans may become accidental intermediate hosts for *E. vogeli*, probably by ingesting eggs from domestic dogs. Polycystic hydatid disease has been reported in Central and South America, from Panama to Paraguay.

Echinococcosis is most common in the liver but also involves the lung and, less commonly, the brain, kidney, spleen, muscle, soft tissues, and bone. The larvae enlarge in situ to become cysts, which grow "silently" for years, usually producing no symptoms until they reach a size of 10 cm or more.

The inflammatory cell infiltrate around cysts in the liver or lung includes lymphocytes, plasma cells, and eosinophils. The cyst wall exhibits an inner hyalinized layer and outer vascular fibrous tissue. Because of their size hydatid cysts of the liver often produce hepatomegaly, and since they compress adjacent structures, such as intrahepatic bile ducts, they may lead to obstructive jaundice. Rupture of a cyst may provoke an acute hypersensitivity reaction, including anaphylaxis, to released antigens. A major complication of rupture is the seeding of adjacent tissues with brood capsules and scolices. When these "seeds" grow, they produce many additional cysts, each with the growth potential of the original cyst. Traumatic rupture of hydatid cysts of abdominal organs results in severe diffuse pain resembling that of peritonitis, and a ruptured cyst in the lung may cause pneumothorax and empyema.

The "unilocular" hydatid cyst of *E. granulosus* is a gelatinous fluid-filled sphere that varies from a few millimeters to many centimeters in diameter. Microscopically, the 1-mm, finely laminated cyst wall is lined internally by a germinal layer from which brood capsules and scolices develop. Fluid aspirated from the cyst often contains "hydatid sand" consisting of free daughter cysts and free scolices. "Multilocular" cysts of *E. multilocularis* involve only the liver. Their laminated membrane is not confining (in contrast to the unilocular cysts of *E. granulosus*), and the cysts spread by budding infiltrative growth, the "alveolar" pattern. This infection may clinically be mistaken for hepatocellular carcinoma. These multilocular cysts grow very slowly, and infected persons may remain asymptomatic for decades. At surgery, the hepatic cysts in early cases appear as yellow-gray masses, whereas in advanced cases pus-filled cysts occupy a large part of the liver. The multilocular cysts are usually sterile and display only an external laminated membrane, without a germinal layer, brood capsules, or scolices.

"Polycystic" hydatid cysts of *E. vogeli* have been found in the liver, lung, heart, intercostal muscles, diaphragm, stomach, omentum, and mesentery. Clinical symptoms include hepatomegaly, jaundice, and palpable peritoneal masses. Radiography demonstrates polycystic structures in the peritoneal cavity with diffuse mineralization. These cysts have been misdiagnosed as hepatic tumors or abscesses, cirrhosis, gastric tumors, and chondrosarcomas of the rib. The larvae reside in fluid or gel-containing polycystic structures. Individual cysts are about 1 cm in diameter, and aggregates several centimeters across may form. The cysts may be so extensive that they replace most of the liver. Microscopically, multiple vesicles (a few millimeters to a few centimeters across) are partitioned by septa formed from the hyaline laminated membrane. This endogenous proliferation of the germinal membrane to form septa is unique to *E. vogeli* (proliferation of germinal membrane is exogenous for *E. multilocularis*). A germinal membrane that lines the septum contains calcareous corpuscles. Brood capsules bud internally from the septate germinal membrane, and scolices develop from the walls of the brood capsules. Portions of the cysts are frequently necrotic and mineralized, and hooklets and calcareous corpuscles may be the only larval structures that can be identified.

The diagnosis of echinococcosis is made by identifying the unilocular, multilocular, or polycystic hydatid cyst. No effective drug has been established for echinococcosis, although mebendazole has shown mixed results. The treatment of choice is surgical removal of the hydatid cyst(s), taking special care to avoid rupture of the cysts to reduce the chances of seeding and recurrence. Cysts should be sterilized with dilute formalin before drainage or extirpation to prevent anaphylactic shock.

Cysticercosis

Cysticercosis, an infection by the larval stage (bladder worm) of *Taenia solium*, the pork tapeworm, prevails where undercooked pork is eaten. The adult *T. solium* is acquired by eating pork infected with cysticerci—that is, measly pork. Pigs acquire cysticerci by ingesting eggs of *T. solium* shed in human feces. **This normal cycle, although a public health problem, is essentially benign for both humans and pigs. However when humans accidentally ingest the eggs from human feces and become infected with cysticerci, the consequences may be catastrophic.** The eggs release oncospheres, which penetrate the wall of the

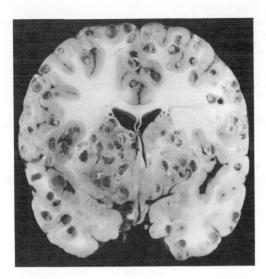

Figure 9-85. Cysticercosis, brain, caused by larvae of the tapeworm *Taenia solium*. The patient died of convulsions caused by the many cysticerci concentrated in the gray matter of the brain.

gut, enter the bloodstream, lodge in tissue, encyst, and differentiate to cysticerci. The cysticercus, a spherical, milky white cyst about 1 cm in diameter, contains fluid and an invaginated scolex with birefringent hooklets. The cysticerci remain viable for an indefinite period and provoke no inflammation but compress adjacent tissue as they grow. The cysticercus dies, leading to a granulomatous reaction with eosinophils, after which the lesion becomes scarred and calcified. Cysticerci in the retina blind the patient. Massive cysticercosis of the brain causes convulsions and death (Fig. 9-85), and in the heart may cause arrhythmias and sudden death.

An aberrant cysticercus, called racemose cysticercus, can also be fatal. It is sterile (without a scolex) and limited to the brain, and has an arborizing growth that produces a large, grapelike mass several centimeters in diameter.

The diagnosis is made from the morphology of the excised cyst. Serologic tests are helpful but do not exclude echinococcosis. A history of tapeworm infection in the patient is significant because autoinfection is possible. Treatment of muscle disease is with praziquantel.

Diseases Caused by Arthropods

The phylum Arthropoda contains many animals of medical importance. As previously discussed, mosquitos, for example, cause millions of deaths each year by spreading malaria; fleas altered the history of medieval Europe by spreading plague.

Our focus here, however, is not on arthropods as vectors but as animals that bite, sting, suck, and invade man. Arthropod taxonomy is shown in Table 9-3.

Arachnids (Scorpions, Spiders, Ticks, and Mites)

Scorpions

Scorpions envenomate when accidentally brushed. They invade human dwellings and lurk in shoes, clothing, towels, sinks, and tubs. Most scorpions cannot kill adults, but children may die if stung by a large scorpion. In most cases only local pain results, but severe envenomations cause acute neurologic symptoms, and those who die suffer respiratory paralysis.

Spiders

Spiders are responsible for two distinct entities: systemic arachnidism, caused by tarantulas and black widow spiders; and necrotic arachnidism, caused by brown recluse spiders. Envenomation by a large "hairy" tarantula is more frightening than dangerous. Only the black widow spider (*Lactrodectus* species) inflicts potentially life-threatening bites, but even its bite is usually nonlethal. The victim develops acute local pain and later headaches and dizziness. Abdominal cramps and convulsions follow. Severe cases are characterized by vomiting, cyanosis, irregular heartbeat, and shock. The venom is a nonhemolytic proteinaceous neurotoxin that acts at both adrenergic and cholinergic junctions. Treatment is with antivenom.

The brown recluse spiders, *Loxoceles reclusa* and several other species, are common in South America and the American south and midwest and have a

Table 9-3 Arthropod Taxonomy

Phylum **Arthropoda**
  Subphylum **Chelicerata**
    Class **Arachnida**—spiders, scorpions, ticks, and mites
  Subphylum **Mandibulata**
    Class **Insecta**
      Order **Anoplura**—sucking lice
      Order **Hemiptera**—true bugs
      Order **Coleoptera**—beetles
      Order **Hymenoptera**—bees, wasps, hornets, and ants
      Order **Lepidoptera**—moths and butterflies
      Order **Diptera**—true flies
      Order **Siphonaptera**—fleas
    Class **Diplopoda**—millipedes
    Class **Chilopoda**—centipedes
    Class **Pentastomida**—tongue worms

distinctive violin-shaped mark over the top of the thorax. The spider lives in closets, basements, porches, barns, and sheds. The victims are often women cleaning house. There is an immediate intense pain at the site of the bite. The skin becomes edematous, ischemic, blackened, and dry, after which cutaneous and extensive subcutaneous necrosis occurs over several square centimeters over a period of 20 to 30 days. Healing is slow and disfiguring, a potentially tragic event, since many bites are on the face.

Ticks and Mites

Female ticks feeding on the skin along the spinal column may inject a neurotoxin that causes difficulty in swallowing and breathing, flaccid paralysis, and, rarely, death. Most patients recover when the tick is removed, but deaths within 1 to 4 days have been reported. Little is known of the pathology of "tick paralysis."

Mites cause a variety of dermatoses. One of the most common human parasites is *Demodex folliculorum*, a minute mite that lives in hair follicles of the face. Chiggers, known to most campers, are bright red mites that are barely visible to the naked eye. They take a meal of tissue juices and provoke intensely pruritic inflammatory lesions at the belt line or at other sites where clothing is pulled tightly. *Sarcoptes scabei*, the mites of human sarcoptic mange, live in cutaneous burrows, where rapidly succeeding generations and their feces provoke intense inflammation and, eventually, secondary bacterial infections.

Insects

Anoplura (Sucking Lice)

There are three distinct lice, namely head, body, and pubic lice. These are *Pediculus humanus capitis, P. humanus humanus,* and *Phthirus pubis,* respectively. Each louse causes a unique pediculosis and rarely invades other areas of the body. Head lice deposit nits (eggs) on hair shafts around the back of the neck. Pubic lice place nits on hair of the pubic region and occasionally the axilla, chest, or eyebrows. Body lice lay nits in clothing and bedding. Lice puncture the skin to feed. Each wound, of which there may be many, becomes an intensely pruritic elevated papule. Without treatment, the skin acquires the appearance of sarcoptic mange and may become secondarily infected with bacteria.

The infestation is common among prisoners, wartime soldiers, and the indigent, and is passed from person to person by casual contact, fomites, or sexual intercourse.

Hemiptera (True Bugs)

Bedbugs (Cimicidae) and cone-nosed bugs (Reduviidae, *Triatominae* sp.) are medically important hemipterans. Bedbugs crawl out of hiding places in floors and walls and suck blood from sleeping victims. The bite causes local edema and itching. Some patients develop asthma. Cone-nosed bugs are most important as vectors of South American trypanosomiasis (Chagas' disease), but they also inflict a painful wound in taking a blood meal.

Coleoptera (Beetles)

Beetles cause a variety of human complaints. Canthariasis is temporary infestation of the digestive tract with beetles. Larval beetles have also been seen in the nares, eyes, or urinary tract. More often beetles create a vesicating lesion of skin. So-called blister beetles (Meloidae) contain cantharidin, a volatile terpene. The substance is obtained commercially from *Lytta vesicatoria* and is sold as an aphrodisiac, so-called Spanish fly. Beetles of another family (Staphylinidae), the rove beetles, contain an alkaloid toxin that causes necrotizing cutaneous lesions.

Lepidoptera (Moths and Butterflies)

Lepidopterism is caused by poison hairs that remain on the adult moth after metamorphosis. "Dust" from moths contains these hairs and causes irritation of the eyes, upper respiratory tract and skin. Urticarial skin lesions are produced when the "hairs" penetrate the skin. Dozens of species of caterpillars are armed with poisonous hairs—gypsy moth, nun moth, flannel moth, hickory tiger, and others.

Hymenoptera (Bees, Wasps, Hornets and Ants)

Most people know the sharp pain that follows envenomation by a hymenopteran. The sting subsides within an hour and there are no lingering effects, although in some victims the afflicted limb may swell. The greatest medical significance of stinging hymenopterans is anaphylactic shock in hypersensitive persons. In fact more people in the United States die from bee, wasp, or hornet stings than from any other envenomation.

Ants are also important stinging insects. Fire ants from South America have spread across the southeastern United States during the past 40 years, attacking animals and people who disturb their mounds. Their hemolytic toxin produces a sharply painful burning sensation and later a blister. The toxin is pyogenic and the wound weeps pus. Aggressive stinging ants abound in the tropics. A large black ant in South America (*Paraponera clavata*) produces a 20-cm swelling and agonizing pain.

Diptera (True Flies)

The diptera are divided into blood suckers and non–blood suckers. This is not a taxonomic division, and often divides males and females of the same species. Among the diptera are the vectors of malaria, leishmaniasis, onchocerciasis, mansonelliasis, loiasis, trypanosomiasis, filariasis, and dozens of arboviral diseases. The same dipterans also can afflict humans directly, often attacking in droves and causing an annoying dermatitis. Mosquitos, gnats, and horse flies are serious pests in many parts of the world.

Although filth flies do not suck blood, they are important pests because they act as fomites, carrying diseases from garbage heaps to food. Defecation by humans in open spaces produces a culture medium for maggots, and fecal-borne diseases are made available for transfer.

Myiasis is infection with the larvae of filth flies. Larvae introduced into the subcutis through bites or wounds provoke an intense inflammatory response and are soon surrounded by an eosinophilic abscess, the so-called warble.

Siphonaptera (Fleas)

Although fleas are important vectors of disease they are themselves only a bothersome infestation. However, one species, *Tunga penetrans*, causes a debilitating infection. The 1-mm female burrows into the epidermis and swells to a diameter of 7 mm or more. It feeds on blood and causes an exquisitely painful inflammatory sore, usually on the feet and beneath the toe nails. Secondary infection with tetanus or gas gangrene may be fatal.

T. penetrans is native to South and Central America, where it prefers dry sandy soil, especially beaches. The flea thrives in Africa today. It was purportedly exported to Africa in the sand ballast of an empty slave ship.

Diplopoda (Millipedes)

Millipedes are distinguished from centipedes by having two pairs of legs per segment, whereas centipedes have only one pair. They do not bite, but spray their venom over a distance of several centimeters. On contact with the skin the venom causes acute burning and necrosis of epidermis. Some millipedes have turned up in the gastrointestinal or urinary tracts.

Chilopoda (Centipedes)

Centipedes have fangs on each leg with which they introduce a mild and only moderately painful toxin. Some centipedes occasionally crawl up the nose and become lodged in frontal sinuses. Others have invaded gastrointestinal or urinary tracts, always accidentally. These infections probably occur while the victim is sleeping.

Diseases Caused by Stinging Microorganisms

Marine Invertebrates

The phylum Cnidaria, the coelenterates, contains the hydras, jellyfish, anemones, and corals. The hydras (class Hydrozoa) and jellyfish (class Scyphozoa) include members that cause lesions in humans. Most of these animals cause only minor stings, but a few are capable of killing an adult in a matter of minutes.

Hydrozoa

The hydrozoa are colonies of single-cell organisms that appear as a single animal; the Portuguese Man-O'-War is an example. It is composed of specialized reproductive, digestive, structural, and offensive organisms. Humans are stung when they accidentally brush against this colony, often while it is being destroyed in the surf. Sedentary hydroids ("stinging seaweed") also cause lesions to those coming into contact with the surfaces on which they grow, for example rocks and swimming rafts. Most hydrozoa cause a dermatitis by injecting venom through the offensive cells, the cnidoblasts. The triggered cnidoblast ejects a nematocyst, a barbed threadlike structure that penetrates skin and introduces the toxin, causing the urticarial rash of hydrozoan stings. More severe attacks may be characterized by high fever and eosinophilia.

Table 9-4 Organisms Causing Opportunistic Infections in Patients with AIDS

Protozoa

Pneumocystis carinii	*Cryptosporidium* spp.
Entamoeba histolytica	*Giardia lamblia*
Toxoplasma gondii	*Isospora belli*

Viruses

Cytomegalovirus	Epstein-Barr
Herpes simplex	Molluscum contagiosum (poxvirus)
Varicella-zoster	Polyoma

Fungi

Candida spp.	*Histoplasma capsulatum*
Coccidioides immitis	*Histoplasma duboisii*
Cryptococcus neoformans	*Sporothrix schcenckii*

Bacteria and Mycobacteria

Campylobacter spp.	*Mycobacterium-avium-intracellulare*
Legionella pneumophila	*Mycobacterium tuberculosis*
Listeria monocytogenes	*Actinomyces* spp
Salmonella spp	*Nocardia* spp
Shigella spp	

Scyphozoa (Jellyfish)

The stings of many jellyfish cause local pain, erythema and vesiculation, and, in severe cases, systemic symptoms. Medically, the most important jellyfish are the Cubomedusae ("box-jellies" or "sea wasps"), two species of which, *Chironex fleckeri* and *Chiropsalmus quadrigatus,* cause fatal stings. The lethal box-jellies are most common in shallow waters around North Queensland and the Philippines, where dozens of deaths are recorded. Immediate excruciating pain is followed by death in a few minutes. In survivors the local effects are severe, with edema and vesiculation progressing to full-thickness skin necrosis.

Opportunistic Infections in the Acquired Immune Deficiency Syndrome (AIDS)

The pandemic of acquired immune deficiency syndrome (AIDS), which is characterized by a progressive irreversible depletion of T-helper lymphocytes, predisposes its victims to opportunistic infections and unusual cancers. The cause of the immune dysfunction is the human immunodeficiency virus (HIV—formerly known as human T-cell lymphotropic virus type III/lymphadenopathy-associated virus [HTLV-III/LAV]), which appears to be transmitted by homosexual and, less frequently, heterosexual contact, from mother to child during the perinatal period, and through parenteral exposure to blood or blood products.

Because of the profound defect in cell-mediated immunity, patients with AIDS are susceptible to a wide variety of viral, fungal, bacterial, and parasitic infections (Table 9-4). These opportunistic infections, often numerous and simultaneous, are typically severe, persistent, or relapsing, despite specific therapy.

The pathology of AIDS is divided into three general categories: lymphoid hyperplasia; unusual tumors, most frequently Kaposi's sarcoma or high grade lymphomas; and opportunistic infections.

More than half of the patients develop *P. carinii* pneumonia, and this is often the first opportunistic infection detected. The pneumonia is usually subacute, but in untreated patients it is ultimately fatal.

Persistent or recurrent diarrhea is common, ranging in severity from several loose stools a day, to copious watery diarrhea that may reach 15 liters a day. Causative agents include *Cryptosporidium, Isopora belli, Entamoeba histolytica, Giardia lamblia, Salmonella, Shigella,* and *Campylobacter.* Furthermore, persistent bacteremia is associated with salmonellosis and shigellosis, cryptosporidiosis with sclerosing cholangitis, and isosporiasis with disseminated extraintestinal infections.

T. gondii, an intracellular protozoal coccidian, causes acute, subacute, or chronic necrotizing encephalitis in patients with AIDS. Characteristically, single or multiple intracerebral defects appear on CT scans of brain. Other focal lesions of the brain include lymphomas and infections with mycobacteria, cytomegalovirus, and nocardia species.

Patients with AIDS frequently have clinically significant disseminated cytomegalovirus infections, characterized by pneumonia, enteritis, and chorioretinitis, and other viral diseases, including herpes simplex, herpes zoster, and molluscum contagiosum. Although many patients with AIDS have serologic evidence of reactivated infections with the Epstein-Barr virus (EBV), there are no recognized histopathologic patterns of infection by EBV in these patients. AIDS patients may also develop progressive multifocal leukoencephalopathy, a demyelinating disorder of the central nervous system caused by polyomaviruses.

Patients with AIDS often have oral and esophageal candidiasis. Although candidiasis may be a serious disseminated disease in any debilitated or immunosuppressed patient, widespread visceral dissemination is infrequent in patients with AIDS. Other diseases affecting AIDS patients are relapsing meningoencephalitis caused by *Cryptococcus neoformans,* disseminated histoplasmosis, coccidioidomycosis, and sporotrichosis.

Mycobacterium avium-intracellulare is a ubiquitous environmental saprophyte that rarely caused disseminated infection in adults, regardless of immunologic status, until the AIDS epidemic. Even patients with malignant tumors who developed atypical mycobacterial infections usually were infected by species other than *M. avium-intracellulare.* In AIDS patients, however, disseminated disease caused by *M. avium-intracellulare* is common. Infections with *M. tuberculosis* may also be seen, particularly in patients in less developed countries.

SUGGESTED READING

BOOKS

Baker RD (ed): Human Infection With Fungi, Actinomycetes and Algae. New York, Springer-Verlag, 1971

Beaver PC, Jung RC, Cupp EW: Clinical Parasitology, 9th ed. Philadelphia, Lea & Febiger, 1984

Benenson AS (ed): Control of Communicable Diseases in Man, 14th ed. Washington, DC, The American Public Health Association. 1985

Berquist LM: Changing Patterns of Infectious Diseases. Philadelphia, Lea & Febiger, 1984

Binford CH, Connor, DH (eds): Pathology of Tropical and Extraordinary Diseases. Washington, DC, Armed Forces Institute of Pathology, 1976

Braude AI, Davis CE, Fierer J (eds): Infectious Diseases and Medical Microbiology, 2nd ed. Philadelphia, WB Saunders, 1986

Chandler FW, Kaplan W, Ajello L: Color Atlas and Text of the Histopathology of Mycotic Diseases. Chicago, Year Book Medical Publishers, 1980

Emmons CW, Binford CH, Utz JP, et al: Medical Mycology, 3rd ed. Philadelphia, Lea & Febiger, 1977

Holt JG, Krieg NR (eds): Bergey's Manual of Systematic Bacteriology, vol. 1. Baltimore, Williams & Wilkins, 1984

Holt JG, Sneath PHA (eds): Bergey's Manual of Systematic Bacteriology, vol 2. Baltimore, Williams & Wilkins, 1986

Joklik WK, Willett HP, Amos DB (eds): Zinsser Microbiology, 18th ed. Norwalk, CT, Appleton-Century-Crofts, 1984

Marcial-Rojas RA (ed): Pathology of Protozoal and Helminthic Diseases, with Clinical Correlation. Baltimore, Williams & Wilkins, 1971

Meyerowitz RL: The Pathology of Opportunistic Infections—With Pathogenetic, Diagnostic and Clinical Correlations. New York, Raven Press, 1983

Mims CA: The Pathogenesis of Infectious Disease. New York, Grune & Stratton, 1976

Mulligan HW (ed): The African Trypanosomiases. New York, John Wiley & Sons, 1970

Rippon JW: Medical Mycology: The Pathogenic Fungi and the Pathogenic Actinomycetes, 2nd ed. Philadelphia, WB Saunders, 1982

Sasa M: Human Filariasis: A Global Survey of Epidemiology and Control. Baltimore, University Park Press, 1976

Strickland GT (ed): Hunter's Tropical Medicine, 6th ed. Philadelphia, WB Saunders, 1984

ARTICLES

Britigan BE, Cohen MS, Sparling PF: Gonococcal infections: A model of molecular pathogenesis. N Engl J Med 312:1683, 1985

Connor DH, George GH, Gibson DW: Pathologic changes of human onchocerciasis—implications for future research. Rev Infect Dis 7:809, 1985

Gibson DW, Heggie C, Connor DH: Clinical and pathologic aspects of onchocerciasis. Pathol Annu 15(2):195, 1980

Reichert CM, O'Leary TJ, Levens DL, et al: Autopsy pathology in the acquired immune deficiency syndrome. Am J Pathol 112:357, 1983

Van Meirvenne N, Le Ray D: Diagnosis of African and American trypanosomiases. Br Med Bull 41:156, 1985

Wear DJ, Margileth AM, Hadfield TL, et al.: Cat scratch disease: A bacterial infection. Science 221:1403, 1983

Winn WC, Myerowitz RL: The pathology of the *Legionella* pneumonias. Hum Pathol 12:401, 1981

10

Blood Vessels

Earl P. Benditt and Stephen M. Schwartz

Structure and Development
of the Vascular System

Diseases of the Large Blood
Vessels

Hypertensive Vascular
Disease

Inflammatory Disorders of
Blood Vessels

Aneurysms

Veins

Lymphatic Vessels

Tumors of Blood Vessels

Figure 10-1. Subdivisions and histologic structure of the vascular system. Each subdivision is subject to a set of pathologic changes conditioned by the structure–function relationship of that part of the system. For example, the aorta, an elastic artery subject to great pressure, frequently shows a pathologic dilatation (aneurysm) if the supporting elastic media is damaged. Muscular arteries are the most significant sites of atherosclerosis. Small arteries, particularly arterioles, are sites of hypertensive changes. Capillary beds, venules, and veins each display their own types of pathologic changes.

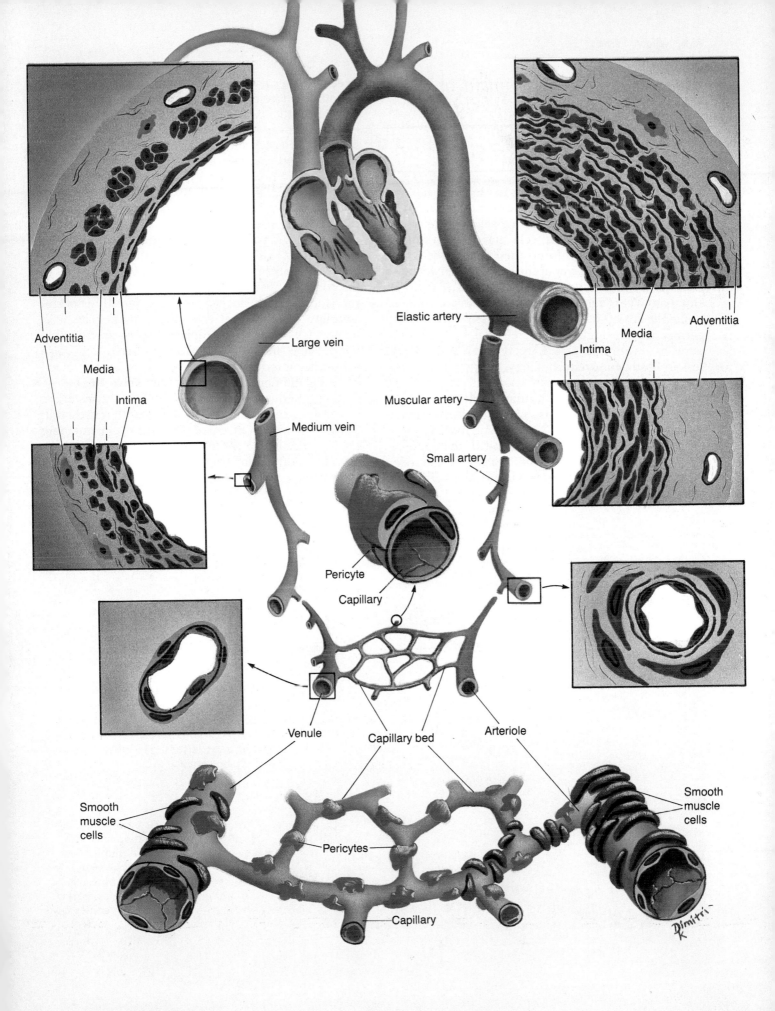

Adventitia

Media

Intima

Elastic artery

Large vein

Muscular artery

Medium vein

Small artery

Intima

Media

Adventitia

Pericyte

Capillary

Venule

Capillary bed

Arteriole

Smooth muscle cells

Smooth muscle cells

Pericytes

Capillary

Dimitri K

Structure and Development of the Vascular System

Cells of the Vessel Wall

The vascular system is complex, but individual blood vessels are among the simplest tissue structures in the body (Fig. 10-1). A blood vessel consists of but two cell types: endothelial cells and smooth muscle cells. The endothelium forms the lining of the tunica intima, a single cell layer at the interface between the blood and the extravascular fluid spaces (Fig. 10-2). Not many years ago the endothelium was considered a simple structural barrier that merely modulated permeation through the vessel wall by providing pores of appropriate size. Largely as a result of progress in tissue culture technology, we now know that endothelial cells accomplish a long list of metabolic functions (Table 10-1). In a number of diseases, endothelial dysfunction is associated with the subendothelial accumulation of blood-borne materials. For example, the accretion of lipid beneath the endothelium in atherosclerotic lesions reflects the failure of the endothelium to serve as an effective barrier between tissue and plasma. Thus, a modern view of endothelium holds that the metabolic and endocrine functions of its cells play a critical role in disease.

The discovery that endothelial cells are the major source of prostacyclin (PGI$_2$) has led to a new concept of the endothelium as an endocrine organ. For example, endothelial cells synthesize endothelial-derived relaxing factor (EDRF), the chemical nature of which is still undefined. EDRF relaxes smooth muscle cells in response to a number of physiologic and pharmacologic agents that were formerly thought to be direct vasodilators. Similarly, there is evidence that endothelial cell–derived factors are important in the control of the inflammatory response. Like macrophages, endothelial cells express class II histocompatibility antigens and are able to participate with monocytes—or even to replace them—in activating lymphocyte transformation. Endothelial cells also synthesize interleukin-1 and several factors involved in coagulation and thrombosis (see Table 10-1).

Less is known about the metabolic functions of the other major cell of the vessel, the smooth muscle cell. These cells have a mechanical function, maintaining the integrity of the vessel wall by providing support for the endothelium. They also control blood flow by contracting or dilating in response to specific stimuli.

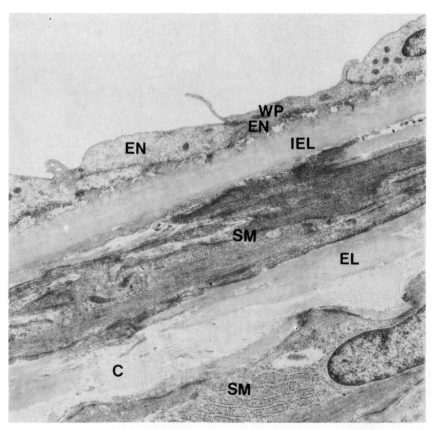

Figure 10-2. Luminal side of the rat aorta. Electron micrograph shows endothelial cells (*EN*) with Weibel-Palade bodies (*WP*), internal elastic (*IEL*), smooth muscle cells (*SM*), collagen (*C*), and elastic lamellae (*EL*).

Table 10-1 Functions of Endothelial Cells of the Blood Vessels
Permeability barrier
Antithrombic agent production: Prostacyclin (PGI₂), adenine metabolites
Prothrombic agent production: Factor VIIIa (von Willebrand factor)
Anticoagulant production: Thrombomodulin, other proteins
Fibrinolytic agent production: Tissue plasminogen activator, urokinase-like factor
Procoagulant production: Tissue factor, plasminogen activator/inhibitor, Factor V
Inflammatory mediator production: Interleukin-1
Provision of receptors for Factor IX, Factor X, LDL, modified LDL, thrombin
Replication
Growth factors: Blood cell colony stimulating factor, insulin-like growth factors, fibroblast growth factor, platelet-derived growth factor
Growth inhibitors: Heparin

In addition, smooth muscle cells synthesize the connective tissue matrix of the vessel wall, which includes elastin, collagen, and proteoglycans. Perhaps the most characteristic component of smooth muscle cells are the proteins that make up the cytoskeleton and provide the contractile force, namely forms of actin and myosin specific for smooth muscle.

Embryonic Development of Blood Vessels

The earliest embryonic vascular primordia are clusters of endothelial cells that arise on the yolk sac between the splanchnic mesoderm and entoderm. These early structures, called **blood islands** (Fig. 10-3), soon separate into peripheral cells that become endothelium and more centrally located cells that produce a short-lived line of primitive blood cells. The vascular primordia arising on the yolk sac consolidate into a plexus, which eventually connects with a system of endothelial tubes arising independently within the body of the embryo. The original capillaries, represented by bare endothelial tubes, recruit the mesenchymal cells that become the smooth muscle cells of the media and the fibroblasts of the adventitia. These cells differentiate into phenotypes appropriate for their locations in the vessel wall and secrete the appropriate extracellular matrix. In the fourth fetal month the three coats of the arterial wall become clearly evident. Once the embryonic vascular system is fully established, it extends by forming new branches, a process called **angiogenesis.** The signals controlling this process are called **angiogenic factors.** For example, fibroblast growth factor, a polypeptide that is mitogenic for several cell types, is angiogenic.

The properties of adult vessels vary depending on location. For example, the endothelium of the brain does not permit the passage of plasma proteins, although the renal glomerular endothelium is moderately permeable. The contractile properties of smooth muscle cells also vary according to site. In the differentiation of the walls of various blood vessels, it is not clear whether developmental factors or reversible adaptations to local conditions are more important. Nevertheless, it is clear that some of these differences must underlie the disparate susceptibilities to vascular diseases among different vascular beds. For example, the local characteristics of the vasculature in the coronary tree seem to play a role in the development of pathologic changes—particularly the sites of predilection for the development of atherosclerosis and, hence, the patterns of myocardial infarction.

Structure of Blood Vessels

Arteries

The simple two-cell structure of blood vessels is made more complex by the organization of the vessel wall into layers called "tunica" (see Fig. 10-1). The largest blood vessels in the body, including the aorta, are the **elastic arteries**. These arteries function as conduits to smaller arterial branches for blood from the heart. Many of the pathologic changes in elastic arteries develop in the innermost layers of these vessels, the **tunica intima.** Atherosclerosis, for example, is a disease of the tunica intima. This layer is defined as **the combination of endothelium and connective tissue on the luminal side of the internal elastic lamina.** The tunica intima of the aorta is thick and contains a matrix of collagen, proteoglycans, and small amounts of elastin. The major cell type in the normal intima is the smooth muscle cell. Other cells are occasional resident lymphocytes, macrophages, and other inflammatory cells derived from the blood.

Proceeding outward, the vessel wall displays layers of smooth muscle cells called the **tunica media.** In the elastic arteries, elastic layers interposed between smooth muscle cells provide a means of minimizing energy loss during the pressure changes of systole and diastole. A breakdown of the media, particularly its elastic layers, leads to a dilatation of the artery, called an **aneurysm.** Much of the disease that occurs in arteries (e.g., atherosclerosis) involves proliferation of medial smooth muscle cells. Alternatively, during normal aging and in hypertension smooth muscle cells may "endoreplicate"—that is, they replicate their DNA without cell division, becoming tetraploid, octaploid, or showing even higher ploidy (Fig. 10-4). This phenomenon is accelerated in the aorta, at least in the hypertensive rat.

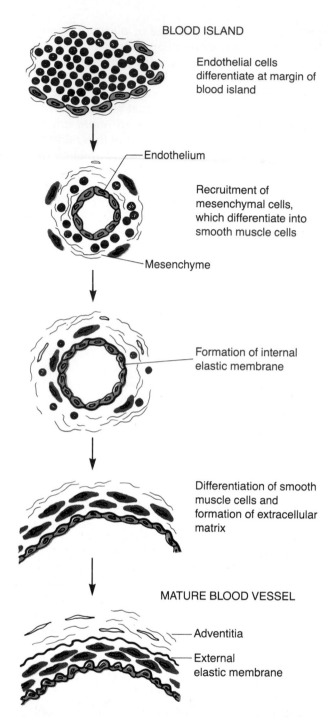

BLOOD ISLAND

Endothelial cells differentiate at margin of blood island

Endothelium

Recruitment of mesenchymal cells, which differentiate into smooth muscle cells

Mesenchyme

Formation of internal elastic membrane

Differentiation of smooth muscle cells and formation of extracellular matrix

MATURE BLOOD VESSEL

Adventitia

External elastic membrane

Figure 10-3.   Differentiation of vessels in early embryos. The course of events from the development of blood islands on the chorioallantoic membrane starts with differentiation of endothelium and proceeds to fully developed arteries or veins.

Medial smooth muscle cells also undergo degenerative changes, often leading to cell death, because they do not receive adequate nutrients or cannot effectively exchange wastes with the circulating blood. In smaller vessels, particularly those with fewer than 30 layers of smooth muscle cells, nutrient exchange for the media is provided only from the lumen of the blood vessel through the endothelium and layers of smooth muscle. However, in larger blood vessels with more layers of smooth muscle, this supply is apparently inadequate. Blood vessels having more than 28 layers of smooth muscle cells typically have a vasculature of their own—the vasa vasorum, which develop from surrounding small capillaries and penetrate from the exterior of the vessel wall. In addition to this external vascular supply, the structure of the tunica media is made even more intricate by the presence of autonomic nerve fibers that influence vascular contractility.

The most external layer of the vessel wall, the **tunica adventitia,** is a connective tissue sheath composed of fibroblasts, small vessels that give rise to the vasa vasorum, and nerves. This region is particularly involved in syphilitic aortitis, a disorder in which monocytes and lymphocytes invade the walls of small vessels and obliterate the lumina. The resulting ischemia of the vessel wall impairs the ability of medial smooth muscle to provide mechanical support, which in turn leads to an aneurysm. Syphilitic vasculitis affecting the root of the aorta results in aortic valvular insufficiency.

The blood conducted by the elastic arteries is distributed to individual organs through large **muscular arteries** (Fig. 10-5). Although atherosclerosis afflicts both the elastic arteries and the larger muscular arteries, most clinical disease is characterized by occlusion of muscular arteries. The tunica media of a muscular artery consists of layers of smooth muscle cells without prominent bands of elastin. However, the wall does have a prominent internal elastic lamina and usually has an identifiable external elastic lamina. The absence of the heavy elastin layers allows for better contraction of the muscular arteries. The intima of the muscular arteries, like that of the aorta, is composed of a prominent layer of intimal smooth muscle cells, their associated connective tissue, and occasional inflammatory cells. Vasa vasorum penetrate the walls of the thicker muscular arteries but are not seen in the smaller ones. As the vascular tree branches further, the tunica media becomes thinner, and the tunica intima totally disappears. Because of this lack of intima, the smaller muscular arteries do not develop atherosclerosis.

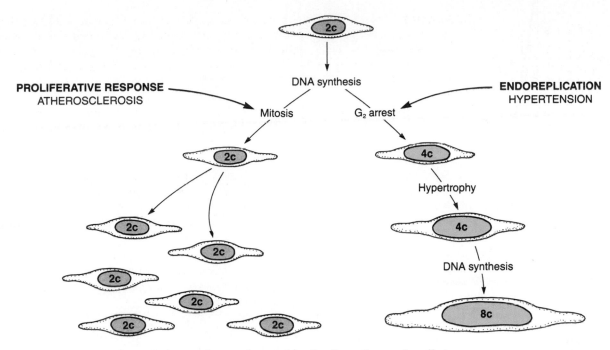

Figure 10-4. Replication of arterial smooth muscle cells. Smooth muscle cells in large arteries undergo two distinct forms of replication. Typical responses to injury, including atherosclerosis or traumatic injury, provoke diploid replication (hyperplasia). By contrast, both aging and hypertension result in DNA replication without cell division (endoreplication). Endoreplication increases the DNA content of individual cells without causing an increase in the number of cells in the vessel wall.

The small muscular arteries play an important role in the regulation of blood flow. The narrow lumen of these vessels produces an increased resistance, thereby reducing blood pressure to levels appropriate for the exchange of water and plasma constituents across the thin-walled capillaries. In addition to reducing pressure to capillary levels the small muscular arteries—sometimes called **resistance vessels**—maintain systemic pressure by regulating total peripheral resistance. Changes in these vessels—specifically, pathologic increases in the ratio of wall thickness to lumen size—are a central feature of hypertension.

Arterioles are the smallest elements of the arterial vascular tree. A typical arteriole consists of an endothelial lining surrounded by one or two layers of smooth muscle cells. No elastic layers are evident. The smallest arterioles provide a dynamic regulation of blood flow by controlling the distribution of blood in the capillary tree. The minute size of these vessels makes them susceptible to mechanical damage and rupture.

The smallest blood vessels, the **capillaries,** consist of endothelium supported only by sparse smooth muscle cells. The capillary endothelium provides for the interchange of solutes and cells between the blood and the extracellular fluid. A necessary feature of this exchange is a great reduction of pressure from that prevailing in the feeding arteries and arterioles. Without that change the filtration pressure across the capillaries would be so high that all of the vascular fluid would be quickly extravasated into the extracellular space. On the other hand, if the capillary wall had a thick tunica media, no exchange would occur, because the distance between the exchange surface of the endothelium and the extravascular tissue would be excessive. The compromise is a low-pressure capillary adapted to exchange across the endothelium by filtration and diffusion.

The endothelium acts as a charged semipermeable membrane, in which the exchange of plasma solutes with extracellular fluid is controlled by molecular size and charge. The endothelium also plays an active metabolic role by (1) synthesizing factors that influence the surrounding cells, (2) modifying molecules in transit across the endothelium, and (3) participating in the inflammatory response by synthesizing

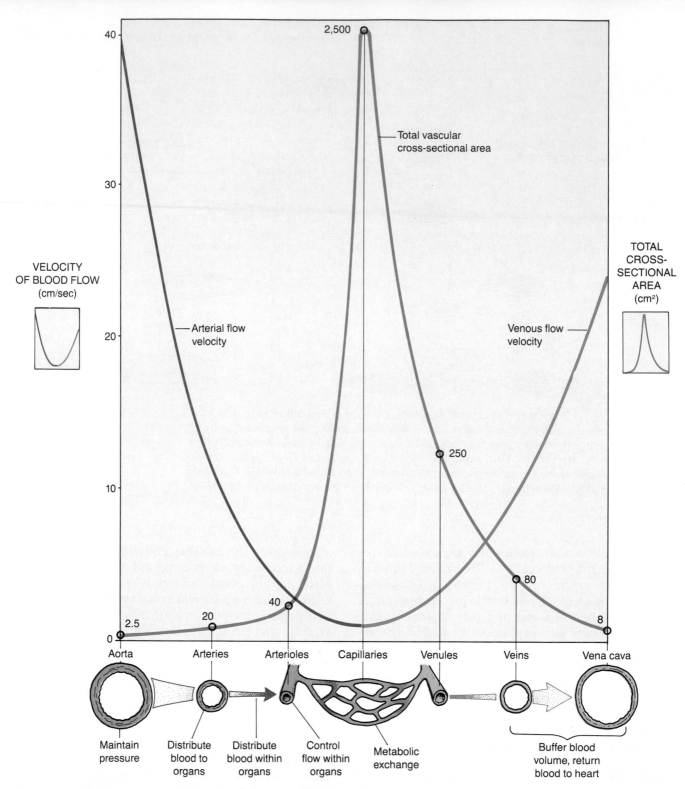

Figure 10-5. Relationship between velocity of blood flow and cross-sectional area in the vasculature. The vascular tree is a circuit that conducts blood from the heart through large-diameter, low-resistance conducting vessels to small arteries and arterioles, which lower blood pressure and protect the capillaries. The capillaries are thin-walled and allow the exchange of nutrients and waste products between tissue and blood, a process that requires a very large surface area. The circuit back to the heart is completed by the veins, which are distensible and provide a volume buffer that acts as a capacitance for the vascular circuit.

inflammatory mediators (see Table 10-1). A few isolated smooth muscle cells, sometimes called pericytes, surround the capillaries (see Fig. 10-1). Despite the special name, pericytes are actually smooth muscle cells, the functions of which are largely unknown. The adventitia of the capillary merges with the surrounding connective tissue and cannot be distinguished from it.

The permeability of capillaries depends on the ultrastructure of the capillary endothelial cells. Brain capillaries are highly impermeable because their endothelium has tightly sealed junctions between individual cells that prevent the exchange of proteins across the vessel wall. Transport in other capillary beds is mediated either by passage of molecules through incomplete cell junctions or by **micropinocytosis,** a process in which molecules traverse the cytoplasm "bucket brigade" fashion, via vesicular transport.

Some believe that little transport occurs by way of micropinocytosis; rather, they contend that vesicles are connected with each other, thereby providing a channel for direct transport of plasma proteins across the cytoplasm. The endothelium itself may be fenestrated—that is, it may have prominent channels across the endothelium, or it may exhibit discontinuous gaps between endothelial cells. Fenestrated capillaries in the renal glomerulus are specifically adapted to filter plasma. The liver sinusoids, which are not true capillaries, also show a fenestrated endothelium, which permits free access of the plasma to the liver cell.

Pathologic changes in the structure of the capillary and venular endothelium result in the accumulation of excess fluid in the interstitial space—that is, in **edema.** For example, histamine causes local edema by opening the intercellular junctions of venules. Other forms of injury or the release of inflammatory mediators lead to increased micropinocytosis. In some instances the endothelium is actually lost. As a result of protein leakage, the difference between the colloid osmotic pressure in the plasma and in the intracellular fluid is diminished. As discussed in Chapters 7 and 12, the change in the net balance of osmotic and hydrostatic pressures in the microvasculature results in an increased flux of water out of the vessels. Edema occurs when the loss of water through the capillaries and postcapillary venules exceeds the drainage capacity of the lymphatics.

Veins

The **venules** collect blood from the capillaries and transport it to a collecting system that returns to the heart. The thin media of the venule is appropriate for a vessel that is not required to withstand a high luminal pressure. Only a few pericytes are associated with the venules.

Venules merge into **small and medium-sized veins,** which in turn converge into **large veins.** The walls of large veins do not display the characteristic elastic lamellae of elastic arteries, and even the internal elastic lamina is well-developed only in the largest veins. Many veins, particularly those in the extremities, have valves formed by endothelium-lined folds of the tunica intima, which assist in the transport of blood under the low-pressure conditions of the venous circulation. The venous system in human lower extremities is only marginally adapted to its function. In many people the superficial veins of the legs become tortuous, dilated, and scarred, and the valves become thickened and ineffective. This set of changes, called **varicose veins,** leads to stasis, further venous injury, and edema. While larger veins are rarely the site of thrombosis, blood clots formed in the deep veins of the legs, in the venous supply of the prostate, or around some tumors may detach and migrate through the veins and the right side of the heart to the lung, where they lodge as life-threatening **pulmonary emboli.**

Lymphatics

The **lymphatic system,** a third set of vessels, is composed essentially of endothelium. This set of channels drains fluid filtered through the capillary and venular endothelium from the plasma, and acts as a pathway to the regional lymph nodes for cells, foreign material, and microorganisms.

Diseases of Large Blood Vessels

Atherosclerosis

The complications of atherosclerosis, which include ischemic heart disease, myocardial infarction, stroke, and gangrene of extremities, account for more than half of the annual mortality in the United States. Ischemic heart disease is by itself the leading cause of death. The incidence of ischemic heart disease in the United States and other western countries rose progressively from the turn of the century to a peak in the late 1960s, but in the past 20 years it has fallen dramatically (by more than 30%).

There are wide geographic and racial variations in the incidence of ischemic heart disease. For example, the mortality from ischemic heart disease is eight times higher in Sweden than in Japan. Study of these regional variations lends support to the hypothesis that death from myocardial infarction is related to underlying atherosclerosis: The extent of coronary atherosclerosis found at autopsy in particular populations shows a direct correlation with mortality from ischemic heart disease in those populations.

Pathogenesis

The most common acquired abnormality of blood vessels is the atherosclerotic lesion, which develops in the intima against a background of smooth muscle cells, blood-derived white blood cells, and a variable amount of connective tissue. This lesion has two critical features: the proliferation of intimal smooth muscle cells and the accumulation of lipid in the intima. The expansion of this common lesion produces the final clinical result: thrombosis and occlusion of a distributing artery.

A major unsolved puzzle in the study of atherosclerosis is that no current theory can account for the ability of blood vessels in some people to conduct blood for a lifetime with little or no evidence of arterial disease, whereas in others vascular lesions develop early, sometimes with catastrophic consequences. Another puzzling problem is the fact that lesions develop much more frequently in some anatomic regions than in others.

Processes

At least five hypotheses have been proposed to explain the origins of atherosclerotic plaques. We wish to emphasize that these hypotheses are **not** mutually exclusive. Viewed in this light, most of the controversy lies in individual opinions as to which process is most important in the initiation of the lesions or their progression into clinically significant disease.

Insudation Hypothesis   Conventional wisdom has for some years asserted that the critical events in atherosclerosis center on the focal accumulation of fat in the vessel wall. The insudation hypothesis states that the lipid in these lesions is derived from plasma lipoproteins, a view consistent with the role of blood lipids as risk factors for myocardial infarction. The insudation hypothesis is now widely accepted, but there is controversy over how the lipid enters the wall.

The form of lipid in the plasma that has been most closely associated with accelerated atherosclerosis is **low-density lipoprotein (LDL).** The LDL particle is far too large (20 nm in diameter) to penetrate the tightly closed endothelial cell junctions. However, endothelial cells have receptors for LDL and for modified forms of LDL. Transport may occur across intact

endothelium either by receptor-mediated uptake of lipoprotein or by nonspecific uptake into micropinocytic channels. Alternatively, lipid may be engulfed by macrophages in the blood and then transported into the vascular wall inside these cells.

Recent studies of atherosclerosis in fat-fed animals have demonstrated that macrophages play a major role in the early stages of lipid accumulation. Little is known about the mechanisms that control the flux of macrophages into and out of atherosclerotic plaques. Although the insudation hypothesis explains the source of plaque lipid, it does not provide a complete explanation for the pathogenesis of the atherosclerotic lesion. Even if we understood the mechanisms underlying the insudation of lipid, many other clinically important features of the plaque, such as smooth muscle proliferation and thrombosis, would remain unexplained.

Encrustation Hypothesis   A theory first suggested in the 19th century asserted that material from the blood is deposited on the inner surface of arteries and is the basis of the thickening of the inner lining. At the time that this suggestion was made, the details of the clotting mechanisms and the functions of platelets in thrombosis were unknown. A modern version of this idea holds that small mural thrombi represent the initial event in atherosclerosis. Organization of these thrombi leads to the formation of plaques, and the expansion of these lesions reflects repeated episodes of thrombosis and organization.

We now know from experimental studies of hyperlipidemic animals and from autopsy studies of children that the mural thrombus is not the initial event in atherogenesis. However, mural thrombosis is a critical part of the later progression of the lesion and probably is the major event leading to vascular occlusion.

Reaction to Injury Hypothesis   Another theory attempts to explain the accumulation of smooth muscle cells in atherosclerotic lesions. It proposes that smooth muscle proliferation depends on the release of polypeptide growth factors by platelets and monocytes that accumulate at sites of injury.

This "reaction to injury" hypothesis evolved from the discovery that the growth of smooth muscle cells in culture requires one or more platelet-derived polypeptides. The best known of these is called **platelet-derived growth factor (PDGF).** PDGF not only is mitogenic for smooth muscle cells, it is also chemotactic for them. Thus, in addition to stimulating the proliferation of cells already in the intima, PDGF may recruit smooth muscle cells from the media. Not only platelets, but smooth muscle cells and endothelial cells as well synthesize growth factors that stimulate the growth of smooth muscle cells. The same mechanism is probably important in the responses of the medial smooth muscle cells when vessels are injured surgically—for example, when plaques are removed by endarterectomy.

Although the "reaction to injury" hypothesis points to a mechanism for smooth muscle proliferation, it does not explain lipid accumulation. Nor does this hypothesis shed light on the initial events that lead to the monoclonality of lesions (discussed below).

Monoclonal Hypothesis The monoclonal concept is also focused on smooth muscle proliferation and was originally derived from the observation that the so-called fibrous caps of atherosclerotic plaques are composed of smooth muscle cells. Furthermore, these cells appear to migrate from the underlying media and then proliferate. Can the lesion, therefore, arise as an aberration of growth control in one or—at most—a few cells, in a manner analogous to a benign smooth muscle tumor such as a leiomyoma? On the other hand, might it not arise from the proliferation of many cells, as would be expected in a healing wound? Based on studies of women who are mosaic for X-linked markers, it has been established that many plaques are monoclonal—that is, they originate from one or, at most, a few smooth muscle cells. Any satisfactory explanation of the early stages of smooth muscle proliferation must account for this evident monoclonality. The only other monoclonal proliferations are neoplasms, both benign and malignant. Thus the monoclonality of the fibrous cap suggests that some unknown etiologic factor, perhaps circulating mutagens or viruses, might induce atherosclerotic plaque formation by altering some genomic features of growth control in the smooth muscle cells of the arterial wall.

Intimal Cell Mass Hypothesis The third smooth muscle hypothesis relates the location of atherosclerotic lesions to the focal accumulation of smooth muscle cells in the normal intima at branch points and other sites in certain vessels, particularly the coronary arteries. Intimal cell masses are found in infancy, are more pronounced in male infants, and occur in the vessels of people of varying ethnicity and location irrespective of the incidence of atherosclerosis. The distribution of intimal cell masses in children resembles the distribution of atherosclerotic lesions in adults. This suggests that the intimal cell mass is either the early lesion of atherosclerosis or a precursor of it. Intimal cell masses in experimental animals fed high-fat diets develop into lesions that display many of the characteristics of fully developed human lesions. Little is known about the development of the intimal cell mass, its growth potential, or its clonality. If the intimal cell mass is indeed the precursor of

atherosclerosis, it is probable that all mankind is susceptible to this disease. In that case, we would view other factors, such as hyperlipidemia, as critical for the progression of the disease to a clinically significant state.

A Unifying Hypothesis We can try to construct a scheme to tie the foregoing hypotheses together:

1. In such a hypothetical sequence, the initial lesion is the intimal cell mass, which arises by the trapping of isolated smooth muscle cells in the intima during development or by mutation and migration of pre-existing smooth muscle cells. If the intimal mass arose either as a mutation or from a few cells trapped in the intima, then monoclonality would be intrinsic to the early plaque.
2. Lipid accumulation in these foci might depend on properties of the intimal smooth muscle cells. The types of connective tissue synthesized by the cells in the intima may render these sites prone to lipid accumulation.
3. Lipid insudation in these benign accumulations of intimal cells would produce cell injury, thereby leading to the accumulation of macrophages and platelets.
4. In turn, the macrophages and platelets could release growth factors, as proposed in the "reaction to injury" hypothesis. Monocytes would play a central role by participating in lipid accumulation and releasing growth factors, thus stimulating further accumulation of smooth muscle cells.
5. As the lesion progresses, endothelial injury may lead to the loss of the anticoagulant properties of the normal wall. The resulting mural thrombosis would lead to the release of platelet-derived growth factors and further acceleration of smooth muscle proliferation. If the thrombus is large, it can directly lead to infarction of a vital organ.

Whether or not this particular hypothetical scenario is correct, aspects of these five hypotheses probably do operate as distinct processes during different phases of atherosclerosis. Figure 10-6 shows how these five hypotheses might interact over the course of lesion development.

Initial Lesion of Atherosclerosis

Two distinct lesions have been proposed as the initial structural abnormality of atherosclerosis. In young children the intima contains focal accumulations of intracellular and extracellular lipid, called **fatty spots**

INTIMAL CELL MASS

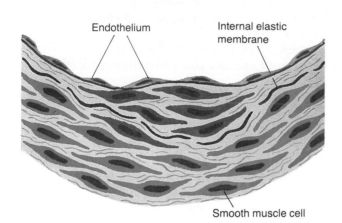

Endothelium

Internal elastic membrane

Smooth muscle cell

INSUDATION

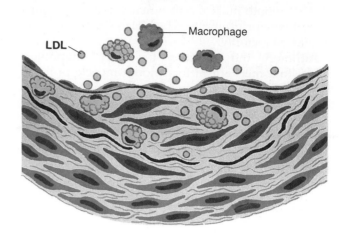

LDL

Macrophage

RESPONSE TO INJURY

Damaged endothelium

Platelets

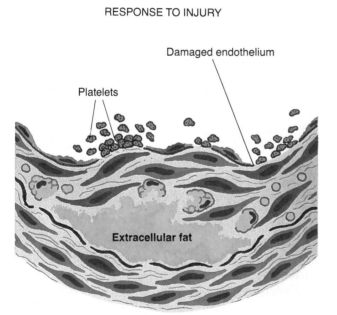

Extracellular fat

ENCRUSTATION AND THROMBOSIS

Blood clot

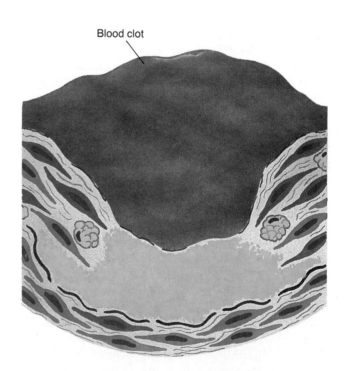

or **fatty streaks.** In these simple focal lesions (Fig. 10-7), cells filled with lipid droplets ("foam cells") accumulate. Originally, the fat-containing cells were thought to be macrophages, but it has been established that many of them are modified smooth muscle cells. A balanced view is that although those cells with the greatest amount of lipid are indeed macrophages, smooth muscle cells also contain fat.

Children who die accidentally usually show significant numbers of fatty spots in many parts of the arterial tree, but these do not correspond well to the distribution of atherosclerotic lesions in adults. For example, fatty spots are common in the thoracic aorta in children, but atherosclerosis in adults is typically prominent in the abdominal aorta. Nonetheless, many believe that fatty infiltration represents the initial lesion of atherosclerosis, and that other factors control the distribution of the later, more clinically significant lesions.

As we have already proposed, an alternative candidate for the initial lesion is **intimal thickening** or an **intimal cell mass.** The location of intimal cell masses, particularly in structures called "cushions" located near arterial branch sites, correlates well with the sites of later development of atherosclerotic lesions.

The concept of the intimal cell mass as the initial lesion is controversial. First, if it is indeed the initial lesion of atherosclerosis, then the very early stages of lesion development should be common to everyone, regardless of age. However, a gradual increase in the thickness of the intima occurs diffusely throughout large arteries as a normal part of aging, and for this reason many prefer to distinguish intimal thickening from atherosclerosis. Furthermore, it has been difficult to establish an animal model to test this hypothesis, since the intimal cell mass seems to arise only in man. By contrast, fatty lesions similar to those in man can be induced in animals. The resulting experimental bias probably exerts an influence on the opinions of many engaged in the study of atherosclerosis. In any event, as was illustrated in Figure 10-6, there is a general agreement that fat accumulation and monoclonal smooth muscle proliferation are the critical processes that lead to the characteristic lesion of atherosclerosis.

Characteristic Lesion of Atherosclerosis

Animals that have been fed lipids for weeks to months develop changes in their vessels that resemble the characteristic lesion of human atherosclerosis. This fibro-fatty lesion consists of two morphologic components (Fig. 10-8). The first, a thick layer of fibrous connective tissue called the **fibrous cap,** is much thicker and less cellular than the normal intima and contains fat-filled macrophages and smooth muscle cells. The second component is the **atheroma,** a necrotic mass of lipid that forms the middle part of the lesion. The term "atheroma" originally referred only to the fatty mass, but it is now used for the entire atherosclerotic lesion.

Other features of the characteristic lesion remain controversial. For example, in human lesions it is difficult to determine the point at which endothelial integrity is lost. In man the endothelium may be damaged during the removal of tissue at surgery or in the period between death and autopsy. The progress of atherosclerotic lesions is easier to follow experimentally. Virtually all studies show that there is some loss of endothelial continuity during progression to the characteristic lesion of atherosclerosis. Importantly, the characteristic lesion may contain blood-borne cells in addition to monocytes. These cells have received little attention in experimental animals, but advanced lesions in man show numer-

Figure 10-6. Unifying hypothesis for the pathogenesis of atherosclerosis. Monoclonality and the intimal cell mass occur very early in plaque development and are good candidates for the initial event. A single smooth muscle cell (*red*) proliferates in the intima, either as a result of a mutation or as part of an "intimal cushion," to form an intimal cell mass. Insudation of plasma lipids into the intimal cell mass occurs by direct passage of LDL across the endothelium and via macrophages that engulf LDL in the blood or in the intima. For reasons that are not clear, the expanding early atherosclerotic lesion is complicated by damage to the endothelium. As a result, platelets adhere to the exposed subendothelial collagen. Platelets and macrophages release growth factors, stimulating a polyclonal proliferation of smooth muscle cells (*blue*) to form the characteristic fibrous plaque. The continued insudation of lipid and its release by degenerating macrophages leads to further accumulation of extracellular lipid. Eventually the surface of the plaque ulcerates, and a thrombus forms on the injured luminal surface.

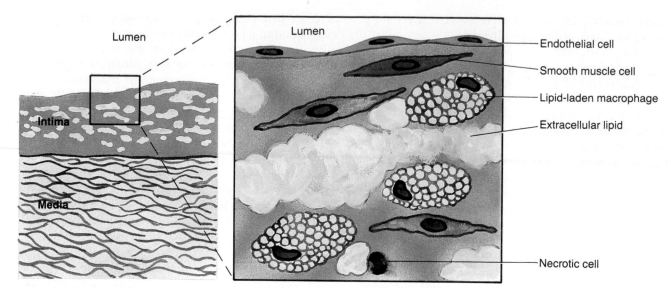

Figure 10-7.   Fatty streak of atherosclerosis. The fatty streak, composed largely of foamy macrophages, is presumed to be an early stage in the formation of atherosclerotic lesions. Note the intimal thickening in the left panel and the infiltrating cells in the enlargement on the right.

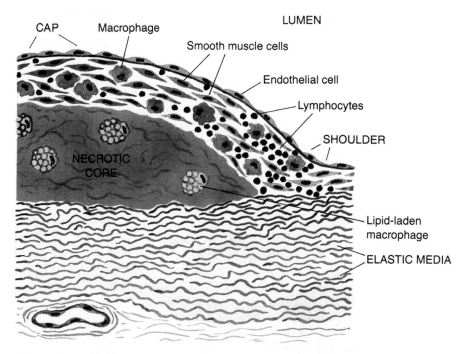

Figure 10-8.   Fibrous plaque of atherosclerosis. In this fully developed fibrous plaque the core contains lipid-filled macrophages and necrotic smooth muscle cell debris. The "fibrous" cap is composed largely of smooth muscle cells, which produce collagen, small amounts of elastin, and glycosaminoglycans. Also shown are infiltrating macrophages and lymphocytes. Note that the endothelium over the surface of the fibrous cap frequently appears intact.

ous activated T cells. The pathologic significance of these cells remains to be established.

Complicated Lesions of Atherosclerosis

Characteristic lesions of the sort described are of little significance in impairing blood flow. However, their distribution and their similarity to more advanced lesions suggest a progression to the final, clinically significant lesion. The critical changes that characterize complicated lesions are thrombosis, upon and within the fibrous cap; neovascularization of the cap and shoulders of the lesion; thinning of the underlying tunica media; calcification within the atheroma and fibrous cap; and ulceration of the fibrous cap. It is likely that thrombosis on the surface of the final, complicated lesion leads to vascular occlusion and clinical cardiovascular disease. Unfortunately, perhaps because of the long time required for such a progression, animal studies have rarely produced progression of atherosclerotic lesions to clinically significant disease.

Progression from the simple characteristic lesion to the more complicated, clinically significant lesion can be found in some people still in their twenties and, in our society, in virtually everyone by age 50 or 60.

Mechanisms of Lesion Progression in Atherosclerosis

The sequence of events in the development of atherosclerosis possibly begins as early as the fetal stage, with the formation of intimal cell masses, or perhaps shortly after birth, when fatty spots evolve. However, the characteristic lesion that is not clinically significant requires as much as 20 to 30 years to form, and the clinically important complicated lesions emerge after several more decades of development (Fig. 10-9). Preventive measures that may affect the long-term development of lesions should be considered primarily for younger people.

The factors that contribute to the progression of simple lesions to complicated ones are not well understood, but are the subject of intense study. A prominent factor in lesion progression could be the macrophage, a cell that may play a role even in the earliest events. A large part of the lipid that accumulates in lesions of fat-fed animals is found in the monocyte-macrophage. Once the macrophages are in the lesion, progression may depend on the inflammatory activities of the monocytes. For example, the monocyte synthesizes platelet-derived growth factor, fibroblast growth factor, epidermal growth factor, interleukin-1, tumor necrosis factor, alpha-interferon,

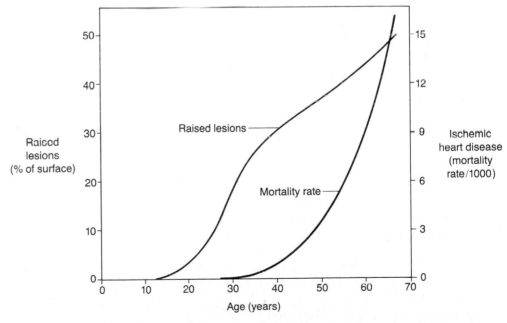

Figure 10-9. Raised lesions in coronary arteries and the mortality rate from ischemic heart disease as a function of age. There is a protracted incubation period of about 25 years between the appearance of raised lesions in the coronary vessels and their lethal complications.

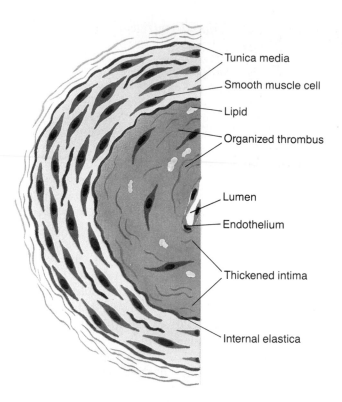

Tunica media
Smooth muscle cell
Lipid
Organized thrombus
Lumen
Endothelium
Thickened intima
Internal elastica

Figure 10-10. Organizing thrombus in the muscular artery. The original platelet mass is augmented by masses of red blood cells and white blood cells. Such a thrombus becomes organized by the ingrowth of endothelial cell sprouts and smooth muscle cells from the intima or inner media. Some lipid and cholesterol crystals may become evident as red blood cells break down.

and transforming growth factor beta. Each of these can either positively or negatively modulate the growth of smooth muscle or endothelial cells. Interferon and tumor growth factor beta inhibit cell proliferation and could account for the failure of endothelial cells to maintain continuity over the lesion. Alternatively, such growth inhibitors could exert a negative feedback effect in the presence of large amounts of growth stimulatory peptides.

Mediators secreted by monocytes and macrophages also are thought to change the functions of overlying endothelial cells in ways that may be important for lesion progression. Of particular interest is the recent discovery that interleukin-1 and tumor necrosis factor stimulate endothelial cell expression of platelet-activating factor, tissue factor, and plasminogen activator inhibitor. **Thus, the combination of monocytes and endothelial cells may be capable of transforming the normal anticoagulant vascular surface to a procoagulant surface.** A further complication is that atherosclerotic plaques also contain T cells. The expression of HLA-DR antigens on both endothelial cells and smooth muscle cells in plaques implies that these cells have undergone some kind of immunologic activation, perhaps in response to gamma interferon released by activated T cells in the plaque. It is possible that these T cells reflect an autoimmune response that is important for the progression of atherosclerotic lesions.

A loss of endothelial continuity is another potential antecedent of plaque progression. The loss of endothelial continuity would (a) increase the permeability of the wall to lipoproteins and, therefore, accelerate lipoprotein accumulation; (b) permit platelet interaction with the vessel wall and the subsequent release of growth factors, resulting in more rapid lesion progression; and (c) allow the formation of a thrombus on the surface of an atherosclerotic lesion. We know from clinical studies that the formation of a thrombus (Fig. 10-10) is the most common clinical event that leads to myocardial infarction. An intervention aimed at dissolving such a thrombus can prevent or limit the size of an evolving myocardial infarction. Recent studies have shown that many occlusive thrombi can be dissolved by enzymes capable of activating plasma fibrinolytic activity, including streptokinase and tissue plasminogen activator (Fig. 10-11).

Risk Factors

The concept of risk factors has emerged from studies of ischemic heart disease in human populations. Any factor associated with a 100% increase in the incidence of ischemic heart disease has been defined as a "risk factor." **The most frequently noted risk factors for ischemic heart disease are hypertension, elevated serum cholesterol levels, cigarette smoking and diabetes (glucose intolerance).** In addition, it is well established that the rates of myocardial infarction increase with age and are greater for men than for women at all ages, although the rate for the latter rises precipitously after the menopause. Hence, **age and sex are considered risk factors.**

Lipid Metabolism

In the 19th century, Virchow identified cholesterol crystals in atherosclerotic lesions. Since that time there has evolved a large body of information on lipoproteins and their role in lipid transport and metabolism.

The insolubility of cholesterol and other lipids (mainly triglycerides) that are important as energy sources and structural elements in cell membranes necessitates a special transport system, whose func-

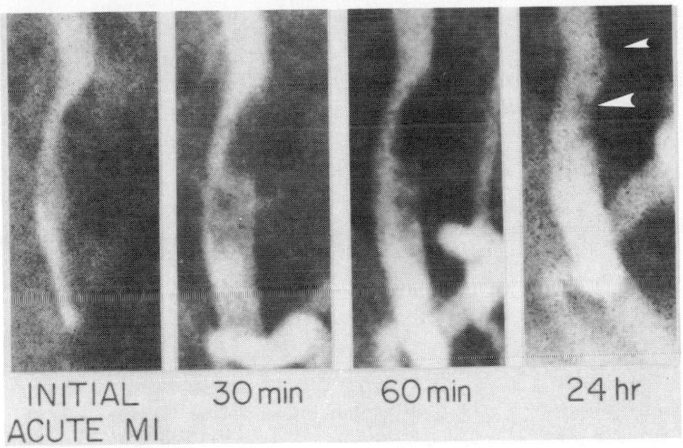

Figure 10-11. Dissolution of coronary artery thrombus. These coronary angiograms show a thrombus (*initial*) in the coronary artery of a 48-year old man, 3 hours after the onset of the symptoms of acute myocardial infarction. He was immediately infused with recombinant human tissue plasminogen activator. Successive frames show stages of dissolution of the thrombus. By 60 minutes after the beginning of infusion, the thrombus is distinctly smaller. The infusion was continued for 6 hours, and at 24 hours the thrombus is almost completely lysed. The lower arrow indicates a small remaining portion of plaque or thrombus; the apparent bulge indicated by the upper arrow is interpreted as an ulceration of the plaque.

INITIAL ACUTE MI   30 min   60 min   24 hr

tion is subserved by a system of lipoprotein particles (Table 10-2, Fig. 10-12). The lipoproteins have been divided into classes according to the density of the solvent in which they remain suspended when centrifuged at high speed (100,000 g or greater). **The major classes of particles are chylomicrons, very-low-density lipoproteins (VLDL), low-density lipoproteins (LDL), and high-density lipoproteins (HDL).** Each of these particles consists of a lipid core with associated proteins, the apolipoproteins. A number of the latter have been described, and each is designated by a letter (and frequently a number) as indicated in Table 10-2.

Lipid Metabolic Pathways, Cholesterol Transport, and Metabolism

The metabolic pathways for lipoproteins containing the B apolipoproteins are two major lipoprotein cascades, one originating from the intestine and the other from the liver (Fig. 10-13). The **exogenous pathway** consists of chylomicrons containing ApoB-48 secreted by the intestine. Following secretion, chylomicrons rapidly acquire ApoCII and ApoE from HDL. These triglyceride-rich lipoproteins primarily transport lipid from the intestine to the liver. The triglycerides in chylomicrons are hydrolyzed by lipoprotein lipase, which is attached to the endothelial cells of the capillary walls. ApoCII activates lipoprotein lipase and causes removal of triglycerides. Thus, chylomicrons are converted to "remnants" and finally to intermediate-density lipoproteins (IDL). The chylomicron remnants are removed by the hepatocyte via an ApoE-mediated (remnant) receptor process.

The **endogenous pathway** involves triglyceride-rich lipoproteins containing ApoB-100 secreted by the liver. As with the chylomicrons, shortly after their secretion the liver VLDL particles acquire ApoCII and

(*Text continued on page 470.*)

Table 10-2 The Apolipoproteins

APOLIPOPROTEIN	APPROX. MOLECULAR WEIGHT	MAJOR DENSITY CLASS	MAJOR SITES OF SYNTHESIS IN MAN	MAJOR FUNCTION IN LIPOPROTEIN METABOLISM
AI	28,000	HDL	Liver, intestine	Activates lecithin: cholesterol acyltransferase
AII	18,000	HDL	Liver, intestine	
AIV	45,000	Chylomicrons	Intestine	
B-100	250,000	VLDL IDL LDL	Liver	Binds to LDL receptor
B-48	125,000	Chylomicrons VLDL IDL	Intestine	
CI	6,500	Chylomicrons VLDL HDL	Liver	Activates lecithin: cholesterol acyltransferase
CII	10,000	Chylomicrons VLDL HDL	Liver	Activates lipoprotein lipase
CIIIO-2	10,000	Chylomicrons	Liver	Inhibits lipoprotein uptake by the liver
D	20,000	HDL		Cholesteryl ester exchange protein
E2-4	40,000	Chylomicrons VLDL HDL	Liver, macrophage	Binds to E receptor system

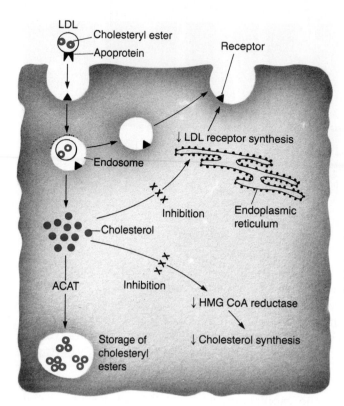

Figure 10-12. The relationship between circulating LDL-cholesterol, LDL receptors, and the synthesis of cholesterol. The LDL, which contains cholesteryl esters, is taken up by cells into vesicles by a receptor-mediated pathway to form an endosome. The receptor and lipids are dissociated, and the receptor is returned to the cell surface. The exogenous cholesterol, now in the cytoplasm, causes a reduction in receptor synthesis in the endoplasmic reticulum and inhibits the activity of HMG CoA reductase in the cholesterol synthesizing pathway. Excess cholesterol in the cell is esterified to cholesteryl esters and stored in vacuoles.

Figure 10-13. Exogenous and endogenous cholesterol transport pathway. In the exogenous pathway cholesterol and fatty acids from food are absorbed through the intestinal mucosa. Fatty acid chains are linked to glycerol to form triglycerides. The triglycerides and the cholesterol are packaged into chylomicrons that are returned via the lymph to the blood. In the capillaries (mainly of fat tissue and muscle, but also other tissues) the ester bonds holding the fatty acids in triglycerides are split by lipoprotein lipase. Fatty acids are removed, leaving cholesterol-rich lipoprotein remnants. These bind to special remnant receptors and are taken up by liver cells. The cholesterol of the remnant is either secreted into the intestine, largely as bile acids, or packaged as very low density lipoprotein particles (VLDL), which are then secreted into the circulation. This is the first step in the endogenous cycle. In fat or muscle tissue the triglyceride is removed from the VLDL with the aid of lipoprotein lipase. The IDL (intermediate density lipoprotein particles [*not shown*]) remain in the circulation. Some IDL is immediately taken up by the liver via the mediation of LDL receptors for ApoB/E. The remaining IDL in the circulation is either taken up by non-liver cells or converted to low density lipoproteins (LDL). Most of the LDL in the circulation bind to hepatocytes or other cells and are removed from the circulation. High density lipoproteins (HDL) take up cholesterol from cells. This cholesterol is esterified by the enzyme lecithin: cholesterol acyltransferase (LCAT), after which the esters are transferred to LDL and taken up by cells.

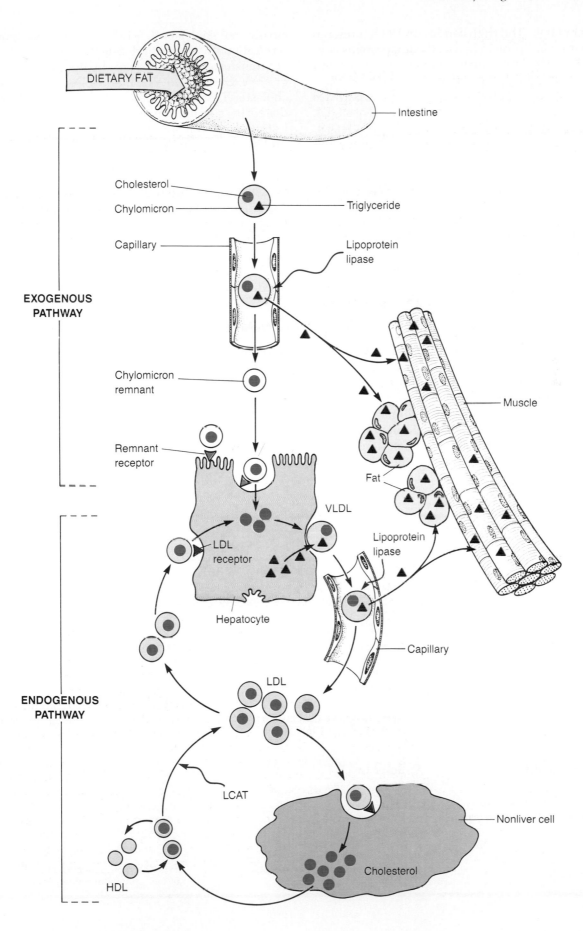

ApoE from HDL. The triglycerides on VLDL undergo hydrolysis by lipoprotein lipase; the lipoproteins containing ApoB-100 are initially converted to IDLs and finally to LDLs. With the conversion of IDL to LDL, most ApoCII and ApoE dissociates from the particles and reassociates with HDL. The conversion of IDL to LDL may, in part, be mediated by hepatic lipase, an enzyme that functions both as a triglyceride hydrolase and, more importantly, as a phospholipase. The LDL, which contains ApoB-100, interacts with high-affinity receptors on the liver and on the peripheral cells, including smooth muscle cells, fibroblasts, and adrenal cells (see Fig. 10-12). The interaction of LDL with its receptor initiates receptor-mediated endocytosis and the catabolism of LDL.

The HDLs containing ApoAI and ApoAII are synthesized by several pathways, including direct secretion by the intestine and liver, and transfer of lipid and apolipoprotein constituents released during the lipolysis of triglyceride-rich lipoproteins that contain ApoB. HDL has been proposed to have two major functions: serving as a reservoir for apolipoproteins, particularly ApoCII and ApoE, and interacting with cells in the uptake and transport of cholesterol from extrahepatic cells to the liver for ultimate removal from the body as cholesterol or bile acids. The latter function has been termed "reverse cholesterol transport." The cholesterol removed from the cells is principally free cholesterol, which rapidly undergoes esterification to cholesteryl esters. Cholesteryl esters are transferred to the core of the lipoprotein particle, or are exchanged to VLDL and LDL. The transfer of cholesteryl esters between lipoprotein particles is mediated by specific transfer proteins. Defects in cholesteryl ester transfer and exchange lead to dyslipoproteinemias, increased intracellular cholesteryl esters, and premature atherosclerosis.

Clinical Disorders of Lipoprotein Metabolism

A number of biochemical defects that produce dyslipoproteinemias are now recognized (Table 10-3). Current and evolving knowledge of the biochemical and molecular defects in patients with dyslipoproteinemias forms the basis for a systematic approach to the diagnosis of the disorders.

Genetic Factors in Atherosclerosis

Although familial clustering of ischemic heart disease has been recognized for several decades, it is only in recent years that genetic studies have made significant strides toward understanding the factors that cause this cluster. It is now recognized that a defect in LDL receptors is a key factor in certain genetic dyslipoproteinemias. In addition, polymorphisms are present in apolipoprotein AI and AII. Apolipoprotein

Table 10-3 Molecular Defects in Patients with Dyslipoproteinemia

	DEFECT	CLINICAL FEATURES
Apolipoprotein Defects		
ApoAI$_{Milano}$	Amino acid change (Arg$_{173}$→Cys)	Reduced HDL
ApoAI + ApoCII deficiency (kindred 1)	Rearrangement in ApoAI and ApoCIII gene	Virtual absence of HDL, severe atherosclerosis
ApoAI + ApoCII deficiency (kindred 2)	Unknown	Virtual absence of HDL, severe atherosclerosis
ApoB-100 and ApoB-48 absence	Unknown	Ataxia malabsorption, visual defects, hemolytic anemia
ApoB-100 absence	Unknown	Mild ataxia, malabsorption
ApoCII deficiency	Structural defect in ApoCII	Type 1 hyperlipidemia, severe hypertriglyceridemia
ApoE$_3$ variants	ApoE$_2$ (Arg$_{158}$ → Cys) ApoE$_2$ (Arg$_{145}$ → Cys) ApoE$_2$ (Lys$_{146}$ → Gln)	Type III hyperlipidemia, elevated plasma cholesterol and triglycerides, premature cardiovascular disease
Enzyme Defects		
Lipoprotein lipase deficiency	Unknown	Type I hyperlipidemia, hypertriglyceridemia
Hepatic lipase deficiency	Unknown	Type IV hyperlipidemia, mild elevations of IDL and HDL
Lecithin cholesterol acyltransferase deficiency	Unknown	Corneal opacities, mild hypertriglyceridemia, and reduced levels of HDL
Receptor Defects		
LDL excess	Absence of or defective receptor	Type II hyperlipidemia, severe elevations of LDL, premature atherosclerosis

E polymorphisms have also been found, accompanied by alterations in LDL levels.

Apolipoprotein E (ApoE) is one of the main protein constituents of VLDL and of a subclass of HDL. The gene locus that codes for ApoE is polymorphic; three common alleles, E2, E3, and E4, code for three major ApoE isoforms, respectively, and determine the six ApoE phenotypes. The several polymorphic forms have a significant influence on serum cholesterol levels and on lipoprotein variation. About 20% of the variability of serum cholesterol has been attributed to ApoE polymorphism. In men, the ApoE 3/2 phenotype is associated with a 20% lower LDL than the most common phenotype, ApoE 3/3. The E4 allele is associated with elevated serum cholesterol. It is interesting to note that there is an increased frequency of the E2 allele and a decreased frequency of E4 among male octogenarians.

An inverse correlation between ischemic heart disease and HDL cholesterol levels has been established. This has been extended by studies of apoprotein levels and polymorphisms of the principal apoproteins associated with HDL. From these studies emerges the fact that the genes for apolipoproteins AI and CIII reside in human chromosome 11 and are physically linked. Polymorphisms of ApoAI have been associated with hypertriglyceridemia and premature atherosclerosis. Other defects in this complex have been associated with **Tangier's disease,** a malady in which low levels of HDL and ApoAI result from faulty post-translational processing of pre- or proforms of ApoAI. Other defects that alter gene expression and are associated with the atherosclerosis of diabetes have been found in chromosome 11.

Viruses and Atherosclerosis

In chickens, an avian herpes virus responsible for the neurolymphomatous neoplasm called Marek's disease causes a fatty proliferative lesion in muscular arteries. The Marek's disease virus, when infecting chicken cells, and the herpes simplex virus, when infecting human smooth muscle cells in culture, alter the lipid and cholesterol metabolism of these cells. Herpes viruses have also been found in human lesions.

A viral etiology for at least some cases of atherosclerosis is compatible with the importance of cell proliferation in the formation of atheromatous plaques. Furthermore, it could explain several hitherto puzzling features of atherosclerosis and thrombosis, namely (a) intimal cell proliferation in the absence of certain common risk factors, (b) the monoclonal nature of cell populations found in many human atherosclerotic lesions, and (c) the role of certain environmental factors in eliciting vascular occlusive disease.

Hemostasis and Thrombosis

Hemostasis—the arrest of hemorrhage—is a normal response to vascular injury that involves vasoconstriction, tissue turgor, coagulation, and thrombosis. Whereas coagulation can occur *in vitro* solely as a result of the activation of the clotting cascade, thrombosis (i.e., the formation of a blood clot in situ) also involves the adherence and aggregation of platelets, the participation of cellular elements of the monocyte–macrophage system, and endothelial cell functions. Although thrombosis is a crucial element of hemostasis, in some circumstances—for instance, in atherosclerosis or a hypercoagulable state—it is often responsible for significant morbidity and mortality.

The effectiveness of thrombolytic agents in the therapy of myocardial infarction clearly shows that thrombotic occlusion is frequently the major event leading from atherosclerosis to occlusive cardiovascular disease. Less severe occlusion, in which blood flow is restricted by a gradual increase in the size of an atherosclerotic lesion or by mural thrombosis and organization, can produce ischemia of an organ. We do not know to what extent this narrowing of the vessel is due to thrombosis, lipid accumulation, or smooth muscle proliferation. Ischemia in the coronary circulation results in **angina pectoris**—chest pain from the heart. Similarly, occlusion of arteries supplying the brain, gut, or legs causes infarction or ischemia. A common form of vaso-occlusive disease in the legs produces muscle pain, termed **intermittent claudication,** on exercise of the leg muscles. Finally, ischemia of one organ can have marked systemic effects. The best-known example is the result of renal artery narrowing by atherosclerosis. The kidney compensates for poor perfusion by elevating its secretion of renin, an enzyme that elevates blood pressure; the result is "renal" hypertension.

Atherosclerosis also causes tissue injury distal to a plaque by **embolus formation**—that is, loss of parts of a plaque into the circulation, with lodgment of the debris in a critical smaller vessel. Emboli from plaques in the carotid artery are one cause of **cerebral vascular occlusion,** also called **stroke.** The weakened wall of an atherosclerotic vessel may also lead to **aneurysm formation** and subsequent hemorrhage.

The circulating cellular element most intimately involved with injury to the blood vessel is the platelet. When vessels are injured, platelets interact with one another to form a platelet thrombus—that is, an aggregate of activated platelets (Fig. 10-14). These

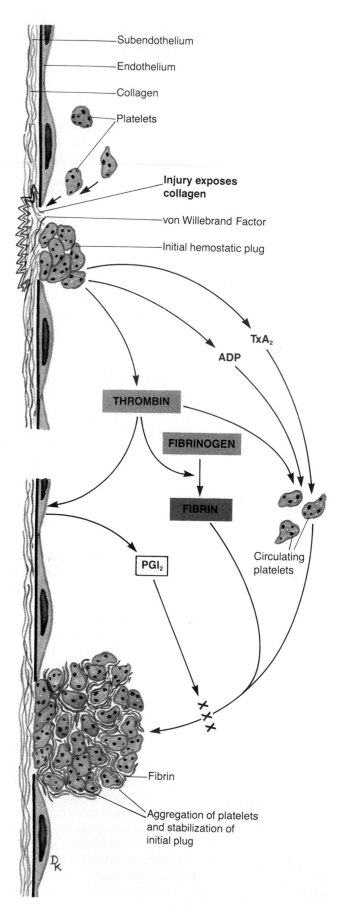

Subendothelium

Endothelium

Collagen

Platelets

Injury exposes collagen

von Willebrand Factor

Initial hemostatic plug

TxA$_2$

ADP

THROMBIN

FIBRINOGEN

FIBRIN

PGI$_2$

Circulating platelets

Fibrin

Aggregation of platelets and stabilization of initial plug

platelet aggregates occlude vessels and prevent the leakage of blood from injured small vessels. The materials released from platelets can stimulate both wound healing and the formation of proliferative lesions in the vessel wall. The latter include both the smooth muscle proliferation seen in the atherosclerotic lesion and, as described below, the proliferative lesions of smooth muscle cells of small vessels in malignant hypertension.

Thrombus formation is normally prevented by blood flow and the anti-thrombotic properties of the endothelium. Thrombi can form when endothelial function is altered, when endothelial continuity is lost, or when blood flow is altered or becomes static. **Simple endothelial loss or injury in a vessel with good flow produces platelet pavementing but not thrombosis (Fig. 10-15).** The presence of a thrombus may lead to further complications when it breaks down. Fragments of thrombi, called emboli or thromboemboli, may circulate to distal vessels and occlude them. When those fragments originate in the venous circulation, the result is often a pulmonary embolism—a major life-threatening event. Emboli may arise from other sources. For example, the disruption of the fatty part of the atherosclerotic lesion may produce a fat or a cholesterol crystal embolus.

Platelet Aggregation

While we have emphasized thrombosis in atherosclerosis, adhesion and aggregation of platelets are critical to repair at normal wound sites. Thrombosis is also an important event in any situation in which endothelial integrity and function are lost or blood flow is obstructed. The aggregation of platelets and the activation of the clotting cascade are exquisitely sensitive to alterations in the microenvironment. The major initiating event for most thrombosis and coagulation *in vivo* is almost certainly some form of injury to the endothelium (see Fig. 10-14). Activated platelets, in turn, release factors that initiate clotting, resulting in the formation of a complex thrombus on

Figure 10-14. The role of platelets in thrombosis. Following vessel wall injury and alteration in flow, platelets adhere and then aggregate. ADP and thromboxane A$_2$ are released and, along with locally generated thrombin, recruit additional platelets, causing the mass to enlarge. The growing platelet thrombus is stabilized by fibrin. Other elements, including leukocytes and red blood cells, are also incorporated into the thrombus. The release of prostacyclin (PGI$_2$) by endothelial cells regulates the process by inhibiting platelet aggregation.

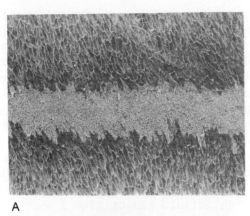

A

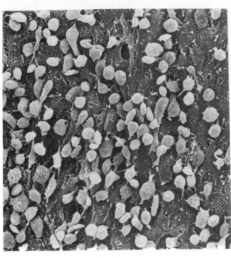

B

Figure 10-15. Scanning electron micrograph of the endothelial surface of a rat aorta 1 hour after the endothelial cells were removed by scraping with a nylon filament. (*A*) Intact endothelium and scratched portion. (*B*) Higher-power view of the scratched area showing a pavement of intact platelets that adheres to the underlying connective tissue in the high-velocity arterial stream.

the vessel wall (see Figs. 10-10 and 10-14). For thrombosis to occur, endothelial continuity must be disrupted or the endothelial cell surface must change from an anticoagulant to a procoagulant surface. Both processes are believed to occur. The most common denuding endothelial injury is the progressive endothelial disruption of an advancing atherosclerotic lesion. Denuding endothelial injury has also been described in homocystinuria, as a response to the injection of radiologic contrast dyes, and in hypoxia and endotoxemia. In addition, the interactions of a thrombus with the underlying subendothelium may cause a further disturbance of endothelial integrity. For example, fibrin applied to the superficial surface of an endothelial cell in culture causes a marked change in cell shape. Finally, inflammatory agents

released from monocytes are able to activate procoagulant activities on the surface of an intact endothelium.

Consideration of how vessels become prothrombotic requires asking why vessels are normally not thrombogenic. The simplest view is that subendothelial thrombogenic molecules are covered by a nonthrombogenic cell layer—the endothelium. According to this view, in the same way that platelets do not aggregate with other blood elements, they also do not aggregate with endothelial cells, and there is thus no need for a specific inhibitory mechanism.

It is now apparent, however, that the endothelium plays an active rather than a passive role in the control of thrombosis. It has been suggested that the major antithrombotic mechanism of the endothelium is the secretion of PGI_2, also known as prostacyclin. However, prostacyclin may actually have a minor role; several other features of the endothelium support its antithrombotic activity. Endothelial cells metabolize adenosine diphosphate (ADP). This is important both because ADP is a strong promoter of thrombogenesis and because its metabolites are antithrombogenic. The luminal surface of the endothelium is coated with heparan sulfate. Although there is no direct evidence that this substance participates directly in the inhibition of clotting of blood, as does exogenous heparin, heparan sulfate does bind a number of clotting factors, including the antiprotease alpha-2 macroglobulin. Endothelial cells also synthesize plasminogen activators, and thus may dissolve some clots as they form. In addition, endothelial cells at the site of thrombosis may take up vasoactive amines released from platelets. Similarly, these cells may limit coagulation by consuming thrombin created during the procoagulant process. There are several other more specific endothelial anticoagulant mechanisms. A cofactor on the endothelial cell surface inactivates thrombin by forming a complex with it and antithrombin 3, a plasma antiprotease. Thrombin itself activates protein C via an interaction with its receptor, called thrombomodulin, which is located on the surface of endothelial cells. Both protein C and thrombomodulin are synthesized by endothelial cells. Activated protein C destroys coagulation Factors V and VII. The extent to which these antithrombotic mechanisms are normally active in the endothelium *in vivo* is unknown.

The presence of these antithrombotic mechanisms on the endothelial surface has raised the intriguing possibility that endothelial dysfunction might lead to thrombosis *in vivo*. There is also evidence that endothelial cells have prothrombotic functions. At least in culture, endothelial cells synthesize von Willebrand factor, which promotes platelet adherence, and

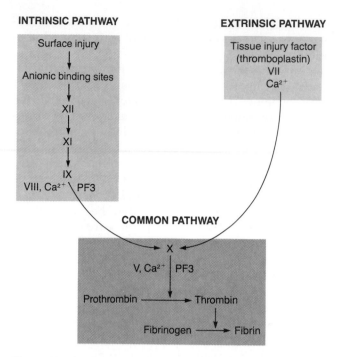

INTRINSIC PATHWAY

Surface injury

↓

Anionic binding sites

↓

XII

↓

XI

↓

IX

VIII, Ca²⁺ ∖ PF3

EXTRINSIC PATHWAY

Tissue injury factor
(thromboplastin)
VII
Ca²⁺

COMMON PATHWAY

X

V, Ca²⁺ | PF3

Prothrombin ⟶ Thrombin

Fibrinogen ⟶ Fibrin

Figure 10-16. Intrinsic and extrinsic pathways for coagulation.

clotting Factor V. The cultured endothelial cell also binds Factors IX and X, a process that may promote coagulation on the endothelial surface *in vivo*. Finally, endothelial cells treated with interleukin-1 or tumor necrosis factor present thromboplastin to the plasma, potentially initiating coagulation via the extrinsic pathway.

Thus, one can envision that prothrombotic, procoagulant injuries at the surface of blood vessels are produced either by the loss of a normal endothelial function or by the stimulation of an abnormal function.

Once platelets are stimulated to adhere to the vessel wall, their contents are spontaneously released. In turn, these contents promote aggregation with new platelets. Aggregation is enhanced by the release of von Willebrand factor; this substance is adhesive for the GP1$_b$ membrane protein and for fibrinogen. The activated platelets also release ADP and thromboxane A$_2$, which recruit additional platelets, thereby causing changes in platelet shape, release of granule contents, and more aggregation. The platelet membrane proteins GP2$_b$ and GP3$_a$ adhere to fibrin and fibrinogen, a process that tends to stabilize the forming thrombus.

The generation of thrombin is probably the most important factor in the progression and stabilization of the thrombus through coagulation. Thrombin is generated at the site of injury by either the intrinsic or extrinsic coagulation pathway. The extrinsic co-

agulation pathway begins with the release of thromboplastin from injured cells. The intrinsic pathway starts with the activation of Factor XII (Hageman factor), an event that depends on the binding of this factor to a component of injured cells. Thrombin itself is sufficient to stimulate further release of platelet-granule contents and the subsequent recruitment of new platelets. As coagulation proceeds, fibrin is formed by the action of thrombin on fibrinogen, and forges cross-bridges bound to the GP2$_b$ and GP3$_a$ receptors on platelets. These links stabilize the aggregation of the platelets and their adherence to the underlying denuded surface.

Blood Coagulation and Clot Lysis

Coagulation of blood depends on a cascade of enzyme activations that reflect the sequential actions of proteases (Fig. 10-16, Table 10-4). Each coagulation factor acts first as a substrate and then as an enzyme. The net result is a powerful, autocatalytic, biologic amplifier.

Coagulation is initiated by two distinct pathways. In the **intrinsic pathway** the initial event is the interaction of Factor XII with any of several biologic surfaces, including products of necrotic cells. The normal endothelium ordinarily prevents Factor XII from interacting with such surfaces. The activated form of Factor XII, namely Factor XII$_a$, is a protease that initiates subsequent interactions among the other factors involved in the intrinsic pathway. These include prekallikrein, Factor IX, and Factor VIII.

The **extrinsic pathway** begins with tissue factor, also a product of cell injury. Tissue factor is a cell surface protein, the gene for which has recently been cloned. The interaction between tissue factor and circulating Factor VII initiates the extrinsic pathway. Activated Factor VII and activated Factor IX (from the intrinsic pathway) both act on Factor X to produce activated Factor X (Factor X$_a$). In turn, Factor X$_a$ interacts with Factor V, calcium, and platelet factor 3, a component of the platelet membrane. Platelet factor 3 only becomes available on the platelet surface during platelet activation. Thus, **coagulation and thrombosis are closely intertwined.** The interaction of Factors X$_a$, V, calcium, and platelet factor 3 leads to thrombin formation. Thrombin activates fibrinogen to form fibrin, and the clot is formed.

The combination of platelet thrombus and clot is unstable because of the activation of plasmin, a fibrinolytic enzyme (Fig. 10-17). During clot formation, plasminogen is bound to fibrin and, therefore, is an integral part of the forming platelet mass. Endothelial cells synthesize plasminogen activator, but in larger thombi circulating plasminogen may also be con-

Table 10-4 Coagulation Factor Designations

FACTOR	STANDARD NAME	ALTERNATIVE DESIGNATIONS
I	Fibrinogen	
II	Prothrombin	
III	Tissue factor	Thromboplastin
IV	Calcium ions	
V	Proaccelerin	Labile factor, accelerator globulin (AcG), thrombogen
(VI)		No longer considered in the scheme of hemostasis
VII	Proconvertin	Stable factor, serum prothrombin conversion accelerator (SPCA)
VIII	Antihemophilic factor (AHF)	Antihemophilic globulin (AHG), antihemophilic factor A, platelet cofactor 1, thromboplastinogen
IX	Plasma thromboplastin (PTC)	Christmas factor, antihemophilic factor B, autoprothrombin II, platelet cofactor 2
X	Stuart factor	Prower factor, autoprothrombin III, thrombokinase
XI	Plasma thromboplastin antecedent (PTA)	Antihemophilic factor C
XII	Hageman factor	Glass factor, contact factor
XIII	Fibrin stabilizing factor (FSF)	Laki-Lorand factor (LLF), fibrinase, plasma transglutaminase, fibrinoligase
—	Prekallikrein	Fletcher factor
—	HMW kininogen	High molecular weight kininogen, contact activation cofactor, Fitzgerald factor, Williams factor, Flaujeac factor, Reid factor, Washington factor

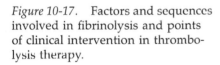

Figure 10-17. Factors and sequences involved in fibrinolysis and points of clinical intervention in thrombolysis therapy.

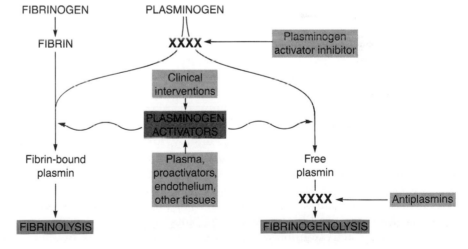

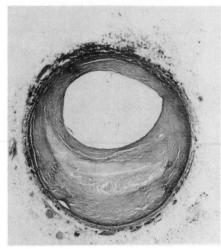
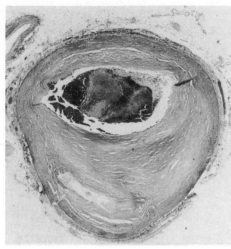

A   B

Figure 10-18.   Atherosclerotic coronary occlusion. (*A*) Coronary artery with atherosclerotic plaque in a 54-year-old man. (*B*) Downstream of the plaque is the occluding thrombus that caused the man's death.

verted to plasmin by products of the coagulation cascade. Plasminogen activator bound to fibrin activates plasmin; in turn, by digesting fibrin, plasmin lyses the clot and disrupts the thrombus. The synthesis of plasminogen activator represents still another antithrombotic mechanism of the endothelial cell. Endothelial cells also synthesize an inhibitor of plasminogen activator. Thus, again this cell possesses pro- and anticoagulant properties.

Coronary Artery Occlusion

It is useful to consider the sequence of events that might occur in a 50-year-old man undergoing the initial events in a myocardial infarction.

The primary process involves a coronary artery wall that is roughened by the underlying atherosclerotic plaque (Fig. 10-18). At this point the surface is not thrombogenic and the endothelium is intact. **Some change occurs in the lesion to make it thrombogenic.** Perhaps the lesion ulcerates. Possibly, toxic products released by macrophages alter endothelial cell viability, so that the cells are sloughed. Vasa vasorum may hemorrhage into the plaque. Any of these circumstances will lead to exposure of the connective tissue of the vessel wall to the circulating blood.

Alternatively, activated macrophages in the lesion may secrete tumor necrosis factor or interleukin-1, causing endothelial cells to secrete thromboplastin. In any event, platelets are stimulated to interact with collagen, fibronectin, or fibrin on the injured surface, after which they adhere and become activated. The activated platelets stimulate platelet aggregation by releasing thromboxane A₂ and ADP. Von Willebrand factor is liberated from platelet alpha granules and possibly from injured endothelial cells, a process

which further accelerates platelet aggregation. The platelet alpha granule contributes to the stabilization of the forming aggregate by liberating fibrinogen and fibronectin. Platelet granules release ADP and vasoactive elements, including histamine, epinephrine, and serotonin. Calcium discharged by the platelets helps to stimulate the coagulation sequence.

Activation of the platelet surface also promotes coagulation by the intrinsic pathway because it leads to binding of Factor X, Factor V, and calcium. In addition to stimulating platelet aggregation, thromboxane A₂ also provokes constriction of the surrounding vessels, thus worsening the occlusion of the lumen. The initiation of the intrinsic clotting cascade results in the release of thrombin. In addition to stimulating the formation of fibrin, thrombin itself is a powerful promoter of platelet aggregation. Thus, the initial aggregate of platelets becomes converted to a mixture of platelets and thrombus. Injury to surrounding smooth muscle and endothelial cells results in the release of tissue factor, which then initiates the extrinsic coagulation pathway.

The interaction between thrombosis and coagulation results in the formation of layers of fibrin and platelets within arterial thrombi. These layers, which are visible when the thrombus is sectioned, are called **lines of Zahn.** The formation of lines of Zahn depends on a high flow rate; thrombi formed in areas of sluggish blood flow, such as veins or atrial appendages, do not show a layered structure. If the thrombus does not progress, it remains attached to the wall and is called a **mural thrombus.** A mural thrombus that becomes sufficiently large occludes the vessel, and is labeled an **occlusive thrombus.**

The organized structure of a thrombus, which reflects a tight interaction between platelets and fibrin, differs in appearance from the **postmortem clot** or the clot formed in a test tube. The lines of Zahn stabilize the thrombus formed during life, whereas the postmortem clot is a more gelatinous structure. Postmorten clots occur in stagnant blood, where gravity fractionates the erythrocytes. The part of the clot that contains many red blood cells is called **current jelly.** The overlying clot, which represents coagulated plasma without red blood cells, is called **chicken fat** because of its color and consistency.

The mural thrombus overlying an atherosclerotic plaque is a rich source of chemotactic factors and mitogens. These agents stimulate the smooth muscle cells in the plaque to grow, secrete collagen, and convert a labile structure into a more permanent one. The thrombus is invaded by smooth muscle cells and connective tissue, and the resulting **organized thrombus** is a permanent structure. New vessels may invade and provide some blood flow across the organized thrombus, a process called **canalization** of the thrombus. Unfortunately, these new vessels are almost always too small to maintain a clinically significant level of blood flow.

A thrombus over a vascular plaque may propagate and eventually occlude the vessel. The observation is important because this mechanism is probably the most common cause of occlusion of the coronary arteries, and because the recent introduction of thrombolytic therapy has in many cases permitted the reestablishment of the lumen. It is now possible to dissolve an early thrombus by injecting enzymes that activate plasmin. If this is done very soon after thrombus formation, the treatment may prevent myocardial infarction.

An interesting example of mural thrombus formation has been documented in a number of deaths following the intravenous or intranasal use of cocaine. The deaths have been associated with acute myocardial infarction or with arrythmias. In these case reports, coronary lesions have been described and fall into three categories: fresh mural platelet thrombi; lesions involving proliferation of smooth muscle cells in the intima; and organized, recanalized thrombi. In some instances, fresh thrombi occur on top of older organized thrombi. These lesions occur in young individuals (21 to 44 years) who are frequently without evidence of atherosclerosis or vasculitis elsewhere. The older lesions have been described as "nonatherosclerotic intimal proliferations." This form of obstructive coronary disease could be primarily due to mural thrombosis and organization. It is possible that coronary spasm leads to an alteration of blood flow, with endothelial injury being followed by thrombus formation.

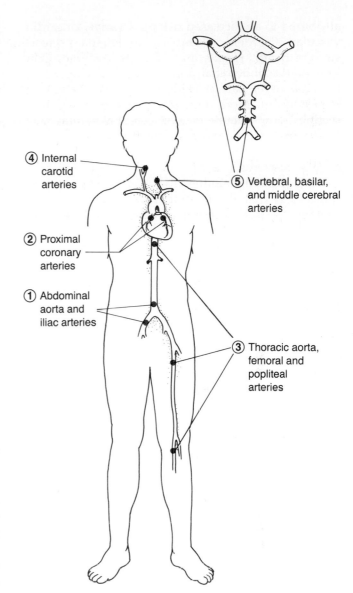

Figure 10-19. Sites of severe atherosclerosis in order of frequency.

The ultimate result of thrombotic vascular occlusion of a coronary artery is myocardial infarction. The same sequence of events occurs in other organs, such as the kidney and brain (Fig. 10-19).

Hypertensive Vascular Disease

Hypertension, with its associated atherosclerotic vascular disease, is a common cause of death in the United States. Among black Americans, hypertension is also the most common fatal heritable disease. Most of the disease associated with hypertension is attributed to an increased risk for a variety of cardiovascular disorders. Examples are angina pectoris, sudden death, stroke, and atherothrombotic occlusion of the abdominal aorta or its branches. More than half of the patients with these diseases also have hypertension. More than 70% of patients with dissecting aortic aneurysm, intracerebral hemorrhage, or rupture of the myocardial wall have an elevated blood pressure. Hypertension is a major risk factor for atherosclerosis, as shown in both epidemiologic and experimental studies. In recent years it has become clear that the treatment of hypertension can prolong life. It is disturbing to realize that the etiology of most hypertension remains unknown: 95% of patients display no identifiable etiology. Thus, the large majority of hypertensive people are described as having **essential** or **primary hypertension.**

Diagnosis

The diagnosis of hypertension depends on a statistical estimate of the relationship of individual blood pressure to the distribution of pressure in our society. Over the course of the day, blood pressure varies over a large range, depending on exertion, emotional state, and other poorly understood factors. Thus, it is important that blood pressure be measured at several different times and under consistent circumstances before a diagnosis of hypertension is made. A greater problem is the variation in blood pressure with age in our population. The mean systolic blood pressure in 20-year-old men is about 130 torr, but the 95% confidence limits include a range from 105 to 150 torr. With age, the average systolic blood pressure increases, so that in 80-year-olds it is approximately 170 torr, with the 95% confidence limits including a range from 125 to 220 torr. Against this background, the "diagnostic level" of blood pressure remains controversial. The World Health Organization has defined systemic hypertension as a systolic pressure greater than 160 torr or a diastolic pressure greater than 90 torr, or both.

Etiology

Attempts to identify a single etiology for primary hypertension have been frustrating. We know from family studies that genetic factors are likely to be important. For example, there is a familial association of hypertension with alterations in membrane transport of sodium and lithium. Interestingly, spontaneous hypertension can be produced in rats in as few as six generations of inbreeding for elevated blood pressure. However, no specific genetic defect has been shown to be causal in rat or man.

The most widespread hypothesis holds that primary hypertension results from an imbalance in the interactions between the mechanisms for controlling cardiac output, renal function, peripheral resistance, and sodium homeostasis (Fig. 10-20). A complex endocrine axis centers on the renin–angiotensin system. As previously noted, renal artery occlusion or dietary salt restriction results in an elevation of the renal secretion of renin. Renin is a protease that lyses angiotensinogen to a decapeptide, angiotensin I. In turn, angiotensin I is converted to angiotensin II by angiotensin converting enzyme, a protein found on the surface of the endothelial cell. Although angiotensin II was originally thought of primarily as a vasoconstrictor, it is now recognized that it also has major effects on centers in the central nervous system that control sympathetic outflow and stimulate aldosterone release from the adrenal gland. Aldosterone acts on renal tubules to increase sodium reabsorption. The net effect is to increase total body fluid volume. Thus, the **renin–angiotensin system** elevates blood pressure by three mechanisms: increased sympathetic output, increased mineralocorticoid secretion, and direct vasoconstriction. The renin–angiotensin–aldosterone axis is antagonized by a hormone, **atrial natriuretic factor,** secreted by specialized cells in the atria. This factor, acting via its own receptors, increases the urinary excretion of sodium and opposes the vasoconstrictor effects of angiotensin II. Secretion of atrial natriuretic factor may be controlled by atrial distension, a consequence of increased volume, or by as yet undefined endocrine interactions.

The importance of this axis of hormones in regulating blood pressure in hypertension is demonstrated by the therapeutic success of antisympathetic agents, diuretics, and angiotensin antagonists. Nonetheless, there is no clear evidence that a specific defect in the renin–angiotensin axis is the essential lesion of primary hypertension. It has proved difficult to identify a crucial defect in this axis or a critical genetic lesion, because the vascular system responds quickly to changes in the effective rates of flow through tissue beds by **autoregulation** (see Fig. 10-20). **In the case of hypertension, the end result of autoregulation is always increased peripheral resistance.** For example, hypertension can be induced in dogs by surgical resection of large amounts of kidney tissue, followed by increased sodium and water intake. Cardiac output, and therefore blood pressure, is rapidly increased as a result of the rapid change in blood volume. Within a few days, however, pressure-induced diuresis results in a return to near-normal cardiac output and plasma volume. At this point, blood pressure is maintained by increased peripheral

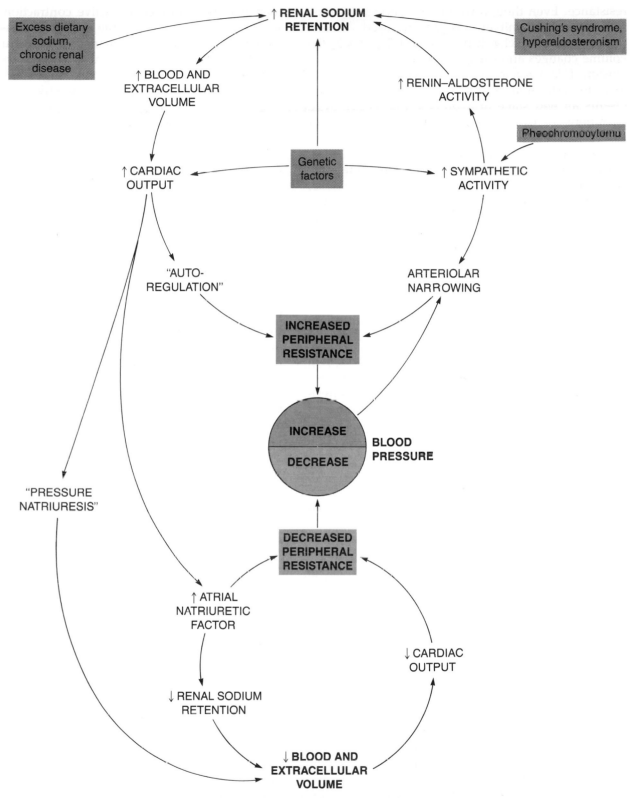

Figure 10-20. Factors contributing to hypertension and the counter-regulatory factors that lower blood pressure. An imbalance in these factors results in the increased peripheral resistance that is responsible for most cases of idiopathic (primary) hypertension. Note the central role of peripheral resistance.

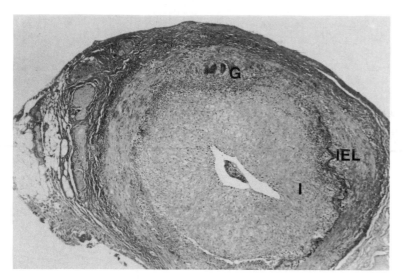

Figure 10-24. Temporal (giant cell) arteritis. A temporal artery shows a fully developed lesion with giant cells in the media (*G*), a thickened intima (*I*), and a few inflammatory cells. *IEL*, internal elastica.

ally benign and self-limited, the symptoms subsiding in 6 to 12 months. In a minority of cases the disease has serious complications, such as blindness, and may even be fatal. The response to corticosteroid therapy is usually dramatic, with symptoms subsiding in a matter of days.

The etiology of giant cell arteritis is obscure, and no bacterial or viral cause has been found. The morphologic alterations suggest an immunologic reaction, and a cell-mediated response to arterial antigens has been reported in some cases. The generalized muscle aching and widespread distribution of its manifestations suggest a relationship to rheumatoid disease.

Wegener's Granulomatosis

Wegener's granulomatosis is a rare necrotizing vasculitis characterized by granulomas of the upper respiratory tract (the nose, sinuses, and lungs) and renal disease. Men are affected more often than women, usually in the fifth and sixth decades of life. The most prominent clinical feature is a persistent bilateral pneumonitis, with nodular infiltrates that undergo cavitation in a manner similar to tuberculous lesions. Chronic sinusitis and ulcerations of the nasopharyngeal mucosa are common. The kidney shows a focal or diffuse necrotizing glomerulitis. Skin rashes, muscular pains, joint involvement, and neuritis occur. Fever is observed in about half the patients. The disease carries a very high mortality: 80% of patients die within a year of onset, with a mean survival of 5 to 6 months. Immunosuppressive therapy (cyclophosphamide) is often highly effective.

The granulomatous lesions of the respiratory tract, which may be as large as 5 cm across in the lung,

appear tuberculoid, with a surrounding fibrous zone containing giant cells and a leukocytic infiltrate. Vasculitis involving small arteries and veins may be found anywhere, but is seen most frequently in the respiratory tract (Fig. 10-25), kidney, and spleen. The vascular lesions of Wegener's granulomatosis closely resemble those of the acute phase of polyarteritis nodosa, showing acute inflammation and fibrinoid necrosis. The kidney exhibits focal necrotizing glomerulonephritis or crescentic glomerular proliferative lesions. Hematuria and proteinuria are common, and the glomerular proliferative disease can progress to renal failure. The etiology of this disease is not clear, and no infectious agent has been uncovered. Its resemblance to other vasculitides, coupled with its response to immunosuppression by cyclophosphamide, suggests an immunologic origin.

Kawasaki's Disease (Mucocutaneous Lymph Node Syndrome)

Kawasaki's disease is an acute vasculitis of infancy and early childhood characterized by high fever, rash, conjunctival and oral lesions, and lymphadenitis. Acute necrotizing vasculitis of small and medium-sized coronary arteries occurs in as many as 70% of patients and is a cause of death in 1% to 2% of cases.

Like many childhood viral diseases, Kawasaki's disease is usually self-limited, and although microbial causes have been sought, none has been conclusively proved. A DNA polymerase with properties suggesting a dependence on the RNA template has been found in peripheral blood mononuclear cells of patients with this malady, and electron microscopy has revealed viral particles in these cells.

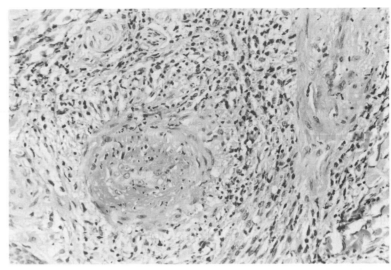

Figure 10-25. Wegener's granulomatosis. A section of lung shows destruction of pulmonary parenchyma, which in part is replaced by fibrous tissue. This fibrous tissue is still infiltrated by a mixed population of inflammatory cells. A small artery displays a cellular infiltrate and proliferation of the arterial smooth muscle cells.

Thromboangiitis Obliterans (Buerger's Disease)

Thromboangiitis obliterans occurs almost exclusively in young and middle-aged men who smoke heavily. The symptoms usually start between the ages of 25 and 40 years and take the form of intermittent claudication (cramping pains in muscles following exercise, which are quickly relieved by rest).

The blood vessels of the legs are most frequently affected, but those of the arm are not uncommonly involved. Rarely are other sites affected, although involvement of coronary, cerebral, and mesenteric arteries has been noted. However, some of these cases may simply represent complications of atherosclerosis.

The process appears earliest as an acute inflammation, with infiltration of medium-sized and small arteries by neutrophils (Fig. 10-26). The inflammation extends to involve neighboring veins and nerves. Small microabscesses of the vessel wall distinguish the process from thrombosis associated with atherosclerosis. These abscesses consist of a central area of neutrophils surrounded by fibroblasts and Langhan's giant cells. The early lesions are further complicated by thrombosis of veins and arteries, often severe enough to result in gangrene of the extremity, for which the only treatment is amputation. Late in the course of the disease the thrombi are completely organized and partly canalized.

The etiologic role of smoking in Buerger's disease is emphasized by the observation that cessation of smoking can be followed by a remission, and resumption of smoking by an exacerbation. Yet the mechanism of action of tobacco smoke is obscure. Although carbon monoxide has been postulated as a

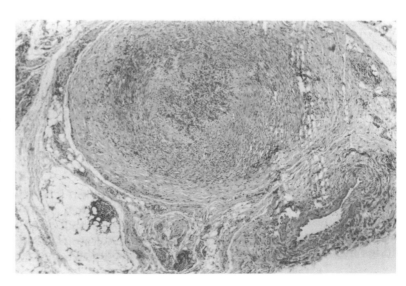

Figure 10-26. Thromboangiitis obliterans (Buerger's disease). An artery from an amputated limb of a 55-year-old male cigarette smoker shows an organized thrombus that has completely occluded the artery. Some inflammatory cells are evident in the adventitial fat. In this instance the adjacent vein has been largely spared.

11

The Heart

Donald B. Hackel and Robert B. Jennings

Functional Anatomy of the Heart

Heart Failure

Congenital Heart Disease

Ischemic Heart Disease

Rheumatic and Other Hypersensitivity Diseases

Hypertensive Heart Disease

Inflammatory Diseases of the Heart

Nutritional, Endocrine, and Metabolic Diseases of the Heart

Cardiomyopathy

Luetic Heart Disease

Cardiac Tumors

Figure 11-1. The coronary circulation. The right coronary artery (*green*) supplies the back of the left ventricle and gives rise to the posterior descending artery. The left main coronary artery divides into the anterior descending (*red*) and the circumflex (*orange*) branches. (*Inset*) Postmortem coronary arteriogram.

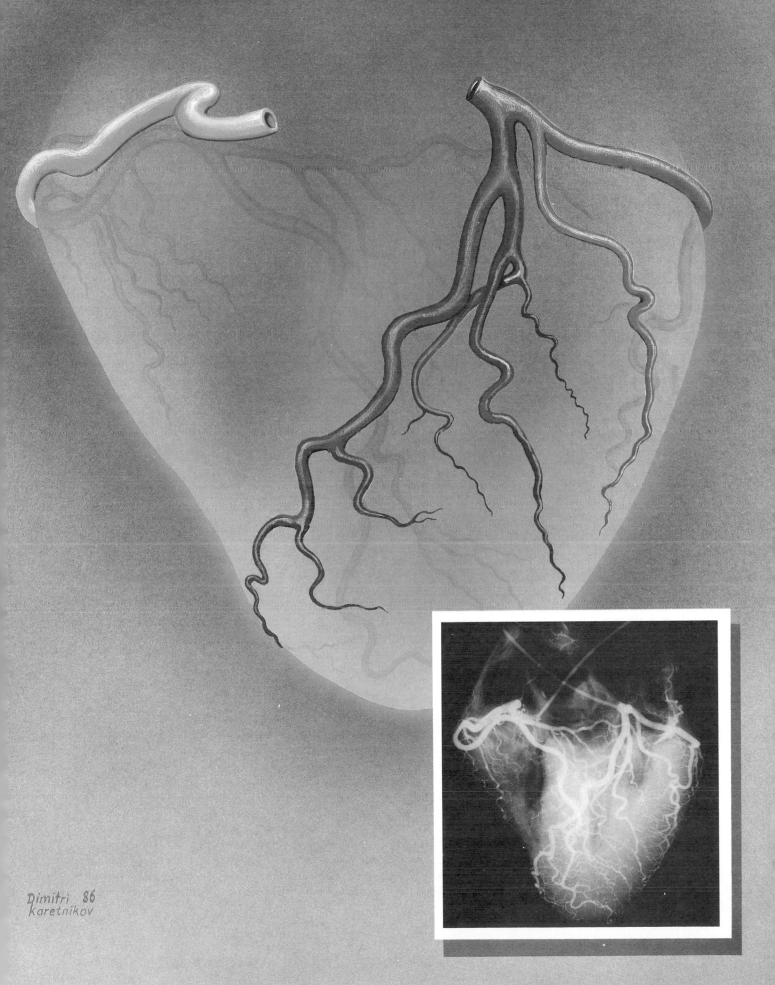

Dimitri 86
karetnikov

Functional Anatomy of the Heart

The heart is a fist-sized muscular pump that has a remarkable ability to work without letup or prolonged rest for the 70- to 80-year span of a human lifetime. Furthermore, it has the ability to increase its output many fold, as demand requires. This is made possible, in part, by the coronary circulation's ability to respond to an increased need for oxygen by increasing coronary blood flow to a rate more than 10 times normal. In addition, in accordance with Starling's law of the heart, the ventricles can respond to an acute increase in their workload by dilating. Thus, the most apparent indication that a patient died in heart failure is the finding at autopsy of dilatation of the ventricles. When an increased workload is imposed for a longer period—as it is in patients with essential hypertension—the heart hypertrophies, an adaptation that increases its capacity for work. However, this compensatory mechanism has its limits, which will be described later.

Because of the unrelenting work demand, the heart also requires much more energy than does skeletal muscle. The presence of a more concentrated mass of mitochondria in cardiac muscle permits this high level of aerobic energy production.

The Coronary Arteries

The right and left main coronary arteries supply the heart with oxygenated blood. These vessels originate in or just above the sinuses of Valsalva at the aortic valve. The epicardial portion of each artery fills and dilates during systole and narrows during diastole. The intramyocardial arteries have the opposite action and are constricted by the systolic muscular pressure, so that flow, especially to the subendocardial regions of the ventricle, is decreased or absent during systole.

Epicardial coronary arteries usually are arranged in the so-called right coronary dominant distribution, although about 10% of hearts are left-dominant. Dominance is determined by the coronary artery that supplies the posterior descending coronary artery (Fig. 11-1). The left anterior descending artery supplies the anterior left ventricle, the adjacent anterior right ventricle, and the anterior two-thirds of the interventricular septum, except in the apical region, where it supplies the ventricles circumferentially (Fig. 11-2B). The left circumflex coronary artery supplies the lateral wall of the left ventricle (Fig. 11-2A). The right coronary artery usually supplies the remainder of the right ventricle and the posteroseptal region of the left ventricle (Fig. 11-2C), including the posterior third of the interventricular septum at the base of the heart (also referred to as the "inferior" or "diaphragmatic" wall). From these distributions one can predict the location of the infarct that would follow occlusion of any of the three coronary artery branches.

It is enlightening to look at the arrangement of the coronary arteries as they pass through the ventricular walls at right angles to the epicardial vessels (Fig. 11-3). Some of these small coronary arteries branch as they pass through the ventricular wall, whereas others maintain a large diameter and pass to the endocardial surface without branching. This route through the myocardium accounts for the fact that infarcts usually occur first in the subendocardial region and then in the epicardial zone. More severe and prolonged ischemia leads to transmural involvement.

The Cardiac Myocyte

The myocardium is made up of branching myocytes, each of which has a single nucleus and is separated from adjacent cells by intercalated discs. The fine structural details of the myocytes can be seen in electron micrographs (Fig. 11-4), which show the sarcolemma, the sarcoplasmic reticulum, the T system of tubules, the nucleus, and numerous mitochondria. The myocyte contains myofilaments made up of sarcomeres. **The sarcomere is the basic functional unit of the contractile apparatus.** It extends from Z line to Z line and contains myosin (thick filament), which is limited to the A band. It also contains filaments of actin (thin filament) which, associated with tropomyosin and troponin, extend from the Z line through the I band and into the A band (Fig. 11-4). The interactions of these myofilaments generate the force for shortening the muscle. The amount of force that can be generated is proportional to the length of the adjoining myofilaments, and is at a maximum when the sarcomeres are between 2 and 2.2 microns in length. When the sarcomere length is less than 2 microns, the thin filaments slide across each other and overlap, decreasing the potential for force-generating cross links; when the sarcomere is stretched beyond 2.2 microns, there is a drop in force that is proportional to the widening H zone. It is apparent that this mechanism is the basis for **Starling's law of the heart.**

In the normal myocyte, troponin acts as an inhibitor of actin–myosin interaction. The small amount of calcium influx that accompanies the action potential stimulates a larger release of calcium from the sarcoplasmic reticulum. This in turn represses troponin,

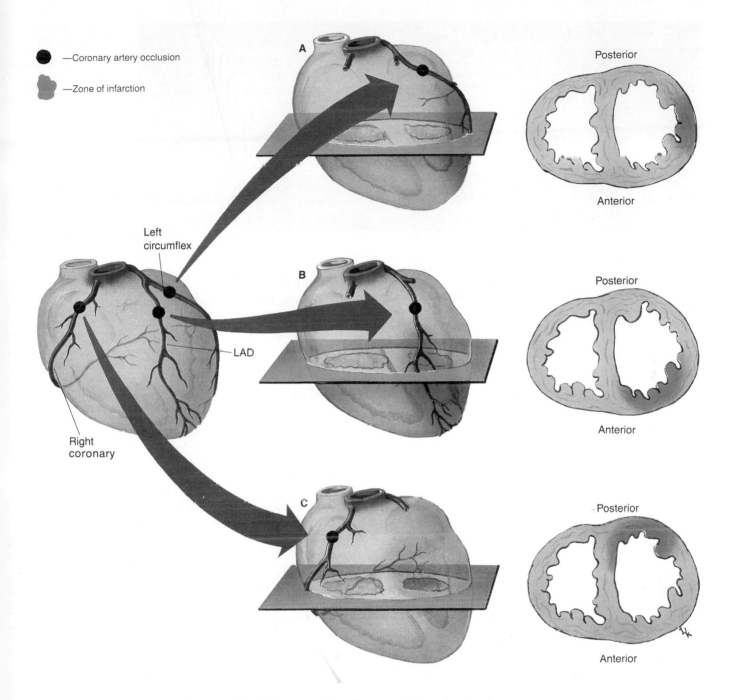

Figure 11-2. Position of left ventricular infarcts resulting from occlusion of each of the three main coronary arteries. (*A*) Posterolateral infarct, which follows an occlusion of the left circumflex artery and is present in the posterolateral wall. (*B*) Anterior infarct, which follows occlusion of the anterior descending branch (*LAD*) of the left coronary artery. The infarct is located in the anterior wall and adjacent two-thirds of the septum, in the apical three-quarters of the left ventricle. It involves the entire circumference of the wall near the apex. (*C*) Posterior ("inferior" or "diaphragmatic") infarct, which results from occlusion of the right coronary artery and involves the posterior wall, including the posterior third of the interventricular septum and the posterior papillary muscle in the basal half of the ventricle. Note the lateral displacement of the posterior papillary muscle caused by the expansion (i.e., stretching) of the infarct region of the left ventricle.

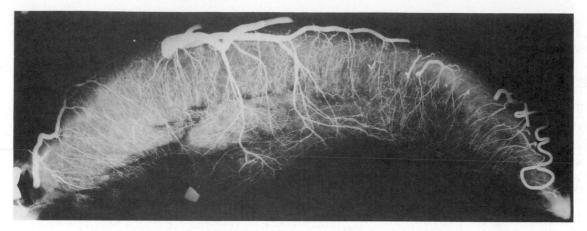

Figure 11-3.   Arteriogram of a longitudinal segment of the posterior wall of the left ventricle, including the posterior papillary muscle. Note the two types of branches passing into the myocardium at right angles to the epicardial artery (*top*). Class A, which quickly divide into a fine network; and class B, which maintain a large diameter and pass with little branching into the subendocardial region and the papillary muscle.

thereby triggering the contraction process. The number of contractile sites activated and the resulting force that is generated are directly proportional to the concentration of calcium in the vicinity of the myofibrils.

The Conducting System

The cardiac conducting system consists of specialized myocytes that have two major functions: (1) They initiate the heartbeat through their automatic rhythmicity, which is stronger in the sinoatrial node than in the more distal parts of the system, and (2) they conduct at a faster rate than the contractile fibers, with the exception of myocytes in the atrioventricular node, which act to delay the passage of the impulse. **Thus, the heartbeat originates in the sinoatrial node.** This site has the most rapid automatic rhythmicity. If it is prevented from functioning as the pacemaker

for the heartbeat, more distal parts of the system become the pacemaker; the slower the rate of the beat, the more distal the pacemaker site. On leaving the sinoatrial node, the impulse continues through the atrioventricular node, passing through the common bundle (bundle of His) and along the left and right bundle branches to the apex of the ventricles, which is the region that is first stimulated to contract. In the normal adult heart the common bundle is the only electrical connection between the atria and the ventricles. Occasionally, however, additional bypass pathways are present, including lateral accessory atrioventricular pathways (bundles of Kent), nodoventricular and fasciculoventricular pathways (Mahaim fibers), and intranodal and atriofascicular pathways (James fibers). Bypass fibers are often found in patients with certain arrhythmias. They can probably function to permit preexcitation of the ventricles and can also establish circus movements that result in tachycardia. The bypass pathways have also been postulated as the basis for Wolff-Parkinson-White syndrome, in which preexcitation is manifested by the delta wave and a short P–R interval.

It is often possible to identify at autopsy specific lesions of the conducting fibers that explain the arrhythmias that were present during life. Examples of these lesions are listed in Table 11-1. Such lesions may cause irregularity of the cardiac rhythm, slowing or speeding up of the heart rate, or partial or complete heart block. These functional defects may be transient or permanent, depending on the conditions

---

Table 11-1 Anatomic Causes of Conducting System Defects

Congenital: Lack of continuity of conducting system fibers (Often occurs with maternal systemic lupus erythematosus)
Traumatic: Surgically induced trauma
Vascular: Myocardial infarct
Inflammatory disease: Myocarditis; sarcoidosis; rheumatoid arthritis
Neoplastic: Primary (mesothelioma) or metastatic cancer
Metabolic: Amyloidosis, hemochromatosis
Aging effects: "Wear and tear"

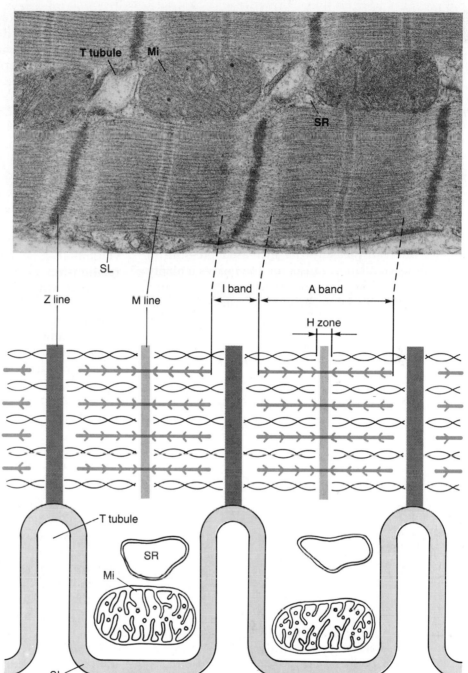

Figure 11-4. Ultrastructure of the myocardium. (*Top*) Electron micrograph of normal dog left ventricle in the longitudinal plane, showing the sarcolemma (*SL*); the sarcomeres of the myofibrils, which are delimited by Z lines; A-bands; I-bands; H-zones; and M-lines. Also present are mitochondria (*Mi*), sarcoplasmic reticulum (*SR*), and T tubules. The I-bands and H-zones are absent when the myofibrils are shortened. (*Bottom*) The structural basis for the banding shown in the electron micrograph. The fine threads that extend at right angles to the thick (myosin) filaments are the cross bridges that form the force-generating crosslinks with actin. The amount of force that can be generated is proportional to the length of the adjoining myofilaments, and is at a maximum when the sarcomeres are between 2 μm and 2.2 μm in length. When the sarcomeres are less than 2 μm in length, the thin filaments slide across each other and overlap, decreasing the potential for force-generating crosslinks; similarly, when the sarcomeres are stretched beyond 2.2 μm, there is a drop in force that is proportional to the widening of the H-zone. It is apparent that this mechanism can be invoked as the basis for Starling's Law of the Heart.

of the injury. For example, acute myocardial infarction or surgical trauma may so injure the conducting fibers that heart block results. However, normal sinus rhythm is often restored as the local inflammatory and hemorrhagic changes subside.

Heart Failure

A common result of various cardiac diseases is heart failure, which is the inability of the heart to pump blood at a rate that is adequate for the body's needs. The functional capacity of the heart to do work can be assessed clinically in a number of ways. For example, one can measure the increased pressure in the venous circulation caused by the heart's inability to propel all of the blood returned to it by the veins. This produces the clinical picture of **backward heart failure**. A rough indication of the severity of this

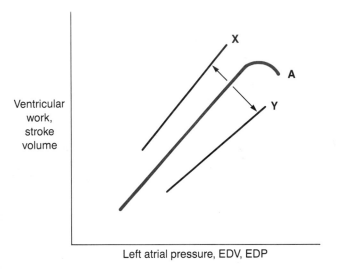

Figure 11-5. The relation of the work of the heart (or stroke volume) to the level of venous inflow, as measured by atrial pressure, or by ventricular end-diastolic volume or end-diastolic pressure. Curve *A* indicates that as the ventricular end-diastolic volume (EDV), end-diastolic pressure (EDP), or left atrial pressure increases, the amount of work done by the heart increases linearly up to a point. Beyond this point there is a decrease in the work done, and the heart fails. However, the downslope of this curve is reached only at very high left atrial pressures. The curve may shift up to position *X* or down to position *Y*, depending on whether the heart is more contractile (e.g., because of the action of norepinephrine) or is less contractile (i.e., in failure), respectively. The failing heart usually functions on the ascending limb of a depressed curve.

condition can be obtained by measuring the jugular venous pressure directly, by observing jugular venous distension with the patient in the upright position, or by determining the size of the liver and spleen, which are enlarged when they are congested with blood. One can also measure the ability of the heart to propel blood forward. For example, cardiac stroke volume may be decreased, a defect that results in so-called **forward heart failure**. The work of the heart can also be measured as the product of the cardiac output and the blood pressure. This calculation is more meaningful if the work is related to a measure of the venous inflow, such as the left or right atrial pressure (Fig. 11-5). The end-diastolic pressure of the ventricle—or better, its end-diastolic volume—can be substituted for atrial pressure. **This relationship is the expression of Starling's law of the heart, which states that the stroke volume of the heart is a function of the diastolic fiber length and that within certain limits, the heart will pump whatever volume of blood is brought to it from the venous circulation.** Thus, cardiac muscle contracts more forcefully when stretched, and an increasing preload (as indicated by elevated end-diastolic ventricular volume) provides a reserve mechanism to augment the performance of the heart.

Effects of Heart Failure

The effects of heart failure are seen in all the organs of the body. They become congested and edematous, and show changes indicative of acute and chronic anoxia. A hypertensive patient who has been in "left-sided heart failure" for a prolonged period will show pulmonary passive congestion, edema, and fibrotic thickening of the alveolar septa. In passive congestion the capillaries fill with blood, and the alveoli contain many hemosiderin-filled macrophages from the phagocytosis of hemoglobin released from red blood cells that have leaked into the alveoli. The edema may be massive, with alveoli being "drowned" in a transudate (Table 11-2). Fibrosis results from chronic anoxia, which causes parenchymal damage and subsequent repair. In earlier and more acute episodes of the same process, the findings may consist mainly of massive edema of the lungs (Fig. 11-6) together with acute vascular congestion. The liver of a patient who has had "right-sided heart failure" displays marked congestion. Distended central vein areas stand out as dark red foci against the yellow of the cells in the periphery of the lobule, giving the liver a gross appearance that has been

Table 11-2 Comparison of Characteristics of a Transudate and an Exudate

	TRANSUDATE	EXUDATE
Protein Content	Low <3g/dl Smaller mol. wt. proteins	High >3g/dl Larger mol. wt. proteins
Specific Gravity	Under 1.015	Over 1.020
Vascular Permeability	Usually normal	Increased
Cellular Content	Few or none	Many red and white blood cells

compared to the cut surface of a nutmeg (hence the term "nutmeg liver") (Fig. 11-7). Microscopically, the sinusoids are distended most prominently in the central regions of the liver lobules; as a result, this is the location of the most severe anoxic effects. After frequent bouts of congestive failure, as occur in patients with long-standing heart disease, the centrilobular regions of the liver develop fine collagen deposits in a process that leads to so-called cardiac cirrhosis.

In heart failure the changes in the heart are non-specific. Conspicuous dilatation of the chambers and hypertrophy of the cardiac muscle are usual.

Causes of Heart Failure

Almost anything that causes the heart to increase its workload for a prolonged period or produces anatomic damage making it more difficult for the heart to function may eventuate in myocardial failure. The most important of these conditions are:

1. Congenital heart disease
2. Ischemic heart disease
3. Rheumatic heart disease and other "immune" diseases, including:

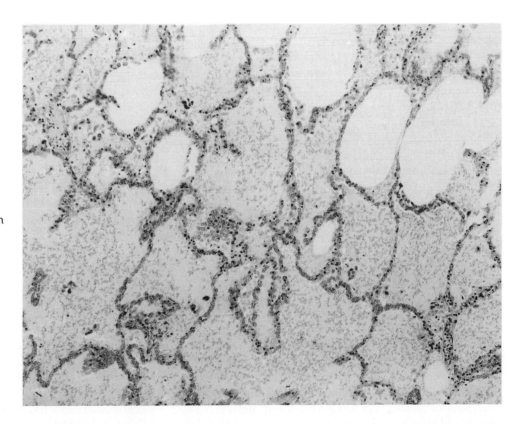

Figure 11-6. Pulmonary edema. Microscopic appearance of an edematous lung, showing the alveoli filled with granular and hyaline eosinophilic edema fluid.

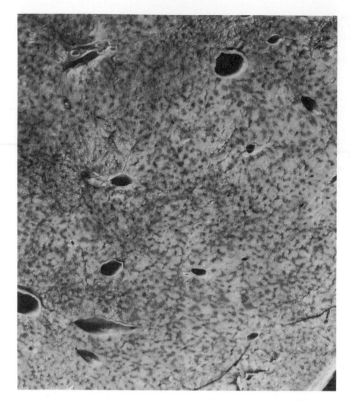

Figure 11-7.   Chronic passive congestion of the liver. The gross appearance of the surface of the liver in a patient with congestive heart failure, showing severe passive congestion, with engorged central veins standing out as darker zones ("nutmeg" appearance).

- Lupus erythematosus
- Rheumatoid arthritis
- Scleroderma

4. Hypertensive heart disease
5. Inflammatory diseases of the heart
6. Nutritional, endocrine, and metabolic diseases, including:

- Thyrotoxicosis
- Myxedema
- Beriberi
- Carcinoid syndrome
- Storage diseases (lipid, carbohydrate)
- Amyloidosis

7. Cardiomyopathy

The most common type of heart disease in this list by far is ischemic heart disease, accounting for more than 80% of deaths due to heart disease. Between 1% and 3% of deaths are due to hypertensive heart dis-

ease, about 1% are due to rheumatic heart disease, and the remaining types account for less than 1% each.

Factors in the Production of Congestive Heart Failure

Although numerous conditions are known to predispose an individual to heart failure (e.g., hypertension, ischemia, valvular disease), the molecular mechanisms of failure remain unknown. However, in the hearts of patients in congestive heart failure there are some changes that may be significant, including a decrease in the beta-adrenergic receptor sites in the myocardium. It also has been demonstrated that the failing heart contains isozymes of myosin with less than normal ATPase activity. Some studies have demonstrated decreases in the capacity of the sarcoplasmic reticulum to transport Ca^{2+} in experimental heart failure (Fig. 11-8).

Congenital Heart Disease

Incidence

The incidence of congenital heart disease is usually cited as being between 0.3% and 1% of all live births. This figure does not include certain common defects that are not functionally significant, such as an anatomically patent foramen ovale that is functionally closed by the flap that covers it. The foramen ovale, therefore, remains closed as long as the left atrial pressure is higher than that in the right atrium. A common bicuspid aortic valve is also clinically insignificant.

The figures for the incidence of particular types of cardiovascular anomaly in patients with congenital heart disease vary depending on many factors, but a range derived from several sources provides the following figures:

Ventricular septal defect, 25% to 30%
Atrial septal defect, 10% to 15%
Patent ductus arteriosus, 10% to 20%
Tetralogy of Fallot, 6% to 15%
Pulmonic stenosis, 5% to 7%
Coarctation of the aorta, 5% to 7%
Aortic stenosis, 4% to 6%
Complete transposition of the great arteries, 4% to 10%
Truncus arteriosus, 2%
Tricuspid atresia, 1%

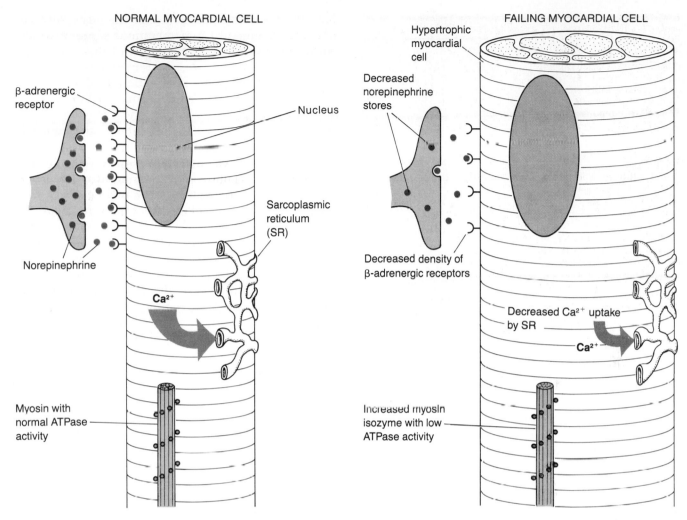

NORMAL MYOCARDIAL CELL

β-adrenergic receptor

Nucleus

Norepinephrine

Sarcoplasmic reticulum (SR)

Ca²⁺

Myosin with normal ATPase activity

FAILING MYOCARDIAL CELL

Hypertrophic myocardial cell

Decreased norepinephrine stores

Decreased density of β-adrenergic receptors

Decreased Ca²⁺ uptake by SR

Ca²⁺

Increased myosin isozyme with low ATPase activity

Figure 11-8. Biochemical characteristics of congestive heart failure.

Etiology

The etiology of congenital cardiac defects is usually not determinable. However, it is worthwhile to ascertain whether the defect in any one case can be recognized as being mainly of genetic or mainly of acquired origin, since this is of obvious importance to the parents in planning future pregnancies. The best evidence for an intrauterine influence on the occurrence of congenital cardiac defects relates to maternal infection with rubella virus during the first trimester, especially during the first 4 weeks of gestation. An association with other virus infections is suspected but is not as well documented. Similarly, thalidomide ingestion early in pregnancy results in a variety of severe congenital lesions, including congenital heart defects in a small number of patients. The maternal use of other drugs (e.g., aspirin) in early pregnancy is also associated with an increased number of cardiac defects in the offspring. An interesting association also has recently been recognized between maternal systemic lupus erythematosus and congenital complete heart block in the offspring.

Classification

There are several ways to categorize hearts with congenital defects. One of the earliest clinically useful schemes was proposed by Maude Abbott, who grouped cases into three categories according to the presence or absence of cyanosis: the acyanotic group (no abnormal communication between the two circulations), the cyanose tardive group (left-to-right shunt with late reversal of flow), and the cyanotic group (permanent right-to-left shunt). As examples of the acyanotic group Abbott described coarctation

Table 11-3 Classification of Congenital Heart Disease

Initial Left to Right Shunt

Ventricular septal defect
Atrial septal defect
Patent ductus arteriosus
Persistent truncus arteriosus
Anomalous pulmonary venous drainage

Right to Left Shunt

Tetralogy of Fallot

No Shunt

Complete transposition of the great vessels
Coarctation of the aorta
Pulmonary stenosis
Aortic stenosis
Coronary artery origin from pulmonary artery
Ebstein's malformation
Complete heart block
Endocardial fibroelastosis

of the aorta, right-sided aortic arch, Ebstein's anomaly, and congenital tricuspid insufficiency. She illustrated the cyanose tardive group with cases of patent ductus arteriosus, patent foramen ovale, and ventricular septal defect. In these patients cyanosis occurs late (i.e., tardive) because the shunt, which is at first from left to right, later becomes a right-to-left shunt (Eisenmenger's complex). This shift occurs because of the development of pulmonary vascular changes that increase pulmonary vascular resistance. (In a protective surgical procedure, the pulmonary artery is banded, thus decreasing the pulmonary blood flow.) As examples of the cyanotic group, Abbott described the tetralogy of Fallot, truncus arteriosus, and complete transposition of the great vessels.

Since Abbott's groupings, numerous classification schemes have been developed to provide the detail necessary to meet clinical requirements—especially those of the surgeon. It is simpler and more pertinent to divide the cases into groups shown in Table 11-3.

The following examples of the most common congenital cardiac defects are, for the most part, straightforward.

Ventricular Septal Defects

(Initial Left-to-Right Shunt)

The fetal heart consists of a single chamber until approximately the fifth week of gestation, after which it is divided by the development of the interatrial and interventricular septa, and by the formation of the atrioventricular valves from the endocardial cushions. A muscular interventricular septum develops

from the apex toward the base of the heart (Fig. 11-9A). This is joined by a membranous septum, which grows downward as an extension of the spiral septum, thus accomplishing the separation into right and left ventricles. **The most common defect is related to failure of this membranous portion to form in whole or in part.** In addition, there may be defects in the muscular portion of the ventricular septum; these are more common in the anterior region but can occur anywhere in the muscular septum.

Ventricular septal defects vary, and may occur as a small hole in the region of the membranous septum, large defects involving more than the membranous region (perimembranous defects), or complete absence of the muscular septum (leaving a single ventricle). Defects occur most commonly at the base of the heart, usually below the crista supraventricularis (infracristal) and behind the septal leaflet of the tricuspid valve, with the common bundle (bundle of His) lying just below the defect (inlet type). Less commonly, the defect occurs above the crista supraventricularis (supracristal) and just below the pulmonary valve (infra-arterial). The supracristal variety is often associated with other defects, such as an overriding pulmonary artery (the Taussig-Bing type of double outlet right ventricle), transposition of the great vessels, or persistent truncus arteriosus. **A small defect may have little functional significance and may actually close spontaneously as the child matures.** Closure is accomplished by either hypertrophy of the adjacent muscle or adherence of the tricuspid valve leaflets to the margins of the defect. **In larger defects there is an initial left-to-right shunt that produces an increased pulmonary blood flow, eventually resulting in pulmonary arteriolar thickening and increased pulmonary vascular resistance.** This resistance may be so great that the direction of the shunt flow is reversed, and goes from right to left **(Eisenmenger's complex).** A patient with this condition displays a late onset of cyanosis (i.e., tardive cyanosis).

Complications of ventricular septal defects include heart failure, ventricular hypertrophy, pulmonary hypertension (with reversal of shunt flow and resulting cyanosis), infective endocarditis, paradoxical emboli, brain abscesses, and prolapse of an aortic valve cusp (with resulting aortic valve insufficiency).

Atrial Septal Defects

The embryologic development of the atrial septum occurs in a sequence that permits the continued passage of oxygenated placental blood across the right atrium. The eustachian valve directs blood through the atrial septal opening into the left atrium. The developing atrial septum is programmed to permit this right-to-left shunt to continue until birth. Beginning at the fifth week of intrauterine life, the septum primum extends downward from the roof of the atrium to join with the endocardial cushions, closing the incomplete segment, or "ostium primum" (Fig. 11-9*A*). Before this closure is complete, the midportion of the septum primum develops a defect, or "ostium secundum," so that the right-to-left flow continues (Fig. 11-9*B*). During the sixth week, a second septum (septum secundum) develops to the right of the septum primum, passing from the roof of the atrium toward the endocardial cushions. This leaves a patent foramen at about the midpoint of the septum. This defect, known as the foramen ovale, persists after birth until it is sealed off by the fusion of the septum primum and septum secundum, after which it is termed the fossa ovalis. However, it remains patent in over 25% of all adults (a "probe-patent foramen ovale"), although it does not normally function as a shunt after birth. The higher pressure in the left atrium normally keeps the valve-like mechanism of the foramen closed.

There are four sites at which the atrial septum may be defective (Fig. 11-9). The first is the upper portion above the fossa ovalis near the entry of the superior vena cava; this defect is known as a **sinus venosus defect.** It is usually accompanied by drainage of the right pulmonary veins into the right atrium. This is an uncommon defect, occurring in only about 5% of atrial septal defects (Fig. 11-9*C*). The second site is the middle portion, where the defect is called an **atrial septal defect, ostium secundum type. This is by far the most common of the four sites, accounting for about 90% of atrial septal defects.** It varies in size, ranging from a patent foramen ovale (which is recognizable as patent only if tested with a probe) to a large defect of the entire fossa ovalis region. When the defect is only probe patent (25% of adult hearts) it is not normally functional; however, it may become a real shunt if circumstances elevate the right atrial pressure, as can occur with recurrent pulmonary thromboemboli. If this situation develops, a right-to-left shunt will be produced, and particles (e.g., thromboemboli) from the right-sided circulation will pass directly into the systemic circulation. These **paradoxical emboli** can produce infarcts in many parts of the body, most commonly in the brain, heart, spleen, intestines, kidneys, and legs. If the atrial septal defect is larger, it may result in an increase in blood flow on the right side of the heart sufficient to dilate and hypertrophy the right atrium and right ventricle, causing the pulmo-

nary artery to become larger in diameter than the aorta. The third defect site is the region adjacent to the endocardial cushion. This anomaly is termed an **atrial septal defect, ostium primum type** (Fig. 11-9*D*). This condition is also rare, accounting for about 7% of all atrial septal defects. There are usually clefts in the anterior leaflet of the mitral valve and the septal leaflet of the tricuspid valve, which may be accompanied by an associated defect in the adjacent interventricular septum. The fully developed combined defect is called a **persistent common atrioventricular canal** (also an endocardial cushion defect, an atrioventricular septal defect, or an atrioventricularis communis). Although rare, it is more frequent in patients with Down's syndrome. The endocardial cushion may form with a single atrioventricular ring and leaflets that cross the midline (complete atrioventricular canal) (Fig. 11-9*E*). The cushion may also join in the midline to form two intact valve rings (incomplete atrioventricular canal). The fourth type of atrial septal defect is the **coronary sinus** type. This abnormality is the rarest of the four. It is situated in the posteroinferior part of the interatrial septum at the site of the coronary sinus ostium and is associated with a persistent left superior vena cava, which drains into the roof of the left atrium.

A variant of the ostium secundum type of atrial septal defect is known as **Lutembacher's syndrome,** an anomaly defined as the combination of mitral stenosis (either congenital or as a result of rheumatic fever) and an ostium secundum type of atrial septal defect. It is thought likely that increased left atrial pressure secondary to the mitral valve obstruction influences the continued patency of the atrial septum.

Complications from atrial septal defects include heart failure, right ventricular hypertrophy, pulmonary vascular sclerosis, cyanosis (if the shunt reverses from right to left), paradoxical emboli, and brain abscess.

Patent Ductus Arteriosus

Early in its development the embryo supposedly recapitulates an ancestral evolutionary stage, with six aortic arches connecting the ventral and dorsal aortas as part of the branchial cleft system (Fig. 11-10). The left sixth aortic arch is partly preserved as the pulmonary arteries, and the arterial continuation on the left to the descending thoracic aorta is retained as the "ductus arteriosus." After birth the ductus contracts in response to the increased arterial oxygen content and becomes fibrotic. Although it may thus be functionally closed immediately after birth, it is not con-

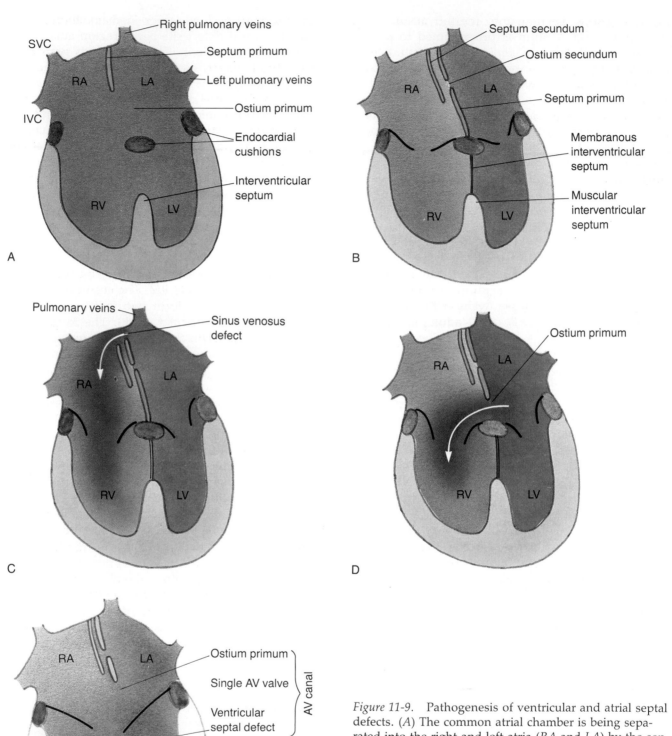

Figure 11-9. Pathogenesis of ventricular and atrial septal defects. (A) The common atrial chamber is being separated into the right and left atria (RA and LA) by the septum primum. Because the septum primum has not yet joined the endocardial cushion material, there is an open ostium primum. The ventricular cavity is being divided by a muscular interventricular septum into right and left chambers (RV and LV). SVC, superior vena cava; IVC, inferior vena cava.

sidered abnormal if it is anatomically patent for 1 to 2 months.

The persistence of a patent ductus arteriosus is one of the most common congenital cardiac defects, and it is especially common in babies whose mothers have had a rubella infection in early pregnancy. When present as an isolated anomaly (rather than as a component of a group of associated anomalies) it can be clinically diagnosed and surgically corrected, usually with complete success. The lumen of a patent ductus may vary greatly in size from patient to patient. A small shunt has little long-term effect on the heart and often will close spontaneously. A large shunt, on the other hand, produces a strain on the heart because of the markedly increased workload required to pump the augmented cardiac output. As a consequence, cardiac hypertrophy, a dilated pulmonary artery (with pulmonary hypertension), and eventual heart failure may supervene. Pulmonary hypertension may develop, with a subsequent reversal of shunt flow to a right-to-left direction.

It is of interest that the ductus arteriosus can be kept open by administration of prostaglandins (PGE$_2$), an effect that can be utilized in treating patients born with a cardiac defect that requires the presence of a left-to-right shunt to survive. Examples include patients with isolated pulmonary stenosis and those with a complete transposition of the great vessels. Conversely, in cases in which the ductus arteriosus is persistently and abnormally patent, it can be caused to contract and then close by inhibitors of prostaglandin synthesis (e.g., indomethacin).

A defect between the base of the aorta and the pulmonary artery is known as an "aortopulmonary window." It is a rare condition that is difficult to differentiate clinically from a patent ductus arteriosus.

Heart failure, cardiac hypertrophy, infective endarteritis, and pulmonary vascular sclerosis complicate the course of uncorrected patent ductus arteriosus.

Other abnormalities of the aortic arch system can be predicted by studying the appearance of the complete aortic arch system and visualizing the possible variations that could occur in its development (Fig. 11-10). For example, the right side of the aortic arch system may be retained rather than the left, resulting in the condition known as a "right aortic arch." This variant is seen in about 25% of patients with tetralogy of Fallot, and in 50% of patients with a truncus arteriosus. A right aortic arch is innocuous, unless it comes as a surprise to the cardiac surgeon.

Persistent Truncus Arteriosus

Persistent truncus arteriosus is a congenital cardiac defect that can be explained as the result of absent or incomplete partitioning of the truncus arteriosus by the spiral septum, thus leaving a common trunk for origin of the aorta, pulmonary arteries, and coronary arteries.

There are several variants of this lesion. Type 1, which is the most common, consists of a common trunk that gives rise to a common pulmonary artery and to the ascending aorta. In type 2 truncus arteriosus the right and left pulmonary arteries originate from a common site in the posterior midline of the truncus. In type 3 the separate pulmonary arteries originate laterally from the common trunk. There are other more rare variants (sometimes called type 4) in which there is no pulmonary trunk, and in which the pulmonary circulation is supplied from the aorta by enlarged bronchial arteries. This type is difficult to differentiate from tetralogy of Fallot with pulmonary artery atresia. The truncus always overrides a ventricular septal defect and receives blood from both ventricles. The valve of the truncus usually has three semilunar cusps, but may have as few as two or as

---

(*B*) The septum primum has joined the endocardial cushions, but at the same time has developed an opening in its mid-portion (the ostium secundum). This opening is partly overlain by the septum secundum, which has now grown down to cover the foramen ovale in part. Simultaneously, the membranous septum joins the muscular interventricular septum to the base of the heart, completely separating the ventricles. (*C*) The sinus venosus type of atrial septal defect is located in the most cephalad region and is adjacent to the inflow of the right pulmonary veins, which thus tend to open into the right atrium. (*D*) The ostium primum defect occurs just above the valve ring, sometimes in the presence of an intact valve ring. It may also, in conjunction with a defect of the valve ring and ventricular septum, form an atrioventricular canal, as shown in *E*. This common opening allows free communication between atria and ventricles.

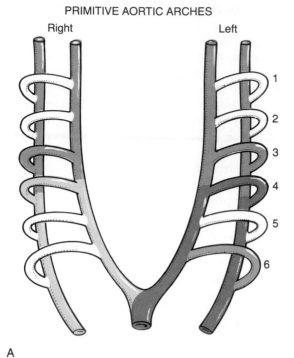

PRIMITIVE AORTIC ARCHES

Right   Left

1
2
3
4
5
6

A

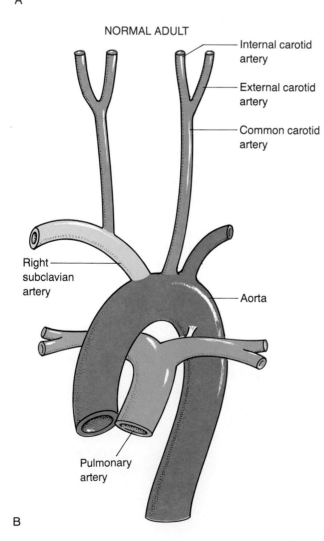

NORMAL ADULT

Internal carotid
artery

External carotid
artery

Common carotid
artery

Right
subclavian
artery

Aorta

Pulmonary
artery

B

many as six, and the coronary arteries arise from its base.

In addition to heart failure, ventricular hypertrophy, and pulmonary vascular sclerosis, these patients may exhibit stenosis or insufficiency of the truncus valve.

Anomalous Pulmonary Vein Drainage

The pulmonary veins form a network of veins in the dorsal mesoderm. A bud from the region of the atrium joins this pulmonary venous confluence. Failure of the correct junction of these tissues can result in various venous anomalies.

Total anomalous pulmonary vein drainage may occur as an isolated defect, or it may be part of the **asplenia syndrome** (splenic agenesis, congenital heart defects, and situs inversus of abdominal organs). Most commonly the pulmonary veins drain into a common pulmonary venous chamber, and then, via a persistent left superior vena cava (the persistent left precardinal vein), into the innominate vein or into the right superior vena cava. A second route for the common pulmonary vein drainage leads into the coronary sinus. A third drainage route consists of persistent posterior and subcardinal veins, which form a mid-dorsal trunk that crosses the diaphragm and enters the portal vein, a gastric vein, or the ductus venosus. Some pulmonary venous obstruction is often present in this third type of drainage.

Less severe impairment may result from partial anomalous pulmonary venous drainage. This may involve one or two pulmonary veins, especially in association with a sinus venosus type of atrial septal defect.

Heart failure, severe anoxemia, and pulmonary venous obstruction result from this anomaly.

Tetralogy of Fallot

(Right-to-Left Shunt)

The four anatomic changes that define the tetralogy of Fallot are pulmonary stenosis, ventricular septal defect, dextroposition of the aorta so that it overrides the ventricular septal defect, and right ventricular hypertrophy (Fig. 11-11). The ventricular septal defect is the result of incomplete closure of the mem-

---

Figure 11-10.   Derivatives of the aortic arches. (*A*) Complete primitive aortic arch system. (*B*) In the normal adult the left fourth aortic arch is preserved as the arch of the adult aorta and the left sixth arch is represented by the pulmonary artery and ductus arteriosus.

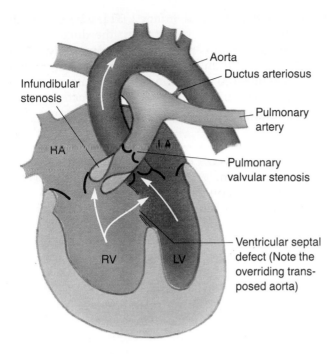

Infindibular stenosis

Aorta

Ductus arteriosus

Pulmonary artery

Pulmonary valvular stenosis

RA

LA

Ventricular septal defect (Note the overriding transposed aorta)

RV

LV

Figure 11-11. Tetralogy of Fallot. Note the pulmonary stenosis, which is due to infundibular hypertrophy as well as to pulmonary valvular stenosis. The ventricular septal defect involves the membranous septum region. Dextroposition of the aorta and right ventricular hypertrophy are shown. Because of the pulmonary obstruction the shunt is from right to left, and the patient is cyanotic.

branous septum and involves both the muscular septum and the endocardial cushions. In addition, the development of the spiral septum, which normally divides the common truncus region into an aorta and pulmonary artery, is probably abnormal, with resulting distortion of the aorta into a more dextral position overlying the septal defect.

Tetralogy of Fallot is the most common type of cyanotic congenital heart disease in older children and adults, and is usually accompanied by clubbing of the fingers. The heart is hypertrophied in such a way as to give it a boot shape. The septal defect is just below the overriding aorta. Pulmonary stenosis is usually due to subpulmonary muscular hypertrophy, with an enlarged infundibular muscle obstructing blood flow into the pulmonary artery. However, in about one-third of these hearts the valve itself is the main cause of the stenosis; in such cases the valve is usually funnel shaped, with the narrow part being more distal. The aortic arch is on the right side in about 25% of cases of tetralogy of Fallot—an incidence that is of importance to the surgeon. In addition to the hazard of being surprised by a right aortic

arch, the surgeon must remember that a large branch of the right coronary artery may cross the pulmonary conus region, which is the cardiotomy site. It should be noted that patency of the ductus arteriosus is protective, since it provides a source of blood to the otherwise deprived pulmonary vascular bed. Increasing cyanosis and shortness of breath are often signs that this beneficial shunt has spontaneously closed.

Uncorrected tetralogy of Fallot is usually a fatal disorder, and leads to heart failure, polycythemia, increased blood coagulability and thrombotic tendency, cerebral infarction, infective endocarditis, and brain abscess.

Transposition of the Great Arteries
(No Shunt Present)

The normal division of the truncus arteriosus into the aorta and pulmonary artery is dependent on the normal development of the spiral septum. Its abnormal development can produce an aberrant positioning of the great arteries, so that the aorta is anterior to the pulmonary artery (which is the opposite of normal) and connects with the right ventricle, while the pulmonary artery drains the left ventricle (Fig. 11-12). This situation can be described as involving atrioventricular concordance and ventriculo-arterial discordance.

The aorta normally curves to the right of the pulmonary artery in its approach to the heart and curves behind the pulmonary artery to reach its cardiac source in a posterior position. In transposition of the great arteries, the aorta is anterior to the pulmonary artery and to its right ("d" transposition) all the way to its origin. This contrasts with **congenitally corrected transposition,** in which the aorta is anterior to, but passes to the left of, the pulmonary artery ("l" transposition). This latter anomaly is "corrected" in the sense that there is an inversion of the ventricles relative to the atria. Although the aorta may be anterior to the pulmonary artery and connects with the anatomic right ventricle (which is in the position of the usual left ventricle and receives the pulmonary venous blood), it still receives the oxygenated blood that is appropriate for it. It is therefore not functionally abnormal at all unless—as is usually the case—there are other complicating anomalies present. The congenitally corrected transposition of the great vessels can be described as having atrioventricular discordance and ventriculo-arterial discordance.

Other variants of transposition of the great arteries include a **double outlet right ventricle,** an anomaly in which the aorta is rotated far to the right and, together with the pulmonary artery, arises from the right ventricle. The **Taussig-Bing malformation** is a

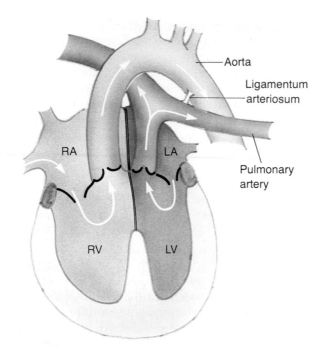

Aorta

Ligamentum arteriosum

Pulmonary artery

RA

LA

RV

LV

Figure 11-12. Complete transposition of great arteries, regular type. The aorta is anterior to, and to the right of, the pulmonary artery ("D-transposition") and arises from the right ventricle. Since there are no interatrial or interventricular connections and no patent ductus arteriosus, this anomaly is incompatible with life.

double outlet right ventricle, in which the ventricular septal defect is above the crista supraventricularis and directly beneath an overriding pulmonary artery.

The regular complete transposition is incompatible with survival, unless there is a large enough shunt to permit mixing of the blood between the two sides of the heart. In the absence of such a shunt severe anoxemia and heart failure supervene.

Coarctation of the Aorta

The arch of the aorta is formed from the left fourth aortic arch (see Fig. 11-10). In the developing fetus, the segment of the aorta distal to the origin of the left subclavian artery and proximal to the ductus arteriosus tends to be narrower than the aorta distal to the ductus arteriosus. If this narrow segment of aorta is so small after birth that it produces a gradient of blood pressure between its proximal and distal segments, it is referred to as a **tubular hypoplastic aorta** or as a **coarctation of the aorta** (Fig. 11-13). A coarctation with this elongated, narrowed segment in the proximal location between the left subclavian artery and the ductus is termed an **infantile (tubular) coarctation,** because this type of defect usually does not

permit survival beyond infancy (Fig. 11-13*A*). With this type of preductal coarctation, the ductus arteriosus usually remains patent. More commonly, however, the coarctation is abrupt, and occurs at or immediately distal to the origin of the ductus arteriosus from the aorta (true coarctation). The ductus is usually closed when this **adult coarctation** is present (Fig. 11-13*B*). However, the terms "infantile" and "adult" types of coarctation are probably best avoided, since there is disagreement as to their exact definition; indeed, some exclude the tubular hypoplastic aorta from the term "coarctation." It is preferable to describe the coarctation as being either pre-, post-, or paraductal in position, and to indicate whether the ductus is open or closed. Occasionally, there is a dilated region distal to the coarctation.

The pressure gradient produced by the coarctation causes hypertension and, occasionally, aortic dilatation proximal to the narrowed focus. The blood pressure measured in the arm is higher than that measured in the leg. The elevated pressure in the upper part of the body results in ventricular hypertrophy and may produce symptoms of dizziness, headaches, and nosebleeds. The lower pressure below the coarctation leads to weakness, pallor, and coldness of the lower extremities. Collateral vessels enlarge in an attempt to bridge the gap between the upper and lower aortic segments. Radiologic examination of the chest shows **notching of the inner surfaces of the ribs** due to pressure from the markedly dilated intercostal arteries. Other developmental abnormalities of the cardiovascular system are associated with the coarctation of the aorta, including bicuspid aortic valves and, in the brain, berry aneurysms of the circle of Willis. The adult type of coarctation can be treated surgically. Recently, noninvasive balloon angioplasty has been used to dilate the narrowed segment of aorta.

The prognosis of uncorrected severe coarctation of the aorta is dismal. Complications include heart failure, rupture of a dissecting aneurysm (secondary to cystic medial necrosis of the aorta proximal or distal to the coarctation), infective endarteritis at the point of narrowing or at the site of jet stream impingement on the wall immediately distal to the narrowing, cerebral hemorrhage, and stenosis or infective endocarditis of a bicuspid aortic valve.

Pulmonary Stenosis (Isolated or "Pure")

Pulmonary stenosis occurs because of developmental deformities arising from the endocardial cushion region of the heart (with involvement of the pulmonary valves), from an abnormality of the right ventricular

PREDUCTAL COARCTATION OF AORTA

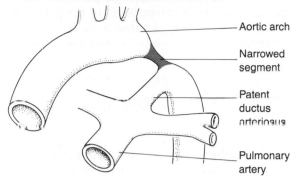

Aortic arch

Narrowed segment

Patent ductus arteriosus

Pulmonary artery

A

POSTDUCTAL COARCTATION OF AORTA

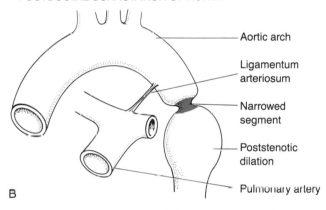

Aortic arch

Ligamentum arteriosum

Narrowed segment

Poststenotic dilation

Pulmonary artery

B

Figure 11-13. Coarctation of the aorta. (A) Preductal ("infantile") type, showing elongated narrow segment ("tubular hypoplasia") proximal to the widely patent ductus arteriosus. (B) Postductal ("adult") type, showing narrowed segment occurring just at or distal to the ductus, which is usually, but not always, closed. A small post-coarctation aneurysm is shown.

infundibular muscle (subvalvular or infundibular stenosis, especially with tetralogy of Fallot), or from abnormal development of the more distal parts of the pulmonary artery tree (peripheral pulmonary stenosis). This third type of pulmonary stenosis is much less common than the other two; it may produce "coarctation" of the pulmonary arteries at one or several sites.

Isolated pulmonary stenosis usually involves the valve cusps, which are fused to form an inverted funnel type of constriction. The artery distal to the valve may develop poststenotic dilatation after several years. In contrast to tetralogy of Fallot, infundibular stenosis with subvalvular muscular hypertrophy is rare in isolated pulmonary stenosis. Clinically,

these patients—like those with tetralogy of Fallot—have clubbing of the fingers and cyanosis. These patients may suffer from heart failure, right ventricular hypertrophy and dilatation, hypertrophy of the right atrium, patent foramen ovale with right-to-left shunt, polycythemia, and endocardial fibroelastosis. The symptoms become worse when the ductus arteriosus begins to close.

Aortic Stenosis

Three types of aortic stenosis are recognized: valvular, subvalvular, and supravalvular. **Subvalvular aortic stenosis** is caused by the abnormal development of a band of subvalvular fibroelastic tissue or a muscular ridge. The basis for the much rarer **supravalvular aortic stenosis** is not known, and the origin of **valvular aortic stenosis** is related to abnormal endocardial cushion development.

The functional significance of the supravalvular type of stenosis differs from that of the other two forms (i.e., valvular and sub-valvular) because of the relation of the stenoses to the coronary artery ostia. Thus, the valvular and subvalvular stenoses increase the work of the heart and at the same time decrease the coronary artery pressure head. The supravalvular stenoses increase the coronary artery perfusion pressure at the same time as they increase the work of the heart—thus, it is reasonable that the supravalvular type of stenosis would be less damaging to heart function over the long run.

Congenital valvular aortic stenosis usually is due to the fusion of two of the three semilunar cusps (the right coronary cusp with the adjacent two cusps), with a resulting bicuspid valve that tends to become calcified over the years. The supravalvular type of aortic stenosis may be part of a syndrome ("supravalvular aortic stenosis syndrome" or "Williams' syndrome") in which there are also several other systemic anomalies, including peripheral pulmonary artery stenoses, idiopathic hypercalcemia, and an abnormal facial appearance ("elfin facies"). Severe aortic valvular stenosis or atresia may be the main defect underlying the occurrence of **hypoplastic left heart syndrome,** in which there is hypoplasia of the ascending aorta, the left ventricle, and the mitral valve. Thickened left ventricular coronary arteries have been found in patients with this condition, and are related to the large arterioventricular channels that persist, presumably because of high intraventricular pressures. Endocardial fibroelastosis is also often present. If the mitral valve is atretic rather than hypoplastic, the left ventricle may consist of only a thin slit, with no endocardial fibroelastosis.

Congenital aortic stenosis is characterized by left ventricular hypertrophy, low blood pressure and consequent fainting spells, endocardial fibroelastosis, and sudden death.

Origin of a Coronary Artery from the Pulmonary Artery

One or, rarely, both coronary arteries may originate from the pulmonary artery rather than from the aorta. When one coronary artery is abnormal, anastomoses usually develop between the two coronary arteries, producing an arteriovenous fistula through which retrograde flow moves from the artery with higher pressure to that with lower pressure. Such patients may exhibit failure of the involved ventricle and myocardial infarction, fibrosis and calcification of the dilated wall, and endocardial fibroelastosis.

Ebstein's Malformation

The tricuspid valve forms from the endocardial cushions, which are derived from the "cardiac jelly" that fills the myoendocardial space and separates the visceral celomic wall from the endocardium. Thus, a defect in the visceral celomic wall where the tricuspid valve is scheduled to develop could produce a malformation in the valve. **In Ebstein's malformation one or more of the tricuspid valve leaflets is abnormal, being plastered down to the right ventricular wall for a variable distance below the right atrioventricular annulus.** Usually the septal and posterior leaflets are involved; they are irregularly elongated and adherent to the right ventricular wall, so that the upper part of the right ventricular cavity (inflow region) functions separately from the distal chamber. The anterior leaflet is usually the least involved of the three and may be essentially normal. In addition, the valve ring may or may not be displaced downward from its usual position. In any event, there is downward displacement of the effective tricuspid valve orifice into the ventricle. The ventricle is thus divided by the displaced tricuspid valve into two separate parts: the atrialized ventricle (proximal ventricle) and the functional right ventricle (distal ventricle). Conspicuous dilatation of the functional ventricle occurs in about two-thirds of such cases. As a result, the right ventricle is often unable to pump the blood efficiently through the pulmonary arteries. There is also insufficiency of the tricuspid valve, the degree of which depends on the severity and configuration of the defect of the leaflets.

Ebstein's malformation leads to heart failure, massive right ventricular dilatation, arrhythmias with palpitations and tachycardia, and sudden death. The anomaly can also be left-sided in patients with a congenitally corrected transposition of the great vessels, in which the tricuspid valve is on the left side in association with the inverted ventricles.

Congenital Complete Heart Block

Congenital complete heart block usually occurs in association with other congenital cardiac anomalies. The disruption of continuity of the cardiac conduction system is probably caused by the major developmental defect. However, in cases of primary (or isolated) congenital complete heart block (i.e., those occurring in otherwise normal hearts) the lack of continuity of the atrioventricular conducting system is thought to be due to the failure of regression of the sulcus tissue, which entirely encloses the conducting tissue during early development.

The hearts of patients with congenital complete heart block generally show a lack of continuity between the atrial myocardium and the atrioventricular node. Alternately, the defect may consist of a fibrous separation of the atrioventricular node from the ventricular conducting tissue. It is of interest to note the high incidence of congenital complete heart block in infants whose mothers have systemic lupus erythematosus. Antinuclear antibodies of the IgG class, which cross the placental barrier, may produce fibrosis in the region around the conducting tissue.

Patients with isolated congenital complete heart block may have little functional difficulty, although their heart rate will, of course, be abnormally slow. Later in life they may develop attacks of Stokes-Adams syncope (i.e., dizziness and unexpected fainting), heart failure, arrhythmias, and cardiac hypertrophy.

Endocardial Fibroelastosis

Although the etiology of endocardial fibroelastosis is not known, it has an interesting correlation with the presence of antibody to the mumps virus antigen. Its similarity to "round heart disease" in turkeys is also of interest, because virus particles have been demonstrated in the hearts of turkeys with this type of endocardial fibroelastosis.

Endocardial fibroelastosis occurs in association with other congenital anomalies, especially aortic atresia and coarctation of the aorta, and in patients with anomalous origin of a coronary artery from the pulmonary artery. However, the isolated occurrence of endocardial fibroelastosis is not uncommon. Hearts showing this condition are dilated and large, weighing two to four times what is expected for the age. The endocardium is porcelain-like, thickened, grayish white, and opaque. The left ventricle is the most commonly involved chamber, although the right ventricle, the left atrium, and the mitral and aortic valves occasionally become thickened. The valves may exhibit fusion of their leaflets, and mitral insufficiency is often present.

Patients with isolated fibroelastosis develop cardiac hypertrophy and succumb to heart failure.

Ischemic Heart Disease

Ischemic heart disease is by far the most common and most important type of heart disease in the United States and other industrialized lands (e.g., Scandinavia, England, Germany, etc.). In contrast, ischemic heart disease is rare in parts of the world that are less well developed, such as India, Africa, and China. This dramatic geographic difference in incidence has important implications, which will be considered later in this chapter.

The term **ischemic heart disease** is applied when **clinical signs and symptoms of myocardial ischemia are present and persistent, and when the supply of oxygen in the coronary arterial blood is inadequate to provide for the oxygen demands of the heart.** The major cause of ischemic heart disease is **coronary atherosclerosis,** a condition that narrows the coronary arterial lumina and limits the ability of these arteries to supply blood to the heart. Coronary atherosclerosis can progress clinically without any symptoms, but usually becomes manifest by a variety of clinical conditions.

Angina Pectoris A typical patient with angina pectoris has recurrent episodes of chest pain, usually brought on by increased physical activity or emotional excitement, although attacks of some types of angina pectoris may also originate during rest or sleep. The pain is of limited duration (1 to 15 minutes) and is usually relieved by decreasing the activity or by sublingual nitroglycerine treatment. The pain may vary in position and may radiate from the chest to involve an arm, the jaw, and/or upper abdomen. Although the most common cause of this condition is severe and extensive coronary atherosclerosis, the limited coronary blood supply is occasionally due to other factors, including coronary vasospasm, aortic stenosis, or aortic insufficiency. There is not necessarily any characteristic anatomic change in the myocardium, although the ischemia borders on causing anatomic damage. In a type of angina pectoris that occurs at rest, the electrocardiogram shows ST segment elevations rather than the depression usually found during attacks of pain in the typical type of angina pectoris. This atypical type of angina pectoris is called "variant angina" or **Prinzmetal's angina,** and reflects **coronary artery spasm.**

Preinfarction Angina Also called **unstable angina, accelerated angina, "crescendo" angina, or coronary insufficiency,** a clinical diagnosis of preinfarction angina is made when a patient complains of progressively increasing frequency and duration of an angina pectoris type of pain that develops over three to four days but displays no evidence of myocardial necrosis. The electrocardiographic changes are not characteristic of infarction, and the serum levels of creatine phosphokinase and lactic dehydrogenase do not become elevated. Most of these patients progress to a frank myocardial infarction, although in some the symptoms may regress.

Myocardial Infarct A **myocardial infarct** is another important manifestation of ischemic heart disease. **It is defined as a focus of old or recent myocardial necrosis having a diameter of over 2.5 cm and caused by an insufficient oxygen supply.** This definition excludes patchy foci of necrosis that may have been caused by various toxins (e.g., adrenalin, allylamine, isoproterenol, alcohol, etc.) or by viruses. It also excludes patchy foci of subendocardial necrosis, such as those caused by global myocardial ischemia, hypotension, cardiopulmonary bypass procedures, or aortic stenosis.

Sudden Death It is not uncommon for the initial manifestation of ischemic heart disease to be an unexpected arrhythmia that may result in sudden death. The arrhythmia is most commonly ventricular fibrillation, an irregularity that often can be converted to a normal rhythm by controlled electric shock, provided treatment is given quickly.

There are a number of different causes of sudden cardiac death, depending on the definition that is used for "sudden death." Some consider death sudden if it occurs immediately, or within an hour of the onset of any symptoms. In other definitions death is sudden if it supervenes within 24 hours of the onset of symptoms. There are also some differences based on the requirement that sudden death be diagnosed only if it is unexpected, as contrasted with other studies in which there is no such requirement. **By far the most common underlying condition of sudden death is coronary atherosclerosis.** There is a large number of other conditions that have been described as the basis for sudden cardiac death, including calcific aortic stenosis, dissecting aneurysm, conduction system abnormality, myxomatous degeneration of the mitral valve, idiopathic hypertrophic subaortic stenosis, anomalous coronary artery origin, and the effects of certain drugs, such as the phenothiazine antidepressants.

Table 11-4 Causes of Ischemic Heart Disease

Decreased Supply of Oxygen

CONDITIONS THAT INFLUENCE THE SUPPLY OF BLOOD

Atherosclerosis and thrombosis
Thromboemboli
Coronary artery spasm
Collateral blood vessels
Blood pressure, cardiac output, and heart rate
Miscellaneous: arteritis (e.g., periarteritis nodosa), dissecting
  aneurysm, luetic aortitis, anomalous origin of coronary artery,
  muscular bridging of coronary artery

CONDITIONS THAT INFLUENCE THE AVAILABILITY OF OXYGEN IN THE
  BLOOD

Anemia
Shift in hemoglobin-oxygen dissociation curve
CO
Cyanide

Increased Oxygen Demand (i.e., Increased Cardiac Work)

Hypertension
Valvular stenosis or insufficiency
Hyperthyroidism
Fever
Thiamine deficiency
Catecholamines

Personality Type

Etiology

Ischemic heart disease is caused by an imbalance between the oxygen demands of the myocardium and the supply of oxygenated blood (Table 11-4). An understanding of this ratio of supply to demand is important in order to understand the various aberrations that can lead to myocardial infarction.

Conditions Influencing the Supply of Blood

Atherosclerosis and Thrombosis

Atherosclerosis is the most common cause of ischemic heart disease. Its nature and pathogenesis are described in detail in Chapter 10, but it is discussed here to point out the features that are of special importance in relation to the coronary arteries. Atherosclerosis initially involves primarily the intima, in which deposition of mucopolysaccharides, lipid, collagen, and calcium occurs. Platelets and fibrin are deposited on the luminal surface. This is followed by the ingrowth of medial smooth muscle cells and capillaries, and eventual hemorrhage and inflammation in the enlarging intimal plaque (Fig. 11-14). In this way the lumen of the artery is progressively encroached upon. **The reduction in coronary blood flow becomes critical when the luminal cross sectional area is decreased by 90%. An acute ischemic**

event is precipitated by the sudden thrombotic occlusion of the narrowed lumen. The stimulus for this sudden occlusion may be the rupture of an atheromatous plaque and exposure of the underlying collagen, a material which is thrombogenic.

Over 80% of patients who are studied by coronary angiography shortly after the onset (within 4 hours) of an acute myocardial infarction show thrombotic occlusion of a coronary artery, whereas only about half of patients studied between 12 and 24 hours after onset of symptoms have a thrombus. In many cases the thrombus can be lysed by the infusion of thrombolytic enzymes, such as streptokinase, tissue plasminogen activator. These findings underlie the conclusion that **coronary artery thrombosis is the event that usually precedes and precipitates a myocardial infarct,** and that its frequent absence at autopsy is due to the lysis in situ of the thrombus by thrombolysins in the blood or endothelium.

Thromboemboli

Thromboembolism is a rare cause of myocardial infarction and the embolus is usually traced to a cardiac source. For example, it occurs in patients with atrial fibrillation and old rheumatic mitral valve disease who have mural thrombi in the left atrial appendage (Fig. 11-15). Thromboembolism is seen in patients with mural thrombi in the left ventricle secondary to infarction, aneurysm, or congestive cardiomyopathy. The most common source of thromboembolism from the heart is valvular vegetations, caused either by infectious endocarditis or by nonbacterial thrombotic endocarditis.

Coronary Artery Spasm

Myocardial infarction occurs in patients whose coronary arteries are apparently normal, as determined by angiography. In a few of these cases coronary artery spasm has been demonstrated by angiography, and it has been suggested that the spasm can cause infarction. The Prinzmetal type of angina pectoris is probably caused by coronary artery spasm and can be treated with alpha-adrenergic blockade.

Collateral Blood Vessels

The normal coronary arteries essentially function as end-arteries. However, most normal hearts have some intercoronary anastomoses, which may be as large as 40 μm in diameter. Hearts that are chronically ischemic due to coronary atherosclerosis develop extensive collateral connections that protect the myocardium from the effects of acute complete occlusion. In pigs and dogs, the gradual occlusion of a coronary artery over 1 to 2 days results in a higher survival rate and less myocardial necrosis than occurs in an-

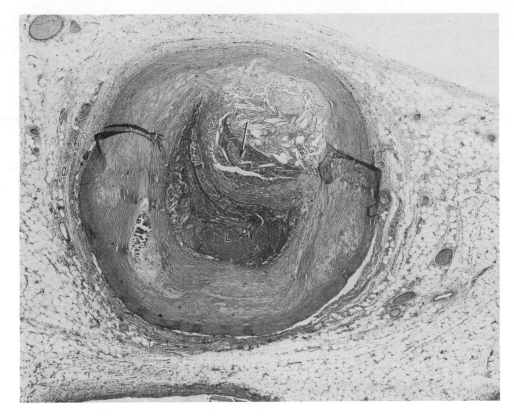

Figure 11-14. Coronary atherosclerosis. Cross section of an epicardial coronary artery showing marked atherosclerosis, with calcium deposits (*lower left, black*), cholesterol clefts (*clear, needlelike spaces, upper right*), hemorrhage (*arrow*) into an intimal plaque, and thrombotic occlusion of the lumen (*L*).

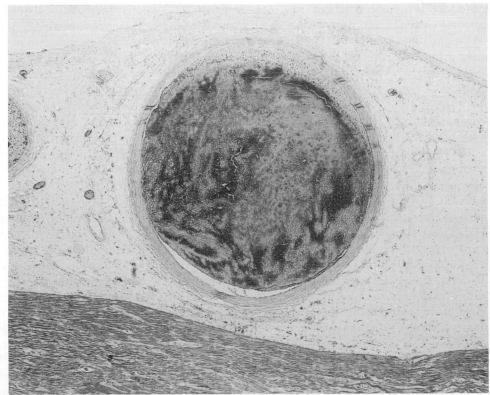

Figure 11-15. Thromboembolus in the left anterior descending coronary artery of a man who suffered from old rheumatic heart disease and who had mitral stenosis and a mural thrombus in the left atrial appendage.

imals after abrupt coronary artery ligation. The presence of coronary collateral vessels can explain certain unusual situations, such as an anterior infarct after recent thrombotic occlusion of the right coronary artery. This result reflects the presence of coronary collaterals that develop between the left anterior descending and right coronary arteries in response to occlusive atherosclerosis of the left anterior descending artery. The myocardium distal to the left anterior descending coronary artery becomes dependent on the right coronary artery blood flow via the collateral connections. As a result, an acute thrombosis of the right coronary artery results in the paradoxical infarction of the anterior left ventricle rather than infarction of the posterior basal left ventricle ("infarction at a distance").

Blood Pressure, Cardiac Output, and Heart Rate

A normal heart accommodates large changes in blood pressure, cardiac output, and heart rate. When the ability of the coronary arteries to dilate is limited by coronary artery sclerosis, however, an increase in heart rate or a sudden decrease in blood pressure or cardiac output may decrease the blood flow through a previously narrowed artery. The region perfused by this artery becomes ischemic and eventually necrotic.

Other Conditions

Coronary artery obstruction may also occur on the basis of coronary **arteritis,** a disorder usually caused by periarteritis nodosa. Another rare cause of coronary artery obstruction is extension of a **dissecting aneurysm** of the aorta into the coronary arteries. Occasionally, medial necrosis and dissecting aneurysm are confined to the coronary artery. The thickened intima of **luetic aortitis** may extend to a coronary artery orifice and obliterate it. An additional basis for a decreased supply of oxygen to the myocardium is a congenitally **anomalous origin of a coronary artery.** The anomalous coronary artery may arise from the pulmonary artery, or it may arise from the aorta at an abnormal site. Sudden death has been reported in patients whose left coronary artery arose from the right sinus of Valsalva and passed to the left between the aorta and the pulmonary artery.

Other situations in which myocardial ischemia and sudden death have been described are related to an **intramural course of the left anterior descending coronary artery.** This artery normally runs in the epicardial fat, but in some hearts it dips into the myocardium for a short distance. The muscular bridge over the left anterior descending coronary artery may result in systolic compression of the vessel.

Conditions Limiting Oxygen Availability in the Blood

Anemia is a common cause of decreased oxygen supply to the myocardium. Although a heart with normal circulation can survive severe anemia, in the presence of coronary atherosclerosis the capacity to increase coronary blood flow may be limited, and cardiac necrosis may result. An additional problem in patients with anemia is the added burden on the heart of an increased workload, secondary to the increased cardiac output needed to supply the other organs with adequate oxygen.

Another example of decreased oxygen delivery to the tissues is **carbon monoxide poisoning.** The high affinity of hemoglobin for CO results in its replacement of oxygen, in turn resulting in oxygen deprivation of the tissues. Cigarette smoking has been shown to lead to a significant CO level in the smoker's blood. **Cyanide poisoning** also results in tissue anoxia. In this instance the defect is due to the binding of cyanide to cytochrome oxidase, an effect that blocks mitochondrial respiration. A **shift of the hemoglobin–oxygen dissociation curve,** caused by cigarette smoking, may also result in decreased oxygen release to the tissues.

Increased Oxygen Demand

Anything that increases the workload of the heart also increases its need for oxygen. Conditions that **increase the blood pressure or the cardiac output,** such as exercise or pregnancy, result in an increased oxygen demand by the myocardium, and so contribute to angina pectoris or myocardial infarction. Disorders that fall into this category include valvular disease (mitral or aortic insufficiency, aortic stenosis), infection, and conditions such as hypertension, coarctation of the aorta, idiopathic hypertrophic subaortic stenosis, and luetic aortitis (which results in aortic valve insufficiency). The effect of any of these is magnified when added to coronary artery narrowing. The increased metabolic rate and tachycardia in patients with **hyperthyroidism** is accompanied by an increase in oxygen demand as well as an increase in the workload of the heart, both of which contribute to myocardial ischemia. This is especially important to recognize clinically, because treatment of the underlying thyroid disease is the most effective treatment for a thyrotoxic patient with symptoms of ischemic heart disease. **Fever also produces an increase in the basal metabolic rate and an increase in cardiac output and heart rate. Excess catecholamines** in the blood result in focal myocardial necrosis, probably on the basis of an increased oxygen demand.

Personality Type

It has been reported that hard driving, aggressive, time conscious, executive type individuals ("type A" personality) have a higher incidence of heart disease than do more easygoing, relaxed people ("type B" personality). "Coronary-prone" individuals—those of the type A behavior pattern—tend to differ biochemically from those of type B; type A individuals have higher plasma triglycerides and cholesterol levels and greater urinary catecholamine excretion. However, there is some controversy as to the relationship between coronary artery disease and the presence of the type A personality, with no correlation between the two being shown in some studies.

Pathology of Myocardial Infarction

Location of Infarcts

Transmural infarcts are usually located in the distribution of one of the three major coronary arteries (see Fig. 11-2). An occlusion of the proximal portion of the right coronary artery results in an infarct of the posterior basal region of the left ventricle and the posterior third of the interventricular septum ("inferior" infarct). An occlusion of the left anterior descending coronary artery produces an infarct of the apical anterior and septal wall of the left ventricle. An occlusion of the left circumflex coronary artery—the least common site—results in an infarct of the lateral wall of the left ventricle. When more than one coronary artery is significantly narrowed, the resulting infarct reflects the combined region of myocardium that is perfused by each involved vessel.

Infarcts may involve predominantly the subendocardial portion of the myocardium or they may be transmural. There are important differences between these two types of infarction (Table 11-5). The subendocardial (nontransmural) infarct is present in the inner one-third to one-half of the ventricle; it is commonly circumferential, so that it is not necessarily in the distribution of any one coronary artery. Coronary artery thrombosis is not usually a cause of subendocardial infarcts. They generally occur as a result of hypoperfusion of the heart in disorders such as aortic stenosis or hemorrhagic shock, or as a result of hypoperfusion during the course of cardiopulmonary bypass. Since the necrosis is limited to the inner layers of the heart, fibrinous epicarditis is not present, as it is with transmural infarcts. Most infarcts are transmural, but ocasionally, owing to the presence of extensive collateral vessels, the infarct is limited to the subendocardial region. In circumferential subendocardial infarcts, usually the result of global myocardial ischemia, secondary to hypotension,

Table 11-5 Differences Between Subendocardial and Transmural Infarcts

SUBENDOCARDIAL INFARCTS	TRANSMURAL INFARCTS
Multifocal	Unifocal
Patchy	Solid
Circumferential	In distribution of a specific coronary artery
Coronary thrombosis rare	Coronary thrombosis common
Often **result** from hypotension or shock	Often **cause** shock
No epicarditis	Epicarditis common
Do not form aneurysms	May result in aneurysm

shock, aortic stenosis plus tachycardia, and so on, the coronary arteries may be normal. In patients who die, transmural infarcts are more common than subendocardial infarcts.

Infarcts involve the left ventricle much more commonly and extensively than they do the right ventricle. This may be partly due to the greater workload imposed on the left ventricle and the greater thickness of the left ventricular wall. Thus, conditions that tend to increase the work of the right ventricle, such as pulmonary hypertension, are more likely to lead to an infarct of that ventricle. Careful postmortem examination of the heart shows that infarction of the right ventricle in posterior myocardial infarcts is actually not uncommon, occurring in about a third of such infarcts. However, most of these are extensions of a transmural left ventricular infarct; infarction limited to the right ventricle is rare.

Gross Characteristics of Infarcts

The early stages in the evolution of a myocardial infarct can be observed in a live animal. When a coronary artery is tied off, the region of myocardium supplied by that coronary artery beats more weakly, then stops beating and bulges outward during systole. If the occlusion is released after only a short time, the beat will return and no anatomic damage will be recognizable. This reversible stage continues for 20 to 60 minutes of complete ischemia, beyond which progressively more extensive permanent cell injury results.

Macroscopically, an acute myocardial infarct is usually not identifiable less than 12 hours from its time of onset. By 24 hours an infarct can be recognized on the cut surface of the involved ventricle either by its pallor or by a reddish-blue color, the latter reflecting the congestion of blood vessels in the infarcted region. After three to five days the infarct is mottled and more sharply outlined, with a central pale, yellowish, necrotic region bordered by a hy-

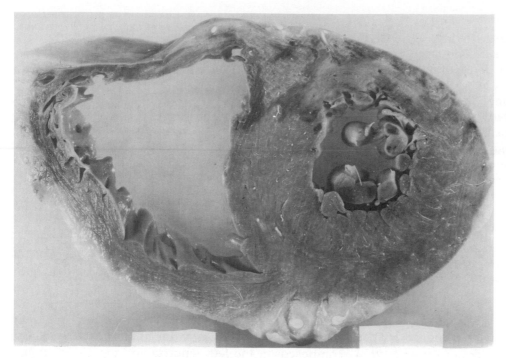

Figure 11-16. Cross section of the ventricles of a man who died 5 days after the onset of chest pain. The infarct is in the posterior and septal regions of both right and left ventricles, is mottled, and has a dark hemorrhagic border. The right coronary artery (*not shown*) was narrowed by severe atherosclerosis and was completely occluded by a recent thrombus. Note the "expansion" of the posterior left ventricular wall, which causes the position of the posterior papillary muscle to become more lateral.

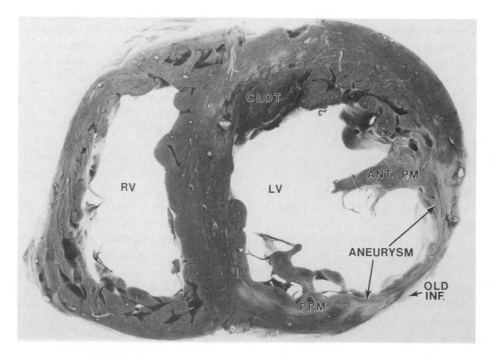

Figure 11-17. Healed myocardial infarct. Cross secton of the ventricles of the heart from a man who had long-standing ischemic heart disease. The posterior and lateral left ventricular walls are replaced by scar tissue (*below*). This old transmural infarct (*old inf.*) is thinned and bulges to form an aneurysm. There is an old, patchy, nontransmural infarct in the anterior subendocardial left ventricle (*above*), which has an adherent mural thrombus (clot). *Ant. PM,* anterior papillary muscle; *PPM,* posterior papillary muscle.

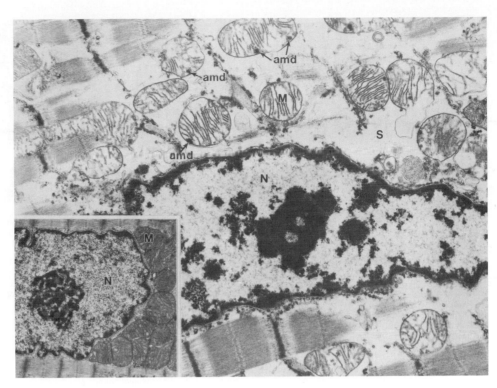

Figure 11-18. Ultrastructure of myocardial ischemia. Electron micrograph of an irreversibly injured myocyte from a dog heart subjected to 40 minutes of low flow ischemia, induced by proximal occlusion of the circumflex branch of the left coronary artery. A nonischemic control myocyte from the same heart is shown in the insert (also compare Fig. 11-4). The affected myocyte is swollen and has abundant clear sarcoplasm (S). The mitochondria (M) also are swollen and contain amorphous matrix densities (*amd*), which are characteristic of lethal cell injury. The sarcolemma of this myocyte (*not shown*) exhibited small areas of disruption. The chromatin of the nucleus (N) is aggregated peripherally, in contrast to the uniformly distributed chromatin in normal tissue.

peremic zone (Fig. 11-16). Occasionally, the infarcted region is hemorrhagic. By two to three weeks the infarcted region is usually depressed and soft, with a refractile, gelatinous appearance. Older infarcts are firm and have the pale gray appearance of scar tissue (Fig. 11-17).

Microscopic Characteristics of Infarcts

The earliest microscopic evidence of an infarct is seen best by electron microscopy (Fig. 11-18). At first the myocyte shows some evidence of edema, with swelling of the sarcoplasmic reticulum and mitochondria, and loss of glycogen. After 30 to 60 minutes of ischemia the mitochondria contain amorphous matrix densities, the nucleus shows clumping and margination of chromatin, and there are some discontinuities in the sarcolemma of the myocyte. After 2 to 6 hours of ischemia the cells in the infarcted zone exhibit loss of lactic dehydrogenase, creatine phosphokinase, and other enzymes. At about the same time, the

tissue potassium concentration decreases, "wavy fibers" can be seen, and contraction bands are demonstrated at the periphery of the infarct. Equivocal alterations in the staining characteristics of the necrotic cells include an increased eosinophilia (Fig. 11-19) and fuchsinophilia and an increase in nonglycogen material stained with the periodic acid-Schiff reaction.

After **one to two days** coagulation necrosis (Fig. 11-19) leads to an infiltrate of polymorphonuclear leukocytes, interstitial edema, and often hemorrhage. By **two to three days** the muscle cells are more clearly necrotic, nuclei disappear, and striations become less prominent. There are more polymorphonuclear leukocytes, which begin to undergo karyorrhexis. Lipid droplets appear in the sarcoplasm. By **five to seven days** the acute inflammatory leukocytic response has abated, so that few, if any, polymorphonuclear leukocytes are present. The infarcted region shows clearing of the dead muscle and inflammatory cells, and intercellular edema is prominent. New collagen

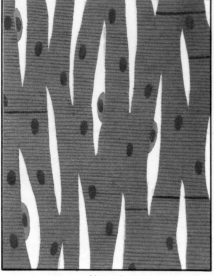
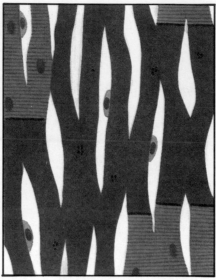
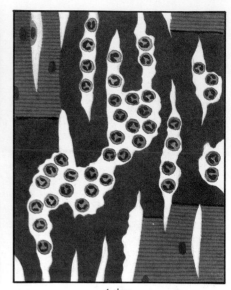

Normal   12-18 hours   1 day

Figure 11-19.   Development of a myocardial infarct. (*A*) Normal myocardium. (*B*) After about 12 to 18 hours the infarcted myocardium shows eosinophilia (red staining) in sections of the heart stained with hematoxylin and eosin. (*C*) About 24 hours after onset of the infarct, polymorphonuclear neutrophils infiltrate around the necrotic myocytes.

formation is evident, lymphocytes and monocytes are present, and the number of fibroblasts and small capillaries is increased. This process begins at the periphery of the infarct and gradually extends toward the center. Collagen deposition proceeds, so that by **three to four weeks** there is considerable fibrous tissue. Thereafter, debris is progressively removed and the scar becomes more solid and less cellular.

It should be recognized that this timetable of the usual sequence of events following a coronary artery occlusion can be altered by local or systemic events. For example, the acute extension of an infarct into a region that previously was partly infarcted may not show the expected changes. A large infarct usually does not mature in its center as rapidly as a smaller infarct. In large infarcts, healing proceeds from periphery to center. Thus, in estimating the age of a large infarct, it is more accurate to base the interpretation on the outer border rather than on the central region. In addition, the use of drugs such as steroids may alter the inflammatory process, thus delaying scar formation and resulting in "mummification" of the central portion of the infarct.

A special type of microscopic alteration of the myocytes is called **contraction band necrosis** or **myofibrillar degeneration** (Fig. 11-20). This is prominent in regions where some blood flow persists, such as at the margins of an acute infarct. It also is seen in situations where reflow occurs—for example, in patients who have had coronary artery bypass grafts or who have been treated by percutaneous transluminal coronary angioplasty. In such cases of restored flow, myofibrillar degeneration is seen in the territory supplied by the grafted or dilated artery. **Contraction band necrosis consists of thick, irregular contraction bands in the myocyte.** Electron microscopy shows disruption of the architecture of the myocyte, dense transverse bands, and swelling of the mitochondria, which contain amorphous matrix densities and calcium phosphate

Clinical Diagnosis of Acute Myocardial Infarction

The clinical diagnosis of acute myocardial infarction is based first on the clinical history. The onset may be sudden, with severe crushing pain that is usually substernal or precordial, but which may present as epigastric burning (simulating indigestion). The pain may extend into the jaw or down the inside of either arm. It is often accompanied by sweating, nausea, vomiting, and shortness of breath. The onset is occasionally preceded by several days of preinfarction angina, in which case the patient suffers from an increased frequency and severity of anginal pain. This prodrome is followed by the sudden onset of characteristically severe pain. About half of the cases of myocardial infarction are clinically silent—that is, they occur without any symptoms and are unrecognized by the patient. Such infarcts are later identified by electrocardiographic changes or at autopsy.

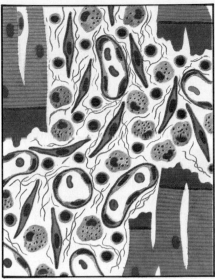 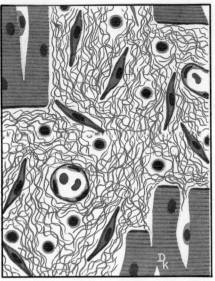

3 weeks   3 months

(*D*) After about 3 weeks the infarct contains granulation tissue with prominent capillaries, fibroblasts, lymphoid cells, and macrophages. The necrotic debris has been largely removed and a small amount of collagen has been laid down. (*E*) After 3 months or more the infarcted region has been replaced by scar tissue.

The diagnosis of acute myocardial infarction is confirmed by electrocardiography. The characteristic changes involve new Q waves and changes in the ST segment and T wave.

The finding of serum enzyme changes further supports the diagnosis of myocardial infarction. The most widely used enzymes for this purpose are the isoenzymes of lactic dehydrogenase (LDH) and a creatine phosphokinase (CPK). There are five different subspecies of LDH, with LDH-1 being in the highest concentration in the heart. After myocyte death, the normally low serum level of LDH-1 is elevated within 6 to 12 hours as a result of leakage of the enzyme from the cells. The level of LDH-2 is not proportionally increased, so that the ratio of LDH-1 to LDH-2 is reversed. A more reliable system for the diagnosis is based on the level of the MB isoenzyme of CPK, which is increased in the period between 7 and 48 hours after the onset of symptoms (reaching its peak in 20 hours), and which is produced almost exclusively by the myocardium. A small amount of CPK-MB enzyme may be derived from other sources.

Complications of Myocardial Infarction

Arrhythmias

Virtually all patients who have a myocardial infarct suffer from some form of cardiac arrhythmia, a complication which accounts for about half of the deaths from coronary heart disease. Premature ventricular beats, sinus bradycardia, ventricular tachycardia, ventricular fibrillation, paroxysmal atrial tachycardia, and partial or complete heart block occur. In cases that respond to atropine treatment, the arrhythmia probably reflects vagal hyperactivity. Second or third degree heart block is seen in 10% to 15% of cases. The heart block is usually transient, especially in patients with posterior infarction.

Cardiogenic Shock

Now that ventricular fibrillation can be effectively treated by electric shock resuscitation, the most feared complication in the hospital is shock. Cardiogenic shock is most likely to occur when the infarct involves more than 40% of the left ventricle; the mortality rate in these cases is as high as 90%.

Rupture

Myocardial rupture may occur within the first 21 days of an acute myocardial infarction, and especially between the second and 10th days, when the infarcted wall is at its weakest. After this time the scar becomes progressively stronger, so that rupture becomes less likely. External rupture of the ventricle produces pericardial tamponade in about 10% of patients with acute myocardial infarction—more commonly in women and in patients with hypertension. In rare cases a ruptured ventricle may be walled off, and the

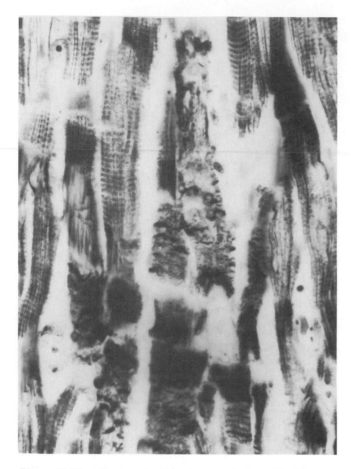

Figure 11-20.   Contraction band necrosis (myofibrillar degeneration). Note the thick abnormal banding and the overall disruption of the myocytes.

patient can thus survive. The result is a false aneurysm (Fig. 11-21).

In a few patients the interventricular septum ruptures. Uncommonly, a papillary muscle is involved, with subsequent rupture of the muscle and massive mitral regurgitation.

Aneurysms

Following an acute transmural myocardial infarct, the ventricular wall tends to bulge outward during systole in one-third of all patients. As the infarct matures, the collagenous scar tissue is susceptible to stretching. The occurrence of myocardial thinning and stretching in the region of an acute myocardial infarction is termed "infarct expansion." This is actually an early aneurysm; patients with this condition exhibit an increase in the incidence of myocardial rupture and have a poorer prognosis. Ventricular aneurysms are seen in 12% to 20% of patients with old myocardial infarcts (Fig. 11-21). Intra-aneurysmal thrombi, which are present in half of these cases, are a source of systemic emboli.

A distinction should be made between "true" and "false" aneurysms (Fig. 11-21). True aneurysms, which are much more common than false aneurysms, are caused by bulging of the weakened, but intact, left ventricular wall. In contrast, false aneurysms result from the rupture of a portion of the left ventricle that has been walled off by pericardial scar tissue. Thus, the wall of a false aneurysm is composed of pericardium and scar tissue, and not the original left ventricular muscle.

Mural Thrombosis and Embolism

The endocardial damage in an infarct predisposes it to adhesion of platelets and to fibrin deposition. Thus, peripheral embolization and infarcts of various organs are a potential hazard after the occurrence of a myocardial infarct, and may justify anticoagulant therapy as a preventive measure.

Pericarditis

Pericarditis usually occurs on the area of the heart surface that overlies the necrotic muscle in transmural infarcts. The deposition of fibrin may be limited to the locality of the myocardial necrosis, or it may occasionally be diffuse. In contrast to this form of pericarditis, which occurs shortly after the onset of the infarction, **postmyocardial infarction syndrome (Dressler's syndrome)** may develop as early as two weeks and as late as two years after infarction. A similar disorder may be seen after cardiac surgery. Circulating antibodies to heart muscle appear in patients with this late-developing pericarditis, and the symptoms are ameliorated by steroid therapy. Thus, this condition may reflect an autoimmune reaction.

Metabolic and Biochemical Effects of Myocardial Ischemia

The heart is an organ that is exquisitely dependent on an uninterrupted supply of oxygen. When the coronary artery blood flow is inadequate to support the aerobic needs of the heart, or when the arterial oxygen content is too low, a series of events leads to depletion of high energy phosphate compounds (e.g., ATP). Unlike skeletal muscle, the heart is unable to develop a significant oxygen debt. When its oxygen supply is suddenly severed it shifts to anaerobic metabolism, a process that cannot adequately supply the metabolic needs of the working myocardium. The biochemical consequences of sudden coronary artery occlusion include the following conditions that could contribute to cell death: ATP depletion, cellular acidosis, lactate accumulation, activation of intracellular proteases, and elevated intracellular calcium levels.

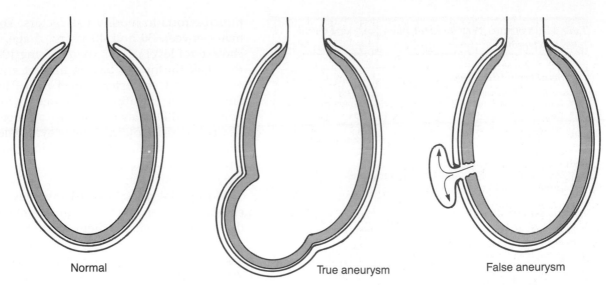

Normal   True aneurysm   False aneurysm

Figure 11-21. True and false aneurysms of the left ventricle. (*Left*) Normal heart. The left ventricular wall (*shaded*) is enclosed by a pericardial sac. (*Center*) True aneurysm shows an intact wall (*black*), which bulges outward. (*Right*) False aneurysm shows a ruptured infarct, which is walled off externally by adherent pericardium. Note that the mouth of the true aneurysm is wider than that of the false aneurysm.

Limitation of Infarct Size

Infarct size can often be limited by clinical treatment directed toward the rescue of jeopardized—but still viable—marginal cells at the border of the infarct. The onset of myocardial ischemia is not immediately followed by cell death, but rather by a period of reversible injury, which is then followed by irreversible injury. During the earlier reversible phase, reperfusion might prevent or limit infarction. However, important experimental studies have not confirmed the concept of a broad lateral zone of injured-but-viable cells. Instead, they have pointed to the transmural area of the infarct as the salvageable region. Experimental studies and clinical trials of strategies to limit infarct size are summarized in Table 11-6.

Reperfusion of Ischemic Myocardium

Several techniques result in early reperfusion of the ischemic myocardium. Surgeons may insert bypass grafts from the aorta to the distal segments of the coronary arteries, in some cases restoring blood flow within four to five hours. Coronary blood flow can also be restored by nonsurgical techniques, such as percutaneous transluminal coronary angioplasty. In this technique a balloon catheter is inserted into the occluded coronary artery, which is then dilated by inflation of the balloon. A third method is the infusion of a fibrinolytic substance into the coronary ar-

tery or peripheral vein, which leads to dissolution of the thrombus. In dogs the use of these techniques can result in a decrease in infarct size and in an improvement of ventricular function. However, after eight hours it is unlikely that any salvageable myocardium remains; reperfusion after this interval frequently produces hemorrhage because of microvascular damage in the ischemic zone.

Prevention of Ischemic Heart Disease

Since the major cause of ischemic heart disease is coronary atherosclerosis, preventing ischemic heart disease is best accomplished through efforts to decrease the severity of atherosclerosis. **The major elements that predispose an individual to heart attacks are an elevated blood cholesterol level, the presence of hypertension, and cigarette smoking.** Any one of these factors significantly increases the risk of heart attacks, and the presence of all three augments the risk more than sevenfold.

In the United States there has been a reversal in what had been a trend of progressively increasing mortality from ischemic heart disease; an actual decrease of about 30% has occurred in the past 10 years. Whether this shift is due to a decrease in smoking, to the use of less fat (especially saturated fat) in the average diet, or to the effective treatment of hypertension is still unknown, but the findings justify con-

Table 11-6 Potential Ways to Limit Infarct Size or Prevent Infarct Extension

Decrease Energy Utilization

Reduce hemodynamic work
- Reduce heart rate—β blockade, carotid sinus stimulation
- Reduce contractility—β blockade, Ca^{++} flux inhibition (verapamil), prostaglandins
- Reduce afterload—intra-aortic balloon counterpulsation
- Reduce preload—nitrates, digitalis (in failing heart)

Reduce cell metabolism directly
- Reduce Ca^{++} influx—β blockade, verapamil, nifedipine
- Induce hypothermia

Increase the Potential Energy Production

Restore or preserve existing perfusion of ischemic myocardium
- Perform emergency revascularization
- Alter coagulation
  Lyse existing thrombi—streptokinase, urokinase, tissue-type plasminogen activator
  Prevent microthrombi—aspirin, prostaglandins
- Improve or preserve collateral blood flow
  Increase diastolic blood pressure
  Balloon counterpulsation
  α-Adrenergic stimulation—methoxamine, norepinephrine
  Vasodilators—verapamil, nifedipine, nitrates, α-adrenergic blockade, prostaglandins, dipyridamole
  Decrease diastolic wall tension (reduce preload)—nitrates
  Prevent myocardial edema—osmotic agents (mannitol), hyaluronidase
- Prevent coronary venous retroperfusion or intermittent coronary sinus occlusion

Increase Blood Oxygen or Substrate Content Despite Persistent Ischemia

- Increase oxygen—correct hypoxemia and anemia, hyperbaric oxygen
- Increase substrates—glucose-insulin-potassium: hypertonic glucose, ATP, pyruvate, amino acids, ribose, adenosine
- Enhance tissue diffusion—hyaluronidase

Reduce Catabolism

- Inhibit adenine nucleotide catabolism—allopurinol
- Inhibit lipolysis—β-pyridyl carbinol, prostaglandins
- Increase acidosis
- Induce hypothermia

Stabilize Cell Structure or Cytosolic Composition

- Reduce electrolyte shifts/prevent cell swelling—β blockade, Ca^{++} flux inhibition (verapamil, nifedipine), osmotic agents (mannitol)
- Stabilize cell membranes (plasmalemma, lysosomes)—steroids, prostaglandins
- Prevent free radical production (allopurinol) or introduce free radical scavengers (superoxide dismutase)

Prevent Microvascular Damage or Obstruction

- Prevent endothelial swelling—osmotic agents (mannitol)
- Prevent platelet aggregation—prostaglandins
- Prevent free radical injury—allopurinol, free radical scavengers (superoxide dismutase)

Reduce Inflammatory Response

- Anti-inflammatory agents—steroids, nonsteroidal anti-inflammatory drugs (ibuprofen)

tinued efforts to modify risk factors. For example, a man between 30 and 40 years of age with a blood cholesterol level of less than 175 mg/100 ml has less than half the risk of having a heart attack than one with a blood cholesterol level over 240 mg/100 ml. Similarly, an elevation of the serum low-density lipoprotein (LDL) level indicates an increased risk of heart disease. However, an elevated level of high-density lipoprotein (HDL) may indicate some resistance to atherosclerosis and a lessened risk of coronary artery disease.

Most populations in which men have a high serum cholesterol level exhibit a high rate of coronary heart disease, and the usual diet is high in fat. By contrast, in most countries whose populations have low cholesterol levels and low rates of coronary artery disease, the diet is low in fat, which is mainly derived from unsaturated fish and vegetable oils. A study comparing Japanese men in Japan to those living in Hawaii and in San Francisco found that the risk of heart attack increased progressively from Japan to Hawaii to the mainland United States—a difference probably related to the dietary differences among these groups. The "dramatic geographic difference in incidence" of atherosclerosis is probably a result of dietary differences from region to region, and underscores the importance of altering those dietary elements that have been linked to a high incidence of heart disease in industrialized Western countries.

In addition, the risk of ischemic heart disease positively correlates with the level of blood pressure; a person with a pressure of 160/95 mmHg has twice the risk of ischemic heart disease as a person with a blood pressure of 140/74 or less, the risk increasing with increasing blood pressure levels. The risk of ischemic heart disease also is increased in cigarette smokers proportional to the number of cigarettes smoked.

Other risk factors for ischemic heart disease include the following:
- Diabetes mellitus (a fivefold greater risk in women between ages 30 and 39)
- Obesity (the higher rates of heart attacks may be only indirectly related to obesity; risk may be augmented because obese persons have higher blood pressure, blood fat, and blood sugar levels)
- Age (risk is greater with increasing age, up to age 80)
- Gender (before age 65, men are more susceptible than women)
- Family history of premature arteriosclerosis
- Use of oral contraceptives
- Sedentary life habits
- Stressful occupation

Although most investigators agree with the importance of many of these risk factors, the significance of obesity, sedentary habits, and oral contraceptives remains controversial.

Rheumatic and Other "Hypersensitivity" Diseases

Rheumatic Heart Disease

Rheumatic heart disease is the result of cardiac involvement by rheumatic fever. Rheumatic fever occurs equally in both sexes and at all ages, but it is more common in children, with the peak incidence occurring between ages 5 and 15. The **clinical diagnosis** of rheumatic fever is made when two major—or one major and two minor—criteria ("the Jones criteria") are met. If this diagnosis is supported by evidence of a preceding streptococcal infection, the probability of rheumatic fever is high.

The **major clinical manifestations** include carditis (murmurs, cardiomegaly, pericarditis, and congestive heart failure), polyarthritis, chorea, erythema marginatum, and subcutaneous nodules. The **minor manifestations** include a previous history of rheumatic fever, arthralgia, fever, certain laboratory tests indicative of an inflammatory process (e.g., elevated sedimentation rate, positive test for C-reactive protein, leukocytosis), and electrocardiographic changes.

Incidence

The incidence of rheumatic fever has decreased dramatically in the United States. The death rate from rheumatic fever has fallen from 14.5 to 6.8 per 100,000 in the period from 1950 to 1972. Although this decline might have been partly the result of antibiotic treatment, such therapy cannot account for the entire decline, since the death rate had begun to fall well before the availability of antibiotics. It is probable that improved socioeconomic conditions in the United States have contributed to the decrease. There is some suggestion, however, that the disease may now be increasing; one study found a marked increase in incidence in the Salt Lake City, Utah, region over the 5 years to 1987, and there is evidence of an increased incidence of rheumatic fever in several other cities of this country. In other countries, rheumatic fever is still very common; it is the most common cause of heart disease in many less developed countries, such as Thailand, Uganda, and Pakistan.

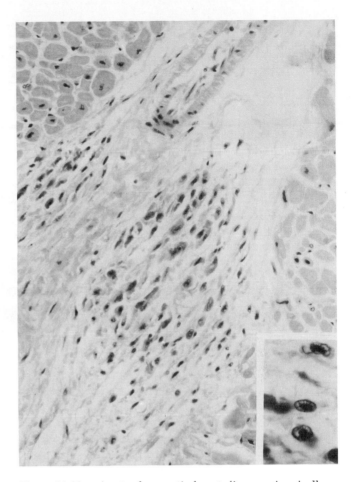

Figure 11-22. Acute rheumatic heart disease. A spindle-shaped Aschoff body is located interstitially in the myocardium. A blood vessel is seen at the top. Within the Aschoff body are noted collagen degeneration, lymphocytes, and Anitschkow cells. (*Insert*) Nuclei of Anitschkow cells, showing "owl eyed" cross sectional appearance and "caterpillar" longitudinal appearance.

Anatomic Features

Acute Rheumatic Carditis

Acute rheumatic heart disease is a pancarditis, involving all three layers of the heart. The myocardium is most typically involved in the acute stage of the disease. A diffuse nonspecific **myocarditis** is present in some cases, together with a unique type of interstitial inflammation—**the Aschoff body** (Fig. 11-22). The Aschoff body's morphologic feature consists of a perivascular focus of swollen eosinophilic collagen, referred to as "fibrinoid necrosis." Surrounding this abnormal collagen are collections of lymphocytes, plasma cells and monocytes. Also present are **Anitschkow cells,** which are characterized by nuclei that have a central band of chromatin. In cross section

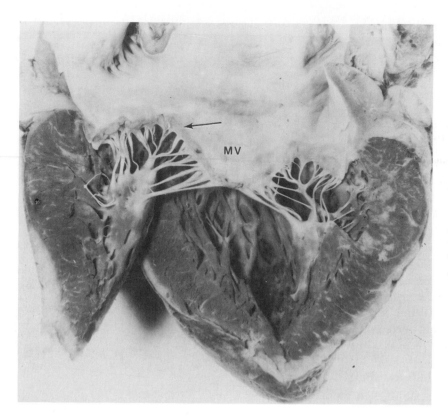

Figure 11-23. Acute rheumatic mitral valvulitis. Opened left ventricular and left atrial cavities showing the anterior mitral valve leaflet (*MV*) in the center with prominent nodular verrucous vegetations aligned just within the valve margins at the point of valve closure (*arrow*). The left ventricular cavity is dilated because of cardiac failure caused by the myocarditis.

these nuclei have an "owl-eye" appearance, and a "caterpillar" appearance when cut longitudinally. Some of these cells may become multinucleated, in which case they are called Aschoff myocytes.

The main cause of death in the acute stage of rheumatic heart disease is heart failure from the myocarditis. Also seen during the acute stage of the disease is a prominent **pericarditis,** characterized by tenacious deposits of fibrin that resemble the shaggy, irregular surfaces of two slices of buttered bread that have been pulled apart—the so-called bread-and-butter appearance. The pericarditis may be recognized clinically by a friction rub, but the involvement has little functional effect and only rarely leads to constrictive pericarditis. During the acute stage, an **endocarditis** involves mainly the valves, which show a finely nodular "verrucous" appearance at the line of closure (Fig. 11-23). Areas of focal collagen degeneration in the valve are surrounded by inflammation, with ulceration of the valve endocardial surface and deposition of fibrin on the surface.

Chronic Rheumatic Heart Disease

A patient who has had an attack of rheumatic fever is more susceptible to recurrent episodes following infections by beta-hemolytic streptococci. **Such recurrent attacks result in repeated and progressively increasing damage to the heart valves. Thus, in chronic recurrent rheumatic heart disease the valve involvement, which was of little clinical significance during the acute attack, becomes the major problem.** For example, the mitral valve, which is the most frequently and severely involved valve, shows conspicuous, irregular thickening and calcification of its leaflets, often with fusion of its commissures and thickening and fusion of the chordae tendineae (Fig. 11-24). As a result, the valve is often severely stenotic and, when viewed from the atrial aspect, has a narrowed orifice described as having a "fish mouth" appearance (Fig. 11-25). The aortic valve, the second most commonly involved valve, shows typical fusion of the commissures and, later, pronounced thickening and calcification of the cusps, with resulting stenosis or insufficiency. The tricuspid valve is similarly involved, although less frequently than the mitral and aortic valves, and the pulmonary valve is the least frequently involved.

Etiology

Although the exact etiology of rheumatic fever is still controversial, several concepts are generally accepted (Fig. 11-26). **The disease occurs after a latent period of two to three weeks following an infection with a group A beta-hemolytic streptococcus, typically a**

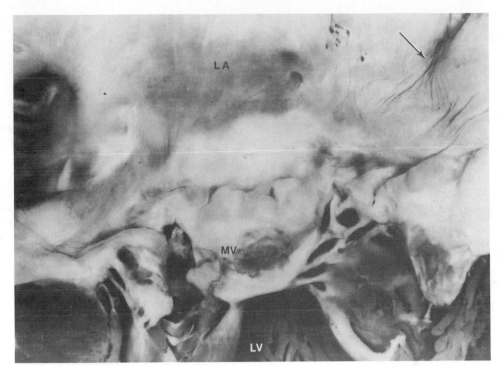

Figue 11-24. Old rheumatic mitral valvulitis. The valve leaflets (*MV*) and chordae tendineae are thickened. This valve was stenotic and also somewhat insufficient. The wrinkled atrial endocardium represents a MacCallum's patch (*arrow*). *MV*, anterior leaflet of mitral valve; *LA*, left atrial cavity; *LV*, left ventricular cavity.

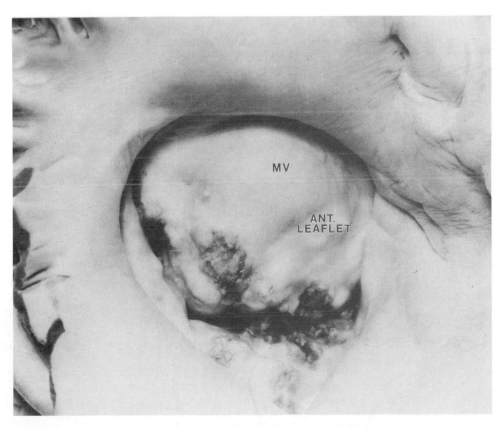

Figure 11-25. Rheumatic mitral stenosis. The mitral valve (*MV*) is seen from the atrial cavity. The anterior mitral leaflet is above, and the posterior leaflet is below. Both are irregular, thickened, and calcified, and the mitral orifice is narrowed. This appearance of the valve orifice is sometimes described as "fish mouth."

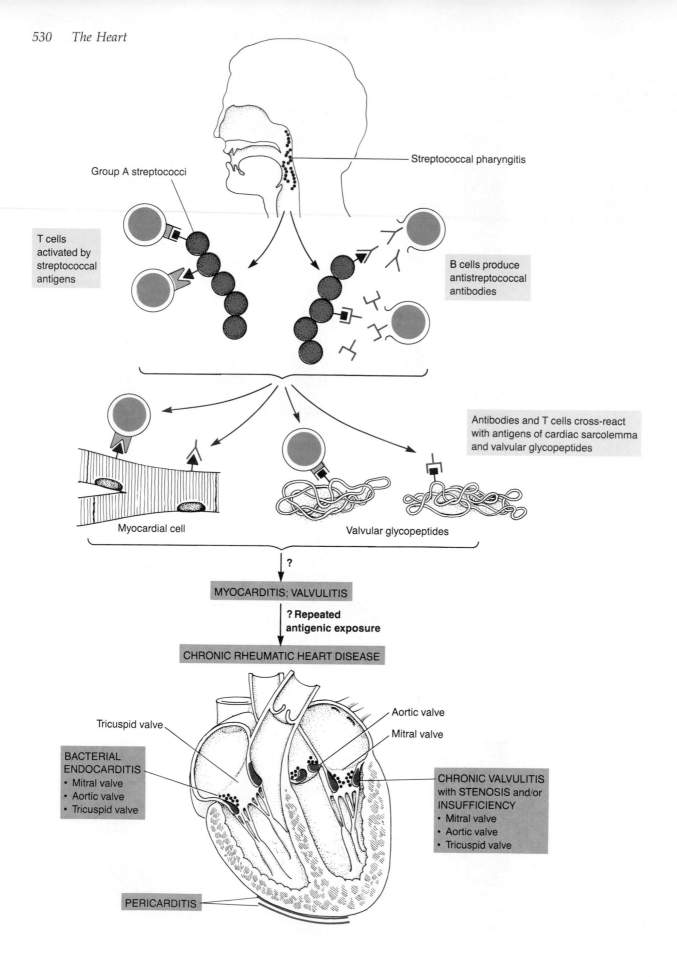

Streptococcal pharyngitis

Group A streptococci

T cells activated by streptococcal antigens

B cells produce antistreptococcal antibodies

Antibodies and T cells cross-react with antigens of cardiac sarcolemma and valvular glycopeptides

Myocardial cell

Valvular glycopeptides

?

MYOCARDITIS; VALVULITIS

? Repeated antigenic exposure

CHRONIC RHEUMATIC HEART DISEASE

Tricuspid valve

Aortic valve

Mitral valve

BACTERIAL ENDOCARDITIS
• Mitral valve
• Aortic valve
• Tricuspid valve

CHRONIC VALVULITIS with STENOSIS and/or INSUFFICIENCY
• Mitral valve
• Aortic valve
• Tricuspid valve

PERICARDITIS

pharyngitis. By the time the symptoms of rheumatic fever appear, the throat culture is usually negative. However, streptococci are considered the cause of the pharyngitis because of elevated titers of antibodies to streptococcal antigens, such as streptolysin O, hyaluronidase or streptokinase in the serum. The more severe the initial streptococcal infection, the greater the likelihood of subsequent rheumatic fever. The treatment of the initial pharyngitis with antibiotics greatly decreases the risk of later rheumatic fever, and prophylactic therapy with penicillin practically eliminates the chance of recurrent rheumatic fever. In some epidemics of Group A streptococcal pharyngitis the incidence of rheumatic fever has been as high as 3%, and in patients who have had a previous attack of rheumatic fever without penicillin prophylaxis the incidence has climbed as high as 30%.

Some streptococcal antigens cross-react with heart antigens, an observation that raises the possibility of an autoimmune etiology. There seems to be an additional hereditary factor for susceptibility to rheumatic fever after streptococcal infection.

Sequelae of Rheumatic Fever

Complete recovery after an acute attack of rheumatic fever is possible. However, there usually remain certain stigmata of prior rheumatic fever. **Adhesive pericarditis,** which follows the fibrinous pericarditis of the acute attack, almost never results in constrictive pericarditis. Probably the most significant late result of rheumatic fever is **scarring of the valves.** One of the most important sequelae of rheumatic heart disease is the **increased susceptibility to the localization of infectious agents on the heart valves.** The irregular, scarred nature of these valves provides an attractive environment to bacteria that would ordinarily pass by. The organisms settle down to establish a **bacterial endocarditis.** Because bacteremia frequently

follows a tooth extraction or a urethral catheterization, a person who has had a prior diagnosis of rheumatic heart disease should be treated prophylactically with penicillin before performance of either of these procedures.

Mural thrombi can form in the atrial or ventricular chambers and give rise to thromboemboli and infarction of various organs. Atrial thrombosis occurs in about 40% of patients with rheumatic valvular disease; rarely, a large thrombus in the left atrial appendage develops a stalk and acts as a **ball valve** that obstructs the mitral valve orifice. A focus of rough, wrinkled endocardium in the posterior aspect of the left atrium, referred to as a "MacCallum's patch," can serve as a clue to previous rheumatic involvement.

Certain noncardiac sequelae of rheumatic heart disease result from disease of the valves. In cases of mitral disease or congestive failure associated with aortic valve involvement, the lung is usually congested. Many hemosiderin-laden "heart failure" cells are seen within alveoli, together with fibrosis of the alveolar septal walls. In addition, there is usually some pulmonary vascular change, principally muscular and intimal arteriolar thickening. Right ventricular hypertrophy (*cor pulmonale*) may develop as a result of a reactive pulmonary hypertension. The characteristic lesion of the liver in such cases is a severe central passive congestion (see Fig. 11-7) that can eventually result in "cardiac cirrhosis," a condition in which the hepatic central vein areas are fibrotic.

Other "Hypersensitivity" Diseases

Lupus Erythematosus

Systemic lupus erythematosus may involve the heart with a pericarditis (usually with an effusion), myocarditis, or endocarditis. The endocarditis is the most

Figure 11-26. Etiologic factors in rheumatic heart disease. The upper portion illustrates the initiating beta-hemolytic streptococcal infection of the throat, which introduces the streptococcal antigens into the body and may also activate cytotoxic T-cells. These antigens lead to the production of antibodies to various antigenic components of the streptococcus, which can cross-react with certain cardiac antigens, including those from the myocyte sarcolemma and from the glycoproteins of the valves. This may be the mechanism for the production of the acute inflammation of the heart in acute rheumatic fever that involves all cardiac layers (endocarditis, myocarditis, and pericarditis). This inflammation becomes apparent after a latent period of 2 to 3 weeks. The insult may progress to chronic stenosis or insufficiency of the valves. These lesions involve the mitral, aortic, tricuspid, and pulmonary valves, in that order of frequency.

striking lesion. Warty (verrucous) vegetations on the valve surfaces are termed **Libman-Sacks endocarditis**. Rarely, they may contain microscopic nuclear fragments ("hematoxylin bodies"), but they are otherwise indistinguishable from the acute lesions of rheumatic mitral valvulitis.

Rheumatoid Arthritis

The heart is rarely involved in patients with rheumatoid arthritis. Characteristic rheumatoid granulomatous inflammation, with fibrinoid necrosis and palisaded lymphocytes and monocytes, may occur in the pericardium, myocardium, or valves. In patients with ankylosing spondylitis, thickening and shortening of the aortic valve cusps may result in insufficiency or stenosis.

Scleroderma Heart Disease

Patients with scleroderma may occasionally have arrhythmias or symptoms of heart failure—associated with interstitial patchy fibrosis of a nonspecific type—without coronary artery disease.

Polyarteritis Nodosa

The heart is involved in about 75% of cases of classic polyarteritis nodosa. The arterial lesions may be acute, healing, or healed, and may result in myocardial infarction, arrhythmias, or heart block. It is likely that some cases of Kawasaki disease (mucocutaneous lymph node syndrome) have been misdiagnosed as polyarteritis nodosa. There are some similarities, and cardiac involvement occurs in about 20% of children with true Kawasaki disease.

Hypertensive Heart Disease

Hypertension is not usually considered to be a primary disease of the heart, and is described in detail in Chapter 10. This section is concerned with the effects of persistently high systemic blood pressure on the heart, especially on the left ventricle. The effects of pulmonary hypertension on the right ventricle are also important, and result in a condition called **cor pulmonale**.

Systemic hypertension is defined, perhaps simplistically, as the persistent presence of blood pressure greater than 140 mmHg systolic or 90 mmHg diastolic. The term **hypertensive heart disease** is used when the heart is enlarged in the absence of an apparent cause other than the hypertension (Fig. 11-27); thus, a diagnosis of hypertensive heart disease is not appropriate for patients with congenital or valvular heart disease.

Hypertension is common in the United States, having an overall prevalence of 20% to 35%. Both the prevalence and the severity of the disease are greater in blacks than in whites. The prevalence of hypertension is greater in women than in men, and it increases progressively with age. There has been a striking decrease in the number of deaths due to hypertension in the last 10 years (including those due to hypertensive heart disease), a decline similar to that seen in the case of coronary heart disease.

Effects of Hypertension on the Heart

The main effect of hypertension on the heart is left ventricular hypertrophy, owing to the increased workload imposed on the heart (Fig. 11-27). The left ventricle is thickened and the overall weight of the heart is increased, exceeding 375 grams in men and 350 grams in women. (The normal heart weight is 300 to 350 grams in men and 250 to 300 grams in women.) Although the association between hypertension and myocardial hypertrophy is generally recognized, some inconsistencies in this correlation raise doubts about a simple cause-and-effect relationship. For example, left ventricular hypertrophy has been recognized as a surprisingly early finding in some patients with mild hypertension. Furthermore, the degree of hypertrophy is often poorly correlated with the level of blood pressure. The difficulty in distinguishing hypertensive heart disease from the cardiomyopathies adds to the uncertainty of a simple explanation for the origin of hypertensive heart disease.

Left ventricular hypertrophy is a compensatory response to the increased workload imposed on the heart by high blood pressure. Myocardial hypertrophy clearly adds to the ability of the heart to handle an increased workload up to a point, beyond which additional hypertrophy is damaging to the heart. This upper limit to useful hypertrophy reflects the increasing diffusion distance between the interstitium and the center of each myofiber, a change that eventually leads to an inadequate supply of oxygen to the myofiber.

An additional effect of hypertension on the heart is the increased severity of atherosclerosis of the coronary arteries. The combination of increased cardiac workload and narrowed coronary arteries leads to a greater risk of myocardial ischemia, infarction, and heart failure.

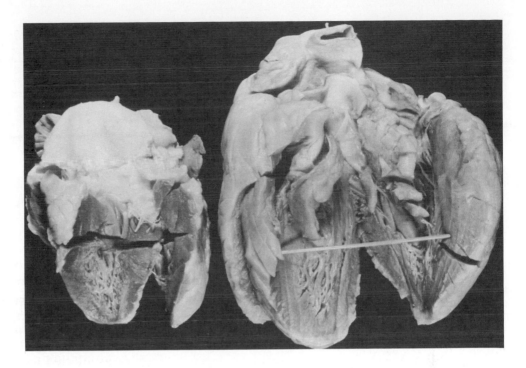

Figure 11-27. Hypertensive heart disease. (*Left*) Normal heart (weight, 300 g). (*Right*) Hypertrophic heart (weight, 650 g) from a patient with longstanding hypertension.

Causes of Death in Patients with Hypertension

The most common cause of death in hypertensive patients is **congestive heart failure,** a complication diagnosed in about 40% of cases. Death may also occur as a result of coronary arteriosclerosis, dissecting aneurysm of the aorta, or ruptured berry aneurysm of the cerebral circulation. A common cause of death is related to the arteriolar nephrosclerosis that results in **renal failure. Intracerebral hemorrhage** also is a frequent fatal complication.

Cor Pulmonale

Cor pulmonale is defined as right ventricular hypertrophy that results from a disorder of the lungs. The term **acute cor pulmonale** is applied to the sudden occurrence of pulmonary hypertension, most commonly caused by pulmonary emboli, with resulting dilation of the right ventricle. This may lead to right heart failure and death if the obstruction occurs rapidly and the right sided pressure is high. Chronic pulmonary hypertension (and **chronic cor pulmonale**) may be caused by a number of conditions that increase pulmonary vascular resistance, including recurrent pulmonary emboli, pulmonary fibrosis, or chronic lung disease, such as pulmonary emphysema. Severe kyphoscoliosis may deform the chest wall and interfere with its function as a bellows,

resulting in hypoxemia and pulmonary vasoconstriction. A small number of cases of cor pulmonale are attributed to "primary pulmonary hypertension," a disorder of unknown etiology. Of course, right ventricular hypertrophy is also caused by disorders that are not primary in the lung—for example, certain congenital heart defects.

Inflammatory Diseases of the Heart

Infective Endocarditis

Etiology

The endocardium may develop focal infections with bacteria or fungi in any region, but the valves are the sites most frequently involved by infective endocarditis. The infection may localize on a normal valve if the organism is especially virulent (e.g., *Staphylococcus aureus*) or if the immune system is impaired (e.g., due to diabetes mellitus, treatment with immunosuppressive agents, etc.). Sites of old valvular disease, however, are predisposed to the localization of bacteria—especially the less virulent types, such as alpha-hemolytic streptococci. Scarred valves provide cracks and crevices that serve as places for organisms to get a "toehold." A prosthetic valve is also a site predisposed to infection because it provides a protected environment for the organisms. The normal "wear and tear" of aging may result in minor endo-

Table 11-7 *Comparison of Acute and Subacute Bacterial Endocarditis*

	ACUTE	SUBACUTE
Duration of Clinical Symptoms	<6 weeks	>6 weeks
Most Common Organisms	Staphylococcus aureus, β-streptococci	α-Streptococci
Virulence of Organism	Highly virulent	Less virulent
Condition of Valves	Usually previously normal	Usually previously damaged
	Perforations common	Perforations rare

cardial damage to the valve surface, so that adherent fibrin–platelet aggregates can form a nidus for circulating organisms. The sources of these organisms are commonly infections of the teeth and gums, the urinary tract (including pyelonephritis and acute prostatitis), the skin, and the lung.

Other conditions that predispose the heart to localization of organisms include myxomatous degeneration of the mitral valve ("floppy valve" or mitral valve prolapse syndrome), nonbacterial thrombotic endocarditis, congenital heart disease (patent ductus arteriosus, tetralogy of Fallot, ventricular septal defect, coarctation of the aorta), and intravenous injection of organisms (especially by drug addicts).

It is important for persons with conditions that predispose them to bacterial infection of the heart to be treated prophylactically with antibiotics when they are exposed to transient bacteremias, particularly after dental extractions or urethral catheterization.

Anatomic Features

The classification of bacterial endocarditis as acute and subacute forms has been largely discarded; antibiotic treatment has so altered the clinical course that the previous distinguishing features have largely disappeared. However, they are still worth describing for didactic purposes, because they illustrate several important features of this condition (Table 11-7).

The mitral valve is most commonly involved with bacterial endocarditis. The vegetations usually form on the atrial surface at the point of closure of the leaflets. The lesions are composed of platelets, fibrin, and masses of organisms. The underlying valve is edematous and inflamed, and may eventually be so damaged that it becomes insufficient. The lesions may vary in size from a small superficial deposit on the valve to exuberant vegetations (see Fig. 11-28). **Infected thrombi** travel to multiple systemic sites, causing infarcts or abscesses in the brain, kidneys,

intestines, spleen, etc. The infective process may spread locally to produce abscesses of the valve rings or of the adjacent mural endocardium and chordae tendineae. The aortic valve is also commonly involved with endocarditis (Fig 11-28). Drug addicts who "mainline" infected drugs have a high incidence of infective endocarditis of the tricuspid valve; in such cases infected thrombi go to the lungs. Addicts may also have cardiac conduction system disturbances, due to the extension of the endocarditis to the membranous interventricular septum and the adjacent common bundle.

Another complication of infective endocarditis is so-called **focal embolic glomerulonephritis.** This is probably not an "embolic" process at all, but rather a result of a hypersensitivity phenomenon similar to diffuse glomerulonephritis, which is also sometimes present in these patients. The patchy hemorrhagic appearance of such kidneys has been described as "flea-bitten."

Nonbacterial Thrombotic Endocarditis (Marantic Endocarditis)

Nonbacterial thrombotic endocarditis is similar in gross appearance to infective endocarditis. However, it does not result in valve perforation, and its microscopic appearance is strikingly different. Infective endocarditis produces a thickened, edematous, and inflamed valve, with clumps of bacteria within the vegetation. By contrast, the nonbacterial lesion is bland, and no inflammation or organisms are found.

Nonbacterial thrombotic endocarditis usually occurs in a patient with increased blood coagulability. It may be part of the disseminated intravascular coagulation syndrome, and is frequently related to a carcinoma—most often a mucinous adenocarcinoma of the pancreas. The endocarditis, therefore, is often a terminal event in patients with wasting diseases,

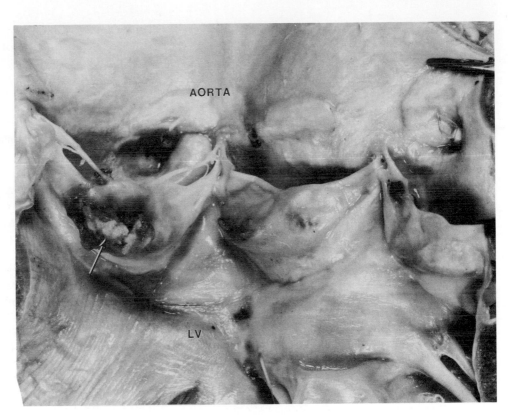

Figure 11-28. Bacterial endocarditis. Aortic valve, with aorta (*above*) and left ventricle (*LV*) (*below*) opened to show a vegetation (*arrow*) on the ventricular surface of the right coronary cusp. The three valve cusps are slightly thickened and have fenestrations (holes) in their free margins, but are otherwise normal. This is from a patient who had bacterial endocarditis caused by *Staphylococcus aureus*. The condition cannot be differentiated grossly from nonbacterial thrombotic endocarditis.

which accounts for the term "marantic." It is clinically manifested by infarcts of the brain, kidneys, spleen, intestines, and extremities that result from embolic fragments of the sterile vegetation in the heart. It has been suggested that this disorder may sometimes precede the development of infective endocarditis and may establish the implantation site of bacteria.

Myocarditis

Although the term "myocarditis" can be applied to any inflammatory involvement of the myocardium, it is usually defined so as to exclude conditions caused by ischemic heart disease. Defined in this way it is found in less than 1% of autopsies.

Etiology

Possible causes of myocarditis are listed in Table 11-8. At one time, the most common diagnosis was in the idiopathic category. With the better diagnostic techniques that are now available, many of the cases that would have been previously diagnosed as idiopathic are determined to be due to viruses—especially those of the coxsackie A and B groups. Almost

any viral infection appears to have the potential of producing myocarditis, and many minor viral diseases of the myocardium are probably clinically unsuspected.

Anatomic Features

Myocarditis is suggested grossly by dilatation of the ventricles, an appearance which also characterizes

---

Table 11-8 Causes of Myocarditis

Idiopathic
- Giant cell myocarditis (Fiedler's myocarditis)

Infectious
- Viral: Coxsackievirus, ECHO, influenza, poliomyelitis
- Rickettsial: Typhus, Rocky Mountain spotted fever
- Bacterial: Diphtheria, staphylococcal, streptococcal, meningococcal, and leptospiral infection
- Fungi and protozoan parasites: Chagas disease, toxoplasmosis, aspergillosis, cryptococcal and monilial infection
- Metazoan parasites: *Echinococcus, Trichina*

Noninfectious
- Hypersensitivity and immunologically related diseases: Rheumatic fever, systemic lupus erythematosus, scleroderma, drug reaction (e.g., to penicillin or sulfonamide), rheumatoid arthritis
- Radiation
- Miscellaneous: Sarcoidosis, uremia

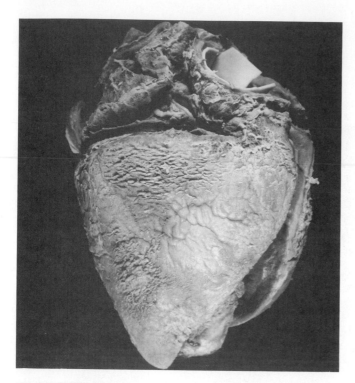

Figure 11-29. Purulent pericarditis. Epicardial surface of right ventricle, showing a shaggy, diffuse fibrinopurulent exudate. The patient was a 25-year-old man who had a bicuspid aortic valve that contained vegetations produced by *Staphylococcus aureus* infection.

heart failure. Microscopically, the most common findings are those of "acute nonspecific myocarditis." Such histologic changes are caused by most infectious agents; they also occur in most of the idiopathic and hypersensitivity cases. Some interstitial edema is usually seen, along with an infiltrate consisting of lymphocytes, monocytes, and variable numbers of plasma cells, neutrophils, and eosinophils. There may be slight to severe myofiber necrosis, and cases of several months duration show considerable interstitial fibrosis. Some cases of myocarditis display a histologic reaction that is better termed "granulomatous." These include cases of tuberculosis of the myocardium (tuberculomas), sarcoidosis, and fungal myocarditis. One idiopathic category is referred to as "giant cell myocarditis" or "Fiedler's myocarditis."

Without multiple sections from different regions of the heart, it is occasionally difficult to distinguish myocarditis from myocardial infarction. The best anatomically differentiating feature is the diffuse involvement of the myocardium in myocarditis, in contrast to the localization of specific vascular beds in myocardial infarction. A diagnosis of acute myocardial infarction is suggested by the presence of a thin uninfarcted subendocardial zone, which is preserved due to the absorption of oxygen from the ventricular cavity.

Pericarditis

Any inflammatory disease of the visceral or parietal pericardium is termed pericarditis. If it is accompanied by myocardial involvement, the diagnosis of "myopericarditis" is appropriate. The clinical incidence of pericarditis is difficult to determine, and the diagnosis is made much more frequently at autopsy. The causes of pericarditis are similar to those for myocarditis (see Table 11-8) and can be grouped under the same headings (idiopathic, infectious, and noninfectious). Metastatic neoplasms also may induce a serofibrinous or hemorrhagic exudation and inflammatory reaction when they involve the pericardium. Pericarditis associated with myocardial infarction and rheumatic fever has been discussed above.

Anatomic Features

Pericarditis can be classified according to its gross morphologic characteristics. For example, it can be described as being **fibrinous, purulent** (Fig. 11-29), **hemorrhagic, adhesive, or constrictive.** Uremia is frequently the cause of the fibrinous type, which has a tendency to become hemorrhagic because of the prominent pericardial granulation tissue. Viral infection also produces a fibrinous pericarditis, as do myocardial infarcts. Pericardial infection by bacteria such as *Staphylococcus aureus* is usually purulent, and may occur secondary to bacterial endocarditis (Fig. 11-29). Adhesive pericarditis is commonly an incidental finding at autopsy; it is the sequel of many different types of pericarditis that have healed and left only relatively minor fibrous adhesions. **Constrictive pericarditis** is rare, and is caused by a previous severe infection that was either purulent or tuberculous in origin. Even though tuberculosis is much less common than it was, it is still the major identifiable cause of constrictive pericarditis. The scar may be so thick (up to 3 cm) that it replaces the layers of the pericardium with a rigid mass of fibrous tissue and narrows the orifices of the venae cavae (Fig. 11-30). The fibrous envelope may contain deposits of calcium. Patients with this type of involvement have a small, quiet heart, in which there is restriction of venous inflow and limitation of diastolic filling. These patients have high venous pressure, low cardiac output, small pulse pressure, and fluid retention, with ascites and peripheral edema.

Nutritional, Endocrine, and Metabolic Diseases of the Heart

Thyrotoxic Heart Disease

Hyperthyroidism has profound effects on the cardiovascular system. Marked tachycardia and an increased workload, due to the lowered peripheral resistance and increased cardiac output, result in high output failure. The diagnosis is apparent if the patient has the classic signs of thyrotoxicosis. Not infrequently, and especially in older patients, the thyrotoxic signs and symptoms are obscure, and thyroid disease is not recognized as the basis for heart failure. The alterations in cardiovascular hemodynamics reflect an increased level of adrenergic activity as well as the direct effects of the thyroid hormone. Thus, in addition to specific treatment for thyroid disease, therapy with beta-adrenergic blocking drugs is indicated.

An additional complicating factor in hyperthyroid patients is the nutritional deficiency that often accompanies the disease. Thus, a patient not only has a heart that is hard pressed by an excessive workload, but often also has an inadequate nutritional intake. Specific vitamin deficiencies may result, especially a deficiency of thiamine, which can further embarrass the heart by limiting its metabolic capacity.

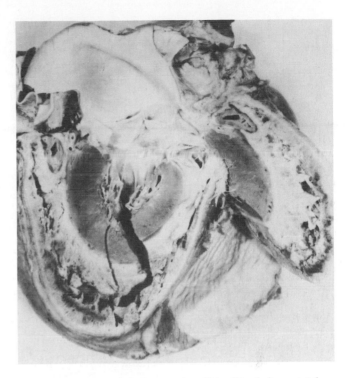

Figure 11-30. Constrictive pericarditis. The left ventricle and aortic valve are illustrated. The atrophic heart (250 g) is solidly encased by a thick, dense, fibrous sheath. The visceral and parietal layers of pericardium are distorted by fibrous and fibrinous bands, and bloody gelatinous material is present in the pericardial sac.

Myxedema and the Heart

Patients with hypothyroidism usually have a decreased cardiac output, decreased heart rate, and decreased myocardial contractility. There may be a pericardial effusion, which can be misinterpreted on radiologic examination as a large heart. The pulse pressure is decreased because of increased peripheral resistance and decreased blood volume. The hearts of patients with myxedema are usually flabby and dilated. The myocardium exhibits some myofiber swelling, and basophilic (or mucinous) degeneration is common. This alteration of the myofiber, which is also seen in other conditions, is well demonstrated by the periodic acid-Schiff reaction.

Thiamine Deficiency (Beriberi) Heart Disease

Beriberi heart disease has been seen in the Orient in patients whose diet is inadequate in vitamins, especially diets including shelled rice and white bread. In the United States it is occasionally seen in alcoholic patients. Thiamine deficiency results in decreased peripheral vascular resistance and increased cardiac output, a combination like that produced by hyperthyroidism, and which leads to high output failure. In addition, the metabolic abnormality resulting from vitamin deficiency affects energy production by the heart.

Carcinoid Heart Disease

Patients with carcinoid tumors that have metastasized to the liver often have right-sided changes of the endocardium. These consist of deposits of pearly gray, uniform, fibrous tissue, without elastic fibers, on the tricuspid and pulmonary valves and on the endocardial surface of the right ventricle. Microscopically, these deposits have a "tacked on" appearance. They result in tricuspid insufficiency or stenosis, and in pulmonary valve stenosis. It is thought that they are caused by high concentrations of tumor-produced serotonin (5-hydroxytryptamine), a compound metabolized in the lungs by monoamine oxidase. As a result, the effect of the serotonin is predominantly

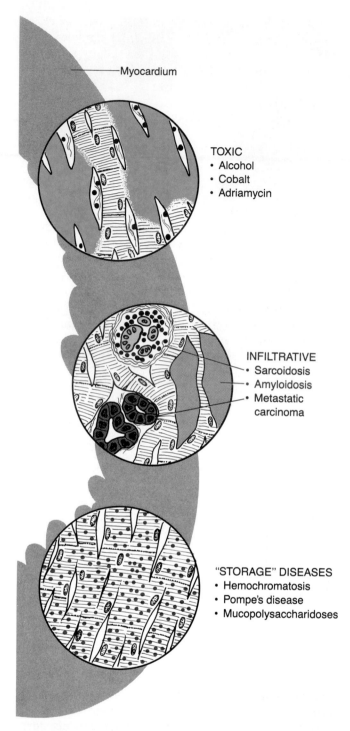

—Myocardium

TOXIC
• Alcohol
• Cobalt
• Adriamycin

INFILTRATIVE
• Sarcoidosis
• Amyloidosis
• Metastatic
  carcinoma

"STORAGE" DISEASES
• Hemochromatosis
• Pompe's disease
• Mucopolysaccharidoses

Figure 11-31.   Degenerative diseases of the myocardium. (*Top*) direct toxic effects of alcohol, cobalt, or doxorubicin (Adriamycin) on the myocytes. The dark-red fibers are necrotic. (*Center*) Infiltrative conditions, exemplified by the inflammatory lesions of sarcoidosis, the interstitial deposits of amyloidosis surrounding the myofibers and capillaries, and metastatic adenocarcinoma. (*Bottom*) "Storage" diseases show myocardial lysosomes containing stored hemosiderin (in hemochromatosis), glycogen (in Pompe's disease), and mucopolysaccharides (in mucopolysaccharidosis).

on the right side of the heart, although it occasionally affects the left side, especially when there is right-to-left shunting of blood across a defective atrial or ventricular septum.

Storage Diseases

Glycogen Storage Disease

Of the various forms of glycogen storage disease, types II (Pompe's disease), III (Cori's disease), and IV (Andersen's disease) affect the heart (Fig. 11-31). The most common and severe cardiac involvement occurs with type II glycogen storage disease. In patients with this condition, the heart is markedly enlarged (up to seven times normal), and some endocardial fibroelastosis is seen in about 20% of patients. The myofibers are vacuolated as a result of the large amounts of stored glycogen. The usual cause of death is cardiac failure.

Mucopolysaccharidosis

Type I mucopolysaccharidosis (Hurler's syndrome) involves the endocardium (causing valve thickening), the myocardium, and the coronary arteries, which are thickened and have narrowed lumens (Fig. 11-31).

Sphingolipidosis

The sphingolipidoses that involve the heart include Fabry's disease and Gaucher's disease. **Fabry's disease,** characterized by a deficiency of a lysosomal hydrolase, is complicated by deposits in the myocardium, cardiac conduction system, and coronary arteries. Valvular deposits may produce stenosis or insufficiency.

Gaucher's disease only rarely involves the heart. There may be deposits in the cardiac myocytes, and the heart may show cor pulmonale secondary to pulmonary alveolar capillary involvement.

Gangliosidosis

The infantile (type I) and the juvenile (type II) forms of generalized (GM_1) gangliosidosis can involve the heart, with cardiomegaly and with swollen histiocytes in the mitral, aortic, and tricuspid valves. Of the two types of GM_2 gangliosidosis, Tay-Sachs disease does not usually involve the heart, but Sandhoff's disease often shows cardiomegaly, endocardial fibroelastosis, mitral and tricuspid valve thickening, and irregular coronary artery narrowing.

Amyloidosis

Details of the nature and of the systemic involvement by amyloidosis are described in Chapter 23; the condition is presented here only in terms of its cardiac involvement. The heart is affected in most of the generalized forms of this disease (Fig. 11-31). Many of these hearts have distinct clinical functional abnormalities that result directly from the amyloid deposits, including electrocardiographic abnormalities, symptoms of congestive failure, enlarged heart, and decreased interventricular septal movement (seen on echocardiogram). The clinical diagnosis can be made with assurance only by endomyocardial biopsy.

At autopsy the enlarged heart is firm and rubbery. Amyloid deposits are nodular, waxy, endocardial deposits in the atria; they also cause thickening of the cardiac valves. Amyloid deposits are seen interstitially in the endocardium and in the walls of intramural coronary arteries. In rare cases the cardiac involvement is limited to the small arteries and causes angina pectoris and sudden death.

The most common cardiac involvement in amyloidosis occurs in cases classified as "primary"—those in which there is no evidence of another preceding or coexisting disease. Another variety of amyloidosis involves the hearts of the aged and is termed **senile cardiac amyloidosis**. This disorder is usually clinically unsuspected, and is most often found only incidentally at autopsy.

Cardiomyopathy

Defined literally, the term "cardiomyopathy" could apply to any heart muscle disease, but for practical reasons the definition is limited so as to exclude myocardial disease caused by ischemic, hypertensive, congenital, valvular, or pericardial abnormalities. It also excludes cases with "specific heart muscle disease." Some cardiologists divide the cardiomyopathies into primary and secondary forms. The **primary** type consists of those cases in which the basic and major process involves the myocardium, and in which the cause of cardiomyopathy is unknown. The **secondary** type is seen in association with another type of heart disease or is secondary to a systemic disease. Cardiomyopathy is classified as congestive (dilated), hypertrophic, or restrictive.

The **congestive cardiomyopathies** include diseases of different etiologies, and it is likely that the initiating event is a viral myocarditis, Chagas' disease, alcoholism, or any one of numerous potential toxins that have not been identified. Anatomic features include cardiomegaly, dilated ventricles, and a high incidence of mural thrombi in the ventricular chambers. The microscopic changes in the myocardium are nonspecific and include myocyte hypertrophy, focal necrosis (usually slight), mitochondrial abnormalities, and myofiber degenerative changes (e.g., fat accumulation).

Many cases of congestive cardiomyopathy occur in chronic alcoholics. Although a specific diagnosis of **alcoholic cardiomyopathy** cannot be made with certainty, it is likely that congestive failure in an alcoholic patient with a large heart, in whom no other cause of heart failure is apparent, is related to the toxic effect of alcohol on the heart muscle. Other directly toxic effects on the myocardium are produced by various agents, such as cobalt (**beer drinker's cardiomyopathy**) and phenothiazine (Fig. 11-31). The cardiac toxicity of Adriamycin limits the dose of this chemotherapeutic drug.

A second common category of cardiomyopathies is called **hypertrophic cardiomyopathy,** defined as **a cardiomyopathy that exhibits cardiomegaly but no ventricular dilatation.** Various other terms have been applied to this condition, some of which are not appropriate because they refer only to variably present features of the condition. The terms that are sometimes used as synonyms for hypertrophic cardiomyopathy are idiopathic hypertrophic subaortic stenosis, asymmetric septal hypertrophy, hypertrophic obstructive cardiomyopathy, idiopathic myocardial hypertrophy, and subaortic muscular stenosis. Several anatomic features are common and characteristic of the condition, although none of them is diagnostic or essential for the diagnosis. These include asymmetric hypertrophy of the ventricular septum and myofiber disarray. **There is evidence that hypertrophic cardiomyopathy is transmitted as an autosomal dominant genetic trait.**

The hearts of such patients show hypertrophy and small ventricular chambers. Terminal heart failure may occasionally produce some ventricular dilation, creating difficulty in differentiating the condition from a congestive cardiomyopathy. However, **asymmetric septal hypertrophy and myofiber disarray are almost invariable.** Although this abnormal myofiber configuration can occur in other conditions (e.g., congenital heart disease), it is not as extensive. Another commonly found lesion in the hearts of patients with hypertrophic cardiomyopathy is endocardial thickening in the left ventricular outflow region.

Restrictive cardiomyopathies are much rarer than the congestive and hypertrophic types. They include those conditions in which there is increased wall stiffness (e.g., amyloidosis) and in which diastolic ventricular volume and stretch are sufficiently impaired to cause a restriction in filling.

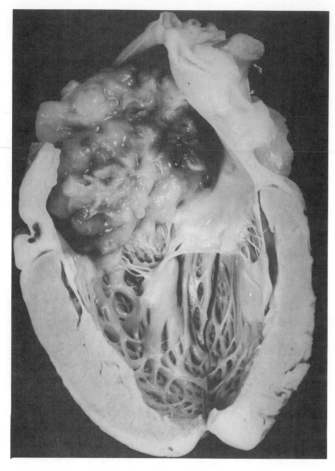

Figure 11-32.   Left atrial myxoma. The heart is from a 33-year-old woman who had symptoms of congestive heart failure that had progressively worsened. The clinical diagnosis was "rheumatic mitral stenosis." The woman died after suffering a stroke caused by a tumor embolus. The grapelike gelatinous nodules of the tumor fill the left atrium and obstruct the mitral valve orifice, producing symptoms similar to those of mitral stenosis.

Luetic Heart Disease

The cardiovascular effects of tertiary syphilis are largely on the aorta. A discussion of these effects is included here mainly because of their former importance as a cause of heart disease. This condition has almost disappeared in the United States, although antibiotic-resistant strains of the spirochete are appearing, and there have been some indications of an increasing incidence of the disease.

Tertiary syphilis causes heart disease by two mechanisms:

- Aortic medial scarring may extend to the aortic valve ring and aortic valve cusps. This widens the valve ring and separates the commissures of the cusps, which become thickened and shortened, and display rolled margins. The effect is severe aortic valve insufficiency. The volume workload of the heart is thus increased, an effect that eventually leads to heart failure.
- The changes characteristic of luetic aortitis, which thicken the aortic intima, may extend from the ascending aorta to involve and obstruct the coronary artery ostia. This can produce myocardial ischemia which, added to the increased workload imposed on the heart by aortic valve insufficiency, gives added impetus to the development of cardiac failure or infarction.

A third possible manner of cardiac involvement by syphilis is the very rare occurrence of a gumma in the myocardium. This lesion can produce cardiac malfunction either by its stimulation of an arrhythmia or by a mechanical effect on the heart's pumping ability.

Cardiac Tumors

Primary cardiac tumors are rare. The most common primary tumor is the **myxoma** (Fig. 11-32), accounting for 35% to 50% of all primary cardiac tumors. **Most myxomas arise in the left atrium, although they can occur in any cardiac chamber or on a valve.** They appear as a gelatinous polyp with a short stalk, but may sometimes be mobile and large enough to obstruct the mitral valve orifice. Microscopically, they have a loose myxoid matrix containing much acid mucopolysaccharide. Within this matrix are polygonal, stellate cells, occurring singly or in small clusters. Some myxomas have been said to represent organized thrombi, but the majority of typical myxomas are true neoplasms.

Another type of primary tumor, which is most common in infants and young children, is the **rhabdomyoma**. These tumors form nodular masses in the myocardium. The cells show small central nuclei and fibrillar processes that radiate to the margin of the cell. The resulting appearance is the basis for the name "spider cell." Rhabdomyomas often occur in association with tuberous sclerosis.

The so-called **mesothelioma** is a rare primary cardiac tumor that occurs in the interatrial septum in the region usually occupied by the atrioventricular node. The tumor encroaches upon the node, leading to heart block or arrhythmia and sudden death. These tumors are composed of cysts lined by bland cuboidal or squamous cells. Although the term "mesothelioma" was first applied to these tumors because of their supposed similarity to the pericardial or pleural tumor of the same name, it is more likely that they are derived from an endodermal source. They have been termed "congenital endodermal heterotopia" or "congenital polycystic tumors" of the atrioventricular node.

The growth of papillary fronds on the heart valves is referred to as a **papillary fibroelastoma**. A fragment can break off to become an embolus to another organ, or the tumor may occlude a coronary artery orifice and produce myocardial ischemia. These tumors are not neoplasms, but are more appropriately termed **hamartomas**. The fronds have a central dense core of collagen surrounded by looser connective tissue, and are covered by a continuation of the endothelial cells of the valve on which the tumor originates. There are some similarities between these papillary fibroelastomas and large Lambl's excrescences, but the two lesions are probably not of the same origin.

Other primary tumors of the heart are even rarer than those described above. These include angiomas, fibromas, lymphangiomas, neurofibromas, and the sarcomatous counterparts of these tumors. Lipomatous hypertrophy of the interatrial septum and encapsulated lipomas are reported.

The most common metastatic tumors of the heart derive from cancer of the lung, breast, and gastrointestinal tract. Lymphomas and leukemia may involve the heart. For some reason, many malignant melanomas metastasize to the heart.

SUGGESTED READING

BOOKS

Becker AE, Anderson RH: Cardiac Pathology. New York, Raven Press, 1983

Bloor CM: Cardiac Pathology. Philadelphia, J B Lippincott, 1978

Braunwald E (ed): Heart Disease, 2nd Ed. Philadelphia, W B Saunders Co, 1984

Fozzard HA, Haber E, Jennings RB et al (eds): The Heart and Cardiovascular System. New York Raven Press, 1986

Pomerance A, Davies M: The Pathology of the Heart. Boston, Blackwell, 1975

Silver MD: Cardiovascular Pathology. New York, Churchill Livingstone, 1983

ARTICLES

Aretz HT, Billingham ME, et al: Myocarditis. Am J Cardiovasc Pathol 1:3, 1987

Ayoub EM: The search for host determinants of susceptibility to rheumatic fever: The missing link. Circulation, 69:197-201, 1984

Bulkley B: The cardiomyopathies, Hospital Practice, 19:59-73, 1984

Forrester JS, Litvack F, Grundfest W: A perspective of coronary disease seen through the arteries of living man. Circulation 75:505-513, 1987

Friedman M, Thoreson CE, Gill JJ et al: Alteration of type A behavior and reduction in cardiac recurrences in post myocardial infarction patients. Am Heart J 108:237-248, 1984

Grundy SM, Arky R, Bray GA, et al: Coronary risk factor statement for the American public. Circulation, 72:1135A-1139A, 1985

Jennings RB, Reimer KA, Steenbergen C: Myocardial ischemia revisited: The osmolar load, membrane damage, and reperfusion. J Mol Cell Cardiol 18:769, 1986

Roberts WC: Coronary thrombosis and fatal myocardial infarction. Circulation 49:1-3, 1974

Shekelle RB, Gale M, Norusis M: Type A score and risk of recurrent coronary heart disease in the aspirin myocardia infarction study. Am J Cardiol 56:221-225, 1985

Tarazi RC: Editorial: The heart in hypertension. N Engl J Med 312:308-309, 1985

Veasy LG, Wiedmeier SE, Orsmund GS et al: Resurgence of acute rheumatic fever in the intermountain area of the United States. N Engl J Med 316:421, 1987

Williams RC: Host factors in rheumatic fever and heart disease. Hospital Practice, 17:125-138, 1982

Zierler S, Rothman KJ: Congenital heart disease in relation to maternal use of Bendectin and other drugs in early pregnancy. N Engl J Med 313:347-352, 1985

12

The Respiratory System

William M. Thurlbeck and Roberta R. Miller

Normal Structure and
Function

Pathology of the Larynx and
Trachea

Lesions in Conducting
Airways

Neoplasia

Lesions Affecting the Lung
Parenchyma

Disease Processes Unique to
the Lung

Diseases of the Pleura

Diseases of Pulmonary
Vasculature

Figure 12-1. Anatomy of the lung. The conducting structures of the lung include (1) the trachea, which has horseshoe-shaped cartilages; (2) the bronchi, which have plates of cartilage in their walls (both the trachea and bronchi have mucus-secreting glands in their wall); and (3) the bronchioles, which do not have cartilage in their walls. The most distal is the terminal bronchiole. The gas-exchanging components comprise the unit distal to the terminal bronchiole, namely, the acinus. Alveoli are lined by type I cells, which are large, flat cells that cover most of the alveolar wall, and by type II cells, which secrete surfactant and are the progenitor cells of the alveolar epithelium. The alveolar capillaries exchange gas in the alveolar wall.

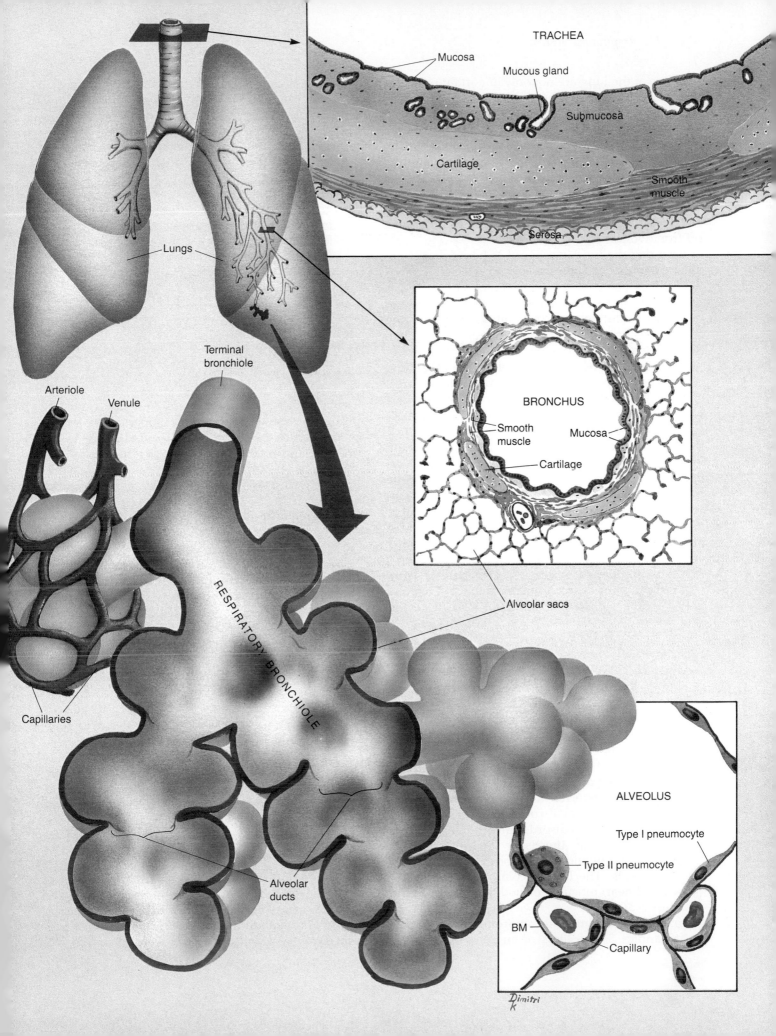

TRACHEA

Mucosa

Mucous gland

Submucosa

Cartilage

Smooth muscle

Serosa

Lungs

Terminal bronchiole

Arteriole

Venule

Capillaries

RESPIRATORY BRONCHIOLE

Alveolar ducts

BRONCHUS

Smooth muscle

Mucosa

Cartilage

Alveolar sacs

ALVEOLUS

Type I pneumocyte

Type II pneumocyte

BM

Capillary

Dimitri
k

Diseases of the lung are not only important problems for individual patients, but major public health concerns. Cancer of the lung causes more deaths than any other cancer—over 100,000 a year in the United States. Chronic airflow obstruction represents the single greatest cost to the Veterans Administration. The adult respiratory distress syndrome is responsible for 75,000 deaths a year in the United States. Humble respiratory tract infections, mostly benign and self-limited, are the most common cause of time off from work.

Each day the lung is exposed to harmful environmental agents, the most obvious of which are found in the workplace, where inhalation of such materials as asbestos and silica results in serious disability or death. Air pollution is also a significant factor in lung disease. Although its effects are less serious than those of asbestos or silica, air pollution is more widespread, and may aggravate or help cause other lung conditions. It may have been responsible for such epidemics as that in the London smog of 1952, which was associated with some 3000 deaths. Most people spend much of their lives inside the home, where the environment is affected by both the external environment and substances generated in the home (e.g., vapors from gas cooking or urea formaldehyde foam). Both cancer and chronic airflow obstruction are overwhelmingly related to tobacco smoking, mostly cigarettes. This unique toxic product has a direct effect on the lung and an indirect one on other organs, notably those of the cardiovascular system.

Although the lung shares with other organs many responses to injuries (e.g., inflammation and neoplasia), we shall emphasize conditions specific to the lung itself:

Chronic airflow obstruction. The major function of the lung is gas exchange; it follows that obstruction to airflow has serious consequences.

Pneumoconiosis (diseases due to respirable inorganic substances). Mining and the processing of minerals require that workers be exposed to minerals and associated dust that produce specific lung lesions.

Restrictive lung disease (infiltrative lung disease). A syndrome referred to as restrictive lung disease is the functional counterpart of infiltrative lung disease. This disorder involves the interstitium of the lung, the tissue around the blood vessels, lymphatics and bronchi; and the airspace walls. The lung becomes stiff and small, with a linear, reticular, or nodular pattern in the chest radiograph.

Infections in the immunocompromised host. Since it handles 5 to 8 liters of air each minute, the lung is exposed to infectious agents more than most organs. Treatment of cancer with immunosuppressive and cytotoxic agents compromises the host's defense mechanisms. In these circumstances lung infections that are often not serious in normal persons may become life-threatening.

Rare and interesting diseases of the lung. A rare group of conditions affects the lung particularly but may be related to diseases in other organs. In this group are such diseases as noninfectious angiitis and granulomatosis.

Normal Structure and Function

Anatomy and Histology

The Larynx

The larynx (Fig. 12-2) is the most superior, expanded portion of the respiratory tract, specialized for the production of the voice. It is bounded above by the pharynx and oral cavity and below by the first tracheal ring. The supporting structures, or "skeleton," of the larynx consist of four cartilaginous structures:

The **epiglottic cartilage,** the most superior cartilage, which supports the epiglottis. The epiglottic tip is the most superior part of the larynx, projecting upward into the pharynx behind the base of the tongue.

The **thyroid cartilage,** the largest laryngeal cartilage, located anteriorly and composed of bilateral plates, fused in the midline to form the laryngeal prominence ("Adam's apple").

The **arytenoid cartilages,** which are paired triangular cartilages located posterolaterally at the level of the thyroid cartilage but which are considerably smaller than the thyroid cartilage. The vocal cords are attached to the arytenoid cartilages, and movement of the cords is facilitated by movement of these cartilages.

The **cricoid cartilage,** which is the most inferior laryngeal cartilage. Anteriorly, it is located between the inferior aspect of the thyroid cartilage and the first tracheal ring. Posteriorly, it is expanded upward to form a synovium-lined joint articulating with the arytenoid cartilages.

The **epiglottis** forms the most superior aspect of the internal structure of the soft tissues of the larynx. Laterally and extending downward, the arytenoepiglottic folds separate the tubular larynx from the piriform sinuses, which are a part of the pharynx. Approximately midway between the epiglottis and the first tracheal ring are paired, abrupt, groovelike outpouchings of the lumen of the larynx, termed the ventricles. The superior borders of the ventricles consist of the vestibular folds, or "false cords," which have no important function in the production of voice. Immediately below the ventricles are the vocal folds, or true cords, which are responsible for laryngeal speech. The **glottis** is composed of the false cords, ventricles, and true cords. The tissue above the false cords is termed the **supraglottis,** and the tissue below the true cords is termed the **infraglottis.**

The superior aspect of the epiglottis, the arytenoepiglottic folds, and the true cords are lined by squamous mucosa. The remainder of the surface of the larynx is normally lined by ciliated respiratory mucosa. The submucosa throughout most of the larynx is composed of loose fibrous stroma and compound mucus-secreting glands, similar to those seen in the trachea and bronchi, which correspond to minor salivary glands of the oropharynx. The submucosa of the true cords is composed of skeletal muscles fibers from the thyroarytenoid muscle.

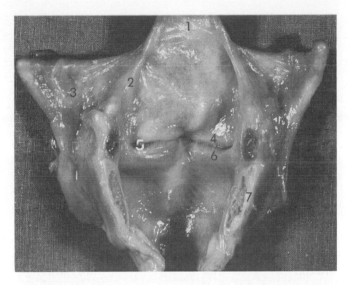

Figure 12-2. The normal larynx. Note the epiglottis (*1*), aryteno-epiglottic folds (*2*), piriform sinuses (*3*), false cords (*4*), ventricles (*5*), true cords (*6*), and cricoid cartilage (*7*). The larynx has been opened posteriorly and margins pinned.

The Lung and Airways

The trachea is approximately 22 cm long, with a cross-sectional area of 2 cm. At the tracheal carina it divides into the two major bronchi (see Fig. 12-1). **The right bronchus diverges at a lesser angle from the trachea, which is why foreign material is more frequently aspirated on the right side.** On entering the lung the bronchi divide into lobar bronchi and then into segmental bronchi, which supply the 19 segments of the lung. Because the segments are individual units with their own bronchovascular supply, they can be resected individually. The number of further ramifications of the bronchi depends on the distance from the hilum. Thus, there is a substantial number of ramifying bronchi in **axial pathways** that traverse the long distance to the periphery of the lung, such as the posterior basal segment, whereas there are far fewer in **lateral pathways** supplying the lung close to the hilum.

The tracheobronchial tree has cartilage and tracheobronchial mucous glands in the wall. The glands are compound tubular glands that display both mucous (pale cells) and serous cells (granular, more basophilic cells). Between them, both types of cell secrete most of the mucus that is found in the tracheobronchial tree. The tracheobronchial tree is lined by a pseudostratified epithelium, which appears as layers, although all cells reach the basement membrane. Most of the cells are ciliated, but mucus-secreting (goblet) cells also exist, as well as basal cells that do not reach the surface. The basal cells are thought to be precursor cells that differentiate to form the more specialized cells of the tracheobronchial epithelium. K (for *Kulchitsky-like*) cells, which resemble the argentaffin and argyrophil cells found in the gut and elsewhere, are neuroendocrine cells that contain a variety of hormonally active polypeptides and vasoactive amines. Although at one time these cells were thought to derive from the neural crest and migrate to the epithelium of the bronchus, it is now clear that they share a common stem cell with other cells of the bronchus and gut.

Succeeding the bronchi are the (membranous) **bronchioles,** which differ from bronchi in that they contain neither cartilage nor mucus-secreting glands. As with bronchi, the number of branchings and their length depend on the pathway from the hilus to the periphery of the lung. In axial pathways there may be up to 25 branchings of conducting airways and a length of approximately 23 cm, whereas in lateral pathways there are only seven generations and a total length of about 8 cm. The epithelium of the bronchioles becomes thinner, until only one cell layer is apparent. The last purely conducting structure is the **terminal bronchiole,** after which the airways have alveoli in their walls. A major change then occurs as the gas-exchanging unit, the **acinus,** is encountered. This unit consists of, in series, first, respiratory bronchioles, airways with both alveolated and nonalveolated epithelium in their walls; second, alveolar ducts, conducting structures with only alveoli in their walls; and third, alveolar sacs, terminal structures lined entirely by alveoli. **The acinus is the unit of gas exchange in the lung.** Understanding this structure is critical to understanding the very important condition known as emphysema.

Alveoli, the gas-exchanging structures of the lung, are lined by two types of epithelium. **Type I cells cover 95% of the alveolar surface, although they comprise only 40% of all the epithelial cells of the alveolus.** They are thin and have a large surface area, a combination that facilitates gas exchange. **Type II cells comprise 60% of the alveolar lining cells,** but because they are more cuboidal they contribute only a small part to the total alveolar surface area. These cells secrete the surfactant material of the alveolar surface that maintains the patency of alveoli. It should be noted that bronchioles are also lined by surfactant and that displacement of surfactant by inflammatory exudate leads to bronchiolar instability and thus impairs their function. Type I cells are very vulnerable to injury, and when they die, type II cells multiply and differentiate to form type I cells, thereby reconstituting the alveolar surface area.

The alveolar epithelial cells are connected by tight junctions that prevent the passage of even small molecules through the epithelial surface. The alveolar wall contains a dense network of capillaries, each alveolus having approximately 1000 capillary segments, about 15 μm long and 8 μm in diameter. The capillaries are lined by endothelial cells that resemble type I epithelial cells in that they have abundant flat cytoplasm but differ in that their junctions are "leaky" or "semitight." Because the junctions are tighter on the arterial side and looser in the small venules, molecules the size of albumin can pass through the capillary endothelium. Both the endothelium and epithelium have basal laminae, and when they are adjacent they fuse into a single basal lamina that forms the thin side of the alveolar capillary membrane, where gas exchange is most efficient. On the opposite side (the thick side), the basal laminae are separate, and collagen, elastin, and proteoglycans are found there. In addition, fibroblasts, some of which contain muscle filaments (myofibroblasts), are also found on the thick side of the alveolar capillary membrane. This region, which constitutes the interstitial space of the alveolar wall, is where significant fluid and molecular exchange occurs and where edema begins.

The pulmonary arteries accompany the airways in a sheath of connective tissue known as the bronchovascular bundle. The more proximal arteries are elastic and then become transitional (four or fewer elastic laminae in their walls). They are succeeded by arteries whose walls have two elastic laminae with a layer of muscle between them. In vessels about 100 μm in diameter or less, muscle extends in a spiral fashion between the elastic laminae, so that the arterial wall is partly muscular and partly nonmuscular where the elastic laminae fuse. The smallest arteries have no muscle.

The smallest veins, which resemble the smallest arteries, join with other veins and drain into the lobular septa, connective tissue partitions that subdivide the lung into small respiratory units. The veins then continue in the lobular septa, joining other veins to form a network that is separate from the bronchovascular bundles.

There are no lymphatics in most alveolar walls. The lymphatics commence in alveoli at the periphery of the acinus, which lies along a lobular septum, the bronchovascular bundle, and the pleura. The lymphatics of the lobular septa and bronchovascular bundle accompany these structures, and the pleural lymphatics drain toward the hilus via the bronchovascular lymphatics.

A crucial concept in understanding lung pathology is that of the **interstitium of the lung.** This is composed of the connective tissue that surrounds the veins and bronchovascular bundle and the tissue on the thick side of the alveolar capillary membrane. Repeated reference will be made to it and to interstitial lung disease.

Embryology

The respiratory system—that is, the larynx, trachea, airways, and alveolar surface—develops as an outpouching of the foregut. The surrounding mesoderm is responsible for development of the interstitial tissue and the vascular system. The tracheobronchial bud divides and redivides to form the airways, which are complete to the segmental level by day 52, the end of the embryonic phase. Further subdivision occurs until week 16, when all conducting airways, up to the terminal bronchiole, are present. This is the end of the pseudoglandular phase. The next stage involves the development of the vascular system and further development of the airways, which now develop a thinned epithelium. The framework of the gas-exchanging unit of the lung, the acinus, is now laid down, the vascular system develops, capillaries reach the epithelium, and gas exchange becomes possible. This phase, the canalicular stage, terminates at about 26 to 28 weeks and fetal viability becomes possible. Further development, referred to as the saccular phase, occurs in the lung periphery as the terminal structures, the primary saccules, become subdivided by secondary crests, a process that results in greater complexity of the gas-exchanging surface and thinning of airspace walls. At 36 weeks the appearance of alveoli indicates the transition from the saccular to the alveolar stage. At birth the number of alveoli is highly variable, ranging from 20 million to 150 million. Most alveoli develop in the first 2 years of life.

Defense Mechanisms

Being exposed to air that is usually at a lower temperature than that of the body, of variable humidity, dirty, and laden with infectious agents, the lung has developed very effective defense mechanisms. The nose and trachea constitute an efficient air conditioning system, which ensures that the air entering the lung is at body temperature and fully saturated with water. The nose traps almost all particles more than 10 μm in diameter and about half of all particles with an aerodynamic diameter of 3 μm (Fig. 12-3). (Aerodynamic diameter refers to the way particles behave in air rather than to their actual size.) **The airway epithelium is protected by the mucociliary blanket.** The ciliary beat drives the mucous blanket toward the trachea, and particles that land on it are thus removed from the lungs and swallowed or coughed up. The mucociliary blanket is effective in disposing of particles 2 to 10 μm in diameter. **The protector of the alveolar space is the alveolar macrophage.** Alveolar macrophages are derived from the bone marrow, probably undergo a maturation division in the interstitium of the lung, and then enter the alveolar space. Unlike macrophages elsewhere they depend on oxidative metabolism. They are particularly effective in dealing with particles whose aerodynamic diameter is less than 2 μm. Very small particles behave as a gas and are exhaled.

Pathology of the Larynx and Trachea

Developmental Anomalies

The commonest serious anomaly of the larynx and trachea is **tracheal–esophageal fistula.** Many variants are known, the simplest of which is a fistula between the trachea and esophagus that allows swallowed food to be aspirated into the trachea and bronchi.

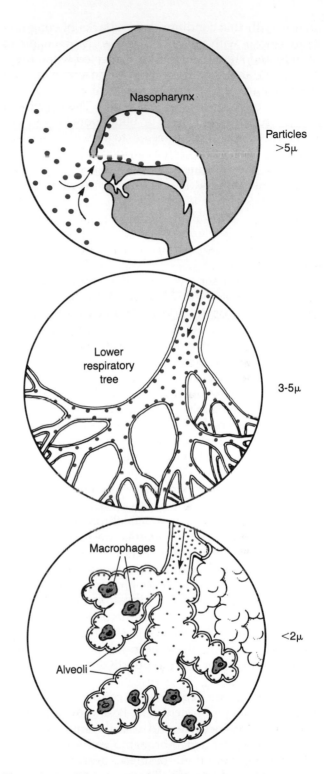

Figure 12-3. Deposition of particles in the respiratory tract. Large particles are trapped in the nose. Intermediate-sized particles deposit on the bronchi and bronchioles and are removed by the mucociliary blanket. Smaller particles terminate in the airspaces and are removed by macrophages. Very small particles behave as a gas and are breathed out.

Infants with this condition have attacks of coughing and cyanosis with feeding. It is readily amenable to surgery and should always be suspected when these symptoms are encountered. A more common and more serious condition is esophageal atresia associated with tracheal–esophageal fistula. The upper end of the esophagus ends in a blind pouch, and the lower esophagus is connected to the trachea. This situation, in which all ingested food and esophageal secretions are aspirated, leads to more severe pulmonary disease, and surgical correction is more difficult.

Infections of the Larynx and Trachea

Epiglottitis is a serious condition, most commonly caused by *Haemophilus influenzae,* type B. Occurring in infants and young children, it may be a life-threatening emergency. Swelling of the acutely inflamed epiglottis produces obstruction to airflow. Inspiratory stridor (a loud wheezing sound on inspiration) occurs, and the onset of cyanosis may indicate airway obstruction so severe as to require tracheostomy. Similar symptoms may be encountered in viral infections of the larynx and trachea, which are most commonly due to infection with para-influenza viruses.

Epiglottitis and laryngotracheobronchitis in children are associated with **croup,** a syndrome characterized by inspiratory stridor, cough, and hoarseness resulting from varying degrees of laryngeal obstruction. Croup due to laryngotracheobronchitis is a complication of an upper respiratory tract infection and is marked by edema of the larynx.

Both **laryngitis,** which causes hoarseness, and **tracheitis,** associated with cough, are common at all ages. Both are caused by viral infections, varying from the common cold to influenza. The systemic effects of fever and malaise are usually more troublesome to the patient than the respiratory symptoms, and anything other than supportive treatment is ineffective.

A variety of rare **degenerative** conditions affect the trachea and major bronchi. The best known, because of its unpronounceable and usually imprecisely recallable name, is tracheo-bronchio-pathica-osteoplastica. In this condition, ossified cartilage is found adjacent to, and sometimes separate from, tracheobronchial cartilage. It leads to "fixed" airway obstruction, in which resistance to flow is equal in inspiration and expiration. Amyloid deposition in the trachea and bronchi may lead to a similar syndrome, and some think the two conditions are closely related.

Neoplastic Conditions

Tumors of the larynx are common. A frequently encountered benign lesion, which is **reactive** rather than neoplastic, is the laryngeal nodule **(singer's nodule).** This lesion, usually single but sometimes multiple, consists of a small polypoid structure, with a simple fibrous stroma and squamous mucosa on the true vocal cords. It occurs most commonly in those who use their voice more than most, particularly singers. Changes in timbre of the voice and hoarseness are the main symptoms. Although a trivial biological lesion, such a nodule may jeopardize a singer's career. Although surgery is curative, the quality of the voice may be impaired.

Squamous papillomas occur in the larynx as either single or multiple lesions and may extend into the trachea and bronchi. Although their etiology is likely viral, they behave like neoplasms in the sense that they may cause life-threatening respiratory obstruction and, rarely, may evolve into an overt squamous cell carcinoma.

The vast majority of laryngeal cancers are **squamous cell carcinomas,** tumors strongly related to cigarette smoking. Based on the location of the lesion laryngeal carcinomas are divided into four groups that have relevance to treatment and prognosis.

A **glottic tumor** is a carcinoma limited to one or both true vocal cords. These tumors are slow to metastasize to lymph nodes and have a good prognosis, at least in the early stage. Radiotherapy or voice-saving surgery is usually curative.

Transglottic carcinomas, by definition, involve the true and false cords. These tumors are likely to metastasize to lymph nodes and often require total laryngectomy (Fig. 12-4).

Supraglottic carcinomas arise in the ventricle, false cords, or epiglottis and do not, by definition, involve the true cords. Nodal metastases are more common than in glottic tumors. Voice-saving surgical treatment is often possible.

Infraglottic carcinomas either are located below the true cords or involve the true cords, with considerable infraglottic extension. Nodal metastases are common, and total laryngectomy is generally required.

Cancers other than squamous cell carcinomas are rare and include tumors of minor salivary gland type, sarcomas, adenocarcinomas, and malignant melanomas.

An unexplained mystery is the rarity of tumors of the trachea. Logically, since potent carcinogens in

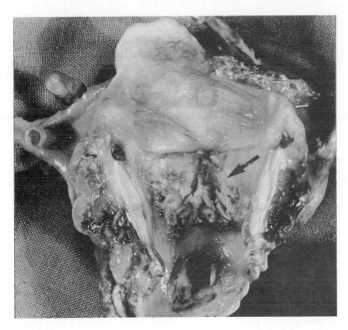

Figure 12-4. Carcinoma of the larynx. The tumor (*arrow*) involves the glottis (ventricle and true cords) and extends below the true cords into the infraglottis. Compare with Figure 12-2.

tobacco smoke should reach the trachea in highest concentration, cancer should be common in this location. The reverse is actually true; cancer of the trachea is distinctly uncommon. Most of the rare tumors encountered are mucoepidermoid carcinomas and adenoid cystic tumors that arise from tracheal mucous glands analogous to the salivary glands. The tumors have characteristics similar to salivary gland tumors.

Trauma

Most serious trauma to the trachea is iatrogenic. When a tracheostomy is performed, the stomal site and the area where the cuffed endotracheal balloon presses on the trachea are both injured. Stomal injury is largely a function of the tube itself. The larger the tube size compared with the size of the trachea, the greater the damage to the anterior tracheal wall. Injury at this site results in late tracheal stenosis, which endoscopically has the appearance of a gothic arch, formed by the collapse of the anterolateral tracheal tissues. These strictures can be minimized by the routine use of small tracheostomy tubes.

Injury at the cuff site is manifested by necrosis of the mucosa, submucosa, and cartilage when the capillary blood flow is interrupted by excessive pressure in the tracheostomy tube balloon. This injury was common in the early days of assisted ventilation, but the condition has now almost disappeared with the advent of high-volume, low-pressure cuffs. Endoscopically, these strictures appear as a circumferential constriction, about 2 cm below the stomal site.

Strictures need early dilatation for control of symptoms, and many of the advanced lesions require surgical excision, with end to end anastomosis of the tracheal components. Laser surgery is effective in treating these strictures.

Tracheobronchial damage may be a complication of burns due to smoke inhalation. Occasionally, direct heat is the source of tracheal injury, and in these cases there are also severe burns of the face and mouth.

Tracheal Compression

External compression of the trachea is most commonly caused by lesions of the thyroid. It is important to remember that both the trachea and the thyroid have an intrathoracic component, and the thyroid lesion may not be readily recognized on physical examination. A variety of other inflammatory and neoplastic lesions of the neck also compress the trachea. As in tracheal stenosis, fixed flow resistance is a complication.

Foreign Bodies

A lodged foreign body may totally occlude the trachea and result in suffocation. Large pieces of food, often steak, lodge in the trachea, classically in a restaurant when the sufferer has had too much to drink (the "Miami Beach syndrome"). The simplest action is the Heimlich maneuver, in which one stands behind the victim, wraps one's arms around him, makes a double clenched fist over the upper abdomen just below the rib cage, and gives a quick, forceful, upward squeeze. Alternatively, the occluding object may be reached via the pharynx, or an emergency tracheostomy may be necessary.

Lesions in Conducting Airways

We deal here with lesions of conducting airways (bronchi and bronchioles) other than those associated with chronic airflow obstruction, which are treated as a separate category later.

Congenital Anomalies

Minor deviations in the arrangement of the bronchial tree, such as variants of the bronchial segments, are common but insignificant. A significant abnormality is **bronchial atresia,** which most often occurs in the bronchus to the apical posterior segment of the left upper lobe. In infants this may result in an overexpanded part of the lung, and, in later life, in an overexpanded lobe that may also be emphysematous. Bronchial mucus, accumulating distal to the atretic region, may appear on radiologic examination as a mass.

Infections

There is clearly an overlap between infections of the trachea and those of the bronchi, and in many instances the term "tracheobronchitis" is appropriate. It is also true that many infections involve the airways and lung parenchyma. Although we have adopted the distinction between airways and parenchyma for reasons of classification and convenience, this division should not be thought of as rigid. Influenza is a characteristic example of tracheobronchitis, and in the occasional patient who dies with this infection, the appearance of the bronchi is dramatic. The surface of the airway is fiery red, reflecting acute inflammation and congestion of the mucosa.

Other infectious agents that involve the intrapulmonary airways more specifically usually affect the more peripheral airways (bronchiolitis). The classic examples are adenovirus, measles, and respiratory syncytial virus. All appear to most seriously affect malnourished children and populations not usually exposed to these agents. Severe symptomatic illnesses are usually confined to infants and children, and recovery is the rule. Symptoms include cough, a feeling of tightness in the chest, and, in extreme cases, shortness of breath and even cyanosis. **Adenovirus infection** produces the most serious sequelae, including extensive inflammation of bronchioles and subsequent healing by fibrosis that obliterates bronchioles or occludes them with loose fibrous tissue. Subsequent collapse of the lung (atelectasis) leads to permanent dilation of the bronchi (bronchiectasis).

Respiratory syncytial virus infection is curious in that it tends to occur in epidemics in nurseries and elsewhere. It is usually a self-limited illness, but rare fatal cases are characterized by peribronchiolar inflammation and disorganization of the histologic appearance of the epithelium. Severe overdistension of the lung parenchyma may be found without obvious bronchiolar obstruction, possibly because of displacement of surfactant from the bronchiolar surface. At one time, **measles** was a major cause of bronchiolitis, but, with the advent of measles vaccine, this is no longer true in developed countries. However, measles-induced bronchiolitis still remains a serious problem elsewhere, particularly in populations seldom exposed to measles. Like adenovirus, it may result in bronchiolar obliteration and bronchiectasis.

Whooping cough, caused by *Haemophilus pertussis,* was a common bacterial infection of the airways. Although rare in the United States, it is becoming increasingly common in Britain, where vaccination is no longer compulsory. Clinically it is typified by fever and severe prolonged bouts of coughing, followed by characteristic deep "whooping" inspiration. Severe bronchial and bronchiolar inflammation have been found in fatal cases. Whooping cough has been implicated as a significant cause of bronchiectasis in the past, but this no longer appears to be the case.

H. influenzae and *Streptococcus pneumoniae* have been implicated in exacerbations of chronic bronchitis (described later). Although these episodes are a nuisance to patients with bronchitis and do not respond particularly well to antibiotic therapy, they have no serious sequelae.

Fungi may also involve bronchi, with aspergillus species being the most common offenders. Aspergilli and other fungi may grow in preexisting cavities, such as those caused by tuberculosis or bronchiectasis. They proliferate to form masses (**"fungus balls"** or **mycetomas**) within the cavities. Radiologic examination shows that a large mass is present within a cavity and is separated from the wall by air. As the patient changes position the ball falls to the most dependent position. In most instances the fungus ball is asymptomatic and represents merely an interesting radiologic finding. However, sometimes it becomes symptomatic, the most important symptom being hemoptysis, due either to the underlying condition or, less commonly, to fungal infection of the cavity wall. Another presentation is **allergic bronchopulmonary aspergillosis.** In this condition patients have severe asthma and cough up thick mucus plugs. Eosinophilic pneumonia (see the following discussion) is a well-documented complication, and eosinophilia of the blood is common. Radiologically, thickened bronchial walls and mucus plugs in the bronchi are visualized. Morphologically, bronchiectasis (dilatation of bronchi) involves segmental bronchi and the next two to four orders of subsegmental bronchi, although the peripheral airways remain normal. The pathogenesis of allergic bronchopulmonary aspergillosis, which is closely related to bronchocentric granulomatosis (discussed later), is poorly understood, but it is presumably related to an immunologic mechanism in response to an aspergillus antigen. Surface invasion of the bronchi may occur, but usually only in an immunocompromised patient. **Candidiasis** (also known as **moniliasis**) is probably the most common fungal lesion of the bronchial epithelium. *Candida albicans* is a normal commensal in the oral cavity, gut, and vagina and is best known for its infection of those regions, often in the immunocompromised host. It may also affect the lungs, usually as a noninvasive growth only on the surface epithelium of the airways, where it may produce surface ulceration.

Irritant Gases

Of the irritant gases in the atmosphere the important ones are oxidants (ozone, oxides of nitrogen) and sulfur dioxide. Oxidants are particularly related to the action of sunlight on automobile exhaust fumes and are notably of importance in major urban areas that experience temperature inversions. Sulfur dioxide is mainly derived from the burning of fossil fuels. Although the precise effects of these agents in low concentration is not certain, and although they clearly have a high nuisance value, it seems likely that they are not a major cause of serious respiratory disease. They may compound the adverse effects of tobacco smoke and emissions created within the home. There is also little doubt that persons living in urban and more polluted areas have worse pulmonary function, as expressed by expiratory flow rates, than those who reside in cleaner environments. Respiratory infections are also more common in young children in regions of high pollution. However, the decrement in function and increase in symptoms is small in the healthy population. In persons with respiratory disease the story is different. Of particular relevance is the experimental observation that ozone makes the airways more reactive, an effect caused by airway inflammation. Thus, air pollution may exacerbate the symptoms of asthmatic individuals and those with established respiratory disease. However, there is no evidence of an increased frequency of lesions in the respiratory tract in persons exposed to high levels of environmental pollution.

In high concentrations irritant gases produce serious morphologic and functional effects. **Nitrogen dioxide** exposure is associated with severe bronchiolar inflammation and occurs classically in two situations. In **silo-filler's disease**, nitrogen dioxide is generated in decomposing silage and inhaled by the person who enters the silo. Severe respiratory distress, and even death, is caused by pulmonary edema secondary to the damage of the alveolar epithelium. Lower levels of NO_2 lead principally to inflammation of the peripheral airways, a process followed by exudation into the airways, with organization of the exudate and bronchiolitis obliterans (filling of the bronchioles with loose fibrous tissue). Surprisingly, this lesion resolves and long-term effects have not been documented. The other source of high levels of NO_2 is the burning of nitrocellulose, the classic example being x-ray film. The other major oxidant, **ozone,** also involves the periphery of the acinus, and exposure to high concentrations may result in pulmonary edema. **Sulfur dioxide,** a highly soluble gas, when inhaled chronically by experimental animals, produces lesions in the more central airways that resemble chronic bronchitis and that may progress to squamous metaplasia. In man, exposure to very high concentrations of SO_2 has been associated with severe inflammation and bronchiolitis.

Unlike sulfur dioxide and oxidants, **chlorine** and **ammonia** are not significant environmental pollutants, but they are released in high concentrations in industrial accidents, where they may produce widespread epithelial damage and death from pulmonary edema. The effects of lower levels of chlorine exposure are not well documented. Ammonia produces extensive bronchial and bronchiolar inflammation, eventually culminating in extensive bronchiectasis, in part from bronchiolar obliteration and in part from direct damage to the bronchi.

Bronchial Obstruction and Aspiration

As previously indicated, aspiration of solid material into the trachea may be rapidly fatal. Aspiration into the bronchial tree is much more common and normally occurs during sleep, when nasopharyngeal secretions are aspirated. Since bronchial obstruction may be a sequel to aspiration, it is appropriate to consider the other effects of bronchial obstruction at this point.

Atelectasis

Atelectasis refers to the collapse of expanded lung tissue. If the supply of air is obstructed, the transfer of gas from the alveoli to the blood leads to a loss of

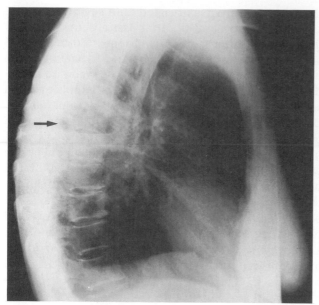

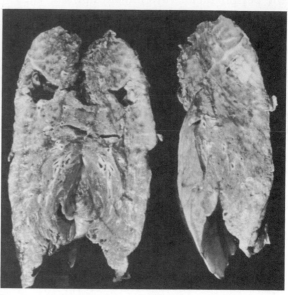

A   B

Figure 12-5.   Lung abscess. A 41-year-old alcoholic woman vomited in bed while stuporous. She developed fever and coughed up copious amounts of sputum. (*A*) A lateral chest radiograph shows an abscess in the superior segment of the right lower lobe (*arrow*). A fluid level is apparent. (*B*) The lower lobe was resected and cut into sagittal slices. The walls of the abscess are thin.

alveolar air and collapse of the involved region. Atelectasis is an important postoperative complication of abdominal surgery, occurring because of mucous obstruction of a bronchus and diminished respiratory movement resulting from postoperative pain. It is often asymptomatic, but when severe it results in hypoxemia. Another important cause of atelectasis, particularly significant in young children, is aspiration of foreign bodies.

Atelectasis may also result from occlusion of a bronchus by a tumor or, less commonly, by lymph nodes containing metastatic cancer. The classic site for the latter is the right middle lobe, because it is long and slender and surrounded by lymph nodes. The term **right middle lobe syndrome** is applied to this condition. At one time the most common cause of this syndrome was tuberculous lymphadenitis, but now lung cancer is the most common cause. In long-standing atelectasis the collapsed lung becomes fibrotic and the bronchi dilate, in part because of infection distal to the bronchus. Permanent bronchial dilatation (i.e., bronchiectasis) results.

Although atelectasis is usually caused by bronchial obstruction, it may also result from direct compression of the lung (e.g., hydrothorax or pneumothorax). Such compression, if severe enough, seriously compromises the function of the affected lung.

Diffuse Alveolar Damage

Aspiration of gastric acid and of water in near drowning results in diffuse alveolar damage and is an important cause of the adult respiratory distress syndrome (discussed in detail later).

Lung Abscess

Lung abscess due to aspiration is most often found in alcoholics, especially those who suffer from poor dental hygiene. The right side of the lung is more frequently affected than the left, because the right main bronchus follows the direction of the trachea more closely at its bifurcation. The site of the abscess is determined by the position the subject was in when the aspiration occurred. If the subject was supine, the superior segment of the right lower lobe (Fig. 12-5) is most likely to be involved, since this is the most direct route of aspiration. If the subject was in the lateral position, the "pectoral" segment (the anterior part of the posterior segment and the posterior part of the anterior segment) of the upper lobe is most often involved, and either the right or the left lung can be affected. The organisms involved are classically anaerobes from the oropharynx, and their effect is compounded by aspiration of vomitus. Acute pneumonia with necrosis of lung tissue ensues. Because of the indolent nature of the process, a fibrous wall forms around the margin. Lung abscesses differ from those elsewhere in their capacity for spontaneous drainage. The cavity thus contains air, necrotic debris, and inflammatory exudate, forming a fluid level, easily visualized radiographically (Fig. 12-5). The lining of the cavity becomes covered with regenerating squamous epithelium. One of the most characteristic symptoms is the production of large amounts of foul-smelling sputum. The differential diagnosis of lung abscess includes lung cancer and cavitary tuberculosis. Cancer is now a more common cause of cavitation than lung abscess. About half of all cases of cavitation due to cancer reflect necrosis of the tumor; the other half follow obstruction of the bronchi and subsequent infection. The walls of a cavitated cancer are characteristically thicker and more irregular in shape than those of a lung abscess (Fig. 12-6); when cavitation is secondary to obstruction, the primary tumor is usually readily visible. A tuberculous cavity is usually associated with considerable fibrosis of the surrounding lung, is nearly always in the upper lobe, and is often bilateral.

Aspiration of Mineral Oil

A now uncommon lung lesion is the paraffinoma, or exogenous lipid pneumonia. Mineral oil was used as the carrier for medications in nose drops, and aspiration of this material produced lung damage. The aspiration of mineral oil is now seen mainly in mental institutions or chronic care facilities, in which mineral oil is used as a laxative. In the lung mineral oil elicits fibrosis, a process that leads to a gray, poorly demarcated greasy lesion. Microscopic examination shows that large oil droplets are surrounded by a foreign body granulomatous response. Some of the droplets may be the size of an alveolus and may be regarded as such by the unwary microscopist.

Endogenous ("Golden") Lipid Pneumonia

Lipid pneumonia may be a sequel to bronchial obstruction. It is seen as a localized condition distal to an obstructed large airway, or it may be widespread when it is secondary to extensive bronchiolar obliteration, such as that found in extrinsic allergic alveolitis. The pneumonia has a characteristic golden yellow color, which reflects the accumulation of fine lipid droplets within alveolar macrophages. The disorder is generally accompanied by mild chronic inflammation and fibrosis. It has been suggested that obstruction induces exudation of plasma into the airspaces; although the protein component can be readily resorbed, the same is not true for the lipid, which then becomes phagocytosed by macrophages.

Neoplasia

Primary Cancer of the Lung

Primary cancer of the lung is the most common cause of death from cancer; more than 100,000 people die each year in the United States from this disease. Regarded as a rare tumor as late as 1945, it now occurs in epidemic proportions. In men the incidence has reached a plateau or may even be decreasing. By contrast, the incidence of lung cancer in women, which lagged behind that in men, has risen alarmingly in the last two decades. The ratio of male to female cases has changed from 10 to 1 to 4 to 1 and is approaching 3 to 1. In fact, the mortality due to lung cancer in women now exceeds that due to breast cancer. The reason for the enormous increase in lung cancer is tobacco smoking in general, and cigarette smoking in particular. Cigarette smoking became particularly common in Great Britain during World War I, and the increase in lung cancer became apparent

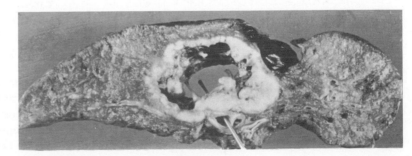

Figure 12-6. Cavitated squamous cell carcinoma. A 55-year-old heavy smoker presented with hemoptysis. In the resected specimen the probe passes from a lobar bronchus into a cavity. Note the thick wall.

in that country in the 1930s and 1940s. In the United States, cigarette smoking became common in men during World War II, and hence the rise in the frequency of lung cancer occurred somewhat later in the United States. Similarly, the present epidemic of lung cancer in women reflects the later acceptance of smoking in the female population. There are some occupational causes of lung cancer, notably uranium mining in North America. Asbestos workers who smoke cigarettes exhibit a much higher incidence of lung cancer than similar workers who do not smoke. It is worth emphasizing that the number of people exposed to other agents that cause lung cancer is small compared with the cigarette smoking population. Lung cancer is, therefore, the most preventable of cancers, a concept that should be stressed, in view of the dismal prognosis for this disease. The five-year survival rate for lung cancer is about 6% and has remained essentially unchanged over the last 30 years.

Problems in Classification

The term bronchogenic carcinoma is often used for primary lung cancer but is perhaps too specific a term, implying an origin from the bronchi. A substantial proportion, perhaps one quarter, of primary lung cancers do not have an obvious bronchial origin. Primary carcinoma of the lung is classified according to the appearance by light microscopy, although it is now apparent that many tumors have a mixed appearance when examined by electron microscopy. Although these observations have important histogenetic implications, their clinical significance is uncertain. The mixed nature of lung cancers is also apparent by light microscopy, and up to 25% have a mixed appearance. The frequency of the different types also depends on the source of study. For example, squamous cell carcinomas are common in surgical specimens, but small cell carcinomas are rare. Since squamous cell cancers are often operable but small cell cancers are not usually treated by surgery, it is not surprising to find a variation in the reported incidence of squamous cell carcinoma of 6% to 60%.

Features Common to Most Forms of Primary Lung Cancer

Lung cancer is more common in men than in women (4:1), except for bronchoalveolar carinomas, carcinoids, and adenoid cystic carcinomas, in which there are no sex differences. Cancers occur more often on the right side than on the left, (52.5% versus 47.5%), reflecting the larger volume of the right lung and are commoner in the upper lobe than in the lower. Metastases occur to the regional intrapulmonary lymph nodes and then to the mediastinal nodes. There are certain sites of predilection for metastasis, notably the adrenals (an unexplained phenomenon), brain, liver, and bone. Clubbing of the fingers may be a presenting feature. A variety of metabolic effects also occurs as a result of secretions from the tumor (described later).

Types of Primary Lung Cancer

Squamous Cell Carcinoma (Epidermoid Carcinoma)

By light microscopy the diagnosis of squamous cell carcinoma requires the presence of intercellular bridges and keratin formation. Keratin occurs either as pearls (a central, brightly eosinophilic aggregate of keratin surrounded by onion-skin layers of squamous cells) or as individual cell keratinization (the cytoplasm of the cell assumes a glassy, intensely eosinophilic appearance). Ultrastructurally, intercellular bridges are seen as intercellular junctions of the classic desmosome type. The ultrastructural counterpart of keratin is tonofilaments. The term "squamous cell carcinoma" (squama = "scale" or "platelike structure") has been adopted by the World Health Organization and is more commonly used than the alternate term, "epidermoid carcinoma" (epidermoid = "resembling epidermis"), since the latter term evokes a fully differentiated structure of several cell types, which is obviously not the case for malignant tumors. **Squamous cell carcinomas, characteristically tumors of the major bronchi, are slow-growing** (Fig. 12-7). They present with symptoms related to their bronchial origin: persistent cough, hemoptysis, or bronchial obstruction, the last accompanied by pulmonary infections (recurrent pneumonias, lung abscesses) or atelectasis. Lymph node metastases are often sufficiently limited to allow surgical resection of the tumor. Tumor cells may be readily found in the sputum and the diagnosis may be made by exfoliative cytology, even when the tumor is not radiologically apparent or invasive (carcinoma in situ). Squamous cell carcinoma is the most common type of lung cancer to undergo central cavitation, and thus, on occasion, must be differentiated from an abscess or tuberculosis (see Fig. 12-6).

The histogenesis of squamous cell carcinoma is of interest because respiratory epithelium normally displays no squamous differentiation. Following injury to the epithelium, such as occurs with cigarette smoking, regeneration from the pluripotential basal layer in the form of squamous metaplasia commonly oc-

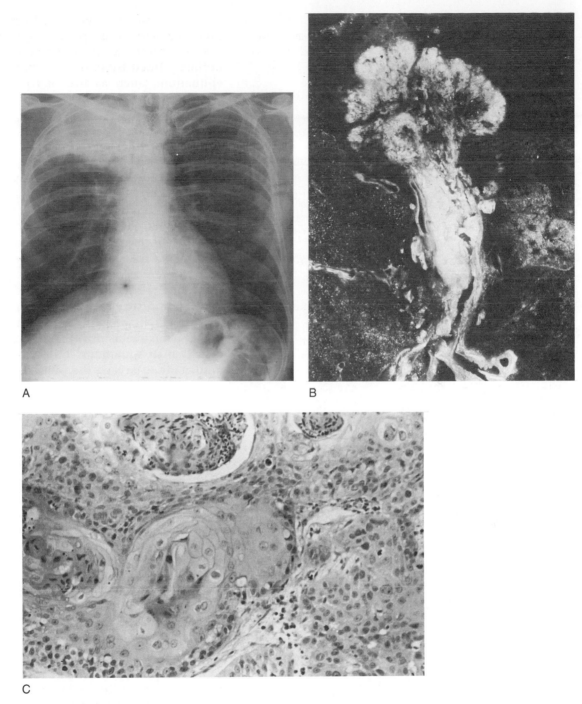

Figure 12-7. Squamous cell carcinoma of the lung. A 62-year-old man had repeated chest infections over a 6-month period. (*A*) A chest radiograph shows a right upper lobe lesion and atelectasis. (*B*) In the resected specimen a large endobronchial tumor is apparent in the right upper lobe bronchus and its segments. This lesion caused the atelectasis. The tumor also invades the lung parenchyma. (*C*) Microscopically, the tumor is a well-differentiated squamous carcinoma.

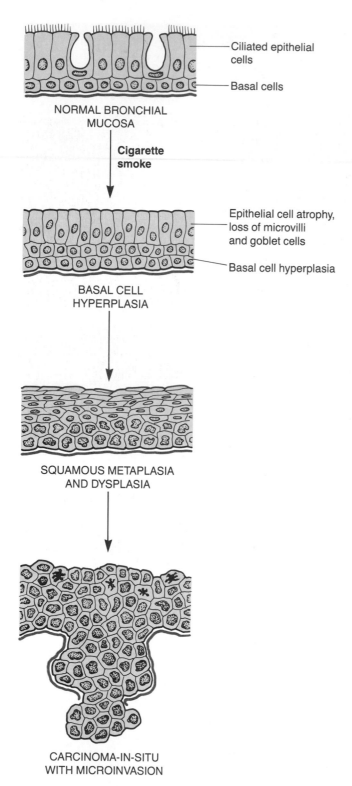

NORMAL BRONCHIAL
MUCOSA

—— Ciliated epithelial
cells

—— Basal cells

**Cigarette
smoke**

BASAL CELL
HYPERPLASIA

—— Epithelial cell atrophy,
loss of microvilli
and goblet cells

—— Basal cell hyperplasia

SQUAMOUS METAPLASIA
AND DYSPLASIA

CARCINOMA-IN-SITU
WITH MICROINVASION

Figure 12-8.   The development of squamous cell carcinoma. First, minor changes occur in the bronchial epithelium (basal cell hyperplasia), followed by squamous cell metaplasia with dysplasia. Then carcinoma in situ ensues, first localized to the epithelium and then extending to bronchial glands and penetrating the basement membrane. Extensive invasion and metastases follow.

curs. **This squamous metaplastic mucosa follows the same sequence of dysplasia, carcinoma in situ, and invasive tumor as that observed in sites that are normally lined by normal or metaplastic squamous epithelium, such as the cervix, oral cavity, vocal cords, esophagus, and skin** (Fig. 12-8).

Adenocarcinoma

Adenocarcinomas of the lung, characterized by a glandular appearance and the secretion of mucus, are commonly peripheral (i.e., beyond an obvious bronchial origin), but a substantial proportion have a bronchial origin (Fig. 12-9). The relative increase in frequency of adenocarcinoma over the last 20 years in part reflects changes in diagnostic criteria. Many tumors that would previously have been called large cell undifferentiated carcinomas are now diagnosed as adenocarcinoma on the basis of a positive mucin stain or ultrastructural examination, in spite of the absence of obvious glandular differentiation. **Adenocarcinomas metastasize readily, tend to grow more rapidly than squamous cell carcinomas, and have a propensity to invade the pleura.**

Large Cell Undifferentiated Carcinoma

Large cell undifferentiated carcinomas are so poorly differentiated that they elude classification as squamous or adenocarcinoma. Many tumors classified as large cell carcinoma by light microscopy show ultrastructural evidence of squamous or glandular differentiation and should be reclassified. Thus, the frequency of this diagnosis depends on the availability of special diagnostic techniques. The behavior of this category of tumors is similar to that of poorly differentiated adenocarcinoma.

Small Cell Carcinoma

Small cell carcinomas, a highly malignant form of lung cancer, are characterized by sheets of small tumor cells (Fig. 12-10C) and include both classic oat cell carcinoma and the intermediate cell variant. In both subtypes, there is minimal architectural differentiation and a great deal of necrosis, often with the deposition of bluish nuclear material in the walls of blood vessels. The nuclei in both subtypes are dense and hyperchromatic. The oat cell subtype has such scant cytoplasm that the tumor cells are only twice the size of lymphocytes, whereas the intermediate cell subtype is characterized by somewhat more cytoplasm. **The clinical behavior of the two subtypes is comparable; both usually metastasize so early (Fig. 12-10A,B) that the lesions are not amenable to surgery.** Chemotherapy is the common treatment, and recent advances have led to a dramatic improvement in prognosis. Small cell carcinomas exhibit neu-

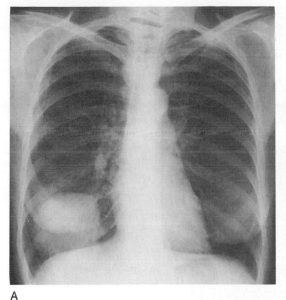

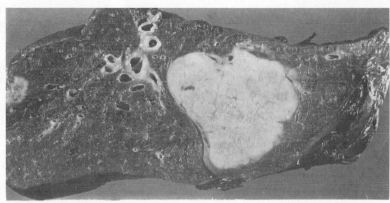

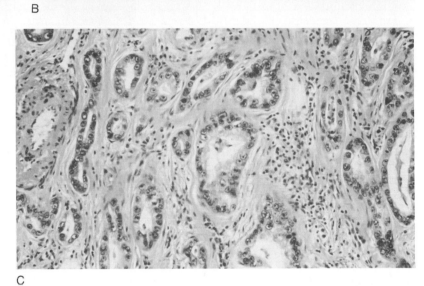

Figure 12-9. Adenocarcinoma of the lung. (*A*) A chest radiograph shows a circumscribed mass in the lower portion of the right middle lobe. (*B*) The resected specimen (transverse section) shows no apparent bronchial origin of the major tumor. A smaller, separate tumor is seen in the lower lobe at the far left. (*C*) The tumor is glandular; special stains demonstrate intracellular and extracellular mucus.

roendocrine differentiation and produce a variety of endocrine peptides. Ultrastructurally, the cells contain scattered dense-core neurosecretory granules, a feature that suggests a relation to Kultchitsky cells.

Bronchioloalveolar Tumors

Bronchioloalveolar tumors are always peripheral in origin and, as the name indicates, derive from bronchiolar or alveolar epithelium. As such, the tumor may originate from mucus-secreting cells, nonciliated (Clara) cells, or type II pneumocytes. Ciliated cells are not encountered. Bronchioloalveolar tumors are well differentiated and characteristically grow along alveolar walls. At their peripheral margins the alveolar architecture is apparent. This form of growth has been described as "lepidic."

Although the distinction between peripheral ad-

enocarcinomas and bronchioloalveolar tumors is hotly debated, the simplest approach is to regard them as the same tumor. If one limits the diagnosis of bronchioloalveolar tumors to those with lepidic growth throughout the tumor mass, it becomes vanishingly rare. More realistically, as the tumor grows, the lepidic growth becomes less apparent in the more central portions of the tumor, and fibrosis becomes more prominent. With further fibrosis a central scar develops, in which the tumor cells become less differentiated and resemble an adenocarcinoma. The important features of bronchioloalveolar carcinoma are as follows:

The prognosis, when limited to a single lesion, is good. In the absence of lymph node metastases, the cure rate is more than 50%.

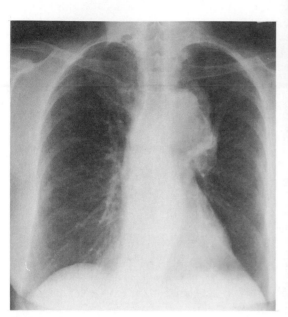

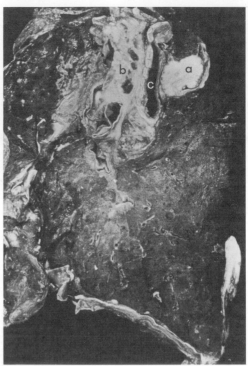

A   B

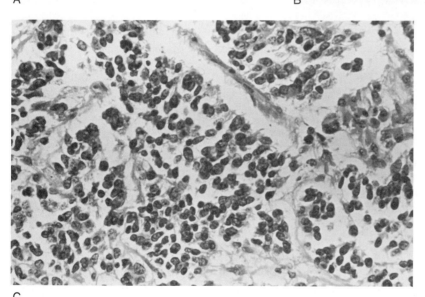

C

Figure 12-10.   Small (oat) cell carcinoma of the lung. A 48-year-old man presented with symptoms of water intoxication, which were caused by inappropriate secretion of antidiuretic hormone. (*A*) A chest radiograph shows a large central mass that represents extensive lymph node metastases. (*B*) An autopsy specimen shows a small lung tumor (*a*). Note the extensive lymph node metastases (*b*) and tumor around the trachea and major bronchi (*c*). The lung is cut in a sagittal plane. (*C*) Microscopically, the tumor consists of small cells with hyperchromatic nuclei and little cytoplasm.

Because of the central scar, the question of origin from a preexisting scar arises (scar cancer), a derivation that is seldom possible to document. Rarely, a previous lesion, such as a granuloma, can be shown, in which case the tumor may be any sort of carcinoma. It is preferable to think of a bronchioloalveolar tumor as not arising from a scar.

It is impossible to distinguish by light microscopy between a bronchioloalveolar tumor and a single metastasis from an adenocarcinoma elsewhere. Statistically, however, solitary metastases almost always occur in the context of a history of a previously excised primary carcinoma, or in a patient with overt symptoms related to the primary cancer.

There is no sex predilection, nor is there a relationship to tobacco smoking.

The usual clinical presentation is as a "coin lesion" (described later).

In addition to the single peripheral bronchoalveolar tumor, a second gross pattern exists, characterized by multiple bilateral nodules or bilateral infiltrates that grossly and radiographically simulate pneumonia. Such patients present with shortness of breath and, occasionally, with the production of large amounts of mucoid sputum (bronchorrhea). The ultimate prognosis is hopeless, although the course may be prolonged and the disease may still be limited to the thorax at the time of death. Metastases from other organs, notably the stomach and pancreas, occasionally present with identical pathologic, clinical, and radiologic features.

Other Carcinomas

Several other categories of lung cancer are recognized in the World Health Organization classification of lung tumors. These are all considerably less common than bronchogenic carcinoma.

Carcinosarcomas

Occasionally cancers of the lung have the appearance of both a carcinoma and a sarcoma in different parts of the tumor, and the two are usually intimately mingled. The sarcoma is usually a fibrosarcoma, but the histologic appearance of a chondrosarcoma or an osteosarcoma may be present. Most commonly, the epithelial component is a squamous carcinoma, although it may be any other form of epithelial malignancy. Whether the sarcomatous component is truly of mesodermal origin or whether these cells are simply abnormal-appearing epithelial cells is an unanswered question. The prognosis of these tumors is similar to that of the epithelial component. A related tumor, the pulmonary **blastoma,** resembles embryonal lung, with a glandular epithelial component consisting of poorly differentiated columnar cells arranged in tubules, without mucus secretion. The intervening tumor is formed by spindle cells that resemble embryonal mesoderm. There is a histologic overlap between blastoma and carcinosarcoma, and the clinical features are similar, although blastomas occur more commonly in younger people, even children.

Carcinoid Tumor

Classically, the carcinoid tumor (Fig. 12-11) was classified as a **bronchial adenoma,** a term implying that it is a benign tumor and glandular in appearance. Both of these assumptions are incorrect. **Classic carcinoids are like small cell carcinomas in being neuroendocrine tumors, but are much better differentiated.** The nuclei have an open chromatin pattern rather than hyperchromasia, the cytoplasm is more abundant, and there is a definite organoid arrangement of cells in ribbons, tubules, and clusters in a richly vascular stroma (Fig. 12-11C). Carcinoids also produce a variety of endocrine peptides and vasoactive amines. Dense-core neurosecretory granules are plentiful, necrosis is absent, and mitotic activity is negligible. The majority of classic carcinoids are central and involve large bronchi; thus, they present with symptoms of obstruction. In contrast to small cell carcinoma, a substantial proportion of carcinoid tumors occur before the age of 40 years, women are affected as commonly as men, and the tumor is not related to smoking. The vast majority of cases are cured by resection. Often the intrabronchial component is small and much of the tumor extends into the lung (iceberg tumor) (see Fig. 12-11). Since nodal metastases are seen in 5% to 10% of resected specimens, the malignancy of the tumor is viewed as low grade; death from classic lung carcinoid is unusual.

Atypical carcinoid tumors resemble classic carcinoid tumors in terms of cell type and general architectural arrangement, but necrosis and mitotic activity are obvious. Nodal metastases are found in approximately half of these tumors, and distant metastases and death, although not nearly so common as in small cell carcinoma, are not rare. Thus, the behavior of the atypical carcinoid tumor is intermediate between that of the classic carcinoid tumor and small cell carcinoma.

Adenoid Cystic Carcinomas and Mucoepidermoid Carcinoma

Adenoid cystic carcinomas and mucoepidermoid carcinomas resemble their namesakes in the salivary glands and are derived from the tracheobronchial mucous glands, structures analogous to the salivary glands. They often present with obstructive symptoms and tend to be locally invasive, although adenoid cystic carcinomas quite often metastasize. Both, especially mucoepidermoid carcinomas, have the distinction of involving the trachea.

Paraneoplastic Syndromes

As neuroendocrine tumors, small cell carcinomas secrete a variety of vasoactive amines and polypeptides that are similar or identical to the normal hormones. These are frequently found in the blood of patients with tumors and may become clinically symptomatic. Inappropriate secretion of antidiuretic hormone is characterized by water intoxication and hyponatremia. Cushing's syndrome is a known complication of the secretion of ACTH or ACTH-like substances.

A

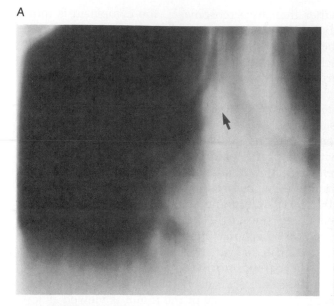

B

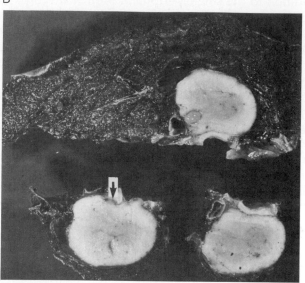

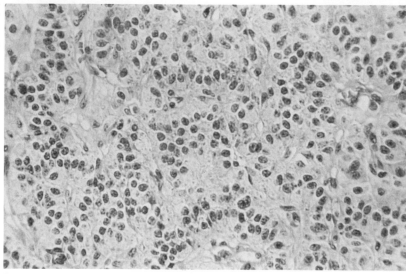

C

Figure 12-11.   Carcinoid tumor of the lung. A 34-year-old nonsmoking woman coughed up blood. (*A*) A tomogram (radiograph of a sagittal slice of lung *in vivo* without computer assistance) illustrates an intrabronchial tumor (*arrow*) in the right mainstem bronchus close to the trachea. (*B*) Gross examination of three slices of the lung illustrates a small intrabronchial tumor (*arrow*) and a more substantial invasive tumor. (*C*) Microscopically, the tumor has an organoid appearance, abundant cytoplasm, and regular nuclei (compare with Figure 12-10C).

Although paraneoplastic Cushing's syndrome may lack some of the overt features of Cushing's syndrome, it always includes hypokalemia and alkalosis. Hypercalcemia is caused by parathormone secretion, but unlike the other paraneoplastic syndromes, it is usually associated with squamous cell carcinoma. Clubbing of the fingers is also associated with lung cancer of all types, but the reason is not known. The carcinoid syndrome is unusual in either classic or atypical pulmonary carcinoid tumors.

Metastatic Tumors

The most common malignant neoplasm of the lung is metastatic tumor. In about a third of all fatal cancers, pulmonary metastases are evident at autopsy.

Metastatic tumors in the lung are typically multiple and circumscribed (Fig. 12-12). Traditionally, metastatic sarcomas are described as the most circumscribed, producing the so-called cannon ball tumors, but this appearance may be found with any metastatic tumor. Single metastases may present a problem in clinical and pathologic diagnosis, particularly when they are adenocarcinomas. Such tumors may resemble primary adenocarcinomas of the lung and may not be distinguishable from them on histologic grounds alone. Uncommonly, metastatic tumors mimic widespread brochoalveolar carcinoma, the usual primary site being the pancreas or stomach. Under these circumstances the primary tumor may be asymptomatic. On rare occasions metastases to the bronchi occur.

An interesting form of metastasis is **lymphangitic**

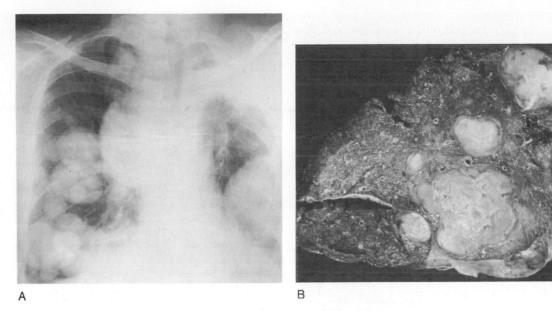

A   B

Figure 12-12. Metastatic tumor in the lung. A 53-year-old man who had a liposarcoma excised from his thigh 2 years previously presented to his physician with shortness of breath. (*A*) A chest radiograph shows multiple discrete masses in both lung fields. (*B*) Gross examination of the lung confirms the discrete nature of the "cannonball" metastases.

carcinoma, a condition in which the tumor is thought to reach the lung via the bloodstream, since it is also found in the small pulmonary arteries. As the name indicates, the cancer spreads widely through the pulmonary lymphatic channels to form a sheath of tumor around the bronchovascular tree and the veins. Clinically, the patients present with shortness of breath and a diffuse reticulonodular pattern on the chest radiograph. The common primary sites are the breast, stomach, pancreas, and colon. The prognosis is hopeless.

Benign Tumors

Benign tumors of the lung are uncommon, and the only one that is found with any frequency is the **hamartoma** (Fig. 12-13). Although the term *hamartoma* implies a malformation, hamartomas are true tumors, occurring most often in middle age and progressively increasing in size. The tumor, which consists of elements usually present in the lung, displays a connective tissue component, with prominent cartilage, some fibrous tissue, and occasionally smooth muscle or fat. These are interspersed with clefts lined by respiratory epithelium. The tumor is well circumscribed and shells out from the surrounding lung parenchyma. It is usually peripheral, but lesions of cartilage, fat, and connective tissue may be found in

the major bronchi and are thought to represent variants of peripheral hamartomas.

The Problem of "Coin" Lesions

A "coin" lesion, defined as a well-circumscribed radiopacity in the periphery of the lung less than 2.5 cm in diameter, is a common clinical problem. Characteristically, the lesion is an incidental finding on a routine chest radiograph (see Fig. 12-13) and poses the clinical problem of a benign or malignant diagnosis. The reported frequency of cancer in coin lesions, as assessed from surgical specimens, ranges from 10% to 70%, a variation that primarily reflects patient selection. In the management of coin lesions, simple clinical observations, such as age and smoking history, are important but not definitive. A past history of tuberculosis, histoplasmosis, or coccidioidomycosis is important, because healed granulomas are the commonest cause of a benign coin lesion. Well-circumscribed and calcified lesions are much less likely to be malignant. If preexisting radiographs are available, they should be studied to assess the rate of growth of the lesion. Lesions that do not grow are unlikely to be malignant, whereas those that show significant growth are more worrisome. When clinical and radiologic features make cancer a serious consideration, sputum cytologic examination and bron-

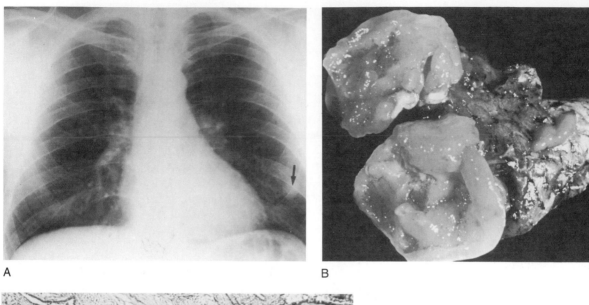

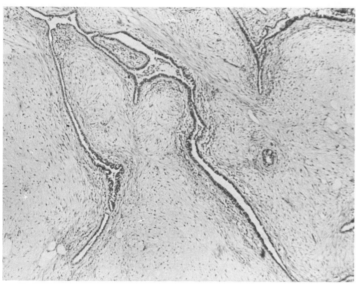

Figure 12-13.   Hamartoma of the lung. (*A*) A routine chest radiograph in a 45-year-old man revealed a small circumscribed parenchymal nodule ("coin lesion") in the left lower lobe (*arrow*). (*B*) Grossly, the cut section shows a well-circumscribed, lobulated lesion. (*C*) Microscopically, the hamartoma consists of cartilage and myxoid and fibrous tissue, separated by spaces lined by respiratory epithelium.

choscopy are valuable. Needle biopsy and aspiration cytology of the nodule have become important modalities and, in some hands, 90% to 95% of malignant nodules can be definitively diagnosed by these techniques.

Lesions Affecting the Lung Parenchyma

Congenital Lesions

The most common congenital lesion of the lung is hypoplasia, a condition that may be accompanied by hypoplasia of the bronchi and pulmonary vessels if the insult occurs early in gestation, as in congenital diaphragmatic hernia. Hypoplastic lungs, characterized by diminished weight, volume, and cell number, are immature for the gestational age. Three major factors have been implicated as causes of pulmonary hypoplasia: (1) Compression of the lung is usually caused by a congenital diaphragmatic hernia. These hernias usually occur on the left side and are due to failure of the pleuroperitoneal canal to close. Varying degrees of herniation of abdominal viscera are present in the affected hemithorax, and the degree of hypoplasia is variable. At one extreme the lung on the affected side is reduced to a small nubbin of tissue, and the lung on the opposite side is severely hypoplastic. At the other extreme, the degree of hypoplasia is so slight that the infant has no symptoms, the abnormalities being noted incidentally on a routine chest radiograph. Other causes of hypoplasia in this category include abnormalities of the chest wall, pleural effusions, and ascites, as in hydrops fetalis. (2) A reduction in the amount of amniotic fluid (oligohydramnios), usually due to genitourinary anomalies, is another important cause of pulmonary hypoplasia. (3) Decreased respiration has been shown experimentally to produce hypoplastic lungs, which may be caused by a lack of repetitive stretching of the lung.

Congenital adenomatoid malformation is a disorder in which lung parenchyma is converted into multiple glandlike spaces lined by bronchiolar epithelium, separated from each other by loose fibrous tissue. The condition is usually unilateral and often unilobar and is often associated with other congenital abnormalities.

Bronchogenic cysts, found in the lung parenchyma and the mediastinum, are lined by respiratory epithelium and delimited by walls which contain muscle and cartilage. Cartilage in the wall distinguishes them from gastroenteric cysts of the mediastinum. They are usually asymptomatic and are found on a routine chest radiograph.

Intralobar sequestration is a congenital abnormality in which a part of the lung is supplied by an abnormal systemic artery that arises from the aorta. All parts of the lung may be involved, but the most common is the left lower lobe. The sequestered portion of the lung is usually accessory—that is, the other segments of the lung are complete. The condition is rarely recognized in the neonatal period and usually presents as recurrent bronchopulmonary infection in childhood. The diagnosis of this disorder, which must be distinguished clinically from bronchiectasis, is made on the basis of a localized area of involvement and is confirmed by the radiographic demonstration that the region is supplied by a systemic artery. The precise diagnosis is important because the systemic artery supplying the intralobular sequestration must be identified. Although it usually arises from the thoracic aorta, it may arise from the abdominal aorta. In the latter circumstance, during surgery the aberrant artery may retract into the abdomen, an event that results in potentially catastrophic abdominal bleeding.

Infections

Viral Infections

Viruses are a common cause of airway lesions, but those that primarily affect the airways may also severely affect the lung parenchyma. The best example

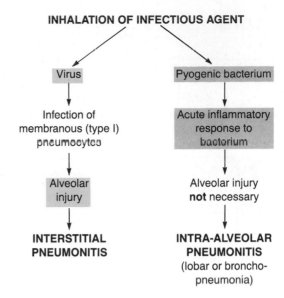

Figure 12-14. Pathogenesis of interstitial and intra-alveolar pneumonitis.

of a disease caused by viruses that affect the airways is influenza; the best example of one caused by viruses that affect both is measles. **It is important to note that viral lung infections produce interstitial (rather than alveolar) pneumonia and diffuse alveolar damage.** Initially, viral infection affects the alveolar epithelium and results in a mononuclear infiltrate in the interstitium of the lung (Figs. 12-14, 12-15). Depending on the severity of the insult, there is necrosis of the type I epithelial cells and formation of hyaline membranes, an appearance that is indistinguishable from diffuse alveolar damage due to other causes. In other instances, the alveolar damage may be indolent and may be characterized by hyperplasia of type II cells and interstitial inflammation. This appearance contrasts with that of most bacterial infections, in which an intra-alveolar exudate predominates and in which the interstitium is only incidentally involved (Figs. 12-14, 12-16).

A characteristic interstitial pneumonia is that produced by the **cytomegalovirus.** Initially described in infants, it is now well recognized in the immunocompromised host (e.g., patients treated with cytotoxic agents or those who suffer from AIDS). In this form of pneumonia there is an intense interstitial exudate of lymphocytes, and the alveoli are lined by type II cells, which have regenerated to cover the epithelial defect left by the necrosis of type I cells. The infected alveolar cells are large (*cytomegalo*) and have a dark-blue inclusion within the nucleus, clumps of basophilic material along the nuclear margin (orbital bodies), and cytoplasmic basophilic inclusions. Their large size makes it easy to recognize them by low-power microscopic examination.

(Text continued on page 566.)

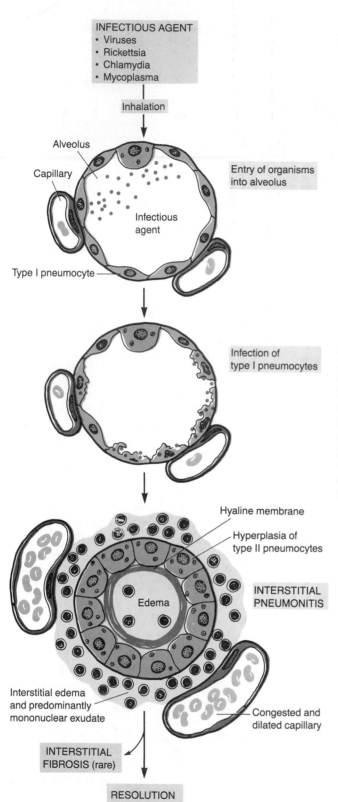

INFECTIOUS AGENT
• Viruses
• Rickettsia
• Chlamydia
• Mycoplasma

Inhalation

Alveolus

Capillary

Entry of organisms into alveolus

Infectious agent

Type I pneumocyte

Infection of type I pneumocytes

Hyaline membrane

Hyperplasia of type II pneumocytes

Edema

INTERSTITIAL PNEUMONITIS

Interstitial edema and predominantly mononuclear exudate

Congested and dilated capillary

INTERSTITIAL FIBROSIS (rare)

RESOLUTION

Figure 12-15. Pathogenesis of interstitial pneumonitis. Although interstitial pneumonia is most commonly caused by viruses, other organisms may also cause significant interstitial inflammation. Type I cells are the most sensitive to damage, and loss of their integrity leads to intra-alveolar edema. The proteinaceous exudate and cell debris form hyaline membranes, and type II cells multiply to line the alveoli. Interstitial inflammation is characterized mainly by mononuclear cells. The disease generally resolves completely but occasionally progresses to interstitial fibrosis.

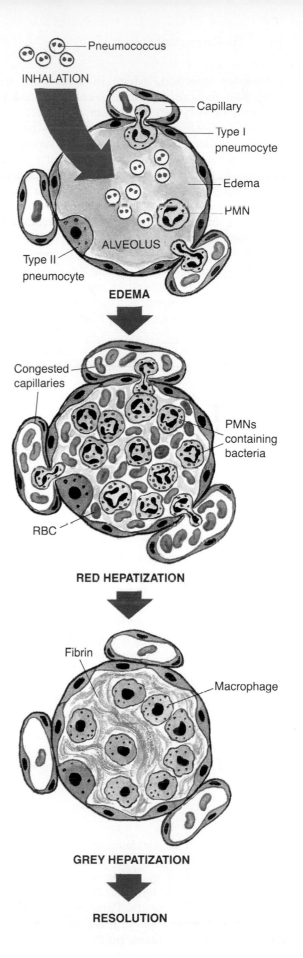

Figure 12-16. Pathogenesis of lobar pneumococcal pneumonia. Pneumococci, characteristically in pairs (diplococci), multiply rapidly in the alveolar spaces and produce extensive edema. They incite an acute inflammatory response, in which polymorphonuclear leucocytes and congestion are prominent (red hepatization). As the inflammatory process progresses, macrophages replace the polymorphonuclear leucocytes and ingest debris (gray hepatization). The process usually resolves, but complications may ensue.

Measles infection, which involves both the airways and the parenchyma, is characterized by the presence of very large (100-μm diameter) multinucleated giant cells that have inclusions in the nucleus. Before it was possible to culture the virus, measles pneumonia was diagnosed as Hecht's giant cell pneumonia and was recognized in children with leukemia. Although interstitial pneumonia is a well-recognized complication of measles, it is rarely fatal, except in immunocompromised, previously unexposed people.

Varicella (both chicken pox and herpes zoster) infection produces disseminated, focally necrotic lesions in the lung, as well as interstitial pneumonia. Pulmonary involvement is usually asymptomatic, except in immunocompromised hosts, in whom it may be fatal. A curious, but rare, sequela in normal people is the occurrence of multiple punctate calcified opacification throughout both lung fields.

Chlamydia

Ornithosis

Ornithosis, an infection with *Chlamydia psittaci*, results from inhaling dust contaminated with excreta from birds, usually pets and often parrots (in which case it is known as psittacosis). Ornithosis is characterized by severe systemic symptoms, with fever, malaise, and muscle aches, but surprisingly few respiratory symptoms, other than cough. Chest radiographs may be negative, and when abnormal show irregular consolidation and an interstitial pattern. The morphologic patterns in most cases are unknown, but the disease is likely to be an interstitial pneumonia. In fatal cases varying degrees of diffuse alveolar damage are present, together with edema, intra-alveolar pneumonia, and necrosis.

Chlamydia Trachomatis

Primarily thought of as a genitourinary pathogen in adults, *Chlamydia trachomatis* causes pneumonia in the neonatal period and is contracted during birth. It leads to both an interstitial and an intra-alveolar pneumonia and may also cause pneumonia in adult immunocompromised patients.

Coxiella Burnetii

Infection with *Coxiella burnetii* was originally described as Q (query) fever. Its usual host is farm animals and thus it is a disease of farm workers or meat packers, but it has also been described in immunocompromised hosts. Patients present with severe systemic symptoms of fever, myalgia and headaches, and, in a few cases, pulmonary complications.

The radiologic features are those of an interstitial and patchy intra-alveolar pneumonia.

Mycoplasma

An important clinical concept is the syndrome of **atypical pneumonia.** In contrast to lobar pneumonia, the onset is insidious, leukocytosis is absent or slight, and the course is prolonged. Respiratory symptoms may be minimal and the chest radiograph shows a patchy intra-alveolar pneumonia or interstitial infiltrate. The common cause of the syndrome is *Mycoplasma pneumoniae*, but other agents include viruses, chlamydia, coxiella, and legionella. It is rarely fatal and is often thought of as a classic example of interstitial pneumonia. The cases that have been examined at autopsy have shown a bronchiolar component, with microatelectasis beyond the bronchiolitis, and interstitial and patchy alveolar pneumonia.

Bacterial Infections

The traditional pathologic classification of **lobar pneumonia** and **bronchopneumonia** has little clinical relevance. Pulmonary bacterial infection should be classified etiologically, but in reality, this is usually impossible. Pneumococcal pneumonia, the classic example of lobar pneumonia, is characterized by a massive purulent exudate in the alveolar spaces (Figs. 12-16, 12-17). It is called lobar because a single lobe may be involved, and that involvement may be complete. More often the involvement is incomplete and more than one lobe is involved. Bronchopneumonia is a favorite term of pathologists because it is so often found at autopsy. It occurs in terminally ill patients and is usually found in the dependent (usually posterior) portions of the lung (Fig. 12-18). Scattered irregular foci of pneumonia are centered on bronchioles and respiratory bronchioles. Bronchiolitis and respiratory bronchiolitis are present, with exudation of polymorphonuclear leukocytes into the adjacent alveoli. Large continuous areas of alveolar involvement do not occur. No single bacterial organism is responsible, and several may be present, often ones not regarded as important pathogens.

Bronchopneumonia has been referred to as the "old man's friend" because it was regarded as the terminal event that spared prolonged suffering. In modern medicine this is not necessarily the case, since successful medical intervention may be the rule rather than the exception. Bronchopneumonia is now almost randomly confused with pulmonary embolism in the terminally ill on the basis of chest radiographs, nuclear scanning, and clinical findings and may be treated inappropriately.

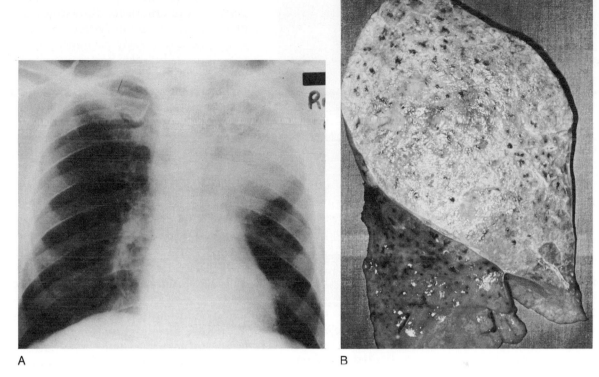

A   B

Figure 12-17. Pneumococcal pneumonia. A 54-year-old alcoholic had a "flulike" illness and several days later developed high fever and chest pain. (*A*) A chest radiograph shows extensive consolidation and alveolar filling of the left upper lobe shortly after the beginning of the illness. (*B*) Some days later gross examination of the lungs at autopsy shows almost complete consolidation of the upper lobe in the phase of gray hepatization.

It is important to classify bacterial pneumonias on the basis of the etiologic agent, because clinical and morphologic features, and therapeutic implications, often vary with the causative organism.

Pneumococcal Pneumonia

Now of diminishing significance because of prompt response to treatment, pneumococcal pneumonia is still a significant illness in industrialized nations; in the nonindustrialized world it is still a major cause of mortality. It is commonly a disease of healthy young to middle-aged adults, is rare in infants and the elderly, and is considerably more common in men than in women. Alcoholics appear to be particularly vulnerable. Pneumococcal pneumonia typically follows a viral infection, often influenza. The onset is acute, with fever and chills. Chest pain due to pleural involvement is common, as is hemoptysis, which is characteristically "rusty," since it is derived from altered blood in alveolar spaces.

Radiologic examination shows alveolar filling in large areas of lung, producing a solid appearance that extends to entire lobes or segments (Figs. 12-16, 12-17). Although the symptoms of pneumonia respond rapidly to antibiotic therapy, radiologically the lesion still takes several days to resolve. Before antibiotic therapy the clinical course was characterized by severe fever, dyspnea, debility, and even loss of consciousness. The dramatic event was the "crisis," when the patient, who appeared moribund, would suddenly become afebrile and return from death's door. The satisfactory resolution of the crisis was the result of a good immune response to the infection. However, all too often the outcome was not favorable and the patient died.

In the earliest stage of pneumococcal pneumonia, protein-rich edema fluid containing numerous organisms (*Streptococcus pneumoniae*) fills the alveoli. Marked congestion of the capillaries is typical. Shortly after this congestion occurs there is a massive outpouring of polymorphonuclear leukocytes accompanied by intra-alveolar hemorrhage. Many of the red blood cells undergo lysis. These cells, together with polymorphonuclear leukocytes, produce the rusty sputum. Because the firm consistency of the affected lung is reminiscent of the liver, this stage

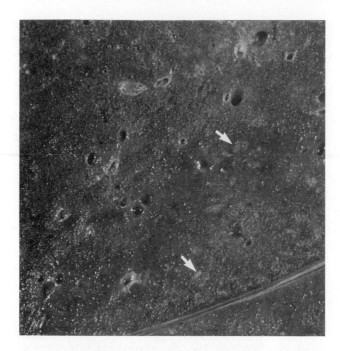

Figure 12-18. Bronchopneumonia. A 67-year-old man had a cerebral tumor (glioblastoma multiforme) and entered the hospital for terminal care. Scattered focal pneumonia is seen adjacent to distal bronchioles (*arrows*).

has been aptly named "red hepatization" (Fig. 12-16).

The next phase, occurring after 2 or more days, depending on the success of treatment, involves the lysis of polymorphonuclear leukocytes and the appearance of macrophages, which phagocytose the fragmented polymorphonuclear leukocytes and other inflammatory debris. The lung is now no longer congested but still remains firm in this stage of "gray hepatization" (Figs. 12-16, 12-17). The alveolar exudate is then removed and the lung gradually returns to normal.

A number of complications may ensue. A painful pleuritis is common because the pneumonia often extends to the pleura. There is usually a small pleural effusion, which resolves. However, this may occasionally be large and purulent (**pyothorax**) and may heal with extensive fibrosis. Rarely, the purulent exudate persists and leads to a loculated collection of pus with fibrous walls (**empyema**). Bacteremia is usually present in the early stages and may result in endocarditis or meningitis. Rarely, the alveolar lesion proceeds to fibrosis, in which case the intra-alveolar exudate becomes organized as fibroblasts proliferate. Gradually, increasing alveolar fibrosis leads to a shrunken and firm lobe, a rare complication known as "carnification." Another uncommon outcome is a lung abscess.

Surprisingly little is known about the precise pathogenesis of pneumococcal pneumonia. The frequency of a previous respiratory tract infection suggests that impairment of airway clearance mechanisms may be important. It has also been suggested that the organisms can multiply rapidly in the increased airway mucus and may then be aspirated into the periphery. The remarkably severe acute inflammation with spreading edema has led to speculation that immunologic mechanisms may be involved.

Klebsiella Pneumonia

The only other organism that causes lobar pneumonia with any degree of frequency is *Klebsiella pneumoniae.* The disease is commonly associated with alcoholism and is seen most frequently in middle-aged men. The onset is less dramatic than that of pneumococcal pneumonia, but the prognosis is considerably worse, because of the patient's underlying condition and because antibiotic therapy is less effective. Radiologic examination shows the evolution of the lesion to be less rapid than that of pneumococcal pneumonia, both in its development and in its regression. A characteristic feature of Klebsiella pneumonia is an increase in size of the affected lobe, so that the fissure "bulges" toward the unaffected region.

The stages in Klebsiella pneumonia are not as well described as those in pneumococcal pneumonia, but the congestion and hemorrhage in the acute phase is less pronounced. There is a greater tendency toward necrosis of tissue and abscess formation. A serious complication is **bronchopleural fistula,** which is a communication between the bronchial air and the pleural space. *K. pneumoniae* has a thick, gelatinous capsule, a feature that is responsible for the characteristic slimy appearance of the cut surface of the lung.

Staphylococcal Pneumonia

Pulmonary infection with *Staphylococcus aureus* commonly occurs as a superinfection following influenzal infections. In the 1957 influenza pandemic it was a major cause of death. Like staphylococcal infection elsewhere, it is characterized by the development of abscesses. In contrast to the classic lung abscess, which is single, the multiple foci of staphylococcal pneumonia produce many small abscesses. In infants, and to a lesser extent in adults, these may lead to **pneumatoceles,** thin-walled cystic spaces lined primarily by respiratory tissue. Pneumatoceles may expand rapidly and compress the surrounding lung, or they may rupture into the pleural cavity, thereby causing a tension pneumothorax. It is thought that a small abscess forms near a bronchus or bronchiole and that the airway forms a flap valve into the abscess, which then has a tendency to expand.

Streptococcal Pneumonia

Streptococcal pneumonia is thought to have been the common superinfection in the 1918–1919 influenza pandemic. It is uncommon and was rare in the 1957 pandemic. It usually occurs in the debilitated and is characterized by a diffuse hemorrhagic pneumonia. Caused by beta-hemolytic streptococci of Lansfield group B, this pneumonia is characteristic of newborn infants, who are infected in the birth canal. The clinical symptoms are similar to those of the infantile respiratory distress syndrome. However, the infants are often full term, have severe toxemia, and die within a few hours. As with the infantile respiratory distress syndrome, the lungs are firm, congested, and airless. In infants who die shortly after birth, hyaline membranes are seen without conspicuous inflammatory reaction. Where death occurs after about 12 hours of life there is a more characteristic appearance of pneumonia.

Gram-Negative Pneumonia

The two common causes of gram-negative pneumonia are *Escherichia coli* and *Pseudomonas aeruginosa*. *E. coli* pneumonia is a recognized complication of gastrointestinal surgery and may be seen in the immunocompromised patient. It presents as a bronchopneumonia and responds poorly to treatment. Pseudomonas pneumonia is most often seen in the immunocompromised person, in patients with burns, and in those with cystic fibrosis. In the first two, the infection reaches the lung by the bloodstream. Often an infectious vasculitis, in which large numbers of organisms can be seen, results in infarction. Pseudomonas infection is common in cystic fibrosis, probably because of the favorable environment provided by the abnormal bronchial secretions. In cystic fibrosis the infection is airborne and usually produces bronchiolitis, with subsequent bronchial obliteration and bronchiectasis. Infection often extends to the lung parenchyma, where it produces a bronchopneumonia that is often fatal. Antibiotic treatment of pseudomonas infections is often unsatisfactory.

Anaerobic Organisms

Many anaerobic organisms are normal commensals of the oral cavity, especially in patients with poor dental hygiene. In stuporous alcoholics, massive aspiration of these organisms leads to necrotizing pneumonia, which may be complicated by a lung abscess. The most dramatic complication is gangrene of the lung, a result of thrombosis of a branch of the pulmonary artery and consequent infarction. The resultant lesion is a large mass of necrotic lung tissue. This is regarded as a medical emergency and requires resection of the affected lung.

Mixed Floral Pneumonias and Pneumonias of Unknown Origin

In a substantial proportion of pneumonias, the majority in some reports, a precise microbiologic diagnosis is not made, and the patients are treated empirically. Many of these correspond to a clinical diagnosis of "bronchopneumonia," as described earlier, and may be caused by any of several organisms, often more than one. An important distinction is that between a "community-acquired" and a "hospital-acquired" pneumonia. The first is usually of sudden onset, often accurately diagnosed, and responsive to treatment. The nosocomial infections (those acquired in the hospital) are complications of treatment, difficult to diagnose (as indicated, often confused with pulmonary embolism), and poorly responsive to therapy.

Legionella Infections

In 1976 a mysterious respiratory ailment broke out at an American Legion convention in Philadelphia. This dramatic event, which was responsible for a large number of deaths, was not initially recognized as being caused by an infectious agent. Speculation about its cause centered on toxic environmental agents and even poisoning with paraquat. The agent, whose exact taxonomy is not completely agreed on, was soon identified as a fastidious organism, with special cultural characteristics. It then became apparent from serologic studies and from histologic studies of the lung that several previous epidemics had occurred but that the causative agent had not been recognized. Moreover, outbreaks of pulmonary infection had been recorded in which the symptoms were different and in which related organisms were involved. The organisms responsible have been dubbed *Legionella pneumophila;* six subtypes are now recognized. Characteristically, outbreaks occur in institutions such as hotels, hospitals, and nursing homes and are due to contamination of air conditioning or heating systems in which the organisms multiply in stagnant water. In the case of the Legionnaires' outbreak, the cases occurred in apparently healthy subjects, but in retrospect many of them were found to have had underlying disease. Hospital-acquired infections, by definition, involve subjects with serious disease, particularly immunocompromised patients. No clinical features are diagnostic and the clinical presentation is variable. The onset is usually acute, with malaise, fever, muscle aches and pains, and curiously, abdominal pain. A productive cough is usual, and chest pain due to pleuritis occasionally occurs. The chest radiograph is variable, but the commonest pattern is the presence of foci of alveolar infiltrates, which may be bilateral. The symptomatology is usually less severe than the chest radiographs suggest. Mortality has been high (10% to 20%), especially in immunocompromised patients. The histologic findings are nonspecific and consist of an alveolar pneumonia, which may contain numerous macrophages, lysis of the intra-alveolar exudate, and individual cell necrosis. The organism is difficult to visualize with conventional stains and is best seen with the Dieterle silver stain. Fluorescent or immunoperoxidase-linked antibodies are used as specific stains. Legionella may also be associated with diffuse alveolar damage (see later).

Pontiac fever, also caused by legionella, is mainly a febrile illness, with slight respiratory symptoms and radiologic abnormalities and a good prognosis. It has occurred in epidemics in office buildings and affects apparently healthy people.

Tuberculosis

No chest disease has had so dramatic a history as tuberculosis. Known since ancient Egypt, it became the scourge of nineteenth-century Europe and North America and during that time was the most common cause of death. There has been an exponential decline in the prevalence of tuberculosis throughout much of the twentieth century. This is probably due as much to decreased overcrowding, which was widespread in the nineteenth century and which facilitated transmission of the infection, as to the introduction of streptomycin and other antituberculosis drugs. The major effect of modern antituberculosis treatment has been to prevent reactivation of the disease, making death from it uncommon.

Pathogenesis Tuberculosis is caused by *Mycobacterium tuberculosis,* a slender, acid-fast aerobic organism. Pulmonary tuberculosis is almost always caused by the human strain of *M. tuberculosis* although atypical mycobacteria may also produce pulmonary infections. The disease has been classically divided into **primary** and **reactivation** tuberculosis; the initial infection is classified as primary tuberculosis and subsequent infections as reactivation tuberculosis. The terms "childhood" and "adult" tuberculosis, respectively, have also been used, but they lack accuracy.

Primary tuberculosis results from the initial exposure to *M. tuberculosis,* most commonly as a result of inhaling droplet nuclei. These are small particles—2

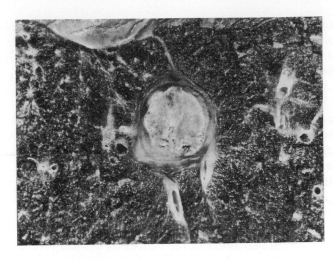

Figure 12-19.   Healed primary tuberculosis. A well-circumscribed pulmonary nodule of healed primary tuberculosis is seen as an incidental finding at autopsy.

µm to 10 µm in diameter—produced by coughing, sneezing, and talking. Primary tuberculosis is usually derived from a subject with "open" (cavitary) tuberculosis who coughs up large amounts of organisms. The bacilli are hardy and can persist for long periods in the environment. When inhaled the viable organism is deposited on the alveolar surface, where it begins to multiply in a previously uninfected person. Little resistance to infection occurs, because phagocytosis of the bacteria by macrophages is ineffective, and even within the macrophages the bacilli replicate.

The clinical and pathologic manifestation of primary tuberculosis is the Ghon complex, which consists of a parenchymal component (Fig. 12-19) and a prominent lymph node component. The parenchymal lesion can occur almost anywhere but is most commonly found in a subpleural location in the middle and lower lobes of the lung. Gross examination reveals a well-circumscribed nodule. Initially these nodules are centrally necrotic but later they become densely fibrotic and calcified. Histologic examination shows an initial acute inflammation followed by an infiltration of macrophages, which eventually appear as epithelioid cells. An immune response is mounted and specifically sensitized T cells liberate a number of lymphokines. Caseous necrosis ensues and the lesion becomes granulomatous, with a peripheral infiltrate of giant cells of the Langerhans type, histiocytes, and lymphocytes, together with a palisaded aggregate of fibroblasts. The central area shows varying features, from caseous necrosis to all degrees of healing, up to dense fibrosis and calcification. The lymph node component of the Ghon complex is found in the draining hilar or intrapulmonary nodes and has microscopic features similar to the pulmonary lesions.

Transmission As mentioned above, most cases of primary tuberculosis in the past were encountered in children, but the sequence of events that leads to the clinical expression of the disease may occur at any age following the first infection. Primary infection is associated with the development of both immunity and hypersensitivity, the latter being recognized by a positive tuberculin test. In animals, immunity and hypersensitivity can be separated experimentally. Immunity limits the development of disease, but hypersensitivity, even to dead organisms or their products, produces extensive necrosis. Surveys of schoolchildren in North America in the 1930s and 1940s showed that the majority of students were tuberculin-positive by the time they left high school. Recent surveys show that only a small minority are now positive; most primary infections occur in adults. A new feature of primary tuberculosis is the occurrence of mini-epidemics in groups living closely together (e.g., submarine crews, teenage groups, and health care workers). This presumably reflects the large proportion of nonimmune, tuberculin-negative persons in the community. Minor epidemics of tuberculosis have occurred in the United States, Canada, Britain, and France with the influx of tuberculous immigrants from nonindustrialized countries.

Complications In most instances, primary tuberculosis is asymptomatic and is found on routine skin testing or on skin testing because of known exposure to tuberculosis. In some instances, mild nonspecific symptoms, such as malaise, fever, and weight loss, may occur. Respiratory symptoms are usually absent. The great majority of primary infections remain localized and heal, but progression or complications do occasionally occur (Table 12-1). **Bacteremia** is probably a common event, and favorite sites of deposition and growth are locations with a high oxygen tension, such as the apices of the lung, growing ends of the long bones, and renal parenchyma. The most serious immediate complication is **miliary tuberculosis,** in which there is invasion of the bloodstream by *M. tuberculosis* and dissemination throughout the body. This occurs when the parenchymal part of the Ghon complex involves a pulmonary artery or vein and discharges its infected contents into the blood. Multiple minute granulomas develop in many organs of the body. The lesions are classically 0.5 mm to 2 mm in diameter, yellowish white, and evenly distributed through the affected organ. (The name "miliary" derives from their supposed resemblance to millet seeds.) A punctate area of necrosis may be seen in the center. Microscopically, the lesions of miliary tuberculosis consist of small granulomas, usually with a central necrotic portion in which numerous organisms are seen. Few organs are spared; those most often involved are the lung (mainly by recirculation of the organisms), spleen, liver, kidney, meninges, and bone marrow. Miliary tuberculosis used to be found most often in young children, but in industrialized countries it has become more common in the elderly and debilitated, in alcoholics, and in high-risk racial groups.

On occasion miliary tuberculosis involves only one organ, and that only focally. Almost any organ can

Table 12-1. Natural Course of Untreated Tuberculosis

COMPLICATIONS AND SEQUELAE	USUAL TIME AFTER CONVERSION	FREQUENCY IN CAUCASIANS
Incubation period 6 weeks (3–8 weeks)		Tuberculin conversion 100% Primary illness 30% Erythema nodosum 5%
Local spread (epituberculosis)	0–6 weeks	5%–10% in young children
Pleural effusion	2–9 months	5%–10% in adults, adolescents, and older children
Miliary tuberculosis and meningitis	2–8 months	5%–10% of children, later dropping to 1%
Extrapulmonary tuberculosis Cervical lymphadenitis	Few weeks to many years later	
Skeletal tuberculosis	First few years	
Genitourinary tuberculosis	Many years later	
Postprimary (reactivation) tuberculosis	At and after puberty	10% in recently infected adolescents, 4% in those infected in early childhood

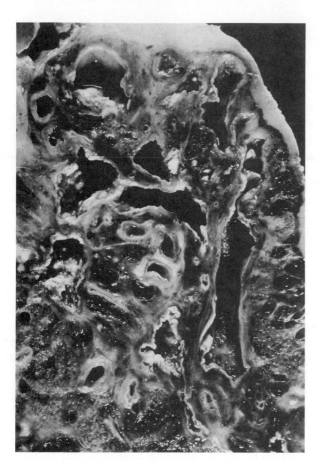

Figure 12-20. Reactivation tuberculosis. An elderly man living in a small city hotel felt unwell for some time, with fever and loss of weight. He was admitted seriously ill and died shortly thereafter. Several of his friends were found to have positive tuberculin skin tests. The lung shows extensive reactivation tuberculosis in the apex, pneumonic consolidation, focal areas of necrosis, and cavity formation.

be involved, most notably the genitourinary organs and bone (although in the latter case, the disease may be bovine tuberculosis, which has a different pathogenesis). A dreaded complication is tuberculous meningitis. In the lung, the parenchymal lesions may rupture into a bronchus causing a rapidly developing pneumonia, primarily lobar or segmental in distribution.

The reasons for progression of infection in a minority of those with primary tuberculosis are not known, but several have been suggested. It has long been known that infants, adolescents, and young adults are especially predisposed. Other factors include (1) the dose, with massive inoculation of organisms likely to produce a progressive lesion; (2) poor nonspecific resistance to infection, as occurs in the elderly or in alcoholics; (3) certain diseases, such as silicosis, or drugs, such as corticosteroids; and (4)

a racial predilection (notable, for example, in native Americans and very important in populations not previously exposed to tuberculosis). Immigrants to North America from Asia, the Philippines, and continental India have a high risk. Tuberculosis has classically been more severe in nonwhite populations, who are thought to have been introduced to the disease by whites. The high incidence and severe mortality of tuberculosis in the nineteenth century, particularly in young people, is thought to have eliminated many susceptible people and to have selected for those with innate resistance. Although colonizers spread the disease to previously unexposed populations, the reverse is now happening, with former colonial people carrying tuberculosis to a nonimmune population of previous colonizers.

Reactivation tuberculosis represents recurrence of pulmonary disease after sensitization to *M. tuberculosis* during primary infection. The term "reinfection tuberculosis," which has also been used, implies that the lesion results from an exogenous reinfection with new organisms. Whether infection occurs from new organisms or old is a contested issue; most believe, however, that the lesions are due to proliferation of preexisting endogenous organisms.

As previously indicated, bacteremia during the primary infection may seed bacteria in the lung. The initial reaction to *M. tuberculosis* is very different in secondary tuberculosis. A cellular immune response occurs after a latent interval and leads to the formation of granulomas and extensive tissue necrosis. Most commonly, the apical and posterior segments of the upper lobe are involved, but the superior segment of the lower lobe is also commonly affected, and no part of the lung can be excluded. A diffuse, fibrotic, poorly defined lesion develops that has focal areas of caseous necrosis (Fig. 12-20). Often these foci heal and calcify, but occasionally the material erodes into a bronchus and is coughed up, after which aspiration may lead to tuberculous pneumonia or a walled tuberculous cavity.

Reactivation tuberculosis is associated with constitutional symptoms—classically, fever, weight loss, night sweats, and malaise. A productive cough is usual, although hemoptysis is infrequent. Pleural involvement leads to pain and pleural effusions. Before the introduction of antituberculosis chemotherapy, cavitary tuberculosis had a mortality rate of about 50%, but the outlook is considerably better today.

Reactivation tuberculosis is uncommon in North America today, except in selected populations, and the predisposing factors are much the same as those involved in the progression of primary tuberculosis. Poverty, diabetes, postgastrectomy status, corticosteroid treatment, immunosuppression, certain malignant diseases, silicosis and other pneumoconioses are implicated. Secondary tuberculosis remains a major problem among native Americans and to a lesser extent among blacks and hispanics.

Atypical Mycobacteria

A number of organisms closely related to *M. tuberculosis* may cause pulmonary disease. These "atypical" mycobacteria are acid-fast and resemble *M. tuberculosis* morphologically, but their growth rates and growth requirements differ. They are not obligate intracellular parasites and exist in the environment. The best known are *M. kansasii* and *M. intracellulare*. The clinical and morphological features of the pulmonary disease are similar to those of *M. tuberculosis* but differ in that primary infections are not usually recognized, the reinfection phase is more indolent, and the organism is less sensitive to antituberculosis drugs. Furthermore, these organisms are not transmitted from person to person, and infection requires some impairment of host defense mechanisms. These atypical mycobacteria are generally considered to be less pathogenic than *M. tuberculosis*.

Actinomycosis

Actinomycosis is caused by infection with actinomycetes, and the usual pulmonary organism is *Actinomyces israelii*. Although actinomycetes resemble fungi in appearance, they are more closely related to bacteria. These weakly (and inconstantly) acid-fast organisms, which normally inhabit the mouth and nose, infect the lung either by massive aspiration or by extension from an actinomycotic subdiaphragmatic or liver abscess. The lung lesions consist of multiple, interconnecting, small lung abscesses. The margin is granulomatous, but the central necrotic area is purulent and contains numerous organisms that grow as colonies of intermingled filaments. Clubbed basophilic filaments are noted at the margins of the colonies, which are visible to the naked eye as small yellow particles ("sulfur granules"). The abscesses invade the pleura and produce bronchopulmonary fistulas and empyema. They may also invade the chest wall.

Nocardiosis

Nocardia asteroides, a gram-positive, acid-fast, aerobic organism, is very similar to actinomyces and is also an oral commensal. The lesions in the lung are similar to those of actinomycosis, but colony-like growth is not seen.

Fungal Infections

Fungal infections of the lung are now common in North America, indeed more common than tuberculosis, but in healthy people they are rarely serious. However, they may be lethal in those who are immunocompromised or debilitated. The most common pulmonary fungal infections are histoplasmosis and coccidioidomycosis.

Histoplasmosis

Histoplasmosis is classically thought of as a disease of the U.S. Midwest and Southeast in general and of the Mississippi and Ohio valleys in particular, with its epicenter in St. Louis. This disease is widespread in the United States, particularly in the Midwest, and extends into Canada. The causative organism is *Histoplasma capsulatum*, a small oval yeast about 3 μm in diameter that rarely shows budding. The disease is caused by inhalation of infected dust, commonly bird droppings. The organism is hardy and survives well in soil.

Histoplasmosis has many clinical and pathologic similarities to tuberculosis. The great majority of infections are asymptomatic and result in lesions similar to the Ghon complex, including a parenchymal granuloma and granuloma formation in draining lymph nodes. The condition is usually recognized only on a routine chest radiograph or a positive histoplasmin skin test. The granulomas are particularly prone to calcify, often with a concentric laminar pattern. The acute phase, in which numerous organisms are seen within macrophages, is followed by granulomatous inflammation with central areas of necrosis in the lesions. These characteristically heal by fibrosis and calcification. The central necrotic area may persist. The organisms are readily recognizable.

In a few cases, the pulmonary lesion progresses or reactivates, which leads to a progressive fibrotic and necrotic lesion that closely resembles reactivation tuberculosis. The lesion has a more fibrotic appearance, and cavitation is less common. The reason for progression is not known, although a large infective dose and poor host response are usually considered to be responsible. Especially in immunocompromised people there may be extensive multiplication of the organisms in macrophages and dissemination through the lungs and to the reticuloendothelial system elsewhere.

Coccidioidomycosis

Coccidioidomycosis is caused by *Coccidioides immitis*, large (30 μm to 60 μm) spherical spores that do not bud but that form endospores within the organism.

Originally known as San Joaquin Valley fever, where the disease has been endemic for many years, coccidioidomycosis is widely spread through the southwestern part of the United States. It shares many of the clinical and pathologic features of histoplasmosis and tuberculosis. In most instances, the lesions are limited to a peripheral parenchymal granuloma, with or without lymph node granulomas, and the disease is recognized by a positive skin test or routine chest radiograph. In a few cases, the lesion is progressive and resembles tuberculosis, although the rate of progression is slow. In dry, dusty conditions the hardy spores that live in the soil are blown into the air and inhaled.

Coccidioidomycosis is a serious condition in dogs, especially those brought into regions where it is endemic. Immunocompromised patients may experience rapid progression of the disease, with release of endospores into the lung, in which case the tissue reaction may be purulent as well as granulomatous.

Cryptococcosis

Cryptococcosis is caused by *Cryptococcus neoformans*, a round, budding yeast that varies in size from 2 μm to 15 μm. It has a thick, mucous gelatinous capsule that shrinks in tissue sections, leaving a halo around the organism. Compared with histoplasmosis and coccidioidomycosis, cryptococcosis is uncommon.

Cryptococcosis results from the inhalation of spores. The organism is frequently encountered in pigeon droppings. A variety of lung lesions is seen, from small parenchymal granulomas that are found only after a search in an autopsy specimen from a patient with cryptococcal meningitis to several large granulomatous nodules (which resemble pulmonary metastases radiologically), pneumonic consolidation, and even cavitation. Most serious pulmonary infections occur in immunocompromised individuals in whom the organisms proliferate extensively within alveolar spaces, with little tissue reaction.

North American Blastomycosis

Blastomycosis is an uncommon condition caused by *Blastomyces dermatitidis*, a budding yeast 8 μm to 15 μm in diameter, that has a thick refractile cell wall. It is mainly concentrated in the basins of the Missouri, Mississippi, and Ohio rivers and in southern Manitoba and northwestern Ontario. The clinical and pathologic features resemble the fungi mentioned earlier and may present as a lesion resembling a Ghon complex or as a progressive, pneumonic condition. The Ghon complex–like lesion is less frequent and differs in that the central necrosis exhibits a purulent reaction, surrounded by the granulomatous

inflammation. In a quarter of the cases the skin is involved, in the form of multiple nodules that slowly increase in size. Exposed areas of the skin may be the primary inoculation site, since most of these lesions are found there. However, the greater frequency of lung involvement without skin lesions has led to the general belief that the primary lesion results from inhalation of airborne spores that are found in the ground.

Branching Fungi

Infection by branching fungi is uncommon in healthy people. Aspergillosis and mucormycosis, seen as branching hyphae in tissue sections, are commonly seen only in the lungs of immunocompromised patients.

Aspergillosis Aspergillosis, usually caused by *Aspergillus niger* and *A. fumigatus,* is the most common and important fungal infection of the lung in this category. Aspergillus, a common mold that thrives in cool, wet conditions, is readily recognized with standard hematoxylin and eosin stains but is best seen on silver-stained section. The hyphae are thin (3 μm to 5 μm) and septate (subdivided by cell walls) and show regular dichotomous branching at a 45° angle (Fig. 12-21*A*). When the fungi grow in cool room temperatures, they have a fruiting head, or terminal structure, in which small cylindrical structures grow from the spherical fruit (Fig. 12-21*B*). In histologic cross section, they resemble an aspergillum (the instrument used for dispensing holy water in the Roman Catholic Church). Aspergilloma, allergic bronchopulmonary aspergillosis, and necrotizing bronchitis have been discussed in the section on conducting airways. **A much more serious manifestation of aspergillus infection occurs in the immunocompromised person, most commonly in leukemic patients treated with cytotoxic agents.** Extensive blood vessel invasion (usually arterial) results in occlusion, thrombosis, and infarction of lung tissue. The involvement is bilateral and widespread and is not amenable to therapy. The extensive blood vessel invasion suggests a hematogenous route, but there is usually no evidence of a primary cutaneous site. The frequent finding of aspergillus in the nasal cavity in patients with aspergillus pneumonia has been suggested as a diagnostic criterion, but aspergillus species are frequently found in nasal secretions and sputum in apparently normal subjects. It may be that the oronasal mucosa is the site of blood-borne infection that occurs in the compromised host. Inhalation may result in fungus balls in the lung.

Mucormycosis (Phycomycosis) Several closely related organisms—*Mucor, Rhizopus,* and *Nisidia*—may

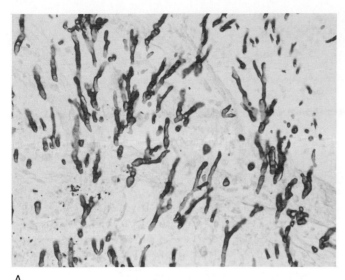

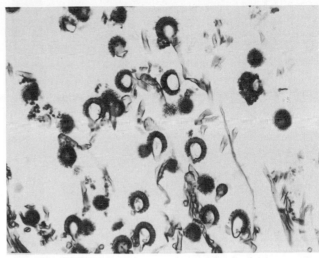

A   B

Figure 12-21.   Pulmonary aspergillosis. (*A*) Invasive aspergillosis is apparent in an immunocompromised man with acute myelogenous leukemia treated with cytotoxic drugs. In this tissue section the fungi are septate and show regular dichotomous branching at angles of approximately 45°. (*B*) When cultured at room temperature, Aspergillus fungi produce a characteristic spherical fruiting head, as shown here.

involve the lung in ways identical to those of aspergillus. These infections also occur as fungus balls or angioinvasive pulmonary lesions in an immunocompromised host. **A classic association is with diabetic ketoacidosis. Infection of the nasal sinuses is characteristic of these fungi.** These organisms have the same staining properties as aspergillus but differ in that the hyphae are not septate and are broader (10 μm to 15 μm), and they branch by irregular dichotomy, usually at right angles.

Candidiasis (Moniliasis)   *Candida albicans* is a normal commensal in the oral cavity, gut, and vagina and is best known for infection in these regions and the skin, often in the immunocompromised host. It also affects the lungs, but usually only the surface epithelium, with noninvasive growth in the airways. Although it may produce surface ulceration, in the lungs it is usually identified only at autopsy in a patient with severe immunosuppression.

Protozoa

Although relatively uncommon in industrialized countries, on a worldwide scale parasitic involvement of the lung is extremely common, most frequently by larval migration through the lung. Those affected either have no symptoms or have systemic symptoms with cough. Lung infiltrates at the bases are accompanied by eosinophilia of the blood. This syndrome is known as **tropical eosinophilia,** and the lesion in the lung is **eosinophilic pneumonia.** A similar uncommon syndrome in temperate zones is thought to be due to the migration of *Ascaris lumbricoides.* Protozoal infection of the lung is uncommon in industrialized countries, and the only significant one is produced by *Pneumocystis carinii.*

Pneumocystis carinii

First recognized as "plasma cell pneumonia," infection with *Pneumocystis carinii* was identified in malnourished infants at the end of World War II (Fig. 12-22). It came into prominence in North America with the advent of renal transplantation and immunosuppression. Since then it has come to be recognized as a major pulmonary complication of chemotherapy for leukemia and lymphoma and of treatment with steroids. It is now also an important cause of death in patients with AIDS. The organism is ubiquitous, and infection is only expressed in the debilitated and immunocompromised.

Clinically and radiologically, the presentation is variable. At one extreme, symptoms may be minimal; at the other there is rapidly progressive respiratory failure. More usually, there are nonspecific respiratory symptoms, including dyspnea and cough. Infection with pneumocystis should be considered in any pulmonary disease in an immunocompromised patient, particularly since it is sensitive to sulfisoxazole–

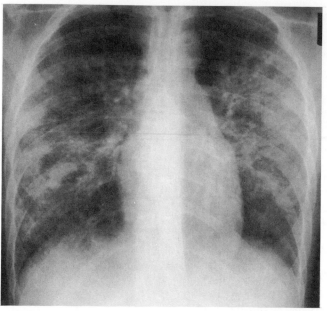

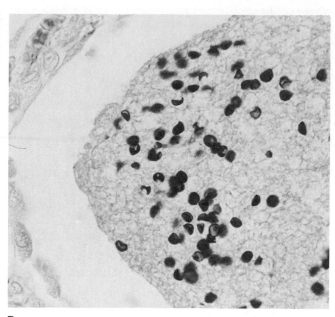

A

B

Figure 12-22.   Pneumocystis carinii infection of the lungs. (*A*) A chest radiograph in a patient with the acquired immune deficiency syndrome shows patchy, bilateral, intra-alveolar and interstitial infiltrates. (*B*) A silver stain shows the characteristic features of the *P. carinii* organisms. Some are round and uniform in size, others are irregular and have a crescentic configuration. The alveolar wall is seen on the left; the alveolar space contains a foamy exudate.

trimethoprim treatment. The diagnosis may be made by recognizing the organism with a variety of procedures, including (in reverse order of success), bronchial brushings, bronchial washings, transbronchial biopsy, needle aspiration of the lung, and open lung biopsy. Most recently, examination of the sputum and bronchoalveolar lavage have shown significant diagnostic accuracy.

The classic lesion is an interstitial pneumonia, with an infiltrate of plasma cells and lymphocytes, diffuse alveolar damage, and Type II cell hyperplasia. The alveoli are filled with a characteristic foamy exudate, the organisms appearing as small "bubbles" in a background of proteinaceous exudate. The organisms are readily recognized by silver stains, which stain the cysts. These are round or indented ("new moon") organisms about 5 μm in diameter (Fig. 12-22B). After sporozoites develop within the cyst, it ruptures and assumes the indented shape. The sporozoites develop into trophozoites, which may be recognized with stains such as Giemsa. In addition to this classic appearance of pneumocystis pneumonia, the infection may present as acute, diffuse alveolar damage, with hyaline membranes, epithelial necrosis, and even pulmonary fibrosis.

Dirofilariasis

Dirofilaria immitis causes dog heart worm infection. Transmitted by mosquito bites, the infection was initially confined to the southeastern United States, but it has now spread widely. An infarct in the lung is produced by the adult worm, which can be recognized in the central necrotic area. Granulomatous inflammation occurs at the periphery and fragments of the worm may be seen in foreign body giant cells.

Metabolic Lesions

Amyloidosis uncommonly involves the lung parenchyma, and two presentations are recognized. Nodular accumulations of amyloid present radiologically as possible multiple pulmonary metastases. Diffuse alveolar amyloidosis, usually associated with cardiac amyloidosis, is characterized by amyloid in the basal lamina of the alveolar capillary membrane. Diffuse interstitial infiltrate is seen radiologically, and the patient may have hypoxemia. In both types of pulmonary amyloidosis there is evidence of systemic amyloidosis elsewhere.

Metastatic calcification in the lung is associated with hypercalcemia, most often due to renal disease. The calcification occurs diffusely in the lung parenchyma and is thought to be due to the intrinsic acidity of the tissue (for the same reason that metastatic calcification occurs in the stomach). It may occur extremely rapidly and is especially well recognized in patients on renal dialysis. Because of the radiopacity of calcium, the radiologic appearance is dramatic. Histologically, calcium is basophilic; therefore, the basal lamina and elastic fibers in alveoli and vessels appear blue with routine stains.

Diffuse Alveolar Damage

The Adult Respiratory Distress Syndrome (ARDS)

The concept of diffuse alveolar damage has been referred to previously, and several known causes have been discussed. **The most important cause of diffuse alveolar damage is the adult respiratory distress syndrome (ARDS). In this syndrome, (Figs. 12-23, 12-24) a patient with apparently normal lungs suffers an insult and then develops rapidly progressive respiratory failure, characterized by hypoxemia and extensive radiologic opacities in both lungs ("white out")** (Figs. 12-24A,B). Over the years there has been considerable debate about the term *ARDS*. Some feel that the definition of rapidly progressive respiratory failure in a patient with apparently normal lungs is too broad, since it obviously encompasses many conditions in which a more specific diagnosis can be made, such as pneumonia of any sort, fat embolism, pulmonary thromboembolism, aspiration, inhalation of toxic gases, and so on. Others have doubted the existence of ARDS related to trauma and have held that the pulmonary lesions are due to known causes, such as oxygen toxicity or hemodynamic pulmonary edema. However, there is now little doubt that ARDS is a useful term and that it is not simply due to oxygen or hemodynamic pulmonary edema. A compromise is easily reached. It should be recognized that the syndrome of ARDS exists and is multifactorial (see Table 12-2) and that it is appropriate to qualify the term as ARDS due to specific conditions, such as nonthoracic trauma, inhalation of toxic gases, aspiration, and so on. In addition, oxygen toxicity produces similar lesions, and an idiopathic category should also be recognized.

ARDS causes about 75,000 deaths a year in the United States. The overall medical costs are enormous, since management requires high technology and intensive care. The syndrome was first recognized as an entity during the Vietnam War as a result of effective resuscitation techniques for seriously injured combatants. (In World War II, effective resuscitation during battle did not occur; in the Korean War, resuscitation was effective but tardy, with the result that many wounded died of acute renal failure.) Typically, nonthoracic trauma or infection (Fig. 12-24) leads to hemodynamic shock, from which the patient is resuscitated. However, recovery is interrupted by respiratory symptoms—namely, tachypnea, dyspnea, and hypoxemia—and a chest radiograph shows diffuse bilateral infiltrates, which progress to virtually complete opacifiction. The patient requires ventilatory assistance and increasing amounts of oxygen. The lungs become stiff (decreased compliance), and increasing end-expiratory pressures are required, until the patient needs 100% oxygen to maintain tissue oxygenation. Half of all patients with ARDS die.

ARDS has been studied in patients and in animal models. The important early event is leakiness of endothelial capillaries, with morphologic loosening of the intercellular junctions. At this stage respiratory failure is not apparent. Then, 24 to 48 hours after the initial insult, pulmonary edema and resultant hypoxemia ensue in the **exudative phase.** The next stage is **diffuse alveolar damage,** in which necrosis of type I epithelial cells and hyaline membranes that line the airspaces are prominent. In the proliferative phase, type II cells multiply to reconstitute the alveolar lining (Fig. 12-24C) and an interstitial inflammatory infiltrate of mononuclear cells is accompanied by proliferation of fibroblasts. All these conditions are present 4 to 7 days after the insult, and the patient usually dies in severe respiratory failure. If the patient survives, the lesions may heal with resorption of the alveolar exudate and hyaline membranes and restitution of the normal alveolar epithelium. Fibroblastic proliferation ceases and the extra collagen is metabolized. It is well documented that patients with ARDS who recover have normal pulmonary function. Alternatively, more fibrous tissue is laid down and the lung then becomes remodeled to produce the "honeycomb lung"—multiple cystlike spaces throughout the lung, separated from each other by fibrous tissue and lined by type II cells, bronchiolar epithelium, or squamous cells (see Fig. 12-39B). The resemblance of the honeycomb lung to the end stage of fibrosing alveolitis is seldom more than superficial. Following ARDS there is more active fibroblastic proliferation and less dense scarring. Bronchiolar epithelium lining is less prominent and secretions are not present in the spaces (see later discussion of fibrosing

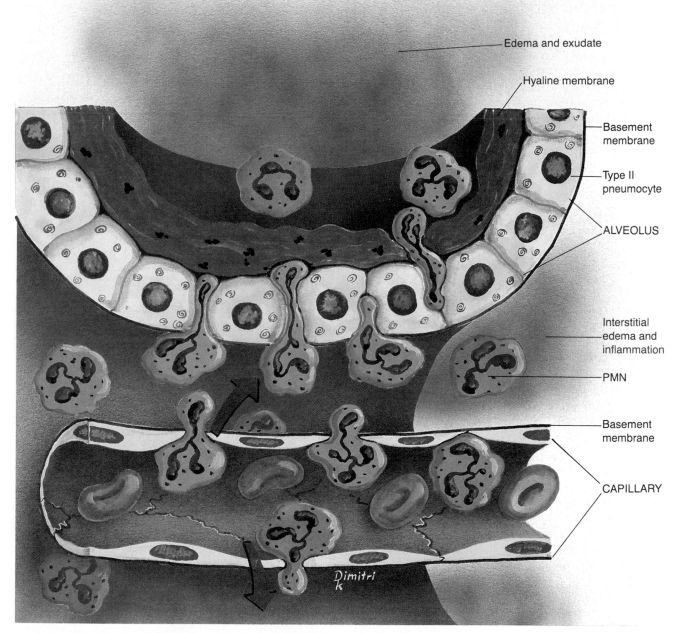

Edema and exudate

Hyaline membrane

Basement membrane

Type II pneumocyte

ALVEOLUS

Interstitial edema and inflammation

PMN

Basement membrane

CAPILLARY

Figure 12-23.   The adult respiratory distress syndrome (ARDS). In ARDS, type I cells die as a result of diffuse alveolar damage. Intra-alveolar edema follows, after which there is formation of hyaline membranes composed of proteinaceous exudate and cell debris. In the acute phase the lungs are markedly congested and heavy. Type II cells multiply to line the alveolar surface. Interstitial inflammation is characteristic. The lesion may heal completely or progress to interstitial fibrosis.

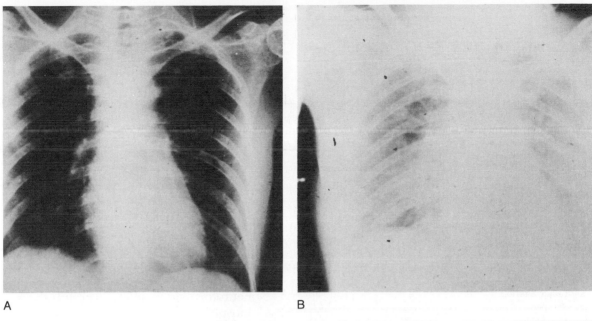

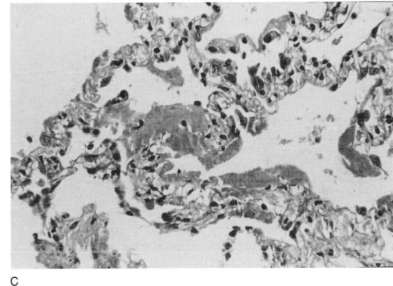

Figure 12-24. Adult respiratory distress syndrome (ARDS). A 24-year-old woman had a criminal abortion and became infected with *Clostridium perfringens* (*Welchii*). (*A*) Initial chest radiograph is normal. (*B*) A chest radiograph 24 hours later shows massive "white out." (*C*) Microscopically, diffuse alveolar damage and hyaline membrane formation are evident.

alveolitis). Occasionally, an appearance similar to bronchopulmonary dysplasia develops.

The pathogenesis of ARDS is not entirely clear. It is thought that activation of the complement system (e.g., by endotoxin in the case of gram-negative septicemia) results in sequestration of neutrophils in the marginating pool. Only a small proportion, perhaps one third, of neutrophils actively circulate in the blood; most of the remainder are found in the lung. Normally, the neutrophils cause no damage, but following activation by complement they release oxygen radicals and hydrolytic enzymes (superoxide and hydrogen peroxide) that damage the endothelium of the lung capillaries. Clinical studies have shown that

a reduced number of neutrophils in the blood of patients with risk factors for ARDS is a good predictor for the development of the syndrome. This finding suggests that increased numbers of neutrophils are sequestered in the pulmonary capillary bed.

In ARDS produced by the inhalation of toxic gases or near-drowning, the damage occurs primarily at the alveolar epithelial surface. As indicated, the alveolar epithelial junctions are usually very tight; damage to the epithelium results in exudation of fluid and proteins from the interstitium into the alveolar spaces. Endothelial damage may or may not occur in ARDS that is due to inhalation of toxic substances, but the sequence of events is similar to that due to

Table 12-2. Important Causes of the Adult Respiratory Distress Syndrome

Nonthoracic trauma
   Shock due to any cause
   Fat embolism

Infection
   Gram-negative septicemia
   Other bacterial infections
   Viral infections

Aspiration
   Near drowning
   Aspiration of gastric contents

Drugs and Therapeutic Agents
   Heroin
   Oxygen
   Radiation
   Paraquat
   Cytotoxic agents

endothelial damage in ARDS that follows trauma or septicemia.

Environmental Causes of Diffuse Alveolar Damage

Ozone

The concentration of **ozone,** a natural constituent of the atmosphere, is increased in areas that suffer from photo-oxidant air pollution. An initial acute inflammatory reaction in the proximal part of the acinus is followed by aggregates of macrophages and epithelial damage. Pulmonary function tests have shown only mild effects of realistic concentrations of ozone, but damage to the alveolar-capillary membrane has been shown in animals and man at concentrations of 5 to 10 parts per million.

Paraquat

The widely used herbicide **paraquat** generates oxygen radicals, which damage chloroplasts, the plant equivalent of mitochondria. As with oxygen, high doses primarily damage the central nervous system. At lower levels this herbicide damages other organs, such as muscle, but the clinical significance is largely related to the lung. The initial lesion caused by the ingestion of paraquat, namely, inflammation and ulceration of the oropharynx and esophagus, is due to direct local toxicity. In man, relatively minor hepatotoxicity and renal toxicity are apparent in the next few days. Pulmonary involvement becomes apparent 4 to 7 days after ingestion, as ARDS develops. Patients rarely recover once pulmonary complications

have evolved. A curious intra-alveolar exudate and organization occurs, as well as the more usual interstitial fibrosis. The intra-alveolar exudate organizes in such a way that the alveolar framework persists and the airspaces are filled with loose granulation tissue.

Iatrogenic Diffuse Alveolar Damage

A variety of therapeutic agents causes diffuse alveolar damage. The evolution of the disease is usually slow; the background implicates specific agents.

Oxygen

Oxygen toxicity has been recognized for nearly 100 years. The lung is the internal organ exposed to the highest ambient partial pressure of oxygen and is thus the most likely to be affected. Pure oxygen is a neurotoxin in animals exposed at more than 1 atmosphere of pressure, causing convulsions and death from nervous system failure. During World War II, since aviators were required to breathe increased concentrations of oxygen at high altitude, experiments with animals were done to study the effects of oxygen on the lung. These studies showed those effects to be harmful. Later observations with patients who were administered high levels of oxygen for respiratory problems led to descriptions of lesions identical to those of ARDS. Pulmonary lesions have developed in patients with long-term exposure to as little as 28% oxygen, but usually it is safe to breathe 40% oxygen (partial pressure of 300 mm Hg) for long periods of time. The mechanism of oxygen toxicity is related to partially reduced oxygen radicals in the same way as that of ARDS due to other causes.

Radiation Pneumonitis

Radiation pneumonitis, the longest recognized form of iatrogenic alveolar damage, is also caused by the generation of oxygen radicals through the radiolysis of water. It is most commonly encountered in irradiation of cancer of the lung, breast, or mediastinum (for lymphoma); the damage is mainly dose related. The initial clinical lesion is diffuse alveolar damage, but experimental studies have shown that the particular susceptibility of the capillary endothelium leads to early widespread capillary occlusion by fibrin thrombi. The acute phase is measured in terms of weeks or months. The result of healing is varied. In extreme cases, which are now uncommon, the affected lung is shrunken and fibrotic, and the lung architecture is largely lost. More usually, **there is diffuse interstitial fibrosis, general retention of lung structure, and bizarre hyperchromatic nuclei of al-**

veolar type II cells. Lipid accumulates within the alveolar capillary endothelium to produce foam cells.

Drug-Induced Diffuse Alveolar Damage

The long list of drugs that cause diffuse alveolar damage includes most chemotherapeutic agents. The best known is **bleomycin,** which is used for the treatment of epithelial cancers, but other frequently used agents, such as methotrexate, 5-fluorouracil, busul fan, and cyclophosphamide, are known causes. As a general rule, all cytotoxic agents should be suspected as a cause of diffuse alveolar damage. With bleomycin, an imprecise dose-dependent relationship has been demonstrated, but such an effect is not apparent with most other drugs. **The morphologic features are similar to those of diffuse alveolar damage from other causes.** Bizarre, atypical, hyperchromatic nuclei in type II cells are particularly common in cases of alveolar damage from chemotherapeutic agents. The bilateral lesions are extensive and most commonly encountered in lung biopsies in the immunocompromised patient. The damage progresses despite withdrawal of the offending agent, although it may be modified by the administration of corticosteroids. Progressive interstitial fibrosis occurs, usually with retention of the lung structure. Methotrexate differs from the other chemotherapeutic agents in that it may sometimes cause a hypersensitivity reaction in the lung. Under these circumstances, the diffuse alveolar damage is reversible after the drug is withdrawn. The lesions that reflect hypersensitivity are characterized by granulomatous inflammation and occasionally vasculitis.

Nonchemotherapeutic agents also cause pulmonary lesions. A good example of such an agent is nitrofurantoin, which is better known as a cause of eosinophilic pneumonia and may also produce a diffuse interstitial pneumonia.

Idiopathic Alveolar Filling Diseases

The concept of idiopathic alveolar filling disease is clinically and pathologically useful. Some conditions primarily produce filling of the alveoli and lead to the radiologic category of "acinar" opacities (i.e., opacified structures similar in size to the acinus are recognized). As more alveolar spaces fill, the air within the conducting airways may be apparent on chest radiographs—the so-called air-bronchogram. **Most alveolar filling diseases have a known etiology, commonly resulting from pneumonia and pulmonary edema.** However, the causes of several conditions are not understood.

Alveolar Lipoproteinosis

Alveolar lipoproteinosis was first described in 1958; its histologic appearance is so distinctive that one wonders why it was not recognized previously. Alveoli are filled with eosinophilic material that resembles edema fluid (Fig. 12-25), with some differences. The material is more deeply eosinophilic and granular than that in pulmonary edema, and there are denser, more eosinophilic bodies, about the size of large cells. These are thought to be cell ghosts (remnants of necrotic cells). By electron microscopy lamellar bodies are seen, together with cellular debris. On gross examination, the material is creamy in color and consistency and has a high lipid content. Although it contains phospholipids similar to surfactant, the material is not surfactive. Classically, the interstitium of the lung is normal, but in some instances there is mild interstitial inflammation and fibrosis and some type II cell hyperplasia. It has been suggested that alveolar lipoproteinosis is due to an excessive secretion of surfactant or to diminished removal of normal surfactant by macrophages. However, the large amount of protein in the material indicates an additional mechanism. A similar appearance has been described in acute silicosis and in children treated for leukemia. In the great majority of cases, no etiologic agent is identifiable, although patients with alveolar lipoproteinosis have a high frequency of occupational exposure to a variety of different substances. Nocardia and other mildly pathogenic organisms have been encountered in fatal cases, but they are thought to be a superinfection rather than causative agents.

The presenting symptoms of alveolar proteinosis are variable and nonspecific. Occasionally there are no symptoms. Generally, however, dyspnea, cough productive of creamy or gelatinous sputum, and repeated respiratory infections are observed. Radiologic examination shows an extensive pneumonia-like, alveolar consolidation, usually bilateral (Fig. 12-25) but sometimes unilateral. Untreated alveolar lipoproteinosis gradually progresses to respiratory failure, but spontaneous remissions do occur. Bronchoalveolar lavage removes the material, and repeated lavage usually cures or halts the progress of the disease.

Pulmonary Hemorrhage

Bilateral extensive pulmonary hemorrhage is generally a complication of other diseases, such as mitral stenosis or, rarely, infection. It also occurs in Goodpasture's syndrome.

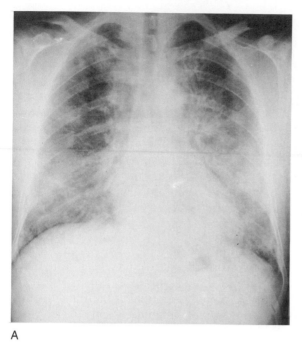
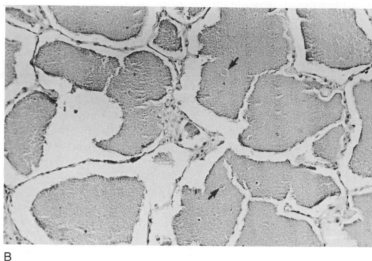

A   B

Figure 12-25.   Alveolar lipoproteinosis. (*A*) A chest radiograph shows widespread alveolar opacities. (*B*) Alveoli are filled with dense, lipoproteinaceous fluid that resembles edema. Note the smaller denser bodies (*arrows*).

Goodpasture's Syndrome

Goodpasture, a Boston pathologist, was investigating the autopsy findings in influenza pandemic deaths just after World War I. In one case in which death occurred several weeks after the attack of influenza, the lung showed extensive bilateral hemorrhage, together with necrotizing angiitis of the systemic vessels and glomerulonephritis. Since then the term *Goodpasture's syndrome* has been applied to the condition of **diffuse bilateral pulmonary hemorrhage accompanied by rapidly progressive glomerulonephritis.**

Antiglomerular Basement Membrane Disease   Goodpasture's disease has now become synonymous with the variant of pulmonary hemorrhage associated with circulating antiglomerular basement membrane antibodies. In this disease antibodies are visualized in the kidneys (and less well in the lung) by immunofluorescence as linear staining of the basement membrane. Although the patients may be adults of any age, they are typically young men and present with hemoptysis, dyspnea, and acute renal disease. Either the renal symptoms or the pulmonary symptoms may come first. As in Wegener's granulomatosis, the renal symptoms are more important than the pulmonary symptoms for the outcome. Anemia from pulmonary bleeding is usual. Radiographic examination reveals diffuse bilateral alveolar filling. The diagnosis is made on the basis of renal biopsy. Histologically, the alveoli are filled with red blood cells and there is suggestive evidence of "alveolitis" in the form of neutrophils in and around alveolar capillaries. Radiologically, the lesions resolve rapidly in a matter of days as the red cells lyse and are then phagocytosed. At this stage hemosiderin-laden macrophages are found in the alveolar spaces and in the interstitium. On gross examination, the lungs are dark red and heavy in the acute phase and rusty brown when the red cells are phagocytosed. Treatment by bilateral nephrectomy has been superseded by the administration of cytotoxic drugs. Plasmapheresis has also been used to remove the antibodies. The disease is no longer uniformly fatal. **The basal laminae of the capillaries in the lungs and the glomeruli are thought to have common antigenic determinants that are targets for antibodies elicited by a primary lung insult or kidney injury.** The resulting damage to the basal laminae produces alveolitis and hemorrhage in the lung and rapidly progressive glomerulonephritis in the kidney.

Other Forms of the Intrapulmonary Hemorrhage Syndrome

An identical clinical and pathologic syndrome occurs in the absence of circulating antiglomerular basement membrane antibodies in about half of the cases of otherwise typical Goodpasture's syndrome. A similar syndrome may also occur in the collagen-vascular diseases. As in Goodpasture's syndrome, necrotizing angiitis may be an associated feature. Wegener's granulomatosis may also have the same presentation as Goodpasture's syndrome but differs in that other evidence of Wegener's granulomatosis is present (e.g., upper respiratory tract lesions or noninfectious granulomas of the lung). Systemic lupus erythematosus may also present as pulmonary hemorrhage.

Evidence of pulmonary hemorrhage, usually old, is commonly found in patients with renal failure. The renal failure may be due to several other causes. Only those with rapidly progressive glomerulonephritis should be regarded as examples of Goodpasture's syndrome.

Idiopathic Pulmonary Hemorrhage (Ceelin's Disease) Primarily of interest to the pediatrician, idiopathic pulmonary hemorrhage presents as hemoptysis and anemia in patients under 20 years of age. The radiologic features are similar to those of Goodpasture's syndrome, but this disease differs in that renal disease is absent, the pulmonary hemorrhages are recurrent and intermittent, and the course is much more protracted or the disease remits spontaneously. Because of the chronicity of the course, the morphologic lesions differ from those in Goodpasture's syndrome. Although the acute lesions are similar, acute alveolitis may not be present, and there may be discontinuity of the alveolar basement membranes. With repeated hemorrhages the elastic tissue of the alveolar walls and blood vessels becomes coated with iron and calcium (presumably dystrophic) and is rendered basophilic. Fragmentation of elastic fibers leads to a foreign body giant cell reaction, an appearance incorrectly described as endogenous pneumoconiosis. The etiology is unknown.

Eosinophilic Pneumonia

Eosinophilic pneumonia, a condition characterized by flooding of eosinophils into alveolar spaces, is encountered in a number of situations.

Tropical Eosinophilia and Löffler's Syndrome
As mentioned previously, migration of tropical parasites through the lung is common. In temperate zones, the migration of *Ascaris lumbricoides* causes a similar condition, in which the pulmonary infiltration of eosinophils is benign and self-limited.

Chronic Eosinophilic Pneumonia
Pulmonary infiltrates with eosinophilia syndrome, also referred to as chronic eosinophilic pneumonia,

is a dramatic condition. Classically, patients suffer severe symptoms, with fever, night sweats, weight loss, cough, and dyspnea. However, symptoms may be minimal. The chest radiograph is usually diagnostic and shows **photographic negative pulmonary edema** (Fig. 12-26)—that is, extensive alveolar filling of the periphery of the lung that spares the central part (the hilum). Often the infiltrates change rapidly in severity and position. About one third of the patients have nasal symptoms and one quarter have asthma. Eosinophilia of the blood is usual, but may be transient. Histologic examination shows the alveolar spaces to be flooded with eosinophils (Fig. 12-26C). There is also interstitial pneumonia and diffuse alveolar damage, with type II cell hyperplasia and an accumulation of macrophages in the airspaces. Vasculitis and bronchiolitis obliterans are also described. The etiology is unknown, but occasionally associated diseases are present. The response to corticosteroids is so dramatic that it may be used as a diagnostic test.

Symptomatic Eosinophilic Pneumonia
An eosinophilic pneumonia resembling the classic chronic eosinophilic pneumonia may be a feature of conditions other than larval migration, including drug hypersensitivity (notably to nitrofurantoin and sulfonamides), rheumatoid arthritis (or a positive rheumatoid factor), and the Churg–Strauss syndrome.

Disease Processes Unique to the Lung

Because of the unique structure and function of the lung, several disease processes are unique to or especially common in that organ.

Chronic Airflow Obstruction

Several diseases are grouped together because they have in common an obstruction to airflow in the lungs. The term "chronic airflow obstruction" is no more specific than anemia, jaundice, or fever.

Little resistance to airflow is encountered in airways less than 2 mm to 3 mm in internal diameter— that is, the smallest bronchi, the bronchioles, and the respiratory bronchioles. This is because as the airways arborize distally their total cross-sectional area increases dramatically. Although airways do narrow slightly with each succeeding generation, the number of generations increases at a faster rate. The summed cross-sectional area is quite large at the level of the

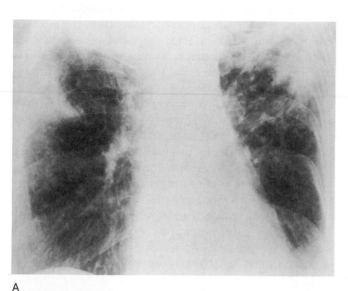

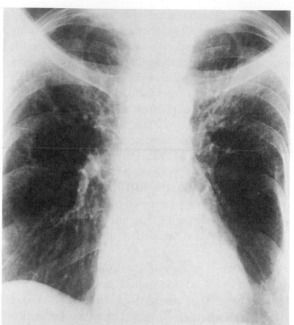

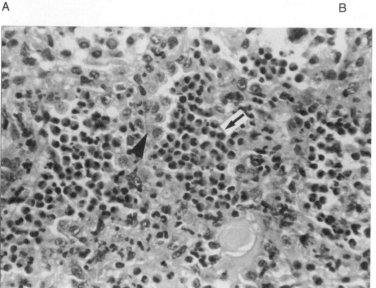

Figure 12-26. Eosinophilic pneumonia. A 50-year-old woman became severely ill with night sweats, malaise, and fever. The peripheral blood showed a high eosinophil count. (*A*) A chest radiograph reveals extensive peripheral infiltrates ("the photographic negative of pulmonary edema"), mostly in the upper zones. (*B*) One week after treatment with corticosteroids the radiograph appears normal. (*C*) Microscopically, the alveolar spaces are flooded with eosinophils (*arrow*). Proliferated type II pneumonocytes line the airspaces (*arrowhead*).

distal bronchi and even larger at the level of the terminal bronchioles. As a result, airway resistance may be normal in spite of considerable morphologic abnormalities in the peripheral airways. For example, it has been calculated theoretically that if every airway less than 2 mm to 3 mm in diameter were destroyed, the resistance in the peripheral airways would only double. Moreover, total airway resistance would theoretically increase by only 10%, a barely detectable change. However, it has now become apparent that the contribution of the peripheral airways

to total resistance is actually greater than originally thought (it may be as high as 40% of total resistance) and that even slight morphologic changes can result in abnormalities of the forced expiratory volume. In patients who died from severe chronic airflow obstruction, the peripheral resistance was increased 30 to 40 times, whereas the central airway resistance was increased only slightly, and inconstantly. Thus, even a modest decrease in forced expiratory volume should alert the physician (and the patient) to the possibility of progressive chronic airflow obstruction and should at least mandate a halt to smoking.

Airflow obstruction has two major causes. Flow has a simple hydraulic basis and can be reduced in only two ways: **by narrowing the tubes or by reducing the pressure to the system. In the lung, narrowed airways produce increased resistance, whereas loss of elastic recoil results in diminished pressure. In simplistic terms, airway narrowing can be thought of as bronchitis, and loss of recoil as emphysema.**

Central Airflow Obstruction

The most important causes of central airflow obstruction are chronic bronchitis, asthma, bronchiectasis, cystic fibrosis, and ciliary dyskinesia syndrome. Although all are associated with abnormalities of the central airways (bronchi), the obstruction to airflow is not necessarily due to these lesions. Chronic bronchitis, a lesion of central airways, may also be associated with peripheral airway narrowing and emphysema. Asthma is primarily a disease of central airways, but in many cases peripheral airway obstruction occurs. In bronchiectasis, cystic fibrosis, and the ciliary dyskinesia syndrome (the last two also have bronchiectasis), the obstruction to flow is actually peripheral to the dilated bronchi. Therefore, these conditions are considered under the rubric of peripheral airway disease.

Chronic Bronchitis
Chronic bronchitis is defined as chronic sputum production and is usually associated with a chronic cough. It is primarily related to tobacco smoking—especially cigarettes; more than 90% of all cases occur in chronic smokers. The frequency of chronic bronchitis is less than 5% in nonsmokers, 10% to 15% in moderate smokers, and more than 25% in heavy smokers. Age is a significant risk factor, although it is hard to distinguish between age and cumulative dose of tobacco smoke. Environment also plays a part; the frequency of bronchitis is higher in urban dwellers than in rural dwellers. Lower socioeconomic class (strictly defined by occupation in Britain) is a significant risk factor, and dusty occupations, such as coal mining, are associated with an increase in the frequency of chronic bronchitis. Finally, although an increased familial frequency of bronchitis has been shown, family clusters tend to share the same risk factors and the same attitude to smoking ("families who smoke together, die together"). Cough and sputum production is usually worse in the morning and more severe in the winter. Recurrent infections with episodes of mucopurulent sputum are typical, often

occurring after viral respiratory tract infections and bacterial superinfections, notably with *Haemophilus influenzae*.

The morphologic counterpart of chronic bronchitis is an increase in the size of the mucus-secreting apparatus (Fig. 12-27). Most mucus is secreted by the subepithelial tracheobronchial mucous glands, which consist of a series of branched tubules that on cross section look like glands and that drain into a duct leading to the epithelial surface. Two types of mucus-secreting cells line the acini, namely, pale mucous cells, which are the most common, and serous cells, which are more basophilic cells containing granules that "cap" the end of the tubules. **Chronic bronchitis is characterized by hyperplasia and hypertrophy of the mucus-secreting cells and an increased proportion of mucous to serous cells.** As a result, both the individual acini and the glands become larger. The increase in size has been measured in a number of ways, but the usual measure is the **Reid index** (Fig. 12-28), that is, the ratio of gland to wall. The thickness of the gland in the plane vertical to cartilage and epithelium is expressed as a proportion of the thickness of the bronchial wall (basement membrane to inner perichondrium) on the same plane. The normal value is 0.4 or less, in chronic bronchitis it is more than 0.5.

Other morphologic changes are also present in chronic bronchitis, but they have not been as well studied. Excess mucus is present in the central and the peripheral airways. "Pits," which may be visualized bronchoscopically in the surface of the bronchial epithelium in the large airways, represent dilated bronchial gland ducts into which several glands may open. Of particular importance, **the bronchial wall is thickened, mainly by mucous gland enlargement, but also as a result of edema of the bronchi.** This leads to encroachment on the bronchial lumen. An increase in inflammatory cells has not been consistently documented in patients with chronic bronchitis. Squamous metaplasia of the bronchial epithelium reflects epithelial damage from tobacco smoke, an effect that is probably independent of chronic bronchitis. An increase in goblet cells of the central airways is apparent in some cases. Increased amounts of muscle are often present and may reflect bronchial hyperreactivity (see Asthma).

Surprisingly, the pathogenesis of chronic bronchitis is not well studied. **The key phenomenon is hypersecretion of mucus in response to chronic injury.** Tracheobronchial glands are under autonomic nervous system (predominantly parasympathetic) control, and disturbances of nervous control may be involved in mucus hypersecretion. Damage to the

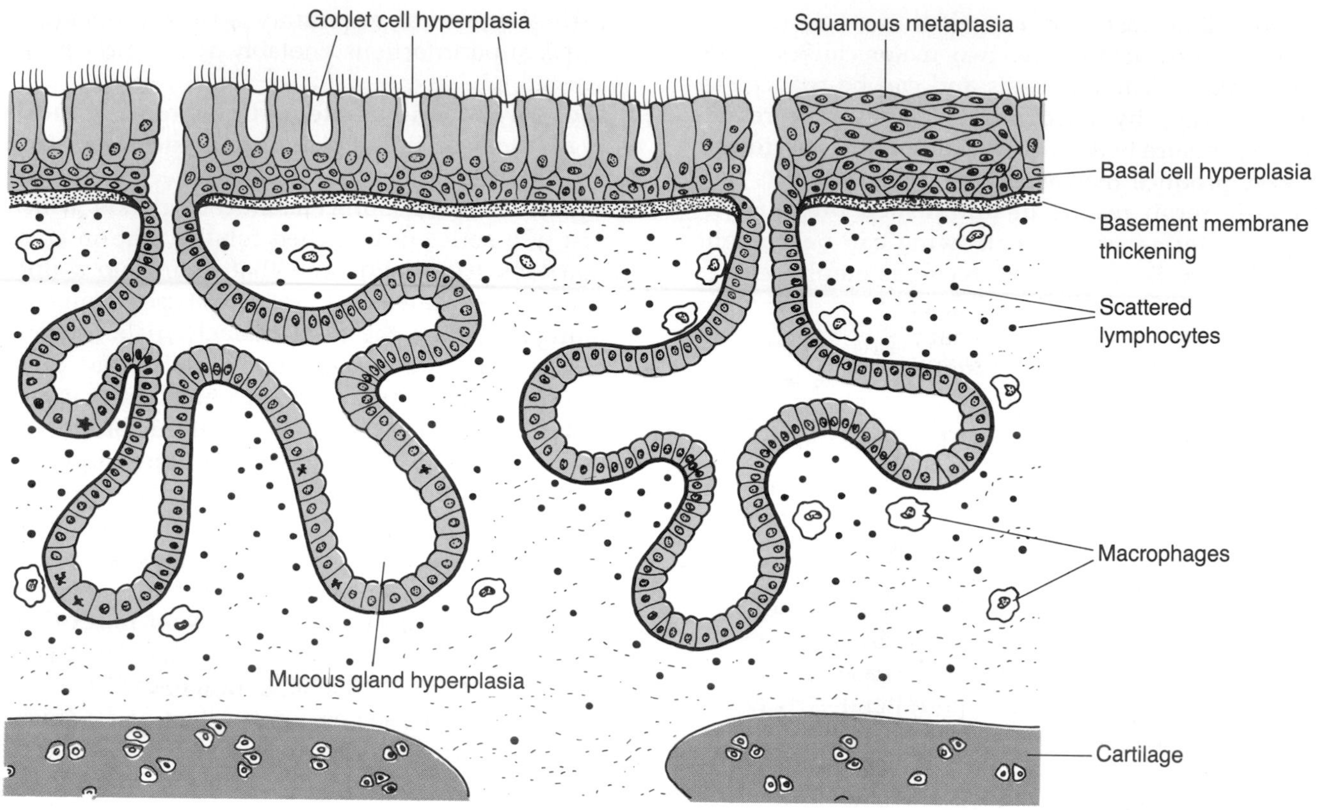

Goblet cell hyperplasia

Squamous metaplasia

Basal cell hyperplasia

Basement membrane thickening

Scattered lymphocytes

Macrophages

Mucous gland hyperplasia

Cartilage

Figure 12-27.   Morphologic changes in chronic bronchitis.

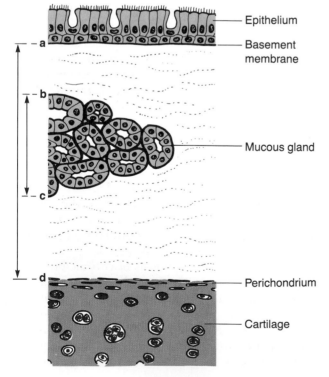

Epithelium

Basement membrane

– a

– b

Mucous gland

– c

– d   Perichondrium

Cartilage

Figure 12-28.   Reid index. The Reid index is the ratio of the thickness of the glands (*b–c*) to that of the bronchial wall (basement membrane to inner perichondrium) (*a–d*). It is increased in chronic bronchitis.

ciliated cells of the surface epithelium leads to increased mitotic activity of the basal cells, which then preferentially differentiate to mucus-secreting (goblet) cells, the product of which is presumably beneficial. When the insult is sufficiently severe, differentiation toward squamous epithelium occurs (see Fig. 12-27).

Asthma

Asthma presents an interesting paradox. Although most physicians correctly feel that they can recognize asthma with accuracy, no committee has defined this disease satisfactorily. Although it is imprecise, the following definition is widely used: "asthma refers to a condition of subjects with widespread narrowing of the bronchial airways which changes in severity over short periods of time, either spontaneously or under treatment, and is not due to cardiovascular disease." The following points are worth noting:

Most asthmatic patients, even when apparently well, have persistent airflow obstruction and morphologic lesions. This explains why asthma is placed in the category of chronic airflow obstruction.

A substantial proportion of patients with the usual clinical features of chronic airflow obstruction, predominantly middle-aged male smokers with chronic bronchitis and airflow obstruction, frequently also have increased airway reactivity—that is, an asthmatic component.

Although increased airway reactivity also occurs following viral bronchial infection or exposure to a substance such as ozone, no one would refer to such patients as having asthma.

With these provisos, **asthma in most patients is readily recognized as acute attacks of airflow obstruction, often easy to treat. Patients are well between attacks. In addition, many patients with chronic bronchitis have evidence of bronchial reactivity, and some may exhibit a distinct overlap with asthma. Finally, any airway insult may produce bronchial hyperreactivity.**

Asthma is classically divided into **extrinsic asthma** and **intrinsic asthma**. Extrinsic asthma is most commonly an immunologic phenomenon and occurs as a response to inhaled antigens. It is strongly related to allergic skin test reactivity and is usually found in children. The prognosis is good. Intrinsic asthma is a disease of adults and its prognosis is significantly worse. The causative factor may not be apparent and skin reactivity is uncommon.

Another way of looking at asthma is to modify the preceding into more specific categories (Fig. 12-29):

Antigen-induced asthma is the most common form of asthma. About one third to one half of all patients with asthma have known or suspected reactions to allergens. Most allergens are airborne and must be present in the environment for a considerable time to induce hyperreactivity. Common allergens include pollens, animal hair or fur, and insect contamination of house dust. Patients with antigen-induced asthma have classic extrinsic asthma.

Asthma may be associated with inhalation of a number of occupation-related substances. More than 80 different occupations have been identified where such a substance occurs. In some instances, these substances may provoke asthma by obvious hypersensitivity mechanisms (e.g., in animal handlers, bakers, and workers with wood and vegetable dusts, metal salts, pharmaceutical agents, and industrial chemicals). In others, the asthma may be due to release of histamine-like substances, a mechanism postulated in byssinosis ("brown lung"), an occupational lung disease in cotton workers. Occupational exposure may directly affect the autonomic nervous system. For example, organic phosphorous insecticides act as anticholinesterases and produce overactivity of the parasympathetic nervous system. Toluene diisocyanate is thought to have a beta-adrenergic antagonist action. Irritant gases, such as hydrochloric acid, ammonia, and heated plastic fumes, have a direct effect on the airways. At high doses almost all those exposed develop acute bronchitis and bronchoconstriction, whereas at low doses these substances produce only bronchoconstriction in sensitive people.

Environmental pollution is associated with bronchospasm, usually during episodes of massive air pollution. Usually patients with preexisting lung conditions are affected, but new cases of asthma do occur. Sulfur dioxide, oxides of nitrogen, and ozone are commonly implicated environmental pollutants.

Although **drug-induced bronchospasm occurs most commonly in patients with known asthma, the agents themselves may produce asthma. The best-known of these is aspirin,** but several other anti-inflammatory agents have been implicated.

Viral respiratory tract infections trigger attacks in young asthmatics and may cause the first attack. In children under the age of 2 years the respiratory syncytial virus is the usual agent, whereas in older children rhinovirus, influenza, and parainfluenza are the common inciting organisms.

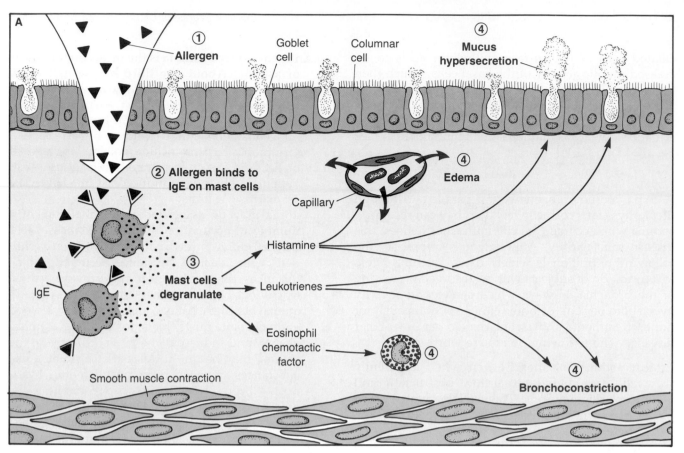

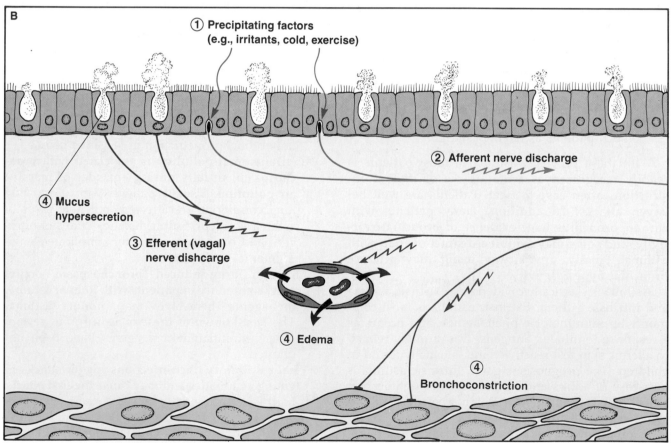

Exercise may induce attacks of asthma in patients who already have the disease; some degree of bronchospasm is usual in such subjects. Exercise may also cause the first attack of asthma. Exercise-induced asthma is related to the magnitude of heat loss from the epithelium of the airways to the intrathoracic gas. The more rapid the ventilation (severity of exercise) and the colder and drier the air breathed, the more likely the asthma is to be precipitated. Thus, an asthmatic playing hockey on an outdoor rink in Canada in winter is more likely to have an attack than one swimming slowly in a pool in summer in Houston.

More patients show a functional resemblance to antigen-induced asthma than have evidence of immunologic involvement. The onset of asthma for such patients is usually after childhood, and they are considered to suffer from "intrinsic asthma."

"Asthmatic bronchitis" is a disputed term and should be confined to patients with chronic airflow obstruction who have clear-cut episodes of acute worsening of airflow obstruction. These may also be regarded as patients with "intrinsic asthma."

As indicated, other patients with typical chronic airflow obstruction have variable airflow obstruction that responds to bronchodilators or have airway hyperreactivity. Such patients are not usually categorized as having asthma. However, occasionally a patient who has otherwise typical chronic airflow obstruction may show unexpected reversibility when treated with bronchodilators or corticosteroids. Such patients, whose number is small, have been referred to as "hidden asthmatics." It is important to recognize them because of the therapeutic implications.

The Importance of Asthma **Asthma is common, affecting 7% to 10% of children and 5% of adults.** It is most common in young children, least common in adolescence, and increases in frequency in adult life. Typically, childhood asthma disappears in adolescence or early adult life and has a good prognosis. Nevertheless, because deaths during acute attacks can occur, acute asthma should be regarded as a medical emergency, and prolonged difficulty in breathing—that is, status asthmaticus—must be terminated.

Anatomic Pathology of Asthma (Fig. 12-30) Most information on status asthmaticus has been derived from autopsies on patients who have died from the disease, and the findings are dramatic. **The airways are filled with thick, tenacious adherent mucous plugs, and the lungs are greatly distended with air.** Histologic examination shows that the mucous plugs contain strips of epithelium and many eosinophils, the extruded granules of which coalesce to form needlelike crystals (Charcot–Leyden crystals). In some cases the mucoid exudate forms a cast of the airways. These casts, which may be coughed up, are known as "Curschmann's spirals." Compact clusters of epithelial cells ("Creola bodies") are also seen in the sputum. The epithelium displays a loss of the normal pseudostratified appearance and may be denuded, with only the basal cells remaining. The basal cells are hyperplastic, and squamous metaplasia is seen. An increase in goblet cells (goblet cell metaplasia) is also apparent. Characteristically, the epithelial basement membrane is thickened, owing to an increase in collagen deep to the true basal lamina. One of the most characteristic features of status asthmaticus is the prominence of bronchial smooth muscle, which reflects muscle hyperplasia. The lamina propria contains numerous eosinophils. Edema and thickening of the bronchial walls are common. All these lesions may also be seen in apparently well asthmatics, but in these patients the lesions are less severe.

Other changes are seen in asthma. Bronchiectasis may occur in unusual locations, such as the upper lobe, probably because of bronchial obstruction by mucous plugs. Although asthma is primarily a disease of the central airways, peripheral airways may be abnormal, with increased airway muscle and goblet cell metaplasia. Emphysema is not a complication

Figure 12-29. Pathogenesis of asthma. (*A*) Immunologically mediated asthma. Allergens interact with IgE on mast cells, either on the surface of the epithelium or, when there is abnormal permeability of the epithelium, in the submucosa. Mediators are released and may react locally or by reflexes mediated through the vagus. (*B*) A variety of other forms of asthma exist that are apparently not immunologically mediated. The morphologic features are the same in the two types of asthma.

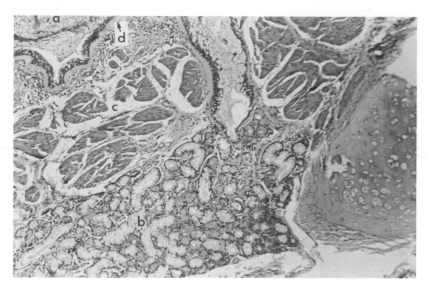

Figure 12-30. Status asthmaticus. A 36-year-old woman developed asthma 2 years previously and had an attack of asthma at home, for which she was treated with bronchodilators. She was admitted to the hospital with severe airflow obstruction and died shortly after. A histologic section shows mucus in the airway (*a*), enlargement of the mucous glands (*b*), an increase in the amount of muscle (*c*), thickening of the basement membrane (*d*), and an increase in inflammatory cells, mostly eosinophils, in both the mucus plug and the bronchial wall.

of long-standing asthma.

A disagreement often arises between pathologists and clinicians concerning the relative importance of mucous plugs and bronchospasm. Pathologists see fatal cases and favor the significance of the dramatic mucous plugs. Clinicians are impressed by the rapid reversibility of airflow obstruction and thus stress the importance of bronchospasm. It seems reasonable to assume that plugs may play a more significant role in status asthmaticus, whereas bronchospasm may be more important in attacks of asthma.

Pathogenesis of Asthma   The etiology and pathogenesis of asthma are clearly complex. **The two primary features of asthma—namely bronchial muscle contraction and mucus secretion—are under nervous system control.** Stimulation of the parasympathetic nervous system, represented by the vagus nerve, leads to bronchial constriction and hypersecretion of mucus. The sympathetic nervous system, through beta-adrenergic receptors, mediates bronchial dilatation and, less certainly, diminished mucus secretion. In addition, there is the nonadrenergic (purinergic) inhibitory system that causes relaxation of the airway smooth muscle.

Numerous mediators released from inflammatory cells or from mast cells result in bronchoconstriction, including histamine; bradykinin; leukotrienes C, D, and E; prostaglandins B_2, F_2, and G_2; and thromboxane A_2. Some of these mediators also increase capillary permeability. Other agents are chemoattractants, for example, eosinophil and neutrophil chemotactic factors of anaphylaxis and leukotriene B_4.

The simplest theory of asthma invokes hypersensitivity. The patient becomes sensitized to an antigen, the antibodies to which are IgE of the mast cells. The inhaled antigen binds to its IgE antibody, after which the mast cells release their contents. These in turn produce bronchial smooth muscle contraction, edema, and release of other mediators that amplify the response. In addition, the products of mast cells stimulate irritant receptors, which induces reflex bronchial constriction and mucus hypersecretion via the vagus nerve. How do the antigens sensitize the mast cells and how do the antigens reach them to trigger the reaction? Since bronchial epithelial cells are connected by tight junctions, loosening of the junctions may be a prerequisite for the appearance of asthma. Such loosening may reflect damage caused by infections, environmental irritants, and tobacco smoke. Mast cells and afferent nerves are present in the surface epithelium. Thus, when the antigen binds to its antibody, epithelial leakiness is amplified and a reflex stimulation occurs. Easier access to the submucosa is then possible, and both direct and reflex actions on smooth muscle occur. Other possible factors are inherent defects, including leakiness of the epithelium; inadequate sympathetic nervous system inhibitory action (beta-adrenergic blockade); and excessive cholinergic reactivity. In summary, one may envisage the pathogenesis of asthma at two extremes. At one extreme, it is mediated entirely through allergens in spite of a healthy epithelium; at the other, a variety of nonspecific stimuli acts on the severely compromised epithelium. In most cases, there is probably a combination of the two. In any event it seems that there is a final common pathway for all types of asthma, as evidenced by the similarity of lesions.

Bronchiolitis

The terms "small airways," "peripheral airways," and "bronchioles" are often considered synonymous, but they are not. Bronchioles are precisely defined as conducting airways that do not exhibit cartilage in the walls and do not contain gas-exchanging structures (the alveoli). The term "small airways" was used to describe both the smallest bronchi and the bronchioles, and "peripheral airways" has a similar but even less precise connotation. Lesions in these airways play a significant role in chronic airflow obstruction; the term "small airways" disease is used to describe them. **We use the term "bronchiolitis" because it involves specific structures and because the lesions are due to inflammation and its consequences. Bronchiolitis is almost always related to cigarette smoking and occurs in patients with the usual features of chronic airflow obstruction.** It is important to recognize that lesions in these airways have been studied chiefly at the two extremes of mild or severe chronic airflow obstruction.

Mild Chronic Airflow Obstruction The lesions are usually studied in lungs resected for cancer, in which case patients with severe chronic obstructive lung disease are excluded. In these specimens the lesions are mild, and **chronic bronchiolar inflammation is the important association with chronic airflow obstruction.** The inflammation is often mild, consisting of an increased number of lymphocytes, which are plasma cells with an occasional neutrophil. The mechanism by which inflammation produces airflow obstruction is unknown. Some have postulated that the inflammatory exudate displaces surfactant; others have suggested that mediators of inflammation produce direct or reflex constriction of bronchioles. **Inflammation may induce fibrosis and narrowing of bronchioles, further compounding airflow obstruction.** Although goblet cell metaplasia is well related to airflow obstruction, it should be regarded as a consequence, not a cause, of inflammation. Increased bronchiolar muscle in smokers with chronic airflow obstruction reflects hyperplasia as a response to inflammation, similar to the situation in asthma. Respiratory bronchiolitis is also a significant cause of mild chronic airflow obstruction (see later).

Severe Chronic Airflow Obstruction Patients with severe chronic airflow obstruction are usually studied at autopsy, and the lesions are different from those in persons with mild chronic airflow obstruction. **The consequences of inflammation, notably severe narrowing of the airways with an excess of very small bronchioles (less than 400 μm in diameter), become more important.** Goblet cell metaplasia is also important, but inflammation, fibrosis, and increased muscle are less significant. In patients with severe emphysema, the bronchioles become distorted by irregular narrowing, a condition that results in airway obstruction.

Special Forms of Bronchiolitis As previously discussed, certain agents other than tobacco smoke produce bronchiolitis, including toxic gases—notably **oxides of nitrogen, ozone, and ammonia.** The first two, which result from photochemical pollution, produce bronchiolitis—in the case of ozone, primarily respiratory bronchiolitis. Most occupational accidents involving nitrogen dioxide are related to the burning of paper or x-ray film or to silo-fillers' disease.

Rheumatoid arthritis is occasionally associated with mild bronchiolitis, but sometimes severe, progressive airflow obstruction occurs. In these circumstances, the smallest bronchi and bronchioles are occluded by loose granulation tissue in a spotty distribution. Other, rare causes of bronchiolitis are graft-versus-host reaction and rejection in heart–lung transplants.

Viral infections are an important cause of bronchiolitis. Although inflammation is usually mild, it may be a life-threatening disease, particularly in children. **Adenovirus** and **measles** bronchiolitis may result in bronchiolar obliteration and bronchiectasis.

Bronchiectasis

Bronchiectasis is usually thought of as a disease of large airways because this is the location of the obvious lesions. However, the origin in most instances lies in the obliteration of peripheral airways. **The disease is defined as permanent abnormal dilatation of bronchi.** Often the cause is clearly obstruction of central bronchi by inhaled foreign bodies, tumor, mucus plugs in asthma, and compressive lymphadenopathy. The last condition is best recognized in the right middle lobe, where the bronchus is long and narrow, has little cartilage support, and is surrounded by a cuff of lymph nodes. Enlargement of these nodes, particularly by tuberculosis, leads to obstruction of the bronchus, atelectasis, and bronchiectasis, a situation described as the "right middle lobe syndrome." However, with the decrease in the incidence of tuberculosis and the increase in lung cancer, the right middle lobe syndrome is now most commonly due to cancer. Bronchiectasis is also a feature of cystic fibrosis and ciliary dyskinesia.

Bronchiectasis was once common, usually resulting from such childhood bronchopulmonary infections as measles and pertussis or from bacterial infections. Vaccines and antibiotics have dramatically

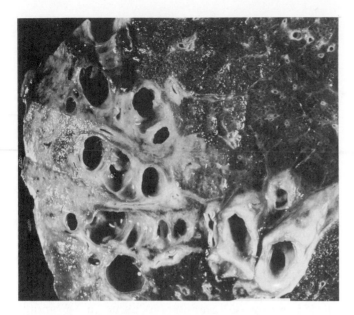

Figure 12-31.   Varicose bronchiectasis. An adolescent boy had cystic fibrosis from birth and died from pulmonary complications. The bronchi are irregularly dilated. Note the distal chronic pneumonitis and fibrosis.

reduced the frequency and the importance of bronchiectasis. Nevertheless, one half to two thirds of all cases of bronchiectasis follow a bronchopulmonary infection, hence the term "post infective bronchiectasis." At present, the most common cause of bronchiectasis is adenovirus infection. The disease is brought about by a severe inflammation of bronchi and bronchioles, which results in destruction of the walls of the central bronchi and obliteration of peripheral bronchi and bronchioles. With the consequent collapse of lung parenchyma (atelectasis), the bronchi dilate. Inflammation in the central airways leads to hypersecretion of mucus and abnormalities of the surface epithelium, including an increased number of goblet cells. A vicious cycle is set up because a pool of mucus is liable to further infection, which leads to progressive destruction of the bronchial walls. On gross examination, the bronchial dilatation is classified as **saccular, varicose,** or **cylindrical.** In the saccular form, the proximal third to fourth branches of the bronchi (the segmental bronchus is the first branch) are severely dilated and end blindly, and there is extensive collapse and fibrosis of lung parenchyma. In varicose bronchiectasis, the bronchi resemble varicose veins when visualized bronchographically, with irregular dilatation and constrictions (Fig. 12-31). Two to eight branchings of bronchi are recognized grossly, bronchiolar obliteration is not as severe, and parenchymal abnormalities are most variable. In cylindrical bronchiectasis, the

bronchi show uniform slight dilatation. Many such cases are examples of bronchitis and emphysema.

Bronchiectasis is most common in the lower lobes, the left more commonly involved than the right, and usually bilateral. The dilated bronchi contain thick, mucopurulent secretions. Microscopically, there is destruction of all components of the bronchial wall, chronic inflammation, a disproportionate number of goblet cells, and squamous metaplasia of the epithelium. Lymphoid follicles are often seen in the bronchial walls. The distal bronchi and bronchioles are scarred and often obliterated. The bronchial arteries increase in size and supply the inflamed bronchial wall and fibrous tissue. Consequently, hemoptysis is a common symptom.

Typically, a patient with bronchiectasis has a history of a severe, recurrent bronchopulmonary infection in childhood and thereafter has chronic productive cough, often with mucopurulent sputum. Radiologically, the affected lung is small, the bronchi are crowded together, and the bronchial walls may be visible. The definitive diagnosis is made bronchographically (by installation of radiographic contrast medium into the lung). Morphologically, the abnormalities are more extensive than visualized radiographically. Surgical resection is more palliative than curative, and although persistence of symptoms and progression of lesions are common, significant functional abnormalities are unusual. It should be noted that acute, reversible dilatation of bronchi may occur as a consequence of bacterial or viral bronchopulmonary infection, and it may take months before the bronchi return to normal size. This is important to recognize because such patients do not require surgery.

Bronchiectasis often complicates **cystic fibrosis.** Pulmonary complications are the most serious manifestation of cystic fibrosis, which is a heritable disorder affecting mucus secretion and eccrine sweat glands. The bronchial mucus is thick and patients are particularly liable to infection with *Pseudomonas aeruginosa.* As a result, bronchial and bronchiolar obliteration lead to bronchiectasis.

Kartegener's syndrome comprises the triad of dextrocardia (with or without situs inversus), bronchiectasis and sinusitis. It is now apparent that the syndrome may be due to a variety of structural and functional abnormalities of cilia (**the immotile cilia, or ciliary dyskinesia, syndrome**). These abnormalities are heritable, the most common of which is deficiency of the dynein arms. Others include radial spoke deficiency (**Sturgess syndrome**) and an abnormal complement of doublets. Since cilia throughout the body are deficient, sterility in both males and females is usual, because of immotility in the vas deferens and the fallopian tube. In the respiratory tract, ciliary defects lead to upper and lower respiratory tract infection in the lung and to bronchiectasis identical with "postinfective bronchiectasis."

Lesions in the Lung Parenchyma

The acinus is distal to the last conducting airway, the terminal bronchiole (Fig. 12-32). It begins with respiratory bronchioles, which have both alveolated and nonalveolated walls, with progressively more alveoli distally. Respiratory bronchioles are succeeded by conducting structures that are entirely alveolated (alveolar ducts), which then end in the alveolar sacs.

Airflow obstruction results from disease of the acinus, including inflammation of respiratory bronchioles (respiratory bronchiolitis), which may be associated with mild abnormalities of expiratory flow in cigarette smokers.

The most important consequence of involvement of the acinus is emphysema, which has been shown to be the most significant cause of chronic airflow obstruction. Airspace enlargement also occurs in conditions other than emphysema, as detailed in Table 12-3.

Simple Airspace Enlargement

Congenital The morphologic changes in the lung in Down's syndrome are as characteristic as the facies. The alveoli and alveolar ducts are enlarged, and there are too few alveoli. A double capillary layer is present in many alveolar walls. It is not clear whether the alveoli are abnormal at birth or whether postnatal development is abnormal. The changes are not associated with abnormalities of pulmonary function.

Congenital lobar overinflation (also referred to, wrongly, as emphysema) is rare. Usually shortly after birth a lobe, or part of a lobe, rapidly overexpands and compresses the remaining normal lung. The infant becomes dyspneic and cyanotic; resection may be required as an emergency, life-saving procedure. This condition is most commonly due to defective development of cartilage in the bronchi, but it may also be caused by mucosal flap valves or pulmonary arterial anomalies that compress the bronchi. In the acute phase there is overexpansion of alveoli, but if the condition persists, true emphysema may result.

Acquired If a lung or part of a lung is removed or collapses, the remaining lung overexpands. Since the orderly arrangement of the acinus is not lost, this is referred to as **compensatory overinflation.**

The changes that occur with age are more com-

plex. Starting at about age 30, the interalveolar wall distance increases. Although the proportion of the lung attributed to alveolar volume decreases, that of the alveolar ducts increases. This change in the geometry of the lung results in a loss of gas-exchanging surface area, roughly 3 m² decade (4%). Alveoli are lost with aging, and muscle decreases in the bronchioles. This change is seen in almost all people, even nonsmokers. Since these changes are thought to reflect normal aging, they are referred to collectively as the **aging lung** rather than as senile emphysema (an abnormal event). Functional changes are minimal, but loss of recoil and diminished expiratory flow rates and diffusing capacity are documented. It is still not clear whether the changes are due to age alone. Wrinkles may provide the best analogy to this situation, for they are characteristic of age but occur mainly in areas exposed to sunlight. It may be that the aging changes in the lung are also influenced by the environment.

Emphysema

Emphysema is defined as **a condition of the lung characterized by abnormal permanent enlargement of the airspaces distal to the terminal bronchiole, accompanied by destruction of their walls without obvious fibrosis.** Emphysema is classified in anatomic terms, but the classification should not obscure the fact that **the severity of emphysema is more important than the type.** In practical terms, as emphysema becomes more severe it becomes more difficult to classify, a situation similar to that of endstage renal disease or cirrhosis of the liver. Emphysema is common, being found in about half of all autopsies, and is easily recognizable.

Proximal Acinar (Centriacinar) Emphysema The proximal part of the acinus (respiratory bronchioles) is selectively or predominantly involved in centriacinar emphysema, of which there are two forms (see

---

Table 12-3. Types of Airspace Enlargement

Simple Airspace Enlargement
  Congenital
  Acquired

Emphysema (Fig. 12-32)
  Proximal acinar (centriacinar) emphysema
  Panacinar (panlobular) emphysema
  Distal acinar (paraseptal) emphysema

Airspace Enlargement with Fibrosis
  Associated with focal scars in the lung
  Associated with interstitial pneumonia and honeycombing

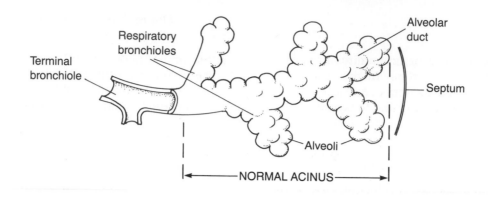

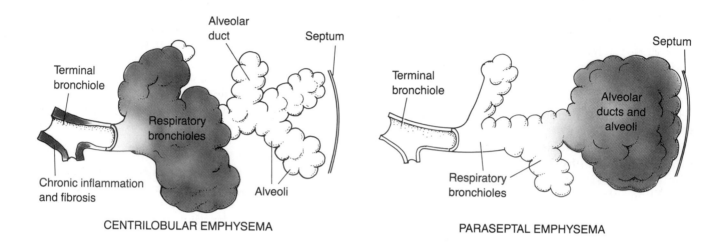

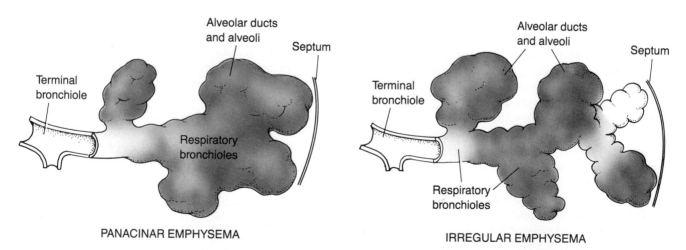

Figure 12-32. Types of emphysema. The acinus is the unit gas-exchanging structure of the lung distal to the terminal bronchiole. It consists of, in order, respiratory bronchioles, alveolar ducts, alveolar sacs, and alveoli. In **centrilobular (proximal acinar) emphysema** the respiratory bronchioles are predominantly involved. In **paraseptal (distal acinar) emphysema** the alveolar ducts are particularly affected. In **panacinar (panlobular) emphysema** the acinus is uniformly damaged. In **irregular emphysema** the acinus is irregularly enlarged and destroyed. There usually is significant fibrosis, so that the condition may be termed **airspace enlargement with fibrosis.**

Fig. 12-32). **Centrilobular emphysema** is the common form of emphysema in nonindustrial populations; **focal emphysema** is recognized in dusty occupations, such as coal mining (coal workers' emphysema or simple pneumoconiosis).

Centrilobular Emphysema Centrilobular emphysema is the form of the disease most frequently encountered and the one usually associated with clinical symptoms (see Fig. 12-32). It involves the central part of the lobule (the smallest portion of the lung bounded by lobular septa, or, more precisely, the cluster of terminal bronchioles near the end of the bronchiolar tree). More exactly, it involves the proximal part of the acinus. **It is associated with, and probably due to, tobacco smoking.** The destroyed and enlarged respiratory bronchioles form airspaces that are separated from each other and from lobular septa by normal alveolar ducts and sacs. As the lesion progresses, these distal structures may also be involved. The bronchioles proximal to the emphysematous spaces are inflamed and narrowed. **Centrilobular emphysema is most common and most severe in the upper zones of the lung (upper lobe and superior segment of lower lobe).** It occurs much more often in men than in women and is commonly associated with chronic bronchitis.

Coal Pneumoconiosis Working with coal, whether as a miner or in other ways, results in an accumulation of coal or other dust in macrophages in and around respiratory bronchioles. Mild dilatation of respiratory bronchioles results, probably from atrophy of muscle. **The lesion resembles centrilobular emphysema but differs in that the enlarged spaces are smaller and more regular, and inflammation of bronchioles is not apparent. Thus, the lesion is primarily distensive rather than destructive.** The anatomic lesion is usually equated with a chest radiograph that shows small nodular densities, although the complete correlation has not been proved. The condition, also referred to as **black lung,** has been considered to cause severe disability. Contemporary evidence, however, suggests that simple coal pneumoconiosis causes only minor impairment of pulmonary function. When coal miners have severe chronic airflow obstruction, it is usually due to other forms of emphysema, notably tobacco-related centrilobular emphysema. Other forms of dust, including iron and urban soot, may also be associated with similar lesions.

Panacinar Emphysema The acinus is uniformly involved in panacinar emphysema (see Fig. 12-32). All parts of the acinus are destroyed and in the final stage a lacy network of supporting tissue is left behind (the "cotton candy lung"). Panacinar emphysema occurs in several different situations.

Familial Emphysema **Familial emphysema is usually due to a defect in circulating α_1-antiproteinase.** Originally described as α_1-antitrypsin deficiency, it is now recognized that the protein has several antiproteinase effects, notably antielastase. The amount and type of α_1-antitrypsin is determined by a pair of codominant alleles, referred to as Pi (proteinase inhibitor). The most common phenotype is PiM (referred to as such since PiMO and PiMM cannot be distinguished). Over 30 different alleles are now recognized. The most serious abnormality is associated with the PiZ allele, which occurs in some 5% of the population, is commoner in those of Scandinavian origin, and is rare in Jews, blacks, and Japanese. The phenotype PiZ (ZZ or ZO) is associated with very low levels of circulating antiproteinase inhibitor, which also has an abnormal electrophoretic mobility. **People with this phenotype often develop cirrhosis of the liver in infancy and emphysema as adults.** The majority of all patients with **clinically** diagnosed emphysema under the age of 40 have α_1-antitrypsin deficiency (PiZ). Symptomatic emphysema is uncommon under the age of 50. Cigarette smoking plays an important role in the causation of emphysema in most affected individuals, but a small number of nonsmokers with PiZ also develop emphysema. PiZ is associated with panacinar emphysema, which is characteristically worse in the lower zones of the lung. Clinically, the patients usually have the "pink puffer syndrome," with greatly enlarged lung volumes and normal blood gases (see later discussion). Other alleles are also associated with emphysema, the most important being PiS, which is found frequently among southern Europeans.

Panacinar Emphysema in Association with Centrilobular Emphysema Panacinar emphysema is often associated with centrilobular emphysema. In such cases, the panacinar form tends to occur in the lower zones of the lung, whereas centrilobular emphysema is seen in the upper ones. The associations are the same as for centrilobular emphysema alone, notably cigarette smoking, chronic bronchitis, and chronic airflow obstruction.

Clinical Features of Emphysema As already noted, when emphysema gets worse it is hard to classify, and experts may classify the same lung differently, as centrilobular, panacinar, or unclassified emphysema. We have also noted that the severity of emphysema is more important than the type in producing chronic airflow obstruction. Curiously, people may have severe emphysema at autopsy without clinical manifestations of chronic airflow obstruction. The frequency of chronic bronchitis increases with the severity of emphysema, and almost all patients

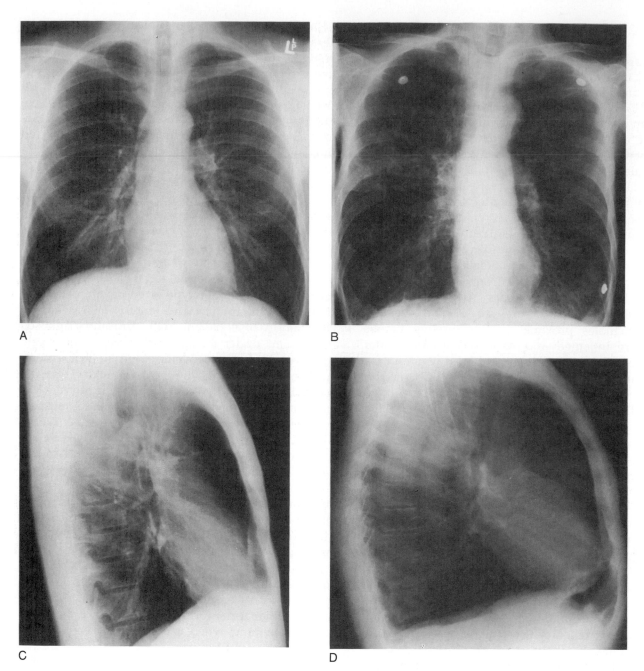

A

B

C

D

Figure 12-33.   Severe emphysema. A 66-year-old former heavy smoker had chronic bronchitis for 30 years. He noted shortness of breath at age 50 and was diagnosed as having emphysema at age 57. A year before death pulmonary function tests showed a reduced forced vital capacity and an increased residual volume. (*A*) A normal chest radiograph. The diaphragm is higher and the lung volumes smaller than in *B*. There is a uniform radiolucency through the lung field, and vessels can be traced well into the outer half of the lung. (*B*) An anteroposterior radiograph of the emphysematous patient shows an overinflated lung, with flattened, depressed diaphragms. The radiolucency of the lung is increased. (*C*) A normal lateral chest radiograph. Note the curved diaphragm, the small retrosternal space, and the vascularization of the lower lobes. (*D*) A lateral chest radiograph of the patient is more dramatic. The lung is overinflated (because total lung capacity is increased), the diaphragm is more obviously depressed, and the retrosternal space is enlarged.

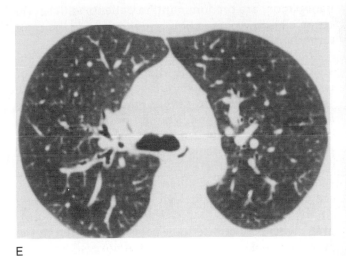

E

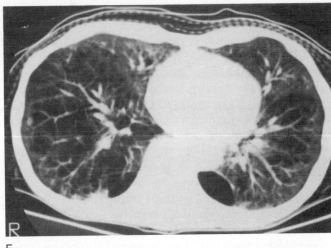

F

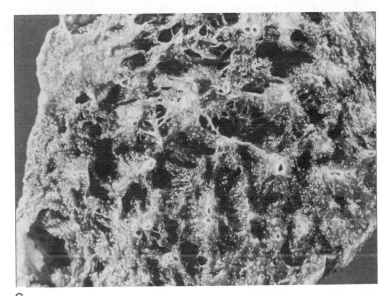

G

Figure 12-33 (continued). (E) A CT scan of normal lung shows a homogeneous gray pattern of lung parenchyma and dense white blood vessels. The major vessels are obvious, and many small vessels are seen in the peripheral lung parenchyma. (F) The CT scan of the patient with emphysema shows numerous radiolucencies that represent emphysematous spaces and diminished vascularity. Lung volume is increased. (G) The gross specimen corresponding to the CT scan shows severe unclassifiable emphysema, which, however, may be mostly centrilobular.

with severe emphysema have chronic bronchitis. Although it was once thought that chronic bronchitis leads to emphysema, **it is now recognized that chronic bronchitis and emphysema share a common etiologic agent, namely tobacco smoke.** Patients usually present to their physician between 55 and 60 years of age with dyspnea of insidious onset. Weight loss is probably due less to lack of calories than to the increased work of breathing. Starvation in animals has been shown to produce emphysema-like changes, and it may be that caloric deficiency aggravates emphysema in man.

The most important radiologic abnormalities include overinflation of the lung, as evidenced by enlarged lungs, depressed diaphragm levels, an inversion of the convexity of the diaphragm and an increased posteroanterior diameter ("barrel chest") (Fig. 12-33). Relative avascularity of the peripheral lung is also described as a sign.

Tests of expiratory flow are poorly related to the severity of emphysema because emphysema is only one cause of chronic airflow obstruction. Tests that reflect the loss of elastic recoil, such as increased functional residual capacity, and particularly total lung capacity, show a better correlation. The best predictor has been the diffusing capacity (transfer factor) for carbon monoxide, although no single test is entirely adequate. It is appropriate to think of chronic airflow obstruction as a multifactorial syndrome, the most important of which is emphysema. The severity of emphysema can be assessed only by an integrated approach. Tests of expiratory flow establish the severity of chronic airflow obstruction. If a patient is young and a nonsmoker, he is unlikely to have emphysema. If he is a middle-aged smoker with chronic bronchitis, he is likely to have emphysema. The chest radiograph provides supplementary evidence, as do the functional tests previously mentioned. In the final analysis, clinical common sense, a chest radiograph, and measurement of the diffusing capacity go a long way in making the assessment.

The "Pink Puffer" and the "Blue Bloater" The literature in the 1960s emphasized that patients with severe chronic airflow obstruction present with two distinct appearances. One type of patient is severely hypoxic and hypercapneic, has peripheral edema because of right ventricular failure, and often has a rate of ventilation less than that suggested by the concentrations of blood gases. Conversely, another patient is thin and has normal blood gas levels because of a sustained high ventilation rate. The former was known as the "blue bloater," and airflow obstruction was thought to be due to chronic bronchitis; the latter was labeled the "pink puffer," and chronic airflow obstruction was attributed to emphysema. These concepts have disappeared from all but the most conservative textbooks, but the fact remains that **the two types of chronic airflow obstruction are still identifiable and represent the opposite ends of a spectrum.** Most patients have features of both. The blue-bloater syndrome is likely to occur in those with diminished response to hypercapnea and perhaps hypoxia. Among such patients, those with the greatest degree of right ventricular hypertrophy have more narrowed peripheral airways. This is a logical observation since those with the blue-bloater syndrome have the greatest ventilation–perfusion inequalities, a situation consistent with severe bronchiolar narrowing.

One should regard chronic airflow obstruction as multifactorial. In the central airways, the bronchioles, and the lung parenchyma, a variety of lesions may contribute to chronic airflow obstruction. They occur together because of a common etiologic agent, namely tobacco smoke. In patients with mild chronic airflow obstruction, bronchiolar lesions, notably inflammation, are predominant; in patients with severe chronic airflow obstruction, emphysema is the most important.

Etiology and Pathogenesis of Emphysema **Conclusive evidence now exists that the major cause of emphysema is tobacco smoking, especially cigarette smoking. Moderate to severe emphysema is rarely found in nonsmokers. The dominant hypothesis concerning the pathogenesis of emphysema is the proteolysis–antiproteolysis theory** (Fig. 12-34). It is now thought that there is a balance between elastin synthesis and catabolism in the lung. If elastolytic activity increases or antielastolytic activity decreases, emphysema results. Increased numbers of neutrophils, which contain serine elastase, are found in the bronchoalveolar lavage fluid of smokers. Smoking also reduces the α_1-antiproteinase activity in the lung, owing to the oxidation of methionine residues in α_1-antiproteinase. In this way, **unopposed and increased elastolytic activity leads to emphysema.** However, although the proteolysis–antiproteolysis theory is attractive, it awaits further confirmation.

Pneumoconiosis

The pneumoconioses are diseases caused by the inhalation of inorganic dusts and represent a subset of occupational lung disease, which also includes disorders caused by the inhalation of gases, vapors, and organic material. The many forms of pneumoconiosis have specific names, depending on the substance inhaled (e.g., silicosis, asbestosis, talcosis). In certain instances the offending agent is uncertain and often the occupation is simply cited (e.g., "arc welder's lung"). Historically, occupations were recognized as predisposing to lung disease before an etiologic agent was recognized. Thus "knife grinder's lung" was used before this malady was recognized as silicosis.

Two major issues complicate the etiology of pneumoconioses. First is the variety of dusts to which the sufferer may have been exposed. Often workers ex-

Figure 12-34.   The proteolysis–antiproteolysis theory of the pathogenesis of emphysema. Cigarette (tobacco) smoking is closely related to the development of emphysema. Some product in tobacco smoke induces an inflammatory reaction. The serine elastase in polymorphonuclear leucocytes, which is a particularly potent elastolytic agent, injures the elastic tissue of the lung. Normally, this enzyme activity is inhibited by α_1-antitrypsin, but tobacco smoke, directly or through the generation of free radicals, inactivates α_1-antitrypsin (proteinase inhibitor).

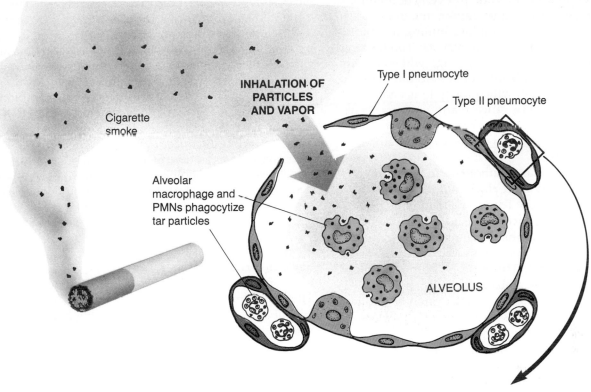

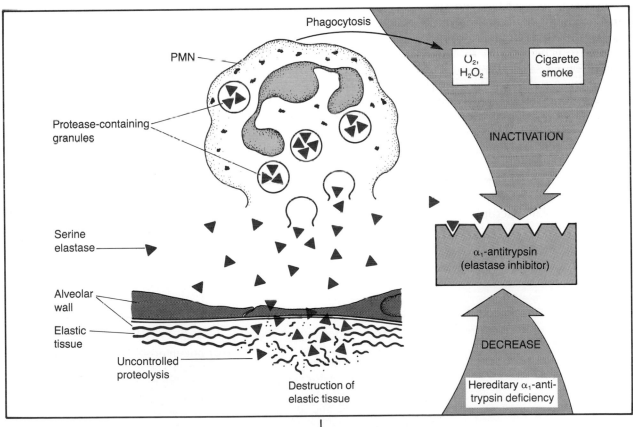

posed to inorganic dusts work in several occupations. It is not unusual for a gold miner, for example, to become a coal miner. In addition, mining of a particular mineral may generate other dusts. The best single example of this is gold mining, where miners' lesions are due to inhalation not of gold but of quartz (silica) from the rock in which the gold is embedded. Second is the difficulty, since many workers smoke cigarettes, in judging the relative contributions of smoking and occupational dusts to respiratory impairment.

The most important pathogenetic feature of inhaled dusts, namely their ability to produce fibrosis, is variable (Fig. 12-35). Thus, small amounts of silica or asbestos may produce extensive fibrosis, but coal and iron are weakly fibrogenic at best. In general, lung lesions reflect the dose and size of the particle delivered to the lung. The dose is a function of the amount of dust in the ambient air and the time spent working in the environment. It is often difficult to calculate the dose because it is unusual for persons to work in precisely the same environmental conditions throughout their working lives. Since particles are often irregular, it is important to express size as **aerodynamic particle diameter,** a parameter that describes the way the particle moves in air. The aerodynamic particle diameter determines where the inhaled dusts deposit in the lung (see Fig. 12-3), the most dangerous being those that reach the peripheral part of the lung, the smallest bronchioles and the acini. The great majority of large particles (more than 10 μm) are filtered by the nasopharynx and never reach the lower respiratory tract. Most particles 2 μm to 10 μm in diameter deposit on the bronchi and bronchioles and are removed by the mucociliary escalator.

Whereas the smaller particles terminate in the acinus, the minute ones behave as a gas and are exhaled. The alveolar macrophages, which ingest the inhaled particles, constitute the primary defense mechanism of the alveolar space. Most of these particles ascend to the mucociliary carpet by an unascertained homing mechanism and are expectorated or swallowed. Others migrate into the interstitium of the lung and then into the lymphatics. A significant number accumulate in the respiratory "sump," in and about respiratory bronchioles and terminal bronchioles. Other particles are not phagocytosed but enter epithelial cells and migrate through them, presumably passively, into the interstitium.

An important concept in the understanding of pneumoconiosis is that of **individual susceptibility,** which reflects differences in airway anatomy and function, particle clearance, defense mechanisms, and immunologic reactivity.

Silicosis

Silicosis is caused by the inhalation of silicon dioxide, of which there are three molecular configurations. The most important is quartz, and the others are crystobalite and trydimite. The earth's crust is composed largely of silicon and its oxides, and these often combine with other minerals to form silicates. Silicon dioxide, often referred to as "free silica," has the distinction of producing the best-known and the most widespread pneumoconiosis.

Silicosis is acquired, notoriously, in sandblasting. Mining also involves exposure to silica, as do numerous other occupations, including stone cutting, polishing and sharpening of metals, ceramic manufacturing, foundry work, and the cleaning of boilers.

Simple Nodular Silicosis

Simple nodular silicosis is the most common form of silicosis and is almost inevitable in any worker chronically exposed to silica. The lungs contain silicotic nodules (always less than 1 cm in diameter, and usually 2 mm to 4 mm in diameter) that, on histologic examination, have a characteristic whorled appearance, with concentrically arranged collagen that forms the largest part of the nodule (Fig. 12-36). At

Figure 12-35. Pathogenesis of pneumoconioses. The three most important pneumoconioses are illustrated. In simple **coal pneumoconiosis,** massive amounts of dust are inhaled and engulfed by macrophages. The macrophages pass into the interstitium of the lung and aggregate around the respiratory bronchioles. Subsequently, the bronchioles dilate. In **silicosis,** the silica particles are toxic to macrophages, which die and release a fibrogenic factor. In turn the released silica is again phagocytosed by other macrophages. The result is a dense fibrotic nodule, the silicotic nodule. **Asbestosis** is characterized by little dust and much interstitial fibrosis. Asbestos bodies are the classic feature.

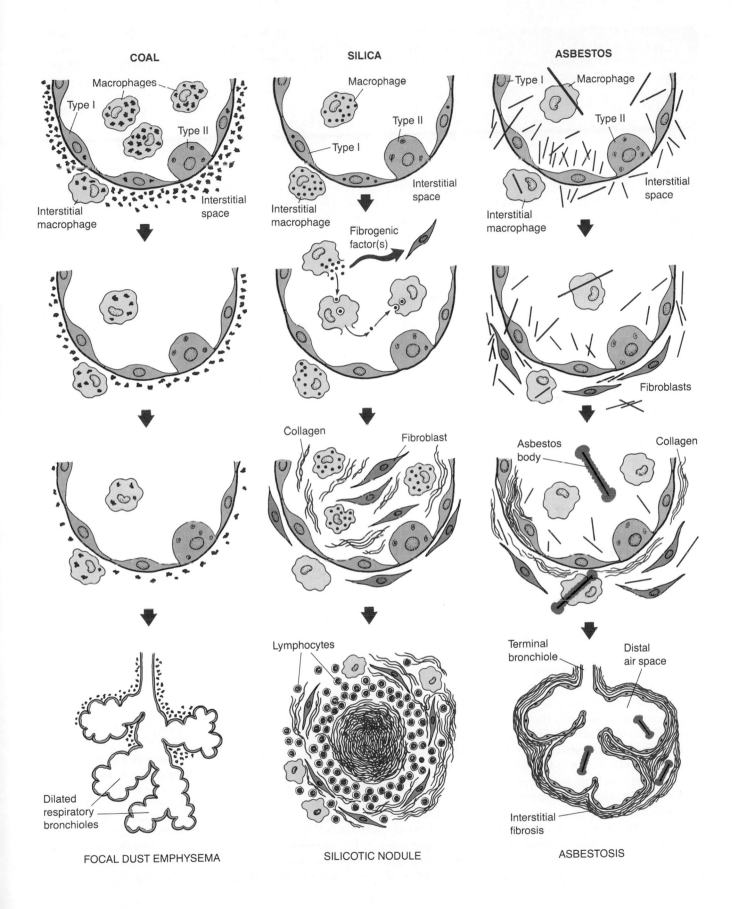

COAL

Macrophages

Type I

Type II

Interstitial macrophage

Interstitial space

FOCAL DUST EMPHYSEMA

Dilated respiratory bronchioles

SILICA

Macrophage

Type II

Type I

Interstitial space

Interstitial macrophage

Fibrogenic factor(s)

Collagen

Fibroblast

Lymphocytes

SILICOTIC NODULE

ASBESTOS

Type I

Macrophage

Type II

Interstitial space

Interstitial macrophage

Fibroblasts

Asbestos body

Collagen

Terminal bronchiole

Distal air space

Interstitial fibrosis

ASBESTOSIS

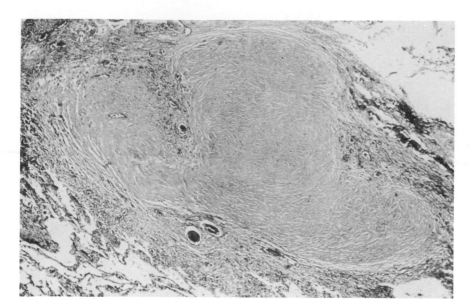

Figure 12-36. Silicotic nodule. The nodule shows central concentric dense collagenous deposition. Mild chronic inflammation is seen at the margin.

the periphery there are aggregates of mononuclear cells, mostly lymphocytes, and fibroblasts. Polarized light reveals doubly refractile silicates within the nodule, but these are not related to the pathogenesis of silicosis (only free silica is responsible). Hilar nodes become enlarged and calcified, often at the periphery of the node ("eggshell calcification"). It has now become apparent that simple silicosis is not usually associated with significant disability, as assessed by pulmonary function.

Progressive Massive Fibrosis

Progressive massive fibrosis (PMF) is defined radiologically as nodular masses of more than 1 cm diameter in a background of simple silicosis. Most of these lesions are considerably larger than 1 cm (5–10 cm) in diameter and are usually located in the upper zones of the lung (Fig. 12-37). Morphologically, the lesions often exhibit central necrosis, although in some instances they consist of aggregates of nodules of simple silicosis ("conglomerate silicosis"). It is well recognized that tuberculosis is much more common in patients with silicosis than in others and that it is a serious complication. This complication was first described in South Africa, where a peculiar situation existed and still exists. Most of the gold miners there are migrant workers who are employed on a short-term contract. During the period of contract they live in barracks. Since the miners come from a background with little immunity and are probably susceptible because tuberculosis is now in the population, and since they live in crowded quarters, one might well expect tuberculosis to be rife, and it is.

Lesions of tuberculosis in the miners closely resemble PMF, hence the notion that PMF is due to tuberculosis. PMF is also common in Welsh coal miners, as is tuberculosis. This is discussed in more detail later.

Most observers give less importance to the tuberculous theory of PMF now than was once the case. Progressive massive fibrosis is related to the amount of silica in the lung. Disability is caused by the destruction of lung tissue that has been incorporated into the nodules.

Acute Silicosis

Now uncommon, acute silicosis results from heavy exposure to finely particulate silica during sand blasting or boiler scaling. It is associated with diffuse fibrosis of the lung in which classic silicotic nodules are not found. Dense eosinophilic material accumulates in alveolar spaces to produce an appearance that resembles alveolar lipoproteinosis. Indeed, experimental administration of finely particulate silica has been used as a model for that condition. The disease progresses rapidly over a few years, in contrast to other forms of silicosis, the progression of which is measured in decades. On radiologic examination, acute silicosis shows diffuse linear fibrosis and a reduction in lung volume. Clinically, there is a severe restrictive defect.

Etiology and Pathogenesis

It was originally thought that the varying degrees of fibrosis associated with different forms of silica reflected differing solubilities. The popular view today

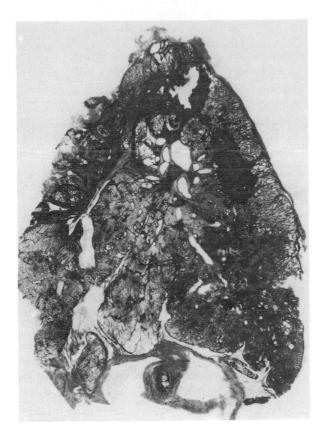

Figure 12-37. Progressive massive fibrosis. A 48-year-old coal worker had increasing shortness of breath, and pulmonary function studies revealed a decreased diffusing capacity. He died of respiratory insufficiency. A sagittal section of lung shows two large masses that represent progressive massive fibrosis with areas of necrosis, mostly at the apex of the lung. A separate mass is present in the superior segment of the lower lobe. Note also the relation of airspace enlargement to the scars. Panacinar emphysema is present in the anterior basal segment of the lower lobe.

is that following the ingestion of silica, macrophages produce a fibroblast stimulating factor. Because of the toxicity of silica, the macrophage dies, thereby releasing the ingested silica and the fibroblast stimulating factor (see Fig. 12-35). The silica is then reingested by macrophages and the process is amplified. The cytotoxicity of silica results from the contact between the mineral particle and the target macrophages. For many years, the death of these cells has been related to the fate of the particles after this contact. In particular, the release of lysosomal enzymes into the cytosol follows rapidly on the phagocytosis of silica particles. It has been suggested that the breakdown of cellular components as a result of the release of lysosomal components produces irreversible cell injury. Although intracellular lysosomal rupture has been documented in silica-treated macrophages, the evidence that it causes cell death is only circumstantial. Experimentally, it has been possible to dissociate intracellular lysosomal rupture from cell death after exposure to silica particles. It is likely that the macrophages are killed because of direct damage to the plasma membrane. Immunologic mechanisms may also be involved in the pathogenesis of silicosis. Immunoglobulins are present in the silicotic nodules, and abnormal serum immunoglobulins (e.g., antinuclear antibodies) are also often present.

Lung Disorders in Coal Workers

Simple Coal Pneumoconiosis

Simple coal pneumoconiosis has been discussed in the section on emphysema. Mild, predominantly distensive enlargement of respiratory bronchioles (see Fig. 12-35) is associated with mild abnormalities of pulmonary function. Radiologic examination shows small nodular opacities or linear opacities.

Progressive Massive Fibrosis

Progressive massive fibrosis was first adequately described in coal miners and has been referred to in the section on silicosis. The size and location of the lesions are similar to those in progressive massive fibrosis of silicosis. It is rare in the United States but common in Wales, where it is thought of as the combined result of coal inhalation and tuberculosis. As previously mentioned, the burden of silica in the lung may play a role in its pathogenesis. The disorder is associated with significant functional disability, and there is usually an obstructive defect, which may or may not be associated with a restrictive defect.

Caplan's Syndrome

Caplan's syndrome was originally described in coal miners as the radiographic appearance of large lung masses together with rheumatoid arthritis. The pulmonary lesions are large (1 cm to 10 cm in diameter), multiple, and bilateral. Histologic examination shows them to be "rheumatoid nodules," but they differ from classic rheumatoid nodules in that the palisading of fibroblasts at the periphery is less apparent and there is necrosis with an acute inflammatory infiltrate. Caplan's syndrome is not confined to coal miners and may occur in silicosis and asbestosis.

Pathogenesis of Coal Pneumoconiosis

The role of silica in coal pneumoconiosis has long been controversial. Coal miners are often exposed to substantial amounts of silica, and the term *anthraco-silicosis* was widely used. (Anthracite is a form of coal.) It was subsequently shown that those who worked only with coal (e.g., trimmers who loaded only coal) developed simple coal pneumoconiosis. It has been suggested that the aggregates of coal particles in macrophages in the walls of respiratory bronchioles weaken the respiratory bronchiolar muscle, thus leading to dilatation. It has recently been shown that the lesions in coal miners who have also been exposed to high levels of silica are different in that the silicotic nodules in the lung are heavily pigmented with coal. In addition, progressive massive fibrosis in these subjects closely resembles conglomerate silicosis. The frequency of coal pneumoconiosis has diminished significantly because of declines in dust levels in underground mines and the increase in strip mining.

Asbestos Pneumoconiosis

Asbestos is a generic term that embraces the silicate minerals that occur as long, thin fibers. They conduct heat poorly and are thus important in insulation. The three major forms of asbestos are crocidolite, which comes mainly from South Africa; chrysotile, the most common form of asbestos, most of which is mined in Quebec; and amosite. **If coal is the classic example of much dust and little fibrosis, asbestos is the prototype of little dust and much fibrosis** (see Fig. 12-35). Most clinically obvious cases occur as a result of the processing and handling of asbestos, rather than in mining, which is a surface operation. Exposure starts with the baggers who package asbestos and continues with those who modify or use it, such as workers who make asbestos products (tiles, cement, insulation material) and those in the construction and shipbuilding industry.

Asbestosis

Classic asbestosis is an interstitial fibrosis of the lung. The features are in general similar to those described in fibrosing alveolitis (usual interstitial pneumonia), as described later. The first lesion is an alveolitis that is directly related to asbestos exposure. Asbestos fibers are long (up to 100 μm) but thin (0.5 μm to 1 μm), so that their aerodynamic particle diameter is small. They deposit particularly at the bifurcations of alveolar ducts. The smallest particles are engulfed by macrophages, but many submicroscopic particles lie free in the interstitium of the lung. The most diagnostic structure is the **asbestos body** (Fig. 12-38), which consists of an asbestos fiber (10 μm to

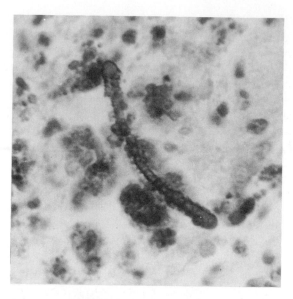

Figure 12-38. Asbestos body. A typical asbestos body has bulbous ends and a beaded body. It is about 75 μm long (for comparison, the visible nuclei are 10 to 15 μm in diameter).

50 μm in length) that has beaded aggregates of iron along its length. By light microscopy it is golden brown with hematoxylin and eosin and stains strongly for iron. The iron staining derives from hemoglobin liberated from microhemorrhages. The fibers are only partly engulfed by macrophages because they are too large for a single macrophage. The macrophages coat the asbestos fiber with protein, mucopolysaccharides, and ferritin. The macrophages also release a fibroblast-stimulating factor that promotes fibrogenesis. In the early stages, asbestosis differs from usual interstitial pneumonia in that the fibrosis occurs in and around alveolar ducts, as well as in the periphery of the acinus. As the lesion progresses, honeycombing (end-stage lung) results, as in terminal usual interstitial pneumonia. Asbestosis is usually more severe in the lower zones of the lung. Pleural thickening is often conspicuous.

Asbestos Bronchiolitis

Asbestos fibers that deposit in the bronchioles and respiratory bronchioles incite a fibrogenic response in these locations and lead to mild chronic airflow obstruction. Thus, asbestos produces an obstructive as well as a restrictive defect, the latter being more serious. At issue is whether such patients should be regarded as having asbestosis, a term that is usually confined to alveolar wall fibrosis. The term *asbestos respiratory bronchiolitis* recognizes this variant.

Pleural Plaques

Pleural plaques are nodular, localized thickenings (2 mm to 3 mm) of the pleura, most often found in the parietal pleura. The margins are irregular and the size varies from a few millimeters to several centimeters across. Microscopically, they are densely collagenous, with interwoven bands of collagen ("basket-weave" pattern), and are sometimes calcified. Pleural plaques are usually an incidental finding in patients with occupational exposure to substantial amounts of asbestos, but such plaques are not uncommon in people with casual exposure.

Asbestos-Induced Pleural Effusion

In some instances a pleural effusion is the only manifestation of asbestos exposure. By definition it is not associated with mesothelioma, is benign and self-limiting, and heals by fibrosis. Such effusions are clinically significant because they are frequently mistaken as evidence of cancer.

Mesothelioma

Mesothelioma may be localized and benign, or it may be malignant. The very existence of this tumor was seriously doubted a few decades ago, **but a clear-cut relationship between asbestos exposure and malignant mesothelioma is now firmly established.** Sometimes the exposure is slight, as in the wives of asbestos workers who wash their husbands' clothes. More often mesothelioma is found in workers heavily exposed to asbestos, predominantly of the crocidolite variety. The clinical and pathologic features of this disease are discussed with diseases of the pleura.

Carcinoma of the Lung and Other Organs

Carcinoma of the lung has been reported to be about three to five times more common in nonsmoking asbestos workers than in nonsmoking workers not exposed to asbestos, although this figure remains to be firmly established. In asbestos workers who smoke, the incidence of carcinoma of the lung is vastly increased, the risk being 60 to 80 times greater than in the general nonsmoking population. It is claimed by some that the incidence of carcinoma of the stomach and perhaps the colon is increased by asbestos exposure because fibers are not only inhaled but ingested. However, the evidence is not convincing at this time.

Asbestos Bodies

Since there are no associated pulmonary lesions, the incidental finding of asbestos bodies in autopsies does not warrant a diagnosis of pneumoconiosis. Digests and concentrates of lung tissue show that asbestos bodies occur in the lungs in virtually all autopsies.

Other Pneumoconioses

More than 40 inhaled minerals cause lung lesions and x-ray abnormalities. Most, such as tin, barium, and iron, are relatively innocuous and accumulate in the lung in the same way as coal, but do not produce morphologic or functional abnormalities. Others are uncommon and may or may not cause disability. Two substances are worth brief mention.

Berylliosis

Beryllium is used in the steel industry and was utilized in fluorescent lamps. It differs from other pneumoconiosis in that the amount and duration of exposure may be small and the lesion may be in part a hypersensitivity phenomenon. The lung lesions are granulomatous and identical to those seen in sarcoidosis.

Talcosis

Talcs are fibrous silicates used in a number of industries and in cosmetic talc. Inhalation of talc results in foreign body granulomas throughout the lung and in interstitial pulmonary fibrosis. Platelike crystals are readily identifiable in the granulomas. A related lesion is found in drug abusers who use talc as the carrier material for drugs injected intravenously.

Restrictive, Infiltrative, or Interstitial Lung Disease

More than 100 disorders are conveniently considered together because they have a similar clinical and radiologic presentation. Clinically, the patients present with shortness of breath, often associated with cough. Clubbing of the fingers is common in the advanced stage. Inspiratory crackles ("Velcro" rales) are heard at the bases. Chest radiographs have small linear and punctate opacities (Fig. 12-39). As the condition progresses, cystlike spaces become apparent. Lung volume is reduced because the lung is stiff (decreased compliance). The fibrosis is associated with increased elastic recoil, a condition that makes the airways more patent and is the driving force to increased flow rates. Diffusing capacity for carbon monoxide is decreased and the alveolar–arterial oxygen gradient is increased. Typically, the latter increases further on exercise, hence the older term "al-

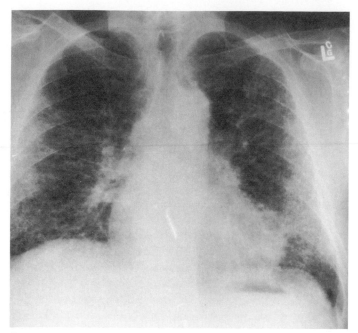

A

Figure 12-39.   Usual interstitial pneumonia. A 54-year-old man suffered from worsening shortness of breath on exertion for 5 years. On physical examination he had clubbing of the fingers and late inspiratory crackles. Pulmonary function tests showed severe impairment. (*A*) A chest radiograph shows increased reticulonodular markings and diminished lung volumes. (*B*) A CT scan obtained through the upper lobes shows peripheral honeycombing, as evidenced by the cystic spaces with dense fibrotic (white) walls and minimal involvement of the central lung parenchyma. Changes in the 10-mm collimation scan (a radiographic slice 10 mm thick) (*a*) are more clearly delineated on the 1.5-mm scan (*b*) because the images are not superimposed. The cystic spaces and fibrotic walls can be seen more clearly in *b*. (*c*) A macroscopic specimen of the right upper lobe cut at the level of the CT scan shows dense peripheral honeycombing. (*d*) A low-power microscopic view of the specimen shows irregular subpleural fibrosis, with cysts 2 to 10 mm in diameter.

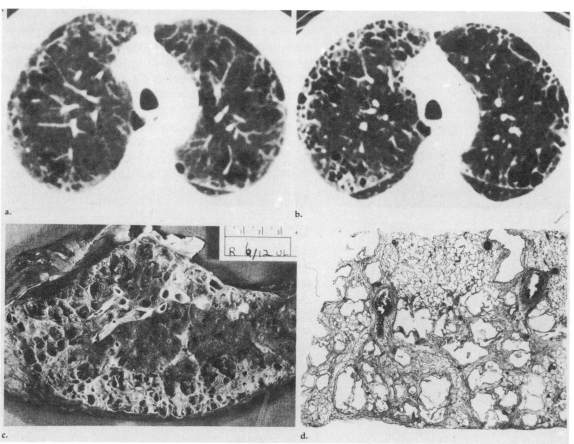

B

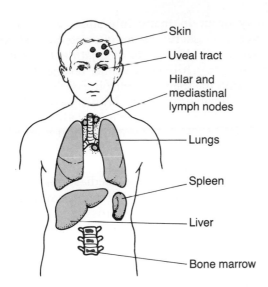

Figure 12-40. Organs commonly affected by sarcoidosis. Sarcoidosis involves many organs, most commonly the lymph nodes and lung.

veolar–arterial capillary block syndrome." Because of the reduction in lung volume, clinicians often refer to the condition as "restrictive lung disease," whereas the radiologic appearance leads radiologists to use the term "interstitial lung disease." Many of the conditions progress to "honeycomb" or "end-stage" lung.

Sarcoidosis

Sarcoidosis, a disease that has eluded a satisfactory definition, is characterized by multiple, uniform, discrete, noncaseating granulomas in almost any organ of the body. The lymph nodes and the lung are most commonly involved (Fig. 12-40). The central part of the granuloma is fibrotic and surrounded by palisaded histiocytes. Giant cells at the periphery resemble those of tuberculosis (Langhan's giant cells). The cuff of lymphocytes that surrounds the histiocytes is inconspicuous, compared with tuberculosis, hence the term "naked tubercle" (Fig. 12-41).

Pulmonary sarcoidosis is apparent by lung and hilar lymph node involvement (the most common), lymph node enlargement alone, or lung disease. Radiologically, there is a diffuse reticulonodular infiltrate, but in occasional cases larger nodules are present, a situation referred to as nodular or alveolar sarcoidosis. Histologically, involvement of both lung and lymph nodes occurs in nearly all instances. Multiple sarcoid nodules are scattered in the interstitium, particularly in relation to lymphatics, that is, in the bronchovascular bundle and in the lobular septa.

There is increased cellularity of the alveolar walls, owing to an infiltrate of mononuclear cells. Granulomas also occur in the airways and occasionally may be so prominent as to lead to airway obstruction (endobronchial sarcoid). The effects on pulmonary function are highly variable. There may be no abnormalities, classic restrictive lung disease, chronic airflow obstruction, or a mixture of restrictive and obstructive lung disease.

In North America sarcoidosis occurs much more frequently in blacks than in whites. It is common in Scandinavian countries. Fever, malaise, and weight loss are characteristic, and erythema nodosum is often seen. Hypercalcemia and small lytic lesions in bones, particularly of the hand, may be observed. Eye complications, such as iridocyclitis and uveitis, also occur. The disease also affects the extrathoracic lymph nodes, spleen, and liver.

Laboratory tests used to diagnose sarcoidosis include subcutaneous injection of Kveim antigen (an extract of spleen from a patient with sarcoidosis) and measurements of the serum level of angiotensin converting enzyme (ACE). About 6 weeks after injection of the Kveim antigen, an indurated granulomatous nodule appears in the skin. The test is seldom used, since the material is scarce. It is also derived from human material and may therefore be hazardous. It is now apparent that raised serum ACE is nonspecific

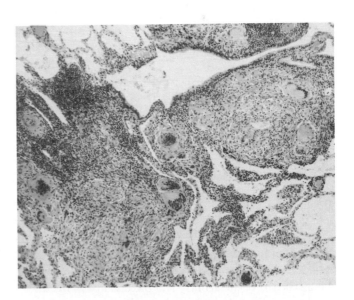

Figure 12-41. Sarcoidosis of the lung. A histologic section of the lung in a case of sarcoidosis shows several noncaseating granulomas that have become confluent. All are approximately the same size, at the same stage of development, and located around peribronchiolar lymphatics.

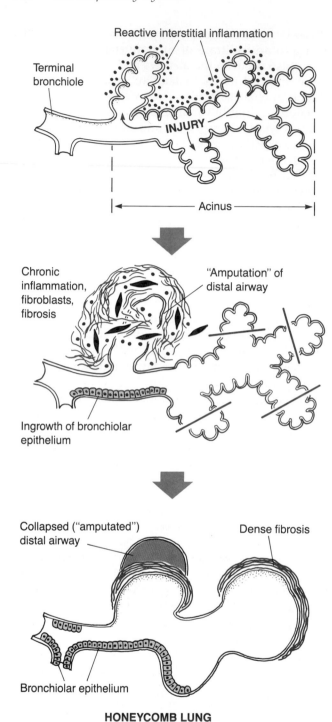

Figure 12-42.   Pathogenesis of honeycomb lung. Honeycomb lung is the end result of a variety of injuries. Interstitial and alveolar inflammation destroys ("amputates") the distal part of the acinus. The proximal parts dilate and become lined by bronchiolar epithelium.

and may occur in many interstitial lung diseases. However, it is useful for monitoring the activity of sarcoidosis and the effects of treatment. Most physicians now use **bronchoalveolar lavage** to monitor the cell content. (Saline is introduced into the distal lung via a flexible fiberoptic bronchoscope and then withdrawn.) The most reliable procedure for the diagnosis of sarcoidosis is **transbronchial lung biopsy,** a procedure in which lung tissue is obtained through a fiberoptic bronchoscope. Occasionally, biopsy of a mediastinal lymph node by mediastinoscopy is diagnostic. Most patients with sarcoidosis respond well to treatment with corticosteroids or spontaneously remit. However, some progress to end stage lung disease with honeycombing.

Pneumoconiosis

The most common cause of infiltrative lung disease is pneumoconiosis, most importantly asbestosis and silicosis. (See discussion above.)

The Interstitial Pneumonias (Fibrosing Alveolitis and Its Variants)

A group of conditions known as the chronic interstitial pneumonias can be regarded as one entity or can be subdivided. Various terms have been used for the group, for example, Hamman–Rich disease, fibrosing alveolitis, idiopathic pulmonary fibrosis, and usual interstitial pneumonia. It is important to note that although the various forms of interstitial pneumonia may be morphologically and, to some extent, clinically distinctive, they all progress to a nonspecific "honeycomb" or "end-stage" lung. Because of alveolitis and subsequent fibrosis, the distal part of the acinus shrinks (Fig. 12-42). In a sense the lesion represents a form of atelectasis and is the reverse of emphysema. With shrinkage of the lung parenchyma, the bronchioles dilate. Because of epithelial damage the bronchiolar epithelium grows into the dilated airspaces that may have been proximal respiratory bronchioles but are no longer recognized as such. The end stage is characterized by multiple cyst-like spaces separated from each other by dense scars (see Figs. 12-39, 12-42). Retraction of the scar, especially of lobular septa, gives the external surface of the lung a hob-nailed appearance, hence the term "pseudocirrhosis."

On histologic examination, the "cysts" (in reality, dilated bronchioles) are found to contain mucus and other debris. Bronchi may also be slightly dilated and irregular. Extensive vascular changes, particularly intimal fibrosis and thickening of the media, are caused by inflammation, fibrosis, and pulmonary hypertension.

Usual Interstitial Pneumonia (Cryptogenic Fibrosing Alveolitis, Idiopathic Pulmonary Fibrosis)

Each of the terms *usual interstitial pneumonia, cryptogenic fibrosing alveolitis,* and *idiopathic pulmonary fibrosis* stresses certain features—the cause is unknown, alveolar inflammation is an important part of the disease, fibrosis is the usual sequel, and there may be unusual forms of interstitial pneumonia. The clinical, radiologic, and functional features are those of restrictive lung disease (Fig. 12-39). A useful classification of usual interstitial pneumonia is as follows, but it should be recognized that the morphologic features are the same in each:

Usual interstitial pneumonia associated with collagen vascular diseases. These include rheumatoid arthritis, systemic lupus erythematosis, and progressive systemic sclerosis. About 20% of cases of usual interstitial pneumonia have overt evidence of a connective tissue disease.
Usual interstitial pneumonia associated with serum abnormalities but not with collagen vascular disease. These include cryoglobulinemia, abnormal serum globulins, positive antinuclear antibodies, and positive rheumatoid factor (rarely positive in the absence of rheumatoid arthritis). These abnormalities have been found in up to 40% of cases.
Usual interstitial pneumonia without overt evidence of collagen vascular disease or serum abnormalities.

The key morphologic feature of usual interstitial pneumonia is heterogeneity of lesions, that is, different appearances in different parts of the lung, in different lung biopsies, and even in different fields of the same lung biopsy. The variation is so great that in some fields the alveolar walls are entirely normal. Inflammation varies from subtle increased cellularity (mainly lymphocytes) of otherwise apparently normal alveolar walls to diffuse alveolar damage with obvious alveolar wall inflammation and hyperplasia of type II cells. Lymphoid aggregates are also seen. By the time a lung biopsy is performed fibrosis is always present, but its severity varies. There may be subtle alveolar wall thickening, detectable only by special stains for collagen. In other cases fibrosis may be obvious but alveolar walls may be maintained, although the acinar structure is somewhat simplified. At the extreme is honeycomb lung, brought about by alveolar wall inflammation and collapse. This condition is characteristically most prominent subpleurally in the lower zones of the lung (Fig. 12-39). Electron microscopic examination reveals gross distortion and infolding of the alveolar basal lamina in the fibrotic areas. Loose granulation tissue in the alveolar spaces leads to alveolar collapse and contraction of fibrous tissue.

Interstitial pneumonia is usually diagnosed in the sixth decade. Dyspnea of gradual onset, often over 5 to 10 years, is customary. About one quarter of all cases date their illness to an acute bronchopulmonary infection, an observation that raises the possibility that the disease is a sequel to viral infection. The classic auscultatory finding consists of fine crackles at the lung bases in late inspiration. The prognosis is bleak, with an average survival of 5 years. The response to treatment, usually corticosteroids, is generally poor.

The etiology of usual interstitial pneumonia is not known, but the condition is usually thought of as an immunologically mediated disorder. Evidence includes the association with collagen-vascular disease and serum protein abnormalities, the presence of circulating immune complexes, the presence of immunoglobulins in alveolar walls, and the release of a lymphokine, migration inhibitory factor, when lymphocytes of patients with the disease are exposed to collagen.

According to one theory, macrophages play a central role in the pathogenesis of usual interstitial pneumonia, and the initial damage is to collagen, by an unknown agent. Macrophages engulf collagen fragments and secrete a fibroblast-stimulating factor, thereby leading to fibrosis. They also release a chemotactic factor for polymorphonuclear leukocytes, which then do further damage. Histologically, neutrophils are not a prominent feature, except in the infected cystic spaces. However, the bronchoalveolar lavage fluid contains increased numbers of neutrophils.

Desquamative Interstitial Pneumonia

Desquamative interstitial pneumonia (DIP) is an uncommon disease characterized by interstitial inflammation and a striking accumulation of macrophages in the alveoli. Opinion is equally divided on whether it is a separate entity or a stage of usual interstitial pneumonia. However, it is important to recognize that desquamative interstitial pneumonia has distinctive clinical features, prognosis, and response to treatment. The patients are younger than those with usual interstitial pneumonia (mean age of 46 years), the symptoms are of shorter duration (2 to 3 years), and the chest radiographs show a fine density (ground glass opacity), most obvious in the costophrenic angles. Pulmonary function changes are slight, and lung volumes do not change. Most patients respond to corticosteroid therapy, and survival is at least twice that of usual interstitial pneumonia. On histologic examination, desquamative interstitial pneumonia is diagnosed by the presence of airspaces stuffed with macrophages. It was originally thought that the cells in the airspaces are desquamated type II epithelial cells, an interpretation that lent the condition its name. However, electron microscopy has shown that the cells are macrophages. The lung architecture remains intact, so that the alveoli are readily recognized. The walls display a mononuclear infiltrate, and there is type II metaplasia of the alveolar lining cells. Fibrosis is slight or nonexistent. The pathogenesis and etiology of DIP are not understood.

Lymphoid Interstitial Pneumonia

Lymphoid interstitial pneumonia is characterized by an infiltrate of mononuclear cells, mostly lymphocytes, restricted to the interstitium. The lung structure is intact and the cells mainly infiltrate alveolar walls, with lesser involvement of perivascular sheaths and lobular septae. It is an uncommon condition, perhaps one fourth as frequent as desquamative interstitial pneumonia. It is often associated with abnormal serum gammaglobulins, of which IgA and IgG are the most common. Lymphocytic interstitial pneumonia is sometimes associated with Sjogren's syndrome, a disorder characterized by a similar infiltrate in the salivary or lacrimal glands. As in the case of Sjogren's disease, lymphoma has developed in some cases of lymphocytic interstitial pneumonia, but in the great majority of instances the infiltrate remains confined to the lungs. Although the disease may progress to an end stage lung, it is usually an indolent condition that gradually progresses to respiratory failure. It can be a complication of AIDS, especially in children.

Lymphocytic interstitial pneumonia is but one example of **lymphoproliferative disorders of the lung** that belong in the gray zone between inflammation and neoplasia. Well-differentiated lymphocytic lymphoma of the lung has been mentioned, and a condition called *pseudolymphoma of the lung* has been proposed. Although criteria have been established to separate the two entities, in reality their prognosis is the same. A small proportion of patients with well-differentiated lymphocytic lymphoma of the lung develop overt lymphoma; the same is true of pseudolymphoma, and it is easy to regard them as the same condition. Lymphomatoid granulomatosis is discussed later and also falls into this category, but it clearly behaves as a malignant lymphoma.

Bronchiolitis Obliterans and Organizing Pneumonia

Recently, a clearly defined condition, bronchiolitis obliterans and organizing pneumonia, has been recognized by its histologic features, namely, the presence of bronchiolitis obliterans (i.e., loose granulation tissue in respiratory bronchioles); abundant loose granulation tissue in alveolar ducts and sacs, which resemble the Masson bodies of organizing pneumonia; interstitial pneumonia; diffuse alveolar damage; and interstitial fibrosis of varying severity, but usually mild. Often there is a history of preexisting respiratory infection. This disease entity is important to recognize because its prognosis is good and it responds to corticosteroid treatment.

Giant Cell Interstitial Pneumonia and Cellular Interstitial Pneumonia

Giant cell interstitial pneumonia and cellular interstitial pneumonia are inadequately documented conditions. Giant cell interstitial pneumonia was distinguished by the presence in airspaces of numerous giant cells formed by macrophages. Characteristically, neutrophils were found in the giant cells, either phagocytosed or as transient guests. The disorder is probably a variant of desquamative interstitial pneumonia. In **cellular interstitial pneumonia** the heterogeneity of lesions of usual interstitial pneumonia is not present, and severe interstitial pneumonia with diffuse alveolar damage predominates. It has been suggested that cellular interstitial pneumonia may be a feature of a collagen-vascular disease that is rapidly progressive, particularly associated with circulating immune complexes, and equivalent to the original cases described by Hamman and Rich.

Eosinophilic Granuloma of the Lung

The histologic appearance of eosinophilic granuloma in the lung is comparable to that elsewhere, notably in bone. The lesions consist of aggregates of macrophages that have large nuclei with open chromatin and are often notched. When cut longitudinally, the notch appears as a central bar through the nucleus.

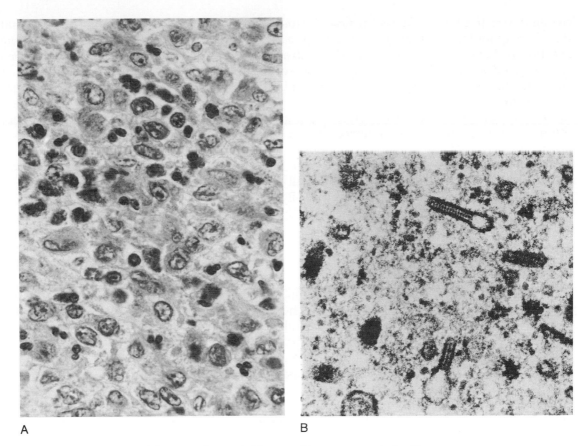

Figure 12-43. Eosinophilic granuloma. A 21-year-old man presented with pneumothorax. (*A*) Microscopically, the characteristic lesions of eosinophilic granuloma contain both Langerhans cells (large, pale macrophages, often with indented nuclei) and eosinophils (dark nuclei). (*B*) An electron micrograph shows intracytoplasmic (Birbeck) granules. Some resemble tennis rackets, with the characteristic structure in the "handle."

The cytoplasm is abundant and eosinophilic, and the cell margins are well defined (Fig. 12-43). Varying numbers of eosinophils are present in the nodular lesion. The combination of histiocytes and eosinophils gives the condition its name. The histiocytes contain inclusions (Birbeck granules; Fig. 12-43) similar to those in the Langerhans cells of the skin. Similar cells are occasionally encountered in the bronchiolar epithelium of the normal lung and in about one third of all cases of usual interstitial pneumonia and its variants. However, in eosinophilic granuloma the cells are more profuse and contain bizarre forms of the granules, which may resemble tennis rackets or even an octopus complete with tentacles (Fig. 12-43B). The presence of these histiocytes and eosinophils and the course of the disease suggest that eosinophilic granuloma is an inflammatory response to an unidentified infectious agent.

In the early stage of the lesion, there is a nodular infiltrate at the center and the periphery of the aci-

nus. It is the latter situation at the pleura that leads to pneumothorax. The lesions excavate and discharge their content into the airways, and the X cells may then be recognized in the sputum. Healing by scarring results in the formation of large cysts.

Eosinophilic granuloma of the lung is primarily a disease of young adults and usually presents as dyspnea. About 20% of patients have spontaneous pneumothorax in the course of the disease. Radiologically, it differs from other forms of infiltrative lung disease in that it is mainly upper zonal and large cystic spaces may be apparent. In fact, it was the first condition described under the heading "honeycomb lung." In most cases, the lesion is limited to the lung, but in some the disease may affect bones (usually the ribs) or may be disseminated. When the base of the skull is affected, particularly the orbit (with proptosis) and pituitary (with diabetes insipidus), eosinophilic granuloma of the lung is regarded as a complication of the Hand–(Weber)–Schüler–Christian syndrome. Involvement of the lung in cases of disseminated eosinophilic granuloma is thought to represent a complication of Letterer–Siwe's disease, although many of the cases are probably lymphomas. Because of the heterogeneity of presentations, despite the similarity of the histologic appearance, the conditions are often collectively referred to as histiocytosis X, and the abnormal Langerhans cells are referred to as X cells.

The prognosis of eosinophilic granuloma of the lung is controversial. When it is limited to the lung and diagnosed by lung biopsy, some 80% of all cases remain the same or improve, 15% gradually get worse, and 5% die of respiratory failure.

Extrinsic Allergic Alveolitis

Extrinsic allergic alveolitis is a response to inhaled allergens, usually large proteins (Fig. 12-44). The prototype is "farmer's lung," caused by the inhalation of thermophilic actinomycetes, notably *Micropolyspora faeni.* These organisms grow in moldy hay. The disease is well documented in the west of England and in the United States, where it is best known in Wisconsin. Classically, a farmworker enters a barn shortly after animals have changed from grazing to eating hay and rapidly develops tightness in the chest, shortness of breath, cough, and mild fever. The lag period is several hours, so the symptoms may only appear after leaving the barn. The symptoms remit but return on reexposure. However, with time the symptoms become chronic. More important, in many instances the initial symptoms may not be noticed or may be attributed to a "virus," and the patient may present with slowly progressive dyspnea, as in usual interstitial pneumonia. In the rare instances in which tissue has been studied in the acute phase, bronchiolar necrosis, eosinophilic infiltrate, vasculitis, and interstitial pneumonia were observed.

More often patients are seen in the subacute or chronic phase, when the biopsy is characteristic. An extensive interstitial pneumonia is characterized by a heavy infiltrate (Fig. 12-45) of lymphocytes and a few plasma cells in the alveolar walls, an appearance resembling that of lymphocytic interstitial pneumonia. Mild diffuse alveolar damage is usually present. Unlike lymphocytic interstitial pneumonia, there is a significant bronchiolar infiltrate, sometimes with bronchiolitis obliterans. As a consequence, focal areas of endogenous lipid pneumonia are seen. **Most characteristic is the presence of scattered, poorly formed granulomas (see Fig. 12-45) that contain foreign body giant cells, some of which exhibit doubly refractile material or needlelike clefts.** The nature of this material is unknown but is thought to be particles in the dusty hay. The lung architecture is usually recognizable, but mild fibrosis may occur, usually in the alveolar walls. In the chronic (end-stage) phase, the interstitial inflammation recedes, but fibrosis is more apparent, the lung architecture is distorted, and honeycombing occurs.

Besides material in moldy hay there are more than 20 other substances that produce extrinsic allergic alveolitis. In pigeon breeder's or bird fancier's lung, the antigen is bird protein. The common bird is the parakeet, but chicken handlers also develop the condition. Other rare causes of extrinsic allergic alveolitis include pituitary snuff, fungi in bark (maple bark stripper's lung), cork (suberosis), malt, mushrooms, and detergents. Ingested drugs, notably methotrexate, also produce a similar lesion. It is important to realize that there may be no apparent antigen exposure and that extrinsic allergic alveolitis may be caused by fungi growing in stagnant water in air conditioners and central heating units. It is essential to distinguish extrinsic allergic alveolitis from usual interstitial pneumonia because removal of the antigen is the only adequate treatment.

Lymphangiomyomatosis

In the rare condition of lymphangiomyomatosis a bizarre proliferation of smooth muscle cells in the lung involves the smooth muscle of lymphatics, arteries, veins, bronchioles, and alveolar walls. The resulting diffuse cystic appearance of the lung differs from the honeycomb lung in that the cysts are large (a few centimeters rather than a few millimeters in diameter), are lined by alveolar epithelium, and con-

Figure 12-44.   Extrinsic allergic alveolitis. In extrinsic allergic alveolitis, an antigen–antibody reaction occurs in the acute phase and leads to acute hypersensitivity pneumonitis. If exposure is continued, this is followed by a cellular or subacute phase, with the formation of granulomas and chronic interstitial pneumonitis.

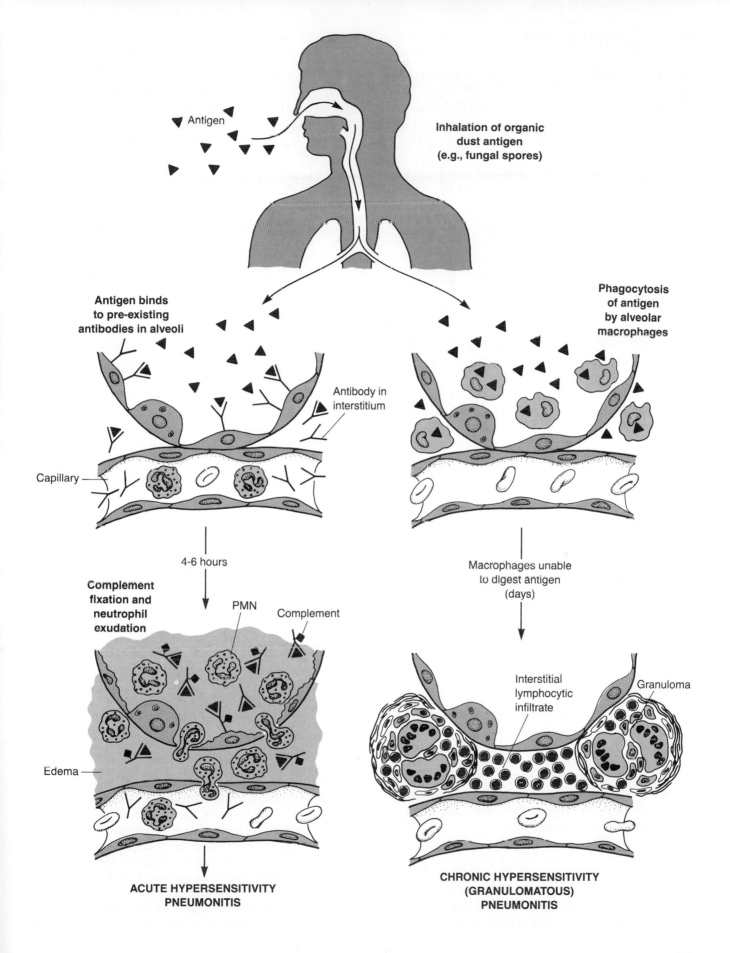

Antigen

Inhalation of organic
dust antigen
(e.g., fungal spores)

Antigen binds
to pre-existing
antibodies in alveoli

Phagocytosis
of antigen
by alveolar
macrophages

Antibody in
interstitium

Capillary

4-6 hours

Macrophages unable
to digest antigen
(days)

Complement
fixation and
neutrophil
exudation

PMN

Complement

Interstitial
lymphocytic
infiltrate

Granuloma

Edema

ACUTE HYPERSENSITIVITY
PNEUMONITIS

CHRONIC HYPERSENSITIVITY
(GRANULOMATOUS)
PNEUMONITIS

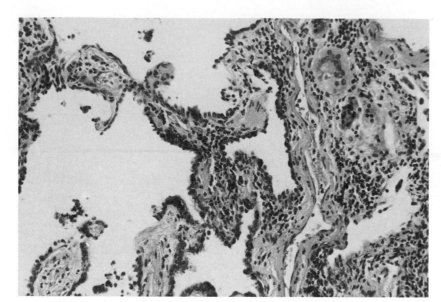

Figure 12-45. Extrinsic allergic alveolitis. A microscopic section of extrinsic allergic alveolitis shows interstitial pneumonia, poorly formed granulomas, and a giant cell containing an inclusion (*top right*). Note the presence of interstitial fibrosis, disorganization of alveolar structures, and type II cell metaplasia. The disease has progressed to end-stage lung.

tain smooth muscle in their walls. The lung is increased in size and loses elastic recoil. The functional effect is thus obstructive rather than restrictive, a situation equivalent to emphysema. The pathogenesis is not clear. Bronchiolar obstruction by smooth muscle may lead to air trapping distortion of the lung, or the proliferated parenchymal smooth muscle may itself distort the lung tissue. The proliferation of venous smooth muscle results in venous occlusion, pulmonary hemorrhage, and hemosiderosis. The involvement of lymphatic channels by smooth muscle proliferation leads to lymph node enlargement in the thorax and elsewhere. Smooth muscle proliferation of lymphatic ducts may lead to their occlusion and to the accumulation of chyle in the pleural cavity (chylothorax). Since identical lesions of the lung and lymph nodes may be seen in tuberous sclerosis, some hold that lymphangiomyomatosis is a *forme fruste* of that disease. However, the other typical brain and skin lesions of tuberous sclerosis are absent, and no evidence exists of a family history.

Lymphangiomyomatosis is exclusively a disease of women, almost always of child-bearing age. Dyspnea is the usual presenting symptom and reflects the pulmonary lesion, chylothorax or pneumothorax. Oophorectomy has produced good results, as has the administration of progesterone.

Noninfectious Angiitis and Granulomatosis

Five rare conditions are traditionally grouped together, although they represent very different disease processes with widely varying prognoses.

Wegener's Granulomatosis

Wegener's granulomatosis is the most common of the five but is rare nonetheless. As originally described, it consisted of a triad of systemic necrotizing vasculitis, necrotizing granulomas of the respiratory tract and glomerulonephritis. It is today regarded as a variant of necrotizing angiitis. Wegener's granulomatosis most commonly affects middle-aged men. The presenting symptoms include sinusitis, middle ear disease, and nonspecific respiratory symptoms. Radiologic examination shows single or, more commonly, multiple intrapulmonary nodules, some of which may cavitate. Ocular and skin lesions are also frequent. When there is no evidence of kidney disease or vasculitis, the term *limited Wegener's granulomatosis* has been used. When left untreated, this variant does not have the invariably fatal course that originally characterized the full-blown syndrome.

Glomerulonephritis is usual in Wegener's granulomatosis and generally rapidly progressive. A dramatic improvement in prognosis has resulted from cytotoxic therapy, changing a formerly fatal condition to one with a 90% to 95% remission rate.

The lesions in the respiratory tract show necrotizing granulomas, characteristically with serpiginous margins, in which there are numerous bizarre giant cells. Necrotizing vasculitis involves the branches of the pulmonary arteries or the systemic arteries in the respiratory tract and helps to establish the diagnosis. Focal glomerular necrosis and crescent formation are seen in the kidneys. The possibility of infectious conditions should be rigorously excluded in patients who have Wegener's granulomatosis limited to the lung.

Churg–Strauss Syndrome (Allergic Angiitis and Granulomatosis)

A subset of patients with asthma have pulmonary infiltrates (primarily due to eosinophilic pneumonia) and vasculitis of both the pulmonary and systemic circulations, characterized by an eosinophilic infiltrate with granulomas. Extravascular granulomas are accompanied by blood eosinophilia. Glomerulitis is also common but is usually asymptomatic. This rare condition is best thought of as a variant of periarteritis nodosa that affects the lung and is thus a relative, albeit a distant one, of Wegener's granulomatosis. It is responsive to corticosteroids.

Necrotizing Sarcoidal Granulomatosis

Necrotizing sarcoidal granulomatosis morphologically resembles sarcoidosis, but it differs in that there is extensive confluent necrosis or multiple punctate necrotic areas in individual granulomas. In addition, pulmonary vasculitis is prominent. Granulomas aggregate about the external elastic lamina of pulmonary arteries or extend through the vessel wall to occlude the lumen. Most authorities consider the disorder to be a variant of sarcoidosis. Radiologically, necrotizing sarcoidal granulomatosis is characterized by numerous well-circumscribed nodules in the lungs, an appearance described in the radiologic literature as "nodular" or "alveolar" sarcoidosis. The prognosis is excellent.

Bronchocentric Granulomatosis

In bronchocentric granulomatosis the airways are filled with cheeselike necrotic material. Granulomatous inflammation extends through and destroys the airway walls. Inflammation involves the adjacent pulmonary arteries, and occlusion of the airways produces lipid pneumonia. Patients with asthma closely resemble those with allergic bronchopulmonary aspergillosis. A substantial proportion of patients diagnosed as having bronchocentric granulomatosis probably suffer really from aspergillosis. Other patients may represent a granulomatous reaction to known infectious agents. However, a significant number of cases with bronchocentric granulomatosis are not due to allergic bronchopulmonary aspergillosis or to infectious granulomatosis.

Lymphomatoid Granulomatosis

Lymphomatoid granulomatosis was first separated from Wegener's granulomatosis on the basis of an angiocentric, angioinvasive infiltrate of pleomorphic lymphoreticular cells. The infiltrate is described as "polymorphous," meaning it is composed of a variety of cells, including lymphocytes, plasma cells, occasional neutrophils, and characteristically abnormal lymphoreticular cells that resemble immunoblasts. Multiple nodules are found in the lung, brain, and kidneys. Involvement of the lymph nodes, spleen, and bone marrow is uncommon. The disease, most common in the middle-aged, has a very poor prognosis, about half of the patients dying within 6 months of diagnosis. It is now apparent that many cases are in reality lymphomas limited to the lung, usually "histiocytic" lymphoma, polymorphous reticulosis, or immunoblastic sarcoma. Newer studies suggest that the disease is probably a T cell lymphoma. However, a few cases seem to be distinct from lymphoma. The term lymphomatoid granulomatosis should be reserved for such cases.

Diseases of the Pleura

Pneumothorax

Pneumothorax is defined as the presence of air in the pleural cavity. It may be due to traumatic perforation of the pleura or may be spontaneous. Traumatic causes include penetrating wounds of the chest wall (e.g., a stab wound and rib fractures). However, traumatic pneumothorax is most commonly iatrogenic and is seen after aspiration of fluid from the pleura, pleural or lung biopsy, transbronchial biopsy, and assisted ventilation with interstitial emphysema. **Spontaneous pneumothorax** is typically encountered in young adults. For example, while exercising vigorously a tall young man develops acute chest pain and shortness of breath. A chest radiograph shows collapse of the lung on the side of the pain and a large collection of air in the pleural space. The condition is due to rupture of emphysematous lesions, usually paraseptal emphysema, through the pleura. These lesions are usually placed superficially and superiorly in the lung. In most cases, spontaneous pneumothorax subsides by itself with or without aspiration of the air. In other instances large amounts of air accumulate in the pleural cavity, and there may be a shift of the mediastinum to the opposite side, with compression of the opposite lung. This situation is referred to as "tension pneumothorax" and implies that the pressure is positive in the pleural space. The condition may be life-threatening and must be relieved by immediate drainage. Spontaneous pneumothorax may also complicate widespread emphysema in the middle-aged and, rarely, other lung conditions, such as tumors.

Bronchopleural fistula, a serious condition in which there is free communication between the airway and the pleura, is usually iatrogenic, caused by the interruption of bronchial continuity by biopsy or surgery. It may also be due to extensive infection and necrosis of lung tissue, in which case the infection is more important than the air.

Pleural Effusion

Normally, only a small amount of fluid in the pleural cavity lubricates the space between the lung and the chest wall. It is thought that fluid is secreted into the pleural space from the parietal pleura and absorbed by the visceral pleura. The conventional explanation is that capillary pressure is higher in the systemic than the pulmonary bed. The visceral pleura also has a rich capillary bed, but "stomata," openings large enough for red cells to enter, are present on the parietal surfaces of both the rib cage and the mediastinum.

Pleural effusion is a term that describes the accumulation of fluid in the pleural cavity and is subdivided according to the appearance of the effusion. The severity varies, from a few milliliters of fluid detected radiologically only as obliteration of the costophrenic angle to a massive accumulation of fluid that shifts the mediastinum and the trachea to the opposite side (see Fig. 12-46A).

Hydrothorax refers to an effusion that resembles water and would be regarded as edema elsewhere. It may be due to increased hydrostatic pressure within the capillaries, as is commonly found in patients with heart failure and in any condition that produces systemic or pulmonary edema. In this form of effusion the protein level is less than 3 g/dl, the number of white cells is low, and the glucose level is close to that of the blood. Similar findings may be found in patients with low serum osmotic pressure, as in renal failure, cirrhosis of the liver, or severe starvation. Whatever the cause, this type of effusion is referred to as a **transudate.** By contrast, fluid that accumulates in the pleural cavity because of increased capillary permeability is referred to as an **exudate.** The common cause of hydrothorax due to exudation is low-grade inflammation, such as that associated with tumor or tuberculosis. Typically, protein levels are more than 3 g/dl, glucose levels are low, and the cellular content is high. The pleural fluid content of lactate dehydrogenase (LDH) is often used as an indicator of inflammation. A ratio of pleural fluid/plasma LDH of more than 0.6 is considered indicative of an exudate. A protein-rich exudate may clot and leave a delicate spiderweb structure. Other important causes of pleural effusion are the collagen-vascular diseases (notably systemic lupus erythematosus and rheumatoid arthritis) and asbestosis.

A turbid effusion that contains many polymorphonuclear leukocytes is referred to as **pyothorax** and results from acute inflammation and infections of the pleura. This may occasionally be caused by an external penetrating wound that brings pyogenic organisms into the pleural space. More commonly, it is a complication of bacterial pneumonia that extends to the pleural surface, the classic example of which is pneumococcal pneumonia. Pyothorax is a rare complication of medical procedures involving the pleural cavity. **Empyema** should be thought of as a variant of pyothorax in which the inflammation is both more severe and chronic, with accumulation of thick pus within the pleural cavity, often with loculation and fibrosis. Empyema has the same causes as pyothorax and was once a dreaded complication of chest infection, since it was often chronic and required prolonged drainage. This is not necessarily the case now.

Hemothorax is the accumulation of blood in the pleural cavity. This may occur because of trauma and is usually due to bleeding from systemic (intercostal) vessels. Most commonly, a pleural effusion is blood-stained. The common causes are tuberculosis, malignancy involving the pleura, and infarction of the lung.

Chyle may accumulate in the pleural cavity (**chylothorax**). This is due to obstruction of lymphatic ducts. The high lipid content renders the fluid turbid and milky. This condition has an ominous portent, because obstruction of the ducts suggests disease of the lymph nodes in the posterior mediastinum. It is thus found as a rare complication of malignant tumor or lymphoma in the mediastinum. It is also a common complication of the rare pulmonary lymphangiomyomatosis (described earlier). In tropical countries chylothorax results from nematode infestations and is responsive to antiparasitic therapy.

Pleuritis

As the name indicates, pleuritis means inflammation of the pleura and is thus frequently associated with pleural effusion. The causes are the same as for pyothorax, but other causes, such as viral infection and pulmonary embolus, are important. Symptoms are usually evident, the most striking being sharp, stabbing chest pain on inspiration. An accumulation of eosinophils in the pleura, as a consequence of pleural rupture and subacute inflammation in spontaneous pneumothorax, is termed eosinophilic pleuritis. Since eosinophilic pleuritis bears a superficial resemblance to eosinophilic granuloma, it is important to recognize it, because eosinophilic granuloma of the lung frequently presents as a spontaneous pneumothorax and has a more serious prognosis

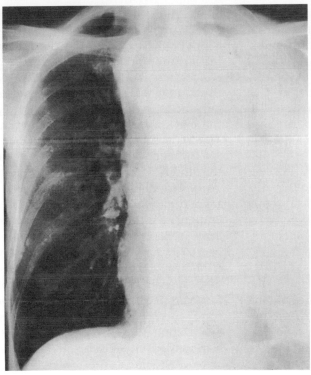
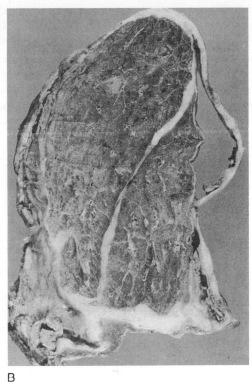

A   B

Figure 12-46. Mesothelioma. A 54-year-old former shipyard worker presented with shortness of breath of 3 months duration. (*A*) A chest radiograph shows a massive left pleural effusion. Note that the trachea and bronchus are displaced to the right, away from the effusion. (*B*) At autopsy extensive mesothelioma surrounds the lung and extends into the major fissure.

than spontaneous pneumothorax of young adults. Eosinophilic pleuritis is confined to the pleura and lacks the characteristic X (Langerhans) cells of eosinophilic granuloma.

Pleural Plaques*

Pleural plaques are dense, hard, white circumscribed lesions, usually of the parietal pleura. These lesions, usually a few millimeters thick and a few centimeters across and sometimes calcified, are most commonly found in the lower chest. Histologically, they show dense collagenous scarring with intersecting bands of collagen (basket-weave pattern). Clinically, they are usually recognized as incidental findings on chest radiographs, and their calcification aids in that recognition. They are common at autopsy, occurring in 1% to 10% of all cases, depending on the population. It is now known that they are usually a manifestation of asbestos exposure, most commonly at a very low level. Thus, they are frequently found in patients

living downwind from asbestos-using plants, in manual laborers not working continuously with asbestos, and in those who live in areas with high asbestos usage.

Mesothelioma

Malignant Mesothelioma*

As mentioned earlier, most cases of pleural malignant mesothelioma are related to asbestos exposure. This disease is most commonly encountered in middle-aged men exposed to asbestos, even for a short time. The patient often presents with a pleural effusion (Fig. 12-46*A*) or a pleural mass, chest pain, dyspnea, and nonspecific symptoms, such as weight loss and malaise. On cytologic examination, aspirated pleural fluid in patients with mesothelioma may be morphologically similar to reactive mesothelial cells associated with inflammation. Biopsy specimens of the pleura may pose similar diagnostic difficulties because metastatic tumors of the pleura may closely mimic mesotheliomas.

*Also see Asbestosis

Characteristically, mesotheliomas exhibit a biphasic histologic appearance. The cells derived from mesothelium form glands and tubules that resemble adenocarcinoma, whereas the malignant cells that originate from the connective tissue deep in the mesothelial surface resemble a fibrosarcoma. The two components are sometimes intimately entwined. In some instances, only the epithelial component is apparent, in which case it is impossible to distinguish mesothelioma from adenocarcinoma. Less commonly, only the connective tissue component is seen, and the histologic appearance is identical to that of a fibrosarcoma. Cell markers and electron microscopy have not provided a clear distinction between mesothelioma and other malignant tumors, notably adenocarcinoma. The most useful criteria for the diagnosis of mesothelioma are the absence of mucin (as evidenced by a negative neutral mucin stain), the presence of hyaluronic acid, and the presence of long microvilli by electron microscopy. Even these are imprecise, and often the diagnosis is made with certainty only at autopsy. On gross examination, the tumor classically encases the lung, extends into fissures and interlobar septa (see Fig. 12-46B), and compresses the lung. Lung invasion is usually limited to the periphery adjacent to the tumor, and lymph nodes are often spared. The lesion may be limited to the thorax, but in about a quarter of the cases metastases appear elsewhere. Treatment is ineffective and the prognosis is hopeless.

Benign (Localized) Mesotheliomas

Benign mesotheliomas are superficial tumors that have a pleural base and resemble benign connective tissue tumors, usually fibromas but occasionally hemangiopericytomas. They are thought to be derived from the submesothelial connective tissue of the pleura. Those benign tumors are well circumscribed and are 3 cm to 10 cm across. Hypoglycemia is a rare associated feature.

Diseases of Pulmonary Vasculature

Pulmonary Embolism

The most common lesion of the pulmonary vasculature is pulmonary embolism, and the most common emboli are thrombi derived from the leg veins. When a careful search is made of the lungs at autopsy, thromboemboli are so frequently encountered that some have regarded them as a normal phenom-

enon. More realistically, thromboemboli are found in one quarter to one third of random autopsies when a thorough search of the pulmonary vasculature is made. They are most common in circumstances in which there is a tendency to increased venous thrombosis, for instance, when venous blood flow is diminished, as in heart failure, prolonged bed rest, traumatic injury, or prolonged sitting in an airplane seat. The commonest sources of thromboembolism are the deep veins of the calf, followed by those of the thigh. Superficial veins are rarely sources. Thromboemboli are also derived from thrombi around indwelling lines in the systemic venous system or the pulmonary artery. Occasionally, they may arise from mural thrombi on the right side of the heart. Emboli are found most often where blood flow is highest, that is, the lower zones of the lung and in the posterior regions, the latter because many patients are recumbent. A variety of consequences may result from thromboembolism, including sudden death, infarction of the lung, and pulmonary embolism without infarction.

Sudden Death

The most dramatic consequence of pulmonary embolism is sudden death. The classic scenario involves a patient who suddenly drops dead, several days after surgery, sometimes while sitting on the toilet. A large embolus is commonly found in the main pulmonary artery, occluding both right and left pulmonary arteries (saddle embolus, Figure 12-47). However, almost as frequently a single pulmonary artery or even a segmental pulmonary artery is occluded. The cause of death in such cases is not clear, since ligation of one pulmonary artery, as in a pneumonectomy, does not cause death. Several suggestions have been made to explain this phenomenon. Reflex constriction of the pulmonary circulation is one.

Infarction of the Lung

As with other organs, occlusion of a pulmonary artery or a branch thereof may result in death of tissue. The lung differs from most other organs in that it has a dual circulation with both systemic (bronchial artery) and nonsystemic (pulmonary artery) contributions. The bronchial arteries supply the airways to about the terminal bronchiolar level, but actual and potential anastomoses exist between the two systems. **As a consequence, pulmonary infarcts are often hemorrhagic in the acute phase because the**

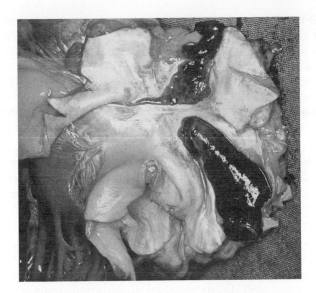

Figure 12-47. Pulmonary embolus. Upon ambulation, several days after surgery, a large embolus at the bifurcation of the main pulmonary artery caused sudden death. The right ventricle and pulmonary valve are at the left. The embolus is in the main pulmonary artery, one branch of which is in the top right-hand corner; the other branch (*bottom right*) contains most of the embolus.

bronchial artery pumps blood into the infarcted area. On gross examination, such infarcts are usually pyramidal (triangular in cross section), with the base at the pleura. Since the end supply of the pulmonary arterial system is at segmental margins as well as pleural surfaces, the infarcts may also occur within the substance of the lung. With the passage of time the blood in the infarct is resorbed and the center of the infarct becomes pale. Vascular granulation tissue forms on the edge of the infarct, after which it is organized to form a fibrous scar. Although the scar may be quite small, it affects a large volume of lung, since there is not only contraction of lung parenchyma but also loss of the air contained in the parenchyma (6 ml to 7 ml of air per gram of lung).

Pulmonary Embolism Without Infarction

Pulmonary thromboemboli are frequently found at autopsy without infarcts. This finding might be anticipated in cases of sudden death from pulmonary embolism, but it also occurs with emboli that reached the lung some time previously. Pulmonary embolism without infarction is explained by the bronchial artery collateral circulation, which keeps lung tissue viable. Similarly, a clinical diagnosis of pulmonary embolism may be made (on the basis of angor animi [a feeling of impending death], chest discomfort, and transient dyspnea) in the absence of radiologic evidence of infarction. Nuclear ventilation/perfusion scans are helpful in thte clinical diagnosis of pulmonary embolism. Regional ventilation is assessed by the inhalation of radioactive gas or aerosols, and perfusions are assessed by the injection of radioactive material; both are detected with an external gamma counter.

In the clinical syndrome of "partial infarction," a patient has the clinical and radiologic findings of pulmonary infarction due to thromboembolism but the lesion resolves instead of contracting to leave a scar. In such cases, hemorrhage and necrosis of the epithelium in the affected area occur but the tissue framework remains. Collateral circulation maintains the viability of the bulk of tissue and enables regeneration of damaged tissue.

Thromboemboli in the lung organize as they do elsewhere. Part of the thrombus is dissolved by thrombolytic activity; the rest is incorporated into the vessel wall, where it eventually is recognized as a small, elevated, fibrous lesion or as a band stretching across the vessel (see the following discussion). Radiologic studies have indicated that about one half of thromboemboli are resorbed and organized, with little narrowing of the vessels, within 8 weeks.

Multiple Recurrent Pulmonary Thromboemboli

Multiple thromboemboli, usually to small pulmonary artery branches, may detach from peripheral veins. They become organized, occlude the pulmonary arterial system, and are a cause of pulmonary hypertension (see later). **Infection of infarcts** produced by thromboemboli is generally mentioned as a complication, but it is rare. **Pleural effusion,** specifically, bloody effusions, may occur following thromboembolism, an event that suggests that infarction has taken place.

Other Forms of Pulmonary Embolism

Substances other than thrombi may traverse the venous system and lodge in the pulmonary circulation.

Fat Embolism

Fat embolism is the most common form of clinically significant embolism other than thromboembolism. Classically, 12 to 24 hours after the fracture of a long bone, often the femur, the patient becomes short of breath. A chest radiograph reveals a diffuse opacity, which may progress to a "white out" resembling that in the adult respiratory distress syndrome. Indeed, **fat embolism is one of the important causes of the adult respiratory distress syndrome.** Petechiae of the skin or conjunctiva occur in some cases. Cerebral symptoms (confusion or even coma) can be caused by fat emboli that have passed through the pulmonary artery into the systemic circulation. In fatal cases, the lungs resemble those in the adult respiratory distress syndrome—that is, they are heavy, hemorrhagic, and edematous. Histologic examination shows the capillaries and small vessels to be distended by spherical globules of fat. These dissolve in the lipid solvents used to prepare tissue for routine histologic examination and appear as empty spaces. The fat can be stained in frozen sections of the lung tissue with oil red O or with osmium tetroxide in formaldehyde-fixed tissue before processing. Studies of battle casualties suggest that fat embolism is a common complication of trauma but is rarely symptomatic.

Fat embolism is usually thought of as a direct consequence of trauma, with fat entering ruptured capillaries at the site of the fracture. However, other evidence suggests that this explanation may be too simplistic. It has been suggested that hemorrhage into the medullary cavity, and perhaps also into the subcutaneous fat, increases tissue interstitial pressure above capillary pressure, so that fat is forced into the circulation. More important, the amount of fat in the pulmonary vascular system is larger than can be accounted for by simple transfer of fat. In addition, the chemical composition of the fat in the lung is different from that in tissue. Finally, bone marrow embolism is usually not prominent.

Bone Marrow Emboli

Bone marrow emboli, complete with hematopoietic cells and fat, are often seen in the lung at autopsy. They are usually the consequence of cardiac resuscitation, a procedure in which fracture of the bones of the thorax, sternum, and ribs is common. No symptoms are attributed to bone marrow embolism.

Air Embolism

Air may enter the venous system if a large vein—for instance, the jugular vein—is transected, an event that may complicate any medical procedure involving the venous system. When blood was administered from bottles, air could enter the blood when the bottle emptied, especially when the blood was forced in under pressure. For an embolism to be fatal, more than 100 cc air has to be introduced into the venous system. Air embolism has also been described as a complication of abortion, usually criminal abortion. It can cause sudden death, in which case frothy blood is present in the right ventricle and pulmonary arteries at autopsy. On histologic examination, bubbles of air, as empty spaces that resemble fat emboli, can be seen in the lung capillaries and small vessels.

Amniotic Fluid Embolism

A rare complication of labor and delivery is severe amniotic fluid embolism, a condition in which amniotic fluid is forced into torn uterine vein sinuses. Sudden collapse and death may ensue; more commonly, diffuse intravascular coagulation results. The latter consequence is caused by the release of thromboplastic substances from amniotic fluid contents. On gross examination the lungs resemble those in the adult respiratory distress syndrome. Microscopically, squames and debris are seen in the small pulmonary arteries and capillaries. Minor amniotic fluid embolism is probably a common asymptomatic event, since autopsies of mothers dying in the perinatal period of other causes frequently find histologic evidence of embolization.

Talc Embolization

Intravenous drug abusers may introduce talc into the lung via the bloodstream. The talc may be the carrier of the drug (as with methadone) or may be used to dilute it. The talc lodges mainly in the small pulmonary arteries and also reaches the capillaries. Occlusion and thrombosis of the vessels ensue, but the talc also escapes through the vessel walls and provokes a granulomatous response. Microscopically, the platelike crystals of talc appear as empty spaces and are brilliantly double refractile. Most often the emboli are asymptomatic, but they may lead to symptoms if the lesions (vascular occlusion, granulomatous inflammation, and fibrosis) are sufficiently widespread and severe.

Tumor Embolism

Tumor emboli are occasionally seen in the lung and are thought to be the source of the lymphangitic form of carcinoma (see preceding discussion).

Schistosomiasis

Schistosomiasis may be associated with the embolization of ova to the lungs from the bladder or gut. The ova occlude small vessels, excite a foreign body reaction, and elicit a granulomatous response. The ova also penetrate through the vessel into the surrounding lung.

Miscellaneous Emboli

A wide variety of substances has been found in the lung. Cotton emboli are surprisingly common and

SMALL PULMONARY ARTERIES

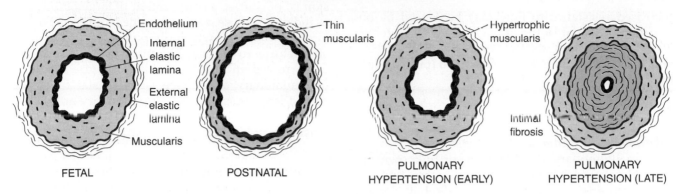

Figure 12-48. Histopathology of pulmonary hypertension. In late gestation the pulmonary arteries have thick walls. After birth the vessels dilate and the walls become thin. Mild pulmonary hypertension is characterized by thickening of the media. As pulmonary hypertension becomes more severe, there is extensive intimal fibrosis and muscle thickening.

are due to cleansing of the skin prior to venipuncture. Emboli of brain matter may be seen in severe cerebral laceration. We have seen a fragment of shrapnel in a segmental pulmonary artery derived from a thigh wound in a veteran of the Spanish Civil War.

Thrombosis of the Pulmonary Arteries

The great majority of thrombi in the pulmonary arterial system are emboli. Spontaneous thrombosis, which is rare, usually occurs in association with congenital cardiac anomalies, particularly atrial septal defects. Angiitis, both infectious and noninfectious, is associated with thrombosis. Thrombi of the small pulmonary vessels also complicate nonthrombotic emboli, such as tumor emboli and talc. Thrombi are also seen in disseminated intravascular coagulation.

Pulmonary Arterial Hypertension

In fetal life the pulmonary arterial walls are thick, but after the third day of life they become thin, mainly because of dilatation (Fig. 12-48). The pressure within the pulmonary arterial system may be increased for one of two reasons—augmented flow or increased resistance within the pulmonary circulation. Whatever the cause, similar morphologic abnormalities result from increased pulmonary artery pressure. **Pulmonary atherosclerosis is seen in the major vessels.** It should be noted that even mild degrees of atherosclerosis are uncommon when pulmonary arterial pressure is normal. **The walls of the small pulmonary vessels thicken, owing to an increase in muscle in the media and an increase in fibrous tissue in the intima (see Fig. 12-48).** An additional change is the development of muscle in vessels that are normally

nonmuscular or partially muscular (arteries generally less than 100 μm in diameter). If the pressure is high and sustained, the arteries dilate and may exhibit curious angiomatoid or plexiform lesions. These nodular lesions, composed of irregular interlacing blood channels, impose a further obstruction in the pulmonary circulation. Necrosis of the arterial wall and pulmonary hemorrhage occur in severe, sustained pulmonary hypertension. Mild structural changes of the pulmonary vasculature are reversible (e.g., with corrective heart surgery). However, severe lesions (plexiform lesions, necrosis, and hemorrhage) indicate that pulmonary arterial hypertension is not correctable. As a result of the increased pressure in the lesser circulation, hypertrophy of the right ventricle of the heart occurs, in which case we speak of cor pulmonale.

Increased Flow

A shunt from systemic circulation (including the heart) to the pulmonary circulation results in increased flow through the lungs. The great majority of cases represents left-to-right shunts in congenital heart disease, although occasional acquired conditions occur, such as rupture of the interventricular septum or an aortic–pulmonary fistula. The severity of the lesions in the pulmonary arteries depends on the severity of the pulmonary hypertension. An additional lesion is present when hypertension exists from birth. At this time the pulmonary artery and the aorta have about the same number of elastic lamellae in their media. In normal infants there is a loss of elastic lamellae in the pulmonary artery after birth, but when pulmonary hypertension is present the fetal pattern persists.

Increased Resistance to Flow

Increased resistance to flow may be caused by obstruction proximal to the lung capillary bed (precapillary hypertension), destruction of the capillary bed, or obstruction distal to the capillary bed (postcapillary hypertension).

Precapillary Pulmonary Hypertension

Primary Pulmonary Hypertension

Primary pulmonary hypertension, of unknown etiology, is caused by increased tone within the pulmonary arteries. It occurs at all ages but is most common in young women in their 20s and 30s. The disorder presents with an insidious onset of dyspnea, and physical signs and radiologic abnormalities are initially slight. As time passes, clinical and radiologic abnormalities become more apparent. Severe morphologic changes of pulmonary hypertension eventually ensue, and the patients die from cor pulmonale and right-sided heart failure. Medical treatment is generally ineffective, and this disease is an indication for heart–lung transplantation.

Multiple Recurrent Pulmonary Emboli

Multiple thromboemboli in the smaller pulmonary vessels gradually restrict the pulmonary circulation. The presenting symptoms are often the same as in primary pulmonary hypertension, but some patients have evidence of peripheral venous thrombosis, usually in the leg veins, or a history of circumstances predisposing to peripheral venous thrombosis. The lesions in the pulmonary vascular system are those of pulmonary hypertension, often severe. Organized thromboemboli are present. Characteristically, these form "webs" in the small pulmonary arteries composed of fibrous bands that extend across the lumen of the vessel. Clinically, it is difficult to distinguish multiple recurrent pulmonary emboli from primary pulmonary hypertension. Lung biopsy is not always helpful, since the lesions in the smallest vessels are identical and vessels of the size that commonly have webs are not included in the biopsy. If the condition is diagnosed during life, plication of, or placement of filters in, the inferior vena cava may prevent further emboli.

Occlusion of Major Vessels

Larger pulmonary arteries than those involved in multiple recurrent pulmonary emboli can also be occluded. Occlusion may be due to thromboemboli in the larger pulmonary arteries or thrombosis of the pulmonary arteries. In these instances the onset is more acute, and specific evidence of classic embolization is often present. Acute pulmonary hypertension is, of course, a concomitant of large emboli but, as indicated, these may be resorbed and incorporated into the wall, after which the pulmonary artery pressure returns to normal. The pulmonary arteries may be narrowed and finally occluded by rare tumors of the pulmonary artery (see later). Distal to the occluded large vessel the small pulmonary arteries are normal, but the classic changes of pulmonary hypertension may be seen in other parts of the lung.

Functional Resistance to Flow

The pulmonary circulation is sensitive to hypoxemia, and any condition that produces hypoxemia results in pulmonary hypertension. This is the most common form of pulmonary hypertension and results from constriction of the small pulmonary arteries. Its causes include chronic airflow obstruction due to any condition that is accompanied by hypoxemia—for instance, infiltrative lung disease, living at high altitude, and alveolar hypoventilation. The last may be due to abnormalities of the chest wall that interfere with the mechanics of ventilation, such as severe kyphoscoliosis and extreme obesity.

Idiopathic hypoventilation is another cause of pulmonary hypertension and in patients with extreme obesity is referred to as the "Pickwickian syndrome." The situation in these subjects is complex. Severe obesity by itself may lead to hypoventilation and abnormal ventilation/perfusion ratios. Obesity may produce obstruction to the upper airway (pharynx) at night, thereby leading to the sleep apnea syndrome. This episodic occlusion during the night results in profound intermittent hypoxemia and disturbances in the pattern of breathing. The disturbance of sleep at night leads to daytime somnolence. Rarely, obesity may be due to hypothalamic dysfunction and may also be associated with a disturbance of the respiratory center and diminished hypoxic drive. In other instances, upper airway obstruction may not be associated with obesity. Such cases are often difficult to recognize, although the characteristic feature is loud and prolonged snoring. All forms of hypoventilation are more common in men than in women. Surgery to the pharynx, pharyngoplasty (in effect, a radical tonsillectomy), may be curative of upper airway obstruction, although a permanent tracheostomy is sometimes required.

In all forms of reactive (functional) pulmonary hypertension the histologic changes in the vessels are slight. They consist of muscularization of the nonmuscular and partially muscular pulmonary arteries and slight medial thickening of the smallest muscular pulmonary arteries. The mildness of the condition is related to the modest degree of hypertension and the often intermittent nature of the hypoxemia.

Capillary Causes of Pulmonary Hypertension

Experimentally, it has been shown that three fourths of the lung can be removed without ensuing pulmonary hypertension. Pneumonectomy in man does not result in pulmonary hypertension, although pulmonary artery pressure may be slightly increased on exercise. Emphysema is commonly cited as a cause of pulmonary hypertension, and it is claimed by some that this is due to the loss of capillary bed. **Pulmonary hypertension in emphysema is mainly due to hypoxemia caused by ventilation/perfusion abnormalities, but it may be that this is compounded by a loss of capillary bed.**

Postcapillary Causes of Pulmonary Hypertension

Postcapillary hypertension differs from the other forms of pulmonary hypertension in that there are venous as well as arterial changes and the parenchyma (alveolar walls) may also be abnormal. The parenchyma is generally normal in precapillary hypertension except in the most severe grades, when pulmonary hemorrhage occurs. In capillary hypertension the parenchyma is by definition abnormal, but not as a consequence of venous hypertension. Venous changes include intimal fibrosis and thickening, or "arterialization," of veins. Veins normally have little elastic tissue and muscle, but with severe venous hypertension extra elastic laminae and new smooth muscle develop.

Cardiac Causes of Pulmonary Hypertension

Left ventricular failure from any cause increases pulmonary venous pressure and hence pulmonary arterial pressure, but the increase is generally quite small. By contrast, mitral stenosis produces severe venous hypertension and significant pulmonary artery hypertension. Although some have argued that pulmonary arterial hypertension reflects reactive vasoconstriction, it is now thought that increased venous resistance is responsible.

Changes in the venous system and parenchyma depend on the severity of the venous hypertension. When severe, as in longstanding mitral stenosis, obvious lesions are present, and mild changes are present in the pulmonary arterial system. The parenchymal changes are included under the rubric of **chronic passive congestion** of the lung. The capillaries are dilated and, because of intermittent hemorrhage, red blood cells are seen in alveolar spaces and in the interstitium. Hemosiderosis, resulting from the breakdown of the red blood cells and phagocytosis of their debris, is prominent. Large macrophages loaded with hemosiderin, so-called heart failure cells, often pack the alveoli. In addition, hemosiderin is seen in the interstitium of the lung and may coat blood vessels. Calcium also accumulates in the elastic fibers of the alveolar walls, which stain blue with hematoxylin, leading to so-called iron and calcium encrustation. Elastic fibers may fragment and elicit a giant cell reaction. There is usually thickening of alveolar walls, with some mild fibrosis. On gross examination, the lungs are brown and firm, an appearance that gives rise to the term **brown induration** of the lung.

Pulmonary Veno-occlusive Disease

Pulmonary veno-occlusive disease is a rare condition characterized by extensive occlusion of the small and medium-sized veins of the lung by loose, sparsely cellular, fibrous tissue. Some larger veins may be involved. Pulmonary veno-occlusive disease produces severe pulmonary venous hypertension and the consequences described previously. The clinical presentation of progressive dyspnea is similar to that of primary pulmonary hypertension but is usually more rapidly progressive. More than half of all cases are encountered in the first three decades of life. In young patients the sex incidence is similar, but beyond the age of 15 it is more frequent in men. Often there is a history of a respiratory infection preceding the onset of dyspnea. Hemoptysis may occur but is infrequent early in the course of the disease. Radiologic examination reveals scattered infiltrates in the lung, representing hemorrhage and hemosiderosis, which increase with the progression of the disease. On gross examination, there is brown induration and atherosclerosis of large pulmonary arteries, as evidence of pulmonary arterial hypertension. Microscopic examination shows partial or total occlusion of small- and medium-sized veins and eccentric intimal thickening of other veins. Arterialization of veins also occurs. The parenchymal changes in the lung, mainly moderate fibrosis of the alveolar walls, are usually obvious. Pulmonary arterial pressure is usually high, so that, histologically, the pulmonary arterial system exhibits severe lesions. Occlusive lesions similar to those seen in the veins are also encountered in the arteries. It is not clear whether the veno-occlusive lesions represent organized thrombi; only rarely can lesions resembling thrombi be found.

The etiology of the condition is unknown, but some have suggested that it is immunologically mediated, resulting from a pulmonary viral infection.

Occlusion of Larger Veins

Major veins may be occluded by sclerosing mediastinitis (sometimes associated with histoplasmosis) or occasionally by a tumor. If all four major veins are involved, the clinical situation is similar to that of veno-occlusive disease. If a single vein or one of its branches is involved, the lesions are localized to the region and pulmonary arterial hypertension does not occur.

Pulmonary Edema

Pulmonary edema, a common clinical and pathologic condition (Fig. 12-49), is defined as increased water within the lung. The key to understanding it is the Starling equation:

$$\text{Fluid movement} = k\left[(P_c - \pi_i) - (P_i - \pi_p)\right]$$

where k is the liquid conductance of the capillary barrier, P is the hydrostatic pressure in the capillary (c) or the interstitium (i) and π is the oncotic pressure of the plasma proteins (p) or interstitial fluid (i).

Although this equation has an admirably scientific appearance, it should be realized that the factors in the equation are not precisely known except for π_p, the capillary oncotic pressure. In more simplistic terms, the outflow of fluid is determined by the difference between the capillary hydrostatic pressure and the interstitial hydrostatic pressure, the hydrostatic pressure being higher. Resorption of fluid is determined by the difference in oncotic pressure between the two compartments. The amount of fluid exuded is modulated by the permeability characteristics of the alveolar capillary membrane. **Thus, there may be hydrostatic, oncotic, or permeability pulmonary edema,** and several forms of edema may be present at the same time.

Endothelial cells are connected to each other by junctions of varying complexity, with varying degrees of "leakiness." The endothelium is thought of as having numerous "small pores," 8 nm in radius, and a few "large pores," 20 nm in radius. This is a theoretical rather than a practical concept; the morphologic counterparts have never been agreed on. The situation is actually more complex, since the passage of macromolecules may be modulated by charged anionic sites on the endothelial surfaces, and charged microdomains on the stomata of endothelial vesicles and the lamina rara of the basal lamina.

Normal passage of fluid and molecules into the interstitium of the lung is thought to occur on the "thick" side of the alveolar wall, where the basal lamina splits to surround the capillary, on the one hand, and underlie the alveolar epithelium, on the other. In this small space there are collagen, elastin, and proteoglycans. Fluid and molecules may also pass from veins into the surrounding interstitium. These circulating components then reenter the circulation via the lymphatics. Lymphatic flow is small, and the ratio of plasma flow to lymphatic flow in the lung is on the order of 5000 to 1. **Pulmonary edema may be interstitial or alveolar. Interstitial edema represents the earliest phase and is an exaggeration of the normal process of fluid filtration.** Lymphatics become distended and fluid accumulates in the interstitium of the lobular septa and around veins and the bronchovascular bundle. Radiologic examination reveals a reticulonodular pattern, more marked in the bases of the lung. Lobular septa become edematous and produce linear shadows (**Kerley B lines**). Edema results in the shunting of blood flow from the bases to the upper lobes of the lungs, and increased airflow resistance occurs because of edema of the bronchovascular tree. Patients are often asymptomatic in this early stage.

When the fluid can no longer be contained in the interstitial space, it spills into the alveoli, a condition termed alveolar edema. At this stage an alveolar pattern is seen, usually worst in the central portions of the lung and in the lower zones (Fig. 12-50). The patient becomes acutely short of breath and bubbly rales are heard. In extreme cases, frothy fluid is coughed up or wells up out of the trachea. Histologic examination shows the airspaces to be filled with eosinophilic material (see Fig. 12-50).

The precise causes of some forms of pulmonary edema are not known. Heroin overdosage and trauma to the brain may lead to fatal pulmonary edema.

Hydrostatic Edema

Hydrostatic edema is due to increased capillary pressure (P_c), usually as a consequence of left-sided heart failure from any cause. Fluid overload during transfusion or resuscitation may also lead to hydrostatic edema.

An interesting but rare form of edema follows rapid aspiration of large pleural effusions and occurs on the side of the aspiration. It has been suggested that the interstitial pressure (P_i) rapidly becomes more negative, drawing fluid into the interstitial space and then the alveoli.

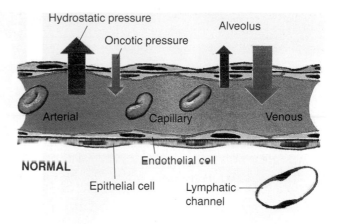

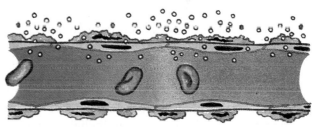

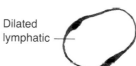

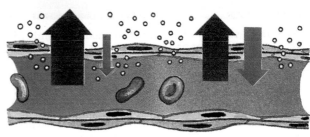

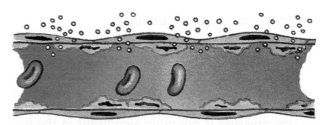

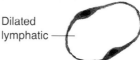

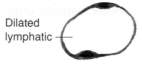

Figure 12-49.   Pathogenesis of pulmonary edema. There is a balance between hydrostatic forces, which tend to make fluid pass out from the capillaries to the interstitium and alveoli, and oncotic forces, which draw fluid in to the capillary bed from the interstitium. Hydrostatic pressure predominates on the arterial side of the capillary and oncotic pressure on the venous side. In hydrostatic edema, the hydrostatic forces dominate, and the fluid is forced into the interstitium of the lung and alveolar spaces. When epithelial damage occurs, the normal tight junctions of epithelial cells are lost and fluid flows freely into alveolar spaces. When there is endothelial damage, the barrier function of the capillary wall is also impaired.

13

The Gastrointestinal Tract

Emanuel Rubin and John L. Farber

The Esophagus
Anatomy
Congenital Disorders
Rings and Webs
Esophageal Diverticula
Motor Disorders
Hiatal Hernia
Esophagitis
Lacerations and Perforations
Neoplasms

The Stomach
Anatomy
Congenital Disorders
Gastritis
Peptic Ulcer Disease
Neoplasms
Mechanical Disorders
Bezoars

The Small Intestine
Anatomy
Congenital Disorders
Infections
Vascular Diseases
Crohn's Disease
Malabsorption
Neoplasms
Pneumatosis Cystoides Intestinalis (Gas Cysts)

The Colon
Anatomy
Congenital Disorders
Infections
Diverticular Disease
Inflammatory Bowel Disease
Vascular Diseases
Radiation Enterocolitis
Neoplasms
Miscellaneous Disorders

The Appendix
Appendicitis
Mucocele
Neoplasms

The Peritoneum
Peritonitis
Retroperitoneal Fibrosis
Neoplasms

Figure 13-1. Mechanisms of nutrient absorption in the small intestine.

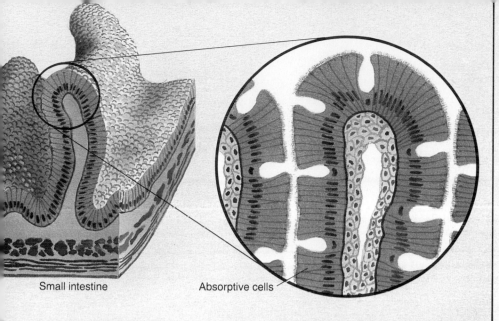

Small intestine

Absorptive cells

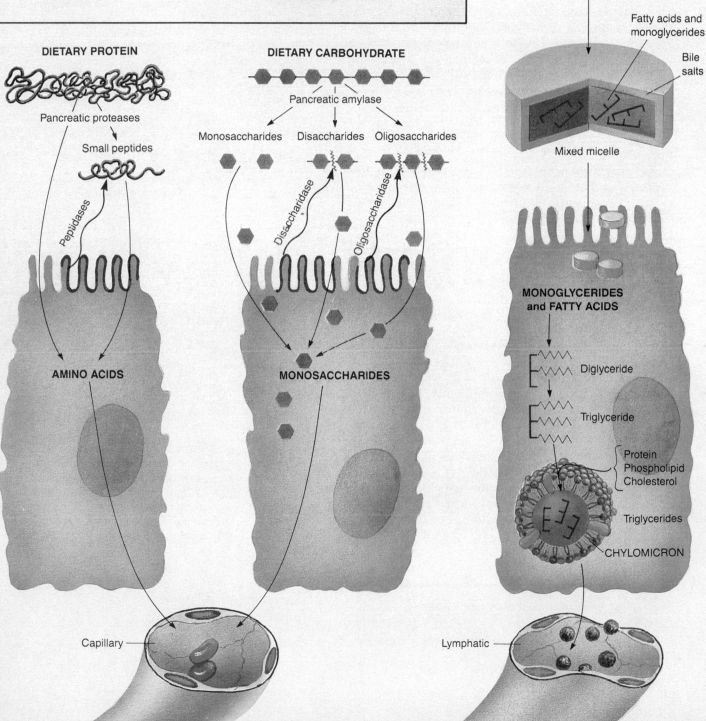

DIETARY FAT

Triglycerides

Glycerol — Fatty acid

Pancreatic lipase

＋ Fatty acids

Bile salts

Fatty acids and monoglycerides

Bile salts

Mixed micelle

DIETARY PROTEIN

Pancreatic proteases

Small peptides

Peptidases

AMINO ACIDS

DIETARY CARBOHYDRATE

Pancreatic amylase

Monosaccharides   Disaccharides   Oligosaccharides

Disaccharidase

Oligosaccharidase

MONOSACCHARIDES

MONOGLYCERIDES and FATTY ACIDS

Diglyceride

Triglyceride

Protein
Phospholipid
Cholesterol

Triglycerides

CHYLOMICRON

Capillary

Lymphatic

The Esophagus
Anatomy

Embryologically, the gut and the respiratory tract arise from the same anlage and comprise a single tube. This structure divides into two separate tubes, the esophagus being dorsal and the future respiratory tract ventral. The initial columnar epithelium, which lines the esophagus in its early development, is replaced by a stratified squamous epithelium.

The adult esophagus is a 25-cm-long tube that contains both striated and smooth muscle in its upper portion and smooth muscle only in its lower portion. The organ is fixed superiorly at the cricopharyngeus muscle, which is considered the upper esophageal sphincter. It courses inferiorly through the posterior mediastinum behind the trachea and the heart and exits the thorax through the hiatus of the diaphragm. The so-called lower esophageal sphincter is not a true anatomic sphincter, but rather a functional one. Tonic muscular contraction at the lower end of the esophagus creates an action similar to that of a one-way flutter valve.

The transition from the normal squamous mucosa of the esophagus to the gastric mucosa at the esophagogastric junction occurs abruptly at the level of the diaphragm. The esophageal submucosa contains mucous glands and a rich lymphatic plexus. The lymphatics of the upper third of the esophagus drain to the cervical lymph nodes, those of the middle third to the mediastinal nodes, and those of the lower third to the celiac and gastric lymph nodes.

The venous drainage of the esophagus is important in portal hypertension, in which esophageal varices occur. These varices are invariably found in the lower third of the esophagus, since the veins of the upper third drain into the superior vena cava and those of the middle third drain into the azygous system. Only the veins of the lower third of the esophagus drain into the portal vein by way of the gastric veins.

The sole function of the esophagus is to serve as a conduit for the passage of food and liquid into the stomach. The act of swallowing, which is not well understood, is remarkably complex and requires precise coordination of a number of separate movements.

Congenital Disorders

The most common esophageal anomaly is the **tracheo-esophageal fistula** (Fig. 13-2). It is frequently combined with some form of **esophageal atresia,** al-

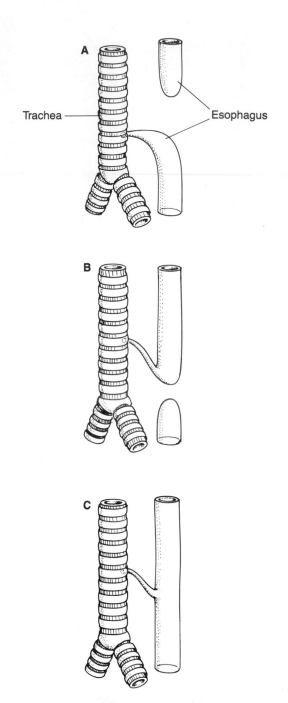

Figure 13-2.   Congenital tracheo-esophageal fistulas. (*A*) The most common type is a communication between the trachea and the lower portion of the esophagus. The upper segment of the esophagus ends in a blind sac. (*B*) In a few cases the proximal esophagus communicates with the trachea. (*C*) The least common anomaly, the H type, is a fistula between a continuous esophagus and the trachea.

though isolated atresia is distinctly uncommon. The cause of esophageal atresia is unknown, but in some cases it has been associated with a complex of anomalies identified by the acronym **Vater syndrome** (*v*ertebral defects, *a*nal atresia, *t*racheo-*e*sophageal fistula, and *r*enal dysplasia). Maternal hydramnios has been recorded in some cases of esophageal atresia and, less commonly, in cases of tracheo-esophageal fistula. Esophageal atresia and fistulas are often associated with congenital heart disease.

In the most common variety of tracheo-esophageal fistula, accounting for about 90% of all such fistulas, the upper portion of the esophagus ends in a blind pouch, and the upper end of the lower segment communicates with the trachea. Since the walls of both the upper and the lower portions of the esophagus are more or less normal, surgical correction is feasible, albeit difficult. In this type of atresia the upper blind sac soon fills with mucus, which the infant then aspirates.

Among the remaining 10% of cases, the most common type involves a communication between the proximal esophagus and the trachea; the lower esophageal pouch communicates with the stomach. Infants with this condition develop aspiration immediately after birth. In another variant, termed an H-type fistula, a communication exists between an intact esophagus and an intact trachea. In some cases the lesion becomes symptomatic only in adulthood, when repeated pulmonary infections call attention to it.

When the proximal and distal portions of the esophagus are separated by a considerable distance, surgical correction is difficult because the ends of the esophageal pouches cannot be approximated. Repeated bouginage (mechanical dilation) of the proximal segment may be successful in elongating it enough to allow approximation of the pouches. In some cases steel dilators have been placed in both upper and lower pouches and subjected to strong magnetic fields. This has led to preoperative approximation of the segments and permitted successful surgical correction.

Congenital esophageal stenosis, which is rare, is surprisingly resistant to mechanical dilation. In some instances elements of pulmonary tissue are found in the stenotic region. An uncommon tracheo-esophageal developmental anomaly consists of a mass of abnormal pulmonary tissue within the lung. Such tissue may be invested by its own separate pleural lining and communicate with the lower esophagus, in which case it is termed **bronchopulmonary foregut malformation.** Passage of esophageal contents into the lung leads to repeated pulmonary infections or an enlarging mediastinal mass.

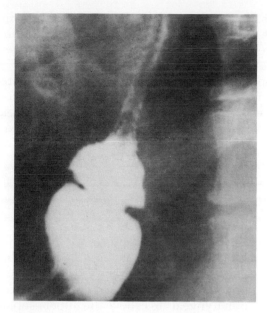

Figure 13-3. Schatzki's mucosal ring. A contrast radiograph illustrates the lower esophageal narrowing.

Rings and Webs

Esophageal webs are defined as thin mucosal membranes that project into the lumen of the esophagus. Usually single, they are occasionally multiple and can be found anywhere in the esophagus. The **Plummer-Vinson (Paterson-Kelly) syndrome** is characterized by a cervical esophageal web, mucosal lesions of the mouth and pharynx, and iron-deficiency anemia. Dysphagia, often associated with aspiration of swallowed food, is the most common clinical manifestation. The Plummer-Vinson syndrome is principally a disease of women, in whom 90% of cases are seen. Carcinoma of the oropharynx and upper esophagus is a recognized complication of the Plummer-Vinson syndrome. The prevalence of this syndrome has significantly declined in recent years, possibly owing to improved nutrition and the addition of supplemental nutrients to food.

Whereas webs in the middle and lower esophagus are distinctly uncommon, **Schatzki's mucosal ring** is a cause of dysphagia that has been noted in as many as 14% of barium meal examinations. The Schatzki ring is a lower esophageal narrowing at the junction of the squamous and columnar epithelium (Fig. 13-3). Typically, patients with narrow Schatzki rings complain of intermittent dysphagia, and a food bolus may lodge in the lower esophagus and require endoscopic intervention. Microscopically, the upper surface of the mucosal ring exhibits stratified squamous epithelium, while the lower is lined by a columnar epithelium. Mild chronic inflammation and fibrosis are common in the submucosa. A few muscle fibers sometimes course through the central portion of the ring. Little is known about the pathogenesis of the Schatzki ring.

Esophageal webs are generally successfully treated by dilation with large rubber bougies; occasionally they can be excised during endoscopy with biopsy forceps. Esophageal bouginage is almost always effective in the treatment of a symptomatic Schatzki ring.

Esophageal Diverticula

A true esophageal diverticulum is an outpouching of the wall that contains all layers of the esophagus. When the sac lacks a muscular layer, it is known as a false diverticulum. Esophageal diverticula occur in the hypopharyngeal area above the upper esophageal sphincter, the middle esophagus, and immediately proximal to the lower esophageal sphincter.

The diverticulum that appears high in the esophagus, known as **Zenker's diverticulum,** was once thought to result from luminal pressure exerted in a structurally weak area and was classed as a **pulsion diverticulum.** Later investigators attributed the lesion to motor incoordination of the cricopharyngeus muscle. Although newer studies have cast doubt on this concept, disordered function of the cricopharyngeal musculature is still generally thought to be involved in the pathogenesis of this false diverticulum.

Zenker's diverticulum is uncommon and affects men more than women. Most affected persons who come to medical attention are over the age of 60 years, an observation that supports the belief that this diverticulum is acquired. The diverticulum can enlarge conspicuously and accumulate a large amount of food. When drugs are trapped in the pouch, their bioavailability may be limited. The typical symptom is regurgitation of food eaten some time previously (occasionally days), in the absence of dysphagia. Recurrent aspiration pneumonia may be a serious complication. When symptoms are severe, surgical intervention is the rule.

Diverticula in the midportion of the esophagus were traditionally termed **traction diverticula** because of their attachment to adjacent mediastinal lymph nodes, usually associated with tuberculous lymphadenitis. However, fibrous adhesions between midesophageal diverticula and diseased mediastinal nodes are uncommon, and it is thought that these pouches often reflect a disturbance in the motor function of the esophagus. A diverticulum in the mid-esophagus ordinarily has a wide stoma, and the pouch is usually higher than its orifice. Thus, such a diverticulum does not retain food or secretions and remains asymptomatic, with only rare complications.

Diverticula immediately above the diaphragm are labeled **epiphrenic diverticula;** unlike other diverticula, they are encountered in young persons. Motor disturbances of the esophagus (e.g., achalasia, diffuse esophageal spasm) are found in two-thirds of patients with this true diverticulum. In addition, it has been speculated that reflux esophagitis plays a role in the pathogenesis of epiphrenic diverticula. The symptoms caused by an epiphrenic diverticulum are difficult to separate from those of the underlying motor abnormalities. However, nocturnal regurgitation of large amounts of fluid stored in the diverticulum during the day is typical. In the face of severe symptoms, surgical intervention directed toward correcting the motor abnormality (e.g., myotomy to correct diffuse esophageal spasm) is appropriate.

Intramural diverticulosis is a rare disorder characterized by numerous small (1-mm to 3-mm) diverticula in the wall of the esophagus, commonly accompanied by a stricture of the upper esophagus. There is evidence that these are not true diverticula, but rather dilated ducts of the submucosal glands. The principal symptom is dysphagia; dilation of the stricture usually ameliorates the condition.

Motor Disorders

The automatic coordination of muscular movement during deglutition results in the free passage of food through the esophagus. Any failure of proper muscular function is included in the concept of motor disorders of the esophagus. The hallmark of motor disorders is difficulty in swallowing, termed **dysphagia.** Dysphagia is often manifested by an awareness of the lack of progression of a bolus of food, and in itself is not painful. Pain on swallowing is termed **odynophagia.** Disordered esophageal motility (for example, spasm) may also cause substernal pain that radiates to the back, arms, neck, and jaw, thereby simulating coronary artery disease.

Dysfunction of striated muscle in the upper esophagus leads to dysphagia. **Systemic diseases of skeletal muscle** also affect the upper esophagus and cause dysphagia. Such diseases include myasthenia gravis, dermatomyositis, amyloidosis, thyrotoxicosis, and myxedema. **Neurologic diseases** that affect nerves to skeletal muscle (e.g., cerebral vascular accidents, amyotrophic lateral sclerosis) may impair swallowing.

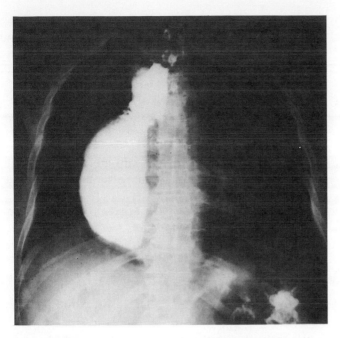

Figure 13-4. Achalasia. A contrast radiograph shows dilatation of the esophagus beginning at the gastroesophageal junction.

Achalasia

Achalasia, at one time termed "cardiospasm," is a disease characterized by the absence of peristalsis in the body of the esophagus and failure of the lower esophageal sphincter to relax in response to swallowing. As a result of these defects in both the outflow tract and the pumping mechanisms of the esophagus, food is retained within the esophagus, and the organ hypertrophies and dilates conspicuously (Fig. 13-4). Dysphagia, occasionally odynophagia, and regurgitation of material retained in the esophagus are common symptoms of achalasia. Aspiration of food may lead to pneumonia.

The cause of achalasia is not well understood, but it is generally agreed that there is a loss or absence of ganglion cells in the myenteric plexus in the area of the lower esophageal sphincter. It has also been suggested that the loss of neurons that release vasoactive intestinal peptide (VIP), which causes relaxation of the lower esophageal sphincter, may play a role. The loss of ganglion cells is occasionally accompanied by chronic inflammation. Electron microscopy demonstrates degeneration of myelin in myelinated fibers and fragmentation of neurofilaments in nonmyelinated fibers. In Latin America achalasia is a common complication of Chagas' disease, the ganglion cells being destroyed by the organisms of *Trypanosoma cruzi*.

Scleroderma (Progressive Systemic Sclerosis)

Scleroderma causes fibrosis in many organs and produces a severe abnormality of esophageal muscle function. The disease affects principally the lower esophageal sphincter, which may become so impaired that the lower esophagus and upper stomach no longer are distinct functional entities and are visualized as a common cavity. In addition, there may be a lack of peristalsis in the entire esophagus. Clinically, patients suffer from dysphagia and heartburn caused by peptic esophagitis due to reflux of acid from the stomach. Microscopically, the smooth muscle is atrophied and submucosal fibrosis and nonspecific inflammatory changes are seen. Intimal fibrosis of the small arteries and arterioles is common and may play a role in the pathogenesis of the submucosal fibrosis.

Peripheral Neuropathy

Peripheral neuropathy associated with diabetes or alcoholism may also interfere with smooth muscle function and can lead to dysphagia.

Hiatal Hernia

"Hiatal hernia" refers to a herniation of the stomach through an enlarged esophageal hiatus in the diaphragm. A common acquired condition, hiatal hernia is in most cases of unknown cause. **Two basic types of hiatal hernia are the sliding, or axial, form, which accounts for most hiatal hernias, and the paraesophageal variety (Fig. 13-5).**

In the **sliding hernia** an enlargement of the diaphragmatic hiatus and laxity of the circumferential connective tissue allow a cap of gastric cardia to move upward to a position above the diaphragm. The condition is so common that, upon appropriate manipulation by the radiologist, more than half the population can be demonstrated to have a small sliding hernia, but only 10% exhibit this abnormality upon routine barium swallow examination. Sliding hiatal hernia is asymptomatic in the large majority of patients, and only 5% of patients diagnosed radiologically complain of symptoms referable to gastroesophageal reflux.

The **paraesophageal hernia** is characterized by herniation of a portion of the gastric fundus alongside the esophagus through a defect in the diaphragmatic connective tissue membrane that defines the esoph-

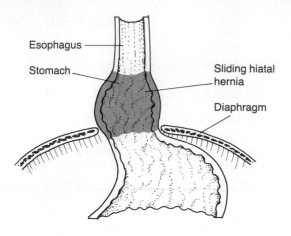

Esophagus

Stomach

Sliding hiatal hernia

Diaphragm

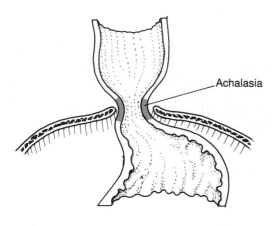

Paraesophageal hiatal hernia

Stomach

Figure 13-5. Disorders of the esophageal outlet.

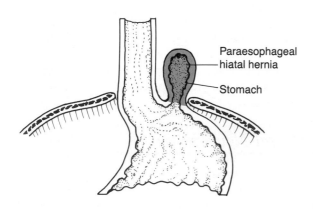

Achalasia

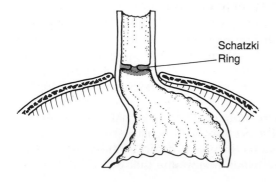

Schatzki Ring

ageal hiatus (see Fig. 13-5). The hernia progressively enlarges, and the hiatus grows increasingly wide. As a result, in extreme cases most of the stomach may herniate into the thorax, and it may even be accompanied by the colon or the small intestine. Interestingly, most large paraesophageal hernias do not cause significant symptoms.

Symptoms of hiatal hernia, particularly heartburn and regurgitation, are attributed to gastroesophageal reflux. However, evidence suggests that the reflux of gastric contents is independent of the hernia and rather is related to incompetence of the lower esophageal sphincter. Classically, the symptoms are exacerbated when the affected person is in the recumbent position, which facilitates acid reflux. Dysphagia, painful swallowing, and occasionally bleeding may also be troublesome. In cases of very large paraesophageal hernias, protrusion of the stomach into the thorax may embarrass respiration. In such large herniations there is a constant risk of gastric volvulus or intrathoracic gastric dilation.

Sliding hiatal hernias do not generally require surgical repair; symptoms are often treated medically. By contrast, an enlarging paraesophageal hernia should be surgically repaired, even in the absence of symptoms.

Esophagitis

Reflux Esophagitis

Reflux esophagitis, formerly termed "peptic esophagitis," results from the regurgitation of gastric contents into the lower esophagus. By far the most common type of esophagitis, it is commonly seen in conjunction with a sliding hiatal hernia, although it often occurs through an incompetent cardia without any demonstrable anatomic lesion.

The principal barrier to the reflux of gastric contents into the esophagus is the lower esophageal sphincter. Although the sphincter is functional rather than anatomic, experimental interruption of the circular smooth muscle of the lower esophagus consistently leads to significant reflux. Agents that cause a decrease in the pressure of the lower esophageal sphincter (e.g., alcohol, chocolate, fatty foods, cigarette smoke) are associated with reflux, as are certain central nervous system depressants (e.g., morphine, diazepam [Valium]) pregnancy, estrogen therapy, and the presence of a nasogastric tube.

Although acid is damaging to the esophageal mucosa, the combination of acid and pepsin may be particularly injurious. Moreover, gastric fluid often contains refluxed bile from the duodenum, which is thought to be harmful to the esophageal mucosa. Alcohol and hot beverages may also damage the mucosa directly.

The earliest alteration produced by gastroesophageal reflux is hyperemia. If reflux is chronic, thickening of the epithelium, termed "leukoplakia," is occasionally seen as irregular greyish white patches. Areas affected by reflux are susceptible to superficial mucosal ulcerations, which appear as vertical linear streaks. Microscopically, the basal layer of the epithelium is thickened, and the rete pegs are elongated and extend toward the surface. A modest increase in lymphocytes is seen in the lamina propria.

If reflux esophagitis is severe enough to damage the esophageal wall deep to the lamina propria, fibrosis is stimulated and may lead to **esophageal stricture.** Such a stricture is usually sharply localized and situated near the lower esophageal sphincter, although it may extend considerably higher. If an esophageal stricture seriously interferes with the passage of food, the esophagus becomes dilated above the narrowing. The most common clinical complaint is progressive dysphagia.

Esophageal ulcers are uncommon complications of reflux esophagitis. They may result in life-threatening hematemesis or, rarely, perforation of the esophagus.

Barrett's epithelium, defined as replacement of the squamous epithelium in the lower third of the esophagus by columnar epithelium, was originally considered to be a congenital lesion. However, it is now recognized that most instances of Barrett's epithelium occur in response to chronic reflux esophagitis. The metaplastic epithelium may occur in patches or may line the entire lower esophagus. The most common histologic pattern is intestinal metaplasia, characterized by villi lined with intestinal goblet cells and sometimes Paneth cells. In other cases gastric epithelium with parietal and chief cells is found. The two types may coexist. Inflammatory changes are usually superimposed upon the epithelial alterations.

The upper border of the metaplastic epithelium is usually adjacent to an ulcerated and inflamed area of the squamous epithelium, and is often the site of a stricture. This suggests that the metaplasia is a protective adaptation by which a glandular epithelium, which is relatively resistant to chemical injury, replaces a more sensitive squamous epithelium. Reversion of Barrett's epithelium to the normal squamous surface has been reported after correction of esophageal reflux. As might be expected of a metaplastic epithelium, **Barrett's epithelium carries a significant risk of malignant transformation to adenocarcinoma.**

In the past, patients with Barrett's epithelium were often recommended for antireflux surgery. However, reflux esophagitis is now usually treated with histamine receptor antagonists, which inhibit gastric acid production, and surgery is reserved for major complications.

Infectious Esophagitis

With the exceptions of **candidiasis** and **herpes simplex,** primary infections of the esophagus are rare.

Infection of the esophagus with Candida species has become commonplace because of an increasing number of immunocompromised persons who receive chemotherapy for malignant disease, who receive immunosuppressive drugs after organ transplantation, or who have contracted AIDS. Esophageal candidiasis also occurs in patients with diabetes and in others with no known predisposing factors. Dysphagia and severe pain on swallowing are usual, and bleeding from the infected site, sometimes severe, is common.

In mild cases of candidiasis a few small, elevated white plaques, surrounded by a hyperemic zone, are present on the mucosa of the middle or lower third of the esophagus. In severe cases confluent pseudomembranes lie on a hyperemic and edematous mucosa. If the pseudomembrane is removed, mucosal ulcerations and hemorrhages result. Microscopically, the candidal pseudomembrane is seen to contain fungal mycelia, necrotic debris, and fibrin. Involvement of the deeper layers of the esophageal wall can lead to fibrosis, sometimes severe enough to create a stricture.

Herpetic esophagitis is most frequently associated with lymphomas and leukemias; indeed, the esophagus is the most common viscus involved with herpes in those diseases. In such cases the infection is often asymptomatic. Herpes infection of the esophagus may also occur in apparently healthy people, in whom it often produces severe pain upon swallowing. The well-developed lesions of herpetic esophagitis are grossly similar to those of candidiasis. In early cases small ulcers or plaques are noted; as the infection progresses, these may coalesce to form larger lesions. Microscopically, the lesions are seen to be superficial, and the epithelial cells exhibit typical herpetic inclusions in their nuclei. Multinucleated giant cells are occasionally encountered. Necrosis of infected cells leads to ulceration, and monilial and bacterial superinfection results in the formation of pseudomembranes. The disease is self-limited in otherwise healthy persons but is protracted in immunocompromised individuals.

Involvement of the esophagus in tuberculosis, syphilis, diphtheria, and histoplasmosis is extremely rare.

Chemical Esophagitis

Chemical injury to the esophagus is usually a result of accidental poisoning in children or attempted suicide in adults. It is produced by the intake of strong alkaline agents (e.g., lye) or strong acids (e.g., sulphuric or hydrochloric acid) used in various cleaning solutions. The alkaline solutions are particularly insidious, because they are generally odorless and tasteless and therefore easily swallowed before protective reflexes come into play. By contrast, acids are immediately painful and, at least in accidental cases, are usually rapidly expelled. Caustic alkaline solids adhere to mucous membranes and penetrate tissue much more rapidly than do acids. Histologically, alkali-induced liquefactive necrosis is accompanied by conspicuous inflammation and saponification of the membrane lipids in the epithelium, submucosa, and muscularis of the esophagus and stomach. Thrombosis of small vessels adds ischemic necrosis to the injury. Severe injury is the rule with liquid alkali, but less than 25% of those who ingest granular preparations have severe complications.

Strong acids produce immediate coagulation necrosis, which results in a protective eschar that prevents injury and limits penetration. Nevertheless, half of patients who ingest concentrated hydrochloric or sulphuric acid suffer severe esophageal injury.

The severity of caustic injury to the esophagus is classified in a manner similar to that of a skin burn. First-degree injury is defined as erythema and edema of the mucosa and submucosa. The mucosa may slough, but no further complications ensue. Second-degree injury refers to penetration of the submucosa and muscularis. Sloughing of the tissue leads to ulceration, the formation of granulation tissue, and eventual fibrosis. Scar formation, which is usually complete within 2 months, but can become severe during the next 6 months, leads to **stricture of the esophagus.** Third-degree injury refers to necrosis of the full thickness of the wall.

Esophagitis in Systemic Illnesses

The squamous mucosa of the esophagus is similar to that of the skin and shares some reactions with that organ. Epidermolysis bullosa and pemphigoid produce bullous lesions in both the skin and esophageal mucosa. In the dystrophic form of epidermolysis bullosa, all organs that are lined by or derived from squamous epithelium are involved, including the skin, nails, teeth, and esophagus. The bullae, which occur episodically, evolve from fluid-filled vesicles to weeping ulcers. Dysphagia and painful swallowing are the rule. Severe cases result in stricture, usually in the upper esophagus. Corticosteroid therapy has been helpful, but not curative. **Pemphigoid** produces subepithelial bullae in the skin and esophagus, but the disease does not lead to scarring.

Graft-versus-host disease in recipients of bone marrow transplants can present as esophageal lesions causing dysphagia, painful swallowing, and symptoms of gastroesophageal reflux. Esophageal webs and strictures may develop. The upper and middle thirds of the esophageal mucosa are friable, and motor function of the esophagus is impaired.

Sarcoidosis of the esophagus is unusual. Unequivocal esophageal **Crohn's disease** has been described.

Esophagitis Produced by Physical Agents

External irradiation for the treatment of thoracic cancers may include portions of the esophagus and lead to esophagitis. Pressure ulcers of the esophageal mucosa are seen in patients who have **nasogastric tubes** in place for prolonged periods of time, although acid reflux also plays a role in such patients.

Lacerations and Perforations

Lacerations of the esophagus result from external trauma, such as automobile accidents and falls from great heights, and from medical instrumentation. However, the most common cause is severe vomiting, during which the intraesophageal pressure may rise as high as 300 torr. The diaphragm descends rapidly, and a portion of the upper stomach is forced up through the hiatus. As a result, forceful retching may cause mucosal tears, beginning in the gastric epithelium and extending into the esophagus. In the **Mallory-Weiss syndrome,** severe retching, often associated with alcoholism, leads to mucosal lacerations of the upper stomach and lower esophagus, which result in the vomiting of bright red blood. Bleeding may be so severe as to require the transfusion of many units of blood. The lacerations may also cause perforation into the mediastinum.

Perforation of the esophagus, whether from trauma or vomiting, can be catastrophic. It is a well-known occurrence in the newborn, in whom it is caused occasionally by suctioning or feeding with a nasogastric tube but in whom it may also occur spontaneously. Rupture of the esophagus as a result of vomiting is known as **Boerhaave's syndrome.**

Figure 13-6 summarizes the major nonneoplastic disorders of the esophagus.

Neoplasms

Benign Tumors

Benign tumors of the esophagus are uncommon and, with the exception of leiomyomas, are curiosities. **Leiomyomas,** which are only 10% as frequent as carcinomas, are usually discovered as an incidental finding during radiologic or endoscopic examination of the upper gastrointestinal tract or at autopsy. The normal mucosa is elevated over an intramural mass, which on microscopic examination is similar to benign smooth muscle tumors in the stomach, described below. Most esophageal leiomyomas are properly treated by being left alone, but if dysphagia or substernal pain is troublesome, simple surgical enucleation suffices.

Squamous cell papillomas of the esophagus are rare and occasionally associated with acanthosis nigricans. They are asymptomatic and have no malignant potential.

Malignant Tumors

Carcinoma of the Esophagus

Epidemiology

Over 90% of cancers of the esophagus are squamous cell carcinomas (Fig. 13-7). The incidence of this tumor in the United States is low, accounting for 7% of all gastrointestinal cancers. However, geographic variations in the incidence of carcinoma of the esophagus are striking, and areas of high incidence are located adjacent to areas of low incidence. There is an esophageal cancer belt extending across Asia from the Caspian Sea region of Northern Iran and the Soviet Union through Soviet Central Asia and Mongolia to Northern China. In parts of China the mortality rate from esophageal cancer in men is reported to be some 70-fold greater than in the United States. By contrast, a nearby Chinese province has a mortality rate comparable to that in the United States. Similarly, the Caspian region of Iran has an incidence of esophageal carcinoma about 30 times greater than the United States, whereas more southern zones of Iran have a low incidence. American blacks have a considerably greater incidence than Caucasians, and

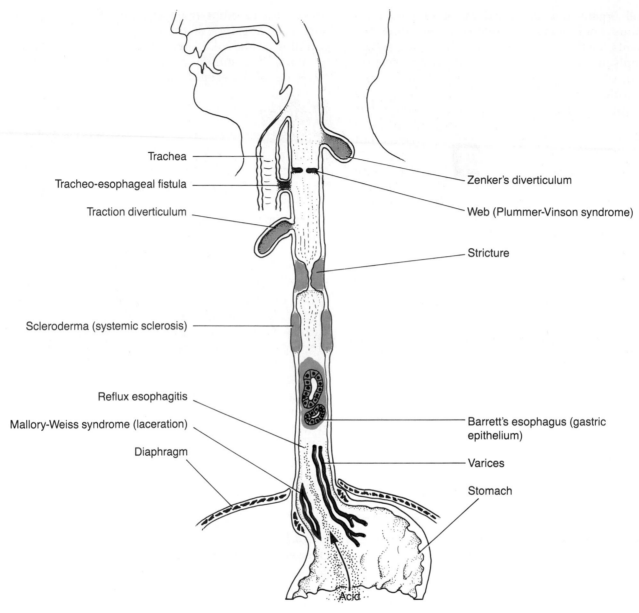

Trachea

Tracheo-esophageal fistula

Traction diverticulum

Scleroderma (systemic sclerosis)

Reflux esophagitis

Mallory-Weiss syndrome (laceration)

Diaphragm

Zenker's diverticulum

Web (Plummer-Vinson syndrome)

Stricture

Barrett's esophagus (gastric epithelium)

Varices

Stomach

Acid

Figure 13-6.   Nonneoplastic disorders of the esophagus.

in the United States urban dwellers are at greater risk than those in rural areas. Cancer of the esophagus is also common in certain regions of France, Finland, Switzerland, Chile, Japan, India, and some parts of Africa. By contrast, other Scandinavian countries, Holland, and Austria have low frequencies. In the United States there is a male predominance of about 3:1.

Etiology
The geographic variations in esophageal cancer, even in relatively homogeneous populations, suggests that **environmental factors contribute strongly to the de-velopment of this disease.** However, no single factor can be incriminated as the cause of esophageal cancer. In the United States **excessive consumption of alcohol** is a risk factor, even when cigarette smoking and degree of urbanization are taken into account. **Cigarette smoking** is also associated with a twofold to fourfold increase in the risk of esophageal cancer, and the number of cigarettes smoked correlates with the presence of dysplasia in the esophageal epithelium. However, the population in the Caspian littoral of Iran, which has one of the highest rates of esophageal carcinoma in the world, neither consumes alcohol nor smokes cigarettes excessively.

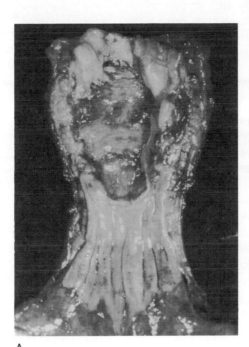

Figure 13.7   Carcinoma of the esophagus. (A) A large, fungating carcinoma of the esophagus is evident above the gastroesophageal junction. (B) Microscopic examination reveals a well-differentiated squamous cell carcinoma.

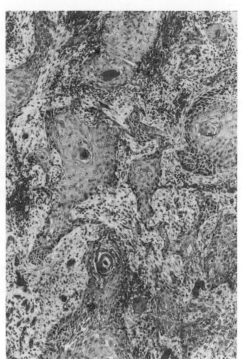

A

B

Nitrosamines and **aniline dyes** produce esophageal cancer in animals. Although high levels of nitrosamines and other potentially carcinogenic compounds have been found in the diets of persons living in high-incidence areas, direct evidence for their contribution to esophageal cancer is lacking. Moreover, such chemical agents have not been detected in many high-risk areas, such as northern Iran.

It has been suggested that the **diets** in areas endemic for esophageal cancer are **lacking in fresh fruits, vegetables, and animal protein,** and in some hyperendemic areas deficiencies of various vitamins and minerals have been claimed. However, the close proximity of endemic and nonendemic areas renders a causative role for these dietary factors unlikely. Improbable and unproved environmental factors include spices, hot foods or liquids, betel nuts, asbestos, air pollution, and radiation. The associations between esophageal cancer and both the Plummer-Vinson syndrome and celiac sprue have not been explained.

Chronic esophagitis, regardless of the cause, predisposes to esophageal cancer in experimental animals and in humans, and areas endemic for esophageal cancer exhibit an increased prevalence of esophagitis. **Achalasia** is a well-known predisposing factor for carcinoma of the esophagus. In fact, as many as 20% of patients with achalasia of more than 25 years' duration can be expected to develop esoph-

ageal cancer. Five percent of individuals who have an esophageal **stricture** after ingestion of lye develop cancer 20 to 40 years later. **Webs, rings, and diverticula** are also associated with a greater risk of esophageal cancer. **Thus, any condition associated with chronic injury to the esophageal mucosa predisposes to squamous cell carcinoma of the esophagus.**

Although the pathogenesis of esophageal cancer is not understood, it is tempting to speculate that irritation of the mucosa by gastric contents, food, alcohol, or other agents stimulates cell proliferation and thereby acts as a promoter for cells initiated by exposure to environmental carcinogens, such as those contained in tobacco smoke.

Clinical Features

The most common presenting complaint is dysphagia, which is usually not recognized until the diameter of the lumen of the esophagus is reduced by 30% to 50%. By this time most tumors are unresectable. Patients with esophageal cancer are almost invariably cachectic, owing to the remote effects of a malignant tumor, anorexia, and difficulty in eating. Painful swallowing occurs in half of the patients, and persistent pain suggests mediastinal extension of the tumor or involvement of spinal nerves. Compression of the recurrent laryngeal nerve produces hoarseness, and tracheo-esophageal fistula is manifested clinically by a chronic cough.

Surgery and radiotherapy are useful for palliation, but the prognosis remains dismal. Only 40% of patients who undergo surgery have tumors that are potentially resectable, and of these one-third die from the operation itself. Of the survivors only 10% (4% of the total) live for 5 years.

Pathology

About half the cases of esophageal cancer involve the middle third of the esophagus; the upper and lower thirds each account for one-fourth of the cases. Grossly, the tumors are of three types: **polypoid,** which project into the lumen (see Fig. 13-7A); **ulcerating,** which are usually smaller than polypoid; and **infiltrating,** the principal plane of growth of which is in the wall. Usually these features overlap. The bulky polypoid tumors tend to obstruct early, whereas the ulcerated ones are more likely to bleed. The infiltrating tumors gradually narrow the lumen by circumferential compression. Local extension of the tumor is commonly a major problem. Microscopically, the neoplastic squamous cells range from well differentiated, with epithelial "pearls" (see Fig. 13-7B), to poorly differentiated. The degree of differentiation does not correlate with the extent of the disease, the presence of metastases, or the prognosis.

The rich lymphatic drainage of the esophagus provides a route for most metastases. The lymphatic vessels of the esophagus follow the blood supply. Accordingly, tumors of the upper third metastasize to the cervical, internal jugular, and supraclavicular nodes. Cancer of the middle third metastasizes to the paratracheal and hilar lymph nodes and to nodes in the aortic, cardiac, and paraesophageal regions. Since the lower third of the esophagus is fed by the left gastric artery, tumors in this portion of the esophagus spread to retroperitoneal, celiac, and left gastric nodes. "Skip" metastases may also involve distant lymph nodes. Visceral metastases to the liver and lung are common, and almost any organ may be involved.

Adenocarcinoma of the Esophagus

Adenocarcinoma of the esophagus accounts for about 5% of malignant esophageal tumors. Most esophageal adenocarcinomas arise in Barrett's epithelium, but a few originate in mucous glands of the esophagus. Some gastric cancers extend upward into the esophagus, and these may be difficult to distinguish from cancers arising in Barrett's epithelium. The symptoms and clinical course are similar to those of squamous cell carcinoma of the esophagus, but a 20% 5-year survival following radical surgery has been reported.

Other Malignancies

Rare primary malignant tumors of the esophagus include melanoma, endocrine tumors, and carcinosarcoma. Metastases to the esophagus from distant tumors are rare, but direct extension from cancers of the lung and thyroid is occasionally encountered.

The Stomach
Anatomy

The stomach, a J-shaped saccular organ with a volume of 1200 ml to 1500 ml, arises as a dilatation of the primitive foregut. It is connected to the esophagus superiorly and to the duodenum inferiorly. Situated in the upper abdomen, the stomach extends from the left hypochondrium across the epigastrium to the region of the umbilicus. The convexity of the stomach, extending leftward from the gastroesophageal junction, is termed the **greater curvature.** The concavity of the right side of the stomach, called the **lesser curvature,** is only about one-fourth as long as the greater curvature. The entire stomach is invested in peritoneum, which descends from the greater curvature as the **greater omentum.**

The interior of the stomach has been divided into five regions (Fig. 13-8): the **cardia,** a small, grossly indistinct zone that extends a short distance from the gastroesophageal junction; the **fundus,** the dome-shaped part of the stomach that is located to the left of the cardia and extends superiorly above a line drawn horizontally through the gastroesophageal junction; the **body,** or **corpus,** which constitutes two-thirds of the entire stomach and descends from the fundus to the most inferior region, where the organ turns right to form the bottom of the J; the **antrum,** the distal third of the stomach, which is positioned horizontally and extends from the body to the pyloric sphincter; and the **pylorus,** the most distal tubular segment of the stomach, which is entirely surrounded by the thick muscular sphincter that governs the passage of food into the duodenum.

The wall of the stomach is composed of a mucosa, submucosa, muscularis, and serosa. The lining of the stomach is disposed in prominent folds, termed the **gastric rugae.** When the stomach is distended, the rugae tend to be flattened and inconspicuous on radiologic examination.

Branches of the celiac, hepatic, and splenic arteries supply blood to the stomach. The gastric veins drain either directly into the portal system or indirectly through the splenic and superior mesenteric veins. A rich plexus of lymphatic channels drains into the gastric and other regional lymph nodes. Both vagal

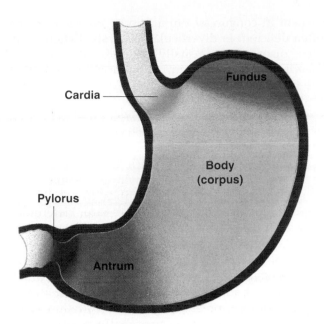

Figure 13-8. Anatomic regions of the stomach.

nerves supply parasympathetic innervation to the stomach, and the celiac plexus supplies sympathetic innervation.

The histologic appearance of the gastric mucosa varies according to the anatomic region. The surface mucosa is a mucus-secreting, columnar epithelium perforated by numerous foveolae, or pits, which represent the orifices of millions of branched, tubular glands. Three types of glands include the **cardiac glands,** located in the cardia; the **gastric (oxyntic, parietal) glands,** in the body and fundus of the stomach; and the **pyloric glands,** in the antrum and the pyloric canal.

The gastric glands, the principal secretory elements of the stomach, are densely arranged perpendicularly to the mucosa and enter the base of the foveola through a narrowed segment termed the neck of the gland. The gastric glands contain four cell types: zymogen (chief) cells, parietal (oxyntic) cells, mucous neck cells, and endocrine cells. The **zymogen,** or **chief,** cells, which reside primarily in the lower half of the gastric gland, are pyramidal, basophilic cells filled with zymogen granules that contain pepsinogen. The basophilia reflects the rich content of ribosomes, a feature characteristic of cells that are actively engaged in protein synthesis. The **parietal,** or **oxyntic,** cells, which occupy the upper half of the gastric gland, are oval or pyramidal eosinophilic cells that secrete hydrochloric acid. The eosinophilia is imparted by the presence of numerous mitochondria, which provide energy for the ion transport necessary for acid secretion. Ultrastructurally, parietal cells exhibit numerous invaginations of the surface membrane, termed "secretory canaliculi," which vastly expand the surface area participating in acid secretion. In addition to being the source of acid, parietal cells are the source of intrinsic factor, which is necessary for the intestinal absorption of vitamin B_{12}.

The **mucous neck cells** are interspersed among the parietal cells in the neck of the gastric gland. These basophilic cells contain considerably more ribosomes and larger mucous granules than do the surface mucous cells, features that suggest more active mucus secretion.

Endocrine cells are scattered in the gastric glands, mostly between the zymogen cells and the basement membrane. These small, round or pyramidal cells are filled with granules that reduce silver salts. Those that reduce silver without prior treatment are termed **argentaffin cells.** These cells also reduce chromium salts and are therefore included in the designation **enterochromaffin cells.** In others, termed **argyrophil cells,** prior reaction with a reducing substance is necessary before the granules stain with silver. The reason for the differences in affinity for silver salts is not understood. Endocrine cells are scattered among the pyloric glands and contain biogenic amines such as serotonin and polypeptide hormones (e.g., gastrin and somatostatin). Vasoactive intestinal peptide is found in neural elements, but not within endocrine cells, of the mucosa.

The pyloric glands, branched and conspicuously coiled structures, empty into foveolae that are substantially deeper than those in other portions of the stomach. The glands are lined by pale cells similar in appearance to mucous neck cells and cells of Brunner's glands in the duodenum.

Cardiac glands are lined by cells that are similar to mucous neck cells and those of the pyloric glands.

Congenital Disorders

Congenital Pyloric Stenosis

Congenital pyloric stenosis, a lesion that obstructs the outlet of the stomach, is the most common indication for abdominal surgery in the initial 6 months of life. It is 4 times more common in males than in females and affects first-born children more often than subsequent ones. It occurs in 1 of 250 to 300 white births but is rare in blacks and Asiatics. The abnormality may have a genetic basis; there is a familial tendency, and the condition is more common in identical than in fraternal twins. Pyloric stenosis has also been recorded in the context of other developmental abnormalities, such as Turner's syndrome, trisomy 18, and esophageal atresia.

Embryopathies associated with rubella infection and maternal intake of thalidomide have been associated with congenital pyloric stenosis. Interestingly, the administration of gastrin, a hormone that stimulates antral contractions, to pregnant bitches leads to pyloric hypertrophy in the litter. The relevance of this finding to the pathogenesis of pyloric stenosis requires further investigation of gastrin levels in the mothers of infants born with this disease and the sensitivity of the offspring to gastrin.

The symptoms of pyloric stenosis usually become apparent within the first month of life, when the infant manifests **projectile vomiting.** Typically, after the stomach has emptied, the infant is ravenous and feeds avidly. The loss of hydrochloric acid in the vomitus results in hypochloremic alkalosis in one-third of the infants. Dehydration and wasting soon ensue. A palpable pyloric "tumor" and visible peristalsis are characteristic of the disorder. Surgical incision of the hypertrophied pyloric muscle is curative.

Gross examination of the stomach shows concentric enlargement of the pylorus and narrowing of the pyloric canal. The only consistent microscopic abnormality is extreme hypertrophy of the circular muscle coat. After pyloromyotomy the "tumor" disappears, although occasionally a small symptomatic mass remains.

Hypertrophic pyloric stenosis is an uncommon disorder in adults. Some cases in adults may be due to prolonged pyloric spasm caused by peptic ulcer disease or gastritis; others represent mild cases of congenital pyloric stenosis. The symptoms and treatment are similar to those in the infant, although no abdominal mass is palpable.

Congenital Diaphragmatic Hernias

Congenital diaphragmatic hernias, of variable size and location, are associated with defective closure of embryologic foramina or abnormalities of the esophageal hiatus. The stomach, together with other abdominal organs, may eventrate into the thoracic cavity. Congenital diaphragmatic hernias are often associated with congenital malrotations of the intestine. Herniation of the abdominal contents into the thorax may be asymptomatic or may lead to severe respiratory embarrassment, necessitating surgical intervention.

Rare Congenital Abnormalities

Duplications, diverticula, and cysts, usually lined by normal gastric mucosa, are distinctly uncommon. Whereas all layers of the stomach wall are usually present in congenital duplications, muscle coats are often deficient in diverticula and cysts. Patients with these disorders are usually asymptomatic. Acquired diverticula caused by inflammatory disorders near the pylorus may produce high (proximal) intestinal obstruction.

In **situs inversus** the stomach is located to the right of the midline, as is the esophageal hiatus. Correspondingly, the duodenum is on the left.

Islands of **aberrant pancreatic tissue** are common in the wall of the antrum and pylorus. Histologically, these pancreatic "rests" are identical to normal pancreatic tissue, except that islets are rare. Heterotopic pancreatic tissue is usually asymptomatic, but pyloric obstruction and epigastric pain have been reported.

Partial gastric **atresias** in the body, antrum, and pylorus have been described, as have cases in which the stomach ends blindly. Congenital pyloric and antral **membranes,** presumably caused by failure of the stomach to canalize, may cause symptoms of obstruction in the neonatal period but more commonly become symptomatic in adults.

Gastritis

The terms "acute" and "chronic gastritis" may be confusing, because to the pathologist they refer only to the morphologic appearance of gastric injury and do not connote a temporal difference. Yet acute gastritis is ordinarily a self-limited disorder, whereas chronic gastritis is typically present for many years. Therefore, it seems preferable to use the term **erosive** for acute gastritis and **nonerosive** for chronic gastritis. Gastritis associated with specific causes, such as infections and hypersensitivity reactions, will be discussed separately.

Erosive Gastritis (Acute Gastritis)

Erosive gastritis is the presence of focal necrosis of the mucosa in an otherwise normal stomach. The erosion of the mucosa may extend into the deeper tissues to form an acute ulcer. The necrosis is accompanied by an acute inflammatory response and often by hemorrhage. In fact, hemorrhage may be so severe as to result in exsanguination.

Causes

Erosive gastritis may be associated with the accidental or suicidal ingestion of corrosive substances, such as those that produce erosive esophagitis. However, more commonly the condition is associated with the intake of **alcohol** or certain drugs, particularly **aspirin** and **other nonsteroidal anti-inflammatory agents.** The oral administration of corticosteroids is also occasionally complicated by erosive gastritis. As with corrosive agents, the injurious effects of alcohol and drugs are, for the most part, topical.

Gastric erosions are also seen in a variety of other clinical situations, the common factor among which appears to be so-called stress. These **stress ulcers,** long known to occur in severely burned individuals **(Curling's ulcer),** commonly result in bleeding, which is occasionally severe. The ulceration may be so severe as to cause perforation of the stomach. Patients occasionally exhibit both gastric and duodenal ulcers. Another cause of stress ulcers is **trauma to the central nervous system,** either accidental or surgical **(Cushing's ulcer).** These ulcers, which may also occur in the esophagus or duodenum, are characteristically deep and carry a substantial risk of perforation. Injury to the brain, particularly if it results in a decerebrate state, often leads to increased acid secretion in the stomach, presumably as a result of increased vagal tone, but also perhaps in part secondary to enhanced production of gastrin. Severe trauma, especially if accompanied by **shock,** prolonged **sepsis,** and **incapacitation** from many debilitating chronic diseases also predispose to the development of erosive gastritis. **The first sign of stress ulcers may be massive, life-threatening hemorrhage.**

Pathology

The typical case of erosive gastritis is characterized grossly by widespread petechial hemorrhages in any portion of the stomach or regions of confluent mucosal or submucosal bleeding. Erosions vary in size from 1 mm to 25 mm across and appear occasionally as sharply punched-out ulcers. Microscopically, patchy mucosal necrosis extending to the submucosa is visualized adjacent to normal mucosa. The necrotic epithelium is eventually sloughed, and deeper erosions and hemorrhage may be present. In extreme cases penetrating ulcers are associated with necrosis extending through to the serosa. Depending on the age of the process, there may be mild inflammation, initially neutrophilic and then mononuclear. Healing is usually complete within a few days.

Pathogenesis

Stress ulcers have been produced experimentally in rats by restraint, forced exertion, and traumatic or hemorrhagic shock. In rats and other species, burns and neurologic trauma also result in erosive gastritis. Certain types of prolonged psychologic stresses have

been reported to produce erosive lesions in the stomach and duodenum. The nonsteroidal anti-inflammatory compounds, corticosteroids, and concentrated ethanol consistently cause gastric erosions in rats.

The role of **hypersecretion of gastric acid** in the pathogenesis of erosive gastritis is not clear. Acid secretion is often increased in some circumstances, such as neurologic trauma, but the development of stress ulcers is not generally accompanied by any such increase. Nevertheless, gastric acid may play a permissive role, since inhibition of gastric acid secretion (e.g., with cimetidine) protects against the development of stress ulcers. **Microcirculatory changes in the stomach induced by shock or sepsis may add ischemic injury as a complication of erosive gastritis.**

Since the contents of the stomach would be highly toxic to any tissue outside the gastrointestinal tract, **it is thought that the protective mechanisms of the gastric mucosa are the important defense against mucosal erosion.** It follows that the pathogenesis of erosive gastritis likely involves, at least in part, impairment of these local defensive factors, which include (a) gastric mucus, (b) tissue prostaglandins, (c) epithelial renewal, and (d) intramural pH.

Each of these defensive factors has been individually investigated as follows:

(a) Experimental administration of corticosteroids and aspirin leads both to **decreased mucus production** and to gastric ulcers. By contrast, certain prostaglandins that stimulate mucus secretion also protect against gastric erosions.

(b) Since most of the pharmacologic effects of nonsteroidal anti-inflammatory agents have been related to inhibition of prostaglandin synthesis, the resulting **prostaglandin deficiency** after administration of these drugs has been postulated to decrease the mucosal resistance to the contents of the stomach.

(c) **The renewal of gastric epithelial cells** is clearly necessary for healing erosions of any etiology. In this respect it is interesting that trophic agents, such as growth hormone, epidermal growth factor, and gastrin, not only stimulate DNA synthesis in the gastric mucosa, but also protect against erosions produced by restraint and by aspirin.

(d) Hemorrhagic shock that produces gastric erosions has been shown to result in a **lowering of the intramural pH of the gastric mucosa,** a sign of back-diffusion of acid and an inability to handle the influx of H^+; acid-induced damage to the gastric mucosa may thus be important in the pathogenesis of certain erosions.

Nonerosive Gastritis (Chronic Gastritis)

Nonerosive gastritis is a chronic inflammatory disease of the stomach of unknown cause that ranges from mild superficial involvement to severe atrophy of the gastric mucosa. By itself the disorder gives rise to few if any symptoms, and the diagnosis is ordinarily made when associated conditions cause the patient to present with clinical complaints. An association between nonerosive gastritis and dyspepsia has not been sustained; thus, **nonerosive gastritis should be considered a histologic rather than a clinical entity.**

A cardinal feature of nonerosive gastritis is the progressive **loss of the capacity to secrete acid (achlorhydria)** as the condition becomes more severe. Achlorhydria arises because of the loss of parietal cells in the body of the stomach. The loss of parietal cells also leads to a deficiency of intrinsic factor, which is necessary for the absorption of vitamin B_{12} in the ileum. As a consequence, **pernicious anemia** develops. Although an increased incidence of gastric ulcers has been reported in association with nonerosive gastritis, it is not certain which is the cause and which is the effect. Certain changes in the character of the mucosal lining cells of the antrum, termed "intestinal metaplasia," have been related to the pathogenesis of **cancer of the stomach** (discussed later).

Pathology

On gross examination nonerosive gastritis displays few if any characteristic alterations; identification of the disorder is made on histologic grounds. On the basis of the primary region of the stomach involved, nonerosive gastritis has been divided into **fundal gastritis** and **antral gastritis,** although the lesions characteristically overlap. The distinction is of more than academic interest, since these disorders do not necessarily have the same cause and the sequelae may be different.

Fundal gastritis typically exhibits a lack of or minimal involvement of the antrum, diffuse gastritis in the body and fundus of the stomach, antibodies to parietal cells, and a significant reduction in or absence of gastric secretion. This form of gastritis may be associated with pernicious anemia, as well as with extragastric "autoimmune" diseases, such as chronic thyroiditis, Addison's disease, vitiligo, and diabetes.

By contrast, antral gastritis, which is considerably more common than fundal gastritis, shows only focal lesions in the body of the stomach, severe involvement of the antrum, a lack of antibodies to parietal cells, and only a modest reduction in gastric secretion. The antral variety of nonerosive gastritis is not associated with pernicious anemia but, like fundal gastritis, carries a significant risk for the development of stomach cancer.

The mildest form of nonerosive gastritis is a **superficial gastritis.** This lesion occasionally reverts to normal but more commonly proceeds to **atrophic gastritis,** a disorder that usually persists indefinitely. In some cases a final stage, **gastric atrophy,** shows few of the inflammatory features of gastritis.

Superficial gastritis typically shows lymphocytes and plasma cells, and occasionally neutrophils, in the lamina propria of the mucosa of the antrum and body of the stomach. The inflammation is most intense around the gastric pits (foveolae), where small foci of neutrophils may also be seen, but the glands are spared. The normal columnar epithelium becomes more cuboidal and contains less mucin than normal. The process may be quiescent, in which case the epithelial cells are little changed and no neutrophils are present. Although superficial gastritis does not involve the gastric glands, histamine-stimulated secretion of acid and pepsin is impaired.

Atrophic gastritis may evolve from superficial gastritis, but there is no sharp distinction between them. Like superficial gastritis, active atrophic gastritis is characterized by prominent chronic inflammation in the lamina propria. However, lymphocytes and plasma cells extend into the deepest reaches of the mucosa as far as the muscularis mucosae. Occasionally, lymphoid cells are arranged as follicles, an appearance that has led to an erroneous diagnosis of lymphoma or pseudolymphoma. Involvement of the gastric glands leads to degenerative changes in their epithelial cells and ultimately a conspicuous reduction in the number of glands; hence the name *atrophic gastritis* (Fig. 13-9). Eventually the inflammatory process may abate, leaving only a thin atrophic mucosa (gastric atrophy).

A common and important histologic feature of nonerosive gastritis is **intestinal metaplasia,** a condition in which the injured gastric mucosa is replaced by an epithelium composed of cells of the intestinal type (Figs. 13-10 and 13-11). Numerous mucin-containing goblet cells and enterocytes line cryptlike glands, and many Paneth cells, which are not normal denizens of the gastric mucosa, are present. However, intestinal villi do not usually form. The various endocrine cells, normally situated on the basement membrane of the gastric glands, are clustered at the base of the crypts, similar to their location in the intestine. Mitoses are more numerous than in the normal gastric mucosa. In most cases islands of metaplastic epithelium alternate with atrophic gastric glands, but in severe cases large areas of the mucosa may resemble colon or small intestine, complete with villi and Paneth cells. Not only are the metaplastic cells morphologically similar to intestinal cells, they also contain enzymes characteristic of the intestine but not of the stomach (e.g., alkaline phosphatase, aminopeptidase). Moreover, whereas gastric secretions contain principally neutral mucins, the goblet cells of the metaplastic epithelium produce the typical intestinal acid mucins.

In the fundus of the stomach with atrophic gastritis, the normal parietal and zymogen cells may be replaced by clear mucous glands similar to those of the cardia or antrum, a change termed "pseudopyloric metaplasia." It is therefore important for the pathologist to know the precise location from which a biopsy was taken, since fundal pseudopyloric metaplasia may be mistaken for gastritis of the antrum.

Pathogenesis and Consequences

Aging

The most common determinant of nonerosive gastritis is aging. Whereas foci of nonerosive gastritis are found in as many as one third of persons aged 30 years, more than half the population over 40 years of age exhibits superficial gastritis. A decade later the same population is affected by mild or moderate atrophic gastritis. Antral gastritis is more severe and occurs earlier than fundal gastritis. These data were obtained in Europe, Japan, and South America, but it is probable that similar patterns obtain in the United States.

Postgastrectomy Gastritis

All individuals subjected to partial gastrectomy develop nonerosive gastritis in the remaining stomach, usually within 2 years. The pattern is typically that of atrophic gastritis with intestinal metaplasia. Despite many theories, the cause remains obscure.

Gastric Ulcers

Chronic gastric ulcers are always accompanied by superficial and atrophic gastritis of the antrum, usually in association with intestinal metaplasia. Less severe gastritis may also affect the body of the stomach. Because the nonerosive gastritis seems to persist after the ulcer heals, it has been postulated that the underlying cause of the gastric ulcer is the gastritis. However, the subject requires further study.

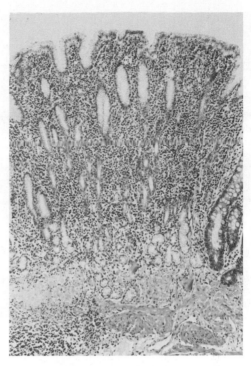

Figure 13-9. Atrophic gastritis. The gastric mucosa is thinned and displays a conspicuous chronic inflammatory infiltrate that separates the atrophic glands. A small focus of intestinal metaplasia is present on the *right*.

Pernicious Anemia

Pernicious anemia, a megaloblastic anemia that is associated with complete achlorhydria, is caused by malabsorption of vitamin B$_{12}$ occasioned by a deficiency of intrinsic factor. The stomach invariably displays atrophy of the fundic glands, accompanied by slight chronic inflammation. Both pseudopyloric and intestinal metaplasia may be prominent. Involvement of the antrum may occur but is generally less severe. In cases in which antral gland activity remains, the number of gastrin-containing cells is increased, and in most cases of pernicious anemia serum gastrin levels are high. Despite the common occurrence of atrophic gastritis among the elderly, only a few aged persons develop pernicious anemia.

Pernicious anemia is suspected to be an autoimmune disease, although the pathogenetic significance of autoantibodies is not fully elucidated. Pernicious anemia is often seen in conjunction with autoimmune diseases of the thyroid and adrenal glands. Half of patients with pernicious anemia have circulating antibodies to thyroid tissue, and about one-third of those with chronic thyroiditis possess gastric autoantibodies. Circulating antibodies to parietal cells are found in 40% to 90% of patients with pernicious anemia. Although up to 20% of persons beyond the age of 60 years exhibit parietal cell anti-

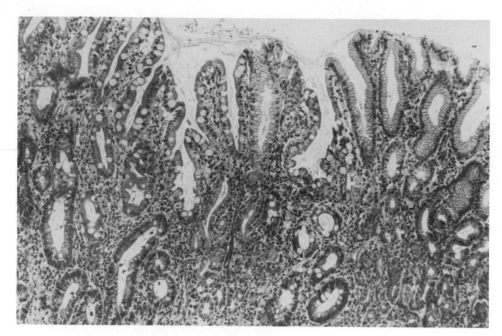

Figure 13-10. Chronic gastritis with intestinal metaplasia. The glands on the *right* are of the gastric type, whereas those in the *center* and on the *left* are of the intestinal type. In the areas of intestinal metaplasia goblet cells are prominent, and rudimentary villi are evident.

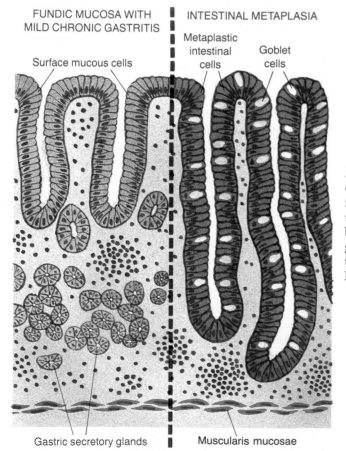

FUNDIC MUCOSA WITH
MILD CHRONIC GASTRITIS

INTESTINAL METAPLASIA

Metaplastic
intestinal
cells

Goblet
cells

Surface mucous cells

Gastric secretory glands

Muscularis mucosae

Figure 13-11. Schematic representation of the pathology of chronic gastritis. In mild gastritis there is chronic inflammation and a reduction in the number and size of the gastric glands. More severe gastritis is accompanied by intestinal metaplasia, a condition in which the normal gastric epithelium is replaced by a metaplastic intestinal-type epithelium containing enterocytes, goblet cells, and Paneth cells.

bodies, few persons under the age of 40 possess them in the absence of pernicious anemia. Moreover, in two-thirds of patients with pernicious anemia, antibodies to intrinsic factor are present. Cell-mediated immunologic abnormalities are also present in most persons with pernicious anemia and are postulated to play a role in the pathogenesis of this disease.

Pernicious anemia shows a familial tendency. Ten percent to 15% of first-degree relatives of patients with pernicious anemia demonstrate severe atrophic gastritis, although they do not suffer from megaloblastic anemia. Moreover, almost all of these relatives have achlorhydria, two-thirds have circulating parietal cell antibodies, and one-fifth manifest antibodies to intrinsic factor. These persons are clearly at high risk of developing pernicious anemia, but it is not known how many actually do so.

Nonerosive Gastritis and Stomach Cancer

It is generally accepted that persons with atrophic gastritis have a higher than normal incidence of carcinoma of the stomach. Reliable statistics about this relationship are difficult to obtain, because atrophic gastritis is usually asymptomatic and therefore does not ordinarily come under medical scrutiny. However, patients with pernicious anemia, who invariably suffer from atrophic gastritis, have a threefold to fourfold increased risk of developing gastric cancer. **Cancer arises in the antrum several times more frequently than in the body of the stomach.** Epidemiologic studies, particularly from Japan, where gastric cancer is common, suggest that antral gastritis is related to the development of carcinoma of the stomach. However, direct evidence for a causal connection has not been firmly established.

Intestinal metaplasia of the stomach has been particularly identified as a preneoplastic lesion for several reasons: stomachs that contain cancer have an increased incidence and severity of intestinal metaplasia; gastric cancer has been shown to arise in areas of metaplastic epithelium; half of all cancers of the stomach are of the intestinal cell type; and many cases of carcinoma of the stomach show aminopeptidase activity similar to that seen in areas of intestinal metaplasia.

Distinct Varieties of Gastritis

Menetrier's Disease (Giant Hypertrophic Gastritis)

Menetrier's disease, an uncommon gastric disorder characterized by giant hypertrophy of the mucosal folds of the stomach, is usually included under the

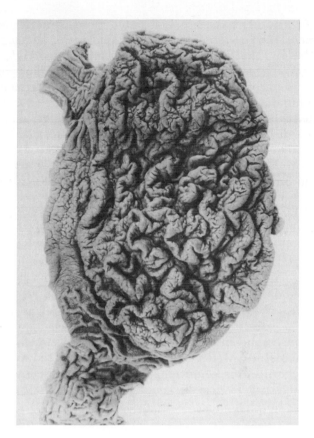

Figure 13-12. Menetrier's disease. The folds of the stomach are increased in height and thickness, forming a convoluted surface.

rubric of inflammatory disorders, although direct evidence for such an etiology is lacking. The cause of the disease is unknown.

Grossly, the stomach is increased in weight as much as 900 g to 1200 g. **The folds of the greater curvature in the fundus and body of the stomach, and occasionally in the antrum, are increased in height and thickness, forming a convoluted surface that has been compared to that of the brain** (Fig. 13-12). Microscopically, the disease is restricted to the mucosa. Hyperplasia of the gastric pits results in a conspicuous increase in their depth and a tortuous (corkscrew) structure. Mucus-secreting cells of the surface or neck type line the foveolae. The glands are elongated, and many appear cystic. These dilated glands, which are lined by superficial-type, mucus-secreting epithelial cells, may penetrate the muscularis mucosae, in which case they resemble the sinuses of Rokitansky-Aschoff in the gallbladder. Pseudopyloric metaplasia is occasionally noted, but intestinal metaplasia does not occur. Lymphocytes, plasma cells, and occasional neutrophils are seen in the lamina propria.

Menetrier's disease is 4 times more common in men than in women and affects persons of all ages. The presenting symptom is usually postprandial pain, relieved by antacids. Weight loss, sometimes of rapid onset, occasionally occurs. Peripheral edema is common, and in some cases ascites and cachexia simulate the presence of cancer. These manifestations of the disease are related to a **severe loss of plasma proteins (including albumin) from the altered gastric mucosa.** The cause of the enormous protein loss into the lumen of the stomach is obscure. Amelioration of protein loss has been reported after treatment with anticholinergic agents or cimetidine. Although gastric acidity is usually low, severe peptic ulceration associated with hyperacidity has occasionally been observed. In such cases the diagnosis of Zollinger-Ellison syndrome is suggested, but this condition can be ruled out by the absence of an elevated serum gastrin level.

The disorder does not usually resolve spontaneously, and in intractable cases partial gastrectomy is necessary. **Menetrier's disease is considered to be a precancerous condition;** therefore, periodic endoscopic surveillance is recommended.

Idiopathic Granulomatous Gastritis

Idiopathic granulomatous gastritis is defined as the presence of epithelioid granulomas in the gastric mucosa when specific granulomatous disorders, such as sarcoidosis, Crohn's disease, and tuberculosis, have been excluded. Occasionally, the granulomas are found in association with mild superficial or atrophic gastritis, but usually little or no additional inflammation is present. By definition the cause is unknown, but granulomas are occasionally found in the vicinity of a peptic ulcer or carcinoma. Sometimes a foreign body giant cell contains food debris. The condition is benign and ordinarily clinically silent.

Eosinophilic Gastritis

Eosinophilic gastritis, often in association with eosinophilic enteritis, is a rare disease in which eosinophilic inflammation involves all layers of the stomach wall or is selectively localized in a single layer. The disease affects principally the antrum and pylorus, where a diffuse thickening of the wall, presumably by muscular hypertrophy, may narrow the pylorus and cause symptoms of obstruction, occasionally severe enough to require surgical relief. In some cases ulceration in the affected area leads to chronic blood loss and anemia. Peripheral eosinophilia and a history of food allergies are common, but many patients have neither. Treatment with corticosteroids may be effective in some patients.

Miscellaneous Causes of Gastritis

Radiation may cause damage to the stomach in the same way that it injures other tissues. Although direct irradiation of the stomach is uncommon, the organ may be included in the field of abdominal radiation for extragastric neoplasms. **Freezing,** once a popular therapy for peptic ulcer disease, has been associated with the development of gastritis; this treatment has been abandoned. As previously mentioned, **Crohn's disease** and **sarcoidosis** on occasion involve the stomach, where they cause symptoms similar to those of gastritis. These disorders may be difficult to distinguish from nonspecific nonerosive gastritis in small gastric biopsy specimens. Specific infections, such as **tuberculosis, syphilis,** and a variety of **fungi,** may also cause inflammation of the stomach. Although cytomegalovirus and herpesvirus are recognized in the stomach, albeit rarely, it is unclear whether these viruses produce mucosal lesions or merely colonize previously injured mucosa.

Peptic Ulcer Disease

"Peptic ulcer disease" refers to breaks in the mucosa of the stomach and small intestine, principally the proximal duodenum, that are produced by the action of gastric secretions. Peptic ulcers of the stomach and duodenum are estimated to afflict 10% of the population of Western industrialized countries at some time during their lives. Although peptic ulcer disease is one of the most common disorders in humans, and despite an enormous number of clinical and experimental studies, it is still unknown why ulcers develop and why they heal. Although peptic ulceration can occur as high as Barrett's esophagus (in addition to ulceration of the squamous mucosa in reflux esophagitis) and as low as Meckel's diverticulum, for practical purposes **peptic ulcer disease affects the distal stomach and proximal duodenum.** Many clinical and epidemiologic features distinguish gastric from duodenal ulcers; the common factor that unites them is the gastric secretion of hydrochloric acid. With rare exceptions, **a person who does not secrete acid will not develop a peptic ulcer anywhere.**

The symptomatologies of gastric and duodenal ulcers are sufficiently similar that the two conditions are generally not distinguishable by history or physical examination. The "classic" case of duodenal ulcer is characterized by burning epigastric pain that is experienced 1 to 3 hours after a meal or that awakens the patient at night. Both alkali and food are said to relieve the symptoms. However, detailed studies have demonstrated that the majority of patients do not conform to the "classic" presentation. Half do not describe their pain as related to meals, and fewer than half report that the pain is relieved by food or alkali. Dyspeptic symptoms commonly associated with gallbladder disease, including fatty food intolerance, distention, and belching, occur in half of patients with peptic ulcers.

Epidemiologic Considerations

Gastric and duodenal ulcers were distinctly uncommon in the 19th century, and those that occurred were usually gastric ulcers in young women. After World War I, the occurrence of duodenal ulcers changed from a rare event to an exceptionally common one, while gastric ulcers decreased in incidence and became a disorder of elderly men and women.

It has been widely perceived that both the incidence and the prevalence of duodenal ulcers have declined substantially during the last 25 years. Certainly, mortality from this disease, as well as the number of admissions to hospitals, have fallen. However, careful population studies in the United States and Europe have not supported the notion that the disease itself is less common today. The decreased hospitalization and mortality may reflect earlier diagnosis, more accurate discrimination of duodenal ulcer disease from other entities that cause ulcer-like symptoms, improved pharmacologic management, and an increase in medical rather than surgical treatment. At the current state of knowledge, **it is inappropriate to draw any firm conclusions regarding trends in the incidence of duodenal ulcer disease.** Only detailed prospective epidemiologic studies can resolve this question. The incidence of gastric ulcers, at least as measured by hospital admissions and outpatient visits, seems to have remained essentially stationary over the last few decades.

The **age profile** of peptic ulcer disease has progressively increased in the last 50 years. The peak incidence of duodenal ulcer disease is now between the ages of 30 and 60, although the disorder may occur in persons of any age, even in infants. Gastric ulcers afflict the middle-aged and elderly more than the young. The **sex distribution** of duodenal ulcers has shown a striking change, from a marked female predominance in the 19th century to a predominantly male predominance today. The incidence of gastric ulcers is the same for men and women. **Racial dif-**

ferences in the incidence of peptic ulcers have been observed, but the studies of different ethnic populations are confounded by variations in many other environmental factors. For example, in Africa duodenal ulcers are rare among blacks, whereas in the United States the incidence is the same in blacks and whites. In India the disease is uncommon in the arid plains but more frequent in certain mountainous areas. The preponderance of evidence suggests that in an urban Western setting all ethnic groups are susceptible.

The common stereotype of the patient with a peptic ulcer is the highly motivated executive operating in a stressful environment. However, careful epidemiologic surveys in the United States and Great Britain have suggested an **inverse relationship between duodenal ulcers and socioeconomic status and education,** although the trends are not marked.

Pathogenesis

Risk Factors

Despite the common wisdom that holds that spicy food and caffeine are ulcerogenic, the evidence to support the contention that the consumption of any food or beverage, including coffee, contributes to the development or persistence of peptic ulcers is surprisingly meager. This lack of evidence for a commonly held assumption extends to alcohol intake, which is also widely considered to be an important determinant in the pathogenesis of peptic ulcer disease. Although high concentrations of alcohol can result in hemorrhagic gastritis and may stimulate acid secretion, there are no data that link the consumption of alcohol to either gastric or duodenal ulcers. However, **cirrhosis** from any cause is associated with an increased incidence of peptic ulcers.

Although close analysis of the epidemiologic data has undermined the strength of some of these associations, it is widely held that the intake of certain drugs leads to peptic ulcers. Both prospective and cross-sectional studies indicate that **aspirin** is an important contributing factor in the genesis of duodenal and especially gastric ulcers. Other **nonsteroidal anti-inflammatory agents** and **analgesics** have been incriminated in the production of peptic ulcers. Prolonged treatment with high doses of corticosteroids has been claimed to increase slightly the risk of peptic ulceration.

Cigarette smoking has been considered a definite risk factor for duodenal and gastric ulcers, particularly gastric ulcers. Recent analysis of the data has weakened, although not eliminated, this association.

The mechanisms by which smoking may predispose to peptic ulcers are controversial.

Genetic Factors

Peptic ulcer disease illustrates the importance of genetic factors and their interaction with environmental mechanisms. First-degree relatives of patients with duodenal ulcers have a threefold increased risk of developing a duodenal ulcer but do not have a similar increase in risk of developing a gastric ulcer. Patients with gastric ulcers similarly "breed true." These data are confirmed by the finding of a considerably higher concordance for these ulcers in monozygotic than in dizygotic twins. (The fact that identical twins show only 50% concordance indicates that genetic factors alone are not sufficient to produce an ulcer; environmental factors must also be involved.)

Further evidence for the role of genetic factors comes from studies of **blood-group antigens.** The risk of duodenal ulcer is about 30% higher in persons with **type O blood** than in A, B, and AB individuals, although patients with gastric ulcers do not exhibit a greater frequency of blood group O. **The quarter of the population that does not secrete blood-group antigens in the saliva and gastric juice is at a 50% increased risk of developing a duodenal ulcer.** The risk of duodenal ulceration is greatly increased (2.5:1) when nonsecretory status is combined with blood group O, a combination that occurs in 10% of the Caucasian population. Associations between certain histocompatibility antigens and peptic ulcers have been claimed but are still debated.

Pepsinogen I is secreted by the chief and mucous neck cells of the gastric mucosa and appears in the gastric juice, blood, and urine. Serum levels of this proenzyme correlate with the gastric capacity for acid secretion and are considered a measure of parietal cell mass. **A person with high circulating levels of pepsinogen I is at 5 times the normal risk of developing a duodenal ulcer.** Hyperpepsinogenemia I is present in half of the children of patients with hyperpepsinogenemia and has been attributed to autosomal dominant inheritance. Thus, not only is hyperpepsinogenemia considered a marker for an ulcer diathesis, it is also thought to indicate a genetically predetermined increase in parietal cell mass.

Many patients with peptic ulcer have normal pepsinogen I secretion, and familial aggregation has also been demonstrated in this group. Familial clustering of duodenal ulcers and **rapid gastric emptying** have been demonstrated, and familial **hyperfunction of gastrin-secreting cells (G cells)** in the antrum is also reported. Patients with a childhood duodenal ulcer are considerably more likely to have a family history of an ulcer diathesis than persons in whom the disease begins when they are adults.

Psychologic Factors

"Stress" has been anecdotally related to peptic ulcers for at least a century, and repressed stress has been considered particularly ulcerogenic. Closer scrutiny of the epidemiologic and experimental evidence supporting these concepts has cast serious doubt on their validity, and many today discount any relationship between stress and ulcers. Whatever the final outcome of this debate may be, **there is no need to incriminate stress in the pathogenesis of peptic ulcers.**

Physiologic Factors

The formation and persistence of peptic ulcers in both the stomach and duodenum require the gastric secretion of acid. This is evidenced principally by the following: all patients with duodenal ulcers and almost all with gastric ulcers are gastric acid secretors; the experimental production of ulcers in animals requires the production of acid; hypersecretion of acid is present in many, but not all, patients with duodenal ulcers (there is no evidence that overproduction of acid by itself is necessary or sufficient to explain duodenal ulceration); and surgical or medical treatment that reduces acid production results in the healing of peptic ulcers. The gastric secretion of pepsin, which may also play a role in the production of peptic ulcers, parallels that of hydrochloric acid.

The maximal capacity for acid production by the stomach is a reflection of total parietal cell mass. Both parietal cell mass and maximal acid secretion are increased up to twofold in patients with duodenal ulcers. However, there is a large overlap with normal values, and **only one third of these patients secrete excess acid.** The increase in parietal cells is paralleled by a comparable increase in chief cells, a situation that is consistent with the increased prevalence of hyperpepsinogenemia in ulcer patients.

The gastric secretion of acid stimulated by food is increased in magnitude and duration in duodenal ulcer patients, although here too there is significant overlap with normal values. In a few patients this may involve, at least in part, an altered response of the G cells to meals. Such individuals exhibit postprandial hypergastrinemia and an increase in the number of G cells in the antrum. The majority of patients with duodenal ulcers, however, show no evidence of G-cell hyperfunction.

Patients with duodenal ulcers may also be more sensitive than normal to gastric secretagogues such as gastrin, possibly as a result of increased vagal tone or a greater than normal affinity of the parietal cells for gastrin. It is further possible that the brisk secretion of acid after a meal is stimulated by increased vagal tone.

The duodenum may also be excessively acidified by the rapid emptying of gastric contents. **Accelerated gastric emptying** has been noted in patients with duodenal ulcers although, as with other factors, there is substantial overlap with normal rates. Normally acidification of the duodenal bulb inhibits further gastric emptying. It has been reported that in the majority of patients with duodenal ulcer this feedback inhibitory mechanism is absent, and duodenal acidification results in continued, rather than delayed, gastric emptying. Evidence suggests that rapid gastric emptying may in some cases be an inherited abnormality.

The pH of the duodenal bulb reflects the balance between the delivery of gastric juice and its neutralization by biliary, pancreatic, and duodenal secretions. The production of duodenal ulcers requires an acidic pH in the bulb—that is, an excess of acid over neutralizing secretions. In ulcer patients the duodenal pH following a meal falls to a lower level and remains depressed for a longer time than in normal individuals. This duodenal hyperacidity certainly reflects the gastric factors discussed above. The role of neutralizing factors, particularly secretin-stimulated bicarbonate secretion by the pancreas and production of bicarbonate by the duodenal mucosa, is uncertain, and the subject remains controversial.

The role of impaired mucosal defenses against peptic ulceration is not well delineated. The mucosal factors, including the function of prostaglandins, may or may not be similar to those protecting the gastric mucosa (considered above in the section entitled Erosive Gastritis).

The various gastric and duodenal factors that have been implicated as possible mechanisms in the pathogenesis of duodenal ulceration are summarized in Figure 13-13.

Although gastric juice is clearly implicated in the production of duodenal ulcers, its role in the formation of gastric ulcers is more difficult to assess. A number of patients with gastric ulcers display hypersecretion of acid, but most secrete not only less gastric acid than patients with duodenal ulcer, but even less than normal people. The genesis of gastric hyposecretion is obscure. The factors implicated include back-diffusion of acid into the mucosa, decreased parietal cell mass, and abnormalities of the parietal cells themselves. Gastric ulcers in patients with acid hypersecretion are usually near the pylorus and are considered variants of duodenal ulceration.

Interestingly, the intense gastric hypersecretion seen in the Zollinger-Ellison syndrome is associated with severe ulceration of the duodenum and even the jejunum, but rarely with gastric ulcers.

The occurrence of gastric ulcers in the face of gastric hyposecretion implies the following possibilities: that the gastric mucosa is in some way particularly sensitive to low concentrations of acid; that some material other than acid damages the mucosa; or that the gastric mucosa is exposed to potentially injurious agents for an unusually long period of time. As discussed in the section entitled Erosive Gastritis, the mucosal barrier to the action of acid, and perhaps to other contents of the stomach, may be impaired in some patients with gastric ulcers, although the evidence is far from conclusive. Reflux of bile (particularly deoxycholic acid and lysolecithin) and pancreatic secretions have been suggested as a cause of gastric ulcers. Although there is some evidence that many patients with gastric ulcers exhibit duodenogastric reflux, there is still debate as to whether the duodenal contents actually cause gastritis and whether this gastritis leads to peptic ulcers of the stomach. Although nonerosive, superficial, and atrophic gastritis often accompany gastric ulcers, it is not known whether the ulcer or the gastritis is the primary event. In some patients who suffer from pyloric obstruction (e.g., persons with adult hypertrophic pyloric stenosis or scarring secondary to a duodenal ulcer) peptic ulcers of the stomach appear to be related to retention of gastric contents. However, the precise elements of the retained gastric contents that precipitate such ulcers have not been elucidated.

There is considerable interest in the possibility that peptic ulcer disease may be caused, at least in part, by colonization of the upper gastrointestinal tract by *Campylobacter pylori*. However, the evidence is contradictory, and a role for this organism in the pathogenesis of peptic ulcers remains controversial.

In summary, the pathogenesis of gastric and duodenal peptic ulcers remains poorly understood. The only certainty is that at least some acid is required for both. The contributions of the mechanisms discussed above are, for the most part, hypothetical, and their relative roles remain to be defined.

Associated Diseases

Cirrhosis is associated with an increased frequency of duodenal ulcers. The incidence of duodenal ulcers in patients with cirrhosis is tenfold greater than in normal persons, and the prevalence after cirrhosis has been established as increased twofold to three-

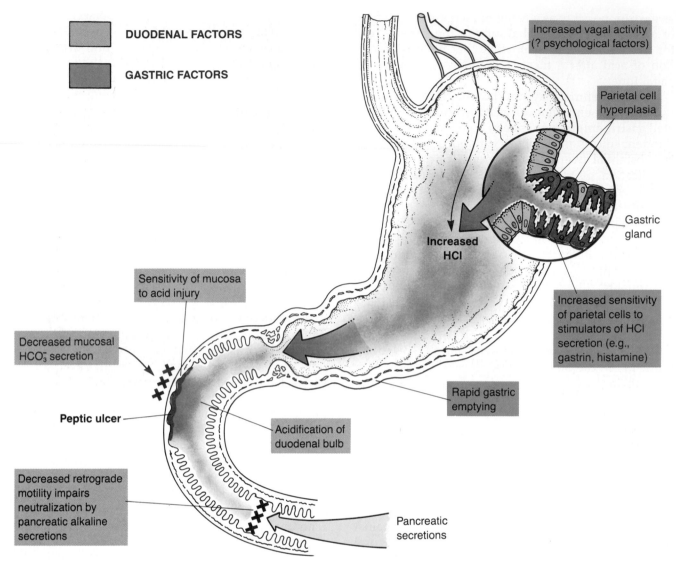

DUODENAL FACTORS

GASTRIC FACTORS

Increased vagal activity (? psychological factors)

Parietal cell hyperplasia

Gastric gland

Increased HCl

Sensitivity of mucosa to acid injury

Decreased mucosal HCO₃⁻ secretion

Increased sensitivity of parietal cells to stimulators of HCl secretion (e.g., gastrin, histamine)

Peptic ulcer

Rapid gastric emptying

Acidification of duodenal bulb

Decreased retrograde motility impairs neutralization by pancreatic alkaline secretions

Pancreatic secretions

Figure 13-13. Gastric and duodenal factors in the pathogenesis of duodenal peptic ulcers.

fold. Moreover, the death rate from duodenal ulcer is increased fivefold in patients with cirrhosis. The mechanisms responsible for this association are unclear.

Patients with **chronic renal failure** maintained on hemodialysis have been reported to be at greater than normal risk for the development of peptic ulcers, although the data are not conclusive. Patients subjected to **renal transplantation** have a substantially increased risk of peptic ulceration and its complications, such as bleeding and perforation. Prophylactic treatment with histamine-receptor antagonists has been reported to reduce this risk.

Peptic ulcers occur in conjunction with a number of hereditary syndromes. There is an increased incidence of peptic ulcers in persons with **multiple endocrine neoplasia, type I (MEN I).** The presence of a functioning parathyroid adenoma and its associated hypercalcemia has been misinterpreted as an association between hypercalcemia and peptic ulcers. It is now recognized that this association is a consequence of the simultaneous occurrence of a gastrinoma and may not necessarily be related to the hypercalcemia itself. The Zollinger-Ellison syndrome (discussed in Chapter 15) is characterized by profound gastric hypersecretion caused by a gastrin-producing islet cell adenoma.

Renal stones are a recognized complication of hyperparathyroidism, and their association in this instance with peptic ulcer also probably reflects an accompanying gastrinoma. However, there seems to be an increased incidence of peptic ulcers in patients with renal stones unassociated with either hypercalcemia (caused by hyperparathyroidism) or an excess intake of milk and antacids for the relief of ulcer symptoms. The underlying mechanism of this association is obscure.

Almost one-third of patients with hereditary **alpha₁-antitrypsin deficiency** have peptic ulcers, and this incidence is even higher in patients who have pulmonary disease as well. Moreover, the number of heterozygotes for alpha₁-antitrypsin deficiency among relatives of patients with peptic ulcer is increased. It has been speculated that in this disorder unopposed proteolytic activity may contribute to peptic ulceration.

Peptic ulcers are found in one-fourth of patients with **chronic lung disease,** and chronic pulmonary disease is increased twofold to threefold in patients who have peptic ulcers. These correlations hold even when the data are corrected for smoking. Although some of these patients with pulmonary disease may have underlying alpha₁-antitrypsin deficiency, the correlation is too strong for this to be the sole explanation. The mechanism for the association has not been established.

Chronic pancreatitis would be expected to predispose to peptic ulcer because of the lack of neutralizing pancreatic juice. However, data regarding such an association are inconclusive.

Pathology

A peptic ulcer should be considered chronic when it does not heal readily and when scarring at the base of the ulcer precludes complete restoration of the normal submucosa and muscularis. Most peptic ulcers arise in the lesser curvature, in the antral and prepyloric regions of the stomach, and in the first part of the duodenum. Gastric ulcers (Fig. 13-14) are usually single and less than 2 cm in diameter, although occasionally they reach a diameter of 10 cm or more, particularly if they are on the lesser curvature. The edges are sharply punched out, with overhanging margins. The flat base is grey and indurated and may exhibit clotted blood or an eroded vessel. Deeply penetrating ulcers produce a serosal exudate, which may cause adherence of the stomach to the surrounding structures. Scarring of ulcers in the prepyloric region may be severe enough to produce pyloric stenosis. On gross examination it may be exceedingly difficult to distinguish chronic peptic ulcer from ulcerating gastric carcinoma. Thus, when

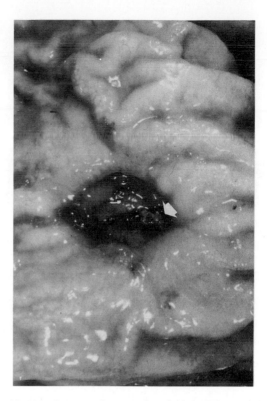

Figure 13-14. Gastric ulcer. A deep peptic ulcer of the stomach has eroded an artery (*arrow*), severe hemorrhage has resulted. The gastric folds converge on the sharply circumscribed ulcer.

examining the stomach, the endoscopist is required to take multiple biopsies from the edges of any gastric ulcer.

Duodenal ulcers (Figs. 13-15 and 13-16) are ordinarily located on the anterior or posterior wall of the first part of the duodenum, within a short distance of the pylorus. The lesion is usually solitary, but it is not uncommon to find paired ulcers on both walls, so-called kissing ulcers.

Microscopically, gastric and duodenal ulcers have a similar appearance (see Fig. 13-16). From the lumen outward, the following are noted: a superficial zone of fibrinopurulent exudate; necrotic tissue; granulation tissue; and fibrotic tissue at the base of the ulcer, which exhibits variable degrees of chronic inflammation. The ulceration typically penetrates the muscle layers, thereby causing them to be interrupted by scar tissue. Blood vessels on the margins of the ulcer may be thrombosed or display obliterating endarteritis. The mucosa at the margins of the ulcer is often hyperplastic and with healing may grow over the ulcerated area as a single layer of epithelium. However, in a large ulcer, this ingrowth of the epithelium may be insufficient to cover the defect completely. Downgrowth of the regenerating epithelium at the

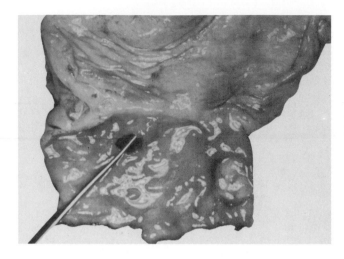

Figure 13-15. Duodenal ulcer. A sharply punched out, perforated peptic ulcer of the duodenum (*probe*) is situated immediately below the pylorus.

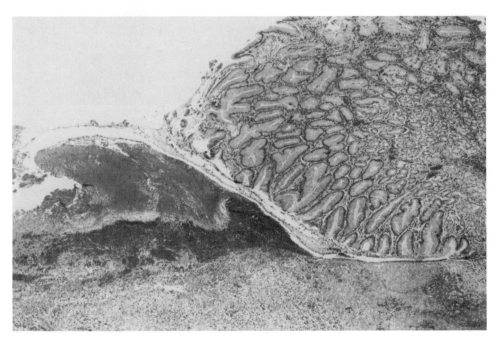

Figure 13-16. Peptic ulcer of the stomach. A photomicrograph demonstrates a sharply demarcated ulcer crater. the bed of the ulcer is covered with a fibrinous and hemorrhagic exudate, below which is inflamed granulation tissue.

margins of the ulcer is visualized in cross section as islands of epithelial cells surrounded by inflamed and fibrotic tissue. This appearance may be confused with that of an infiltrating carcinoma. Gastric ulcers are commonly accompanied by nonerosive gastritis, and the tissue surrounding a gastric or duodenal ulcer is often secondarily inflamed.

Complications

Hemorrhage

The most common complication of peptic ulcers is bleeding, occurring in up to 20% of the patients. In many cases bleeding is occult and, in an otherwise asymptomatic ulcer, may be manifested as iron-deficiency anemia or as occult blood in the stools. Massive life-threatening hemorrhage is a well-recognized danger in patients with active peptic ulcers. Indeed, the first indication that a patient has an ulcer may come from a massive bleeding episode. Disorders of coagulation, whether from a primary clotting disorder or induced by anticoagulant drugs, increase the risk of bleeding from peptic ulcers. Despite improvements in surgical and endoscopic management, transfusion therapy, and the availability of drugs such as H_2-receptor antagonists, mortality from bleeding peptic ulcers has not changed over the last 30 years and remains at about 10%.

Perforation

Perforation is a serious complication of peptic ulcer disease that occurs in 5% or less of patients; in one third of the cases there are no antecedent symptoms referable to peptic ulcer. Perforations occur more commonly with duodenal than with gastric ulcers, the large majority occurring on the anterior wall of the duodenum. Perforations are divided into those in which the luminal contents freely escape into the peritoneal cavity and those in which the penetration is sealed by surrounding structures or peritoneum. Because the anterior walls of the stomach and duodenum are undefended by contiguous tissue, ulcers in these locations are more likely to be complicated by free perforation, which leads to generalized peritonitis and the accumulation of air in the abdominal cavity, a condition called **pneumoperitoneum.** Posterior gastric ulcers perforate into the lesser peritoneal sac, where the inflammatory reaction may be contained. When ulcers penetrate into the pancreas, liver, or greater omentum, they cause intractable symptoms. They may also penetrate the biliary tract and fill it with air.

Perforated ulcers continue to be associated with high mortality. The overall mortality for perforated gastric ulcers is 10% to 40%, 2 to 3 times more than that for duodenal ulcers (5–13%). Perforations are occasionally complicated by hemorrhage, in which case about half of the patients die. Although shock, abdominal distention, and pain are common symptoms, perforations are occasionally diagnosed for the first time at autopsy, particularly in institutionalized, elderly patients.

Pyloric Obstruction (Gastric Outlet Obstruction)

Pyloric obstruction occurs in 5% to 10% of ulcer patients, and peptic ulcer disease is the most common cause of pyloric obstruction in adults. Narrowing of the pyloric lumen by an adjacent peptic ulcer may be caused by muscular spasm, edema, muscular hypertrophy, or contraction of scar tissue; most commonly it is due to a combination of these. Retention of gastric contents results in epigastric distress, anorexia, and early satiety. Eventually obstruction may ensue. In the majority of patients a succussion splash is elicited in the fasting state. Most patients with symptomatic pyloric obstruction eventually require surgical relief.

Development of Combined Ulcers

The simultaneous occurrence of gastric and duodenal ulcers in the same patient is far greater than can be accounted for by chance alone. In the United States almost half the patients with gastric ulcers also have a duodenal ulcer or an ulcer scar. In prospective studies patients with gastric ulcers have been found to have a significantly increased risk of developing a subsequent duodenal ulcer. Individuals with duodenal ulcers are also at higher than normal risk of developing a subsequent gastric ulcer, although their risk is less than that of persons in the reverse situation.

Malignant Transformation of a Benign Gastric Ulcer

It is extremely difficult to distinguish a cancer arising in a preexisting gastric ulcer from an ulcerated primary carcinoma. This difficulty does not complicate the study of duodenal ulcers, since malignant transformation of a duodenal ulcer is virtually unknown. However, although cancers originating in well-recognized benign peptic ulcers probably account for considerably less than 1% of all malignant tumors in the stomach, such cancers have been documented.

Neoplasms

Benign Tumors

Leiomyoma, a benign tumor of smooth muscle cells, is the most common tumor of the stomach (Fig. 13-17). Careful study of autopsy specimens reveals its presence in 25% to 50% of the population over 50 years of age. The tumors range in size from barely detectable to large masses more than 20 cm in diameter. Leiomyomas less than 2 cm in diameter are usually asymptomatic. Larger tumors may ulcerate and bleed or may cause pain, in which case the disorder is clinically indistinguishable from a peptic ulcer. Grossly, the tumors are submucosal and covered by intact mucosa or, when they project externally, by peritoneum. The cut surface has a whorled appearance and often shows cystic spaces. Microscopically, gastric leiomyomas show variable cellularity and are composed of spindle-shaped smooth muscle cells embedded in a collagenous stroma, similar to their appearance elsewhere. The cells are disposed in whorls and interlacing bundles. The nuclei are often arranged in parallel rows, which resemble the palisading of neurilemmomas. The presence of bizarre and giant nuclei is not necessarily a sign of malignancy. Local excision is curative.

Leiomyoblastoma, a variant of leiomyoma, appears macroscopically similar to the usual smooth muscle cell tumor. However, the cells are polygonal

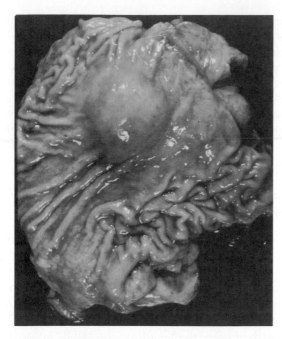

Figure 13-17. Leiomyoma of the stomach. The tumor is submucosal and covered by an intact mucosa.

rather than spindle shaped and have a substantial eosinophilic cytoplasm, a perinuclear clear zone, and no myofibrils. Thus, they are not easily recognized as smooth muscle cells, and the term **epithelioid leiomyoma** has also been suggested for these tumors. For the most part leiomyoblastomas are benign, but metastases have been recorded. The histologic criteria for malignancy, particularly the number of mitoses, are the same as for other smooth muscle sarcomas (see below). Even when metastases are present, the growth of the tumors is often indolent, and long-term survival after resection is common.

Epithelial polyps of the stomach, classed as either **hyperplastic** or **adenomatous,** account for almost half of all benign gastric tumors. The large majority of gastric polyps are found in patients with achlorhydria, and both types occur in association with atrophic gastritis and pernicious anemia, as well as in stomachs that harbor carcinoma. Hyperplastic polyps, which represent the majority of polyps, may be single or multiple and present as small pedunculated or sessile lesions. They are not true neoplasms but are probably a result of chronic inflammation and regenerative hyperplasia of the mucosa. Microscopically, the polyps consist of elongated, branched crypts lined by normal foveolar epithelium, beneath which pyloric or gastric glands mingle with collagen and smooth muscle fibers. Cystic dilatation of the glands and chronic inflammation may be conspicu-ous. **Hyperplastic polyps have no malignant potential.**

Adenomatous polyps are true neoplasms. They occur most commonly in the antrum. Grossly, the polyps range from less than 1 cm in diameter to a considerable size, the average being about 4 cm. Most adenomatous polyps are sessile and more often single than multiple. Microscopically, adenomas are composed of villous structures or a combination of tubular and villous glands, usually lined by intestinal or superficial gastric epithelium. Occasionally, an adenomatous polyp is composed solely of tubular glands, similar to those that arise in the colon.

Adenomatous polyps manifest a malignant potential variably reported at 5% to 75%. The malignant potential increases with the size of the polyp and is greatest for lesions larger than 2 cm in diameter. As in the colon, villous adenomas seem to undergo malignant transformation more frequently than tubular adenomas.

Pseudolymphoma, or benign lymphoid hyperplasia, is a reactive lymphoid infiltrate in the wall of the stomach often associated with a peptic ulcer or gastritis. There is no reason to believe that pseudolymphomas undergo malignant transformation; their clinical importance lies in the need to distinguish them from malignant lymphoma. Grossly, the "tumor" presents as a small, flat, nodular, centrally ulcerated thickening of the gastric wall. Microscopically, follicular lymphoid infiltrates and a few plasma cells are seen in the mucosa and submucosa. Reactive fibrosis in the area of peptic ulceration is common.

Benign lipomas, vascular tumors, fibromas, and heterotopic tissue are occasionally encountered in the stomach.

Malignant Tumors

Carcinoma of the Stomach

As recently as the mid-20th century, carcinoma of the stomach was the most common cause of death from cancer among men in the United States. For reasons that have not been explained, the incidence of gastric carcinoma has steadily decreased. However, it remains the sixth most common cause of cancer death in the United States. The incidence of stomach cancer remains exceedingly high in such countries as Japan and Chile, where the rates are 7 to 8 times that in the United States. Although the cause of gastric cancer is unknown, as discussed in Chapter 5, migrants from high-risk to low-risk areas show a decline in the incidence of cancer of the stomach, an observation that strongly implicates environmental factors in its pathogenesis.

Risk Factors

Dietary factors have been invoked to account for geographic variations in the incidence of gastric cancer. Studies of dietary habits are complicated by the fact that they require retrospective analyses over a very long time, and it is often difficult to isolate nutritional factors from other environmental influences. Nevertheless, carcinoma of the stomach is more common among people who eat large amounts of starch, smoked fish and meat, and pickled vegetables. Benzpyrene, a potent carcinogen, has been detected in smoked foods. Attention has also been focused on the possible role of nitrosamines, powerful animal carcinogens, in the pathogenesis of cancer of the stomach. Secondary amines are converted nonenzymatically to nitrosamines in the presence of nitrates or nitrites. High nitrate concentrations have been found in the soil and water in certain areas where the incidence of gastric cancer is high, and processed meats and vegetables are high in nitrates and nitrites. In addition, certain persons at increased risk of gastric cancer, such as patients with atrophic gastritis and intestinal metaplasia, have a high intragastric pH and high stomach concentrations of bacteria that can convert nitrates to nitrites, a situation that favors the production of nitrosamines.

The decreased incidence of gastric cancer in the United States has been paralleled by the increased use of refrigeration, a practice that inhibits the conversion of nitrates to nitrites and also obviates the need to add such compounds for food preservation. The consumption of whole milk and fresh vegetables rich in vitamin C is inversely related to the occurrence of stomach cancer. Vitamin C has been shown to inhibit the nitrosation of secondary amines *in vivo*.

Genetic factors cannot be identified in most cases of carcinoma of the stomach. A few familial clusters of gastric cancer and several cases in twins have been reported. Whereas 38% of the general population are of **blood type A,** half of patients with gastric cancer display this blood type.

Gastric cancer is uncommon in persons under the age of 30 and shows a sharp peak in incidence in persons over the age of 50 years. However, the age of onset seems to be somewhat lower in Japan, where the disease is endemic. In the United States there is only a slight male predominance, but in countries with a high incidence of this tumor, the male to female ratio is about 2:1. The risk of gastric cancer is particularly high in **low socioeconomic settings,** an observation that has been used to explain the high frequency of the tumor among American blacks and the fact that the incidence of the disease in that population has not declined as rapidly as it has among whites.

Atrophic gastritis, pernicious anemia, subtotal gastrectomy, and **gastric adenomatous polyps** have been discussed above as factors associated with a high risk of stomach cancer.

Pathology

Adenocarcinoma of the stomach, which accounts for more than 95% of all malignant gastric tumors, originates primarily from mucous cells of the normal superficial epithelium or from areas of intestinal metaplasia. The tumors are most common in the distal stomach, on the lesser curvature of the antrum and prepyloric region. They are rare in the fundus but may occur in any location. In occasional cases, particularly in patients with pernicious anemia, tumors may arise at several sites simultaneously.

Advanced Gastric Cancer By the time most gastric cancers in the Western world are detected, they are advanced—that is, they have penetrated beyond the submucosa into the muscularis and may extend through the serosa. The macroscopic appearance of these advanced cancers is of great importance not only to the pathologist, but also to the radiologist and the endoscopist, who may be called upon to distinguish carcinomas from benign lesions and to assess the degree of spread. Advanced gastric cancers are divided into three major macroscopic types. First is the **polypoid (fungating) type,** which accounts for about one-third of the cancers. It is a solid mass, up to 10 cm in diameter, that projects into the lumen of the stomach. The surface may be partly ulcerated, and the deeper tissues may or may not be infiltrated. Second is the **ulcerating type,** which constitutes another third of all gastric cancers. Visualized as a shallow ulcer, it varies in size from 1 cm to 10 cm in diameter (Fig. 13-18). The surrounding tissue is firm, raised, and nodular. Characteristically, the lateral margins of the ulcer are irregular and the base is ragged, in contrast to the benign peptic ulcer, which exhibits punched-out margins and a smooth base. Despite these differences, the radiologic differentiation of these two entities is occasionally difficult. Endoscopic biopsies from the margins of the ulcer usually provide a correct diagnosis, but the absence of malignant cells does not guarantee a benign lesion, since necrotic or reactive tissue may predominate in the areas biopsied. The third type of advanced gastric cancer is the **diffuse or infiltrating type,** which constitutes about one-tenth of all stomach cancers. No

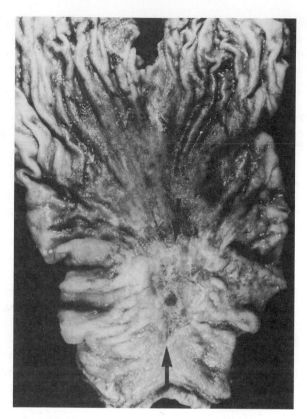

Figure 13-18. Ulcerating carcinoma of the stomach. A centrally ulcerated gastric cancer, characterized by raised, indurated margins (*arrows*), is present in the antrum.

true tumor is seen macroscopically; instead, the wall of the stomach is conspicuously thickened and firm. When the entire stomach is involved, the term **linitis plastica (leather-bottle stomach)** (Fig. 13-19) is applied. In the diffuse type of gastric carcinoma, the invading tumor cells induce extensive fibrosis in the submucosa and muscularis. As a result, the wall is stiff and may be more than 2 cm thick. Whereas the normal stomach has a volume greater than 1 liter, the leather-bottle stomach contains as little as 150 ml. Interestingly, because tumor cells are often scarce in well-developed linitis plastica, this condition was historically not recognized as a tumor; instead it was thought to represent an infectious or inflammatory disease.

Microscopically, the histologic pattern of advanced gastric cancer varies from **well-differentiated adenocarcinoma to a totally anaplastic tumor.** The polypoid variant typically contains well-differentiated glands, whereas linitis plastica is characteristically poorly differentiated. Particularly in the ulcerated type of cancer, the tumor cells may be arranged in cords or small foci. Many tumor cells contain clear mucin that displaces the nucleus to the periphery of the cell, re-

sulting in the so-called **signet ring cell** (Fig. 13-20). Extracellular mucinous material may be so prominent that the malignant cells seem to float in a gelatinous matrix, in which case it is called a **colloid** or **mucinous carcinoma.** Tumors that display papillary infoldings are termed **papillary adenocarcinomas,** and those that form solid tumor masses are referred to as **medullary carcinomas.**

Early Gastric Cancer   In the early 1960s Japanese gastroenterologists, alarmed by the high incidence of stomach cancer in their country, began to screen the adult population endoscopically for early evidence of that disease. They defined **early gastric cancer** as a tumor that is confined to the mucosa or submucosa (Fig. 13-21). An earlier term, **superficial spreading carcinoma,** should be considered synonymous with "early gastric cancer." In Japan early gastric cancer accounts for fully one-third of all stomach cancers, whereas in the United States and Europe it constitutes only about 5% of diagnosed cancers.

Early gastric cancer is strictly a pathologic diagnosis; the term does not refer to the duration of the malignant tumor, its size, the presence of symptoms, the absence of metastases, or the curability. In fact, 5% to 20% of early gastric cancers are already metastatic to lymph nodes at the time of detection.

Similar to advanced cancer, most early gastric cancers are found in the distal stomach and have been classified by Japanese investigators according to their macroscopic appearance. Three major types are recognized. **Type I protrudes into the lumen as a polypoid or nodular mass. Type II is a superficial, flat lesion** that may be slightly elevated or depressed. **Type III is an excavated malignant ulcer** that does not ordinarily occur alone, but rather represents ulceration of type I or type II tumors.

The polypoid and the superficial elevated varieties of early gastric cancer are typically well-differentiated adenocarcinomas. In the flattened or depressed superficial early cancers, the pattern ranges from well differentiated to anaplastic. The excavated lesions have the highest proportion of undifferentiated tumors.

It is generally accepted that many gastric cancers originate from epithelium that has undergone intestinal metaplasia. The endoscopic studies of early gastric cancer have established the validity of this concept and have demonstrated that well-differentiated adenocarcinomas usually arise in the context of intestinal metaplasia, commonly associated with atrophic gastritis, whereas less differentiated and anaplastic tumors are more likely to originate from the normal superficial gastric mucosa. However, considerable overlap occurs, and no firm rules can be applied.

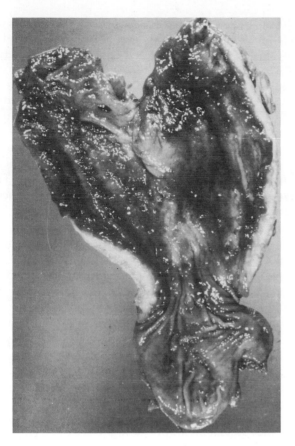

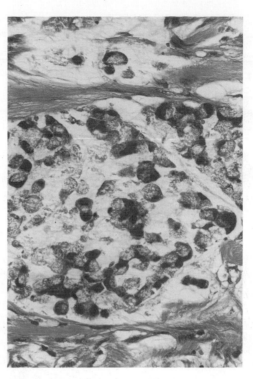

Figure 13-20. Signet ring cells of gastric adenocarcinoma. Intracellular mucin displaces the nuclei to the periphery of the tumor cells.

Figure 13-19. Infiltrating gastric carcinoma (linitis plastica). The wall of the stomach is thickened and indurated by diffusely infiltrating cancer.

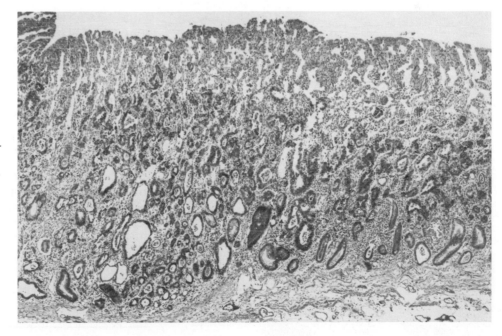

Figure 13-21. Early gastric cancer. Irregular neoplastic glands are seen in the mucosa superficial to the muscularis mucosae.

EARLY GASTRIC CANCER

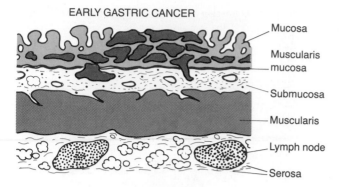

— Mucosa

— Muscularis
  mucosa

— Submucosa

— Muscularis

— Lymph node

— Serosa

POLYPOID CARCINOMA

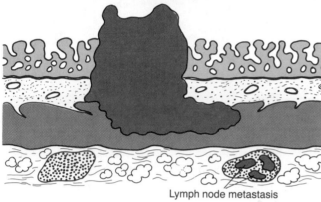

Lymph node metastasis

ULCERATING CARCINOMA

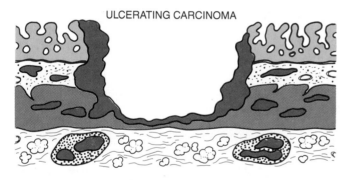

INFILTRATING CARCINOMA (LINITIS PLASTICA)

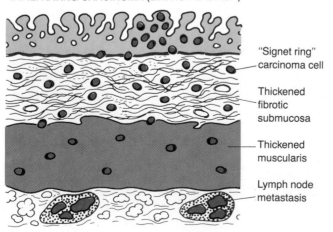

"Signet ring"
carcinoma cell

Thickened
fibrotic
submucosa

Thickened
muscularis

Lymph node
metastasis

Intuitively one would suppose that early gastric cancer would be the precursor of advanced gastric cancer. However, this is not necessarily the case. Early gastric cancer may be a different disease from advanced cancer, and it may exhibit a more benign course and greater curability because of an inherently lower biologic potential for invasion, possibly related to the differences between the intestinal and gastric cell types. For example, early gastric cancer has a considerably better prognosis than advanced cancer, even in the presence of lymph node metastases. The 10-year survival rate for surgically treated advanced gastric cancer is about 20%, compared with 95% for early gastric cancer. Moreover, the mean age of onset of early gastric cancer is uniformly lower than that of advanced cancer, and the early variety shows a striking geographic distribution. Nevertheless, in some cases well-documented early gastric cancer has indeed progressed to advanced cancer.

Gastric cancer metastasizes principally by the lymphatic route to regional lymph nodes of the lesser and greater curvature, the porta hepatis, and the subpyloric region. Distant lymphatic metastases also occur, the most common being an enlarged supraclavicular node, called **Virchow's node** or **sentinal node.** Hematogenous spread may seed any organ, including the liver, lung, or brain. Direct extension to nearby organs is often encountered. Carcinoma of the stomach can also spread to the ovary, where it is termed a **Krukenberg tumor.**

Figure 13-22 schematically depicts the major types of gastric cancer.

Clinical Features

In the United States and Europe, most patients with gastric cancer have metastases by the time they present for examination. Thus, the symptoms and course are usually those of advanced cancer. The most frequent initial symptom is weight loss, usually associated with anorexia and nausea. The majority of patients complain of epigastric or back pain, a symptom that mimics benign gastric ulcer and is often relieved by antacids or H_2-receptor antagonists. However, as the disease advances, symptomatic amelioration with medical therapy disappears. Obstruction of the gastric outlet may occur with large tumors of the antrum or prepyloric region. Massive bleeding is uncommon, but chronic bleeding is often reflected in the finding of occult blood in the stools and anemia. Tumors that involve the cardioesophageal junction result in dysphagia and occasionally mimic achalasia.

Figure 13-22.   The major types of gastric cancer.

Patients with early gastric cancer may be asymptomatic but usually complain of dyspepsia or epigastric pain. Weight loss, melena, and anemia are present in a minority of patients.

Two-thirds of patients with stomach cancer have fasting achlorhydria, compared with less than 25% of normal persons of the same age. Although fewer than one-quarter of gastric cancer patients have achlorhydria after maximal stimulation of gastric acid secretion, achlorhydria that persists despite pentagastrin stimulation in a patient with a gastric ulcer virtually always indicates malignancy.

Whereas **carcinoembryonic antigen** secretion in the normal stomach is low, about one-quarter of patients with advanced gastric cancer have elevated serum levels of this tumor marker. This test has little value in the diagnosis of stomach cancer, but it may be helpful in monitoring the course of metastatic disease or of postoperative recurrence.

Endocrine Cancers

Various endocrine cells in the normal gastric mucosa may give rise to neoplasms, collectively termed **carcinoid tumors.** Many are composed of argentaffin cells, but a few are argyrophilic. It is often difficult on histologic grounds to distinguish between benign and malignant carcinoid tumors. Most of these tumors do not display hormonal function, although an occasional one secretes serotonin, and their metastases can cause the carcinoid syndrome. The features of carcinoid tumors are discussed below.

Gastric Lymphoma

Primary lymphoma of the stomach accounts for less than 5% of all malignant stomach tumors, but it is the most common of all extranodal non-Hodgkin's lymphomas, constituting 20% of such neoplasms. **Clinically and radiologically, gastric lymphoma mimics gastric adenocarcinoma.** The presenting symptoms of gastric lymphoma—weight loss, dyspepsia, and abdominal pain—are similar to those of gastric adenocarcinoma. The age at diagnosis is usually 40 to 65 years, and there is no sex predominance. Radiologically, the tumors often cannot be differentiated from carcinoma, because they may be polypoid, ulcerating, or diffuse. The histologic varieties are similar to those in primary nodal lymphomas, as described in Chapter 20.

The prognosis for gastric lymphoma is considerably better than that for adenocarcinoma. The overall 5-year survival is 40% to 45%, depending on the extent of disease at the time of diagnosis. The treatment of favorable cases is primarily surgical; the value of postoperative radiotherapy is uncertain. More widespread lesions are treated with chemotherapy.

Leiomyosarcoma

Leiomyosarcomas, which constitute about 1% of gastric malignant tumors, present as palpable masses in up to half of patients. The initial symptoms are similar to those of leiomyoma, but weight loss is more common. Although there is no exact correlation between the size of a tumor and prognosis, tumors larger than 8 cm in diameter are more likely to have spread by the time of diagnosis. Macroscopically, the leiomyosarcoma is similar to the benign leiomyoma, except that it is often larger and softer. Microscopically, it is often difficult to predict the biologic behavior of a smooth muscle tumor from its morphologic appearance in the absence of infiltration or metastases. Cellular pleomorphism and hyperchromasia may be present in both benign and malignant tumors, but the number of mitoses is usually greater in leiomyosarcomas than in leiomyomas. In some cases the true nature of the tumor becomes apparent only after long-term follow-up. Metastasis is usually by the hematogenous route to the lungs, and direct spread to adjacent tissues may occur. Treatment is surgical, and the 5-year survival rate is 25% to 30%.

Metastatic Carcinoma

Metastases to the stomach from tumors elsewhere are uncommon. The stomach is occasionally secondarily involved in lymphomas and leukemias. The most common metastases from solid tumors are from malignant melanoma, although examples of many other tumors have occasionally also been recorded. A metastasis may ulcerate and mimic a primary tumor of the stomach.

Mechanical Disorders

Rupture of the stomach is rare and most commonly associated with blunt abdominal trauma from automobile accidents. **Spontaneous gastric perforation** typically occurs in middle-aged women and follows gastric overdistention, severe vomiting, labor and delivery, or production of excess CO_2 after ingestion of sodium bicarbonate or after consumption of unusually large quantities of carbonated beverages. Distention of the stomach during cardiopulmonary resuscitation has resulted in rupture of the stomach. Spontaneous perforation of the stomach in the neonate has also been described. The consequences of rupture and spontaneous perforation are catastrophic, and early surgical repair is crucial for survival. Pneumoperitoneum after endoscopy has been recorded but it is not dangerous.

Volvulus of the stomach refers to torsion of the stomach upon itself. This rare condition may be asymptomatic if the vascular supply of the stomach is not compromised. However, severe abdominal pain, upper gastrointestinal obstruction, and shock accompany interruption of blood flow and blockage of the lumen. A gastric tumor or pressure from an extragastric mass may warp the anatomy of the stomach and allow it to twist. Gastric volvulus has also occurred in association with a large hiatal hernia. Nasogastric decompression and surgical repair are the usual treatment.

Diverticula of the stomach are rare, developing after prolonged stress to the stomach wall from tumors, ulcers, gastritis, and surgery. Diverticula in the cardia are not associated with such conditions; they presumably result from congenital weakness of the wall or perhaps unusual intraluminal pressure at this site. Patients are either asymptomatic or complain of nonspecific symptoms. Hemorrhage and perforation are uncommon complications.

Bezoars

Bezoars are foreign bodies in the stomach of animals and humans that are composed of food or hair that has been altered by the digestive process. Historically, bezoars were esteemed for their alleged therapeutic properties and esthetic value, and one was included in the crown jewels of Queen Elizabeth I. **Phytobezoars** are vegetable concretions that are unusual in the normal stomach, except in persons who eat many persimmons or swallow unchewed bubble gum. Phytobezoars are usually found in persons with conditions that cause delayed gastric emptying, such as peripheral neuropathy of diabetes or gastric cancer, and in persons undergoing therapy with anticholinergic agents. Cimetidine treatment has been causally linked to phytobezoars. **In the last few decades, phytobezoars have been found principally in patients who display delayed gastric emptying and hypochlorhydria after partial gastrectomy, particularly when the surgery has included vagotomy.** Wandering bezoars may cause small intestinal obstruction. Plant bezoars contain vegetable or fruit fibers (e.g., potato skins, corn, celery) and seeds. Unripe pulp or ripe skin of persimmons contains tannin monomers that polymerize at low pH to form a tannin-cellulose-protein complex, which acts as a glue

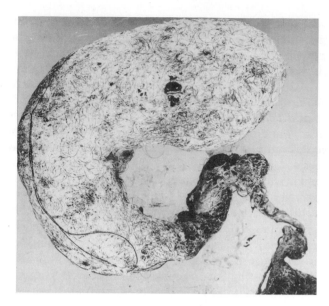

Figure 13-23.   Trichobezoar (hairball). A mass of hair in a gelatinous matrix forms a cast of the stomach.

that binds other material and results in a dark, hard, sticky phytobezoar. The majority of patients with persimmon bezoars have bleeding from an associated gastric ulcer.

The preferred treatment of phytobezoars is chemical attack with cellulase; in some cases manual disruption by endoscopic techniques, including jets of water, has been successful. However, enzymatic therapy is usually not effective for persimmon bezoars, and surgery is required.

A trichobezoar is a hairball within a gelatinous matrix; it is usually seen in long-haired girls or young women who eat their own hair as a nervous habit. Such a bezoar may grow by accretion to form a complete cast of the stomach, reaching a size of up to 3 kg (Fig. 13-23). Strands of hair may extend into the bowel as far as the transverse colon, the so-called Rapunzel syndrome. Most trichobezoars require surgical removal.

The Small Intestine
Anatomy

The intestinal tract begins early in development as a tube that joins the stomach to the cloaca. This tube progressively elongates, and its cephalic portion becomes the segment that extends from the distal duodenum to the proximal ileum. The more caudal portion develops into the distal ileum and the proximal two-thirds of the transverse colon. The vitelline duct, which connects the primitive duct with the yolk sac, may persist as a Meckel's diverticulum. To achieve the final position of the intestine, the fetal gut undergoes a complex series of rotations.

The small intestine extends from the pylorus to the ileocecal valve and, depending on the tone of its muscle, measures from 3.5 m to 6.5 m in length. It is divided into three regions: the **duodenum** is the first 25 cm, the **jejunum** is the proximal 40%, and the **ileum** is the distal 60%. The entire length of the small intestine, which is disposed in redundant loops, is movable, except for the duodenum, which is almost entirely retroperitoneal and therefore fixed. There is no sharp demarcation between the jejunum and ileum, and these two regions merge gradually. The wall of the jejunum is thicker and its lumen wider than that of the ileum.

The C-shaped duodenum surrounds the head of the pancreas and receives the biliary drainage of the liver and the pancreatic secretions through the common bile duct at the ampulla of Vater. The distal duodenum becomes invested by mesentery and merges with the jejunum at the ligament of Treitz. The proximity of the duodenum to its neighbors means that it may be affected by disorders such as cancer of the pancreas and cholecystoduodenal fistulas. Conversely, duodenal ulcers may penetrate into the pancreas or liver.

The **plicae circularis,** the spiral folds that consist of mucosa and submucosa, are most prominent in the distal duodenum and proximal jejunum, usually disappearing in the terminal ileum. **Peyer's patches** are lymphoid aggregates in the submucosa measuring up to 3 cm in diameter. They are located in the antimesenteric aspect of the distal half of the ileum. The ileocecal valve is not a true valve, but rather a muscular sphincter that regulates the flow of intestinal contents into the cecum.

The duodenum is served by the pancreaticoduodenal branch of the hepatic artery, which arises from the celiac artery. The jejunum and ileum are supplied by the superior mesenteric artery (a branch of the aorta), which is arranged in arcades in the mesentery, thereby providing abundant collateral circulation in its distal reaches. The veins draining the small intestine empty into the portal venous system. The lymphatic channels of the duodenum drain to the portal and pyloric lymph nodes, whereas those of the jejunum and ileum communicate with the mesenteric lymph nodes. The lymphatics of the terminal ileum empty into the ileocolic nodes. The small intestine is innervated by sympathetic fibers from the celiac plexus and ganglia and by parasympathetic fibers from the vagus nerve.

An understanding of the microscopic anatomy of the small intestine is crucial for an appreciation of its function in health and disease. Similar to the stomach and the colon, the wall of the small intestine is composed of four layers: the mucosa, the submucosa, the muscularis, and the serosa. In the retroperitoneal duodenum, however, only the anterior wall is covered by a serosa. The serosa consists of loose connective tissue bounded by a single layer of mesothelial cells. The muscularis exhibits an outer longitudinal layer and an inner circular layer, both of which function in a coordinated manner to propel the intestinal contents by peristalsis. The submucosa consists of vascularized connective tissue and a few scattered lymphocytes, plasma cells, and macrophages, with an occasional mast cell and eosinophil. In the duodenum the submucosa is occupied by the Brunner's glands, branched structures that contain mucus and serous cells that secrete mucus and bicarbonate to protect the duodenal mucosa from peptic ulceration. The lymphatic and venous capillaries of the mucosa drain into a highly developed system of lymphatic and venous plexuses in the submucosa. The myenteric nerve plexuses of Auerbach, which lie between the two layers of the muscularis, and the Meissner's plexuses in the submucosa are interconnected, although they are considered to be functionally distinct.

The distinctive feature of the intestinal mucosa is its arrangement in villi, finger-like projections 0.5 mm to 1 mm in length that expand the absorptive area enormously. The macroscopic structure of the villi varies in different regions of the small intestine. In the proximal duodenum the villi tend to be broad and blunted, whereas in the distal duodenum and proximal jejunum they exhibit a more slender, leaf-shaped appearance. Finger-shaped villi are the rule in the distal jejunum and ileum. There are also geographic variations in the normal appearance of villi. For example, the populations of Southeast Asia and the Caribbean tend to exhibit shorter villi, deeper crypts, and increased cellularity of the lamina propria than do those of the United States and Europe. Whether this represents genetic influences or a difference in diet or bacterial flora is not clear.

The villi are composed of a columnar epithelium resting on a basement membrane, a lamina propria, and a muscularis mucosa, which separates the mucosa from the submucosa. The connective tissue of the lamina propria forms the core of the villus and surrounds the crypts of Lieberkuhn at the base of the villi. The normal lamina propria is home to a variety of mesenchymal cells, including lymphocytes, plasma cells, and macrophages. Plasma cells in this location principally secrete IgA into the intestinal lumen or the lamina propria itself. Occasional eosinophils and mast cells are scattered throughout. A few smooth muscle cells and fibroblasts are also present. The cellular composition of the lamina propria suggests that it protects against invasion by bacteria that may penetrate the mucosa and segregates foreign material that breaches the mucosa.

The columnar epithelial cells of the villi are principally absorptive, whereas those lining the crypts are the source of cell renewal and secretion. Four cell types are recognized in the crypts: Paneth, goblet, endocrine, and undifferentiated cells.

The **Paneth cells** at the base of the crypts are similar to the zymogen cells of the pancreas and salivary glands that are actively engaged in exocrine secretion. Within the Paneth cells eosinophilic secretory granules fill a basophilic cytoplasm. The function of these cells and the nature of their secretions are poorly understood.

The **goblet cells** of the lateral walls of the crypts are flask-shaped and filled with mucous granules. They are similar in structure and function to goblet cells elsewhere.

The **undifferentiated cells,** located in the lateral walls of the crypts and interspersed between the Paneth cells at their bases, are the most numerous cells of the crypts. Small glycoprotein secretory granules are grouped in the apical cytoplasm of some of these undifferentiated cells. These cells function as the reserve cells from which all the other mucosal cells are renewed, and thus mitoses are numerous among them.

The **endocrine cells,** both argentaffin and argyrophilic, appear inverted, with an apical nucleus and basal granules. The basal location of the granules implies that they are secreted into the lamina propria rather than the lumen. These cells produce numerous gastrointestinal hormones and peptides, including gastrin, secretin, and cholecystokinin, glucagon, vasoactive intestinal peptide, and serotonin. The secretion of such hormones in response to appropriate stimuli is presumed to regulate many gastrointestinal functions. As in other tissues, primary tumors derived from these cells are often characterized by striking hormone secretion.

The intestinal villi are lined principally by absorptive cells, with an admixture of a few goblet and endocrine cells. The **absorptive cells,** or **enterocytes** (see Fig. 13-1), are tall and display basally situated nuclei. Numerous microvilli extend from the surface into the lumen, thus increasing the absorptive surface some 30-fold. The plasma membrane of the microvilli is covered by a glycocalyx (fuzzy coat) produced by the absorptive cell. Disaccharidases and peptidases

reside in this glycocalyx. Certain receptors, such as that for the intrinsic factor–vitamin B_{12} complex in the ileum, are also present in the membrane-glycocalyx complex. The cytoplasm immediately beneath the microvilli contains a network of actin microfilaments, termed the "terminal web." These filaments, which are also associated with myosin and other contractile proteins, insert into the core of the microvilli and presumably serve as a contractile apparatus. The lateral borders of adjacent plasma membranes form tight junctions that are impermeable to macromolecules but permit passive transport of small molecules by the paracellular route. Absorbed material is transported from the epithelial cell into the intercellular space between absorptive cells through the lateral or basal plasma membranes, after which it penetrates the basement membrane, traverses the lamina propria, and enters a capillary or a lymphatic channel.

Some IgA is produced in the lamina propria as a dimer that diffuses through the basement membrane of the crypt to reach the basal or lateral surface of the epithelial cell, where it combines with the secretory component produced by that cell. The resulting secretory IgA molecule is then taken up by the epithelial cell and secreted into the lumen. Secretory IgA, which is more resistant to proteolysis than is serum IgA, binds food antigens and prevents bacterial adherence to the intestinal epithelial cells. Moreover, IgA can neutralize bacterial toxins and inhibit the replication and mucosal penetration of viruses.

Cell renewal in the small intestine is limited to the crypts, where undifferentiated cells divide. The newly formed cells migrate up the villus, where they terminally differentiate into absorptive cells and are eventually extruded at the tip of the villus. Their absorptive capacity is maximal when the cells reach the upper third of the villus. At the tip of the villus, the cells degenerate and slough into the lumen. The mucosal epithelium of the small intestine is replaced within a period of 4 to 7 days. This rapid cell proliferation explains why the intestinal epithelium is particularly sensitive to radiation and chemotherapeutic agents.

Congenital Disorders

Atresia and Stenosis

Intestinal atresia and stenosis, although rare, are the most frequent causes of neonatal intestinal obstruction. **Atresia** is defined as a complete congenital occlusion of the intestinal lumen, which may be manifested as a thin intraluminal diaphragm, as blind proximal and distal sacs joined by a cord, or as disconnected blind ends. Multiple intestinal occlusions may give the appearance of a string of sausages. Although the majority of cases of congenital atresia are thought to reflect developmental defects, a quarter of the cases are associated with meconium ileus, and cystic fibrosis is discovered in one-tenth of the cases of atresia.

The obstructed fetal intestine is dilated and filled with fluid, a condition detectable with imaging techniques. Twenty percent to 30% of mothers of fetuses with high intestinal atresia develop polyhydramnios during the last trimester, presumably because the fetus does not swallow amniotic fluid.

Congenital stenosis is an incomplete stricture of the small intestine, which narrows, but does not occlude, the lumen. Stenosis may also be caused by an incomplete diaphragm. Although the condition is usually symptomatic in infancy, cases in middle-aged adults have been recorded.

Intestinal atresia or stenosis is diagnosed on the basis of persistent vomiting of bile-containing fluid within the first day of life. Meconium is not passed. Surgical correction is usually successful, but coexistent anomalies often complicate the course.

Duplications

Gastrointestinal duplications (enteric cysts), which may occur from the esophagus to the anus, are spherical or tubular structures attached to the alimentary tract. They may present as cystic structures or may communicate with the lumen of the gastrointestinal tract. Intestinal duplications are most common in the ileum and less so in the jejunum. The duplications have a smooth muscle wall and an epithelium of the gastrointestinal type. Communicating duplications are often lined by gastric mucosa, a situation that may lead to peptic ulceration, bleeding, or perforation. The cystic duplications may cause intestinal obstruction by extrinsic pressure or may be associated with intussusception. Many duplications are silent, but those that become symptomatic require surgical removal.

Meckel's Diverticulum

Meckel's diverticulum, caused by persistence of the vitelline duct, is the most common and the most clinically significant congenital anomaly of the small intestine (Fig. 13-24). The diverticulum is found on the antimesenteric border of the ileum, 60 cm to 100 cm from the ileocecal valve in the adult. However, 60% of patients are under 2 years of age. The diverticulum is about 5 cm in length, with a diameter

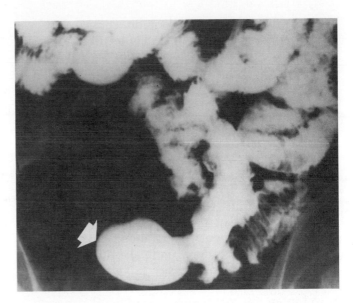

Figure 13-24. Meckel's diverticulum. A contrast radiograph of the small intestine shows a barium-filled diverticulum of the ileum (*arrow*).

slightly less than that of the ileum, but considerably larger than that of the appendix. A fibrous cord may hang freely from the apex of the diverticulum or may be attached to the umbilicus, and fistulas between a Meckel's diverticulum and the umbilicus have been described.

Meckel's diverticulum is a true diverticulum in that it possesses all the coats of the normal intestine and the mucosa is similar to that of the adjoining ileum. Most Meckel's diverticula are asymptomatic and discovered only as an incidental finding at laparotomy for other causes, or at autopsy. Of the minority that become symptomatic, about half contain ectopic gastric, duodenal, pancreatic, biliary, or colonic tissue. Of these, more than three-quarters exhibit gastric ectopic tissue.

Meckel's diverticulum may be complicated by hemorrhage, intestinal obstruction, diverticulitis, and perforation with peritonitis. In cases of fistula, a fecal discharge from the umbilicus may be observed. **The most common complication is bleeding, which is responsible for half of all lower gastrointestinal hemorrhage in children.** Bleeding results from **peptic ulceration** of the ileum adjacent to ectopic gastric mucosa. The diverticulum may act as a lead point for **intussusception** and thus cause intestinal obstruction. Obstruction can also be caused by volvulus around the fibrotic remnant of the vitelline duct. Inflammation of a Meckel's diverticulum—that is, **diverticulitis**—leads to symptoms indistinguishable from those of appendicitis. Thus, the surgeon who operates for acute appendicitis but encounters a normal appendix is well advised to search for a

Meckel's diverticulum. Perforation, complicated by a rapidly spreading peritonitis, may result from peptic ulceration, either in the diverticulum or in the ileum.

Traditionally surgery was recommended even for an asymptomatic Meckel's diverticulum; this advice has now been questioned, because the incidence of surgical complications may be greater than the risk of an untreated diverticulum.

Malrotation

Defective intestinal rotation in fetal life leads to abnormal positions of the small intestine and colon, anomalous attachments, and bands. The clinical importance of such rotational anomalies in children and adults lies in their propensity to cause volvulus of the small and large intestine and incarceration of the bowel in an internal hernia.

Meconium Ileus

The earliest manifestation of cystic fibrosis is often neonatal intestinal obstruction caused by the accumulation of tenacious meconium in the small intestine. The abnormal consistency of the meconium reflects a deficiency in pancreatic enzymes and high viscosity of the intestinal mucus. Usually the distal ileum is contracted beyond the obstruction, whereas the midileum proximal to the inspissated meconium is dilated. In half of affected infants, meconium ileus is complicated by volvulus, perforation with a meconium peritonitis, or intestinal atresia. Meconium ileus must be differentiated from the distal intestinal obstruction syndrome associated with cystic fibrosis, in which a small plug of meconium in the distal colon may eventually be passed, thus relieving the obstruction.

Successful treatment of meconium ileus without complications may be accomplished by means of a hypertonic enema containing a detergent. Complicated meconium ileus always requires surgical intervention and is associated with significant mortality.

Infections

Diarrheal Diseases

Bacterial Diarrhea

Bacterial diarrhea has plagued humans since the dawn of recorded history and continues to be an important clinical problem. Despite advances in the identification of organisms, antibiotic therapy, and fluid and electrolyte replacement, infectious diarrhea still causes many deaths worldwide, particularly in underdeveloped countries and in infants. The normal small bowel has few microorganisms (usually less than 10^4/ml), mostly aerobic bacilli such as lactobacilli. These organisms travel in the food stream and normally do not colonize the small intestine. Infectious diarrheal states are caused by colonization with bacteria such as toxigenic strains of *Escherichia coli* and *Vibrio cholera*. The most significant factor in infectious diarrhea is increased intestinal secretion, stimulated by bacterial toxins and enteric hormones. Decreased absorption and increased peristaltic activity contribute less to the diarrhea.

The colon harbors an abundant bacterial flora, with a concentration 7 orders of magnitude greater than that of the small intestine. In the colon anaerobic bacteria—for example, *Bacteroides* and *Clostridium*—outnumber aerobic organisms by a factor of 1000. With the more rapid transit of intestinal contents during a diarrheal episode, the flora are shifted to a more aerobic population, including *E. coli*, *Klebsiella*, and *Proteus*. Moreover, the offending organisms themselves become conspicuous, and a small intestinal pathogen such as *V. cholera* may be the major isolate in the stools.

The paucity of bacteria in the stomach and small intestine is accounted for by a number of protective mechanisms: gastric acid production is inimical to bacterial growth, an effect that explains the overgrowth of bacteria in the stomach in the presence of achlorhydria; bile has antimicrobial activity; the peristaltic propulsion of intestinal contents limits the time available for bacterial accumulation; the normal flora secrete their own antimicrobial substances to maintain an ecologic balance (indeed, treatment with broad-spectrum antibiotics alters the natural flora and allows overgrowth of ordinarily harmless organisms); and the plasma cells of the lamina propria secrete IgA into the intestinal lumen.

The individual agents responsible for infectious diarrhea have been discussed in Chapter 9, which deals with infectious diseases. Here we only briefly review the major entities. The agents of infectious diarrhea are conveniently classified into **toxigenic** organisms, which produce diarrhea by elaborating toxins, and **invasive** bacteria.

Toxigenic Diarrhea

The prototypic organisms that produce diarrhea by secreting a toxin are *V. cholera* and toxigenic strains of *E. coli*. Toxigenic diarrhea is characterized by the following: damage to the intestinal mucosa is minimal or absent; the organism remains on the mucosal surface, where it secretes its toxin; and, owing to fluid secreted into the small intestine, there is watery diarrhea, which can lead to dehydration, particularly in the case of cholera. Although many organisms have been isolated in so-called **travelers' diarrhea,** the most common pathogen in almost all studies is toxigenic *E. coli.*

Diarrhea Caused by Invasive Bacteria

Invasive bacteria, as their name implies, cause diarrhea by directly injuring the intestinal mucosa. Among these organisms *Shigella, Salmonella,* certain strains of *E. coli, Yersinia,* and *Campylobacter* are the most widely recognized. The invasive organisms tend to infect the distal ileum and colon, whereas the toxigenic bacteria mainly involve the upper intestinal tract. Curiously, despite the obvious morphologic lesions associated with these organisms, the mechanism by which they produce diarrhea has not been clarified. Enterotoxins have been identified, but their role in causing diarrhea has not been established. Invasion of the mucosa by bacteria increases the synthesis of prostaglandins in the affected tissue, and inhibitors of prostaglandin synthesis seem to block fluid secretion. It is also possible that the damaged mucosa is unable to resorb fluid from the lumen.

Shigellosis principally affects the colon, although the terminal ileum is occasionally involved. Microscopically, a granular and hemorrhagic mucosa exhibits numerous shallow serpiginous ulcers. The inflammation, which is especially severe in the sigmoid colon and rectum, is usually superficial. In the early stage the accumulation of neutrophils in damaged crypts (crypt abscesses) is similar to that in ulcerative colitis, and the lymphoid follicles of the mucosa break down to form ulcers. As the infection recedes, the ulcers heal and the mucosa returns to normal.

Typhoid fever (*Salmonella* enteritis), today uncommon in the industrialized world, still presents a problem in underdeveloped countries. Necrosis of lymphoid tissue, principally in the terminal ileum, leads to scattered ulcers. Infection of Peyer's patches results in oval ulcers, the longer dimension of which is in the long axis of the intestine. Occasionally, lymphoid follicles in the large bowel or the appendix are ulcerated. The base of the ulcer is composed of black necrotic tissue mixed with fibrin. Microscopically, the early lesions of typhoid fever contain large basophilic macrophages filled with typhoid bacilli, erythrocytes, and necrotic debris. Necrosis of lymphoid follicles becomes confluent, and mucosal ulceration follows. Similar lymphoid hyperplasia and necrosis are seen in the regional lymph nodes. Healing of the ulcers is complete within a week of the acute symptoms and leaves little fibrosis or other sequelae. Intestinal hemorrhage and perforation, principally in the ileum, are the most feared complications of typhoid fever and tend to occur in the third week and during convalescence.

Nontyphoidal salmonellosis, formerly known as "paratyphoid fever," is an enteritis caused by *Salmonella* strains other than *S. typhi* and is generally a far less serious illness than typhoid fever. In addition to causing diarrhea, bacteremia, and fever, this disorder also involves localized infections at other sites. The principal target is the ileum, although minor involvement of the colon may also take place. The organisms invade the mucosa, which shows mild ulceration, edema, and infiltration with neutrophils. Hematogenous dissemination from the intestine may carry the infection to bones, joints, and meninges. Interestingly, there seems to be a relationship between sickle cell anemia and *Salmonella* osteomyelitis, presumably because phagocytosis of the products of hemolysis prevents further ingestion of the *Salmonella* organisms and allows their dissemination through the bloodstream.

Invasive *E. coli* is an uncommon cause of bloody diarrhea that resembles shigellosis, possibly because it exhibits surface antigens similar to those of Shigella. The disease has been reported principally in Japan and among American troops in Vietnam.

***Yersinia* enterocolitis,** transmitted by pets or contaminated food, is most common in young children. It causes diarrhea, cramps, and fever and lasts 1 to 3 weeks. In addition to causing enterocolitis, *Yersinia* causes acute mesenteric adenitis and pain in the right lower quadrant. Infected children have undergone laparotomy because of a mistaken diagnosis of appendicitis. The ileocecal nodes are enlarged and matted together. On section, small yellow microabscesses are seen, corresponding to epithelioid granulomas with central necrotic zones and infiltration with neutrophils. Langhans' or foreign body–type giant cells are sometimes present. In addition to there being submucosal edema and an inflammatory infiltrate, the ileum and appendix may contain similar granulomas, causing an appearance that has been mistaken for Crohn's disease. Adults, who are less susceptible than children, suffer an acute diarrhea, often followed within a few weeks by erythema nodosum or erythema multiforme. Patients with chronic debilitating diseases may develop a fatal Yersinia bacteremia, which is resistant to antibiotic treatment.

***Campylobacter* infection** has been recognized only recently as an important cause of gastroenteritis. In fact, some investigators have reported a higher incidence of *Campylobacter* than nontyphoidal *Salmonella* and *Shigella* infections in the United States, and in one survey from Great Britain, half of all bacterial diarrhea was caused by *Campylobacter*. Humans are involved mainly by contact with infected domestic animals or through ingestion of poorly cooked or contaminated food. Adults usually recover from the diarrheal illness in less than 1 week.

Food Poisoning

Infectious agents can produce gastroenteritis not only by infecting the bowel directly, but also by elaborating enterotoxins in contaminated food, which is then ingested.

Staphylococcus aureus is a common cause of food poisoning. Symptoms result from the ingestion of food contaminated with strains of *Staphylococcus* that produce an exotoxin that damages the epithelium of the gastrointestinal tract. Within 6 hours of the ingestion of tainted food, severe vomiting and abdominal cramps occur, often followed by diarrhea. Most victims recover in 1 to 2 days.

Clostridium perfringens elaborates an enterotoxin that causes vomiting and diarrhea. Although the organism is anaerobic, it can tolerate exposure to air for as long as 3 days. Maximal activity of the clostridial enterotoxin is in the ileum. In most cases watery diarrhea and severe abdominal pain, which begin 8 to 24 hours after ingestion of the contaminated food, last only about 1 day. However, outbreaks of a necrotizing enteritis with high mortality are associated with the consumption of undercooked pork in New Guinea, where the disease is known as **pigbel.**

Viral Gastroenteritis

Within the last two decades specific viruses have been shown to cause diarrhea. **Rotaviruses** cause self-limited vomiting and watery diarrhea, principally in children less than 2 years of age. Rotavirus infection is a common cause of infantile diarrhea and accounts for about half of the cases of acute diarrhea in hospitalized children under the age of 2 years. The virus has been demonstrated in duodenal biopsy specimens and is associated with flattening of the surface epithelium and impaired intestinal absorption for periods of up to 2 months.

The **Norwalk viruses** account for one-third of the epidemics of viral gastroenteritis in the United States. The agent has not been propagated in culture but has been demonstrated by electron microscopy in the stools. The virus targets the upper small intestine, where it causes patchy mucosal lesions and malabsorption. Vomiting and diarrhea are usual, but the symptoms resolve within 2 days. The morphologic and absorptive alterations require 1 or 2 weeks for reversal.

Other viruses that have been implicated as etiologic agents of infectious diarrhea include echovirus, coxsackie virus, cytomegalovirus, adenovirus, and coronavirus.

Tuberculosis

Historically an important disease, gastrointestinal tuberculosis is now uncommon in industrialized countries, although it is still a problem in underdeveloped countries. At one time a large proportion of intestinal tuberculosis involved infection with *Mycobacterium bovis*, which was principally transmitted by contaminated milk. However, the control of tuberculosis in dairy herds and the pasteurization of milk have made infection with this organism a curiosity. Today virtually all cases of intestinal tuberculosis in Western countries are caused by *Mycobacterium tuberculosis.*

Although there is a strong correlation between the frequency of intestinal tuberculosis and the severity of pulmonary disease, as many as half the patients with intestinal tuberculosis do not have radiologic evidence of pulmonary involvement. **Most cases of intestinal tuberculosis are caused either by ingestion of bacteria in food or by the swallowing of infectious sputum.** After it is ingested, the tubercle bacillus, protected from digestion by its waxy capsule, passes into the small bowel. The bacterium then establishes a locus of infection, usually (in 90% of patients) in the ileocecal region. Infection also occurs in the colon, jejunum, appendix, rectum, and duodenum, in that order of frequency. Esophageal and gastric tuberculosis are rare.

Almost all patients with intestinal tuberculosis complain of chronic abdominal pain, and about two-thirds have a palpable abdominal mass, usually in the right lower quadrant. Weight loss, fever, and weakness are common. Tuberculosis of the appendix has been mistakenly diagnosed as acute appendicitis. Diarrhea occurs in a minority of patients, and about the same number suffer from constipation. The disease is treated medically with antituberculosis drugs.

The macroscopic presentation of intestinal tuberculosis is divided into three categories: ulcerative, hypertrophic, and ulcerohypertrophic. The **ulcerative** form, seen in over half of the patients, is characterized by one or more circular or oval ulcers of varying size in the transverse plane of the bowel. As the ulcers heal, reactive fibrosis may cause a circumferential ("napkin ring") stricture of the bowel lumen. The involved bowel is indurated and the serosa studded with greyish white nodules. Mesenteric lymph nodes are typically enlarged and on cut section display caseous necrosis. Before antibiotic treatment, ulcerative tuberculosis was associated with a particularly high mortality.

In **hypertrophic** disease (10% of patients) the ileocecal region or the colon exhibits an exuberant inflammatory and fibroblastic reaction throughout the thickness of the wall. Adhesions between the bowel, mesentery, and lymph nodes may form a palpable mass, and the mass or a secondary stricture may cause intestinal obstruction. Protrusion of the hypertrophic lesion into the bowel lumen may mimic carcinoma.

The **ulcerohypertrophic** variety of intestinal tuberculosis, seen in about one-third of the patients, combines the features of the ulcerative and hypertrophic forms.

Microscopically, typical tuberculous granulomas are found in all layers of the bowel wall, particularly in the Peyer's patches and lymphoid follicles, and in the mesenteric lymph nodes. Occasionally, tuberculous granulomas are visualized only in the lymph nodes, and the bowel wall displays only nonspecific inflammatory lesions. In old lesions the granulomas become hyalinized and then disappear, leaving only a dense scar containing small foci of lymphocytes. Seen at autopsy or in surgical specimens, old tuberculous strictures are difficult to distinguish from other causes of stricture, such as ischemic enterocolitis or Crohn's disease. Crohn's disease exhibits virtually all the changes produced by intestinal tuberculosis, and indeed these entities have often been confused by pathologists. Unfortunately, the bacilli and caseating granulomas in tuberculous enteritis are often not demonstrable, thereby adding to the difficulty in making a correct diagnosis.

Complications of intestinal tuberculosis include obstruction, fistulas, perforation, and abscess. Anorexia and malabsorption may lead to severe malnutrition.

Fungi

The gastrointestinal tract is not normally a hospitable environment for fungi. The number of commensal organisms is minuscule, and such organisms are restricted to yeasts and anaerobic actinomycetes. Therefore, fungal infection of the gastrointestinal tract occurs almost exclusively in immunocompromised persons or, in the case of actinomycosis, in persons who have suffered trauma to the gut.

Suppression of the normal bacterial flora by antibiotics also favors fungal growth. Under these circumstances the most common mycoses are caused by Candida, Mucor species, and Histoplasma, although other fungi are occasionally described. Mucormycosis and candidiasis typically cause mucosal erosions; these may progress to larger ulcers, which are surrounded by hemorrhage and necrosis. The inflammation is characteristically neutrophilic and may show remarkably little reaction to the administration of cytotoxic agents. Mucormycetes have a tendency to invade blood vessels, but hematogenous dissemination from the intestine is rare. Disseminated histoplasmosis may involve the bowel, where it causes elevated plaques that ulcerate and may even perforate.

Parasites of the Small Intestine

Parasitic diseases of the small bowel are discussed in detail in Chapter 9 and summarized in Figure 13-25. These parasites include **protozoa,** such as *Giardia lamblia,* Coccidia species, and Cryptosporidia, **nematodes (roundworms)** such as Ascaris, Strongyloides, and hookworm, and **flatworms.** The flatworms are divided into tapeworms (cestodes), which include *Diphyllobothrium latum, Taenia solium, Taenia saginata,* and *Hymenolepis nana,* and flukes (trematodes), which include various schistosomes and the giant intestinal fluke, *Fasciolopsis buski.* In addition, trichinosis has an intestinal phase, during which vomiting, diarrhea, and colic mimic acute food poisoning or bacterial enteritis.

Vascular Diseases

Ischemic bowel disease affects the small intestine or large intestine or both, depending on the vessel involved. The gradual occlusion of a large mesenteric artery allows the development of collateral circulation. Therefore, symptoms of chronic ischemic bowel disease do not ordinarily arise unless two or more major arteries are compromised, usually by atherosclerosis. However, narrowing of the celiac axis itself by atherosclerosis can cause chronic ischemia.

Acute Vascular Occlusion

The sudden occlusion of an artery by thrombosis or embolization leads to infarction of the small bowel before collateral circulation comes into play. Depending on the size of the vessel, infarction may be seg-

CATEGORY	ORGANISMS	TRANSMISSION
PROTOZOON	Giardia 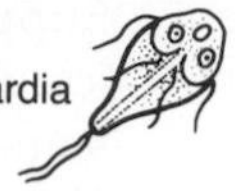	Fecal-oral
ROUND WORMS (NEMATODES)	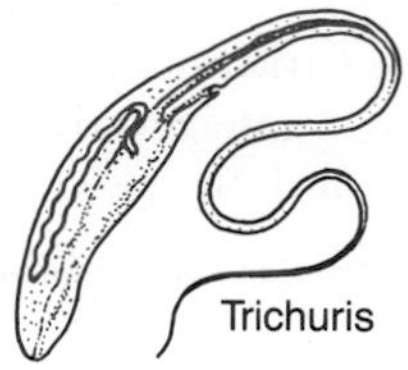 Trichuris 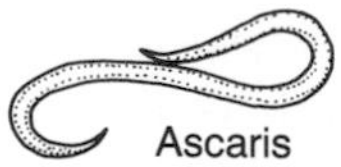 Ascaris	Fecal-oral
	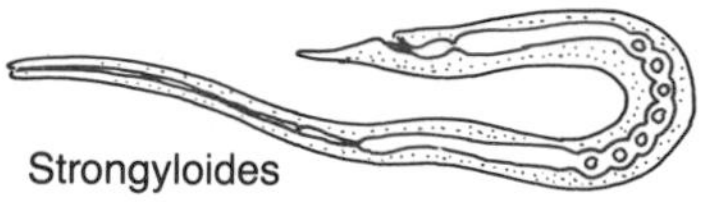 Strongyloides 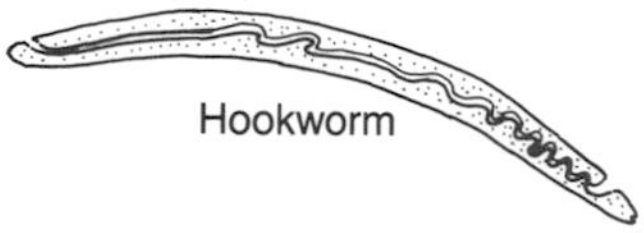 Hookworm	Free-living larvae in soil penetrate skin
TAPEWORMS (CESTODES)	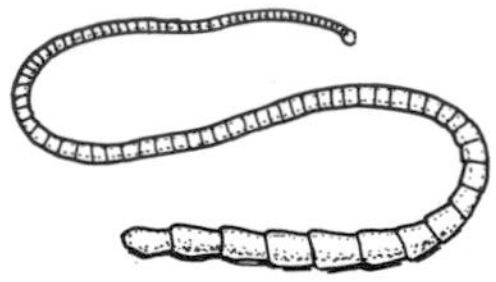 Pork tapeworm *Taenia solium* (2-4 meters) 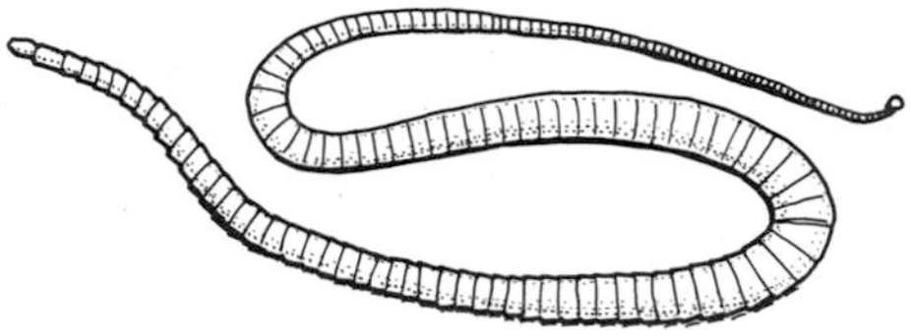 Fish tapeworm *Diphyllobothrium latum* (3-10 meters) 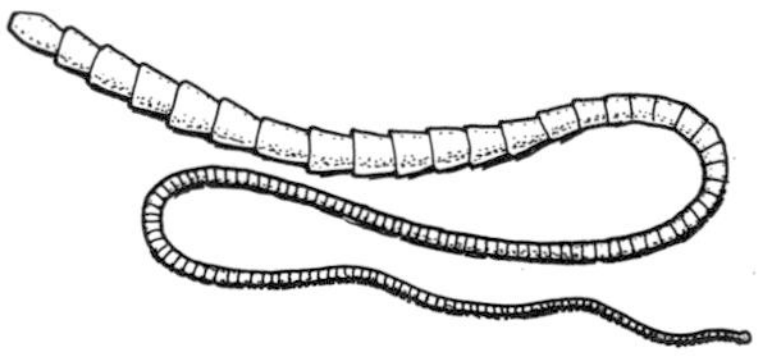 Beef tapeworm *Taenia saginata* (4-8 meters)	Undercooked or raw flesh containing cysts
	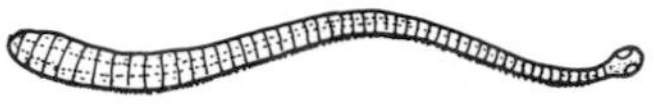 Human tapeworm *Hymenolepis nana* (0.5-5 cm)	Fecal-oral
FLUKE (TREMATODE)	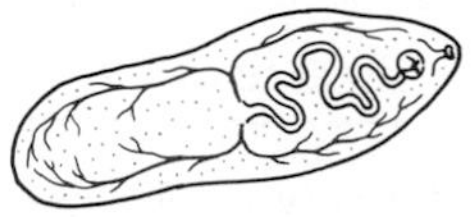 *Fasciolopsis buski*	Fecal-oral (with intermediate host)

Figure 13-25. Parasites of the small bowel.

670

mental (Fig. 13-26) or may lead to gangrene of virtually the entire small bowel. About half of the cases of intestinal infarction are caused by **embolic or thrombotic occlusion of the superior mesenteric artery.** About one-quarter are the result of **inferior mesenteric artery occlusion, mesenteric venous thrombosis,** or **arteritis,** and in the remaining quarter no acute vascular occlusions are demonstrated. Transmural infarction of the colon as a result of embolization to the inferior mesenteric artery is uncommon because of the oblique takeoff of this vessel from the aorta, its relatively smaller caliber, and its richer collateral circulation.

In addition to intrinsic vascular lesions, **volvulus, intussusception,** and **incarceration of the intestine in a hernial sac** may all lead to bowel infarction. Nonocclusive intestinal infarction, which may be extensive, is seen in hypoxic patients with reduced cardiac output from shock or acute myocardial infarction. Reduced cardiac output and shock cause redistribution of blood flow to the brain and other vital organs, thereby reducing mesenteric blood flow. In addition, patients in shock often receive alpha-adrenergic agents, which may further shunt blood away from the intestine. The drastically lowered perfusion pressure in the arterioles leads to their collapse, aggravating the ischemia even more.

Thrombosis of the mesenteric veins occurs under a variety of conditions, including hypercoagulable states, stasis, and inflammation. Almost all thromboses affect the superior mesenteric vein, whereas only 5% of the cases involve the inferior mesenteric vein. The collateral flow in the distribution of the superior mesenteric vein is usually sufficient to preclude infarction of the intestine. However, the thrombosis of smaller veins can also lead to transmural infarction.

Clinically, in mesenteric artery occlusion the abrupt onset of abdominal pain is virtually invariable. Bloody diarrhea, hematemesis, and shock are common, and in untreated cases perforation is frequent. As the infarction progresses, systemic manifestations become more severe, and **death is inevitable without surgical intervention.** In extensive infarction, as a result of occlusion in the proximal portion of the superior mesenteric artery, almost the entire small bowel needs to be resected, a condition that is also not compatible with ultimate survival.

The infarcted bowel is edematous and diffusely purple. The demarcation between infarcted bowel and normal tissue is usually sharp, although venous occlusion may lead to a more diffuse appearance. Extensive hemorrhage is seen in the mucosa and submucosa, the former becoming necrotic. Although

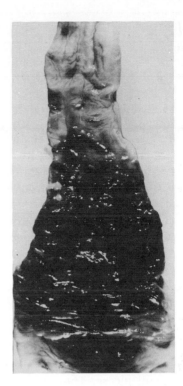

Figure 13-26. Infarct of the small bowel. Occlusion of a branch of the superior mesenteric artery led to hemorrhagic infarction of the small bowel. Note the sharp demarcation between the dilated, infarcted zone and the normal bowel.

the deep muscle layers are initially preserved, they eventually also become necrotic. The mucosal surface shows irregular white sloughs, the wall becomes thin and distended, and bubbles of gas may be present in the mesenteric veins. The serosal surface is cloudy and covered by fibrin.

The death of smooth muscle interferes with peristalsis and leads to **adynamic ileus,** a condition in which the bowel proximal to the lesion is dilated and filled with fluid. Intestinal organisms may pass through the damaged wall and cause **peritonitis** or **septicemia.**

In nonocclusive intestinal ischemia, the principal lesion is restricted to the mucosa. Mucosal changes range from foci of dilated capillaries with a few extravasated erythrocytes to severe hemorrhagic necrosis and bleeding into the lumen. Ulcers of varying size may result. In some cases greenish yellow soft plaques slough into the bowel lumen or are easily scraped off the underlying viable tissue. If the patient survives the episode of hypoperfusion, the bowel may be completely repaired, or it may heal with granulation tissue and fibrosis with eventual stricture formation.

Chronic Ischemia

Atherosclerotic narrowing of the major splanchnic arteries leads to chronic intestinal ischemia. As in the heart, the result is intermittent abdominal pain, termed **intestinal (abdominal) angina.** Characteristically the pain begins within a half hour of eating and lasts for a few hours. Presumably this reflects the need for greater blood flow during periods of active digestion. Many cases of frank infarction of the intestine are preceded by abdominal angina. Recurrent abdominal pain has also been ascribed to pressure on the celiac axis from surrounding structures and has been labeled the **celiac compression syndrome.**

Chronic ischemia of the small bowel may lead to fibrosis and the formation of a stricture. Ischemic strictures of the small bowel, which may be single or multiple, produce intestinal obstruction or, occasionally, malabsorption secondary to stasis and bacterial overgrowth. These strictures are concentric, and the mucosa of this region is atrophic and often exhibits one or more small ulcers. The submucosa is thickened and fibrotic and displays granulation tissue, which may extend into the muscular layers.

Crohn's Disease

Historically, Crohn's disease, a chronic inflammatory disorder of the bowel wall, was considered to be restricted to the small intestine. However, it is now clear that the disease may involve all other parts of the gastrointestinal tract, particularly the colon and anorectal region. Therefore, the subjct is treated together with ulcerative colitis under the rubric of **inflammatory bowel disease,** discussed below.

Malabsorption

Malabsorption is a general term used to describe a number of clinical conditions in which one or more important nutrients are inadequately absorbed by the gastrointestinal tract. Although some nutrient absorption occurs in the stomach and colon, only absorption from the small intestine, mainly in the proximal portion, is clinically important. The two substances that are preferentially absorbed by the distal small intestine are bile salts and vitamin B_{12}.

Normal intestinal absorption is characterized by a **luminal** phase and an **intestinal** phase (see Fig. 13-1). The luminal phase, consisting of those processes that occur within the lumen of the small in-

testine, alters the physicochemical state of the various nutrients such that they can be taken up by the absorptive cells in the small bowel epithelium. The intestinal phase includes those processes that occur in the cells and transport channels of the intestinal wall. Each of the two phases includes several critical components, and derangement of one or more leads to impaired absorption.

In the luminal phase of intestinal absorption it is critical that **pancreatic enzymes** and **bile acids** be secreted into the duodenal lumen in adequate amounts and in a normal physicochemical condition. Two additional factors are important for optimal activity of both pancreatic enzymes and bile salts: a normal and regulated flow of gastric contents into the duodenum and an appropriately high pH of the duodenal contents. Normal pancreatic enzyme excretion into the duodenum requires adequate pancreatic exocrine function and an unobstructed flow of pancreatic juice.

The supply of a normal quantity and quality of bile to the duodenum requires adequate hepatocellular function, unobstructed flow of bile, and an intact enterohepatic circulation of bile salts. The enterohepatic circulation of bile begins with absorption of most of the intestinal bile salts from the distal ileum and ends with their excretion into the duodenum through the bile ducts. Normally, 95% of intestinal bile salts are recycled through the enterohepatic circulation, the remaining 5% being excreted in the stools. The essential conditions for the normal functioning of the enterohepatic circulation are normal intestinal microflora, normal ileal absorptive function, and an unobstructued biliary system.

Thus, **luminal-phase** malabsorption has four major causes:

1. **Interruption of the normal continuity of the distal stomach and duodenum,** as occurs after gastroduodenal surgery (gastrectomy, antrectomy, pyloroplasty).
2. **Pancreatic dysfunction,** as a result of chronic pancreatitis, pancreatic carcinoma, or cystic fibrosis.
3. **Deficient or ineffective bile salts,** which may result from three possible causes. First is **impaired excretion of bile** because of liver disease. Second is **bacterial overgrowth,** which occurs as a result of a disturbance in the motility of the gut. It is seen in such conditions as blind loop syndrome, multiple diverticula of the small bowel, and muscular or neurogenic defects of the intestinal wall (e.g., amyloidosis, scleroderma, diabetic enteropathy). When gastrointestinal motility is defective, bile salts are de-

conjugated by the excess small bowel bacteria. The deconjugated bile salts, although absorbed and cycled normally through the enterohepatic circulation, are ineffective in the process of micelle formation, which is essential for the normal absorption of monoglycerides and free fatty acids. The third cause of ineffective or deficient bile salts is **absence or bypass of the distal ileum** caused by surgical excision, surgical anastomoses, fistulas, or ileal disease (e.g., Crohn's disease, lymphoma).

4. **Abnormally low intraduodenal pH,** as seen in patients with hypersecretion secondary to a gastrinoma (Zollinger-Ellison syndrome).

The **intestinal phase** of absorption may be interrupted at four different points: in the microvilli, in the absorptive area, in the metabolic function of the absorptive cells, and during transport.

1. **Microvilli.** The intestinal disaccharidases and oligopeptidases are integrally bound to the microvillous membranes. Disaccharidases are essential for sugar absorption, since only monosaccharides can be absorbed by the intestinal epithelial cells. Oligopeptides and dipeptides may be absorbed by alternate mechanisms that do not require peptidases. Abnormal function of the microvilli may be **primary,** as in the primary disaccharidase deficiencies, or **secondary,** when there is damage to the villi, as in celiac disease (sprue). The various enzyme deficiencies—for example, that of lactase—are characterized by intolerance for the corresponding disaccharides.

2. **Absorptive area.** The considerable length of the small bowel and the amplification of its surface wall by the intestinal folds (valves of Kerkring) provide a large absorptive surface. Moreover, the presence of villi and microvilli creates an additional absorptive area that is equivalent to the area of a basketball court. If sufficiently severe, a diminution in this area results in malabsorption. The surface area of the small intestinal epithelium may be diminished by small bowel resection (short bowel syndrome), gastrocolic fistulas (bypassing the small intestine), or a number of small intestinal diseases that are associated with mucosal damage (celiac disease, tropical sprue, Whipple's disease).

3. **Metabolic function of the absorptive cells.** Nutrients within the absorptive cells depend for their subsequent transport to the circulation on their metabolism within these cells. There, monoglycerides and free fatty acids are reassembled into triglycerides and coated with proteins (apoproteins) to form chylomicrons and lipoprotein particles. Nonspecific damage to small intestinal epithelial cells occurs in celiac disease, tropical sprue, Whipple's disease, and gastrinoma. Specific metabolic dysfunction is seen in **abetalipoproteinemia** (associated with acanthocytosis), a disorder in which the absorptive cells are unable to synthesize the apoprotein required for the assembly of lipoproteins and chylomicrons.

4. **Transport.** Nutrients are transported from the intestinal epithelium through the intestinal wall by way of blood capillaries and lymphatic vessels. Impaired transport of nutrients through these conduits is probably an important factor in the malabsorption associated with Whipple's disease, intestinal lymphoma, and congenital lymphangiectasia.

Although abnormalities in any one of the four components of the intestinal phase may cause malabsorption, some diseases affect more than one of these components. Figure 13-27 summarizes the major causes of malabsorption.

Clinical Features

Malabsorption may be either specific or generalized. In **specific,** or **isolated malabsorption,** an identifiable molecular defect causes malabsorption of a single nutrient. Examples of this group are the disaccharidase deficiencies (notably lactase deficiency) and deficiency of gastric intrinsic factor, which causes malabsorption of vitamin B_{12}, and consequently pernicious anemia. In **generalized malabsorption** (sometimes referred to as "pan-malabsorption"), the absorption of several or all major nutrient classes is impaired.

Generalized malabsorption, defined as the inadequate absorption of all the major nutrients (proteins, carbohydrates, and fats) leads to generalized malnutrition. In adults this is manifested by weight loss and sometimes cachexia; in children it is expressed as "failure to thrive."

Specific deficiency states may be manifested by anemia secondary to a deficiency of iron, folic acid, or vitamin B_{12}, or by a combination of these three. Patients may have a bleeding diathesis due to vitamin K deficiency, or they may have tetany, osteomalacia (in adults), or rickets (in children) due to malabsorption of vitamin D and calcium. In some patients a deficiency of water-soluble vitamins of the B group is responsible for glossitis, cheilosis, dermatitis, and peripheral neuropathy.

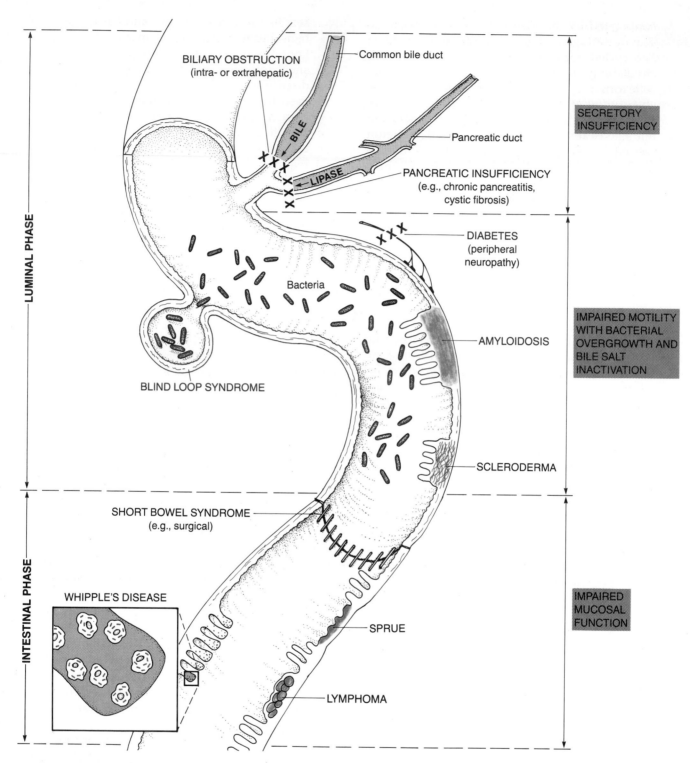

Figure 13-27. Causes of malabsorption.

Secondary effects of nonabsorbed or partially absorbed substances may lead to diarrhea. In disaccharide deficiency the unhydrolyzed sugars in the gut are metabolized by colonic bacteria to lactic acid, CO_2, and water, a process that results in explosive "fermentative" diarrhea. In patients with ileal dysfunction, bile salts that are not absorbed pass into the colon and cause "choleretic diarrhea," a reflection of the stimulation of colonic secretion.

Laboratory Evaluation

Laboratory tests are available to detect specific forms of malabsorption. For example, disaccharidase deficiency is diagnosed by measurement of blood sugar after the oral administration of a standard amount of disaccharide, as in the **lactose tolerance test,** or by measurement of the activity of disaccharidase in a small bowel biopsy specimen. Vitamin B_{12} absorption is assessed by the Schilling test, in which isotopically labeled vitamin B_{12} is administered orally and its blood level then determined. This test also helps distinguish between malabsorption resulting from intrinsic factor deficiency and other causes of vitamin B_{12} malabsorption.

In generalized malabsorption there is almost always impaired absorption of dietary fat. The most reliable and sensitive test of overall digestive and absorptive function is the **quantitative fecal fat analysis,** which serves as a standard for all other tests for malabsorption. **Steatorrhea** is the hallmark of generalized malabsorption, and the two terms are often used interchangeably.

A few of the tests currently in use for the evaluation of various causes of malabsorption merit mention.

d-Xylose Absorption

Xylose is a 5-carbon sugar the absorption of which does not require any of the components of the luminal phase. Blood levels and urinary excretion of this compound after ingestion of a defined amount thus serve as useful tests for the intestinal phase of absorption.

$^{14}CO_2$ Cholyl-Glycine Breath Test

Measurement of $^{14}CO_2$ in exhaled air following oral administration of $^{14}CO_2$-cholyl-glycine is a test of bile salt absorption by the ileum. It is employed in the diagnosis of the blind or stagnant loop syndrome (caused by bacterial overgrowth) and of ileal absorptive function. A newer test to detect bacterial overgrowth is the ^{14}C-xylose breath test.

Schilling Test

Originally devised for the diagnosis of pernicious anemia, the Schilling test has been modified for additional use as a test of ileal absorptive function, bacterial overgrowth, and pancreatic function.

Celiac Disease (Celiac Sprue)

Celiac disease (gluten-sensitive enteropathy, nontropical sprue) is characterized by generalized malabsorption; a typical, but nonspecific, small intestinal mucosal lesion; and a prompt clinical, and slower histologic, response to withdrawal of gluten-containing foods from the diet.

Epidemiology

The prevalence of celiac sprue is highly variable, ranging from 1 in 300 in western Ireland to 1 in 3000 in other countries. The true incidence of the disease is not known because of the high frequency of latent disease. The disorder is worldwide and affects all ethnic groups. There is only a slight female predominance, the sex ratio being 1.3:1. The malady may present at any time after the introduction of cereals into the diet. Most cases are diagnosed during childhood, although the disease may become clinically apparent for the first time as late as the seventh decade of life. The frequency of clinically overt disease among first-degree relatives has been estimated at 8%, but biopsy studies have indicated that the true familial frequency may be over 20%.

Etiology and Pathogenesis

The etiology of celiac disease remains unresolved, but there is a great deal of information about its pathogenesis.

Role of Cereal Proteins

Experiments on successfully treated, asymptomatic patients with celiac disease have shown that the ingestion or instillation into the histologically normal small intestine of wheat, barley, or rye flour is followed by the clinical features and histologic changes typical of celiac sprue. Other grains, such as rice and corn flour, do not have such an effect. Both the water-insoluble portion of wheat flour, namely **gluten,** and an alcoholic extract called **gliadin** have the same ef-

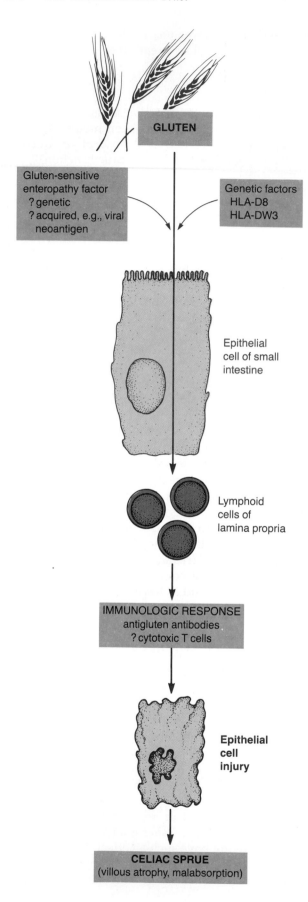

GLUTEN

Gluten-sensitive enteropathy factor
? genetic
? acquired, e.g., viral neoantigen

Genetic factors
HLA-D8
HLA-DW3

Epithelial cell of small intestine

Lymphoid cells of lamina propria

IMMUNOLOGIC RESPONSE
antigluten antibodies
? cytotoxic T cells

Epithelial cell injury

CELIAC SPRUE
(villous atrophy, malabsorption)

fect as whole wheat. Attempts to elucidate the precise molecular structure of the causative agent or the precise mechanisms of its action have been inconclusive.

Genetic and Immunologic Factors

Studies during the past two decades suggest that the pathogenesis of celiac sprue may involve the interplay of complex genetic factors and an abnormal immunologic response to ingested cereal antigens. Although overt celiac sprue and latent disease are frequent among family members, a definite genetic pattern of inheritance has not been established, and both concordance and discordance for celiac sprue have been documented in identical twins.

Approximately 80% of celiac disease patients carry the histocompatibility antigen HLA-B8; a similar frequency has been reported for HLA-DW3. Both of these antigens occur in less than 20% of the adult population, and both are frequent in other diseases associated with an altered immune response. However, these antigens are not carried by all patients with celiac sprue, and not all persons who carry one or both of these antigens develop the disease. Other genetic factors are probably involved; indeed, a higher than normal frequency of additional non-HLA antigens has been found in celiac sprue patients and their parents. Notable among these is the "gluten-sensitive enteropathy (GSE) B-cell antigen," which is segregated independently of HLA antigens. The genetic mechanisms responsible for the development of celiac disease are thus likely to reside in at least two loci, one related to the two HLA antigens and the other related to the B-cell antigen.

The intestinal lesion in celiac disease is characterized by damage to the epithelial cells and a marked increase in the number of plasma cells in the lamina propria and of T-lymphocytes within the epithelial cell layer. *In vivo* gliadin challenge of individuals with treated celiac sprue stimulates local immunoglobulin synthesis. Moreover, gliadin applied to an organ culture of jejunal mucosa *in vitro* induces the proliferation of T cells. An attractive, but unproved, immunologic theory has been proposed for the pathogenesis of celiac disease. According to this hypothesis, celiac disease develops in persons who carry genes that code for gliadin receptors on lymphocytes. The binding of gliadin then activates some process the final result of which is damage to the small intestinal epithelium.

Figure 13-28.   Hypothetical mechanisms in the pathogenesis of celiac disease.

Celiac disease is occasionally associated with **dermatitis herpetiformis,** a vesicular skin disease that typically affects the extensor surfaces and the exposed parts of the body. In this disorder subepidermal neutrophilic infiltration leads to local edema and blister formation. Deposits of IgA are detected in the region of the basement membranes. Almost all patients with dermatitis herpetiformis have a small bowel mucosal lesion similar to that of celiac disease, although only 10% have overt malabsorption. However, only a few patients who suffer from celiac disease develop dermatitis herpetiformis. Treatment with a strict gluten-free diet is followed by improvement of both the gastrointestinal symptoms and the skin lesions. The histocompatibility antigen HLA-B8 is much more frequent in patients with dermatitis herpetiformis than in normal persons.

Malabsorption in celiac disease probably results from multiple factors, including a reduction in the surface area of the intestinal mucosa (due to the blunting of villi and microvilli) and impairment of intracellular metabolism within the damaged epithelial cells. A probable aggravating factor is secondary disaccharidase deficiency, related to damage to the microvilli.

A hypothetical mechanism for the pathogenesis of celiac disease is presented in Figure 13-28.

Clinical Features

Clinically, celiac disease is characterized by generalized malabsorption. Typically, a child comes to medical attention because he ceases to thrive soon after the introduction of cereals into his diet. Not infrequently, overt signs of malabsorption are lacking, and the disease is suspected only because of growth retardation. Less commonly, the symptoms and signs of malabsorption are initially manifested in an adult.

The systemic manifestations of celiac disease are related to the various deficiency states that result from generalized malabsorption. Late complications in some cases include lymphoma of the small bowel, other malignant diseases of the gastrointestinal tract, and an inflammatory entity termed "ulcerative jejunitis." Treatment with a strict gluten-free diet is usually followed by a complete and prolonged clinical and histologic remission.

Pathology

The hallmark of celiac disease is a flat small intestinal mucosa, with blunting or total disappearance of villi, abnormal epithelial cells on the mucosal

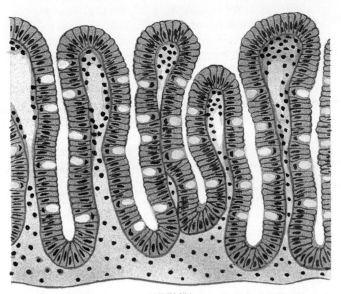

NORMAL

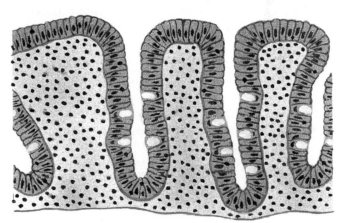

CELIAC DISEASE

Figure 13-29. Celiac disease. Elongation of the crypts, and chronic inflammation of the lamina propria are characteristic. In complete villous atrophy of longstanding disease the mucosa is flat.

surface, and increased cellularity of the lamina propria but not of the deeper layers (Fig. 13-29). The most severe histologic abnormalities in untreated celiac disease usually occur in the duodenum and proximal jejunum. There is a progressive decrease in severity distally; in some cases the ileal mucosa appears virtually normal. The clinical severity of the disease is thought to be related to the length of the affected intestine.

The villi are short and blunt or entirely absent, and the crypts are deeper than normal (see Fig. 13-29). The total thickness of the mucosa is not decreased, because lengthening of the crypts compensates for shortening of the villi. Thus the term "villous atrophy," which has been used to describe this appearance, is considered by many to be inappropriate, particularly since the rates of epithelial cell renewal and migration in celiac disease have been reported to be increased sixfold.

The absorptive cells are flattened and more basophilic than normal, and the basal polarity of their nuclei is lost. Electron microscopic examination reveals shortening and fusion of the microvilli. Some epithelial cells contain cytoplasmic and mitochondrial vacuoles, and large lysosomes have been described in the region of the intercellular tight junctions.

The epithelial cells lining the crypts of Lieberkuhn appear to be normal, but the crypts are longer than usual and contain numerous mitotic figures. The numbers of lymphocytes and plasma cells in the lamina propria are markedly increased. Most of the plasma cells produce IgA (as in the normal small bowel). Polymorphonuclear leukocytes and eosinophils may also be increased in the lamina propria.

Whipple's Disease

Whipple's disease is a rare systemic disorder in which **the small intestine is consistently involved and malabsorption is the most prominent feature.** It most commonly affects white men in their 30s and 40s. Other clinical findings include fever, increased skin pigmentation, anemia, lymphadenopathy, arthritis, pericarditis, pleurisy, endocarditis, and central nervous system involvement.

Etiology and Pathogenesis

Whipple's disease typically shows infiltration of the small bowel mucosa by large macrophages that are packed with small, rod-shaped bacilli. Dramatic clinical remissions occur with antibiotic therapy. Despite the demonstration that Whipple's disease is caused by bacterial infection, the specific causative agent has not been identified, and the pathogenesis is still unclear. Attempts to isolate the responsible organism have yielded conflicting results, and no single organism has been incriminated. Furthermore, the sporadic nature of the disease and the lack of evidence for direct transmission have not permitted the establishment of an epidemiologic pattern. The results of several studies suggest that host susceptibility factors, possibly defective T-lymphocyte function, may be important in predisposing toward the disease.

Pathology

Macroscopically, the bowel wall is thickened and edematous, and the mesenteric lymph nodes are usually enlarged. Histologic examination of the small intestine reveals flat, thickened villi and extensive infiltration of the lamina propria with large macrophages (Fig. 13-30A). **The cytoplasm of these macrophages is filled with large glycoprotein granules that stain strongly with periodic acid-Schiff (PAS).** Importantly, the other normal cellular components of the lamina propria—that is, plasma cells and lymphocytes—are depleted. The lymphatic vessels in the mucosa and submucosa are dilated, and large lipid droplets abound within lymphatics and in extracellular spaces, a finding that suggests obstruction of the lymphatics.

In contrast to the striking distortion of the villous architecture, the epithelial cells show only patchy abnormalities, including attenuation of the microvilli and an accumulation of lipid droplets within the cytoplasm. **Electron microscopic examination reveals numerous small bacilli within macrophages and free in the lamina propria (Fig. 13-30B).** Many bacilli cluster immediately beneath the epithelial basement membrane.

The mesenteric lymph nodes draining the affected segments of small bowel reveal similar microscopic changes. A characteristic infiltration by macrophages containing bacilli may also be found in other organs, notably the lung, heart, spleen, liver, endocrine glands, brain, bone, and synovial membranes. Heart lesions may include vegetations on the heart valves that contain bacilli-laden macrophages, sometimes with superimposed streptococcal endocarditis.

Abetalipoproteinemia

Abetalipoproteinemia is an autosomal-recessive inherited disease characterized by a failure to synthesize apoprotein B, a constituent of the membrane coat of low-density lipoproteins. It is an example of malabsorption resulting solely from a metabolic defect within the absorptive cells. Small intestinal absorptive cells that lack apoprotein B fail to assemble chylomicrons, an essential component of lipid transport out of the cell. The other manifestations of the disease result from defects in cell membrane structure, manifested in erythrocytes as acanthocytosis and in the central nervous system as selective demyelinization, particularly of the posterior columns. Typical neurologic manifestations are loss of deep tendon reflexes, sensory ataxia, and a mild form of retinitis pigmentosa. The serum shows a total ab-

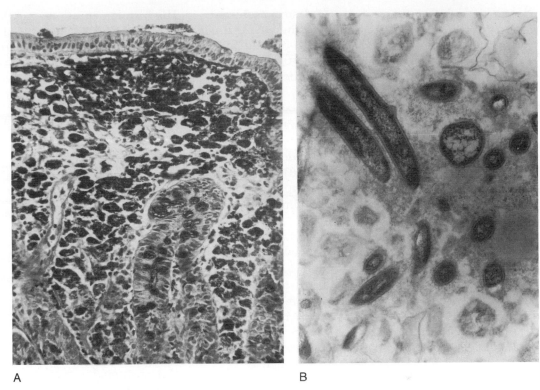

Figure 13-30. Whipple's disease. (*A*) A photomicrograph of a section of jejunal mucosa, stained by the periodic acid-Schiff (PAS) reaction, shows abundant large macrophages filled with cytoplasmic material. (*B*) An electron micrograph of (*A*) demonstrates small bacilli in a macrophage.

sence of chylomicrons, very-low-density lipoproteins (VLDL), and low density lipoproteins (LDL). In addition, serum levels of cholesterol and triglycerides are low, and the bulk of serum lipids are carried within high-density lipoprotein particles.

Malabsorption in abetalipoproteinemia is partially reversed by ingestion of medium-chain (rather than the usual long-chain) triglycerides; these lipids are transported through the absorptive cells without an apoprotein coat.

Histologically, the villi, lamina propria, and submucosa appear normal. The epithelial cells contain lipid vacuoles, but no lipid is seen in the intestinal lymphatics. This lipid probably represents triglyceride, which has been assembled within the cell but which cannot be transported into the basolateral intercellular space because of the lack of apoprotein B.

Hypogammaglobulinemia

Malabsorption occurs frequently in patients with acquired hypogammaglobulinemia. The histologic appearance of the small intestine may be normal (except for a lack of plasma cells in the lamina propria), or nodular lymphoid hyperplasia may be seen. Occasionally there is a flat mucosa, similar to the lesion of celiac sprue except for a lack of plasma cells in the lamina propria; in this case the disorder is termed **hypogammaglobulinemic sprue.**

Most hypogammaglobulinemic patients with malabsorption are found to be infected in the small intestine with *Giardia lamblia.* Appropriate treatment with metronidazole is followed by improved intestinal absorption.

Congenital Lymphangiectasia

Congenital lymphangiectasia is a poorly understood disease that usually begins in childhood and probably reflects a generalized malformation of the lymphatic system. A syndrome of intestinal lymphangiectasia and peripheral lymphedema is known as **Milroy's disease.** In addition to having steatorrhea caused by impaired transport of chylomicrons by intestinal lymphatics, patients with congenital lymphangiectasia suffer from **protein-losing enteropathy,** a condition characterized by excessive loss of plasma proteins into the gut. In this respect protein-losing enteropathy may also occur in association with certain gastrointestinal tumors, Whipple's disease, Crohn's disease, bacterial overgrowth, parasitic infestations of the bowel, and Menetrier's disease.

Other important features of congenital lymphangiectasia are lymphopenia and impaired cell-mediated immunity, caused by the loss of small lymphocytes into the bowel lumen. Chylous ascites (milky, lipid-containing peritoneal fluid) occurs in some cases as a result of leakage of lymph from the mesenteric or serosal lymphatic vessels into the peritoneal cavity.

The lesions of congenital lymphangiectasia are recognized macroscopically as opalescent white spots, microscopically as **dilated subepithelial lymphatics (lacteals).** The submucosal lymphatics also tend to be dilated. The mucosal epithelium is normal, but the villi may be blunted or even absent in areas overlying severe lymphatic dilatation.

Intestinal lymphangiectasia, with all or some of the associated clinical features described above, occurs as a secondary manifestation of small intestinal or retroperitoneal lymphoma, other retroperitoneal tumors, tuberculosis, sarcoidosis, chronic pancreatitis, and retroperitoneal fibrosis.

Tropical Sprue

Tropical sprue is a poorly understood disease of obscure cause that is acquired in certain endemic tropical areas and is characterized by progressively severe malabsorption and nutritional deficiency. Cure, or at least amelioration of the symptoms, usually follows treatment with oral tetracycline and folic acid.

The disease is endemic to Puerto Rico, Cuba, the Dominican Republic, and Haiti but is uncommon in other parts of the West Indies. It also occurs in the northern parts of South America and many Far Eastern countries.

The cause of tropical sprue is not known. Some studies suggest that **long-standing contamination of the bowel with bacteria,** perhaps toxigenic strains of *E. coli*, may be important, and that **folate deficiency** may play a role in pepetuating the intestinal lesion.

Typically, steatorrhea, anemia, and weight loss are followed by progressively severe manifestations of folic acid and vitamin B_{12} deficiencies and hypoalbuminemia. Typical laboratory findings are increased fecal fat, impaired d-xylose absorption, megaloblastic anemia, and decreased disaccharidase activity in the intestinal mucosa.

The histologic findings are variable, ranging from mild widening and blunting of villi to a completely flat mucosa indistinguishable from that seen in celiac sprue. The histologic changes in the epithelium and the inflammation of the lamina propria usually parallel the severity of the alterations in the villi.

Radiation Enteritis

Abdominal irradiation may cause transient damage to the small intestinal mucosa. Anorexia, abdominal cramps, and changes in bowel habits occur frequently during the course of abdominal radiation therapy, and laboratory studies in such patients indicate malabsorption of bile salts and disaccharides. Transient histologic changes in the small bowel include shortening of the villi, increased cellularity in the lamina propria, and submucosal edema. These changes usually revert to normal within 12 days of cessation of radiotherapy.

Chronic radiation damage is less common in the small intestine than in other parts of the gastrointestinal tract, probably because the mobility of the loops of small intestine reduces their continued exposure to the radiation beam.

Occasionally, subacute or chronic radiation damage does occur, especially when the radiation dose is very high, when segments of small bowel become fixed (as a result of postoperative or inflammatory adhesions), when the blood supply to the bowel is impaired, or when the radiation is combined with chemotherapeutic agents that may augment radiation damage. Malabsorption in such situations may result from a combination of mucosal damage and impaired motility, resulting in bacterial overgrowth.

The major histologic features of subacute and chronic radiation damage to the small intestine are similar to those seen elsewhere in the gastrointestinal tract; they include mucosal ulceration, swelling and detachment of endothelial cells of the small arterioles in the submucosa, obliteration by fibrin plugs of the lumina of the arterioles, and the presence of large foam cells beneath the intima. Thickening and fibrosis of the submucosa ensue, together with signs of progressive ischemia.

Neoplasms

The small intestine is curiously resistant to neoplasia, despite the fact that it is the longest portion of the alimentary tract. Tumors of the small intestine constitute less than 5% of all gastrointestinal tumors.

Although many factors have been proposed as the cause of this anomaly, none has been proved, and all are speculative. The following are the most credible of the theories, which are not mutually exclusive. (1) The rapid transit time in the small bowel limits the length of exposure of the mucosa to carcinogens in the food. (2) The concentration of carcinogens may be lower in the large liquid volume of the small intestine than in the more solid contents of the colon. (3) Detoxifying enzymes in the small intestine may be more active than those in the stomach or colon. (4) The bacterial flora of the colon is far more voluminous than that of the small intestine. Moreover, the colonic bacteria are principally anaerobes, which have been shown to convert bile acids into carcinogens. (5) Humoral and cellular immune systems are more active in the small intestine than at other sites in the gastrointestinal tract. IgA has been theorized to protect in some unknown way against the development of neoplasms. The lymphoid nodules of the small bowel contain abundant T-lymphocytes, which may participate in immune surveillance. (6) The kinetics of cell renewal are different in the small intestine than at other sites in the alimentary tract. It has been suggested that fewer cells in the small intestine retain a proliferative potential as they migrate up the villus than do cells of the crypts of the stomach or colon.

Benign Tumors

The most common benign tumors of the small intestine are adenomas, leiomyomas, and lipomas. As in other portions of the gastrointestinal tract, neurogenic tumors, fibromas, angiomas, and hamartomas may be encountered. Benign tumors of the small intestine rarely become malignant.

Adenomas of the small intestine resemble those of the colon (discussed below). As in the colon, adenomas in the small intestine may be tubular, villous, or a mixture of these types. The villous adenoma is rare in the small intestine, usually occurring in the ileum. Although most adenomas remain benign, some, especially the villous type, undergo malignant transformation. Benign adenomas are ordinarily asymptomatic, but bleeding and intussusception are occasional complications.

The **Peutz-Jeghers syndrome** is an autosomal dominant hereditary disorder characterized by intestinal polyps and mucocutaneous melanin pigmentation, particularly evident on the face, buccal mucosa, hands, feet, and perianal and genital areas. Except for the buccal pigmentation, the freckle-like macular lesions usually fade at puberty. The polyps occur most commonly in the proximal regions of the small intestine but are sometimes seen in the stomach and the colon. Patients usually present with symptoms of obstruction or intussusception; in as many as one-quarter of the cases, however, the diagnosis is suggested by pigmentation alone in an otherwise asymptomatic person. Acute upper gastrointestinal hemorrhage and occult bleeding with anemia may complicate the course.

The polyps in Peutz-Jeghers syndrome are not true neoplasms, but rather **hamartomas.** Histologically, a branching network of smooth muscle fibers continuous with the muscularis mucosa supports the glandular epithelium of the polyp (Fig. 13-31). Peutz-Jeghers polyps are generally considered benign; however, 2% to 3% of patients develop adenocarcinoma, although not necessarily in the hamartomatous polyps.

Leiomyomas of the small intestine occur at all levels but are most common in the jejunum. This tumor ordinarily presents as an intramural mass covered by intact mucosa. However, the lesion may protrude into the lumen, where necrosis of tumor tissue and ulceration of the overlying mucosa give rise to bleeding. Intestinal obstruction is uncommon, but volvulus may be a complication. Histologically, leiomyomas of the small intestine are similar to those elsewhere. Surgical removal of large tumors is advisable because of bleeding and the significant risk of malignancy.

Lipomas occur throughout the length of the small intestine but are most common in the distal ileum.

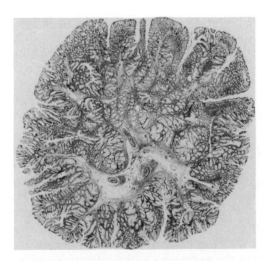

Figure 13-31. Peutz-Jeghers polyp. In this hamartomatous polyp the glandular epithelium is supported by a network of smooth muscle.

Although for the most part asymptomatic, these submucosal tumors may become large and produce intestinal obstruction, usually as a result of intussusception. The overlying mucosa may become ulcerated and bleed.

Malignant Tumors

Adenocarcinoma

Although adenocarcinoma of the small intestine accounts for only a minute proportion of all gastrointestinal tumors, it constitutes half of all malignant small bowel tumors. The large majority of adenocarcinomas are located in the duodenum and jejunum. Most occur in middle-aged persons, and there is a moderate male predominance. Interestingly, the geographic variation in the incidence of small bowel adenocarcinoma correlates with that of colon cancer, but not with that of stomach cancer. For instance, Japanese who migrate to Hawaii have a lower than normal incidence of stomach cancer but a higher than normal incidence of both colon cancer and small bowel adenocarcinoma.

Adenocarcinoma of the small intestine is usually annular; therefore, the symptoms are commonly those of progressive intestinal obstruction. Occult bleeding is common and often leads to iron-deficiency anemia. Acute bleeding and perforation are infrequent. Adenocarcinoma of the duodenum, which is distinct from ampullary carcinoma, may involve the papilla of Vater and cause obstructive jaundice or pancreatitis.

Adenocarcinoma of the small intestine may be polypoid, ulcerative, or simply annular and stenosing. In addition to causing intestinal obstruction directly, a polypoid tumor may be the lead point of an intussusception. Microscopically, adenocarcinomas, which originate from the epithelium of the crypts rather than the villi, resemble colon cancer. By the time the patient becomes symptomatic, most adenocarcinomas have metastasized to local lymph nodes, and overall 5-year survival is less than 20%.

A risk factor for adenocarcinoma is inflammatory disease of the small bowel. Patients with Crohn's disease are known to be at a significantly increased risk, perhaps as high as 100-fold. Moreover, the mean age for the appearance of an adenocarcinoma of the small intestine is 10 years younger than average in patients with Crohn's disease, and the cancer tends to occur in the same area as the inflammatory lesions, namely the ileum. Adenocarcinoma of the terminal ileum has also been reported in a few patients with ulcerative colitis who manifested "backwash ileitis."

Additionally, adenocarcinoma is a rare complication of celiac disease.

Primary Lymphoma

Primary lymphoma, which originates in nodules of lymphoid tissue within the bowel wall, represents the second most common malignant tumor of the small intestine in industrialized countries, where it accounts for about 15% of small bowel cancers. By contrast, another type of primary lymphoma comprises more than two-thirds of all cancers of the small intestine in underdeveloped countries. The latter type of intestinal lymphoma was originally described in Mediterranean populations, but it is now clear that it is distributed throughout the poorer parts of the world. Because these two types of lymphoma have distinct epidemiologic, clinical, and pathological features, they are labeled, respectively, the "Western" type and the "Mediterranean" variety. The small intestine may be secondarily involved in disseminated lymphomas, but symptomatic disease is uncommon. The classification of primary intestinal lymphoma is identical with that of nodal lymphoma, which is discussed in Chapter 20.

The cause of primary lymphoma of the small bowel is unknown, but an association with celiac disease is well documented, occurring in as many as one-tenth of primary lymphoma patients. It is assumed that the persistent activation of lymphocytes in the bowel is related to the subsequent development of lymphoma. However, although a gluten-free diet improves the inflammatory component of the enteropathy, there is no evidence that it prevents the appearance of lymphoma.

The risk of intestinal lymphoma is also increased in conditions that favor the development of nodal lymphoma, particularly immunodeficiency following treatment with immunosuppressive drugs.

Mediterranean lymphoma typically occurs in poor countries in young men of low socioeconomic status; it is therefore thought by some to have an environmental cause. **This neoplasm has been associated with alpha-chain disease, a proliferative disorder of intestinal B-lymphocytes that secrete IgA.** The protein secreted by the malignant cells (into the serum or the intestinal lumen) is an immunoglobulin consisting of incomplete alpha chains without light chains. In fact, Mediterranean lymphoma and alpha-chain disease are thought by some to be the same disorder, termed **immunoproliferative small intestinal disease.**

Mediterranean intestinal lymphoma, which typically affects men under the age of 30, predominantly

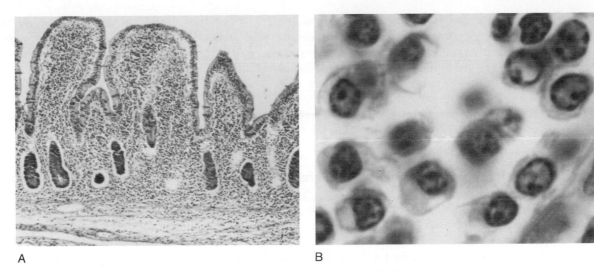

A   B

Figure 13-32. Mediterranean intestinal lymphoma. (*A*) The villi are short and blunted, and the lamina propria is filled with lymphoid cells. (*B*) A high-power view of (*A*) shows plasma cells and plasmacytoid lymphocytes.

involves the duodenum and proximal jejunum. A long segment of small intestine, or even the entire small bowel, is characteristically affected. The lymphoma typically presents as a diffuse infiltration of the mucosa and submucosa by plasmacytoid lymphocytes or plasma cells (Fig. 13-32). Lymphomatous infiltration of the mucosa leads to mucosal atrophy and severe malabsorption, as previously discussed.

The **Western type of intestinal lymphoma** usually affects adults over the age of 40 years and children under the age of 10 years. It is most common in the ileum, where it presents as a fungating mass that projects into the lumen, an elevated ulcerated lesion, a diffuse segmental thickening of the bowel wall, or plaquelike mucosal nodules. As a result, intestinal obstruction, intussusception, and perforation are important complications. Occult bleeding is common, although massive acute hemorrhage may also occur. Microscopically, all varieties of non-Hodgkin's lymphoma are encountered. When the disease is localized and confined to the small intestine, it does not recur after surgical removal in over half the patients. When extraintestinal spread is present, the 5-year survival rate is less than 10%.

Chronic abdominal pain, diarrhea, and clubbing of the fingers are the most frequent clinical signs of intestinal lymphoma. Diarrhea and weight loss reflect the underlying malabsorption. Chemotherapy and occasionally radiotherapy are employed as treatment, since the disease is usually too diffuse to permit surgery. This primary therapy often requires additional antibiotic treatment to control bacterial overgrowth in the diseased intestine. Patients with Mediterranean lymphoma tend to survive longer than those with the Western type of lymphoma.

Carcinoid Tumor

Carcinoid tumors of the gastrointestinal tract arise from argentaffin cells, which are part of the neuroendocrine system of the gut, at the base of the mucosal crypts. These cells are included in the amine precursor uptake and decarboxylation (APUD) system found in many other organs, as described in Chapter 21. The carcinoid tumors are capable of secreting all the peptides and amines produced by their normal counterparts, namely the argentaffin cells, although not all such tumors readily stain with silver salts. The most commonly secreted hormone is **serotonin.**

Whereas carcinoid tumors constitute less than 1% of all gastrointestinal tumors, **they are the most common benign tumors of the small intestine and account for 20% of all malignant tumors.** Since argentaffin cells are most numerous in the appendix and terminal ileum, it is not surprising that carcinoid tumors are most frequent at these sites. In fact, **35% to 40% of all carcinoid tumors are found in the appendix,** and almost as many are found in the ileum. Interestingly, 2% of carcinoid tumors of the small bowel arise in a Meckel's diverticulum.

Carcinoid tumors can occur anywhere in the gastrointestinal tract, from the esophagus to the anal canal. Most of these tumors are minute and are found only incidentally, often in an appendectomy specimen. Such very small growths are almost invariably benign. **For practical purposes carcinoid tumors of the appendix less than 2 cm across do not metastasize.** In general, the malignant potential of intestinal carcinoid tumors appears to be related to their size. Tumors of less than 1 cm in diameter are rarely malignant, 50% of those between 1 cm and 2 cm in diameter metastasize, and 80% of those larger than 2 cm in diameter metastasize.

Carcinoid tumors of the gastrointestinal tract, especially those of the small intestine, are often multicentric; that is, multiple primary tumors arise, either simultaneously or at different times. They are also seen in association with the multiple endocrine neoplasia (MEN) syndromes, most commonly with type I. Since APUD cells are widespread, carcinoid tumors are found in a variety of locations, including the pancreas, bronchus, gallbladder, ovary, and testis. Carcinoid tumors of the gastrointestinal tract are also associated with a significantly increased frequency of nonendocrine malignant tumors, both in the alimentary tract and elsewhere.

Macroscopically, small carcinoid tumors present as yellowish submucosal nodules covered by intact mucosa. Large tumors may grow in a polypoid, intramural, or annular pattern (Fig. 13-33A) and often undergo secondary ulceration. The cut surface is firm and bright yellow. Microscopically, the neoplasms appear as nests, cords, and rosettes of uniform small, round cells (Fig. 13-33B). Occasional glandlike structures are also encountered. The nuclei exhibit a remarkable regularity, and mitoses are rare. In the solid nests the cells on the periphery tend to have small, more hyperchromatic nuclei than those in the center. An abundant eosinophilic cytoplasm contains cytoplasmic granules, which by electron microscopy are typically of the neurosecretory type.

As they enlarge, carcinoid tumors invade the muscular coat and penetrate the serosa, often causing a conspicuous desmoplastic reaction. This fibrosis is responsible for peritoneal adhesions and kinking of the bowel, which may lead to intestinal obstruction. These neoplasms metastasize first to regional lymph nodes. Subsequently, hematogenous spread leads to metastases at distant sites, particularly the liver. Surgical resection, the only therapy for the primary tumor, accomplishes a 5-year cure in half the cases of small bowel carcinoid tumors.

Carcinoid tumors are marked by a unique clinical condition, termed the **carcinoid syndrome,** that is caused by the release of a variety of active tumor products. Although most carcinoids are to some extent functional, this syndrome is ordinarily seen only in cases with extensive hepatic metastases. **The classic symptoms of the carcinoid syndrome include diarrhea (often the most distressing symptom), episodic flushing, bronchospasm, cyanosis, telangiectasia, and skin lesions.** About half of the patients also suffer from right-sided cardiac valvular disease. Diarrhea is thought to be caused by serotonin, but the tumor secretory products involved in the other symptoms have not been clearly identified.

After its release into the blood, serotonin is metabolized to 5-hydroxyindoleacetic acid (5-HIAA) by monoamine oxidase either in the tumor or in other tissues. The presence of 5-HIAA in the urine is a diagnostic test for the carcinoid syndrome. Whereas the liver, lung, and brain all have high levels of activity of monoamine oxidase and (presumably) of enzymes that inactivate other tumor secretions, the right side of the heart is exposed to the full effects of tumor products that have been released into the vena cava from hepatic metastases. As a result, endocardial fibrosis, probably a reaction to endothelial damage, occurs. Fibrous plaques form on the tricuspid and pulmonic valves, the endocardium of the right-sided cardiac chambers, the vena cava, the coronary sinus, and the pulmonary artery. Distortion of the valves leads to **pulmonic stenosis** and **tricuspid regurgitation.**

Leiomyosarcoma

Leiomyosarcomas in the small intestine, similar clinically and pathologically to those in the stomach, are rare. This cancer has a slower course than small bowel adenocarcinoma, and the 5-year survival rate has been reported to be better than 50%. Rare instances of other cancers of mesenchymal origin have been reported in the small intestine.

Pneumatosis Cystoides Intestinalis (Gas Cysts)

Pneumatosis cystoides intestinalis is an uncommon disorder in which numerous pockets of gas are found in the wall of the gut anywhere in the gastrointestinal tract. About 85% of cases are associated with an underlying gastrointestinal disease, including intestinal obstruction, peptic ulcers, Crohn's disease, mesenteric ischemia, volvulus, and neonatal necrotizing enterocolitis. The remaining cases, in which no other lesions are found, are idiopathic. The idiopathic variety is found primarily in adults and usually affects the colon, whereas the secondary type is more frequent in the small intestine. Pneumatosis

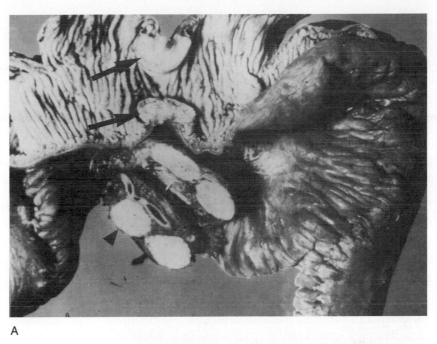

A

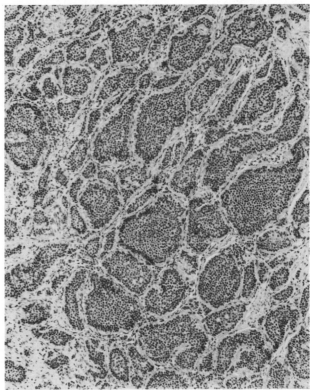

B

Figure 13-33. Carcinoid tumor of the small intestine. (*A*) An annular carcinoid tumor (*arrows*) constricts the lumen of the small intestine. Lymph node metastases (*arrowhead*) are evident. (*B*) A photomicrograph of (*A*) demonstrates nests and cords of uniform small, round cells.

in adults is ordinarily benign, depending on the underlying disease. However, intestinal pneumatosis associated with neonatal necrotizing enteritis has a high mortality.

The cause of intestinal pneumatosis is not clear. One theory holds that a mechanical break in the continuity of the mucosa allows the entry of air from the lumen to the submucosa. Alternatively, there is some evidence that the gas is a product of bacterial action, particularly in neonatal necrotizing enterocolitis.

Macroscopically, the cysts appear as bubbles under the serosa of the intestine, and the bowel wall feels spongy. In some cases the air cysts are located principally in the submucosa, in which case the cut surface of the bowel wall appears to be honeycombed. The cysts vary from a few millimeters to several centimeters in diameter. In addition to appearing in the small and large intestines, cysts may occur in the stomach and the mesentery. Microscopic examination reveals cystic spaces in the submucosa or beneath the serosa, and these spaces are lined by large macrophages and multinucleated giant cells. Little or no other inflammation is elicited by the cysts. The mucosa overlying submucosal cysts is attenuated and may contain small hemorrhages.

Clinically, most patients have episodic diarrhea. Constipation and diminished caliber of the stools may be related to intestinal obstruction by the cysts. There is often blood in the stools, and rectal bleeding may be brisk. When intestinal pneumatosis is a complication of neonatal necrotizing enterocolitis, bowel perforation and peritonitis are frequent; these complications are rare in adults.

Gas cysts may disappear spontaneously or may persist for years. Relief of symptoms may be obtained by oxygen inhalation or treatment with the antimicrobial agent metronidazole.

The Colon
Anatomy

The colon, defined as the portion of the gastrointestinal tract from the ileocecal valve to the anus, is 90 cm to 125 cm in length. The proximal part shares a common embryologic origin with the small intestine, both being derived from the embryonic midgut and supplied by the superior mesenteric artery. The distal half of the colon is embryologically distinct. It is derived from the embryonic hindgut, is supplied by the inferior mesenteric artery, and serves principally as a storage organ.

The colon is traditionally divided into six regions in a sequence that proceeds from the ileocecal valve distally: cecum, ascending colon, transverse colon, descending colon, sigmoid colon, and rectum. The bend between the ascending and transverse colon in the right upper quadrant is termed the "hepatic flexure," and that between the transverse and descending segments in the left upper quadrant is termed the "splenic flexure." The caliber of the lumen progressively diminishes from the cecum to the sigmoid colon.

Similar to the small intestine, the colon is endowed with outer longitudinal and inner circular muscle coats. However, in the colon the longitudinal muscle constitutes three separate bundles, termed the **taeniae coli**. Evaginations of the colonic wall between the taeniae, called the haustra, are separated by the semilunar folds. The appendices epiploicae are small serosal masses of fat, invested by peritoneum. The vermiform appendix arises at the apex of the cecum and terminates as a blind tube; it averages about 8 cm in length but occasionally measures up to 20 cm.

The ileocecal valve functions as a sphincter to regulate the flow of intestinal contents into the cecum. However, it is an incompetent sphincter, and reflux of cecal contents into the ileum is usual, a situation that may account for so-called **backwash ileitis** in ulcerative colitis. The internal sphincter of the anal canal is continuous with colonic smooth muscle. The external anal sphincter, the major mechanism by which continence of the bowel is maintained, surrounds the anal canal with a layer of skeletal muscle.

Histologically, the surface of the colonic mucosa is flat, and punctuated by numerous pits, termed "crypts" or "glands" of Lieberkuhn. The mucosa of the surface and crypts is lined by a tall columnar epithelium. The surface epithelium consists primarily of simple columnar cells and occasional goblet cells. The crypts are lined mostly by goblet cells, except at their bases, where undifferentiated cells and a variety of endocrine cells are located. The basal undifferentiated cells constitute the reserve cell population of the colonic mucosa and exhibit numerous mitoses. Mucosal cells migrate from the bases of the crypts toward the luminal surface, from where they are sloughed. The ultrastructural appearance of the mucosal cells is similar to that in the small intestine, except that the microvilli of the absorptive cells are much shorter and narrower in the colon.

The lamina propria of the colonic mucosa contains lymphocytes, plasma cells, macrophages, and fibroblasts. An occasional neutrophil or eosinophil may also be encountered. Lymphoid follicles interrupt the continuity of the muscularis mucosae, and extend into the mucosa, where they are grossly visualized as small nodules. The submucosa is similar to that in the small intestine, but lymphatic channels are far less prominent. The lymphatics drain into paracolic nodes in the serosal fat, intermediate nodes located along the course of the colic blood vessels, and central nodes clustered near the aorta. Parasympathetic and sympathetic innervations terminate in Meissner's and Auerbach's enteric plexuses.

Congenital Disorders

Congenital Megacolon (Hirschsprung's Disease)

Hirschsprung's disease is an uncommon, but not rare, familial disorder in which colonic dilatation (Fig. 13-34) results from a defect in the innervation of the rectum. **The lesion is a congenital absence of ganglion cells in the wall of the rectum** (Fig. 13-35). In about one-fourth of the cases, ganglion cells are deficient in more proximal portions of the colon, and in unusual cases the lesion may extend as far as the small intestine.

The pathogenesis of Hirschsprung's disease can be traced to an interruption of the developmental sequence that leads to innervation of the colon. The normal caudal migration of cells from the neural crest that eventually gives rise to the intramural ganglion cells is interrupted. Because the internal anal sphincter marks the terminus of this migration, the aganglionic segment always includes the rectum and may extend for variable distances proximally, depending on the point at which the primitive neuroblasts are halted. Given that the aganglionic rectum and occasionally the adjacent colon are permanently contracted, the fecal contents do not readily enter this stenotic area, and the proximal bowel becomes dilated.

The incidence of congenital megacolon is 10 times higher than normal in infants with **Down's syndrome,** and 2% of patients with Down's syndrome are born with Hirschsprung's disease. Although most cases of aganglionosis of the colon are uncomplicated by other lesions, the disorder has also been reported in conjunction with a number of other congenital abnormalities, including anomalies of the kidneys and lower urinary tract, imperforate anus, ventricular septal defect, and the Laurence-Moon-Biedl syndrome.

The clinical signs are delayed passage of meconium by the neonate and the development of vom-

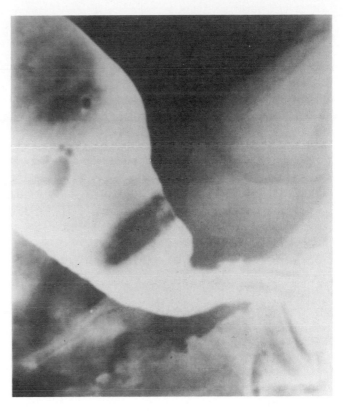

Figure 13-34. Hirschsprung's disease. A contrast radiograph shows marked dilatation of the rectosigmoid colon.

iting in 2 to 3 days. In some cases complete intestinal obstruction requires immediate surgical relief. In others repeated enemas ameliorate the obstruction; however, fulminant enterocolitis has occasionally followed treatment with multiple enemas. In children who have short rectal segments lacking ganglion cells, and who suffer only partial obstruction, constipation, abdominal distention, and recurrent fecal impactions characterize the clinical course.

The most serious complication of congenital megacolon is an enterocolitis, in which necrosis and ulceration affect the dilated proximal segment of the colon and may extend into the small intestine. The cure for Hirschsprung's disease is surgical removal of the aganglionic segment.

The definitive diagnosis of Hirschsprung's disease is made on the basis of absent ganglion cells in a transmural rectal biopsy. Additionally, there is a striking increase in nonmyelinated cholinergic nerve fibers in the submucosa and between the muscle coats. The absence of ganglion cells leads to an accumulation of acetylcholine and its corresponding enzyme, acetylcholinesterase. The histochemical demonstration of this enzyme, which is not visualized in the normal rectal wall, has been reported to

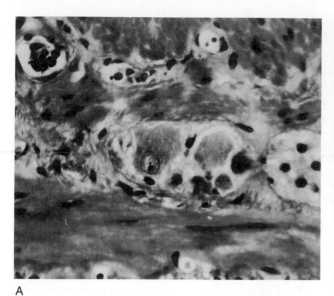
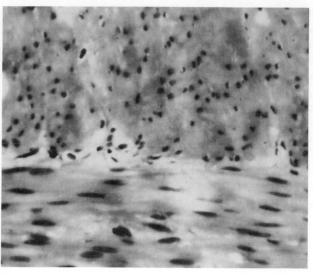

A   B

Figure 13-35.   Hirschsprung's disease. (*A*) A photomicrograph of normal ganglion cells in the wall of the rectum. (*B*) A rectal biopsy from a patient with Hirschsprung's disease shows an absence of ganglion cells.

enhance the reliability of the diagnosis based upon rectal biopsy.

Acquired megacolon in children often has a psychogenic background and frequently is associated with the prolonged use of laxatives. However, some cases in which ganglion cells are demonstrated by rectal biopsy begin in infancy and are associated with fecal incontinence. The cause of this apparently organic disturbance is not well understood, but the disorder is thought to represent a functional abnormality of colonic motility. Acquired megacolon in adults can result from disorders that interfere with the innervation of the bowel or smooth muscle function. Examples include diabetic neuropathy, parkinsonism, myotonic dystrophy, scleroderma, amyloidosis, and hypothyroidism. Interestingly, similar to achalasia, which causes the destruction of esophageal ganglion cells, Chagas' disease may cause aganglionic megacolon.

Anorectal Malformations

Anorectal malformations, among the most common developmental defects, vary from minor narrowing to serious and complex anomalies. These lesions result from arrested development of the caudal region of the gut in the first 6 months of fetal life. The classification of these defects is based on the relationship of the terminal bowel to the levator ani muscle. The classes are high or supralevator deformities, in which the bowel ends above the pelvic floor; inter-

mediate deformities; and low or translevator deformities, in which the bowel ends below the pelvic floor. **Anorectal agenesis** and **rectal atresia** are supralevator deformities, whereas **anal agenesis** and **anorectal stenosis** are classed as intermediate ones. **Imperforate anus** is a low or translevator deformity in which the opening is covered by a cutaneous membrane behind which meconium is visible. A variant of imperforate anus is **anal stenosis.** All types of anorectal anomalies occur with and without **fistulas** between the malformation and the bladder, urethra, vagina, or skin. On occasion a **pilonidal cyst** in a young adult must be distinguished from an anorectal fistula. This acquired lesion in the gluteal cleft superior to the anus consists of cysts or sinus tracts containing hair and is thought to be initiated by the penetration of hair beneath the skin. However, its location and the absence of a tract leading to the anus clearly mark it as an entity distinct from anorectal fistula.

Abnormal positions of the colon are principally the result of **malrotation** of the small intestine. The cecum may come to lie in the left lower quadrant or may be located in the middle of the abdomen, in which case it remains attached to its mesentery.

Infections

The principal bacterial and parasitic infections that affect the colon, including shigellosis, amebiasis, and tuberculosis, have been discussed either in Chapter 9 or above in the context of infectious diarrhea. Most of the remaining infectious diseases are transmitted sexually, principally affect male homosexuals, and primarily involve the anorectal region. These diseases, popularly referred to in medical parlance as the **gay bowel syndrome,** are transmitted by anal intercourse and oral-anal or oral-genital contact. Such diseases include gonorrhea, syphilis, lymphogranuloma venereum, anorectal herpes, and venereal warts (condylomata acuminata). There is also a high incidence of colonic infections, such as amebiasis and shigellosis, among male homosexuals.

Pseudomembranous Colitis

Pseudomembranous colitis is an inflammatory disease of the colon characterized by exudative plaques superimposed on a congested and edematous mucosa. Before the antibiotic era, pseudomembranous colitis was considered primarily a complication of intestinal surgery. After the introduction of antibiotics in the early 1950s, the administration of these drugs, principally tetracycline and chloramphenicol, was recognized to predispose to pseudomembranous colitis. At that time it was thought that the eradication of certain bacteria in the gut allowed the overgrowth of *Staphylococcus aureus*, and the term "staphylococcal enterocolitis" was used synonymously with "pseudomembranous enterocolitis." However, in studies dating to the early 1970s, it became clear that *S. aureus* contributes little or not at all to the pathogenesis of antibiotic-associated colitis. It is now recognized that *Clostridium difficile*, which has also been implicated in neonatal necrotizing enterocolitis, is the offending organism. *C. difficile* is not invasive, but it produces toxins that damage the colonic mucosa. Interestingly, although almost all antibiotics have been incriminated in colitis associated with *C. difficile*, particularly ampicillin, clindamycin, and the cephalosporins, the bacteria usually remain sensitive to these antibiotics.

Although most cases of pseudomembranous colitis are today associated with antibiotic therapy, gastrointestinal surgery remains a risk factor. Other predisposing conditions include various diseases of the colon (e.g., adenocarcinoma, obstruction, ischemic colitis, Crohn's disease, Hirschsprung's disease, shigellosis), shock, spinal fractures, burns, uremia, heavy metal poisoning, and therapy with antineoplastic agents.

The mechanism by which *C. difficile* becomes pathogenic is not entirely clear. Only 2% to 3% of healthy adults harbor the organism, whereas 10% to 20% of individuals who have recently been treated with antibiotics are infected. By contrast, the microbe can be isolated from the stools of 95% of patients with antibiotic-associated pseudomembranous colitis. About half of healthy neonates are colonized by *C. difficile*, but the isolation rate falls to adult levels by 1 year of age. The low prevalence of colonization by *C. difficile* in normal adults suggests that the pathogen is transferable. Indeed, outbreaks of pseudomembranous colitis associated with this organism in hospitalized patients have been traced to contaminated sigmoidoscopes, toilets, bed pans and floors, and treatment of hospitalized carriers with vancomycin has helped control the disease.

Antibiotic-associated infections with *C. difficile* are virtually always accompanied by diarrhea, but in most cases the disorder does not progress to colitis. In patients who develop pseudomembranous colitis, fever, leukocytosis, and abdominal cramps are superimposed on the diarrhea. In the preantibiotic era, this form of colitis was a catastrophic event, and many patients died within hours or days from ileus and irreversible shock. Today pseudomembranous colitis, although still a serious disease, is usually controlled with oral vancomycin therapy (also metronidazole and bacitracin) and supportive fluid and electrolyte therapy.

Macroscopically, the colon, particularly the rectosigmoid region, exhibits raised yellowish plaques of up to 2 cm in diameter that adhere to the underlying mucosa (Fig. 13-36). The intervening mucosa appears congested and edematous but is not ulcerated. In severe cases the plaques coalesce to form extensive pseudomembranes. Microscopic examination of the lesions discloses a loss of the superficial epithelium, thought to be the initial pathologic event. Subsequently, the crypts become disrupted and are expanded by mucin and neutrophils, an appearance similar to that of the crypt abscesses of ulcerative colitis. The pseudomembrane consists of the debris of necrotic epithelial cells, mucus, fibrin, and neutrophils.

The lesions are occasionally restricted to the small intestine, in which case the term **pseudomembranous enteritis** is applied. When both the small and the large bowel are involved, the condition is referred to as **pseudomembranous enterocolitis.** Pseudomembranes are occasionally encountered in other enteric infections, such as those involving *S. aureus* and Candida.

Diverticular Disease

Diverticulosis is an acquired herniation (diverticulum) of the mucosa and submucosa through the muscular layers of the colon. The presence of nec-

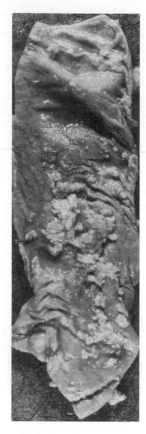

Figure 13-36.   Pseudomembranous colitis. The mucosal surface of the colon is covered by raised, irregular plaques composed of necrotic debris and an acute inflammatory exudate.

rotizing inflammation in diverticula is called **diverticulitis,** and its complications are included under the rubric of **diverticular disease.**

Diverticulosis shows a striking geographic variation, being common in Western societies and infrequent in Asia, Africa, and underdeveloped countries. Within the same geographic area, high socioeconomic groups exhibit a considerably higher prevalence than do their poorer neighbors, and migrants from a low-incidence area to a high-incidence one acquire the increased predilection for the disorder. Diverticulosis is unusual in persons under 40 years of age and increases in frequency with age. Although the true prevalence of diverticulosis is difficult to ascertain, it appears that some 10% of people in Western countries are afflicted. Interestingly, this disorder was distinctly uncommon in the last century but now has been demonstrated in one-third to one-half of persons over the age of 60 years.

The striking variation in the prevalence of diverticulosis implies that environmental factors are primarily responsible for the disease. Western pop-ulations consume a diet in which refined carbohydrates and meat have replaced crude cereal grains, and it is widely assumed that the lack of indigestible fibers in some way predisposes to the formation of diverticula in susceptible persons. In this respect the larger fecal mass in those who ingest a high-fiber diet diminishes spontaneous motility and intraluminal pressure in the colon. This concept has been supported by the observation that in a carefully matched British population, vegetarians had a three-fold lesser prevalence of diverticulosis than their meat-eating counterparts.

Humans are the only species to develop diverticulosis coli. Although the colons of some other mammals, such as rabbits, horses, and subhuman primates, also have discontinuous bundles of longitudinal muscle—that is, the taeniae coli—these animals are all herbivorous and clearly ingest large amounts of indigestible fiber. According to the fiber hypothesis, a lack of dietary residue in the Western diet leads to sustained bowel contractions and a consequent **increase in intraluminal pressure.** Such prolonged elevated pressure is thought to lead to a herniation of the superficial coats of the colon through the muscular layers into the serosa.

It is probable that, in addition to pressure, **defects in the wall of the colon** are required for the formation of a diverticulum. The circular muscle of the colon is interrupted by connective tissue clefts at the sites of penetration by the nutrient vessels that supply the submucosa and mucosa. In persons of advancing age this connective tissue loses its resilience and, therefore, its resistance to the effects of elevated intraluminal pressure. This concept is supported by the observation that persons with heritable disorders of collagen (e.g., the Marfan syndrome or Ehlers-Danlos syndrome) acquire precocious diverticulosis.

The abnormal structures that characterize diverticulosis are not true diverticula that contain all layers of the intestinal wall, but rather **pseudodiverticula,** in which only the mucosa and submucosa are herniated through the muscle layers. **The sigmoid colon is affected in 95% of the cases,** but diverticulosis can affect any segment of the colon, including the cecum. When more proximal segments of the colon are involved, it is almost always in association with diverticula of the sigmoid.

Diverticula vary in number from a few to several hundred (Fig. 13-37*A*). Most appear in parallel rows between the mesenteric and lateral taeniae. The diverticula, which measure up to 1 cm in greatest dimension, are connected to the intestinal lumen by necks of varying length and caliber. Hardened fecal material (fecaliths) is frequently present in the diver-

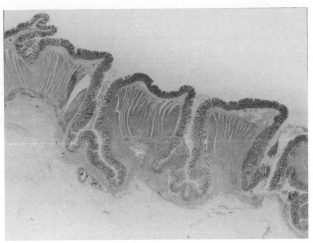

B

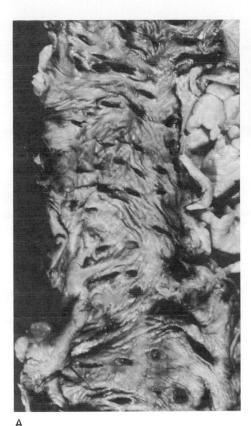

A

Figure 13-37. Diverticulosis of the colon. (*A*) Numerous diverticula open on the mucosal surface of the colon. (*B*) A low-power photomicrograph of (*A*) shows that the mucosa of the diverticula, which extends through the muscle layers, is in continuity with the surface mucosa.

ticula but does not signify diverticulitis. The muscular wall of the affected colon is consistently thickened, but whether this thickening precedes the diverticulosis or results from it is unknown.

Microscopically, a diverticulum characteristically presents as a flasklike structure that extends from the lumen through the muscle layers (Fig. 13-37*B*). The wall of the diverticulum is in continuity with the surface mucosa and therefore displays an epithelium and a submucosa. The base of the diverticulum is formed by serosal connective tissue.

Diverticulosis is generally asymptomatic, and 80% of affected persons remain symptom free. However, a significant number of those with diverticulosis complain of episodic colicky abdominal pain. Both constipation and diarrhea, sometimes alternating, may occur, and flatulence is common. **Sudden, painless, and severe bleeding** from colonic diverticula is a cause of serious lower gastrointestinal hemorrhage in the elderly, occurring in as many as 5% of persons with diverticulosis. Chronic blood loss may lead to anemia.

Although the large majority of persons with diverticulosis remain asymptomatic, in 10% to 20% diverticulitis supervenes at some time in their lives. Low-grade chronic inflammation begins at the base

of the diverticulum, presumably in response to the irritation produced by retained fecal material. This process produces necrosis of the wall of the diverticulum, an event that results in perforation and the release of fecal contents containing bacteria into the peridiverticular tissues. The resulting abscess is usually contained by the appendices epiploicae, the pericolonic fat, the mesentery, or adjacent organs, but infrequently free perforation leads to **generalized peritonitis.** Fibrosis in response to repeated episodes of diverticulitis may constrict the lumen of the bowel, thereby causing **intestinal obstruction. Fistulae** may form between the colon and adjacent organs, including the bladder, vagina, small intestine, and skin of the abdomen.

The most common symptoms of diverticulitis are persistent lower abdominal pain and fever. Changes in bowel habits, ranging from diarrhea to constipation, are frequent, and dysuria indicates irritation of the bladder. Most patients exhibit tenderness in the left lower quadrant, and a mass in that area is not infrequently palpated. Leukocytosis is the rule.

Antibiotic treatment and supportive measures are usually successful in alleviating acute diverticulitis, but about 20% of patients eventually require surgical intervention.

Inflammatory Bowel Disease

"Nonspecific inflammatory bowel disease" is a term that describes two diseases, Crohn's disease (regional enteritis) and ulcerative colitis. Although these two disorders usually differ sufficiently to be clearly distinguishable, they have many common features, and it is still debated whether they are two distinct entities or merely ends of a single spectrum. Until more definitive information becomes available, it is convenient to consider both diseases within a single conceptual framework because of the following common features: inflammation of the bowel, lack of a proved causal agent, pattern of familial occurrence, and systemic manifestations. **Similarities apart, Crohn's disease and ulcerative colitis have different clinical courses and natural histories.**

Crohn's Disease

Crohn's disease has acquired a multitude of names, owing to the confusion that has resulted from its varied anatomic and clinical features. It has variously been referred to as "terminal ileitis" and "regional ileitis" when it involves mainly the ileum, and "granulomatous colitis" and "transmural colitis" when it principally affects the colon. Today the eponym "Crohn's disease" is most commonly used because the disorder may involve any part of the gastrointestinal tract and even tissues in other organs.

Epidemiology

Crohn's disease occurs throughout the world, with an annual incidence of 0.5 to 5 per 100,000. Reports from various countries indicate that the incidence has risen dramatically over the past 25 years. The disease usually appears in adolescents or young adults and is most common among people of European origin, with an apparently higher frequency among Jews. There is a slight female predominance (up to 1.6:1). A family history of inflammatory bowel disease (Crohn's disease or ulcerative colitis) has been found in up to 40% of cases. The greatest frequency is among siblings, suggesting that environmental factors play a role, although Crohn's disease has only rarely been described in both a husband and a wife.

Etiology and Pathogenesis

Intensive research since the disease was first described in 1932 has failed to elucidate the etiology and pathogenesis of Crohn's disease. Several infec-tious agents have been suggested as possible causative agents. Bacteria that have been cultured from tissue involved with Crohn's disease include a variant of Pseudomonas and atypical mycobacteria. The possibility of a viral cause has also been raised. None of these studies has given consistently reproducible results, and the excitement that has accompanied each new discovery of a possible causal pathogen has waned with failure to confirm the initial results.

If an infectious agent is not responsible for the disease, perhaps altered host susceptibility plays a role. Several studies have shown impairment of **cell-mediated** immunity in patients with Crohn's disease. Some investigators have suggested increased suppressor T-cell activity, and others have claimed impaired phagocytic function. None of these findings has been confirmed. Inconsistent results have also been reported from studies of histocompatibility antigens in this disease.

The possibility that Crohn's disease might be caused by immune-mediated damage to the intestine has been suggested by the chronic and recurrent nature of the inflammation and by the occurrence of systemic manifestations that are frequently associated with "autoimmune" diseases. However, no consistent evidence has been produced in favor of abnormal humoral immune responses or of circulating immune complexes as a cause of the disease. In recent years most immunologic studies have been concerned with the possible role of cell-mediated cytotoxicity. Some studies support the hypothesis that cytotoxic T cells sensitized to bacterial or other antigens damage the intestinal wall.

The possibility that dietary factors or emotional stress may play a role in the pathogenesis of Crohn's disease has led to a number of studies that have again produced inconsistent results.

The understanding of the fundamental nature of Crohn's disease is not much better today than it was more than a half century ago, when the disease was first described.

The clinical manifestations and the natural history of Crohn's disease are extremely variable and are related to the anatomic localization of the disease. The most frequent symptoms are abdominal pain and diarrhea, seen in over 75% of patients, and recurrent fever, seen in 50%. The onset of the disease is usually insidious, although symptoms may occur acutely. When the disease involves mainly the ileum and cecum, the sudden onset may mimic appendicitis, and the diagnosis of Crohn's disease is occasionally made for the first time at the time of abdominal surgery. If the disease involves the ileum predominantly, the major clinical features are right lower quadrant pain, intermittent diarrhea and fever, and frequently a tender mass in the right lower quadrant of the abdomen. Crohn's disease of the colon leads to diarrhea and sometimes colonic bleeding. In cases of diffuse small intestinal involvement, malabsorption and malnutrition may be the major features. Lipid malabsorption may also result from interruption of the enterohepatic cycle of bile salts because of ileal disease. In 10% to 15% of cases the major site of involvement is the anorectal region, and recurrent anorectal fistulas are the presenting sign. When Crohn's disease begins in childhood, its major manifestation may be retardation of growth and physical development. The most frequent extraintestinal inflammatory features are in the eye (episcleritis or uveitis), the medium-sized joints (arthritis), and the skin (erythema nodosum).

The most common intestinal complications of Crohn's disease are **intestinal obstruction and fistulas.** Occasionally, free perforation of the bowel occurs. **The risk of intestinal cancer is at least threefold higher than normal in patients with Crohn's disease.** Systemic complications (in addition to the eye, joint, and skin lesions mentioned above) include liver disease (pericholangitis, sclerosing cholangitis), cholelithiasis, oxalate stones in the kidneys, and amyloidosis.

No curative treatment is available for Crohn's disease. Several medications are effective in suppressing the inflammatory reaction, including corticosteroids, sulfasalazine, metronidazole, and 6-mercaptopurine. Surgical resection of obstructed areas or of severely involved portions of intestine and drainage of abscesses caused by fistulas are required in some cases.

Pathology

Two major features characterize the pathology of Crohn's disease and serve to differentiate it from other inflammations of the gastrointestinal tract. First, the inflammation usually involves **all** layers of the bowel wall and is therefore referred to as **transmural** inflammatory disease. Second, the inflammation of the intestine is **discontinuous**—that is, segments of inflamed tissue are separated by apparently normal intestine. The inflamed areas are frequently (and paradoxically) referred to as "skip" areas by surgeons and endoscopists.

It is convenient to classify Crohn's disease into four broad macroscopic patterns, although many patients do not fit precisely into any one of them: the disease involves mainly the ileum and cecum in 50% of cases, only the small intestine in 15%, only the colon in 20%, and principally the anorectal region in

15%. Crohn's disease is occasionally observed in the duodenum and stomach, and more rarely in the esophagus and oral cavity, almost always in association with small intestinal Crohn's disease. In women with anorectal Crohn's disease, the inflammation may spread to involve the external genitalia.

Macroscopically, the bowel affected by Crohn's disease appears thickened and edematous, as does the adjacent mesentery (Fig. 13-38). Mesenteric lymph nodes are frequently enlarged, firm, and matted together. The lumen is narrowed by edema in early cases and by a combination of edema and fibrosis in long-standing disease. Nodular swelling, fibrosis, and ulceration of the mucosa lead to a "cobblestone" appearance. Ulcers vary in depth. In early cases the ulcers have an "apthous" or "serpiginous" appearance; later they become deeper and appear as linear clefts or fissures.

The cut surface of the bowel wall shows the transmural nature of the disease, with thickening, edema, and fibrosis of all layers. Within the submucosal and muscular layers, ulcers coalesce to form large intramural channels. Involved loops of bowel often become adherent, and fistulas between such segments are frequent. These fistulas, presumably a late result of the deep mural ulcers, may also penetrate from the bowel into other organs, including the bladder, uterus, vagina, and skin. Most fistulas end blindly, forming abscess cavities within the peritoneal cavity, in the mesentery, or in retroperitoneal structures. Lesions in the distal rectum may create perianal fistulas, a well-known presenting feature of Crohn's disease.

Microscopically, the disease appears as a **chronic inflammatory process that extends through all layers of the bowel wall** (Fig. 13-39). During early phases of the disease small, superficial mucosal ulcerations are seen, together with mucosal and submucosal edema and an increase in the number of lymphocytes, plasma cells, and histiocytes. Endothelial swelling in small blood vessels and lymphatics is usually prominent. Later, long, deep, fissure-like ulcers are seen, and vascular hyalinization and fibrosis become apparent.

The microscopic hallmark of Crohn's disease is the appearance of discrete, noncaseating granulomas, mostly in the submucosa. Indistinguishable from those of sarcoidosis, these granulomas consist of focal aggregates of epithelioid cells, vaguely limited by a rim of lymphocytes. Multinucleated giant cells may be present, and the center of the granulomas usually displays hyaline material but no caseation. Birefringent **Schaumann bodies** are occasionally seen.

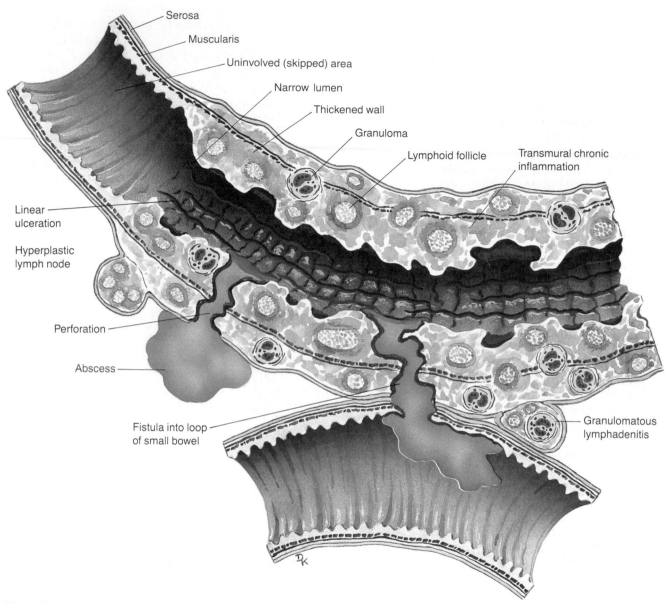

Figure 13-38. Crohn's disease. A schematic representation of the major features of Crohn's disease in the small intestine.

Although the presence of discrete granulomas is strong evidence in favor of the diagnosis of Crohn's disease, **the absence of granulomas by no means excludes the diagnosis.** Indeed, only half the cases show the typical granulomas, while the others show either a diffuse granulomatous reaction or nonspecific transmural inflammation. Thus, the diagnosis of Crohn's disease is made principally on the basis of the **transmural** nature of the inflammation rather than on the basis of the presence of granulomas.

In the differential diagnosis of Crohn's disease one must consider the possibility of ulcerative colitis; bacterial infections, especially Campylobacter, Yersinia enterocolitica, and tuberculosis; amebic colitis; schis-

tosomiasis; and, less commonly, inflammation due to Chlamydia. Other conditions that may mimic Crohn's disease (especially Crohn's colitis) are pseudomembranous colitis, radiation injury, and lymphoma.

Ulcerative Colitis

Ulcerative colitis is common in the Western world, occurring principally, but not exclusively, in young adults. The terms "nonspecific" and "idiopathic" have also been applied to this condition. The disease is characterized by chronic diarrhea and rectal bleeding, with a pattern of exacerbations and remissions, and with the possibility of serious local and systemic complications.

Epidemiology

In Europe and North America, ulcerative colitis has an annual incidence of 4 to 7 per 100,000 population and a prevalence of 40% to 80%. There appears to be no sex predominance. The disease usually begins in early adult life, with a peak incidence in the third decade of life. However, it also occurs in childhood and in old age. In the United States, whites are affected more commonly than blacks. It has been reported that the disease is especially common among Jews in the United States, although a study in Israel has shown a lower incidence and prevalence of the disease in Tel Aviv than in Baltimore, Copenhagen, or Oxford.

Etiology and Pathogenesis

The cause of ulcerative colitis is not known. Attempts to implicate a viral or bacterial agent have given only inconsistent results. It has been suggested that there may be an association between exacerbations of ulcerative colitis and infection with *Clostridium difficile*, the organism implicated in the pathogenesis of antibiotic-associated diarrhea and pseudomembranous enterocolitis. However, subsequent studies have failed to confirm the involvement of this organism.

The higher than normal incidence of ulcerative colitis in first-degree relatives of patients with the disease (up to 40% familial incidence) points to a possible genetic predisposition. Indeed, in some families as many as six patients with this disease have been described, and concordance has been reported in monozygotic twins. However, available family studies do not suggest any distinct mode of genetic transmission, and studies of HLA distribution in patients with ulcerative colitis have not demonstrated a consistent pattern.

A possible role for so-called "psychosomatic" factors in the pathogenesis of ulcerative colitis was entertained for many years, but several well-planned studies during the past 20 years have failed to incriminate specific psychologic traits, other than those to be expected in any long-term chronic disease.

The possibility that an abnormal immune response may play a role in the pathogenesis of ulcerative colitis has been extensively studied. The presence of abundant lymphoid tissue throughout the colon has made such a possibility attractive, as has the documented association of this disorder with immunore-

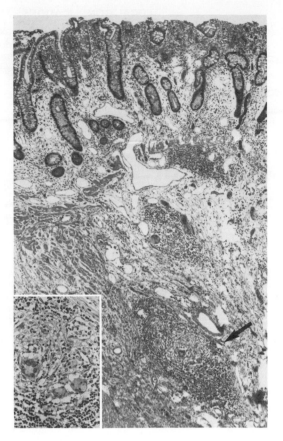

Figure 13-39. Crohn's disease. A photomicrograph of the small intestine shows transmural inflammation and a giant cell granuloma deep within the wall (*arrow*). (*Inset*) High-power view of the granuloma.

lated features, such as uveitis, erythema nodosum, and vasculitis. Several studies have demonstrated an increased frequency of circulating antibodies against antigens in colonic epithelial cells and against cross-reacting antigens in enterobacteria (particularly the "Kunin antigen"). Furthermore, *in vitro* studies of cell-mediated immune function have shown that mononuclear cells from the colonic mucosa and from the blood of ulcerative colitis patients are toxic for autologous colonic epithelial cells. However, these abnormalities are not found exclusively in patients with ulcerative colitis, nor are any of these changes a prerequisite for the development of ulcerative colitis. It is therefore possible that all of these features are merely epiphenomena—that is, the result, rather than the cause, of the mucosal damage.

Clinical Features

The clinical course and manifestations of ulcerative colitis are highly variable. Most patients (70%) have intermittent attacks, with partial or complete remis-

LOCAL COMPLICATIONS

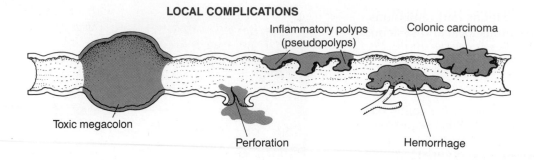

Inflammatory polyps
(pseudopolyps)

Colonic carcinoma

Toxic megacolon

Perforation

Hemorrhage

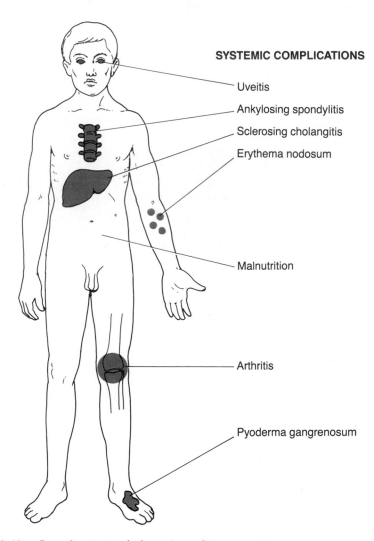

SYSTEMIC COMPLICATIONS

Uveitis

Ankylosing spondylitis

Sclerosing cholangitis

Erythema nodosum

Malnutrition

Arthritis

Pyoderma gangrenosum

Figure 13-40.   Complications of ulcerative colitis.

sion between attacks. A small number (less than 10%) have a very long remission (several years) following their first attack. The remaining 20% have continuous symptoms without remission.

It is convenient to classify the disease into three arbitrary clinical categories: mild, moderate, and severe (fulminant).

Approximately 50% of patients with ulcerative colitis suffer from "mild" disease. Their major symptom is rectal bleeding, sometimes accompanied by tenesmus (rectal pressure and discomfort). The disease in these patients is usually limited to the rectum but may extend to the distal sigmoid colon. Extraintestinal complications are uncommon, and in most patients in this category, the disease remains mild throughout their lives.

About 40% of patients are categorized as having "moderate" ulcerative colitis. They usually suffer from recurrent episodes, lasting days or weeks, of loose bloody stools, crampy abdominal pain, and frequently low-grade fever. Moderate anemia is a common result of chronic fecal blood loss.

Ten percent of patients have "severe" or "fulminant" ulcerative colitis, usually, but not always, apparent from its onset. These patients have more than 6, and sometimes more than 20, bloody bowel movements daily, frequently accompanied by fever and other systemic manifestations. The loss of blood and fluids rapidly leads to anemia, dehydration, and electrolyte depletion. Massive hemorrhage is occasionally life-threatening. A particularly dangerous complication is **"toxic megacolon"**, in which extreme dilatation of the colon occurs. Patients with this condition are at high risk for perforation of the colon. Fulminant ulcerative colitis is a medical emergency requiring immediate, intensive medical therapy and, in some cases, prompt colectomy. About 15% of patients with fulminant ulcerative colitis die of the disease.

Extraintestinal Manifestations

Various complications of ulcerative colitis are shown in Figure 13-40.

Arthritis is seen in 25% of patients with ulcerative colitis. **Eye inflammation** (mostly uveitis) develops in about 10%, and **skin lesions** occur in about the same number. The most common cutaneous lesions are erythema nodosum and pyoderma gangrenosum, the latter being a serious, noninfective disorder characterized by deep, purulent, necrotic ulcers in the skin.

Liver disease occurs in up to 3% of patients, the most common pathologic findings being pericholangitis and fatty liver. Chronic active hepatitis is occa-

sionally encountered in conjunction with ulcerative colitis, and **sclerosing cholangitis** and **carcinoma of the bile ducts** are both associated with the intestinal disease. **Thromboembolic phenomena,** mostly deep vein thromboses of the lower extremities, occur in about 6% of ulcerative colitis patients.

Pathology

Three major pathologic features characterize ulcerative colitis and help differentiate it from other inflammatory conditions.

First, ulcerative colitis is a **diffuse** disease, usually extending from the most distal part of the rectum for a variable distance proximally. When the disease involves the rectum alone, it is referred to as **"ulcerative proctitis."** When the inflammatory process extends as far as the splenic flexure, the term **"left-sided colitis"** is applied. **"Universal colitis"** or **"pancolitis"** describes disease involving the entire colon, from the anorectal junction to the ileocecal valve. Sparing of the rectum or involvement of the right side of the colon alone is rare and suggests the possibility of another disorder, such as Crohn's disease.

Second, the inflammatory process of ulcerative colitis is **limited to the colon** and does not involve the small intestine, stomach, or esophagus. When the cecum is affected, the disease ends at the ileocecal valve, although minor inflammation of the adjacent ileum is sometimes seen ("backwash ileitis").

Third, histologically, ulcerative colitis is **essentially a disease of the mucosa.** Involvement of deeper layers is uncommon, occurring only in fulminant cases, usually in association with toxic megacolon.

The macroscopic appearance of the mucosa throughout the colon has been extensively documented through the increasingly widespread use of fiberoptic colonoscopy. Early in the course of the disease the mucosal surface appears raw, red, and granular. It is frequently covered with a yellowish exudate and bleeds easily when touched by an instrument or a cotton swab. Later, small, superficial ulcers appear. These ulcers coalesce to form irregular, shallow, ulcerated areas that appear to surround islands of intact mucosa (Fig. 13-41). Subsequently, raised areas of mucosa, corresponding to inflammatory polyps or "pseudopolyps," can be seen. In cases of toxic megacolon the lumen is widely dilated, and the wall is thin and friable. Single or multiple perforations are common in toxic megacolon, and the serosal surface is often covered by a fibrinopurulent exudate.

The microscopic features of ulcerative colitis correlate well with the colonoscopic appearance. Although they are not specifically diagnostic, they rep-

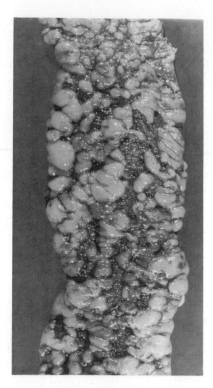

Figure 13-41. Ulcerative colitis. The mucosal surface of the colon exhibits irregular ulcerated areas that surround islands of colonic mucosa.

resent a highly characteristic pattern of injury. The early microscopic signs are mucosal congestion, edema, microscopic hemorrhages, a diffuse inflammatory infiltrate in the lamina propria, variable loss of the surface epithelium, and damage to the intestinal crypts, which are often surrounded and infiltrated by neutrophils (Fig. 13-42). Suppurative necrosis of the crypt epithelium gives rise to the characteristic **"crypt abscess"**, which appears as a dilated, degenerated crypt filled with neutrophils.

Later in the course of the disease, lateral extension and coalescence of crypt abscesses undermine the mucosa, leaving areas of ulceration adjacent to hanging fragments of mucosa. Such mucosal excrescences surrounded by ulceration are seen by endoscopy or roentgenographic examination as **inflammatory polyps.** Tissue destruction is accompanied by manifestations of tissue repair. Highly vascular granulation tissue develops in denuded areas (Fig. 13-43). Collagen deposition is sparse and patchy, and fibrosis is not a prominent feature. Importantly, the strictures characteristic of Crohn's disease are absent. Microscopically, the intestinal crypts may appear tortuous, branched, and shortened in the late stages, or the mucosa may be diffusely atrophic.

In long-standing cases the large bowel is almost invariably shortened, especially in the left side. The haustral markings are indistinct and are replaced by a granular mucosal pattern. Microscopically, advanced ulcerative colitis is characterized by mucosal atrophy and a chronic inflammatory infiltrate in the mucosa and submucosa (see Fig. 13-42).

Ulcerative Colitis and Colon Cancer

It is generally agreed that **people with long-standing, extensive ulcerative colitis have a higher risk of colon cancer than the general population.** The risk is related to the extent of colonic involvement and the duration of the disease. Because of differences in patient selection and analysis of the data in various studies, the true cumulative risk for the development of colon cancer is not known. Some estimates of this risk have been very high; 60% was reported in the United States and 34% was reported in Sweden among persons who have had ulcerative colitis for 25 to 30 years. By contrast, a retrospective study in Denmark reports a risk of less than 1.4% after 18 years, and investigators in Czechoslovakia and Israel describe even lower risks. The true value in the Western world is probably intermediate; a recent well-controlled study in the United States places the cumulative risk of colon cancer after 25 years of ulcerative colitis at about 12%. Young age at the onset of colitis does not seem to be an independent risk factor, but since patients in whom ulcerative colitis develops at a young age have a longer duration of disease, they also have a relatively high cumulative incidence of cancer.

The greatest frequency of colon cancer is in patients with involvement of the entire colon; in patients with disease limited to the rectum, colon cancer is no more common than in the general population. In 15% of cases the cancer is multicentric.

Epithelial Dysplasia

Epithelial dysplasia is a common finding in the colon and rectum of patients with long-standing ulcerative colitis (Fig. 13-44). The cytologic criteria, which are comparable to those for dysplasia in tubular or villous adenomas, include variation in the size, shape, and staining qualities of the nuclei; stratification of nuclei; an increase in the number of mitoses; and abnormal goblet cells. It is thought that severe epithelial dysplasia reflects a high probability of cancer elsewhere in the colon or an increased risk of development of such a cancer. In resected colons from patients with ulcerative colitis that contained colon cancer, distant dysplasia was present in almost three-quarters of the specimens, and half showed severe dysplasia distant from the tumor. Conversely, in patients who underwent colectomy because of severe dysplasia, cancer

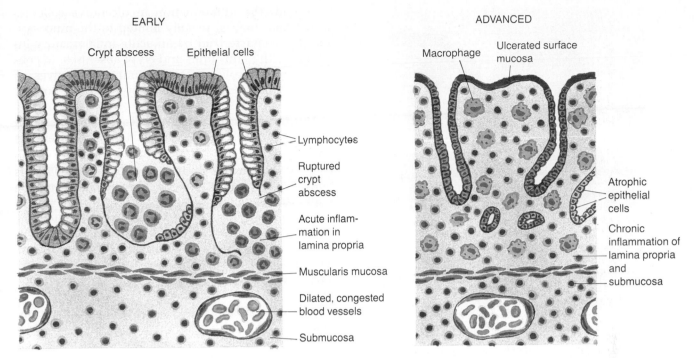

EARLY

ADVANCED

Crypt abscess   Epithelial cells

Macrophage   Ulcerated surface mucosa

Lymphocytes

Ruptured crypt abscess

Acute inflammation in lamina propria

Muscularis mucosa

Dilated, congested blood vessels

Submucosa

Atrophic epithelial cells

Chronic inflammation of lamina propria and submucosa

Figure 13-42. Ulcerative colitis. Schematic representation of the major microscopic features of early and advanced ulcerative colitis.

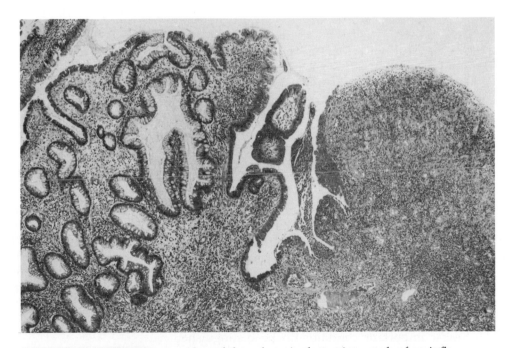

Figure 13-43. Inflammatory polyp of the colon. A photomicrograph of an inflammatory polyp in a case of ulcerative colitis shows an excrescence of granulation tissue (*right*) and polypoid glandular mucosa (*left*).

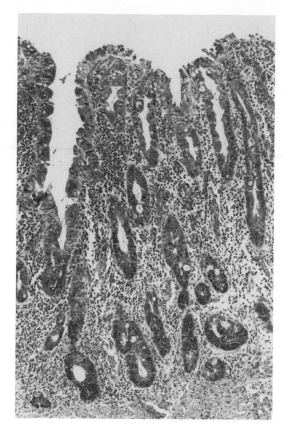

Figure 13-44. Epithelial dysplasia in ulcerative colitis. The colonic mucosa exhibits severe chronic inflammation and irregular and atypical epithelial cells.

was discovered in almost half of the resected colons. Because of the strong association between severe epithelial dysplasia and colon cancer, routine surveillance by colonoscopic biopsy of all patients with ulcerative colitis has been recommended by some, although the cost/benefit ratio of this procedure is controversial. Once severe dysplasia has been detected, a careful search for cancer elsewhere in the colon is certainly warranted. Whether colectomy should be advised without the demonstration of frankly malignant tissue is still debated.

Differential Diagnosis

The most important condition to be distinguished from ulcerative colitis is Crohn's disease of the colon (Crohn's colitis, granulomatous colitis). The distinction between the two conditions is based on the difference in anatomic localization and histologic appearance.

First, ulcerative colitis is a diffuse process, usually more severe distally. By contrast, Crohn's colitis is a patchy disease, with frequent sparing of the rectum.

Second, the inflammation in ulcerative colitis is superficial—that is, usually limited to the mucosa—and it is characterized by an acute inflammatory infiltrate, with neutrophils and crypt abscesses. In contrast, Crohn's colitis is transmural and involves all layers, with granulomas in many, though not all, specimens.

Third, demarcation of the disease at the ileocecal valve, or in the colon distal to it, favors ulcerative colitis. Involvement of the terminal ileum, a cobblestone-like gross appearance, discrete ulcers, and fistulas favor Crohn's colitis.

In approximately 10% of cases a precise diagnosis of ulcerative colitis versus Crohn's colitis cannot be made. Other conditions that should be considered in the differential diagnosis of ulcerative colitis are bacterial infections (e.g., Shigella, Salmonella, Campylobacter) and amebic colitis, especially in endemic areas.

When the inflammation is limited to the rectum, other infectious agents, including viruses, Chlamydia, fungi, and other parasites should be considered. Proctitis due to these agents is common in male homosexuals, and a variety of opportunistic infections of the bowel are encountered in patients with the acquired immunodeficiency syndrome (AIDS).

Other conditions that may mimic ulcerative colitis are ischemic colitis, antibiotic-associated colitis, radiation injury, and the "solitary rectal ulcer syndrome."

Treatment

In the absence of a proved cause or a well-understood pathogenesis, no specific therapy is available for ulcerative colitis. Treatment is aimed at improving the general condition of the patient, suppressing the inflammatory response with corticosteroids and other anti-inflammatory agents, and maintaining the state of remission for as long as possible. Selected patients benefit from a total colectomy, and new surgical techniques that make possible the sparing of the anal sphincter may lead to more widespread use of surgical treatment.

Vascular Diseases

Ischemic Colitis

As already discussed, the colon is subject to the same types of ischemic injury as the small intestine. Extensive infarction of the colon, unlike the small bowel, is uncommon; chronic segmental disease is the rule. The most vulnerable areas are those between adjacent arterial distributions, so-called watershed areas. For example, the splenic flexure lies between the regions supplied by the superior and inferior mesenteric arteries, and the rectosigmoid area shares the blood from the inferior mesenteric and internal iliac arteries.

Because the cause of most cases of ischemic colitis is atherosclerosis, the intestinal disease usually occurs in persons over the age of 50 years. Colonic ischemia also occurs in about 2% of patients undergoing aortoiliac reconstruction and has been reported in association with hypercoagulable states, vasculitis, and colorectal cancer.

Some patients present with the symptoms and complications of bowel infarction and require immediate surgical intervention. However, in the majority of patients the acute signs stabilize, and radiographic examination shows only the pattern associated with intramural hemorrhage and edema. Such patients may recover completely or may develop a colonic stricture, in which case surgical removal of the affected segment becomes necessary. Segments of ischemic stricture show variable mucosal ulceration and inflammation, as well as widening of the submucosa by granulation tissue and fibrosis. Hemosiderin-laden macrophages are a common feature, and patchy fibrosis of the muscular coats may also be present. Submucosal arterioles are characteristically thick walled and tortuous.

Ischemic disease of the rectosigmoid area is typically manifested by abdominal pain, rectal bleeding, and a change in bowel habits. Upon sigmoidoscopy multiple ulcers, hemorrhagic nodular lesions, or a pseudomembrane is seen. The rectal biopsy exhibits the characteristic changes of ischemic necrosis of the bowel: mucosal ulcerations, crypt abscesses, and submucosal inflammation and fibrosis. Recovery is often associated with narrowing of the rectosigmoid lumen.

On clinical grounds alone, ischemic colitis often cannot be distinguished from nonspecific ulcerative colitis, Crohn's disease of the colon, or certain forms of infectious colitis.

Angiodysplasia (Vascular Ectasia)

Angiodysplasia, a recently recognized cause of lower intestinal bleeding, is characterized by localized arteriovenous malformations, predominantly in the cecum and ascending colon. The mean age at presentation is 60 years. Younger persons preferentially exhibit lesions at other sites, including the rectum, stomach, and small bowel. Interestingly, angiodysplasia is associated with aortic valve disease in one-quarter of the cases. It has been suggested that the

disorder may be secondary to chronic circulatory insufficiency of the intestine, intestinal muscle hypertrophy, and resulting venous obstruction. Patients typically complain of multiple bleeding episodes, although the lesions may also cause chronic occult bleeding. Radiologic studies and examination at laparotomy are usually negative. Thus, the diagnosis is difficult and often requires selective mesenteric arteriography or colonoscopy. Surgical removal of the affected segment is curative.

The resected specimen displays small, often multiple hemangiomatous lesions, usually less than 0.5 cm in diameter. Microscopically, the veins and capillaries of the submucosa are tortuous, thin-walled, and dilated. The attenuated walls of these vessels are presumably responsible for their propensity to bleed. Upon resection of the colon, the ectatic vessels tend to collapse; their demonstration is facilitated by vascular injection with silicone rubber or radiographic contrast materials.

Hemorrhoids

Hemorrhoids are dilated venous channels of the hemorrhoidal plexuses that result from the downward displacement of the anal cushions. These cushions are composed of submucosal connective tissue and are thought to aid in anal continence. **Internal hemorrhoids** arise from the superior hemorrhoidal plexus above the pectinate line, whereas **external hemorrhoids** originate from the inferior hemorrhoidal plexus below that line. The fact that bleeding from hemorrhoids is bright red—that is, arterial—has suggested the possibility that these vessels are not truly varicose veins, but rather a form of arteriovenous shunts similar to those of the corpus cavernosum of the genitalia.

Hemorrhoids are common, to some degree afflicting at least half the population over the age of 50 years in Western countries. By contrast, they are infrequent in populations that consume high-fiber diets. Hemorrhoids are common in pregnancy, presumably because of the increased abdominal pressure. Contrary to historical assumptions, hemorrhoids are now reported not to be more frequent than usual in patients with portal hypertension, although such patients may have rectal varices.

Clinically, the salient feature of hemorrhoids is **bleeding,** and chronic blood loss may lead to **iron-deficiency anemia. Rectal prolapse** often develops in patients with hemorrhoids. Prolapsed hemorrhoids may become irreducible, a situation that leads to painful "strangulated" hemorrhoids. **Thrombosis** of external hemorrhoids is exquisitely painful and requires evacuation of the vascular clot.

Microscopic examination of hemorrhoidectomy specimens discloses dilated vascular spaces with excess smooth muscle in their walls. Hemorrhage and thrombosis of varying severity are common. Squamous metaplasia of the overlying transitional zone may be noted. The result of thrombosis and the organization of an internal hemorrhoid is a **fibrous polyp of the anal canal;** a similar process in an external hemorrhoid results in an **anal tag.**

Radiation Enterocolitis

Radiation therapy for malignant disease of the pelvis or abdomen is not uncommonly complicated by injury to the small intestine and colon. The lesions produced by radiotherapy range from a reversible injury of the intestinal mucosa to chronic inflammation, ulceration, and fibrosis of the intestine. Complications include perforation and the subsequent development of internal fistulas, hemorrhage, and stricture, occasionally severe enough to lead to intestinal obstruction. Clinically significant radiation colitis is most common in the rectum.

Acutely, radiation results in decreased mitoses and, in the small bowel, shortening of the villi. Mucosal inflammation is conspicuous, and in the colon crypt abscesses may be seen. Failure of epithelial renewal may lead to ulceration. Subacute changes, occurring 2 to 12 months after radiotherapy, are noted after the mucosa has healed. Damage to submucosal vessels leads to thrombosis, and the submucosa becomes fibrotic, often containing bizarre fibroblasts. As a result of radiation vasculitis, progressive ischemia further injures the bowel. A slightly increased risk of colon cancer has been reported in persons who have undergone radiotherapy.

Neoplasms

Benign Tumors

Polyps

A gastrointestinal polyp is defined as a mass that protrudes into the lumen of the gut. Polyps are subdivided according to their attachment to the bowel wall (e.g., sessile or pedunculated), their histologic

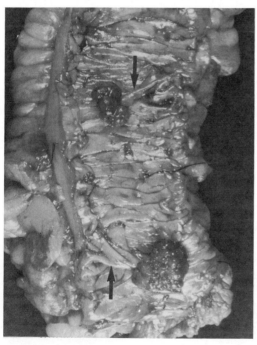
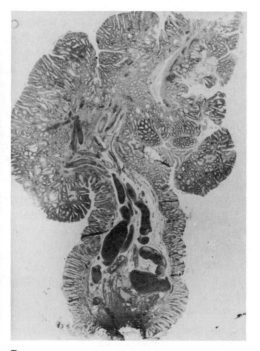

A   B

Figure 13-45.   Tubular adenoma of the colon. (*A*) Two pedunculated tubular adenomas are attached to the mucosa by fibrovascular stalks (*arrows*). (*B*) A low-power photomicrograph of a tubular adenoma of the colon shows closely packed epithelial tubules. The fibrous stalk is highly vascular and lined by normal colonic epithelium.

appearance (e.g., hyperplastic or adenomatous), and their neoplastic potential (i.e., benign or malignant). By themselves benign polyps are only infrequently symptomatic, and their clinical importance lies in their potential for malignant transformation.

Colonic polyps are classified broadly as neoplastic and nonneoplastic. The neoplastic polyps are adenomas and carcinomas; the nonneoplastic ones include hyperplastic, juvenile, inflammatory, hamartomatous, and others.

Adenomatous Polyps

Adenomatous polyps, which arise from the mucosal epithelium, are composed of undifferentiated crypt cells that have accumulated beyond the needs for replacement of the surface cells sloughed into the lumen. The precise prevalence of adenomatous polyps of the colon is difficult to ascertain worldwide, but it is certainly highest in Western countries. As in diverticular disease, the only consistent environmental difference between high-risk and low-risk populations that has been identified is the diet. Compared with high-risk regions, low-risk areas are characterized by staple diets rich in indigestible fiber and low in animal fat. In the United States it appears that at least one adenomatous polyp is present in half of the adult population, a figure that rises to more than two-thirds among persons over the age of 65 years. There is a modest male predominance, the sex ratio being 1.4:1. In about one-quarter of those who harbor at least one polyp, two or more polyps are present.

Almost half of all adenomatous polyps of the colon are located in the rectosigmoid region and can therefore be detected by digital examination or by sigmoidoscopy. The remaining half are evenly distributed throughout the rest of the colon. The macroscopic appearance of an adenoma varies from a small, pedunculated tubular adenoma to a large, sessile villous adenoma. Many adenomatous polyps share features of both, in which case they are referred to as "tubulovillous adenomas."

Tubular adenomas, which constitute two-thirds of benign large bowel adenomas, are typically smooth-surfaced spheres; they usually measure less than 2 cm in diameter and are attached to the mucosa by a stalk (Fig. 13-45*A*). About 4% are reported to be larger than 2 cm across. Some tubular adenomas are sessile, and a few pedunculated polyps show typical villous features. Microscopically, the tubular adenoma exhibits closely packed epithelial tubules, which may be uniform or may be irregular and excessively branched (Fig. 13-45*B*). The tubules are embedded in a fibrovascular stroma similar to the normal lamina propria. Often the tubules show focal cystic dilatation. The

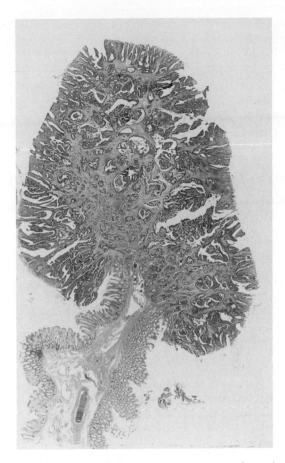

Figure 13-46. Adenocarcinoma arising in a pedunculated adenomatous polyp. A low-power photomicrograph shows irregular neoplastic glands invading the stroma. The stalk is uninvolved.

stalk of the pedunculated tubular adenoma is lined by normal colonic mucosa, and its interior is composed of fibrovascular tissue similar to that of the normal submucosa.

Although the majority of tubular adenomas display little epithelial atypia, one-fifth, particularly the larger tumors, show a range of dysplastic features that vary in severity from mild nuclear pleomorphism to frank invasive carcinoma (Fig. 13-46). Dysplastic changes include hyperchromatic and pleomorphic nuclei, which have lost their basal polarity and exhibit increased numbers of mitoses. In severe dysplasia the glands become crowded and highly irregular in size and shape and show papillary or cribriform (sievelike or perforated) growth patterns.

The neoplastic glands must remain superficial to the muscularis mucosae for the polyp to be considered benign. Penetration of this muscle layer, which is considered evidence of malignant transformation, brings the tumor cells into the region of the lymphatic

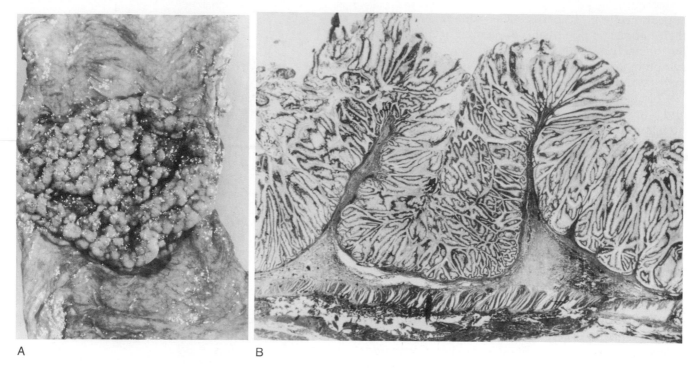

A   B

Figure 13-47.   Villous adenoma of the colon. (*A*) The colon contains a large, broad-based, elevated lesion that has a cauliflower-like surface. (*B*) A low-power photomicrograph of (*A*) shows finger-like processes that resemble the villi of the small intestine. The villi are supported by cores of fibrovascular connective tissue.

plexus of the submucosa and thus provides an avenue for metastasis.

Intramucosal lesions that are severely dysplastic are classed by some pathologists as **carcinoma in situ.** They are found in about 10% of resected tubular adenomas. The natural history of such lesions is poorly defined, and it is not clear whether they become invasive, and if so, with what frequency and over what time period. **However, as long as the dysplastic focus remains superficial to the muscularis mucosae, the lesion is invariably cured by resection of the polyp.** The risk of invasive carcinoma correlates with the size of the tubular adenoma. Only 1% of tubular adenomas less than 1 cm across contain invasive carcinoma at the time of resection; among those between 1 cm and 2 cm, 10% are found to be malignant, and among those greater than 2 cm, 35% are malignant. Given that only few tubular adenomas are more than 2 cm in diameter, the overall risk of invasive carcinoma in these growths is still small.

Villous adenomas, which constitute about one-tenth of adenomatous polyps and are found predominantly in the rectosigmoid region, are typically large, broad-based, elevated lesions that grossly display a shaggy, cauliflower-like surface (Fig. 13-47*A*). More

than half are greater than 2 cm in diameter and on occasion reach a size of 10 cm to 15 cm across. Microscopically, villous adenomas are composed of thin, tall, finger-like processes that superficially resemble the villi of the small intestine; they are lined externally by epithelial cells and supported by a core of fibrovascular connective tissue corresponding to the normal lamina propria (Fig. 13-47*B*). About one-quarter of adenomatous polyps manifest both tubular and villous features; they are classed as **tubulovillous adenomas.** Tubulovillous adenomas tend to be intermediate in distribution and size between the tubular and villous forms, one-quarter to one-third being larger than 2 cm across.

In contrast to tubular adenomas, **villous adenomas commonly contain foci of carcinoma.** In tumors less than 1 cm, the risk is 10 times higher than that for comparably sized tubular adenomas. Of greater importance is the fact that villous adenomas greater than 2 cm in size have a 50% incidence of invasive carcinoma at the time of resection. Given that 60% of these neoplasms measure more than 2 cm in greatest dimension, **more than one-third of all resected villous adenomas contain invasive cancer.** Tubulovillous adenomas are again intermediate between tu-

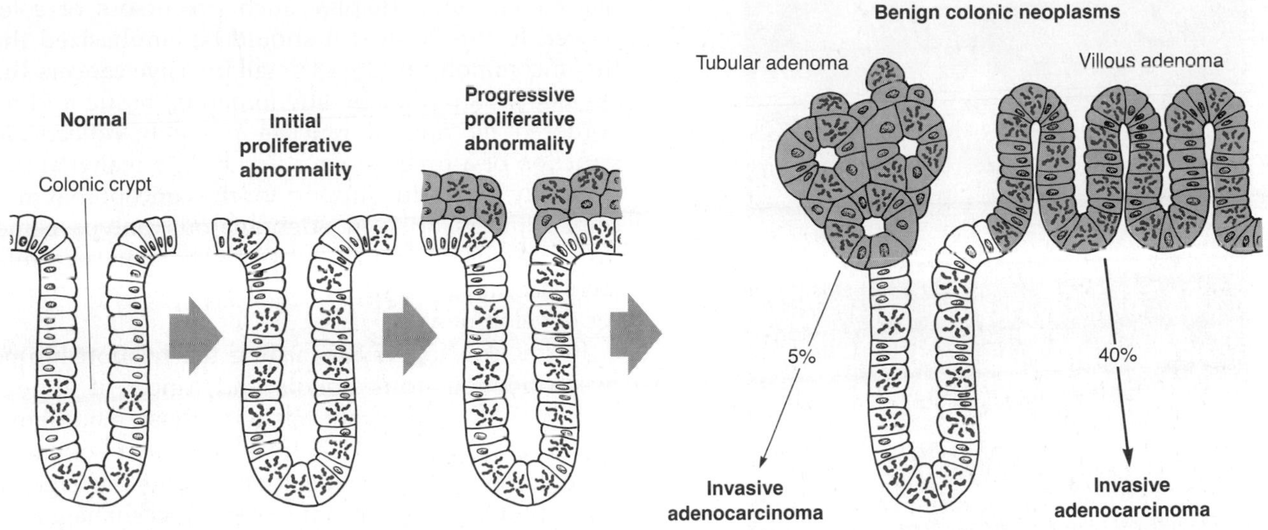

Figure 13-48. The histogenesis of adenomatous polyps of the colon. The initial proliferative abnormality of the colonic mucosa, the extension of the mitotic zone in the crypts, leads to the accumulation of mucosal cells. The formation of adenomas may reflect epithelial-mesenchymal interactions.

bular and villous adenomas in the risk of invasive carcinoma. The cytologic indicators of dysplasia and malignant transformation in villous and tubulovillous adenomas are the same as those for tubular adenomas.

The histogenesis of adenomatous polyps involves a failure of maturation or, conversely, a persistence of cell replication, in the epithelial cells that migrate toward the surface of the crypts (Fig. 13-48). Normally, DNA synthesis ceases when the cells reach the upper third of the crypts, after which they mature, migrate to the surface, become senescent, and are sloughed into the lumen. The adenomatous polyp is thought to arise from a focal disruption of this orderly sequence, such that the epithelial cells maintain their proliferative capacity throughout the entire depth of the crypt. Thus, mitotic figures are initially visualized not only along the entire length of the crypt, but also on the mucosal surface. As the lesion evolves, cell proliferation exceeds the rate of sloughing, and the cells begin to accumulate on the surface. Eventually, the accumulated cells on the surface of the mucosa form tubules or villous structures.

The differences in histogenesis between tubular and villous adenomas have been theorized to result from differences in mesenchymal cell proliferation in the lamina propria. It has been postulated that, in the absence of mesenchymal cell proliferation beneath the altered mucosa, the proliferating epithelial cells fold in to form tubules. The resistance to outward expansion could also explain why tubular adenomas remain small. By contrast, if growth of the lamina propria is stimulated parallel to that of the epithelium, the latter folds outward to produce villous structures. Without the constraint of an immobile lamina propria, the lesion can grow to a larger size.

Adenomatous Polyps and Colorectal Cancer Although it is now generally accepted that invasive carcinoma can arise in an adenomatous polyp, there has been controversy as to whether such benign tumors are necessary precursors of colon cancer. A better question is not whether adenomatous polyps are the **only** precursors of cancer, analogous to the relationship between epithelial dysplasia in the uterine cervix and squamous cell carcinoma, but whether **most** colon cancers arise in preexisting polyps. The weight of evidence, which tends to support such a hypothesis, can be summarized as follows.

First, the **geographic coincidence** in the frequencies of adenomatous polyps and colorectal cancer suggests a causal relationship. For example, the prevalence of both adenomatous polyps and colon cancer is extremely low in African blacks; polyps and cancer are both more frequent in American blacks. Moreover, Japanese born in Hawaii display a higher frequency of both diseases than those born in Japan. In geographic regions in which there is a high risk of

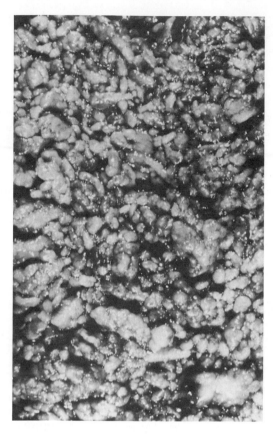

Figure 13-49. Familial polyposis. The mucosal surface of the colon is carpeted by innumerable adenomatous polyps.

colorectal cancer, adenomatous polyps tend to be larger, are more often villous, and display more severe dysplasia than those in low-risk areas.

Second, the difference in the **age of onset** between adenomatous polyps and colorectal cancer suggests that the latter follows the former. Adenomatous polyps tend to antedate colon cancer by 10 to 15 years.

Third, adenomas are commonly found in colons that harbor a carcinoma, and one-third of colons resected for cancer contain an adenomatous polyp. Moreover, the presence of an adenomatous polyp in the same specimen resected for cancer doubles the risk that another carcinoma will develop in the remaining colon.

An argument can be made that the preceding points simply reflect the fact that the same stimulus that promotes the growth of adenomatous polyps independently leads to cancer in an otherwise normal mucosa. However, epithelial dysplasia, carcinoma in situ, and early invasive cancer are simply not found arising from normal mucosa, even in colons that harbor frank invasive carcinoma or many adenomatous polyps. By contrast, adenomatous polyps in cancer-

ous colons often display such precursors of colon cancer. In this context it should be emphasized that the uncommon finding of small invasive cancers that are not surrounded by adenomatous tissue and are bordered by normal mucosa probably reflects destruction of a preexisting polyp by the malignancy.

Finally, powerful support for the concept that most colon cancers arise in adenomatous polyps comes from studies in which prophylactic polypectomies have drastically reduced the risk of subsequent cancer development.

In this controversy regarding the relationship between adenomatous polyps and cancer, it appears that the burden of proof lies with those who deny a causal connection. Before the availability of operative endoscopy, when polypectomy above the sigmoid colon entailed a laparotomy, the proper management of polyps discovered radiologically was hotly debated. Today it is common practice to avoid discussion and simply remove all clinically detected polyps through a colonoscope.

Inherited Adenomatous Polyposis Syndrome

Familial Polyposis Coli

Familial polyposis coli, inherited as an autosomal dominant trait, is characterized by the progressive development of innumerable adenomatous polyps of the colon, particularly in the rectosigmoid region. Although young patients have only few polyps, in a matter of a few years the colonic mucosa becomes carpeted, sometimes throughout its length, with thousands of adenomas (Fig. 13-49). These are mostly tubular adenomas, although tubulovillous and villous adenomas are also present. Microscopic polyps, sometimes involving a single crypt, are even more numerous. **Carcinoma of the colon is inevitable, nearly always by age 40, unless a total colectomy is performed.**

Although a few polyps are usually present by 10 years of age, the mean age for the occurrence of symptoms is 36 years, by which time cancer is already present in more than half of the patients. In addition to having colonic polyps, some persons with familial polyposis suffer from polyps in the small intestine and stomach, although malignant transformation at these sites is rare. Children of an afflicted parent have an even chance of developing polyposis; other relatives exhibit a 10% risk of manifesting the disease.

Gardner's Syndrome

Gardner's syndrome is an autosomal dominant, familial disorder characterized by gastrointestinal polyposis, principally in the colon, but commonly in the stomach and in the vicinity of the ampulla of Vater; osteomas of the skull, mandible, and long bones; and soft tissue tumors of the skin. The disease ultimately progresses to cancer of the colon. It is thought that Gardner's syndrome may not be a distinct entity, but rather a variant of familial adenomatous polyposis.

Turcot's Syndrome

The rare combination of familial polyposis of the colon with malignant tumors of the central nervous system is called "Turcot's syndrome." There is insufficient evidence to conclude that the disorder is an autosomal recessive trait, as has been claimed, or that the syndrome is truly a distinct entity. A number of cases of colon cancer have been reported in association with Turcot's syndrome.

Nonneoplastic Polyps

Whereas all adenomatous polyps, and possibly colon cancer, may be considered to occupy places on the same developmental spectrum, the nonneoplastic polyps are entirely different entities from one another and are grouped together solely because of their gross appearance as raised lesions of the colonic mucosa.

Hyperplastic Polyps (Metaplastic Polyps)

Hyperplastic polyps, the most common polypoid lesions of the colon, are particularly frequent in the rectum. Since the polyps are benign, and since the term "hyperplastic" carries a connotation of neoplastic growth, the term "metaplastic polyp" has also been used to emphasize the fact that this type of polyp is not a forerunner of cancer.

These polyps present macroscopically as small, sessile, raised mucosal nodules that are usually up to 0.5 cm in diameter but occasionally larger. They are almost always multiple, and have even been mistaken for familial polyposis coli. Histologically, the crypts of the hyperplastic polyp are elongated and may exhibit cystic dilatation (Fig. 13-50). The overall appearance is superficially similar to that of a villous adenoma. The epithelium is composed of well-differentiated goblet cells and absorptive cells, without any atypical features. Focal infolding of the crowded epithelium imparts a saw-toothed appearance to the mucosal lining. The lamina propria is also unremarkable.

The pathogenesis of the hyperplastic polyp is thought to involve a defect in the maturation of the normal mucosal epithelium. In a hyperplastic polyp cell renewal at the base of the crypt is retarded, and the upward migration of the cells is slowed. Thus, the epithelial cells differentiate and acquire absorptive characteristics lower in the crypts. Moreover, they persist on the surface mucosa longer than normal cells.

Hyperplastic polyps are remarkably common, being present in 40% of rectal specimens in persons under the age of 40 years and in 75% of older individuals. The association of hyperplastic polyps with rectal cancer is striking; 90% of specimens removed

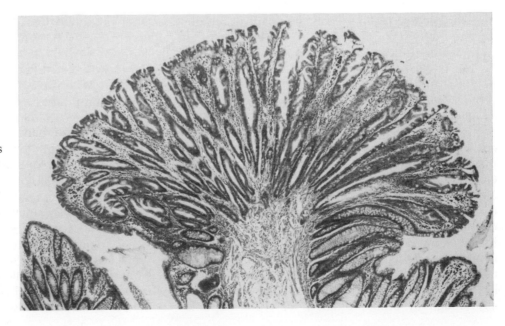

Figure 13-50. Hyperplastic polyp of the colon. A low-power photomicrograph shows elongated crypts, which create an appearance superficially similar to that of a villous adenoma.

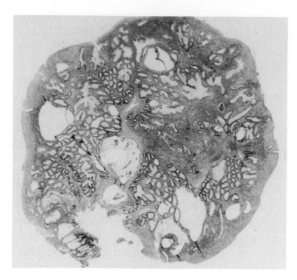

Figure 13-51.   Juvenile polyp of the colon. A low-power photomicrograph shows cystic epithelial tubules embedded in a fibrovascular stroma.

for cancer contain such polyps. Moreover, hyperplastic polyps seen in association with rectal cancer are often grouped around the tumor. In addition, hyperplastic polyps are more common than usual in colons that contain adenomatous polyps and in populations with higher than normal rates of colon cancer. Thus, although these asymptomatic lesions are not themselves preneoplastic, they reflect an increased risk of colon cancer.

Juvenile Polyps (Retention Polyps)

Juvenile polyps, as their name implies, are most common in children below the age of 10 years, but about one-third occur in adults. They are not observed during the first year of life, and are, therefore, thought to be acquired. Because the lesions are characterized by mucus-filled cysts (hence the name "retention polyp"), and because they do not display epithelial proliferation or atypism, **juvenile polyps are classed as hamartomas.**

Juvenile polyps may be single or multiple and occur most commonly in the rectum, although they may be seen anywhere in the small or large bowel. Grossly, most polyps are pedunculated lesions up to 2 cm in diameter that have a smooth, rounded surface, in contrast to the fissured surface of an adenomatous polyp. Histologically, dilated and cystic epithelial tubules are embedded in a fibrovascular lamina propria (Fig. 13-51). The cells lining the tubules are regular and show no atypical features; the lesion does not progress to cancer. The polyps usually slough by autoamputation or regress spontaneously. Pedunculated juvenile polyps in the rectum may prolapse during defecation, and their ready amputation may deposit them on the toilet paper. Because of their tendency to bleed, juvenile polyps are usually surgically removed.

The polyps of the Peutz-Jeghers syndrome, which may be found in the colon, are also hamartomatous. They were discussed above in the context of small intestinal benign neoplasms.

Inflammatory Polyps

Inflammatory polyps are not neoplasms, but rather elevated masses of regenerating epithelium and granulation tissue over ulcerations caused by an inflammatory disease of the colon. Such polyps are commonly found in association with ulcerative colitis and Crohn's disease; they are also encountered in cases of amebic colitis and bacterial dysentery. Microscopically, inflammatory polyps are composed principally of chronically inflamed granulation tissue intermixed with large, basophilic, proliferating epithelial cells. As healing proceeds, epithelial regeneration restores the mucosal architecture. Although these lesions are themselves not precancerous, they occur in chronic inflammatory diseases associated with a high incidence of cancer (e.g., ulcerative colitis) and must therefore be distinguished from adenomatous and malignant polyps.

Lymphoid Polyps

Lymphoid tissue, in the form of follicles or as scattered lymphocytes or plasma cells in the lamina propria, is normally present in the colonic mucosa. Submucosal accumulations of lymphoid tissue, almost invariably in the rectum, usually present as single, sessile nodules measuring from a pinpoint size to as large as 5 cm in diameter. On occasion multiple lesions impart a cobblestone appearance to the mucosa. Microscopically, these polyps are covered by intact mucosa and are composed of prominent lymphoid follicles with germinal centers. They are more common in females than in males and are seen in persons of any age, including children. The lesions are usually asymptomatic and are unrelated to malignant lymphomas, although in rectal biopsies they may superficially resemble malignant lymphoid tissue.

In **nodular lymphoid hyperplasia,** a condition seen primarily in children, there is an excessive accumulation of the normal follicular lymphoid tissue of the colon. Macroscopically, the mucosa exhibits numerous small sessile or polypoid nodules up to 0.5 cm in diameter. The microscopic appearance is similar to that of lymphoid polyps. The condition is not related to malignant lymphoma, but the radiologic appearance can be mistaken for familial polyposis coli.

Malignant Tumors

Adenocarcinoma of the Colon and Rectum

In Western industrialized societies colorectal cancer is second in incidence only to carcinoma of the lung in men and, except for breast cancer, holds the same rank in women. Although the widely used term "colorectal" implies a common biology, evidence suggests that the differences between cancers of the colon and rectum are more fundamental than simple location. For instance, whereas colon cancer is at least 4 times more common in the United States than in Japan, the incidence of rectal carcinoma in the two populations is virtually the same. In general, rectosigmoid carcinoma accounts for a considerably higher proportion of all large bowel cancers in populations at high risk for cancer of the large bowel than in low-risk populations. Moreover, cancer of the colon shows a slight female preponderance, whereas cancer of the rectum shows a slight male preponderance. In the United States the incidence of cancer has been shifting from a predominance in the rectum to a predominance in the colon. Overall, in the United States about one-third of large bowel cancers occur in the rectum and rectosigmoid regions and an additional one-fourth occur in the sigmoid colon.

Pathogenesis

Assuming that cancer of the colon arises in, or is at least correlated with, adenomatous polyps, factors associated with the development of such polyps are also implicated in the genesis of colorectal cancer. The importance of environmental factors in the pathogenesis of colon cancer is emphasized by the high incidence of the disease in industrialized countries and among migrants from low-risk to high-risk regions. **The major environmental risk factor has been suggested to be the diet, specifically a diet low in indigestible fiber and high in animal fat.** As previously discussed, such a diet has also been incriminated in the etiology of other colonic diseases, including diverticulosis, adenomatous polyps, appendicitis, and ulcerative colitis.

Compared with a high-fiber diet, a **low-fiber diet** is associated with a slower transit of fecal contents through the colon, thereby permitting longer exposure of the mucosa to any chemical in the stools. Moreover, it has been suggested that fiber may bind potential carcinogens and, by increasing the bulk of the stools, dilute their concentration.

An **increase in fat consumption**—for example, that associated with the recent change in dietary habits in Japan—is paralleled by an increased incidence of colon cancer, whereas a reduced content of animal fat in the diet of certain ethnic groups in the United States has been accompanied by a decreased incidence of colon cancer. The ingestion of fat elicits the secretion of bile into the intestine, and some bile acids have been claimed experimentally to enhance the tumorogenicity of intestinal carcinogens. In this context cholecystectomy, a procedure that increases the colonic content of secondary bile acids in the colon, has been shown in some studies (although not in others) to be associated with an increased risk of right-sided colon cancer.

It has also been demonstrated that the feces of persons in high-risk populations have a higher content of **anaerobic bacteria** than those of persons in low-risk populations and that such microorganisms, particularly Bacteroides species, can convert bile salts into compounds that are potentially carcinogenic. Repopulation of the colon with Lactobacillus protects experimental animals against chemically induced colon cancer.

A low prevalence of colon cancer has been correlated with high levels of selenium in the soil and plants of certain geographic areas. The endogenous antioxidant glutathione peroxidase is a selenium-containing enzyme. Exogenous antioxidants (e.g., butylated hydroxytoluene and vitamin E) and a reducing agent such as ascorbic acid have protected animals against the experimental production of colon cancer. Diets rich in cruciferous vegetables—for instance, cauliflower, brussels sprouts, and cabbage—and those that provide vitamin A are said to be associated with a lower incidence of colon cancer.

Risk Factors

Age is probably the single most important risk factor in the general population. The risk is low before age 40 and increases steadily to age 50, after which it doubles with each decade to reach a maximum at age 75.

A **prior colorectal cancer** increases the risk of a subsequent tumor. In fact, 5% to 10% of patients treated for colorectal cancer subsequently develop a second malignant lesion of the colon. Moreover, 2% to 5% of patients in whom a colorectal cancer is discovered harbor another primary (synchronous) malignant tumor of the colon. As previously mentioned, patients who have had an **adenomatous polyp** removed, or who demonstrate the presence of such a polyp, are at increased risk for the subsequent development of colorectal cancer.

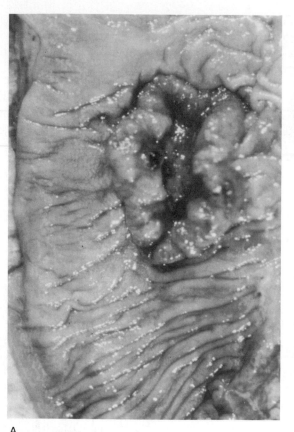

A

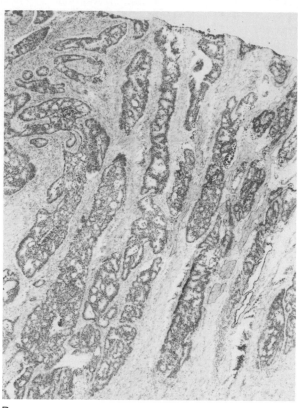

B

Figure 13-52.   Adenocarcinoma of the colon. (*A*) The opened colon contains an elevated, centrally ulcerated, infiltrating mass. (*B*) A photomicrograph of (*A*) reveals moderately differentiated infiltrating adenocarcinoma extending from the ulcerated mucosal surface.

The previously discussed risk of colorectal cancer in **ulcerative colitis** is directly correlated with the duration of this inflammatory disease and its extent within the colon. Disease limited to the rectum seems not to be associated with an increased risk of cancer. Recent studies suggest that the risk of colon cancer in patients with Crohn's colitis may be as high as that in patients with ulcerative colitis. The risk of cancer in patients with Crohn's colitis is also related to the duration and extent of the disease.

Except for Peutz-Jeghers syndrome, the **hereditary polyposis syndromes** are inevitably complicated by colon cancer. Even the Peutz-Jeghers syndrome is not a true exception; its hamartomatous lesions are associated with a higher than normal incidence of adenomatous polyps and, therefore, of colon cancer.

Colon cancer shows a modest increase in frequency among relatives of patients with the disease, a finding that suggests some genetic contribution to the development of colon cancer. Familial kindreds with colorectal cancer have been described, and there is some evidence for inheritance as an autosomal

dominant trait. A previous history of cancer at other sites, particularly breast or genital cancer in women, is associated with a higher than normal frequency of colorectal cancer.

Pathology

The gross appearance of colorectal cancers is similar to that of adenocarcinomas elsewhere in the gastrointestinal tract; they may be **polypoid, ulcerating, or infiltrative, in the last case customarily annular and constrictive** (Fig. 13-52*A*). Polypoid cancers are most common on the right side of the colon, particularly in the cecum, where the large caliber of the colon allows unimpeded intraluminal growth. Annular constricting tumors occur most often in the distal portions of the colon. Ulceration of tumors, irrespective of the growth pattern, is usual.

The vast majority of colorectal cancers are adenocarcinomas (Fig. 13-52*B*), which are microscopically similar to their counterparts in other portions of the gastrointestinal tract. Most are well differentiated and secrete small amounts of mucin. About 10% to

15% secrete considerable quantities of mucin, in which case they are classed as mucinous adenocarcinomas. The degree of differentiation influences the prognosis, the better differentiated tumors being associated with a more favorable outlook. Occasionally, the predominant mucus-producing cell is of the "signet ring" variety, in which case the cancer is associated with a particularly poor prognosis.

The prognosis of colon cancer is more closely related to the extension of the tumor through the wall of the colon than to its histologic characteristics. Colorectal cancers are usually staged according to the Dukes' classification or its variants (Fig. 13-53). Dukes' A cancer (15%) is confined to the mucosa and submucosa and does not penetrate the muscular layers. Dukes' B classification (35%) refers to a tumor that has penetrated the muscle wall and possibly invaded the pericolic fat but has not metastasized to lymph nodes. A Dukes' C tumor (50%) is similar to Dukes' B but shows lymph node metastases. After the establishment of the Dukes' classification, a D category was added to signify distant metastases.

The size of the tumor correlates poorly with prognosis, the depth of invasion described by the Dukes' classification being of greater value. Patients with Dukes' A colon cancer are almost invariably cured by surgical resection. The 5-year survival of patients with Dukes' B tumors is about 60%, while that of patients with stage C disease is about 35%. The original Dukes' classification has been refined by the subdivision of stages B and C into additional categories that are meant to provide greater precision in predicting prognosis. In general, cancers of the distal colon and rectum tend to be more infiltrative than those on the right side and therefore usually present at a more advanced Dukes' stage, with its correspondingly poorer prognosis.

Direct spread of colon cancer is commonly observed in resected specimens. In its penetration of the muscular layers, colon cancer tends to exploit the same gaps that house the penetrating arteries as does the process that results in diverticulosis. The connective tissues of the serosa offer little resistance to the spread of the tumor, and cancer cells are often found in the fat and serosa at some distance from the primary tumor. Characteristically, **colorectal cancer invades lymphatic channels** and initially involves the lymph nodes immediately underlying the tumor. Lymphatic metastases tend to spread to adjacent nodes, and only rarely are so-called "skip" metastases encountered. The **peritoneum** is occasionally

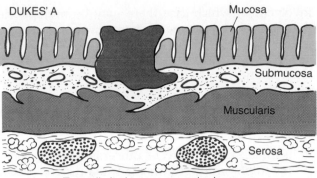

DUKES' A

Mucosa
Submucosa
Muscularis
Serosa

Tumor limited to mucosa and submucosa

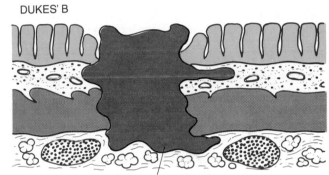

DUKES' B

Extension to all layers

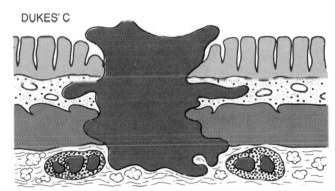

DUKES' C

Metastases to regional lymph nodes

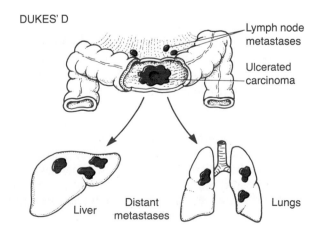

DUKES' D

Lymph node metastases
Ulcerated carcinoma

Liver   Distant metastases   Lungs

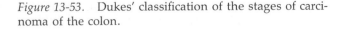

Figure 13-53. Dukes' classification of the stages of carcinoma of the colon.

involved, in which case there may be multiple deposits throughout the abdomen. Venous invasion leads to **blood-borne metastases,** which involve the liver in 75% of patients with metastatic disease. The lungs, bones, and brain are not uncommon sites of metastases.

Clinical Features

In its initial stages colorectal cancer is clinically silent. As the tumor grows, the most common sign is **occult intestinal bleeding** when the tumor is in the proximal portions of the colon or **bright red blood** when the lesion is in the rectum. In the right side of the colon, particularly in the cecum, where the diameter of the lumen is large and the fecal contents liquid, tumors grow to a large size without causing symptoms of obstruction. Chronic asymptomatic bleeding typically causes severe anemia, which is thus often the first indication of colon cancer. By contrast, cancers on the left side of the colon, where the caliber of the lumen is small and the fecal contents more solid, often constrict the lumen, producing **obstructive symptoms** manifested as changes in bowel habits, gaseousness, and abdominal pain. Rectal cancer is often signaled by tenesmus (straining at stool) and a reduction in the caliber of the stools. Occasionally, colon cancer **perforates** early and produces symptoms indistinguishable from those of diverticulitis. When the tumor has extended beyond the confines of the intestine, it may produce enterocutaneous and rectovaginal **fistulas,** tumor masses in the abdominal wall, bladder symptoms, and sciatic nerve pain. Intra-abdominal spread may cause **small intestinal obstruction and ascites.**

The presence of carcinoembryonic antigen (CEA) in the serum was originally suggested to be a valuable test for colorectal cancer. Unfortunately, experience has demonstrated that the test is usually positive only in advanced cancer; it is therefore not an adequate screening test for early, and hence curable, lesions. Fewer than 5% of patients with Dukes' A tumors and only about 25% of those with Dukes' B tumors exhibit elevated circulating levels of CEA. Nevertheless, the test is often employed to evaluate patients with metastases of unknown origin and to monitor patients postoperatively for recurrent disease.

A positive test for occult blood in the feces with reagent-impregnated paper predicts the presence of a cancer or an adenoma in 40% to 50% of the cases. For persons who are inclined to comply with an effective screening program, periodic fiberoptic sigmoidoscopy and testing for occult blood in the feces is thought to improve the prognosis of colorectal cancer, since these methods can often detect the disease at an early stage.

The only curative treatment for colorectal cancer is surgery. Small polyps are easily removed endoscopically; large lesions require segmental resection. Tumors close to the anal verge often necessitate abdominal-perineal resection and colostomy, although newer surgical techniques frequently allow sphincter preservation.

Carcinoid Tumors

Carcinoid tumors of the colon constitute a small proportion of all such tumors in the gastrointestinal tract. They behave similarly to carcinoid tumors of the small intestine, in which malignancy correlates with size. About half of carcinoid tumors of the colon have metastasized by the time they are discovered. The pathologic and clinical features are discussed above in the context of small bowel tumors.

Large Bowel Lymphoma

Primary lymphoma of the colon is distinctly uncommon, constituting only about one-tenth of all primary gastrointestinal lymphomas. The neoplasm may present as segmental involvement of the mucosa, as diffuse polypoid lesions, or as a mass extending beyond the confines of the colon. The presenting symptoms in the case of large tumors are similar to those of other primary intestinal cancers, but the diffuse polypoid form may radiologically resemble the inflammatory polyps of ulcerative colitis.

Cancers of the Anal Canal

Carcinomas of the anal canal, which constitute 2% of cancers of the colon, may arise at or above the dentate line. These tumors occur in both sexes but are more common in women, usually over the age of 50 years. Since the tumors tend to grow upward, they may be misdiagnosed clinically as rectal carcinomas. These epithelial neoplasms have various histologic patterns, such as **squamous, basaloid,** and **cloacogenic.** Bowen's disease of the anus represents carcinoma in situ, whereas extramammary Paget's disease at this site reflects intraepithelial invasion by the tumor. There are few clinical differences in behavior among the different tumor types, and they can be conveniently classed as **epidermoid carcinoma.** Carcinoma of the anus penetrates directly into the surrounding tissues, including the internal and external sphincters, perianal soft tissues, prostate, and vagina. Lymphatic spread carries the tumor to the pelvic and inguinal nodes and hematogenous dissemination may lead to distant metastases.

Chronic inflammatory disease of the anus—for instance, venereal disease—fissures, and trauma produced by anal intercourse predispose to anal cancer. In fact, receptive anal intercourse among male homosexuals is associated with a 30-fold increase in the risk of anal cancer. It has been observed that factors associated with genital carcinoma (cancer of the penis, scrotum, cervix, or vulva)—namely, poor hygiene, indiscriminate sexual practices, and genital warts—also contribute to the development of anal cancer. In addition, cigarette smoking is associated with a significantly increased risk of anal cancer. The usual symptoms include bleeding, pain, and an anal or rectal mass. Often the tumor is not clinically recognized as a malignant lesion and may be discovered only in a hemorrhoidectomy specimen. Abdominal-perineal resection, with or without radiotherapy, is the customary treatment. More than half of the patients survive for at least 5 years.

Malignant melanoma of the anus is rare but well recognized. Because of its location and early metastasis, it is infrequently diagnosed before it has spread distantly.

Miscellaneous Cancers

Malignant counterparts of the various benign mesenchymal tumors—for example, leiomyosarcoma and neurogenic sarcoma—have been occasionally reported but are far less common in the colon than in other parts of the alimentary tract.

Miscellaneous Disorders

Endometriosis

Endometriosis involves the colon and rectum in 15% to 20% of the cases but is ordinarily asymptomatic and is discovered only incidentally during laparotomy for other reasons. When symptoms do occur (abdominal pain, constipation, and even intestinal obstruction), they may be mistaken for those of colorectal cancer. The pathology of endometriosis is described in detail in Chapter 18, which deals with gynecologic pathology. Briefly, endometriomas generally present as indurated tumors of up to 5 cm in diameter in the serosa and muscularis of the bowel, although they may penetrate the submucosa. As a result of repeated hemorrhage, the lesions are surrounded by reactive fibrosis. Symptomatic endometriomas of the colon and rectum usually project into the lumen as polypoid masses covered by intact mucosa.

Melanosis Coli

Melanosis coli is a medical curiosity that refers to the occurrence of **dark brown pigment in the colonic mucosa** of persons who are chronic users of **anthracene-type cathartics,** including cascara sagrada, rhubarb, senna, and aloe. The condition is not associated with symptoms and is entirely reversible. Although melanosis coli has been reported in association with partially obstructing colon cancers, many patients with such cancers use laxatives, and there is little reason to believe that the pigmentation is related directly to the cancer. The gross appearance of the pigmented mucosa of the colon has been likened to tiger or crocodile skin or, as in chronic passive congestion of the liver, a section of natural nutmeg. Microscopically, macrophages in the lamina propria are seen to contain pigment granules. The pigment is lysosomal and, despite the name, is not melanin, but rather lipofuscin.

Cathartic Colon

Women who have used the laxatives listed above and other irritant cathartics, such as castor oil and phenolphthalein, for many years may develop chronic constipation and lower abdominal pain, without diarrhea. Grossly, the transverse colon is pendulous and the sigmoid is dilated. In some cases there is only mild thickening of the terminal ileum or no abnormalities at all. Melanosis coli is often present. Interestingly, there is sometimes a loss of myenteric neurons, which is thought to reflect a neurotoxic effect of the irritant laxative.

Stercoral Ulcers

Incomplete evacuation of the feces, usually in association with debilitating disease or old age, may lead to the formation of a large mass of stool that cannot be passed (fecal impaction). **Stercoral ulcers result from pressure necrosis of the mucosa caused by the fecal impaction.** Although such ulcers are most common in the rectosigmoid region, they have also been reported as high as the transverse colon. The most feared complications are severe, even exsanguinating, rectal bleeding and perforation leading to peritonitis. Chronic blood loss may lead to iron-deficiency anemia.

The Appendix

The vermiform appendix, which is usually 8 cm to 10 cm in length, typically has a retrocecal attachment to the cecum, but its tip is generally not fixed and can therefore move freely. The appendix is invested with a mesentery called the "mesoappendix." The wall of the appendix is composed of the same layers as the rest of the intestine: mucosa, submucosa, muscularis, and serosa. The most prominent microscopic feature is the predominance of submucosal lymphoid tissue, which reaches its largest size during adolescence and then progressively atrophies. Because of its presumed homology with the avian bursa of Fabricius, the appendix is considered by some to have an immune function, although such a role remains to be established. Thus, although the appendix has historically been considered a vestigial structure, its status is a matter of debate.

Appendicitis

Acute Appendicitis

Acute appendicitis, by far the most common disease of the appendix, is the most frequent cause of an abdominal emergency. Although the incidence peaks in the second and third decades, acute appendicitis may occur in persons of any age. For reasons unknown, the incidence of the disease seems to be declining.

The pathogenesis of acute appendicitis is thought to relate to obstruction of its orifice, with secondary distention of the lumen and bacterial invasion of the wall. Mechanical obstruction by fecaliths or solid fecal material in the cecum is demonstrated in one-third of the cases. Occasionally tumors, parasites, or foreign bodies are incriminated. Lymphoid hyperplasia as a result of bacterial or viral stimulation (e.g., by Salmonella or measles) may obstruct the lumen and lead to appendicitis. However, **no obstruction is demonstrated in up to half of patients with appendicitis,** and the factor that precipitates the disease is unknown. The higher incidence of appendicitis in industrialized countries has been attributed to the fact that fecaliths and viscid fecal material are more common in persons who consume a low-fiber diet than in those who consume a high-fiber diet.

As secretions distend the obstructed appendix, the intraluminal pressure rises and eventually exceeds the venous pressure, thereby causing venous stasis and ischemia. As a result, the mucosa ulcerates and permits invasion by intestinal bacteria. The accumulation of neutrophils produces microabscesses, and arterial thromboses aggravate the ischemia. The infected necrotic wall becomes gangrenous and may perforate, often in 24 to 48 hours.

Acute appendicitis is typically manifested by epigastric or periumbilical cramping pain, but the pain may be diffuse or initially restricted to the right lower quadrant. Shortly thereafter, nausea and vomiting occur, and the patient develops a low-grade fever and a moderate leukocytosis. The pain shifts to the right lower quadrant, where point tenderness is the rule. A diseased retrocecal appendix is shielded from the anterior abdominal wall by the cecum and ileum; atypical symptoms are therefore easily misinterpreted because of their poor localization. In the elderly appendicitis may also produce only vague symptoms, and the diagnosis is often not made until perforation occurs. A number of conditions that do not require surgery are not infrequently misdiagnosed as appendicitis; these include mesenteric adenitis in children, Meckel's diverticulitis, mittelschmerz (ovulatory rupture of an ovarian follicle), and acute salpingitis.

Macroscopically, the resected appendix is congested, tense, and covered by a fibrinous exudate. The lumen often contains purulent material, and a fecalith may be evident (Fig. 13-54). Microscopically, early cases show mucosal microabscesses and a purulent exudate in the lumen. As the infection progresses, the entire wall becomes infiltrated with neutrophils, which eventually reach the serosa. Necrosis of the wall leads to perforation and release of the luminal contents into the peritoneal cavity. In patients who escape surgery and survive, the inflammatory process may subside, leaving a narrow, scarred appendix in which the lumen is obliterated.

The complications of appendicitis are principally related to perforation, which is reported to occur in about one-third of children and young adults. Almost all children under the age of 2 have a perforated appendix at the time of operation, as do up to three-quarters of patients over the age of 60. **Periappendiceal abscesses** are common, but abscesses may develop anywhere in the abdominal cavity. **Fistulous tracts** may appear between the perforated appendix and adjacent structures, including the small and large bowel, bladder, vagina, or abdominal wall. Because venous blood from the appendix drains into the superior mesenteric vein, **pylephlebitis** (thrombophle-

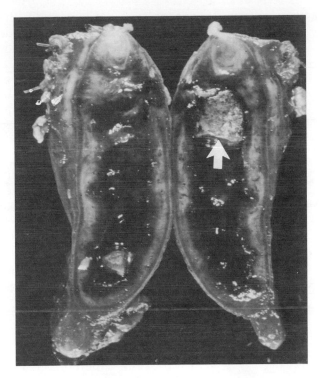

Figure 13-54. Acute appendicitis. The lumen of the appendix is dilated and contains a purulent and hemorrhagic exudate. A fecalith (*arrow*) obstructs the proximal lumen.

bitis of the intrahepatic portal vein radicals) and **hepatic abscesses** are feared complications. **Diffuse peritonitis** and **septicemia** are dangerous sequelae. The most common complication of acute appendicitis is **wound infection** following surgery; it occurs in up to one-quarter of patients with perforation and in one-third of those who develop a periappendiceal abscess.

The treatment of acute appendicitis is surgical in the vast majority of cases. Because perforation carries a much higher risk of death than does laparotomy, early surgical intervention is warranted even when the diagnosis of acute appendicitis is not entirely secure. In fact, even in the best hands 10% of all resected appendices can be expected to be normal. In remote locations where surgical facilities are not available, or when accompanying illnesses prohibit laparotomy, antibiotic treatment has occasionally been attempted.

Chronic Appendicitis

Chronic appendicitis is either rare or nonexistent, depending on the need to explain the removal of an uninflamed appendix. However, recurrent appendicitis, although uncommon, is documented.

Other Causes of Appendicitis

Crohn's disease of the terminal ileum involves the appendix in about one-quarter of the cases and may affect the appendix even when it is localized to distant sites in the small intestine or colon. **Ulcerative colitis** also may spread to the mucosa of the appendix. **Tuberculous appendicitis** is usually found in association with tuberculous enteritis, and rare cases of **actinomycotic infection** are recorded. **Yersinia** infection of the ileum may also involve the appendix.

Mucocele

Obstruction of the appendix may lead to distention of the lumen by secreted mucus, a condition termed "mucocele" (Fig. 13-55). The mucus-filled appendiceal mass may be large enough to be palpable and require exploratory laparotomy. A mucocele may be-

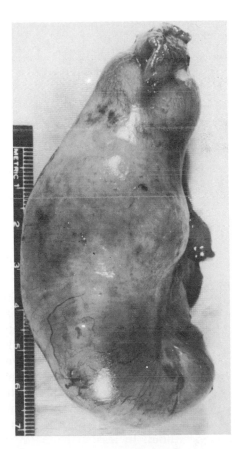

Figure 13-55. Mucocele of the appendix. The appendix is markedly distended by mucus.

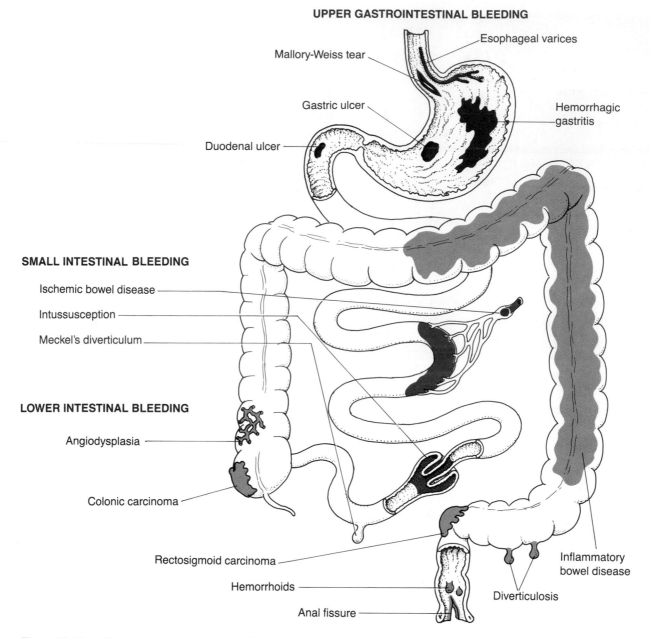

Figure 13-56. Causes of gastrointestinal bleeding.

come secondarily infected and rupture, thereby discharging mucin and debris into the peritoneal cavity. This material may be mistaken at laparotomy for tumor implants on the peritoneum, but it will invariably be reabsorbed without incident. However, when the mucocele results from mucus secretion by a cystadenocarcinoma of the appendix, perforation may lead to seeding of the peritoneum by malignant mucus-secreting tumor cells, a condition known as **pseudomyxoma peritonei.** In less than one-third of the cases this malignant disease of the peritoneum is caused by disease of the appendix; in half it originates from ovarian mucinous cystadenocarcinoma.

Neoplasms

The most common neoplasm of the appendix is the carcinoid tumor, which is almost invariably benign in that location. As in the other parts of the gastrointestinal tract, leiomyomas, fibromas, lipomas, and benign neurogenic tumors are encountered. Benign epithelial tumors (e.g., cystadenomas, adenomatous polyps) are rare. The appendix infrequently gives rise to adenocarcinoma, mucinous cystadenocarcinoma, lymphosarcoma, malignant carcinoid tumors, and sarcomas.

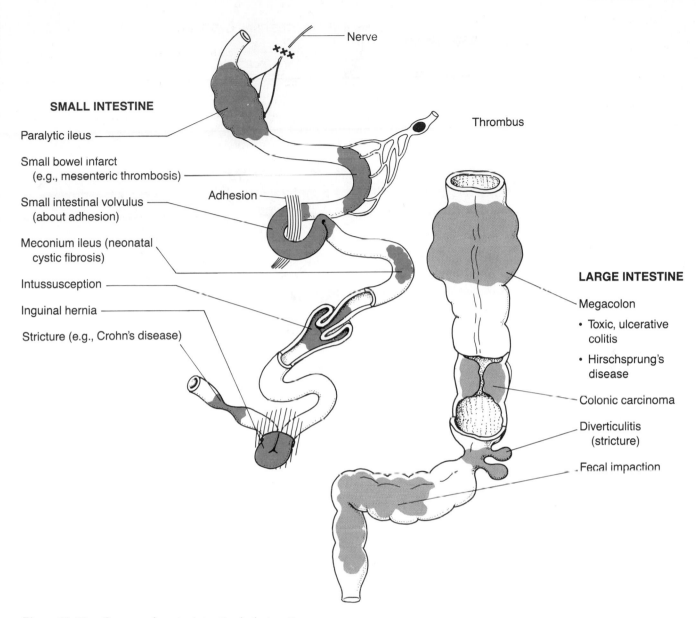

SMALL INTESTINE

Paralytic ileus

Small bowel infarct
(e.g., mesenteric thrombosis)

Small intestinal volvulus
(about adhesion)

Meconium ileus (neonatal
cystic fibrosis)

Intussusception

Inguinal hernia

Stricture (e.g., Crohn's disease)

Nerve

Adhesion

Thrombus

LARGE INTESTINE

Megacolon
- Toxic, ulcerative
  colitis
- Hirschsprung's
  disease

Colonic carcinoma

Diverticulitis
(stricture)

Fecal impaction

Figure 13-57. Causes of gastrointestinal obstruction.

Figures 13-56 through 13-59 summarize the causes of gastrointestinal bleeding and obstruction and the major benign and malignant tumors of the gastrointestinal tract.

The Peritoneum

The peritoneum is the mesothelial lining of the abdominal cavity and its viscera. As the name implies, the visceral peritoneum invests the gastrointestinal tract from the stomach to the rectum and encircles the liver. The parietal peritoneum lines the abdominal wall and the retroperitoneal space. The omentum, formed by a double layer of peritoneum, encloses blood vessels and a variable amount of fat.

Peritonitis

Bacterial Peritonitis

The most common cause of bacterial peritonitis is perforation of an abdominal viscus, as in an inflamed appendix, peptic ulcer, or colonic diverticulum. The clinical presentation is often that of an acute abdomen, in which severe abdominal pain and ten-

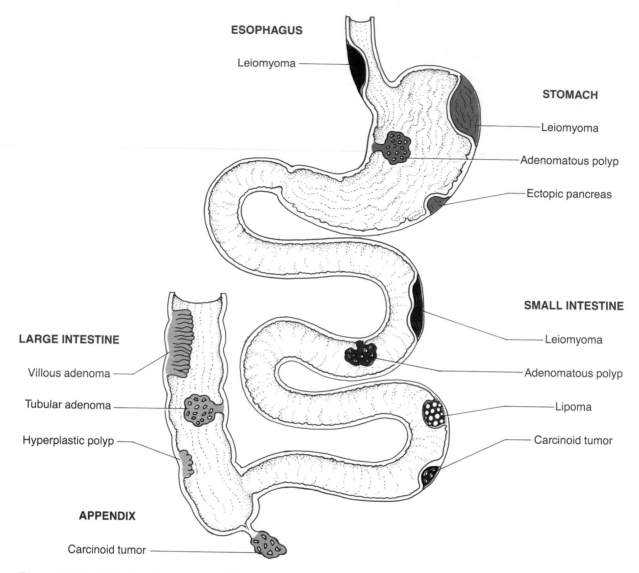

Figure 13-58.   Major benign tumors of the gastrointestinal tract.

derness predominate. Nausea, vomiting, and a high fever are usual, and in severe cases generalized peritonitis, paralytic ileus, and septic shock ensue. Often the perforation becomes "walled off," in which case a peritoneal abscess results.

The bacteria released into the peritoneal cavity from the gastrointestinal tract vary according to the site of perforation and the duration of the peritonitis. Often several aerobic and anaerobic species are cultured, including *E. coli*, Bacteroides species, various Streptococcus species, and Clostridium. Despite treatment with antibiotics, surgical drainage and debridement, and supportive measures, generalized peritonitis is still associated with a mortality of 50% and is especially dangerous in the elderly.

The macroscopic appearance of bacterial peritonitis is similar to that of purulent infection elsewhere. A fibrinopurulent exudate covers the surface of the intestines, and upon organization, fibrinous and fibrous adhesions form between loops of bowel, which become joined to each other. Such adhesions may eventually be lysed, or they may lead to **volvulus** and **intestinal obstruction.** Bacterial salpingitis, usually gonococcal, may lead to pelvic peritonitis and adhesions, a characteristic of **pelvic inflammatory disease.**

Chronic **peritonal dialysis** is today a frequent cause of bacterial peritonitis, owing to contamination of instruments or dialysate. The clinical course is usually more mild than that seen with a perforated

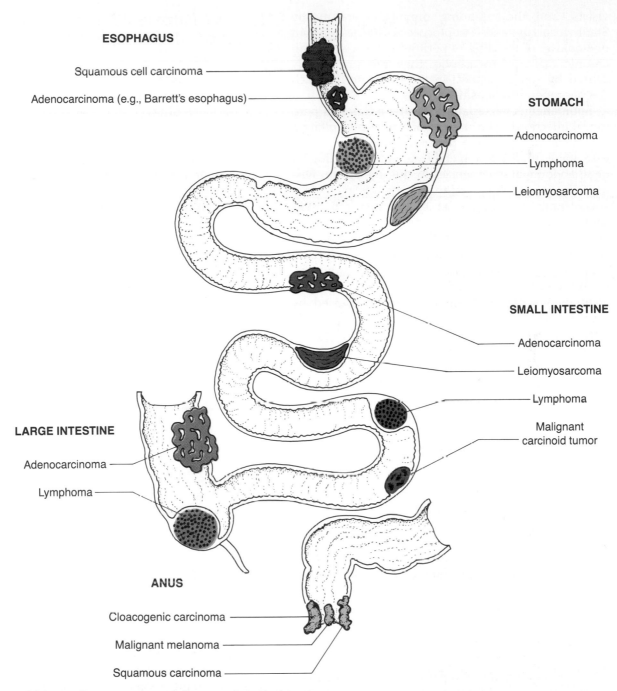

Figure 13-59. Major malignant tumors of the gastrointestinal tract.

viscus, and the offending organisms are mostly Staphylococcus and Streptococcus species. About one-quarter of the cases of peritonitis associated with chronic dialysis are aseptic; they are presumably caused by some chemical in the dialysate to which the peritoneum is sensitive.

Spontaneous bacterial peritonitis refers to a peritoneal infection in the absence of a clear precipitating circumstance, such as a perforated viscus. The disease is not uncommon in children, accounting for 2% of all abdominal emergencies in this age group. Historically, spontaneous bacterial peritonitis in children was usually a complication of the **nephrotic syndrome** and was principally caused by pneumococci or streptococci. Even today the majority of children who develop peritonitis with gram-positive organisms suffer from the nephrotic syndrome. However, since the advent of the antibiotic era, most cases of spontaneous peritonitis in children are caused by gram-negative organisms, usually derived from urinary tract infections. The disease causes symptoms of an acute abdomen and ordinarily leads to surgical intervention, unless the child is known to have the nephrotic syndrome. Even with antibiotic treatment, the mortality remains at 5% to 10%.

The most common cause of spontaneous peritonitis in adults (occurring in about 10% of such patients) is cirrhosis complicated by portal hypertension and ascites.

Tuberculous peritonitis is an unusual form of bacterial peritonitis. It is rarely seen in industrialized countries but occasionally complicates tuberculosis in developing countries. Many patients with tuberculous peritonitis do not suffer from concurrent pulmonary or miliary tuberculosis, an observation that suggests the activation of latent tuberculous foci in the peritoneum derived from previous hematogenous dissemination.

Chemical Peritonitis

The escape of bile into the peritoneum, usually from a perforated gallbladder but sometimes from a needle biopsy of the liver, produces **bile peritonitis,** an insult that may lead to shock. **Hydrochloric acid** from a perforated peptic ulcer of the stomach or duodenum, **hemorrhage,** and **foreign materials,** such as talc, may also elicit an inflammatory reaction in the peritoneum. **Acute pancreatitis** causes the release and activation of potent lipolytic and proteolytic enzymes, which produce a severe peritonitis and fat necrosis. Shock is common and may be lethal unless adequately treated.

Familial Paroxysmal Polyserositis (Familial Mediterranean Fever)

Familial paroxysmal polyserositis, an inherited autosomal recessive disorder, is characterized by recurrent episodes of fever and abdominal pain reflecting an aseptic peritonitis. The disease presents as a peritonitis in about half of the cases and as arthritis in about one-quarter. Pleuritis is the initial complaint in only 5% of patients. However, almost all affected individuals eventually manifest peritonitis, and more than half develop arthritis and pleuritis at some time. The disease predominates in Sephardic Jews and other Mediterranean populations, such as Armenians, Turks, and Arabs. The cause of familial paroxysmal polyserositis remains obscure, but in the absence of complications the prognosis is good. Unfortunately, secondary amyloidosis, which results in renal failure, is a frequent complication. Colchicine taken at the time of prodromal symptoms often aborts an acute attack of the disease.

Retroperitoneal Fibrosis

Idiopathic retroperitoneal fibrosis, an uncommon fibrosing condition of the abdomen, becomes symptomatic when it causes **obstruction of the ureters.** Although no cause is discernible in most cases, the disorder has been linked to treatment of migraine headaches with methysergide. A similar idiopathic fibrosis has also been described in the mediastinum and may affect the mesentery.

Neoplasms

Mesenteric and Omental Cysts

Mesenteric and omental cysts are generally of lymphatic origin but may derive from other embryonic tissues. Usually a slowly enlarging, painless mass is discovered in a child over the age of 10 years. The cyst may come to medical attention because of rupture, bleeding, torsion, or intestinal obstruction. Surgical excision is curative.

Mesothelioma

One-quarter of all mesotheliomas arise in the peritoneum, and mesotheliomas are the most common primary tumor of that tissue. Like pleural mesotheliomas, most of these malignant tumors are associated with exposure to asbestos. The pathologic characteristics of peritoneal mesotheliomas are identical to those of their pleural counterparts, described in Chapter 12.

By far the most common malignant disorder of the peritoneum is **metastatic carcinoma,** although peritoneal involvement is also common in intestinal lymphoma. Ovarian and pancreatic carcinomas are particularly likely to seed the peritoneum, but any intra-abdominal carcinoma can spread to the peritoneum.

Rarely, large retroperitoneal soft tissue tumors, such as lipomas, fibromas, myxomas, and mixtures of these mesenchymal elements, are encountered. They may attain a very large size and are not uncommonly sarcomatous.

SUGGESTED READING

Books

Berk JE, Haubrich WS, Kalser MH, et al (eds): Bockus Gastroenterology, 4th ed. Philadelphia, WB Saunders, 1985

Enterline H, Thompson J: Pathology of the Esophagus. New York, Springer-Verlag, 1984

Morson BC, Sawson IMP: Gastrointestinal Pathology, 2nd ed. Oxford, Blackwell Scientific, 1979

Sleisenger MH, Fordtran JS (eds): Gastrointestinal Disease, 3rd ed. Philadelphia, WB Saunders, 1983

Spiro HM: Clinical Gastroenterology, 3rd ed. New York, Macmillan, 1983

Review Articles

Calkins BM, Mendeloff AI: Epidemiology of inflammatory bowel disease. Epidemiol Rev 8:60, 1986

Cole SG, Kagnoff MF: Celiac disease. Annu Rev Nutr 5:241, 1984

Collins RH Jr., Feldman M, Fordtran JS: Colon cancer, dysplasia, and surveillance in patients with ulcerative colitis. A critical reveiw. N Engl J Med 316:1654, 1987

Correa P, Haenszel W, Tannenbaum S: Epidemiology of gastric carcinoma. Natl Cancer Inst Monogr 62:129, 1982

Green PH, O'Toole KM, Weinberg LM, et al: Early gastric cancer. Gastroenterology 81:247, 1981

Guth PH: Pathogenesis of gastric mucosal injury. Annu Rev Med 33:183, 1982

Janowitz HD: Crohn's disease—50 years later. N Engl J Med 304:1600, 1981

Joint Iran/IARC Study Group: Oesophageal cancer studies in the Caspian Littoral of Iran. Results of population studies—a prodrome. J Natl Cancer Inst 59:1127, 1977

Kritchevsky D: Diet, nutrition and cancer. The role of fiber. Cancer 58:1830, 1986

Mayberry JF: Some aspects of the epidemiology of ulcerative colitis. Gut 26:968, 1985

Mayberry JF, Rhodes J: Epidemiological aspects of Crohn's disease: A review of the literature. Gut 25:886, 899, 1984

Szabo S: Pathogenesis of duodenal ulcer disease. Lab Invest 51:121, 1984

14 The Liver and Biliary System

Emanuel Rubin and John L. Farber

The Liver

Anatomy

Functions

Bilirubin Metabolism and the Mechanisms of Jaundice

Hepatic Failure

Acute Viral Hepatitis

Chronic Hepatitis

The Pathology of Acute and Chronic Hepatitis

Alcoholic Liver Disease

Primary Biliary Cirrhosis

Cirrhosis

Portal Hypertension

Toxic Liver Injury

Vascular Disorders

Nonviral Infections of the Liver

Neonatal Hepatitis

Neoplasms

The Pathology of Liver Transplantation

The Gallbladder and Extrahepatic Bile Ducts

Anatomy

Congenital Anomalies

Cholelithiasis

Acute Cholecystitis

Chronic Cholecystitis

Cholesterolosis

Primary Sclerosing Cholangitis

Neoplasms

Figure 14-1. Microanatomy of the liver.

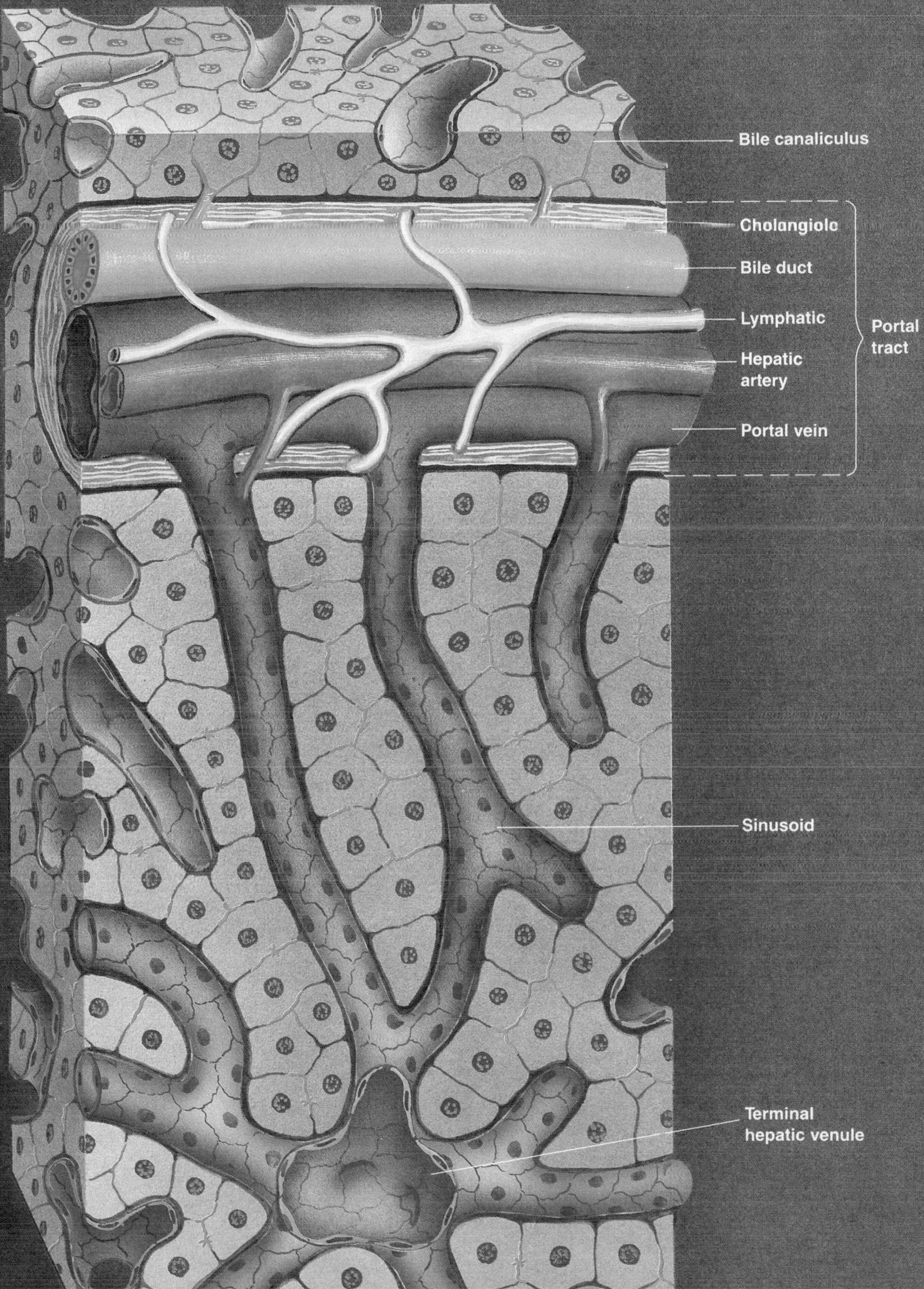

Bile canaliculus

Cholangiole

Bile duct

Lymphatic

Hepatic artery

Portal vein

Portal tract

Sinusoid

Terminal hepatic venule

Dimitri
k

The Liver
Anatomy

The liver arises from the embryonic foregut as an entodermal bud that differentiates into the hepatic diverticulum. Strands of entodermal cells mingle with proliferating mesenchymal cells to form all the structures of the adult liver, the gallbladder, and the extrahepatic biliary ducts.

The liver is the largest visceral organ in the body; in the average adult man it weighs about 1500 g. Situated in the right upper quadrant of the abdomen immediately below the diaphragm, it consists of two lobes, a larger right lobe and a smaller left lobe, separated on the surface by the falciform ligament. Inferiorly, the right lobe exhibits lesser segments, the caudate and quadrate lobes. The gallbladder is located inferiorly in a fossa of the right hepatic lobe and normally extends slightly beyond the inferior margin of the liver.

The liver has a dual blood supply consisting of the hepatic artery, a branch of the celiac axis, and the portal vein, formed by the convergence of the splenic and superior mesenteric veins. The hepatic veins drain into the inferior vena cava, which is in intimate contact with and partly surrounded by the posterior surface of the liver. The hepatic lymphatics drain principally into lymph nodes of the porta hepatis and the celiac axis. The hepatic nerve plexus is innervated from the vagus and phrenic nerves and the lower thoracic sympathetic ganglia.

The common hepatic duct, formed by the union of the right and left hepatic ducts, receives the cystic duct from the gallbladder to form the common bile duct. Just before entering the duodenum, the common bile duct joins with the pancreatic duct. It terminates in the ampulla of Vater, where its lumen is guarded by the sphincter of Oddi.

An understanding of the microscopic structure of the liver is crucial for an appreciation of liver pathology. **The basic unit is the polyhedral lobule** (Figs. 14-2, 14-3), classically depicted as a hexagon. **Portal**

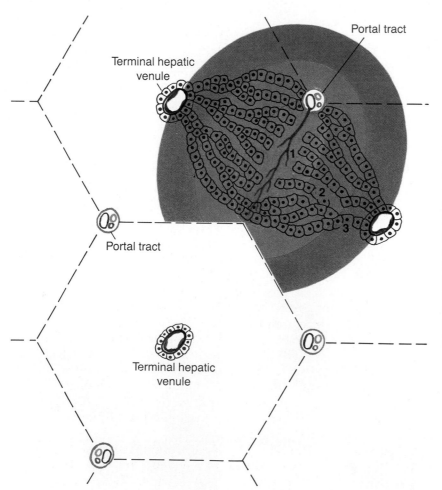

Figure 14-2. Morphologic and functional concepts of the liver lobule. In the **classic,** morphologic liver lobule, the periphery of the hexagonal lobule is anchored in the portal tracts, and the terminal hepatic venule is in the center. The **functional** liver lobule is an acinus derived from the gradients of oxygen and nutrients in the sinusoidal blood. In this scheme the portal tract, with the richest content of oxygen and nutrients, is in the center (*zone 1*). The region most distant from the portal tract (*zone 3*) is poor in oxygen and nutrients and surrounds the terminal hepatic venule.

Portal tract

Terminal hepatic venule

Portal tract

Terminal hepatic venule

triads (or portal tracts) are found peripherally at the angles of the polygon. These portal triads—so named because they contain intrahepatic branches of the **bile ducts, hepatic artery, and portal vein**—are collagenous zones surrounded by an adjacent circumferential layer of hepatocytes called the limiting plate. As its name implies, the **central vein** (also known as the terminal hepatic venule) resides in the center of the lobule. Radiating from it are **one-cell-thick plates of hepatocytes,** which extend to the perimeter of the lobule, where they are continuous with the plates of other lobules. Between the plates of hepatocytes are the hepatic sinusoids, which are lined by endothelial cells and Kupffer cells.

The large blood vessels that enter the liver at the porta hepatis eventually divide into the small interlobular branches of the hepatic artery and portal vein in the portal triads. From the portal triads the interlobular vessels distribute blood to the hepatic sinusoids, where it flows centripetally into the central vein. The central veins coalesce to form sublobular veins, which eventually merge into the hepatic veins.

Bile flows in the opposite direction to the blood. Bile is secreted by hepatocytes into the bile canaliculi, formed by the apposed lateral surfaces of contiguous hepatocytes. From the canaliculi the bile flows into the bile ductules (canals of Hering or cholangioles) at the border of the portal tract, and then enters a branch of the intrahepatic bile duct. Within each lobe of the liver, smaller bile ducts progressively merge, eventually forming the right and left hepatic ducts.

The classic lobule described above is depicted as arranged around the central vein simply because of the histologic appearance of the liver. However, from a functional point of view, **the lobule can also be thought of as an acinus with its center in the portal tract** (see Fig. 14-2). Such a concept takes into account the functional gradients that exist within the lobule. Concentrations of oxygen, nutrients, and hormones in the blood are highest at the portal tracts and progressively decline as the blood courses through the sinusoids to the central vein. This functional heterogeneity of the liver lobule can be expressed in terms of concentric functional zones around portal tracts. Zone 1, the most highly oxygenated zone, encircles the portal tracts, whereas zone 3, which surrounds the central veins, is oxygen-poor. The intermediate or mid-lobular area is referred to as zone 2. For convenience, pathologic changes in the liver are usually designated in relation to the classic histologic lobule. For example, centrilobular necrosis refers to a lesion around the central veins, whereas periportal fibrosis is seen at the periphery of the classic lobule.

About 80% of the total cell population of the liver

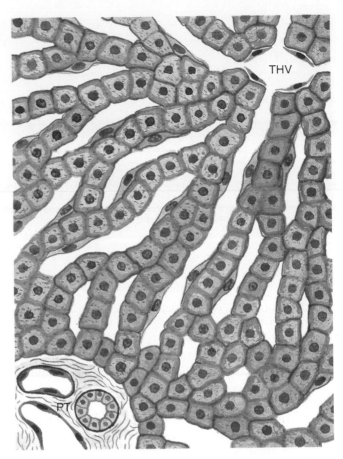

Figure 14-3. Schematic representation of the normal liver lobule. The portal tract (*PT*) contains branches of the hepatic artery, portal vein, and interlobular bile duct. The liver cells plates converge to the terminal hepatic venule (*THV*).

consists of hepatocytes. The hepatocyte, roughly 30 μm across, has three specialized surfaces, sinusoidal, lateral, and canalicular. Each cell has two sinusoidal surfaces, which exhibit numerous slender microvilli. The sinusoidal surface is separated from the endothelial cells that line the sinusoids by the space of Disse (Fig. 14-4). The canalicular surfaces of adjacent hepatocytes form the **bile canaliculus,** a collecting structure that is actually an intercellular space without a separate and distinct wall. The canalicular surface displays microvilli extending into the lumen. Leakage of bile from the canaliculus is prevented by a tight junctional complex between adjacent hepatocytes. The lateral, or intercellular, surfaces of adjacent hepatocytes are in close contact and contain gap junctions.

The centrally placed, spherical nucleus of the hepatocyte exhibits one or more nucleoli. The nuclei vary in size in ratios of 2, 4, and 8—values that

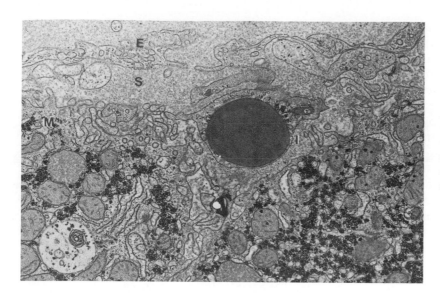

Figure 14-4. The space of Disse. An electron micrograph shows the space of Disse (*S*) outlined on one side by a fenestrated endothelial cell (*E*) and on the other by the surface microvilli (*M*) of two hepatocytes and a portion of an Ito cell (*I*).

correspond to differences in ploidy (DNA content). About half of the nuclei are polyploid, and about one-quarter of the hepatocytes are binucleate. The cytoplasm is rich in organelles and shows prominent rough and smooth endoplasmic reticulum, Golgi complexes, mitochondria, lysosomes, and peroxisomes. In addition, in the fed state, abundant glycogen and occasional fat droplets are evident.

The sinusoid is lined by a sheet of endothelial cells, which is penetrated by numerous holes called fenestrae. Unlike their counterparts in other tissues, adjacent endothelial cells do not form junctions and leave many gaps between them. The result is a sieve-like structure that affords free communication between the sinusoidal lumen and the space of Disse. Free access of sinusoidal plasma to the hepatocyte is further facilitated by the absence of a basement membrane between the endothelial and liver cells.

The phagocytic Kupffer cells, which lack fenestrae, are located either in the gaps between adjacent endothelial cells or on their surface. (The Kupffer cells belong to the monocyte-macrophage system derived from the bone marrow. For that reason, after liver transplantation, the Kupffer cell population eventually originates from the recipient rather than the donor.) Beneath the endothelial cells in the space of Disse are found occasional cells with specialized storage capacities (Ito cells). These cells contain fat, vitamin A, and other lipid-soluble vitamins. The most abundant extracellular matrix component in the space of Disse is fibronectin. Occasional bundles of type I collagen fibers provide the scaffold of the liver lobule. There is no continuous connective tissue barrier between the plasma and the surface of the hepatocyte, although by light microscopy reticulin stains impart the false impression of a continuous membrane.

Functions

Although the hepatocyte is clearly a highly differentiated cell, it subserves a wide variety of functions. These can be broadly categorized as metabolic, synthetic, storage, catabolic, and excretory functions, with the understanding that there is substantial overlap between these divisions. The following are representative functions in each category.

Metabolic Functions   The liver is the central organ of glucose homeostasis, and responds rapidly to fluctuations in the concentration of blood glucose. In the fed state excess blood glucose is shunted to the liver to be stored as glycogen; in the fasting state the liver maintains blood glucose levels by glycogenolysis and gluconeogenesis. For gluconeogenesis the liver uses amino acids; the nitrogenous portion is converted to urea. In the fasting state, during which energy is derived from the oxidation of fat, free fatty acids are taken up by the liver, converted to triglycerides, and secreted in the form of lipoproteins to be used elsewhere.

Synthetic Functions   Most serum proteins, with the major exception of the immunoglobulins, are synthesized in the liver. Albumin is the principal source of plasma oncotic pressure, and its decrease in chronic liver disease contributes to the development of edema and ascites. Blood coagulation depends on the continuous production of clotting factors, most of which, including prothrombin and fibrinogen, are synthesized by hepatocytes. Liver failure is thus characterized by a severe and often life-threatening bleeding diathesis. It is also interesting that endothelial cells of the liver manufacture Factor VIII, and hemophilia has been reported to be ameliorated by liver transplantation. Complement and other acute-phase reactants are also secreted by the liver, as are numerous specific binding proteins—for example, the binding proteins for iron, copper, and vitamin A. Again, Wilson's disease, a disorder of copper metabolism that is associated with deficient ceruloplasmin production by the liver, is cured by liver transplantation.

Storage Functions   The liver is an important storage site for glycogen, triglycerides, iron, copper, and lipid-soluble vitamins. Severe liver disease can result from excessive storage—for instance, glycogen in type IV glycogenosis and excess iron in hemochromatosis.

Catabolic Functions   Endogenous substances, including hormones and serum proteins, are catabolized by the liver in order to maintain a balance between their production and their elimination. Thus, in chronic liver disease impaired catabolism of estrogens contributes to feminization in men. The liver is also the principal site for the detoxification of foreign compounds (xenobiotics), such as drugs, industrial chemicals, environmental contaminants, and perhaps products of bacterial metabolism in the intestine.

Excretory Functions   The principal excretory product of the liver is bile, a material that not only provides a repository for the products of heme catabolism but also is vital for fat absorption in the small intestine.

Bilirubin Metabolism and the Mechanisms of Jaundice

Normal Bilirubin Metabolism

Bilirubin, the major end product of heme catabolism, has no known physiologic function, although a role as an antioxidant has been suggested. Up to 85% of bilirubin is derived from senescent red blood cells, which are removed from the circulation by mononuclear phagocytes of the spleen, bone marrow, and liver. The remaining bilirubin arises from the degradation of heme produced from other sources, the most important of which is the premature breakdown of hemoglobin in developing erythroid cells in the bone marrow. The amount of bilirubin produced from the turnover of non-hemoglobin hemoproteins—for instance, the mitochondrial and microsomal cytochromes—is small and does not ordinarily contribute to the development of jaundice.

Bilirubin is released from phagocytes and other cells into the circulation, where it is bound to albumin for transport to the liver. Albumin in the circulation and the extracellular space constitutes a large binding reservoir for bilirubin and ensures a low extracellular concentration of free (unbound) bilirubin. Free bilirubin, unlike that bound to albumin or conjugated with glucuronic acid, is toxic to the brain. In this respect, it is important to note that certain drugs that compete with bilirubin for binding sites on albumin—for example, sulfonamides and salicylates—tend to shift bilirubin from the plasma into tissues and thereby increase its cytotoxicity.

On reaching the sinusoidal plasma membrane of the hepatocyte, the albumin-bilirubin complex is dissociated by a mechanism that is poorly understood. It is still debated whether the albumin-bilirubin complex dissociates to release unbound bilirubin for transport across the plasma membrane or binds to a recognition site on the membrane and then transfers bilirubin directly to the membrane transport system. Within the cell free bilirubin is again bound to protein, in this case two cytoplasmic proteins termed **ligandin** and **fatty-acid binding protein.** These anion-binding or "carrier" proteins transfer bilirubin to the endoplasmic reticulum, which contains the UDP-glucuronyltransferase system responsible for the conjugation of bilirubin with glucuronic acid. This reaction principally forms water-soluble bilirubin diglucuronide and a small amount (less than 10%) of the monoglucuronide. The conjugated bilirubin diffuses through the cytosol to the bile canaliculus, where it is excreted into the bile by a carrier-mediated process that is the rate-limiting step for overall transhepatic transport of bilirubin.

After its excretion into the small intestine in bile, conjugated bilirubin is not absorbed and remains intact until it reaches the distal small bowel and colon, where it is hydrolyzed by the bacterial flora to free bilirubin. In turn, the unconjugated bilirubin is reduced to a mixture of pyrroles, known collectively as **urobilinogen.** While most of the urobilinogen is excreted in the feces, a small proportion is absorbed in the terminal ileum and colon, returned to the liver, and re-excreted into the bile; this entire process is termed the **enterohepatic circulation of bile.** Some urobilinogen escapes reabsorption by the liver and reaches the systemic circulation, after which it is excreted in the urine.

An increased concentration of bilirubin in the blood (> 1.0 mg/dl) is termed **hyperbilirubinemia.** When the circulating bilirubin concentration attains levels greater than 2.0 mg/dl to 2.5 mg/dl, the skin and sclerae become yellow, in which case the condition is known as **jaundice** or **icterus.** As shown in Figure 14-5, many conditions are associated with hyperbilirubinemia. Overproduction of bilirubin, interference with hepatic uptake or intracellular metabolism of bilirubin, and impairment of bile excretion are all causes of jaundice.

Overproduction of Bilirubin

An increased production of bilirubin results from **increased destruction of red blood cells**—that is, hemolytic anemia—or ineffective erythropoiesis (dyserythropoiesis). In unusual circumstances the breakdown of the erythrocytes in a large hematoma may also provide excess bilirubin.

In the adult even severe hemolytic anemia does not produce a sustained rise in serum bilirubin concentration beyond 4.0 mg/dl, provided that hepatic bilirubin clearance remains normal. However, the combination of prolonged hemolysis, as in sickle cell anemia, and intrinsic liver disease, such as viral hepatitis, leads to extraordinarily high levels of circulating bilirubin and pronounced jaundice. The hyperbilirubinemia of uncomplicated hemolytic disease principally involves unconjugated bilirubin, whereas in parenchymal liver disease both conjugated and unconjugated bilirubin participate. Although the unconjugated hyperbilirubinemia of hemolytic disease is of little clinical significance in the adult, in the newborn it may be catastrophic. As discussed in Chapter 6, which deals with genetic and childhood diseases, hemolytic disease of the newborn may result in concentrations of unconjugated bilirubin high enough to cause damage to the brain **(kernicterus).** Kernicterus has generally been associated with bilirubin concentrations over 20 mg/dl, but subtle degrees of psychomotor retardation may follow considerably lower bilirubin concentrations.

In disorders characterized by ineffective erythropoiesis—for example, megaloblastic and sideroblastic anemias—the fraction of bilirubin derived from the bone marrow may be increased to the point that hyperbilirubinemia develops. A rare hereditary disease of unknown etiology, **primary shunt hyperbilirubinemia,** or **idiopathic dyserythropoietic jaundice,** is characterized by massive overproduction of bilirubin in the bone marrow and is associated with chronic unconjugated hyperbilirubinemia. The bone marrow shows conspicuous erythroid hyperplasia and erythrophagocytosis, and iron turnover is augmented.

Decreased Hepatic Uptake

Hyperbilirubinemia can result from impaired hepatic uptake of unconjugated bilirubin. Such a situation is seen in generalized liver cell injury, exemplified by viral hepatitis. Certain drugs—for example, rifampin and probenecid—interfere with the net uptake of bilirubin by the liver cell and may produce a mild unconjugated hyperbilirubinemia.

Decreased Bilirubin Conjugation

Crigler-Najjar Disease

The closest condition to a pure inherited defect in bilirubin conjugation is **Crigler-Najjar disease,** Type I. In this recessively inherited malady, little or no bilirubin is conjugated in the hepatocyte and the patients suffer from **unremitting unconjugated hyperbilirubinemia.** The defect resides in a **complete absence of UDP-glucuronyltransferase activity.** Patients with this disorder cannot synthesize the missing enzyme: treatment with phenobarbital, an inducer of microsomal enzymes, is without effect. Infants with Crigler-Najjar disease invariably develop bilirubin encephalopathy and usually die in the first year of life. A few patients have reached adolescence, only to develop inexplicably a fatal bilirubin encephalopathy. The bile in this condition, which contains no conjugated bilirubin and no more than trace amounts of unconjugated bilirubin, is colorless. The liver is histologically normal, although, for reasons unknown, occasional canalicular bile thrombi are present. The hepatocytes also appear normal by electron microscopy, except for minor nonspecific changes.

Figure 14-5.   Mechanisms of jaundice at the level of the hepatocyte. Bilirubin is derived principally from the senescence of circulating red blood cells, with a smaller contribution from the degradation of erythropoietic elements in the bone marrow, myoglobin, and extraerythroid cytochromes. Jaundice results from overproduction of bilirubin (hemolytic anemia) or defects in its hepatic metabolism. The locations of specific blocks in the metabolic pathway of bilirubin in the hepatocyte are illustrated.

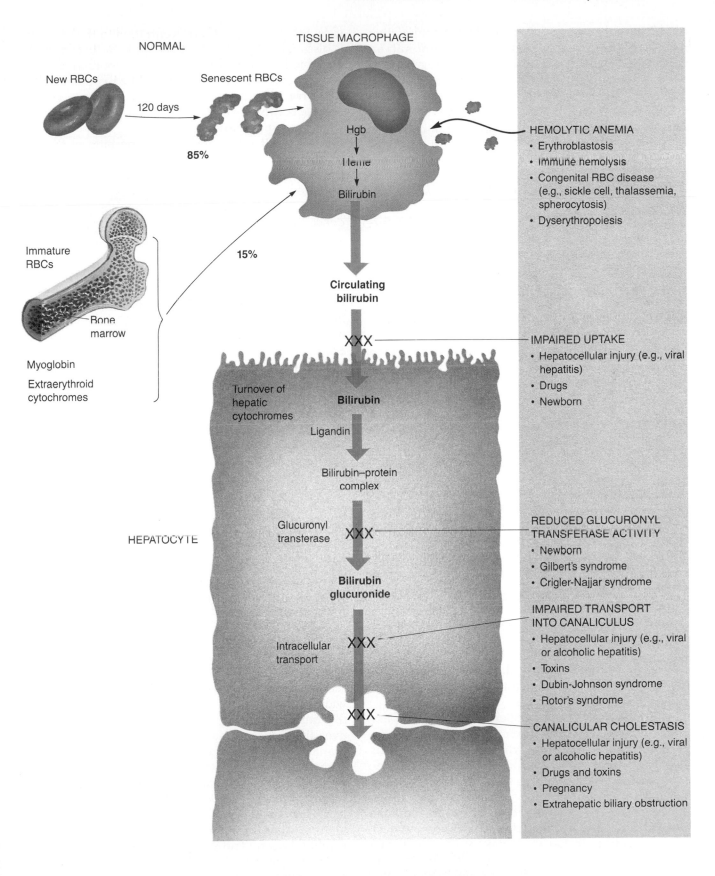

NORMAL

TISSUE MACROPHAGE

New RBCs

Senescent RBCs

120 days

85%

Hgb

Heme

Bilirubin

Immature RBCs

Bone marrow

Myoglobin

Extraerythroid cytochromes

15%

Circulating bilirubin

XXX

Turnover of hepatic cytochromes

Bilirubin

Ligandin

Bilirubin–protein complex

HEPATOCYTE

Glucuronyl transferase

XXX

Bilirubin glucuronide

Intracellular transport

XXX

XXX

HEMOLYTIC ANEMIA
- Erythroblastosis
- Immune hemolysis
- Congenital RBC disease (e.g., sickle cell, thalassemia, spherocytosis)
- Dyserythropoiesis

IMPAIRED UPTAKE
- Hepatocellular injury (e.g., viral hepatitis)
- Drugs
- Newborn

REDUCED GLUCURONYL TRANSFERASE ACTIVITY
- Newborn
- Gilbert's syndrome
- Crigler-Najjar syndrome

IMPAIRED TRANSPORT INTO CANALICULUS
- Hepatocellular injury (e.g., viral or alcoholic hepatitis)
- Toxins
- Dubin-Johnson syndrome
- Rotor's syndrome

CANALICULAR CHOLESTASIS
- Hepatocellular injury (e.g., viral or alcoholic hepatitis)
- Drugs and toxins
- Pregnancy
- Extrahepatic biliary obstruction

Much information relating to bilirubin conjugation has been obtained from studies in the Gunn rat, an animal that exhibits an inherited unconjugated hyperbilirubinemia virtually identical to Crigler-Najjar disease, Type I. These animals have no detectable hepatic UDP-glucuronyltransferase activity, suffer lifelong jaundice, and develop bilirubin encephalopathy. Like patients with Crigler-Najjar disease, Type I, these rats do not respond to phenobarbital treatment.

Type II Crigler-Najjar disease is similar to but less severe than Type I, and manifests only a partial decrease in the activity of UDP-glucuronyltransferase. Hepatocytes in affected persons have some capacity to synthesize this enzyme, and treatment with phenobarbital induces a decrease in unconjugated hyperbilirubinemia. This feature is the most reliable criterion for distinguishing Type II from Type I Crigler-Najjar disease. Almost all patients with Type II disease develop normally, but in some, kernicterus may lead to bilirubin encephalopathy. Type II disease is unquestionably familial, but the exact mode of inheritance is unclear.

Gilbert's Syndrome

Gilbert's syndrome is defined as an **inherited, mild, chronic unconjugated hyperbilirubinemia (< 6 mg/dl) that is caused by impaired clearance of bilirubin in the absence of any detectable functional or structural liver disease.** Gilbert's syndrome occurs in 3% to 7% of the population, more often in men than women, and is usually recognized after puberty. The sex differences and the age at onset suggest that hormones influence the modulation of bilirubin metabolism in the liver. It has long been known that factors that increase serum bilirubin concentrations in normal people, such as fasting or an intercurrent illness, produce an exaggerated increase in serum bilirubin levels in persons with Gilbert's syndrome. This effect probably reflects the initially higher bilirubin level rather than any intrinsic difference in the physiologic response to stress.

Although most cases of Gilbert's syndrome appear to be inherited in an autosomal dominant fashion, sporadic cases also occur in which there is no familial history of the disease. The precise defect in the hepatic clearance of bilirubin in Gilbert's syndrome has not been defined, but the disease is most likely caused by an **inherited defect in bilirubin conjugation.** A number of early studies were interpreted as showing defects in hepatic uptake of bilirubin, but newer evidence does not support such a contention for either Gilbert's syndrome or Crigler-Najjar dis-

ease. Since the ligandin concentration in the liver cell is also normal, it does not seem likely that intracellular binding of bilirubin or its transport to the endoplasmic reticulum is impaired. **The hypothesis that defective bilirubin conjugation is the cause of the disease is strongly buttressed by the observation that UDP-glucuronyltransferase activity is reduced in practically all cases.** As a result the ratio of the diglucuronide to the monoglucuronide conjugates in the bile is conspicuously decreased, a change that is also observed in Crigler-Najjar disease, Type II, and the heterozygous Gunn rat. Despite the strong evidence for a defect in bilirubin conjugation, however, a number of puzzling observations remain to be explained. Most of these center on the lack of a correlation between UDP-glucuronyltransferase levels and hyperbilirubinemia in other diseases, and the fact that phenobarbital, the administration of which ameliorates the hyperbilirubinemia of Gilbert's syndrome, does not necessarily lead to increased enzyme activity.

Gilbert's syndrome is, for the most part, asymptomatic, although vague symptoms of lassitude and weakness are common. These symptoms are possibly related to the anxiety engendered by the discovery of a chronically elevated bilirubin level rather than to the disease itself. Mild hemolysis is thought to occur in more than half of those with Gilbert's syndrome, but the mechanism is unclear.

Decreased Intracellular Transport of Conjugated Bilirubin

Dubin-Johnson Syndrome

Dubin-Johnson syndrome is a familial disease recognized by chronic or intermittent jaundice, accompanied by a "black" liver. The conjugated hyperbilirubinemia is caused by a defect in the transport of conjugated bilirubin from the hepatocyte to the canalicular lumen. This defect probably reflects a wider impairment of organic anion excretion, since the transhepatic transport of a number of anionic dyes (bromsulfophthalein [BSP], rose bengal, indocyanine green) is also diminished. In addition, there is an accompanying defect in the hepatic excretion of coproporphyrins. The color of the liver reflects the accumulation of a dark-brown pigment in the hepatocytes. Interestingly, a mutant Corriedale sheep exhibits a syndrome indistinguishable from human Dubin-Johnson syndrome.

The syndrome is inherited in an autosomal recessive fashion. It is rare among most populations, but

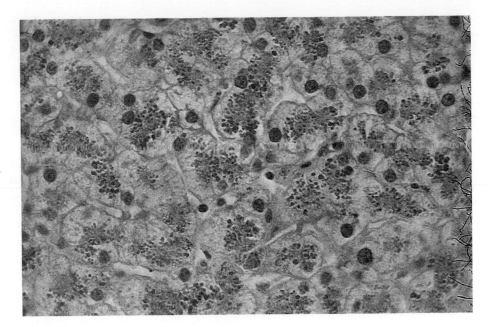

Figure 14-6. Dubin-Johnson syndrome. The hepatocytes contain coarse, iron-free, dark-brown granules.

certain groups that tend to have high rates of intermarriage, such as Iranian Jews and Japanese in remote areas, have a considerably higher incidence. Except for mild intermittent jaundice, most patients do not complain of any symptoms. As in Gilbert's syndrome, vague nonspecific complaints are common. Half of those affected have dark urine. In women the disease may be discovered when jaundice appears during pregnancy or as a result of the use of oral contraceptives. The serum bilirubin varies from 2 mg/dl to 5 mg/dl, although it may be much higher transiently. About 60% of the increased bilirubin in the serum is conjugated.

The microscopic appearance of the liver is entirely normal, except for the accumulation of coarse, iron-free, dark-brown granules in hepatocytes and Kupffer cells, primarily in the centrilobular zone (Fig. 14-6). By electron microscopy the pigment is seen in enlarged lysosomes. The nature of the pigment is not conclusively established, but available evidence suggests that it is related to melanin.

Rotor's Syndrome

Rotor's syndrome, a familial conjugated hyperbilirubinemia, is similar to the Dubin-Johnson syndrome but there is no associated pigmentation of the liver. Moreover, there are significant differences in the excretion of dyes and coproporphyrins. As in the Dubin-Johnson syndrome, patients with Rotor's syndrome have few symptoms and lead normal lives.

Benign Recurrent Cholestasis

Self-limited, periodic episodes of intrahepatic cholestasis preceded by malaise and itching constitute the hallmarks of benign recurrent cholestasis. Symptoms may last from several weeks to several months, although periods of several years have been reported. The mean number of attacks in a lifetime is three to five, but a significant proportion of affected persons have as many as ten attacks. Recurrences have been noted at intervals of weeks to years. Serum bilirubin level during the acute episodes is in the range of 10 mg/dl to 20 mg/dl, and most of the bilirubin is conjugated. Serum alkaline phosphatase activity is significantly increased, while that of aminotransferase is only slightly elevated. The liver shows centrilobular cholestasis and a few mononuclear inflammatory cells in the portal tracts. All the structural and functional alterations disappear during remissions, and no permanent sequelae have been reported. The cause is unknown.

Familial Fatal Intrahepatic Cholestasis (Byler Disease)

Familial fatal intrahepatic cholestasis was originally described among several Amish families, all of whom were named Byler. Since then, other familial cases have been reported. The disorder is inherited as an autosomal recessive trait. Infants develop cholestatic jaundice, after which cirrhosis gradually develops. There is an associated high incidence of retinitis pigmentosa, and the children are often mentally retarded. Death from liver disease usually supervenes by the time of adolescence. The pathogenesis is not understood.

Neonatal Jaundice

In the fetus the transhepatic clearance of bilirubin is negligible; hepatic uptake, conjugation, and biliary excretion are all much lower than in children and adults. Hepatic UDP-glucuronyltransferase activity is only 10% of that in adults, and ligandin levels are low. Nevertheless, fetal bilirubin levels remain low because bilirubin traverses the placenta, after which it is conjugated and excreted by the maternal liver.

The liver of the neonate assumes the responsibility for bilirubin clearance before its conjugating and excretory capacities are fully developed. Moreover, the demands on the liver in the neonate are actually increased, because of an augmented destruction of circulating red blood cells during this period. As a consequence **the normal neonate exhibits a transient, physiologic, unconjugated hyperbilirubinemia.** This physiologic jaundice is more pronounced in premature infants, both because the hepatic clearance of bilirubin is less developed and because the turnover of red blood cells is more pronounced than in the term infant. The hepatic bilirubin conjugating capacity reaches adult levels about 2 weeks after birth; the ligandin level takes somewhat longer to reach adult values. As a result of this hepatic maturation, serum bilirubin levels rapidly decline to adult values shortly after birth.

In cases of maternal-fetal blood group incompatibilities that lead to erythroblastosis fetalis (see Chapter 6), a striking overproduction of bilirubin in the fetus results from immune-mediated hemolysis. However, although newborns with erythroblastosis fetalis display increased bilirubin levels in cord blood, jaundice only becomes severe after birth, because maternal metabolism of bilirubin no longer compensates for the immaturity of the neonatal liver.

Impairment of Canalicular Bile Flow

The secretion of bile into the canaliculus and its passage into the biliary collecting system is an active process that depends on a number of factors, including (a) the functional and structural characteristics of the canalicular microvilli, (b) the permeability of the canalicular plasma membrane, (c) the intracellular contractile system surrounding the canaliculus (mi-

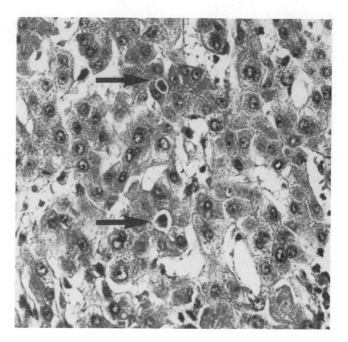

Figure 14-7.   Bile stasis. A photomicrograph of liver shows prominent bile plugs (*arrows*) in dilated bile canaliculi. The hepatocytes around the bile plugs are arranged in an acinar fashion.

crofilaments, microtubules), and (d) the interaction of bile acids with the secretory apparatus.

Cholestasis is defined by three distinct criteria: morphologic, clinical, and functional. **The pathologist defines cholestasis as the morphologic demonstration of visible biliary pigment within bile canaliculi and hepatocytes (Fig. 14-7).** The clinical diagnosis is based on the accumulation in the blood of materials normally transferred to the bile, including bilirubin, cholesterol, and bile acids, and the presence in the blood of elevated activities of certain enzymes, typically alkaline phosphatase. **Functionally, cholestasis represents a decrease in bile flow through the canaliculus and a reduction in the secretion of water, bilirubin, and bile acids by the hepatocyte.** Cholestasis may be produced by intrinsic liver disease, in which case the term **intrahepatic cholestasis** is used, or by obstruction of the large bile ducts, a condition known as **extrahepatic cholestasis.** In any event, cholestasis represents a defect in the transport of bile across the canalicular membrane.

Cellular Mechanisms of Cholestasis

The biochemical basis of cholestasis is not entirely clear, but a number of abnormalities in the formation and movement of bile have been described.

Lobular Distribution of Cholestasis   Both intrahepatic and extrahepatic cholestasis are characterized by an initially preferential **localization of visible bile pigment in the centrilobular zone** (Fig. 14-8). Although the basis for this distribution remains enigmatic, it may relate to both the gradient from portal tract to central zone in the formation of bile acids and the increased levels of microsomal mixed function oxidases in pericentral hepatocytes. Fluid secretion into the canalicular bile is divided into two components: one dependent on the secretion of bile acids and the other independent of bile acid secretion. Since the periportal hepatocytes secrete most of the bile acids, the fluid content in the periportal zone of the canaliculus is greater than that in the central zone, a condition that tends to keep bilirubin in solution. Moreover, the bile acids themselves, which act as detergents in the intestine, also solubilize aggregates of bilirubin. These properties may serve to limit the extent of peripheral, as opposed to central, bile deposition in cholestatic conditions. To the above factors is added the higher activity of microsomal mixed function oxidases in the central zone, which predisposes central hepatocytes to injury by activated oxygen species formed during the biotransformation of drugs and other toxins. Such an effect may promote the deposition of bile in the centrilobular areas in cholestatic disorders.

Damage to the Canalicular Plasma Membrane   The canalicular plasma membrane is the site of sodium (and therefore fluid) secretion into the bile. In addition, this membrane participates in the secretion of bile acids and bilirubin. The secretion of fluid is under the control of the Na^+–K^+–ATPase of the canalicular membrane. Alterations in the canalicular membrane by agents capable of perturbing its lipid structure (e.g., chlorpromazine) inhibit Na^+–K^+–ATPase and decrease bile flow. Similarly, ethinyl estradiol increases the cholesterol content of the canalicular membrane, inhibits ATPase, and interferes with bile flow. Both chlorpromazine and ethinyl estradiol may cause cholestasis in some people. Morphologic alterations in the canalicular membrane—for example, those associated with the infusion of certain monohydroxy bile acids, such as taurolithocholate—are also accompanied by a decreased bile flow. Although correlations between the physical structure and chemical composition of the canalicular membranes and bile flow are imperfect, the evidence suggests a causal relationship.

Alteration in the Contractile Properties of the Canaliculus   It has been shown by cinematography that bile is propelled along the canaliculus by a **peristalsis-**

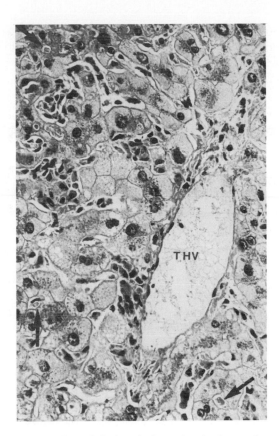

Figure 14-8.   Centrilobular cholestasis. A photomicrograph in the area of a terminal hepatic venule (*THV*) shows ballooned hepatocytes that contain prominent bile pigment granules. Bile plugs (*arrows*) in dilated bile canaliculi are evident. Foci of macrophages that have ingested bile are conspicuous.

like contractile activity of the hepatocytes. Agents that interact with the pericanalicular actin microfilaments (e.g., cytochalasin, phalloidin, and possibly chlorpromazine) inhibit this peristalsis and may cause cholestasis.

Alterations in the Permeability of the Canalicular Membrane   It has been suggested that certain agents that produce cholestasis, including estrogens and taurolithocholate, permit back-diffusion of bile components by making the canalicular membrane more permeable, or "leaky."

The effects of extrahepatic biliary obstruction clearly begin with increased pressure in the bile ducts. However, in the early stages the biochemical and morphologic events at the canalicular level are similar to those that occur with intrahepatic cholestasis, including **a centrilobular predilection for the appearance of canalicular bile plugs.**

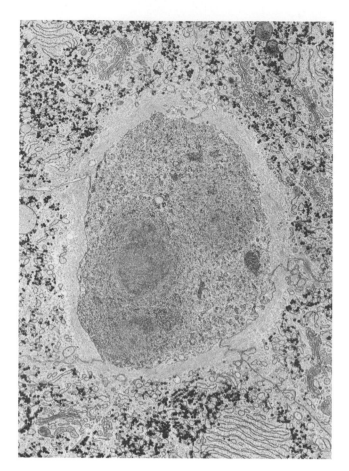

Figure 14-9. Cholestasis. An electron micrograph shows a distended bile canaliculus that has a thickened, filamentous ectoplasmic zone and encloses a granular bile plug.

The invariable presence of bile constituents in the blood of individuals with cholestasis implies a regurgitation from the hepatocyte into the bloodstream. The hepatic clearance of unconjugated bilirubin in cholestasis is normal, and the rise in the levels of bile pigments in the plasma is due to a reflux of monoconjugates and diconjugates of bilirubin into the blood. Even in the face of complete bile duct obstruction, the serum bilirubin level rises only as high as 30 mg/dl to 35 mg/dl. Renal excretion of bilirubin prevents further accumulation.

The Morphology of Cholestasis

The morphologic hallmark of cholestasis is the presence of brownish bile pigment within dilated canaliculi and in hepatocytes. By electron microscopy the canaliculus is enlarged, and the microvilli are usually blunted and decreased in number or even absent (Fig. 14-9). Although back-diffusion of bile may occur, the canalicular tight junctions are almost invariably preserved. By light microscopy, the biliary concretions appear homogeneous, but at the ultrastructural level they may have a variable appearance, including lamellar, crystalline, and granular forms. The pericanalicular zone of the hepatocyte is widened by an apparent increase in the number of microfilaments. Bile stasis in the hepatocyte is reflected in the presence of large, inhomogeneous, bile-laden lysosomes.

When cholestasis persists, secondary morphologic abnormalities develop. Scattered necrotic hepatocytes probably reflect a toxic effect of excess intracellular bile. Within the sinusoids, macrophages and lymphoid cells appear. The macrophages and resident Kupffer cells contain bile pigment and cellular debris. In general, these changes parallel the severity and duration of the cholestasis. **Whereas early cholestasis is restricted almost exclusively to the central zone, chronic cholestasis is marked by the appearance of bile plugs in the periphery of the lobule as well.** Cholestasis in the periphery of the lobule may reflect mechanical obstruction of the canaliculi by secondary proliferation of and damage to the bile ductules, which link the canaliculi with the smallest branches of the portal bile ducts. Periportal fibrosis further aggravates obstruction to bile flow into the biliary ducts. Although the exact mechanism responsible for this fibrosis in chronic cholestasis is not clear, injury to the ductular cells, ductular proliferation, and the escape of bile may contribute.

In longstanding cholestasis (usually the result of extrahepatic biliary obstruction), groups of hepatocytes manifest hydropic swelling accompanied by a diffuse impregnation with bile pigment and a reticulated appearance, a triad termed **feathery degeneration.** The necrosis of such cells, together with the accumulation of extravasated bile in the area, results in a golden-yellow focus of extracellular pigment and debris known as a **bile infarct** or **bile lake** (Fig. 14-10).

The sites of obstruction to the flow of bile in the liver are depicted in Figure 14-11.

Hepatic Failure

When either the mass of liver cells is sufficiently diminished or their function is impaired, hepatic failure ensues (Fig. 14-12). For instance, hepatic failure may result from the replacement of liver cells by metastatic carcinoma. By contrast, the liver cell mass is adequate in many cases of cirrhosis, but the associated vascular disorganization and consequent perfusion deficits result in impaired hepatocyte function and liver failure. Thus, the term "hepatic failure" does not refer to one specific morphologic change, but rather to a clinical syndrome that results from inadequate liver function. The consequences of acute and chronic failure are depicted in Figure 14-41, which deals with the complications of cirrhosis, the most common cause of hepatic failure.

Jaundice

Hepatic failure is always associated with jaundice as a result of an inadequate clearance of bilirubin by the diseased liver. The hyperbilirubinemia is for the most part conjugated, but on occasion increased erythrocyte turnover may lead to unconjugated hyperbilirubinemia, thereby aggravating the jaundice.

Hepatic Encephalopathy

Patients who suffer chronic liver failure, or in whom the portal circulation is diverted, show a variety of neurologic signs and symptoms collectively termed **hepatic encephalopathy.** With unrelenting liver failure, hepatic encephalopathy may progress from sleep disturbance, irritability, or personality changes in Stage I, to lethargy and disorientation in Stage II, deep somnolence in Stage III, and coma in Stage IV. This sequence may occur over a period of many months or evolve rapidly in days or weeks in cases of fulminant hepatic failure. Associated neurologic symptoms include a flapping tremor of the hands, called **asterixis,** and hyperactive reflexes in the earlier stages, extensor toe responses later, and a decerebrate posture in the terminal stages.

The pathogenesis of hepatic encephalopathy remains elusive. It is probable that the encephalopathy is caused in part by toxic compounds absorbed from the intestine that have escaped hepatic detoxification because of hepatocyte dysfunction or the existence of structural or functional vascular shunts. The latter mechanism is particularly evident after the surgical construction of a portal-systemic anastomosis (portal vein to inferior vena cava or its equivalent) for the relief of portal hypertension, which accounts for the synonym **portasystemic encephalopathy.**

Ammonia levels are usually increased in the blood and brain of patients with hepatic encephalopathy. Most of the body's ammonia is of dietary origin, coming from ingestion of ammonia in foods, digestion of proteins in the small intestine, and bacterial catabolism of dietary protein and urea secreted into the intestine. The hypothesis that ammonia has an important role in the pathogenesis of hepatic en-

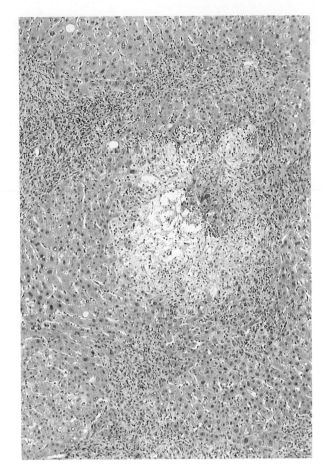

Figure 14-10. Bile infarct (bile lake). A photomicrograph of the liver in a patient with extrahepatic biliary obstruction shows an area of necrosis and the accumulation of extravasated bile.

cephalopathy is supported by the finding that patients with cirrhosis or a portacaval shunt can display the symptoms and signs of hepatic encephalopathy after ingesting ammonium salts, urea, or protein. However, the correlation between the increased concentration of blood ammonia and the severity of hepatic encephalopathy is inexact. In the brain, ammonia is converted to glutamine by astrocytes, and the glutamine concentration in cerebrospinal fluid correlates better with the degree of hepatic encephalopathy than does the blood level of ammonia.

Other substances may also be involved in the pathogenesis of hepatic encephalopathy. Among these are **mercaptans,** which result from the breakdown of sulfur-containing amino acids. The characteristic breath odor of patients with hepatic failure, termed **fetor hepaticus,** reflects the presence of mercaptans in saliva. Patients with cirrhosis who are fed methionine develop hepatic encephalopathy and the odor

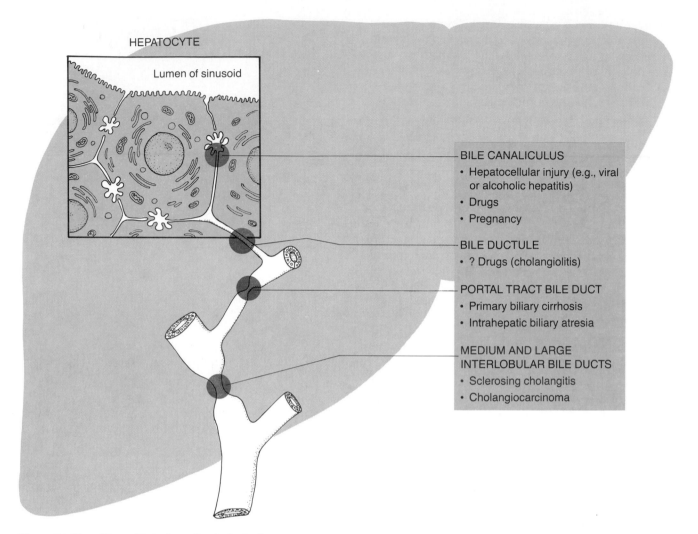

HEPATOCYTE

Lumen of sinusoid

BILE CANALICULUS
• Hepatocellular injury (e.g., viral or alcoholic hepatitis)
• Drugs
• Pregnancy

BILE DUCTULE
• ? Drugs (cholangiolitis)

PORTAL TRACT BILE DUCT
• Primary biliary cirrhosis
• Intrahepatic biliary atresia

MEDIUM AND LARGE INTERLOBULAR BILE DUCTS
• Sclerosing cholangitis
• Cholangiocarcinoma

Figure 14-11.   Sites of intrahepatic cholestasis.

of mercaptans, both of which regress after methionine withdrawal. One of the major inhibitory neurotransmitters in the brain, **gamma-aminobutyric acid (GABA),** is also produced by bacteria in the colon, and its blood and cerebrospinal fluid levels are elevated in hepatic failure. A role for GABA in the pathogenesis of hepatic coma is attractive, though unproved. Another hypothesis for the pathogenesis of hepatic encephalopathy holds that increased blood levels of aromatic amino acids, typical of hepatic failure, lead to decreased synthesis of normal neurotransmitters, such as norepinephrine, and augmented production of **false neurotransmitters,** such as octopamine. A toxic effect of **phenols** and **fatty acids** on the brain has also been postulated. Finally, there is experimental evidence for a disturbance in the blood–brain barrier in hepatic failure.

Morphologic changes in the brain of patients with acute or chronic hepatic encephalopathy are not large enough to account for the functional disturbances. In autopsy studies of patients who have died with chronic liver disease and hepatic coma, **the most striking changes are found in the astrocytes.** These cells are increased in number and size, and show the swelling, nuclear enlargement, and nuclear inclusions characteristic of **Alzheimer Type II astrocytes.** Interestingly, such changes can be produced in animals by portacaval shunts and chronic administration of ammonia. The deep layers of the cerebral cortex and subcortical white matter, the basal ganglia, and the cerebellum exhibit a laminar necrosis and a spongiform appearance.

In patients with fulminant hepatic failure, cerebral edema is commonly found at autopsy, often in con-

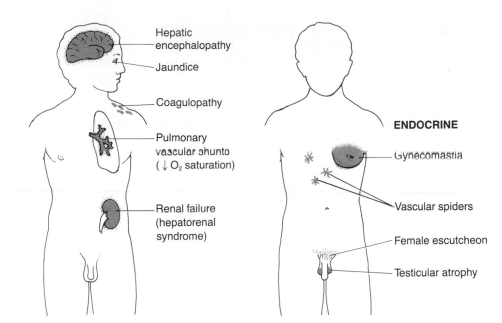

Figure 14-12. Complications of hepatic failure.

junction with uncal and cerebellar herniation. This edema is not regarded as simply a terminal event, but rather is considered a specific lesion associated with hepatic coma, although the precise mechanism is unclear.

Hepatorenal Syndrome

Acute hepatic failure is commonly marked by an associated renal failure characterized by azotemia, often with oliguria or anuria. Although the severity of renal failure does not necessarily parallel the extent of hepatic failure, renal failure usually indicates a poor prognosis. Curiously, the kidneys appear normal histologically and clearly maintain the ability to function normally. Kidneys from patients who have died of the hepatorenal syndrome function well when transplanted into recipients with chronic renal failure. Moreover, in patients with the hepatorenal syndrome, liver transplantation can restore renal function. Although no intrinsic renal disease can be demonstrated morphologically, at autopsy jaundiced patients with the hepatorenal syndrome show bile staining of renal tubular cells and bile casts in the lumina: the so-called **biliary nephrosis.** However, these morphologic alterations are not thought to contribute to the renal dysfunction.

The **major determinant of the hepatorenal syndrome seems to be a decrease in renal blood flow and a consequent reduction in glomerular filtration rate.** It is thought that a reduction in the effective circulating blood volume leads to compensatory renal vasoconstriction. The resulting decrease in renal perfusion and the shunting of blood from the cortex to the medulla lead to reduced glomerular filtration. It is also suspected that vasoactive substances produced by the failing liver, or inadequately cleared by it, contribute to the renal hemodynamic changes. Possible mediators are prostaglandins, renin and angiotensin, vasoactive intestinal peptide, endotoxin, and other poorly characterized vasoactive agents.

Defects of Coagulation

Bleeding often accompanies hepatic failure, in part because of defects in hemostasis that parallel the severity of the liver disease. The impairment of hemostasis is caused principally by **reduced hepatic synthesis of coagulation factors and by thrombocytopenia.** The decreased production of clotting factors (fibrinogen, prothrombin, and Factors V, VII, IX, and X) reflects the generalized impairment of protein synthesis by the liver. The prolonged prothrombin time is most closely related to the decrease in the plasma concentration of Factor VII.

Disseminated intravascular coagulation (DIC) may also occur in liver failure, and at least mild DIC may be universal in severe end-stage liver failure. Intravascular coagulation may reflect necrosis of liver cells, activation of Factor XII (Hageman factor) by endotoxin, or inadequate hepatic clearance of activated clotting factors from the circulation.

A low platelet count (less than 80,000 μl) occurs commonly in hepatic failure and is accompanied by qualitative abnormalities in platelet function. The thrombocytopenia may result from hypersplenism, bone marrow depression, or the consumption of circulating platelets by intravascular coagulation.

Hypoalbuminemia

Decreased levels of circulating albumin almost invariably complicate hepatic failure. Hypoalbuminemia is an important factor in the pathogenesis of the edema often seen in chronic liver disease. Impaired synthesis of albumin by the injured liver is the most common cause of hypoalbuminemia. Occasionally, albumin synthesis is normal, but in such cases the rate of albumin production does not correlate well with the concentration of albumin in the blood. Alcohol appears to inhibit albumin synthesis.

Pulmonary Complications

Changes in pulmonary hemodynamics result in decreased arterial oxygen saturation in about half of those with chronic liver disease. Occasionally, this is severe enough to result in cyanosis. Several explanations of the decrease in arterial oxygen saturation have been advanced: (a) microscopic arteriovenous fistulas with a right-to-left shunt; (b) a shift in the hemoglobin dissociation curve to the right (reduced affinity for oxygen); (c) alveolar hypoventilation; (d) a reduction in pulmonary diffusion capacity; and (e) alterations in ventilation-perfusion ratios. Of these proposed explanations, arteriovenous shunts and a shift in the hemoglobin dissociation curve have been shown to exist (arterial desaturation is responsible for the clubbing of the fingers occasionally encountered in chronic liver disease), although the reduction in oxygen affinity is not large enough to explain the arterial desaturation by itself. The other mechanisms remain speculative.

Endocrine Complications

In assessing endocrine changes associated with chronic hepatic failure, it is important to distinguish between the direct effects of alcohol abuse, a common cause of liver disease, and changes that are better attributed to hepatic dysfunction. Chronic hepatic failure of any etiology in males is associated with feminization, a condition characterized by gynecomastia, a female body habitus, and a female distribution of pubic hair (female escutcheon). In addition, vascular manifestations of hyperestrogenism are common, and include spider angiomas in the territory drained by the superior vena cava (upper trunk and face) and palmar erythema. **Feminization is attributed to a reduction in the hepatic catabolism of estrogens and weak androgens, such as androstenedione and dehydroepiandrosterone.** The weak androgens are converted to estrogenic compounds in peripheral tissues, thereby adding to the burden of circulating estrogens. Moreover, the extrahepatic portasystemic shunts that spontaneously develop as a result of portal hypertension in cirrhosis permit the estrogens and weak androgens excreted in the bile to bypass the liver when they are reabsorbed from the intestine. It is also possible that an increase in the sensitivity of estrogen-responsive tissues may contribute to the feminization of men with chronic liver disease.

Men who suffer from alcoholic liver disease are more likely to be feminized than those with liver disease from other causes, and the severity of feminization is usually greater. The reason for this increased tendency to feminization in alcohol-induced liver disease is not clear. However, there is evidence to suggest that alcohol, either directly or as a consequence of alcohol-induced hypogonadism, reduces the content in the liver of an estrogen-binding protein that may protect the cell from excess estrogenic stimulation.

In addition to feminization, the large majority of chronic alcoholic men also suffer hypogonadism, manifested by testicular atrophy, impotence, and loss of libido. Alcoholic women also exhibit gonadal failure, presenting as oligomenorrhea, amenorrhea, infertility, ovarian atrophy, and loss of secondary sex characteristics. These effects of alcohol on gonadal function in both sexes reflect a direct toxic action independent of chronic liver disease.

Acute Viral Hepatitis

Viral hepatitis is defined as a viral infection of hepatocytes that produces necrosis and inflammation of the liver. The disease has been recognized as "epidemic jaundice" for millenia. Many viruses and other infectious agents are capable of producing hepatitis and jaundice (Table 14-1), but in the industrialized world more than 95% of the cases of viral hepatitis involve a limited number of hepatotropic viruses, known as the hepatitis A, hepatitis B, and so-called non-A, non-B hepatitis viruses. A fourth virus, found only in association with hepatitis B, is known as the hepatitis D virus. The following discussion will emphasize the illnesses caused by these four viruses, and the reader is referred to Chapter 9 for consideration of the other agents.

Table 14-1. Infectious Agents That Cause Hepatitis

Hepatitis A virus
Hepatitis B virus
Non-A, non-B hepatitis virus(es)
Yellow fever virus
Epstein-Barr virus (infectious mononucleosis)
Lassa, Marburg, and Ebola viruses
Rubella virus
Herpes simplex virus
Cytomegalovirus
Enteroviruses other than hepatitis A virus
Leptospires (leptospirosis)
Entamoeba histolytica (amebic hepatitis)

The outbreaks of jaundice that were recorded in association with military campaigns from ancient times to the modern era were almost certainly caused by the hepatitis A virus. Historical evidence for transmission of hepatitis by inoculation with human serum dates to the mid-nineteenth century, when shipyard workers in Germany experienced jaundice after being vaccinated against smallpox with a vaccine that contained human lymph. During and after World War II, two distinct modes of transmission of human hepatitis were conclusively established, one spread in epidemic form and the other parenterally, especially by blood transfusion or inoculation by contaminated needles. The identification in the 1960s of an antigen in an Australian aborigine (Australia antigen) that was later shown to be a component of the virus associated with parenteral transmission of hepatitis led directly to the identification of the hepatitis B virus. Subsequently, the hepatitis A virus was identified in human feces by immune electron microscopy. It soon became apparent that the elimination of blood containing the hepatitis B virus from donor blood did not insure against post-transfusion hepatitis. This remaining form of hepatitis, the agent of which has yet to be characterized, has been termed non-A, non-B hepatitis.

Hepatitis A

The Hepatitis A Virus (HAV)

Hepatitis A virus can be demonstrated in the feces of patients with hepatitis A by its immune precipitation with convalescent serum or immune serum globulin (Fig. 14-13). HAV is a small RNA-containing **enterovirus** of the picornavirus group. Only a single antigenic strain of the virus is recognized. The hepatocyte is the sole site of viral replication, and presumably shedding of progeny virus into the bile accounts for its appearance in the feces. On the basis of indirect evidence, it has been assumed that, like other enteroviruses, HAV is directly cytopathic. However, other mechanisms may also be operative, as is suggested by the observation that viral shedding in the feces, a consequence of the release of virus from the hepatocytes into bile, occurs before the onset of necrosis in the liver. Moreover, a role for immune-mediated damage to hepatocytes is suggested by the observation that, *in vitro*, natural killer (NK) cells preferentially kill monkey kidney cells infected with HAV.

Clinical Features

Following an incubation period of 3 to 6 weeks, with a mean of about 4 weeks, patients develop nonspecific symptoms, including fever, malaise, and anorexia. Concomitantly, liver injury is evidenced by a rise in the serum aminotransferase activity (Fig. 14-14). As the activity of aminotransferase begins to decline, usually 5 to 10 days later, jaundice may appear. It remains evident for an average of 10 days but may persist for more than a month. In most cases the elevated aminotransferase activity returns to normal by the time jaundice has disappeared. **Hepatitis A never pursues a chronic course. There is no carrier state, and infection provides lifelong immunity.** Moreover, virtually all patients recover without he-

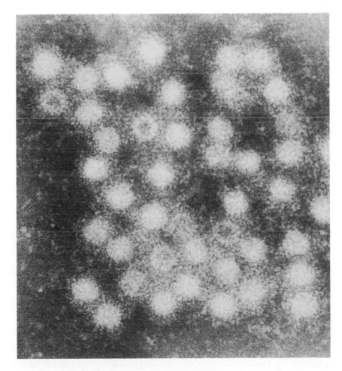

Figure 14-13. Electron micrograph of hepatitis A virus (HAV). A fecal extract was treated with convalescent serum containing anti-HAV.

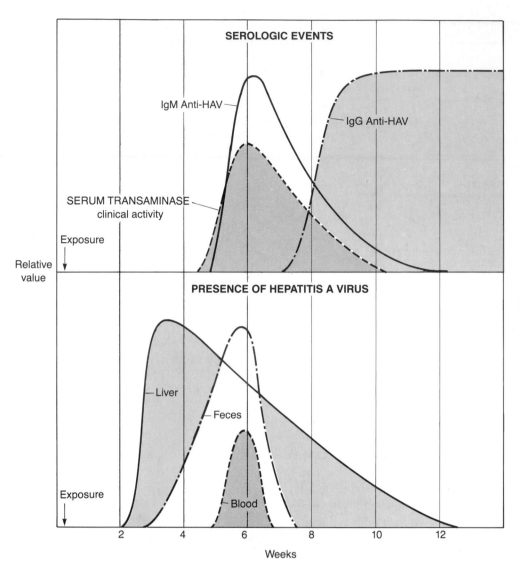

Figure 14-14. Typical serologic events associated with hepatitis A.

patic encephalopathy, and fatal fulminant hepatitis occurs only rarely.

HAV can be detected in the liver about 2 weeks after infection, reaches a maximum in another 2 weeks, and disappears shortly thereafter (see Fig. 14-14). Fecal shedding of HAV follows its appearance in the liver by about a week and lasts for only a brief time. The period of viremia is also short, occurring early in the course.

The first detectable antibody response to HAV infection is the appearance of IgM anti-HAV in the blood during the acute illness (see Fig. 14-14). The antibody titer begins to fall within a few weeks and generally disappears by 3 to 5 months. IgG anti-HAV appears as the patient recovers and the IgM anti-HAV titer has begun to fall; it maintains peak levels after the IgM antibody has disappeared and persists for life. The finding of IgM anti-HAV in the serum of a patient with acute hepatitis confirms HAV as the cause.

Epidemiology of Hepatitis A

In the United States the relative contributions of the different viral types to the total number of cases of hepatitis are not adequately defined. The uncertainty arises, in part, because fewer than 5% of persons who have serologic evidence of previous hepatitis caused by HAV recall a prior episode of jaundice or any other liver ailment, which indicates that the large majority of infections are anicteric. Among hospitalized patients, a population clearly selected for more severe disease, hepatitis A accounts for about 10% to 25% of all cases of viral hepatitis. By contrast, in the less developed countries hepatitis A is hyperendemic and rates of inapparent infection in children are extremely high. As a result, adult cases of hepatitis A are unusual in those regions. Childhood hepatitis A is also common in institutions for the mentally retarded and in daycare centers in the United States.

For hepatitis A, as for other viral diseases that do not lead to a chronic carrier state, the only reservoir for the disease seems to be the acutely infected individual. **Transmission depends primarily on serial transmission from person to person by the fecal-oral route.** Epidemics of hepatitis A also depend on person-to-person spread and occur under crowded and unsanitary conditions, such as exist in warfare, or by fecal contamination of water and food. Edible shellfish concentrate the virus in contaminated waters and may also transmit the infection if inadequately cooked. Although hepatitis A is not ordinarily a sexually transmitted disease, the infection rate is particularly high among male homosexuals, as a result of oral-anal contact.

Hepatitis B

The Hepatitis B Virus (HBV)

HBV is a hepatotropic DNA virus which was the first of the so-called hepadnaviruses. Other members of this family include hepatotropic viruses that affect woodchucks, ground squirrels, and Pekin ducks. The DNA of HBV consists of one long circular strand, containing the entire genome, and a shorter complementary strand, which varies from 50% to 85% of the length of the longer strand. Thus, the DNA is predominantly double-stranded, with a variable single-stranded segment (Fig. 14-15). The core of the virus contains a DNA polymerase and immunologically reactive elements, called the **core antigen (HBcAg)** and the **"e" antigen (HBeAg)**. HBeAg is a soluble antigen closely associated with HBcAg, and may be a degradation product of the latter. The core of the virus is enclosed in a coat that contains lipid, protein, and carbohydrate and expresses an antigen termed **hepatitis B surface antigen (HBsAg)**.

The surface coat, corresponding to the original Australia antigen, is synthesized by the infected hepatocyte independently from the viral core, and is secreted into the blood in vast amounts. This material is visualized by electron microscopy in centrifuged serum as two distinct particles (see Fig. 14-15), one a 22-nm sphere and the other a tubular structure 22

nm in diameter and 40 nm to 400 nm in length. **HBsAg particles are immunogenic but not infectious.** The **intact and infectious virus** is also found in the same preparations as a 42-nm sphere **(Dane particle)**, consisting of a 27-nm inner core and an outer shell 7 nm in thickness.

HBV is not directly cytopathic, and the mechanism underlying necrosis of hepatocytes remains under study. This lack of a direct cytopathic action is reflected in the fact that asymptomatic chronic carriers of the virus maintain a large burden of infectious virus in the liver for years without functional or biochemical evidence of liver cell injury. Therefore, it has been postulated that the destruction of virus-infected hepatocytes is mediated by immunologic responses. However, neither the relevant antigens nor the mediators of immunologic injury are defined.

Clinical Features

In contrast to hepatitis A, there are four well recognized clinical courses associated with HBV infection (Fig. 14-16): **acute, self-limited hepatitis; fulminant hepatitis; chronic hepatitis; and a chronic, asymptomatic carrier state.** The large majority of patients have an acute, self-limited hepatitis similar to that produced by HAV, in which complete recovery and lifelong immunity is the rule. More often than hepatitis A, but still only rarely, acute hepatitis B pursues a fulminant course characterized by massive liver cell necrosis, hepatic failure, and a high mortality. In a small minority of patients the virus is not eradicated following the acute infection, and the hepatitis becomes chronic. In the fourth group, the patients become chronic, asymptomatic carriers of HBV after having recovered from a mild acute hepatitis.

Acute, Self-Limited Hepatitis B

The acute onset and symptoms of hepatitis B are for the most part similar to those of hepatitis A, although acute hepatitis B tends to be somewhat more severe. In addition, the incubation period is considerably longer. Typically, symptoms do not appear for about 2 to 3 months after exposure, but incubation periods of less than 6 weeks and as long as 6 months are occasionally encountered. As in hepatitis A, serologic studies have shown that many cases, including virtually all infections in infants and children, are anicteric and not, therefore, clinically apparent.

HBsAg is the first marker to appear in the serum of patients with acute hepatitis B, being detected 1 week to 2 months after exposure and 2 weeks to 2 months before the onset of symptoms (see Fig.

(Text continues on page 744)

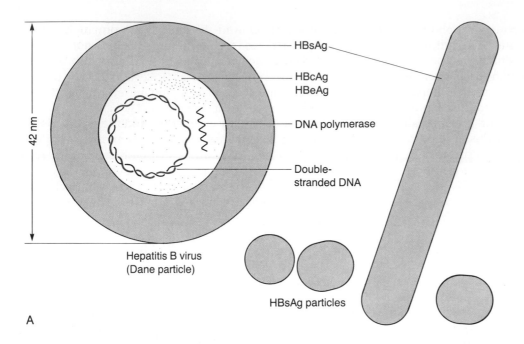

Hepatitis B virus
(Dane particle)

HBsAg particles

A

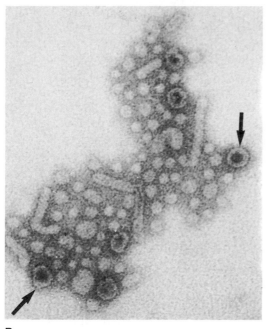

B

Figure 14-15. (*A*) Schematic representation of the hepatitis B virus (HBV) and serum particles associated with HBV infection. (*B*) Electron micrograph of particles from centrifuged serum in a case of hepatitis B. Rodlike and spherical particles containing HbsAg are evident. The complete virion, composed of the viral core and its surrounding envelope, is represented by Dane particles (*arrows*).

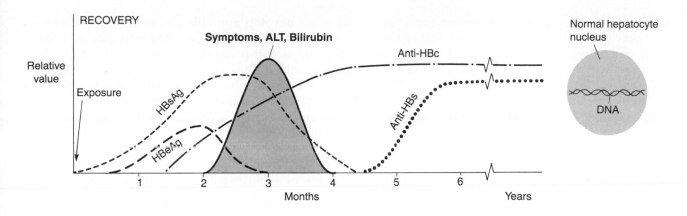

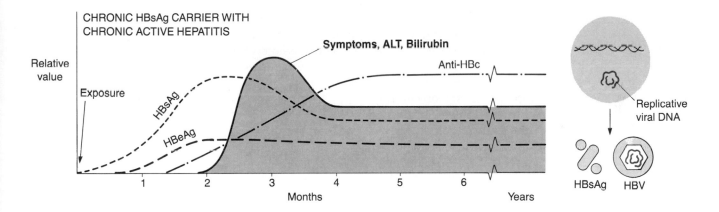

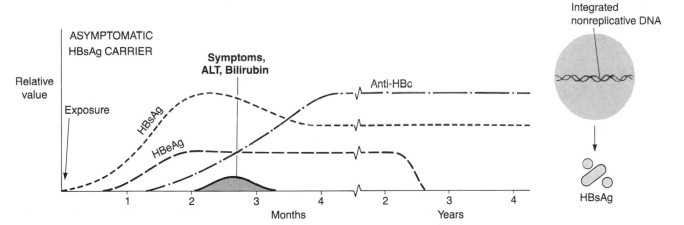

Figure 14-16. Typical serologic events in three distinct outcomes of hepatitis B. (*Top panel*). In most cases the appearance of anti-HBs assures complete **recovery.** Viral DNA disappears from the nucleus of the hepatocyte.

(*Middle panel*) In about 10% of cases of hepatitis B, HBs antigenemia is sustained for longer than 6 months, owing to the absence of anti-HBs. Patients in whom viral replication remains active, as evidenced by sustained high levels of HBeAg in the blood, develop **chronic active hepatitis.** In such cases the viral genome persists in the nucleus but is not integrated into the host DNA.

(*Lower panel*) Patients in whom active viral replication ceases or is attenuated, as reflected in the disappearance of HBeAg from the blood, become **asymptomatic carriers.** In these individuals the HBV genome is integrated into the host DNA.

14-16). HBsAg disappears from the blood during the convalescent phase in patients who recover rapidly from the acute hepatitis. It should be noted that an occasional patient with unquestionable hepatitis B is consistently negative for HBsAg in the blood. Nevertheless, such individuals display considerable HBsAg in the liver. In this situation the clinical course tends to be mild and brief. Simultaneous with or shortly after the disappearance of HBsAg, antibody to HBsAg (anti-HBs) is found in the blood. Its appearance heralds complete recovery, and its presence provides lifelong immunity. Antibody to HBcAg (anti-HBc) appears shortly after anti-HBs, roughly at the time that serum aminotransferase activity begins to rise. HBcAg itself does not circulate freely in the serum of infected persons. Anti-HBc also remains elevated for life and is a useful marker of previous HBV infection, although, unlike anti-HBs, it does not seem to play a role either in clearing the virus or in protecting against reinfection.

HBeAg, the second circulating antigen to appear in hepatitis B, is seen before the onset of clinical disease and after the appearance of HBsAg. HBeAg generally disappears within about 2 weeks, while HBsAg is still present. Anti-HBe appears shortly after the disappearance of the antigen and is detectable for up to 2 years or more after resolution of the hepatitis. The presence of HBeAg in the serum correlates with a period of intense viral replication and, hence, maximal infectivity of the patient.

Circulating HBsAg–anti-HBs immune complexes cause a variety of extrahepatic ailments. Among these are arthritis, polyarteritis, glomerulonephritis, rash, urticaria, pancreatitis, and cryoglobulinemia. Although aplastic anemia is most commonly associated with non-A, non-B hepatitis, on rare occasions it has been encountered following acute hepatitis B infection.

The Chronic Carrier State

In 5% to 10% of cases of hepatitis B, the patients do not develop anti-Hbs and consequently do not resolve HBs antigenemia. Accordingly, the infection persists, the patients do not recover, and the disease progresses to chronic hepatitis B. Newer studies suggest that if high-risk groups (male homosexuals, intravenous drug addicts, and so on) are excluded from consideration, the risk of chronic hepatitis is considerably lower than previously estimated. **Clinically, HBs antigenemia that is sustained for longer than 6 months and is accompanied by hepatic dysfunction indicates chronic hepatitis.** A few of these patients eventually develop anti-Hbs—often after many years—clear the virus, and are restored to full health. Others (no more than 3% of patients with hepatitis

B) never develop anti-HBs and suffer from a relentless and progressive chronic hepatitis that may lead to cirrhosis. All patients with persistent HBV infection develop anti-HBc, and chronic hepatitis B is characterized by the presence of this antibody and HBsAg. Hepatitis associated with persistent HBs antigenemia is often accompanied by the continued presence of HBeAg.

Some of the patients who do not produce anti-HBs have at first only an inapparent or mild, transient episode of acute hepatitis, after which they remain asymptomatic despite the presence of high levels of HBsAg in the blood. The hepatocytes of these chronic asymptomatic carriers remain infected with HBV, and both the liver and blood contain infective virus.

As will be discussed in detail under the heading of hepatocellular carcinoma, chronic hepatitis B is associated with a significant risk of liver cancer.

The possible outcomes of infection with the hepatitis B virus are summarized in Figure 14-17.

Epidemiology of Hepatitis B

It is estimated that there are about 200 million chronic carriers of HBV in the world, constituting an enormous reservoir of infection. Depending on the incidence of primary infection with HBV, the carrier rates vary from as little as 0.3% (United States and Western Europe) to 20% (Southeast Asia, sub-Saharan Africa, and Oceania). In the latter populations an important avenue by which the high carrier rate is sustained is vertical transmission of the virus from a carrier mother to her newborn.

Before the advent of routine screening of blood for HBsAg, chronic HBV carriers posed a public health hazard as a source of post-transfusion hepatitis. The threat of HBV-positive post-transfusion hepatitis has been largely eliminated by routine screening for HBsAg, although 5% to 10% of post-transfusion hepatitis is still attributed to hepatitis B.

There is some evidence to support a genetic predisposition to the carrier state, since it has been reported to cluster in families, possibly as an autosomal recessive trait, and appears with considerably greater frequency in some ethnic groups. Whereas no more than 10% of adults infected with HBV become carriers, neonatal hepatitis B is, as a rule, followed by persistent infection. Males exhibit an increased tendency to become carriers. It has been suggested that immunosuppressed individuals are more susceptible to persistent HBV infection, and the carrier state is more common in renal dialysis patients and persons afflicted with Down's syndrome, leprosy, and chronic lymphocytic leukemia. In the United States chronic HBV carriers are particularly common among

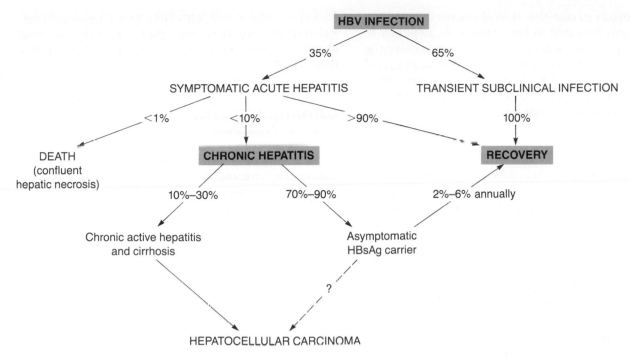

Figure 14-17. Possible outcomes of infection with the hepatitis B virus.

male homosexuals, drug addicts, certain health-care workers, and institutionalized mentally retarded children. Of particular public health concern is the fact that paid blood donors are far more likely to harbor HBV than is the general population.

The only significant reservoir of HBV is man. Unlike hepatitis A, hepatitis B is not transmitted by the fecal-oral route, nor does it contaminate food and water supplies. Although HBsAg is found in most secretions, **infectious virus has been demonstrated only in blood, saliva, and semen.** Historically, transmission of hepatitis B was thought to be limited to direct transfer of blood products, either by transfusion or by the use of contaminated needles. However, it is now clear that the large majority of cases of hepatitis B result from transmission associated with intimate contact. The routes by which contact-transmission occurs are not entirely defined, but it seems probable that a direct transfer of the virus via breaks in the skin or mucous membranes is most common. In this respect, sexual contact, heterosexual or homosexual, is an important mode of transmission.

Hepatitis B Vaccine

The immunogenicity of HBsAg and the fact that anti-HBs protects against HBV infection have allowed the development of effective vaccines against hepatitis B. The original vaccine was prepared by purifying HBsAg particles from the blood of HBV carriers. Synthetic vaccines, composed of HBsAg or its immunogenic epitopes, have been produced using recombinant DNA. It is likely that that worldwide use of these vaccines will eventually reduce the prevalence of HBV infection and relegate hepatitis B to the status of a minor disease. It will also serve to prevent the major cause of hepatocellular carcinoma in the world.

Hepatitis D

A distinct hepatotropic virus, hepatitis D virus (HDV, delta agent), is associated exclusively with HBV infection. It was first described in 1977, but studies of immune globulin obtained in the United States in 1944 have shown that the virus has been present at least since that date, and presumably earlier. HDV is an RNA virus, visualized in hepatocytes as a 25-nm particle that is present predominantly in the nucleus. In the blood HDV is coated with HBsAg and appears as a 37-nm particle. **HDV is likely a defective virus for which HBV is the helper.** Assembly of HDV in the liver requires the synthesis of HBsAg, and, therefore, infection with this virus is limited to persons (and sub-human primates) infected with HBV. HDV infection may occur either simultaneously with HBV infection (coinfection) or following HBV infection (superinfection). In cases of coinfection, the replication of HDV is limited to the period of HBsAg synthesis. HDV and HBsAg are cleared together, and the clinical course is generally no different from that of the usual acute hepatitis B. However, it has been reported that in some cases the presence of HDV leads to severe, fulminant, and often fatal hepatitis. On the other hand, superinfection of an HBV carrier typically increases the severity of an existing chronic hepatitis.

Non-A, Non-B Hepatitis

The advent of routine screening of blood for HBsAg led to an expectation that post-transfusion hepatitis would virtually disappear. This prediction proved inaccurate, as the incidence of post-transfusion hepatitis was only modestly reduced. It was discovered that there is a form of hepatitis that is not associated with HAV or HBV, or any of the serologic markers for these viruses. This form of the disease has been termed **non-A, non-B hepatitis. Today, about 90% of post-transfusion hepatitis in the United States is classed as non-A, non-B.** About 20% of sporadic cases of hepatitis (those not associated with a known epidemiologic risk) also represent non-A, non-B hepatitis. It is now thought that there are three or four transmissible agents that produce non-A, non-B hepatitis. Although non-A, non-B hepatitis is linked to blood transfusions and the administration of blood products, one non-A, non-B agent is transmitted enterically and is known to cause an epidemic, often water-borne, form of hepatitis in some parts of the world. In the United States the groups at higher risk for hepatitis B seem also to be more likely to contract non-A, non-B hepatitis.

Although numerous candidate viruses and particles have been proposed, none is accepted as the etiologic agent of non-A, non-B hepatitis. Moreover, no serologic markers for the disease exist. Thus, at the present time, non-A, non-B hepatitis remains a diagnosis of exclusion.

The clinical course and mode of transmission of most cases of non-A, non-B hepatitis are similar to those of hepatitis B. The incubation period of parenterally transmitted disease averages 7 to 8 weeks, but the range is wide. The acute illness tends to be less severe than that in hepatitis B, but may also lead to fulminant hepatitis. Since non-A, non-B hepatitis is associated with the transfusion of blood and blood products, it is clear that a carrier state exists. Chronic liver disease is a more frequent complication in non-A, non-B hepatitis than in hepatitis B. In contrast to hepatitis B, in which no more than 10% of patients have elevations of serum aminotransferase for more than 6 months, about half of patients with post-trans-

fusion non-A, non-B hepatitis have persistently elevated levels for more than 1 year. Up to 20% of these chronic carriers of non-A, non-B hepatitis eventually develop cirrhosis.

Chronic Hepatitis

Chronic hepatitis refers to the presence of inflammation and necrosis in the liver for more than 6 months. The proportion of cases of chronic hepatitis attributable to persistent viral hepatitis is not precisely known, particularly since the diagnosis of non-A, non-B hepatitis remains exclusionary. Only about 15% of patients with chronic hepatitis in the United States display HBs antigenemia, whereas the prevalence in Italy is about 50%, and in parts of Asia it may be even higher. HBsAg-negative chronic hepatitis is probably caused in large part by other viruses, collectively termed non-A, non-B, but it may also result from the use of drugs such as isoniazid and methyldopa. Chronic hepatitis may also be a feature of certain systemic diseases, including Wilson's disease and α_1-antitrypsin deficiency.

A clinically distinct form of chronic hepatitis, termed **"lupoid," or "autoimmune," hepatitis,** occurs in young and middle-aged women and is accompanied by hypergammaglobulinemia, autoantibodies, the lupus erythematosus (LE) cell phenomenon, and multi-system involvement of other organs of a kind commonly attributed to autoimmune mechanisms. Those affected often exhibit histocompatibility antigens that have been associated with other autoimmune diseases, notably HLA-B8. Whether undetected viruses play an etiologic role is unclear, and the autoimmune basis of this disease cannot be considered firmly established. Whereas the response to corticosteroid therapy in other forms of chronic hepatitis is generally unsatisfactory, patients with "autoimmune" hepatitis often respond favorably to such treatment. Untreated patients, or those who are refractory to therapy, have a high risk of developing liver failure and cirrhosis.

While the aforementioned mechanisms (viruses, drugs, and "autoimmunity") account for many cases of chronic hepatitis, it is fair to say that a significant proportion of cases are of unknown etiology.

About 90% of patients with **chronic hepatitis B** are male, whereas chronic hepatitis of unknown etiology that has "autoimmune" features shows a female predominance. In chronic hepatitis B the disease characteristically begins as typical acute hepatitis, but in contrast to the usual course of the disease the hepatitis does not resolve within 6 months. However, the large majority of patients who present initially with chronic hepatitis B, with or without cirrhosis, do not have a history of jaundice or acute liver disease. In these cases it is assumed that the episode of acute hepatitis B was clinically inapparent. **Chronic active hepatitis B carries a high risk for the development of cirrhosis. Furthermore, chronic hepatitis B seems to be the major predisposing cause of primary hepatocellular carcinoma worldwide.**

In addition to nonspecific constitutional symptoms of anorexia and malaise, patients with chronic hepatitis B display variable degrees of jaundice and hepatosplenomegaly. Serum aminotransferase activity is consistently elevated, and mild increases in alkaline phosphatase are common. Extrahepatic manifestations are similar to those in acute hepatitis B. HBeAg is more common in patients with chronic active hepatitis B than in asymptomatic carriers and is associated with more severe disease and greater infectivity of the blood. HBe antigenemia also correlates with the presence of the complete HBV virion, HBV DNA, and HBV DNA polymerase activity in the blood.

It appears that, at least in part, the severity of chronic hepatitis B is related to the degree of viral replication, as indicated by the presence in the blood of HBeAg, HBV DNA, and HBV DNA polymerase. As noted previously, the replication of HBV is dissociated from the production of HBsAg. At one extreme is the asymptomatic carrier, who continues to synthesize large amounts of HBsAg, but in whom there is little viral replication. In these apparently healthy patients, the HBV genome seems to be integrated into the host DNA. By contrast, those carriers of HBV in whom viral replication is particularly active suffer from persistent liver cell necrosis, expressed clinically as chronic active hepatitis. In these patients the HBV persists in the nucleus but is not integrated into the host DNA.

In view of the fact that HBV is not directly cytopathic to hepatocytes, it is thought that cell-mediated immunity underlies the pathogenesis of chronic hepatitis B. Recent evidence suggests that the tissue injury in chronic active hepatitis B may be mediated by cytotoxic T lymphocytes directed against HBcAg on the surface of the hepatocyte in association with a histocompatibility antigen. However, findings from other studies are at such variance with this concept or so equivocal that the precise mechanism by which liver cells are injured in chronic hepatitis B is far from clear.

Chronic non-A, non-B hepatitis tends to be a milder disease than either chronic hepatitis B or chronic hepatitis of unknown etiology. Extrahepatic manifestations and autoantibodies are rare. Most patients do not develop symptoms or signs of chronic liver disease, and liver failure is distinctly uncommon. Nevertheless, as noted previously, cirrhosis ultimately develops in up to 20% of such patients.

The Pathology of Acute and Chronic Hepatitis

Acute Viral Hepatitis

The morphologic appearance of the liver in acute viral hepatitis is similar in hepatitis A, hepatitis B, and non-A, non-B hepatitis. The hallmark of viral hepatitis is liver cell injury and necrosis (Fig. 14-18). Within the hepatic lobule, scattered necrosis of single cells or small clusters of hepatocytes is seen. A few necrotic liver cells appear as small, **deeply eosino-**

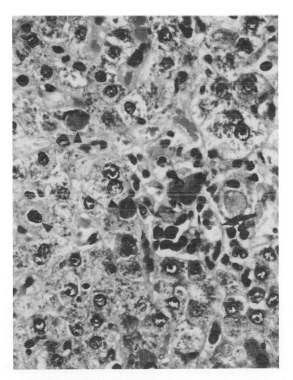

Figure 14-18. Acute viral hepatitis. A photomicrograph shows disarray of liver cell plates, focal drop-out of hepatocytes (*arrow*) and replacement by lymphoid cells, and scattered mononuclear inflammatory cells. The remnants of necrotic hepatocytes have been extruded into the sinusoids, where they appear as acidophilic, or Councilman, bodies (*arrowheads*).

philic bodies (Councilman or acidophilic bodies), sometimes containing pyknotic nuclear material, that have been extruded from the liver cell plate into the sinusoid (see Fig. 14-18). Although acidophilic bodies are characteristic of viral hepatitis, they are also occasionally encountered in other diseases associated with liver cell necrosis. In acute viral hepatitis many liver cells appear normal, but others show varying degrees of hydropic swelling (balloon cells) and differences in size, shape, and staining qualities. Concomitantly, regenerative liver cells, which display a larger nucleus and an expanded basophilic cytoplasm, are also seen. The resulting irregularity of the liver cell plates is termed lobular disarray.

Chronic inflammatory cells, principally lymphoid, infiltrate the lobule diffusely, surround individual necrotic liver cells, and accumulate in areas of focal necrosis. In addition to the lymphoid cells, macrophages may be prominent, and eosinophils and polymorphonuclear leukocytes are not uncommon. These changes tend to be somewhat more pronounced in the centrilobular zones, although they are present throughout the lobule. Characteristically, lymphoid cells infiltrate between the wall of the central vein and the liver cell plates, an appearance termed central phlebitis. Swelling and proliferation of the endothelial cells of the central vein (endophlebitis) often develop. The Kupffer cells are enlarged, project into the lumen of the sinusoid, and contain lipofuscin pigment and phagocytosed debris (seen particularly well with the PAS reaction), including fragments of acidophilic bodies. Cholestasis is sometimes seen, in which case the term cholestatic hepatitis is applied. In this variant of acute viral hepatitis, and occasionally in the more classic case, many liver cells are arranged around a lumen, thus presenting an acinar or glandular appearance. The lumen of such an "acinus" may contain a large bile plug.

The portal tracts are almost always enlarged and edematous. As a rule chronic inflammatory cells accumulate within the portal tracts, but the severity of this inflammatory reaction varies from mild to pronounced. The inflammatory cells in the portal tracts mirror the distribution of those in the lobule. Infrequently, aggregates of lymphoid cells within the portal tracts assume a follicular form. The limiting plate of hepatocytes around the portal tracts is usually intact and presents a sharp border with the portal tract. In some instances of acute viral hepatitis that resolve without complications, the inflammatory infiltrate extends from the portal tracts into the lobular parenchyma, thereby disrupting the limiting plate and simulating the appearance of chronic hepatitis. The portal tracts commonly exhibit only a few prolif-

erated bile ductules, although occasionally this phenomenon may be more conspicuous. During recovery, hepatic regeneration is reflected in the presence of mitotic figures in the liver cell plates. All of the pathologic changes are gradually reversed and the normal hepatic architecture is completely restored.

Hepatic Localization of HBV Antigens

During the incubation period and after the onset of symptoms in cases of acute hepatitis B, HBcAg can be demonstrated in the nucleus and HBsAg in the cytoplasm and occasionally in the plasma membranes of hepatocytes. During the active stage of the disease, only scattered cells exhibit these antigens. By contrast, in immunocompromised individuals and in immunologically tolerant infants, most hepatocyte nuclei stain for HBcAg. In these patients membrane-associated HBsAg is present only in a few cells that stain for HBcAg. Asymptomatic HBsAg carriers show a uniform cytoplasmic distribution of HBsAg in many hepatocytes, but few or no HBcAg-positive nuclei are seen. This is consistent with the lack of HBeAg and HBV DNA-polymerase in the blood, and points to limited viral replication in asymptomatic carriers, as discussed above. In severe cases of acute hepatitis B, the majority of hepatocytes may show HBcAg, a finding in agreement with the high titers of HBeAg that may be in the blood (active viral replication). About half of these HBcAg-containing cells display membrane-associated HBsAg.

Confluent Hepatic Necrosis

The term "confluent hepatic necrosis" refers to a severe variant of acute viral hepatitis, which is characterized by the death of a large number of hepatocytes and, in extreme cases, of almost all the liver cells. In contrast to the most common form of acute viral hepatitis described above, in which the necrosis of hepatocytes appears to be random and patchy, confluent hepatic necrosis typically affects whole regions of the lobule (Fig. 14-19). At one end of the spectrum of lesions are bands of necrosis (bridging necrosis), which stretch between adjacent portal tracts, between adjacent central veins, and between portal tracts and central veins. These bands of necrosis are not necessarily uniform throughout the liver, and lobules that have retained the normal architecture may be situated next to severely affected ones. Curiously, the lobular inflammatory infiltrate is often scanty, although the portal tracts are generally inflamed and often contain an appreciable number of polymorphonuclear leukocytes. The death of adja-

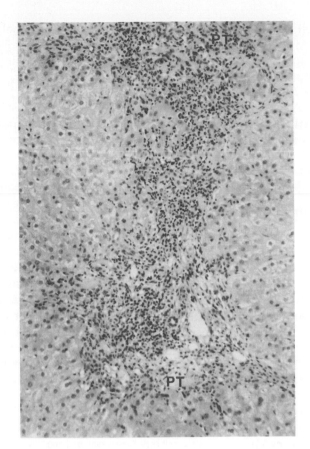

Figure 14-19. Confluent hepatic necrosis. A photomicrograph shows a zone of hepatic necrosis that bridges the portal tracts (*PT*) of adjacent lobules.

cent plates of hepatocytes results in the collapse of the collagenous stroma to form bands of connective tissue, best visualized with a reticulin stain. Increased collagen synthesis may also contribute to the formation of these connective tissue bands. When such bands encircle an area of liver cells, a nodular pattern, similar to that seen in cirrhosis, may be suggested. The presence of bridging necrosis in younger persons (under 30 years of age) has no adverse prognostic significance. However, when this lesion is evident in patients over the age of 40, as many as half eventually die in hepatic failure. This type of acute viral hepatitis was formerly termed **subacute hepatitis,** but the term is inappropriate, since it has a temporal, rather than a purely morphologic, connotation.

Submassive confluent necrosis defines an even more severe injury involving necrosis of entire lobules or groups of adjacent lobules. Clinically, these patients manifest severe hepatitis, which may rapidly proceed to hepatic failure, in which case the disease is classed as **fulminant hepatitis.** In about one-fifth of the cases that eventually prove fatal, the course is

protracted, death from hepatic failure occurring in 2 to 5 months.

Massive hepatic necrosis (acute yellow atrophy), although uncommon, is the most feared variant of acute viral hepatitis, because it is a form of fulminant hepatitis that is almost invariably fatal. Grossly, the liver is shrunken to as little as 500 g (one third of the normal weight). The capsule is wrinkled, and the mottled, red-tan parenchyma is soft and flabby. Microscopic examination reveals that virtually all the hepatocytes are dead (Fig. 14-20), and the hepatic lobule is represented only by the reticulin framework, which in many areas has collapsed. Often the only viable hepatocytes are disposed as a thin rim surrounding the portal tracts. Macrophages, erythrocytes, and necrotic debris fill the sinusoids and impinge on the necrotic remnants of the liver cell plates. For unknown reasons the massive necrosis does not elicit a vigorous inflammatory response in either the parenchyma or the portal tracts. A few proliferated bile ductules are common, and occasionally small ductular structures lined by altered hepatocytes are present in the remnants of the lobules.

Young patients who survive submassive or massive confluent hepatic necrosis generally do not develop cirrhosis and, in the case of hepatitis B, do not become HBsAg carriers. By contrast, older persons who recover from fulminant hepatitis are more likely to progress to chronic hepatitis and cirrhosis.

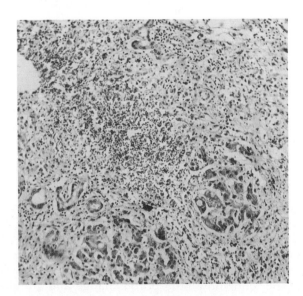

Figure 14-20. Massive hepatic necrosis. A photomicrograph shows the loss of virtually all hepatocytes. The reticulin framework has collapsed, and the area in the center of the field is hemorrhagic. A sparse chronic inflammatory infiltrate is evident throughout the affected lobules.

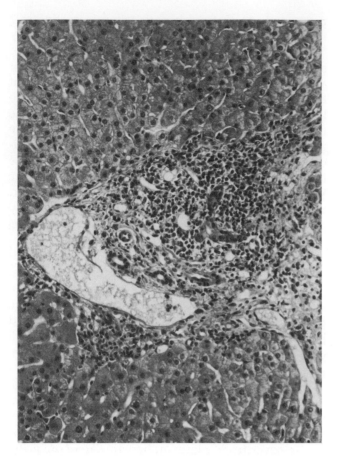

Figure 14-21. Chronic persistent hepatitis. A photomicrograph shows the portal tract infiltrated by mononuclear inflammatory cells. The lobular parenchyma is essentially intact.

Chronic Hepatitis

There are two basic morphologic types of chronic hepatitis that have prognostic significance: chronic persistent hepatitis and chronic active hepatitis.

Chronic Persistent Hepatitis

Chronic persistent hepatitis is a mild form of chronic hepatitis that does not progress to more severe disease. About half of those clearly identified as having chronic HBV infection demonstrate **lymphocytic infiltration limited to the portal tracts** (Fig. 14-21). The others, who show little portal change and are often referred to as "normal" or "asymptomatic" HBV carriers, show only minimal or sporadic increases in serum aminotransferase. **Thus, the so-called asymptomatic carrier simply represents the most inactive extreme of the spectrum of persistent viral hepatitis.** Characteristically, the limiting plate is intact. Liver cell necrosis and lobular inflammation are minimal, and the Kupffer cells appear normal. Scattered cells display a large granular cytoplasm, which contains abundant HBsAg (**"ground-glass hepatocytes"**) (Fig. 14-22).

A morphologic distinction between chronic persistent hepatitis caused by HBV infection and that caused by the non-A, non-B agent(s) cannot be reliably made. "Ground-glass hepatocytes" are not present in the latter.

Chronic Active Hepatitis

Chronic active hepatitis is a necrotizing inflammatory disease that may progress to cirrhosis. Inflammation and focal necrosis early in the course of the disease are distributed irregularly among the lobules, without the predominantly centrilobular localization characteristic of acute viral hepatitis. Later the portal tracts become densely infiltrated by lymphocytes, macrophages, and occasional plasma cells (Fig. 14-23). **The inflammation characteristically penetrates the limiting plate and surrounds individual hepatocytes and groups of hepatocytes on the borders of the portal tracts.** The resulting irregular appearance of the periportal zone has been termed "piecemeal necrosis" and has been considered a hallmark of progressive disease. However, it is now recognized that piecemeal necrosis is present in other chronic liver diseases, and even in some cases of acute hepatitis. Thus, its diagnostic value is dubious, and reliance on it may lead to error. The expanded portal tracts often show a mild to severe proliferation of bile ductules, which probably represents a nonspecific response to chronic liver injury. It is not uncommon to observe intralobular changes similar to those of acute hepatitis, including single-cell necrosis, acidophilic bodies, ballooned hepatocytes, and central phlebitis. When seen in the context of chronic active hepatitis, confluent hepatic necrosis, in the form of bridging necrosis, is an ominous predictor of rapid progression to cirrhosis.

Strands of connective tissue extend from the portal tracts into the lobules, giving the former a stellate (star-shaped) appearance. Threads of connective tissue also envelop single hepatocytes and groups of cells, particularly adjacent to the portal tracts. In patients with chronic active hepatitis B, "ground-glass" cells are scarce in areas of necrosis and inflammation, presumably because they are destroyed by an immune reaction.

The end stage of chronic active hepatitis is characterized by dense collagenous septa, which destroy the lobular architecture and divide the liver into

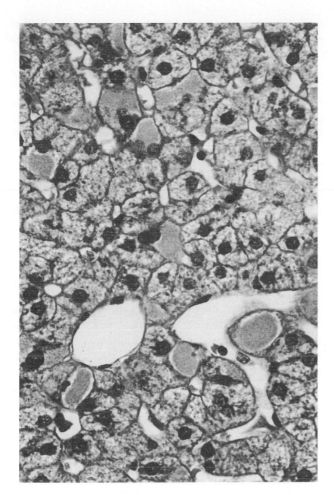

Figure 14-22. "Ground-glass" hepatocytes. A photomicrograph of a case of chronic persistent hepatitis B shows scattered hepatocytes with an abundant granular cytoplasm containing HBsAg.

hepatocellular nodules, an appearance termed cirrhosis (Fig. 14-24). In the cirrhotic stage the activity of the hepatitis is evidenced by continued inflammation and liver cell necrosis.

In evaluating patients with chronic active hepatitis, it is important to realize that the clinical activity of this disease does not necessarily correlate with the morphologic appearance of the liver. Individuals with only mild symptoms and modest elevations of serum aminotransferase activity may display severe chronic active hepatitis with progression to cirrhosis on liver biopsy. **Thus, although imperfect and subject to sampling errors, the liver biopsy remains the most important predictor of the course of chronic hepatitis.**

A schematic comparison of the morphologic features of acute and chronic viral hepatitis is shown in Figure 14-25. Table 14-2 compares the major features of the common forms of viral hepatitis.

Alcoholic Liver Disease

The deleterious effects of excess alcohol (ethanol, ethyl alcohol) consumption have been recognized since the early days of recorded history. The prophet Isaiah warned "Woe to him that is mighty to drink wine." The specific association of alcohol abuse and cirrhosis was noted by the English physician Thomas Heberden in 1699, when he linked "scirrhous livers" with the consumption of "spirituous liquors." Until the middle of the 20th century, the high incidence of liver disease in alcoholics was generally attributed to a toxic effect of ethanol. Subsequently, however, the similarity between the experimental nutritional liver disease in rats induced by dietary choline deficiency and human alcoholic liver disease, and the fact that some alcoholics are malnourished, led to the assumption that alcohol per se is not hepatotoxic. Rather, it was thought that the nutritional deficiencies associated with alcohol abuse are responsible for the liver disease commonly seen in alcoholics. This notion was subsequently questioned on clinical

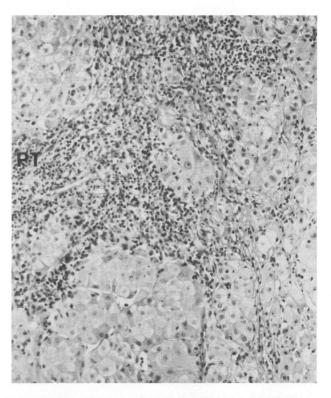

Figure 14-23. Chronic active hepatitis. A photomicrograph shows a mononuclear inflammatory infiltrate in an expanded portal tract (*PT*). The inflammation penetrates the limiting plate and surrounds groups of hepatocytes on the border of the portal tract.

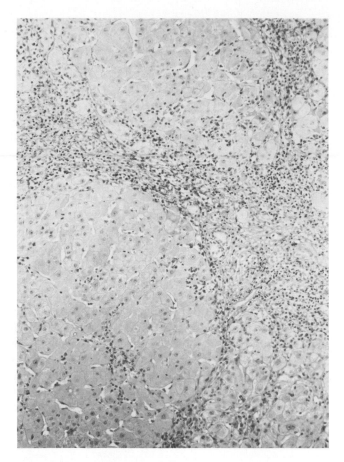

Figure 14-24. Cirrhosis in chronic active hepatitis. A photomicrograph of the liver from a patient with long-standing chronic active hepatitis B shows hepatocellular nodules and chronically inflamed fibrous septa.

grounds, when it became clear that only a very small proportion of all alcoholics are socially deteriorated ("skid row" alcoholics) and that the majority are apparently adequately nourished or even obese. Experiments in which alcohol was given together with nutritionally adequate diets to rats, subhuman primates, and human volunteers demonstrated that alcohol is indeed toxic to the liver, as evidenced by the production of fatty liver and ultrastructural changes in the hepatocytes. Moreover, cirrhosis was produced in baboons fed alcohol with a diet containing all essential nutrients. Thus, today alcohol is again recognized as a direct hepatotoxic agent.

The Epidemiology of Alcoholic Liver Disease

As in the relationship between smoking and cancer, **the evidence linking alcoholism to cirrhosis of the liver in man is derived from epidemiologic data.** The prevalence of cirrhosis is highest in those countries with the highest per capita consumption of alcohol. This relationship between alcohol consumption and chronic liver disease is valid regardless of the specific nature of the preferred beverage (e.g., wine in France, beer in Australia, and spirits in Scandinavia). A quantitative correlation between alcohol consumption and death from cirrhosis of the liver has also been established in the various states of the United States. When the consumption of alcoholic beverages is restricted, as occurred during the Prohibition era in the United States and during World War II in France, deaths from cirrhosis of the liver decline. Although only a minority of chronic alcoholics develop cirrhosis, a dose-response relationship between the duration of exposure and the amount of alcohol consumed and the appearance of cirrhosis has been established (Fig. 14-26).

It is estimated that in the United States about 7% of the total population is alcoholic. However, when one considers only the population at risk, eliminating children, the aged, institutionalized persons, and ethnic or religious groups that abjure the use of alcohol, the prevalence of alcoholism is considerably higher. **About 15% of alcoholics can be expected to develop cirrhosis, and many of these individuals die in hepatic failure or from the extrahepatic complications of cirrhosis.** In fact, in many urban areas of the United States with high alcoholism rates, cirrhosis of the liver, about 70% of which is associated with alcoholism, is now the third or fourth leading cause of death.

The amount of alcohol required to produce chronic liver disease varies widely depending on body size, age, sex, and race, but the lower range seems to be about 80 g/day (235 ml of 86-proof alcoholic beverage) for men, and probably lower for women. In fact, there is some evidence that women are constitutionally more susceptible to the ravages of alcoholism than men, and the threshold dose for the development of cirrhosis in women has been claimed to be as low as 20 g/day, although this value seems unrealistically low. The daily amount of alcohol in established cirrhotic patients is usually in the range of 160 g to 220 g/day. In general, more than 10 years of alcoholism are required to produce cirrhosis, although a few cirrhotic patients give shorter histories of heavy alcohol use. It has been suggested that, for practical purposes, a pint of whiskey a day for 15 years is a threshold for the development of cirrhosis.

The Metabolism of Ethanol

Ethanol is rapidly absorbed from the stomach, and is eventually distributed in body water space. Almost all of the ethanol consumed is metabolized by the

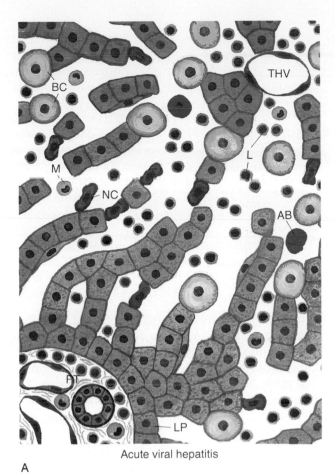

A Acute viral hepatitis

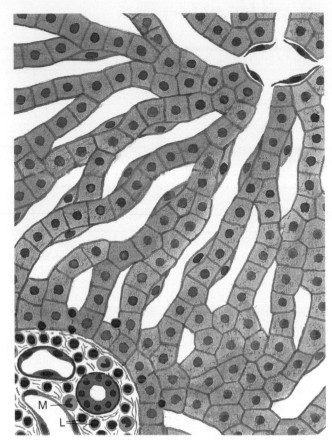

B Chronic persistent hepatitis

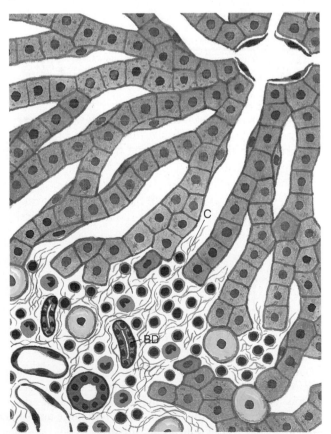

C Chronic active hepatitis

Figure 14-25. Schematic representation of the major morphologic features of acute and chronic viral hepatitis.

(*A*) **Acute viral hepatitis** is characterized by scattered necrosis of single hepatocytes and small clusters of hepatocytes, ballooned cells (*BC*), necrotic cells (*NC*), and acidophilic bodies (*AB*) free in the sinusoids. The inflammation in the lobules and portal tracts (*PT*) is predominantly lymphocytic (*L*), although a few macrophages (*M*) are also seen. The limiting plate (*LP*) is intact. (*THV*, terminal hepatic venule).

(*B*) In **chronic persistent hepatitis,** chronic inflammation is confined to the portal tracts, and the limiting plate is intact. The lobular parenchyma appears normal.

(*C*) **Chronic active hepatitis** is marked by severe chronic inflammation in the portal tracts. Periportal necrosis of hepatocytes is conspicuous, ballooned cells are present, and the limiting plate is eroded. The inflammation extends into the lobular parenchyma and is accompanied by periportal fibrosis. The expanded portal tracts often display proliferated bile ductules (*BD*). (*C*, collagen)

Table 14-2. Comparative Features of the Common Forms of Viral Hepatitis

	HEPATITIS A	HEPATITIS B	NON-A, NON-B HEPATITIS
Genome	RNA	DNA	Unknown
Incubation period	3–6 weeks	6 weeks to 6 months	7–8 weeks (average)
Transmission	Oral	Parenteral	Parenteral (rarely, oral)
Blood	No	Yes	Yes
Feces	Yes	No	Rare
Vertical	No	Yes	Unknown
Fulminant hepatic necrosis	Very rare	Yes	Yes
Chronic hepatitis	No	10%	50%
Carrier state	No	Yes	Yes
Liver cancer	No	Yes	Unknown

liver to acetaldehyde and acetate. Between 5% and 10% is excreted unchanged, principally in the urine and in the expired breath. The principal route of ethanol oxidation in the liver (Fig. 14-27) is via cytosolic alcohol dehydrogenase (ADH), an NAD-dependent enzyme. A minor but nevertheless important metabolic pathway is a microsomal ethanol oxidizing system (MEOS) in the smooth endoplasmic reticulum, which is a mixed function oxidase and utilizes NADP as a cofactor. Since the K_m of ADH is only about 1 mM, and that of MEOS about 7 mM, at clinically significant blood alcohol concentrations (20–100 mM), both enzyme systems are saturated. Thus, for practical purposes, in contrast to most drugs, the clearance of alcohol from the body is linear—that is, a fixed quantity is metabolized per unit time. A rough guide for the average man is about 7 g to 10 g of alcohol eliminated per hour. However, chronic alcoholics metabolize ethanol at a substantially higher rate, provided that they do not suffer from active liver disease. The precise explanation for this accelerated rate of ethanol oxidation is still debated.

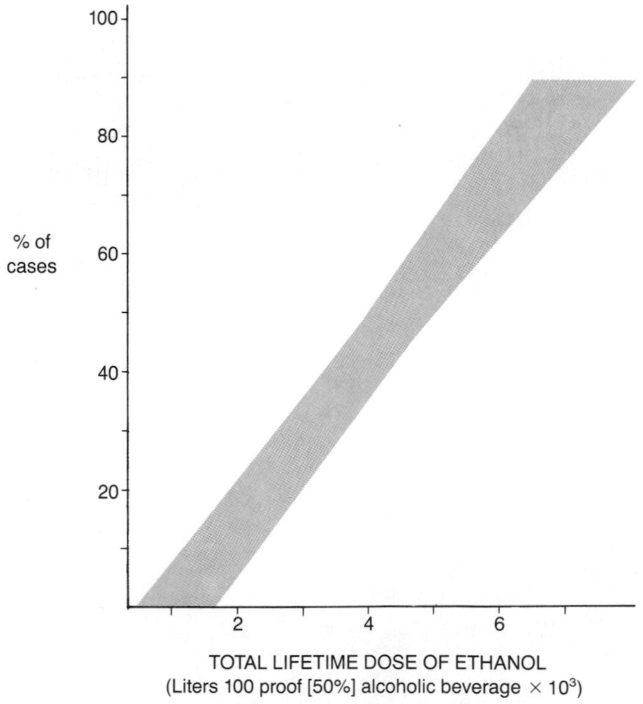

Liver Diseases Produced by Alcohol Consumption

The spectrum of alcoholic liver disease spans three major morphologic and clinical entities: **fatty liver, alcoholic hepatitis, and cirrhosis.** Although these lesions usually occur sequentially, they may coexist in any combination and may be independent entities.

Fatty Liver and Associated Lesions

Virtually all chronic alcoholics accumulate fat in hepatocytes (steatosis). As a result the liver becomes yellow and enlarged—sometimes massively, to as much as 3 times the normal weight. The increased weight does not reflect fat accumulation alone, since protein and water content are also increased. Microscopically, the extent of visible fat accumulation varies from minute droplets scattered in the cytoplasm of a few hepatocytes to distention of the entire cytoplasm of most cells by coalesced droplets (Fig.

Figure 14-26. Dose-response relationship between the amount of alcohol consumed in a lifetime and the incidence of cirrhosis. Only a minority of all alcoholics develop cirrhosis, but those who drink very large amounts are at a high risk of developing the disease.

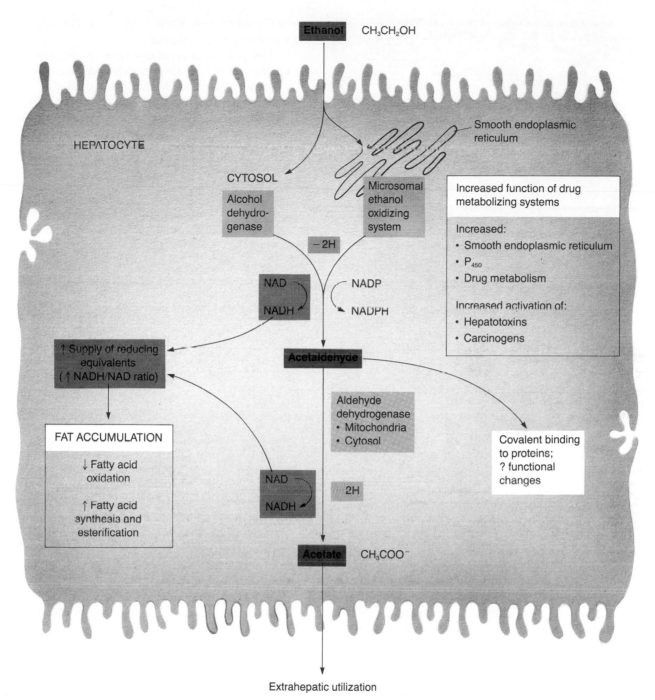

Figure 14-27. The metabolism of ethanol and its hepatocellular effects.

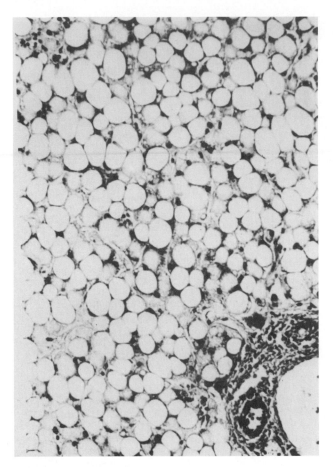

Figure 14-28. Alcoholic fatty liver. A photomicrograph shows the cytoplasm of almost all the hepatocytes to be distended by fat, which displaces the nucleus to the periphery. Note the absence of inflammation and fibrosis.

14-28). In the latter situation, the liver cell is scarcely recognizable as such, and bears a resemblance to an adipocyte, the cytoplasm being represented by a distended clear area, and the nucleus flattened and displaced to the periphery of the cell. When the steatosis is mild, centrilobular hepatocytes are preferentially affected, but as the lesion progresses the entire lobule is involved. A few thin strands of connective tissue may extend from the portal tracts or the central veins, **but usually there is no increase in connective tissue.** Occasionally, cholestasis is observed in the fatty liver, although the pathogenesis is unclear.

The ultrastructural appearance of the hepatocyte in alcohol-induced fatty liver reflects the cytotoxicity of ethanol, rather than an effect of the fat per se. The mitochondria are enlarged, with occasional bizarre giant forms. The smooth endoplasmic reticulum exhibits hyperplasia resembling that produced by other inducers of microsomal drug-metabolizing enzymes. Initially, the fat accumulates as globules, which even-tually merge to form large, cytoplasmic bodies of variable electron density.

The ultrastructural changes in mitochondria and endoplasmic reticulum produced by chronic ethanol ingestion are paralleled by functional alterations. Hepatic mitochondria show decreased rates of substrate oxidation (e.g., of fatty acids) and impaired formation of ATP. The hyperplasia of the smooth endoplasmic reticulum is accompanied by an increase in the activity of the cytochrome P_{450}-dependent mixed-function oxidases. Not only is the microsomal ethanol-oxidizing system induced, but the metabolism of a wide variety of drugs is also enhanced. The increased microsomal function also augments the metabolism of potential hepatic toxins and carcinogens. This results in an exaggeration of the toxicity of agents such as carbon tetrachloride and acetaminophen, and may play a role in the association of alcoholism with certain cancers. In contrast to chronic alcohol consumption, which promotes microsomal functions, the presence of ethanol in the blood and hepatocytes after acute alcohol ingestion inhibits the activity of mixed-function oxidases and acutely reduces the rate of clearance of drugs from the body.

The pathogenesis of fatty liver is not precisely understood, and the relative contributions of different pathways may vary, depending on the amount of alcohol consumed, dietary lipid content, body stores of fat, hormonal status, and other variables. Nevertheless, the accumulation of fat clearly depends on the presence of ethanol, since it is fully and rapidly reversible upon discontinuation of alcohol ingestion. To understand the factors that may be involved in the accumulation of lipid, it is helpful to review briefly lipid metabolism in the liver. Dietary fat, in the form of chylomicrons and free fatty acids, is transported to the liver, where it is taken up by the hepatocyte. Triglycerides are then hydrolyzed to free fatty acids. These, in turn, undergo beta-oxidation in the mitochondria, or are converted to triglycerides in the endoplasmic reticulum. The newly synthesized triglyceride is secreted in the form of lipoproteins or retained for storage.

It has been shown that most of the fat deposited in the liver after chronic alcohol consumption is derived from the diet. However, in the fasting state, much of the fat in the liver has been accumulated from endogenous fat depots. Ethanol increases lipolysis and thus the delivery of free fatty acids to the liver, possibly through hormonal mechanisms, for example, via epinephrine, ACTH, or prostaglandins. Within the hepatocyte, ethanol increases fatty acid synthesis, decreases mitochondrial oxidation of fatty acids, increases the production of triglycerides, and impairs the release of lipoproteins (Fig. 14-29). Col-

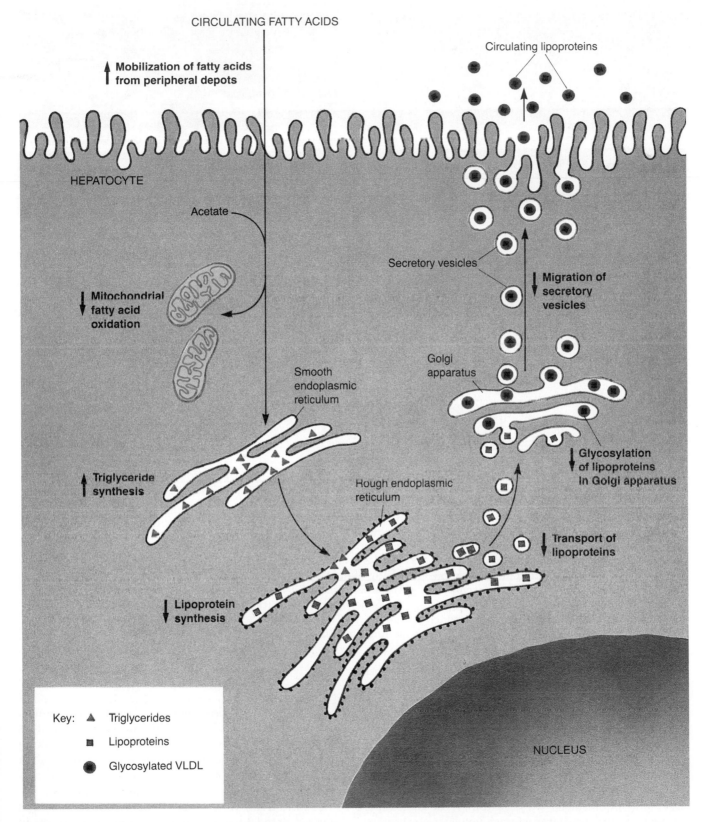

Figure 14-29.   Pathogenesis of alcoholic fatty liver.

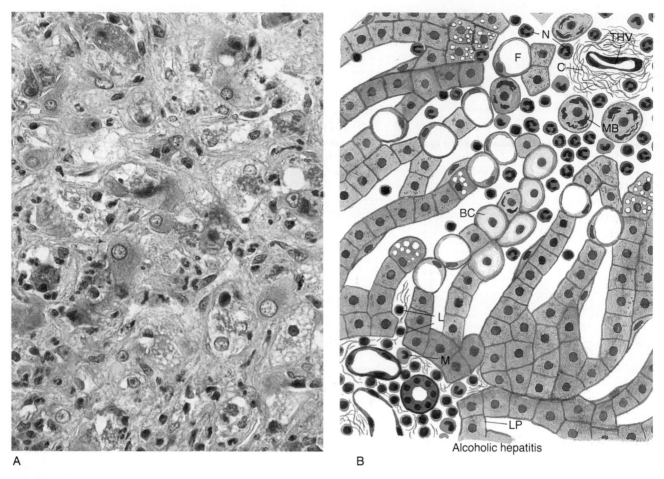

A   B

Alcoholic hepatitis

Figure 14-30. Alcoholic hepatitis. (*A*) A photomicrograph shows necrosis and degeneration of hepatocytes, Mallory bodies (eosinophilic inclusions) in the cytoplasm of injured hepatocytes, and infiltration by neutrophils. (*B*) Schematic representation of the major pathologic features of alcoholic hepatitis. The lesions are predominantly centrilobular, and include necrosis and loss of hepatocytes, ballooned cells (*BC*), and Mallory bodies (*MB*) in the cytoplasm of damaged hepatocytes. The inflammatory infiltrate consists predominantly of neutrophils (*N*), although a few lymphocytes (*L*) and macrophages (*M*) are also present. The central vein, or terminal hepatic venule (*THV*), is encased in connective tissue (*C*) (central sclerosis). Fat-laden hepatocytes (*F*) are evident in the lobule. The portal tract displays moderate chronic inflammation, and the limiting plate (*LP*) is focally breached.

lectively, these metabolic consequences produce a fatty liver, but the quantitative role for each is not established and may be variable.

Clinically, patients with uncomplicated alcoholic fatty liver have surprisingly few symptoms of liver disease. Except for the unusual combination of fatty liver and cholestasis, the bilirubin level is normal, and the serum aminotransferase levels are only minimally elevated—up to twice normal at most. Sudden death has been reported in alcoholics with fatty livers, but in most cases this is probably due to extra-

hepatic disease, such as sudden cardiac arrhythmias, to which alcoholics are notoriously susceptible. It is important to recall that, despite the striking morphologic change in the liver, alcoholic fatty liver is a fully reversible lesion and does not by itself progress to more severe disease, notably cirrhosis.

A fatty liver, while characteristic of alcoholism, is not restricted to that condition, and is also seen in obesity, uncontrolled diabetes, and kwashiorkor, and following prolonged administration of corticosteroids.

Alcoholic Hepatitis

The classic clinical features associated with alcoholic hepatitis are malaise and anorexia, fever, right upper quadrant abdominal pain, and jaundice. A mild leukocytosis is common. The serum aminotransferase activity, particularly that of glutamic-oxaloacetic transaminase (GOT), is moderately elevated, but not to the levels often seen in viral hepatitis. Serum alkaline phosphatase activity is usually increased. The sudden onset of jaundice, leukocytosis, and an elevated serum alkaline phosphatase has on occasion led to the erroneous diagnosis of obstructive jaundice. In severe cases the prothrombin time may be prolonged to such an extent that liver biopsy is not feasible, a situation associated with an ominous prognosis.

The pathogenesis of alcoholic hepatitis is mysterious. Alcoholics may have mild fatty liver for many years and, without any change in drinking habits, suddenly develop acute alcoholic hepatitis. The basis for the conversion of the benign fatty liver into the necrotizing lesion of alcoholic hepatitis may be the key to the eventual solution of the riddle of alcoholic liver injury.

Alcoholic hepatitis is an acute necrotizing lesion characterized by necrosis of hepatocytes, predominantly in the central zone, cytoplasmic hyaline inclusions within hepatocytes, a neutrophilic inflammatory response, and perivenular fibrosis (Fig. 14-30). In the typical case of acute alcoholic hepatitis, the hepatic architecture is basically intact, with a normal relationship of portal tracts to central venules. The hepatocytes show variable hydropic swelling, which gives them a heterogeneous appearance. Isolated necrotic liver cells, or clusters of them, exhibit pyknotic nuclei and karyorrhexis. Scattered hepatocytes contain so-called Mallory bodies—that is, alcoholic hyaline (see Fig. 14-30). These cytoplasmic inclusions, which are more common in visibly damaged, swollen hepatocytes, are visualized as irregular skeins of eosinophilic material or as solid eosinophilic masses, often in a perinuclear location. Ultrastructurally, they are composed of aggregates of intermediate (cytokeratin) filaments (Fig. 14-31). The damaged, ballooned hepatocytes, particularly those containing Mallory bodies, are surrounded by neutrophils, although a more diffuse, intralobular inflammatory infiltrate is also present. Cholestasis, varying from mild to severe, is present in as many as one-third of the cases. An important point is that alcoholic hepatitis is usually superimposed on an existing fatty liver, although there is no evidence that fat accumulation predisposes or contributes to the development of alcoholic hepatitis.

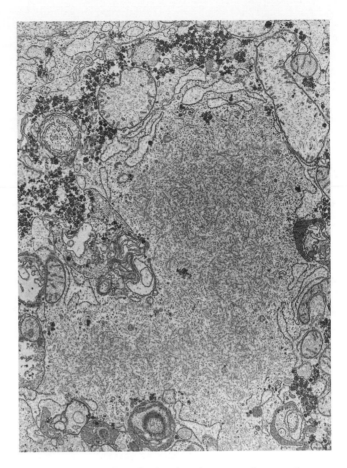

Figure 14-31. Mallory body. An electron micrograph shows an aggregate of filamentous material in the cytoplasm of a hepatocyte. The mass displaces the cytoplasmic organelles peripherally.

Collagen deposition is a constant feature of alcoholic hepatitis, especially around the central vein (terminal hepatic venule). In severe cases the venule and perivenular sinusoids are obliterated and surrounded by dense fibrous tissue, in which case the lesion has been termed **central hyaline sclerosis** (Fig. 14-32). This fibrotic lesion may persist after recovery from an episode of alcoholic hepatitis, and is, therefore, occasionally seen in a liver that does not display the other morphologic stigmata of alcoholic hepatitis. This finding may also explain the presence of portal hypertension in some alcoholics who do not have cirrhosis. Small strands of collagen may also be seen in the sinusoidal walls and in the periphery of the portal tracts. Characteristically, threads of connective tissue surround individual or groups of damaged hepatocytes.

The appearance of the portal tracts is highly variable. In some instances they appear virtually normal, whereas in others they are enlarged and contain a mononuclear infiltrate and proliferated bile ductules.

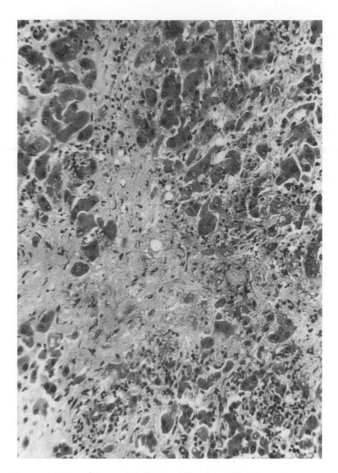

Figure 14-32. Central hyaline sclerosis. A photomicrograph from the liver of a patient with alcoholic liver disease shows the obliteration of the terminal venule by fibrous tissue.

The altered portal tracts often display spurs of fibrous tissue that penetrate the lobules. The inflammation may be so severe that it spills over into the lobule and obscures the limiting plate, an appearance similar to that of so-called piecemeal necrosis in chronic active hepatitis.

The histologic appearance of the liver in alcoholic hepatitis, when combined with an appropriate history, presents no diagnostic problem. However, a similar pattern of liver injury is occasionally seen in other conditions, including Wilson's disease, diabetes, and Indian childhood cirrhosis, and after jejunoileal bypass for morbid obesity. In addition, Mallory bodies are also occasionally encountered in primary biliary cirrhosis, extrahepatic biliary obstruction, drug-induced hepatic injury, and primary hepatocellular carcinoma.

The prognosis in patients with alcoholic hepatitis

correlates with the severity of the liver cell injury. In some patients the disease rapidly progresses to hepatic failure and death. The mortality in the acute stage of alcoholic hepatitis ranges from 10% to 30%. If the patient survives and continues to drink, the acute stage may be followed by a persistent alcoholic hepatitis, and more than a third of such patients progress to cirrhosis in only 1 or 2 years. Among those who abstain from alcohol after recovery from acute alcoholic hepatitis, only about a quarter have no morphologic residuals by 6 months, and about one in five progresses to cirrhosis. Recovery in the remaining abstainers is slow, and most show histologic lesions more than a year after the initial episode.

Alcoholic Cirrhosis

In about 15% of alcoholics, hepatocellular necrosis, fibrosis, and regeneration eventually lead to the formation of fibrous septa surrounding hepatocellular nodules, the two features that define cirrhosis (Fig. 14-33). The other lesions of alcoholic liver disease—namely, fatty liver and acute or persistent alcoholic hepatitis—are often seen in conjunction with cirrhosis. It is an open question whether typical alcoholic hepatitis—that is, an acute, inflammatory and necrotizing hepatic injury—is a necessary precursor of cirrhosis. **However, some form of persistent necrosis clearly precedes the development of cirrhosis.** Although epidemiologic data are conflicting, the weight of evidence suggests that the prognosis in cases of alcoholic cirrhosis is better in those who abstain from alcohol abuse.

Primary Biliary Cirrhosis

Primary biliary cirrhosis is a chronic liver disease that occurs principally in middle-aged women and whose clinical course is characterized by progressive cholestasis. The use of the term "cirrhosis" in the designation of this malady is misleading in that the cirrhosis is actually a late complication of the disease. **The basic lesion is a chronic, destructive disease of the intrahepatic bile ducts (nonsuppurative, destructive cholangitis).**

Primary biliary cirrhosis accounts for up to 2% of deaths from cirrhosis. It shows no apparent ethnic predilection, but several familial clusters of the disease have been reported. A hereditary predisposition is also suggested by the finding of characteristic immunologic abnormalities in some unaffected relatives.

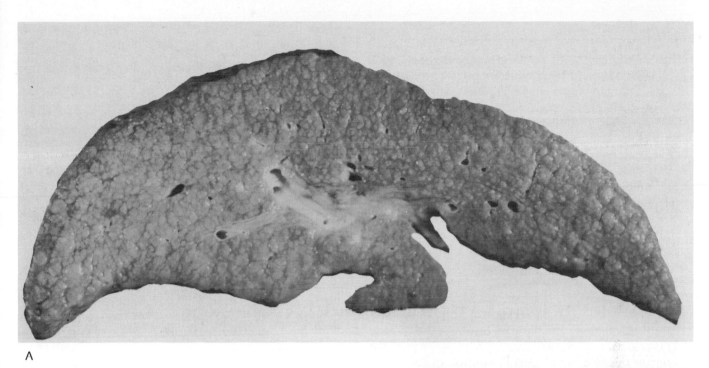

A

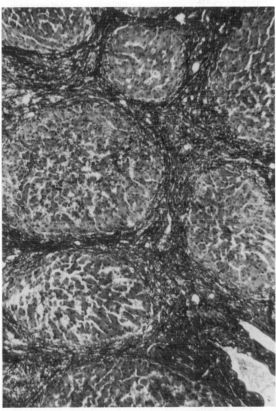

B

Figure 14-33. Alcoholic cirrhosis. (*A*) The cut surface of the liver is divided into innumerable small, regular nodules, separated by connective tissue septa. The pattern is predominantly micronodular. (*B*) A photomicrograph shows small regular nodules surrounded by uniform fibrous septa.

Clinical Features

Of those afflicted with primary biliary cirrhosis, 90% to 95% are women, usually between 30 and 65 years of age. In many patients the initial symptoms are fatigue and pruritus without jaundice, although about one-fifth of patients have jaundice when first seen. The cause of the severe pruritus is unknown, but it is relieved by oral treatment with resins (for example, cholestyramine) that bind bile acids and other anions. On the other hand, a substantial proportion of patients with primary biliary cirrhosis have no symptoms during the early stages of the disease; some of these patients remain asymptomatic and appear to have an excellent prognosis, whereas others ultimately present with advanced cirrhosis and its complications.

In a typical case, a high serum alkaline phosphatase activity is accompanied by a normal or only slightly elevated serum bilirubin level. As the disease advances, most patients have a progressive increase in serum bilirubin level. Serum aminotransferase activities are only moderately elevated. The serum cholesterol level is strikingly increased, and an abnormal lipoprotein, known as lipoprotein-X, which is seen in many forms of chronic cholestasis, appears. In the precirrhotic stages, most of the excess cholesterol is in the high density lipoprotein fraction, a fact that may account for the rarity of atherosclerosis in these patients. Nevertheless, cholesterol-laden macrophages accumulate in the subcutaneous tissues, where they appear as localized lesions termed **xanthomas.** Because of the impairment in the excretion of bile into the intestine, severe **steatorrhea** due to fat malabsorption is common. Because of associated malabsorption of vitamin D and calcium, **osteomalacia** and **osteoporosis** are important complications of primary biliary cirrhosis. Those patients who eventually develop cirrhosis die in hepatic failure or of the complications of **portal hypertension.**

The disease generally pursues an indolent course. Patients who develop cirrhosis usually survive 10 to 15 years, while in those without symptoms life expectancy may not be curtailed.

The Pathology of Primary Biliary Cirrhosis

Microscopically, three major stages in the evolution of primary biliary cirrhosis are recognized. These are characterized, respectively, by ductal lesions, scarring, and cirrhosis.

Stage I: The Duct Lesion

Stage I primary biliary cirrhosis is characterized by a unique lesion, namely a **chronic destructive cholangitis** affecting the intrahepatic small and medium-sized bile ducts (Fig. 14-34). The injury to the bile ducts is segmental and therefore appears focal in histologic sections. The bile ducts are surrounded principally by lymphocytes, but plasma cells and macrophages are also seen. In some patients eosinophils are conspicuous in the portal tracts, but neutrophils are rare. Characteristically, the bile duct epithelium is irregular and hyperplastic, with stratification of epithelial cells and occasional papillary ingrowths. Foci of necrotic epithelial cells and ulceration of the epithelium are not uncommon. In some portal tracts, lymphoid follicles, occasionally containing germinal centers, are present. Discrete epithelioid granulomas often occur in the portal tracts and may impinge on the bile ducts. In Stage I the lobular parenchyma tends to be normal, but in a minority of cases, mild central cholestasis is present.

Stage II: Scarring

As a result of the destructive inflammatory process characteristic of Stage I primary biliary cirrhosis, the small bile ducts virtually disappear, and scarring of medium-sized bile ducts is common. Such scarring constitutes Stage II disease. Chronic inflammation persists in the portal tracts but is not as severe as in Stage I. The chronic inflammatory infiltrate, both in Stage I and Stage II, may spill over into the periportal parenchyma, disrupt the limiting plate, and create a ragged border between portal tracts and the hepatic parenchyma—an appearance that may be mistaken for chronic active hepatitis. The presence of large amounts of copper and occasional Mallory bodies in the peripheral zone of the lobule assists in the differentiation from chronic active hepatitis. Proliferation of bile ductules within the portal tracts is usual and may be florid. Relatively acellular collagenous septa extend from the portal tracts into the lobular parenchyma and begin to encircle some lobules. Cholestasis, when present, may be severe, and is now located at the periphery of the portal tracts.

Stage III: Cirrhosis

The disease terminates as **end-stage liver disease**— that is, **cirrhosis**—characterized by fibrous septa that encompass regenerative nodules. Grossly, the bile-stained liver is dark green and exhibits a fine nodularity. Microscopically, small bile ducts are scarce and

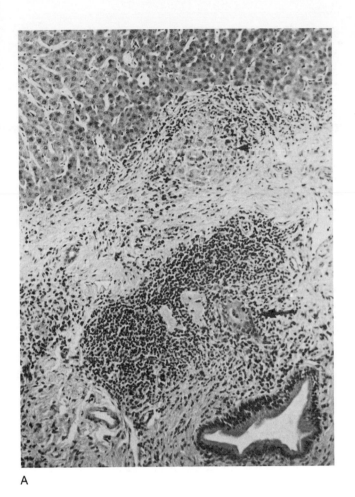

A

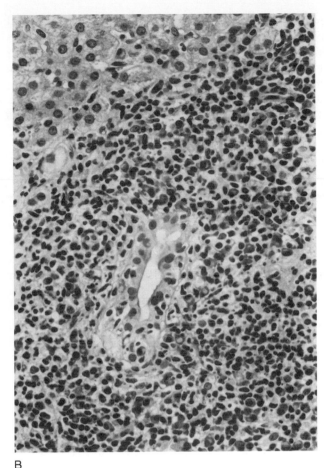

B

Figure 14-34. Primary biliary cirrhosis, Stage 1. (*A*) A photomicrograph shows a portal tract expanded by a lymphocytic infiltrate. A large interlobular bile duct (*lower right*) exhibits an irregular and hyperplastic epithelium. A smaller duct (*arrow*) shows severe degenerative changes. An epithelioid granuloma (*arrowhead*) is present within the portal tract. The hepatocytes appear normal. (*B*) A higher-power view of a portal tract shows a dense infiltrate of lymphoid cells surrounding a damaged interlobular bile duct (chronic destructive cholangitis).

medium-sized ducts conspicuously reduced in number. There is little inflammation within either the fibrous septa or the parenchymal nodules.

Immunopathogenesis of Primary Biliary Cirrhosis

Primary biliary cirrhosis is associated with many immunologic abnormalities and is, therefore, widely held to be an autoimmune disease. Although this may be probable, it should be stated at the outset that direct proof for this conjecture is lacking. Almost all (85%) of patients with primary biliary cirrhosis have at least one other disease usually classed as autoimmune, and almost half (40%) have two or

more such ailments. Among these disorders are chronic thyroiditis, rheumatoid arthritis, scleroderma, and Sjögren's syndrome.

Both humoral and cellular immunity appear to be altered. Serum immunoglobulin levels are increased, especially the level of IgM. More than 90% of the patients have circulating anti-mitochondrial antibodies, a finding commonly used in the diagnosis of primary biliary cirrhosis. Despite the fact that this antibody reacts with several antigens of the inner mitochondrial membrane, it has no inhibitory effect on mitochondrial function and plays no known role in the pathogenesis or progression of the disease. Other circulating autoantibodies are anti-nuclear, anti-thyroid, anti-platelet, anti-acetylcholine receptor and anti-ribonucleoprotein antibodies. The complement system is chronically activated, the increased complement turnover reflecting activation of the classical pathway. The reported decreases in the number of circulating T lymphocytes is not thought to be related to the pathogenesis of the disease.

The most attractive explanation for the initial destruction of bile ducts in primary biliary cirrhosis is an attack on the biliary epithelial cells by cytotoxic T lymphocytes. The infiltrating lymphocytes in the portal tracts are mostly T cells, both helper and suppressor. The ductal epithelial cells of patients with primary biliary cirrhosis express unusually large amounts of the Class I histocompatibility antigens HLA-A, B, and C. Moreover, unlike normal bile duct epithelial cells, they also express Class II HLA-DR antigens. Thus, the membranes of these bile duct epithelial cells appear to be an inviting target for sensitized cytotoxic T lymphocytes. The provocative suggestion has been made that the bile duct lesion of primary biliary cirrhosis is akin to the lesions of both graft-versus-host disease and the rejection of transplanted livers. The reasons for the antigenic alterations in the membranes of the bile duct epithelial cells, and the precise mechanism of T lymphocyte activation, remain to be elucidated.

Cirrhosis

The end stage of chronic liver disease is cirrhosis, defined as the destruction of normal hepatic architecture by fibrous septa that encompass regenerative nodules of hepatocytes. This morphologic pattern invariably results from persistent liver cell necrosis. Advanced cases of cirrhosis all tend to have a similar appearance, and often the etiology can no longer be ascertained by morphologic examination alone. During earlier stages, on the other hand, the characteristic features of the inciting pathogenic insult may be evident, as, for example, the fat and Mallory bodies typical of alcoholic liver injury or the chronic inflammation and periportal necrosis characteristic of chronic active hepatitis. Histologic examination of the liver may also allow the diagnosis of primary biliary cirrhosis, extrahepatic biliary obstruction, α_1-antitrypsin deficiency, glycogen storage disease Type IV, hemochromatosis, and chronic hepatic venous obstruction.

Morphologic Classification of Cirrhosis

The number of terms applied to the different forms of cirrhosis rivals the number of etiologic agents incriminated in chronic liver disease. Out of this ap-

parent complexity, we can extract a simple spectrum of nodular patterns. At one end of this spectrum, usually in the early evolution of cirrhosis, is the **micronodular** type, characterized by small, uniform nodules separated by thin fibrous septa (see Fig. 14-33). At the other end of the spectrum, ordinarily late in the course of the disease, is **macronodular cirrhosis**, in which grossly visible, coarse, irregular nodules are mirrored histologically by large nodules of varying size and shape that are encircled by bands of connective tissue that also vary conspicuously in width (Fig. 14-35). Between these two extremes are many cases which show features of both types, and for which the term **mixed cirrhosis** is appropriate.

Micronodular cirrhosis was previously termed Laennec's, portal, septal, or nutritional cirrhosis. With the exception of the term Laennec's cirrhosis, which honors the French physician who provided the first accurate description of this disease, these terms have little to recommend them, and the last is actually misleading. Micronodular cirrhosis exhibits nodules scarcely larger than a lobule, measuring less than 3 mm in diameter.

The micronodules show no landmarks of lobular architecture in the form of portal tracts or central venules. The connective tissue septa separating the nodules are usually thin, but irregular focal collapse of parenchyma may lead to the presence of wider septa. In active stages of the cirrhotic process, numerous mononuclear inflammatory cells and proliferated bile ductules inhabit the septa. The close approximation within the septa of capillaries and venules, fibroblasts, mononuclear inflammatory cells, and young connective tissue is similar to the appearance of granulation tissue in other organs. It is reasonable to assume that the same mechanisms that control the healing of wounds by granulation tissue in extrahepatic sites are also operative in the cirrhotic liver. The prototype of micronodular cirrhosis is alcoholic cirrhosis, but this pattern may also be observed in primary and secondary biliary cirrhosis, hemochromatosis, Wilson's disease, chronic obstruction to the venous outflow of the liver (Budd-Chiari syndrome), and certain inherited metabolic disorders.

Macronodular cirrhosis was formerly labeled postnecrotic, posthepatitic, or multilobular cirrhosis. The large, irregular nodules often contain portal tracts and efferent venous channels, evidence that the original process was characterized by multilobular necrosis that healed with the formation of large scars surrounding more than a single lobule. **However, it is now recognized that the micronodular pattern can be converted into a macronodular one by continued**

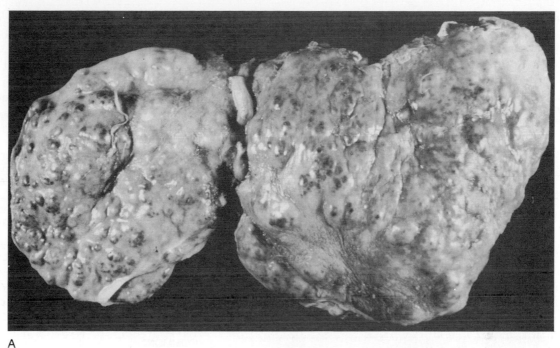

A

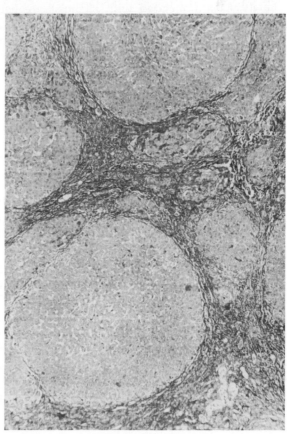

B

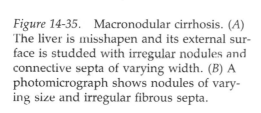

Figure 14-35. Macronodular cirrhosis. (*A*) The liver is misshapen and its external surface is studded with irregular nodules and connective septa of varying width. (*B*) A photomicrograph shows nodules of varying size and irregular fibrous septa.

regeneration and expansion of existing nodules. This is particularly the case in alcoholics who abstain from drinking after the diagnosis of cirrhosis has been made. Given sufficient time almost all (90%) cases of micronodular cirrhosis, even in those who continue to drink, will be converted to the macronodular pattern, usually within 2 to 3 years. The connective tissue septa in macronodular cirrhosis are characteristically broad and contain elements of pre-existing portal tracts, mononuclear inflammatory cells, and proliferated bile ductules. In a variant, formerly termed posthepatitic cirrhosis, the macronodules are separated by slender strands of connective tissue that join widely separated portal tracts. Macronodular cirrhosis is classically associated with chronic active hepatitis. It is also occasionally a result of submassive hepatic necrosis, in which case the liver may be grossly misshapen.

Etiology of Cirrhosis

The diseases associated with cirrhosis are listed in Table 14-3. It is clear that they have little in common, except for the fact that they are all accompanied by persistent liver cell necrosis. Most cases of cirrhosis are attributable to alcoholism and chronic viral hepatitis, although a significant contribution from unexplained chronic active hepatitis is a factor. The following discussion will focus on less common causes of cirrhosis.

Extrahepatic Biliary Obstruction

The extrahepatic biliary system may be obstructed by gallstones passing through the cystic duct to lodge in the common bile duct, cancer of the bile duct or

Table 14-3. Causes of Cirrhosis

Alcoholic liver disease
Chronic active hepatitis
Primary biliary cirrhosis
Extrahepatic biliary obstruction
Hemochromatosis
Wilson's disease
Cystic fibrosis
α_1-Antitrypsin deficiency
Glycogen storage disease, Types III and IV
Galactosemia
Hereditary fructose intolerance
Tyrosinemia
Hereditary storage diseases: Gaucher's, Niemann-Pick, Wolman's, mucopolysaccharidoses
Zellweger's syndrome
Indian childhood cirrhosis

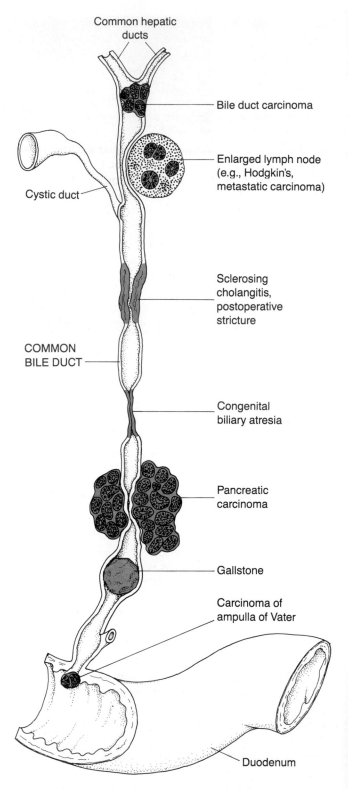

Figure 14-36.   Major causes of extrahepatic biliary obstruction.

surrounding tissues (pancreas or ampulla of Vater), external compression by enlarged neoplastic lymph nodes in the porta hepatis (as in Hodgkin's disease), benign strictures (postoperative or primary sclerosing cholangitis), and congenital biliary atresia (Fig. 14-36).

Early in the precirrhotic stage of extrahepatic biliary obstruction, the liver is swollen and bile-stained. In prolonged obstruction the bile becomes almost colorless ("white bile"), because of the suppression of the secretion of bilirubin, although the liver remains green. Initially, centrilobular cholestasis is accompanied by edema of the portal tracts, and in biopsy specimens early extrahepatic obstruction is difficult to differentiate from the various forms of intrahepatic cholestasis. As obstruction proceeds mononuclear inflammatory cells infiltrate the portal tracts. Tortuous and distended bile ductules, characterized by a high cuboidal epithelium, proliferate (Fig. 14-37). These stand in contrast to the bile ductules seen in other chronic liver diseases, in which the cells are flattened. The cholestasis eventually extends to the periphery of the lobule. Dilated bile ducts may rupture, leading to the formation of **bile lakes, a feature diagnostic of extrahepatic biliary obstruction.** Leakage of bile into the portal tracts also causes the appearance of foamy, lipid-laden macrophages, often aggregated as **granulomas.** Damaged hepatocytes containing large amounts of bile show **feathery degeneration.** Single-cell necrosis within the lobules is common, and periportal necrosis, associated with the portal inflammatory reaction, may be prominent. Infection of the obstructed biliary passages often leads to a superimposed suppurative cholangitis, intraluminal pus, and even intrahepatic abscesses. Within bile ducts and proliferated ductules, biliary concretions may be conspicuous, again a diagnostic feature of extrahepatic biliary obstruction.

With time the portal tracts become enlarged and fibrotic. Typically, the **periductal fibrosis** is concentric, giving rise to the term **"onion skin" fibrosis.** As in other forms of cirrhosis characterized by periportal necrosis, in about 10% of cases of cirrhosis caused by extrahepatic biliary cirrhosis, septa eventually extend between the portal tracts of contiguous lobules and form a micronodular cirrhosis. In the early stage of this cirrhotic phase, the portal-to-portal linkage distinguishes this disease from the portal-to-central pattern typical of alcoholic cirrhosis or from that of macronodular cirrhosis. However, in the late stage of extrahepatic biliary obstruction, further alterations make the distinction difficult.

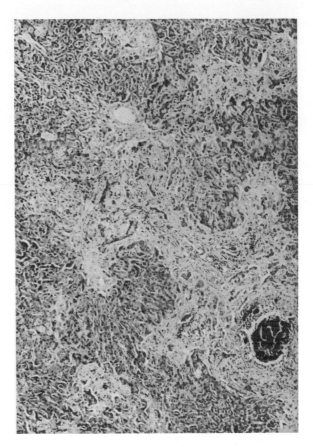

Figure 14-37. Secondary biliary cirrhosis. A photomicrograph of the liver from a patient with carcinoma of the pancreas that obstructed the common bile duct is shown. Irregular fibrous septa extend from an enlarged portal tract (*lower right*). Numerous proliferated bile ductules are seen within the septa. A dilated interlobular bile duct contains a dense biliary concretion.

Hemochromatosis

Hemochromatosis is defined pathologically as the accumulation of very large amounts of iron in the parenchymal cells of a variety of organs and tissues. The liver is always affected, contains more than 0.5 g iron per 100 g wet weight, and is usually cirrhotic. Siderosis refers to the accumulation of excess iron without tissue injury. **Primary hemochromatosis** is an inherited error of metabolism in which the absorption of iron is in excess of body needs. **Secondary hemochromatosis** arises as a consequence of certain inherited and acquired refractory anemias (e.g., thalassemia) that are characterized by the ineffective utilization of iron for erythropoiesis. In secondary hemochromatosis the intestinal absorption is also inappropriately high, but in this case it reflects a

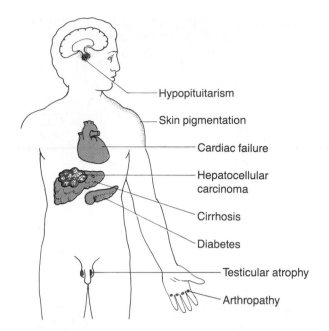

- Hypopituitarism
- Skin pigmentation
- Cardiac failure
- Hepatocellular carcinoma
- Cirrhosis
- Diabetes
- Testicular atrophy
- Arthropathy

Figure 14-38.   Complications of hemochromatosis.

response to the persistent anemia. In such circumstances iron overload is aggravated by multiple blood transfusions. In addition, secondary hemochromatosis may also result from excessive amounts of iron in the diet, when continued for years.

The body of a normal man contains 3 g to 4 g iron, two-thirds of which is present in hemoglobin, myoglobin, and iron-containing enzymes. The remainder is represented by storage iron, which exists in two forms, namely soluble ferritin and insoluble hemosiderin. Ferritin, the primary iron storage protein, is present in the cytoplasm of all cells and, in small amounts, in the circulation. Hemosiderin is a product of the degradation of ferritin, and, unlike the latter, is visualized by light microscopy as golden-yellow granules that stain with the Prussian blue reaction. The liver is an important organ for the storage of iron, although a comparable amount of storage iron exists in the bone marrow.

The absorption of iron from the gastrointestinal tract is controlled by the need to maintain appropriate iron stores. In the normal adult the iron stores remain constant, and consequently iron absorption is relatively constant. The obligatory daily iron loss through the urine and desquamated cells of the gut and skin is about 1 mg in men. Women suffer extra losses during menstruation and pregnancy. The possible range of daily iron absorption is from less than 0.5 mg a day in the individual with a normal iron bal-

ance, to an upper limit of 4 mg in those with iron deficiency. Dietary ascorbate is important in iron absorption, because ferric iron in the diet is reduced by ascorbic acid to ferrous iron, the form in which it can be absorbed by the small intestine. The absence of dietary vitamin C significantly decreases the amount of iron that can be absorbed. Ferrous iron is toxic and is readily converted to the ferric ion within the intestinal mucosal cell, where it is either complexed with transferrin for transport in the blood or stored as ferritin. When body stores of iron are high, intestinal storage is favored, and excess iron is sloughed into the gut with the extrusion of the villous epithelial cells. By contrast, when body iron stores are deficient, or if a defect in iron regulation is present within the mucosal cells, most of the iron is routed through the transferrin pathway and absorbed into the bloodstream.

Primary Hemochromatosis

In primary hemochromatosis, 20 g to 40 g of iron—that is, up to ten times the normal content—accumulates in the body. **The clinical hallmarks of advanced hemochromatosis are cirrhosis, diabetes, skin pigmentation, and cardiac failure (Fig. 14-38).** The disease is most often manifested clinically in patients between 40 and 60 years of age, and men are afflicted 10 times as often as women. This striking male predilection may be attributed to the increased loss of iron in women during the reproductive years. However, given sufficient time to absorb additional iron, postmenopausal women also seem to be at risk for the development of hemochromatosis. The excess iron is located exclusively within the storage compartment, and thus iron stores are increased up to 50 times normal. Since maximum iron absorption is about 4 mg per day, it is clear that hemochromatosis takes years to develop.

Primary hemochromatosis appears to be inherited as an autosomal recessive disorder. Although the genetic defect is common, it has become clear that not all patients who exhibit this genetically determined increase in iron absorption develop hemochromatosis. While only a few families have been reported in which more than one member has hemochromatosis, lesser degrees of iron overload are often found in relatives of those with the disease. The histocompatibility antigens A3, B7, and B14 occur more commonly in patients with hemochromatosis than in the normal population. In one study the haplotype A3B14 carried a relative risk of 23. It is thought that the gene for hemochromatosis is located on the short arm of chromosome six near the HLA-A locus. It now appears that this iron-loading gene is far more common than previously suspected, at least in white populations. It has been estimated that the heterozygous frequency is between 10% and 15%, and that 1 person in 200 to 400 is homozygous. Yet, only 1 in 5 homozygotes develops clinically apparent hemochromatosis.

The mechanisms underlying the increased deposition of iron of parenchymal organs in primary hemochromatosis are obscure, but an increased uptake of iron by the duodenal mucosa has been documented. Although an increased affinity of the liver for iron was postulated, this theory is no longer tenable, particularly since the hepatic iron stores are readily mobilized by venesection or by treatment with iron chelators. In addition, ferritin structure and synthesis are normal in hemochromatosis.

Currently, the most attractive hypothesis postulates a central role for abnormal regulation of iron storage in both the intestinal epithelial cell and the monocyte-macrophage system. This theory is buttressed by the demonstration that, despite the large amounts of iron in parenchymal cells of many organs, intestinal epithelial cells and reticuloendothelial cells have a low iron content. As noted above, the absorption of iron by the intestinal epithelial cell seems to be controlled by its content of storage iron. A decrease in this pool normally facilitates iron absorption; a portion of absorbed iron, carried on transferrin, is then stored in reticuloendothelial cells. However, in primary hemochromatosis the excess iron no longer finds a home in the reticuloendothelial cells, but rather is transferred to parenchymal cells, such as the hepatocyte.

Secondary Hemochromatosis

Hemochromatosis may also occur in persons who do not carry the gene for primary hemochromatosis. Within certain limits, the amount of iron absorbed bears a relation to the amount of iron ingested. For example, a low iron content in the diet renders the development of hemochromatosis unlikely. Whether excess dietary iron can produce iron overload in a normal person is still debated. Many patients with hemochromatosis (up to 40%) have a long history of alcohol abuse, and it is thought that alcohol may enhance both the accumulation of iron and its associated cell injury. The possible mechanisms are not clear, but the high iron content of many alcoholic beverages, the increased iron absorption in some patients with cirrhosis, and a putative synergism between two hepatotoxins (i.e., alcohol and iron) have been suggested.

An interesting example of secondary hemochromatosis is presented by the well-recognized iron accumulation in blacks of sub-Saharan Africa, commonly misnamed **"Bantu" siderosis.** These populations show a high incidence of siderosis without tissue damage, presumably because of the consumption of large amounts of iron-containing alcoholic beverages. A small proportion of these individuals show both severe siderosis and tissue injury, an appearance similar to that of primary hemochromatosis. With the recent replacement of "home-brewed" beverages of low alcoholic but high iron content by Western spirits of higher alcohol but lower iron content, the incidence of siderosis has fallen, while that of alcoholic cirrhosis has increased. Thus, under some conditions, excess dietary iron appears to play a role in the development of secondary hemochromatosis, although the contributions of other exogenous and genetic factors have not been fully elucidated.

Massive iron overload occurs in patients with certain anemias such as thalassemia major, sideroblastic anemias, and other anemias associated with ineffective erythropoiesis. As a result **secondary hemochromatosis** may develop even in children and adolescents. The source of the excess iron is the patient's diet or transfused blood. Increased iron absorption occurs despite the saturation of transferrin; the release of iron by intravascular hemolysis adds a further burden of iron. It is important to note that patients with thalassemia often develop hemochromatosis whether or not they have received blood transfusions. On the other hand, multiple blood transfusions alone are generally insufficient to produce secondary hemochromatosis, even in patients with hypoplastic anemia given many transfusions (250 mg iron/500 ml unit of blood). In these patients iron is concentrated principally in reticuloendothelial cells, and cirrhosis is rare.

Pathology of Hemochromatosis

The Liver   **The liver in hemochromatosis is enlarged and reddish brown, and exhibits a uniform micronodular cirrhosis (see Fig. 14-38).** In most respects the pattern is similar to that of alcoholic cirrhosis, which may explain the occasional confusion in the differentiation of these entities when alcoholic cirrhosis is accompanied by superimposed iron accumulation. The hepatocytes and bile duct epithelium are filled with iron granules, and lipofuscin pigment is increased (Fig. 14-39). Late in the disease, many Kupffer cells contain large deposits of iron de-

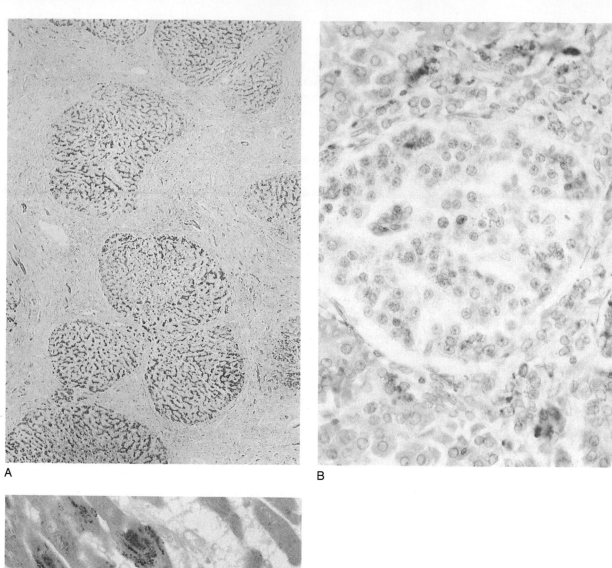

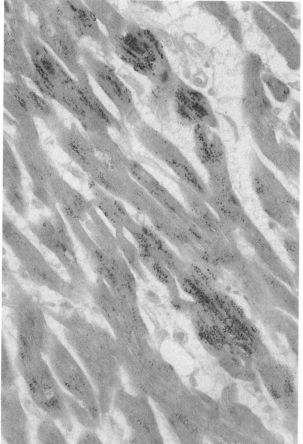

Figure 14-39. Hemochromatosis. A Prussian blue stain for iron demonstrates considerable iron in a cirrhotic liver (*A*), in an islet of Langerhans from the pancreas of the same patient (*B*), and in the myocardium (*C*).

rived from the phagocytosis of necrotic hepatocytes. Within the fibrous septa iron is conspicuous in proliferated bile ductules and macrophages. Eventually, as in micronodular cirrhosis of other causes, the pattern is transformed to that of a macronodular cirrhosis.

The liver disease in hemochromatosis generally pursues an indolent and prolonged course, but a quarter of patients eventually die in hepatic coma or from gastrointestinal hemorrhage. Hepatocellular carcinoma is a significant late complication of hemochromatosis, occurring in up to 15% of cases. Unfortunately, in patients who have already developed cirrhosis, this risk does not appear to be reduced by the removal of iron by venesection or chelators.

Cirrhosis with secondary iron overload shows varying degrees of iron accumulation, but the iron deposition is generally less extensive than in hemochromatosis, and is often restricted to the periphery of the nodules. The absence of iron deposition in the septa suggests that the cirrhosis preceded the iron accumulation. Transfusional and other types of siderosis are characterized by the uniform, initial deposition of iron in Kupffer cells, with eventual spillover into the hepatocytes.

In hemochromatosis ferric iron is stored predominantly in lysosomes. As noted in Chapter 1, iron is an essential factor in the cell injury mediated by activated oxygen species. It is reasonable to speculate that the presence of excess iron in cells renders them more susceptible to injury by partially reduced oxygen species generated during the normal metabolism of oxygen.

Extrahepatic Manifestations The **skin** in patients with primary hemochromatosis is typically pigmented, but only half exhibit increased iron deposition in the skin. Most patients display increased melanin in the basal melanocytes. The accumulation of hemosiderin pigment is particularly severe in the sweat glands.

Diabetes, a common complication of hemochromatosis, results from the **deposition of iron in the pancreas.** Grossly, the organ appears rust-colored and is firm, reflecting underlying fibrosis. Both the exocrine and endocrine cells are affected, particularly the former. Frequently, there is degeneration of acinar cells and a reduction in the number of islets of Langerhans. The combination of pigmented skin and glucose intolerance in patients with hemochromatosis is often referred to as "bronze diabetes."

Congestive heart failure is a common cause of death in patients with hemochromatosis. The heart is often enlarged, sometimes weighing more than twice normal. Microscopically, the myocardial fibers contain iron pigment, which is more extensive in the ventricles than in the atria. Necrosis of cardiac myocytes and accompanying interstitial fibrosis are common.

The endocrine system is typically involved in hemochromatosis. Iron is deposited in the pituitary, adrenal, thyroid, and parathyroid glands. However, tissue damage is not a usual feature in these organs, except for the pituitary, in which the release of gonadotropins is impaired. As a result, **testicular atrophy** is seen in a quarter of the male patients, even without iron deposition in the testes. The disturbance in the pituitary-gonadal axis is characterized by loss of libido and amenorrhea in women, and impotence and sparse body hair in men. These effects are often manifested well before the onset of symptoms of liver disease.

Arthropathy, most severe in the fingers and hands, occurs in 25% to 75% of patients with hemochromatosis, and is sometimes the initial symptom. When arthritis affects the larger joints, such as the knee, it may be severe enough to be disabling. Although deposits of hemosiderin may be seen in the synovium and articular cartilage, the pathogenesis of the arthritis is unclear.

Laboratory Diagnosis of Hemochromatosis

The normal value for plasma iron is 80–100 μg/dl, and transferrin is normally about one-third saturated. In patients with primary hemochromatosis, the serum iron concentration is more than doubled and transferrin is entirely saturated. The concentration of circulating transferrin, like that of other proteins whose synthesis is impaired in chronic liver disease, is reduced. The concentration of ferritin in the blood, which parallels the amount of storage iron, is greatly increased in hemochromatosis. Urinary excretion of iron after the administration of an iron chelator (deferoxamine) is a useful diagnostic test.

Treatment

The treatment of hemochromatosis is based on the removal of iron from the body, most effectively by repeated phlebotomy. Weekly phlebotomies for 2 to 3 years can remove 20 g to 40 g of iron, after which phlebotomies every 2 to 3 months maintain iron balance. The beneficial effect of repeated phlebotomies is impressive. The 10-year survival of untreated patients with hemochromatosis is a mere 6%, whereas in those treated by phlebotomy, it is more than five times as great. In patients with refractory anemias, continuous intravenous administration of iron chelators has been helpful.

Heritable Disorders Associated With Cirrhosis

Wilson's Disease (Hepatolenticular Degeneration)

Wilson's disease is a hereditary disorder of copper metabolism in which injury to the liver and brain is associated with deposition of excess copper. The disease is transmitted by an autosomal recessive gene thought to be located on chromosome 13. The carrier rate is in the vicinity of 1 in 100, and the incidence of clinical disease is about 30 per million, with a slight predilection for males. The gene appears to have a worldwide distribution.

Copper Metabolism

In the fetus most of the body copper is contained in the liver, principally in lysosomes and bound to metallothionein. After birth the hepatic copper concentration falls, and by age 3 months the liver copper reaches adult concentrations (about 8% of total body copper). The daily copper requirement for the normal adult is between 1 mg and 2 mg. Since the intake of copper in the diet is ordinarily considerably greater, copper balance is easily maintained. Unlike iron absorption, body copper homeostasis is not regulated at the level of the intestine. Copper absorbed from the intestine is bound to albumin and amino acids and transported to the liver. Within the hepatocyte, copper is utilized for the synthesis of copper-containing enzymes (e.g., cytochrome oxidase and superoxide dismutase); bound to metallothionein for storage in lysosomes; complexed with the copper-binding protein ceruloplasmin for return to the blood; and excreted into the bile. Biliary excretion of copper is the primary mechanism by which body copper balance is maintained, since negligible amounts of copper are reabsorbed by the intestine. As a result copper accumulates in the liver during prolonged cholestasis from any cause, such as, for example, primary biliary cirrhosis or extrahepatic biliary obstruction. About 90% to 95% of circulating copper is bound to ceruloplasmin, from which it is made available to peripheral tissue as well as returned to the liver.

Wilson's disease is characterized by a striking reduction in the serum levels of ceruloplasmin. However, several observations suggest that hepatic copper overload in Wilson's disease cannot be simply attributed to diminished ceruloplasmin levels alone: a few patients with well-documented Wilson's disease and copper overload in the liver have normal ceruloplasmin levels; heterozygotes often exhibit significantly diminished levels of ceruloplasmin, but do not develop copper overload; the severity of the clinical expression of the disease does not correlate with the serum ceruloplasmin concentration; and the administration of ceruloplasmin does not ameliorate the defect in copper metabolism. It is now clear that intestinal absorption of copper is unaltered in Wilson's disease. On the other hand, biliary, and therefore fecal, excretion of copper is reduced to about a quarter of the normal rate. Theories that attribute the defect in copper excretion by the hepatocyte to abnormal copper binding proteins in the liver have met with little support. Thus, although the primary lesion in Wilson's disease is probably related to defective biliary excretion of copper, the exact pathogenesis remains obscure.

The similarity between copper metabolism in Wilson's disease and that in the fetus is interesting, in that both are characterized by low concentrations of copper and ceruloplasmin in the blood and high levels in the liver. It has been suggested that the transition from fetal to adult copper metabolism is regulated by a gene that controls copper excretion from the liver cell, either by influencing biliary copper excretion or by controlling the synthesis and secretion of ceruloplasmin. According to this scenario, Wilson's disease might represent a malfunction of this gene. In any event, the primacy of the liver as the seat of the disease is attested to by its cure with liver transplantation.

Although the total serum copper concentration is low in Wilson's disease, that fraction not bound to ceruloplasmin (albumin-bound or free copper) is greater than normal, both relatively and absolutely. It is possible that this increased concentration of free copper plays a role in the excess deposition of copper in extrahepatic tissues.

The mechanism by which excess copper injures cells remains elusive. Like iron, copper may catalyze the formation of potent oxidizing species from superoxide anions and hydrogen peroxide produced by normal oxygen metabolism. In this regard, copper can replace iron in the Fenton reaction, in which ferrous iron and hydrogen peroxide generate hydroxyl radicals (see Chapter 1).

Clinical Features

Half of the patients with Wilson's disease display some symptoms by adolescence, and the remainder become ill in their early adult years. A few instances have been recorded in which the disease did not become apparent until middle age. The presenting symptoms are referable to chronic liver disease in about half the patients, while one-third initially present with neurologic complaints, and about one-tenth are seen because of psychiatric manifestations. A quarter of the patients show symptoms related both to the liver and to the central nervous system.

The **liver disease** begins insidiously with nonspecific symptoms and progresses to chronic liver disease indistinguishable from that of other forms of chronic active hepatitis. Wilson's disease should, therefore, be included in the differential diagnosis of HbsAg-negative chronic hepatitis. Eventually chronic hepatitis and cirrhosis result in jaundice, portal hypertension, and hepatic failure. Unlike hemochromatosis, Wilson's disease is not associated with an increased risk of primary hepatocellular carcinoma.

The **neurologic disease** begins with mild incoordination and tremors. In untreated cases dysarthria and dysphagia appear, and in late stages disabling dystonia and spasticity occur. Progressive behavioral abnormalities and dementia may lead to the institutionalization of patients before the diagnosis of Wilson's disease becomes evident.

Ophthalmic manifestations invariably accompany the neurologic disease. The **Kayser-Fleischer ring** is a golden-brown, bilateral discoloration of the cornea, which encircles the periphery of the iris and obscures its muscular pattern. It represents a deposition of copper in Descemet's membrane. This ophthalmic sign is not diagnostic of Wilson's disease unless it is accompanied by neurologic disease. Kayser-Fleischer rings may be absent in patients with Wilson's disease who suffer only from hepatic disease and in presymptomatic children. Corneal rings may also be present in other cholestatic liver diseases characterized by copper accumulation, including primary biliary cirrhosis, biliary atresia, and chronic active hepatitis with cirrhosis. In some patients the Kayser-Fleischer rings are accompanied by **sunflower cataracts,** green discs of copper deposition in the anterior capsule of the lens.

Skeletal lesions are commonly found on radiographic examination. They include osteomalacia, osteoporosis, spontaneous fractures, and various arthropathies. Clinical symptoms are less common, but are occasionally the presenting complaint.

Renal glomerular and tubular dysfunction, manifested by proteinuria, lowered glomerular filtration, aminoaciduria, and phosphaturia, is common in Wilson's disease. Although it was proposed that the aminoaciduria represents a primary gene defect in Wilson's disease, it is now thought to be secondary to copper deposition in the renal tubules. This concept is supported by the observation that the renal disease disappears with removal of excess copper by chelating agents.

Transient **acute hemolytic episodes,** presumably related to a sudden release of free copper from the liver, occur in as many as 15% of patients with Wilson's disease. This hematologic complication commonly precedes the development of overt liver disease, and therefore, Wilson's disease should be included in the differential diagnosis of nonimmune hemolytic anemia in young people. With the development of severe liver disease, hypersplenism and coagulation defects often supervene.

Pathology

The initial alterations in the liver of children are nonspecific and include mild to moderate fat accumulation, lipofuscin deposition, and glycogen in the nuclei of hepatocytes. Subsequently, the disease progresses from mild to severe chronic active hepatitis with all of the typical histologic features of that disease. The periportal hepatocytes often contain Mallory bodies, and cholestasis, with bile casts in proliferated bile ductules, is not infrequent. Occasional acidophilic bodies may be present. Kupffer cells are enlarged and contain hemosiderin, derived from phagocytosis during episodes of intravascular hemolysis. Cirrhosis may develop rapidly, even in childhood. An initial micronodular cirrhosis eventually assumes a macronodular pattern. **In young adults the presence of fat, Mallory bodies, hepatocellular necrosis, and cholestasis may lead to an erroneous diagnosis of alcoholic liver disease.** By electron microscopy, the hepatocytes exhibit large, distorted mitochondria and numerous vacuolated and enlarged lysosomes.

The staining of the liver with rubeanic acid or rhodanine demonstrates copper granules in hepatocytes in some patients; most cases do not stain positively, however, even when hepatic copper concentrations are high. Copper stains are also positive in cholestatic states and neonatal livers, in which hepatic copper levels are also high. Chemical measurement of liver copper in unfixed tissue demonstrates more than 250 μg copper per gram dry weight.

In the brain the corpus striatum and occasionally the subthalamic nuclei display a reddish-brown discoloration. The central white matter of the cerebral or cerebellar hemispheres may manifest spongy softening or cavitation, in which case the overlying cortex is atrophic. The astrocytes proliferate in the putamen, and the number of neurons is decreased.

Treatment

Treatment of Wilson's disease not only prevents the accumulation of tissue copper but also extracts copper that has already been deposited. d-Penicillamine, a copper-chelating agent, augments the excretion of copper in the urine. Both central nervous system dysfunction and the symptoms of liver disease are often reversed by treatment. When d-penicillamine treatment is initiated during the early, asymptomatic phase, the clinical disease is entirely prevented. Liver transplantation is curative, even after neurologic symptoms have developed.

Cystic Fibrosis

Historically, cystic fibrosis was almost invariably fatal in childhood, as a result of repeated pulmonary infections and respiratory insufficiency. However, the advent of antibiotic therapy and techniques for respiratory toilet have allowed many patients to survive into adult life. Concomitantly, hepatic complications of cystic fibrosis have become far more common. Cystic fibrosis is discussed in detail in Chapter 6, which deals with genetic diseases.

Newborn infants with cystic fibrosis may present with obstructive jaundice within the first few weeks of life. Biliary obstruction results from the accumulation of tenacious mucous plugs in the intrahepatic biliary tree, and in that sense is analogous to the meconium ileus found in half of these patients. Recovery typically occurs in 1 to 6 months, but some infants die in hepatic failure.

In children who survive to adolescence, clinically symptomatic liver disease develops in as many as 15%, and cirrhosis is found in 10% of patients who survive beyond the age of 25 years. The pattern of cirrhosis closely resembles that seen with extrahepatic biliary obstruction, but the lesions characteristically are focally accentuated in different parts of the liver. The cirrhosis is assumed to result from the obstruction of fine biliary passages by inspissated mucus. The interlobular bile ducts are focally dilated and contain eosinophilic, PAS-positive material. Since this focal lesion may be missed in a needle biopsy of the liver, establishment of the diagnosis often depends on the clinical history. Portal hypertension and splenomegaly may accompany the cirrhosis, and may indeed be the basis of the presenting complaints.

α_1-Antitrypsin Deficiency

α_1-Antitrypsin deficiency, inherited as an autosomal recessive trait, was initially described as a cause of emphysema (see Chapter 12). Thereafter, cases of liver disease without pulmonary involvement were described, and disease of both organs has also been recognized. α_1-Antitrypsin is synthesized in the liver,

and the deficiency syndromes result from a defect in the secretion of the protein, possibly owing to abnormal glycosylation or biosynthesis.

The clinical expression of liver disease in α_1-antitrypsin deficiency is highly variable, ranging from a rapidly fatal neonatal hepatitis to an absence of any hepatic dysfunction. **Of those infants with the ZZ genotype—that is, those who are susceptible to the development of clinical disease—about 10% develop neonatal cholestatic jaundice (conjugated hyperbilirubinemia).** This condition is far more common than previously recognized, and accounts for 15% to 30% of all cases of neonatal conjugated hyperbilirubinemia. Most infants recover within 6 months, but a few progress to cirrhosis within 1 or 2 years. Moreover, about half the patients with the ZZ phenotype have other intermittent abnormalities of liver function, and 10% to 20% develop permanent liver disease. The mechanism by which liver cells are injured in α_1-antitrypsin deficiency is not understood.

The characteristic feature in the liver of patients with α_1-antitrypsin deficiency is the presence of faintly eosinophilic, PAS-positive cytoplasmic droplets (Fig. 14-40). These tend to be small in infancy, but may reach the size of the nucleus in older individuals. By electron microscopy, these inclusions are visualized as amorphous material within dilated cisternae of the endoplasmic reticulum. Since cytoplasmic globules resembling those in this condition are occasionally encountered in other disorders, a definitive diagnosis is made by demonstrating their reactivity with antibody to α_1-antitrypsin.

In infants the associated hepatitis cannot be distinguished morphologically from other forms of neonatal hepatitis or from chronic active hepatitis. As in neonatal hepatitis from other causes, hepatocellular giant cells are prominent in some cases and often disappear within 6 to 12 months. Canalicular cholestasis is frequently striking. In infancy, conspicuous proliferation of bile ductules and fibrosis may erroneously lead to a diagnosis of extrahepatic biliary atresia. The increasing portal fibrosis is accompanied by a decrease in the number of bile ducts, again confusing the diagnosis with intrahepatic biliary atresia. Micronodular cirrhosis develops by the age of 2 to 3 years, and may ultimately become macronodular. Children with cirrhosis usually die before the age of 10 years from hepatic failure or other complications of α_1-antitrypsin deficiency.

Some children manifest hepatic dysfunction, but develop cirrhosis only slowly. These patients may be asymptomatic until early adulthood, when they may present with symptoms of cirrhosis as the initial complaint. Another group of affected children recovers

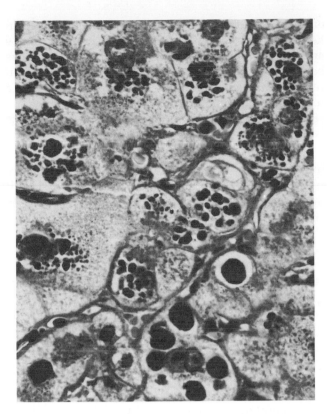

Figure 14-40.   α₁-Antitrypsin deficiency. A photomicrograph of a section of liver stained by the periodic acid-Schiff (PAS) reaction shows the presence of numerous cytoplasmic droplets in the hepatocytes.

entirely from the acute illness in infancy and has no further evidence of liver disease.

The cirrhosis of α₁-antitrypsin deficiency is complicated by a very high incidence of hepatocellular carcinoma.

Inborn Errors of Carbohydrate Metabolism

Glycogen Storage Diseases

The biochemical basis of the glycogen storage diseases has been discussed in Chapter 6. These disorders seem to be inherited as autosomal recessive traits. Only glycogenosis Type IV (brancher deficiency, Andersen's disease) is inevitably complicated by cirrhosis. A slowly developing cirrhosis may be seen in glycogenosis Type III (debrancher deficiency, Cori's disease), but is not inevitable. Glycogenosis Type I (glucose-6-phosphatase deficiency, von Gierke's disease) is associated with striking hepatomegaly, and Type II (acid maltase deficiency, Pompe's disease) with mild hepatomegaly. Neither is complicated by cirrhosis.

In **Type I disease,** the hepatocytes are distended by large amounts of glycogen, which appears pale in sections stained with hematoxylin and eosin. The enlarged liver cells compress the sinusoids and may obscure the normal arrangement of the hepatic cell plates. The PAS stain is heavily positive, and electron microscopy demonstrates masses of glycogen particles in the cytoplasm. Glycogen is present within the nuclei as well. Fat accumulation varies from mild to severe, but fibrosis is usually absent.

Type II disease is characterized by only mild distention of hepatocytes, without fat or fibrosis. The cytoplasm of the hepatocytes contains small clear areas, which by histochemistry and electron microscopy have been shown to be lysosomes distended with glycogen.

Infants with **glycogenosis Type III** show severe hepatomegaly, and the liver morphologically resembles that seen in Type I. Fat is less conspicuous, but fibrosis is present and may progress to cirrhosis.

In **glycogenosis Type IV,** infants present with severe hepatomegaly and die of cirrhosis by the age of 4 years. Sharply circumscribed, PAS-positive inclusions, somewhat resembling those seen in α₁-antitrypsin deficiency by light microscopy, are present in enlarged hepatocytes. By electron microscopy these inclusions consist of fibrillar material. The brancher enzyme deficiency responsible for glycogenosis, Type IV, leads to the synthesis of an abnormal glycogen molecule that has fewer branch points than normal. This glycogen is less soluble than the normal one and therefore has an unusual ultrastructural appearance. Unlike normal glycogen, it is only partially digested by diastase. Deposits of abnormal glycogen are also found in the heart, skeletal muscle, and brain. Extensive fibrosis eventually progresses to cirrhosis, which is initially micronodular but may develop macronodular features.

Galactosemia

Galactosemia, inherited as an autosomal recessive trait, is caused by a deficiency of galactose-1-phosphate uridyl transferase, the enzyme that catalyzes the second step in the conversion of galactose to glucose. As a result of this metabolic defect, galactose and its metabolites accumulate in the liver and other organs. Infants with this disorder who are fed milk rapidly develop **hepatosplenomegaly, jaundice, and hypoglycemia.** Cataracts and mental retardation are common.

Microscopically, within 2 weeks of birth the liver shows **extensive and uniform fat accumulation, and striking proliferation of bile ductules in and around the portal tracts.** Cholestasis is often present in canaliculi and bile ductules. Within several weeks the hepatic cell plates become arranged around a lumen, thus assuming a glandular or acinar appearance. Bile plugs fill many of these pseudoacini. At about 6 weeks of age, fibrosis begins to extend from the portal tracts into the lobule and within 6 months progresses to **cirrhosis**. The institution of a galactose-free diet has been reported to ameliorate the disease and reverse many of the morphologic alterations. The basis of the liver cell injury and necrosis in this disorder is mysterious.

Hereditary Fructose Intolerance

Hereditary fructose intolerance is an autosomal recessive disease caused by a deficiency of fructose-1-phosphate aldolase; rare instances of fructose 1,6-diphosphate phosphatase deficiency have also been recorded. When fructose is fed early in infancy, hepatomegaly, jaundice, and ascites develop. However, the feeding of fructose after the age of 6 months results in far less severe disease, and the only clinical impairment is spontaneous hypoglycemia. **Infants who suffer from liver disease show the changes of neonatal hepatitis**—namely, hepatocellular necrosis, giant hepatocytes, inflammation, ductular proliferation, and cholestasis. Fat accumulation may be marked. **Progressive fibrosis culminates in cirrhosis.**

Tyrosinemia

Tyrosinemia is an autosomal recessive disease that interferes with the catabolism of tyrosine to fumarate and acetoacetate. The precise biochemical defect is controversial, but it appears reasonable to assume that damage to the liver and kidney is caused by the accumulation of succinyl acetone and succinyl acetoacetate, both of which are potent electrophiles that can react with the sulfhydryl groups of glutathione and proteins. Tyrosinemia occurs in acute and chronic forms. In the acute disease, which begins within a few weeks or months of birth, hepatosplenomegaly is associated with **liver failure and death, usually before the age of 12 months.** The appearance of the liver is remarkably similar to that of galactosemia, including progression to **cirrhosis.** The chronic disease begins in the first year of life, and is characterized by **growth retardation, renal disease, and hepatic failure.** Death usually supervenes before the age of 10 years. The incidence of **hepatocellular carcinoma** associated with tyrosinemia is extraordinarily high. In one series of patients who survived beyond 2 years of age, 37% manifested neoplastic transformation in the liver.

Miscellaneous Inherited Causes of Cirrhosis

A wide variety of inborn errors of metabolism have been associated with cirrhosis, including storage diseases, such as Gaucher's disease, Niemann-Pick disease, mucopolysaccharidoses, neonatal adrenoleukodystrophy, and Wolman's disease. Zellweger's syndrome, in which peroxisomes are lacking, has been linked with cirrhosis. Cirrhosis has also been reported in association with hereditary hemorrhagic telangiectasia.

Indian Childhood Cirrhosis

Indian childhood cirrhosis is a fatal disorder largely restricted to India and parts of Southeast Asia, although an occasional case with similar morphologic and clinical features has been reported from the United States. The disorder affects children, mostly boys, between the ages of 1 and 4 years. The liver in this **micronodular cirrhosis** displays hydropic swelling of hepatocytes, focal necrosis, and fibrosis connecting portal tracts and central venules. Diffuse fibrosis around injured hepatocytes and groups of cells is usual. Characteristically, Mallory bodies are abundant, but little fat is present. **This constellation of morphologic features is almost identical to that seen in alcoholic liver disease.** The etiology and pathogenesis are entirely unknown. Familial cases have been reported, but no hereditary pattern has been established. A search for viruses, toxins, and nutritional deficits has been fruitless.

Portal Hypertension

The portal vein, arising at the junction of the superior mesenteric vein with the splenic vein, carries the major venous drainage from the gastrointestinal tract, the pancreas, and the spleen into the liver. The portal vein delivers two-thirds of the hepatic blood flow, but accounts for less than half of the total oxygen supply, the remainder being supplied by the hepatic artery. Normally, the pressure in the portal vein is only 5 to 10 mm Hg. For practical purposes, **portal hypertension, defined as a sustained increase in portal venous pressure, is almost always a result of obstruction to blood flow somewhere in the portal circuit,** and complications arise from the increased pressure and dilatation of the venous bed behind the obstruction. **The major complications of this increased pressure and the opening of collateral channels are bleeding from gastroesophageal varices, ascites, and splenomegaly.**

For the sake of convenience, obstruction to the flow of portal blood can be pictured as **prehepatic** (occurring before the blood enters the hepatic sinusoids); **intrahepatic** (occurring during transit through the portal tracts and lobules); or **posthepatic** (occur-

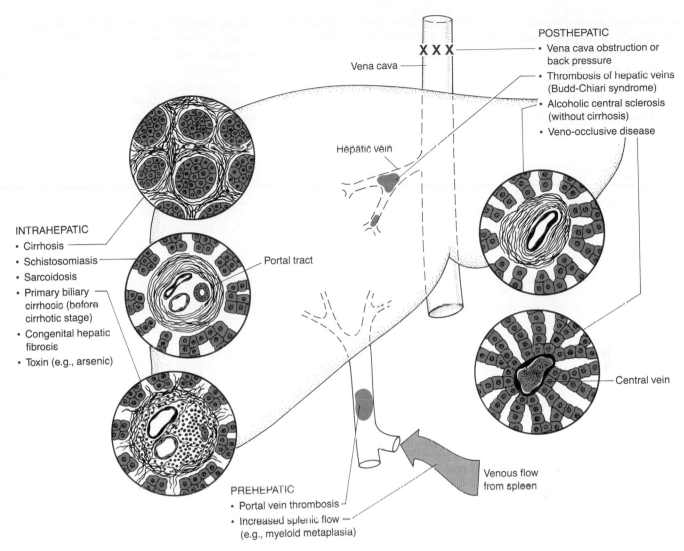

POSTHEPATIC
- Vena cava obstruction or back pressure
- Thrombosis of hepatic veins (Budd-Chiari syndrome)
- Alcoholic central sclerosis (without cirrhosis)
- Veno-occlusive disease

Vena cava

Hepatic vein

INTRAHEPATIC
- Cirrhosis
- Schistosomiasis
- Sarcoidosis
- Primary biliary cirrhosis (before cirrhotic stage)
- Congenital hepatic fibrosis
- Toxin (e.g., arsenic)

Portal tract

Central vein

Venous flow from spleen

PREHEPATIC
- Portal vein thrombosis
- Increased splenic flow (e.g., myeloid metaplasia)

Figure 14-41. Causes of portal hypertension.

ring after exit of the blood from the lobules) (Fig. 14-41). In this scheme the term "hepatic" refers to the lobule rather than the entire liver.

Intrahepatic Portal Hypertension

By far the most common cause of portal hypertension is cirrhosis. Regenerative nodules impinge upon and deform the **hepatic veins,** thereby obstructing blood flow distal to the lobules. The small **portal veins and venules** are trapped, narrowed, and often obliterated by scarring of the portal tracts. Moreover, blood flow through the hepatic artery is increased, and small **arteriovenous communications** become functional. In this way, portal hypertension due to obstruction of blood flow distal to the sinusoid is augmented by the increase in arterial blood flow. Moreover, an increase in splanchnic arterial blood flow, the cause of which is unclear, is an important factor in the maintenance of portal hypertension. Central vein sclerosis and sinusoidal fibrosis contribute to the development of portal hypertension in alcoholic liver disease. In fact, portal hypertension can result from alcoholic central sclerosis even in cases that do not progress to cirrhosis.

In addition to cirrhosis, intrahepatic portal hypertension can be caused by other conditions that interfere with the flow of blood through the liver, including cystic disease of the liver (see Chapter 16, which includes a discussion of cystic disease of the kidney), partial nodular transformation of the liver in the region of the porta hepatis, nodular regenerative hyperplasia (small regenerative nodules without fibrosis that compress the intervening hepatic parenchyma), and metastatic or primary carcinoma of the liver. In rare instances sarcoidosis involving the liver has been associated with portal hypertension, either because the granulomas directly obstruct blood flow by compressing the portal venules or sinusoids or because portal and periportal scarring distort the portal vein radicals.

Worldwide, hepatic schistosomiasis (*S. mansoni* and *S. japonicum*) is a major cause of portal hypertension. The ova released from the intestinal veins traverse the portal system and lodge in the portal venules, where they elicit a granulomatous reaction that heals by scarring. Hepatic function is well maintained, but the intrahepatic presinusoidal vascular obstruction leads to severe portal hypertension.

Occasional cases of portal hypertension with splenomegaly occur in the absence of any demonstrable intrahepatic or extrahepatic disease, in which case the term **idiopathic portal hypertension** is applied. Historically, increased portal blood flow from the enlarged spleen was incriminated, but this now seems unlikely. In some cases portal fibrosis and compression of portal veins, together with the deposition of collagen in the space of Disse, have been described. In prolonged idiopathic portal hypertension, portal fibrosis may be conspicuous. However, as the name indicates, the etiology is still being sought. In some countries (England, Japan) idiopathic portal hypertension accounts for 15% to 35% of all cases that require surgery to decompress the portal circulation.

Prehepatic Portal Hypertension

The classic example of **prehepatic portal hypertension** is **portal vein thrombosis,** which may be caused by tumors, infections, hypercoagulability states associated with oral contraceptive use and pregnancy, pancreatitis, and surgical trauma. Some cases are without known cause, but **the most common association in portal vein thrombosis is with cirrhosis.** Primary hepatocellular carcinoma characteristically invades branches of the portal vein, and occasionally reaches and occludes the main portal vein. When the portal vein is obstructed by a septic thrombus, bacteria may seed the intrahepatic branches of the portal vein **(suppurative pylephlebitis)** and cause multiple hepatic abscesses.

Occlusion of the portal vein may be manifested in the neonatal period or in early childhood. In some cases umbilical sepsis is an important cause, but other local and systemic infections may also play a role.

Often the portal or the splenic vein is replaced by a fibrous cord or interlacing vascular channels, a process termed **cavernous transformation.**

The liver normally offers little resistance to the outflow of blood through the sinusoids and can, therefore, accommodate substantial increases in blood flow without a secondary increase in pressure. However, under some uncommon circumstances increased portal venous blood flow can be associated with, or increase the severity of, portal hypertension. An **arteriovenous fistula**—that is, an abnormal communication between an artery and the portal vein—may lead to portal hypertension. It generally arises from trauma or rupture of an aneurysm of the splenic or hepatic artery. Such a fistula may also be found in association with hereditary hemorrhagic telangiectasia **(Osler-Weber-Rendu syndrome).** Portal hypertension also occasionally occurs in patients with splenomegaly from a variety of causes, including polycythemia vera, myeloid metaplasia, and chronic myelogenous leukemia. Although increased blood flow is the etiologic factor in this form of portal hypertension, the liver also responds with increased resistance to blood flow, particularly with sclerosis of the smaller portal vein radicals. In cirrhosis, the accompanying splenomegaly may further aggravate portal hypertension.

Posthepatic Portal Hypertension

Posthepatic portal hypertension can be defined as any obstruction to blood flow through the hepatic veins beyond the liver lobules, either within or distal to the liver. **Occlusion of the hepatic veins,** commonly known as the **Budd-Chiari syndrome,** was originally described in the large hepatic veins, but is now known to occur in venous tributaries of any size, including central hepatic venules. The principal cause of the Budd-Chiari syndrome is thrombosis of the hepatic veins, in association with such diverse conditions as polycythemia vera, hepatocellular carcinoma, tumor metastases from the adrenals and kidneys, bacterial infections, the use of oral contraceptives, pregnancy, and trauma. However, in more than half the cases, no specific etiology for the Budd-Chiari syndrome is evident. Thrombosis is most common in the large hepatic veins close to their exit from the liver and in the intrahepatic portion of the inferior vena cava. In parts of Africa and the Orient, membranous webs of unknown etiology, presumably congenital, compromise the vena cava above the orifices of the hepatic veins and commonly cause the Budd-Chiari syndrome. Increased back pressure in the venous system caused by severe congestive heart failure, tricuspid stenosis or regurgitation, or constrictive pericarditis may mimic the Budd-Chiari syndrome, although such complications of heart disease have been rendered uncommon by contemporary medical and surgical treatment.

A variant of the Budd-Chiari syndrome is represented by occlusion of the central venules and small branches of the hepatic veins, a condition termed **hepatic veno-occlusive disease.** Most commonly this disorder is traced to the ingestion of toxic pyrrolizidine alkaloids present in plants of the *Crotalaria* and *Senecio* families that are used in the formulation of "bush tea" in primitive societies. It is also seen in patients treated with certain antineoplastic chemotherapeutic agents, after hepatic irradiation, and in association with bone marrow transplantation, possibly as a manifestation of graft-versus-host disease.

Thrombosis of the hepatic veins, when total, presents as an acute illness characterized by abdominal pain, enlargement of the liver, ascites, and mild jaundice. Acute hepatic failure and death often occur rapidly. The more usual course, in which the obstruction of the hepatic venous circulation is incomplete, is marked by similar symptoms, but may pursue a protracted course over periods ranging from 1 month to a few years. More than 90% of these patients develop ascites, usually severe, and splenomegaly is seen in over 30%. The liver is usually enlarged. Typically, the serum bilirubin and aminotransferase activities are only modestly increased. Most patients eventually die in hepatic failure or from the complications of portal hypertension. Liver transplantation has been successful in curing the disease.

In the early acute stage of hepatic vein thrombosis, the liver is swollen and tense, and the cut surface exhibits a mottled appearance and oozes blood. In the chronic stage, the cut surface is paler, and the liver is firm, owing to an increase in connective tissue. Microscopically, the hepatic veins display thrombi in varying stages of evolution, from recent clots to well-organized thrombi that have been recanalized (Fig. 14-42). In veno-occlusive disease similar thrombotic occlusions are present within the terminal hepatic venules, although some investigators have claimed that the proliferation of endothelial cells, rather than thrombosis, represents the initial lesion. Acutely, the sinusoids of the central zone are dilated and packed with red blood cells. The liver cell plates are compressed, and necrosis of centrilobular hepatocytes is accompanied by the deposition of fibrin. In longstanding venous congestion, fibrosis of the central zone radiating into the more peripheral portions of the lobules is conspicuous. The sinusoids are dilated, and the central to midzonal hepatocytes show pressure atrophy. Red blood cells may be dislocated

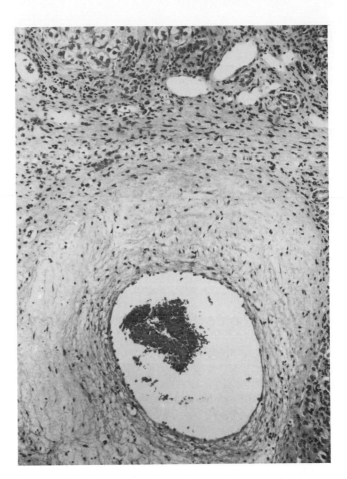

Figure 14-42. Budd-Chiari syndrome. A photomicrograph shows a recanalized hepatic vein. Perivenous fibrosis and a markedly thickened intima are evident.

into the space of Disse, and may be grouped in areas of hepatocyte necrosis. Eventually, connective tissue septa link adjacent central zones to form nodules with a single portal tract in the center, a process known as reverse lobulation. The fibrosis is usually not severe enough to justify a label of cirrhosis, although on rare occasions nodular transformation of the architecture is significant enough to warrant this appellation.

Complications of Portal Hypertension

Portal hypertension leads to several systemic complications (Fig. 14-43). The classic complications are esophageal varices, splenomegaly, and ascites.

Esophageal Varices

The most important complications of portal hypertension arise from the opening of portal-systemic collaterals as an adaptation to decompress the portal

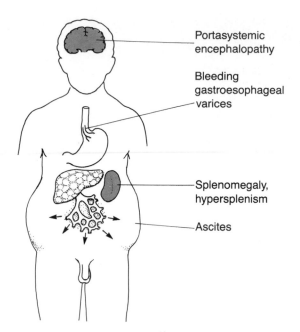

Figure 14-43. Complications of portal hypertension.

venous system. The collaterals of most clinical significance, located in the submucosa of the lower esophagus and upper stomach, are a result of communications between the portal vein and the gastric coronary vein. Because of the increased blood flow and higher pressure that follow the opening of these collaterals, the submucosal veins in the vicinity of the esophagogastric junction become dilated and protrude into the lumen. One of the most common causes of death in patients with cirrhosis and other disorders associated with portal hypertension is exsanguinating upper gastrointestinal hemorrhage from **bleeding esophageal varices.** Surprisingly, the precise cause of this bleeding is uncertain, since there is no simple correlation between portal venous pressure and the risk of variceal bleeding. The prognosis in cases of bleeding esophageal varices is poor, and the acute mortality may be as high as 40%. In patients who survive an initial episode of variceal bleeding, long-term survival is poor because of a high risk of rebleeding or a worsening of liver failure. Patients in whom the portal hypertension is caused by a prehepatic block, such as hepatic schistosomiasis, have a much better prognosis than those with cirrhosis, because of the absence of underlying liver dysfunction. Importantly, death associated with bleeding esophageal varices is frequently not attributable directly to exsanguination and shock, but rather is the result of **hepatic failure** precipitated by the stress, ischemic necrosis of the liver, and the encephalopathy caused by the acute nitrogenous load imposed by the exsanguinated blood in the intestinal tract.

Acute variceal hemorrhage may be treated by direct tamponade with an inflatable balloon, injection of varices with sclerosing agents through an endoscope, or intravenous administration of vasopressin to reduce splanchnic blood flow and portal venous pressure. For patients with repeated episodes of variceal bleeding, permanent decompression of the portal circulation can be achieved by surgically constructed portasystemic shunts. These procedures divert blood from the high-pressure portal circulation to the lower-pressure systemic venous circulation. Portasystemic shunt surgery is generally reserved as a last resort for patients who continue to bleed from varices, in part because of the high operative mortality and in part because of the risk of portasystemic encephalopathy following diversion of the portal blood from the liver. The surgical diversion of portal blood from the liver may also increase the risk of subsequent hepatic failure.

The back pressure in the portal vein is also transmitted to its tributaries, including the inferior hemorrhoidal veins, which become dilated and tortuous, resulting in **anorectal varices.** Although the umbilical vein in the falciform ligament does not carry blood in the adult circulation, it remains probe-patent. In portal hypertension blood flows from the portal vein through this channel to the epigastric veins of the anterior abdominal wall. Clinically, visible collateral veins radiating from the umbilicus produce the pattern known as **caput medusae.** On occasion, the left renal vein also becomes enlarged through anastomoses from the splenic vein or other channels.

Splenomegaly

The spleen in portal hypertension enlarges progressively, and splenomegaly is considered by some as the single most important diagnostic sign of portal hypertension. The enlarged spleen often gives rise to the syndrome of **hypersplenism**—that is, a decrease in the life span of all of the formed elements of the blood and, therefore, a reduction in their circulating numbers. Hypersplenism is attributed to an increased rate of removal of red blood cells, white blood cells, and platelets because of the prolonged transit time through the hyperplastic spleen. Grossly, the spleen is firm and enlarged, up to 1000 g, and its cut surface is uniformly deep red, with an inapparent white pulp. Microscopically, the sinusoids are dilated and their walls are thickened by fibrous tissue and lined by hyperplastic reticuloendothelial cells. Focal hemorrhages lead to the deposition of iron in the form of siderotic nodules, known as **Gamna-Gandy bodies.**

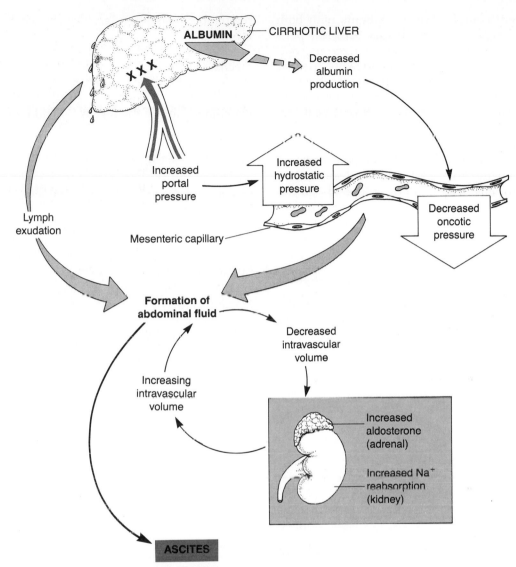

Figure 14-44. Pathogenesis of ascites.

Ascites

Ascites—that is, the accumulation of fluid in the peritoneal cavity—often accompanies portal hypertension, most commonly in patients with decompensated cirrhosis. The amount of fluid may be so great, frequently many liters, that it not only distends the abdomen, but also interferes with breathing. The onset of ascites in cirrhosis is associated with a poor prognosis.

The pathogenesis of ascites remains a subject of investigation, but it is generally thought that the increased formation of hepatic and intestinal lymph is important (Fig. 14-44). In addition, an increase in sinusoidal pressure in the liver results in an imbalance in Starling forces and drives serum proteins into the interstitial space. Eventually, the rate of formation of hepatic lymph exceeds the capacity of the lymphatics to remove it, and the liver "weeps" fluid into the peritoneal cavity. Impaired reabsorption of ascitic fluid by the peritoneum is also thought to play a role in the pathogenesis of ascites. Hypoalbuminemia in patients with cirrhosis also contributes to the formation of ascites, because of the decreased plasma oncotic pressure.

The sequestration of fluid in the peritoneal cavity leads to a decrease in the effective plasma volume, which in turn leads to renal sodium and fluid retention through a number of possible mechanisms, including decreased glomerular filtration, increased aldosterone activity, and increased sodium reabsorption. The increased renal retention of sodium and fluid aggravates ascites formation, and creates a vicious cycle.

An important complication in patients with both cirrhosis and ascites is **spontaneous bacterial peritonitis.** The infection is extremely dangerous, and carries a 60% to 90% mortality, even when treated with antibiotics. Presumably, the ascitic fluid is seeded with bacteria from the blood or lymph, or by the passage of bacteria through the bowel wall. No underlying infectious source is found, and the pathogenesis remains obscure. Typically, the white blood cell count in the ascitic fluid of spontaneous bacterial peritonitis is greater than 500/mm³, and more than half are neutrophils. The diagnosis depends on the presence of bacteria, principally *E. coli* and group D streptococci, in the ascitic fluid or on culture.

Toxic Liver Injury

The spectrum of acute chemically-induced hepatic injury is so broad that it spans the entire spectrum of liver disease, from clinically trivial, transient cholestasis, to fatal fulminant hepatitis. Chronic toxic injury to the liver is equally diverse, being expressed, at one extreme, as a mild persistent hepatitis and, at the other, as an active cirrhosis. Although hepatic injury caused by drugs accounts for less than 5% of all cases of jaundice, it comprises up to 25% of fulminant hepatic necrosis.

The multiplicity of drugs that cause liver injury, the differences in their chemical structure and metabolism, and the diverse patterns of injury all preclude a simple classification of toxic injury. In general, certain hepatotoxic chemicals invariably produce liver cell necrosis—that is, their action is entirely **predictable.** Among such agents are substances as diverse as yellow phosphorus, the organic solvent carbon tetrachloride, the mushroom poison phalloidin, and the analgesic acetaminophen. The defining characteristics of the liver injury produced by "predictable" hepatotoxins are as follows:

- The agent, in sufficiently high doses, always produces liver cell necrosis.
- The extent of hepatic injury is dose-dependent. Although exceptions exist, these compounds produce the same lesions in different species.
- The liver necrosis is characteristically zonal—often, but not exclusively, centrilobular.
- The period between administration of the toxin and the development of liver cell necrosis is brief.

Historically, predictable hepatic necrosis was encountered principally in an industrial or occupational context, but today a greater awareness of the potential danger of liver damage and better occupational safety regulations have rendered such accidents uncommon.

Chapter 1 includes a discussion of the possible mechanisms by which these toxins produce liver necrosis. Briefly, toxic liver necrosis is, in most (though not all) cases, a consequence of the metabolism of the compound by the mixed function oxidase system of the liver, by which activated oxygen species and reactive metabolites are produced. The rate of drug metabolism is influenced by many factors, including age, sex, nutritional status, interactions with other drugs, and prior induction of hepatic drug metabolizing activity.

In contrast to the aforementioned classic poisons, **most reactions to drugs are unpredictable** and seem to represent **idiosyncratic** events or manifestations of unusual sensitivity to a dose-related side effect. Sensitive individuals may be predisposed to idiosyncratic reactions either because they possess metabolic pathways different from those of the general population, or because they are unusually sensitive to a uniform pharmacologic effect of the drug other than the desired therapeutic response. For example, chlorpromazine, a drug administered because of its effects on the central nervous system, reproducibly inhibits bile flow in experimental animals. On the other hand, when chlorpromazine is given chronically to patients in the usual therapeutic dose range, only a small proportion of patients develop cholestatic jaundice. Under these circumstances, it is not clear whether the jaundice in man results from a qualitative differ-

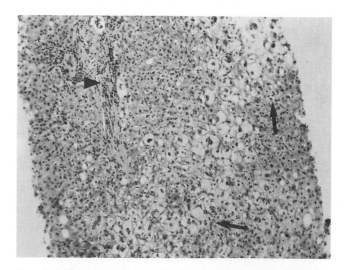

Figure 14-45. Toxic centrilobular necrosis. A liver biopsy specimen from a young woman who had ingested a large amount of acetaminophen in a suicide attempt shows centrilobular ballooning and necrosis of hepatocytes (*arrows*). The area surrounding the portal tract (*arrowhead*) appears normal.

ence in the response of the hepatocyte to chlorpromazine or simply reflects an exaggerated inhibition of bile flow. An immunologic reaction to drugs, their metabolites, or modified liver cells has not been ruled out, although direct evidence is weak. **Drugs that are principally cholestatic do not necessarily depend upon metabolism for their action.**

With these considerations in mind, we shall discuss toxic liver injury in terms of the morphologic patterns of the resulting reaction.

Zonal Hepatocellular Necrosis

Drugs and chemicals that are predictable hepatotoxins and act via their metabolites typically cause centrilobular necrosis (Fig. 14-45), presumably because of the greater activity of drug-metabolizing enzymes in the central zones. Examples of such agents are carbon tetrachloride, acetaminophen, and the toxins of the mushroom *Amanita phalloides*. A minority of predictable hepatotoxins cause periportal necrosis, including yellow phosphorus, allyl alcohol, and ferrous sulfate. In the affected zones hepatocytes show coagulative necrosis, hydropic swelling, and variable amounts of fat. Occasional acidophilic bodies, the remnants of necrotic hepatocytes, are free in the sinusoids. Inflammation is often sparse, although, if the patient survives, a secondary inflammatory response becomes more conspicuous. If the dose of the hepatotoxin is sufficiently large, necrosis may extend to involve the entire lobule, leaving only a thin rim of viable hepatocytes surrounding the portal tracts. Patients die in acute hepatic failure or recover without sequelae. The chronic administration of hepatotoxins that cause zonal necrosis, exemplified by carbon tetrachloride, produces cirrhosis in experimental animals. However, this is generally not a problem in man: Once the acute toxic injury has been recognized, measures are usually taken to preclude reexposure to the offending agent.

Fatty Liver

The accumulation of triglycerides within the hepatocytes—that is, hepatic steatosis or fatty liver—occurs in response to a variety of hepatotoxins, generally in a predictable fashion. Although substantial overlap may exist, two morphologic patterns are seen; namely, **macrovesicular and microvesicular steatosis** (Fig. 14-46). In macrovesicular steatosis, light microscopy shows the cytoplasm of the liver cell to be occupied by fat, seen as a large clear area that distends the cell and displaces the nucleus to the

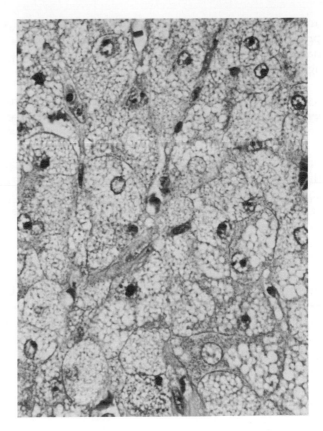

Figure 14-46. Microvesicular fatty liver. A liver biopsy specimen in a case of Reye's syndrome shows small droplet fat in hepatocytes and a centrally located nucleus.

periphery. In the microvesicular variety, small fat vacuoles are dispersed throughout the cytoplasm, and the nucleus retains its central position. In addition to its association with chronic ethanol ingestion, macrovesicular fat results from the experimental administration of, or accidental exposure to, such direct hepatotoxins as carbon tetrachloride and the poisonous constituents of certain mushrooms. Moreover, corticosteroids and some antimetabolites, such as methotrexate, may cause macrovesicular steatosis. There is no reason to believe that the presence of fat, per se, is in any way injurious to the hepatocyte. Rather, its accumulation reflects the underlying liver cell damage. In many, but not all, instances of toxic steatosis, the basis for fat accumulation is impaired secretion of lipoproteins as a consequence of an interference with protein synthesis.

A puzzling variant of toxic macrovesicular steatosis resembles **alcoholic hepatitis,** not only in the distribution of fat but also in the presence of **Mallory bodies** and an acute inflammatory response. This unusual combination has been associated with the administration of the antiarrhythmic agent amiodarone, the coronary vasodilator perhexilene maleate, and synthetic estrogens used in the treatment of prostatic carcinoma. Experimentally, Mallory bodies have also been produced in mice with the antifungal agent griseofulvin.

In contrast to macrovesicular steatosis, which by itself is in general clinically inconsequential, microvesicular fatty liver is commonly associated with severe, and sometimes fatal, liver disease, although milder forms are recognized. Again, it is not the presence of fat but the underlying metabolic defects that produce the liver dysfunction. Perhaps the most common and widely feared example of liver disease associated with microvesicular steatosis is **Reye's syndrome, an acute disease of children characterized by hepatic failure and encephalopathy.** The symptoms usually begin after a febrile illness, commonly influenza or varicella infection, and have recently been claimed to correlate with the administration of **aspirin.** Clearly, Reye's syndrome is more complex than simple aspirin toxicity, because it almost always occurs only after a febrile illness, and the doses of aspirin consumed are far too small to produce liver injury in otherwise normal children. These observations suggest a possible synergism between aspirin and viral infection in the causation of Reye's syndrome, but the precise mechanisms remain to be elucidated. In any event, with the decline in the use of aspirin in children, and possibly a reduced incidence of influenza, Reye's syndrome is now distinctly uncommon.

Under the light microscope, the liver in Reye's syndrome displays a typical microvesicular steatosis without accompanying hepatocellular necrosis or inflammation. Electron microscopy demonstrates **characteristic alterations in mitochondria of the liver and brain,** including large budding and branching forms. Mitochondrial dysfunction, characterized principally by a decrease in intramitochondrial enzymes, leads to impaired oxidation of fatty acids and hyperammonemia. Cerebral edema and fat accumulation are reported in the brain.

Reye's syndrome has been compared with **Jamaican vomiting illness,** caused by the ingestion of **hypoglycin,** a poison in the unripened fruit of the ackee tree. The toxic principal binds to coenzyme A, thereby inhibiting fatty acid oxidation. A toxic microvesicular steatosis that is similar morphologically and functionally to Reye's syndrome has been associated in Thailand with the intake of **aflatoxin,** a fungal product (*Aspergillus*) that contaminates the diet. Intravenous administration of **tetracycline** in high doses, particularly in pregnant women, has also resulted in microvesicular steatosis and hepatic failure.

Microsteatosis, not infrequently associated with hepatic failure, is a feature of the so-called **fatty liver of pregnancy,** the pathogenesis of which is unknown. In this condition the morphologic appearance of the liver is similar to that in Reye's syndrome, but the characteristic mitochondrial abnormalities of the latter are not present. Many of the patients exhibit pre-eclampsia, and some cases have occurred in association with accompanying disorders—for example, pancreatitis and disseminated intravascular coagulation. The condition ordinarily improves upon delivery, although in some cases progressive hepatic failure could not be averted. Women who have suffered fatty liver of pregnancy may complete subsequent pregnancies without untoward effects.

Triglycerides are not the only lipids that can accumulate in the liver in response to toxic injury. **Phospholipidosis,** which resembles certain heritable disorders of lipid metabolism (for instance Niemann-Pick and Tay-Sachs diseases), occurs after the administration of drugs such as perhexilene maleate and amiodarone. By light microscopy, both hepatocytes and Kupffer cells are enlarged and show a foamy cytoplasm. By electron microscopy, crystalloid or lamellated inclusions are found within distended lysosomes. Drugs that cause phospholipidosis are amphiphilic and bind to phospholipids, thereby inhibiting their catabolism. Changes similar to those in the liver occur in extrahepatic sites, include the lung, bone marrow, and lymphoid tissues.

Intrahepatic Cholestasis

Acute intrahepatic cholestasis is one of the most frequent manifestations of idiosyncratic types of drug-induced liver disease. A few drugs, principally sex steroids of the contraceptive or anabolic type, cause **bland centrilobular cholestasis** with virtually no hepatocellular necrosis or inflammation. Except for mild jaundice, pruritus, and an elevated serum alkaline phosphatase level, the patients feel well.

Many other drugs, of which chlorpromazine is the prototype, are associated with **centrilobular cholestasis, slight to moderate inflammation, and mild hepatocellular injury.** Eosinophils are often conspicuous in the portal tracts, a feature that suggests a hypersensitivity reaction to chlorpromazine or its metabolites. In addition, as previously noted, chlorpromazine has been shown in animals to inhibit bile flow directly.

An unusual pattern of cholestatic liver injury is characterized by the **proliferation of bile ductules** in the portal tracts and the appearance of **inspissated bile within the lumina.**

In some cases continued administration of a drug that has produced acute cholestasis may lead to a chronic cholestatic syndrome resembling primary biliary cirrhosis, although the long-term prognosis is clearly more favorable than that of primary biliary cirrhosis if the drug is discontinued.

Mild Intralobular Hepatitis

A wide variety of drugs (e.g., aspirin and synthetic penicillins) may produce a mild liver injury, frequently dose-dependent, that is rapidly reversible upon discontinuation of the drug. Small foci of liver cell necrosis are scattered throughout the lobule and are associated with a few mononuclear inflammatory cells. A sparse infiltrate in the portal tracts is common. The morphologic characteristics of viral hepatitis, such as lobular disarray, acidophilic bodies, hydropic swelling, cholestasis, and significant inflammation, are lacking, and the disease does not become chronic. A similar pattern is not uncommon in systemic diseases that do not primarily affect the liver, such as sepsis and ulcerative colitis.

Lesions Resembling Viral Hepatitis

All the typical clinical and morphologic features of acute viral hepatitis can be seen after the administration of some drugs that cause idiosyncratic (unpredictable) liver injury. The most widely appreciated examples are the inhalation anesthetic halothane, the anti-tuberculosis agent isoniazid, and the anti-hypertensive drug methyldopa. Although the incidence of these viral-hepatitis–like reactions is low, they are far more dangerous than viral hepatitis itself, causing more severe disease and a much higher mortality rate. The entire range of acute liver injury, from mild anicteric hepatitis to rapidly fatal fulminant hepatic necrosis, is encountered. It deserves repetition that, for practical purposes, the pattern of liver injury is morphologically indistinguishable from that of documented acute viral hepatitis. As in viral hepatitis, when the offending agent is removed—that is, when the virus is cleared or the drug is withdrawn—complete recovery is the rule.

The fact that hepatitis caused by halothane is typically more severe after a second or third exposure suggests that an allergic or immunologic mechanism mediates the injury. The frequent occurrence of peripheral eosinophilia and eosinophils in the liver in cases of halothane hepatitis supports this concept. However, it has not been definitively established that an immunologic mechanism plays a role in halothane hepatitis. Alternatively, exposure to halothane may alter the response of the liver to subsequent exposures.

Chronic Active Hepatitis

Persistent intake of hepatotoxic drugs can lead to a syndrome indistinguishable from chronic active hepatitis. Like chronic active hepatitis caused by persistent viral infection, drug-induced chronic active hepatitis may progress to cirrhosis. On discontinuation of drug administration, the lesion usually resolves, although this may require many months. In cases that have progressed to cirrhosis, the scarring remains, but the inflammatory and necrotizing activity is halted. Among the drugs incriminated in the production of chronic active hepatitis are the laxative oxyphenisatin, the antihypertensive agent methyldopa, the anti-tuberculosis drug isoniazid, and certain sulfonamides.

Granulomatous Hepatitis

A number of drugs occasionally associated with hepatotoxicity may also induce noncaseating, "sarcoid-like" granulomas in the portal tracts and the lobular parenchyma. In some instances other organs also display granulomas. Focal necrosis and minimal intrahepatic cholestasis may complicate the granulomatous hepatitis. The liver damage is transient and does not lead to chronic lesions. Among the many drugs that have been associated with granulomatous hepatitis are the anti-inflammatory agent phenylbutazone, the anti-arrhythmic drug quinidine, and allopurinol, used in the treatment of gout.

Vascular Lesions

As noted in the discussion of portal hypertension, occlusion of the hepatic veins (**Budd-Chiari syndrome**) has been reported to follow the use of oral contraceptive agents, presumably a reflection of the general hypercoagulable state associated with the use of these steroids. Obstruction at the level of the terminal venules (central veins), termed **veno-occlusive disease,** may result from the ingestion of certain alkaloids in "bush teas" or from the administration of some agents used in the chemotherapy of cancer.

Anabolic sex steroids, and occasionally contraceptive steroids, sometimes produce a peculiar hepatic lesion, **peliosis hepatis,** characterized by cystic, blood-filled cavities that are not lined by endothelial cells (Fig. 14-47). In some cases, peliosis caused by anabolic steroids, such as methyltestosterone and norethandrolone, is associated with mild intrahepatic cholestasis. Other agents that have been associated with peliosis are the anti-estrogen tamoxifen and excess vitamin A.

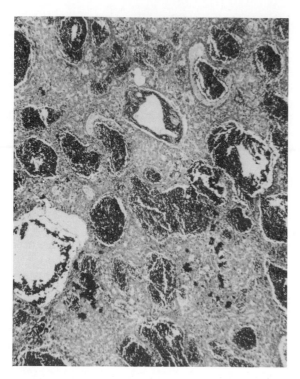

Figure 14-47. Peliosis hepatis. The liver contains numerous large, irregular, blood-filled spaces.

Hyperplastic and Neoplastic Lesions

The spectrum of hepatic lesions caused by chemicals extends to benign and malignant tumors. Although preneoplastic hepatic nodules and hepatocellular carcinoma are regularly produced by chemicals in experimental animals, examples in man are few. Today, it is recognized that the use of oral contraceptives, and uncommonly anabolic steroids, may be associated with the development of **hepatic adenomas,** benign tumors of hepatocytes whose greatest danger lies in their propensity to rupture and then bleed profusely. A few cases of primary hepatocellular carcinoma have been reported in persons taking oral contraceptives or anabolic steroids, but an etiologic association is controversial. **Focal nodular hyperplasia,** a solitary mass of apparently normal hepatocytes traversed by fibrous septa, was suggested as a complication of oral contraceptive use, but subsequent studies have cast doubt on this association.

Hemangiosarcomas of the liver appeared many years after the intravenous administration of Thorotrast (thorium dioxide), a radioactive compound used in the past to visualize the liver. This particulate material is engulfed by Kupffer cells, where it remains inert indefinitely, emits local radiant energy, and thereby produces neoplastic transformation. Chronic

exposure to inorganic arsenic, usually in the form of insecticides, and the inhalation of vinyl chloride in an industrial setting have also been linked to the development of hemangiosarcoma of the liver.

Vascular Disorders

Congestive Heart Failure

Acute Passive Congestion

At autopsy it is common for the liver to be acutely congested, presumably because of a failing heart in the agonal period. On cut section, the liver is diffusely speckled with small red foci, which microscopic examination reveals to be centrilobular zones with moderately dilated and congested sinusoids and terminal venules. These changes are not clinically significant.

Chronic Passive Congestion

In the face of **persistent congestive heart failure,** the pressure in the peripheral venous circulation increases, impeding venous outflow from liver and producing chronic passive congestion of that organ. Unlike acute congestion, in which it is somewhat enlarged, with chronic congestion the liver is often reduced in size. On gross examination the cut surface of the liver exhibits an accentuated lobular pattern, with a mottled appearance of alternating light and dark areas (Fig. 14-48). Because this pattern is reminiscent of a cut nutmeg, it has been termed **"nutmeg liver."** In severe cases the centrilobular terminal venules and adjacent sinusoids are conspicuously dilated and filled with red blood cells. The liver cell plates in this zone are thinned by pressure atrophy, and may even be absent, leaving a collapsed reticulin framework. In extreme cases, frank hemorrhagic necrosis of the hepatocytes in the centrilobular zones is conspicuous. These changes are far less prominent in the periphery of the lobule, but the hepatocytes in this area often contain increased amounts of fat. Chronic passive congestion of the liver is of more pathologic than clinical interest, since the condition has little effect on hepatic function. However, moderate increases in serum aminotransferase activity are common. Serum bilirubin levels may be mildly elevated, but jaundice is only partly of hepatic origin. This jaundice may also be caused in part by pulmonary infarcts, which are often found in jaundiced patients suffering from cardiac failure. Features of portal hypertension, including splenomegaly and ascites, sometimes accompany chronic passive conges-

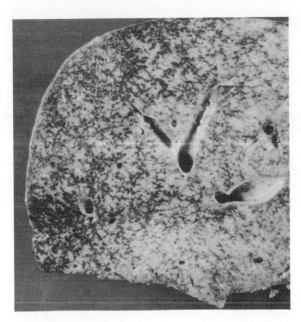

Figure 14-48. Chronic passive congestion of the liver. The surface of the liver exhibits an accentuated lobular pattern, termed "nutmeg" liver.

tion of the liver, but bleeding from esophageal varices is distinctly uncommon.

Cardiac Fibrosis of the Liver

In cases of particularly severe and longstanding **right-sided heart failure**—for example, tricuspid valvular disease of constrictive pericarditis—chronic passive congestion progresses to varying degrees of hepatic fibrosis. Delicate fibrous strands envelop terminal venules, and septa radiate from the centrilobular zones. The walls of the terminal venules and occasionally the sublobular veins may be thickened (phlebosclerosis). In prolonged cases of heart failure, the septa may link adjacent central veins, thereby producing a "reverse lobulation." Pressure atrophy of the centrilobular hepatocytes remains prominent. The older term "cardiac cirrhosis" is inappropriate, since the complete septa and regenerative nodules of true cirrhosis are rarely encountered.

Shock

Shock from any cause results in decreased perfusion of the liver, and often leads to ischemic necrosis of the centrilobular hepatocytes. The centrilobular zone, referred to as zone 3 in the functional concept of the hepatic acinus (see Fig. 14-2), is most distal to the blood supply from the portal tracts, and normally has a low oxygen tension. As a consequence centri-

lobular hepatocytes are most vulnerable to the ischemia of hypoperfusion. Microscopically, coagulative necrosis of centrilobular hepatocytes is accompanied by frank hemorrhage. If the shock is prolonged, or the patient survives, acute inflammatory cells accumulate in the necrotic zones. The lesion superficially resembles chronic passive congestion, but is distinguished from it by a lack of dilatation and congestion of the veins and an absence of pressure atrophy.

Infarction

Infarcts of the liver are uncommon because of its dual blood supply and the anastomotic structure of the hepatic sinusoids. Acute occlusion of the hepatic artery or its branches is unusual, but can occur as a result of embolism, polyarteritis nodosa, or accidental ligation during surgery. Under such circumstances, irregular pale areas, often surrounded by a hyperemic zone, reflect the underlying ischemic necrosis.

Thrombosis of the extrahepatic portal vein and the hepatic veins has been discussed in the context of portal hypertension. The acute occlusion of intrahepatic branches of the portal vein, generally in the presence of elevated hepatic venous pressure, classically produces the **"Zahn infarct,"** a dark-red, triangular area with its base on the surface of the liver. There is a surprising discrepancy between this distinctive gross appearance and the paucity of microscopic changes. In particular, hepatocellular necrosis is absent, and the only abnormality is dilatation and congestion of the sinusoids. Thus the traditional term "infarct" is actually a misnomer. The interruption of portal blood flow through the sinusoids allows a backflow of venous blood into the sinusoids and perhaps stimulates a compensatory increase in arterial flow, thereby creating stasis in and distention of the sinusoids.

Nonviral Infections of the Liver

Bacterial Infections

Bacterial infections are uncommon causes of liver disease in the industrialized countries, and when seen are for the most part complications of infections elsewhere. **The characteristic reactions in the liver are granulomas, abscesses, and diffuse inflammation.** Infections associated with granulomatous inflammation elsewhere—for instance, tuberculosis, tularemia, and brucellosis—also cause granulomatous hepatitis. Staphylococci, streptococci, and gram-negative enterobacteria produce **pyogenic hepatic abscesses.** It

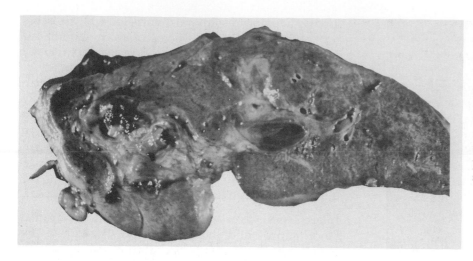

Figure 14-49. Cholangitic abscesses of the liver. The cut surface of the liver shows a large irregular abscess cavity in the right lobe and smaller ones in the other areas. The patient died of pancreatic carcinoma, which had obstructed the common bile duct.

is increasingly recognized that anaerobic inhabitants of the gastrointestinal tract, particularly *Bacteroides* species and microaerophilic streptococci, are a common cause of liver abscesses. Organisms reach the liver in arterial or portal blood or through the biliary tract. Seeding of the liver with organisms from distant sites in cases of septicemia is through the arterial blood. By contrast, intra-abdominal suppuration, as in peritonitis or diverticulitis, is transmitted to the liver in portal blood, where it typically causes **pylephlebitic abscesses** (Fig. 14-49). At one time pylephlebitis was the most common cause of hepatic abscesses, but the control of abdominal sepsis with antibiotics has rendered this route of infection uncommon. Biliary obstruction from any cause is often complicated by bacterial infection of the biliary tree, termed **ascending cholangitis**. The retrograde biliary dissemination of organisms (usually *E. coli*) leads to the formation of **cholangitic abscesses** in the liver—today the most common form of hepatic abscess in Western countries. Nevertheless, in about half of all cases of hepatic abscess, the source of infection cannot be demonstrated. Hepatic abscesses are more commonly located in the right lobe of the liver, presumably because of its larger mass. Diffuse inflammation of the liver from bacterial infection is distinctly uncommon today, but may be encountered in various septicemic states, particularly in immunocompromised patients.

Clinically, patients with a hepatic abscess typically present with high fever, rapid weight loss, right upper quadrant abdominal pain, and hepatomegaly. Jaundice occurs in a quarter of the cases, but the serum alkaline phosphatase level is almost always elevated. The abscess is localized by radiographic imaging of the liver. The morphologic appearance of a pyogenic abscess in the liver is similar to that in other sites. Solitary abscesses are treated with surgical drainage and antibiotics, but multiple abscesses present a difficult therapeutic problem. The complications of hepatic abscess relate principally to rupture and direct spread of the infection. Pleuropulmonary fistulas, from the rupture of an abscess through the diaphragm, and peritonitis, from leakage into the abdominal cavity, occur. The dissemination of organisms in the blood may lead to septicemia and metastatic abscesses in other parts of the body. The mortality from hepatic abscess, even in treated cases, remains high, ranging from 40% to 80%. However, early diagnosis and aggressive treatment can significantly reduce the mortality.

Parasitic Infections

Parasitic infestations of the liver are a serious public health problem worldwide, although they are uncommon in industrialized countries. These diseases are discussed in Chapter 9, which deals with infectious diseases. Here we summarize the major parasitic diseases that involve the liver.

Protozoal Diseases

Amebiasis

In the United States the carrier rate for *Entamoeba histolytica* is probably less than 5%, but a prevalence up to 35% has been reported in homosexual men. Amebiasis of the liver, the most common extra-intestinal complication, leads to amebic abscesses, which are multiple in about half of the cases (Fig. 14-50). The symptoms are similar to those that characterize pyogenic abscesses, but are ordinarily less severe. Secondary infection of an amebic abscess with pyogenic organisms is common. With appropriate treatment (tissue amebicides) the abscess may heal and leave only residual scar tissue. Alternatively, if the abscess continues to grow, it may rupture into the peritoneal cavity, where it produces peritonitis, a complication associated with a mortality as high as 40%. The amebae may also invade the blood, in which case abscesses of the brain and lung may ensue.

On gross examination, the abscesses typically range from 8 to 12 cm in diameter, appear well-circumscribed, and contain thick, dark material, which has been likened to "anchovy paste" or "chocolate." Microscopically, the border between the necrotic abscess and the surrounding liver parenchyma is not as sharp as implied by the gross appearance. The trophozoites are not apparent in the necrotic debris, but may be visualized in the periphery.

Malaria

The hepatic involvement in malaria is a frequent cause of hepatomegaly in endemic areas, and reflects Kupffer cell hypertrophy and hyperplasia secondary to the phagocytosis of the debris resulting from the rupture of parasitized erythrocytes. The Kupffer cells are heavily pigmented and protrude into the sinusoidal lumen, which is often congested with parasitized erythrocytes. This hepatic involvement does not give rise to significant hepatic dysfunction.

Visceral Leishmaniasis (Kala-Azar)

As in malaria, the hepatomegaly of chronic visceral leishmaniasis results from reticuloendothelial hyperplasia in the liver. In leishmaniasis, however, in contrast to malaria, the Kupffer cells ingest the parasitic organism itself, which appears as "Donovan bodies." These organisms are demonstrated in almost three-quarters of liver biopsies. Macrophages containing Donovan bodies are often present in the portal tracts, where lymphocytes and eosinophils also accumulate. Clinically, there is little evidence of hepatic dysfunction.

Helminthic Diseases

The major helminthic infestations of the liver are ascariasis, liver flukes, echinococcosis, and schistosomiasis. *Hepatic schistosomiasis* has already been discussed in the context of portal hypertension.

Ascariasis

From the duodenum the worms of *Ascaris lumbricoides* gain access to the biliary tree, where they may produce an acute biliary colic. When the parasites retreat or are endoscopically removed from the common bile duct, the symptoms subside. However, when the worms lodge in the intrahepatic biliary passages,

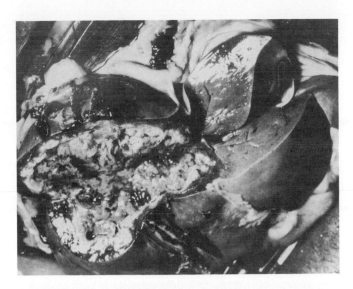

Figure 14-50. Amebic abscess of the liver. The liver has been incised to reveal a large amebic abscess of the right lobe.

their disintegration results in the liberation of innumerable eggs, which precipitate a severe, suppurative cholangitis. As in the usual pyogenic abscess, the resulting cholangitic abscesses may rupture into the peritoneal cavity or into the pleural space. Spread of the infection into the hepatic or portal veins causes pylephlebitis, a highly dangerous complication. Ascaridic cholangitis, in general, carries a grave prognosis.

At autopsy, the liver is enlarged and numerous irregular cavities contain foul-smelling material, in which the remnants of degenerated parasites are found. The periphery of the abscess often displays a granulomatous response and sometimes an eosinophilic infiltrate.

Liver Flukes

The major parasitic flukes that involve the human liver are *Clonorchis sinensis* and *Fasciola hepatica*. Man is the definitive host for *C. sinensis*, whereas sheep and cattle are the principal reservoir of *F. hepatica*. Both parasites lodge in the intrahepatic biliary tree, where they provoke hyperplasia of the biliary epithelium, particularly severe in clonorchiasis. Although periductal fibrosis is common, most patients remain asymptomatic. However, in severe infestation with *C. sinensis*, the accumulation of material from degenerated worms, parasite eggs, and viscid mucus secreted by metaplastic goblet cells in the biliary epithelium obstructs intrahepatic bile flow and leads to intrahepatic pigment gallstones. Secondary infection of the bile with *E. coli* causes cholangitis and cholangitic abscesses, common causes of surgical emergencies in some oriental countries. Migration of *C. sinensis* into the pancreatic duct produces pancreatitis. Biliary infestation with *C. sinensis* is an etiologic factor in the development of cholangiocarcinoma.

Echinococcosis (Cystic Hydatid Disease)

Infection with the tapeworms of the genus *Echinococcus*, principally *E. granulosus*, is an important zoonosis that involves the human liver. Larvae, termed **onchospheres**, pass from the intestine into the portal circulation and lodge in the liver, where they encyst. In a few days a germinal membrane develops, from which brood capsules, containing innumerable scolices (the future head of the adult worm), arise. The cyst expands slowly, and produces symptoms only after many years. Within the liver the cyst behaves as a space-occupying lesion; systemic manifestations reflect toxic or allergic reactions to the absorption of constituents of the organisms. Mechanical obstruction of intrahepatic bile ducts may be complicated by secondary infection, namely cholangitis. Rupture of the cysts into the bile ducts commonly leads to pain and jaundice.

Leptospirosis (Weil's Disease)

Infection of man with organisms of the genus *Leptospira* is accidental, the reservoir being a wide variety of domestic animals. However, fewer than one-fifth of patients who contract leptospirosis give a history of direct contact with animals. **Weil's syndrome** refers to leptospirosis complicated by prolonged fever and jaundice, and often azotemia, hemorrhages, and altered consciousness. Weil's syndrome occurs in only 1% to 6% of all cases of leptospirosis. The morphologic alterations of the liver in fatal cases are nonspecific, and include focal necrosis, enlarged Kupffer cells, and centrilobular cholestasis. The organisms are generally not demonstrable in the liver.

Syphilis

Hepatic lesions from syphilis were at one time common, but with effective antibiotic treatment of the initial infection, they are now rarely encountered. Congenital syphilis causes neonatal hepatitis, which results in diffuse fibrosis in the portal tracts and around individual liver cells or groups of hepatocytes. Up to 10% of patients with **secondary syphilis** develop a hepatitis that is clinically similar to viral hepatitis. Focal necrosis of hepatocytes, Kupffer cell hyperplasia, and mild portal and parenchymal inflammation are present. The organisms are demonstrated in the liver in about half of these cases. **Tertiary syphilis** is characterized by single or multiple hepatic gummas—focal lesions resembling granulomas, which heal with a dense scar. Retraction of the scars in severe cases with multiple gummas produces deep clefts and a gross pseudolobation of the liver, termed **hepar lobatum,** a condition that should not be confused with cirrhosis.

Neonatal Hepatitis

Neonatal hepatitis is a poorly defined clinical and pathologic entity of multiple etiologies, which have in common **prolonged cholestasis morphologic evidence of liver cell injury, and inflammation.** In about 50% of all cases of neonatal hepatitis, the cause is discernible (Table 14-4), and about 30% of cases are assigned to α_1-antitrypsin deficiency alone. Most of

Table 14-4. Causes of Neonatal Hepatitis

Idiopathic

Idiopathic neonatal hepatitis
Prolonged intrahepatic cholestasis
  1. Arteriohepatic dysplasia (Alagille's syndrome)
  2. Paucity of intrahepatic bile ducts not associated with specific syndromes
  3. Zellweger's syndrome (cerebrohepatorenal syndrome)
  4. Byler disease

Mechanical Obstruction of the Intrahepatic Bile Ducts

Congenital hepatic fibrosis
Caroli's disease (cystic dilation of intrahepatic ducts)

Metabolic Disorders

Defects of carbohydrate metabolism
  1. Galactosemia
  2. Hereditary fructose intolerance
  3. Glycogenosis Type IV
Defects of lipid metabolism
  1. Gaucher's disease
  2. Niemann-Pick disease
  3. Wolman's disease
Tyrosinemia (defect of amino acid metabolism)
α_1-Antitrypsin deficiency
Cystic fibrosis
Parenteral nutrition

Hepatitis

Hepatitis B
TORCH agents
Varicella
Syphilis
ECHO viruses
Neonatal sepsis

Chromosomal Abnormalities

Down's syndrome
Trisomy 18

Extrahepatic Biliary Atresia

the other cases with known causes can be attributed to viral hepatitis B and infectious agents such as the TORCH group (toxoplasmosis, rubella, cytomegalovirus, and herpes simplex). A few cases represent hepatic injury associated with metabolic defects, for instance galactosemia or fructose intolerance. Occasional cases of neonatal hepatitis are seen in association with Down's syndrome and other chromosomal disorders. The remaining 50% of all cases of neonatal hepatitis are of unexplained etiology, but it is likely that as yet unidentified viruses and metabolic defects will be recognized. Rare familial cases of neonatal hepatitis have been reported.

The characteristic hepatic lesion of neonatal hepatitis is giant cell transformation of hepatocytes, hence the former term "giant cell hepatitis" (Fig. 14-51). The giant cells contain as many as 40 nuclei and may appear detached from other cells in the liver plate. The pale, distended cytoplasm contains large amounts of glycogen and, for unexplained reasons, iron. The number of giant cells decreases with time, and they are rare in children over 1 year of age. Bile pigment is often prominent within canaliculi and hepatocytes. Ballooned hepatocytes, acinar transformation, and acidophilic bodies are also typical of neonatal hepatitis. Extramedullary hematopoiesis is often conspicuous. Chronic inflammatory infiltrates are seen in the portal tracts as well as in the lobular parenchyma. Pericellular fibrosis around degenerating hepatocytes, singly or in groups, is common, and fibrous tissue septa extend from the portal tracts.

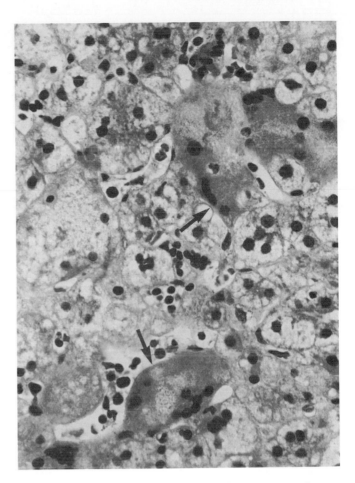

Figure 14-51. Neonatal hepatitis. A photomicrograph shows multinucleated giant hepatocytes (*arrows*), liver cell injury, and a mild chronic inflammatory infiltrate.

Biliary Atresia

The confusion surrounding the concept of neonatal hepatitis is aggravated by its association with both intrahepatic and extrahepatic biliary atresia. It has been suggested that biliary atresia in the neonate, whether intrahepatic or extrahepatic, is secondary to neonatal hepatitis. Alternatively, the etiologic agent of neonatal hepatitis may independently cause biliary atresia. At one end of the spectrum are cases in which a striking paucity of intrahepatic bile ducts is seen in a liver that exhibits little cell injury and inflammation, while at the other extreme, a comparable scarcity of bile ducts is accompanied by severe neonatal hepatitis. Moreover, the cordlike remnant of the common bile duct in cases of extrahepatic biliary atresia often displays chronic inflammation. Instances have been recorded in which a chronically inflamed but patent bile duct has closed and scarred. Lastly, extrahepatic biliary atresia, like pure intrahepatic biliary atresia, is often associated with full-blown neonatal hepatitis. Since embryologically the bile ducts differentiate from hepatocytes, it is possible that primary liver cell

damage in the fetus retards or prevents the development of intrahepatic biliary passages. These observations support the concept that neonatal hepatitis, intrahepatic biliary atresia, extrahepatic biliary atresia, and possibly choledochal cyst **all result from a common inflammatory process** ("infantile obstructive cholangiopathy") and are not true congenital anomalies.

Both intrahepatic and extrahepatic biliary atresia lead to a proliferation of bile ductules in the portal tracts (more severe in extrahepatic atresia). Such proliferation may be inconspicuous in classic neonatal hepatitis. Intrahepatic biliary atresia is demonstrated quantitatively by counts of bile ducts in histologic sections.

Most patients who have uncomplicated neonatal hepatitis recover without sequelae. Intrahepatic biliary atresia associated with neonatal hepatitis carries a much poorer prognosis, and in many children progresses to biliary cirrhosis. Uncorrected extrahepatic biliary atresia invariably results in progressive sec-

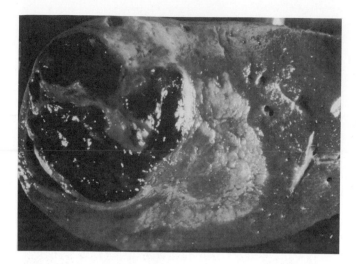

Figure 14-52.   Hepatic adenoma. The cut surface of the liver shows a large vascular and hemorrhagic mass in the right lobe.

ondary biliary cirrhosis and is incompatible with survival. While surgical correction has been successful in some anatomically favorable cases, the majority of cases of extrahepatic, as well as intrahepatic, biliary atresia can only be cured by liver transplantation.

Arteriohepatic Dysplasia

Arteriohepatic dysplasia **(Alagille's syndrome)** is characterized by the association of intrahepatic bile duct paucity with a constellation of congenital anomalies, including broad forehead, widely spaced eyes, defects of the vertebrae, peripheral pulmonic stenosis, short stature, and mental retardation. The morphologic characteristics of neonatal hepatitis appear during the first few months of life. Although mild fibrosis of the portal tracts occurs, the syndrome does not progress to cirrhosis and the prognosis is good. An autosomal recessive transmission has been suggested in most cases, but reports of a high frequency of the disorder in successive generations of a single kindred support an autosomal dominant inheritance in some cases.

Neoplasms

Benign Tumors and Tumor-like Lesions

Hepatic Adenoma

Hepatic adenomas are benign tumors of hepatocytes that occur almost always in women in the reproductive years, usually as a solitary, sharply demarcated mass up to 40 cm in diameter and 3 kg in weight

(Fig. 14-52). In a quarter of the cases, smaller multiple adenomas are present. On gross examination, the tumor is encapsulated and paler than the surrounding parenchyma. Hemorrhage and necrosis in the center of the tumor are common and account for episodes of sudden abdominal pain. However, in about a third of patients with hepatic adenomas—particularly pregnant women who have previously used oral contraceptives—the tumors bleed into the peritoneal cavity and require treatment as a surgical emergency.

Microscopically, the neoplastic hepatocytes resemble their normal counterparts, except that they are not arranged in a lobular architecture (Fig. 14-53). Portal tracts and central venules are not present. The cells composing the adenoma may be very large and eosinophilic, or filled with glycogen, which makes the cytoplasm appear clear. By electron microscopy, the neoplastic hepatocytes have a "simplified" appearance. The tumor is circumscribed by a fibrous capsule of variable thickness, and the adjacent hepatocytes appear compressed. Large, thick-walled ar-

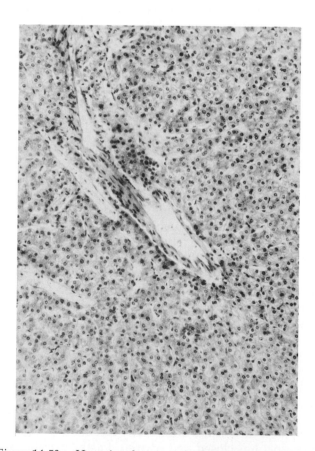

Figure 14-53.   Hepatic adenoma. A photomicrograph of the mass illustrated in Figure 14-52 shows plates of highly differentiated, neoplastic hepatocytes without discernible hepatic architecture. A large blood vessel is evident in the center.

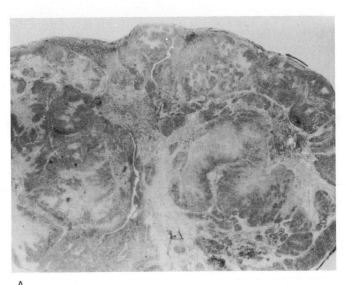

A

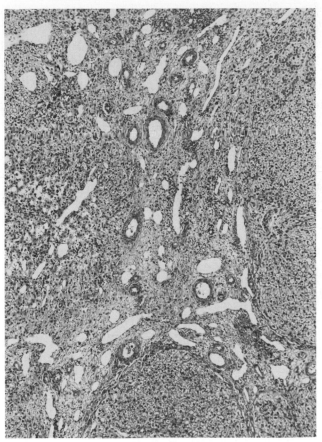

B

Figure 14-54. Focal nodular hyperplasia. (*A*) A low-power photomicrograph reveals irregular fibrous septa and a disorganized hepatic parenchyma. (*B*) A higher-power photomicrograph shows hepatocellular nodules and irregular, highly vascularized, and chronically inflamed fibrous septa.

teries are often seen in the vicinity of the capsule, and arteries and veins traverse the tumor.

Hepatic adenomas were exceedingly rare before the availability of oral contraceptives, but since their introduction, many such tumors have been reported, and they are today a well-recognized, although uncommon, complication. Even large adenomas have been reported to disappear after discontinuation of oral contraceptives. A few adenomas are encountered in men, and they have occasionally been reported in association with the use of anabolic steroids. Despite isolated reports of progression to hepatocellular carcinoma, hepatic adenoma is not generally thought to be a premalignant lesion.

Focal Nodular Hyperplasia

Focal nodular hyperplasia is a nodular liver mass varying in size from 5 cm to 15 cm in diameter and weighing as much as 700 g. On occasion, it protrudes from the surface of the liver, and it may even be pedunculated. The cut surface exhibits a characteristic central scar from which fibrous septa radiate. The division of the mass by multiple fibrous septa accounts for the older term "focal cirrhosis." Micro-

scopically, hepatocytic nodules are circumscribed by fibrous septa (Fig. 14-54), which contain numerous tortuous bile ducts and mononuclear inflammatory cells. Within the nodules, lobular architecture is absent. The lesion exhibits large arteries and veins in the septa, but hemorrhage is uncommon. The mass is not truly encapsulated, although the border is distinct on gross examination.

Focal nodular hyperplasia shows a female predominance, although not as marked as that of hepatic adenoma. While some authors have suggested that focal nodular hyperplasia is related to the use of oral contraceptives, others question this conclusion, because the lesion occurs in children and older people, including men, and its incidence has apparently not increased since the advent of oral contraceptives. The lesion does not progress to cancer.

Nodular Transformation (Partial Nodular Transformation, Nodular Regenerative Hyperplasia)

Nodular transformation occurs in noncirrhotic livers and is characterized by small, hyperplastic nodules without fibrosis. The lesion may be partial and located predominantly in the perihilar region or may be diffuse throughout the liver. The clinical importance of nodular transformation relates to portal hypertension, which accounts for the older term "non-cirrhotic portal hypertension." The nodules, composed of liver cells arranged in plates that are two and three cells thick, compress the surrounding parenchyma. Liver cell dysplasia—that is, enlargement of the cells, nuclear pleomorphism, and the presence of multinucleated hepatocytes—is occasionally noted within the nodules. The etiology of nodular transformation is unknown, but it has been reported in association with the use of oral contraceptives or anabolic steroids, extrahepatic infections, neoplasms, and chronic inflammatory disorders. The lesion is not considered to be preneoplastic.

Hemangioma

Hemangiomas, occurring at all ages and in both sexes, are the most common benign tumors of the liver, being found in up to 7% of autopsy specimens. They are ordinarily small and asymptomatic, although larger tumors have been reported to cause abdominal symptoms and even hemorrhage into the peritoneal cavity. Grossly, the tumor is usually solitary and less than 5 cm in diameter, but multiple hemangiomas and giant forms have been described. Microscopically, the tumor is similar to cavernous hemangiomas found elsewhere.

Infantile hemangioendothelioma, a rare cellular tumor that appears during the first 2 years of life, and sometimes at birth, contains arteriovenous shunts that may be large enough to cause congestive heart failure. Malignant transformation has been reported in a few cases.

Cystic Disease of the Liver

Bile duct microhamartomas (von Meyenburg complexes) consist of anomalous, small cystic bile ducts embedded in a fibrous stroma. They are usually multiple, and vary from barely visible greyish-white foci to nodules 1 cm in diameter. Microscopically, the cysts are lined by bile duct epithelium and sometimes contain inspissated bile. It is thought that these clinically inapparent lesions represent one end of the spectrum of cystic disease of the liver.

Solitary and multiple simple cysts lined by cuboidal to columnar epithelium are often associated with adult polycystic disease of the kidney, and are not infrequently seen in livers that contain von Meyenburg complexes.

Congenital hepatic fibrosis is marked by enlarged portal tracts, which exhibit extensive fibrosis and nu-

merous bile ductules that communicate with the biliary tree. The bile ductules may be so dilated that they resemble microcysts, but even in these cases they retain their communication with the biliary system. The area involved by congenital hepatic fibrosis is sharply demarcated from the normal liver parenchyma, and regenerative nodules are absent, an appearance that distinguishes this condition from cirrhosis. The origin of the lesion, which is an inherited congenital malformation, is unknown, but it has been postulated that the initial lesion may arise from von Meyenburg complexes. The principal complication of this disorder is severe portal hypertension, with recurrent bleeding from esophageal varices.

Malignant Tumors

Hepatocellular Carcinoma

Hepatocellular carcinoma occurs in all parts of the world, but its incidence shows a striking geographic variability. In Western industrialized countries the tumor is uncommon; in sub-Saharan Africa, Southeast Asia, and Japan, the rates are up to 50 times greater. For example, in Mozambique, which seems to have the highest incidence in the world, two-thirds of all cancers in men and one-third in women are hepatocellular carcinomas.

An association between hepatocellular carcinoma and infection with the hepatitis B virus (HBV) is now clearly established. The geographic incidence of this tumor correlates strongly with the prevalence of the carrier state for HBV. Moreover, in areas of high incidence, HBV infection is documented in 80% to 90% of patients with hepatocellular carcinoma, and is probably present, but undetected, in many of the others. Indeed, a significant proportion of patients classified as HBsAg-negative on the basis of serologic studies have been shown to contain HBcAg in the nuclei of liver cells at autopsy. Most patients have had chronic HBV infection for many years, the disease often being transmitted from an infected mother to her newborn child perinatally. The carrier state is indeed dangerous, since such individuals are estimated to have as much as a 200-fold increased risk of developing hepatocellular carcinoma. About a quarter of those with chronic hepatitis B acquired at or near birth ultimately develop hepatocellular carcinoma.

Although most cases of hepatocellular carcinoma associated with HBV infection occur in patients with cirrhosis, numerous cases in non-cirrhotic livers have also been reported. However, in most instances of hepatocellular carcinoma in non-cirrhotic, HBsAg-positive individuals, the liver shows some degree of chronic active hepatitis, which suggests that persistent cell injury may be crucial in the pathogenesis of hepatocellular carcinoma. Further evidence that HBV has an important role in the development of hepatocellular carcinoma comes from the demonstration that **the genome of HBV is integrated into the host DNA of both the non-neoplastic liver cells and the tumor cells.** According to the multistep concept of carcinogenesis in the liver discussed in Chapter 5, integration of the HBV genome into host DNA would be considered the initiating event, while chronic hepatitis would represent the promoting mechanism. Woodchucks infected with a hepadnavirus corresponding to HBV also develop hepatocellular carcinoma.

In industrialized countries that have a low incidence of both HBV infection and hepatocellular carcinoma, the principal predisposing condition to hepatocellular carcinoma is alcoholic cirrhosis. However, unlike HBV-associated cancer, hepatocellular carcinoma in alcoholics is ordinarily restricted to those with advanced macronodular cirrhosis. Indeed, many, if not most, of the alcoholic patients with hepatocellular carcinoma have been abstinent long before the detection of the neoplasm in the liver. Presumably, these patients have survived long enough for regenerative activity in the liver to convert a micronodular cirrhosis to the macronodular variety, thereby contributing to the development of hepatocellular carcinoma. It is of interest that many patients with alcoholic cirrhosis who develop hepatocellular carcinoma also display markers of HBV infection, and that many have integrated HBV DNA in the genome of their liver cells. It is not clear whether HBV infection simply contributes to the evolution of the cirrhosis, or whether integration of viral DNA into the host genome serves as an initiating event, which is promoted to hepatocellular carcinoma by alcoholic cirrhosis.

Other forms of cirrhosis are also associated with a high incidence of hepatocellular carcinoma. Liver diseases occurring in conjunction with hemochromatosis and α_1-antitrypsin deficiency carry a substantial risk of hepatocellular carcinoma: about 10% of patients with hemochromatosis may be expected to develop the tumor. On the other hand, hepatocellular carcinoma is rare in patients with "autoimmune" chronic active hepatitis and cirrhosis, Wilson's disease, and primary biliary cirrhosis. Hepatitis A has not been incriminated as a predisposing factor for hepatocellular carcinoma. Whether chronic non-A, non-B hepatitis predisposes to liver cancer is not clear.

Aflatoxin B_1, a contaminant of many foods, particularly in less developed countries, produces hepatocellular carcinoma in a number of mammalian species. The incidence of liver cancer in man has been roughly correlated with the content of aflatoxin in the diet, although significant exceptions have been found. Since areas in which the diet is heavily contaminated with aflatoxin are also areas in which hepatitis B is endemic, the contribution of this toxin to the development of hepatocellular carcinoma in man remains enigmatic.

Hepatocellular carcinoma is considerably more common in men than in women, presumably a reflection of the increased occurrence of both the HBV carrier state and alcoholism in men. The tumor usually presents as a painful and enlarging mass in the liver. Ascites, portal vein thrombosis, occlusion of hepatic veins, and hemorrhage from esophageal varices are common. The prognosis is dismal, and patients die of malignant cachexia, rupture of the tumor with catastrophic bleeding into the peritoneal cavity, bleeding esophageal varices, or hepatic failure.

Hepatocellular carcinoma may be associated with a variety of paraneoplastic manifestations (e.g., polycythemia, hypoglycemia, hypercalcemia) as a result of hormone production by the tumor. α-Fetoprotein, a circulating marker produced by hepatocellular carcinomas, is particularly important because of its diagnostic value. Normally, this fetal protein falls to very low levels (less than 10 ng/ml) by 1 year of age. In patients with hepatocellular carcinoma, levels above 4000 ng/ml are reported, and in most cases the value is over 400 ng/ml. Since elevated levels of α-fetoprotein are also encountered in other neoplastic and non-neoplastic liver diseases and in some extrahepatic disorders, the finding of high concentrations of this oncofetoprotein is not absolutely diagnostic of hepatocellular carcinoma. Nevertheless, it remains an excellent screening measure for detection of this tumor, and is used to monitor treated patients for recurrence.

Hepatocellular carcinomas appear grossly as soft and hemorrhagic tan masses in the liver. Occasionally, a green color is present, indicating bile staining. In some cases a very large solitary tumor occupies a large portion of the liver, whereas in other cases many smaller tumors are found. Multiple lesions are thought to indicate a multicentric origin of the tumor, although intrahepatic metastases from a single hepatocellular carcinoma cannot be excluded. The tumor has a tendency to grow into portal veins, and may extend to the vena cava, and even the right atrium, through the hepatic veins. A number of histologic patterns are recognized, but no prognostic

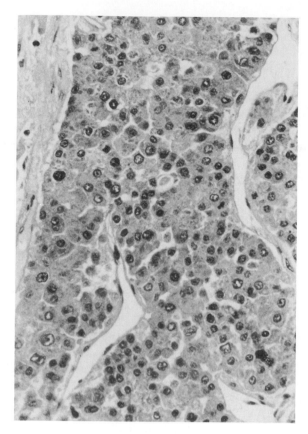

Figure 14-55. Hepatocellular carcinoma. A photomicrograph shows a trabecular pattern of malignant hepatocytes.

significance can be attributed to any of them. Most hepatocellular carcinomas exhibit a **trabecular** pattern—that is, the tumor cells are arranged in trabeculae or plates that resemble the normal liver (Fig. 14-55). The plates are separated by endothelium-lined sinusoids, but Kupffer cells are absent. Occasionally, tumor growth in the trabecular variant compresses the sinusoids to such an extent that the lesion appears solid. A second histologic variant is termed the **pseudoglandular (adenoid, acinar)** pattern. In this variety the malignant hepatocytes are arranged around a lumen, and thus resemble glands. The lumen may contain bile, and biliary canaliculi are often seen between the tumor cells. Endothelium-lined sinusoids are interspersed between the pseudoglandular structures. It is important to bear in mind that the acini formed by the tumor cells are not true glands, and the lesion should not be confused with adenocarcinoma. Some hepatocellular carcinomas contain a considerable fibrous stroma, which separates tumor cell plates, accounting for the term "scirrhous" carcinoma.

A distinctive histologic appearance has been noted in hepatocellular carcinomas arising in an apparently normal liver, principally in adolescents and young adults. Termed **fibrolamellar hepatocellular carcinoma,** the tumor is composed of large, eosinophilic, neoplastic hepatocytes arranged in clusters surrounded by delicate collagen fibers. As with oncocytes in other tumors, the eosinophilic character of the cytoplasm reflects an accumulation of mitochondria. The prognosis is better than in other varieties of hepatocellular carcinoma.

Cytologically, some tumors are highly **pleomorphic** and exhibit conspicuous variation in the size and staining properties of the tumor cell nuclei, multinucleated cells, and giant cells. These changes may lead to disarray of the tumor cell plates, so that the trabecular pattern is obscured. Other hepatocellular carcinomas may be partly or entirely composed of clear cells, which usually contain glycogen but may contain fat. Such clear cell tumors have been on occasion mistakenly identified as metastatic renal cell of adrenal carcinomas. Mallory bodies are seen in a minority of hepatocellular carcinomas, although in some cases they are particularly conspicuous. Occasional carcinomas exhibit eosinophilic globules in the cytoplasm of tumor cells, some of which contain α-fetoprotein or α_1-antitrypsin.

Hepatocellular carcinomas may reach a large size before metastasizing. Metastases occur widely, but the most common sites are the lungs and portal lymph nodes. Surgical resection of the primary tumor has rarely effected a cure, but in cases where the tumor has not extended beyond the confines of the liver, hepatic transplantation is a promising therapy.

Cholangiocarcinoma (Bile Duct Carcinoma)

Cholangiocarcinomas, defined as malignant hepatic tumors of biliary epithelium, arise anywhere from the large intrahepatic bile ducts at the porta hepatis to the smallest bile ductules at the periphery of the hepatic lobule. Tumors that arise at the lobular level are termed **peripheral cholangiocarcinomas,** and frequently occur in association with cirrhosis. Tumors of the larger intrahepatic ducts are rare. Lesions arising at the convergence of the right and left hepatic ducts are known as **hilar cholangiocarcinomas,** and produce symptoms of extrahepatic biliary obstruction.

The peripheral cholangiocarcinomas are composed of small cuboidal cells arranged in a ductular or glandular configuration (Fig. 14-56). Characteristically, they show substantial fibrosis, and on liver biopsy

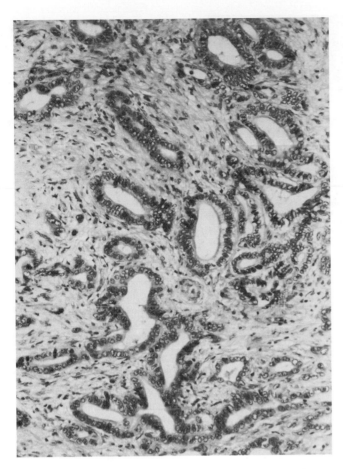

Figure 14-56.   Cholangiocarcinoma. Neoplastic glands are embedded in a dense fibrous stroma.

they may be confused with metastatic scirrhous carcinoma of the breast or pancreas. A combined form of hepatocellular carcinoma and peripheral cholangiocarcinoma has been labeled **cholangiohepatocellular carcinoma.** Since both components of this tumor are associated with cirrhosis, some of the cholangiohepatocellular carcinomas may actually represent the collision of two independent carcinomas. On the other hand, evidence of transition between the two types of cells has been described within single tumors.

Hilar cholangiocarcinomas present three histologic patterns: a small sclerosing tumor that obliterates the duct; a tumor that spreads within the wall of the duct; and a rare intraductal papillary variant.

Cholangiocarcinomas show a lesser tendency to invade the portal and hepatic veins than hepatocellular carcinomas. They metastasize to a wide variety of extrahepatic sites, and show a greater predilection for the portal lymph nodes than do hepatocellular carcinomas.

Hepatoblastoma

Hepatoblastoma is a rare malignant tumor of children, found from birth to the age of 3 years. Attention is called to the tumor by enlargement of the abdomen, vomiting, and failure to thrive. The serum α-fetoprotein level is almost invariably elevated, and occasionally secretion of ectopic gonodotropin leads to sexual precocity. Some of these children also exhibit congenital anomalies, including cardiac and renal malformations, hemihypertrophy, and macroglossia.

The tumor presents as a partially necrotic and hemorrhagic circumscribed mass up to 25 cm in diameter. Microscopically, cells of epithelial and mesenchymal appearance are seen, but occasionally the latter are missing. The epithelial component includes cells resembling embryonal and fetal cells. The "embryonal" cells are small and fusiform, and are arranged in ribbons or rosettes. The "fetal" cells more closely resemble hepatocytes, contain glycogen and fat, and are arranged in trabeculae with intervening sinusoids. Extramedullary hematopoiesis is usually seen in the area populated by "fetal" cells. Foci of squamous epithelium are occasionally encountered. The mesenchymal elements include those often present in teratomas, including connective tissue, cartilage, and osteoid.

Untreated hepatoblastomas are invariably fatal, but surgical resection by partial hepatectomy has been curative in many instances.

Sarcomas of the Liver

Hemangiosarcoma is the only significant sarcoma of the liver. As noted above, it may result from exposure to thorium dioxide, vinyl chloride, or inorganic arsenic. Patients with this malignant tumor present with hepatomegaly, jaundice, and ascites. Hematologic abnormalities, including pancytopenia and hemolytic anemia, are often prominent, and in many cases reflect splenomegaly from noncirrhotic portal hypertension. The tumor may rupture and bleed vigorously into the abdominal cavity. The prognosis is poor.

On gross examination, hemangiosarcoma is characteristically multicentric, presenting as multiple hemorrhagic nodules, which may coalesce. Microscopic examination reveals spindle-shaped, neoplastic, endothelial cells that line the sinusoids and compress the liver cell plates. The tumor may form cavernous blood spaces and solid masses of neoplastic cells. Extramedullary hematopoiesis is almost invariable. Hemorrhage, thrombosis, and infarction of-

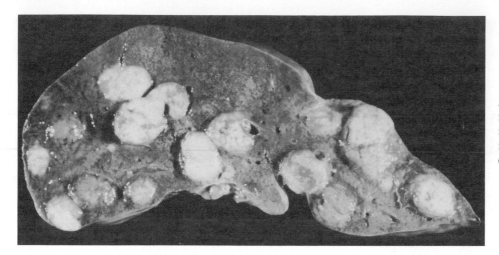

Figure 14-57. Metastatic carcinoma in the liver. The cut surface of the liver shows many firm, pale masses of metastatic colon cancer.

ten complicate the morphologic pattern of this tumor. The tumor metastasizes widely, but it has been suggested that, at least in some cases, these deposits represent independent primary tumors.

Other rare malignant mesenchymal tumors of the liver include embryonal rhabdomyosarcoma, leiomyosarcoma, fibrosarcoma, and malignant mesenchymomas.

Metastatic Cancer

Metastatic cancers are by far the most common malignant neoplasms of the liver. The liver is involved in a third of all metastatic cancers, including half of those of the gastrointestinal tract, breast, and lung. Other tumors that characteristically metastasize to the liver are pancreatic carcinoma and malignant melanoma. The liver may show only a single nodule of tumor or may be virtually replaced by metastases (Fig. 14-57), and liver weights of 5 kg or more are not uncommon. In fact, liver metastases are the commonest cause of massive hepatomegaly. Metastatic carcinomas are often seen on the surface of the liver as umbilicated masses, a reflection of central necrosis and hemorrhage. The metastatic deposits are often histologically similar to the primary tumor, but on occasion are so undifferentiated that the primary site cannot be determined.

Clinically, weight loss is a common early finding. Portal hypertension with splenomegaly, ascites, and gastrointestinal bleeding may occur. Obstruction of the major bile ducts or replacement of most of the liver parenchyma leads to jaundice. If the patient lives long enough, hepatic failure may ensue. Often the first indication of metastatic tumor in the liver is an unexplained increase in the serum alkaline phosphatase level. The majority of patients die within a year of the diagnosis of liver metastases.

The Pathology of Liver Transplantation

The increasing availability of hepatic transplantation, and the accompanying problems related to allograft rejection, have focused attention on the morphologic criteria by which the outcome can be assessed and therapy recommended. In this respect, it is clear that serial liver biopsies are the best means of clinical

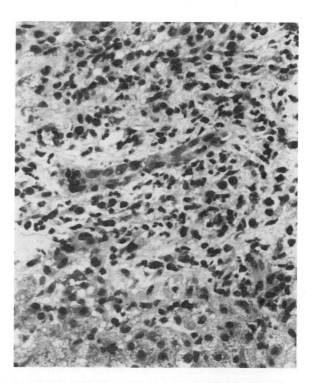

Figure 14-58. Bile duct injury in liver allograft rejection. A photomicrograph of a portal tract shows lymphocytes surrounding and infiltrating the wall of a small branch of the portal bile duct.

assessment after liver transplantation. Despite immunosuppressive therapy, about three-quarters of patients subjected to hepatic transplantation may be expected to develop some morphologic evidence of graft rejection in as little as 2 days or as long as 6 months.

Early rejection is characterized by chronic inflammation and enlargement of the portal tracts. Large and small lymphocytes, plasma cells, and macrophages are present, and a few neutrophils and eosinophils are common. Occasionally, the inflammatory infiltrate extends beyond the borders of the portal tracts and is associated with necrosis of periportal hepatocytes, an appearance similar to that of the so-called piecemeal necrosis of chronic active hepatitis. Early rejection results in distortion of the bile ducts by the portal inflammatory infiltrate, atypism of bile duct epithelial cells, and often inflammation of the ductal epithelium itself (Fig. 14-58). Hyperplasia and chronic inflammation of bile ductules within the portal tracts may be conspicuous. Most cases exhibit moderate cholestasis, principally in the centrilobular zones.

In almost all cases of early rejection, lymphocytes are adherent to the endothelium of terminal venules and small branches of the portal veins, with or without subendothelial inflammation (Fig. 14-59). Varying degrees of centrilobular necrosis are accompanied by collapse of the reticulin framework; in severe cases collapsed zones may link adjacent central venules.

This combination of mixed portal inflammation, mononuclear infiltration of venous endothelium, and injury to intrahepatic bile ducts has been compared to graft-versus-host disease. Intensive treatment with immunosuppressive agents generally causes most of these changes to subside.

Allograft rejection persisting for more than 2 months generally exhibits a less intense inflammatory reaction, although in some cases it may remain severe. Periportal hepatocellular necrosis, however, is usually more conspicuous. **Damage to interlobular bile ducts** is now more prominent. As the lesion progresses, these small bile ducts are destroyed and persistent cholestasis, similar to that seen in primary biliary cirrhosis, ensues.

On occasion, even in early rejection, medium-sized arteries in the porta hepatis display a vasculitis, with fibrinoid necrosis, disruption of the elastic lamina, and an infiltrate of lymphocytes and macrophages. Within several months subintimal foam cells, intimal sclerosis, and myointimal hyperplasia may narrow or occlude these arteries.

A serious complication is the occasional occurrence of viral hepatitis B or infection with cytomegalovirus or herpes simplex, type I, in the transplanted liver.

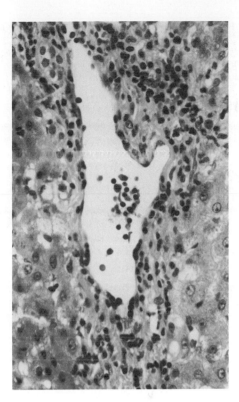

Figure 14-59.   Portal vein phlebitis in liver allograft rejection. A photomicrograph shows lymphocytes surrounding a portal vein and adherent to its endothelium.

The Gallbladder and Extrahepatic Bile Ducts

Anatomy

The gallbladder originates from the same foregut diverticulum that gives rise to the liver. In about a week the gallbladder and cystic duct are discernible. The lumen of the gallbladder is formed in the twelfth week.

The adult gallbladder, a thin elongated sac about 8 cm in length and about 50 ml in volume, occupies a fossa on the inferior surface of the liver between the right and the quadrate lobes. The primary function of the gallbladder is the storage, concentration, and release of bile. The cystic duct, which empties the gallbladder into the hepatic duct, is about 3 cm long. Its mucosa is arranged in a series of folds, termed the valves of Heister. Dilute bile from the hepatic duct passes into the gallbladder via the cystic duct, where it is concentrated and subsequently discharged into the common bile duct. The gallbladder is usually supplied by a branch of the right hepatic

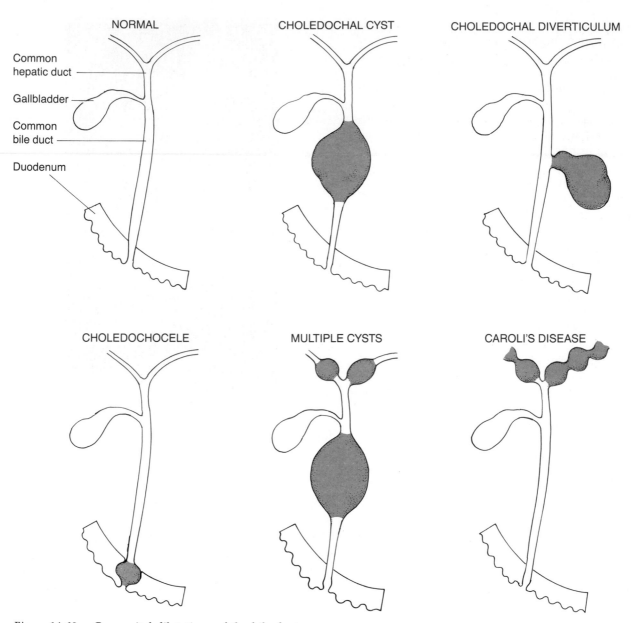

NORMAL

Common hepatic duct

Gallbladder

Common bile duct

Duodenum

CHOLEDOCHAL CYST

CHOLEDOCHAL DIVERTICULUM

CHOLEDOCHOCELE

MULTIPLE CYSTS

CAROLI'S DISEASE

Figure 14-60.   Congenital dilatations of the bile ducts.

artery. Anatomic variations in the vascular anatomy may bring the parent artery into the surgical field of a cholecystectomy, in which case the surgeon must take great care not to ligate it. A similar caution must be exercised to avoid ligation of the common bile duct. A rich plexus of lymphatics drains the gallbladder and serves as a convenient route for metastases from gallbladder carcinoma.

The wall of the gallbladder is composed of a mucous membrane, a muscularis, and an adventitia, and is covered by a reflection of the visceral peritoneum. The mucosa is thrown into folds, and consists of a columnar epithelium and a lamina propria of loose connective tissue. Dipping into the wall of the gall-

bladder are mucosal diverticula, termed **Rokitansky-Aschoff sinuses.** Branched mucous glands are found near the neck of the gallbladder. The **ducts of Luschka,** presumably remnants of aberrant embryonic bile ducts, are located in the connective tissue between the liver and the gallbladder, and connect with the cystic duct.

Congenital Anomalies

Developmental anomalies of the gallbladder are rare and of little clinical significance, except for the surgeon. **Agenesis** and **atresia** occur, and **duplication** is occasionally noted. **Heterotopic tissue,** including gastric, adrenal, pancreatic, and thyroid elements, has been recorded in the gallbladder, usually in conjunction with cholelithiasis and cholecystitis. Although the gallbladder is usually partially embedded in the liver, it floats free in about 4% of the normal population. Ectopic locations of the gallbladder, including the left lobe of the liver and the falciform ligament, are seen uncommonly.

The cystic duct may be absent or duplicated. On occasion it is abnormally long and enters the bile duct close to its termination, or it may join the right hepatic duct. Again, these are important considerations for the surgeon.

Anomalies of the bile duct include **duplication** and **accessory bile ducts. Extrahepatic biliary atresia** is thought to be part of the spectrum of disease associated with neonatal hepatitis and, accordingly, has been discussed above. Congenital dilatations of the bile duct include **choledochal cyst** (85% of all cases), **choledochal diverticulum,** and **choledochocele** (Fig. 14-60). Multiple cysts may occur as segmental dilatations in the entire extrahepatic biliary tree. Similar multiple dilatations in the intrahepatic portion of the biliary tree, termed **Caroli's disease,** predispose to bacterial cholangitis. It has been suggested that choledochal cysts form part of the same complex as neonatal hepatitis and biliary atresia.

Cholelithiasis

Cholelithiasis is defined as the presence of stones within the lumen of the gallbladder or in the extrahepatic biliary tree. About three-quarters of gallstones in the industrialized countries consist primarily of cholesterol, while the remainder are composed of calcium bilirubinate and other calcium salts (pigment gallstones). Pigment stones predominate in the tropics and the Orient. Most gallstones are not radiopaque, but about 15% (usually pigment stones) can be visualized radiographically. With the use of contrast medium concentrated in the gallbladder, most stones can be recognized radiographically as negative images. Gallstones are frequently asymptomatic, but may cause mild to severe pain ("biliary colic") as a result of impaction in the cystic duct.

Cholesterol Stones

Cholesterol stones are round or faceted, yellow to tan, single or multiple, and vary from 1 mm to 4 cm in greatest dimension (Fig. 14-61). Between 50% and 100% of the stone is composed of cholesterol; the rest consists of calcium salts and mucin. Cholesterol gall-

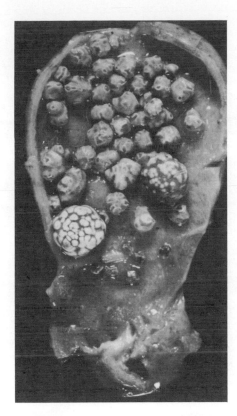

Figure 14-61. Cholesterol gallstones. The gallbladder has been opened to reveal numerous yellow cholesterol gallstones. The gallbladder wall is thickened as a result of chronic cholecystitis.

stones are common in the U.S. population: 20% of American men and 35% of women over the age of 75 years have gallstones at autopsy. However, during their reproductive period, **women are three times more likely to develop cholesterol gallstones than men,** the incidence being higher in users of oral contraceptives and in women with several pregnancies. Interestingly, cholesterol gallstones are exceedingly common in Pima Indian women of the American Southwest, among whom three-quarters are affected by age 25, and 90% above the age of 60 years. This occurrence is thought to reflect genetic factors. Blacks in the United States have a lower incidence of gallstones than whites, but a higher incidence than blacks in Africa. This difference probably reflects environmental influences, although a role for genetic admixtures is also possible.

Pathogenesis

The pathogenesis of cholesterol stones relates principally to the composition of the bile (Fig. 14-62). Normally, cholesterol, a compound highly insoluble in water, is secreted by the hepatocytes into the bile, where it is held in solution by the combined action

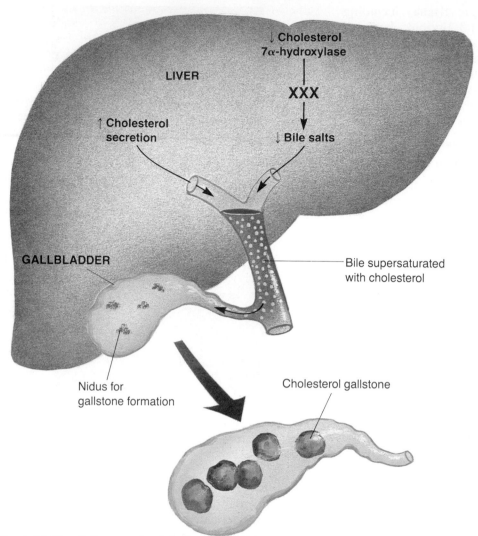

Figure 14-62. Pathogenesis of cholesterol gallstones.

of bile acids and lecithin and carried in the form of mixed lipid micelles. If the bile contains excess cholesterol or is deficient in bile acids, the bile becomes supersaturated, and under some circumstances the cholesterol precipitates as solid crystals. **The bile of persons afflicted with cholesterol gallstones has more cholesterol as it leaves the liver than that of normal individuals, pointing to the liver, rather than the gallbladder, as the culprit in the genesis of cholesterol stones.** The hepatocytes of patients with cholesterol gallstones are deficient in 7α-hydroxylase, the enzyme involved in the rate-limiting step by which bile salts are formed from cholesterol. As a result, **the total size of the bile salt pool is reduced.** The resulting decrease in bile salt secretion contributes to

the stone-forming (lithogenic) properties of the bile. Furthermore, **in obese people, cholesterol secretion by the liver is augmented,** further adding to the supersaturation of the bile with cholesterol.

Although cholesterol supersaturation of the bile is apparently required for gallstone formation, additional factors are also required. Cholesterol does not precipitate from saturated bile obtained from patients without gallstones, even after prolonged incubation. On the other hand, bile from persons without gallstones, but with properties similar to those in the bile of patients with gallstones, crystallizes without difficulty. It is thought that the mucinous glycoproteins secreted by the gallbladder epithelium provide the necessary nidus for crystallization.

Risk Factors

The higher prevalence of gallstones in premenopausal women has been attributed to the fact that estrogens stimulate the formation of lithogenic bile by the liver. Estrogens increase the hepatic secretion of cholesterol and may decrease the secretion of bile acids. These effects are augmented during pregnancy, because the gallbladder empties more slowly in the last trimester, thereby causing stasis and increasing the opportunity for precipitation of cholesterol crystals. Indeed, progesterone has been shown to inhibit discharge of bile from the gallbladder. These mechanisms are also invoked to explain the increased incidence of gallstones in users of oral contraceptives.

Other major risk factors for the development of cholesterol gallstones can be divided into those that relate to increased biliary cholesterol secretion, those that relate to decreased secretion of bile salts and lecithin, and those that relate to a combination of the two.

Risk factors associated with increased biliary cholesterol secretion include the following:

Increasing age
Obesity
Membership in certain ethnic groups (e.g., Chilean women, some northern European groups)
Familial predisposition
Diets high in calories and cholesterol
Certain metabolic abnormalities associated with high blood cholesterol levels, for instance, diabetes, some genetic hyperlipoproteinemias, and primary biliary cirrhosis.

Decreased secretion of bile salts and lecithin occurs in nonobese Caucasians who develop gallstones. Gastrointestinal absorptive disorders that interfere with the enterohepatic circulation of bile acids—for instance, pancreatic insufficiency secondary to cystic fibrosis and Crohn's disease—also decrease secretion of bile acids and favor gallstone formation.

Cholesterol synthesis is increased while that of bile salts and lecithin is reduced in American Pima Indians and in those who take certain drugs (e.g., clofibrate).

Pigment Stones

Pigment stones are classed as **black** or **brown** stones, which have different characteristics. Black stones are irregular and measure less than 1 cm across. On cross section, the surface appears glassy. Black stones contain calcium bilirubinate, bilirubin polymers, calcium salts, and mucin. The incidence of black stones is increased in old and undernourished people, but no correlations with gender, ethnicity, or obesity have been made. Chronic hemolysis, such as occurs with sickle cell anemia and thalassemia, predisposes to the development of black pigment stones. Cirrhosis, either because it leads to increased hemolysis or because of damage to liver cells, is also associated with a high incidence of black stones. However, in most **instances no predisposing cause for the formation of black pigment stones is evident.**

The pathogenesis of black pigment stones is related to an increased concentration of unconjugated bilirubin in the bile. Unconjugated bilirubin is insoluble in bile and is usually present in only trace amounts. When increased amounts are secreted by the hepatocyte, the unconjugated bilirubin precipitates as calcium bilirubinate, probably around a nidus of mucinous glycoproteins. For unexplained reasons, patients without known predisposing factors who develop black pigment stones have increased concentrations of unconjugated bilirubin in the bile.

Brown pigment stones are spongy and laminated, and contain principally calcium bilirubinate mixed with cholesterol and calcium soaps of fatty acids. In contrast to the other types of gallstones, brown pigment stones are found more frequently in the intrahepatic and extrahepatic bile ducts than in the gallbladder. These stones are almost always associated with bacterial cholangitis, in which *E. coli* is the predominant organism. Rare or uncommon in the West, brown stones are almost entirely restricted to Asians infested with *Ascaris lumbricoides* or *Clonorchis sinensis*, helminths that may invade the biliary tract. In the rare cases in Western countries, these stones are found only in patients with mechanical obstruction to the flow of bile, as in sclerosing cholangitis or as a result of a catheter in the common bile duct after common bile duct surgery.

The pathogenesis of brown pigment stones also relates to an increased concentration of unconjugated bilirubin in the bile. It has been proposed that conjugated bilirubin is hydrolyzed to unconjugated bilirubin by the action of bacterial beta-glucuronidase or other hydrolytic enzymes.

Clinical Course of Gallstones

Gallstones may remain "silent" in the gallbladder for many years, and few patients ever die of cholelithiasis itself. One study that followed patients with initially asymptomatic gallstones for up to 11 years found that half remained asymptomatic, one-third developed significant symptomatology, and fewer than 20% developed serious complications. The incidence of severe complications rose with increasing age. However, more recent studies indicate that the 15-year cumulative probability that asymptomatic stones will lead to biliary pain or other complications is less than 20%. These statistics bear upon the question of whether to perform cholecystectomy for asymptomatic gallstones. In some otherwise healthy individuals, the small risk associated with cholecystectomy may justify elective surgery. However, when diseases that increase the operative risk, such as cardiac or pulmonary disorders, are present there is little reason not to manage "silent" gallstones conservatively. On the other hand, more cautious physicians recommend that *all* asymptomatic patients be treated medically unless symptoms supervene. Diabetics present a special case, because acute cholecystitis in these patients carries a high risk of serious complications, and cholecystectomy during the acute disease is far more dangerous than elective surgery. Medical treatment of gallstones has now become a possibility. Oral intake of a bile acid, chenodeoxycholic acid (and more recently taurocholic acid), and percutaneous instillation of a cholesterol solvent into the gallbladder have dissolved radiologically documented gallstones. Lithotripsy has also been used.

Most of the complications of cholelithiasis relate to the obstruction of the cystic duct or common bile duct by stones. Passage of a stone into the cystic duct often, but not invariably, causes severe biliary colic and may lead to acute cholecystitis. Repeated episodes of acute cholecystitis may lead to chronic cholecystitis. The latter condition can also result from the presence of stones alone. Gallstones may pass into the common duct **(choledocholithiasis)**, where they may lead to obstructive jaundice, cholangitis, and pancreatitis. In fact, in populations where alcoholism is not a factor, gallstones are the most common cause of acute pancreatitis. Passage of a large gallstone into the small intestine may cause intestinal obstruction, a condition called **gallstone ileus.** In obstruction of the cystic duct, with or without acute cholecystitis, the bile in the gallbladder is reabsorbed, to be replaced by a clear mucinous fluid secreted by the gallbladder epithelium. The term **hydrops of the gallbladder (mucocele)** is applied to the distended and palpable gallbladder, which may become secondarily infected.

Acute Cholecystitis

In 90% to 95% of cases acute cholecystitis is associated with the presence of gallstones, while the remaining cases **(acalculous cholecystitis)** occur in conjunction with sepsis, severe trauma, infection of the gallbladder with *Salmonella typhosa*, and polyarteritis nodosa. The initial symptom of acute cholecystitis is abdominal pain in the right upper quadrant, and most patients have already experienced episodes of biliary colic. In about a third of the cases, the gallbladder is palpable. Mild jaundice, caused by stones in or edema of the common bile duct, is evident in about 20% of patients. In most cases the acute illness subsides within a week, but persistent pain, fever, leukocytosis, and shaking chills indicate progression of the acute cholecystitis and the need for cholecystectomy.

The external surface of the gallbladder in acute cholecystitis is congested and layered with a fibrinous exudate. The wall is remarkably thickened by edema, and opening the viscus reveals a fiery-red or purple mucosa. Gallstones are usually found within the lumen, and a stone is often seen obstructing the cystic duct. On rare occasions, when obstruction of the cystic duct is complete and bacteria have invaded the gallbladder, the cavity may be distended by cloudy, purulent fluid, a condition termed **empyema of the gallbladder.** However, in some cases, fluid that grossly appears purulent actually consists simply of an emulsion of cholesterol crystals. Microscopically, edema and hemorrhage in the wall are striking, but neutrophilic infiltration is ordinarily only modest. Secondary bacterial infection may lead to true suppuration in the gallbladder wall. The mucosa shows focal ulcerations or, in severe cases, widespread necrosis, in which case the term **gangrenous cholecystitis** is applied. A feared complication in severe cases, which may occur after secondary bacterial infection, is **perforation,** most commonly of the fundus. Discharge of bile into the abdominal cavity results in **bile peritonitis.** More commonly, the contents of the perforated gallbladder are localized by inflammatory adhesions, a lesion known as a **pericholecystic abscess.** The gallbladder contents may also erode into the small or large intestine, creating a **cholecystenteric fistula.** The prognosis for acute acalculous cholecystitis is not as favorable as that associated with stones, perforation and other complications being more frequent.

As the inflammatory process resolves, the gallbladder wall becomes fibrotic and the mucosa heals. However, the function of the gallbladder is usually impaired, so that it no longer concentrates contrast materials and is no longer visualized radiographically. Dystrophic calcification of the injured gallbladder produces the so-called **porcelain gallbladder.**

The pathogenesis of acute cholecystitis is related to the presence of concentrated bile and gallstones within the gallbladder. Bacterial infection is secondary to biliary obstruction, rather than a primary event. It has been theorized that obstruction of the cystic duct by a gallstone leads to the release of phospholipase from the epithelium of the gallbladder. In turn, this enzyme may hydrolyze lecithin and release lysolecithin, a membrane-active cellular toxin. At the same time, disruption of the mucous coat of the epithelium renders the mucosal cells vulnerable to damage by the detergent action of concentrated bile salts. It has also been suggested that bile supersaturated with cholesterol is toxic to the epithelium.

Chronic Cholecystitis

Chronic cholecystitis, almost invariably associated with gallstones, is the most common disease of the gallbladder. It may result from repeated attacks of acute cholecystitis, or, more often, from longstanding gallstones. In the latter case, the pathogenesis probably relates to chronic irritation and chemical injury to the gallbladder epithelium. Many patients with chronic cholecystitis complain of nonspecific abdominal symptoms, although it is not at all clear that these are necessarily related to the gallbladder disease. On the other hand, pain in the right hypochondrium is typical, and often episodic. The diagnosis is best made by ultrasonography, which demonstrates gallstones in a thick, contracted gallbladder. Cholecystectomy is the definitive treatment.

Grossly, the wall of the gallbladder is thickened and firm, and the serosal surface may show fibrous adhesions to surrounding structures as a result of previous episodes of acute cholecystitis. Gallstones are usually found within the lumen, and the bile often contains "gravel"—that is, fine precipitates of calculous material. The bile is infected with coliform organisms in about half of the cases. The mucosa may be focally ulcerated and atrophic, or may appear intact. Microscopically, the wall is fibrotic and often penetrated by sinuses of Rokitansky-Aschoff. Chronic inflammation of variable degree may be seen in all layers. In longstanding chronic cholecystitis, the wall of the gallbladder may become calcified, in which case the term "porcelain gallbladder" is used.

Cholesterolosis

Cholesterolosis of the gallbladder, defined as the accumulation of cholesterol-laden macrophages within the submucosa, is a common incidental finding at autopsy, but is not ordinarily associated with symptoms. It often is seen in conjunction with cholesterol gallstones and is therefore thought to reflect the presence of bile supersaturated with cholesterol. Grossly, the appearance of scattered, yellow mucosal flecks accounts for the term "strawberry gallbladder." Microscopically, the mucosal folds are swollen with large, foamy macrophages, in which a small nucleus is displaced to the periphery.

Primary Sclerosing Cholangitis

Primary sclerosing cholangitis is an inflammatory and fibrosing process that narrows and eventually obstructs the extrahepatic and intrahepatic bile ducts. The diagnosis is made only after other causes of fibrosis—for example, choledocholithiasis, tumors, or surgical trauma—have been excluded. However, the presence of cholelithiasis does not necessarily negate the diagnosis of primary sclerosing cholangitis, since the conditions may coexist. The majority of patients are men under the age of 40 years. Clinically, progressive biliary obstruction leads to persistent obstructive jaundice and eventually to secondary biliary cirrhosis.

The cause of primary sclerosing cholangitis is unknown, but **about two-thirds of the patients also have ulcerative colitis.** A few cases have been described in patients with colonic involvement by Crohn's disease. Primary sclerosing cholangitis has also been reported in association with retroperitoneal fibrosis, lymphoma, and the fibrosing variant of chronic thyroiditis, Riedel's struma. Theories of immune pathogenesis have been entertained, but no firm evidence for such an explanation is at hand.

Grossly, the wall of the common bile duct is thickened and the lumen is stenotic, either uniformly or segmentally. When the intrahepatic bile ducts are involved, a segmental pattern is the rule. Microscopically, diffuse fibrosis and moderate chronic inflammation are noted. The mucosa remains normal. The wall of the gallbladder is often thickened, possibly because it is affected by the same inflammatory process. The histologic appearance varies with the duration of the illness. The sequence of changes is basically the same as that encountered with other causes of chronic extrahepatic biliary obstruction. The end stage of the disease is characterized by typical secondary biliary cirrhosis.

Primary sclerosing cholangitis has a poor prognosis; the mean survival after the appearance of symptoms is 6 years. Surgical dilatation of the common bile duct, insertion of a stent, and biliary bypass operations have been successful in a few cases, but liver transplantation is the most promising option.

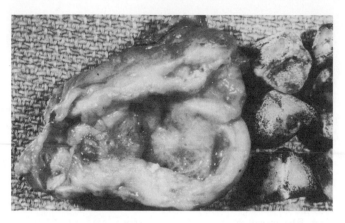

Figure 14-63.   Carcinoma of the gallbladder. The gallbladder wall is infiltrated by firm, greyish-white tumor. The lumen contains cholesterol gallstones.

Neoplasms

Benign Tumors

Benign tumors of the gallbladder and extrahepatic biliary ducts are rare. In the gallbladder, **papillomas** are the most common and may be single or multiple. In three-quarters of the cases, they are associated with gallstones. Mucous gland **adenomas** in the infundibulum are reported and are also often associated with gallstones. The combination of smooth-muscle proliferation and an adenoma has been termed **adenomyoma.** Fibromas, lipomas, leiomyomas, and myxomas have also been recorded.

The bile ducts are affected by the same benign tumors that occur in the gallbladder. Such tumors are clinically more important, since they may obstruct biliary flow and cause jaundice.

Malignant Tumors

Carcinoma of the Gallbladder

The most common tumor of the gallbladder is **adenocarcinoma** (Fig. 14-63). Although it is not one of the more frequent cancers, it is not rare, being incidentally found in 2% of patients who undergo gallbladder surgery. **Because this cancer is usually associated with cholelithiasis and chronic cholecystitis, it is considerably more common in women than men.** In addition, populations that have a high incidence of cholelithiasis, such as Native Americans, have a higher risk of carcinoma of the gallbladder.

The calcified gallbladder (porcelain gallbladder), which represents an extreme variant of chronic cholecystitis, is particularly prone to the development of gallbladder cancer. The symptoms produced by the tumor are similar to those encountered with gallstone disease. However, by the time the tumor becomes symptomatic, it is almost invariably incurable, the 5-year survival rate being less than 3%. For practical purposes, surgical cure is obtained only in patients who undergo cholecystectomy for gallbladder disease and in whom the cancer is an incidental finding.

Gallbladder carcinoma may occur anywhere in the gallbladder but most frequently appears in the fundus. **The tumor is characteristically an infiltrative, well-differentiated adenocarcinoma.** It is usually **desmoplastic,** and thus the wall of the gallbladder becomes thickened and leathery. **Squamous metaplasia** may be so conspicuous that the tumor is thought to be a squamous carcinoma. Occasionally, the tumor grows into the lumen of the gallbladder and assumes a **papillary** configuration. Anaplastic, giant cell, and spindle cell forms of gallbladder carcinoma are reported. The rich lymphatic plexus of the gallbladder provides the most common route of metastasis, but vascular dissemination and direct spread into the liver and contiguous structures occurs.

Carcinoma of the Bile Duct and the Ampulla of Vater

Cancer of the extrahepatic bile ducts, almost always adenocarcinoma, typically presents as obstructive jaundice. The tumor is less common than gallbladder cancer, and the female predominance of gallbladder cancer is not evident. The cause of bile duct cancer is unknown, but gallstones are frequently found in those affected, and there is an association with idiopathic inflammatory disease involving the colon. The tumor has also been reported to arise in choledochal cysts and in Caroli's disease. In the Orient, bile duct carcinoma is associated with biliary infestation by the fluke *Clonorchis sinensis.* As in carcinoma of the gallbladder, growth may be endophytic (into the lumen) or diffusely infiltrative. The prognosis is poor, but because symptoms arise early in the course of the disease, the prognosis is somewhat better than that of gallbladder carcinoma.

The bile duct may also be obstructed by **adenocarcinoma of the ampulla of Vater.** The initial symptom is again obstructive jaundice, although a few patients present with pancreatitis. In contrast to bile duct carcinoma, surgical treatment of cancer of the ampulla of Vater leads to a 35% 5-year survival rate.

SUGGESTED READING

BOOKS

Czaja AJ, Dickson ER: Chronic Active Hepatitis: The Mayo Clinic Experience. New York, Marcel Dekker, 1986

Farber E, Phillips MJ, Kaufman N: Pathogenesis of Liver Diseases. Baltimore, Williams & Wilkins, 1987

MacSween RNM, Anthony PP, Scheuer PJ: Pathology of the Liver. Edinburgh, Churchill Livingstone, 1979

Peters RL, Craig JR: Liver Pathology. Edinburgh, Churchill Livingstone, 1986

Schiff L, Schiff ER (eds): Diseases of the Liver, 6th ed. Philadelphia, JB Lippincott, 1987

Sherlock S: Diseases of the Liver and Biliary System, 7th ed. Oxford, Blackwell Scientific Publications, 1985

Zakim D, Boyer TD (eds): Hepatology: A Textbook of Liver Disease. Philadelphia, WB Saunders, 1982

Zimmerman HJ: Hepatotoxicity: The Adverse Effects of Drugs and Other Chemicals on the Liver. New York, Appleton Century Crofts, 1978

REVIEW ARTICLES

Balistreri WF: Neonatal cholestasis. J Pediatr 106:171-184, 1985

Frei JV, Ghent CN (eds): First International Workshop and Colloquium on the Pathology of Liver Transplantation. May 28, 1986, London, Ontario, Canada. Transplant Proc 18 (suppl 4):119–173,1986

Friedman LS, Dienstag JL: Recent developments in viral hepatitis. Disease-A-Month 32: 313–385, 1986

Gallan JL, Knapp AB: Bilirubin metabolism and congenital jaundice. Hosp Pract 17:83–106, 1985

Kaplan MM: Primary biliary cirrhosis. New Engl J Med 316:521, 1987

MacSween RN, Burt AD: Histologic spectrum of alcoholic liver disease. Semin Liver Dis 6:221–232, 1986

Mezey E: Alcoholic liver disease. Progr Liver Dis 7:555-572, 1982

Rubin E: Iatrogenic liver injury. Hum Pathol 11:312–331, 1980

ORIGINAL ARTICLES

Blumberg BS: Polymorphisms of serum proteins and the development of isoprecipitins in transfused patients. Bull NY Acad Med 40:377–386, 1964

Mallory FB: Cirrhosis of the liver: Five different types of lesions from which it may arise. Bull Johns Hopkins Hosp 22:69–75, 1911

Rubin E, Lieber CS: Alcohol-induced hepatic injury in non-alcoholic volunteers. New Engl J Med 278:869–876, 1968

15

The Pancreas

Dante G. Scarpelli

Anatomy

Embryology

Developmental Defects

Pancreatitis

Neoplasms of the Exocrine
Pancreas

Neoplasms of the Endocrine
Pancreas

Figure 15-1. Protein synthesis in the pancreatic acinar cell. An electron microscopic autoradiograph of a rat pancreatic acinar cell 30 minutes after a pulse
label of [³H] leucine shows serpentine silver grains that delineate the localization of (1) synthesis, (2) intracellular transport, (3) concentration, and (4) storage of digestive proenzymes. The arrows show the vectorial movement of the
secretory product.

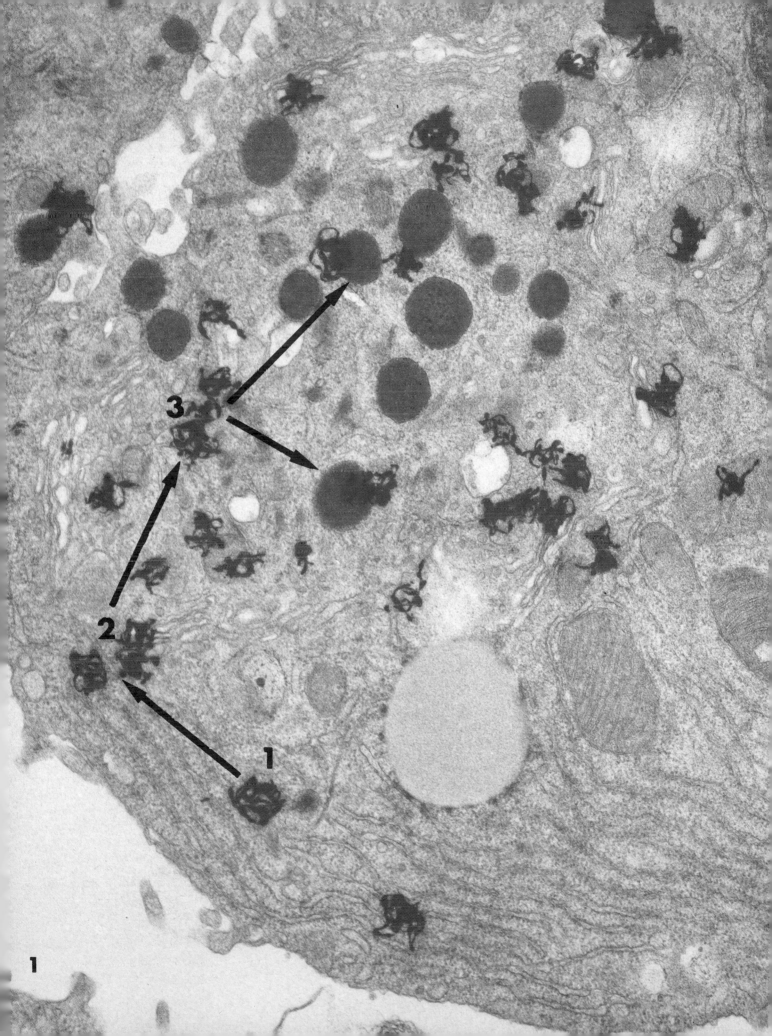

Anatomy

The pancreas is a mixed exocrine–endocrine gland that extends transversely in the upper abdomen and is cradled between the loop of the duodenum and the hilum of the spleen. It is retroperitoneal, behind the lesser omental sac and the stomach, a location that renders it largely inaccessible to physical examination and other modalities of direct clinical assessment. The adult pancreas is 10 to 15 cm long and weighs from 60 to 150 g. It is divided into three anatomic subdivisions: the head, which lies in the concavity of the duodenum and extends to the superior mesenteric vessels immediately behind the organ; the body, which includes most of the gland; and a tapered tail, which ends at the hilum of the spleen. The secretions of the exocrine pancreas drain via the duct of Wirsung, which begins by the convergence of several small ducts in the tail and extends into the head, collecting secretions from ductal tributaries along the way. It then turns downward and backward, where it empties into the duodenum at the ampulla of Vater. Occasionally, in addition to the major duct, an accessory duct of Santorini represents the duct of the embryonic ventral pancreas. The major pancreatic duct may enter the duodenum directly or, more commonly, drain into the common bile duct immediately proximal to the ampulla of Vater. The common channel that carries bile and pancreatic secretions is invested with a circular complex of smooth muscle fibers, which condense as they pass through the duodenal wall into the sphincter of Oddi.

Exocrine tissue, comprising 80% to 85% of the pancreas, consists of secretory cells organized in acini that connect with ductules. These in turn merge into small ducts that empty into medium and large ducts, and finally form the main pancreatic duct. **Acinar cells synthesize some 20 different digestive enzymes, which are secreted into the intestine following both neural and hormonal stimulation.** Stimulation of the vagus nerves increases the flow of pancreatic juice. Amino acids and a duodenal–jejunal pH of less than 3 trigger the release of the polypeptide hormone cholecystokinin, and antral distension stimulates that of secretin. Cholecystokinin and secretin bind to surface receptors on acinar and duct cells, respectively, stimulating the secretion of digestive enzymes from the acinar cells and of bicarbonate ions and water from the duct cells. Bicarbonate ions serve to neutralize the highly acidic gastric chyle in the intestine and to achieve an optimum pH for the function of pancreatic digestive enzymes. The daily secretion of about 1.5 to 3 liters of pancreatic juice attests to the remarkable synthetic and secretory capacity of acinar cells and the transport of ions and water by ductal cells.

The endocrine pancreas consists of cells organized into islets that are distributed throughout the organ. These endocrine islets comprise only about 2% of the total pancreas. Islets contain several cell types, each of which synthesizes one or more hormones, including insulin and glucagon, among others. Following the proper stimulus the hormones are secreted directly into the blood. The structure and function of pancreatic endocrine cells are discussed in detail in Chapter 21.

Embryology

The pancreas begins as two outpouchings of the entodermal lining arising on the dorsal and ventral sides of the embryonic duodenal tube. These hollow bulges grow as a result of the proliferation of entoderm-deprived epithelial cells, an effect induced by their close association with the mesenchyma that surrounds the primitive gut tube. Mesenchyma also induces orientation of pancreatic epithelium to form branching ducts within the bulge. The dorsal pancreas grows more rapidly than the ventral, and at the sixth week of embryonic development, it becomes an elongated structure. The ventral pancreas is rotated dorsally by unequal growth of the duodenal wall and brought into approximation with the dorsal anlage, with which it ultimately fuses during the seventh week to become a single organ. Most of the adult pancreas is derived from the dorsal pancreas, except for the head, which arises largely from the ventral rudiment. The duct systems of the two embryonic pancreata also fuse, giving rise to a single duct, the precursor of the major pancreatic duct (the duct of Wirsung). The unfused segment of the duct of the ventral pancreas remains to become the smaller accessory duct of Santorini, which enters the duodenum through a separate orifice. When fusion is complete, Santorini's duct is absent.

Cytologic differentiation of the pancreas begins with the appearance of ducts, which arise from nests of entodermal cells surrounded by mesodermal mesenchyma. The ducts, consisting of a single layer of cuboidal cells, branch into enlongate ductules that arborize to form a complex duct system. At the third month of development acinar cells arise from the ductules in terminal and lateral buds. The acinar cells differentiate and 5 weeks later acquire their complement of distinctive zymogen granules. Factors produced by mesodermal mesenchyma are obligatory for the synthesis of digestive proenzymes, the hallmark of acinar cell differentiation. This is a prime example of the critical importance of cell–cell interaction in normal development and differentiation.

Islet cells are also derived from larger ducts, about a month earlier than acinar cells. Islets arise as elongated and serpentine lateral extensions and consist of solid masses of cells that rapidly acquire the spectrum of small, dense, secretory granules characteristic of endocrine pancreas. The sequence of acinar and islet cell development and differentiation, once accomplished, has generally been considered to be fixed. However, recent studies suggest that this may not be so and that pancreatic acini may, under the proper stimuli, convert to structures indistinguishable from preexisting ductules. Such plasticity of differentiation of pancreatic cells in the adult has interesting implications when one considers the pathogenesis of some pancreatic diseases, especially cancer of the pancreas.

Developmental Defects

Developmental defects of the pancreas include (1) **aberrant or accessory pancreas,** in which pancreatic tissue is present outside its normal location; (2) encirclement of the duodenum, and less frequently, the bile duct or portal vein, by pancreatic tissue—the so-called **annular pancreas;** (3) still more infrequently, a variety of failures of fusion of the two pancreatic anlages, including the ducts, termed **pancreas divisum;** (4) absence of the parts of adult gland derived from the dorsal pancreas, namely, the body and tail; and (5) congenital cysts.

Aberrant (ectopic) pancreas, which is incidentally encountered in 2% of autopsies and is not rare, is most commonly localized in the wall of the duodenum, stomach, and jejunum. More rarely, it has been found in Meckel's diverticulum of the ileum, the common bile duct, gall bladder, liver, spleen, and various other foci in the abdominal cavity. In the wall of the gastrointestinal tract, pancreatic nodules localize immediately below the mucosa, in the muscularis, beneath the serosa, or in small diverticula. The tissue contains all the components of normal pancreas, namely, acini, ducts, and islets. The most plausible theories of the origin of aberrant pancreas are (1) incomplete atrophy of the left ventral anlage; (2) regression to a more primitive pattern of differentiation reminiscent of that seen in lower vertebrates, especially certain fish in which exocrine and endocrine pancreatic tissue are diffusely distributed in

liver, intestinal wall, and peritoneum; (3) inappropriate expression of the pluripotent developmental capacity of the embryonic gut; and (4) buds of embryonic pancreatic tissue that have penetrated the intestinal wall and have become isolated from the main mass and thus misplaced by rapid longitudinal growth of the intestine. Of these theories, the last two (3 and 4) seem most probable.

Annular pancreas is a fairly uncommon condition in which the head of the gland surrounds the second portion of the duodenum; encirclement may be complete or incomplete. Annular pancreas may be associated with duodenal atresia, an anomaly that requires surgery very soon after birth. Such infants infrequently have other congenital anomalies, including trisomy 21 (Down syndrome). Many patients with annular pancreas do not require surgery in early life but develop symptoms at 60 or 70 years of age. More commonly, the diagnosis is made incidental to radiologic studies for a duodenal ulcer. This anomaly is probably due to a failure of the ventral anlage to migrate behind the duodenum. Since this migration is due to increased focal growth of the duodenal wall, the annular pancreas reflects impaired development of the duodenum. Failure of fusion of the rudiments of the pancreas leads to two separate glands, each with its separate duct draining into the duodenum.

True cysts of the pancreas are thought to arise from faulty development of pancreatic ducts. Although their mode of origin is not understood, it is postulated that cysts are caused by the failure of embryonic ducts to regress as they are replaced by more permanent ones. Remnants of persistent ducts are presumed to become obstructed and form cysts that fill with fluid. Congenital cysts can be single or multiple and range in size from a few millimeters to large cysts that may fill the upper abdomen. Such cysts are lined by cuboidal-to-flat epithelium and contain fluid with both amylase and proteolytic enzyme activity.

Pancreatitis

Pancreatitis is defined as an inflammatory condition of the exocrine pancreas that results from injury to acinar cells. Depending on its severity and duration, pancreatitis presents in a variety of clinical forms. These range from a mild, self-limited disease, consisting of acute inflammation and edema of the stroma with little or no acinar cell necrosis, to the more severe and sometimes fatal acute hemorrhagic pancreatitis with massive necrosis. A debilitating form, chronic relapsing pancreatitis, is characterized

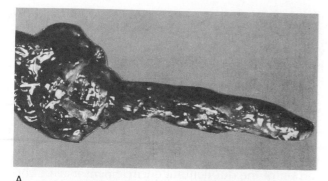

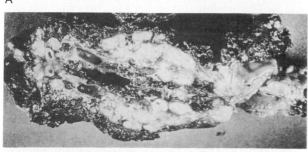

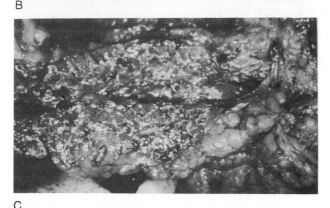

Figure 15-2.   Acute hemorrhagic pancreatitis. (*A*) The head, body, and tail of the pancreas are intensely hemorrhagic. (*B*) The longitudinal cut surface shows large areas of confluent hemorrhagic necrosis that are clearly demarcated from pale nodular foci of nonnecrotic pancreas. (*C*) Numerous yellow-white foci of fat necrosis are present on the surface and in the substance of a necrotic pancreas at a stage somewhat later than that shown in *B*.

by recurrent attacks of severe abdominal pain and progressive fibrosis, ultimately leading to pancreatic insufficiency.

Acute Pancreatitis

The mild and presumably reversible form of acute pancreatitis, termed *interstitial* or *edematous pancreatitis,* has not been extensively studied because of its brief and benign clinical course. An infiltrate of poly-

morphonuclear leukocytes and edema of the connective tissue between lobules of acinar cells constitute the initial lesion. There is no necrosis of acinar cells, fat necrosis, or hemorrhage. Acute hemorrhagic pancreatitis is a condition of middle age, with a peak incidence at 60 years. It is often associated with chronic biliary disease and alcohol abuse and erupts abruptly, usually following a heavy meal or excessive alcohol intake. It is more common in men than in women, especially when it is associated with the chronic abuse of alcohol. Clinically, the patient presents with severe epigastric pain that is referred to the upper back and is accompanied by nausea and vomiting. Within a matter of hours catastrophic peripheral vascular collapse and shock ensue. When shock is sustained and profound, pancreatitis may be complicated within the first week of onset by the adult respiratory distress syndrome and acute renal failure, a situation that is fatal in 7% of cases. Early in the disease, pancreatic digestive enzymes are released from injured acinar cells into the blood and the abdominal cavity. Elevation of serum amylase and lipase levels as early as 24 to 72 hours is diagnostic, as are high enzyme levels in the abdominal ascitic fluid.

Initially, the pancreas is edematous and hyperemic. Within a day, pale, gray foci appear, rapidly becoming friable and hemorrhagic. As the disease progresses, **these foci enlarge and become so numerous that most of the pancreas is converted into a large retroperitoneal hematoma, in which pancreatic tissue is barely recognizable** (Fig. 15-2 *A, B*). Yellow-white areas of fat necrosis appear at the interface between necrotic foci and fat tissue in and around the pancreas, including the adjacent mesentery (Fig. 15-2 *C*). These nodules of necrotic fat have a pasty consistency, which becomes firmer and chalk-like as more calcium and magnesium soaps are produced. Saponification reflects the interaction of cations with free fatty acids released by the action of activated lipase on triglycerides in fat cells. As a result, the level of blood calcium may be depressed—sometimes to the point of causing neuromuscular irritability, such as facial tics. Extrapancreatic fat necrosis, arising as a consequence of the release of lipase from the injured pancreas into the blood, has been reported in subcutaneous fat, skeletal muscle, and bone marrow.

The most prominent tissue alterations in acute pancreatitis are acinar cell necrosis, an intense acute inflammatory reaction (Fig. 15-3*A*), **and foci of necrotic fat cells** (Fig. 15-3*B*). Late sequelae in patients who survive the shock and its systemic complications include the formation of pancreatic abscesses and

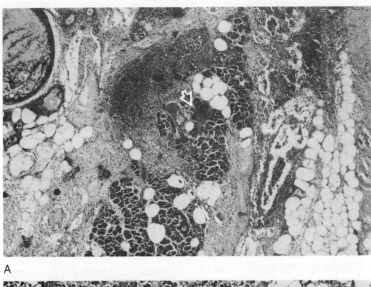

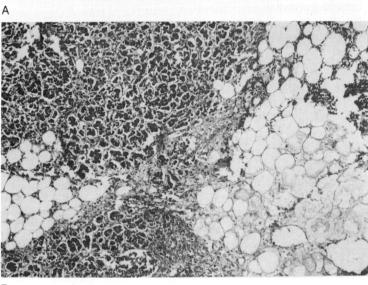

Figure 15-3. Acute hemorrhagic pancreatitis. (*A*) Hemorrhage is evident in the center and right of the microscopic field. The pancreatic lobule in the center shows a focus of acinar cell necrosis (*arrow*). (*B*) A later stage of acute pancreatitis. A focus of fat necrosis (*right*) can be compared with normal fat tissue (*left*).

pseudocysts. In the latter structures, large spaces limited by connective tissue contain degraded blood, debris of necrotic pancreatic tissue, and fluid rich in pancreatic enzymes. Pseudocysts may enlarge enough to compress and obstruct the duodenum. They may become secondarily infected and form an abscess. Rupture is a rare complication that leads to a chemical or septic peritonitis, or both.

Pathogenesis of Acute Pancreatitis

Autopsy studies at the turn of the century established the association of chronic cholecystitis and cholelithiasis with acute hemorrhagic pancreatitis. In some cases gallstones were found lodged near the orifice of the common duct beyond the point where it is joined by the pancreatic duct. Since a stone impacted at this site obstructs both ducts, it would be expected to cause the reflux of bile into the pancreas. There-

fore, it was theorized that such obstruction was the etiologic factor in the development of acute hemorrhagic pancreatitis. This notion was prevalent for many years and gained support from experimental studies in animals in which hemorrhagic pancreatitis was induced by retrograde infusion of a mixture of pancreatic juice and bile into the main pancreatic duct. However, in recent years it has become increasingly apparent that although pancreatitis is often accompanied by conditions that serve to impair normal duct secretion, frank obstruction of the common duct or pancreatic duct is often not present. The foregoing must be tempered by the fact that studies in monkeys, involving simultaneous fluoroscopic visualization of contrast medium in the biliary tree and the measurement of pressures in the common bile duct, have established that intermittent reflux into the pancreatic duct can occur in the absence of obstruction.

Increasingly, studies suggest that failure of one or more of the complex systems of physiologic checks and balances that exist in the blood, the pancreas, and other tissues that serve to prevent the inappropriate activation of pancreatic enzymes and to protect the host from their deleterious effects may also contribute to the development of acute pancreatitis. Although the mechanisms that initiate the various forms of pancreatitis have been the focus of much study and research, they continue to elude us and are the subjects of speculation. From the foregoing consideration of the various types of pancreatitis, **it is clear that a breakdown of intracellular compartmentation of digestive proenzymes synthesized by the acinar cell and inappropriate and premature activation of these proenzymes are common to all variants of pancreatitis.** Differences in the severity and duration of membrane damage may in part determine the type of pancreatitis that ultimately develops.

The pancreas is protected from the harmful effects of its lytic enzymes by a series of highly compartmented systems of intracellular membranes. These membranes effectively isolate the pancreatic enzymes from their synthesis by the rough-surfaced endoplasmic reticulum to their release into the ductular lumen in response to stimulation by the gastrointestinal hormone cholecystokinin. This process involves the extrusion of the nascent proenzyme proteins into the cisternae of the endoplasmic reticulum, from which they are moved progressively by a system of vesicles to the *cis* and *trans* elements of the Golgi complex, and from that site to condensing vacuoles, from which the zymogen granules are ultimately derived. On secretion the membrane of the granule fuses with the plasma membrane before its extrusion by exocytosis. At each step of their formation and secretion the enzymes are totally sequestered in a membrane-bound space. The various potent inhibitors of proteolytic enzymes present in many body fluids and tissues constitute a second line of protection, defending the organism against inappropriate activation of the digestive proenzymes of the pancreas. However, this defense is not total. Four potent protease inhibitors have been identified in human plasma: α_1-antitrypsin, α_2-macroglobulin, C_1 esterase inhibitor, and pancreatic secretory trypsin inhibitor. Although collectively these can inhibit two types of trypsin in addition to chymotrypsin and elastase, they are without effect on two other potent proteases, carboxypeptidases A and B. These inhibitors bind strongly to the proteases and render them inactive. Although α_2-macroglobulin reduces the capacity of either of the trypsin molecules to digest protein, it

does not completely prevent them from cleaving small synthetic peptides. Thus, tryptic activity is demonstrable in plasma, even when trypsin is bound by the inhibitor. Further, a trypsin inhibitor in human pancreatic juice is unable to inhibit the enzyme completely, even when the inhibitor is present in excess. Apparently the inhibitor is digested by the trypsin to which it is bound, a reaction that requires calcium ions. Thus, despite the variety of inhibitors of trypsin in different body compartments, the protection they render is less than complete. Since it turns out that activated trypsin is also able to activate other pancreatic proenzymes, such as chymotrypsinogen, proelastase, prophospholipase, and procarboxypeptidase, its incomplete inhibition in pancreatic juice and plasma poses a hazard.

Secretion by acinar cells delivers fluid rich in proenzymes to the ductules, where they are activated almost immediately. **Although most of the secretion is discharged into the duct system and enters the duodenum, a small amount diffuses back into the periductular extracellular fluid and eventually the plasma.** This happens because normal ducts contain fluid under some, albeit low, pressure. Thus, any condition that tends to diminish the patency of pancreatic ducts or the easy outflow of exocrine secretion could be expected to exacerbate back-diffusion across the ducts, which can trigger a massive inappropriate activation of digestive proenzymes. If the obstruction is sufficiently severe, this process could even involve the acinar cells. Well-documented causes of pancreatic duct obstruction include gallstones, frequently in association with chronic cholecystitis, and chronic alcohol abuse. Although ethanol is well recognized as a chemical toxin, a direct toxic effect on pancreatic acinar or duct cells has yet to be demonstrated. **However, ethanol can adversely affect the pancreas by causing spasm or acute edema of the sphincter of Oddi, especially following an alcoholic binge, and by stimulating the secretion of secretin from the small intestine, which in turn triggers the exocrine pancreas to secrete pancreatic juice.** When these effects occur together (i.e., enhanced secretion into an obstructed duct), the results may be disastrous. The transudation of pancreatic secretion into periductal pancreatic tissues and eventually peripancreatic tissue leads to chemical injury. The activated enzymes digest proteins, lipids, and carbohydrates of cell membranes. Phospholipase A causes lysis of cell membranes, and when mixed with bile converts lecithin to the potent cytotoxin lysolecithin. Damage to the capillaries leads to hemorrhage and local anoxia, which further intensifies and extends tissue damage.

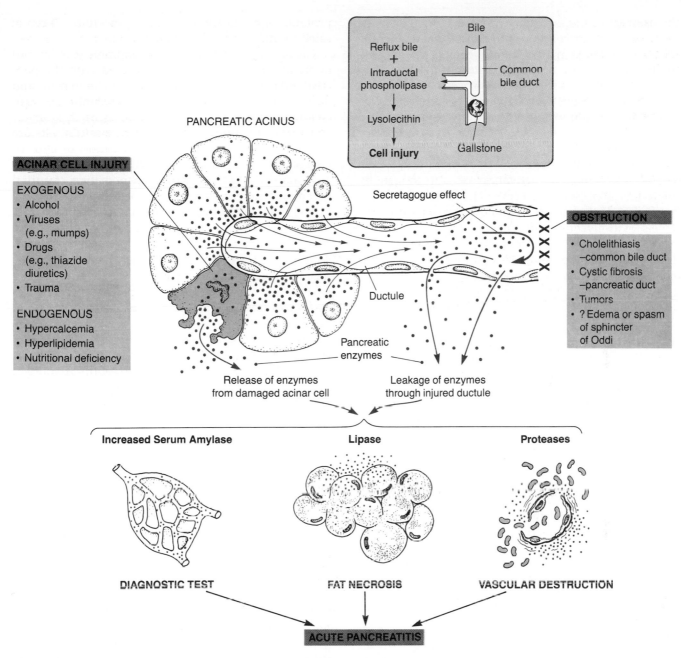

ACINAR CELL INJURY

EXOGENOUS
- Alcohol
- Viruses
  (e.g., mumps)
- Drugs
  (e.g., thiazide
  diuretics)
- Trauma

ENDOGENOUS
- Hypercalcemia
- Hyperlipidemia
- Nutritional deficiency

Reflux bile
+
Intraductal
phospholipase
↓
Lysolecithin
↓
Cell injury

Bile
Common
bile duct
Gallstone

PANCREATIC ACINUS

Secretagogue effect

Ductule

Pancreatic
enzymes

OBSTRUCTION
- Cholelithiasis
  —common bile duct
- Cystic fibrosis
  —pancreatic duct
- Tumors
- ?Edema or spasm
  of sphincter
  of Oddi

Release of enzymes
from damaged acinar cell

Leakage of enzymes
through injured ductule

Increased Serum Amylase **Lipase** **Proteases**

DIAGNOSTIC TEST **FAT NECROSIS** **VASCULAR DESTRUCTION**

ACUTE PANCREATITIS

Figure 15-4. The pathogenesis of acute pancreatitis. Injury to the ductules or the acinar cells leads to the release of pancreatic enzymes. Lipase and proteases destroy tissue, thereby causing acute pancreatitis. The release of amylase is the basis for a test for acute pancreatitis.

In addition to the foregoing, other factors that cause pancreatic acinar cell injury and pancreatitis include viruses, endotoxemia, ischemia, drugs, trauma, hypertriglyceridemia, and hypercalcemia. The mechanisms by which some of these induce injury are known, but those for others—such as corticosteroids, estrogens, azathioprine, hypertriglyceridemia, and hypercalcemia—remain unclear. In hypertriglyceridemia and hypercalcemia, it is thought that toxic fatty acids are formed by the action of pancreatic lipase on triglycerides and the activation of trypsinogen by high levels of serum calcium. Experimentally, the perfusion of the isolated canine pancreas with high levels of triglycerides induces edema, hemorrhage, and a striking release of free fatty acids into the perfusate. The pathogenesis of acute hemorrhagic pancreatitis is outlined in Figure 15-4.

Chronic Pancreatitis

Chronic pancreatitis is thought to result from recurrent bouts of acute pancreatitis, which lead to a progressive destruction of acinar cells, followed by healing and fibrosis. As a result, exocrine and endocrine functions are lost. Like acute pancreatitis, chronic pancreatitis is associated with alcoholism and, less commonly, with biliary tract disease, hypercalcemia, or hyperlipidemia. About one half of cases are seen in patients without any of these risk factors. In the acute phase, focal pancreatic necrosis is accompanied by a polymorphonuclear infiltrate, which is replaced by lymphocytes and plasma cells. Healing is characterized by the removal of necrotic tissue by macrophages, a proliferation of capillaries and fibroblasts, and finally the deposition of collagen. In advanced cases, large areas of the pancreas are replaced by fibrosis, and the exocrine and endocrine tissues become atrophic. **The most common type of chronic pancreatitis is chronic calcifying pancreatitis, a disorder most frequently associated with alcoholism.** Intraductal protein plugs eventually calcify and lead to the formation of stones in the ducts (Fig. 15-5). In chronic pancreatitis following sustained alcohol abuse, ductules and ducts are so often filled with thick proteinaceous secretion that some have concluded that such secretions may be an important mechanism of obstruction. Since alcohol is a potent secretagogue for the exocrine pancreas, one can visualize a situation of secretion against obstruction. In another form of this disease, chronic obstructive pancreatitis, stenosis of the sphincter of Oddi is associated with gallbladder stones. Although in this condition the pancreatic ducts are filled with thick proteinaceous secretions, they are rarely the focus of calcification or stone formation.

Chronic pancreatitis is more common in men, and in about 10% of cases it is associated with the pancreas divisum (incomplete fusion of the ventral and dorsal pancreatic anlage). **Diabetes mellitus, pancreatic insufficiency with its attendant steatorrhea and malabsorption, and pancreatic pseudocysts are frequent complications in the late stages of chronic pancreatitis** (Fig. 15-6, Fig. 15-7).

A rare variant of chronic pancreatitis, **familial hereditary pancreatitis,** merits special mention. It occurs with increased frequency in certain families, predominantly in girls, and becomes apparent in early childhood. Its pattern of inheritance is autosomal dominant, and in some instances the disease is associated with an aminoaciduria, in which the pattern of excretion resembles that of the recessive form of cystinuria. A second biochemical abnormality in some cases is hypercalcemia, secondary to hyperplasia or adenomas of the parathyroid glands. Hereditary pancreatitis is not associated with alcohol abuse or chronic biliary disease. It is noteworthy that about 20% of such patients have subsequently developed ductal adenocarcinoma of the pancreas; however, in view of the rarity of this disease, these data must be interpreted with caution. Except for the features noted previously, hereditary pancreatitis is indistinguishable from chronic relapsing pancreatitis, including its associated late complications.

Neoplasms of the Exocrine Pancreas

Benign Tumors

Benign tumors of the exocrine pancreas are rare. The most common one, which presents as a large cystic tumor, deserves mention because it is important that it be differentiated diagnostically from the various congenital and acquired cysts that are not true neoplasms.

Cystadenomas of the pancreas are large, multiloculated, cystic tumors, usually localized in the body or tail. They occur most frequently in women between ages 50 and 70. Cystadenomas, which constitute about 10% of cystic lesions of the pancreas, are of two types, depending on whether they are lined by serous or mucinous epithelium. Serous cystadenomas consist of numerous cysts of varying size, lined by a cuboidal epithelium with a clear glycogen-rich cytoplasm. The microcystic variant consists of uniformly small cysts, which on gross examination

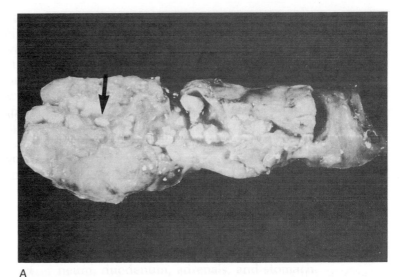

A

Figure 15-5. Chronic calcifying pancreatitis. (*A*) A gross photograph shows numerous calculi in the pancreatic duct (*arrow*). The gross architecture of the organ is severely distorted by fibrosis. (*B*) Atrophic lobules of acinar cells are surrounded by dense fibrous scar tissue infiltrated by lymphocytes. To the right of the lumen (*L*) a major duct contains granular deposits of calcified material, and to the left, a dilated medium-sized duct is partially denuded of its epithelial lining and has dense linear calcific deposits at its periphery (*arrow*). (*C*) At a higher magnification, lymphocytic infiltration and scarring are evident in part of an acinar cell lobule. Calcific material occludes its draining ductule (*arrow*).

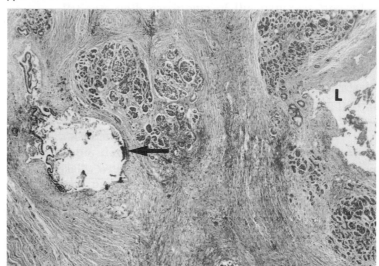

B

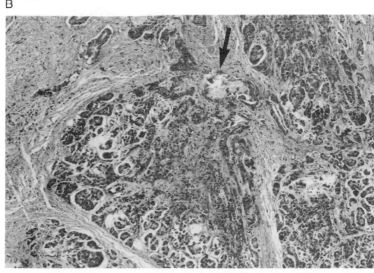

C

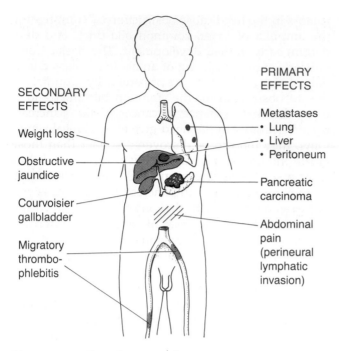

SECONDARY EFFECTS

Weight loss

Obstructive jaundice

Courvoisier gallbladder

Migratory thrombophlebitis

PRIMARY EFFECTS

Metastases
• Lung
• Liver
• Peritoneum

Pancreatic carcinoma

Abdominal pain (perineural lymphatic invasion)

Figure 15-8. Complications of pancreatic carcinoma.

retroperitoneal space and may invade the adjacent spleen and the splenic vein, showering the liver with metastases. Intraperitoneal metastases appear as small, grayish, firm nodules in the mesentery and on the surface of intraperitoneal organs.

More than 75% of ductal adenocarcinomas of the pancreas are well differentiated, secrete mucin, and stimulate a florid synthesis and deposition of collagen by the host, a process referred to as a desmoplastic reaction (Fig. 15-9C). Histologically, such carcinomas resemble mucinous adenocarcinoma of the lung, stomach, gallbladder, colon, ovary, and other organs. Thus, in the absence of symptoms referable to the pancreas, the identification of distant foci of metastatic cancer as pancreatic in origin is difficult. The remaining 25% of carcinomas that originate from pancreatic ducts and ductules include giant cell carcinoma, adenosquamous carcinoma, microadenocarcinoma, and a few other rare types.

Etiology and Pathogenesis

The factors involved in the causation of pancreatic cancer are obscure. Epidemiologic studies have implicated both host and environmental factors as of possible etiologic significance. **Notable among the host factors is chronic gallbladder disease, particularly that associated with cholesterol gallstones, diabetes mellitus, and chronic hereditary pancreatitis. Environmental factors that have been implicated in-**clude cigarette smoking, diets high in meat and fat, and occupational exposure to chemicals, namely, β-naphthylamine, benzidine, and coal tar derivatives.

The association of obstructive gallbladder disease with pancreatic cancer is of special interest because it may serve to explain how carcinogenic chemicals, if they are indeed involved in pancreatic carcinogenesis, may reach the pancreas. As previously discussed, the liver is one of the major organs involved in the oxidative metabolism of foreign compounds, including carcinogens and other potentially toxic chemicals. Metabolites of such reactive intermediates are released into the bile and the blood and could gain direct access to the pancreas either by the reflux of bile into the pancreatic duct or from the blood.

Diabetes mellitus, especially in women, is an important risk factor for the development of carcinoma of the pancreas, the incidence being two times higher in diabetics than in the rest of the population. In fact, it is the most frequent cancer encountered in diabetics. It may be significant that those ethnic groups that appear to be particularly susceptible to diabetes mellitus—namely, American Indians, blacks, Jews, Hawaiians, and Maoris—also have a high incidence of pancreatic cancer. Furthermore, proliferative lesions of the pancreatic ducts, such as papillary hyperplasia and metaplasia, are frequently encountered in diabetics.

Epidemiologic studies have shown a significant increase in risk of pancreatic cancer in cigarette smokers. A causal relationship is further implied by an apparent dose response related to the number of cigarettes smoked per day, and the demonstration of hyperplastic pancreatic ducts in autopsy studies of smokers. Since the preponderance of pancreatic cancer in men is thought by some to be due to the greater number of smokers among men, it will be of interest to see if the incidence of this disease increases in women as a consequence of their greater adoption of the smoking habit in the past few decades. This has already occurred with lung cancer.

Experimental studies lend support to a role for chemical carcinogenesis in pancreatic cancer. 7,12-dimethylbenz[a]anthracene, a polycyclic hydrocarbon carcinogen, and a number of β-oxidized dipropylnitrosamines, among other carcinogens, are pancreatic carcinogens in rodent species. The nitrosamines are of particular interest because they induce adenocarcinoma of pancreatic ducts, the predominant type of pancreatic cancer in man.

Epidemiologic studies also suggest that dietary factors are involved in the development of pancreatic cancer. Although a positive correlation has been shown to exist between the consumption of a variety of foodstuffs and mortality from pancreatic cancer, a

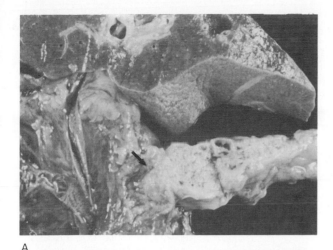

A

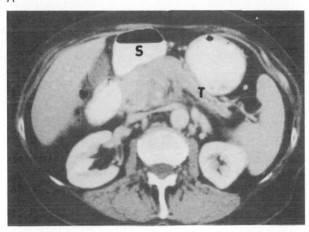

B

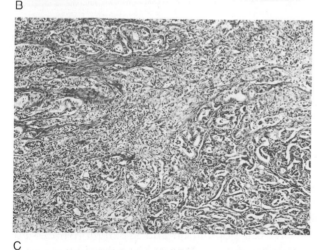

C

Figure 15-9. Carcinoma of the head of the pancreas. (A) Local invasion of the adjacent duodenum is evident (*arrow*). The common bile duct is dilated. The liver is free of metastases. (B) A CT scan at midabdominal level shows a carcinoma of the head of the pancreas compressing the stomach (S) anteriorly; also note the atrophy of the tail (T) at the right. (C) A tissue section of adenocarcinoma of pancreas reveals markedly atypical neoplastic glands that infiltrate the connective tissue of the pancreas.

high intake of meat and fat appears to be of particular significance, especially the latter. In Japan, for example, where pancreatic cancer was a rare disease, its incidence has increased steadily over the past 25 years. This coincides with the period of westernization of Japanese dietary practices, in which consumption of meat and fat has increased. Similar relationships between the consumption of meat and fat and pancreatic cancer have also been identified in affluent Western societies. Experimental dose–effect relationships between the level of fat consumption and carcinogenesis support the etiologic role of dietary factors.

Recent studies have shed new light on the pathogenesis of pancreatic cancer. Chronic exposure of experimental animals to chemicals known to induce pancreatic cancer causes a metaplasia of acini to duct-like structures, which betray their origin by the occasional presence of acinar cells rich in zymogen granules. In the hamster, an animal model that develops a ductal adenocarcinoma bearing a striking resemblance to that encountered in man, the metaplastic ducts proliferate and develop preneoplastic changes and frank malignant tumors simultaneously with similar proliferative and preneoplastic changes in the epithelium of medium and large pancreatic ducts. These findings were given further support by the discovery at autopsy of comparable lesions in some ostensibly normal pancreatic glands, especially those of cigarette smokers, and in the noncancerous portions of the pancreas of patients with ductal adenocarcinoma. The metaplastic acini in noncancerous pancreatic tissue failed to stain with a monoclonal antibody to a surface antigen present on normal acinar cells. Instead they stained intensely with a monoclonal antibody to a surface antigen expressed on normal duct epithelium. Although this evidence is circumstantial, it suggests that the widely held view that ductal adenocarcinoma arises solely from preexisting ducts and ductules is open to question.

Neoplasms of the Endocrine Pancreas

Benign and malignant tumors of the pancreatic islets are common enough to be encountered occasionally during a lifetime in a busy medical practice. **These tumors secrete large amounts of potent hormones that lead to profound physiologic disturbances that are responsible for distinctive clinical syndromes.** Before considering islet cell tumors, a brief discussion of the development and function of normal islets will serve to set this group of intriguing tumors in perspective.

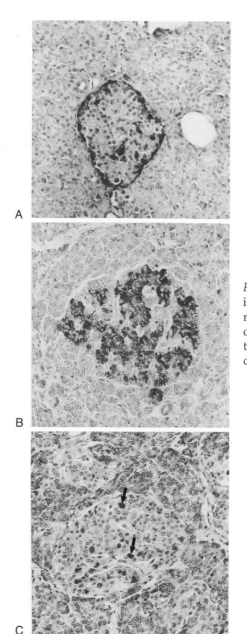

Figure 15-10.   Localization of hormones of the pancreatic islet by specific antibodies. The immunoperoxidase technique reveals (*A*) glucagon in alpha cells at the periphery of the islet; (*B*) insulin in beta cells distributed throughout the islet; and (*C*) somatostatin in sparsely distributed delta cells.

Normal Pancreatic Islets

The islets of Langerhans, which form the endocrine portion of the pancreas, are scattered throughout the organ and consist of richly vascularized globular masses of cells, which in the human pancreas are estimated to total from 200,000 to 2 million cells. Six distinct cell types have been identified and correlated with hormone synthesis and storage. Alpha cells, which contain glucagon, and beta cells, in which insulin is localized, have been best characterized. The two types of delta cells, D and D_1 (which secrete somatostatin and vasoactive intestinal polypeptide, respectively), and pancreatic polypeptide-secreting

cells have been less well studied. The enterochromaffin cells, which secrete the vasoactive amine serotonin (5-hydroxytryptamine), are a minor component of the islet cell population and are demonstrable by their capacity for staining with potassium dichromate. The cellular composition of islets varies in the different anatomic subdivisions as follows: In the head the ratios of the component cells are beta>polypeptide-secreting>delta>alpha as contrasted with the body and tail, where the ratios are beta>alpha>delta>polypeptide–secreting. **Alpha cells are localized in the outer rim of the islets and constitute 15% to 20% of the total islet cell population** (Fig. 15-10A). In the alpha cells, glucagon, like insulin and other hormones, is synthesized as a prohormone, proglucagon, with a molecular weight of 19,000 daltons. Before export the prohormone is cleaved to active hormone, a 3500-dalton product. Glucagon induces glycogenolysis and gluconeogenesis, thereby raising the blood glucose level. Its secretion is stimulated by hypoglycemia, by the ingestion of a low-carbohydrate–high-protein meal, and by an intravenous infusion of amino acids. By virtue of these responses by alpha cells, glucagon, together with insulin, serves to maintain fuel homeostasis. At least two precursor peptides of proglucagon apparently constitute separate regions of the molecule. These are called glicentins 1 and 2 and have been localized to the secretory granules in alpha cells. Radioimmunoassay of glucagon in serum reveals several species, of which only the 3500-dalton variety appears to be biologically active. Larger species, weighing 9000 daltons and 16,000 daltons, respectively, represent forms of the incompletely cleaved prohormone. It is noteworthy that in patients with a rare condition called familial hyperglucagonemia, in whom the level of serum glucagon may be 10 times normal, 85% of the hormone consists of molecular forms higher than 9000 daltons.

Beta cells comprise the largest proportion, 60% to 70%, of cells in islets. They are distributed throughout the islet when visualized by their affinity for certain stains, such as aldehyde fuchsin or pseudoisoocyanin, or by specific antibody to insulin (Fig. 15-10B). By electron microscopy the insulin is resolved into characteristic polygonal and rhomboidal crystals enclosed in secretory vesicles. The synthesis and secretion pathway for insulin can be considered as a general model for the other islet cell types. Insulin is synthesized in the rough endoplasmic reticulum of beta cells as a single chain precursor molecule, termed *proinsulin*, with a molecular weight of about 9000 daltons. This molecule is transferred by an ATP-dependent process to the Golgi membrane system, where it is packaged into smooth-surfaced microvesicles, the precursors of storage granules. Beginning in the microvesicles and continuing in the secretory granules, Zn^{2+} is added to the proinsulin molecule, after which it is progressively cleaved by membrane-bound proteases into equimolar amounts of insulin and the peptide that connects the A and B chains of insulin (C-peptide). The mature secretory granules, guided by the microtubules, migrate centripetally in the cytoplasm until they fuse with the plasma membrane and are extruded into the extracellular space, a process termed *exocytosis*. The final release involves an influx of Ca^{2+} ions into the cell. As is true for a large number of other intracellular processes, cAMP participates in the insulin secretory process. However, the major obligatory stimulus for insulin secretion is the binding of glucose to glucose receptors on surface of the beta cell. These events are summarized in Figure 15-11.

Delta cells are fewer in number and slightly larger than alpha cells; like alpha cells, delta cells tend to be localized at the periphery of islets (Fig. 15-10C). They are situated between the alpha and the beta cells so that the three cell types are often contiguous. Delta cells secrete somatostatin, a 1600-dalton peptide identical to that discovered earlier in the hypothalamus that inhibits the pituitary release of growth hormone. Somatostatin synthesized in the islets inhibits secretion by alpha and beta cells and one type (D_1) of delta cell, acinar cells of the exocrine pancreas, and certain hormone-secreting cells in the gastrointestinal tract. Coupled with the topographical cell–cell relations noted earlier, these hormonal interactions suggest that somatostatin plays a regulatory role in alpha and beta cell secretion, which is reflected in the high stability of glucose homeostasis. **D_1 cells are smaller than the other islet cell types and are rare in the islets of normal human pancreas.** They synthesize a 3800-dalton peptide termed vasoactive intestinal polypeptide, a molecule that has also been localized in ganglion cells and nerve fibers of the pancreas, gut, and brain. Vasoactive intestinal polypeptide induces glycogenolysis and hyperglycemia, as does glucagon, and in addition regulates the tone, motility, and ion and water secretion by epithelial cells of the gastrointestinal tract. The latter function is mediated by its ability to activate adenyl cyclase, thus leading to the production of cAMP.

Pancreatic polypeptide-producing cells are located primarily in the islets of the head of the pancreas and synthesize a 4300-dalton polypeptide, which appears to have variable and opposed functions. These include stimulation of the secretion of enzymes from the gastric mucosa and inhibition of a variety of functions, such as smooth muscle contraction in the intestine and gallbladder, production of gastric acid, and secretion by the exocrine pancreas and biliary system. Enterochromaffin cells, identified by their capacity for reducing ammoniacal silver and for staining by potassium dichromate, are rare components of the islet cell population in the head of the pancreas. They synthesize serotonin, a vasoactive amine that causes vasodilatation and increased permeability of the venular capillaries, and the 2700-dalton peptide motilin, which stimulates motility of gastric smooth muscle and increases the tone of the sphincter at the gastroesophageal junction.

The various types of islet cells, the products they secrete, and their physiologic actions are summarized in Table 15-1.

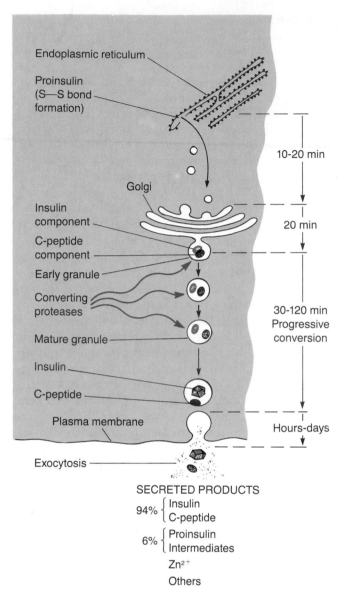

Endoplasmic reticulum

Proinsulin
(S—S bond
formation)

10-20 min

Golgi

Insulin
component

C-peptide
component

20 min

Early granule

Converting
proteases

30-120 min
Progressive
conversion

Mature granule

Insulin

C-peptide

Plasma membrane

Hours-days

Exocytosis

SECRETED PRODUCTS

94% { Insulin
      C-peptide

6% { Proinsulin
     Intermediates

Zn^{2+}

Others

Figure 15-11.   Synthesis and secretion of insulin. Proinsulin is synthesized in the endoplasmic reticulum of beta cells and transferred to the Golgi apparatus. There it is packaged into microvesicles, and cleaved into insulin and C-peptide. Finally, the mature secretory granule is extruded into the extracellular space and its contents are released.

The APUD Concept

Tinctorial and histochemical properties shared by cells of the pancreatic islets and endocrine cells of the gastrointestinal system suggest that they are phylogenetically related. This notion is strengthened by the fact that with the exception of alpha and beta cells, which are restricted to the islets, all the other cells of the islets are also present to varying extents in the intestinal mucosa. The uptake of amine precursors and their decarboxylation is a shared property that has led to a concept that links the islets and the gastrointestinal endocrine cells with other parts of the endocrine system and the autonomic nervous system. A large and diffuse system, assigned the acronym APUD (amine precursor uptake and decarboxylation), currently consists of over 40 different cell types. The APUD concept postulates that the component cells of the system have a common derivation from the neural crest and neuroectoderm; recently, this has been expanded to include the neuroendocrine-programmed epiblast. In support of this concept, many of the polypeptides synthesized by APUD cells are also synthesized in the brain, peripheral ganglia, and cells of the adrenal medulla. As in many unifying concepts the APUD theory has been tested experimentally, and some of the results have been contradictory. For example, complete excision of the

Table 15-1. Secretory Products of Islet Cells and Their Physiologic Actions

CELL	SECRETORY PRODUCT	MOL. WT. (DALTONS)	PHYSIOLOGIC ACTIONS
Alpha	Glucagon	3500	Catabolic, stimulates glycogenolysis and gluconeogenesis, raises blood glucose.
Beta	Insulin	6000	Anabolic, stimulates glycogenesis, lipogenesis, and protein synthesis, lowers blood glucose.
Delta	Somatostatin	1600	Inhibits secretion of alpha, beta, D_1, and acinar cells.
D_1	Vasoactive intestinal polypeptide (VIP)	3800	Same as glucagon, also regulates tone and motility of GI tract and activates cAMP of intestinal epithelium.
PP	Human pancreatic polypeptide (hPP)	4300	Stimulates gastric enzyme secretion, inhibits intestinal motility and bile secretion.
EC	Serotonin substance P (motilin)	176	Induces vasodilation, increases vascular permeability, stimulates motility of gastric muscle and tone of lower esophageal sphincter.

ectoderm in rat embryos did not alter the normal development of islets, nor their content of insulin. Recently, quail-chick chimeras were produced by implanting the neural crest from quail embryos into the region of previously excised neural crest of chicken embryos. Elements identified as quail cells by virtue of their characteristic nucleus were not present in the entoderm of the chick, the precursor of the pancreas and gut, nor were they found as enterochromaffin cells of the gut. These results do not negate the APUD concept but suggest that although some APUD cells arise from neuroectoderm, others originate in the entoderm. Alternatively, they may, indeed, all derive from neuroectoderm, but migrate so early in gastrulation that the experiments with chimeras did not detect them. The APUD concept has certainly served to broaden our concept of the "endocrine system" and its complex biology, and our understanding of the histogenesis and function of tumors of the so-called gastroenteropancreatic system.

Islet Cell Tumors

Alpha Cell Tumors (Glucagonomas)

Glucagon-secreting tumors of the pancreatic islets (glucagonomas) are rare and have been encountered mainly in perimenopausal and postmenopausal women. **These tumors are associated with a syndrome consisting of mild diabetes, a necrotizing, migratory, erythematous rash of the lower body, and anemia.** Since mild diabetes, dermatitis, and anemia are not infrequent in older adults, the syndrome is often missed until its persistence and severity suggest that it may be associated with an unsuspected un-

derlying disease. Late diagnosis, together with a possibly increased propensity for malignant behavior of alpha cell tumors, may serve to explain why more than half of the more than 40 cases reported have been malignant and have metastasized to regional lymph nodes and liver. The diagnosis is firmly established by the finding of elevated levels of glucagon in the serum and the localization of glucagon in the tumor. However, not all cases of alpha cell tumor stain for glucagon. Some are positive for glicentin peptides, and those that are not stained by antibodies to glucagon and the glicentins may contain abnormal molecular variants that do not possess the antigenic determinants recognized by antibodies to the normal molecules. The secretory granules of alpha cell tumors sometimes differ ultrastructurally from their normal counterparts, but they are often indistinguishable from normal (Fig. 15-12). Recently, it has been reported that in addition to glucagon some alpha cell tumors contain other hormones, such as insulin, somatostatin, and pancreatic polypeptide.

In patients with alpha cell tumors, plasma glucagon levels are elevated, up to 30 times above normal. In addition to the characteristic hyperglycemia, fasting plasma amino acid levels are decreased to levels as low as 20% of normal. Experimental animal studies have shown that in hepatocytes high levels of glucagon induce autophagy, proteolysis, and lipolysis, the last leading to an increase in gluconeogenesis. Surgical removal of benign, functional alpha cell tumors is followed by a rapid and complete remission of clinical symptoms. In patients with the malignant variant and metastases, surgical removal of the bulk of the tumor leads to a marked amelioration of symptoms, which return as the metastases grow to sufficient size to raise the serum level of glucagon.

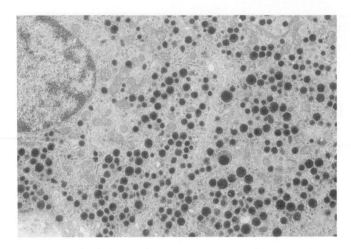

Figure 15-12.   Alpha cells in a functional glucagonoma. The granules are indistinguishable from those of normal alpha cells.

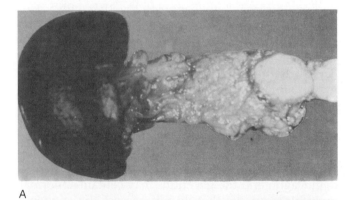

A

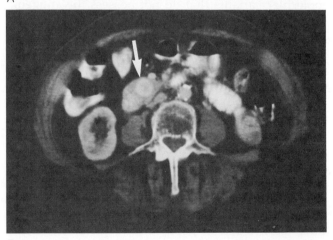

B

Figure 15-13.   Insulinoma. (*A*) An insulinoma in the tail of the pancreas. The tumor has been bisected. (*B*) A CT scan of the abdomen shows a solitary insulinoma (*arrow*).

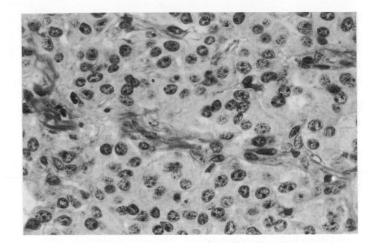

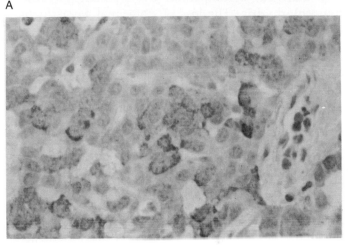

Figure 15-14. A functional insulinoma. (*A*) Nests of tumor cells resembling normal islet cells are surrounded by numerous capillaries. (*B*) The cytoplasm of the tumor cells stain with insulin antibody as demonstrated by the immunoperoxidase technique.

Beta Cell Tumors (Insulinomas)

Beta cell tumors are the most common of the islet cell neoplasms. The functional variant releases sufficient insulin to induce severe hypoglycemia (<40 mg/dl) and a syndrome of sweating, nervousness, and hunger, which may progress to confusion, lethargy, and coma. Since these symptoms are relieved by eating, it is common for patients to be overweight. Frequently, the diagnosis is delayed by the prominence of symptoms of abnormal behavior that cause some patients to be under psychiatric care. Most cases are characterized by only a mild hypoglycemia, and in some the tumor is not functional, which may delay the diagnosis. Neoplastic beta cells, unlike their normal counterparts, are not regulated by the blood glucose level and continue to secrete insulin autonomously even when the level of glucose is very low. **Most beta cell tumors are benign single lesions in the body or tail of the pancreas** (Fig. 15-13), some as small as 1 mm in diameter. Only 5% demonstrate

malignant behavior and in the majority surgical enucleation is accompanied by a rapid disappearance of symptoms. Histologically, the insulinoma cells usually resemble normal beta cells (Fig. 15-14*A*). The diagnosis is established by the demonstration of high levels of insulin in the blood and in the tumor cells (Fig. 15-14*B*). Electron microscopy of the tumor usually shows the pleomorphic, paracrystalline cores surrounded by a clear halo that are typical of insulin stored in normal beta cells. Rarely, the insulin granules are atypical.

Delta Cell Tumor (Somatostatinoma)

This rare tumor is worthy of mention because the clinical findings are so nonspecific that its diagnosis is almost always missed preoperatively. The syndrome consists of mild diabetes mellitus, gallstones, steatorrhea, indigestion, and hypochlorhydria. These conditions result from the inhibitory actions of somatostatin on other cells of the pancreatic islets and

APUD cells of the gastrointestinal tract that secrete insulin, cholecystokinin, glucagon, and gastrin. Thus, the levels of insulin and glucagon in blood are decreased. In addition to producing somatostatin some delta cell tumors also secrete calcitonin or ACTH. The tumor is usually solitary and slow growing, and in about one-half of the cases it exhibits malignant behavior with hepatic metastases.

D_1 Tumors (VIPomas)

D_1 tumors consist of the islet cells that synthesize and secrete vasoactive intestinal polypeptide (VIP). **They give rise to the Verner–Morrison syndrome, which is characterized by explosive and profuse watery diarrhea, accompanied by hypokalemia and hypochlorhydria.** The loss of water may be as high as 5 liters per day, with an attendant excretion of up to 300 mmol potassium. Severe dehydration and debility are frequent complications, which, together with the intractable diarrhea, has led to the term *pancreatic cholera*. These profound effects are due to the excessive activation of adenyl cyclase in the mucosal cells of the small intestine by vasoactive intestinal peptide. In turn, high levels of cAMP drive the active secretion of intracellular electrolytes, including potassium and water. The tumors are usually solitary and benign, and there are few reports of malignant behavior. High levels of circulating vasoactive intestinal peptide and severe diarrhea have also been encountered in patients with a variety of nonpancreatic neoplasms containing different types of APUD cells, for example, ganglioneuroma, pheochromocytoma of the adrenal medulla, medullary thyroid carcinoma, and bronchogenic carcinoma. In some patients the Verner–Morrison syndrome is caused by the multiple endocrine neoplasia (MEN) syndrome, Type 1. This familial disorder is characterized by neoplasms in several endocrine organs simultaneously, especially adenomatous tumors of the pituitary and parathyroid glands.

Pancreatic Polypeptide-Secreting Tumors

Pancreatic polypeptide-producing tumors are rare and are not associated with a clinical syndrome, despite the fact that they are functional and secrete high levels of pancreatic polypeptide in the blood. The tumors are usually single and benign, although a few have metastasized to the liver. Pancreatic polypeptide is also secreted by other islet cell tumors in addition to their specific hormones, especially after stimulation by a meal, and it has been suggested that it may be a useful adjunct marker to detect islet cell tumors.

Enterochromaffin Cell (Carcinoid) Tumors

True enterochromaffin cell tumors of pancreatic islets that elaborate serotonin are rare; the benign variant induces the so-called atypical carcinoid syndrome, consisting of a severe facial flush, hypotension, periorbital edema, and lacrimation. The malignant variant metastasizes to the liver and causes the classic carcinoid syndrome, which is additionally associated with endocardial fibrosis of the right heart. Some islet cell tumors with the histologic features of carcinoid tumors have contained products other than serotonin, such as insulin, gastrin, vasoactive intestinal peptide calcitonin, and prostaglandins.

Pancreatic Gastrinoma (Ulcerogenic Islet Cell Tumors)

Pancreatic gastrinoma is an islet cell tumor consisting of so-called G-cells that synthesize and secrete gastrin, a potent hormonal stimulus for the secretion of gastric acid. The location of this tumor in the pancreas is curious, because gastrin-containing cells have not demonstrated in normal islets. The tumor is thought to arise from multipotent endocrine stem cells that have undergone inappropriate differentiation to form gastrin-secreting islet cells (G-cells) in the endocrine pancreas. By electron microscopy G-cells bear a strong resemblance to the gastrin-secreting cells that normally reside in the duodenal mucosa. The capacity of islet cells to secrete gastrin, a duodenal hormone, is another example of the surprising plasticity of cells of the APUD system. This tumor was incriminated some 30 years ago as the cause of **intractable gastric hypersecretion and severe peptic ulceration of the duodenum and jejunum, the so-called Zollinger–Ellison syndrome,** named after the two surgeons who first described it. The reason for the "ulcerogenic potential" of this peculiar islet cell tumor was eventually established when the development of highly specific antisera to gastrin made possible the demonstration of high levels of gastrin in the blood and in the tumor. **Among islet cell tumors, pancreatic gastrinomas are second in frequency only to insulinomas.** Fifteen percent of cases of the Zollinger–Ellison syndrome are due to gastrinomas outside the pancreas, particularly in the duodenum. Malignant gastrinomas are more common than the benign variant, and multiple adenomas are more frequent than single ones. Metastases to regional lymph nodes and liver are often functional. In cases of this syndrome due to multiple functional adenomas of G-cells, the symptoms are disturbances of physiology that are so chronic and debilitating,

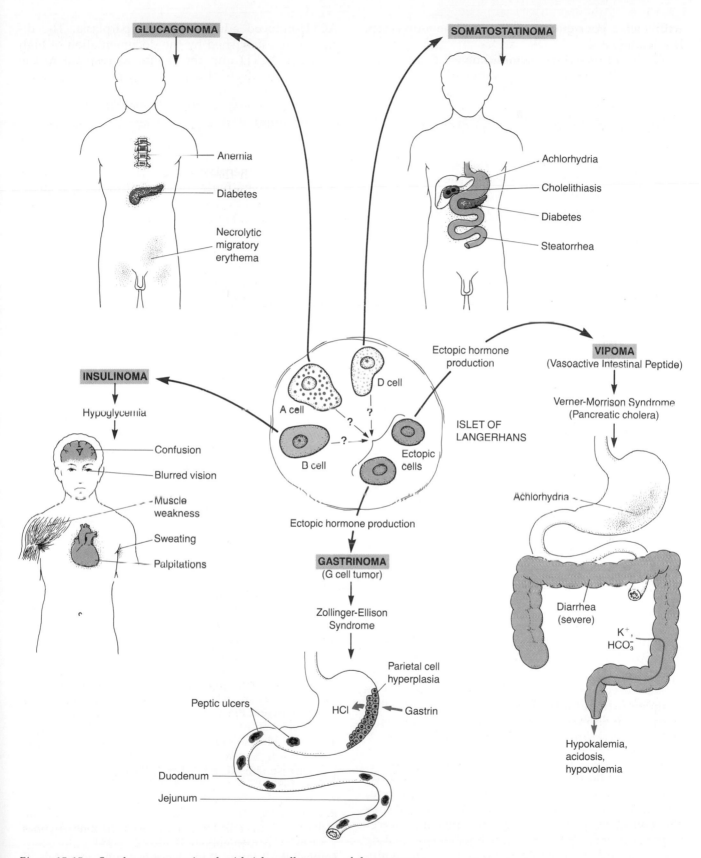

Figure 15-15.   Syndromes associated with islet cell tumors of the pancreas.

with such a poor quality of life, that the term *benign* is a relative one.

The syndromes and complications of the major types of islet cell tumors are summarized in Figure 15-15.

Multiple Endocrine Neoplasia (MEN) Syndromes

The occurrence of multiple adenomas of the endocrine system was first reported at the turn of this century. The condition is infrequent, has a familial distribution, and is characterized by **adenomatosis of the pituitary, parathyroids,** and **pancreas** (MEN type I). It is frequently associated with the Zollinger–Ellison syndrome, in which case gastrin-secreting islet cell tumors are usual. The syndrome reflects the functional state of the neoplastic glands and may be quite complex. Such diverse conditions as acromegaly, pituitary dwarfism, hypogonadism, hyperparathyroidism, hyperinsulinism, hyperadrenocorticism, hyperthyroidism, and the carcinoid syndrome have been described either alone or in various combinations. Multiple endocrine neoplasia with peptic ulceration is inherited as an autosomal dominant gene with a high level of penetrance. Since abnormal growth of different tissues is the major common feature of this condition, the gene abnormality has been described as pleiotropic. The syndrome has been documented in various ethnic groups, including Italian, Swiss, Mexican, and Puerto Rican families.

A variant of the multiple endocrine neoplasia syndrome—**Sipple's syndrome, or MEN type II**—consists of multiple tumors of the adrenal medulla (pheochromocytomas), medullary carcinomas of the thyroid (calcitonin-secreting tumors), and parathyroid hyperplasia or adenoma. In this condition the pancreas is normal, and hypergastrinemia and peptic ulceration are absent. A variant of Sipple's syndrome presents with mucocutaneous neuromas of the eyelids, lips, tongue, bronchus, intestines, and urinary bladder.

This discussion of islet cell tumors would not be complete without a brief consideration of two interesting, though rare, functional tumors, namely, pancreatic corticotropinoma and parathyrinoma.

Corticotropinoma (Ectopic ACTH Syndrome)

Corticotropinoma is an islet cell tumor that secretes both low- and high-molecular-weight ACTH. It may also simultaneously secrete gastrin, insulin, corticotropin-releasing hormone, melanocyte-stimulating hormone, and other peptides and amines. The symptoms reflect high blood levels of cortisol from an ACTH-induced adrenocortical hyperplasia. The diagnosis is established by the documentation of high levels of ACTH and the failure to respond to the suppressive effects of dexamethasone.

Parathyrinoma (Ectopic Hypercalcemia Syndrome)

Parathyrinoma is an islet cell tumor that causes signs and symptoms indistinguishable from those seen in parathyroid hyperplasia and adenoma. The peptides secreted by parathyrinomas are structurally heterogeneous and differ immunologically from parathyroid hormones. Thus, they cannot be measured by the usual radioimmunoassay, which makes the diagnosis difficult. Surgical removal of the islet cell tumor, or chemotherapy with streptozotocin in cases in which the tumor is not amenable to resection, causes a prompt lowering of blood calcium levels and the disappearance of symptoms.

SUGGESTING READING

BOOKS

Bloodworth JMB Jr, Greider MH: The endocrine pancreas and diabetes mellitus. In Bloodworth JMB Jr (ed): Endocrine Pathology: General and Surgical, 2nd ed, pp 586–613. Baltimore, Williams & Wilkins, 1982

Brandborg LL: Acute pancreatitis. In Sleisenger MH, Fordtran JS (eds): Gastrointestinal Disease, 2nd ed, vol. 2, pp 1409–1421. Philadelphia, WB Saunders, 1978

Cubilla AL, Fitzgerald PJ: Cancer (non-endocrine) of the pancreas. A suggested classification. In Fitzgerald PJ, Morrison AB (eds): The Pancreas, pp 82–110. Baltimore, Williams & Wilkins, 1980

Sarles H, Figarella C, Tiscornia O, et al: Chronic calcifying pancreatitis (CCP). Mechanism of formation of the lesions. New data and critical study. In Fitzgerald PJ, Morrison AB (eds): The Pancreas, pp 48–66. Baltimore, Williams & Wilkins, 1980

Schmidt H, Creutzfeldt W: Etiology and pathogenesis of pancreatitis. In Bockus HL (ed): Gastroenterology, vol. 3, pp 1005–1019. Philadelphia, WB Saunders, 1976

Sindelar WF, Kinsella TJ, Mayer RJ: Cancer of the pancreas. In DeVita VT Jr, Hellman S, Rosenberg SA (eds): Cancer: Principles and Practice of Oncology, 2nd ed, pp 691–739. Philadelphia, JB Lippincott, 1985

Snodgrass PJ: Pathophysiology of the pancreas. In Sodeman WA Jr, Sodeman WA (eds): Pathologic Mechanisms of Disease, 7th ed, pp 922–963. Philadelphia, WB Saunders, 1985

REVIEW ARTICLES

Mallory A, Kern F Jr: Drug-induced pancreatitis: A critical review. Gastroenterology 78:813–820, 1980

Trapnell JE: Patterns of incidence in acute pancreatitis. Br Med J 2:179–183, 1975

ORIGINAL ARTICLES

Fraumeni JF Jr: Cancers of the pancreas and biliary tract: Epidemiological considerations. Cancer Res 35:3437–3446, 1975

Friesen SR: Tumors of the endocrine pancreas. New Engl J Med 306:580–590, 1982

Greider MH, Rosai J, McGuigan JE: The human pancreatic islet cells and their tumors. II. Ulcerogenic and diarrheogenic tumors. Cancer 33:1423 1443, 1974

Levin DL, Connelly RR, Devesa SS: Demographic characteristics of cancer of the pancreas: Mortality, incidence, and survival. Cancer 41:1456–1468, 1981

Opie EL: The etiology of acute hemorrhagic pancreatitis. Johns Hopkins Hosp Bull 12:182–188, 1901

Parsa I, Longnecker DS, Scarpelli DG, et al: Ductal metaplasia of human exocrine pancreas and its association with carcinoma. Cancer Res. 45:1285–1290, 1985

Solcia E, Capella C, Buffa R, et al: Pathology of the Zollinger-Ellison Syndrome. Prog Surg Pathol 1:119–133, 1980

Wermer P: Endocrine adenomatosis and peptic ulcer in a large kindred. Am J Med 35:205–212, 1963

Wynder EL, Mabuchi K, Maruchi N, et al: Epidemiology of cancer of the pancreas. J Natl Cancer Inst 50:645–667, 1973

16

The Kidney

Benjamin H. Spargo and James R. Taylor

Anatomy

Clinical Syndromes in Renal Disease

Congenital Abnormalities

Cystic Disease of the Kidney

Noninflammatory Lesions Associated with the Nephrotic Syndrome

Inflammatory Glomerular Lesions

Renal Diseases Associated with Systemic Disorders

Tubulointerstitial Diseases

Vascular Diseases

Toxemia of Pregnancy

Hydronephrosis

Renal Stones

Tumors of the Kidney

Figure 16-1. The renal vascular system. A scanning electron micrograph of a corrosion cast of the renal vasculature shows the terminal arborizations of the blood vessels and the capillaries of the glomerular tufts.

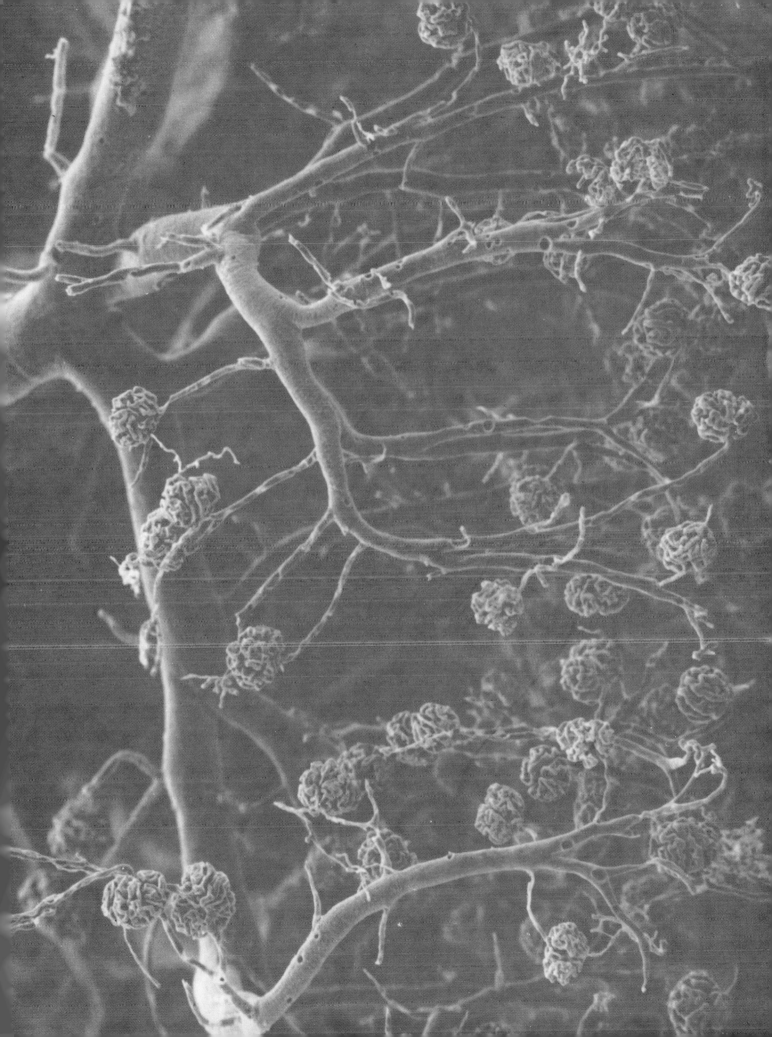

Anatomy

The adult kidney, a paired organ that weighs on average 150 g, consists of a cortex and medulla. The medulla is composed of approximately 12 pyramids, the bases of which are at the corticomedullary junction. Each pyramid consists of an inner and outer zone. The inner zone, called the papilla, empties into a minor calyx. The outer zone is divided into the outer stripe and inner stripe. Medullary rays are faint vertical striations that consist of collecting ducts and ascending thick limbs. Each lobe of the cortex is subdivided by an interlobular artery, which branches from the arcuate artery. The inner and outer zones of the cortex have their own characteristic capillary plexuses. The outer cortex receives branches from the efferent arterioles of the superficial glomeruli, whereas the deeper zones are nourished by the efferents of the juxtamedullary glomeruli. Within the cortical substance are the proximal and distal tubules and collecting ducts (Fig. 16-1). The proximal tubule is longer and is more conspicuous in histologic sections. The common forms of acute renal failure primarily reflect disordered renal hemodynamics. These changes in blood flow, now termed *vasomotor nephropathy*, relate to an almost total cessation of ultrafiltration at the glomerulus because of shunting of the cortical blood flow from the cortex; medullary flow remains unchanged. The wall of the afferent arteriole, as it approaches the glomerulus, exhibits characteristic granulated cells. This area, the adjacent hilar cells, and the macula densa form the juxtaglomerular apparatus that secretes renin and is active in the regulation of glomerular blood flow.

The glomerulus is a specialized tuft of capillaries with an arteriole at either end (Figs. 16-2, 16-3, and 16-4). The most interesting features of these capillaries are the lack of a continuous basement membrane, the provision of a specialized and highly organized epithelial covering, and the system of mesangial phagocytosis. The glomerular basement membrane, a continuation of the arteriolar basement membrane, merges at the hilus with the membrane of Bowman's capsule. In turn, Bowman's capsule is continuous with the basement membrane of the proximal tubule. There are, however, differences between the chemical composition of the glomerular basement membrane and that of other basement membranes, and the former does not completely surround each capillary. The part of the capillary facing the mesangium is separated from the mesangial cell network only by endothelial cell cytoplasm. Therefore, there is a potential pathway through the mesangium for capillary blood to interact with the juxtaglomerular apparatus,

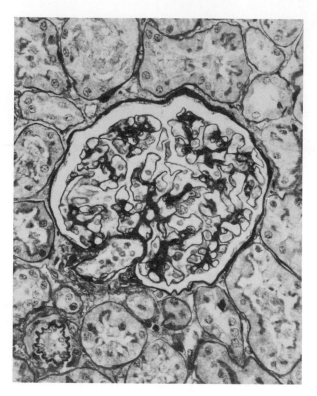

Figure 16-2.   Normal glomerulus, light microscopy.

a feature that may contribute to the control of arteriolar tone. Glomerular capillaries have an attenuated endothelial layer, approximately 40 nm thick, with numerous holes, some of which are closed by a thin membrane (Fig. 16-5). The existence of this sievelike structure suggested to early workers that permeability was controlled at this level, but the fenestrae are too large (up to 100 nm in diameter) and the endothelium appears to play a largely passive role in filtration. The glomerulus is supported by a mixed cellular and stromal mesangial network, which is similar in some respects to the mesentery of the intestine. Important functions of the mesangium other than support include phagocytosis, maintenance of the glomerular basement membrane, and (probably) contractility. Although morphologically similar to many other basement membranes, the glomerular basement membrane is functionally and chemically distinctive. By classic morphologic techniques, it is approximately 300 nm thick and has three definable layers: a central dense zone, the lamina densa, sandwiched between paler zones; the lamina rara interna; and the lamina externa (Fig. 16-5). The glomerular basement membrane has a strong negative charge, owing to the presence of the polyanionic proteoglycan heparan sulfate. This property allows charge-

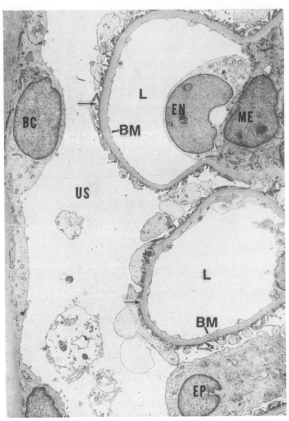

Figure 16-3. Normal glomerulus, electron micrograph. The normal glomerular capillary is covered by epithelial cells (*EP*) with foot processes (*arrows*) in contact with the basement membrane (*BM*). The endothelial cell (*EN*) has large pores and surrounds the capillary lumen (*L*). The mesangial cell (*ME*) is bordered by the endothelial cell on the luminal surface and the stalk basement membrane on the lateral areas. (*US*, urinary space, *BC*, Bowman's capsule)

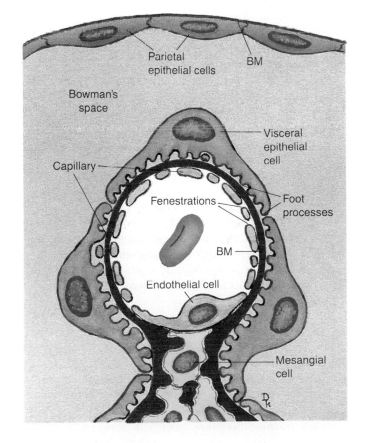

Figure 16 4. Normal glomerulus. The relation of the different glomerular cell types to the significant stroma is illustrated using a single glomerular loop. The entire outer aspect of the glomerular basement membrane (*BM*) (peripheral loop and stalk) is covered by the epithelial cell foot processes. The outer portions of the endothelial cell, which surrounds the capillary lumen, are in contact with the inner surface of the basement membrane, whereas the central part is in contact with the mesangial cell of the stalk. The relationship of the mesangial cell to its stroma is unique to the glomerulus and has not been entirely clarified.

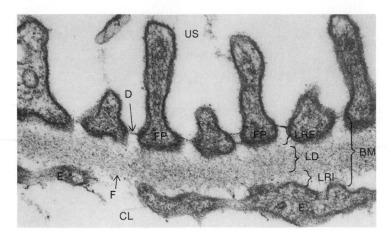

Figure 16-5. The glomerular filter, electron micrograph. Molecules that pass from the capillary lumen (*CL*) to the urinary space (*US*) pass through the fenestrations (*F*) of the endothelial cell (*E*), the trilaminar basement membrane (*BM*)—made up of the lamina rara interna (*LRI*), the lamina densa (*LD*), and the lamina rara externa (*LRE*)—and the slit pore diaphragm (*D*) that connects podocyte foot processes (*FP*).

selective filtration of electrically neutral and cationic molecules and relative exclusion of negatively charged molecules such as albumin (Fig. 16-6). The glomerular basement membrane also discriminates between molecules on the basis of size. It is freely permeable to molecules with radii less than 2 nm and virtually impermeable to those with radii greater than 4 nm. Fine fibrils are apparent within the glomerular basement membrane, raising the possibility that molecules are sieved through a fibrillar-gel matrix. However, it is thought that these fibrils are probably artifacts of fixation. Recent studies indicate that the glomerular basement membrane is formed predominantly by epithelial cells, and that a smaller component (lamina rara interna) may be contributed by endothelial cells.

Clinical Syndromes in Renal Disease

The general availability in recent years of renal dialysis and transplantation programs has dramatically reduced the mortality rate ascribed to renal diseases. The 35,000 annual deaths attributed to kidney disease in the United States is a small number compared with the 750,000 and 400,000 who succumb to heart disease and cancer, respectively, each year. However, the morbidity associated with diseases of the kidney continues to be substantial.

Traditionally, kidney diseases have been divided into one of four morphologic components: glomerular, tubular, interstitial, and vascular. For example, the nephrotic syndrome, which is characterized by the loss of large amounts of protein in the urine, is almost invariably the result of a glomerular disease. The tubules, interstitium, and blood vessels are often entirely normal morphologically, at least early in the course of the disease. Ultimately, damage in one of these components results in changes in the others. With progression to advanced disease it may become impossible to ascertain which component was initially involved. Thus, so-called end stage renal disease is the sequel to a broad spectrum of chronic renal diseases. Because diseases involving different components of the kidney have different clinical presentations, several major syndromes have been described.

The **nephrotic syndrome** is characterized by heavy proteinuria, at a rate of 3.5 g or more of protein lost per 24 hours. These patients usually display a low serum albumin level, edema, and hypercholesterolemia.

The **nephritic syndrome** is characterized invariably by microscopic hematuria and often by gross blood in the urine. Variable degrees of proteinuria, a decreased glomerular filtration rate, and oliguria are usual. Salt and fluid retention often result in edema and hypertension. A clinicopathologic entity called **rapidly progressive glomerulonephritis** is a severe form of the nephritic syndrome in which a rapid and progressive decline in renal function is observed clinically. Oliguria is usually severe. Histologically, glomerular crescents are usually seen.

Acute renal failure is characterized by oliguria (a 24-hour urine volume less than 400 ml) and a rapid onset of azotemia, without a substantial amount of proteinuria. The cause may be an inadequate perfusion of the kidneys (e.g., prerenal azotemia), intrarenal parenchymal disease (e.g., acute tubular necrosis, interstitial nephritis), or a postrenal obstruction of the urinary tract. **Chronic renal failure**, which can be the end stage of a number of renal diseases, is characterized by prolonged symptoms and uremia.

Chronic interstitial nephritis is a term used to describe tubular atrophy and renal scarring in association with an inflammatory infiltrate. In patients

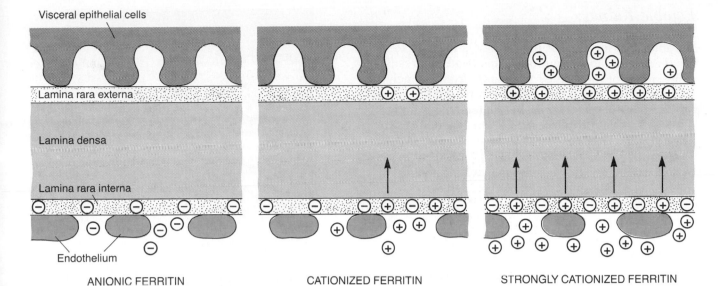

Figure 16-6 Effect of molecular charge on capillary wall permeability is illustrated using ferritin as a marker. Ferritin particles pass without resistance through the 100-nm endothelial pores. Anionic ferritin does not enter the glomerular basement membrane, because it is excluded by the polyanionic charge on the lamina rara. Cationic ferritin binds to the anionic sites in the lamina rara interna and externa. Strongly cationized ferritin saturates these anionic sites and enters the urinary space.

with this disease impaired tubular function results in an inability to concentrate the urine, obligatory sodium wasting, and reduced acid secretion. A number of disorders, including repeated chronic infections (chronic pyelonephritis), chronic reflux of urine, and chronic exposure to certain drugs (analgesic nephropathy), can lead to this condition.

Hypertension, if longstanding, results in renal parenchymal destruction ("benign" nephrosclerosis and "malignant" nephrosclerosis). It can be secondary to acute and chronic renal diseases.

Congenital Abnormalities

Renal Agenesis

The absence of both kidneys is clearly not compatible with life. The majority of infants born with this anomaly are stillborn, and in most cases the mother suffers from oligohydramnios. Bilateral renal agenesis is often associated with other congenital anomalies, including low-set ears, receding chin, beaklike nose, and pulmonary hypoplasia. Associated congenital anomalies of the genitalia are common, as are lower-limb anomalies.

Unilateral renal agenesis is not a serious matter if there are no associated anomalies, because the single kidney hypertrophies sufficiently to assure normal renal function. However, such a situation is a contraindication for renal biopsy. Moreover, it poses an embarrassment for the surgeon who performs a nephrectomy without having ruled out unilateral renal agenesis.

Horseshoe Kidney

Occasionally, the renal anlage does not divide adequately and the infant is born with fusion of the two kidneys, usually at the lower poles, a condition appropriately called *horseshoe kidney*.

Renal Hypoplasia

Renal hypoplasia is a reduction in renal mass without parenchymal malformation, with a decrease of more than 50% in the number of renal lobules. A form of segmental hypoplasia, known as the Ash–Upmark kidney, presents in early adolescence with severe hypertension and may also be complicated by pyelonephritis and renal insufficiency. In these cases a sclerotic hypoplastic lobule is related to an abnormal vasculature between functioning groups of nephrons.

Ectopic Kidney

An abnormal location of the kidney is referred to as renal ectopia. Most commonly, this condition results from failure of the kidney to migrate from the pelvis to the flank in the fetus. Renal ectopia may involve only one kidney or it may be bilateral. The ureters drain into the appropriate side of the bladder in **simple ectopia**. By contrast, in **crossed ectopia**, the ectopic kidney is on the same side as its normal mate, in which case its ureter crosses the midline and drains into the contralateral side of the bladder.

Cystic Disease of the Kidney

Cystic disease of the kidney comprises a heterogeneous group of congenital, developmental, and acquired disorders, many of which are inherited. Their study is important because some forms of adult polycystic disease are important causes of morbidity and mortality and represent a diagnostic problem for clinicians, pathologists, and radiologists.

Cystic Renal Dysplasia

Cystic renal dysplasia is defined as an abnormality of differentiation in the kidney, or a part of the kidney, that results in the persistence of abnormal structures, such as cartilage and undifferentiated mesenchyme. This sporadic lesion, which does not exhibit a familial tendency, is usually unilateral, but on occasion is bilateral. **Renal dysplasia is the most common cystic disorder in children and is the most frequent cause of an abdominal mass in newborn infants.** Malformations of other organs (e.g., ventricular septal defects, tracheoesophageal fistulas, and lumbosacral meningomyeloceles) occasionally occur in conjunction with renal dysplasia.

Grossly, a dysplastic kidney reveals a disorderly mass of cysts that vary in size from microscopic to several centimeters in diameter. The kidney does not show the usual beanlike shape but rather resembles a mass of grapes. Frequently, an associated ureteral malformation, which is sometimes obstructive, is found. This finding suggests that obstruction in early fetal life is important in the development of at least some cases of renal dysplasia. Dysplasia is recognized histologically by focally dilated ducts that are lined by a cuboidal or columnar epithelium. These are surrounded by mantles of undifferentiated mesenchyme (Fig. 16-7), which sometimes contain smooth muscle and islands of hyaline cartilage.

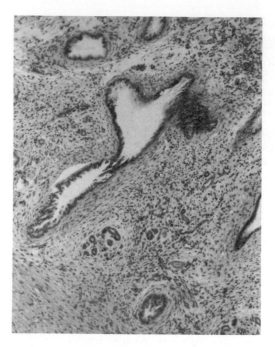

Figure 16-7. Cystic renal dysplasia. A light micrograph shows one large duct and many very immature renal tubules surrounded by undifferentiated cellular mesenchyme.

Polycystic Kidney Disease

Polycystic kidney diseases (Fig. 16-8) are conditions in which portions of the renal parenchyma are converted to cysts of varying sizes. Traditionally, two forms have been described, one primarily in adults and the other in children. These are differentiated on the basis of their mode of inheritance, clinical manifestations, and morphologic manifestations.

Adult Polycystic Disease

Adult polycystic disease, an important cause of renal failure, is responsible for 8% to 10% of all end-stage kidney disease. It is usually inherited as an autosomal dominant trait, although there is a significant incidence of spontaneous mutation. Patients typically present with symptoms by the fourth decade. These include a sense of heaviness in the loins, the presence of bilateral frank masses, and the passage of blood clots in the urine. Azotemia (elevated blood urea nitrogen) progresses to uremia (clinical renal failure) over a period of several years. Involvement is nearly always bilateral.

Grossly, the kidneys in adult polycystic disease are markedly enlarged bilaterally; each kidney may

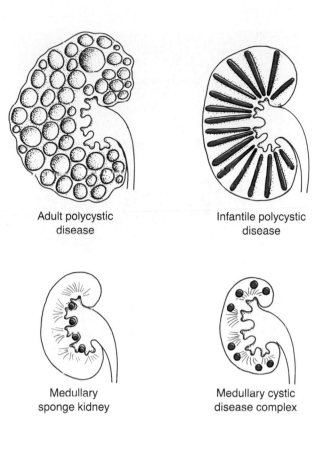

Adult polycystic
disease

Infantile polycystic
disease

Medullary
sponge kidney

Medullary cystic
disease complex

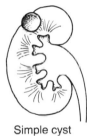

Simple cyst

Figure 16-8. Cystic diseases of the kidney.

thelium. Cysts are also seen occasionally in the spleen and pancreas. Fifteen percent of patients have an associated cerebral aneurysm; subarachnoid hemorrhage is the cause of death in many of these patients.

The pathogenesis of adult polycystic disease is not understood. The metanephric anlage, which gives rise to the nephrons, fuses with the ureteric bed to connect them with the collecting ducts and calyces. It has been proposed that in polycystic kidney, the ureteric bud and metanephric anlage fail to fuse, resulting in abnormal cystic development of nephrons. Others have theorized that the disorder represents a failure of the first generation of metanephric nephrons to involute; still others have claimed that focal polypoid hyperplasia of the epithelial lining of tubules leads to dilatation of nephrons.

Infantile Polycystic Disease

Infantile polycystic disease is rare, compared with the adult variety. It is found primarily in infants and small children, although exceptional cases present in adults. Inheritance in most cases appears to be autosomal recessive, and the involvement of several generations within the same family, seen in the adult form, has not been reported in infantile polycystic disease. Two clinical presentations are seen in this condition; the more frequent is in the newborn, who suffers from congenitally enlarged, spongy kidneys and renal insufficiency. Less frequently, older chil-

weigh as much as 4500 g (Fig. 16-9). The external contour of the kidney is distorted by numerous cysts, which may be as large as 5 cm in diameter. These are usually filled with a clear to straw-yellow fluid, although occasionally there is hemorrhage into a cyst. Microscopically, the cysts are lined, for the most part, by a nondescript cuboidal and columnar epithelium. The cysts appear to arise from virtually any point along the nephron, and some contain glomeruli. Areas of normal renal parenchyma are found between the cysts. As the cysts progressively expand, they exert pressure on the normal areas, which leads to increasing loss of renal parenchyma.

About one-third of patients with adult polycystic disease also have hepatic cysts lined by biliary epi-

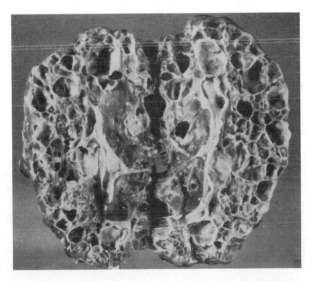

Figure 16-9. Adult polycystic disease. The kidney is strikingly enlarged and the parenchyma almost entirely replaced by cysts of varying size.

dren present with enlarged kidneys that have small cysts, tubular atrophy, and interstitial fibrosis. The involvement is invariably bilateral. There are usually associated liver changes, termed *congenital hepatic fibrosis*, which are characterized by enlargement of portal areas, an increase in connective tissue and a proliferation of bile ducts. Most infants with polycystic disease die in the perinatal period, often because the large kidneys compromise expansion of the lungs.

In contrast to adult polycystic disease, the external surface in the infantile disorder is smooth. The kidneys are often so large that the delivery of the infant is impeded. The fusiform cysts are dilatations of cortical and medullary collecting ducts that have a striking radial arrangement (Fig. 16-10). Interstitial fibrosis and tubular atrophy are common, particularly in children who present at an older age. As in the adult form, the calyceal system is normal.

Medullary Sponge Kidney

Medullary sponge kidney is a disorder characterized by small (< 5 mm in diameter) cysts in one or more of the renal papillae (see Fig. 16-8). The disease has no effect on renal function and is, therefore, asymptomatic in young people. When symptomatic, it is usually discovered between the ages of 30 and 60, when the affected person complains of flank pain, dysuria, hematuria, or gravel in the urine. In 75% of such patients the disease is bilateral, and cortical cysts are characteristically absent. The cysts are customarily lined by cuboidal or columnar epithelium and communicate with the collecting ducts in the renal papillae. Although the disease itself does not pose a threat to health, secondary stones may form in the cysts and predispose to pyelonephritis. This disorder has not been conclusively shown to be hereditary, even though familial cases have been described.

Nephronophthisis—Medullary Cystic Disease Complex

The medullary cystic disease complex is a group of related diseases that display both recessive and dominant modes of inheritance. The primary disturbance is in the tubules. This disease complex accounts for 10% to 20% of renal insufficiency seen in childhood. Clinically, these patients present with evidence of deteriorating tubular function. A defect in the concentrating ability of the tubules is reflected in polyuria, polydipsia, and enuresis (bed wetting). Progressive azotemia and uremia follow. The kidneys

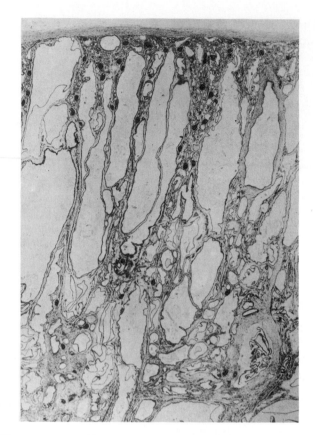

Figure 16-10.   Infantile polycystic disease. There is prominent dilatation of the nephrons in both the cortex and the medulla. Note the characteristic radial arrangements of the cysts.

are small. When they are sectioned, multiple, variable-sized cysts (up to 1 cm in diameter), which arise from the distal portions of the nephron, are seen at the corticomedullary junction (see Fig. 16-8). Atrophic tubules with markedly thickened basement membranes and tubular loss out of proportion to the glomerular loss are the first histologic features of the disease. At this stage the kidneys may not yet be cystic; in fact, variants of this disorder that remain noncystic have been described. Eventually the corticomedullary cysts accumulate, and the remainder of the parenchyma becomes increasingly atrophic. Secondary glomerular sclerosis, interstitial fibrosis, and a nonspecific inflammatory infiltrate dominate the histologic picture.

Simple Renal Cysts

Simple renal cysts are very common acquired lesions, found in about half of people over the age of 50 years. They are usually incidental findings and rarely produce clinical symptoms unless they are very large.

These cysts, which may be solitary or multiple, are found in the outer cortex, bulging the capsule, or in the medulla. Microscopically, they are lined by a nondescript flat epithelium. Although the cysts are entirely benign, they may be confused clinically with renal cell carcinoma.

Noninflammatory Lesions Associated with the Nephrotic Syndrome

Any process that interferes with the structural integrity of one of the three components of the glomerular capillary wall—that is, the endothelial cell, the basement membrane, and the epithelial cell—can result in the abnormal loss of protein in the urine. This discussion of glomerular pathology begins with a discussion of five noninflammatory lesions that frequently produce the pure nephrotic syndrome, defined as massive proteinuria, hypoalbuminemia, and peripheral edema.

Epithelial Cell Disease (Minimal Change Disease, Lipoid Nephrosis)

The appearance of "normal" or "minimally changed" glomeruli in the majority of children with the nephrotic syndrome puzzled early investigators of renal pathology. It was not until ultrastructural studies showed diffuse obliteration of the epithelial cell foot processes that speculation about a nonglomerular origin of proteinuria in these patients came to an end. This morphologic alteration, with the concomitant exclusion of other abnormalities, remains one of the major contributions of electron microscopy to routine diagnosis of renal disease. Neither the cause nor the pathogenesis of epithelial cell disease is known. Experimental administration of the aminonucleoside puromycin to rats produces proteinuria with an ultrastructural appearance identical to that of the human minimal change disease. The precise site of damage in the experimental model is obscure, and there is no evidence of exposure to toxic chemicals in patients with epithelial cell disease.

In human disease there is a significant association between an allergic history and the onset of the nephrotic syndrome, which sometimes follows infection or exposure to allergens. Involvement of the immune system has, therefore, been postulated. The occasional association of a similar morphologic lesion with Hodgkin's disease, a condition associated with

T cell dysfunction, has led to the postulate that this lesion may be due to a disorder of T lymphocyte function. Numerous studies have disclosed several alterations of T lymphocyte function in patients with epithelial cell disease, but clear evidence of a role for cell-mediated immunity is not yet available. The recent detection of circulating immune complexes in both children and adults with epithelial cell disease has revived interest in humoral immune mechanisms. These complexes, which are present only during relapse, do not bind complement and are not detected by assays that depend on complement fixation. The lack of complement binding might explain the typically negative or minimal findings by immunofluorescence, but the significance of these complexes and the mechanisms by which they might cause proteinuria are uncertain. Clearly, the morphologic lesion may represent the endpoint of several pathogenetic pathways. Epithelial cell disease is predominantly a disorder of children, in whom it is the major cause of the nephrotic syndrome. However, the disorder also occurs in adults with significant frequency (18% of adults with the nephrotic syndrome). Most patients are boys who present initially below the age of 6 years. The initial presentation does not differ significantly from that of the nephrotic syndrome caused by other disorders, although a history of recent exposure to an antigen in a child with an atopic diathesis is suspicious for epithelial cell disease.

Most adults and children with epithelial cell disease show complete remission of proteinuria within 8 weeks of initiation of corticosteroid therapy. However, after the withdrawal of corticosteroids about half of the patients suffer intermittent relapses for up to 10 years. Each relapse is responsive to corticosteroid therapy, and **there is no tendency to progress into chronic renal failure.** A subgroup of patients shows only partial remission with corticosteroid therapy and continues to lose protein in the urine, the degree of proteinuria frequently depending on the dosage of steroids. A yet smaller group is totally resistant to corticosteroid therapy. Finally, a small group of patients achieves complete remission without any therapy.

Death from infection was frequent before antibiotics and corticosteroids became readily available. A fatal outcome or progression to renal failure is now exceptional. The development of azotemia in a patient diagnosed as having epithelial cell disease should always suggest an incorrect diagnosis, usually focal segmental glomerulosclerosis, or sometimes a complication such as interstitial nephritis or renal vein thrombosis. In the absence of complications, the

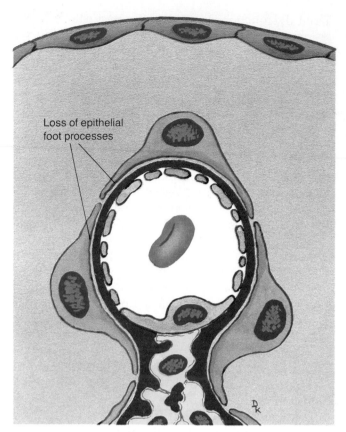

Loss of epithelial
foot processes

Figure 16-11.   Epithelial cell disease. This condition is characterized predominantly by epithelial cell changes, particularly the effacement of the foot processes. All other glomerular structures appear intact.

eventual outlook for patients with epithelial cell disease is probably no different from that of the general population.

By definition, by light microscopy **the glomeruli in minimal change (epithelial cell) disease appear entirely normal.** In actuality, however, there is often some irregular prominence of epithelial cells, and minor degrees of mesangial enlargement are common. The presence of any glomerular abnormality is always an indication to search carefully for segmental sclerosing lesions. Although occasional globally sclerotic glomeruli are present at all ages, more than one or two sclerotic glomeruli raises a suspicion of potentially progressive disease.

The lowered oncotic pressure of the plasma leads to increased lipoprotein secretion by the liver and a consequent hyperlipemia. The presence of lipid in the proximal tubular cells and in the urine reflects the loss of lipoproteins through the glomeruli and is responsible for the term *lipoid nephrosis,* which was used previously for this condition.

Characteristically, **electron microscopic examina-**tion reveals total effacement of epithelial cell foot processes, the basement membrane being covered by sheets of cytoplasm** (Fig. 16-11). No electron-dense deposits are seen. The visceral epithelial cells show prominent intracytoplasmic organelles, an appearance that suggests increased cytoplasmic activity, and also frequently contain large vacuoles. Numerous microvilli protrude from the surface of the epithelial cells (Fig. 16-12). Scanning electron microscopy of these lesions shows that the loss of foot processes is due to their retraction into the parent cell bodies rather than to actual fusion. This retraction is presumably the result of extensive cell swelling. **Since all of these changes are completely reversible during remission, the diagnosis of epithelial cell disease can only be confirmed when there is significant proteinuria.**

Immunofluorescence studies for antibodies or complement in epithelial cell disease are negative, but weak mesangial reactions for IgM and the C3 component of complement are occasionally seen. This is probably a manifestation of increased mesangial uptake of macromolecules rather than a localization of immune complexes. The localized deposition of IgM and C3 in glomerular tufts is important, because it may represent the first indication of a focal segmental sclerosing lesion, before it is evident by light microscopy. As mentioned earlier, an experimental disease, which mimics epithelial cell disease both morphologically and functionally, can be produced by the administration of puromycin aminonucleoside to rats. In this experimental model, heavy proteinuria has been related to a loss of polyanionic sites on the glomerular basement membrane. This loss allows anionic proteins, particularly albumin, to pass easily through the normal barrier. The loss of basement membrane polyanionic sites is thought to reflect toxic injury to the epithelial cell by the aminonucleoside, a postulate that is supported by other manifestations of epithelial injury. In particular, swelling and retraction of the foot processes, together with cytoplasmic vacuoles, are found.

Focal Segmental Glomerulosclerosis

Focal segmental glomerulosclerosis accounts for 10% of the nephrotic syndrome in children and 10% to 20% in adults, with a slight male predominance. This morphologic pattern is seen in many types of glomerular disease; therefore, it is questionable whether it is a distinct entity. The pathogenesis of this morphologic lesion is obscure. Early studies of experimental aminonucleoside-induced proteinuria showed that repeated administration of the drug caused segmental glomerular lesions, which then

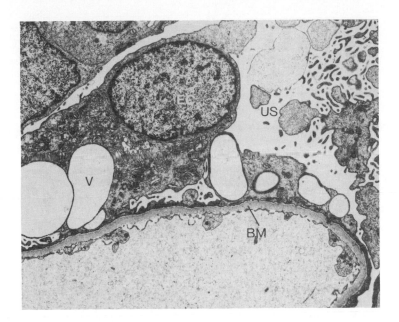

Figure 16-12.   Epithelial cell disease. In this electron micrograph the epithelial cells (*EC*) display foot process effacement, "villous" hyperplasia, and numerous vacuoles (*V*). *BM*, basement membrane, *US*, urinary space

progressed in the absence of the toxin. In addition, aging rats of several species develop increasing proteinuria and glomerular lesions identical to those of focal segmental glomerulosclerosis. Similar experimental lesions develop after removal of one kidney, in which case protein overload and consequent proteinuria are caused by hyperfiltration. There is, therefore, considerable evidence to suggest an association between chronic proteinuria and focal segmental glomerulosclerosis, although a causal relationship remains to be established. As in epithelial cell disease, the finding in many patients with focal segmental glomerulosclerosis of significant depression in the responsiveness of their lymphocytes to various mitogens suggests a possible defect in cellular immunity.

Most patients with the diagnosis of focal segmental glomerulosclerosis present with the insidious onset of the nephrotic syndrome and a nonselective proteinuria. Many of these patients are hypertensive; microscopic hematuria is also frequent. In a minority of patients lesions of focal segmental glomerulosclerosis develop after an extended history of proteinuria that has been variably sensitive to the administration of corticosteroids. Many of these patients have had a previous kidney biopsy that was read as epithelial cell disease. These patients do somewhat better than those in whom focal segmental glomerulosclerosis was diagnosed initially. Corticosteroids are rarely of benefit in adults with an initial biopsy diagnosis of focal segmental glomerulosclerosis, and their effect in children is variable. It is probable that the typical focal glomerulosclerosis that occurs soon after the onset of the nephrotic syndrome is an indication of

a progressive course at all ages. Most patients suffer a progressive decline in renal function for a period of up to 10 years, although a few, often those with a more severe degree of proteinuria at presentation, progress to end-stage renal failure in fewer than 3 years. Although renal transplantation has been successful in many of these patients, the disease recurs with some frequency in the transplanted organ.

By light microscopy varying numbers of glomeruli show segmental areas of capillary loop collapse (Fig. 16-13) and adjacent synechial adhesions to Bowman's capsule. Lipid-containing foam cells are located in the mesangial area of involved glomeruli. The frequent accumulation of a PAS-positive material in the affected areas produces the lesion referred to as *hyalinosis*. This is a valuable finding in the differentiation of focal segmental glomerulosclerosis from a segmentally scarred focal glomerulonephritis. Uninvolved glomeruli appear entirely normal, although on occasion a diffuse, global mesangial hypercellularity is superimposed on all the glomeruli. By electron microscopy diffuse effacement of the epithelial cell foot processes is identical to the lesion of minimal change nephropathy. In addition, folding and thickening of the basement membrane (Fig. 16-14) and capillary collapse are present in sclerotic glomeruli. In more advanced lesions an extensive accumulation of granular, electron-dense material throughout the affected segments represents insudative trapping of plasma proteins. Deposits of immune complexes are not found.

Immunofluorescence studies show segmental trapping of IgM or C3 in the segmental areas of sclerosis and hyalinosis. IgG, C4, and C1q are less fre-

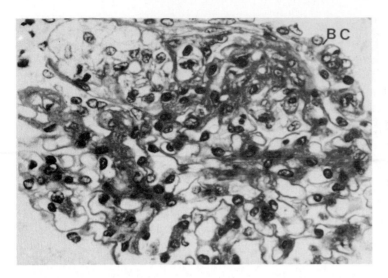

Figure 16-13. Focal segmental glomerulonephritis. Light microscopy shows areas of collapse of the capillary loops with loss of vascular lumina and adjacent adhesions to Bowman's capsule (*BC*).

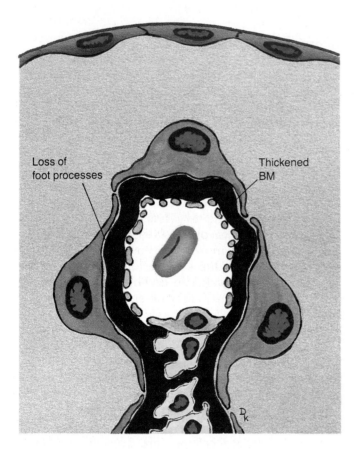

Figure 16-14. Focal segmental glomerulosclerosis. This disorder typically displays epithelial cell change and thickening of the basement membrane. The epithelial cells show effacement of the foot processes and distension of the cytoplasm. The basement membrane is thickened and folded. The glomeruli located deep within the cortex are the earliest to demonstrate these pathognomonic changes, at a time when the other glomeruli may show only the minimal change described in Figure 16-11.

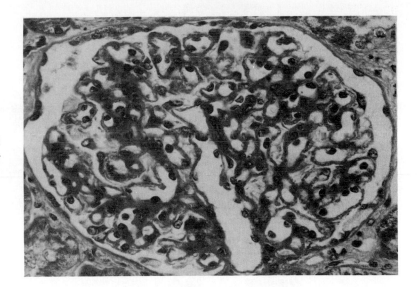

Figure 16-15. Membranous nephropathy, light micrograph. The glomerulus is slightly enlarged and shows slight diffuse thickening of the capillary walls. There is no hypercellularity.

quently found. These segmental reactions may precede light microscopic evidence of damage. This trapping of material is nonspecific and presumably is not related to the pathogenetic mechanisms of the disease.

Membranous Nephropathy

Membranous nephropathy, characterized by a distinct morphologic pattern, reflects a diverse etiology. Although many associated precipitating factors have been described, most cases are idiopathic. **Membranous nephropathy is the most frequent cause of the nephrotic syndrome in adults (30% of the cases).** Because of the electron-dense immune complex deposits in this condition and the demonstration by immunofluorescence of immunoglobulins and complement, **membranous nephropathy is thought to be caused by the deposition of immune complexes.** Two diseases in animal models that are mediated by immune complexes support this concept. Repeated injections of soluble antigens (chronic serum sickness model) in experimental animals produces a lesion that, like membranous nephropathy, has subepithelial deposits without inflammation. Similarly, membranous nephropathy is also produced by the administration of endogenous antigen (kidney emulsion with adjuvant) in the model of active **Heyman nephritis.** In this experimental disease, antibody directed against an antigen in the proximal convoluted tubule cross-reacts with an antigen on the glomerular epithelial cell membrane, followed by complement activation and in situ deposits.

Most patients have the primary, idiopathic form of membranous nephropathy. However, a number of associated conditions predispose to the development of "secondary" membranous nephropathy. In adults, **one of the most frequent associations is with epithelial neoplasms, which have been found in up to 10% of patients.** Certain drugs, such as gold and penicillamine (used in the treatment of rheumatoid arthritis), can cause the lesion. **Membranous nephropathy has been seen in association with various systemic infections, most frequently the hepatitis B virus. Up to 10% of patients with systemic lupus erythematosus may present with a membranous lesion.** When these predisposing conditions are recognized, their removal or treatment often results in the eradication of the membranous lesion and clinical remission of the nephrotic syndrome.

By light microscopy the glomeruli are slightly enlarged, yet normocellular (Fig. 16-15). Depending on the length of time the patient has had the disease, the capillary walls are normal or thickened. In the early stages of the disease silver stains reveal multiple projections, or "spikes," of argyrophilic material on the epithelial surface of the basement membrane. As the disease progresses, there is encroachment on the capillary lumina and eventually glomerular obsolescence. This lesion is classified as noninflammatory because there is no cellular proliferation. However, in advanced disease irregular capillary collapse may result in the erroneous impression of mesangial hypercellularity. Late in the course of the disease, with advanced stages of glomerular sclerosis, this lesion cannot be distinguished from other forms of chronic glomerulonephritis. Tubular loss and focal prominence of the interstitial tissue parallel the degree of glomerular sclerosis.

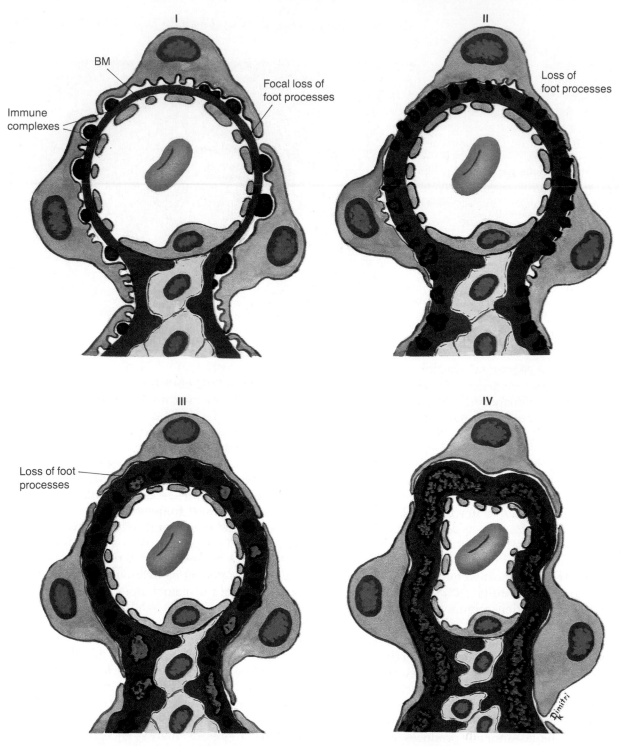

Figure 16-16. Membranous nephropathy. Membranous nephropathy is related to the extracapillary deposition of immune complexes and the accompanying changes in the basement membrane. Stage I exhibits marked, diffuse subepithelial deposits in both the peripheral capillaries and the stalk. The outer contour of the basement membrane remains smooth and foot process effacement is focal. Stage II disease has a spike and dome pattern. The domes are the deposits that gradually extend into the basement membrane. Reactive spikes of newly formed basement membrane tent up the epithelial cells, the foot processes of which are extensively effaced. In Stage III disease newly formed basement membrane has sequestered intramembranous deposits. Variations in density of trapped deposits relate to light areas where the deposit has disappeared, leaving the spongy-appearing and thickened basement membrane. With Stage IV disease there is further loss of deposits and even greater widening of the now diffusely spongy basement membrane.

In the early phase of the disease (Stage I), small granular subepithelial deposits (Fig. 16-16) are seen along the basement membrane. Intracapillary mesangial and subendothelial deposits are not present. A progression of the disease over time can often be documented with serial biopsies. Stage II is characterized by protrusion of "spikes" of basement membrane between deposits of electron-dense material (Fig. 16-17). By Stage III, these deposits are incorporated into the widening basement membrane. In Stage IV the basement membrane is markedly distorted, and mobilization of the deposits has imparted a moth-eaten appearance to the membrane.

With resolution of the lesion the basement membrane is reconstituted and assumes an essentially normal appearance, except for the increased thickness.

Immunofluorescence reveals peripheral granular staining for IgG and C3 in a membranous pattern. Mesangial deposits are not seen in the idiopathic variety of membranous nephropathy, but they are frequent in the membranous lesion of systemic lupus erythematosus.

The usual course in adults is chronic proteinuria and slow deterioration into renal failure within 10 to 15 years. The rapidity of deterioration is variable and cannot be accurately predicted at the time of diagnosis. Recent evidence suggests that corticosteroids are beneficial in patients with idiopathic membranous nephropathy who have begun treatment before there has been deterioration of renal function. Overall the prognosis is better in children, owing to the greater frequency of permanent remission.

Diabetic Glomerulosclerosis

Only the glomerular lesion of diabetes mellitus is discussed here. A more general discussion of diabetes is found in Chapter 22. The term *diabetic glomerulosclerosis* (Kimmelstiel–Wilson syndrome) embraces the glomerular changes seen in diabetes. These alterations are an expression of the diabetic microangiopathy that is seen in many systemic arterial small vessels and capillaries. As in the systemic vessels, glomerular sclerosis is caused by the progressive accumulation of basement membrane material, a deposit that results in an enlargement of the glomeruli. The pathogenesis of the lesion is controversial, but it appears to be related to the severity and duration of hyperglycemia. The extent to which physical factors, such as hyperfiltration, also play a role is not known.

The proteinuria in diabetic glomerulosclerosis is initially mild and may remain so. Hematuria is usu-

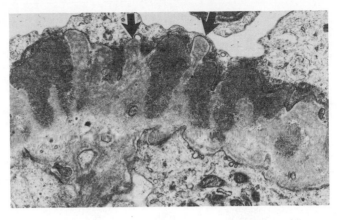

Figure 16-17. Diffuse membranous nephropathy of long duration. An electron micrograph shows deposits of electron-dense material between spikes (*arrows*) of widened glomerular basement membrane.

ally not present. Patients who have proteinuria in the nephrotic range (> 1g/24 hours) usually progress to renal failure within 6 years. It is unusual to have a significant degree of azotemia without proteinuria. Significant proteinuria is usually accompanied by other signs of advanced microangiopathy, such as diabetic retinopathy.

The earliest detectable lesion of diabetic glomerulosclerosis is a diffuse widening of mesangial areas by the accumulation of a PAS-positive matrix. With progression the capillary basement membrane appears thicker and the mesangium becomes increasingly prominent (Fig. 16-18). The glomerulus becomes enlarged and may appear hypercellular. **Diffuse glomerulosclerosis,** the term that refers to this state of enlarged glomeruli with diffusely thickened basement membranes, may occur alone or may be mixed with **nodular glomerulosclerosis.** In the latter condition the nodules in the glomeruli are rounded, homogeneous, eosinophilic masses that appear in centrilobular areas (Fig. 16-19). They may be single or multiple within the same glomerulus. With time the nodules become acellular, in which case only a rim of peripheral mesangial nuclei is visible. Silver stains reveal a pattern of concentric lamination. Concomitant with the development of glomerulosclerosis, insudative changes occur in both the adjacent arterioles and the glomerular tufts. These are manifested by hyaline arteriolosclerosis (Fig. 16-19), which **in diabetics uniquely involves both the afferent and efferent arterioles.** Insudative lesions in the glomeruli are recognized as rounded nodules situated between Bowman's capsule and the parietal epithelium ("capsular drops") or as subendothelial accumula-

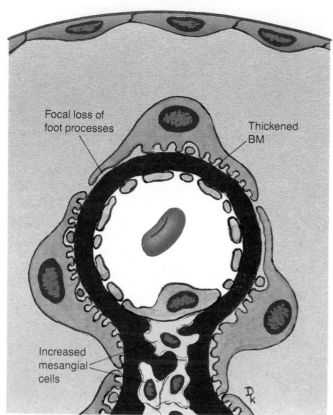

Figure 16-18.   Diabetic glomerulosclerosis. The glomerular tuft is enlarged and displays a thickened basement membrane that retains a normal texture and density with smooth inner and outer contours. Focal effacement of the epithelial cell foot processes is common. An accumulation of basement membrane–like stroma in the mesangium parallels the diffuse widening of the basement membrane.

tions along the capillary loops ("fibrin caps"). Lipid-filled foam cells (Fig. 16-19) may also be seen in late stages of the disease. The thickening of the capillary wall is caused by a widening of the basement membrane, which may be many times its normal width. An accumulation of basement membrane–like stroma in the mesangium parallels the diffuse widening of the basement membrane and may become nodular and acellular (Fig. 16-20). The insudative lesions consist of granular, electron-dense masses that often contain lipid material and debris. There are no deposits of immune complexes.

Diffuse linear trapping of IgM, C3, and fibrin is seen by immunofluorescence. This is thought to be a result of nonspecific absorption of these and other plasma proteins into the thickened glomerular basement membrane rather than a consequence of the deposition of immune complexes.

Amyloidosis

Amyloidosis is actually a group of diseases, all of them characterized by the extracellular deposition of a proteinaceous material in a variety of tissues (see Chapter 23). The accumulation of this material results in the obliteration of tissue structure and disturbed function. Amyloid is conventionally defined as an eosinophilic, amorphous material by light microscopy that shows a fibrillar ultrastructure and a beta-pleated sheet configuration by x-ray diffraction analysis. By light microscopy, the most secure identification is made by the presence of a characteristic apple-green color in sections stained with Congo red and examined under polarized light. Amyloid fibrils are actually composed of polypeptide fragments of normal serum proteins. The two major forms of amyloid are termed the AL and AA proteins. The AL protein is a portion of the light chain of the immunoglobulin molecule. Extracellular deposition of this protein is seen in association with plasma cell dys-

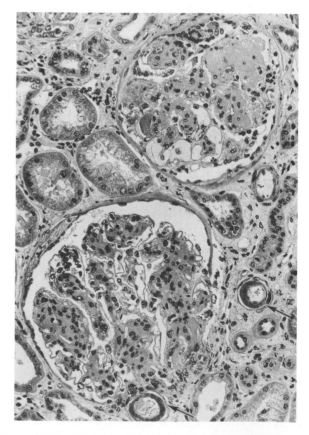

Figure 16-19.   Diabetic glomerulosclerosis. A light micrograph shows a prominent increase in the mesangial matrix. Capillary dilatation and the presence of foam cells are conspicuous features. The arrows indicate "hyalinized" arterioles.

crasias in so-called primary amyloidosis. Secondary amyloidosis involves the deposition of a protein that is normally found in the serum and that is called the AA protein. This protein is elevated in disorders associated with chronic inflammation (e.g., tuberculosis or rheumatoid arthritis). Both the AL and AA forms of amyloidosis are systemic. A rarer form of systemic amyloidosis, called heredofamilial amyloidosis, involves the tissue deposition of prealbumin. Finally, localized forms of the disease exist both in endocrine glands and in the heart and brain of older people (senile amyloidosis).

Renal involvement is frequent in most systemic forms of amyloidosis. The glomeruli are most frequently affected, a situation that results in alterations in permeability and leads to proteinuria. This proteinuria is nonselective and in 60% of patients is severe enough to produce the nephrotic syndrome. Generally, there is no hematuria, and the urinary

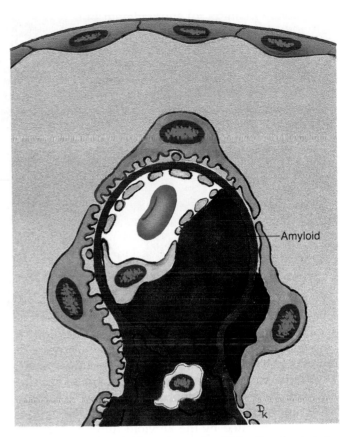

Figure 16-21. Amyloid nephropathy. This disorder is initially associated with the accumulation of characteristic fibrillar deposits in the mesangium. These inert masses, which are fibrillar by electron microscopy, extend along the inner surface of the basement membrane, frequently obstructing the capillary lumen. Focal extension of amyloid through the basement membrane may elevate the epithelial cell, in which case irregular spikes along the outer surface of the basement membrane are seen.

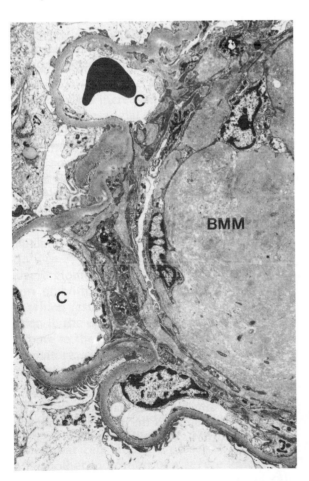

Figure 16-20. Advanced nodular glomerulosclerosis. An electron micrograph shows an aggregate of basement membrane material (*BMM*). The peripheral capillary (*C*) demonstrates diffuse basement membrane widening but a normal texture.

sediment is bland. Severe infiltration of the glomeruli and renal vasculature results in renal failure. Only glomerular amyloidosis is discussed here.

Amyloid deposition is initially mesangial, producing diffuse widening of axial areas (Fig. 16-21). However, it progressively spreads to obliterate capillary lumina (Fig. 16-22). With increasing deposition of amyloid, the glomeruli become enlarged and the hyaline mesangial pattern becomes nodular. This appearance may be confused with diabetic glomerulosclerosis, but the nodules of amyloid are not PAS positive, as they are in diabetic glomerulosclerosis. Finally, the glomerular structure is obliterated, and the glomeruli appear as large hyaline balls.

Electron microscopy provides the most secure method for the identification of amyloid. It appears as fibrils composed of randomly arranged non-

charged barrier in the glomerulus. The antigens in clinically important forms of circulating immune complex nephritis may be either exogenous or endogenous. Examples of immune complex nephritis induced by exogenous antigens include **bacterial antigens** in the glomerulonephritis associated with streptococcal infections and bacterial endocarditis, and **viral antigens** in glomerulonephritis induced by hepatitis B. **DNA** acts as an endogenous antigen in the pathogenesis of lupus nephritis. **Tumor-associated antigens** have been implicated in the development of cases of glomerulonephritis.

In addition to the injury produced by the trapping of preformed antigen–antibody complexes, the glomerulus may be damaged by the binding of circulating antibody to an antigen that has already deposited in the glomerular basement membrane (**in situ immune complex formation**). The best-known example is Goodpasture's syndrome, in which the basement membrane acts as an endogenous antigen to which circulating antibasement membrane antibodies bind. Immunofluorescence shows a linear localization of IgG along the basement membrane. The combination of antigen with antibody results in the activation of complement, and a rapidly progressive glomerulonephritis usually results. Another example of in situ immune complex formation (Heyman nephritis) has already been discussed in the section on the nephrotic syndrome. In some patients, membranous nephropathy is thought to be a consequence of the combination of circulating antibody with a discontinuously distributed subepithelial antigen. Other examples of in situ immune complex formation may involve "planted" antigens that are not intrinsic to the glomerulus—for instance, DNA, bacterial and viral products, and immunoglobulins themselves.

The **alternate complement pathway** is important in the pathogenesis of a lesion called **membranoproliferative glomerulonephritis.** In some forms of this disease, only complement C3 is found in the glomeruli by immunofluorescence, and immunoglobulins are absent. The alternate pathway for complement activation is also important in focal glomerulonephritis due to IgA deposition.

Although there is no direct evidence that cell-mediated processes cause any form of human glomerulonephritis, there are occasional cases of what appears to be immunologically mediated disease in which the accumulation of mononuclear cells and the absence of immunoglobulins suggest a delayed type (cell-mediated) reaction. Indirect evidence that cell-mediated immunity plays a role in human disease is that lymphocytes from a patient with glomerulonephritis exhibit reactivity in vitro to a glomerular antigen, which is presumed to be a target.

Once immune complexes have localized within a glomerulus, a number of secondary pathogenetic mechanisms appear to play a role in effecting immunologic injury. These include the complement-neutrophil system, monocytes and macrophages, and the coagulation system. The role of complement activation in the recruitment of polymorphonuclear leukocytes is well established, and neutrophils are conspicuous in many glomerular diseases. The dependence of various forms of glomerular injury on both complement and neutrophils is illustrated by the changes in the expression of glomerular lesions in experimental animals depleted of these components. Monocytes and macrophages infiltrate the glomerulus in many forms of renal disease and contribute to the cellularity of the glomerular tufts and the surrounding crescents. Activated macrophages release a number of biologically active molecules that are probably important in tissue damage. Fibrin can usually be demonstrated in Bowman's space early in the formation of crescents and is probably partly responsible for subsequent epithelial cell proliferation and crescent formation. Finally, platelets may be activated by sensitized mast cells and basophils on exposure to antigen or immune complexes. There is growing evidence to suggest that platelet-derived polycationic proteins disturb the polyanionic character of the glomerular wall and contribute to its damage.

With this background of the terminology and the pathogenesis of the glomerulonephritides, a description of several of the more important forms of glomerulonephritis can begin. The following examples to be discussed in greater detail are selected either because of the frequency with which they are encountered clinically or because of their value in illustrating the pathogenesis of glomerular injury.

Acute Glomerulonephritis (Postinfectious Glomerulonephritis)

Although acute glomerulonephritis has been documented as a sequel to a variety of infectious agents—such as staphylococci, pneumococci, spirochetes, and viruses—the most frequent association is with **group A streptococci.** Although not seen as frequently now as in the past, this disorder is still one of the most common renal diseases in childhood.

The exact mechanism by which the infection brings about the characteristic proliferative changes is still not completely characterized, although the similarities with the experimental model of acute serum sickness are striking. Both have a latent period of 9 to 14 days between the time the patient is exposed to a new antigen and the occurrence of prolif-

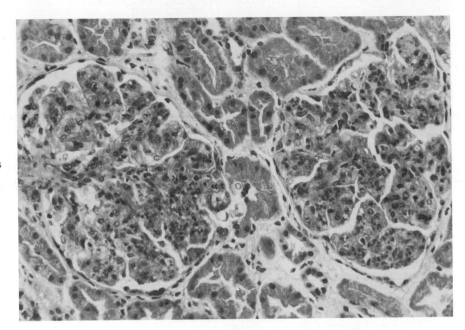

Figure 16-24. Acute poststreptococcal glomerulonephritis. A light micrograph shows enlarged glomerular tufts and obstructed capillaries. Mesangial and endothelial cells are proliferated. Scattered neutrophils are present.

erative glomerulonephritis. The pattern of immunofluorescence is identical, as is the ultrastructural appearance of subepithelial "humps." Streptococcal antigen has been difficult to demonstrate in the glomeruli of patients with this disease, possibly because the antigen is quickly removed from the inflamed glomeruli or is "masked" by immunoglobulin and complement. Circulating immune complexes are demonstrable in half of the patients with acute poststreptococcal glomerulonephritis, and there is recent evidence to support an in situ binding of antibody to planted subepithelial bacterial antigen.

Only certain strains of group A streptococci are nephritogenic. The primary infections may be in either the pharynx or, especially in hot and humid environments, the skin. Because the organisms may not be recoverable at the time of the nephritis, the diagnosis depends on the serologic evidence of a rise in titers to streptococcal products. The disease most commonly affects children. The nephritic syndrome typically begins abruptly with oliguria, hematuria, facial edema, and hypertension. Usually there is a depression of serum C3 during the acute syndrome. This returns to normal within 1 to 2 weeks, as does the clinical condition of most patients. However, in a minority of patients an abnormal urinary sediment persists for years after the acute episode. Exacerbations of the disease may occur on reinfection with another nephritogenic organism.

By light microscopy, a diffuse enlargement and hypercellularity of the glomeruli is present if the biopsy is taken within the first 3 weeks of the onset of acute glomerulonephritis (Fig. 16-24). The hypercel-

lularity is due to the proliferation of both endothelial and mesangial cells (Fig. 16-25) and to infiltration of neutrophils. The proliferation of mesangial cells results in an exaggeration of the normal lobular pattern. Crescents may be present, but they are usually sporadic and segmental. Tubulointerstitial damage and inflammation occur in parallel with the glomerular changes. The blood vessels generally show no changes.

The characteristic ultrastructural features of acute postinfectious glomerulonephritis are the subepithelial "humps." These deposits are invariably accompanied by intracapillary, mesangial, and subendothelial deposits, although the latter two may be much more difficult to find in the acute phase. The humps are variably sized, dome-shaped deposits, which are situated on the epithelial aspect of the basement membrane (Figs. 16-25 and 16-26). They tend to collect over the mesangial regions and are not as diffusely distributed as the epimembranous deposits of membranous nephropathy. The presence of numerous humps is often correlated with unusually severe inflammation and delayed resolution. Frequently, basement membrane irregularities are seen.

Immunofluorescence typically reveals granular peripheral reactions for IgG and C3 along the basement membrane, in locations corresponding to the humps. Short strips of mesangial and intramembranous linear staining may also be seen. Later on in the course, C3 may be present without IgG.

The typical morphologic features of acute inflammation usually have resolved by 8 weeks from the onset of the nephritis (Fig. 16-27). However, a pattern

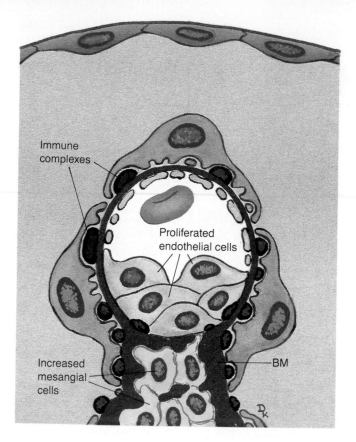

Figure 16-25. Postinfectious glomerulonephritis. Trapping of immune complexes in a subepithelial pattern ("lumpy-bumpy") is seen, together with focal effacement of foot processes. Less prominent subendothelial immune complexes are associated with endothelial cell proliferation and are related to increased capillary permeability and narrowing of the lumen. Frequently, proliferation of mesangial cells and a thickened mesangial basement membrane result in widening of the stalk and conspicuous trapping of immune complexes.

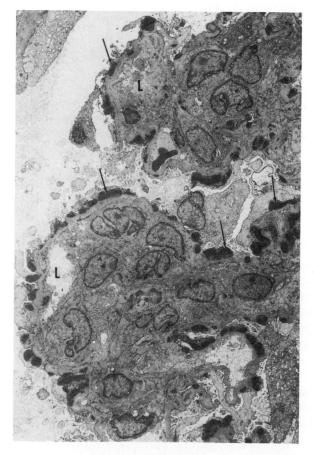

Figure 16-26. Postinfectious glomerulonephritis. An electron micrograph demonstrates numerous subepithelial humps (*arrows*). The capillary lumina (*L*) are markedly narrowed.

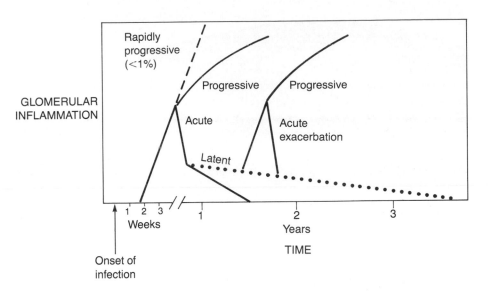

Figure 16-27. The natural history of acute poststreptococcal glomerulonephritis. In typical acute poststreptococcal glomerulonephritis, the inflammation begins to subside after a month and disappears after two months to 1½ years, although in latent cases full resolution may require up to 3 years. In a few cases relentless progression of the disease occurs. Acute exacerbations follow the same course as the initial episode. Rapidly progressive cases are uncommon.

of diffuse prominence of the mesangial matrix, which reflects mesangial hypercellularity, may persist for years. Generally, those patients who recover completely will have done so both clinically and histologically by 3 years from onset. A small number of patients present with an unusually severe lesion that displays many crescents and progresses quickly to renal failure, a condition termed **rapidly progressive glomerulonephritis.**

The issue of the long-term prognosis in acute glomerulonephritis has generated considerable controversy. The incidence of clinically detectable renal disease in long-term studies of patients with poststreptococcal glomerulonephritis has varied dramatically. Some investigators claim an overall complete recovery in more than 95% of patients, whereas others report that more than 50% of their patients developed chronic renal insufficiency, hypertension, or proteinuria. The reasons for this remarkable disagreement are not entirely clear but may reflect the fact that the study in which the patients showed more progressive disease included a large number of adults with severe initial disease. Thus, although some degree of caution must remain with respect to the long-term prognosis of renal function, most data suggest that complete recovery, particularly in children, is the rule.

Crescentic Glomerulonephritis

Crescentic glomerulonephritis is an ominous morphologic pattern (Fig. 16-28) in which the majority of glomeruli are surrounded by an accumulation of cells in Bowman's space. The crescent is an expression of fulminant glomerular damage and always leaves severe residual scarring. Crescentic glomerulonephritis is associated with a number of underlying conditions and should always prompt a search for other diagnostic features that allow a subclassification (Table 16-1). Clinically, most patients with a substantial number of crescents suffer a rapid and progressive decline in renal function. Irreversible renal failure with severe oliguria or anuria occurs within weeks unless adequate therapy is administered.

The escape of fibrin into Bowman's space seems to be important for the formation of glomerular crescents. **Fibrin can invariably be demonstrated by immunofluorescence in active crescentic glomerulonephritis.** Anticoagulation prevents both fibrin accumulation and crescent formation in experimental forms of crescentic glomerulonephritis. Fibrin and other plasma proteins that may be important in crescent formation presumably gain access to Bowman's space through breaks in the inflamed glomerular basement membrane. In the past, crescents were thought to consist primarily of epithelial cells. Recent evidence, however, suggests that macrophages contribute to the cellularity of young "cellular" crescents at least as much as epithelial cells. Cells that have the light microscopic and ultrastructural appearance of fibroblasts are the major cellular constituent in older "fibroepithelial" crescents.

Although the crescent is a nonspecific morphologic lesion, it is always a complication of severe underlying glomerular disease, rather than a primary event. The crescents range from small groups of cells filling only a segment of Bowman's space (Fig. 16-29) to circumferential masses of cells

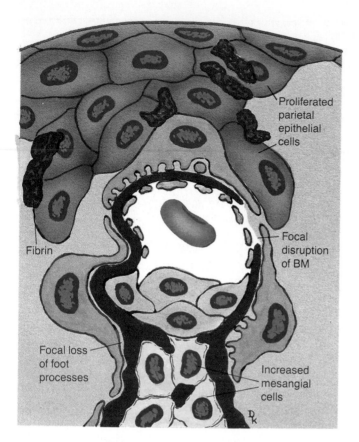

Proliferated parietal epithelial cells

Fibrin

Focal disruption of BM

Focal loss of foot processes

Increased mesangial cells

Figure 16-28.   Crescentic (rapidly progressive) glomerulonephritis. This severe variety of glomerulonephritis shows not only changes in the glomerular tuft but also conspicuous proliferation of parietal epithelial cells, the latter forming the "crescent." Fibrin is often prominent between the proliferating epithelial cells. White blood cells may also be present in active cellular crescents. Focal disruption of the peripheral capillary basement membrane may result in red blood cells in Bowman's space. Crescentic glomerulonephritis is not a specific diagnostic entity, but describes the morphologic counterpart of a maximally active process, as, for example, crescentic poststreptococcal, crescentic IgA, and crescentic lupus glomerulonephritis.

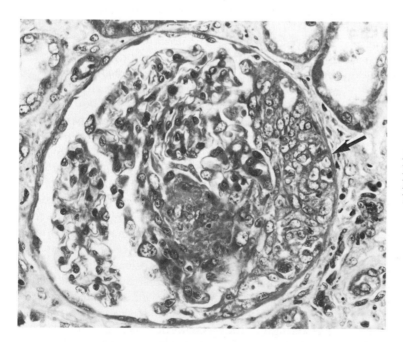

Figure 16-29.   Crescentic glomerulonephritis. A light micrograph shows prominent sheets of proliferating epithelial cells (*arrow*) that fill much of Bowman's space.

Table 16-1. Differential Diagnosis of Crescentic Glomerulonephritis

CONDITION	LIGHT MICROSCOPY	ELECTRON MICROSCOPY	IMMUNOFLUORESCENCE
Idiopathic cresentic glomerulonephritis	Crescents and tuft proliferation	Negative	Negative
Anti–glomerular basement membrane disease	Crescents and segmental tuft proliferation	Negative	Linear IgG and C3
Poststreptococcal glomerulonephritis	Crescents, tuft proliferation, exudative changes	Intracapillary deposits, subepithelial "humps"	Peripheral, granular IgG and C3
Membranoproliferative glomerulonephritis	Crescents, lobular distortion of the tuft, mesangial interpositioning	Subendothelial deposits, mesangial interpositioning	Peripheral, granular C3, properdin
IgA nephropathy/Henoch–Schönlein purpura	Crescents, tuft proliferation	Mesangial deposits	Mesangial IgA, with variable C3, IgG IgM
Systemic lupus erythematosus	Crescents, wire loops, hematoxylin bodies	Subendothelial and mesangial deposits, "fingerprinting" of deposits, peritubular deposits	"Full house" pattern of both mesangial and peripheral IgG, IgA, IgM, C3, C4, Clq
Systemic vasculitis	Crescents, focal arteritis	Negative	Negative

that completely surround the glomerulus. They evolve from a cellular to a fibrocellular form; eventually they scar and form the foundation of a fibrous crescent. The shapes of the cells in a cellular crescent range from spindle to ovoid, and they are often intermingled with neutrophils and fibrin. Mitotic figures are frequently seen, and multinucleated giant cells may also be found. Within several weeks, enough organization has taken place in the crescent so that a connective tissue matrix, which stains with silver, is mingled with the cells. Eventually, segmental crescents become incorporated in Bowman's capsule as a segmental fibrous collar, or in the glomerulus as a segmental glomerular scar. Circumferential crescents result in globally scarred glomeruli. There are frequently discontinuities in Bowman's capsule in the later stages. The glomeruli are by definition inflamed in crescentic glomerulonephritis, although, in the idiopathic forms of the disease and those associated with vasculitis, the cellular proliferation in the tuft may be segmental, and much of the tuft may only appear collapsed. Assignment into one of the specific entities listed in Table 16-1 requires careful examination of the glomerular lesions in crescentic glomerulonephritis.

Idiopathic crescentic glomerulonephritis is essentially a diagnosis of exclusion that is made when there is no ultrastructural or immunohistochemical evidence of immune complex localization or vasculitis. As mentioned in the discussion of poststreptococcal glomerulonephritis, a few patients present after a pharyngitis with a rapid downhill course and a renal biopsy shows a crescentic glomerulonephritis. The changes typical of poststreptococcal glomerulonephritis are found by electron microscopy and immunofluorescence. Other specific systemic diseases that can cause crescentic glomerulonephritis are membranoproliferative glomerulonephritis, IgA nephropathy, Henoch–Schonlein purpura, systemic small vessel arteritis, and systemic lupus erythematosus.

Anti–glomerular basement membrane disease is a rare condition in which the patient develops an antibody directed against his own glomerular basement membrane (Fig. 16-30). This immune attack results in a rapidly progressive, crescentic glomerulonephritis. Eighty percent of these patients are male, with an average age of 29 years at the onset of disease. Many simultaneously suffer from pulmonary hemorrhages and recurrent hemoptysis—sometimes severe enough to be life threatening—because of a cross reactivity of the antibodies with the alveolar basement membranes. The clinical spectrum of anti–glomerular basement membrane disease includes patients with symptoms of glomerulonephritis with or without evidence of pulmonary hemorrhage. A small number of patients exhibit only pulmonary symptoms. When both the lungs and kidneys are involved, the eponym **Goodpasture's syndrome** is used in honor of the investigator who first described the association during the American influenza epidemic at the time of World War I. Anti–glomerular basement membrane antibody is revealed by the presence of a linear binding of IgG and C3 with immunofluorescence (Fig. 16-31), and by the identification of circulating anti-basement membrane antibodies. There are no diagnostic ultrastructural or light microscopic findings.

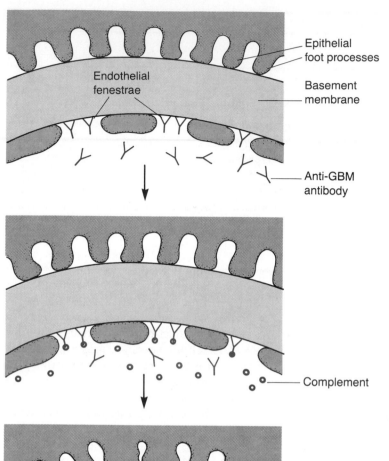

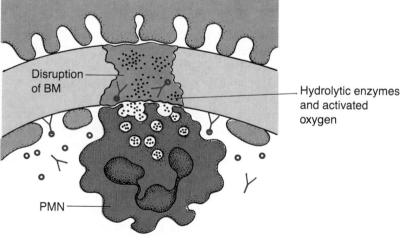

Figure 16-30. Pathogenesis of anti–glomerular basement membrane (*anti-GBM*) antibody glomerulonephritis.

Membranoproliferative Lesions

Membranoproliferative lesions are inflammatory lesions whose name comes from the **characteristic combination of basement membrane thickening and endothelial and mesangial cell proliferation.** In the initial description, children and young adults presented with either the nephrotic or nephritic syndrome and persistently low levels of the third component of complement (C3). The patients did not have poststreptococcal glomerulonephritis or other systemic inflammatory conditions that could account for the hypocomplementemia. The vast majority of these patients progressed to end-stage renal failure. It is now clear that not all patients with this group of diseases have low complement levels, and this is no longer required for diagnosis. Furthermore, although the light microscopic appearance of the renal lesion in the majority of these patients is very similar, **there are sufficient distinctions both ultrastructurally and immunologically to warrant the division of the disease into two predominant groups. These are called membranoproliferative type I and type II.**

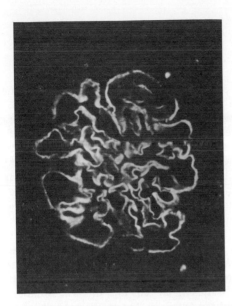

Figure 16-31. Acute anti–glomerular basement membrane antibody glomerulonephritis. In this fluorescence micrograph uniform linear IgG localizes along the capillary walls. Anti–human IgG was used to demonstrate the presence of the anti–basement membrane antibody.

Type I membranoproliferative glomerulonephritis (also called membranoproliferative glomerulonephritis with subendothelial deposits) (Fig. 16-32) has been associated with a number of conditions, including, most importantly, hepatitis B antigenemia, infection of ventriculoatrial shunts (for the treatment of hydrocephalus), bacterial endocarditis, streptococcal infections, and cancer. **However, the great majority of cases are idiopathic.** Circulating immune complexes have been found in some patients with this disease, and there is evidence that they may play a role in the activation of complement via the classical pathway. By light microscopy, diffusely enlarged glomeruli, with a marked centrilobular, mesangial cell proliferation, produce a lobular distortion to the glomeruli (Fig. 16-33). This pattern has in the past been called lobular glomerulonephritis. Silver stains characteristically show a double contour to the peripheral basement membrane in this disease. This feature, which has been erroneously described previously as "splitting" of the basement membrane, is a consequence of the marked inflammatory expansion of the mesangial area. As a result, the cytoplasm and matrix of the mesangium are forced peripherally into the capillary loops and insinuate themselves between the endothelial cells and the basement membrane. This process is called **mesangial interpositioning** and is characteristic of, but not limited to, the membranoproliferative lesions. The expansion of the mesangial areas and subsequent interpositioning is easily appreciated with the electron microscope. Typically, there is a continuous layer of mesangial cytoplasm around the entire capillary. Subendothelial and mesangial electron-dense deposits are present in type I disease (Figs. 16-32 and 16-34). Subepithelial humps may also be seen. Immunoglobulins and complement are demonstrated in the majority of cases by immunofluorescence.

Another term for **type II membranoproliferative glomerulonephritis** is **dense deposit disease.** The clinical presentation and course are similar to type I membranoproliferative glomerulonephritis. Circulating immune complexes are infrequently found in type II patients. However, nearly all patients have a circulating immunoglobulin of the IgG class (C3 nephritic factor) that causes continued activation of the alternative complement pathway by altering the delicate balance between activator and inactivator enzymes (Fig. 16-35). The role of C3 nephritic factor in the pathogenesis of glomerulonephritis remains obscure, particularly since complement activation by the alternative pathway has not produced glomerular disease in laboratory animals. However, the recurrence of type II disease in renal transplants suggests that glomerular injury is mediated through some humoral factor.

The light microscopic appearance of type II disease is identical to that of type I, although the degree of cellularity may be more variable between glomeruli. The pathognomonic feature of this form of the disease is the characteristic ribbonlike zone of increased density located centrally within the thickened basement membrane (Fig. 16-36). Areas of density may also be found in the membranes of peritubular capillaries and in the elastic laminae of arterioles. In contrast to type I disease, immunofluorescence shows only weak, discontinuous reactions for C3 along the basement membrane. Immunoglobulins are not found.

Recently, a third type of membranoproliferative lesion, **type III,** has been described. By light microscopy, it is identical to types I and II. However, ultrastructurally there is a marked distortion of the basement membrane by massive amounts of electron-dense deposits that occur on both sides of the basement membrane. As in type II disease, C3 in the absence of immunoglobulins is most frequently demonstrated by immunofluorescence.

Focal Glomerulonephritis

Focal glomerulonephritis is a morphologic term that is used when only some of the glomeruli are involved. In conditions that produce this lesion, the

(Text continues on p. 862)

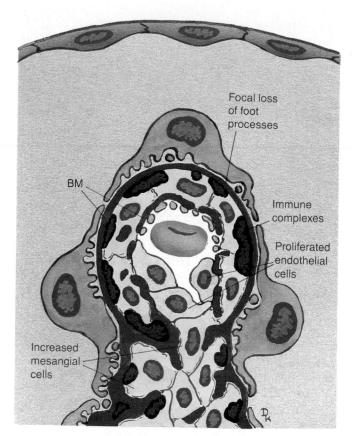

Focal loss
of foot
processes

BM

Immune
complexes

Proliferated
endothelial
cells

Increased
mesangial
cells

Figure 16-32. Membranoproliferative glomerulonephritis, type I. In this disease the glomeruli are enlarged. Hypercellular tufts and narrowing or obstruction of the capillary lumen are seen. Large subendothelial deposits of immune complexes extend along the inner border of the basement membrane. The mesangial cells proliferate and migrate peripherally into the capillary. Basement membrane material accumulates in a linear fashion parallel to the basement membrane in a subendothelial position. The interposition of mesangial cells and basement membrane between the endothelial cells and the original basement membrane creates a double-contour effect. The accumulation of mesangial cells and stroma in the tufts narrows the capillary lumen. The stalk is also widened by the proliferation of mesangial cells and the accumulation of basement membrane stroma. The entire process leads progressively to lobulation of the glomerulus, consolidation of the lobules, and eventually a "cannonball" effect. Note the proliferation of endothelial cells and focal effacement of foot processes.

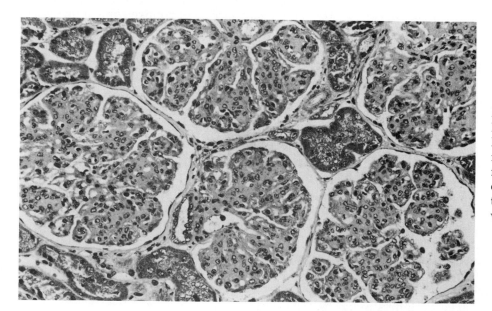

Figure 16-33. Membranoproliferative glomerulonephritis, type I. A light micrograph shows glomerular lobulation and diffuse mesangial proliferation. Peripheral extension of mesangial matrix material obstructs the lumina and widens the capillary walls.

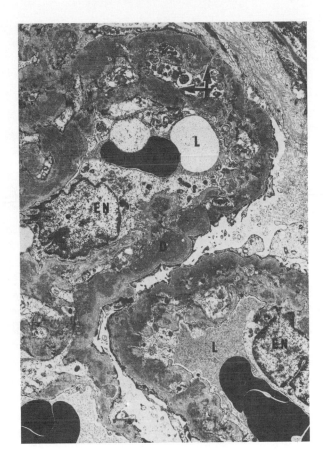

Figure 16-34. Membranoproliferative glomerulonephritis, type I. An electron micrograph demonstrates double contour basement membrane (*arrows*) with mesangial interposition and prominent subendothelial deposits. *EN*, endothelial cell; *L*, capillary lumen

Figure 16-35. Complement activation by C3 nephritic factor in membranoproliferative glomerulonephritis, type II. The alternative pathway of complement activation involves the conversion of C3 to C3b. This conversion is mediated by the activity of a C3 convertase (C3bBb), which in turn is stimulated by the product of the reaction, namely C3b. This positive feedback system is normally restrained by two inhibitory factors (C3b inactivator and β-1 H). C3 nephritic factor (an IgG autoantibody against C3 convertase) in the serum of patients with type I membranoproliferative glomerulonephritis stabilizes C3 convertase, thereby increasing its activity and augmenting the alternative complement pathway.

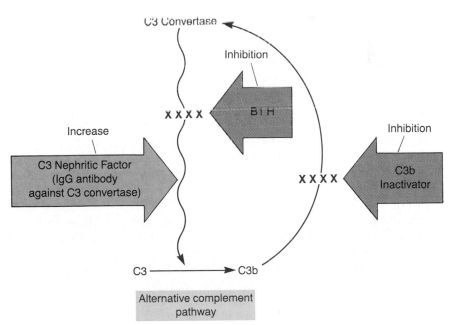

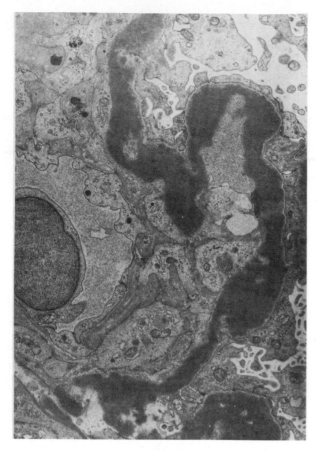

Figure 16-36. Membranoproliferative glomerulonephritis, type II (dense deposit disease). An electron micrograph demonstrates thickening of the basement membrane and increased density of the lamina densa.

inflammation is frequently also limited to segmental portions of the glomerular tufts. This disorder must be distinguished from the focal sclerosing lesions seen in focal segmental glomerulosclerosis. Focal glomerulonephritis may occur as an early or mild manifestation of a systemic disease that usually affects all glomeruli or as a nonsystemic primary glomerulonephritis. Thus, as in crescentic glomerulonephritis, the light microscopic appearance of focal glomerulonephritis may be produced by a number of conditions (Table 16-2). The lesion is subclassified by immunofluorescence and electron microscopy (see Table 16-2).

IgA nephropathy (also known as **Berger's disease**) is an important newcomer to the list of focal glomerulonephritides that merit special consideration. With the more widespread use of immunofluorescence, it has become clear in recent years that this condition, which was once considered a "French disease," is actually **the most common type of adult primary glomerulonephritis in many parts of the world, ac-**

counting for over 20% of cases in France, Italy, Australia, Japan, and Singapore. In the United States the incidence is lower, ranging from 3% to 10%. IgA nephropathy is primarily a disease of young men, with a peak age of 15 to 30 years. The pathogenesis is not understood. The occasional development of IgA nephropathy in patients who have chronic inflammatory lesions of IgA-containing mucosal surfaces, such as gluten enteropathy, Crohn's disease, and chronic bronchitis, suggests an increased entry of exogenous mucosal antigens (e.g., those of viruses or bacteria) into the general circulation, where they complex with IgA. This concept is supported by the occurrence of IgA nephropathy in patients with chronic liver disease, who have an impaired ability to clear such immune complexes from the blood. Thus, an increased formation of IgA immune complexes may eventually lead to asymptomatic proteinuria and microscopic hematuria in some patients and more severe renal disease in others, including acute or chronic renal failure, nephrotic range proteinuria, and malignant hypertension. Although it was once felt that this was a benign disease, **it is now becoming clear that up to 20% of these patients develop end-stage renal failure.** Once diagnosed, the lesion does not spontaneously resolve and is unresponsive to therapy. IgA nephropathy (Fig. 16-37) is a mesangial proliferative lesion, meaning that mesangial cell proliferation is the sole or predominant abnormality in many of the cases. The involvement is highly variable and may be either focal or diffuse. In most young children and in patients with mild disease, the mesangial proliferation is mild and is accompanied by a prominence of the mesangial stroma (Fig. 16-38). Frequently, hyaline material, representing mesangial deposits, can be seen, particularly in those patients destined to progress to renal failure, who exhibit segmental necrosis of the glomerular tufts, crescents, and scarring. Ultrastructural examination confirms the mesangial cellularity and increased stroma. In addition, there is a variable amount of finely granular, electron dense deposits, located primarily in the mesangium (Fig. 16-39). These are typically in a position immediately beneath the basement membrane, which bulges because of their presence. Immunofluorescence microscopy, which is pivotal in the diagnosis of this entity, reliably shows a diffuse mesangial reaction with IgA, usually accompanied by IgG, IgM, and C3. The early-acting complement components, such as C1q and C4, are not seen.

A close relationship exists between IgA nephropathy and the renal lesion of **Henoch–Schonlein (allergic purpura) nephritis**. The latter usually presents

Table 16-2. Differential Diagnosis of Focal Glomerulonephritis

Condition	Light Microscopy	Electron Microscopy	Immunofluorescence	Other
Idiopathic focal glomerulonephritis	Focal glomerulonephritis, often segmental	Negative	Negative	—
IgA nephropathy	Mesangial cell proliferation	Mesangial deposits	Mesangial IgA, C3	Intermittent hematuria
Henoch–Schönlein glomerulonephritis	Mesangial cell proliferation, frequently crescentic	Mesangial deposits	Mesangial IgA, C3	Purpura, arthritis, abdominal pain
Anti-glomerular basement membrane disease	Frequently segmental, often necrotizing	Negative	Linear IgG and C3	± pulmonary hemorrhage
Lupus glomerulonephritis	Mesangial and endothelial proliferation	Various deposits, "fingerprinting" of deposits, tubulovesicular bodies	"Full house" pattern of immune complex deposits	± systemic syndrome, anti-nuclear factor, etc.
Bacterial endocarditis	Mesangial and endothelial proliferation, segmental	Variable	Variable	Cardiac murmur, fever
Systemic vasculitis	Often crescentic, segmental necrosis, focal arteritis	Negative	Negative	Systemic symptoms

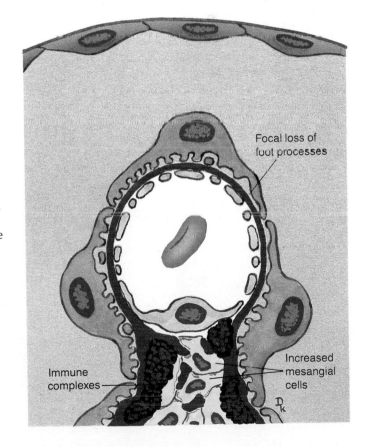

Figure 16-37. IgA nephropathy. Significant accumulation of IgA is seen in the stalk, most commonly between the mesangial cells and the basement membrane. The disease is associated with a variable inflammatory reaction.

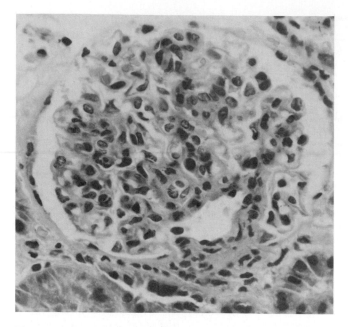

Figure 16-38. IgA nephropathy. A light micrograph shows mesangial cell proliferation and the mesangial accumulation of hyaline material.

with a more severe degree of inflammation. Clinically, these two entities are distinguished on the basis that IgA nephropathy is manifested as a primary glomerulonephritis involving only the kidneys. However, Henoch–Schonlein purpura is a systemic disease, usually seen in children, that presents with purpura of the lower extremities, arthritis, and abdominal pain. It is likely that these two conditions are, in fact, opposite poles of a single disease process.

Renal Diseases Associated with Systemic Disorders

Systemic autoimmune and metabolic diseases may involve the kidney. In many of these diseases, the renal damage is a major cause of morbidity and mortality.

Systemic Lupus Erythematosus

Systemic lupus erythematosus is an autoimmune disorder that primarily affects young women. Of the 5000 new patients a year in the United States with this disease, as many as 70% will develop clinically significant renal disease. Such patients usually have a number of serologic abnormalities, including circulating antibodies to nuclear components and depressed complement components, although these are not invariably present and do not always correlate with the progression of the renal lesion. The variety of renal lesions in systemic lupus erythematosus is reflected in a wide spectrum of clinical manifestations, including the nephritic and nephrotic syndromes. On occasion, lupus nephropathy presents primarily with dysfunction of the renal tubules, which reflects the interstitial inflammation of glomerulonephritis.

Systemic lupus erythematosus is the prototypic example of a human immune complex disease. Unlike many of the putative immune complex diseases already discussed, the role of such complexes in this disease is well characterized. There is a generalized

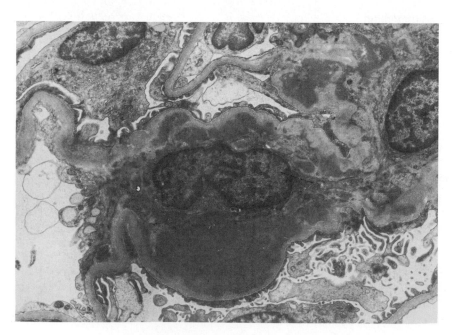

Figure 16-39. IgA nephropathy. An electron micrograph demonstrates prominent IgA deposits in the widened mesangial stalk.

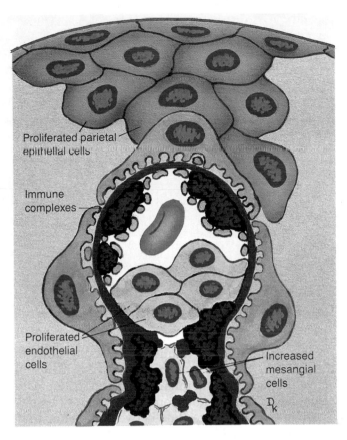

Figure 16-40. The glomerulonephritis of systemic lupus erythematosus. The glomerulus in this disease is characterized by conspicuous intercapillary immune complexes. The mesangial deposits separate the basement membrane from the proliferating mesangial cells and extend into the peripheral capillary as subendothelial deposits. Severe cases not only show changes in the glomerular tuft but also exhibit conspicuous proliferation of capsular epithelial cells and formation of cellular crescents.

hyperactivity of the B-cell system, with an outpouring of antibodies to a variety of nuclear and nonnuclear antigens, including native, double-stranded and single-stranded DNA, RNA, and nucleoproteins. In contrast to the increased B-cell activity, T-cell function is diminished, an effect that is probably related, in part, to the presence of lymphocytotoxic antibodies. The underlying cause for these abnormalities is not known, although an underlying genetic predisposition appears likely. It is clear that the trapping of circulating immune complexes, probably those containing double-stranded DNA, is responsible for much of the renal damage in this disease. A more detailed discussion of systemic lupus erythematosus is found in Chapter 4.

A description of the morphologic alterations in lupus nephritis centers on the glomeruli, because they bear the brunt of the immunologic assault. Cellular proliferation in lupus glomerulonephritis is typically mesangial and often irregular. Mild glomerular involvement is characterized by diffuse mesangial expansion, with or without hypercellularity, and there is often a superimposed, segmental endothelial cell proliferation. More severe inflammation is manifested by enlarged, hypercellular glomeruli; enhanced lobulation; segmental areas of tuft necrosis;

karyorrhexis; polymorphonuclear cell infiltration; and crescent formation (Fig. 16-40). Immune complexes, which are particularly prominent in this disease and may display unusual crystalline patterns, localize in mesangial, subendothelial, or epimembranous areas (Fig. 16-40). Often IgG, IgA, and IgM and C3, C4 and C1q are present in the same glomerulus—the so-called full house pattern. By electron microscopy the deposits of immune complexes display a whorled pattern, which has been likened to fingerprints. There is a correlation between the site of the deposits and the pattern and severity of the inflammatory change. Exclusively mesangial deposits elicit no inflammatory response at all. Heavy subendothelial deposits can usually be recognized at the light microscopic level by a marked thickening of the involved capillary wall, which results in a characteristic formation that has been called a "wire loop" (Fig. 16-41). Hyaline thrombi are also seen as eosinophilic plugs of material that seem to occlude the lumina of involved capillary loops. In areas of segmental necrosis, hematoxylin bodies, which are lilac-tinged fragmented nuclei, may be found. **The hematoxylin bodies are considered to be the only pathognomonic light microscopic feature of tissue damage of lupus erythematosus in the kidney and other**

are multiple myeloma, primary amyloidosis, Waldenstrom's macroglobulinemia, and cryoglobulinemia. The renal complications of paraproteinemia are diverse in both morphology and pathogenesis. Glomerular deposits of paraproteins may cause capillary occlusion or glomerular sclerosis, with or without amyloid formation. They may also activate complement and cause cellular proliferation. If the paraproteins are small (e.g., circulating light chains) and not polymerized, they can be filtered freely and result in tubular lesions.

Multiple myeloma is a disease of the immunoglobulin-producing B lymphocyte that occurs predominantly in the fifth decade and later. More than half of all multiple myeloma patients have renal involvement at some point in the course of their disease. In addition to the circulating paraproteins, other factors, such as hypercalcemia, hyperuricemia, and frequent renal infections, also contribute to the incidence of renal failure in these patients. The renal lesions of multiple myeloma are divided into three types: that associated with the excretion of large amounts of light chains (called Bence–Jones proteins), in which there is primarily tubular destruction, and two types of tissue deposition of immunoglobulin fragments—in the form of amyloid fibrils and, rarely, in kappa light-chain glomerulosclerosis.

"Myeloma cast nephropathy" is the term used to describe the renal lesion associated with the excretion of large amounts of light chains. **The characteristic lesions consist of multiple, dense, lamellated, and fractured casts in the distal and collecting tubules** (Fig. 16-42). These casts are brightly eosinophilic and refractile and are frequently surrounded by multinucleated giant cells. Immunohistochemical staining of this material shows that they are usually composed of kappa light chains. A latticelike configuration of the more crystalloid casts is demonstrated ultrastructurally.

Tissue deposition is favored in cases of circulating paraproteins that are polymerized into larger aggregates and have a high isoelectric point. (At pH 7.4 they are negatively charged and are thus repelled by the negative charge of the basement membrane.)

The more common type of tissue deposition of immunoglobulin fragments is in the form of **amyloid fibrils.** The nature and staining properties of these fibrils, which are composed in part of immunoglobulin light chains, is described in the section on the nephrotic syndrome and in Chapter 23. The accumulation of amyloid fibrils often begins in the mesangial area and then extends peripherally, with subsequent occlusion of the capillary loop (see Fig. 16-21). Amyloid is also found in the basement mem-

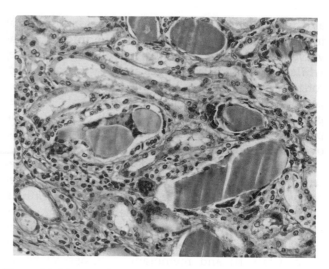

Figure 16-42.   Myeloma of the kidney. A light micrograph shows the broad casts and multinucleated giant cells that are characteristic of obstructive light chain nephropathy.

brane of the tubules and around interstitial vessels, although the degree of proteinuria correlates better with the amount of glomerular amyloid and the degree of glomerular epithelial cell disruption. Lambda light chains are demonstrated more frequently than kappa chains in amyloid deposits.

The third form of tissue deposition of paraprotein is rare and has only recently been recognized. It is referred to as **kappa light-chain glomerulosclerosis**, although the tubules and interstitium are also infiltrated with the deposits. The glomeruli are enlarged, with thickening of the capillary walls by intensely PAS-positive material. This process results in a nodular mesangial expansion of the glomeruli, in a manner similar to the lesion of nodular diabetic glomerulosclerosis. The similarity continues in that there is a diffuse refractile thickening of the basement membrane of the tubules. Immunofluorescence microscopy reveals a diffuse deposition of kappa light chains in the regions outlined by the PAS-positive material. Ultrastructurally, there is a uniform, finely granular electron-dense material distributed along the glomerular and tubular basement membranes and throughout the mesangial matrix. Amyloid fibers are not present, and the usual histochemical stains for amyloid are negative.

Waldenstrom's macroglobulinemia is a lymphoproliferative syndrome that is characterized by a high serum concentration of monoclonal IgM, which causes marked elevation of viscosity and may be associated with Bence–Jones proteins in the urine. Renal involvement is uncommon. The most frequent finding is partial or complete occlusion of glomerular capillaries by PAS-positive "thrombi," which can be shown to be monoclonal IgM by immunofluorescence. Proliferative glomerulonephritis and membranous nephropathy have also been associated with Waldenstrom's macroglobulinemia.

A similar spectrum of renal lesions is associated with **cryoglobulinemia.** Cryoglobulins are monoclonal immunoglobulin molecules (usually IgM), or mixtures of immunoglobulin classes, which are defined by their capacity to precipitate at 4°C. They are found in a wide variety of autoimmune, lymphoproliferative, and inflammatory conditions. A lesion of diffuse mesangial and endothelial cell proliferation, with brightly eosinophilic PAS-positive thrombi, is most frequently present. Characteristic organized annular structures are seen ultrastructurally in about half of these cases. A membranous nephropathy has also been described in this setting.

Hereditary Nephritis

A hereditary form of glomerulonephritis is referred to by the eponym **Alport's syndrome.** The disease affects both sexes, but is more severe in men, who usually die of renal failure before the age of 40. Even though affected women show signs of the disease, and some die prematurely, others live a normal life span. Variable proteinuria and hematuria are the rule, and the nephrotic syndrome complicates the course of the disease. Thirty percent to 50% of patients exhibit high-frequency nerve deafness, and some suffer from abnormalities of the eyes, including disorders of the lens and the macula.

By light microscopy the glomerulonephritis is patchy and its severity varies across the entire spectrum of glomerular disease, from a mild focal proliferative form to a full-blown crescentic glomerulonephritis. Focal loss of tubules and interstitial fibrosis accompany the glomerular lesions. An alteration in the glomerular basement membrane is seen with the electron microscope. The basement membrane is thickened by a splitting of the lamina densa into interlacing lamella that surround electron-lucent domains. However, these changes are not pathognomonic of hereditary nephritis, having been described in other forms of glomerulonephritis. There is no deposition of immune complexes or other apparent cause for the glomerular lesions.

A defect in the chemical composition of basement membranes remains a likely basis of the renal disease, as well as of the abnormalities occurring in the eye and ear, in Alport's syndrome. Supporting such a hypothesis is the observation that the glomerular basement membranes of Alport's patients lack the Goodpasture antigen and therefore do not bind antiglomerular basement membrane antibodies.

Tubulointerstitial Diseases

Renal diseases that are initially limited to the tubules and interstitium are usually grouped together. Because a disorder that affects the tubules causes an immediate reaction in the interstitium, and vice versa, it is often difficult to discern which of these morphologic components is injured as the primary event. Tubulointerstitial diseases are caused by many different etiologic agents. This group of disorders is distinguished clinically from the glomerular diseases by the absence of symptoms typically referable to the glomerulus, such as the nephrotic syndrome or an active nephritic sediment. These patients often demonstrate defects in tubular function, such as an inability to concentrate urine, salt wasting, and a metabolic acidosis. Like the glomerulonephritides, tubulointerstitial diseases tend to resemble each other in the advanced stages of disease. Thus, the clinicopathologic entity of **chronic interstitial nephritis,** a term that describes marked tubular atrophy with interstitial fibrosis, is the result of a number of pathologic processes.

Pyelonephritis and Urinary Tract Infection

Infection is a major cause of tubulointerstitial disorders. Pyelonephritis—defined as a combined inflammation of the parenchyma, calyces, and renal pelvis—occurs in two forms: acute pyelonephritis, which is always a result of a bacterial infection of the kidney, and chronic pyelonephritis, the pathogenesis of which is controversial. The latter may be the result of chronic infection, with or without obstruction.

Acute Pyelonephritis

The development of ascending acute pyelonephritis depends on four factors: a source of pathogenic microorganisms, infection of the urine, reflux of the infected urine up the ureters into the renal pelvis and calyces, and entry of the bacteria through the papillae into the renal parenchyma.

Normally, the urine is sterile, a condition that reflects the absence of bacteria in the urinary tract. However, the distal portion of the urethra is commonly colonized by commensal organisms, which pose no threat of infection. In some women who seem to be unusually vulnerable to recurrent attacks of acute pyelonephritis, this flora is replaced by organisms from the gastrointestinal tract that gain entry to the urethra from the perineum and vestibule of the vagina. Thus, the most common offending organism is *Escherichia coli*. The factors responsible for this change in bacterial flora are not well understood but may reflect poor hygiene, hormonal effects, and genetic predisposition. Moreover, the female urethra lacks the antibacterial action of prostatic secretions.

The entry of urethral bacteria into the bladder often occurs without any known preceding cause. The higher incidence of urinary tract infections in women may be related, in part, to the short urethra. In some cases, catheterization of the urinary bladder carries organisms into the bladder. Initial sexual intercourse in women who have not previously been sexually active is implicated in cases of acute cystitis ("honeymoon cystitis"). The infection has been attributed to trauma to the distal urinary tract with mechanical transfer of organisms into the urethra and bladder.

During micturition the bladder normally empties completely except for 2 ml or 3 ml of residual urine. The subsequent addition of sterile urine from the kidneys ordinarily dilutes any bacteria that may have found their way into the bladder. However, under some circumstances the residual urine volume is increased (e.g., in cases of prostatic obstruction or an atonic bladder caused by neurogenic disorders, such as paraplegia or the neuropathy of diabetes). As a result the bladder contents are not sufficiently diluted with sterile urine from the kidneys to prevent the accumulation of bacteria. The glycosuria of diabetes further predisposes to infection by providing a rich medium for bacterial growth. Asymptomatic bacteriuria occurs in up to 10% of pregnant women, one quarter of whom develop acute pyelonephritis. This increased incidence of acute pyelonephritis in pregnancy can also be attributed to an increased residual urine volume. Under the influence of high levels of progesterone, the bladder musculature becomes flaccid and does not expel the urine with customary efficiency. It should be noted that, even with normal dilution of the residual urine, sufficient organisms may be present to allow the development of acute pyelonephritis, and indeed most cases of acute pyelonephritis occur in women with normal residual volumes. Bacteria in the bladder urine usually do not gain access to the kidneys. The ureter commonly inserts into the bladder wall at a steep angle (Fig. 16-43) and courses parallel to the bladder wall between the mucosa and muscularis in its most distal portion. The intravesicular pressure produced by micturition occludes the distal lumen of the ureter, thereby pre-

venting reflux of urine. In many individuals who are particularly susceptible to ascending pyelonephritis, an abnormally short passage of the ureter within the bladder wall is associated with an angle of insertion that is more perpendicular to the mucosal surface of the bladder. Thus, on micturition, rather than occluding the lumen, intravesicular pressure forces urine into the patent ureter. This reflux is sufficiently powerful to force the urine into the renal pelvis and calyces.

Even when present in the calyces, bacteria are not necessarily carried into the renal parenchyma by the reflux pressure. The simple papillae of the central calyces are convex and do not readily admit reflux urine (see Fig. 16-43). By contrast, the concave shape of the peripheral compound papillae allows easier access to the collecting system. However, if the pressure is prolonged, as in obstructive uropathy, even the simple papillae are eventually rendered vulnerable to retrograde entry of urine. From the collecting tubules the bacteria gain access to the interstitial tissue of the kidney.

The vast majority of cases of acute pyelonephritis stem from ascending infection, but under some circumstances and with certain organisms, blood-borne pathogens can become resident in the kidney. For example, gram-positive organisms, such as staphylococci, can disseminate from the infected valve of a bacterial endocarditis and establish a focus of infection in the kidney. In such cases, the cortex is more commonly the site of the infection than the medulla and pyramids, and abscesses are more likely to be seen than in ascending pyelonephritis. The kidney is commonly involved in miliary tuberculosis. Even fungi, such as aspergillus, can seed the kidney in an immunocompromised host. Experimentally, the normal kidney is highly resistant to infection by circulating gram-negative bacteria. However, in the face of urinary tract obstruction (e.g., by ligation of the ureter), the kidney becomes more vulnerable to hematogenous pyelonephritis. Although the relevance of these experimental findings to the pathogenesis of acute pyelonephritis in man is unclear, there are clinical reasons to believe that any damage to the kidney (e.g., that associated with the interstitial nephritis of chronic analgesic abuse) renders it more susceptible to infection by the hematogenous route. Symptoms of acute pyelonephritis include costovertebral angle tenderness and systemic evidence of infection, such as fever and malaise. The peripheral white blood cell count is often elevated. The differentiation of upper from lower urinary tract infection is often clinically difficult, but the finding of white blood cell casts in the urine is diagnostic of pyelonephritis.

Grossly, the kidneys of acute pyelonephritis may

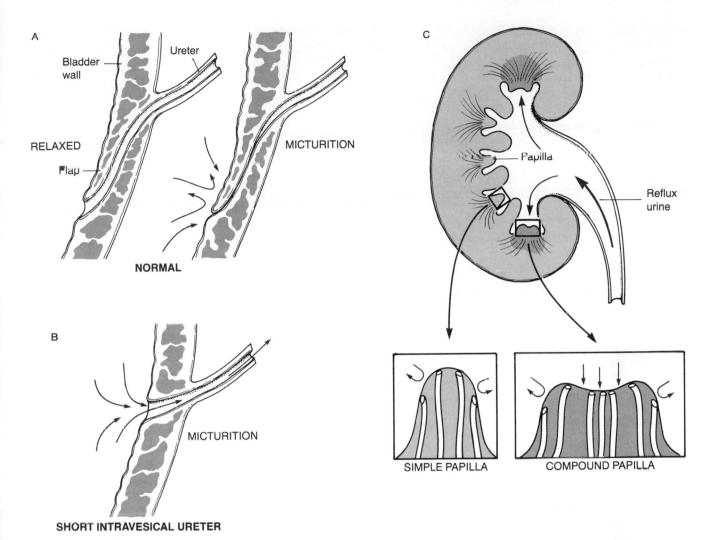

Figure 16-43. Anatomic features of the bladder and kidney in pyelonephritis caused by ureterovesical reflux. **Bladder.** (*A*) In the normal bladder the distal portion of the intravesical ureter courses between the mucosa and the muscularis of the bladder. A mucosal flap is thus formed. On micturition the elevated intravesicular pressure compresses the flap against the bladder wall, thereby occluding the lumen. (*B*) Persons with a congenitally short intravesical ureter have no mucosal flap, because the entry of the ureter into the bladder approaches a right angle. Thus, micturition forces urine into the ureter. **Kidney.** (*C*) The so-called simple papillae of the central calyces are convex and do not readily allow reflux of urine. By contrast the peripheral compound papillae are concave and permit entry of refluxed urine.

have small abscesses on the subcapsular surface. In areas where there has been severe reflux or obstruction, the cortex is thinned and the papillae blunted. Most infections involve only one or two papillary systems. The parenchyma, particularly the cortex, may be extensively destroyed by the acute inflammatory process (Fig. 16-44), although vessels and glomeruli often show some resistance to infection. A modest number of polymorphonuclear leukocytes may also be seen. In severe cases, necrosis of the papillary tip may occur. Acute and chronic pyelonephritis are focal diseases and much of the kidney often appears normal.

Chronic Pyelonephritis

Chronic pyelonephritis is a chronic tubulointerstitial disorder in which there is gross, irregular, and often asymmetric scarring, together with deformation of the calyces and the overlying parenchyma. It often

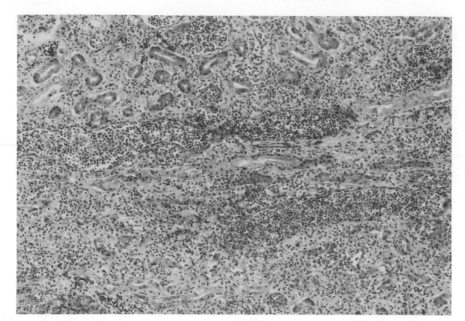

Figure 16-44.   Acute pyelonephritis. A light micrograph shows an extensive infiltrate of neutrophils in the collecting tubules and interstitial tissue.

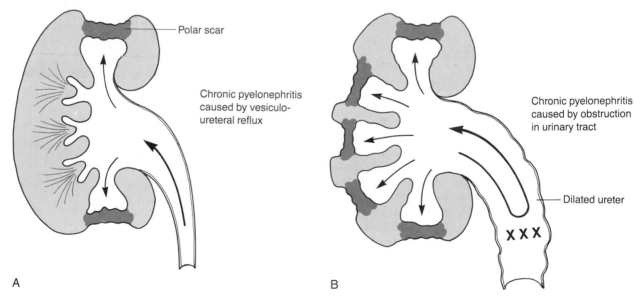

Polar scar

Chronic pyelonephritis caused by vesiculo-ureteral reflux

Chronic pyelonephritis caused by obstruction in urinary tract

Dilated ureter

A

B

Figure 16-45.   The two major types of chronic pyelonephritis. (*A*) Vesicoureteral reflux causes infection of the peripheral compound papillae and, therefore, scars in the poles of the kidney. (*B*) Obstruction of the urinary tract leads to high-pressure backflow of urine that causes infection of all papillae and diffuse scarring of the kidney and thinning of the cortex.

progresses to so-called end-stage kidney—that is, a shrunken and fibrotic kidney that is insufficient to maintain renal function. In fact, about 15% of patients referred for renal dialysis or transplants suffer from chronic pyelonephritis. **The relationship of the tubulointerstitial damage to the calyx in this disease cannot be overemphasized.** Tubular atrophy and interstitial fibrosis can result from a number of conditions, but only chronic pyelonephritis and analgesic nephropathy (see later) produce this combination of calyceal deformity with overlying corticomedullary scarring. The role of bacterial infection in chronic pyelonephritis is less secure than in the acute form of the disease, although in most cases infection is thought to play a role. Primary infections in the kidney that produce the lesions of chronic pyelonephritis are almost invariably associated with either obstruction or vesicoureteral reflux, or both. Whether reflux of sterile urine in the absence of infection can produce the focal scars typical of chronic pyelonephritis is a controversial issue.

Chronic pyelonephritis is divided into cases with some form of obstruction and those without (Fig. 16-45). The vast majority of cases without obstruction are associated with vesicoureteral reflux (so-called **reflux nephropathy**). In cases with mechanical obstruction, the pathologic changes are due to a combination of obstruction and infection; all of the calyces and the renal pelvis are dilated and the parenchyma is uniformly thinned (Fig. 16-46). In cases associated with vesicoureteral reflux, the calyces at the poles of the kidney are preferentially expanded and are associated with overlying discrete, coarse scars that cause an indentation of the renal surface.

Microscopically, the scars are composed of atrophic dilated tubules, which are surrounded by interstitial fibrous tissue (Fig. 16-47). The glomeruli may be completely uninvolved, may have periglomerular fibrosis, or may be sclerotic. The most characteristic tubular change is severe atrophy of the epithelium with diffuse eosinophilic hyaline casts. In cross section such tubules resemble colloid-containing thyroid follicles. The pattern is called thyroidization. A mixed lymphocytic and histiocytic inflammatory infiltrate is seen, especially early in the course of the disease.

Tubulointerstitial Nephritis Caused by Drugs

An ever-expanding list of drugs has been associated with the development of renal damage. That the kidneys are uniquely susceptible to drug-induced injury

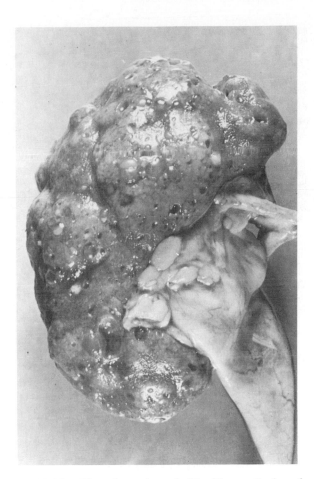

Figure 16-46. Chronic pyelonephritis. The cortical surface of this small kidney contains many irregular, depressed scars. Note the dilated ureter. The gross appearance illustrated here corresponds closely to that depicted graphically in Figure 16-45 and illustrates the type of chronic pyelonephritis caused by urinary tract obstruction.

is not surprising in view of the fact that they receive 25% of the cardiac output and the tubules concentrate the drug locally to high levels. Drug-induced parenchymal injury is produced by three general mechanisms: An acute interstitial nephritis may be induced by a predominantly allergic mechanism; acute renal failure can result from direct nephrotoxicity of a drug; and chronic, slowly progressive renal damage may be caused by prolonged ingestion of certain analgesic compounds.

Acute drug-induced tubulointerstitial nephritis of the hypersensitivity type is now a well-recognized clinicopathologic reaction to an increasing number of drugs. It is characterized clinically by acute renal insufficiency, microscopic or macroscopic hematuria, fever, nausea, vomiting, and an elevated erythrocyte sedimentation rate. It has most frequently been as-

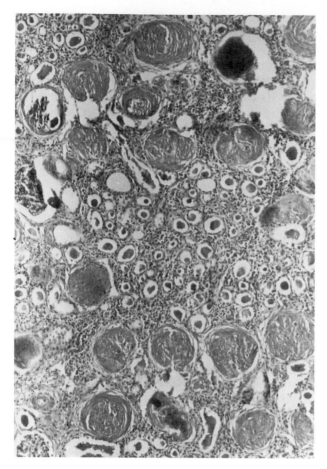

Figure 16-47.   Chronic pyelonephritis. A light micrograph illustrates a cluster of atrophic tubules containing casts in their lumina (so-called thyroidization), surrounded by sclerotic glomeruli.

sociated with synthetic penicillins (methicillin, ampicillin), but other antibiotics, diuretics, and nonsteroidal and anti-inflammatory agents have also been implicated. The symptoms typically begin about 2 weeks after drug administration has begun. The histologic findings, which are not specific, include a lymphohistiocytic inflammatory widening of the interstitium and interstitial edema. Granulomas may be seen, especially when the lesion is associated with the use of sulfonamides or methicillin. Although eosinophils may be prominent, they are not necessary for the diagnosis. In severe cases the tubules show swelling of epithelial cells, exfoliation, and necrosis. The glomeruli are generally uninvolved.

Antibiotics, such as the aminoglycoside gentamicin, and antifungal agents, such as amphotericin B, often cause renal insufficiency by a direct nephrotoxic effect. They produce an acute tubular necrosis that is

indistinguishable from that seen in shock or mercuric chloride poisoning. This type of injury, which is limited to the tubules and the interstitium, is usually dose related.

Chronic tubulointerstitial renal disease can be caused by the heavy usage of analgesic compounds that contain phenacetin. This disease is prevalent in Australia and western Europe but accounts for less than 2% of patients with end-stage renal failure in the United States. Analgesic nephropathy is seen most frequently in middle-aged women who have a history of personality disorders and chronic headaches. The minimal requirement for the development of renal damage is the consumption of 2 kg to 3 kg of phenacetin over a period of 3 years. Symptoms, which tend to occur only in the late stages of the disease, include premature aging, a brownish discoloration of the skin, an inability to concentrate the urine, metabolic acidosis, and anemia. Sloughing of necrotic papillary tips into the renal pelvis may result in colic. Radiographically, bilateral papillary necrosis in different stages of development can be detected.

In advanced stages of chronic tubulointerstitial disease caused by analgesic abuse, both kidneys are shrunken equally. Retracted cortical scars overlie necrotic papillae. Nearly all the papillae exhibit a variably dense consistency and brownish discoloration, evidence of different stages of necrosis. Early microscopic changes, which are confined to the papillae and the inner medulla, consist of patchy necrosis of the cells of the loops of Henle and focal widening of the interstitium. These necrotic areas eventually become confluent and extend to the corticomedullary junction, after which the collecting ducts become involved. There are characteristically few inflammatory cells around the necrotic foci. Eventually the entire papilla becomes necrotic, often remaining in place as a structureless mass. In such circumstances, dystrophic calcification of the necrotic papilla is common. Other papillae show incomplete detachment of the clefts at the demarcation zone, or they may be completely sloughed. There is an associated secondary tubular atrophy in the overlying cortex, as well as diffuse interstitial fibrosis. A distinctive feature in this condition is a homogeneous thickening of the walls of the capillaries immediately beneath the transitional epithelium of the entire urinary tract. In addition, the mucosal membranes of the lower urinary tract display a brownish discoloration.

The pathogenesis of analgesic nephropathy is not clear. Possibilities include a direct nephrotoxicity of the agents ingested or ischemic damage as a result of drug-induced vascular changes.

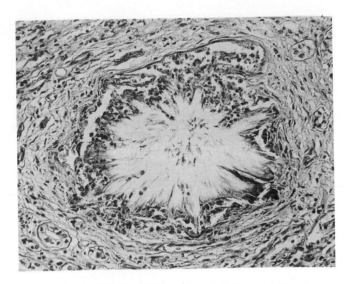

Figure 16-48. Urate nephropathy. A light micrograph shows radially arranged urate crystals that are surrounded by a chronic inflammatory reaction that includes foreign body giant cells at the periphery.

Urate Nephropathy

Any condition associated with elevated levels of uric acid in the blood may lead to a urate nephropathy. The classic disease in this category is primary gout, in which the biochemical basis of the hyperuricemia has not been established. At least as common today are those disorders in which hyperuricemia reflects an increased cell turnover (e.g., leukemia and polycythemia). Chemotherapy for malignant tumors can result in a sudden increase in blood uric acid, owing to the massive necrosis of cancer cells. Diseases that interfere with the excretion of uric acid can also result in hyperuricemia, as after the chronic intake of certain diuretics. Chronic lead intoxication also interferes with the proximal tubular secretion of uric acid and leads to saturnine gout.

Urate nephropathy can present as either acute renal failure or as chronic tubulointerstitial disease. The acute form is often associated with the treatment of malignant diseases with cytotoxic agents. The catabolism by the liver of large amounts of purines released from the DNA of necrotic cells leads to hyperuricemia. Acute renal failure reflects the obstruction of the collecting ducts by precipitated crystals of uric acid. The precipitated uric acid in the collecting ducts is seen grossly as yellow streaks in the papillae. Histologically, the tubular deposits appear amorphic, but in frozen sections the crystalline structure is apparent. The tubules proximal to the obstruction are

dilated. Some collecting ducts are penetrated by uric acid crystals, which provoke a foreign body giant cell reaction (Fig. 16-48).

Chronic gout can result in chronic tubulointerstitial nephropathy caused by the tubular and interstitial deposition of crystalline monosodium urate. The basic disease process is similar to that of acute urate nephropathy, but the prolonged course results in a more substantial deposition of urate crystals in the interstitium, interstitial fibrosis, and cortical atrophy. Although renal lesions are found in most individuals with chronic gout, a significant compromise of renal function is seen in fewer than half of such cases. It should be noted that chronic renal disease itself may lead to hyperuricemia and secondary gout.

Uric acid stones occur in 20% of patients with chronic gout and in 40% of those with acute hyperuricemia. Uric acid stones are not uncommon, accounting for one tenth of all cases of urolithiasis.

Nephrocalcinosis

Calcium deposits in the kidney are not uncommon, having been reported in as many as one fifth of kidneys at autopsy and in many renal biopsies, particularly in children. These incidental deposits are usually insignificant morphologically and are not associated with any functional alterations. By contrast, significant degrees of calcification are seen in conditions associated with hypercalcemia or with injury localized to the kidney (Table 16-3). The extent

Table 16-3. Causes of Nephrocalcinosis

Increased resorption of calcium from bone
Primary hyperparathyroidism
Multiple myeloma
Bone metastases
Paraneoplastic hypercalcemia (bronchogenic carcinoma, renal cell carcinoma)

Increased absorption of calcium from the gastrointestinal tract
Sarcoidosis
Hypervitaminosis D
Milk-alkali syndrome
Idiopathic hypercalcemia

Renal osteodystrophy

Dystrophic calcification
Previous toxic renal injury
Previous acute vascular injury (cortical necrosis, acute tubular necrosis)
Renal tubular acidosis

of calcification varies from mild, microscopically visible deposits to marked calcium accumulation visible grossly and radiologically. Nephrocalcinosis secondary to hypercalcemia may be accompanied by calcium deposition elsewhere in the body (e.g., in alveolar walls and blood vessels).

In conditions that produce hypercalcemia—namely, those associated with either increased resorption of calcium from bone or an increased intestinal absorption of calcium—the accompanying nephrocalcinosis reflects the increased filtration and concentration of calcium by the kidneys. The calcification seen after necrosis caused by drugs or vascular insults is probably due to dystrophic calcification of dead tissue. In the face of severe hypercalcemia, typified by primary hyperparathyroidism, gross examination characteristically reveals wedge-shaped scars adjacent to normal renal tissue. These scars do not result from vascular obstruction but reflect tubular atrophy and dilatation with interstitial fibrosis secondary to obstruction of the larger collecting tubules by calcium concretions. Microscopically, there is also a striking calcification of the basement membranes of the renal tubules, particularly those of the proximal convoluted tubules. Surrounding the tubules the interstitial tissue also displays calcium deposits. Scattered glomeruli show calcification of Bowman's capsule, and the walls of intrarenal arteries may be similarly affected. With hematoxylin, renal calcium deposits are deeply basophilic, and with the more specific von Kossa stain, they are black. By electron microscopy the mitochondria of renal tubular epithelial cells contain abundant calcium deposits.

Some patients with nephrocalcinosis caused by hypercalcemia have impaired renal function, but the relative contributions of renal calcification and hypercalcemia have not been resolved. The focal tubular obstruction and cortical scarring make the kidney more vulnerable to pyelonephritis.

Hypokalemic Nephropathy

Renal function is impaired in hypokalemic states, whether complicating intrinsic renal disease or resulting from gastrointestinal disorders, overproduction of adrenal hormones, or other causes (e.g., diabetic ketoacidosis or the use of certain diuretics). The cause of renal malfunction in hypokalemia is a disturbance in the tubular concentrating mechanism.

The most frequently described morphologic abnormality is the appearance of large, clear vacuoles

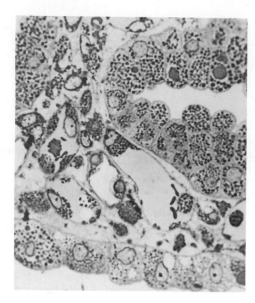

Figure 16-49.   Hypokalemic nephropathy in the rat. A light micrograph demonstrates prominent lysosomes that fill the cytoplasm of all the cells at the tip of the papilla. The lysosomes contain phospholipid and regress rapidly on potassium repletion.

in the epithelial cells of the proximal convoluted tubule. This lesion is nonspecific and is not present in many cases. There continues to be debate as to whether it actually represents an artefact of inadequate fixation. In contrast, potassium-depleted rats display a distinctive renal lesion. Prominent, phospholipid-filled lysosomes are present in all cells at the tips of the papillae (Fig. 16-49). The appearance of this lesion is associated with an impaired ability to concentrate the urine. Lowered concentrations of sodium in the medullary interstitium presumably interferes with the countercurrent exchange mechanism, an alteration that results in a dilute urine. The morphologic and functional changes are rapidly reversible on the resupply of potassium.

Acute Tubular Necrosis

Acute tubular necrosis is the most frequent cause of the clinical syndrome of acute renal failure. Clinical recognition of the condition is important because in less severe cases it is reversible. In the majority of patients it results in a rapid deterioration of renal function characterized by oliguria that may last from 4 days to 4 weeks. This is followed by a diuretic stage, in which there is relief of the oliguria but persistent severe tubular dysfunction. Classic microdissection

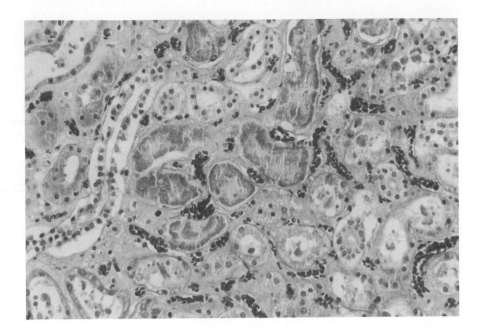

Figure 16-50. Acute tubular necrosis. A light micrograph illustrates early necrosis with a pattern of variable nuclear disruption. The casts in the lumina are disrupted cells.

studies have suggested that there are two patterns of tubular injury: ischemic (tubulorrhexic) necrosis and nephrotoxin-induced injury. It is usually not possible to distinguish between these two patterns in routine biopsy material, despite the fact that they occur by different mechanisms. Any event that precipitates shock, either hypovolemic or endotoxic shock, often results in ischemic acute tubular necrosis. Such events include trauma, hemorrhage, burns, dehydration, and sepsis. Toxic acute tubular necrosis was historically associated with acute mercuric chloride poisoning as a form of suicide. More recently, the disorder has been caused by a number of antibiotics and cancer chemotherapeutic agents, and ethylene glycol, a potent tubular toxin, has been used to adulterate wine, causing a number of deaths in Austria and Italy.

The morphologic changes in ischemic tubular necrosis and in most cases of nephrotoxin-induced injury are subtle, and the absence of substantial morphologic changes led early investigators to propose that the damage actually was in the medulla. The condition was therefore termed "lower-nephron nephrosis". In fact, most of the tubular changes, which may be quite patchy, are seen in the border zone between the outer medulla and the cortex. Both the straight terminal portion of the proximal convoluted tubule and the medullary thick ascending limb of Henle's loop show morphologic changes. These alterations include shedding and necrosis of epithelial cells (Fig. 16-50) and sloughing of cellular debris into the tubular lumina, which results in the formation of hyaline and granular casts in the distal tubules and the collecting ducts of the papillae. Differentiation of proximal from distal tubules becomes difficult because of dedifferentiation of the injured tubules and loss of the PAS-positive brush border. More severe lesions that have resulted in a substantial amount of atrophy may exhibit tubular dilatation. Later in the development of the lesion, re-epithelialization of the tubules is manifested by a flat, cuboidal epithelial lining that has frequent mitotic figures. Since this regenerated epithelium is functional, therapy is directed toward supporting the vital functions of the patient until this stage is reached. Finally, there is a distinct morphologic feature, the origin of which is unknown, which consists of lymphocytes, monocytes, and neutrophils in the vasa recta of the medulla.

Although the correlation between the clinical course and the morphologic changes is not perfect, in general a more severely oliguric patient shows more severe tubular necrosis, and in the most severe case, complete renal cortical necrosis.

The cause of the decreased renal function and oliguria in acute tubular necrosis is not well understood. In all probability a combination of the following is important: leakage of tubular fluid back through the damaged epithelial lining, tubular obstruction due to sloughing of necrotic epithelial cells, and arteriolar vasoconstriction, which shunts blood away from the cortex (Fig. 16-51).

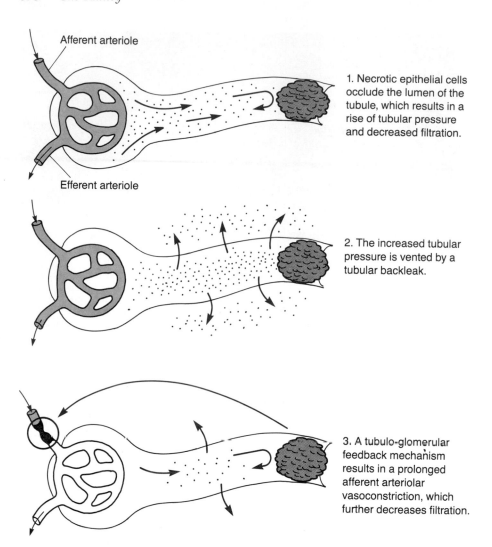

Afferent arteriole

Efferent arteriole

1. Necrotic epithelial cells occlude the lumen of the tubule, which results in a rise of tubular pressure and decreased filtration.

2. The increased tubular pressure is vented by a tubular backleak.

3. A tubulo-glomerular feedback mechanism results in a prolonged afferent arteriolar vasoconstriction, which further decreases filtration.

Figure 16-51.   Pathogenesis of oliguria in acute tubular necrosis.

Vascular Diseases

Hypertension

Like many clinical phenomena seen with renal disorders, hypertension is the single expression of many pathogenetic pathways. Some degree of renal vascular disease is usual in patients with prolonged hypertension, and it may be severe enough to cause renal failure. No definition is completely accepted for hypertension, but a diastolic reading of 95 mm Hg has been suggested as an indication for therapy.

Hypertension is separated into benign and malignant forms. **Malignant hypertension** occurs more frequently in men than in women, typically around the age of 40. Blacks are particularly susceptible to this form of accelerated hypertension. The diastolic pressure is generally above 115 mm Hg. Headache and unusual mental disturbances occur frequently, as does a characteristic retinopathy. Acute and chronic renal failure are common. The pathologic changes of benign nephrosclerosis relate to the consequences of ischemia. Ischemic glomeruli display irregular changes that are distinctly different from those of intrinsic glomerular disease (e.g., glomerulonephritis). Moreover, totally obliterated glomeruli may be located beside completely normal ones. Initially, the glomerular capillaries are thickened and shriveled. Cells of the glomerular tuft are progressively lost, and collagen and matrix material are deposited within Bowman's space, most prominently, distant from the hilus. Eventually the glomerular tuft is rep-

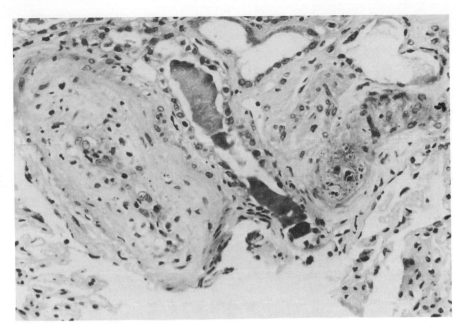

Figure 16-52. Malignant hypertension. A light micrograph illustrates interlobular arteries that show a near-obliteration of the lumina with marked intimal thickening. There is a prominent fluid and cellular exudate in the vessel wall.

resented by a dense, eosinophilic globular mass enclosed in a scar, all within Bowman's capsule. Tubular atrophy, a consequence of the obsolescence of the glomerulus, is associated with fibrosis of the related interstitium. The pattern of change in the blood vessels depends on the size of vessel involved. Large arteries down to the size of the arcuate arteries show arteriosclerotic changes of the intima, splitting of the internal elastic lamina, and partial replacement of the muscular coat with fibrous tissue. Interlobular arteries show medial hypertrophy, in addition to similar changes. Arterioles display hyaline thickening of the entire wall.

Malignant nephrosclerosis shows many of the same sclerotic changes described previously, but in addition the glomeruli frequently exhibit fibrinoid necrosis, sometimes in continuity with a necrotizing lesion of the preglomerular arteriole. Subtotal infarction of glomeruli, with dilated capillaries stuffed with red blood cells, is common. Usually less than half of the glomeruli show acute, necrotizing, inflammatory lesions. The arterioles exhibit fibrinoid necrosis, whereas in the larger arteries the lumen is markedly reduced in size by profuse intimal thickening, owing to cellular proliferation and the accumulation of a myxoid matrix (Fig. 16-52). Morphologic diagnosis of these hypertension-related lesions is usually straightforward, but the vascular changes can be mimicked by those seen with extensive parenchymal loss, as in vascular sclerosis of disuse in advanced kidney disease.

Renal Vasculitis

Vasculitis is a general descriptive term that, like *glomerulonephritis*, is used in both a clinical and pathologic sense. The diagnosis is generally made by the recognition of a vasculitis syndrome, which is further defined by biopsy pathology and the radiologic features. The clinical course of the systemic vasculitis of polyarteritis is variable. More than half of those affected have an aggressive disease, but in many the disease exhibits a self-limited course if they survive the initial onslaught. About 25% of patients have chronic or relapsing disease, and late deaths are frequently due to vascular catastrophies in a number of organs, complications of hypertension, or renal failure.

Treatment remains controversial, and the administration of corticosteroids is ineffective in many cases. Sustained remissions have been reported with immunosuppression by cyclophosphamide. Newer therapy includes plasmapheresis and cytotoxic drugs and emphasizes the importance of an early vigorous approach to the treatment of systemic vasculitis. The morphologic features that aid in classification emphasize the size and type of involved vessels. Medium-sized arteries exhibit the major lesions (Fig. 16-53) in classic **polyarteritis nodosa.** The small arteries are characteristically involved in the **hypersensitivity vasculitides.** Renal involvement may entail focal or diffuse glomerulonephritis, frequently with crescents and a rapidly progressive glomerulonephritis. A fea-

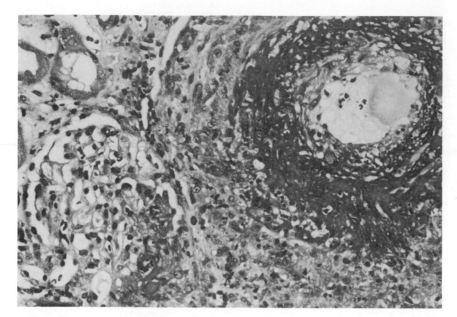

Figure 16-53. Polyarteritis nodosa. A light micrograph demonstrates the focal arterial lesion of polyarteritis. A large area of fibrinoid necrosis is surrounded by a cellular exudate rich in neutrophils.

ture that may help to distinguish this condition from other forms of glomerulonephritis is the focal arteritis that affects interlobular arteries and, frequently, arterioles (Fig. 16-53). Fibrinoid change is conspicuous in areas of acute focal necrosis, and there are neutrophils and eosinophils in the damaged areas. Arterial thrombosis results in infarction. Fibrin is conspicuous in areas of necrosis, in crescents, and in the lumens of affected arteries, as well as in the reactive media of the arteries.

Wegener's granulomatosis, a condition related to polyarteritis nodosa, is characterized by a necrotizing granulomatous lesion and vasculitis of the upper and lower respiratory tract, crescentic glomerulonephritis, and disseminated small vessel arteritis. The untreated disease is rapidly fatal and death from renal failure occurs within a few months. Recently, the use of cyclophosphamide has appreciably improved the prognosis of Wegener's granulomatosis.

Microangiopathic Hemolytic Anemia

Microangiopathic hemolytic anemia occurs in a number of conditions, including the hemolytic uremic syndrome, thrombotic thrombocytopenic purpura, and systemic scleroderma. This type of nonimmune (Coomb's negative) hemolytic anemia is characterized by misshapen and disrupted red blood cells, thrombocytopenia, and fibrin deposition in the walls and lumina of small arteries and arterioles in many organs, but particularly prominent in the kidney. The red cell abnormalities and accompanying hemolysis, as well as the thrombocytopenia, are probably related to trauma within the damaged blood vessels.

Hemolytic Uremic Syndrome

Historically, the hemolytic uremic syndrome was considered to affect infants and children. Shortly after a nonspecific respiratory or gastrointestinal illness, the child suddenly develops anemia, bleeding, renal failure, neurologic abnormalities, and cardiovascular symptoms. No specific etiologic agent has been demonstrated. A major factor in the pathogenesis of this syndrome is endothelial damage associated with a deficiency of prostacyclin activator—a vasodilator and a potent inhibitor of platelet aggregation. Another important factor is intravascular coagulation, which also may relate to endothelial damage. In this respect thrombi composed of varying combinations of fibrin and platelets are often found within glomerular capillaries, arterioles, and small arteries. An additional, familiar childhood form with an autosomal dominant mode of inheritance has been reported. Since the original descriptions, the disease has been reported in adults, commonly in women who have used oral contraceptives or who suffer acute renal failure in the postpartum period. Treatment with drugs such as mitomycin and cyclosporin has also been implicated.

The glomerulus appears to be the principal site of damage in the kidney. Endothelial swelling is prominent, and foci of epithelial cell proliferation and even crescents appear. Mesangial cell proliferation may occur but is inconspicuous. By electron microscopy, a clear area of subendothelial widening, a foamy mesangial matrix, and some aneurysmal capillary dilation are prominent (Fig. 16-54). Thrombi are variably present in glomeruli. The preglomerular arterioles display focal damage, with insudation of fibrin and red blood cells and thrombosis. Neutrophils may be present but are not prominent. The reasons for the preferential localization of this disease to the kidney have not been elucidated. If, as seems likely, endothelial damage is the initiating event, then the specialized endothelium of the glomerulus may be particularly vulnerable.

The infantile and childhood type, which frequently has only glomerular lesions, is associated with complete recovery in the large majority of cases, with a mortality of less than 5%. The adult and postpartum type usually presents with involvement of glomeruli, afferent arterioles, and interlobular arteries. The prognosis is more guarded, and a fatal outcome is seen in 60% of the cases. Recent attention has been focused on the beneficial effect of plasma exchange, a procedure that is assumed to supply the missing plasma component.

Thrombotic Thrombocytopenic Purpura

Thrombotic thrombocytopenic purpura is a microangiopathic disease that is morphologically difficult, if not impossible, to distinguish from the adult form of the hemolytic uremic syndrome. It differs in that it is generally seen in an older age group, has a lesser involvement of the kidney, affects many organs (particularly the central nervous system), and has a worse prognosis. The characteristic clinical features of thrombotic thrombocytopenic purpura include a low platelet count with bleeding (skin, gastrointestinal tract, genitourinary tract, and retina), hemolytic anemia, neurologic abnormalities, fever, and renal disease. As in the adult hemolytic uremic syndrome, women are more commonly affected than men. The disease is usually fatal, but an occasional patient survives. Although many subtle renal changes have been described, the lesions of thrombotic thrombocytopenic purpura are, at best, difficult to differentiate from those of the hemolytic uremic syndrome.

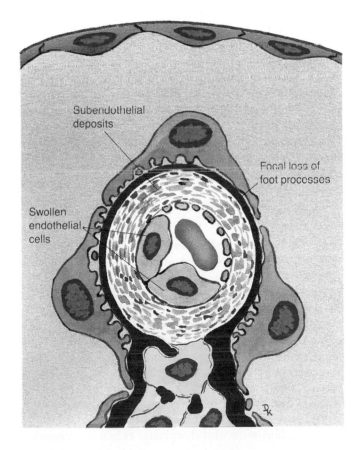

Figure 16-54. Hemolytic uremic syndrome. A wide band of subendothelial electron-lucent material narrows the capillary lumen. Moderate endothelial cell proliferation and focal irregular areas of endothelial cell swelling contribute to narrowing of the lumen. Focal effacement of epithelial foot processes is noted.

Systemic Scleroderma (Progressive Systemic Sclerosis)

Systemic scleroderma is a disease in which there is deposition of collagen, typically in the skin but also in other organs such as the gastrointestinal tract, lungs, and heart. Vascular changes, particularly in the fingers (Raynaud's phenomenon) and the kidney, virtually always develop. The disease shares certain immunologic abnormalities with systemic lupus erythematosis, dermatomyositis, and mixed connective tissue disease, but an immune pathogenesis has not been proved.

In scleroderma complicated by renal involvement, microangiopathic hemolytic anemia is related to vascular changes in the kidney. Azotemia, severe hypertension, and renal failure are common and indicate a grave prognosis.

The smaller arterial vessels—namely, the interlobular and afferent arterioles—are the sites of the characteristic lesions. In the interlobular arteries, the lumen is narrowed by loose fibrous tissue in which nuclei are disposed in a concentric fashion. The proliferated tissue shows a mucinous appearance, which reflects the presence of hyaluronic acid. Fibrin is deposited within the thickened intima. Small fibrin thrombi are occasionally seen in the lumen. Conspicuous fibrin deposition, severe enough to be termed fibrinoid necrosis, is seen in the afferent arterioles. These vascular changes may result in small infarcts. Changes in the glomeruli are variable. Some are intensely congested and even infarcted, whereas other glomeruli appear normal. The glomerular capillary basement membrane may be thickened. No consistent pattern of immune deposits has been documented.

Renovascular Hypertension

The total occlusion of a main renal artery produces a type of hypertension that is potentially curable by reconstitution of the arterial lumen. The initial experiments that led to the understanding of this syndrome were carried out in rats a half century ago by Goldblatt, and since that time the kidney totally deprived of vascular supply has been known as the Goldblatt kidney. Ninety percent to 95% of the cases are caused by lesions of atherosclerosis. This lesion is two times more likely to occur in men than in women and is seen in older age groups (average 55 years). The other major lesion that produces this syndrome is fibromuscular dysplasia. When the vascular occlusion is related to atherosclerosis, aortic plaques impinge on the ostium and narrow the proximal portion of the renal artery, more frequently on the left than on the right. Occasionally, atherosclerotic aneurysms of the abdominal aorta compromise the origin of the renal arteries. By contrast, the lesion of renal artery dysplasia consists of a fibrous and fibromuscular stenosis of the renal artery that is not atherosclerotic, is more common in women, and occurs at a younger age (average age 35 years). In this variety of vascular occlusion, the involvement of arterial branches often makes revascularization impossible.

There are several patterns of renal artery involvement that are conveniently lumped under the heading of fibromuscular dysplasia. The most common variety is characterized by bilateral fibrosis of the media of the distal two-thirds of the renal artery and its main branches. In some cases, the fibrosis is principally in the other one-third to two-thirds of the media, and the irregular pattern results in a beaded appearance on an angiogram. In these cases, which may be bilateral or unilateral, the intima is typically spared. In about 10% of cases hypercellularity in short lengths of the media of the renal artery results in marked stenosis while the other layers of the artery are not affected. Although the condition frequently does not worsen in those individuals who display principally fibrosis, the subgroup with medial hyperplasia often exhibits clinical progression. Rarely, the principal lesion is intimal fibroplasia, which consists of an accumulation of loose, cellular fibrous tissue. Reduplication of the internal elastic lamina is common.

Whether vascular occlusion is caused by atherosclerosis or by fibromuscular dysplasia, the involved kidney typically is reduced only slightly in size. The glomeruli, the arteries, and the arterioles all appear normal. Focal tubular atrophy is often noted. The juxtaglomerular apparatus is prominent and demonstrates hyperplasia, increased granularity, and a greater length.

The pathogenesis of hypertension in cases of renal artery stenosis relates to the hyperplasia of the juxtaglomerular apparatus (Fig. 16-55) and the resulting increase in the production of renin, angiotensin II, and aldosterone. Whereas plasma renin activity is conspicuously increased in the renal vein from the compromised kidney, the renin content of venous blood from the contralateral kidney is reduced. The ischemic kidney secretes excess renin and retains sodium and water, but the intact one loses both. However, the predominant effect is exerted by the ischemic kidney and is related to an elevation of blood

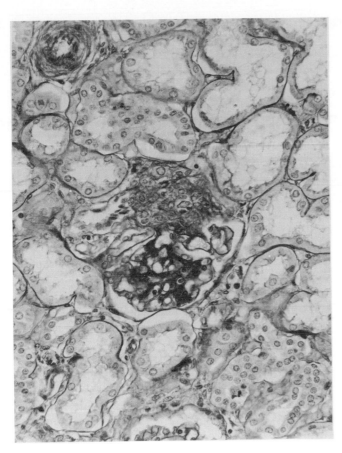

Figure 16-55. Hyperplasia of the juxtaglomerular apparatus in a patient with renovascular hypertension.

pressure. The hypertension is reversible on reconstitution of the blood supply to the ischemic kidney, and in about half of the cases, hypertension is cured either by surgical revascularization or nephrectomy. Yet, in long-standing renovascular hypertension, even the unprotected kidney may be sufficiently damaged by hypertensive vascular changes to sustain hypertension.

Renal Infarcts

Renal infarcts for the most part are caused by arterial obstruction, and the majority represent embolization to the branches of the main renal artery. Typically, an acute infarct is manifested clinically as sharp flank or abdominal pain and hematuria. The size of the infarct varies with the size of the occluded vessel. Common sources of emboli include mural thrombi overlying myocardial infarcts or, in longstanding fibrillation, located on the atrial wall; infected valves in bacterial endocarditis; and complicated atherosclerotic plaques in the aorta. Occasionally, a branch of

the renal artery is occluded by thrombosis superimposed on an underlying atherosclerosis or polyarteritis nodosa. The lumina of the small branches of the renal artery may be so severely compromised in malignant hypertension, scleroderma, or the hemolytic uremic syndrome that the blood supply is insufficient to maintain the viability of the tissue. Occlusion of small vessels by sickled erythrocytes in sickle cell anemia commonly causes infarcts, especially in the papillae. Hemorrhagic renal infarction caused by renal vein thrombosis may complicate severe dehydration, particularly in small infants, but is also seen in adults with septic thrombophlebitis and conditions associated with hypercoagulability.

Variably sized, wedge-shaped areas of ischemic necrosis with the base on the capsular surface are typical. All structures within the affected zone are necrotic. Acute infarcts are bordered by a hemorrhagic zone. Healed infarcts are sharply circumscribed and depressed cortical scars containing obliterated glomeruli, atrophic tubules, interstitial fibrosis, and a mild chronic inflammatory infiltrate. Dystrophic calcification is occasionally encountered in old infarcts. At the margins of a healed infarct, the viable tissue resembles that seen in chronic ischemia or in chronic pyelonephritis. In some cases, proliferation of glomerular epithelial cells is common and may be so severe as to form a crescent. These changes may be confused with an intrinsic glomerular disease in renal biopsies.

A distinctive form of embolization is that characterized by the presence of debris from complicated aortic atherosclerotic plaques, especially from aneurysms of the abdominal aorta. The atherosclerotic origin of the emboli is evidenced by needle-shaped clefts of cholesterol crystals within the occluding embolus.

Infarction of an entire kidney by occlusion of the main renal artery is uncommon. When the main renal artery is occluded, it is more common for the kidney to remain viable because of collateral circulation. Clearly, in such a circumstance renal function ceases.

Recurrent infarction may lead to a shrunken end-stage kidney difficult to distinguish from that of chronic pyelonephritis. If enough renal parenchyma is lost, hypertension and renal failure may ensue.

Bilateral Cortical Necrosis

Bilateral cortical necrosis refers to necrosis of part or all of the renal cortex with sparing of the medulla. Historically, the most common clinical circumstance

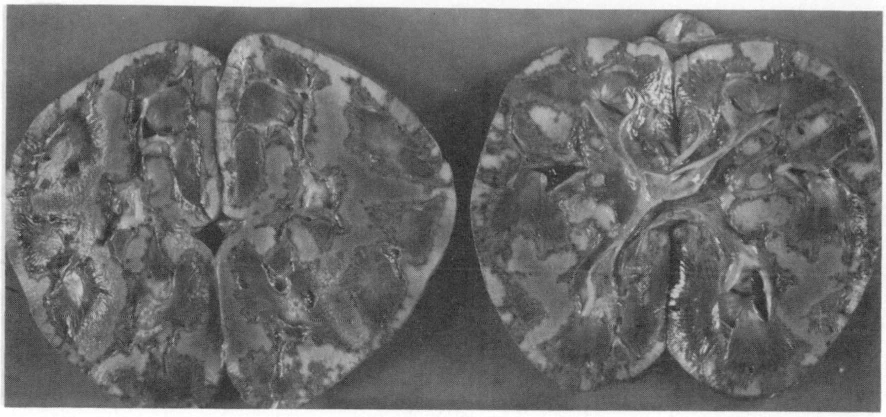

Figure 16-56. Bilateral cortical necrosis in a 22-year-old woman who died from gram-negative septicemia complicating a septic abortion. The necrotic cortex is paler than the rest of the parenchyma.

associated with renal cortical necrosis has been the premature separation of the placenta (abruptio placentae), a complication of the third trimester of pregnancy. Renal cortical necrosis can also complicate any clinical condition associated with hypovolemic or endotoxic shock, and it has been reported with ethylene glycol (antifreeze) poisoning. Since all forms of shock are associated with acute tubular necrosis, it is not surprising that there is an overlap between this syndrome and cortical necrosis, both clinically and pathologically.

In cortical necrosis the lesion is ischemic in origin. The vasa recta that supply arterial blood to the medulla arise from the arcuate and juxtamedullary interlobular arteries proximal to the vessels supplying the outer cortex. Occlusion of the outer cortical vessels by vasospasm or fibrin thrombin will lead to cortical necrosis and spare the medulla. Experimentally, vasoconstrictors, such as vasopressin and serotonin, produce cortical necrosis. The experimental Shwartzman phenomenon, which is characterized by disseminated intravascular coagulation with widespread fibrin thrombi, also causes cortical necrosis. The relative contribution of each of these factors to the pathogenesis of human cortical necrosis is not entirely clear, and it may vary, depending on the cause of the disease.

The extent of the necrosis varies from focal to patchy to confluent. In the mildest variety, scattered areas of cortical necrosis less than 1 mm in diameter are seen. Within these foci necrosis of some of the glomeruli with thrombosis of the vascular pole occurs. The proximal convoluted tubules are invariably necrotic, as are most of the distal tubules. In the viable portions of the cortex, the glomeruli and distal convoluted tubules are unaffected, but many of the proximal convoluted tubules are necrotic. In the confluent case, the cortex is diffusely necrotic (Fig. 16-56) bilaterally except for thin rims of viable tissue immediately beneath the capsule and at the corticomedullary junction. In patients who survive, striking dystrophic calcification of the necrotic areas may develop.

Clinically, severe cortical necrosis leads to acute renal failure, which is indistinguishable from that produced by acute tubular necrosis. Recovery is determined by the extent of the disease, but there is a significant incidence of hypertension in those who survive.

Sickle Cell Nephropathy

Apart from the hematologic abnormalities, the most common manifestations of sickle cell disease and sickle cell trait are renal changes. The interstitial tissue in which the vasa recta course is hypertonic and has a low oxygen tension. As a result the erythrocytes in the vasa recta tend to sickle and occlude the lumen. Infarcts in the medulla and papilla ensue, sometimes severe enough to cause papillary necrosis. Hematuria frequently accompanies these events, and in most cases tubular concentrating ability is impaired. The glomeruli are conspicuously congested with sickle cells. A membranoproliferative glomerulonephritis, seen in occasional patients, may be accompanied by the nephrotic syndrome. Some have attributed this glomerulonephritis to the deposition of immune complexes containing tubular epithelial antigens, but this is controversial. Ischemic scarring of the medulla leads to focal tubular loss and atrophy. Iron deposits may be present in epithelial cells of the tubules, and regenerating epithelial cells exhibit mitoses.

Toxemia of Pregnancy

Pre-eclampsia is a complication of the third trimester of pregnancy and is defined by the triad of hypertension, proteinuria, and edema. When these are complicated by convulsions, the term *eclampsia* is applied. These two conditions are subsumed under the rubric of toxemia. The pathogenesis is discussed in the chapter on gynecologic pathology (Chapter 18).

The kidney is invariably involved in pre-eclampsia. The glomeruli are uniformly enlarged, and the endothelial cells are swollen (Fig. 16-57), which results in an apparently bloodless glomerular tuft. An increase in the number and size of mesangial cells is usual. By electron microscopy the swollen endothelial and mesangial cells contain large, irregular vacuoles. Vacuoles are also present in the foot processes and the trabeculae of the epithelial cells. Fibrin can be demonstrated along the inside of the capillary walls between the endothelial cell and the basement membrane.

In the past, pre-eclampsia and eclampsia were feared complications of pregnancy. The disease is uncommon today, presumably because of improved prenatal care and management of hypertension. When pre-eclampsia does occur, the lesions are usually entirely reversible.

Hydronephrosis

Hydronephrosis is defined as dilatation of the renal pelvis and calyces, flattening of the papillae, and atrophy of the renal cortex. Hydronephrosis is always the result of urinary tract obstruction, whether from tumors, stones, vesicoureteral reflux, or other obstruction. The causes of urinary tract obstruction are discussed in detail in the chapter on urologic pathology (Chapter 17).

In early hydronephrosis, the most prominent finding is dilatation of the collecting ducts, followed by dilatation of the proximal and distal convoluted tubules. Eventually the proximal tubules become widely dilated, and loss of tubules is common. Interestingly, the glomeruli are usually spared. As discussed previously, the hydronephrotic kidney is more susceptible to pyelonephritis.

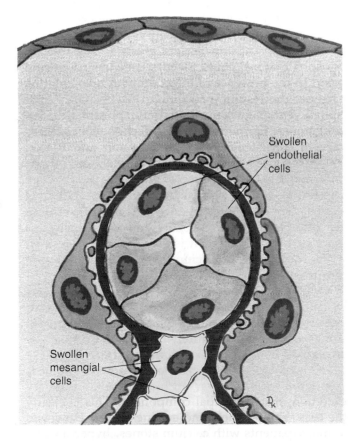

Figure 16-57. Pre-eclamptic nephropathy. Pre-eclamptic nephropathy, or pregnancy-induced nephropathy, exhibits marked swelling of endothelial cells with narrowing of the lumina. Both endothelial and mesangial cells are enlarged and have multiple vacuoles and vesicular structures.

17

The Urinary Tract and Male Reproductive System

Robert O. Petersen

Renal Pelvis and Ureter

Urinary Bladder

Urethra

Testis

Testicular Adnexa

Prostate

Penis

Scrotum

Figure 17-1. Embryologic development of the urinary tract and male reproductive system.

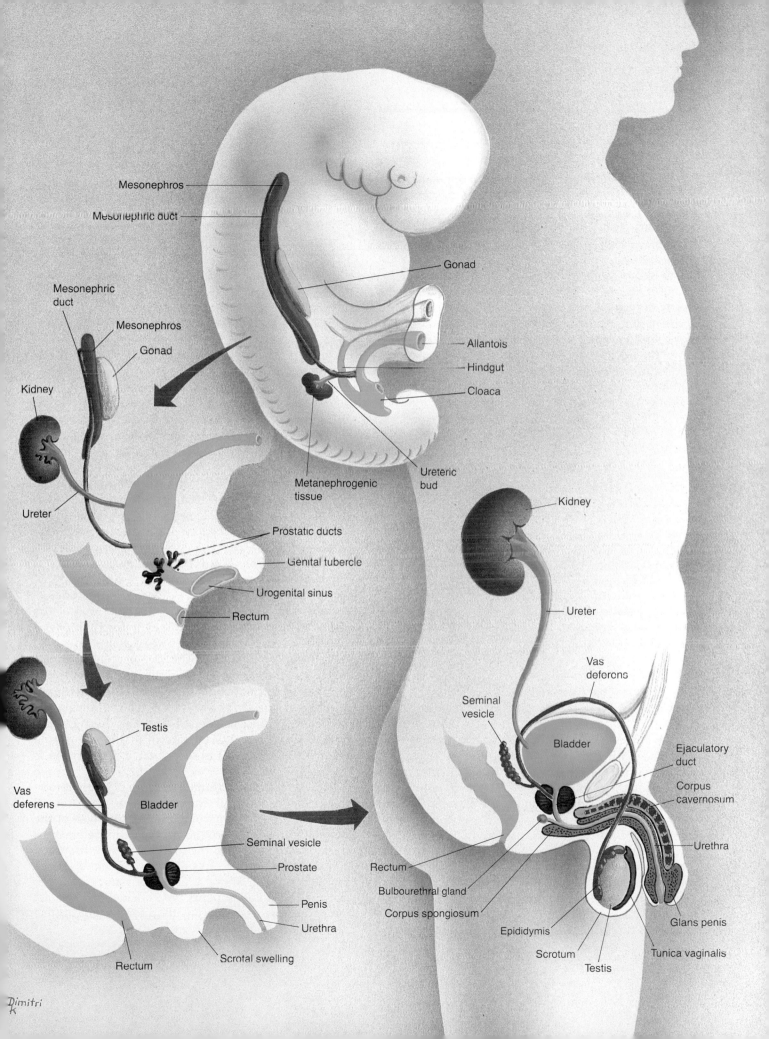

Mesonephros

Mesonephric duct

Gonad

Mesonephric duct

Mesonephros

Gonad

Allantois

Hindgut

Cloaca

Kidney

Ureter

Metanephrogenic tissue

Ureteric bud

Kidney

Prostatic ducts

Genital tubercle

Urogenital sinus

Rectum

Ureter

Vas deferens

Seminal vesicle

Testis

Bladder

Ejaculatory duct

Corpus cavernosum

Vas deferens

Bladder

Seminal vesicle

Prostate

Penis

Urethra

Rectum

Bulbourethral gland

Corpus spongiosum

Urethra

Glans penis

Epididymis

Scrotum

Testis

Tunica vaginalis

Rectum

Scrotal swelling

Dimitri
K

Renal Pelvis and Ureter

Normal Structure

The mucosa of the caliceal system and renal pelvis is composed of a transitional epithelium of two to three cell layers, increasing to three to five cell layers in the ureter. The epithelium is attached to a basement membrane. The lamina propria is evident only in the ureters, where it is composed of loose collagenous fibers and thin-walled vessels. In the renal pelvis the tissue immediately subjacent to the basement membrane is the renal pelvic smooth muscle, which is arranged in a spiral continuous with the musculature of the ureter. Historically, the ureteral smooth muscle has been described as consisting of two layers: the inner longitudinal and the outer circular. More recent studies, using serial cross sections of the ureter, describe the muscles as organized in interlacing spirals without well-defined layers. In the distal ureter an additional longitudinal muscle layer is observed between the circular muscle bundles and the adventitia. Contraction of the muscle layers of the ureter produces the stellate lumen characteristic of cross sections of this structure. External to the muscularis of both the renal pelvis and the ureter is a well-vascularized, loose fibroadipose tissue of the adventitia within the retroperitoneum.

The vascular supply to the renal pelvis and ureter is from branches of the renal, gonadal, and common iliac arteries, which have numerous anastomoses. The lymphatic drainage of the renal pelvis and proximal ureter is to the regional periaortic lymph nodes (lateral lumbar nodes); that of the distal ureter is to the internal iliac lymph nodes.

Embryology

The structure that ultimately develops into the ureter and renal pelvis—the metanephric duct—emerges from the distal mesonephric duct at a point near its entrance into the cloaca (Fig. 17-1). The metanephric duct, beginning as the metanephric diverticulum, grows cephalad after a mass of mesenchyme (metanephrogenic mesenchyme) envelops its blind end. The metanephric duct induces the development of nephrons in this metanephric mesenchyme. The metanephric duct and the differentiating metanephric mesenchyme migrate cephalad as a unit. The metanephric mesenchyme induces the blind end of the metanephric duct to subdivide, progressively forming the major and minor calices. The latter give rise to the collecting tubules, which ultimately connect with the tubular system of the nephron.

After the metanephric duct has developed, the distal mesonephric duct from which it arose is partially absorbed into the lateral wall of the urogenital sinus, thus separating the ostia of the metanephric duct (which becomes the ureter) and the mesonephric duct (which becomes the male ejaculatory duct system). Ureteral muscle appears at twelve weeks of gestation and is present throughout the length of the ureter at eighteen weeks.

Congenital Disorders

A number of congenital disorders affect the renal pelvis and ureter. **Agenesis of a ureter** results from the failure of the metanephric diverticulum to develop from the mesonephric duct. It is associated in all cases with agenesis of the ipsilateral kidney. Conversely, the more common condition of **ureteral duplication** results either from formation of multiple metanephric buds (complete duplication) or from a premature bifurcation of a single bud (incomplete duplication). Most of such anomalies are unilateral.

Ectopic ureters reflect anomalous development of the distal mesonephric duct as it and the metanephric duct are absorbed into the lateral urogenital sinus. Because the distal mesonephric duct ultimately forms part of the proximal urethra, ejaculatory duct, seminal vesicle, and vas deferens, any abnormal juxtaposition of it and the ostium of the metanephric duct (which forms the ureter) may result in termination of the ureter into any of these mesonephric structures.

Diverticula are observed rarely in both the renal pelvis and ureter. A caliceal diverticulum is characterized by a cystic dilatation of a single calix of the kidney, which retains continuity with the uninvolved caliceal system through a narrow distal channel. In most instances, a calix of the upper pole of the affected kidney is involved. A congenital defect in the embryologic formation of the calix is the most probable underlying cause. Most caliceal diverticula are identified through incidental findings during retrograde pyelography. Only rarely do the diverticula enlarge to such a magnitude that a flank mass is observed.

A **ureteral diverticulum** is truly rare. True ureteral diverticula contain all components of the ureteral wall, including the muscularis within the wall of the diverticulum, and are round to oval extraureteral sacs that communicate with the ureteral lumen through a stoma. Such cases are regarded as congenital in origin. By contrast, those ureteral outpouchings that lack structural components are considered to be acquired defects associated with prior trauma, infection, calculi, or distal stricture.

Congenital ureteral valves, also rare, must be differentiated from acquired valves present in dilated, tortuous ureters, which are usually secondary to distal ureteral obstruction. True congenital ureteral valves show transverse folds of ureteral mucosa containing smooth muscle, and ureteral obstructive changes above the valve, with normal ureteral structure below it.

The term **congenital megaloureter** is a description applied to many distinct entities that have only recently been classified on the basis of etiology and pathogenesis. Regardless of the underlying cause, the markedly enlarged ureter is associated with hydronephrosis and ultimate renal function impairment if the structural defect is left uncorrected. No single pathologic abnormality is observed and the underlying causes are diverse.

Amyloidosis

Localized submucosal deposits of amyloid, unassociated with a plasma cell dyscrasia, have been reported in the renal pelvis and, more frequently, in the ureter. In most instances the distal ureter is involved. The clinical presentation generally relates to obstructive symptoms that result from the amyloid deposits. Occasionally such deposits are associated with foci of dystrophic calcification, a combination which assists in the radiologic diagnosis. The underlying cause remains unexplained.

Endometriosis

Endometriosis of the ureter is rare, and no equivalent lesions have been identified in the renal pelvis. The disorder is most commonly encountered in the fourth and fifth decades of life, but has been reported in women as young as 21 years of age. Rare examples have been observed in postmenopausal women in their sixth and seventh decades. Although ureteral involvement by endometriosis is usually unilateral, rare bilateral examples have been reported. When it occurs, endometriosis most commonly involves the lower one-third of the ureter, and concurrent involvement of the genital organs is frequent.

Endometriosis sufficiently severe to cause ureteral obstruction—and thus secondary obstruction with hydroureter and hydronephrosis (Fig. 17-2)—is usually extrinsic, with the lesion in the periureteral adventitia. Regardless of location, a focus of endometriosis invariably displays endometrial glands and stroma. Evidence of recent and old hemorrhage, in the form of hemosiderin, is frequently seen. The clin-

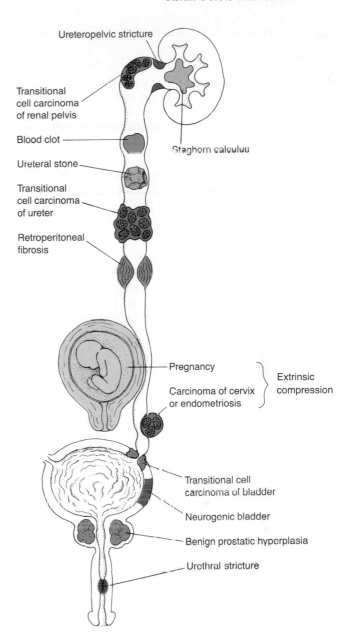

Figure 17-2. Causes of ureteral obstruction.

ical significance of ureteral endometriosis is the resultant ureteral obstruction. The treatment is surgical excision of the affected ureteral segment.

Inflammatory Disorders

Inflammatory disorders of the renal pelvis and ureter are most commonly associated with ascending infection, often as a complication of partial ureteral obstruction or associated with lithiasis. Frequently, inflammatory changes of the ipsilateral kidney (pyelonephritis) are observed, especially in association with intrapelvic lithiasis. In most instances gram-negative organisms are implicated. Uncommon causes of pyelitis and ureteritis include fungal organisms, schistosomiasis, radiation injury, and malacoplakia. The histologic findings are usually nonspecific and include a chronic inflammatory cell infiltrate of variable intensity in the lamina propria of the affected urinary tract segment. On occasion, mucosal ulceration is observed. With chronicity, associated changes of the urothelium include Brunn's buds, Brunn's nests, pyelitis cystica and glandularis, and ureteritis cystica and glandularis. (Metaplastic and proliferative variants of urothelium are discussed later in this chapter.) The histologic features of malacoplakia involving the renal pelvis and ureter are identical to those in the more common locations of malacoplakia, specifically the urinary bladder. The characteristic inclusions of malacoplakia, the Michaelis-Gutmann bodies, are identified by the PAS and von Kossa stains.

Fibroepithelial Polyps

Fibroepithelial polyps arise in the renal pelvis and the ureter, although rarely. These lesions are usually observed at the ureteropelvic junction or in the proximal one-third of the ureter. Fibroepithelial polyps have been variously regarded as congenital, inflammatory, hamartomatous, or neoplastic; synonyms include inflammatory polyp, fibroma, and hamartoma. Although most common in early adulthood, examples have been observed in children and in the elderly. A female predilection has been reported. Patients present with flank pain with or without hematuria.

Fibroepithelial polyps are smooth nodules or, alternatively, filiform projections, varying in size from a few millimeters to several centimeters. Their exophytic growth produces smooth-contoured filling defects when examined by retrograde pyelography. Histologically, the urothelium covering the centrally edematous stromal stalk is either normal or hyperplastic. The stroma contains collagen fibers, variable numbers of small blood vessels, and, on occasion, smooth muscle fibers. Acute and chronic inflammatory cells, focal hyalinization of the stroma, and calcification are all inconstant features. The absence of clinical and histologic evidence of inflammation in many cases suggests that the polyps do not have an inflammatory origin. The presence of smooth muscle in some lesions suggests that they may represent hamartomatous proliferations rather than true neoplasms. It is possible that some of these lesions evolve in a manner analogous to polypoid cystitis with stromal fibrosis.

Proliferative and Metaplastic Variants of Urothelium

The metaplastic and proliferative variants of urothelium, observed throughout the urinary tract (including the renal pelvis and ureter), have been the subject of considerable study, but their pathogenesis and clinical significance remain unsettled. These lesions are classified into two groups, characterized either by hyperplasia or by combined hyperplasia and metaplasia. The group that demonstrates only hyperplasia includes simple hyperplasia, Brunn's invaginations and nests, and pyelitis (or ureteritis) cystica. The urothelial changes that combine hyperplasia and concurrent metaplasia include pyelitis (or ureteritis) glandularis, mucinous metaplasia, nephrogenic metaplasia, and squamous metaplasia.

The etiology of these lesions has been variously regarded as neoplastic or inflammatory. Indeed, all have been found in association with chronic inflammation. However, the frequency with which they are observed in the absence of previous and concurrent inflammation supports the interpretation that these lesions are proliferative and metaplastic variants, which arise from the urothelium spontaneously.

Simple hyperplasia refers to an increase in the number of cell layers of the mucosal transitional epithelium. This change has a flat configuration, with neither papillary features nor invaginations into the lamina propria.

Bulbous invaginations of the surface urothelium into the lamina propria are characteristic of **Brunn's buds.** Alternatively, solid, round nests of urothelial cells, apparently detached from the surface and seen within the lamina propria, are termed **Brunn's nests.** The cells within these buds and nests are similar to those of the surface epithelium.

Small slits or round spaces are commonly present in otherwise solid Brunn's nests. The size of the central lumen varies, as does the number of surrounding cell layers. Eosinophilic, proteinaceous material is present within the lumen. Such structures are called pyelitis (or ureteritis) cystica and may achieve sufficient size to be apparent on gross examination.

Pyelitis glandularis is characterized by glandular structures lined by mucus-secreting columnar epithelial cells. The glands are haphazardly arranged or are clustered within the lamina propria, frequently in proximity to Brunn's nests and pyelitis cystica. The latter structures differ from pyelitis glandularis only in the nature of the lining cells. Structures with cytologic features of both pyelitis cystica and pyelitis glandularis (which represent incomplete metaplastic change) are not uncommon. In most cases the overlying surface epithelium remains composed of transitional cells, but metaplastic squamous epithelium or mucus-secreting columnar cells, similar to those observed in the underlying glandularis structures, occur. Although pyelitis (or ureteritis) glandularis is usually focal, rare examples of a diffuse glandular type of metaplasia have been reported. When pyelitis glandularis is extensive and demonstrates columnar cell metaplasia on the surface, its resemblance to colonic mucosa is striking. Paneth cells have been observed in rare cases.

Nephrogenic metaplasia, the most recently described urothelial proliferative alteration, has not been described in the renal pelvis. However, rare examples have recently been reported within the ureter. This metaplastic alteration is most commonly observed in the bladder trigone. The exact pathogenesis of nephrogenic metaplasia is unknown. Multiple small tubular structures, surrounded by a well-defined basement membrane, are clustered together within the lamina propria and bear a superficial resemblance to adenocarcinoma.

Squamous metaplasia of the upper urinary tract has also been observed. Many cases, but not all, are associated with recurrent urinary tract infections and lithiasis. Thus, squamous metaplasia usually is observed in the context of established inflammation, but can develop spontaneously in the absence of identifiable injury to the urothelium.

The clinical significance of the proliferative and metaplastic variants of the urothelial mucosa of the renal pelvis and ureter is unclear. Although commonly found in association with urinary tract infection, these changes are known to occur in the absence of inflammation. These changes are also observed in association with primary neoplasms of the urothelium, but there is no substantial evidence to suggest that a urothelium that demonstrates these lesions is at a greater risk of neoplastic transformation. The occurrence of squamous cell carcinoma and adenocarcinoma in the renal pelvis or ureter, although rare, has been reported. It is not unreasonable to assume that squamous cell carcinomas may arise in a urothelial surface that has undergone squamous metaplasia. Similarly, adenocarcinomas likely arise from a urothelial surface that contains pyelitis or ureteritis glandularis. Such neoplastic transformation may be explained by the continued action of the offending agent on the metaplastic cell population. However, simply because neoplastic transformation may ultimately occur, it is inappropriate to regard the metaplastic epithelium as inherently at a greater risk for cancer. In rare cases, extensive squamous metaplasia of the renal pelvis and ureter has led to keratin production of such magnitude as to obstruct the ureters.

Neoplasms of the Renal Pelvis and Ureter

Most neoplasms of the renal pelvis and ureter are carcinomas. Mesenchymal tumors, both benign and malignant, are distinctly rare. Benign transitional cell papillomas in the urinary tract are currently regarded as uncommon.

Carcinoma of the Renal Pelvis and Ureter

Carcinoma of the upper urinary tract is of the transitional cell variety in 90% of cases. Of the remainder, squamous cell carcinomas far outnumber primary adenocarcinomas of the renal pelvis and ureter.

All histologic types of renal pelvic and ureteral carcinomas show a definite male predilection, with a peak frequency in the sixth and seventh decades of life. Patients present with hematuria and flank pain. A detectable mass on physical examination is uncommon. A history of lithiasis is occasionally reported.

The gross and microscopic features of each of the three histologic types of carcinoma affecting the renal pelvis and ureter allow for a specific diagnosis. Transitional cell carcinomas are usually exophytic, with papillary projections evident on gross examination (Fig. 17-3). The extent of invasion of the underlying wall of the renal pelvis or ureter is variable at the time of surgical excision. Squamous cell carcinomas tend to be more infiltrative and exhibit a lesser exophytic component. Surface ulceration and an association with lithiasis are also more frequent with squamous cell carcinomas. Adenocarcinomas are characteristically mucinous, a feature detected on gross inspection of the opened specimen.

The World Health Organization classification of transitional cell carcinoma comprises three grades. Grade 1 carcinoma is composed of papillary projections lined by neoplastic transitional cells that show minimal nuclear pleomorphism and mitotic activity. The papillae are long and delicate, and fusion of papillae is focal and limited. Grade 3 carcinoma is characterized by significant nuclear pleomorphism, frequent mitosis, and fusion of the papillae. Occasional bizarre cells may be present, and focal sites of squamous differentiation are often seen. Although invasion of the underlying renal pelvic and ureteral wall occurs in all grades of transitional cell carcinoma, it is consistently more frequent in grade 3 neoplasms. The histologic and cytologic features of grade 2 transitional cell carcinomas are intermediate between those of grade 1 (the best differentiated) and grade 3 (the most poorly differentiated).

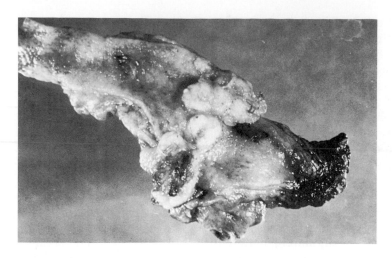

Figure 17-3. Transitional cell carcinoma of the ureter. The neoplasm is an irregular raised lesion with central ulceration.

Squamous cell carcinomas are identified by the presence of widespread and uniform squamous differentiation; adenocarcinomas are characterized by gland formation, frequently with abundant mucin production.

Metaplastic and dysplastic changes in the urothelium adjacent to the overt neoplasm may include foci of sufficient atypism to be labeled carcinoma in situ. Such changes may be observed in association with urothelial tumors of all three histologic types.

The development of multiple similar urothelial neoplasms is integral to the natural history of transitional cell carcinomas, but not the other types. Patients with transitional cell carcinomas of the renal pelvis show similar ureteral tumors in 20% of cases, and 13% suffer from simultaneous tumors in the urinary bladder. Moreover, an additional 20% develop independent transitional cell carcinomas of the bladder after removal of the original tumor by radical nephrectomy. A similar multiplicity of urothelial neoplasms is observed with primary tumors of the ureter: 10% of patients show simultaneous bladder transitional cell carcinomas, and an additional 27% develop these neoplasms in the bladder following primary surgical treatment for the ureteral tumor. From these figures it becomes clear that close long-term follow-up is obligatory for patients with previously diagnosed transitional cell carcinomas in any part of the urinary tract.

The ultimate survival of patients with primary transitional cell carcinomas of the renal pelvis and ureter is closely related to both the stage and grade of the tumor. Neoplasms confined to the mucosa, as well as those in which invasion is limited to the lamina propria, have a good prognosis. A progressive decrease in survival at 5 years is observed with all tumors that show greater local infiltration. Few patients with local invasion beyond the ureter or with distant metastases survive 5 years. The poor survival rates observed with primary renal pelvic or ureteral squamous cell carcinomas and adenocarcinomas are attributable to the consistently higher stage of these tumors at the time of primary surgical therapy.

Mesenchymal Neoplasms

Rare primary benign and malignant mesenchymal neoplasms occur in the wall of the renal pelvis and ureter. Those occurring most frequently are of smooth muscle origin (e.g., leiomyoma, leiomyosarcoma). The histologic features of these mesenchymal tumors are identical to those of corresponding neoplasms in more common sites.

Metastatic Neoplasms

Metastatic neoplasms to the renal pelvis are distinctly rare, and those of the ureter only slightly more common. The principal complication is urinary tract obstruction, a phenomenon most frequent in those cases showing metastases to the ureters. Metastases to the ureter from distant sites are considerably less frequent than involvement of the ureter by the contiguous spread of neoplasms from adjacent organs, such as the ovary, bladder, cervix, and colon.

Urinary Bladder

Normal Structure and Embryology

The urinary bladder develops in two stages from the cloaca and the urogenital sinus. The latter results from the partitioning of the cloaca into the dorsal rectum and the more ventral urogenital sinus (see Fig. 17-1). The urogenital sinus serves as the origin of the urachus, urinary bladder, and proximal urethra. Progressive attenuation of the urachus forms the umbilical ligament in the adult, which retains an attachment to the bladder dome.

The caudal urogenital sinus makes contact with an ectodermal invagination at the urogenital membrane, thereby forming the complete urethral lumen. Thus, **the bladder and the urethral urothelium are of endodermal origin, with the exception of the most distal segment, which is of ectodermal origin. Each ureter, originating from the mesonephric duct in the form of a metanephric diverticulum, is of mesodermal origin.** The incorporation of the mesonephric duct into the bladder wall in the region of the trigone results in a transient localized mesonephric contribution to the bladder mucosa. This mesonephric urothelium is replaced by urothelium of endodermal derivation from the urogenital sinus. With the growth and enlargement of the bladder, the mesonephric duct is absorbed into the wall of the urogenital sinus at a location that ultimately becomes the proximal urethra. The muscular investments of the ureters, bladder, and urethra are of mesodermal origin.

The mucosal lining of the urinary bladder is composed of urothelial cells, with five to seven layers from the basal cells to the surface. The urothelium is continuous with that of the ureters and the urethra, which tend to have fewer layers. A basal lamina beneath the urothelium separates it from the richly vascularized subjacent lamina propria. The most superficial cells, the so-called umbrella cells, are large and flat. Each covers several smaller cells of the intermediate layer.

The lamina propria, composed principally of loose collagen, overlies the interweaving bundles of smooth muscle—the muscularis layer. The anatomic areas of the bladder include the dome, anterior and posterior walls, lateral walls, trigone regions, and the bladder neck. Urachal remnants are commonly observed in the bladder wall, usually in the region of the dome, and less frequently in the anterior wall.

Congenital Malformation of the Urinary Bladder

Uncommon congenital malformations of the urinary bladder include agenesis, complete and incomplete duplication, hourglass deformity, and diverticulum. Two disorders are of major clinical significance: exstrophy and complications of persistent urachus.

Exstrophy

Exstrophy is a congenital vesicocutaneous fistula that remains after the incomplete closure of the anterior abdominal wall and the underlying anterior bladder wall, and results from an overgrowth of the cloacal membrane. The normal mesodermal structures develop around the central diversion, which ultimately ruptures, exposing the bladder mucosa to the exterior around and through the defect of the anterior abdominal wall. Abrasion by clothing and the continuous escape of urine results in chronic infection of the involved area. The estimated frequency of this congenital anomaly is one per 50,000 births. Associated anomalies are common and, among others, include failure of fusion of the labia in girls and epispadias in boys.

The externalized bladder mucosa exhibits acute and chronic inflammation and metaplastic changes, most frequently squamous and glandular metaplasia (Fig. 17-4). Fibrosis and chronic inflammation are present in the muscularis in all patients older than 1 year. Although the congenital defect may be surgically repaired, the inflammation and the established metaplastic changes in the bladder mucosa tend to persist.

The condition of the patient with an uncorrected exstrophic bladder is lamentable. There is continuous leakage of urine, persistent or recurrent local infection, and an increased risk of ascending urinary tract infection. Moreover, there is an increased risk of neoplastic transformation of the metaplastic urothelium, with resultant adenocarcinoma, squamous cell carcinoma, and, least frequently, transitional cell carcinoma. The median age of all patients with a cancerous complication of exstrophy is the fifth decade, with 75% of patients aged 30 to 59 years.

Bladder Diverticulum

Bladder diverticula are common and require surgical excision only infrequently. Some studies indicate that diverticula are produced by increased intravesical pressure secondary to bladder outlet obstruction, while some regard bladder diverticula as congenital. The majority are observed in men older than 50 years and are commonly associated with obstruction secondary to prostatism. Diverticula occasionally are encountered in infants and children who have no evidence of obstruction. The most common location is the vicinity of the ureteral orifices, frequently immediately superior to the opening. In this location, enlargement of the diverticulum results in secondary ureteral obstruction or vesical reflux. Small saccules

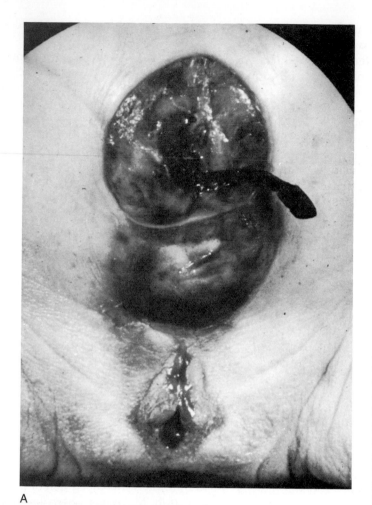

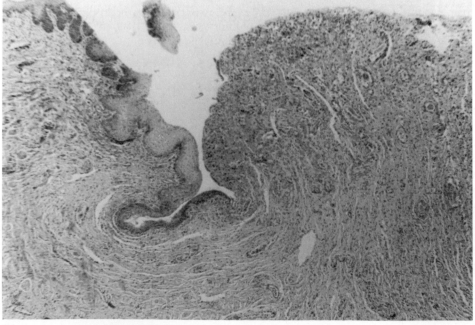

Figure 17-4.   Exstrophy of the urinary bladder. (*A*) A defect in the anterior abdominal wall with exstrophy of the urinary bladder is present in a 2-month-old girl. (*B*) A histologic section shows that the exstrophic urinary bladder (*right*) is continuous with the epidermis of the skin (*left*). Abundant inflammation and fibrosis are present in the lamina propria of the exstrophic urinary bladder.

and diverticula are without symptoms or clinical significance. Progressive enlargement leads to stagnation of urine, infection, and the formation of bladder stones—conditions that indicate a need for surgical intervention.

The excised bladder diverticulum has a narrow orifice that opens into a larger cavity. The diverticulum distorts the outside contour of the urinary bladder. The narrow intramural neck is found between bundles of the inner layer of the bladder muscle. The distended wall of the diverticulum contains attenuated muscle fibers, which are most commonly observed in young patients. This difference in the frequency with which smooth muscle is seen has led to the impression that congenital diverticula are identified by the presence of this structural component and that acquired diverticula have no muscle within the diverticular wall. In practice, all diverticula with long-standing chronic inflammation show fibrosis of the wall that may have replaced the original muscle. This observation is independent of a patient's age. Superimposed chronic inflammation, with or without squamous metaplasia, is observed in the majority of excised specimens.

The most serious complication of a bladder diverticulum, fortunately rare, is the development of cancer within it. Transitional cell and squamous cell carcinomas are the most frequently encountered types. The prognosis is poor because of the occult location of the growth and the ease of invasion into the attenuated wall of the diverticulum.

Persistent Urachus

The urachus is a tapered cephalic extension of the urogenital sinus (which later becomes the urinary bladder) that is contiguous with the allantois. Following birth, this tubular structure normally undergoes progressive fibrous atrophy as it descends caudally with the urinary bladder, to which it remains attached. The point of attachment is most commonly in the vesical dome. The regressive changes that result in closure of the cephalad end at the umbilicus and the caudal end at the bladder wall obliterate the intervening segment and convert it to a solid fibrous cord.

The clinical disorders associated with persistent urachus relate to the extent and location of the urachus that remains patent. Persistence of the entire urachus from the bladder to the umbilicus results in drainage of urine from the umbilicus, and supervening infection is common. Alternatively, incomplete persistence of the urachus forms a blind pouch, open either to the skin at the umbilicus or to the urinary bladder. Segmental persistence of the lumen with closure at both ends leads to a urachal cyst. The least common—but most serious—complication of persistent urachal segments is cancer: 90% are adenocarcinomas, although transitional and squamous cell carcinomas are encountered. Patients with such malignant tumors in the urachus have hematuria and a mid-anterior wall mass. Mucus in an umbilical discharge or in the urine may be observed in some patients with urachal mucinous adenocarcinomas.

Diagnostic criteria have been established to support a diagnosis of cancer of urachal origin as opposed to cancer of bladder origin. Such criteria include the following:

- The neoplasm should be located within the dome or anterior wall of the bladder.
- The bulk of the tumor must be located within the muscularis, without involvement of the mucosa of the urinary bladder.
- The bulk of tumor infiltration must be external to the bladder wall and involve the anterior abdominal wall.
- The presence of a urachal remnant associated with the tumor is supportive of the diagnosis.

The practical application of these criteria to distinguish tumors of urachal origin from those of vesical origin is often difficult, especially with large tumors that show extensive vesical ulceration of the bladder mucosa in addition to extensive intramural infiltration. Patients with urachal carcinomas have a poorer survival rate than those with the corresponding histologic type of bladder cancer.

Proliferative and Metaplastic Variants of Bladder Cancer

A spectrum of hyperplastic and metaplastic changes of the urothelium is commonly observed in the urinary bladder. Indeed, these same mucosal changes are observed throughout the urinary tract, as was discussed earlier in this chapter.

The hyperplastic urothelial changes include simple hyperplasia of the surface urothelium and focal proliferative mucosal invaginations—termed Brunn's buds or Brunn's nests—and cystitis cystica. The metaplastic proliferations include cystitis glandularis, squamous metaplasia, and nephrogenic metaplasia. **These alterations are observed in circumstances characterized by urothelial inflammation, including**

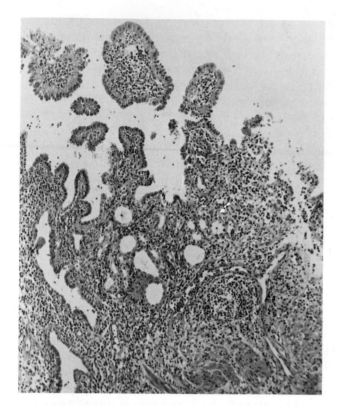

Figure 17-5. Nephrogenic metaplasia (adenoma) of the bladder. Papillary and simple tubular structures in the mucosa and superficial lamina propria are lined by epithelium similar to that of the renal tubular epithelium. Numerous inflammatory cells infiltrate the adjacent lamina propria.

urinary tract infections, bladder stones, neurogenic bladders, and exstrophy.

The finding of cystitis cystica in 60% of normal bladders suggests that, along with Brunn's nests, it represents a spontaneous normal proliferative variant of urothelium. Cystitis glandularis, per se, seems not to be associated with an inherently greater risk of neoplastic transformation, but the persistent injurious factors related to its development are probably implicated in the neoplastic transformation that leads to adenocarcinoma.

Although squamous metaplasia has traditionally been attributed to reactive urothelial proliferations associated with inflammation, apparently spontaneous squamous metaplasia is seen in about half of normal bladders in adult women and in approximately 10% of those in adult men. The question of whether there is an increased risk of neoplastic conversion of this metaplastic squamous cell population remains problematic. Therapeutic efforts to eliminate

a cause of inflammation, if present, coupled with prolonged follow-up, is appropriate.

The most recently described metaplastic change of urothelium, called **nephrogenic metaplasia,** occurs most frequently in the urinary bladder, but has been reported in rare instances in the urethra and the ureter. Numerous small tubules clustered in the lamina propria produce a papillary exophytic nodule (Fig. 17-5). Nephrogenic metaplasia is commonly found in the clinical context of chronic cystitis; it has no age predilection, with cases reported from infancy to the eighth decade. There is a pronounced male predominance (75% of cases occur in men). These lesions are usually in the trigone region, but they have been observed in all locations within the bladder. Transurethral resection is the most common form of therapy, but recurrences are not uncommon. The histogenesis of these lesions remains unsettled. Ultrastructural studies confirm the epithelial nature of the tubular lining cells, which show microvilli, complex intracellular interdigitations, and tight junctions. These features have been variously interpreted as recapitulations of different segments of the renal tubules, including the proximal convoluted tubules, the thin limb of Henley's loop, and the collecting tubules.

Inflammatory Disorders

The vast majority of cases of acute and chronic cystitis are caused by coliform bacteria and are treated successfully with antibiotics. Cystitis is classified according to its cause, duration (acute or chronic), and histologic appearance. The histologic features are characteristic of acute and chronic inflammatory responses elsewhere, but in other respects are nonspecific. Exceptions to this nonspecific appearance include tuberculosis, gas-forming bacterial infections (cystitis emphysematosa), schistosomiasis, papilloma virus infections (condyloma acuminatum), eosinophilic cystitis, gangrenous cystitis, polypoid cystitis, hemorrhagic cystitis, malacoplakia, plasma cell granuloma, and eosinophilic granuloma.

Polypoid Cystitis

Polypoid cystitis is a reversible inflammatory lesion of the bladder mucosa characterized by papillary, polypoid, exophytic mucosal projections (Fig. 17-6). Histologically, there is vascular congestion, stromal edema, and an inflammatory cell infiltrate within the lamina propria. When these mucosal elevations are

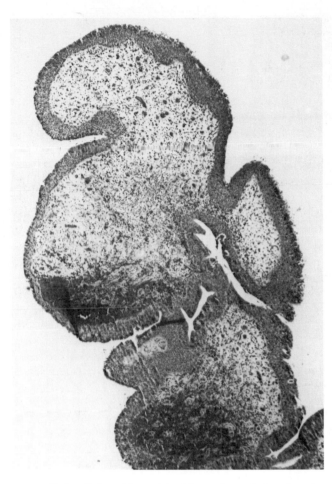

Figure 17-6. Polypoid cystitis. The polypoid structure is lined by a focally hyperplastic urothelial surface devoid of dysplastic changes. The underlying lamina propria has a chronic inflammatory cell infiltrate against a background of marked stromal edema.

broad based (wider than they are tall), they are described as bullous cystitis.

Most cases of polypoid cystitis are associated with indwelling catheters, an association that explains the disease's predilection for the posterior wall and dome of the bladder. Some lesions persist for long periods of time following removal of the catheter and are associated with increased stromal fibrosis. The histologic appearance resembles that described for the same entity elsewhere in the urinary tract. The deposition of collagen within the stalk of these polypoid lesions transforms an initially reversible lesion of the mucosa into a permanent one. These benign papillary or polypoid inflammatory lesions must not be misinterpreted as papillary neoplasms arising in the bladder mucosa.

Eosinophilic Cystitis

Eosinophilic cystitis is a descriptive term that accurately describes the predominant cell in the inflammatory infiltrate of this enigmatic form of cystitis. The lesion is rare and its cause is unknown. Patients frequently, but not invariably, have clinical evidence of an allergic diathesis involving the lungs or gastrointestinal tract. A peripheral eosinophilia may accompany the bladder lesion. This type of cystitis is usually seen in middle-aged adults, but has been observed in all age groups. The clinical presentation, with dysuria, frequency, and occasional hematuria, is similar to that in other forms of cystitis.

Chronic Interstitial Cystitis (Hunner's Ulcer)

Chronic interstitial cystitis, an inflammatory disorder of unknown etiology, is classically associated with a mucosal ulcer (Hunner's ulcer), although it is not required for the diagnosis. The typical case is chronic and involves a middle-aged woman, but the lesion has been observed in adult men and, rarely, in children. The most common symptoms are long-standing suprapubic pain, frequency, and urgency, with or without hematuria. At cystoscopy, mucosal edema, focal petechiae, and irregular hemorrhagic areas are characteristic. The lesions are most prevalent in the dome and posterior wall. The negative urine cultures are both characteristic and confounding when attempting to determine the underlying cause. Various forms of therapy have been employed in interstitial cystitis, but none has been entirely satisfactory.

Histologically, the mucosal ulcer displays an intense acute inflammatory reaction. The predominant findings in the lamina propria are vascular dilatation and edema, but importantly, a chronic inflammatory cell infiltrate composed of lymphocytes and mast cells is commonly observed within the muscularis, which frequently also shows fibrosis.

Malacoplakia

Malacoplakia, an inflammatory disorder of unknown cause, was originally described in the gastrointestinal tract, but more recently has been reported in a wide variety of organs. **The inflammatory lesions are characterized by a predominance of histiocytes,** the so-called von Hansemann cells, which have diagnostic intracytoplasmic inclusions, the Michaelis-Gutmann bodies (Fig. 17-7).

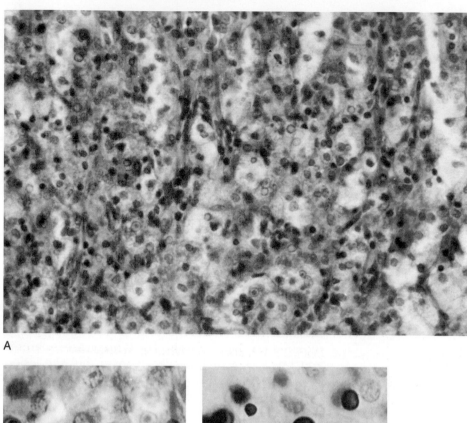

A

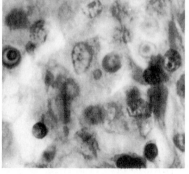
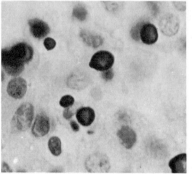

B

Figure 17-7.   Malacoplakia. (*A*) Numerous Michaelis-Gutmann bodies are seen as well-defined spherical structures, some of which have a central inclusion. The background inflammatory cells are composed principally of histiocytes, with fewer lymphocytes. (*B*) Michaelis-Gutmann bodies are seen at high magnification following special staining procedures.

The histologically distinct inflammatory lesion is commonly associated with an infection of the urinary tract by *E. coli*. A direct causal relationship between these bacteria and malacoplakia is dubious, primarily because of the high frequency of urinary tract infections caused by these bacteria and the rarity of malacoplakia.

The urinary bladder is the single most common site of this enigmatic disorder, with approximately half of all reported cases occurring in this organ.

Malacoplakia is found in all age groups, with the peak frequency occurring in the fifth to the seventh decades. There is a marked preponderance of cases in women, regardless of the site of occurrence. A clinical background of intercurrent disease, including immunosuppression, chronic infectious disorders, and cancer, is not uncommon. The clinical symptomatology is nonspecific and suggests cystitis. At cystoscopy the typical lesions appear as multiple yellow-tan plaques, some with central umbilication. There is no site of predilection within the bladder. Early investigators regarded malacoplakia either as a reflection of a neoplastic process or as an infectious disorder, but an acquired functional impairment of monocytes is currently considered a likely cause. The ultrastructural identification of fragments of bacteria within the histiocytes of the malacoplakia lesions may reflect an acquired defect in lysosomal degradation of the bacteria.

Iatrogenic Cystitis

Cystitis as a complication of radiation therapy or chemotherapy, most commonly treatment with cyclophosphamide, has received increasing attention. The typical features of all radiation-induced lesions—endothelial proliferation, subendothelial accumulation of histiocytes, and atypical fibroblasts within the stroma—are also seen in the bladder. The histologic changes associated with cyclophosphamide produce a form of hemorrhagic cystitis, commonly in association with cytologic atypia of the urothelial cells. The bladder lesions result not from cyclophosphamide itself, but from its metabolic breakdown products in the urine.

Amyloidosis

Amyloid deposits within the wall of the urinary bladder are rare, but they may be confused with cancer clinically and may also cause life-threatening hematuria. Most cases of vesical amyloidosis are of the localized type, but the secondary variety does occur. The patient usually presents with gross hematuria, at which time cystoscopic examination reveals plaques, nodules, or masses, often ulcerated, randomly scattered within the bladder. The diagnosis requires microscopic detection of the characteristic amorphous deposits of amyloid fibrils, which are most abundant within the lamina propria but also involve the muscularis. Depending on the extent of hematuria, surgical excision of the involved areas of the bladder is sometimes required, and recurrent episodes of hematuria are typical.

Endometriosis

The urinary bladder is the most common site of endometriosis of the urinary tract. The symptoms usually appear anytime from the second to the fifth decade of life, with a peak frequency in the fourth

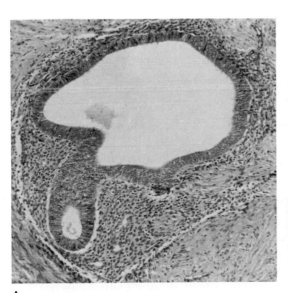
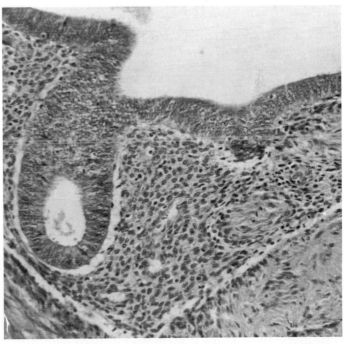

A   B

Figure 17-8. Endometriosis of the bladder. (*A*) Endometrial glandular epithelium with associated endometrial stromal cells within the muscularis layer of the bladder is diagnostic. (*B*) Higher magnification of (*A*).

decade. Patients present with pelvic pain, frequency, and urgency. Hematuria is reported in only one-fourth of the patients. The fact that about 60% of the patients have a history of pelvic surgery (hysterectomy, cesarean section, and other procedures capable of disseminating fragments of endometrium) suggests an implantation pathogenesis. The cause of endometriosis in the absence of prior surgery remains controversial.

The diagnosis of vesical endometriosis requires the identification of endometrial glandular epithelium in association with endometrial stromal cells (Fig. 17-8). Past hemorrhage is identified by the presence of hemosiderin in the stromal tissue.

Neoplastic Disorders

The urinary bladder is the site of origin of benign or malignant epithelial and mesenchymal neoplasms. **Epithelial neoplasms, virtually all of which are transitional cell carcinomas, comprise more than 98% of all primary tumors.** Benign epithelial tumors and all mesenchymal neoplasms are rare. The metaplastic potential of the bladder urothelium is reflected in a variety of epithelial neoplasms other than the transitional cell type, including squamous cell carcinoma, adenocarcinoma, and carcinomas with mixed differentiation. The bladder is also, albeit rarely, host to carcinoid tumors, primary malignant melanoma, small-cell undifferentiated carcinoma, and uncommon variants of adenocarcinoma (mucinous, signet ring, and clear cell carcinoma).

Benign Epithelial Neoplasms of the Urinary Bladder

Inverted papillomas, rare tumors of the urothelial mucosa, typically present exophytic proliferations that appear as nodular papillomas. Inverted papillomas are most commonly observed in the urinary bladder, but have also been reported in the renal pelvis, ureter, and urethra. They are covered by normal urothelium, from which endophytic cords grow into the subjacent lamina propria in a manner reminiscent of exaggerated Brunn's nests (Fig. 17-9). The localized nature of the endophytic columns or cords of urothelium produces the cumulative effect of an exophytic mass. In the urinary bladder, inverted papillomas are most common in the trigone region. They are more frequent in men, with a peak incidence in the sixth and seventh decades. Hematuria of recent onset is the usual clinical presentation. Recent reports

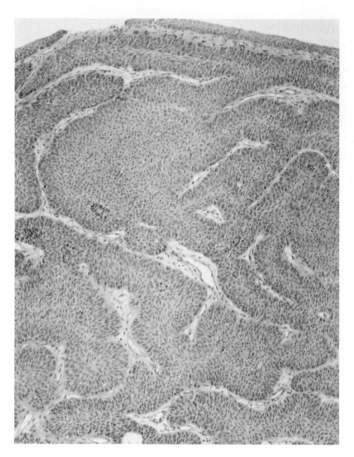

Figure 17-9. Inverted papilloma of the bladder. Interweaving cords of transitional epithelium originating from the surface mucosa dominate the exophytic bladder lesion.

of apparent malignant change have appeared, but the true frequency of malignant transformation is unknown.

Transitional cell papillomas of the urinary bladder exhibit a normal urothelial mucosal epithelium seven layers thick or less. Papillary neoplasms that meet these criteria are uncommon, and their acceptance as papillomas, rather than as low-grade transitional cell carcinomas, has occurred only within the last two decades. These neoplasms comprise 2% to 3% of bladder epithelial neoplasms and occur most frequently in men over the age of 50 years. Patients typically present with painless hematuria. The majority of cases show single lesions 2 to 5 cm in diameter, but multiple lesions are not unusual. **"Recurrences" are common (70% of patients) and the development of invasive carcinoma occurs in about 7% of patients.**

Although there is no evidence that papillomas are malignant, they arise in a urothelial mucosa that is not at rest, and evolving neoplasms can be detected only by repeated evaluations for many years. In most instances, "recurrences" represent new tumors that develop elsewhere in the urinary bladder.

Transitional Cell Carcinoma In Situ

The term "carcinoma in situ" is reserved for full-thickness dysplastic changes in flat (nonpapillary) urothelium (Fig. 17-10). The term is not applied to noninvasive papillary transitional cell carcinoma, in spite of the fact that the lesion is, by definition, confined to the mucosal surface. Carcinoma in situ is characterized by a urothelium of variable thickness, which exhibits nuclear abnormalities involving the entire mucosa from the basal layer to the surface. These include nuclear enlargement, hypochromatism, irregular shape, prominent nucleoli, and coarse chromatin. Occasional multinucleated cells are present. Variation in nuclear polarity, which produces a disorganized appearance, is a constant feature.

Vesical carcinoma in situ, occurring in the absence of papillary carcinoma, is associated with the subsequent development of invasive carcinoma in one-third of the cases. The majority of invasive transitional cell carcinomas arise from flat lesions of carcinoma in situ, rather than from papillary transitional cell carcinomas.

Papillary Transitional Cell Carcinoma

The incidence of bladder carcinoma shows significant geographic and racial differences throughout the world. The highest frequencies are recorded among Caucasians in the United States and Western Europe, whereas a low prevalence is reported in Japan and among blacks in the United States. Men are affected three to four times as often as women. Bladder carcinoma may be encountered at any age, but most patients (80%) fall within the range of 50 to 80 years old.

The association of bladder cancer with occupational exposure to certain organic chemicals has been known since its original observation in 1895. The increased frequency of bladder cancer noted among workers in the German dye industry was subsequently confirmed by observations among dye industry workers in the United States. The experimental production of bladder carcinomas in dogs by the administration of beta-naphthylamine, one compound to which the dye industry workers were exposed, was subsequently reported. These experiments proved that bladder carcinoma can be initiated by the exposure of the bladder mucosa to urine containing the carcinogen. Subsequently the association of occupational exposure to carcinogens with an increased risk of bladder cancer has been identified in the leather, rubber, paint, and organic chemical industries. Smoking has also been associated with an increased incidence of bladder carcinoma. There is no evidence that viruses or radiation are etiologically linked to bladder cancer.

The elucidation of the metabolic pathways of the naphthylamines has clarified the organ specificity of their carcinogenic action. The arylamines are oxidized and conjugated with glucuronic acid in the liver, after which the conjugates are excreted in the urine. In the bladder epithelium, beta-glucuronidase hydrolyzes the glucuronic acid conjugate at the acidic pH of urine, thereby producing arylnitrenium ions, which bind to the guanine moiety of DNA in the bladder mucosal cells.

Transitional cell carcinoma of the bladder typically presents with sudden hematuria, and less frequently with dysuria. Cystograms reveal a filling defect that is confirmed by cystoscopy. Multiple tumors are not uncommon. The sites of origin for vesical transitional cell carcinoma, in order of frequency, are the lateral walls, followed by the posterior wall. In low-grade neoplasms the papillary pattern, evident on histologic examination, is apparent grossly at the time of cystoscopy. These patterns present a range of appearances, from small, delicate papillary lesions that are apparently limited to the surface, to larger, solid, invasive masses that frequently show surface ulceration. As was discussed for other locations, transitional cell carcinomas of the bladder show growth patterns that are exophytic and papillary, infiltrating, or both. The lower grade (more differentiated) neoplasms tend to be predominantly, if not exclusively, papillary and exophytic; the predominantly infiltrating neoplasms are more typically high grade—that is, less differentiated. These lesions lack both the surface desquamation of keratin characteristic of squamous cell carcinoma and the mucinous features commonly observed in adenocarcinomas. Transitional cell carcinomas of the bladder are classified according to the World Health Organization grading system previously described in the discussion of these neoplasms in the renal pelvis and ureter.

The extent of transitional cell carcinoma is described according to a staging classification (Fig. 17-11). Tumors that are limited to the mucosa, without evidence of invasion, are regarded as stage O. Stage A tumors are those that invade the lamina propria. Invasion of muscle is designated as stage B.

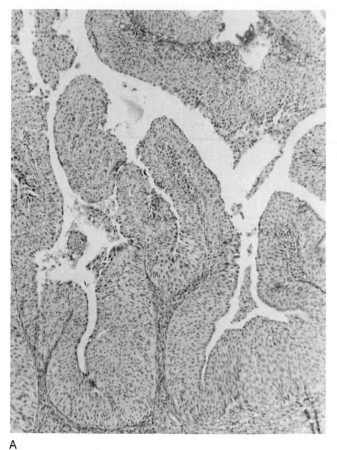

A

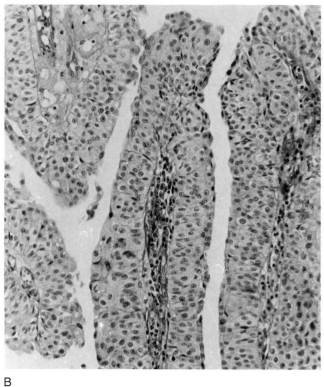

B

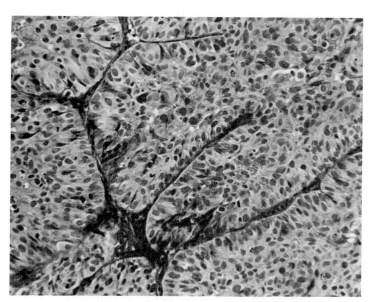

C

Figure 17-10.   Transitional cell carcinoma, grades 1 through 3. (*A*) Grade 1: The papillary structures are covered by a thickened urothelium demonstrating only mild nuclear atypism; mitotic figures are rare. (*B*) Grade 2: This papillary neoplasm is characterized by nuclear pleomorphism and uncommon mitoses; most tumor cells have prominent nucleoli. (*C*) Grade 3: Marked nuclear pleomorphism and frequent mitoses, associated with blunting and fusing of the papillae, are present in this tumor.

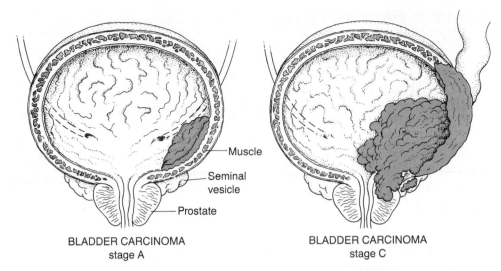

BLADDER CARCINOMA
stage A

BLADDER CARCINOMA
stage C

Figure 17-11. Clinical staging of bladder carcinoma. Carcinoma of the bladder, stage A, is restricted to the mucosa and lamina propria. Advanced carcinoma, stage C, exhibits a larger intravesical mass and invasion of the bladder wall, where it may obstruct the ureter and produce hydroureter. In this stage the tumor extends beyond the bladder to the prostate and seminal vesicles.

If only superficial muscle invasion is noted, the stage is termed B1; if the invasion is deep, it is classified B2. Perivesical invasion is considered stage C, and metastatic tumors are regarded as stage D. **At the time of initial presentation, 85% of patients have tumor confined to the urinary bladder (stages O to C), and 15% have regional or distant metastases (stages D1 and D2, respectively).**

Therapeutic decisions referable to bladder carcinoma are intimately related to the accurate determination of tumor stage. Papillary lesions limited to the mucosa (stage O) or lamina propria (stage A) are commonly treated conservatively with transurethral resection. Close follow-up is obligatory to detect "recurrences"—that is, the development of new tumors. Radical cystectomy is performed on patients who demonstrate muscle invasion (stages B1 and B2), and occasionally on those with clinically evident stage C tumor. In addition, the growing respect for the aggressive natural history of carcinoma in situ of the urinary bladder has prompted advocacy of radical cystectomy for such lesions.

An increased probability of tumor progression and subsequent recurrences is associated with a number of factors, including:

- large tumor size
- high-stage tumor
- high-grade tumor
- the presence of multiple tumors
- vascular or lymphatic invasion
- urothelial dysplasia, including carcinoma in situ

Overall, tumor progression has been reported in as many as 30% of patients who initially present with superficially invasive or noninvasive neoplasms. These neoplasms are not treated aggressively. It has been appreciated only recently that 80% to 90% of all patients with muscle wall invasion already had such invasion at the time of initial presentation. The remaining 10% to 20% of patients with tumors that invade the muscle wall have had a history of noninvasive transitional cell carcinoma that recurred and progressed, with ultimate demonstration of deep invasion into the muscle. Such patients with invasion of muscle or worse tumor conditions, such as invasion of the perivesical adipose tissue, have a significant frequency of regional lymph node metastases at the time of initial diagnosis—that is, stage D1 tumors. The median survival of such patients is approximately 1 year, but recent advances in chemotherapy have significantly improved survival rates. Metastases of bladder carcinoma are most frequent in regional lymph nodes and periaortic lymph nodes, liver, lung, and bone, in order of decreasing frequency. The most common immediate causes of death in patients with bladder carcinoma are uremia, carcinomatosis, and pneumonia, in that order.

Uncommon Histologic Types of Bladder Carcinoma

Squamous Cell Carcinoma

In the United States, squamous cell carcinoma of the urinary bladder is distinctly uncommon. By contrast, the frequency of this histologic type is significantly higher in the Middle East, where it is epidemiologically related to the prevalance of schistosomiasis. The clinical presentation of patients with this type of bladder carcinoma is similar to that seen in the more common transitional cell carcinoma. However, **at the time of initial presentation, virtually all patients with squamous cell carcinoma demonstrate invasion of the bladder wall, and therefore have a poorer prognosis than those with transitional cell carcinoma.** The histologic features of vesical squamous cell carcinoma are similar to those in more common locations. Squamous metaplasia of the nontumorous vesical urothelium is common in cases of squamous cell carcinoma.

Adenocarcinoma

Adenocarcinoma is the third most frequent histologic type of bladder carcinoma, but is not often encountered. Approximately 80% of reported cases have appeared in the literature within the last two decades. As with the other histologic forms of bladder carcinoma, there is a pronounced male predilection. The presenting symptoms are not specific for vesical adenocarcinoma, and most patients experience hematuria, with or without dysuria. Rarely, the passage of mucous material at micturition is associated with a mucin-producing adenocarcinoma of the urinary bladder. The diagnosis of vesical adenocarcinoma requires a differentiation of this neoplasm from urachal adenocarcinomas and from the more frequent adenocarcinomas that involve the bladder by metastatic spread or by direct extension. Like patients with squamous cell carcinoma, most of those with vesical adenocarcinoma present with invasive tumors.

The histologic patterns encountered in primary adenocarcinoma of the bladder include the papillary, glandular, mucinous, adenoid cystic, signet ring cell, and clear cell types. Focal areas of transitional cell carcinoma, with or without squamous cell carcinomatous foci admixed with the predominant adenocarcinoma, may be observed. An association with cystitis cystica and cystitis glandularis has been reported in a minority of cases of bladder adenocarcinoma.

Miscellaneous Rare Epithelial Cancers

Rare primary vesical carcinoid tumors, small cell undifferentiated carcinomas (oat cell carcinomas), and malignant melanomas have been reported. Each is identified by its unique morphologic features, which are similar to those of corresponding tumors found in more common locations. In all instances the diagnosis of primary neoplasms of these types in the urinary bladder requires differentiation from the more frequently found metastatic tumors in the urinary bladder.

Mesenchymal Neoplasms

A variety of benign mesenchymal tumors, including leiomyomas, hemangiomas, granular cell tumors, and neurofibromas, have been reported within the urinary bladder. The histologic features of these intravesical neoplasms are similar to their respective counterparts seen more commonly in other locations.

Malignant mesenchymal tumors are equally uncommon, most frequently represented by rhabdomyosarcomas and leiomyosarcomas. In contrast to all other sarcomas of the urinary bladder, rhabdomyosarcomas occur most commonly in children, and 90% occur in patients under the age of 40 years. The lesion is usually an embryonal rhabdomyosarcoma. The typical rhabdomyosarcoma of childhood in the urinary bladder is an edematous mucosal polypoid mass, which has been likened to a cluster of grapes. The diagnosis of these neoplasms has been improved with the increased application of immunohistochemical staining techniques and with election microscopy. In addition, recent advances in combined treatment with radiation and chemotherapy have resulted in greatly increased survival rates.

Miscellaneous Tumors

Unusual tumors arising in the urinary bladder include vesical pheochromocytomas, malignant lymphomas, and plasmacytomas. More commonly, the urinary bladder is secondarily involved in systemic malignant lymphoma and plasmacytoma. Leukemic involvement of the urinary bladder is also seen, although it is rarely a clinical problem. Mixed tumors (carcinosarcomas) of the urinary bladder have been reported, but many of these are probably collision tumors.

Metastatic Tumors

The overall frequency of metastases to the urinary bladder, as observed at autopsy, is less than 5%. The most common primary carcinomas that disseminate to the urinary bladder, in order of decreasing frequency, are malignant melanoma, stomach, breast, and lung. Only rarely does a metastatic lesion in the bladder produce gross hematuria that requires surgical intervention.

Urethra

Normal Structure

The male urethra is divided into the proximal (posterior) urethra and the distal (anterior) urethra. In men, the posterior urethra begins at the internal urethral orifice of the prostatic urethra and continues to the membranous urethra. Throughout the length of this prostatic urethra, prostatic duct ostia are present on the posterior and lateral walls. The distal urethra is divided into the proximal portion, called the bulbous urethra, and the more distal penile urethra, which terminates in the fossa navicularis, immediately internal to the external orifice (meatus). The transitional cell epithelium lining the male proximal urethra, which is continuous with the bladder urothelium, gradually changes to stratified columnar epithelium in the membranous and bulbous portions of the urethra. The more distal portion of the urethra, the fossa navicularis, is lined by stratified squamous epithelium continuous with the external urethral orifice. The bulbourethral (Cowper's) glands, which are mucus-secreting glands of the tubular alveolar type, are situated in the bulbous portion of the anterior urethra.

The proximal urethra in women, as in men, has transitional epithelium in continuity with the bladder lining. The proximal urethral lining gradually changes to stratified columnar epithelium, which in turn makes a transition to stratified squamous epithelium near the external urethral orifice. Mucosal invaginations, with minimal penetration of the periurethral tissue, are more common in the proximal urethra.

Congenital Disorders

Congenital disorders of the urethra are uncommon, and include abnormalities of the location of the external urethral orifice: in **hypospadias** the urethra opens on the underside of the penis; in **epispadias** the urethra opens on the upper side of the penis. **Urethral valves,** with associated bladder outlet obstruction, are also rarely encountered. Rare urethral duplication and urethral enlargement (megalourethra) have been recorded.

Inflammatory Disorders

Among the most frequently seen and clinically important inflammatory disorders of the urethra are those caused by *Neisseria gonorrhoeae* and *Chlamydia trachomatis*. The pathogenesis and pathologic features of these infections are discussed in Chapters 9 and 18.

Less common infections include those caused by streptococci, *M. tuberculosis*, and human papillomavirus (type 6). The last is the etiologic agent for condyloma acuminatum. Rare cases of malacoplakia have been reported; the histologic features of malacoplakia in the urethra are similar to those described for the urinary bladder.

Diverticulum

Diverticula of the urethra are virtually limited to women, in whom they are most frequently diagnosed in the third to the sixth decade. The dorsal lateral wall of the mid-urethra is their characteristic location. Patients present with postmicturition dribbling, urinary frequency, and urgency. Physical examination reveals a compressible bulge in the anterior vaginal wall. The pathogenesis of these lesions is unsettled, but the majority are probably acquired secondary to trauma or obstruction of a periurethral duct.

On occasion, a urethral diverticulum is the site of stone formation, endometriosis, or nephrogenic metaplasia. Histologic features of the diverticulum include focal ulceration with associated inflammation, overlying attenuated circumferential smooth muscle, and fibrosis of the urethral wall.

Rare cancers in urethral diverticula have been reported. Adenocarcinomas constitute the majority of such malignant complications, with fewer examples of transitional cell carcinoma and squamous cell carcinoma.

Proliferative and Metaplastic Changes of the Urethral Urothelium

The metaplastic and proliferative changes described in the renal pelvis, ureter, and urinary bladder also are observed in the urethra. In most instances their discovery is incidental, most frequently in fragments from a transurethral resection of the prostate. The histologic features of these urothelial changes are identical to those already described.

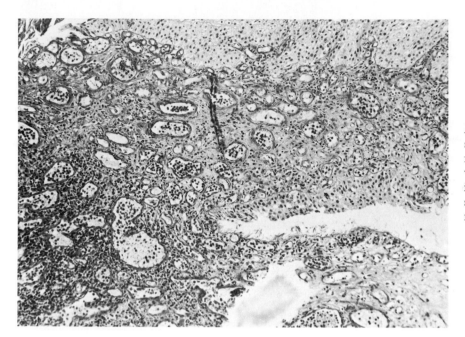

Figure 17-12.   Urethral caruncle. The submucosa of the distal urethral segment contains many thin-walled blood vessels. Numerous acute and chronic inflammatory cells are present in the stroma. Hyperplasia of the overlying mucosa can be seen at the top.

Urethral Polyps

Various types of polypoid and papillary lesions, both non-neoplastic and neoplastic, may occur in the urethra. Such lesions include nephrogenic metaplasia, fibroepithelial polyps, polypoid urethritis, condyloma acuminatum, caruncle (unique to the female urethra), adenomatous polyps with prostatic epithelium (unique to the male urethra), squamous papilloma, transitional cell papilloma, and papillary transitional cell carcinoma. All of the above lesions have histologic features identical to their more common counterparts in other locations within the urinary tract.

Caruncle

Urethral caruncles are inflammatory lesions near the urethral meatus that produce pain and bleeding. They occur exclusively in women, most frequently after menopause. The etiology and pathogenesis are unclear, but prolapse of the urethral mucosa and associated chronic inflammation have been suggested.

The constant features of caruncles are intense acute and chronic inflammation involving the mucosa and lamina propria (Fig. 17-12). The mucosa is either squamous or transitional cell epithelium, and exhibits ulceration, hyperplasia, and hyperkeratosis. Complex patterns of papillomatosis and occasional dysplastic epithelium may give this inflammatory lesion a superficial resemblance to carcinoma. The severe inflammation and associated stromal edema produce an exophytic polypoid mass. There is no evidence that caruncle leads to subsequent urethral cancer.

Adenomatous Polyp with Prostatic Epithelium

Adenomatous polyps are exophytic, villous, and glandular proliferations of prostatic tissue in the prostatic urethra (Fig. 17-13). The pathogenesis of this lesion is obscure. Ectopic prostatic tissue, metaplasia of urethral urothelium, prolapse of prostatic ducts, and developmental anomalies of the prostate have all been suggested. Patients present with hematuria, hemospermia (blood in the semen), or both. The peak age frequency is the second to the fourth decade. Microscopically, these polyps are lined by typical prostatic acinar epithelium. Corpora amylacia have been observed in acini within the villous structures. Positive staining for prostate-specific antigen confirms the prostatic origin of the epithelium of these polyps. The lesions are not premalignant, and treatment is by conservative transurethral resection.

Epithelial Neoplasms

Benign epithelial tumors of the urethra are uncommon and include squamous cell papillomas, transitional cell papillomas, and inverted papillomas. The histologic features of these benign urothelial neoplasms are identical to their counterparts in the urinary bladder.

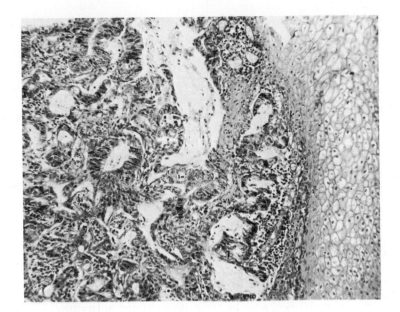

Figure 17 13. Adenomatous polyp of the urethra. The polypoid structure is covered with transitional cell urothelium *(right)*. Prostatic acinar structures are scattered throughout the fibromuscular stroma.

Carcinoma of the urethra is unusual, with a female predominance of 2:1. In order of decreasing frequency, squamous cell carcinoma, transitional cell carcinoma, adenocarcinoma, and malignant melanoma have been reported in the urethra. There are rare reports of clear cell carcinoma, cloacogenic carcinoma, adenoid cystic carcinoma, and carcinoid tumors.

The histologic type of urethral carcinoma can often be related to its site of origin. Transitional cell carcinomas tend to arise in the proximal urethra, squamous cell carcinomas in the distal urethra, and adenocarcinomas in the mid-urethra. Malignant melanomas are almost exclusively found in the distal urethra.

The cause of urethral carcinoma is unknown. Disorders frequently associated with this neoplasm include urethral stricture, prior instrumentation, venereal disease, and, importantly, prior or concomitant bladder carcinoma. Urethral carcinoma is most frequently observed in the sixth and seventh decades. Most patients present with urethral bleeding and dysuria. The majority of carcinomas of the urethra originate in the distal or anterior portion or, alternatively, involve the entire urethra at the time of presentation. In spite of the accessible location and associated symptoms of these neoplasms, the majority of urethral tumors have spread to adjacent tissues or metastasized to regional lymph nodes at the time of initial presentation.

The primary therapy for urethral malignancies is radical surgery. The prognosis is related to the site of origin, the size of the tumor, and its stage. Those tumors arising in the distal urethra consistently have a higher survival rate than those arising in the proximal urethra, because the latter tend to show more local invasion at the time of initial detection. The frequency of distant metastases from urethral carcinoma is not high (14%).

Mesenchymal Tumors

Primary mesenchymal neoplasms of the urethra are rare. Such tumors include leiomyomas, hemangiomas, and their malignant counterparts.

Metastatic Tumors

Metastatic tumors of the urethra are rare and usually originate in adjacent structures, including the prostate, bladder, and rectum. Pain, hematuria, and urethral obstruction in a patient with a known cancer suggest the diagnosis.

Testis

Normal Structure and Embryology

The testis develops from the undifferentiated cells of the gonadal ridge. During the third gestational week, the germ cells migrate from the yolk sac endoderm to assume residence in the gonadal ridge. Differentiation of the undifferentiated ridge to a testis requires aggregation of germ cells in the sex cords, which later become seminiferous tubules.

The origin of the sex cords containing the Leydig cells and the Sertoli cells is debated. One view regards the Sertoli cells of the seminiferous tubules and the Leydig cells of the gonadal interstitium as derivates of a common gonadal stromal cell precursor. On the other hand, some view the sex cords as resulting from downgrowth of the surface epithelium into the gonad. The unsettled state of this embryologic question is reflected in the World Health Organization classification, in which tumors of these cells are termed "sex cord/stromal neoplasms." During gestation there is a progressive transition of the sex cords to recognizable seminiferous tubules that ultimately connect to the testicular excretory ductal system, which is derived from the mesonephric (wolffian) duct. Within the testis the seminiferous tubules converge and become contiguous with the rete testis tubules that connect to the efferent ductules of the proximal epididymis. The epididymis, in turn, continues as the vas deferens and its distal diverticular outpouching, the seminal vesicles.

The normal descent of the testis from the intraabdominal point of origin progresses in late gestation. At the time of normal term delivery, approximately 96% of all male newborns have intrascrotal testes. Failure of testes to complete their normal descent into the scrotum is called **cryptorchidism.** The size and structure of the adult testis are achieved only after a period of dramatic growth and maturation at puberty under the influence of pituitary gonadotropins. The hormonally-induced changes initiate spermatogenesis, the reemergence of interstitial Leydig cells, and their synthesis of testosterone, the last resulting in a conspicuous increase in circulating testosterone.

The normal adult testis is invested with a layer of mesothelial cells (tunica vaginalis) that covers the outer fibrous capsule of the testis, the tunica albuginea. This capsule has internal septal ramifications that divide the testis into about 250 lobules. Within each of the lobules the coiled seminiferous tubules and interstitium are intermingled. The arterial supply to the testis is through the testicular arteries, which originate from the abdominal aorta. The venous drainage is a dual system: the right internal spermatic vein drains into the vena cava, and the left drains into the ipsilateral renal vein. This anatomical difference has several clinical implications, which are discussed later in this chapter.

Following puberty, active spermatogenesis is apparent within the seminiferous tubules. The time and the extent of physiologic regression of spermatogenesis are variable. Advanced regressive changes as-

sociated with old age are characterized by decreased spermatogenesis, increased interstitial cells (Leydig cells), and tubular and interstitial fibrosis.

The disorders of greatest clinical importance are testicular neoplasms and abnormalities associated with male infertility. Inflammatory disorders are infrequent.

Congenital Disorders

Congenital disorders of the male gonad include abnormalities of location, number, and structure. With the exception of cryptorchidism, all are rare.

Cryptorchidism

The failure of the testes to descend completely into their normal position within the scrotum is termed cryptorchidism (Fig. 17-14). At term, 4% of male

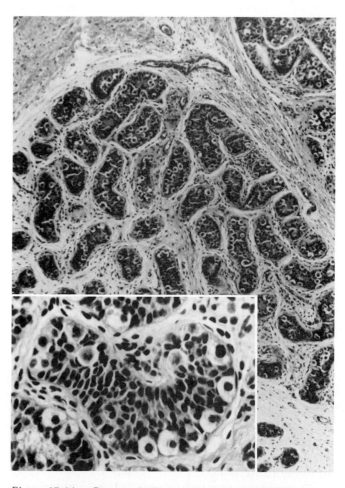

Figure 17-14.   Cryptorchidism. The diameter of the seminiferous tubules is smaller than normal in this testis from a 2-year-old infant. A higher power view (*inset*) shows that the germ cells are reduced in number.

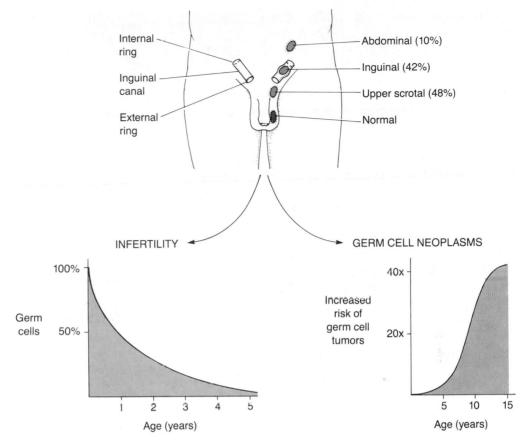

Figure 17-15. Cryptorchidism and associated complications. There is a 50% reduction in germ cell number after the first year of life and virtually a complete loss by 4 to 5 years of age. After age 5 the risk of germ cell tumors increases steeply.

newborns demonstrate one or more cryptorchid testes. Spontaneous descent of the testis occurs in the vast majority of these infants within the first year of life. The prevalence of cryptorchidism among adults is variously reported as 0.03% to 0.4%. Cryptorchidism is most commonly unilateral and is usually an isolated anomaly. Since the mechanisms that determine the normal descent of the testis are obscure, in most instances the cause of testicular maldescent is unknown. **Cryptorchidism is associated with infertility and germ cell neoplasms (Fig. 17-15), and therefore requires therapy.**

The histologic changes observed in the cryptorchid testis are related to age. If orchiopexy (therapeutic repositioning of the testis) is delayed beyond puberty, a decreased number of germ cells, stromal fibrosis, and infertility are observed (Fig. 17-16). The earliest changes in the malpositioned testis, from birth to 5 years of age, are reduced diameters of the seminiferous tubules and decreased numbers of germ cells. Indeed, complete absence of germ cells has been observed in patients as young as 3 years of age.

The risk of developing germ cell tumors (most commonly seminomas and embryonal carcinomas) in cryptorchid testes is increased 35-fold. Virtually all patients who have developed germ cell tumors after orchiopexy had that operation postponed to age 10 years or later. Germ cell tumors have not been reported in patients in whom orchiopexy was performed before age 5.

Disorders of Sexual Differentiation

Disorders of Genetic Sex

Disorders of genetic sex are represented by gonadal dysgenesis (Turner's syndrome), mixed gonadal dysgenesis, and true hermaphrodites.

Patients with **gonadal dysgenesis (Turner's syndrome),** characterized by an abnormal karyotype (45, XO or mosaic patterns), display bilateral streak gonads composed of fibrous stroma devoid of germ cells. In persons with **mixed gonadal dysgenesis** the testis is associated with a contralateral streak gonad, the latter identical to that in Turner's syndrome. Pure

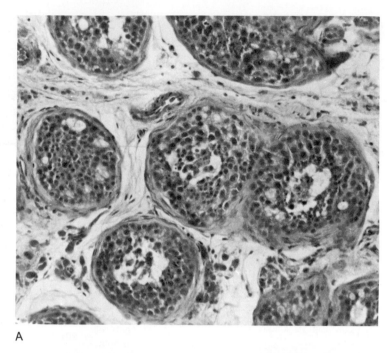

A

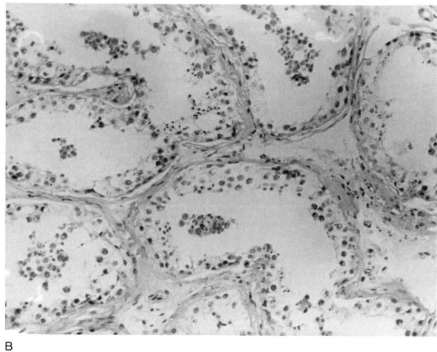

B

Figure 17-16.   Histopathology of the testis in infertility. (*A*) Maturation arrest. The tubules contain only early stage germ cells. There is a complete absence of spermatids and spermatozoa. (*B*) Hypospermia. The number of germ cells is markedly reduced.

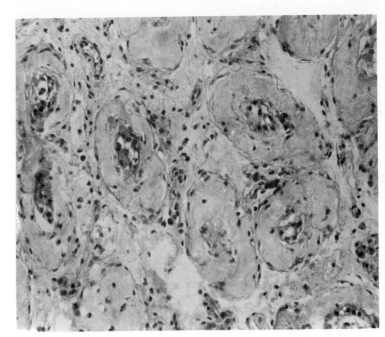

Figure 17-16 (continued). (C) Klinefelter's syndrome. There is marked thickening of the tubular membranes, absence of spermatogenesis, rare Sertoli cells, and clusters of interstitial cells.

C

gonadal dysgenesis, characterized by bilateral streak gonads, is usually associated with a female phenotype and an XX or XY karyotype. The pathogenesis of pure gonadal dysgenesis is not established.

In **true hermaphrodites** the bilateral gonads consist of varying combinations of ovarian and testicular tissue. Such ovotesticular structures show unequivocal testicular seminiferous tubules in proximity to ovarian primordial follicles.

Disorders of Phenotypic Sex

Patients with disorders of phenotypic sex have gonads consistent with the genotype but have ambiguous phenotypic features. Prototypes of phenotypic disorders in the male are the **pseudohermaphroditic states** that result from disorders of testosterone synthesis. In **testicular feminization** the peripheral testosterone receptors are abnormal, a situation that leads to the phenotypic expression of circulating estrogens. In the **female pseudohermaphrodite** (adrenogenital syndrome in a genotypic female), adrenal hypersecretion of adrenal androgens results in the virilization of the genotypic female.

Infertility

Male infertility is broadly classified into pretesticular, testicular and post-testicular causes. Primary testicular disorders are the most common, and post-testic-

ular disorders the least common. Among the pretesticular causes are primary genetic, pituitary, and systemic metabolic disorders, including uremia, cirrhosis, and diabetes. Primary testicular disorders include Kleinfelter's syndrome, varicocele, orchitis, and a variety of injurious physical and chemical agents, including heat, radiation, and exogenous drugs. Post-testicular causes of male infertility involve congenital and therapeutic obliteration of the epididymis or vas deferens, and retrograde ejaculation as a result of transurethral prostatic resection.

Infertile males may exhibit structural immaturity of the seminiferous tubules, hypospermatogenesis, germ cell maturation arrest, intratubular sloughing of germ cells, and peritubular or tubular fibrosis (see Fig. 17-16). Not uncommonly, mixed patterns of testicular abnormalities are observed. Alternatively, morphologic changes in the testis may be enigmatically absent, in which case testicular biopsy provides little information as to the underlying cause of the infertile state. The histologic changes in the testes are not specific, because the reactions of the testes to injury are limited and can be produced by a variety of disorders.

The most common form of male infertility with an underlying cause of abnormal sexual differentiation is Klinefelter's syndrome, a disorder characterized by gynecomastia, hypospermatogenesis, increased FSH secretion, and normal Leydig cell function. The testes show tubular hyalinization and an absence of elastic fibers in the walls of the seminiferous tubules. These histologic features, together with abnormal karyotypes (most commonly XXY), support the diagnosis of Klinefelter's syndrome.

Inflammatory Disorders

Clinically, orchitis takes the form of acute and chronic inflammation, frequently in association with concurrent involvement of the ipsilateral epididymis. Most cases have an underlying gram-negative bacterial infection, frequently in association with urinary tract infection. Orchitis due to viral, fungal, or rickettsial organisms is less common. Testicular involvement by spirochetes in syphilis is discussed in Chapter 9.

The most common viral orchitis is caused by **mumps** and presents with pain and gonadal swelling, most often unilateral. Testicular involvement in mumps occurs in 20% of adult male patients.

Chronic orchitis is uncommon, although gonadal involvement in tertiary syphilis, tuberculosis and a number of fungal infections is well documented.

Two forms of granulomatous inflammation of the testes, currently of unknown etiology, are **malacoplakia** and **granulomatous orchitis.** The histologic features of testicular malacoplakia are similar to those found more commonly elsewhere, particularly in the urinary bladder. The characteristic Michaelis-Gutmann inclusions, identified by appropriate special stains, allow a specific diagnosis. The noncaseating granulomas seen in granulomatous orchitis fail to reveal any organism, nor do they display the presence of sperm or remnants of sperm that may act as inciting agents. This contrasts with sperm granulomas of the epididymis, which characteristically show phagocytosis of sperm in the inflammatory focus. Destruction of variable numbers of seminiferous tubules occurs in both malacoplakia and granulomatous orchitis. Both forms of orchitis are most often seen in middle-aged men, and the diagnosis is rarely made prior to orchiectomy. The enlarged, indurated gonad is clinically similar to a testicular neoplasm, but obviously differs histologically.

Testicular Torsion

Torsion of the spermatic cord, if complete, produces severe pain and ischemic infarction of the testicular germ cells within a few hours. Most commonly, torsion presents shortly after vigorous physical exercise, but it may occur at rest. An abrupt onset of scrotal pain followed by swelling heralds the event. Less frequently, recurrent, incomplete torsion is observed. The swollen, firm, infarcted testis shows the gross and microscopic features of hemorrhagic infarction of the testicular contents. Recurrent, incomplete torsion of the spermatic cord results in a fibrotic testis significantly reduced in size.

Torsion of the spermatic cord is fortunately uncommon, and is frequently associated with congenital abnormalities of the intrascrotal contents that contribute to increased mobility of the testis and epididymis, such as high attachment of the tunica vaginalis on the spermatic cord. Testicular torsion is different from torsion of the testicular or epididymal appendages, which may produce a similar clinical picture.

Testicular Neoplasms

Tumors of the testes comprise three major histogenetic categories: germ cell tumors, gonadal stromal/sex cord tumors, and neoplasms not unique to the gonads (i.e., mesenchymal neoplasms) (Fig. 17-17). In addition, rare examples of metastatic tumors within the testis are observed. The neoplasms of germ cell origin constitute more than 90% of the tumors of the male gonad, and the majority of those remaining are of gonadal stromal/sex cord origin.

Germ Cell Neoplasms

The histogenesis of germ cell neoplasms has been largely clarified as a result of experimental and morphologic studies. Cytologic atypism of germ cells in the context of cryptorchidism progresses to germ cell carcinoma in situ within the seminiferous tubules, an event followed by microinvasion. Similar germ cell tumors in extragonadal sites (primarily in mid-axial locations) are currently thought to reflect neoplastic transformation of germ cells that migrated from the endodermal yolk sac to these extragonadal sites.

The neoplastic transformation of a germ cell gives rise to either a seminoma (an undifferentiated germ cell neoplasm) or an embryonal carcinoma (a neoplasm of totipotential cells). Embryonal carcinoma may undergo somatic differentiation and become a teratoma. Alternatively, extraembryonic differentiation results in a yolk sac tumor (endodermal sinus tumor) or a choriocarcinoma. Direct transformation of cytologically malignant intratubular germ cells to each of these histologic types of germ cell neoplasms

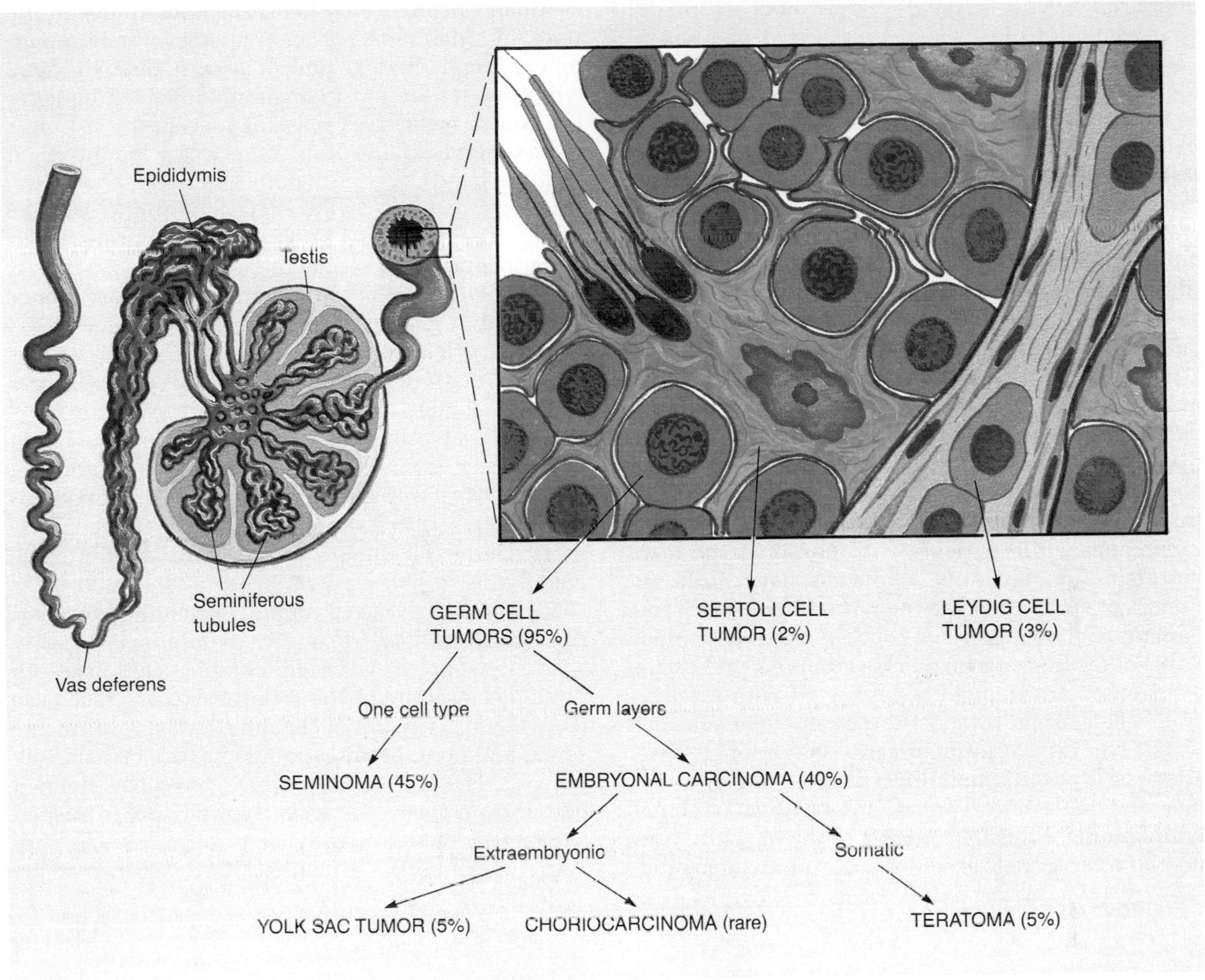

Figure 17-17.   Histogenesis of testicular neoplasms.

has been reported. Not uncommonly, germ cell tumors reflect divergent differentiation, within both the primary testicular neoplasm and the metastatic sites. In addition, metastases of germ cell tumors may show a form of differentiation not present in the primary gonadal tumor. This divergence may reflect a metastasis from an undetected small focus within the primary tumor, or it may be an indication of the capability of seminomas or embryonal carcinomas to differentiate into either somatic or extraembryonic neoplastic tissues in both primary and metastatic sites.

There are intriguing geographic and racial differences in the frequency of testicular germ cell tumors. High rates are observed in the United States, in contrast to low ones in Japan. Incidence rates are consistently reported to be higher in whites than in blacks in all geographic locations. Three peak age groups are observed: infants and children, adults in the third and fourth decades, and men older than 50 years. Genetic influences are apparent in only rare cases of twins or of fathers and sons. A role for previous trauma and infection cannot be entirely excluded, but such a history is rarely elicited. As previously noted, cryptorchidism significantly increases the risk of subsequent germ cell cancer, particularly seminoma. Bilateral germ cell neoplasms are infrequent, and most arise independently. There is little doubt, however, that the development of a germ cell neoplasm in one testis increases the risk of a second germ cell tumor in the contralateral gonad, although the reason remains speculative.

Germ cell tumors present as testicular swelling or pain. Sometimes the first symptoms derive from metastasis. Each of the testicular germ cell neoplasms exhibits specific age predilections, albeit with considerable overlap. **Infants and children are most commonly afflicted with yolk sac tumors and teratomas. Choriocarcinomas are more frequent in the second and third decades, embryonal carcinoma in the third decade, and seminoma in the fourth decade.**

The identification of tumor markers, including human chorionic gonadotropin and α-fetoprotein, both detectable in the serum, significantly assists in the diagnosis and follow-up of patients with germ cell neoplasms. **Elevations of serum chorionic gonadotropin are typically found in patients with choriocarcinoma, while patients with elevations of α-fetoprotein are generally found to have yolk sac tumors or embryonal carcinomas with yolk sac components.** Following orchiectomy, a fall in the serum levels of these tumor markers is observed, and tumor recurrences are frequently associated with a return of elevated serum levels of these same markers.

The clinical evolution of germ cell tumors is characterized by contiguous infiltration of the epididymis and metastatic spread, primarily to regional lymph nodes and subsequently to the lungs. In contrast to other germ cell tumors, **choriocarcinoma disseminates primarily by hematogenous routes to the lung.** In order of decreasing frequency, the retroperitoneal lymph nodes, lungs, liver, and mediastinal lymph nodes are most commonly involved by germ cell tumor metastases. Distant metastases are most often observed in the first 2 years following the initial diagnosis and surgical therapy. As noted above, the histologic features of the metastatic tumor may be divergent from those observed in the primary gonadal neoplasm. The emergence of metastases that are histologically different from the primary tumor has significant therapeutic implications.

Germ cell neoplasms are solid intratesticular growths that tend to bulge from cut surface. Areas of cystic change are not prominent, except in teratomas. Variable amounts of necrosis, commonly with hemorrhage, are observed in virtually all germ cell tumors, especially the largest ones. In choriocarcinoma, hemorrhagic necrosis involves even small tumors. Germ cell tumors may extend directly to the epididymis.

Each of the germ cell tumors is identified by characteristic histologic features. **Seminomas** display solid nests or cords of proliferating cells between randomly scattered, thin, fibrovascular trabeculae (Fig. 17-18). A lymphocytic infiltrate is usual in the septa, and noncaseating granulomas are occasionally present. The tumor cells, which have well-defined borders and clear cytoplasm, typically occur in solid sheets and show no tendency to form tubular, papillary, or glandular structures. Rare variants of the

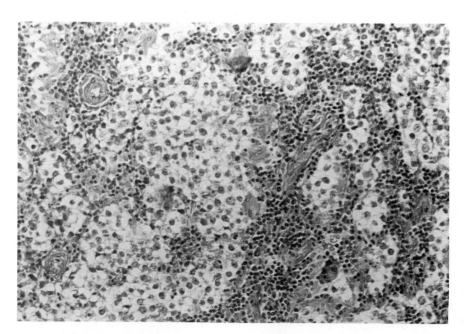

Figure 17-18. Classic seminoma. Nests of tumor cells are confined by fibrous septa containing numerous lymphocytes.

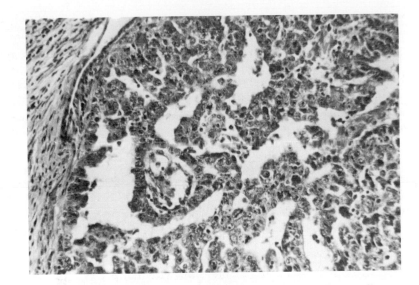

Figure 17-19. Embryonal carcinoma. A cystic space is lined and almost filled with carcinoma cells that lack distinct cell membranes.

classic seminoma include anaplastic seminoma and spermatocytic seminoma; the latter is found in men more than 50 years old.

Embryonal Carcinoma

Embryonal carcinomas typically show variable histologic patterns, such as acinar, tubular, and papillary forms (Fig. 17-19). The cell borders are ill-defined, and the nuclei have prominent nucleoli and coarse chromatin. Variably extensive hemorrhage and necrosis are usual.

Teratomas

Teratomas are identified by the random admixture of tissues derived from the ectoderm, entoderm, and mesoderm (Fig. 17-20). Squamous epithelial mucosa is admixed with gastrointestinal or respiratory epithelium. Occasionally, thyroid and neural elements are also present. The background stroma may contain foci of cartilage, bone, and fat. **The morphologic features of teratomatous germ cell tumors are not directly related to their natural history.** Specifically, morphologically mature teratomas, which would ordinarily be interpreted as benign, commonly behave in a malignant manner and metastasize. By contrast, teratomas in infants and children, including those with foci of undifferentiated cells, are uniformly benign. An explanation for this bewildering clinical behavior has not been established.

Yolk Sac Neoplasms

Yolk sac neoplasms, the most common germ cell tumor of infants, display a reticulated pattern of tumor cells with multiple microcysts and papillary clusters, all in a background of myxoid stroma. The tumor cells surround a characteristic structure, the Schiller-Duval body, which consists of a microcyst with a glomerulus-like structure containing a central fibrovascular core (Fig. 17-21). Immunoperoxidase stains identify α-fetoprotein within tumor cells and within the extracellular eosinophilic globules typical of this tumor. The descriptive names entodermal sinus tumor and yolk sac tumor reflect the histologic similarity of this neoplasm to the structure of the rat placenta.

Choriocarcinoma

Choriocarcinoma, representing germ cell differentiation to an extraembryonic structure, namely the placenta, is composed of neoplastic syncytiotrophoblasts and cytotrophoblasts (Fig. 17-22). These tumors are uncommon in pure form and usually occur as a component of a mixed germ cell neoplasm. The characteristic multinucleated syncytiotrophoblasts are intimately admixed with clusters of cytotrophoblasts. Syncytiotrophoblasts stain positively for chorionic gonadotropin. The tumor cells are typically found in areas of extensive hemorrhage and necrosis.

Mixed Germ Cell Tumors

Mixed germ cell tumors, which exhibit more than one type of neoplastic germ cell, are common. There are more than a dozen possible combinations, but the most frequent are teratoma with embryonal carcinoma (teratocarcinoma) and teratoma with embryonal carcinoma and seminoma. A surprisingly high frequency of yolk sac tumor components has been noted in these tumors.

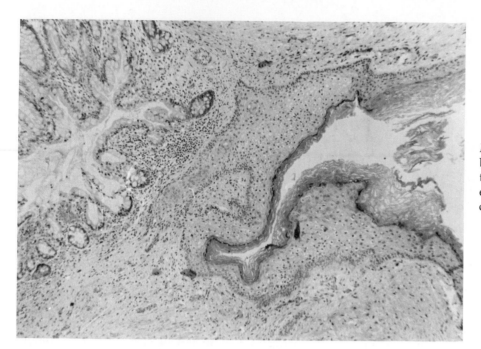

Figure 17-20. Teratoma. A cyst lined by well-differentiated squamous epithelium is in proximity to a focus of entodermal glands that resemble colonic mucosa.

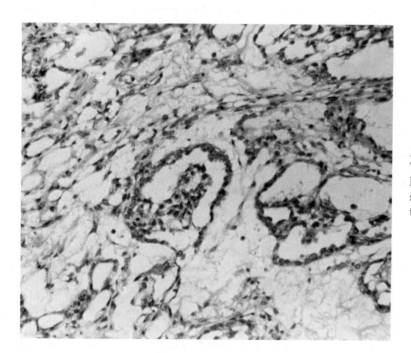

Figure 17-21. Yolk sac (entodermal sinus) tumor. The tumor is composed of dilated tubular spaces lined by flattened cells with an edematous stroma. A glomerulus-like structure is present at the center.

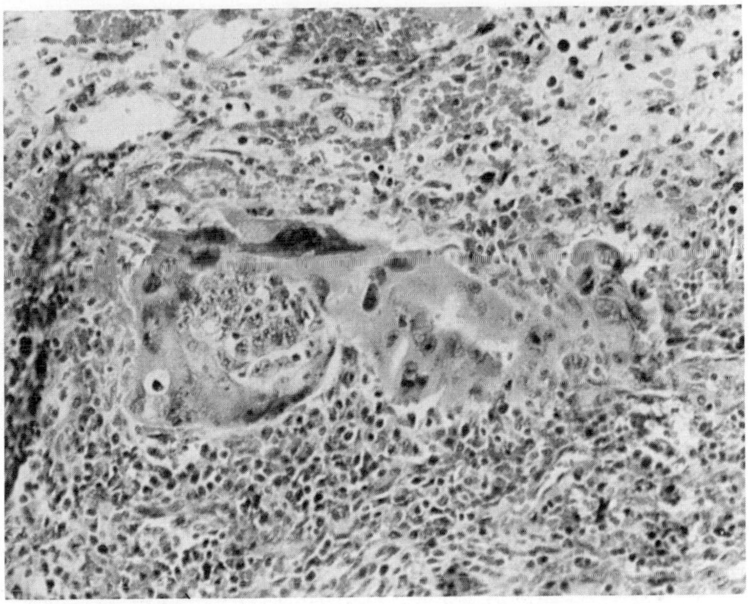

Figure 17-22. Choriocarcinoma. The syncytiotrophoblast cells surround a cluster of cytotrophoblast cells. Hemorrhage is evident in the adjacent tissue.

Gonadal Stromal/Sex Cord Tumors

Primary neoplasms of Sertoli, Leydig, granulosa, and theca cells constitute 5% to 6% of testicular tumors (see Fig. 17-17). These tumors may occur in "pure" form or as mixtures of neoplastic Sertoli and Leydig cells.

Leydig Cell Tumors

Leydig cell tumors are rare and occur in two age groups: boys younger than four years of age and men in the third to sixth decades. The endocrine effects from these interstitial cell (Leydig cell-derived) tumors in prepubertal children lead to precocious physical and sexual development. By contrast, feminization, such as gynecomastia, is observed in some adults with this tumor. Either estrogen or testosterone levels may be elevated, but there is no characteristic pattern. Most cases (90%) are clinically benign.

Leydig cell tumors are well-circumscribed, and some appear encapsulated. The cut surface is yellow to brown, and the larger tumors have grossly apparent fibrous trabeculae, a feature that imparts a lobular appearance.

Microscopically, the tumor reveals sheets of polygonal cells with variably abundant eosinophilic or vacuolated cytoplasm, which may contain lipofuscin pigment (Fig. 17-23). The characteristic cytoplasmic inclusion, the Reinke crystal, observed in almost half of these tumors, is a well-defined, rectangular, eosinophilic structure. The round nuclei are centrally located. Mitoses, hemorrhage, and necrosis are customarily absent. A prediction of biologic behavior of Leydig cell tumors on histologic grounds is hazardous. Of the few reported cases of malignant Leydig cell tumors, 75% showed capsular or vascular invasion. Importantly, 25% of those which proved to be clinically malignant showed neither feature.

Sertoli Cell Tumors

Neoplasms of Sertoli cells are even more infrequent than those of Leydig cells, and 20% have been malignant. These tumors usually develop in the first four decades of life, with only a few cases reported in older patients. Patients most commonly present with a scrotal mass.

Sertoli cell neoplasms are well-circumscribed, solid and yellow-gray. Microscopically, these tumors demonstrate a tubular arrangement, with solid cords of cells and a fibrous trabecular framework (Fig. 17-24). One-third of Sertoli cell tumors have admixed Leydig cells and are regarded as mixed gonadal stromal tumors. Like malignant Leydig cell tumors, malignant Sertoli cell neoplasms present a diagnostic challenge. The malignant variant exhibits greater cellular pleomorphism, areas of necrosis, and a reduced tendency to form cords and tubules.

Gonadoblastoma

Gonadoblastomas are rare neoplasms composed of an admixture of germ cell and immature sex cord/

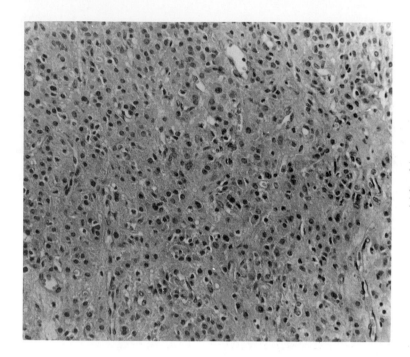

Figure 17-23. Leydig cell (interstitial cell) tumor. The tumor cells, arranged in sheets, are moderately pleomorphic and have abundant cytoplasm. No mitoses are present.

gonadal stromal elements, including Sertoli and, less frequently, Leydig cells. Virtually all arise in dysgenetic gonads. About half of the reported cases are associated with an overgrowth of the germ cell component, and about 10% of these have demonstrated metastatic spread.

Histologically, the diagnostic feature is an intimate admixture of gonadal stromal cells and germ cells. When germ cell overgrowth occurs, the resulting pattern is that of a seminoma.

Mesenchymal Neoplasms

Testicular mesenchymal neoplasms, both benign and malignant, are distinctly rare. These tumors mimic their counterparts in other locations.

Hematopoietic Neoplasms

Rarely, the testis is involved by lymphoma, leukemia, and, least frequently, plasmacytoma. Cases of primary plasmacytoma in the testis are generally accepted. Malignant lymphoma and leukemias usually occur in the context of systemic disease, but a few cases of apparently primary lymphoma of the testis have been reported. Of increasing concern is the increasing frequency of relapse of leukemias in the testes of children following therapy-induced remission. Curiously, the testis may be the first recognized site of relapse.

Metastatic Tumors

Metastatic tumors to the testis are rare, the most common tumors being those of the prostate, lung, skin (melanoma), and colon.

Testicular Adnexa

The testicular adnexa comprise the epididymis, the vas deferens, and the seminal vesicles. All are of mesonephric origin and serve as the excretory ducts, in continuity with the rete testes, in the testicular mediastinum. The epididymis and proximal vas deferens, like the tunica albuginea of the testis, are covered by a mesothelial cell lining, the tunica vaginalis. The seminal vesicles are located posterior to the prostate gland, and their excretory ducts anastomose with the distal vas deferens proximal to its entrance into the prostatic urethra.

Testicular Tunics

Hydrocele

The most common cause of scrotal swelling is hydrocele, a collection of serous fluid in the scrotal sac (Fig. 17-25). Hydroceles either are congenital and associated with a patent processus vaginalis or are acquired because of an inflammatory disorder, usually

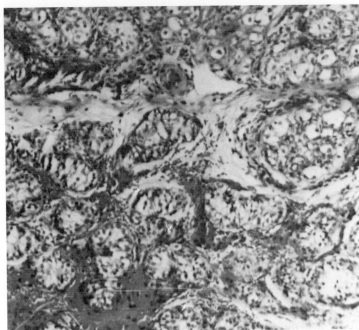

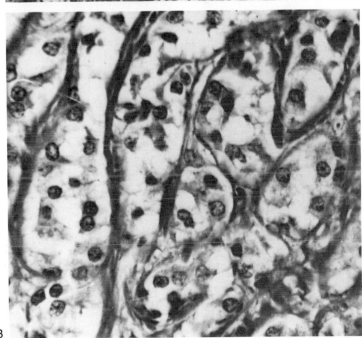

Figure 17-24. Sertoli cell tumor. (*A*) The neoplastic Sertoli cells are arranged in tubules of variable size. (*B*) A higher-power view shows the typical vacuolated cytoplasm, round nuclei, and prominent nucleoli.

A

B

one that involves the epididymis and the testis. The complications of hydrocele include infection (vaginalitis) and hemorrhage (hematocele). Hydroceles are differentiated from **spermatoceles** (cystic enlargements of the epididymis) by the presence of sperm in the cyst fluid of the latter. **Varicoceles** are dilatations of tributaries of testicular veins, a disorder which may have a deleterious effect on fertility.

Fibrous Pseudotumor

Fibrous pseudotumor refers to fibrous plaques or nodules, frequently with dystrophic calcification, involving the tunica albuginea. The lesion is currently regarded as a late result of an inflammatory process. Half of the cases are associated with a hydrocele, and a significant number have a prior history of trauma or orchitis. These lesions are not neoplastic, but their gross features and clinical presentation simulate a testicular neoplasm. Awareness of this entity may prevent unnecessary radical surgery.

Mesothelial Cell Proliferations

Local or diffuse mesothelial cell proliferation as a result of an intrascrotal inflammation is not uncommon. This proliferation is mostly encountered as an incidental finding in surgical specimens, usually in hydrocele sacs. The absence of histologic features of malignancy allows this reparative or reactive proliferative lesion to be differentiated from a rare malignant mesothelioma reported to occur within the scrotum.

Intrascrotal Mesothelial Cell Neoplasms

A nonpapillary form of benign mesothelioma, termed **adenomatoid tumor,** has a controversial histogenesis: origin from endothelial, mesonephric, müllerian, and mesothelial elements has been claimed. Available evidence supports a mesothelial cell derivation. These benign neoplasms are usually located in the upper pole of the epididymis, with fewer cases involving the tunica vaginalis of the testis or the spermatic cord. These tan nodules are well-demarcated and vary in size from a few millimeters to 2 cm, although rare examples have been reported up to 6 cm. Microscopically the histologic picture has been classified into three patterns: plexiform, tubular, and mixed. The lining cells in both tubular and plexiform patterns vary from flat to cuboidal. The lesion resembles a vascular neoplasm, with innumerable small, irregular cysts or tubules and interstitial dense fibrous tissue.

Ultrastructural studies support the view of a mesothelial origin of these neoplasms.

Malignant Mesothelioma of the Tunica Vaginalis

Papillary mesothelial cell proliferation like that usually observed in the pleura or in the peritoneal cavity is rarely observed within the scrotal sac. As in the more common locations, these neoplasms are epithelial, fibrous, or biphasic (exhibiting both epithelial and fibrous components). The epithelial component characteristically assumes a papillary configuration and often displays psammoma bodies. Solid areas of poorly differentiated malignant mesothelial cells, nuclear pleomorphism, and mitoses differentiate the tumors from benign mesothelial proliferation. Patients with malignant mesothelioma of the scrotum experience local invasion and distant metastases.

Epididymis

The epididymis is affected by inflammatory disorders and rare neoplasms. Rare congenital anomalies of the epididymis include abnormal position, failure of fusion of the testis, and adrenal rests. Acquired cysts **(spermatoceles)** are more common and reflect cystic dilatation of the efferent ducts or the more proximal rete testes (see Fig. 17-25). As noted previously, the cystic fluid of a spermatocele contains sperm, a finding that allows the differentiation from hydrocele.

Inflammatory Disorders

Most cases of epididymitis in men younger than 35 years of age are due to *N. gonorrhoeae* and *Chlamydia trachomatis*; in older men, *E. coli* from associated urinary tract infections serves as the most common etiologic agent. The histologic features are nonspecific. Cases of recent origin show the hallmarks of acute inflammation; persistence of infection is associated with increased numbers of plasma cells, histiocytes, and lymphocytes, and ultimately with the fibrotic obstruction of infected ducts. **Epididymal inflammation caused by *N. gonorrhoeae* is a common cause of male infertility.**

Tuberculous involvement of the male genital tract is now uncommon and is usually associated with previously established pulmonary and renal infections. Concurrent prostatic and testicular involvement in these cases is common. Tuberculous epididymitis is clinically manifested by a palpable beading of the vas deferens. Microscopically the tuberculous

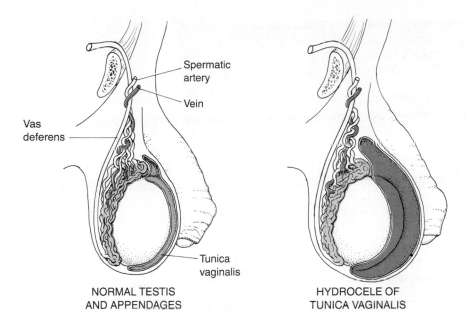

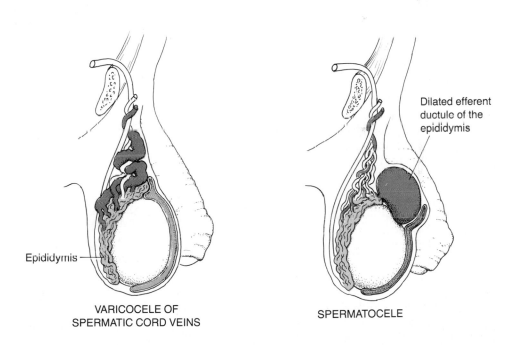

Figure 17-25. Hydrocele, varicocele, and spermatocele.

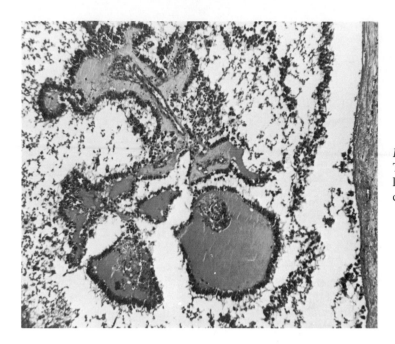

Figure 17-26. Papillary cystadenoma of epididymis. The cystic dilatation of the epididymis contains papillary infoldings lined by benign epithelial cells with clear cytoplasm.

etiology is evidenced by the typical caseating granulomas and Langhans' giant cells. Stains for acid-fast organisms frequently demonstrate the tubercle bacilli in the lesions. Such tuberculous granulomas must be differentiated from other rare granulomatous inflammations of the epididymis and from the more common spermatic granulomas.

Spermatic granulomas result from an intense inflammatory response to sperm that have gained entrance to the interstitium of the epididymis. The underlying cause of this sperm extravasation is obscure, but trauma to or infection of the epididymal ducts may play a role. Patients present with scrotal pain and swelling, frequently of weeks or months duration. Histologically, a mixed inflammatory cell infiltrate is associated with numerous extravasated sperm fragments and phagocytosis of sperm by histiocytes. Ultimately the inflammatory process results in interstitial fibrosis and ductal obstruction.

There are rare reported cases of malacoplakia involving the epididymis, and half of these have concurrent involvement of the testis. Histologic features supporting the diagnosis of malacoplakia are identical to those described in more common sites of involvement.

Neoplasms

The epididymis is a rare site of both benign and malignant neoplasms of epithelial and mesenchymal origin. In addition, the epididymis is affected by metastatic tumors from a variety of primary sites.

Papillary cystadenoma is an unusual benign neoplasm of the epididymis that has been reported in association with von Hippel-Lindau disease, a disorder characterized by cerebellar hemangioblastoma, retinal angioma, hemangiomas of the spinal cord, epidermal cysts, and cystic structures of the lung, pancreas, and kidneys. These cystic neoplasms of the epididymis are characterized by papillary projections arising from the cyst wall (Fig. 17-26). The papillary projections are lined by a layer of secretory and ciliated columnar cells bearing a resemblance to the lining epithelium of the efferent ductules. Cytoplasmic vacuolization is commonly observed, and PAS-positive secretory material can be detected in both intracellular and extracellular locations.

Primary epididymal carcinomas (most frequently adenocarcinomas) are rare, but are highly malignant. Mesenchymal neoplasms of smooth muscle (leiomyoma and leiomyosarcoma) and skeletal muscle (rhabdomyosarcoma) have also been reported in the epididymis. All are extremely rare.

Spermatic Cord

The spermatic cord is composed of the vas deferens and the accompanying arteries, veins, lymphatics, and nerves within a loose fibromuscular and adipose tissue investment. The most frequent clinical disorders involving this structure are dilatation of the venus plexus **(varicocele)**, inflammatory lesions, and a variety of benign and malignant mesenchymal neoplasms.

Vasitis nodosa refers to the presence of sperm-containing ductules within the muscularis and the periadventitial fibroadipose tissue of the vas deferens (Fig. 17-27). These ductules communicate with the central lumen of the vas deferens. Foci of hyperplastic ductules are observed after recanalization of the vas deferens following its segmental resection. The intramural location of these proliferating ductules superficially resembles invasive adenocarcinoma. However, the presence of sperm within the tubules in association with chronic inflammation, including sperm granulomas, suggests the appropriate diagnosis is vasitis nodosa.

Benign mesenchymal neoplasms of the spermatic cord are common in clinical practice, and lipomas constitute more than 90% of all such tumors. All other tumors are individually rare. They include adenomatoid tumors, lymphangiomas, leiomyomas, and a variety of other neoplasms.

Numerous types of malignant mesenchymal neoplasms (sarcomas) also have been observed in the spermatic cord. The most frequent include rhabdomyosarcoma, leiomyosarcoma, and fibrosarcoma. Typical of sarcomas in all locations, these neoplasms tend to disseminate by the hematogenous route. A notable exception is rhabdomyosarcoma of the spermatic cord, which frequently demonstrates regional lymph node metastases.

Seminal Vesicles

The paired seminal vesicles are rarely involved by clinically significant disorders. **Seminal vesicle cysts** are of unknown etiology. They may originate from previously undetected inflammatory processes or may be congenital. The cystically dilated seminal vesicle generally presents as irritative bladder symptoms. These cysts are usually unilocular and, important for their identification, have sperm fragments within the lumen.

Primary adenocarcinoma of the seminal vesicle is extremely rare or nonexistent, and some reported cases may actually have been prostatic carcinoma.

Prostate

Normal Structure and Embryology

The human prostate develops from epithelial evaginations that appear along the prostatic urethra during the third gestational month (see Fig. 17-1). Those evaginations of the proximal urethra undergo minimal development and give rise to simple periurethral glands. Evaginations that arise more distally in the prostatic urethra give origin to the five independent groups of tubules that ultimately grow to form the prostate gland. Between birth and puberty there is little prostatic development. At puberty, under the influence of testosterone, the prostate grows to an average adult weight of 20 grams. Beginning at about 50 years of age the prostate undergoes either progressive atrophy or, alternatively, enlargement from nodular hyperplasia. Frequently, both atrophy and hyperplasia are present in the prostates of elderly men. By the age of 80 years, half of the prostatic acini are obliterated.

Historically, the structural organization of the prostate was described in terms of five lobes: an anterior lobe, a middle lobe, two lateral lobes, and a

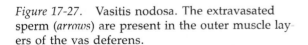

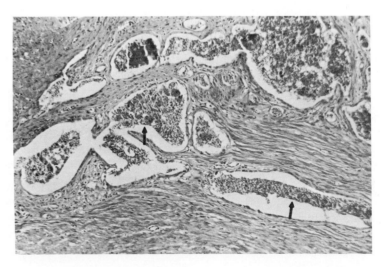

Figure 17-27. Vasitis nodosa. The extravasated sperm (*arrows*) are present in the outer muscle layers of the vas deferens.

posterior lobe. However, more recent studies have failed to identify separate lobes within the prostate. In addition, neither estrogen-induced histologic changes nor prostatic diseases demonstrate any regard for lobe boundaries.

Recently, five histologically distinct regions of the prostate have been identified. An anterior zone, corresponding to the originally described anterior lobe, is composed principally of fibromuscular stroma and few prostatic glands. A peripheral zone, roughly equivalent to the lateral and posterior lobes, constitutes approximately 75% of the glandular component of the prostate and contains simple glands and loose stroma. The majority of prostatic adenocarcinomas originate in this zone. A central zone, located between the ejaculatory ducts, is separated from the peripheral zone by fibrous trabeculae. Its location approximates that of the originally described middle lobe. The periurethral glands, confined to a sleeve of the proximal urethra, comprise a fourth zone. The most recently described zone, the transitional zone, contains glands that terminate in the proximal urethra and grow laterally around the distal end of the internal urethral sphincter. This zone lies anterior to the central zone and is the site of the majority of hyperplastic nodules of the prostate.

Microscopically, the prostate of the newborn exhibits simple tubules radiating from the urethra, with abundant intervening primitive fibromuscular stroma. In the newborn the urethra and distal prostatic ducts frequently show squamous metaplasia induced by maternal estrogen in utero, which gradually disappears in the early postnatal months. Responsiveness to estrogen is retained in the adult prostate, as demonstrated by the squamous metaplasia commonly observed after estrogen therapy for prostatic adenocarcinoma.

During the postnatal growth period the microscopic features of the mature adult prostate are achieved. Tubuloalveolar glands are clustered in a fibromuscular stroma that is continuous with the enveloping fibrous capsule. The acinar epithelium is pseudostratified and columnar, with a basal cell layer adjacent to the basal lamina. Similar epithelium lines the excretory ducts through most of their length to the urethra, where there is a change to transitional cell epithelium continuous with that of the urethra. The fibromuscular stroma contains smooth muscle, collagen, and elastic fibers in circumferential orientation around the acini and ducts. Occasional skeletal muscle fibers are incorporated into the prostate gland, most often in the anterolateral areas of the prostate.

During the period of senescent atrophy of the prostate gland there is progressive acinar obliteration. The remaining acini are smaller and are lined by cuboidal or flattened epithelium, which has diminished secretory activity. The stroma shows replacement of collagenous tissue by smooth muscle. Focal areas of epithelial hyperplasia occur in glands that are otherwise lined by atrophic epithelial cells. These foci of hyperplasia have been variously regarded as secondary hyperplasia or postsclerotic hyperplasia, and they have been considered as possible sites of origin of prostatic acinar carcinoma.

Secretion of neutral epithelial mucins is identified by the PAS stain. Appropriate stains have also identified melanin in both acinar epithelial and stromal cells, but its significance, if any, is unclear. Argyrophil and argentaffin cells have also been observed in the normal adult prostate, arising from differentiation of prostatic epithelial cells rather than by migration from the neural crest. Rare examples of primary prostatic carcinoids have been reported.

Both prostate-specific antigen and prostatic acid phosphatase are found by immunohistochemical techniques in normal, hyperplastic, and neoplastic prostatic glandular epithelium (Fig. 17-28). **These staining techniques are useful diagnostically because they serve to identify the prostatic origin of adenocarcinomas in metastases.** In contrast to the uniform staining for prostate-specific antigen in well-differentiated prostatic adenocarcinomas, in both primary and metastatic sites, many poorly differentiated prostatic carcinomas do not stain positively. Thus, a poorly differentiated metastatic tumor may still be of prostatic origin, even if it is negative for prostate-specific antigen. It is interesting that this antigen appears in prostatic epithelium at the time of puberty, and is absent before that time.

Control of Prostatic Growth

In spite of significant progress in our understanding of the control of prostatic growth, much remains to be clarified. Early studies on experimental animals identified the hormonal influence of testosterone. Subsequently, the therapeutic value of estrogen in controlling the growth of prostatic cancer was established.

Testosterone and Estrogen
The prostatic atrophy induced by castration of young animals is reversed by the administration of exogenous testosterone. Clinically, individuals who had been castrated before puberty, and who failed to

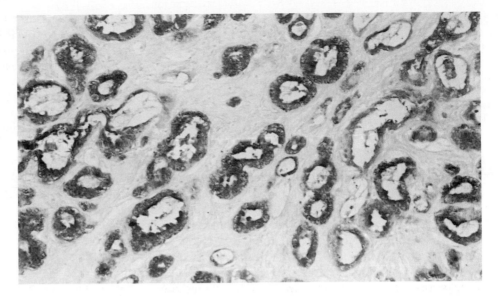

Figure 17-28. Prostatic adeno-carcinoma. The tumor cells, arranged in glands, stain positively for prostate-specific antigen when the immunoperoxidase technique is used.

show the normal prostate of the second and third decades, were observed to be immune to nodular hyperplasia and adenocarcinoma in later years. It is not clear why nodular hyperplasia and carcinoma arise while serum levels of testosterone are decreasing and those of estrogen are increasing.

Testosterone in the prostate is converted to dihydrotestosterone by 5α-reductase. The steroid is then coupled to a receptor protein, and the complex is transferred to the nucleus, where it combines with chromatin. As a result of this combination at specific gene sites, protein synthesis is selectively affected. Investigative interest is thus centered on the regulation of intracellular metabolism of dihydrotestosterone and its possible interrelationships with estrogen metabolism. The well documented influence of estrogens on the progression of prostatic adenocarcinoma has not been matched by an understanding of its effect on the normal growth and function of the prostate.

Inflammatory Disorders

Acute prostatitis characteristically presents as intense discomfort on urination and is associated with fever, chills, and perineal pain. Gram-negative bacteria, especially *E. coli*, are the most common etiologic agents. The pathogenesis of most prostatic infections is thought to involve reflux of the infected urine into the prostatic ducts. Prostatic abscesses are observed in men older than 50 years, but are currently uncommon. The morphologic features of acute prostatitis

are nonspecific, consisting of an acute inflammatory infiltration of the prostatic acini and stroma.

Chronic Prostatitis

Beyond the impression that chronic prostatitis represents a failure of acute prostatitis to resolve, the understanding of this disorder is limited. It is most common in men older than 50 years, but has been reported in virtually all age groups. Most patients with chronic prostatitis are symptomatic and report suprapubic, perineal, and low back discomfort. A clinical history of previous acute prostatitis is not uncommon. However, many patients are asymptomatic, and the diagnosis is rendered after examining prostatic fluid or prostatic tissue removed for other reasons. Gram-negative cocci are implicated most frequently, but some investigators have claimed gram-positive cocci to be the most common etiologic agents. The pathogenesis of chronic prostatitis involves reflux of infected urine into the prostatic ducts. Additional factors such as prostatic calculi, local prostatic duct obstruction, and regional vascular abnormalities may all contribute to the perpetuation of the infection.

Nonspecific Nongranulomatous Prostatitis

Nonspecific nongranulomatous prostatitis is most frequently encountered in specimens of nodular hyperplasia. The histologic features are entirely nonspecific, and the underlying cause is not apparent in routine sections of the lesion. The nonspecific chronic inflammatory lesion demonstrates a dense intraglandular and periglandular infiltrate of lymphocytes, plasma cells, and histiocytes, frequently accompanied by variable numbers of acute inflammatory cells. Focal gland destruction is not uncommon. The etiology and clinical significance of such cases are not understood.

Nonspecific Granulomatous Prostatitis of Unknown Etiology

The symptoms of chronic nonspecific granulomatous prostatitis are vague, and the diagnosis is made histologically. The pathogenesis is not understood but may involve an inflammatory reaction to inspissated secretions or bacterial products, reflecting localized prostatic duct obstruction. Histologically, noncaseating granulomas are associated with localized destruction of prostatic ducts and acini. In later stages the affected area of the prostate demonstrates fibrosis. A rare variant of this type of prostatitis is the eosinophilic variety, identified by numerous eosinophils in a background of noncaseating granulomas. Granulomas with fibrinoid necrosis have been reported, and rare cases are associated with a necrotizing vasculitis. This variant displays a high frequency of associated systemic or pulmonary allergic diathesis.

Granulomatous Prostatitis of Specific Etiology

On rare occasions, granulomatous prostatitis is caused by specific etiologic agents. These include tuberculosis and a wide variety of fungal infections.

Malacoplakia

Rare cases of malacoplakia have been reported to involve the prostate, sometimes associated with the same lesion within the urinary bladder. Most patients present with dysuria or urinary retention, usually in the fifth to the ninth decade. The histologic features of malacoplakia involving the prostate are identical to those described for other locations.

Prostatic Infarct

Infarcts of the prostate, usually focal, are identified incidentally in tissue removed for prostatic hyperplasia, and have a frequency as high as 25%. No primary vascular lesions have been identified, and the cause of prostatic infarcts is unclear. Trauma from previous catheterizations or extrinsic pressure on regional vas-

cular tributaries by enlarging hyperplastic nodules may be involved. Histologically, the infarcts vary in size and age. Recent infarction of ductal or acinar epithelium and surrounding stroma is often associated with interstitial hemorrhage, with neutrophils at the margin. Ducts and acini in the surrounding noninfarcted prostatic tissue show squamous metaplasia or, less frequently, transitional cell or columnar cell metaplasia. Experimentally, these metaplastic changes are apparent within 3 days of prostatic infarction. The natural evolution of focal prostatic infarct leads to a scar, frequently with persisting squamous metaplasia of the adjacent prostatic ducts.

It is important to distinguish infarcts of the prostate from prostatic carcinoma. Thirty percent of prostatic infarcts are associated with transient elevation of serum acid phosphatase. Histologically, the associated squamous metaplasia must not be misdiagnosed as squamous carcinoma in the prostate.

Nodular Prostatic Hyperplasia

Incidence and Epidemiology

Three epidemiologic factors—geography, race, and age—are related to the incidence of prostatic hyperplasia. Prostatic hyperplasia is least frequent in the Orient and most frequent in Western Europe. The prevalence of this disorder in the United States is intermediate between these two extremes, with a higher frequency among American blacks than whites. The peak age of patients with **clinical** prostatism is the seventh decade. By contrast, autopsy studies show no such peak in the age distribution, but rather a progressive increase in frequency with age. The incidence of prostatic hyperplasia in all age groups is far greater at autopsy than is suggested by clinically apparent prostatism (Fig. 17-29). **About 75% of men 80 years of age or older have prostatic hyperplasia, but the disorder is rarely observed in men younger than 40 years of age.**

Pathogenesis

Our current understanding of nodular hyperplasia is summarized in its name. Prior to the recognition of its hyperplastic nature, prostatic enlargement in elderly men was variously interpreted as a neoplastic, hypertrophic, inflammatory, or vascular disorder. The earliest histogenetic events in the evolution of nodular hyperplasia of the prostate are not understood. It has been postulated that stromal-epithelial interactions ultimately give rise to the hyperplastic

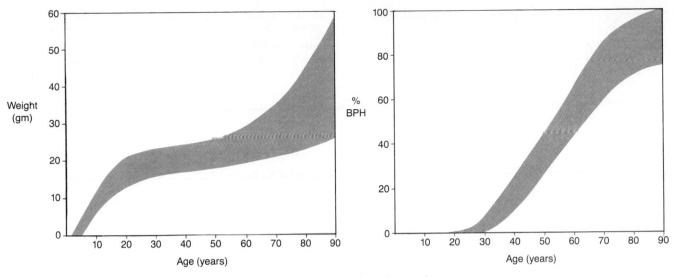

Figure 17-29.   Growth of the prostate (*left*) and frequency of nodular hyperplasia (*right*). By 80 years of age, most men have benign prostatic hyperplasia.

nodules, although it is not clear whether the stroma may induce the epithelial proliferation or vice versa. Pure stromal hyperplasia in a nodular configuration and virtually pure epithelial nodules are both observed, and a relationship between the two remains speculative.

Although the role of testosterone in the hormonal regulation of prostatic growth is well documented, its role in the pathogenesis of prostatic hyperplasia is less clear. The efficacy of castration in treating established prostatic hyperplasia is debatable. Exogenous testosterone has no observable effect either on the histologic appearance of hyperplastic nodules or on the areas of the prostate that evidence senile atrophy. Advancing age is associated with a comparable reduction in circulating testosterone in both normal controls and men with prostatic hyperplasia. No reduction in serum dihydrotestosterone is observed. On the other hand, prostatic hyperplasia has been produced in dogs by the administration of dihydrotestosterone. Serum levels of estrogen increase with advancing age in men, but its role, if any, in the production of prostatic hyperplasia is not understood.

Pathology

Early nodular hyperplasia occurs in the periurethral submucosa of the proximal urethra, recently described as the transitional zone. The developing nodules distort and compress the centrally located ure-

thral lumen and the more peripherally located normal prostate (Fig. 17-30). In examples of well developed nodular hyperplasia, the normal prostate is limited to an attenuated rim of tissue beneath the prostatic capsule. Each nodule is clearly demarcated from adjacent nodules and from normal prostate by an enveloping fibrous pseudocapsule. On cut section, secondary changes of focal hemorrhage and infarction may be present, especially in the larger nodules. On occasion, prostatic calculi are present within the dilated hyperplastic acini. The secondary changes resulting from prostatism are related to bladder outlet obstruction (Fig. 17-31).

Histologically, nodular hyperplasia reflects the proliferation of epithelial cells of the acini and ductules, the smooth muscle cells, and the stromal fibroblasts—all in variable proportions. Five types of nodules have been described: stromal (fibrous), fibromuscular, muscular, fibroadenomatous, and fibromyoadenomatous (the most common type). A rare variant, frequently associated with the development of macroscopic prostate cysts, histologically resembles cystosarcoma phyllodes of the breast; its name, the phyllodes type of hyperplasia, reflects this similarity.

In the typical fibromyoadenomatous nodule, the epithelial (adenomatous) component reveals tall columnar cells overlying the basal cell layer (Fig. 17-32). This epithelium lines acini of various sizes—some of microcystic proportions. Intraglandular papillary hyperplasia is characteristic.

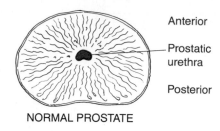

NORMAL PROSTATE

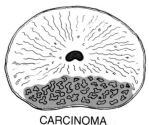

BENIGN PROSTATIC
HYPERPLASIA

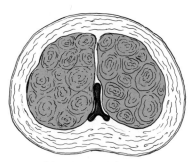

CARCINOMA
OF PROSTATE

Figure 17-30.   Normal prostate, nodular hyperplasia, and adenocarcinoma. In benign prostatic hyperplasia the nodules distort and compress the urethra and exert pressure on the surrounding normal prostatic tissue. Prostatic carcinoma usually arises from peripheral glands, in which case it does not compress the urethra.

The stroma of each type of nodule differs in composition, but common to all is the absence of elastic tissue. The proportion of stroma and glandular epithelium varies over a wide spectrum, with some nodules composed exclusively of fibrous tissue and intermixed smooth muscle. In the most typical hyperplastic nodule, glandular acini are randomly scattered through the stroma of the nodule. Associated histologic features of hyperplastic nodules include cystic dilatation of ducts, chronic inflammatory cells, and corpora amylacea within the glandular acini. The glands of the uninvolved peripheral region of the prostate are frequently atrophic and compressed by the expanding nodules. Immunoperoxidase staining of hyperplastic nodules shows consistently positive staining for prostate-specific antigen and prostatic acid phosphatase in the hyperplastic epithelium.

Incidental foci of prostatic adenocarcinoma are found in about 10% of surgical specimens submitted with the preoperative diagnosis of prostatic hyperplasia.

Neoplastic Disorders

Prostatic Adenocarcinoma

Epidemiology

Prostatic adenocarcinoma is the second most frequent cancer in American men, among whom it causes an estimated 26,000 deaths yearly. The effect of age, geography, and race on the frequency of prostatic carcinoma has been extensively documented. **It is a disease of elderly men; patients younger than 50 years of age constitute less than 1% of cases of prostatic carcinoma in the United States.** At the age of 50 years the estimated lifetime probability of developing clinically apparent prostatic carcinoma is 9.5% for white and 11.4% for black American men. Approximately 75% of all patients with clinically diagnosed prostatic carcinoma are 60 to 79 years old. The true frequency of prostatic carcinoma is significantly higher than that indicated by the clinical frequency and is shown in autopsy studies. The term "latent carcinoma" has been applied to clinically undetected carcinomas, which constitute 67% to 94% of all prostatic carcinomas. **The incidence of prostatic carcinoma at autopsy progressively increases, rising from less than 10% among men 40 to 50 years of age to between one-third and one-half of men over the age of 80 years.**

There is considerable geographic variation in the age-related death rates for prostatic carcinoma throughout the world. The highest frequencies are reported in the United States and the Scandinavian countries, whereas the lowest mortality rates are described in Mexico, Greece, and Japan. Most Western European countries have intermediate rates. Certain ethnic groups, such as Americans of Polish and Japanese descent, demonstrate a higher incidence of prostatic carcinoma than men in their families' respective countries of origin. **The mortality rate from prostatic carcinoma among black American men is among the highest observed in the world, significantly exceeding that of white Americans.** Interest-

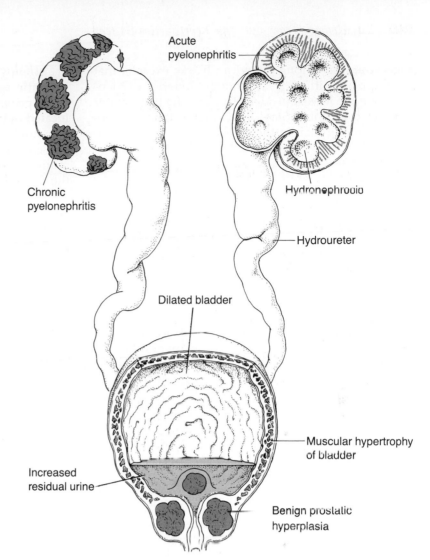

Acute
pyelonephritis

Chronic
pyelonephritis

Hydronephrosis

Hydroureter

Dilated bladder

Muscular hypertrophy
of bladder

Increased
residual urine

Benign prostatic
hyperplasia

Figure 17-31. Complications of benign prostatic hyperplasia.

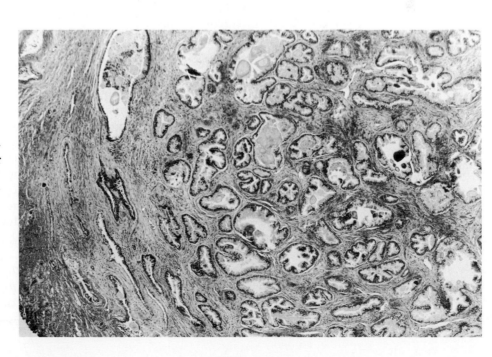

Figure 17-32. Nodular hyperplasia of the prostate. The columnar epithelium lining the acini is composed of two layers. Numerous papillary projections are present in the enlarged acini.

ingly, the rate among American blacks exceeds that among blacks in Africa. Although American Orientals have the lowest incidence among the three major races in the United States, it is higher than that observed among men in the Orient.

Etiology and Pathogenesis

The etiology of prostatic adenocarcinoma is unknown, but the principal focus of research interest is directed toward endocrine influences. Such diverse etiologic agents as cadmium and viruses have been considered as possible etiologic agents, but are without substantive support. The hormonal (testosterone) control of normal prostatic growth and the responsiveness of primary and metastatic carcinomas to therapeutic castration and exogenous estrogens provide supportive evidence for a role of hormones in the production of prostatic adenocarcinoma. Unfortunately, despite considerable research, these empirical observations are not matched by a corresponding increase in our understanding of the role of hormones. Attempts to demonstrate higher levels of serum androgens in patients with prostatic carcinoma have not yielded consistent results. Elevated urinary estrone/androsterone ratios have been reported in patients with prostatic carcinoma. Future studies of tissue dihydrotestosterone, androgen receptors, and 5α-reductase may clarify the role of testosterone in the etiology or progression of prostatic adenocarcinoma.

Until recently, experimental production of prostatic carcinoma has had only limited relevance to the study of the human disease. The experimental tumors were squamous cell carcinomas or sarcomas. In 1982 the first production of adenocarcinoma by a chemical carcinogen in experimental animals was reported following the administration of 3,2'-dimethyl-4-aminobiphenyl (DMAB). More recently, the production of prostatic adenocarcinoma in rats following the prolonged administration of testosterone has been reported.

Histogenesis

The histogenesis of prostatic adenocarcinoma is only slightly clearer than its etiology. The possibility that prostatic adenocarcinoma originates from hyperplastic nodules is without substantive support. **Currently, most investigators believe that the most probable source of prostatic adenocarcinoma resides in foci of hyperplastic acinar cells in otherwise atrophic peripheral glands.** Occasionally, such hyperplastic foci demonstrate atypical cytologic features.

Pathology

Prostatic adenocarcinomas, which account for 98% of all primary prostatic tumors, are most commonly located in the peripheral zones. These neoplasms are commonly multicentric. The cut surface of the prostate characteristically shows irregular, yellow-white, indurated subcapsular nodules. Characteristically, the best-differentiated tumors show uniform medium- or small-sized glands (Fig. 17-33). **Most glands are lined by a single layer of uniform neoplastic epithelial cells.** Progressive loss of differentiation of prostatic adenocarcinomas is characterized by increasing variability of gland size and configuration and by intraglandular patterns of epithelial proliferation. Papillary or cribriform patterns are common in larger neoplastic glandular structures. Uncommonly, a tumor is composed of small undifferentiated cells, growing individually or in sheets, without evidence of any structural organization. In such tumors necrosis of both the tumor and the infiltrated adjacent normal prostate is frequent, in contrast to the infrequency of this finding in the better-differentiated tumors. The majority of prostatic adenocarcinomas of acinar origin are well-differentiated.

The spectrum of differentiation is expressed in a grading system which has prognostic value and is based primarily on an assessment of the degree of the differentiation of the tumor glands. Cytologic features, which are not included in the criteria for grading, also exhibit a spectrum, from minimal to marked nuclear pleomorphism and hyperchromatism. One or two prominent nucleoli in the background of chromatin clumped near the nuclear membrane is the most frequent nuclear feature. The cytoplasm may be vacuolated and may simulate the clear cell variety of renal cell carcinoma, or it may stain as lightly eosinophilic. Cell borders are distinct in the better-differentiated tumors, but are indistinct in the more poorly differentiated examples. **A single layer of cuboidal cells in neoplastic acini is, from a practical standpoint, the most frequently employed criterion to establish the diagnosis of prostatic adenocarcinoma.** The histologic changes produced by endocrine and radiation therapy include tumor acinar atrophy and regressive cytologic features, including nuclear pyknosis, loss of nucleoli and cytoplasmic vacuolization. Estrogen-induced squamous metaplasia of non-neoplastic ductal epithelium is typical.

Extraprostatic Spread of Prostatic Adenocarcinoma

The high frequency of invasion of the prostatic capsule observed with adenocarcinoma is related to the

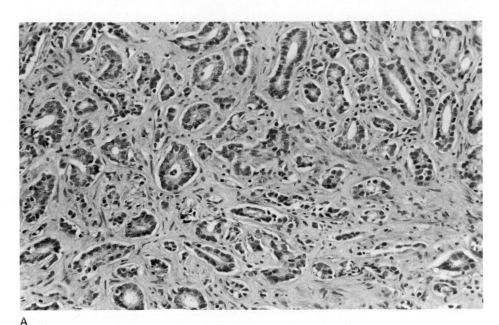

A

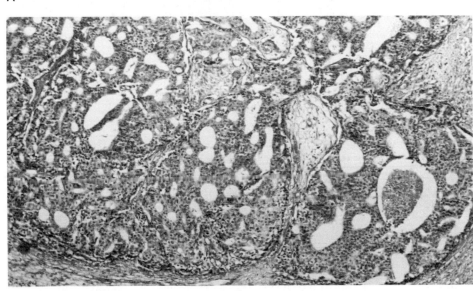

B

Figure 17-33. Adenocarcinoma of the prostate. (*A*) Neoplastic glands lined by a single layer of tumor cells are separated by stroma infiltrated by tumor cells. (*B*) Large nests of tumor cells have a cribriform arrangement.

high frequency of its subcapsular location. In both intraprostatic and periprostatic locations, **perineural invasion by this neoplasm is usual.** This was originally thought to represent perineural lymphatic invasion, but ultrastructural studies have demonstrated that peripheral nerves are devoid of perineural lymphatic vascular channels. This mode of invasion actually represents contiguous spread of the tumor along a tissue space that offers the plane of least resistance.

Contiguous invasion of the seminal vesicles by direct extension is common. Direct invasion of the

urinary bladder is less frequent until late in the clinical course of prostatic carcinoma. Invasion of the rectum occurs, but is distinctly uncommon.

Wide dissemination of prostatic carcinoma is characteristic at the time of death. Accumulating evidence from surgical staging procedures suggests that the earliest metastases occur in the obturator lymph node. Subsequent lymphatic dissemination involves the iliac and periaortic lymph nodes. Metastases to the lung result from further lymphatic spread through the thoracic duct and, independently, through venous dissemination via the prostatic ve-

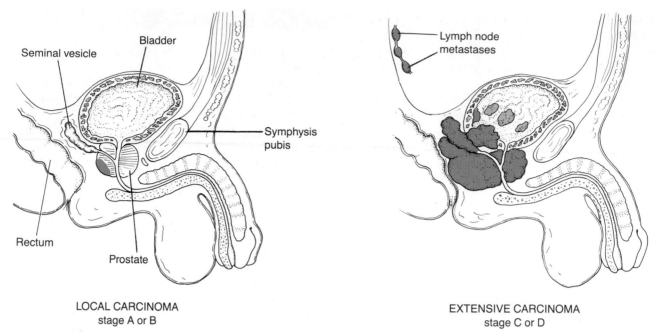

Figure 17-34.   Clinical staging of prostatic carcinoma. In stages A and B the tumor is confined to the prostate. In stage C the carcinoma has extended beyond the prostatic capsule to involve adjacent structures. Lymph node or distant metastases are present in stage D.

nous plexus and the inferior vena cava. Metastases to bone (particularly in the vertebral column, ribs, and pelvic bones) are a thorny clinical problem; they are found in autopsies of almost all patients who have died of prostatic carcinoma.

Natural History

Stage A carcinomas are detected as incidental microscopic foci in clinically benign specimens of prostatic tissue (Fig. 17-34). Substage A1 is the appropriate designation when the tumor foci are focal; if a high proportion of prostatic chips contain tumor, it is designated stage A2. Tumor associated with clinically palpable nodules but still confined to the prostate is termed clinical stage B. Again, focal lesions are stage B1, and if more than one lobe of the prostate is involved, the stage is B2. Stage C is the term applied to prostatic neoplasms that demonstrate local invasion beyond the prostatic capsule, but in which there are no metastases to regional lymph nodes or distant sites. Stage D represents those cases that have metastasized to regional pelvic lymph nodes (D1) or exhibit distant metastases (D2). **About 25% of prostatic carcinomas are detected at the time of microscopic examination of clinically benign prostate tis-** **sue (stage A). An additional 30% of patients present with a clinically detectable prostatic nodule identified by rectal examination.** About 15% of patients have clinical evidence of local spread (stage C) at the time of initial presentation, and the remaining 30% suffer from regional or distant metastases.

Understaging a diagnosis of prostatic carcinoma is a much more common problem than the reverse. It is difficult to detect intraprostatic carcinoma by rectal examination. Furthermore, the ability to detect extraprostatic spread (stage C) by rectal examination has been only recently surpassed by radiologic evaluation (CT scan). Pedal lymphangiography has a limited ability to detect early regional lymph node metastases (stage D1). The more recently developed bone scanning techniques have significantly improved the accuracy of staging of patients with bone metastases. Previously, bone radiographs and serum levels of prostatic acid phosphatase, the latter frequently elevated in the context of metastatic prostate carcinoma, had a significant frequency of false-negative results.

Among patients initially presenting with stage D prostate carcinoma is a subgroup that is diagnostically challenging. The term "occult carcinoma" refers to cases of undiagnosed prostatic carcinoma in which the first clinical manifestations are caused by metastases to organs, such as the lymph nodes, lungs, or bones. Immunohistochemical staining of biopsies of metastatic sites have proved valuable in identifying the prostate as the primary site.

At the time of autopsy, metastases of prostatic carcinoma are observed in the lymph nodes, bones, lung, and liver, in order of frequency. Widespread dissemination of the tumor (carcinomatosis), frequently with terminal pneumonia or sepsis, is the most common cause of death.

Transitional Cell Carcinoma

The distal prostatic ducts, on rare occasions, give origin to transitional cell carcinomas. Because these carcinomas are centrally located, patients present with urinary bladder outflow obstruction. Only rarely is serum acid phosphatase activity elevated. Microscopic features of prostatic transitional cell carcinoma include dilated ducts containing malignant transitional type epithelial cells that proliferate in solid patterns. Occasionally, central necrosis produces a comedo pattern. Infiltration of the prostatic stroma takes the form of cords or small nests and, less commonly, of individual tumor cells.

The diagnosis of primary transitional cell carcinoma of the prostate requires the exclusion of a primary bladder or urethral carcinoma that has spread to involve the distal prostatic ducts. In contrast to typical prostatic adenocarcinoma, which produces osteoblastic metastases, osseous metastases of prostatic transitional cell carcinoma are most frequently osteolytic. Importantly, these neoplasms are not responsive to the usual hormonal manipulation appropriate for prostatic adenocarcinoma. Transitional cell carcinomas of the prostate have a poorer prognosis than adenocarcinomas of acinar origin.

Prostatic Ductal Carcinoma

Rare cases of adenocarcinoma of the prostate have histologic features suggesting an origin from prostatic ductal epithelial cells. These lesions frequently display a papillary configuration. The natural history of these tumors is incompletely understood by virtue of their rarity. A type of ductal carcinoma previously regarded as of müllerian origin, termed "endometrial" carcinoma of the prostate, is now thought to be of prostatic origin rather than from müllerian derivatives in the region of the prostate.

Squamous Cell Carcinoma of the Prostate

Squamous cell carcinoma of the prostate is distinctly rare. None of the reported patients have shown elevated acid phosphatase. The site of origin within the prostate and the histogenesis of these neoplasms are currently unsettled. Histologically, the neoplasm exhibits invasive nests or cords of cytologically malignant squamous epithelial cells. Among the few reported cases, none has benefited from estrogen therapy.

Miscellaneous Rare Carcinomas of the Prostate

There are rare prostatic carcinomas that show a mixed differentiation, including combinations of transitional cell carcinoma, squamous cell carcinoma, and adenocarcinoma. The most common combination is adenocarcinoma with transitional cell carcinoma. The prostatic origin of both histologic forms is documented by positive staining for prostate-specific antigen.

Mucinous carcinoma frequently demonstrates typical signet ring cells. This neoplasm is composed of acini of varying size that are filled with extracellular mucin. Rare examples of adenoid cystic carcinoma and primary carcinoids in the prostate have been recorded. Small cell undifferentiated carcinoma, on occasion associated with ectopic ACTH production and clinical Cushing's syndrome, has been described.

Mesenchymal Neoplasms

Both benign and malignant mesenchymal neoplasms, including those of smooth muscle and skeletal muscle origin, have been reported as primary in the prostate. Skeletal muscle tumors occur usually in children and rarely in men older than 50 years of age. The opposite age distribution has been observed among the few reported patients with prostatic leiomyosarcoma, the majority of whom are older than 50 years of age, with rare examples in children in the first decade.

Metastatic Tumors

Metastatic tumors in the prostate are rare, and contiguous spread—that is, direct invasion from the bladder or urethra—is much more common. Cancer metastatic from distant sites includes leukemic infil-

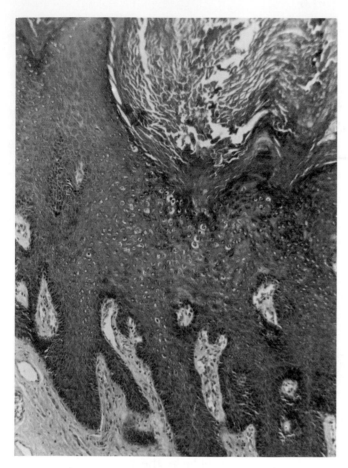

Figure 17-35. Condyloma acuminatum of the penis. The epidermis shows hyperkeratosis, parakeratosis, acanthosis, and papillomatosis.

tration (principally chronic lymphocytic leukemia), melanoma, and carcinoma of the lung.

Penis

The disorders of the penis of greatest clinical frequency are sexually transmitted inflammatory disorders and epithelial neoplasms, principally squamous cell carcinoma in the latter category. Congenital anomalies of the penis (agenesis and duplication) are extremely rare. Balanoposthitis (inflammation of the glans and prepuce) is usually associated with congenital or acquired **phimosis,** which is the inability to retract the prepuce because of an abnormally small preputial orifice. Circumcision is effective therapy for phimosis and the complication of balanoposthitis.

An interesting disease, termed **sclerosing lipogranuloma,** is an inflammatory reactive process directed toward exogenous lipids and waxes that gain access to the dermis. It has been reported most commonly among young men in the penis and scrotum. The exogenous lipids prompt a foreign body giant cell reaction, associated with variable amounts of fibrosis. In most instances, there is a previous history of trauma to the genital region involving the site of injury.

Sexually Transmitted Inflammatory Lesions of the Penis

Sexually transmitted inflammatory lesions of the penis include syphilis, chancroid, granuloma inguinale, lymphogranuloma inguinale, and genital herpes. The causative agents, pathogenesis, and histologic features are discussed in detail in Chapter 9.

The vesicular lesions caused by herpesvirus type II contrast with the epithelial proliferative lesion—wartlike exophytic dermal proliferations—caused by the human papillomavirus in cases of condyloma acuminatum (Fig. 17-35).

Peyronie's Disease

Peyronie's disease, a malady of unknown etiology, is characterized by focal, asymmetric, fibrous induration of the shaft of the penis. The fibrosis results in curvature and discomfort of the penis at the time of erection. Rare examples appear to be inherited, with an autosomal dominant transmission. The typical case appears as an ill-defined induration of the penile shaft, without evidence of significant change of the overlying skin, in a young or middle-aged man. A dense dermal fibrosis is associated with a nonspecific chronic inflammatory cell infiltrate, which tends to diminish in older lesions. Collagen focally replaces muscle in the septum of the corpus cavernosum. No reliable therapy has emerged.

Neoplastic Disorders

Squamous cell carcinoma in situ has been described in three clinical pathologic variants: Bowen's disease, erythroplasia of Queyrat, and the more recently described Bowenoid papulosis. Whether Bowen's disease and erythroplasia of Queyrat indeed represent two separate nosologic entities remains a matter of debate. The clinical distinctiveness of Bowenoid papulosis is unquestioned. Squamous cell carcinoma in situ in these lesions exhibits extensive or patchy parakeratosis and hyperkeratosis, papillomatosis with broad epidermal papillae, thinning of the granular layer, and cytologic atypia of the keratinocytes of all layers of the epidermis. The atypical keratinocytes do not invade the underlying dermis. A chronic inflammatory cell infiltrate within the subjacent dermis is characteristic.

In contrast to the average age of 50 years for Bowen's disease and erythroplasia of Queyrat, Bowenoid papulosis occurs in men two decades younger. In addition, Bowenoid papulosis presents as multiple violet papules in the penile shaft. Bowen's disease and erythroplasia of Queyrat usually involve the glans penis.

The frequency with which Bowen's disease and erythroplasia of Queyrat progress to invasive squamous cell carcinoma remains unsettled. To date, no examples of invasive squamous cell carcinoma have been associated with the reported cases of Bowenoid papulosis.

Squamous Cell Carcinoma of the Penis

The frequency of penile squamous cell carcinoma shows a marked geographic variation, with the highest incidence observed in Asian countries, Africa, and Central America. The lesion is uncommon in the United States. This variation in frequency has been associated with personal, social, and religious practices, including personal hygiene and the practice of circumcision. Fewer than 10 cases of penile cancer have been reported in men who were circumcised at birth. The average age of patients is approximately 60 years.

The etiology of this skin cancer remains unknown. Possible contributions of herpes simplex virus and smegma in the causation of penile cancer are currently unknown.

Clinically, squamous cell carcinoma of the penis is found on the glans or the prepuce, and presents as an ulcerated and hemorrhagic mass. The typical squamous cell carcinoma of the glans penis may evidence both exophytic and infiltrating characteristics. Destruction of the urethral meatus is an occasional observation in patients. Microscopically, the typical features of a well-differentiated, focally keratinizing squamous cell carcinoma are observed. Rare examples are poorly differentiated. An invasive tumor is associated with a dense, chronic inflammatory cell infiltrate in the adjacent dermis, which may show dysplastic changes. The tumor may invade deeply and extensively along the penile shaft.

Appropriate therapy includes partial or complete penectomy. The ultimate prognosis is closely related to the extent of tumor growth at the time of primary surgical excision and to the presence of lymphatic or vascular invasion. Although most penile squamous cell carcinomas are confined to the penis at the time of initial presentation, occult metastases to inguinal lymph nodes are not uncommon. Conversely, half of the patients with clinically enlarged regional lymph nodes have no nodal metastases, but rather reactive changes secondary to the inflammation associated with the primary penile tumor.

The natural history of penile squamous cell carcinoma is dissemination to the inguinal lymph nodes, followed by further spread to the iliac lymph nodes, and ultimately widespread distant metastases. This progression can be expected within 2 years of the initial diagnosis and therapy of the primary tumor. The ultimate survival of patients with penile carcinoma is closely related to the clinical stage and, to a lesser degree, to the histologic grade of the primary squamous cell carcinoma. At 5 years, one-quarter to one-half of patients with stage I penile carcinoma are dead, and the prognosis is progressively worse with more extensive cancer. The disturbingly high mortality rate of clinical stage I tumors leads to the inescapable conclusion that these patients have occult disseminated disease at the time of primary therapy.

Miscellaneous Epithelial Neoplasms

Rare cases of verrucous carcinoma, basal cell carcinoma, and malignant melanoma of the penile skin have been reported in the literature. The histologic features of the latter two carcinomas are identical to those noted in its more common locations. Verrucous carcinoma is seen with greater frequency in the upper respiratory tract, primarily in the larynx. In the penis, it demonstrates indolent growth, with deep encroachment by broad bands of neoplastic epithelial cells, which show minimal atypia. Dissemination of this variant of squamous cell carcinoma to regional lymph nodes is distinctly rare. This observation remains unqualified, even in the presence of very large primary tumors, which on occasion have resulted in complete destruction of the penis. Rare examples of extramammary Paget's disease involving the penis have been reported. The histogenesis of penile Paget's disease remains as controversial as that in all extramammary locations.

Mesenchymal Neoplasms

Mesenchymal neoplasms of the penis, both benign and malignant, are rare. Their histologic features are identical to those observed elsewhere.

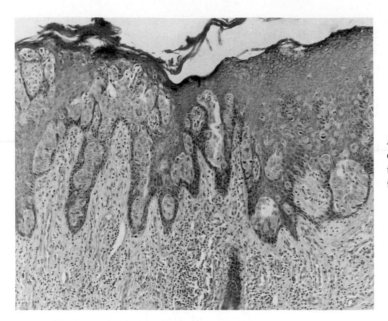

Figure 17-36.   Paget's disease of the scrotum. The enlarged Paget's cells are present as nests adjacent to the basement membrane and as single cells scattered throughout the epidermis.

Metastatic Neoplasms

The penis usually is invaded by contiguous malignant tumors, including carcinoma of the urinary bladder, urethra, and prostate. Metastatic spread to the penis from distant primary sites is distinctly uncommon.

Scrotum

Inflammatory disorders of the scrotum are generally of minor clinical significance and usually associated with poor personal hygiene. Sclerosing lipogranuloma, most commonly reported in the penile shaft, has also been reported in the scrotum.

Neoplasms

The most common cancer of the scrotum is squamous cell carcinoma. The high frequency of this malignancy among chimney sweeps was originally reported in 1775 by Sir Percival Pott, who is considered by many to be the father of occupational medicine. Pott implicated constant exposure to soot as the causative agent of the scrotal skin tumors. That coal miners did not show the high frequency of scrotal carcinoma observed among chimney sweeps suggested that the carcinogen was produced in the combustion of coal. Indeed, numerous carcinogens were subsequently identified in soot.

Squamous cell carcinoma of the scrotum is most frequently seen in men in their sixth and seventh decades. The lesion is usually single and limited to one side of the scrotal sac, commonly the anterior inferior surface. Typically, the lesion is well-differentiated. At the time of initial clinical presentation, many patients demonstrate invasion and metastases beyond the scrotum, principally to the regional inguinal or ilioinguinal lymph nodes. The principal therapy of scrotal carcinoma is surgical excision.

Miscellaneous Neoplasms of the Scrotum

Rare examples of basal cell carcinoma, malignant melanoma, and **Paget's disease** of the scrotum appear in the literature (Fig. 17-36). These tumors have microscopic features that are identical to those in lesions described elsewhere.

SUGGESTED READING

BOOKS
Petersen RO: Urologic Pathology. Philadelphia, JB Lippincott, 1986
Scully RE: Tumors of the Ovary and Maldeveloped Gonads. Atlas of Tumor Pathology, 2nd Series, Fascicle 16, AFIP, Washington, DC, 1979

REVIEW ARTICLES
Damjanov I, Katz SM: Malakoplakia. Pathology Annual 16:103, 1981
Mostofi FK: Pathology of germ cell tumors of testis: A progress report. Cancer 45:1735, 1980
Wilson JD: The pathogenesis of benign prostatic hyperplasia. Am J Med 68:745, 1980

ORIGINAL ARTICLES

Brawn PN: The origin of invasive carcinoma of the bladder. Cancer 50:515, 1982

Koss LG: Mapping of the urinary bladder: Its impact on the concepts of bladder cancer. Hum Pathol 5:533, 1979

Kunze E, Schauer A, Schmitt M: Histology and histogenesis of two different types of inverted urothelial papillomas. Cancer 51:348, 1983

Marshall VF: The relation of the preoperative estimate to the pathologic demonstration of the extent of vesical neoplasms. J Urol 68:74, 1952

Marshall FC, Uson AC: Neoplasms and caruncles of the female urethra. Surg Gynecol Obstet 110:923, 1960

Martin DC: Germinal cell tumors of the testis after orchiopexy. J Urol 121:422, 1979

Melamed MR, Vousta NG, Grabstald H: Natural history and clinical behavior of in situ carcinoma of the human urinary bladder. Cancer 17:1533, 1964

Melicow MM: Histologic study of vesical urothelium intervening between gross neoplasms in total cystectomy. J Urol 68:261, 1952

Mostofi RK: Potentialities of bladder epithelium. J Urol 71:705, 1954

Muller J, Skakkebaek NE: Abnormal germ cells in maldescended testes: A study of cell density, nuclear size and deoxyribonucleic acid content in testicular biopsies from 50 boys. J Urol 13:730, 1984

Nocks BN, Heney NM, Daly JJ, et al: Transitional cell carcinoma of renal pelvis. Urol 19:472, 1982

Ritchey ML, Novicki DE, Schultenover SJ: Nephrogenic adenoma of bladder. A report of 8 cases. J Urol 131:537, 1984

Utz DC, Hanash KA, Farrow GM: The plight of the patient with carcinoma in situ of the bladder. J Urol 103:160, 1970

Werth DD, Weigel JW, Mebust WK: Primary neoplasms of the ureter. J Urol 125:632, 1981

Wong T-W, Strauss FH II, Warner NE: Testicular biopsy in the study of male infertility. I. Testicular causes of infertility. Arch Pathol 95:151, 1973

18 Gynecologic Pathology

Stanley J. Robboy, Maire A. Duggan,
Robert J. Kurman

Embryology

Infectious Disorders

Vulva

Vagina

Cervix

Body of Uterus
and Endometrium

Fallopian Tube

Ovary

Placenta and Gestational
Trophoblastic Disease

Endometriosis

Figure 18-1.   Menstrual cycle, showing hormonal, ovarian, and endometrial changes.

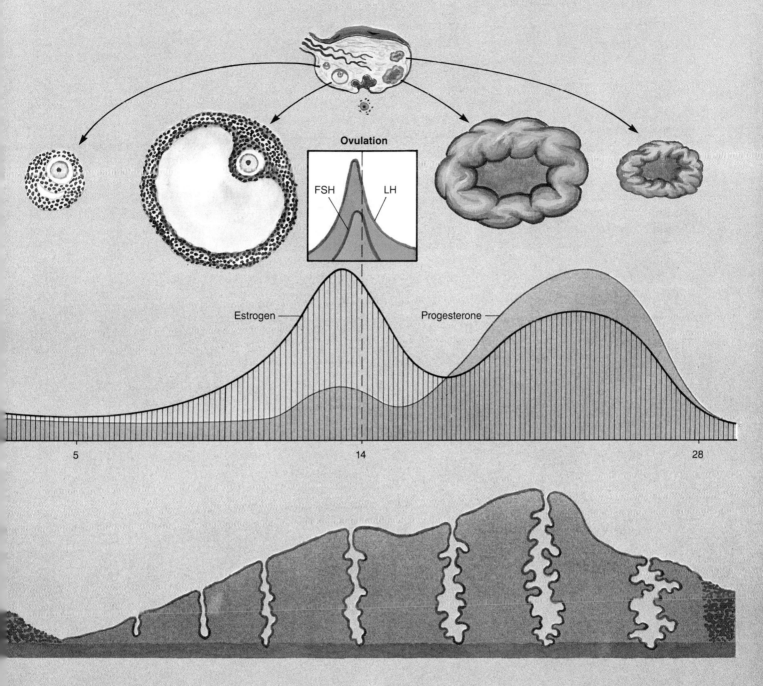

Ovulation

FSH   LH

Estrogen   Progesterone

5   14   28

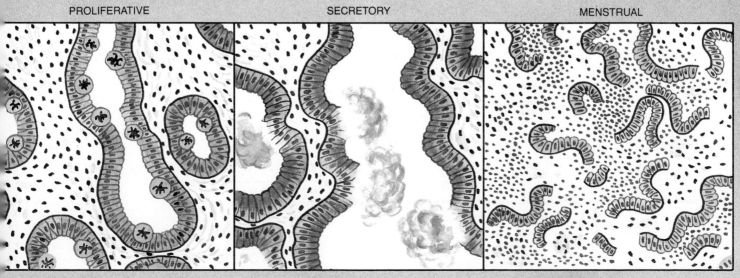

PROLIFERATIVE   SECRETORY   MENSTRUAL

Embryology

In general, fetal development is predominantly female unless subjected to a number of factors that originate in the fetal testis. Both the sex and autosomal chromosomes directly influence the differentiation of the indifferent gonad (urogenital ridge). The sex chromosomes determine whether the gonad will differentiate into testis or ovary. If the gonadal stroma is male, genes associated with the Y chromosome interact with other components of the somatic cells in the primitive gonad and initiate the development of seminiferous tubules. The gene responsible for the expression of the H-Y antigen complex that determines gonadal differentiation is auto-somal, but genes on the X and Y chromosomes have a regulatory influence on H-Y gene expression.

The müllerian ducts in both females and males appear around day 37 as funnel-shaped openings of celomic epithelium. These develop into paired, undifferentiated tubes that later fuse to become a straight uterovaginal canal at about day 54. Sertoli cells of the developing testis produce müllerian inhibiting substance, a polypeptide protein that causes the müllerian (paramesonephric) ducts to regress. In the absence of this substance the müllerian ducts develop passively to form the fallopian tubes, uterus, and wall of vagina. Müllerian inhibiting substance is first secreted in an effective amount 56 to 62 days after fertilization, or about 2 weeks after the testis becomes anatomically distinct. Development of the

Table 18-1 Infectious Diseases of the Female Genital Tract

ORGANISM	DISEASE	DISTINCTIVE FEATURE
Sexually Transmitted Diseases		
GRAM-NEGATIVE RODS AND COCCI		
Calymmatobacterium granulomatis	Granuloma inguinale	Donovan body
Gardnerella vaginalis	Gardnerella infection	Clue cell
Haemophilus ducreyi	Chancroid (soft chancre)	
Neisseria gonorrhoeae	Gonorrhea	
THE SPIROCHETES		
Treponema pallidum	Syphilis	
THE MYCOPLASMAS		
Mycoplasma hominis	Nonspecific vaginitis	
Ureaplasma urealyticum	Nonspecific vaginitis	
THE RICKETTSIAS		
Chlamydia trachomatis, types D-K	Various forms of PID*	
Chlamydia trachomatis, type L (1-23)	Lymphogranuloma venereum	
VIRUSUS		
Papilloma virus	Condyloma acuminatum	Koilocyte
Herpes simplex, type 2	Herpes infection	Multicleate giant cell
Molluscum contagiosum	Molluscum infection	Molluscum body
Cytomegalovirus	Cytomegalic inclusion disease	
PROTOZOA		
Trichomonas vaginalis	Trichomoniasis	
Selected Non-Sexually Transmitted Diseases		
GRAM-POSITIVE BACTERIA		
Staphylococcus aureus	Toxic shock syndrome	
THE ACTINOMYCES AND RELATED ORGANISMS		
Actinomyces israelii	PID (one of many organisms)	Sulfur granules
Mycobacterium tuberculosis	Tuberculosis	Necrotizing granulomas
FUNGI		
Candida albicans	Candidiasis	

* PID, pelvic inflammatory disease

masculine external genitalia is dependent on the local conversion of testosterone (the "prohormone") to dihydrotestosterone. In the absence of stimulation by dihydrotestosterone, the external genitalia remain female. Female internal organs and external genitalia develop partially even in the absence of hormones secreted by the fetal ovary. Female development also occurs when gonads are not present. Unless interrupted by the regressive influence of müllerian inhibiting substance, differentiation of the müllerian ducts proceeds cephalocaudally to form fallopian tubes, a uterus, and a vagina. The genital tubercle develops into the clitoris, the genital folds into the labia minora, and the genital swellings into the labia majora. The basic architecture of the female genital tract is completed by day 120.

Infectious Disorders

Infectious disorders of the female genital tract are common and caused by a wide variety of pathogenic organisms (Table 18-1). Most of these pathogens are acquired during sexual intercourse, and collectively the resulting diseases are called "sexually transmitted diseases."

Sexually Transmitted Diseases

Bacteria

Granuloma Inguinale (Calymmatobacterium granulomatis)

C. granulomatis, a gram-negative, nonmotile, encapsulated rod related to the family *Enterobacteriaceae*, causes granuloma inguinale. The disease occurs with equal frequency in males and females. The primary lesion begins as a painless, ulcerated nodule involving the genital, inguinal, or perianal skin. Extensive local spread and lymphatic permeation occur later. Vacuolated histiocytes are packed with characteristic intracellular bacteria (Donovan bodies). The organism is best seen with a Wright stain and resembles a closed safety pin. The squamous epithelium overlying the involved area may demonstrate severe hyperplasia, sometimes exuberant enough to be misinterpreted as a squamous cell carcinoma.

Gardnerella Infection (G. vaginalis)

G. vaginalis, **a sexually transmitted, gram-negative coccobacillus, accounts for 90% of cases of nonspecific vaginitis.** A biopsy specimen is usually normal, because the organism neither penetrates the mucosa nor elicits an inflammatory reaction. The diagnosis can be established either by direct microscopic examination of the vaginal discharge or by Papanicolaou smear. The squamous cells are covered by coccobacilli (clue cells) and are not accompanied by a significant inflammatory reaction.

Chancroid (Haemophilus ducreyi)

H. ducreyi, a gram-negative, nonmotile bacillus, causes chancroid, also called soft chancre. This disease is rare in the United States. Following a 3 to 5 day incubation period, single (or sometimes multiple), small vesiculopustular lesions appear on the cervix, vagina, vulva, or perianal region. The lesions may discharge to form a purulent ulcer that is painful and bleeds easily. There may be associated inguinal lymphadenopathy, fever, chills, and malaise. Histologic examination reveals a granulomatous inflammatory reaction. The diagnosis is confirmed by culture. A major complication is scar formation during the healing phase, an outcome that may eventuate in urethral stenosis.

Gonorrhea (Neisseria gonorrhoeae)

N. gonorrhoeae, a fastidious, gram-negative diplococcus, is the causative organism of gonorrhea. It is a difficult organism to culture, requiring CO_2 and specially enriched media for growth. **A sexually transmitted disease, its incidence is one million cases a year in the United States. It is a frequent cause of acute salpingitis and pelvic inflammatory disease** (see below). The stratified and cornified layers of the adult vulva and vaginal epithelium are resistant to infection by the organism. The juvenile vulvovaginal tissue, which has thinner epithelial layers and an alkaline vaginal secretion, is more susceptible to infection.

The organism adheres to the mucous membranes of the lower genital tract and reaches the tubal lumen directly by ascending the cervical and endometrial cavities (Fig. 18-2). An acute endometritis results during its passage. The organism attaches to nonciliated cells in the fallopian tube, is engulfed within 3 hours by the microvilli, and elicits a pronounced, acute, fibrinous, inflammatory reaction, which is confined to the mucosal surface. From the tubal lumen the infection may spread to involve the ovary, a course that results in a tubo-ovarian abscess. It may also spread more widely to involve the pelvic and abdominal cavities, with the formation of subdiaphragmatic and pelvic abscesses. Systemic complications include septicemia and septic arthritis. The organism induces a purulent inflammatory reaction at all sites of infection. Resolution is rarely complete and there is for-

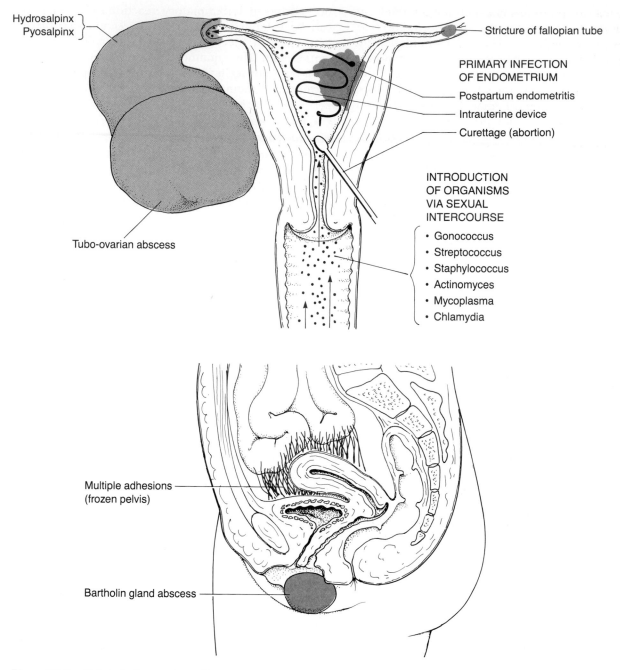

Hydrosalpinx
Pyosalpinx

Stricture of fallopian tube

PRIMARY INFECTION
OF ENDOMETRIUM

Postpartum endometritis

Intrauterine device

Curettage (abortion)

Tubo-ovarian abscess

INTRODUCTION
OF ORGANISMS
VIA SEXUAL
INTERCOURSE

• Gonococcus
• Streptococcus
• Staphylococcus
• Actinomyces
• Mycoplasma
• Chlamydia

Multiple adhesions
(frozen pelvis)

Bartholin gland abscess

Figure 18-2.   Pelvic inflammatory disease.

mation of dense fibrous adhesions. **Healing with distortion and destruction of the tubal epithelium often leads to sterility.**

The Spirochetes

Syphilis (Treponema pallidum)

Syphilis is a venereal disease caused by *T. pallidum,* a thin, motile, spiral-shaped (spirochete) bacterium. It is acquired through sexual contact with an infected individual or *in utero* (congenital syphilis). Because of a complex immunologic reaction to the bacterium, which results in a long-term host–parasite relationship, untreated syphilis may wax and wane, progressing through three stages: primary, secondary, and tertiary (early, infectious, and late syphilis, respectively).

The organism penetrates small abrasions in the skin or normal mucosal membranes. The initial manifestation, the chancre, usually appears at the portal of entry after an incubation period of about 3 weeks. Initially, this lesion is a painless, indurated papule, 1 cm to 2 cm in diameter, surrounded by an inflammatory cuff, which breaks down to form an ulcer. The chancre may persist for 2 to 6 weeks and then heals spontaneously. The secondary stage, which appears after a latent period of several weeks to several months, is characterized by low-grade fever, headache, malaise, lymphadenopathy, and the reappearance of highly contagious syphilitic lesions called condylomata lata (syphilitic warts). After 2 to 6 weeks, the secondary infectious lesions heal and the symptoms disappear spontaneously. Any time thereafter, the tertiary stage, complicated by cardiovascular and nervous system involvement, may develop.

Mycoplasma

Mycoplasma (M. hominis and Ureaplasma urealyticum)

Mycoplasmas are minute pleomorphic organisms that resemble the so-called ''L'' bacterial forms. They are common commensals of the oropharyngeal and urogenital tracts. Colonization of the lower genital tract by both organisms occurs through sexual contact. *M. hominis* is responsible for a small proportion of cases of symptomatic cervicitis and vaginitis. It is more frequently cultivated in association with *Gardnerella vaginalis* or *Trichomonas vaginalis*, which are well-recognized causes of vaginitis. Although the role of mycoplasmas in genital tract infection is not completely understood, the organisms are encountered in pelvic inflammatory disease (see below), acute salpingitis, spontaneous abortion, puerperal fever, and low birth weight. The histologic appearance of the affected tissue is usually unremarkable.

Rickettsia

Chlamydia and Lymphogranuloma Venereum (Chlamydia trachomatis)

C. trachomatis, a rickettsial organism, is a common venereally transmitted organism. It is an obligate, gram-negative, intracellular bacterium that, because it is small and replicates only within susceptible cells, was previously considered to be a virus. Fifteen serotypes are known, and they result in a wide variety of clinical conditions, including trachoma, mucopurulent conjunctivitis, and lymphogranuloma venereum. In the more common form of genital infections, the cervical mucosa is inflamed and the endocervical metaplastic squamous cells reveal small inclusion bodies. Complications include ascending infection of the endometrium, fallopian tube, and ovary, with consequent pelvic inflammatory disease (see below), tubal occlusion, and infertility. Infants who are delivered vaginally may become infected and develop conjunctivitis.

A second form of sexually transmitted disease caused by *C. trachomatis* is **lymphogranuloma venereum.** The infection is indigenous to tropical countries. In the first stage of the disease a small painless vesicle forms after 3 to 30 days at the site of inoculation. It heals in a few days and in many instances is unrecognized. The second stage presents with the development of bilateral enlargement of inguinal lymph nodes, which may rupture and form suppurative fistulas. The inguinal nodes in men and perirectal nodes in women become matted and painful. **In a few untreated patients, a third stage is characterized by scarring, which may cause lymphatic obstruction, with resultant genital elephantiasis and rectal strictures.** Infected tissues show necrotizing granulomas, neutrophilic infiltrates, and, occasionally, inclusion bodies within histiocytes.

Viruses

Condyloma Acuminatum (Human Papilloma Virus)

The human papilloma virus is a DNA virus. Over 40 types are recognized, five of which are associated with genital tract disease. Types 6 and 11 are usually seen with **condyloma acuminatum** (venereal warts), lesions that are being increasingly recognized as **a common form of sexually transmitted disease.** Of particular concern with these diseases is their **association with and possible etiologic role in the development of cervical dysplasia, carcinoma in situ, and squamous cell carcinoma.** Types 16, 18, and 31 have been found in the vast majority of high-grade precancerous lesions and invasive carcinomas (see below).

Large condylomas, which are entirely benign, are evident on visual examination, but many are small and require colposcopic detection. The lesions occur on the vulva, perianal region, perineum, vagina, and cervix and may involve the distal urethra and rectum. They grow as papules, plaques, or nodules and eventually as spiked or cauliflower-like excrescences. The most striking finding on microscopic examination is a papillomatous proliferation of squamous epithelium. The characteristic epithelial cell is the koilocyte, a cell with a wrinkled nucleus that contains viral particles. The morphologic changes of condyloma are common in dysplastic epithelial cells of the cervix. The presence of viral DNA sequences in the preneoplastic lesions, in cancers, and even in the metastases of squamous cell cancers provides strong evidence of an etiologic role for the **papilloma virus in the development of cervical cancer** (see below).

Herpes Simplex (H. Simplex, Type 2)

Herpes simplex, serotype 2, an intranuclear, double-stranded DNA virus, is a common cause of sexually transmitted, genital infection. After an incubation period of 1 to 3 weeks, many small vesicles develop on the vulva, vagina, and cervix. The vesicles develop into painful ulcers. In the latent state the virus remains in the sacral ganglia. Diagnosis is made by cytologic interpretation of a vaginal or cervical smear or by tissue biopsy. Characteristic cytologic features include multinucleated giant cells and, occasionally, large nuclei with eosinophilic inclusions. Intraepithelial vesicles show ballooning degeneration of the adjacent epithelial cells, many of which contain large nuclei with eosinophilic inclusions. The inclusions are not pathognomonic of herpes simplex, type 2, as similar inclusions are found in varicella and herpes zoster. Complications include a **possible oncogenic role in the development of cervical cancer** (see below) and transmission of the virus to the neonate during birth. **Neonatal infection is often fatal.**

Molluscum Infection (M. contagiosum)

M. contagiosum, a highly contagious poxvirus, is characterized by multiple, smooth, gray-white nodules that are centrally umbilicated and exude a cheesy material. They occur predominantly in the genital region, but may be found elsewhere on the body. Characteristic large, cytoplasmic viral inclusions ("molluscum bodies") are found in the infected epithelial cells.

Cytomegalic Inclusion Disease (Cytomegalovirus)

The cytomegalovirus (CMV) is a rare pathogen in the female genital tract. It causes endocervicitis, endometritis, and oophoritis. Infection of the endometrium may result in spontaneous abortion or infection of the neonate. Infected cells exhibit characteristic large, eosinophilic, intranuclear inclusions and, occasionally, cytoplasmic inclusions.

Protozoa

Trichomoniasis (Trichomonas vaginalis)

T. vaginalis is a large, pear-shaped, flagellated protozoan that is **a common cause of vaginitis.** The disease is sexually transmitted; about 25% of women are asymptomatic carriers. The infection presents as a heavy, yellow-gray, thick, foamy discharge accompanied by severe itching, dyspareunia (painful intercourse), and dysuria (painful urination). The diagnosis is confirmed by a wet mount preparation in which the motile trichomonads are seen or by demonstrating the organisms in a Papanicolaou-stained cervical smear.

Diseases not Transmitted Sexually

Bacteria

Toxic Shock Syndrome (Staphylococcus aureus)

The toxic shock syndrome was first identified in 1978 in women using tampons. Symptoms include high fever, vomiting, diarrhea, a diffuse rash, and shock. At the peak incidence of the disease in 1980, 90% occurred in women at the time of menstruation. The fatality rate is about 6%. The risk of contracting the disease is increased by the use of **magnesium-absorbing fibers, which until recently were used in superabsorbent tampons.** *S. aureus* colonizes the damaged vaginal mucosa and releases exotoxins that are responsible for the major manifestation of the syndrome. Low levels of magnesium provide an ideal condition for production of toxins by the bacteria. Pathologic features include perivasculitis in many organs and changes associated with shock.

The Actinomyces and Related Organisms

Tuberculosis (Mycobacterium tuberculosis) M. tuberculosis may infect any segment of the genital tract. Most cases of genital infection result from localized dissemination of the mycobacterium from a focus in the fallopian tubes, infection of which reflects spread from the lung. Large quantities of exudate may form and distend the fallopian tube, conditions labeled **pyosalpinx** and **hydrosalpinx.** The adjacent ovary may be involved in the process. **Tuberculous salpingitis** often results in fibrinous adhesions and scarring, complications that cause a multiplicity of functional abnormalities—infertility, ectopic gestation, and pelvic pain.

The microscopic feature typical of tuberculosis is the necrotizing granuloma. The endometrium, because it sheds cyclically, exhibits granulomas before they have sufficient time to necrotize; caseous necrosis, therefore, is not seen.

Actinomycosis (Actinomyces israelii) Genital tract actinomycosis is uncommon but has been increasingly reported in association with intrauterine devices, although other foci may exist. *A. israelii*, the causative organism, is a gram-positive rod that is thought to enter the uterine cavity via the tail of the IUD. It ascends to infect the fallopian tube, ovary, and broad ligaments to form a tubo-ovarian abscess. Suppurating lesions display drainage tracts that contain dense microcolonies of the organism ("sulfur granules.") Actinomycosis results in extensive fibrosis and scarring.

Fungi

Candidiasis (Candida albicans)

Approximately 10% of women are asymptomatic carriers of vulvovaginal fungi, *C. albicans* being the most common. About 1% to 2% of nonpregnant and 5% to 10% of pregnant women present with clinically apparent **vulvovaginitis.** Pregnancy, diabetes mellitus, and the use of oral contraceptives promote vaginal candidiasis. The infection presents as vulvar itching and a whitish discharge. Clinical examination reveals firmly adherent, small white plaques. The diagnosis can be made by finding characteristic spores and pseudohyphae in a wet mount preparation or with a Papanicolaou stain. Tissue biopsy discloses considerable submucosal edema and a chronic inflammatory infiltrate. The fungus generally does not penetrate the epithelium and the white patches correspond to foci of desquamated, necrotic epithelial cells, cellular debris, bacterial flora, and the spores and pseudohyphae of *C. albicans*. Untreated, the infection waxes and wanes, and it frequently disappears following delivery.

Diseases of Multiple Causes (Polymicrobial)

Pelvic Inflammatory Disease

Pelvic inflammatory disease (PID) describes an infectious process of the pelvis and pelvic organs that usually follows extension of bacteria present in the vagina at the time of menses (see Fig. 18-2). *N. gonorrhoeae* **is the principal single organism causing PID, but most infections are polymicrobial.** Patients usually present with lower abdominal pain. Because the salpingitis is almost always bilateral, there is bilateral adnexal tenderness and marked discomfort when the uterus and cervix are palpated. **Infection with chlamydia, which is typically silent, is one of the most common infectious causes of infertility due to tubal damage.** In the later stages of PID, the ovaries may become involved with abscess formation. **Rupture of a tubo-ovarian abscess is a life-threatening complication.** It is believed that intrauterine devices are also associated with a higher frequency of PID because they permit the introduction of the causative organism. Actinomycosis should be suspected when a patient with a long-standing IUD develops a low-grade, chronic fever, dull ache, and pelvic mass.

Vulva

Anatomy

The vulva is composed of the mons pubis, labia majora and minora, clitoris, and vestibule. With the onset of puberty, the mons pubis and the lateral borders of the labia majora acquire increased subcutaneous fat and develop coarse hair. The sebaceous and apocrine glands in these regions develop concomitantly. The paired external openings of the paraurethral glands (Skene's glands) lie on either side of the urethral meatus. Bartholin's glands, which are located immediately posterolateral to the introitus, are branching, mucus-secreting, tubuloalveolar glands, drained by a duct 2.5 cm long. In addition, scattered through the vulva are microscopic mucous glands. The femoral and inguinal lymph nodes provide the primary lymph drainage routes, except for the clitoris, which shares the lymphatic drainage of the urethra.

Dystrophy

Dystrophy, a term that refers to a group of lesions **without malignant potential,** is defined as a disorder of epithelial growth that often presents as a white lesion of the vulva, resulting in otherwise unclassified alterations of the epithelial and dermal architecture. The dystrophies—**hyperplastic dystrophy and lichen sclerosus**—occur in women of any age but are most frequent in middle age.

Hyperplastic dystrophy is characterized by a proliferation of squamous epithelium (acanthosis) that results in enlargement and confluence of the epidermal rete ridges. Commonly, the thickened epithelium displays a marked increase in superficial keratin, a condition called hyperkeratosis. This thickened layer of epithelium, previously termed "leukoplakia," imparts a white appearance to the vulva. Since carcinomas may also be keratinized and appear white, the term has caused considerable confusion and is, therefore, no longer used. Biopsy is required to distinguish hyperplastic dystrophy, which is benign, from dysplasia and carcinoma.

Lichen sclerosus comprises **hyperkeratosis, blunting or loss of rete ridges, and a homogeneous, acel-**

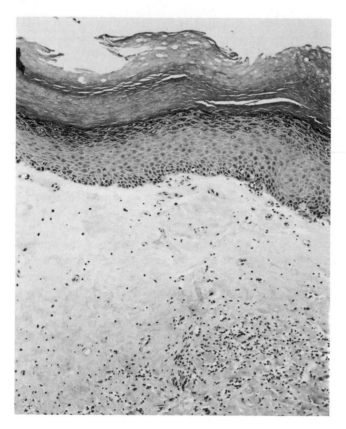

Figure 18-3.   Lichen sclerosus of the vulva. The epidermis shows loss of the normal ridged pattern, hyalinized dermis, chronic inflammatory infiltrate, and hyperkeratosis.

lular, subepithelial zone (Fig. 18-3). This acellular zone results from swelling and splitting of the collagen bundles into individual fibers and fibrils, which become enveloped by a gel-like matrix. A band of chronic inflammatory cells typically lies beneath this layer. The term "lichen sclerosus et atrophicus" was once applied to this condition. However, kinetic studies have shown that the lesion is not atrophic but has remarkable metabolic activity. Itching is the most common symptom, and dyspareunia is often troublesome. There is no association with cancer.

Cysts

Bartholin's gland cyst. The paired Bartholin's glands produce a clear mucoid secretion that continuously lubricates the vestibular surface but does not contribute significantly to vaginal secretion prior to intercourse. The ducts are prone to obstruction and consequent cyst formation. The cysts may become infected, which leads to the formation of abscesses. Bartholin's gland abscess is often associated with gonorrhea but can be caused by *Staphylococcus* and some anaerobic organisms. Treatment consists of incision, drainage, marsupialization, and appropriate antibiotics.

Keratinous cysts, also termed epithelial inclusion cysts, are frequently seen on the vulva, especially the labia majora. They contain a white cheesy material and are typically lined by stratified squamous epithelium. The cyst may represent occluded sebaceous glands that have undergone squamous metaplasia.

Mucinous cysts are derived from obstructed mucinous glands. Despite theories of "dysontogenic" development, detailed anatomic studies in newborns have found that mucinous glands are normally present throughout the vulva, including the region of the urethra. Since the glands are lined by mucinous columnar cells and produce mucinous secretions, obstruction and infection may occur.

Benign Tumors and Tumor-Like Conditions

Ectopic breast tissue, in the form of small, isolated nodules, may extend in the "milk line" to the vulva and enlarge during pregnancy.

Hidradenoma is an unusual benign tumor of apocrine sweat gland origin that develops in the labia majora or, sometimes, the labia minora as a sharply circumscribed nodule under 2 cm in diameter. Microscopically, the lesion is papillary and composed of tubules and acini lined by two layers of cells; an inner, apocrine columnar cell layer and an outer, myoepithelial cell layer.

Syringoma is an adenoma of eccrine glands. They are flesh-colored papules arising within the dermis of the labia majora that are usually asymptomatic. The ducts are lined by two layers of cells, the outer being myoepithelial.

Connective tissue tumors are of several types. Senile hemangiomas (cherry hemangiomas) are small, red-to-purple skin papules of no clinical significance. Excessive surface trauma may induce bleeding and necessitate excision. Histologic examination reveals numerous dilated capillaries in the connective tissue. The pyogenic granuloma, previously thought to be a reaction to superficial wound infection, is a variant of hemangioma. Secondary infection occurs, because the surface of the lesion is easily traumatized. Soft-tissue tumors found elsewhere in the body also occur in the vulva, including granular cell tumor (a tumor of Schwann cell origin), leiomyoma, fibroma, lipoma, and histiocytoma.

Malignant Tumors and Premalignant Conditions

Squamous Cell Lesions

Dysplasia and Carcinoma in Situ

Vulvar dysplasia was in the past an uncommon disease. During the past two decades, dysplasia and carcinoma in situ (also called vulvar intraepithelial neoplasia) have increased in frequency, especially in the young. **The epidemiologic characteristics of patients with vulvar intraepithelial neoplasia and cancer are similar to those of women with cervical intraepithelial neoplasia and cancer, an association that suggests that a venereally transmitted agent may play a role in the genesis of squamous neoplasia in both sites.** Moreover, the fact that women with condyloma acuminatum ("venereal warts") and associated dysplasia are approximately 15 years younger than those with only dysplasia suggests that papilloma virus may trigger the development of dysplasia.

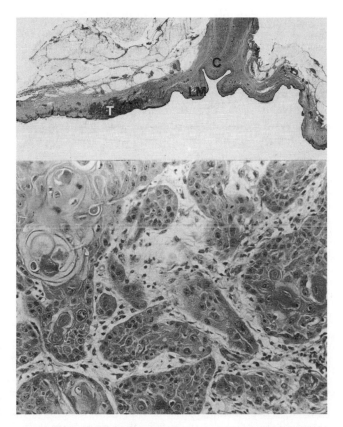

Figure 18-4. Squamous cell carcinoma of the vulva. (*Top*) A 1-cm tumor (*T*) confined to the dermis. The specimen shows left and right halves of the perineum, including the labia minora (*LM*) and clitoris (*C*). (*Bottom*) Small nests of neoplastic squamous cells, some with keratin pearls, are invasive in the stroma.

Table 18-2 Clinical Staging of Carcinoma of the Vulva

STAGE	DESCRIPTION
0	Carcinoma in situ
I	Tumor 2 cm or less in diameter, confined to vulva
II	Tumor greater than 2 cm in diameter, confined to vulva
III	Tumor of any size extending to urethra, vagina, perineum, or anus, or lymph nodes obviously involved but mobile
IV	Tumor invading bladder, rectum, or bone; or any fixed nodes; or any distant metastases

Papilloma virus, usually HPV-16, is found in over 80% of the lesions of vulvar intraepithelial neoplasia. Following local excision, dysplasia often persists or recurs (25%) or progresses to invasive carcinoma involving the vulva, vagina, or anus (20%).

Criteria for distinguishing the various grades of dysplasia or carcinoma in situ are less precise for the vulva than for the cervix. As in the cervix, degrees of severity are based on a consideration of qualitative as well as quantitative changes. Bowen's disease, a term that still sometimes appears in the dermatologic literature, is a synonym for carcinoma in situ.

Squamous Cell Carcinoma

Squamous cell carcinoma of the vulva (Fig. 18-4) accounts for 3% of all genital cancers in women and is **the most common primary malignant neoplasm of the vulva (90%).** In the past it affected mainly older women (over age 60), but like dysplasia, it now occurs more frequently in younger women. Approximately two-thirds of vulvar carcinomas are exophytic; the others are ulcerative and endophytic. Itching of long duration is commonly the first symptom; with ulceration, bleeding and secondary infection may develop. The tumors grow slowly, extend to the contiguous skin, vagina, and rectum, and metastasize to inguinal, femoral, and pelvic lymph nodes.

A staging system for vulvar cancer employs 2 cm in greatest dimension as the critical size that differentiates Stage I from Stage II lesions (Table 18-2). Patients with involvement of the pelvic lymph nodes on microscopic examination have a 5-year survival rate of less than 25%. When only the inguinal nodes are involved, the survival rate is 65%. The survival rate approaches 90% when the nodes are uninvolved. Tumor differentiation also affects prognosis, the more differentiated cancers being associated with a longer mean survival.

"Microinvasive cancer of the vulva" is a concept that was employed until recently in an attempt to identify the minimum diameter and depth below

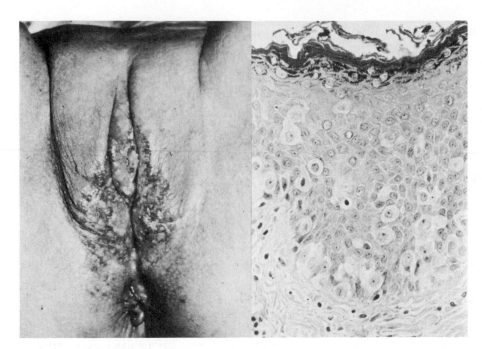

Figure 18-5. Paget's disease of the vulva. The neoplastic cells are single, infiltrate the epithelium, and have copious pale cytoplasm, which easily distinguishes them from surrounding keratinocytes.

which tumors do not metastasize. Tumors invasive to less than 5 mm have an 11% rate of metastasis. Tumors with a depth of invasion of 1 mm or less have virtually no metastatic potential. **Carcinomas are now described in terms of depth of invasion without specifying "microinvasion."**

Verrucous carcinoma is a distinct variety of squamous cell carcinoma that presents as a large fungating mass, resembling a giant condyloma acuminatum. Recurrence usually results from inadequate prior excision. **The tumor is unusually well differentiated,** being composed of large nests of squamous cells with copious cytoplasm and relatively small, bland nuclei. Squamous pearls are uncommon and mitoses are rare. The tumor invades with broad tongues, and at the stromal interface is commonly accompanied by a **heavy lymphoplasmacytic infiltrate. This cancer typically invades locally but does not metastasize.** Wide local surgical excision is the treatment of choice.

Paget's Disease

Paget's disease is primarily an integumentary neoplasm found in the milk line, from the axilla to the vulva. It occurs most often in the nipple, where it is almost always associated with an underlying ductal adenocarcinoma. In the vulva, Paget cells arise de novo in the epidermis or in epidermally derived adnexal structures, but the exact cell origin is still unknown. Paget's disease of the vulva is an intraepithelial neoplasm that may become invasive. Paget cells are usually confined to the epidermis and appear

as large single cells or, less commonly, as clusters of cells that lack intercellular bridges and have a pale, vacuolated cytoplasm (Fig. 18-5). The cytoplasm contains neutral and acid mucopolysaccharides, which stain with PAS and mucicarmine. **Paget's disease is often far more extensive than is apparent on preoperative biopsy. Treatment requires wide local excision with generous borders or simple vulvectomy.**

Malignant Melanoma

Malignant melanoma accounts for approximately 5% of malignant vulvar neoplasms. It occurs most commonly in the sixth and seventh decades but occasionally is seen in younger women. The tumor is highly aggressive and is associated with a low overall survival rate.

Vagina

Anatomy

The vagina extends from the uterus to the vestibule at an angle of more than 90°. It is approximately 7 cm along the ventral wall and 9 cm along the dorsal wall. The squamous epithelial lining is responsive to sex hormones. Estrogen supports the synthesis of intracellular glycogen, which gives the epithelium a characteristic appearance in both tissue sections and Papanicolaou smears. Lymph drains through the perivaginal plexus situated laterally. The lymphatics from the vaginal vault and upper anterior vagina communicate with branches from the cervix and drain into the iliac lymph nodes. Lymph from the posterior upper vagina drains into the region of the inferior gluteal, sacral, and anorectal nodes. The lower vagina drains to the femoral, inguinal, and pelvic lymph nodes.

Non-Neoplastic Conditions

Senile Atrophic Vaginitis

Senile atrophic vaginitis is a superimposed **secondary infection of an atrophic squamous epithelium, a consequence of postmenopausal estrogen deficiency.** The epithelium becomes thin and, as a result, a poor barrier to infection or abrasion. Common symptoms are dyspareunia or vaginal spotting. The latter must be distinguished from signs of uterine malignancy, which also occurs in older women.

Cysts

The paired mesonephric (wolffian) ducts, which may have multiple branchings and lie lateral to the vagina, degenerate during fetal life. Rarely, cysts may develop at any point along their course. Most cysts are less than a few millimeters in diameter, but on occasion they may be more than 1 cm across. The lining cells lack cilia and have a pale luminal cytoplasm and nuclei with bland chromatin. Mesonephric cysts are frequently confused with the cystic form of adenosis, a lesion of young women usually associated with prenatal exposure to diethylstilbestrol (DES).

Vaginal Adenosis and Squamous Metaplasia (DES-Related Changes)

Exposure during prenatal life to DES is associated with the subsequent development of clear cell adenocarcinoma of the vagina, adenosis (presence of glandular tissue in the vagina), squamous metaplasia, cervical ectropion, gross structural changes in both the vagina and cervix, and upper genital tract abnormalities. It has been estimated that up to two million women were exposed *in utero* between 1940 and 1971; the vast majority were exposed during the 1940s and 1950s. In addition to the DES-related cases, adenosis has been also found on occasion in older women who were born before the DES era.

The development of adenosis has an embryologic basis. In the normal sequence of development, just before the 8th week of gestation, the müllerian ducts fuse into the common uterovaginal canal. At the 10th

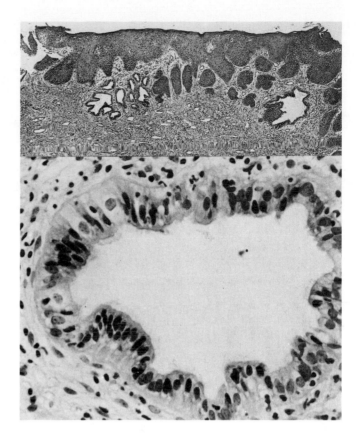

Figure 18-6. Vaginal adenosis. (*Top*) Glands lined by ciliated dark cells resembling tubal or endometrial (tuboendometrial) epithelium are present in the inflamed lamina propria. In areas outside the photograph they merge with the squamous pegs. The surface epithelium is composed of glycogen-free squamous cells, which account for the abnormal iodine staining. (*Bottom*) Higher-power view of tuboendometrial cells.

week, the glandular epithelium is replaced by squamous epithelium, a process believed to involve an upgrowth of urogenital sinus–type epithelium, which undermines and replaces the glandular tissue. The process is complete by the 18th week. Given any time during the period of about the 8th through the 18th week, DES inhibits this process of transformation from glandular to squamous epithelium and some glandular tissue remains. This residual glandular tissue constitutes the area of adenosis (Fig. 18-6).

The frequency of DES-related adenosis is greater the earlier the time during pregnancy when the mother first began the drug and the larger the total dosage of the drug taken. About one-third of all exposed women have adenosis or show evidence of squamous metaplasia, which is a physiologic healing response of the vagina to the presence of the adenosis (i.e., to the glandular tissue). Both conditions are usually asymptomatic in exposed daughters. Occasionally, the glands become infected or produce cop-

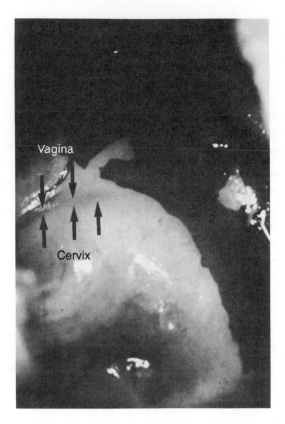

Figure 18-7. Abnormal iodine (Schiller) stain. The aglycogenated (nonstraining) areas in both the vagina and cervix identify the areas of squamous metaplasia (the "transformation zone"). The normal glycogenated epithelium stains deep brown. Arrows demarcate the cervicovaginal boundary.

ious mucus; both of these circumstances lead to symptoms.

The lesions of adenosis are composed of one of two types of cells: mucinous columnar cells that resemble the normal cells lining the endocervix, and cells that resemble the normal ones lining the endometrium or fallopian tube. The metaplastic squamous cells that line the surface of the vagina are immature and glycogen-poor and therefore do not stain with iodine; glycogen of the normal, mature vaginal and cervical squamous cells stains mahogany brown with iodine, a property that forms the basis of the Schiller test (Fig. 18-7).

Benign Tumors and Tumor-Like Conditions

Fibroepithelial Polyp

Vaginal polyps are rare, usually single, and less than 1 cm in diameter. Not uncommonly, polyps occur in pregnant women. The whitish, connective tissue polyp is short and rubbery and is covered by squamous epithelium. Polyps are benign and must be differentiated from embryonal rhabdomyosarcoma, a highly malignant tumor.

Miscellaneous Mesenchymal Growths

A number of benign tumors in the vagina resemble those in other parts of the gynecologic tract. These include tumors of smooth muscle (leiomyoma) and striated muscle (benign rhabdomyoma), and neurofibroma. These solid submucosal tumors tend to be less than 2 cm in diameter. An unusual neoplasm is the **granular cell tumor.** Clusters of cells up to 5 cm in diameter have copious **granular cytoplasm and ill-defined borders.** The tumors are now recognized as benign lesions of **Schwann cell origin.** Granular cell tumors that impinge on the overlying squamous epithelium can elicit pseudoepitheliomatous hyperplasia and may be confused with squamous cell carcinoma.

Malignant Tumors

Primary malignant tumors of the vagina are rare, constituting less than 2% of all genital tract tumors.

Squamous Cell Carcinoma
Squamous cell carcinoma develops most commonly in the posterior wall of the upper one-third of the vagina, where it usually presents as an exophytic mass. It is a disease of older women, the peak incidence lying between the ages of 60 and 70 years. Vaginal dysplasia and carcinoma in situ occur, and may precede the development of invasive carcinoma. Not infrequently, squamous cell carcinoma of the vagina develops some years after cervical or vulvar carcinoma, a sequence that supports the concept of a field effect of carcinogenesis in the lower genital tract. The prognosis is related to the clinical stage of the tumor (Table 18-3). The 5-year survival rate is 80% to 90% for Stage I tumors, 50% for Stage II tumors, and 20% for Stage III and IV tumors.

Clear Cell Adenocarcinoma
Approximately 0.1% of women exposed *in utero* to DES develop **clear cell adenocarcinoma,** most frequently on the anterior wall of the upper third of the vagina (Fig. 18-8). The tumor rarely appears before age 13 and is most common between ages 17 and 22. **Although almost all clear cell adenocarcinomas are associated with vaginal adenosis, very few women with adenosis develop this cancer.** Atypical adenosis is suspected of being the precursor lesion. The co-

pious clear cytoplasm, reflecting the presence of glycogen, accounts for the name "clear cell" adenocarcinoma. With more frequent screening programs, more tumors are detected when they are small and asymptomatic. At this stage the overall survival rate approaches 100%. In more advanced stages, the tumors may spread hematogenously (first occurrence in the lung) or by lymphatic spread.

Embryonal Rhabdomyosarcoma (Sarcoma Botryoides)

Embryonal rhabdomyosarcoma is an exceedingly rare vaginal tumor that occurs almost exclusively in children under the age of 4 years. The tumor is of stromal (mesenchymal) origin and arises in the lamina propria. **It appears as confluent polypoid masses resembling a bunch of grapes**—hence the name sarcoma botryoides (Greek *botrys* grapes) (Fig. 18-9). The tumor is composed of poorly differentiated spindle and round cells (rhabdomyoblasts), some of which display the cross striations of striated muscle. A dense zone of round cell rhabdomyoblasts, referred to as the cambium layer, is present beneath the vaginal epithelium. Deep to this, the stroma is myxomatous and shows scattered rhabdomyoblasts. The prognosis is poor; the 5-year survival rate is less than 15%.

Endodermal Sinus Tumor

Endodermal sinus tumor, a rare germ cell neoplasm, occurs almost exclusively in children, and presents as a mass filling the lumen of the vagina and protruding through the introitus. Consequently, it may be confused with embryonal rhabdomyosarcoma. The neoplasm histologically resembles its counterpart in the ovary or testis. It is characterized by the presence of Schiller-Duval bodies (resembling endodermal sinuses of the rat placenta) and eosinophilic hyaline globules. The tumor synthesizes α-fetoprotein, which can be measured in the serum and serves as a tumor marker in diagnosis and follow-up.

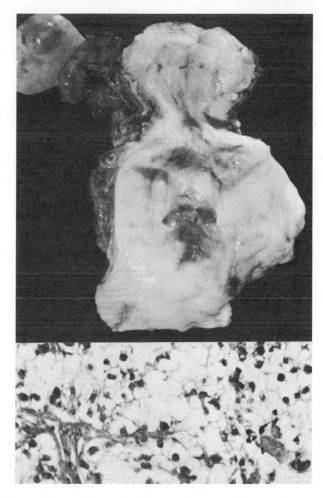

Figure 18-8. Clear cell adenocarcinoma of the vagina (*top*). Microscopic pattern of clear cell tumor (*bottom*).

Malignant Melanoma

Malignant melanoma is a rare neoplasm composed of malignant melanocytes and forming a dark, pigmented mass, which may project extravaginally. Its features are those of malignant melanoma as described elsewhere. It occurs in elderly women, and the prognosis is poor.

Cervix

Anatomy

The cervix (Latin *cervix* neck) is the most caudal portion of the uterus and protrudes into the upper vagina. Its exposed portion, called interchangeably "exocervix," "ectocervix," or "portio vaginalis," is covered by squamous epithelium, which contains glycogen. The endocervix, the canal leading to the corpus, is lined by longitudinal mucosal ridges,

Table 18-3 Clinical Staging of Carcinoma of the Vagina

STAGE	DESCRIPTION
0	Carcinoma in situ
I	Tumor limited to vaginal wall
II	Tumor involving subvaginal tissue, but not extending to pelvic wall
III	Tumor extending to pelvic wall
IV	Tumor extending beyond true pelvis or involving mucosa of bladder or rectum
IVA	Spread to adjacent organs
IVB	Spread to distant organs

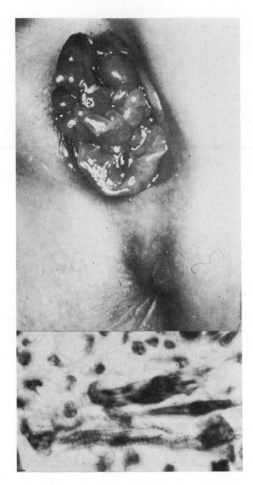

Figure 18-9. Embryonal rhabdomyosarcoma (sarcoma botryoides) of the vagina. (*Top*) The tumor appears as a bunch of grapes protruding through the introitus. (*Bottom*) Rhabdomyoblasts (striated muscle) with cross striations.

which are composed of fibrovascular cores lined by a single layer of mucinous columnar cells. The external os is the macroscopically visible junction between the exocervix and endocervix. The squamocolumnar junction is the anatomic junction between the squamous and mucinous columnar epithelia. The area between the endocervix and endometrial cavity is called the isthmus or lower uterine segment.

The Transformation Zone

The cervix remodels continuously during life. During prenatal life and infancy, the columnar epithelium that is normally present within the cervical os may extend onto the exocervix or vagina, a feature resulting in the original squamocolumnar junction being located on the exocervix. The columnar epithelium later regresses into the endocervical canal and is replaced by squamous epithelium. **The area between** the original squamocolumnar junction and the new squamocolumnar junction is termed the "transformation zone."** The glandular tissue, in response to a variety of stimuli (local pH, hormones), undergoes replacement by metaplastic squamous cells. Cells normally present deep to the mucinous epithelium (reserve cells) begin to proliferate. Initially, the layer of squamous cells is thin and immature and is characterized by large nuclei and small amounts of cytoplasm. Over time, these cells stratify and displace the glandular columnar cells. The immature metaplastic squamous epithelium displays progressive nuclear maturation and increasing amounts of glycogen-free cytoplasm toward the surface. Subsequently, the cells glycogenate and are indistinguishable from the original squamous epithelium.

Inflammatory Disease

Acute and chronic cervicitis result from infection by any number of microorganisms, particularly *Streptococcus*, *Staphylococcus*, or *Enterococcus*, and, less commonly, *Neisseria gonorrhoeae* and *Chlamydia trachomatis*. Some of these microorganisms are sexually transmitted, whereas others may be introduced by foreign bodies, such as residual fragments of tampons and pessaries. Purulent, malodorous vaginal discharge is a clinical sign of acute cervicitis. The inflamed cervix becomes congested and edematous. Since biopsy samples from the cervix frequently exhibit some degree of nonspecific chronic inflammation, the diagnosis of chronic cervicitis should be made only when numerous lymphoid cells are present.

Benign Tumors and Tumor-Like Conditions

Endocervical Polyp

The endocervical polyp is the most common cervical growth. It often presents with vaginal bleeding or discharge and appears as a single, smooth, or lobulated mass, typically less than 3 cm in diameter. The lining epithelium is mucinous, with varying degrees of squamous metaplasia, and the stroma is edematous and contains thick-walled blood vessels. Carcinoma rarely arises in polyps (0.2% of cases).

Microglandular Hyperplasia

Microglandular hyperplasia, usually an asymptomatic lesion, is caused by progestogen stimulation. For that reason it occurs during pregnancy and the postpartum period and in women taking oral contraceptives. It may be confused with a well-differentiated adenocarcinoma, since the glands are closely packed and have no intervening stroma. The lesion is benign, and there have been no recorded cases of malignant transformation. It is less commonly encountered now than in the past because the progestin content of oral contraceptives has diminished.

Leiomyoma

Leiomyoma of the cervix accounts for 8% of all uterine leiomyomas. It can become symptomatic by bleeding or prolapsing into the endocervical canal, an event that leads to uterine contractions and pain resembling the early phases of labor. The gross and microscopic appearances of cervical leiomyomas are similar to those of the leiomyomas described below.

Miscellaneous Benign Connective-Tissue Tumors

A number of benign tumors occur in the cervix that resemble those found in other parts of the body. Among these are hemangioma, neurofibroma, ganglioneuroma, adenofibroma, and adenomyoma.

Malignant and Premalignant Neoplasms

Squamous Cell Diseases

Dysplasia and Carcinoma in Situ

Dysplasia and carcinoma in situ are encompassed in the classification of **cervical intraepithelial neoplasia (CIN).** Since the introduction of mass screening programs using Papanicolaou-stained cervical smears, the frequency of detection of cervical dysplasia and carcinoma in situ has increased dramatically, with a corresponding decrease in the incidence of invasive carcinoma. *Dysplasia,* **which means abnormal growth, implies an alteration in the morphologic and constitutional character of a cell such that it has acquired the potential for malignant transformation.** *Carcinoma in situ,* **abbreviated CIS, refers to a malignant lesion that is confined to the epithelium— that is, one that has not invaded the underlying stroma.** The term cervical intraepithelial neoplasia, abbreviated CIN, was introduced to emphasize that dysplasia and CIS are points on a continuum rather than separate entities. **CIN is defined as a spectrum of intraepithelial change that begins with minimal overall atypia and progresses through stages of more marked intraepithelial abnormality to invasive squamous cell carcinoma.** The following classification has been adopted: CIN I, mild dysplasia; CIN II

moderate dysplasia; CIN III severe dysplasia and carcinoma in situ.

It is believed that half of all dysplasias regress, only 10% progress to carcinoma in situ, and fewer than 2% progress to invasive cancer. The rate of progression to a higher grade depends on the degree of preexisting dysplasia: higher degrees of dysplasia require shorter transit times to carcinoma in situ. It is thought that the average time for all dysplasias to progress to carcinoma in situ is on the order of ten years.

Epidemiology and Etiology **Multiple sexual partners and early age at first coitus are the most important factors that correlate with the development of CIN.** Recent epidemiologic studies indicate that cigarette smoking is an independent risk factor. As a consequence, dysplasia and carcinoma in situ are considered within the context of sexually transmitted diseases. There is no evidence to support the contentions that low socioeconomic status, syphilis, gonorrhea, spermatozoon DNA, or certain contraceptive methods are themselves causative of CIN. **Instead, most investigative work points to a virus in association with a cocarcinogen as the responsible agent.** In part, this concept is based on the well-known, carcinogenic potential of viruses. The most frequently implicated viruses are the herpes simplex virus, type 2, (HSV 2) and the human papillomavirus (HPV).

Herpes Simplex Virus, Type 2 (HSV 2) The evidence linking HSV to cervical neoplasia is based on seroepidemiologic studies showing elevated HSV 2 antibody titers in women with cervical neoplasia. Certain viral subgenomes cause transformation of cells in vitro and induce tumor formation in nude mice. In addition, HSV DNA has been identified in CIN lesions of all grades and in tissue culture of squamous cell carcinomas. These subgenomes have been recognized in 40% of cervical carcinomas. Although the exact role of the virus in cervical carcinogenesis is not clear, it has been suggested that herpes and HPV may be synergistic.

Human Papillomavirus Human papillomavirus has recently been recognized as a likely etiologic agent for cervical squamous carcinoma. Although only a small percentage of women infected with the virus develop CIN, **80% of early dysplastic lesions demonstrate cytologic features of HPV infection. Moreover, epithelial cells in almost all grades of CIN and invasive carcinoma contain HPV DNA.** Recently, HPV DNA has also been identified within cultured cell lines of cervical cancer and in lymph node metastases of patients with cervical cancer.

The classic benign condyloma contains either HPV 6 or HPV 11; these are regarded as low-risk HPV types. By contrast, cells in the vast majority of severe

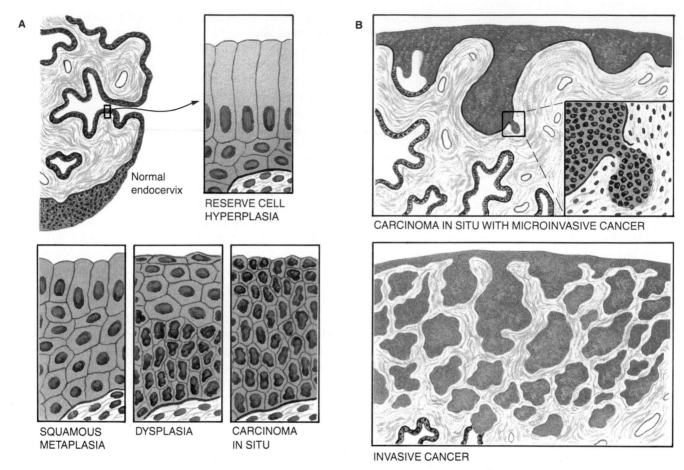

Figure 18-10.   Pathologic sequence of states leading to squamous cell carcinoma of the cervix. (*Upper left*) Reserve cell hyperplasia in an endocervical gland in the region of the squamocolumnar junction. (*Lower left*) The reserve cell hyperplasia becomes more extensive and is called squamous metaplasia. The metaplastic cells undergo changes leading to mild abnormalities (mild dysplasia) and more severe changes (carcinoma in situ). (*Upper right*) Focus of microinvasive (early invasive) cancer arising in carcinoma in situ. (*Lower right*) Invasive squamous cell carcinoma.

dysplasias and invasive cancer contain HPV 16, 18, or 31; these are therefore considered to be high-risk HPV types. The lower grades of dysplasia contain a heterogeneous distribution of all HPV types. **Thus, it appears that cervical dysplasia is a manifestation of HPV infection.** Most of these dysplasias are produced by low-risk HPVs and are benign infections, while a small proportion contain high-risk HPVs and are therefore considered precursors of cervical cancer.

Histology (Fig. 18-10)   **In mild dysplasia (CIN I), the most pronounced changes are in the basal third of the epithelium,** but cells with abnormal nuclei migrate toward the surface; these latter cells are sloughed and are the dysplastic cells detected in Papanicolaou smears. **Generally, substantial cytoplasmic differentiation occurs in cells in the upper two-thirds of the epithelium. In moderate dysplasia**

(CIN II), the most profound changes are found in the lower and middle thirds of the epithelium. Cytodifferentiation occurs in cells in the upper third but is less than in mild dysplasia. In severe dysplasia and carcinoma in situ (CIN III), the nuclear changes involve all layers of the epithelium, and cytodifferentiation is minimal.

Dysplasia and carcinoma in situ can be detected on colposcopic examination by signs associated with their altered vasculature and epithelial changes. The latter begin in the transformation zone and are believed to be unicellular in origin. The dysplastic process occurs more commonly on the anterior than the posterior lip of the cervix, and often extends to involve the endocervical glands.

Treatment   All women should have annual cervical smears beginning at age 18 or when sexual activity begins, whichever comes first. The frequency of subsequent examination is guided by the Papanicolaou smear and biopsy findings. Colposcopic examination is often used to delineate the extent of the lesion and indicate the areas to be biopsied. Some gynecologists follow women with mild dysplasia (CIN I) conservatively (i.e., repeated smears plus close follow-up), whereas others treat the patient. High-grade lesions are treated on the basis of extent of disease. Cryosurgery, which can be performed in the office, is commonly used. In certain situations cervical conization, laser vaporization, and (rarely) hysterectomy are performed. Follow-up smears should continue for life, since vaginal or vulvar squamous cancer may later develop.

Microinvasive Squamous Cell Carcinoma
Microinvasive carcinoma is an early stage in the spectrum of cervical cancer (Stage IA), and is characterized by **minimal invasion of the stroma by neoplastic cells.** Small clusters of cells or solid lesions invasive to less than 3 mm without vascular invasion are not associated with lymph node metastases. Therefore, such lesions do not require radical treatment. Therapy consists of a simple hysterectomy.

Squamous Cell Carcinoma
Squamous cell carcinoma of the cervix has become an uncommon disease in the United States, where the incidence is 15 new cases annually per 100,000 women. In Central and South America, parts of Asia, and Africa, it remains a leading cause of cancer death. In some high-risk areas, the incidence has reached 1 new case per 1000 women a year. The age of presentation peaks at 51 years, or about 10 to 20 years after the peak of carcinoma in situ. Invasive carcinoma and CIN share similar epidemiologic factors.

The most frequent complaint is vaginal bleeding after intercourse or douching. The cancer, which occurs predominantly within the transformation zone, may be exophytic or endophytic. Three main microscopic patterns occur. **Large cell nonkeratinizing carcinoma,** accounting for two-thirds of the cases, is characterized by solid nests of large malignant epithelial cells with no more than individual cell keratinization. **Large cell keratinizing carcinoma** shows nests of keratinized cells organized in concentric whorls—the so-called keratin pearls. The third and least common pattern, **small cell carcinoma,** is composed of infiltrating masses of small, cohesive, malignant cells without evidence of keratinization. Some of the small cell carcinomas are now recognized as carcinoid tumors. With newer techniques of radiotherapy the prognosis is similar for the different tumor patterns.

Cervical cancer spreads by direct extension and via lymphatic vessels, and only rarely by the hematogenous route. Local extension into surrounding tissues results in ureteral compression; the corresponding clinical complications are hydroureter, hydronephrosis, and renal failure, the last being the most common cause of death (50% of patients). Bladder and rectal involvement lead to fistula formation. Metastasis to regional lymph nodes involves the paracervical, hypogastric, and external iliac nodes.

The clinical stage of the tumor is the best prognostic indicator of survival (Table 18-4, Fig. 18-11). The overall 5-year survival rate for all tumors combined is 60%. Survival rates are as follows: Stage I, 90%; Stage II, 75%; Stage III, 35%; and Stage IV, 10%. Approximately 15% of patients will develop recurrences on the vaginal wall, bladder, pelvis, or rectum within 2 years of appropriate therapy.

Verrucous Carcinoma
Verrucous carcinoma, a rare variant of well-differentiated squamous cell carcinoma, occurs more commonly on the vulva but occasionally arises in the cervix.

Adenocarcinoma
Endocervical adenocarcinoma has increased in frequency in recent years and now accounts for about 10% of cervical malignant tumors. The mean age at presentation is 56 years, and the most common presenting sign is vaginal bleeding. Most adenocarci-

Table 18-4 Clinical Staging of Carcinoma of the Cervix Uteri

STAGE	DESCRIPTION
0	Carcinoma in situ (cervical intraepithelial neoplasia III)
I	Carcinoma confined to cervix (corpus extension disregarded).
IA	Preclinical carcinoma (Diagnosed by microscopy only)
IA1	Minimal microscopic stromal invasion
IA2	Measurable lesions detected microscopically (max 5 mm)
IB	All lesions greater than Stage Ia2
II	Invasive carcinoma extending beyond the cervix but not reaching lateral pelvic wall; involvement of vagina limited to upper two-thirds.
IIA	Paracervical extension not suspected.
IIB	Paracervical extension suspected.
III	Invasive carcinoma extending to lateral pelvic wall or lower third of vagina.
IIIA	No extension to the pelvic wall.
IIIB	Extension to pelvic wall, hydronephrosis, or nonfunctioning kidney.
IV	Extended spread involving:
IVA	Mucosa of urinary bladder or rectum.
IVB	Extension beyond true pelvis.

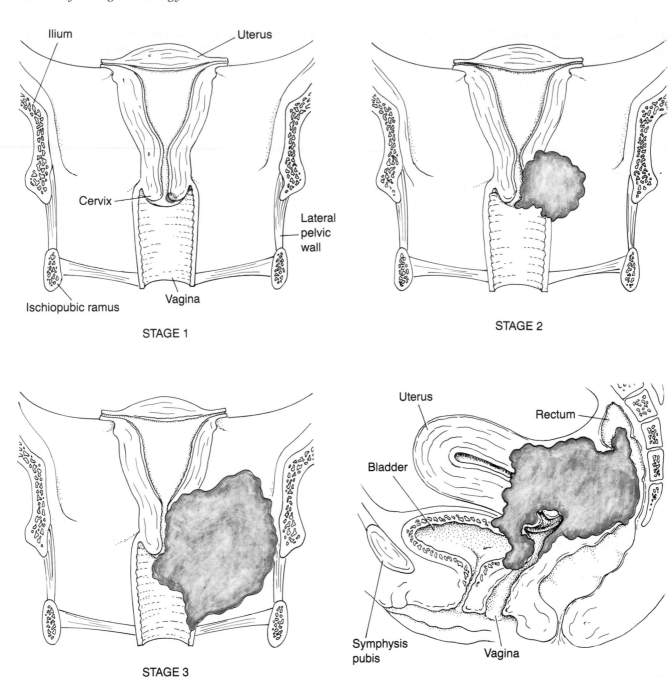

Figure 18-11. Stages of cervical cancer. (*Upper left*) Stage I: tumor is confined to the cervix. (*Upper right*) Stage II: tumor involves the upper vagina. (*Lower left*) Stage III: tumor is fixed to the bones of the pelvic sidewall. (*Lower right*) Stage IV: tumor involves the mucosa of the bladder and rectum.

nomas are of the endocervical cell (mucinous) type. On gross examination they have a fungating polypoid or papillary appearance. It is important to differentiate adenocarcinoma arising in the endocervix from adenocarcinoma of the endometrium extending into the cervix, because the treatment differs. Carcinoembryonic antigen (CEA) is present in 80% of endocervical adenocarcinomas but in only 8% of endometrial adenocarcinomas. However, overlap precludes its use as a significant discriminating factor. The tumor spreads in a fashion similar to squamous cell carcinoma of the cervix, and the overall 5-year survival rate is about 50%.

Body of Uterus and Endometrium

Anatomy

The uterine corpus (body) is smaller than the cervix at birth and during childhood but increases rapidly in size after puberty. The endometrium is composed of glands and stroma (see Fig. 18-1). It is thin at birth and consists of a continuous surface of cuboidal epithelium, which dips to line a few sparse tubular glands. After puberty, the endometrium thickens. The upper two-thirds is responsive to hormones and is shed with each menstrual phase. The lower third, the basal layer, is the germinative portion and with each cycle regenerates a new functional zone. The endometrium is supplied by the arcuate arteries, which traverse the outer myometrium and give off two sets of vessels, one to the myometrium and the other, the radial arteries, to the endometrium. In turn, the radial arteries branch into basal arteries to the basal endometrium and spiral arteries to the superficial two-thirds of the endometrium.

Physiologic Changes

Normal Menstrual Cycle

The normal endometrium undergoes changes that support the growth of the implanted fertilized ovum (zygote). During the first 14 days of the menstrual cycle, the endometrium, under estrogenic stimulation, exhibits proliferation of both tightly coiled epithelial glands and stroma. The glands produce a watery alkaline secretion, which provides a "friendly" fluid medium to facilitate passage of sperm through the uterus and tubes. The passage from cervical canal through the fallopian tube occurs in about 1 hour. At about the 14th day a ripened graafian follicle in the ovary discharges a single ovum, which over the day becomes fertilized in the fallopian tube. Implantation on the endometrium occurs 4 to 5 days later. During this time, the granulosa cells of the corpus luteum (the graafian follicle that has given up its ovum) begin to secrete substantial amounts of progesterone, the hormone that stimulates transformation of the endometrium from a proliferative to a secretory state. The endometrial glands, which have been long and tightly coiled, now begin to enlarge. All the cells that line the glands develop abundant, glycogen-rich, subnuclear vacuoles (day 17–19).

Over the next several days the endometrial glandular cells produce copious secretions, which bathe the implanted zygote and support it while it develops tentacles to parasitize the endometrium for its nourishment. During days 20 to 22, the endometrium displays prominent glandular secretions and stromal edema. The glands now appear dilated, have serrated borders, and are less coiled. On day 23 the stromal cells become enlarged and rounded. These cells, which normally appear first about the arterioles, are the precursors of the decidual cells of pregnancy and are therefore referred to as "predecidual." By the 27th day the entire stroma has become decidualized.

In the absence of pregnancy, a series of regressive events occurs. Trophoblastic cells are not formed and chorionic gonadotropin (hCG) is not secreted. Without stimulation by hCG, the newly formed luteinized granulosa and thecal cells of the corpus luteum degenerate. The corpus luteum is responsible for progesterone production, a process that maintains the decidualized endometrium. As the corpus luteum degenerates, progesterone levels fall, the endometrium breaks down, and menses ensue.

Pregnancy

Under the progestational influence of the corpus luteum of pregnancy, the endometrial stroma undergoes a marked decidual change. The endometrial glands become hypersecretory and exhibit widely dilated glands lined by cells with abundant glycogen. Even if the pregnancy is ectopic or trophoblastic disease is present, an exaggerated hypersecretory response may occur. The nuclei of glandular cells become enlarged, bulbous, and polyploid, because the DNA has replicated but the cells have not divided. The nuclei protrude beyond the apparent cytoplasmic limits of the cell into the gland lumen, an appearance referred to as the **Arias-Stella reaction.** It is important that this change not be confused with adenocarcinoma. The changes can persist for up to 8 weeks after delivery.

Inflammatory Changes

Acute Endometritis

Acute endometritis, characterized by the presence of polymorphonuclear leukocytes, results when an infection ascends from the cervix. The usually impervious cervical barrier is compromised by abortion, delivery, and instrumentation. Curettage is both diagnostic and curative because it removes the necrotic tissue that serves as the nidus of infection.

Pyometra

Pyometra, pus in the endometrial cavity, is associated with any lesion that causes cervical stenosis, such as a tumor or scarring from surgical treatment (conization) of the cervix. Long-standing pyometra may be associated with the development of squamous cell cancer of the endometrium.

Chronic Endometritis

Chronic endometritis is diagnosed by the identification of plasma cells in the endometrium. Lymphocytes and lymphoid follicles are normally found scattered in the normal endometrium, but their presence is not considered diagnostic of chronic endometritis. Chronic endometritis is associated with IUD use, pelvic inflammatory disease, and retained products of conception after an abortion or delivery. Clinically, patients usually complain of bleeding, pelvic pain, or both. The condition is generally self-limiting.

Tuberculosis

Tuberculosis is a specific type of chronic endometritis. It occurs in about half of the cases of genital tuberculosis, usually as a result of seeding from the fallopian tubes. In other areas of the body afflicted with tuberculosis, the granulomas have time to develop the characteristic caseous necrosis and Langhan's giant cells. The granulomas that develop in the endometrium, however, are no more than one cycle old, owing to menstrual shedding, and thus are at an early stage of development. Noncaseating, poorly formed granulomas with rare giant cells constitute the most typical appearance. Occasionally, tuberculosis presents as a nonspecific endometritis confined to the upper or middle third of the endometrium.

Dysfunctional Bleeding

Dysfunctional uterine bleeding is defined as abnormal bleeding in the absence of an organic lesion of the endometrium. It is one of the most common gynecologic disorders of women of reproductive age, but one that is still poorly understood. The bleeding may be due to anovulatory cycles related to excessive and prolonged estrogenic stimulation. Without ovulation, a corpus luteum does not develop and progesterone is not secreted. The endometrium, therefore, fails to proceed through the normal secretory phase, and an abnormal menstrual cycle results.

Organic lesions of the uterus must be excluded before the diagnosis of dysfunctional bleeding can be made. Examples of organic disorders are carcinoma, hyperplasia, polyps, endometritis, complications of intrauterine or ectopic pregnancy, and the effect of an IUD.

Anovulatory Bleeding

Anovulatory bleeding is the most common form of dysfunctional uterine bleeding, particularly during adolescence and the climacteric period. It is believed that estrogen maintains the stromal fluid turgescence, that supports the blood vessels. Anovulatory bleeding is caused by a fall in estrogen levels, which results in loss of fluid from the stroma and hence loss of vascular support. The vascular collapse leads to compression of the vessels, which in turn leads to stasis, thrombosis, infarction, and hemorrhage. On microscopic examination the glands are disordered and appear crowded because of severe stromal necrosis and collapse of the proliferative endometrium.

Abnormalities of the Normal Menstrual Cycle

Dysfunctional bleeding may also be associated with abnormalities of the normal menstrual cycle. **Ovulatory oligomenorrhea** (cycle longer than 45 days) is almost always due to a long follicular phase and may be the prelude to ovarian failure. **Ovulatory polymenorrhea,** in which cycles are less than 18 days in length, is caused by short follicular phases (seen generally in adolescence) or short luteal phases (inadequate luteal phase). The latter may be due to defects in factors that maintain the corpus luteum.

Drug-Induced Endometrial Lesions

Estrogens

Estrogens used for replacement therapy are either conjugated (Premarin) or nonsteroidal (diethylstilbestrol). Despite the dissimilarity in their chemical structures, both are estrogenic and can, in low concentrations, stimulate the endometrium and thereby produce a number of endometrial abnormalities.

Contraceptive Steroids (Progestin-Estrogen Agents)

A variety of estrogens, most of which are not natural hormones, are included as the estrogenic compound in oral contraceptive agents. In the combined preparations, which contain both progestational and estrogenic components, there is potent progestin stimulation but little estrogenic stimulation. The decidual change, therefore, appears early and overshadows the glandular alterations. Over time, the endometrial glands atrophy.

Physically Induced Endometrial Lesions

Intrauterine Device

Disease caused by intrauterine devices has been described in the section on pelvic inflammatory disease.

Asherman's Syndrome

In Asherman's syndrome, intrauterine fibrous adhesions traverse, but do not necessarily obliterate, the endometrial cavity. The etiology of this condition is poorly understood. It may be related to curettage of an infected uterus in which the endometrium becomes denuded. Clinically, the patient complains of hypomenorrhea, amenorrhea, or infertility.

Adenomyosis

Adenomyosis is defined as the presence of endometrial glands and stroma within the myometrium. It affects parous women of reproductive age and regresses after menopause. Patients usually present with varying degrees of dysfunctional uterine bleeding and dysmenorrhea. Because the endometrial–myometrial junction is typically irregular, a diagnosis of adenomyosis is made in hysterectomy specimens only when endometrial glands and stroma are identified at least 3 mm beneath the endometrium. When this definition is employed, adenomyosis is found in about 15% of uteri removed for any indication.

Adenomyosis is believed to develop as a consequence of endometrial implantation during uterine trauma caused by parturition, myomectomy, or curettage. Occasionally, it is found in nulliparous women who have had no instrumentation. In these cases the foci may develop as a consequence of metaplasia of uncommitted mesenchymal cells.

The uterus becomes enlarged because of smooth-muscle hypertrophy around the endometrial foci. On gross examination the myometrium contains small, soft, red areas, some of which are cystic. Microscopic

examination reveals glands lined by mildly proliferative to inactive endometrium and surrounded by endometrial stroma. Secretory changes are rare except during pregnancy and in patients treated with progestins. Varying degrees of hyperplasia may be seen, and occasionally surface endometrial hyperplasia may extend into the foci of adenomyosis. Similarly, adenocarcinoma of the endometrium may extend into these foci, but this does not indicate myometrial invasion, and the prognosis is that of an adenocarcinoma confined to the endometrium.

Infertility

Approximately 15% of couples in the United States are involuntarily infertile. In women, fertility can be impaired by a wide range of anatomic and structural abnormalities, such as congenital anomalies, tumors, pelvic inflammation, and endometriosis. Fertility is also reduced by various physiologic and endocrine disturbances of reproductive tract function, some of which are discussed elsewhere in this chapter. Representative causes are depicted in Figure 18-12.

Abnormal Proliferations of Endometrial Glands and Stroma

Polyps

Endometrial polyps are more common after menopause and typically present with bleeding. Polyps vary in size from several millimeters to large enough to fill and even expand the entire endometrial cavity (Fig. 18-13). They originate at any site in the fundus. Most are solitary, but 20% are multiple. The color varies from tan-pink to white. A red color may be due to surface ulceration or hemorrhagic infarction. Microscopic examination reveals endometrial glands admixed with a normal to fibromatous endometrial stroma and covered by endometrial epithelium. Polyps develop from the zona basalis, and the base contains tortuously dilated blood vessels. The glandular epithelium is usually asynchronous with the adjacent endometrial phase and occasionally undergoes a variety of metaplastic changes. Adenocarcinoma can develop in a polyp—approximately 0.5% to 3.0% of polyps contain adenocarcinoma.

Endometrial Hyperplasia and Adenocarcinoma

A broad **spectrum of proliferative disease, constituting a morphologic and biologic continuum, begins with hyperplasia of endometrial glands and ends**

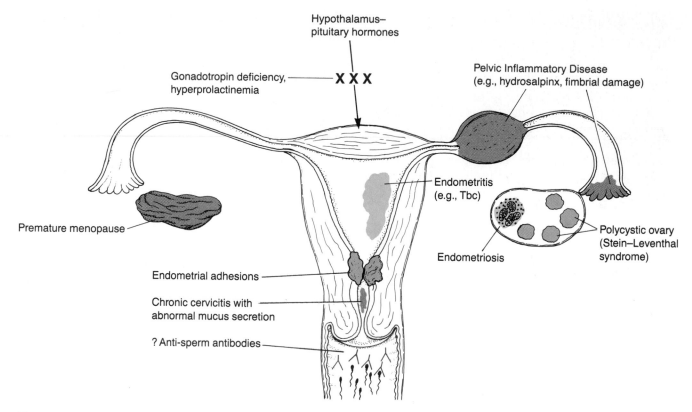

Figure 18-12. Causes of acquired infertility.

with adenocarcinoma. Endometrial hyperplasias and adenocarcinomas are frequently associated with exogenous or endogenous estrogen excess.

Hyperplasias

The problem of classification has been compounded by a terminology that has been consistent only in its lack of consistency. **Cystic hyperplasia,** at the low end of the proliferative spectrum, is the most common form of hyperplasia. **Dilated glands of varying size are lined by columnar epithelium and exhibit some degree of mitotic activity and stratification.** The proliferative activity helps to distinguish it from cystic (senile) atrophy—the so-called Swiss cheese endometrium—which is a regressive change. **The more advanced degrees of hyperplasia, which border on early adenocarcinoma, have been called "adenomatous hyperplasia," "atypical hyperplasia," and "carcinoma in situ,"** but their variable definitions preclude comparison.

One schema in common use designates hyperplasias as mild, moderate, or severe (Fig. 18-14). Newer proposals regard the hyperplasia as simple or complex, with or without atypia. "Mild" or "simple" hyperplasia is a proliferative lesion that displays no evidence of cytologic atypia and minimal glandular

complexity and crowding. About 1% of such lesions progress to adenocarcinoma.

"Moderate" or "complex" hyperplasia, or "simple hyperplasia with atypicality," is a proliferative lesion with cytologic atypia or marked glandular crowding. About 5% of such lesions progress to adenocarcinoma.

"Severe" or "complex atypical" hyperplasia is characterized by a proliferative lesion with cytologic atypia and marked glandular crowding, generally as back-to-back glands. About 30% of such lesions progress to adenocarcinoma.

The duration of progression from the milder degrees of hyperplasia to cancer is about 10 years. The duration from the more advanced degrees with cytologic atypia is about 4 years.

Not infrequently, adenocarcinoma in situ is focal, arising on a background of severe hyperplasia. Even though curettage may disclose only hyperplasia, about one-sixth of uteri nonetheless harbor small foci of adenocarcinoma.

Treatment   The manner in which endometrial hyperplasia is treated depends to some degree on the patient's age, her desire to retain fertility, the severity of the hyperplasia, and the ability to control effectively the risk factors associated with the develop-

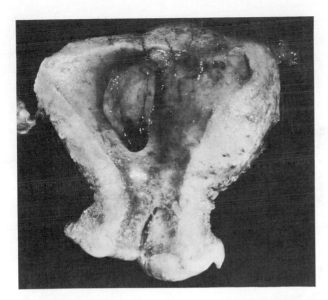

Figure 18-13. Endometrial polyp. Bleeding resulted from the necrotic tip.

ment of endometrial carcinoma. Depending on the woman's age, the hyperplasia may result from anovulatory cycles, polycystic ovarian disease, an estrogen-producing tumor, or even obesity. In each case, therapy aimed at the primary disease may alleviate the estrogenic stimulation. Several studies have shown that treatment with large doses of progestins can produce objective remissions, although substantial numbers of recurrences can be expected. Hysterectomy is usually considered the therapy of choice in a woman who has completed childbearing and has a significant degree of hyperplasia on curettage.

Adenocarcinoma

Adenocarcinoma of the endometrium has several morphologic patterns, each with a different prognosis. **The most common type, accounting for approximately 60% of all endometrial carcinomas, is the pure adenocarcinoma, which is composed entirely of glandular cells.** Adenocarcinomas of the endometrium are divided into three grades: well differentiated (grade 1), moderately differentiated (grade 2), or poorly differentiated (grade 3) (Fig. 18-15). **Secretory carcinoma,** a closely related variant, is characterized by cells with subnuclear vacuolization. It usually occurs in premenopausal women. Secretory carcinoma is associated with excessive progesterone, usually in the form of a newly formed corpus luteum, and has a more favorable outcome than pure adenocarcinoma.

The second most common type of carcinoma contains squamous cells in addition to the glandular element. If the **squamous element is well differentiated,** exhibiting minimal atypia, the tumor is called **adenoacanthoma.** If it is **poorly differentiated,** the tumor is called **adenosquamous carcinoma.**

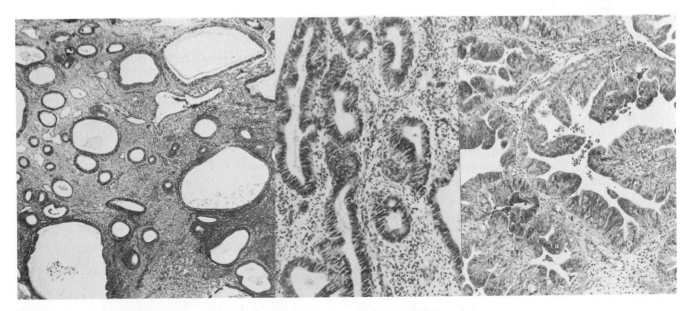

Figure 18-14. Hyperplasia of the endometrium: Mild (*left*), moderate (*middle*), and severe, or markedly atypical (*right*). The glands in mild hyperplasia are dilated, and the lining epithelium is proliferative and has occasional mitoses. Moderate hyperplasia is characterized by more closely packed glands. Severely atypical hyperplasia displays closely packed glands with highly proliferative epithelium and marked architectural abnormality.

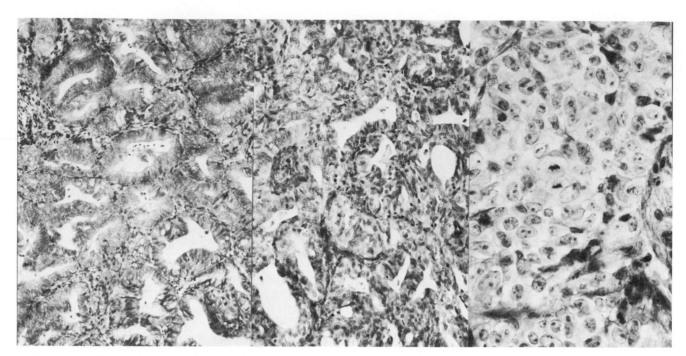

Figure 18-15.   Adenocarcinoma of endometrium, grades 1–3. Grade 1 (*left*): well-differentiated tumor composed entirely of glands. Grade 2 (*middle*): moderately differentiated tumor characterized architecturally by both glands and solid sheets of cells. Grade 3 (*right*): poorly differentiated tumor composed entirely of sheets of cells; no glands are present.

Other types of endometrial cancers are less common. Serous adenocarcinoma of the endometrium, which resembles serous adenocarcinoma of the ovary, has psammoma bodies and has been separated as a distinct entity because it has a worse prognosis than endometrial adenocarcinoma of the usual type. Clear cell adenocarcinoma, a tumor that typically occurs in elderly women, is composed of large cells with copious amounts of cytoplasmic glycogen or "hobnail" cells that line glandular lumens. The serous, clear cell, and adenosquamous carcinomas are associated with poor outcomes.

Survival   The actuarial survival rate of all patients with endometrial cancer following treatment (regardless of history of estrogen usage) is 80% after the second year, 73% after the fifth year, and 64% after 10 years. Tumors that have grown to involve the cervix have a greater potential for lymph node metastasis and a poorer prognosis (Tables 18-5 and 18-6). Tumors that extend outside the uterus have the worst prognosis.

Pathogenesis   **The clinical features associated with endometrial cancer include diabetes mellitus, obesity, hypertension, breast cancer, nulliparity, and late menopause. These factors point to a relatively increased estrogenic milieu.** Women with ovarian agenesis do not develop endometrial cancer unless treated with exogenous estrogens. A higher frequency of endometrial cancer is found in women with granulosa cell tumors (which secrete estrogens) and in women who receive unopposed exogenous estrogens, such as postmenopausal women treated with estrogens for menopausal symptoms.

The age of the patient is closely correlated with the grade, depth of invasion, and stage of the tumor. Women whose tumors are well differentiated, have not yet infiltrated more than superficially into the myometrium, or are confined to the corpus are much younger than women whose tumors are poorly differentiated, deeply invasive, or have spread beyond the corpus.

Clinical Course   **Adenocarcinoma of the endometrium spreads by the lymphatics, the blood vessels, and transperitoneal seeding via the fallopian tubes.** The most common site of metastasis is the lung (41% of cases with metastases), a location that suggests that hematogenous spread may occur early in the course of the disease. Other organs that may harbor metastases, in descending order of frequency, are the peritoneum and omentum; the ovary, liver, and bowel; and the vagina, bladder, and vertebrae. Unlike cervical cancer, endometrial cancer may spread

Table 18-5 Clinical Staging of Carcinoma of the Corpus Uteri

STAGE	DESCRIPTION
I	Tumor confined to corpus
IA	Length of uterine cavity 8 cm or less
IB	Length of uterine cavity more than 8 cm
II	Tumor involving both corpus and cervix, but is not outside uterus
III	Tumor extending beyond uterus but not outside true pelvis
IV	Tumor extending beyond true pelvis or involving the mucosa of bladder or rectum
IVA	Spread to adjacent organs
IVB	Spread to distant organs

Grading (FIGO)*

G1 Highly differentiated
G2 Differentiated with partly solid areas
G3 Predominantly solid or entirely undifferentiated carcinoma

* FIGO, International Federation of Gynecology and Obstetrics

Table 18-6 Stage, Grade, and Survival for all Types of Endometrial Carcinomas

	5-YEAR SURVIVAL (%)				10-YEAR SURVIVAL (%)			
STAGE	FIGO GRADE	1	2	3	FIGO GRADE	1	2	3
	BRODER GRADE	1	2	3	4	BRODER GRADE	1	2	3	4
IA	100	96	66	57	100	90	63	57
IB	100	74	71	44	100	43	71	16
II	—*	80	42	12	—	—	—	—
III, IV	—	25	33	17	—	—	—	—

* — Insufficient numbers

directly to para-aortic lymph nodes without involving the pelvic nodes.

Treatment In general, patients with well-differentiated tumors confined to the endometrium are treated by hysterectomy. Preoperative or postoperative radiation is administered if the tumor is poorly differentiated, the myometrium is more than superficially invaded, or the cervix is involved.

Endometrial Tumors with a Stromal Component

Endometrial stromal tumors display a spectrum of malignant behavior that can be correlated with their histologic features (Table 18-7). The tumors can be divided into two major categories microscopically, based on whether the tumor margin is expansile or infiltrating. Tumors with expansile margins are referred to as stromal nodules and are benign, whereas those with infiltrating margins are classed as stromal sarcomas. The low-grade sarcomas have also been called **endolymphatic stromal myosis** and **endometrial stromatosis.**

Endometrial Stromal Sarcoma Endometrial stromal sarcoma may be polypoid and fill the endometrial cavity, or it may diffusely invade the uterus. **Large masses of spindle cells with scant cytoplasm dissect the myometrium and extensively invade vascular channels. The neoplastic cells resemble endometrial stromal cells in the early and mid proliferative phases.** A characteristic feature of all types of endometrial stromal tumors is a rich vascular supporting framework, with the neoplastic cells concentrically arranged around blood vessels. Nuclear atypism may be minimal to severe and mitotic activity restrained or exuberant, depending on the differentiation of the sarcoma. As these tumors become progressively less differentiated (Fig. 18-16), it may be difficult to recognize a resemblance to endometrial stroma, and consequently they may be classified as undifferentiated sarcoma. These tumors may recur even if confined to the uterus at initial surgery. Recurrences usually involve the pelvis initially and are followed later by pulmonary metastases. In low-grade sarcoma many years may elapse before recurrent disease be-

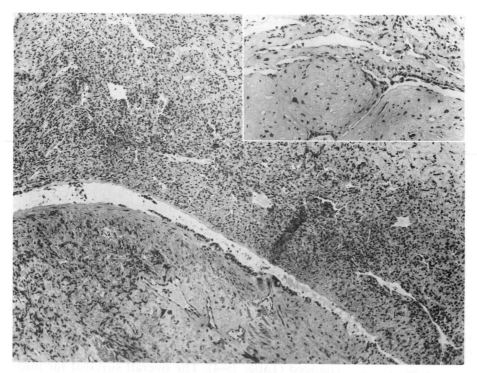

Figure 19-15. Malignant phyllodes tumor (cystosarcoma phyllodes). This tumor has the same overall microscopic stromal and epithelial pattern as fibroadenoma (see Fig. 19-7B). The stroma is more cellular and, as in this case, may be obviously malignant. The inset shows a higher-power view of a chondrosarcomatous area of the tumor.

bles a fibroadenoma may be given the designation of cystosarcoma solely on the basis of increased cellularity and mitotic activity of the stroma. In these cases, the term **"cellular fibroadenoma"** is preferred to benign cystosarcoma. Such tumors are unlikely to metastasize, and are adequately treated by local excision. If incompletely excised, they may recur locally. A clearly malignant phyllodes tumor has an obviously sarcomatous stroma and usually is poorly circumscribed, with invasion into the surrounding breast tissue (Fig. 19-15). The tumors may have various sarcomatous tissue types, such as malignant fibrous histiocytoma, chondrosarcoma, and osteosarcoma. Cystosarcomas preferentially metastasize to distant sites rather than the axillary lymph nodes. For this reason, the initial treatment of the phyllodes tumor consists of wide excisional biopsy if the tumor is small, or a simple mastectomy if the tumor is large. An axillary lymph node dissection is not necessary.

Miscellaneous Tumors

Both benign and malignant neoplasms can originate from the normal mesenchymal elements of the breast. **Lipomas** and, less commonly, **hemangiomas, leiomyomas,** and **fibromas** occur. Of the malignant counterparts, the **angiosarcoma,** although rare, is a particularly pernicious neoplasm.

Neoplasms in which both malignant mesenchymal and malignant epithelial components are found are termed **carcinosarcomas.** These are rare and must be distinguished from cystosarcoma phyllodes in which the epithelial component is always benign.

Malignant lymphoma may involve the breast. Most commonly, the breast involvement is in addition to other, more common sites of involvement. However, occasionally lymphoma may be primary in the breast.

Neoplasms of skin and adnexal structures may arise in the nipple, areola or other skin of the breast. Their biologic behavior and histologic appearance are identical to similar tumors outside of the breast.

Although relatively uncommon, metastases from primary neoplasms in other parts of the body may present in the breast. The most common are carcinomas of the opposite breast and melanoma.

SUGGESTED READING

BOOKS

Azzopardi JG: Problems in Breast Pathology. In Bennington, JL (ed): Major Problems in Pathology, Vol II. Philadelphia, W B Saunders, 1979

Haagensen CD: Diseases of the Breast, 2nd ed. Philadelphia, W B Saunders, 1971

Harris JR, Hellman S, Henderson IG, et al: Breast Diseases. Philadelphia, JB Lippincott, 1987

McDivitt RW, Stewart FW, Berg JW: Tumors of the Breast. In Atlas of Tumor Pathology, 2nd series. Fasc. 2. Washington, Armed Forces Institute of Pathology, 1968

Rosai J,. Ackerman's Surgical Pathology, Vol II. 6th ed. St. Louis, C V Mosby, 1981

REVIEW ARTICLES

American Cancer Society Anatomical Conference: Breast cancer 1983. Cancer 53(suppl):589-832, 1984

Henderson IC, Canellos GP: Cancer of the breast: The past decade. N Engl J Med 302:17-30, 78-90, 1980

Kelsey JL: A review of the epidemiology of human breast cancer. Epidemiol Rev 1:74-109, 1979

ORIGINAL ARTICLES

Bartow SA, Black WC, Waeckerlin RW, Mettler FA: Fibrocystic disease: A continuing enigma. Pathol Annu 17:93-111, 1982

Bloom HJG, Richardson WW: Histological grading and prognosis in breast cancer: A study of 1409 cases which have been followed for 15 years. Br J Cancer 11:359-377, 1957

Fisher B, Bauer M, Margolese R, et al: Five-year results of a randomized clinical trial comparing total mastectomy and segmental mastectomy with or without radiation in the treatment of breast cancer. N Engl J Med 312:665-673, 1985

Fisher E, Gregario R, Fisher B, et al: The pathology of invasive breast cancer: A syllabus derived from findings of the National Surgical Adjuvant Breast Project (Protocol No 4). Cancer, 36:1-84, 1975

Fisher E, Sass R, Fisher B: Pathologic findings from the National Surgical Adjuvant Project for Breast Cancers (protocol No. 4). Discriminance for tenth year treatment failure. Cancer 53:712–723, 1984

Heller KS, Rosen PP, Schottenfeld D, et al: Male breast cancer: a clinicopathologic study of 97 cases. Am Surg 188:60-65, 1978

McGuire WL: Hormone receptors: their role in predicting prognosis and response to endocrine therapy. Semin Oncol 5: 428–433, 1978

Page DL, Dupont WD, Rogers LW, Rados MS: Atypical hyperplastic lesions of the female breast: A long-term follow-up study. Cancer 55:269-2708, 1985

Rosen PP, Lieberman PH, Brown DW, et al: Lobular carcinoma in situ of the breast: Detailed analysis of 99 patients with average follow-up of 24 years. Am J Surg Pathol 2:225-251, 1978

Wellings SR, Jensen HM, Marcum RG: An atlas of subgross pathology of the human breast with special reference to possible precancerous lesions. J Nat Cancer Inst 55:231–275, 1975

The World Health Organization: The World Health Organization histological typing of breast tumors, 2nd ed. Am J Clin Pathol 78:806-816, 1982

20 The Blood and the Lymphoid Organs

Hugh Bonner

Normal Structure and Function

Hemostasis

Anemia

Erythrocytosis (Polycythemia)

Benign Disorders of Polymorphonuclear Leukocytes

Proliferative Disorders of Mast Cells

Benign Disorders of the Mononuclear Phagocyte System

Differentiated Histiocytoses

Benign Disorders of Lymphoid Cells

Disorders of the Spleen

Monoclonal Gammopathy of Unknown Significance

Chronic Myeloproliferative Syndromes

Acute Myeloproliferative Syndromes: The Acute Nonlymphocytic Leukemias

Malignant Disorders of the Mononuclear Phagocyte System

The Lymphocytic Leukemias

The Non-Hodgkin's Malignant Lymphomas

Plasma Cell Neoplasia

Hodgkin's Disease

Bone Marrow: Metastatic Tumors

Lymph Nodes: Metastatic Tumors

Figure 20-1. Cellular differentiation and maturation of the lymphopoietic *(left)* and hematopoietic *(right)* systems.

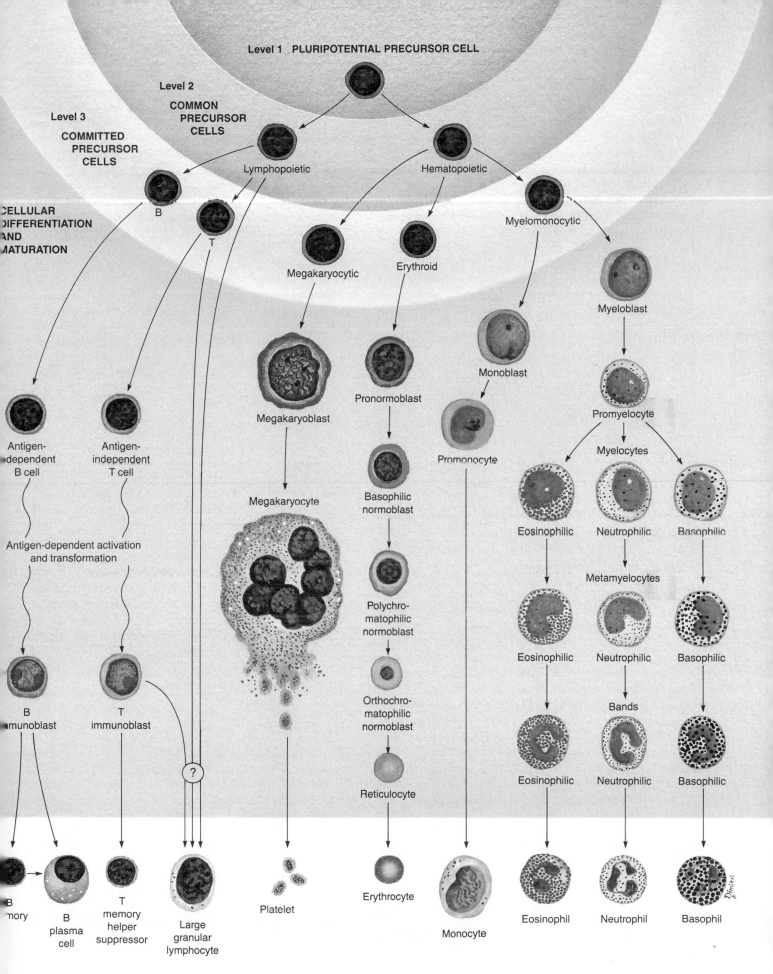

Level 1 PLURIPOTENTIAL PRECURSOR CELL

Level 2
COMMON
PRECURSOR
CELLS

Level 3
COMMITTED
PRECURSOR
CELLS

Lymphopoietic

Hematopoietic

B

T

Myelomonocytic

CELLULAR
DIFFERENTIATION
AND
MATURATION

Megakaryocytic

Erythroid

Myeloblast

Monoblast

Antigen-
dependent
B cell

Antigen-
independent
T cell

Megakaryoblast

Pronormoblast

Promonocyte

Promyelocyte

Myelocytes

Antigen-dependent activation
and transformation

Megakaryocyte

Basophilic
normoblast

Eosinophilic

Neutrophilic

Basophilic

Metamyelocytes

Polychro-
matophilic
normoblast

Eosinophilic

Neutrophilic

Basophilic

B
immunoblast

T
immunoblast

Bands

Orthochro-
matophilic
normoblast

Eosinophilic

Neutrophilic

Basophilic

?

Reticulocyte

B
memory

B
plasma
cell

T
memory
helper
suppressor

Large
granular
lymphocyte

Platelet

Erythrocyte

Monocyte

Eosinophil

Neutrophil

Basophil

Level 4
DIFFERENTIATED FUNCTIONAL BLOOD CELLS

In the bone marrow, a pluripotential precursor cell gives rise to two distinct multipotential hematopoietic and lymphopoietic precursor cells. Pursuing an orderly sequence of differentiation and maturation, the hematopoietic precursor cells develop into erythrocytes, granulocytes, monocytes, and platelets, which are released to the peripheral blood. Monocytes in turn enter the tissues and yield a variety of specialized histiocytes and their functional counterparts, the phagocytic macrophages; together they constitute the mononuclear phagocyte system. Marrow lymphopoietic precursor cells undergo a diphasic differentiation, with subsequent evolution of the B- and T-lymphocytes of the immune system. B cells differentiate in the bone marrow and undergo a maturation sequence in a variety of peripheral lymphoid organs. Differentiation and maturation of T cells require the inductive microenvironment of the thymus gland, probably under the influence of hormones secreted by thymic epithelium. The complex molecular and cellular biology of hematopoietic and lymphopoietic cells is reflected in the heterogeneity of benign and malignant hematopoietic and lymphopoietic disorders.

Normal Structure and Function

The Hematopoietic System

Embryologic Development

Hematopoiesis, or blood cell production, first occurs in the fetal yolk sac. Here "blood islands," consisting of clusters of nucleated erythroblasts, are identified in the third week of embryogenesis. Beginning in the third gestational month and continuing until late in the third trimester, the liver is the principal site of fetal erythrocyte production. From the fifth gestational month, the bone marrow is the principal site of granulocyte and megakaryocyte (platelet) production. During later fetal life, blood cell production also occurs in other extramedullary sites, such as the spleen, lymph nodes, and thymus. At term, hematopoiesis is essentially restricted to the bone marrow.

An important aspect of fetal extramedullary hematopoiesis relates to the potential for postnatal reactivation of these sites of blood cell production in situations of increased demand for erythrocyte production. Such reactivated foci of extramedullary hematopoiesis can be identified in the spleen, lymph nodes, and liver and occasionally appear as unidentified masses, most commonly in the paravertebral soft tissues.

Essentially all bone marrow is hematopoietically active in the fetus and the young child. Such active marrow is called "red" marrow because of its color, imparted by erythroid cells in the sinusoids and by the developing hematopoietic cells. Beginning approximately at age 4 years, there is a gradual retraction of the red marrow to the flat bones of the axial skeleton and to the proximal humerus and femur; this process is completed approximately at age 18 years. In the adult the distal long bones contain fatty, or "yellow," marrow. This inactive marrow is reactivated to active, or red, marrow in situations of increased demand. Such reactivation, combined with enhanced productive capacity of the red marrow of the axial skeleton, may increase erythrocyte production up to seven- to eightfold. Extramedullary hematopoiesis generally does not appear in the spleen, lymph nodes, or liver, unless there is anemia so severe that the bone marrow is unable to compensate.

Structure

The bone marrow consists of a complex network of sinusoids or vascular channels, that are fed by a nutrient artery and that drain into a central longitudinal vein. The sinusoids are separated by an intersinusoidal stroma, which is the site of hematopoiesis. Slender endothelial cells, a basement membrane, and adventitial "reticular" cells separate the sinusoidal lumen from the hematopoietic stroma. Mature red and white blood cells enter the blood through this sinusoidal wall by a poorly understood "release phenomenon." The adventitial cells send out complex cytoplasmic processes which, together with delicate extracellular reticulin fibers, provide a scaffolding for the developing hematopoietic cells. It is thought that the adventitial cells accumulate lipid and become the "fat cells" of the bone marrow.

Function

The three functions of the bone marrow are hematopoiesis (blood cell production), lymphopoiesis (production of uncommitted lymphocytes), and phagocytosis (a component of the mononuclear phagocyte system).

Adventitial reticular cells play an important but poorly understood role in creating the "hematopoietic inductive microenvironment," in which the complex differentiation and maturation of blood cell precursors occur. Specific levels of cellular differentiation are recognized (Fig. 20-1, Table 20-1). The pluripotential precursor cell (level 1), precursor of

Table 20-1 Differentiation of Hematopoietic and Lymphopoietic Cells

LEVEL	HEMATOPOIETIC CELLS	LYMPHOPOIETIC CELLS
1	Pluripotential precursor cells	Pluripotential precursor cells
2	Common hematopoietic precursor cells	Common lymphopoietic precursor cells
3	Committed precursor cells of erythrocytes, granulocytes and monocytes, megakaryocytes	Committed precursor cells of T-lymphocytes and B-lymphocytes
4	Differentiated functional hematopoietic blood cells	Differentiated functional lymphocytes

both the hematopoietic and lymphopoietic precursor cells, is a long-lived and slowly dividing cell. It is only rarely called upon to supplement the more differentiated common hematopoietic and lymphopoietic precursor cells (level 2), which are committed to the dual cell lineages. In hematopoiesis, precursor cells committed to restricted cell lines (level 3) are induced to proliferate and differentiate by specific cytopoietic hormones. These cytopoietins include colony-stimulating factor neutrophil-monocyte, probably derived from T-lymphocytes and from mononuclear phagocytes, which induces the proliferation and differentiation of a common precursor cell of neutrophils and monocytes; and erythropoietin, produced principally in the kidneys, which induces erythroid precursor proliferation and differentiation. Thrombopoietins remain as yet poorly characterized. Differentiated hematopoietic blood cells and lymphocytes constitute the mature or functional cells (level 4).

Bone marrow precursor cells resemble small to medium-sized lymphocytes and are not morphologically distinctive. A functional characteristic of all precursor cells is the capacity for self-renewal as well as for differentiation. Self-renewal is mandatory to maintain the required precursor cell pool and to continuously replenish the mature blood cell elements, which have a finite life span.

Hematopoietic committed precursor cells give rise to "blasts," which are the first morphologically distinctive progenitor cells. Specific subtypes of blasts include erythroblasts (pronormoblasts), myeloblasts, monoblasts, and megakaryoblasts.

Clusters of **erythroid normoblasts** mature in the hematopoietic stroma in close proximity to the sinusoids. A macrophage may be found in the center of such clusters. This functional complex of central mac-

rophage and associated maturing erythroid cells is called the **erythroblastic island.** The macrophage functions to provide iron to the developing normoblasts and to ingest nuclei ejected from orthochromatic normoblasts. Approximately 4 cell divisions in 4 days are required for an erythroblast (pronormoblast) to mature into a reticulocyte, an immature erythrocyte that lacks a nucleus. The reticulocyte migrates through the endothelial cell cytoplasm or between these cells to the sinusoid lumen. Maturation to an erythrocyte occurs after 1 to 2 days in the peripheral blood, with the loss of residual ribosomes and mitochondria.

Granulocytes develop from myeloblasts in the hematopoietic stroma away from the sinusoid wall. Cell division, approximately 3 to 5 mitoses in 3 to 5 days, ceases at the myelocyte stage. At the metamyelocyte stage there is initial migration to the sinusoid, with subsequent maturation and retention in a large marrow storage pool until release to the peripheral blood occurs.

Megakaryocytes develop from large mononucleated megakaryoblasts. Similar to erythroid cells, they mature in close proximity to the sinusoid wall. Following a series of amitotic divisions (nuclear division without cytoplasmic division), mature megakaryocytes with multilobed nuclei are formed. Cytoplasmic fragments are budded directly into the sinusoids, where in turn they become the platelets of the peripheral blood.

Examination of the Bone Marrow

The cellularity of the bone marrow is best evaluated in biopsy sections, in which the normal geographic relationships are preserved (Table 20-2). In the normal adult approximately 50% of the marrow biopsy

Table 20-2 Normal Adult Bone Marrow (age: $\geq 18 \leq 70$ years)

Fat:cell ratio 50:50 ± 10%
Myeloid:erythroid (M:E) ratio 2:1 to 4.5:1

Cell Distribution

    Erythroid series
    10–15% (mean, 12.5%)
    Granulocytic series
    30–45% (mean, 37.5%)
    Fat cells
    40–60% (mean, 50%)

Megakaryocytes 2–5 per high-power field
Plasma cells ≤ 3% (perivascular)
Lymphocytes ≤ 20% (interstitial or in well-defined nonparatrabecular aggregates)
No fibrosis

Table 20-3 Indications for Bone Marrow Examination

Abnormalities of peripheral blood
  Pancytopenia
  Leukopenia
  Thrombocytopenia
  Anemia with reticulocytopenia
  Presence of myeloid precursor cells or abnormal lymphoid
    cells
  Presence of nucleated red blood cells
Evaluation of marrow iron stores
Monoclonal gammopathy
Suspicion of metastatic or primary neoplasm
Suspicion of granulomatous disease
Clinical staging of neoplasia
  Malignant lymphoma
  Hodgkin's disease
  Carcinoma

---

surface area consists of fat cells and 50% of active hematopoietic tissue. The normal ratio of maturing granulocytic (myeloid) to maturing erythroid cells (myeloid:erythroid ratio) is between 2:1 and 4.5:1. Thus, in a normal adult approximately 40% to 60% of the marrow biopsy surface area consists of fat cells, 30% to 45% of maturing granulocytic cells, and 10% to 15% of maturing erythroid cells. In children hematopoietic tissue is relatively increased, with a mean fat:cell ratio of 30:70. In persons over the age of 70 years, hematopoietic tissue is relatively decreased, with a mean fat:cell ratio of 70:30.

Normally, 2 to 5 megakaryocytes per high-power field (40X) are identified in the hematopoietic stroma contiguous to the sinusoidal wall. The normal bone marrow contains less than 3% plasma cells and less than 20% lymphocytes. The reticulin (silver) stain normally reveals only scattered delicate fibers in the hematopoietic stroma. With the trichrome stain for connective tissue, only slight perivascular fibrosis is seen.

Evaluation of bone marrow iron stores is most accurately assessed in Prussian blue–stained aspirate smears. The normal bone marrow contains easily identified scattered granules of stainable iron in the cytoplasm of macrophages. Minute granules of iron in the form of ferritin are found in the cytoplasm of approximately 40% of the erythroid precursor cells.

Examination of the bone marrow is important in the diagnosis and management of a variety of clinical disorders (Table 20-3). Bone marrow infiltrative disorders, such as myelofibrosis with myeloid metaplasia, malignant lymphoma, metastatic carcinoma, granulomatous inflammation, and lipid storage diseases, are best detected by examination of biopsy sections. The cytologic features of hematopoietic and lymphopoietic cells and other cells indigenous or for-eign to the bone marrow are best evaluated in Romanowsky (Wright's or Wright's-Giemsa) stained smears.

The Peripheral Blood

The peripheral blood smear is evaluated systematically, with particular attention to erythrocyte morphology, the white blood cell differential count, the presence of abnormal or immature white blood cells, and the number and size of platelets.

The Mononuclear Phagocyte System

The mononuclear phagocyte system takes origin in the bone marrow from a precursor cell common to both neutrophil and monocyte cell lines, the colony-forming unit neutrophil-monocyte (CFU-NM). The CFU-NM is sensitive to colony-stimulating factor neutrophil-monocyte (CSF-NM), a glycoprotein hormone that regulates granulocyte and monocyte production *in vivo*. CSF-NM is produced both by activated T cells and by monocyte-macrophages. Thus, there is an element of self-regulation in the mononuclear phagocyte system. Following stimulation by CSF-NM, precursor monoblasts first develop into promonocytes in the deeper portions of the hematopoietic stroma. After migrating to the sinusoid wall, they are released to the sinusoidal lumen and then to the peripheral blood, where they are found as mature monocytes.

Circulating monocytes are phagocytic. They leave the blood and enter the tissues randomly—that is, recently matured monocytes are as likely to exit the circulation as are older monocytes. In the tissues mononuclear phagocytes are defined as histiocytes if they are not actively phagocytic, and as macrophages if they are actively phagocytic. A variety of different properties, specialized transformations, and morphologic appearances is observed in macrophages in different sites. Traditionally, a number of names have been applied to these various subpopulations, but all are now included in the term **mononuclear phagocyte system** (Fig. 20-2). Multinucleated giant cells develop either from cell fusion of mononuclear phagocytes or from nuclear endoreduplication. A specialized subpopulation of cells called dendritic reticulum cells and interdigitating reticulum cells is involved in antigen processing and presentation to B- and T-lymphocytes. Dendritic reticulum cells and interdigitating reticulum cells may be derived from Langerhans cells of the skin, which in turn probably originate from bone marrow mononuclear phagocyte precursor cells.

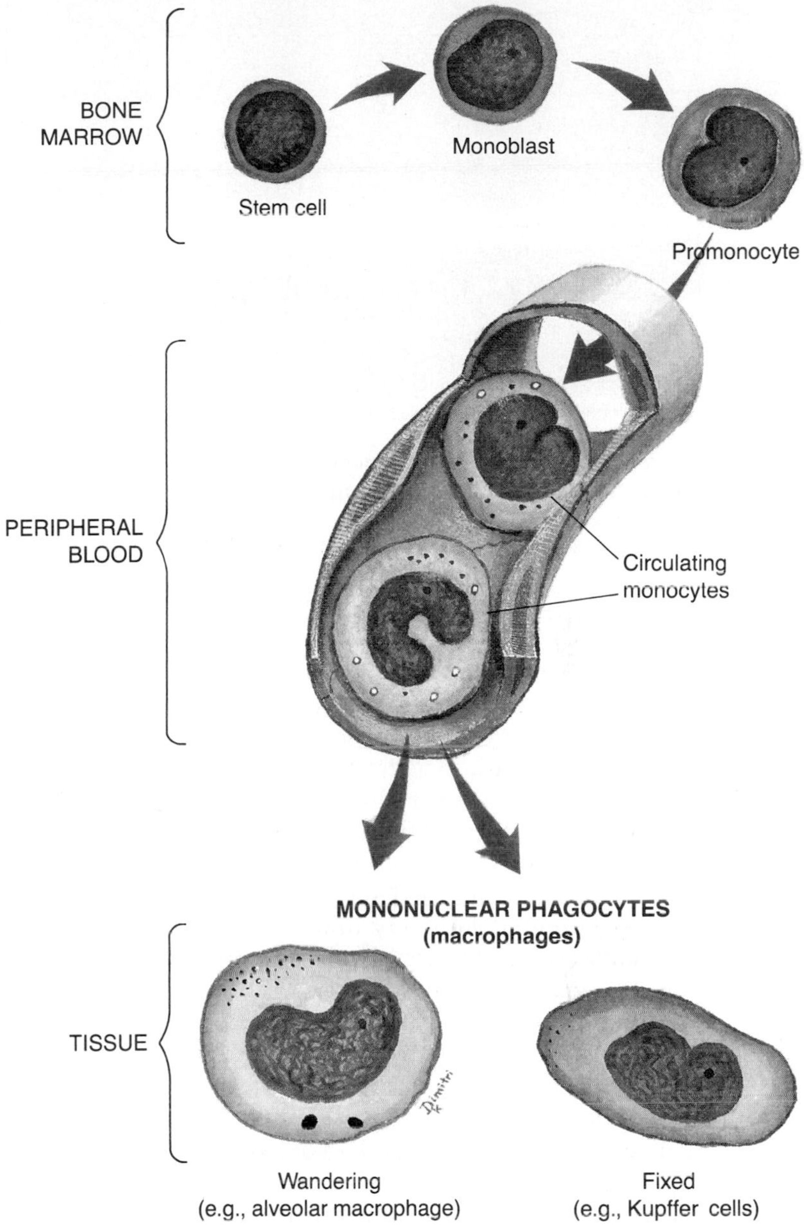

Figure 20-2. The mononuclear phagocyte system. The mononuclear phagocyte system takes origin in the bone marrow from primitive precursor cells, which give rise to monoblasts and then to promonocytes. Promonocytes mature into monocytes, which circulate in the peripheral blood. These monocytes then exit the peripheral blood and enter the tissues, where they become the various specialized histiocytes and functional phagocytic macrophages.

The functions of the mononuclear phagocytes include the following:

- Phagocytic defense against microorganisms
- Antigen pinocytosis, processing, and presentation to B- and T-lymphocytes
- Production of interleukin 1 or T-lymphocyte–activating factor
- Modulation of the inflammatory response by soluble mediators
- Killing of tumor cells
- Regulation of granulocytopoiesis and monocytopoiesis by CSF-NM secretion

- Removal of senescent red blood cells, with breakdown of hemoglobin and presentation of salvaged iron to developing erythroid cells.

The Lymphopoietic System

The lymphopoietic system consists of the primary lymphoid organs, the bone marrow and thymus, the secondary or peripheral lymphoid organs, and the recirculating B- and T-lymphocytes. The bone marrow and thymus are sites of primary antigen-independent differentiation of lymphocytes. Immune re-

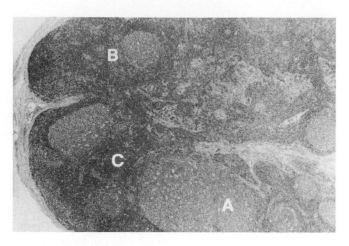

Figure 20-3. B- and T-cell–dependent areas of the lymph node. *A*, B-cell follicle; *B*, B-cell mantle zone; *C*, T-cell paracortex (interfollicular zone).

actions occur in the peripheral lymphoid organs, which include the central and peripheral lymph nodes, spleen, oropharyngeal lymphoid tissue of Waldeyer's ring, Peyer's patches of the terminal ileum, and the bronchus-associated lymphoid tissue. Because the lymphopoietic system is interconnected by two circulatory systems— the lymphatic channels and the bloodstream—circulating sensitized antigen-specific lymphocytes are constantly exposed to antigen that has been trapped in the peripheral lymphoid organs. Humoral antibody and effector T cells are also released into the circulatory system.

Lymph Nodes

The lymph nodes consist of organized collections of lymphoid tissue located along the lymphatic vessels.

Typically gray-white and ovoid or bean-shaped, they vary from approximately 2 mm to 2 cm in greatest dimension. A supporting structure is provided by a fibrous connective tissue capsule and radiating trabeculae. A delicate fibrous tissue network or reticulum provides internal support.

Architecturally, an outer cortex and inner medulla are recognized. Defined B- and T-cell domains characterize the architectural substructure of the cortex (Fig. 20-3). The B-cell–dependent cortex consists of follicles, which may be immunologically inactive (primary follicles) or active (secondary follicles or germinal centers). Primary follicles appear as cohesive aggregates of small, normal-appearing lymphocytes. By contrast, germinal centers contain a spectrum of small, intermediate, and large (transformed) lymphocytes. There are also scattered macrophages—the so-called "tingible body" macrophages—that contain nuclear and cytoplasmic debris. Stellate cells with long cytoplasmic processes—the dendritic reticular cells—are located near the periphery of the germinal centers. These dendritic reticular cells process and present antigen to B cells and induce B-lymphocyte transformation and proliferation, with subsequent germinal center formation. Following transformation, clonal expansion in the germinal centers, and migration to the B-cell–dependent medullary cords of the lymph nodes, B-lymphocytes either become immunoglobulin-secreting plasma cells or exit the lymph nodes as memory B-lymphocytes.

The T-cell–dependent paracortex (deep cortex) is situated between and deep to the B-cell follicles. In addition to T-lymphocytes, scattered histiocytes and interdigitating reticulum cells are found in the paracortex. The interdigitating reticulum cells process and present antigen to T-lymphocytes in a manner analogous to that in which dendritic reticular cells process and present antigen to B-lymphocytes.

Circulating B- and T-lymphocytes enter the lymph nodes by migrating through the tall endothelial cells of postcapillary venules in the paracortex. T-lymphocytes generally remain in the paracortex, whereas B-lymphocytes home to the primary or secondary follicles. Lymph or interstitial fluid enters the lymph nodes through afferent lymphatics in the convexity of the cortex. Percolating through first the subcapsular and then the radial sinuses, lymph exits through efferent lymphatics. The sinuses are lined by cells derived from the mononuclear phagocyte system. The arrangement of the sinuses maximizes exposure of foreign antigen in lymph to macrophages and to immunoreactive B- and T-lymphocytes.

Lymphoid Tissue Associated with the Gut and Bronchi

Aggregates of lymphoid tissue are present along the course of the gastrointestinal tract, with prominent accentuation in the oropharyngeal tonsillar and adenoidal tissue (Waldeyer's ring) and in Peyer's patches of the terminal ileum. Less prominent aggregates of lymphocytes are also distributed in the lamina propria of the bronchial tree. In sites such as the tonsils and Peyer's patches, lymphocytes arrive by migration through tall endothelial cells of vessels comparable to the postcapillary venules of the lymph nodes. Gut- and bronchus-associated lymphocytes play an important role in immunologic protection of the host in areas of vulnerability to potential invaders. IgA secretion is a prominent component of this protective function.

The Spleen

The functions of the spleen relate to both lymphopoietic and hematopoietic cell lineages and are reflected in the distinctive anatomy of the lymphoid white pulp and the erythroid red pulp.

The normal weight of the spleen is 100 g to 170 g. The supporting structure consists of a fibrous capsule, radiating trabeculae, and a delicate stromal framework of reticulin fibers. The splenic artery enters at the hilum and then branches into the trabecular arteries, following the course of the fibrous trabeculae. Leaving the trabeculae, the central arteries become ensheathed by lymphocytes. This lymphoid tissue constitutes the splenic white pulp. The white pulp is further subdivided into a T-cell domain, namely the periarteriolar lymphoid sheath, and a B-cell domain, the follicles (Fig. 20-4). The periarteriolar lymphoid sheath is a narrow cuff of small T-lymphocytes that envelopes the central artery. The B-cell follicles are eccentrically situated in relation to the central artery. Like the lymph nodes, the follicles are either inactive or activated, activated follicles being associated with germinal center formation. Arising from the central artery, follicular arteries enter the B-cell follicles and terminate in a marginal sinus in the region of the marginal zone, the junction between the white and red pulp. Circulating lymphocytes exit the vascular system from the marginal sinus and travel to their respective B- and T-cell locations. Lymphocytes leave the white pulp and enter the red pulp

by way of bridging channels that cross the marginal sinus. The periarteriolar lymphoid sheath extends around the B-cell follicle and continues to ensheath the central arteries until the level of the small penicilliary arteries, which terminate in the red pulp.

The red pulp comprises a network of stromal cords and vascular sinuses. Lining the sinuses are longitudinally oriented slender endothelial cells and radially oriented ring fibers consisting of a discontinuous basement membrane. In the red pulp numerous phagocytic macrophages are found in both the stromal cords and the sinuses. Penicilliary arteries terminate in the sinuses (closed circulation) or, less commonly, in the cords (open circulation). Termination in the cords exposes erythrocytes to the additional hazard of migration through the cord and across the sinus wall to the sinus lumen. In the pulp cords erythrocytes (1) are subjected to the sustained scrutiny of mononuclear phagocytes, (2) must exhibit deformability in order to traverse the thin interstices between the lining endothelial cells, and (3) must be able to survive the hypoxia, hypoglycemia, and acidosis that are characteristic of the stromal cord microenvironment. Most normal erythroid cells do survive, ultimately enter the trabecular veins and leave the splenic hilum by way of the splenic vein.

The splenic white and red pulps have separate functions. As part of the peripheral lymphoid system, effector B- and T-lymphocytes of the white pulp perform an immunologic function for the circulatory system comparable to the localized immunologic function of the lymph nodes. The white pulp is the source of protection from blood-borne infection, is a major site of production of opsonizing IgM antibody,

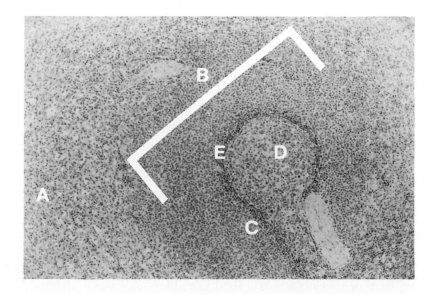

Figure 20-4.   Normal anatomy of the spleen. *A*, red pulp; *B*, white pulp; *C*, T-cell dependent periarteriolar lymphoid sheath; *D*, B-cell follicle; *E*, B-cell mantle zone.

and is also a site of production of lymphocytes and plasma cells.

The red pulp is involved in a number of functions relating to the erythrocyte. First, senescent and damaged erythrocytes are recognized and phagocytosed by splenic macrophages. Under ordinary circumstances, the spleen accounts for the removal of about half of senescent or damaged erythrocytes, the remainder being destroyed in the liver, bone marrow, and other sites of the mononuclear phagocyte system. Following phagocytosis and breakdown of erythrocytes, iron is released from hemoglobin, stored in the macrophage, released, bound to transferrin, and transported to the bone marrow for reutilization in erythrocyte production. Second, abnormal erythrocyte inclusions, such as Howell-Jolly bodies (remnants of nuclear DNA), Heinz bodies (denatured hemoglobin), and siderotic granules (iron) are recognized and removed (pitted) by macrophages without destruction of the erythrocyte. Third, as the erythrocyte matures, removal of membrane lipids occurs, principally in the splenic red pulp cords. In the absence of this function, such as after splenectomy, there is excess erythrocyte membrane in relation to hemoglobin content, a situation that leads to the formation of flat target cells. Target cells are erythrocytes with deficient content of hemoglobin in relation to cell volume. The small amount of hemoglobin "puddles" centrally, creating a target cell appearance.

Under normal circumstances, one-third of the peripheral blood platelet pool is sequestered in the spleen. Normally, no significant sequestration of erythrocytes or granulocytes occurs. As previously noted, the splenic red pulp is a potential site of extramedullary hematopoiesis in situations of chronic demand for increased red blood cell production.

Cell Identification

Maturation Sequence

The primitive hematopoietic precursor cells, less than 1:2000 of the bone marrow nucleated cells, are indistinguishable from small to medium-sized lymphocytes. They are demonstrated only by use of monoclonal antibodies and clonal assays *in vitro*.

Blast Cells   Blast cells are the first identifiable cell type in hematopoietic cell maturation. Blast cells can be assigned to a specific lineage because of their distinctive morphologic features. Erythroid pronormoblasts have intense cytoplasmic basophilia. The cytoplasm of myeloblasts is a light gray-blue, and the

nucleoli are more numerous and the chromatin finer than in pronormoblasts. Monoblasts are identified by their distinctive gray cytoplasm and a slightly coarse, or "ropy," chromatin. Megakaryoblasts are easily recognized by their large size.

The maturation of the erythroid cell series is best evaluated in Wright's- or Wright's-Giemsa–stained smears (see Fig. 20-1). The sequence from pronormoblast to basophilic, polychromatophilic, and finally orthochromatic normoblast involves (1) increasing condensation or density of chromatin, from the delicate loose chromatin of the pronormoblast to the dense hyperchromatic chromatin of the orthochromatic normoblast; (2) decreasing blue and increasing orange-red tint to the cytoplasm, as the cytoplasmic content of ribosomes decreases and the hemoglobin content increases; and (3) decreasing cell size from the pronormoblast to the orthochromatic normoblast.

Reticulocytes   The ejection of the nucleus from an orthochromatic normoblast gives rise to the reticulocyte, an immature erythrocyte slightly larger than a mature erythrocyte. A delicate grayish-blue tint, which reflects the presence of residual ribosomes and mitochondria, is characteristic of the reticulocyte. The reticulocyte matures to a mature erythrocyte in 1 to 2 days in the peripheral blood, with the loss of residual ribosomes and mitochondria.

Granulocytes   The maturation sequence of the granulocytes is also best evaluated in Wright's- or Wright's-Giemsa–stained smears (see Fig. 20-1). The sequence from myeloblast to promyelocyte, myelocyte, metamyelocyte, band, and finally mature polymorphonuclear leukocyte involves (1) the progressive condensation of chromatin; (2) the increasing complexity of the nuclear configuration, from the round nucleus of the myeloblast, promyelocyte, and myelocyte to the slight nuclear indentation of the metamyelocyte, to the prominent nuclear indentation of the band, to the discrete lobes of the mature leukocyte, connected by delicate nuclear threads; and (3) the acquisition of primary (azurophilic) granules at the promyelocyte stage and secondary (specific) granules—neutrophilic, eosinophilic, or basophilic—at the myelocyte stage.

Monocytes   The maturation of monocytic cells progresses from bone marrow monoblast to promonocyte, to peripheral blood mature monocyte, and finally to tissue histiocyte or phagocytic macrophage. This maturation involves the acquisition of an eccentric indented or bean-shaped nucleus at the promonocyte stage and progressively more abundant gray cytoplasm. The chromatin becomes increasingly coarse and "ropy." In the tissues it is difficult to distinguish histiocytes from mesenchymal fibro-

Table 20-4 Mononuclear Phagocyte System: Immunologic and Functional Markers

Immunologic

IgG$_{Fc}$	Fc receptor for heavy-chain IgG
Ia	HLA-DR–linked antigen
EAC	Complement receptor
Lysozyme*	
α_1-antichymotrypsin*	

Functional

In vitro phagocytosis

* Immunohistochemical demonstration utilizing peroxidase-antiperoxidase (PAP) or avidin-biotin-complex (ABC) technique

blasts, since both exhibit elongated nuclei and scanty cytoplasm. Unless there is obvious morphologic evidence for macrophage differentiation and phagocytic function, specific cell markers are required to define cells as components of the mononuclear phagocyte system (Table 20-4).

Megakaryocytes The maturation of megakaryocytes from single-lobed megakaryoblasts to mature megakaryocytes with 16 or 32 nuclear lobes is characterized by increasing hypersegmentation of the nuclei and accumulation of azurophilic cytoplasmic platelet precursors.

Morphologic and Immunologic Evaluation

Precise identification of the cell lineage, the degree of cell differentiation, and cell transformation of lymphopoietic cells is complex and generally requires both morphologic and immunologic evaluation. Primitive antigen-independent B and T cells are morphologically indistinguishable from small to medium-sized lymphocytes. If not exposed to the appropriate sensitizing antigen, antigen-dependent, committed B and T cells appear as small lymphocytes. When ac-

tivated by the appropriate antigen, both B and T cells undergo transformation to large proliferating and protein synthesizing cells. These transformed cells are called "atypical" lymphocytes when identified on the peripheral blood smear and immunoblasts when seen in tissue sections. "Atypical" lymphocytes have abundant blue cytoplasm and frequently multiple nucleoli; immunoblasts have a round to oval nucleus, with clear or vesicular chromatin, one to several eosinophilic nucleoli, and moderately abundant clear to purple cytoplasm. The "atypical" lymphocytes and immunoblasts subsequently modulate to either small memory B-or T-lymphocytes or to effector B plasma cells and T effector cells.

In infections and immune reactions, in which there is commonly lymphocyte transformation and modulation, the sizes and appearances of the lymphocytes vary widely in the peripheral blood smear and occasionally in the tissues. In the peripheral blood there are small, medium-sized, and large, or "atypical," lymphocytes; in the tissues small lymphocytes, partially activated or transformed lymphocytes, and large activated lymphocytes or immunoblasts are seen.

In lymph nodes and in other sites in which B germinal centers are found, four cell types are seen: small cleaved, large cleaved, small noncleaved, and large noncleaved. Plasma cells in tissue sections are identified by a distinctive eccentric nucleus, with marginally clumped chromatin and abundant blue-purple cytoplasm. The precise identification of antigen-independent and antigen-committed B-lymphocytes requires a panel of specific cell markers (Table 20-5). Similarly, the identification of antigen-independent differentiating thymic T-lymphocytes and mature postthymic antigen-independent and antigen-committed T-lymphocytes also requires a complex panel of cell markers (Table 20-6).

Table 20-5 Cell Markers in B-Cell Ontogeny

MARKERS	STEM CELL	PRE-PRE-B	PRE-B	B CELL	B-IMMUNOBLAST	PLASMA CELL
Ig gene rearrangement	−	+	+	+	+	+
Terminal deoxynucleotidyl transferase	+	+	+	−	−	−
Ia HLA-DR immune response linked	+	+	+	+	+	±
CALLA (common acute lymphoblastic leukemic antigen)	±	+	+	−	−	−
Cytoplasmic μ chain	−	−	+	−	−	−
Surface immunoglobulin	−	−	−	+	+	−
Pan B	−	+	+	+	+	−
Cytoplasmic immunoglobulin	−	−	−	−	±	+
Complement receptor	−	−	−	±	±	−
IgG$_{Fc}$ receptor	−	−	−	+	+	−

Table 20-6 Cell Markers in T-Cell Ontogeny

MONOCLONAL ANTIBODY	IMMATURE				MATURE	
	EARLY THYMOCYTE	COMMON THYMOCYTE	LATE THYMOCYTE PROHELPER	LATE THYMOCYTE PROSUPPRESSOR	INDUCER-HELPER	CYTOTOXIC-SUPPRESSOR
Pan T	−	−	+	+	+	+
E-rosette receptor	+	+	+	+	+	+
Inducer/helper	−	+	+	−	+	−
Cytotoxic/suppressor	−	+	−	+	−	+
Common thymocyte	−	+	−	−	−	−
Transferrin receptor	+	−	−	−	−	−
Early dividing cell	+	+	+	+	−	−
Terminal deoxynucleotidyl transferase	+	+	±	±	−	−

In disorders of hematopoietic and lymphopoietic cells, there is an even more striking morphologic and functional diversity of cell types than is appreciated in normal hematopoietic and lymphopoietic cell differentiation. This diversity is characteristic of both nonneoplastic and neoplastic disorders. Morphologic and biochemical identification (Table 20-7) is required for the distinction of primitive cells of the myeloid (granulocytic), monocytoid, and lymphoid cell lineages. Such identification is particularly useful in the differentiation of the various acute leukemias. Subtypes of the leukemias and the malignant lymphomas can also be distinguished by use of labeled monoclonal antibodies directed against cell surface antigens or by use of immunohistochemical techniques to demonstrate cytoplasmic antigens in tissue sections. Additional techniques employed in the study and identification of abnormal hematopoietic and lymphopoietic cell types include electron microscopy, cytogenetics, and demonstration of gene rearrangements.

Hemostasis

Hemostasis, or the arrest of bleeding, is dependent on the proper functioning of three biologic systems: the blood vessels, the platelets, and the plasma coagulation factors.

Table 20-7 Biochemical Identification of Cell Lineage

	MYELOID	MONOCYTOID	LYMPHOID
Enzyme			
MPX—Myeloperoxidase	2^+-4^+ d	$^+$ d	0
CAE—Naphthol AS-D chloroacetate esterase	2^+-4^+ d	0	0
AP—Acid phosphatase	$0-1^+$ d	2^+-4^+ d	$0-1^+$ f
TRAP—Tartrate-resistant acid phosphatase	0	0	Hairy cell
BG—Beta-glucuronidase	0	$0-^+$ d	$+-1^+$ f
ANAE—Alpha-naphthyl acetate esterase	$0-1^+$ d	3^+-4^+ d*	$0-1^+$ f
ANBE—Alpha-naphthyl butyrate esterase	0	3^+-4^+ d*	$0-1^+$ f
NASDA—Naphthol AS-D acetate esterase	$0-1^+$ d	3^+-4^+ d*	$0-1^+$ f
Tdt—Terminal deoxynucleotidyl transferase	0	0	+
Glycogen			
PAS—Periodic acid-Schiff reaction	± d	± d	$0-4^+$ b
Lipid			
SBB—Sudan black B	1^+-3^+ d	$±-2^+$ d	0

* Reaction inhibited by sodium fluoride.
(d, diffuse pattern; f, focal pattern, paranuclear; b, block pattern)
0, nonstaining; 1+, rare positive cells; 2+, mild increase; 3+, moderate increase; 4+ marked increase

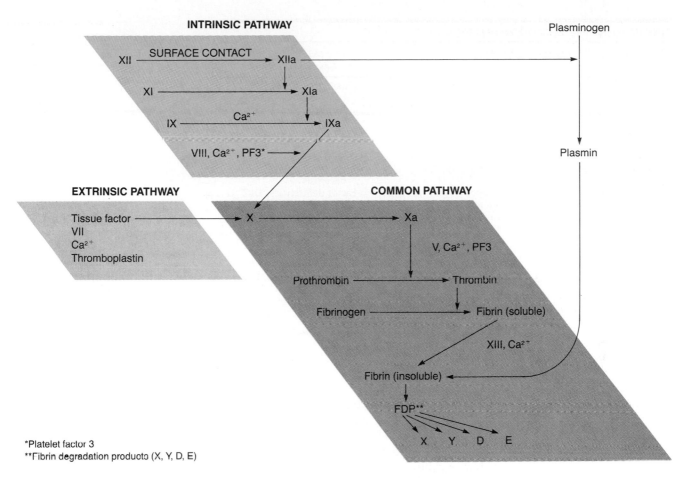

Figure 20-5. The coagulation cascade. Blood coagulation is initiated either by an intrinsic pathway induced by the exposure of Factor XII to negatively charged subendothelial collagen or by an extrinsic pathway induced by the release of tissue factors or thromboplastins. The intrinsic and extrinsic systems then undergo a final common pathway by which fibrinogen is ultimately converted to fibrin, which in turn is stabilized or made insoluble and becomes the stable blood clot.

Normal Hemostasis

Arteriolar vasoconstriction, induced by vasoactive substances such as serotonin and thromboxane A_2, which are secreted by activated platelets and by neurogenic mechanisms, contributes to the arrest of local bleeding. Vasoconstriction alone, however, is usually inadequate to ensure hemostasis.

The participation of platelets and the plasma protein clotting factors is essential to hemostasis. Platelets are responsible for the formation of the primary platelet plug and for the contribution of platelet factor 3. Immediately following damage to the vascular endothelium, platelets adhere to the subendothelial collagen. They then undergo shape change (viscous metamorphosis), with secretion of ADP, fibrinogen, and other platelet granule products (release reaction). Circulating platelets aggregate, and the primary platelet plug, which is responsible for the initial cessation of bleeding, is formed. This process is termed **primary hemostasis.** Platelets also contribute platelet factor 3, a platelet membrane phospholipid complex that potentiates coagulation in conjunction with the plasma protein clotting factors.

The coagulation schema, or cascade (Fig. 20-5), consists of a complex sequence of proteolytic reactions that culminate in the formation of the fibrin clot. Initial activation of the coagulation cascade occurs by two mechanisms: The intrinsic system involves the exposure of factor XII to negatively charged collagen following damage to endothelial cells; and the extrinsic system is triggered by the

Table 20-8 Screening Tests of Hemostasis (Coagulation Tests)

LABORATORY TEST	FACTORS OR FUNCTIONS MEASURED	ASSOCIATED DISORDERS OR ABNORMALITY
Bleeding time	Platelet function	Qualitative (acquired or congenital) disorders of platelets, Von Willebrand's disease
	Vascular integrity	Quantitative disorders of platelets, acquired vascular disorders
Platelet count	Platelet quantitation	Thrombocytopenia, thrombocytosis
Prothrombin time	Evaluation of extrinsic system and common pathway (I, II, V, VII, X)	Factor deficiencies, DIC, liver disease, oral anticoagulant therapy
Partial thromboplastin time	Evaluation of intrinsic system and common pathway (I, II, V, VIII, IX, X, XI, XII)	Factor deficiencies, factor inhibitor, DIC, heparin therapy
Thrombin time	Evaluation of common pathway	Dysfibrinogenemia, DIC, afibrinogenemia, heparin therapy

(*DIC*, disseminated intravascular coagulation)

activation of factor VII following tissue damage, with the release of thromboplastins from procoagulant tissue or endothelial cells. Both the intrinsic and the extrinsic systems then follow a common pathway by which prothrombin is converted to thrombin, which in turn cleaves fibrinogen to fibrin. A soluble blood clot is formed by the initial polymerization of fibrin monomers. This clot is then stabilized by the replacement of hydrogen bonds with covalent bonds, a step that requires thrombin-activated factor XIII.

Simultaneously with the production of the hemostatic plug, the fibrinolytic system, which is responsible for resorption of the blood clot (fibrinolysis), is activated at the site of clot formation. Circulating inactive plasminogen is converted to the active proteolytic enzyme plasmin (fibrinolysin) by the action of factor XIIa or by tissue factors. Plasmin digests fibrin and fibrinogen to form the fibrin and fibrinogen degradation products X, Y, D, and E.

Disorders of Hemostasis

Congenital and acquired disorders of each of the three biologic systems involved in hemostasis predispose either to spontaneous bleeding or to excessive bleeding following trauma. The characteristics of the bleeding episodes provide a clue as to the type of hemorrhagic diathesis. Bleeding due to vascular disorders consists of petechial and purpuric hemorrhages in the skin and in the gastrointestinal and genitourinary tracts. Bleeding due to platelet disorders is also usually petechial, from small vessels in

the skin, mucous membranes, and the serosal surfaces of the body cavities. In platelet disorders bleeding usually occcurs immediately following trauma or a surgical procedure. Bleeding due to coagulation factor deficiencies is seen as large areas of ecchymosis, as hematomas in sites such as the subcutaneous or muscle tissues, and as hemorrhage into the gastrointestinal system, genitourinary tract, and joint spaces (hemarthrosis). There may also be delayed bleeding following trauma or surgery. Evaluation of a bleeding disorder requires a careful personal and family history and the use of common laboratory screening tests (Table 20-8).

Blood Vessel Disorders

Hereditary vascular disorders that may be associated with bleeding include hereditary hemorrhagic telangiectasia (Osler-Weber-Rendu disease) and connective tissue disorders, such as Marfan's syndrome. **Acquired vascular defects** are an uncommon cause of clinical bleeding. In **vitamin C deficiency** (scurvy), collagen synthesis and deposition of intercellular cement are defective, and bleeding occurs in the subcutaneous tissues, skeletal muscle, gingiva, and skin around hair follicles. **Senile purpura** is caused by an age-related atrophy of the connective tissue supporting structures that predisposes to skin hemorrhage, particularly on sun-exposed areas. In **Cushing's syndrome** purpura is related to the catabolic effect of corticosteroids on the perivascular connective tissues. Purpura may also be due to **drug-induced vascular damage.** Serum paraproteins and cryoglobulins may also cause vascular damage and bleeding. **Allergic purpura,** which occurs primarily in children, is usually preceded by an upper respiratory tract infection. Vasculitis, most prominent in small dermal vessels, is seen, histologically characterized by perivascular inflammatory cell infiltrates consisting of neutrophils and eosinophils. Fibrinoid necrosis of the vessel walls and platelet plugging of the vascular lumina are prominent. IgA and complement may be identified in the vessel walls. Clinically allergic purpura is manifested by purpura and generalized vasculitis in the joints, kidneys, and gastrointestinal tract. **Schönlein-Henoch purpura** refers to allergic purpura associated with joint pain and gastrointestinal symptoms.

Disorders of Platelets

Quantitative and qualitative disorders of platelets are important and common causes of hemorrhage.

Quantitative Disorders

Thrombocytopenia is a decrease in the platelet count to less than the normal 150,000 platelets per microliter. A decrease in the platelet count to less than 50,000 per microliter increases the hazard of bleeding from trauma or surgical procedures. Spontaneous bleeding can occur with a platelet count below 20,000, and is especially likely to occur with a count below 5000 per microliter. Thrombocytopenia can result from decreased production of platelets, increased destruction of platelets, and splenic sequestration of platelets.

Decreased production of platelets is due either to a decreased number of megakaryocytes in the bone marrow or to ineffective thrombopoiesis (intramedullary destruction of megakaryocyte-platelets). A decreased megakaryocyte mass occurs in aplastic anemia, bone marrow infiltrative diseases (myelophthisis), and bone marrow hypoplasia caused by x-irradiation, myelotoxic agents (chloramphenicol, thiazide diuretics, alcohol), and viral infections. Bone marrow hypoplasia with megakaryocytopenia also occurs in the congenital disorder **Fanconi's pancytopenia.**

Ineffective thrombopoiesis with increased intramedullary destruction of megakaryocytes and platelets is observed most commonly in the megaloblastic anemias of vitamin B_{12} or folic acid deficiency. The **May-Hegglin anomaly,** a defect in megakaryocyte cell maturation, is characterized by thrombocytopenia, bizarre circulating giant platelets, and Döhle bodies in neutrophils. Döhle bodies are blue–staining portions of cytoplasm, which represent ribosome-associated endoplasmic reticulum.

Increased destruction of platelets occurs both by immune and by nonimmune mechanisms and is accompanied by an increase in bone marrow megakaryocytes. Immune destruction of platelets is seen in idiopathic thrombocytopenic purpura, isoimmune neonatal purpura, posttransfusion purpura, drug-induced thrombocytopenic purpura, and secondary immunologic purpura.

Idiopathic thrombocytopenic purpura (ITP) occurs either as an acute disorder in children or as a chronic disorder in adults. **Acute ITP** usually occurs in children younger than 6 years of age, generally following an acute viral illness. There is a rapid decrease in the platelet count, frequently to less than 20,000 platelets per microliter. Petechial or purpuric hemorrhages of the skin and mucous membranes are conspicuous. The mechanism of the thrombocytopenia may involve the binding of circulating antigen-antibody complexes to platelet Fc receptors. Such coated platelets are vulnerable to destruction by splenic macrophages. Eighty percent of the cases of acute ITP spontaneously remit in weeks or months, and recurrences are unusual.

Chronic idiopathic thrombocytopenic purpura typically is a disorder of middle-aged women. IgG antiplatelet antibody is demonstrated in approximately 85% of the cases. Unlike acute ITP, chronic ITP is not generally precipitated by an infectious episode, and its course is punctuated by relapses and remissions. The hallmark of ITP is an increase in young hyposegmented megakaryocytes in the bone marrow. Platelet destruction in chronic ITP occurs principally in the spleen, which is usually of normal size, and reveals reactive hyperplasia of the white pulp and occasionally an increase in macrophages.

Chronic ITP is sometimes followed by the development of a collagen vascular disease, such as systemic lupus erythematosus, or a malignant lymphoma. Chronic ITP may also develop secondarily in a collagen vascular disease, a malignant lymphoma, or chronic lymphocytic leukemia.

In **isoimmune neonatal purpura,** an immunologically mediated thrombocytopenia develops in the fetus and neonate by a mechanism analogous to the destruction of fetal erythrocytes in erythroblastosis fetalis. In this disorder a Pl^{A1}-negative mother develops anti-Pl^{A1} IgG antibodies, which cross the placenta and destroy the fetal platelets. The severe thrombocytopenia causes a bleeding diathesis. Spontaneous recovery usually occurs in several weeks. In **posttransfusion purpura** the thrombocytopenia is also immunologically mediated. As a consequence of sensitization to Pl^{A1} antigen from a prior blood transfusion or a previous pregnancy, a Pl^{A1}- negative person transfused with Pl^{A1}-positive platelets may develop a severe thrombocytopenia.

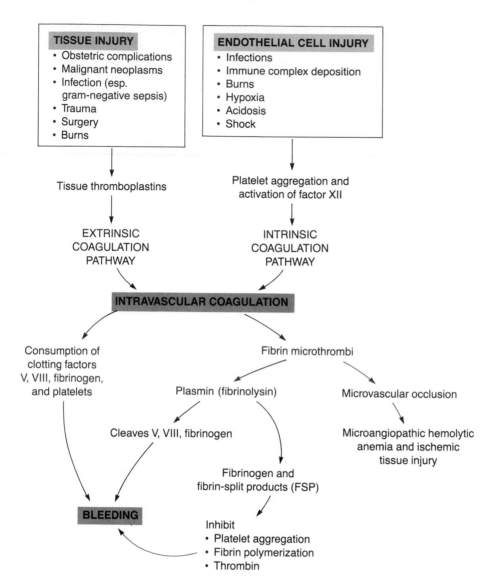

Figure 20-6. The pathophysiology of disseminated intravascular coagulation (DIC). The syndrome of DIC is precipitated either by tissue injury, with release of tissue thromboplastin and activation of the extrinsic coagulation pathway, or by endothelial cell injury, with activation of the intrinsic coagulation pathway. Intravascular coagulation is induced by either or, frequently, both mechanisms. Clinically, there is bleeding from multiple sites and microvascular occlusions or thromboses with secondary microangiopathic hemolytic anemia and ischemic tissue injury.

In **drug-induced thrombocytopenia,** an immunologic mechanism is also postulated. Platelets are destroyed, probably in the spleen, after being coated with drug-antibody complexes. The most commonly incriminated drugs include quinidine, the thiazide diuretics, and meprobamate. A decreased platelet count may also result from an increased nonimmune consumption of platelets, as occurs in disseminated intravascular coagulation, thrombotic thrombocytopenic purpura, and the hemolytic uremic syndrome. Although these disorders are not primary abnormalities of platelets, they are considered here because they involve a reduction in platelet survival.

Disseminated intravascular coagulation (DIC) is a complex acquired disorder characterized by both widespread intravascular coagulation and diffuse hemorrhage. The clinical disease reflects both the thrombotic and particularly the hemorrhagic dia-

thesis. The pathophysiology of DIC (Fig. 20-6) relates to an initial, widespread initiation of microvascular coagulation either by tissue damage, with release of tissue procoagulants or thromboplastins into the peripheral circulation (extrinsic pathway), or by extensive endothelial cell injury, which activates factor XII and initiates platelet aggregation, with release of platelet factor 3 (intrinsic pathway). Both mechanisms are commonly involved. **Widespread intravascular coagulation and fibrin deposition produces ischemia of severely affected organs.** In addition, the red blood cells are fragmented in passage through the intravascular fibrin deposits (**microangiopathic hemolytic anemia**). Schistocytes (fragmented erythrocytes) are identified on the peripheral blood smear in 20% of the cases. **Fibrin-platelet microthrombi are seen in the microvasculature of essentially any organ.** The most commonly involved sites, in decreasing order of frequency, are the brain, heart, lungs, kidneys, adrenal glands, spleen, and liver.

The hemorrhagic diathesis in DIC dominates the clinical symptomatology. It results from the consumption of platelets, clotting factors (V and VIII), and prothrombin (consumption coagulopathy), as well as from the activation of plasminogen to plasmin (fibrinolysin). The presence of plasmin further depresses the serum levels of factors V and VIII and cleaves fibrinogen and fibrin to degradation products. These "split products" impair fibrin polymerization and platelet aggregation.

Disorders commonly associated with DIC include obstetric complications, cancer, massive trauma, and infections, particularly those with accompanying sepsis. The presentation and the clinical course of DIC are determined by the underlying disease process. With certain cancers there is an associated low-grade DIC that is clinically inapparent and detected only by laboratory studies. In DIC secondary to gram-negative sepsis and endotoxemia, a fulminant and frequently lethal clinical course is observed. Laboratory studies in DIC show a low platelet count, low serum fibrinogen, prolonged prothrombin, partial thromboplastin and thrombin times, and elevated fibrinogen-fibrin split products.

Thrombotic thrombocytopenic purpura (TTP) is a rare, acute systemic disorder of the microcirculation, that is most common in young women. The pathogenesis is obscure but appears to be related to immunologically mediated damage to small blood vessels. Fibrin-platelet microthrombi are seen in the lumina of small arterioles and capillaries in essentially any organ or tissue. The clinical syndrome consists of the pentad of fever, thrombocytopenia, microangiopathic hemolytic anemia, renal failure, and fluctuating neurologic deficits.

The hemolytic uremic syndrome, a disease of the microvasculature in infants and young children, is similar to thrombotic thrombocytopenic purpura. The characteristic lesions are fibrin-platelet microthrombi in the renal microvasculature. The clinical syndrome consists of thrombocytopenia, microangiopathic hemolytic anemia, and renal failure. Typically, no neurologic deficits occur.

Thrombocytopenia due to splenic sequestration reflects a redistribution of the peripheral blood platelet pool. A larger than normal proportion, over one-third, of the peripheral blood platelet pool is retained in the spleen. The platelet redistribution is roughly proportional to the size of the spleen. In massive splenomegaly as much as 90% of the peripheral blood platelet pool may be sequestered in the spleen.

Dilutional thrombocytopenia results from massive blood transfusions. Viable platelets are depleted in banked blood that has been stored for more than 24 hours. Massive transfusion of such blood can result in a dilutional thrombocytopenia.

Qualitative Disorders

Qualitative or functional platelet disorders are an uncommon cause of clinical bleeding. Qualitative platelet disorders are characterized by a prolonged bleeding time in conjunction with a normal platelet count. Qualitative platelet disorders may be congenital or acquired. In either case platelets exhibit defects of adhesion, aggregation or release.

The disorders discussed below are illustrative of the three principal qualitative platelet defects. In **Bernard-Soulier** or **giant platelet syndrome,** the platelets which vary widely in shape and size, show a defective adherence to subendothelial collagen owing to a deficient membrane glycoprotein. Severe bleeding may be observed. In **Glanzmann's thrombasthenia** the platelets exhibit a defect in aggregation, probably as a result of a deficiency of several membrane glycoproteins. Because of this deficiency, fibrinogen bridges between platelets are not formed, a lack that results in impaired platelet aggregation. The clinical bleeding disorder is mild, affecting mucosal surfaces. Disorders of platelet release reflect either deficient platelet ADP content or deficient platelet release; although platelet aggregation is impaired, the resulting bleeding disorder is mild.

Acetylsalicylic acid (aspirin) irreversibly acetylates platelets and induces a defect in platelet factor 3 release. Platelet function is therefore impaired for the life span of the circulating platelet (9–11 days), and there is an increased risk of hemorrhage following trauma or surgery. In the laboratory a prolonged bleeding time and abnormal platelet aggregation tests are characteristic.

Disorders of Coagulation Factors

Both quantitative and qualitative defects of all of the plasma protein clotting factors have been identified. These defects may be hereditary or acquired. Only **hemophilia A (Factor VIII deficiency), von Willebrand's disease** and **hemophilia B (Factor IX deficiency),** are common.

Factor VIII is a complex composed of the Factor VIII functional coagulant molecule (VIII:C), the von Willebrand's factor (VIII R:WF), and the ristocetin cofactor (VIII R:RCo). The Factor VIII molecule is synthesized in part by vascular endothelial cells and in part by megakaryocytes or the liver. **Hemophilia A,** or **classic hemophilia,** is a deficiency of Factor VIII:C; it accounts for approximately 85% of the hereditary clotting factor disorders. It is an X-linked recessive trait and therefore common only in males. One-quarter of the cases arise from a *de novo* mutation. Factor VIII levels vary widely. In severe hemophilia a Factor VIII level of only 1% of normal is typical. In moderate hemophilia a Factor VIII level of 1% to 5% is characteristic, and in the mild variety levels vary from 5% to 10% of normal. **Severely affected persons manifest spontaneous bleeding into the weight bearing joints (hemarthrosis).** Repeated hemarthroses eventually lead to joint deformities. Bleeding into the soft tissues and the viscera also occurs. In the laboratory a prolonged partial thromboplastin time (PTT) and decreased Factor VIII levels are noted.

Von Willebrand's disease is due either to qualitative or to quantitative abnormalities of a factor (von Willebrand's factor, Factor VIII–related protein, VIII R:WF) that circulates as a complex with the Factor VIII:C molecule. The two molecules are coded for by separate genes, Factor VIII:C on the X chromosome and Factor VIII R:WF on one or more autosomes. Therefore, von Willebrand's disease is an autosomal dominant disorder.

Von Willebrand's factor is required for the normal adherence of platelets to subendothelial collagen. **In von Willebrand's disease, there is a lack of normal platelet adhesiveness, but there is no intrinsic abnormality of the platelets.** Because of the **functional** platelet defect, however, the bleeding time is prolonged. For poorly understood reasons a mild decrease in Factor VIII coagulative activity is also usually observed, and the PTT is usually prolonged.

In von Willebrand's disease there is also a decrease in or lack of the ristocetin cofactor (VIII R:RCo). Because of this deficiency, upon the addition of the antibiotic ristocetin, aggregation of platelets either is decreased or does not occur. The demonstration of deficient or absent ristocetin-induced aggregation of platelets is a useful screening test for von Willebrand's disease.

The clinical severity of von Willebrand's disease varies. Generally, there is episodic mucosal bleeding, particularly from the gastrointestinal tract. Menorrhagia is also common. There is usually excessive bleeding following trauma. However, unlike hemophilia A, bleeding into the joint spaces is uncommon. The disorder tends to lessen in severity with age.

Hemophilia B, which is the result of Factor IX deficiency, is a less common disorder than either hemophilia A or von Willebrand's disease. Like hemophilia A, it is a sex-linked recessive disorder. The clinical severity of the disorder is dependent on the level of Factor IX. The disorder is severe when the Factor IX level is 1% of normal, moderate when the Factor IX level is 1% to 5% of normal, and mild when the Factor IX level is at 5% to 10% of normal. The clinical syndrome is indistinguishable from that of hemophilia A. Recurrent hemarthroses may result in a crippling deformity of the joints.

Deficiencies of clotting factors other than Factors VIII and IX are uncommon. Since these deficiencies are characteristically autosomal recessive traits both males and females are affected. Clinically, there is usually a mild bleeding disorder. However, deficiencies of Factors V, X, and XIII are occasionally associated with severe bleeding. In acquired clotting factor disorders, there are frequently deficiencies of several clotting factors. For example, **vitamin K deficiency results in decreased hepatic synthesis of Factors II, VII, IX, and X.** Because all clotting factors except Factor VIII are synthesized only by the liver, severe hepatic parenchymal disease is commonly associated with a hemorrhagic diathesis.

Anemia

Anemia is a reduction below the normal range of the hemoglobin concentration in the peripheral blood. The normal hemoglobin concentration is 14 g/dl to 18 g/dl for men and 12 g/dl to 16 g/dl for women. The hemoglobin concentration is higher in men than in women because of the stimulatory effect of androgens on erythropoiesis. Androgens increase erythropoietin production by the renal juxtaglomerular apparatus and increase sensitivity of erythroid precursor cells in the bone marrow to erythropoietin. Normal adult values for the complete blood count are outlined in Table 20-9. The normal hemoglobin concentration in the prepubertal child is 11 g/dl to 13 g/dl.

Disorders associated with anemia are classified according to either pathophysiologic or morphologic criteria (Table 20-10). **The pathophysiologic classification separates disorders associated with anemia into two major categories: those due to bone marrow failure with underproduction of erythrocytes, and those caused by peripheral loss or destruction of erythrocytes.** The clinical history is helpful in distinguishing anemia due to marrow failure from anemia due to peripheral loss of erythrocytes. For example, a history of exposure to a bone marrow toxin, such as benzene, suggests that marrow failure is the cause of the anemia, whereas a history of recent hemorrhage points to peripheral loss of erythrocytes. Objective information is provided by the reticulocyte count (see Table 20-10). In disorders associated with

---

Table 20-9 The Complete Blood Count (CBC): Normal Adult Values

Erythrocytes

Hemoglobin	Male, 14–18 g/dl
	Female, 12–16 g/dl
Hematocrit	Male, 40–54%
	Female, 35–47%
Red blood cell (RBC) count	Male, 4.5–6 × 10^6/µl
	Female, 4–5.5 × 10^6/µl

Indices
  Mean cell volume   82–100 µm³
  Mean cell hemoglobin   27–34 µµg
  Mean corpuscular hemoglobin concentration   32–36%

Leukocytes (WBC)

	ABSOLUTE COUNT/µl	DIFFERENTIAL (%)
Total WBC	4000–11,000	
Neutrophil granulocytes	1800–7000	50–60
Neutrophil bands	0–700	2–4
Lymphocytes	1500–4000	30–40
Monocytes	0–800	1–9
Basophils	0–200	0–1
Eosinophils	0–450	2–3

Platelets

Quantitative normal value: 150,000–400,000/µl
Qualitative estimation on smear: # platelets/oil immersion field × 10,000 = estimated platelet count
Normal ratio of RBC:platelets — 15:1 to 20:1

---

bone marrow failure, the reticulocyte count is decreased because of inadequate erythroid cell production. In diseases caused by hemorrhage or by increased peripheral destruction of erythrocytes (hemolysis), the reticulocyte count is increased, a finding that reflects increased erythropoietin production induced by hypoxia. Erythropoietin stimulates marrow erythroid precursor cells and reticulocyte release to the peripheral blood. Examination of the peripheral blood smear provides clues to the pathophysiology of the anemia (Fig. 20-7).

The morphologic classification of anemia is based on a quantitative assessment of two of the erythrocyte indices: the mean corpuscular volume (MCV) and the mean corpuscular hemoglobin concentration (MCHC). An erythrocyte with a normal cell volume is said to be **normocytic.** An erythrocyte with a normal hemoglobin concentration is termed **normochromic.** On the basis of the erythrocyte indices, the anemias are morphologically classified as (a) normocytic, normochromic; (b) macrocytic, normo-

(Text continues on p. 1034)

Table 20-10 Classification of Anemia

PATHOPHYSIOLOGIC

UNDERPRODUCTION		INCREASED LOSS OR DESTRUCTION	
Bone marrow failure		Hemorrhage	↑ **Reticulocyte**
Deficiency of hematinic factors	↓ **Reticulocyte count**	Hemolysis	**count**
Bone marrow suppression			

MORPHOLOGIC

	MCV	MCHC
Normocytic, normochromic	Normal	Normal
Macrocytic, normochromic	Increased	Normal
Microcytic, hypochromic	Decreased	Decreased
Normocytic, hyperchromic	Normal	Increased

(*MCV*, mean cell volume; *MCHC*, mean corpuscular hemoglobin concentration)

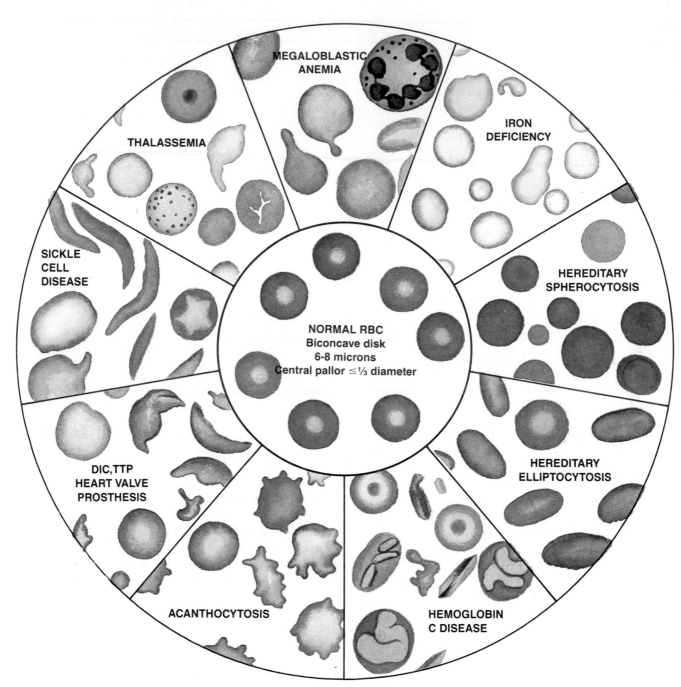

Figure 20-7. The anemias. The pathophysiology and characteristic morphologic features of the various anemias are shown. The morphology of normal erythrocytes is contrasted in the central circle.

DISORDER	PATHOPHYSIOLOGY	MORPHOLOGY
Megaloblastic anemia	Disturbance in DNA synthesis	Oval macrocytes, teardrop poikilocytosis, hypersegmented polys
Iron deficiency	Disturbance in hemoglobin synthesis (lack of iron)	Hypochromic, microcytic
Hereditary spherocytosis	Membrane defect	Spherocytes
Hereditary elliptocytosis	Membrane defect	Elliptocytes
Hemoglobin C disease	Abnormal globin chain	Target cells, rhomboid crystals (HbC)
Acanthocytosis	Membrane lipid defect (abetalipoproteinemia)	Irregular spiculation (similar to spur cells of liver disease)
DIC, TTP, heart valve prosthesis sequela	Mechanical damage to erythrocytes	Schistocytes
Sickle cell disease	Abnormal globin chain	Sickle cells
Thalassemia	Disturbance in hemoglobin synthesis (defect of globin chain)	Hypochromic, microcytic, poikilocytosis, basophilic stippling
Myelophthisic anemia	Marrow replacement or infiltration	Teardrop poikilocytosis, immature WBC and RBC, large platelets
Anemia of chronic disease	Block in utilization of storage iron	Normochromic, normocytic to mild hypochromic, microcytic
Sideroblastic anemia	Defect in porphyrin and heme synthesis	Bimorphic population (normal and microcytic), Pappenheimer bodies
Anemia of renal disease	Multifactorial	Burr cells (uniform marginal scalloping)
Autoimmune hemolytic anemia	RBC destruction mediated by antibodies	Spherocytes
Acute blood loss anemia	Hemorrhage	Polychromasia (increased reticulocytes)

chromic; (c) microcytic, hypochromic; and (d) normocytic, hyperchromic (see Table 20-10). Assigning an anemia to one of these categories is useful in defining the pathophysiology of the underlying disorder. For example, microcytic (small) and hypochromic (pale) cells are observed in iron-deficiency anemia. Large red cells with a normal hemoglobin concentration—that is, macrocytic, normochromic erythrocytes—are characteristic of B_{12} or folic acid deficiency.

Because of the decreased oxygen-carrying capacity of the blood, the physiologic consequence of any anemia is tissue hypoxia. Chronic hypoxia may cause histologic changes, including fat accumulation and, with more severe anemia, ischemic necrosis. Both lesions are prominent in tissues that are especially sensitive to the effects of chronic hypoxia—the cardiac muscle fibers, the renal proximal convoluted tubules, and the hepatic centrilobular cells.

The clinical symptoms of anemia reflect both the severity and the rapidity of onset of the anemia. For example, acute blood loss due to a massive hemorrhage may precipitate shock. By contrast, the insidious development of an anemia of comparable severity is well tolerated because of compensatory increases in plasma volume and cardiac output. In addition, there is a decrease in the oxygen affinity of hemoglobin, mediated by an increase in erythrocyte 2,3-diphosphoglycerate, a change that alters the oxygen dissociation curve of the hemoglobin molecule by a so-called shift to the right. Hence, an increased quantity of oxygen is delivered to the tissues at any pO_2.

In slowly developing anemias clinical symptoms develop when the hemoglobin concentration is less than 7 g/dl to 8 g/dl. These symptoms include weakness, easy fatigability, and dyspnea on exertion. Pallor is the most common clinical sign. There are also signs referable to specific organ systems. Cardiac flow murmurs and a gallop rhythm are cardiovascular signs. Neuromuscular ailments include headache and drowsiness. Gastrointestinal symptoms include glossitis and dysphagia. Certain clinical signs provide clues as to the specific pathophysiologic

---

Table 20-11 Anemia: Pathophysiologic Classification

Underproduction (Impaired Erythrocyte Production)

I. Hematopoietic stem cell proliferation and differentiation abnormality
- Aplastic anemia (aplastic pancytopenia)
- Myelodysplasia (dyshemopoiesis)

II. Erythroid-committed stem cell proliferation and differentiation abnormality
- Pure red cell aplasia
- Anemia of chronic renal disease
- Anemia of endocrine disorders
- Congenital dyserythropoietic anemias

III. Erythroblast proliferation and maturation abnormality
  A. Defective DNA synthesis
- B_{12} deficiency or impaired utilization
- Folate deficiency or impaired utilization
- Inborn errors

  B. Defective hemoglobin synthesis
    1. Heme synthesis abnormality
- Iron deficiency

    2. Globin synthesis abnormality
- Thalassemias

IV. Unknown or multiple mechanisms
- Anemia of chronic disease
- Sideroblastic anemias
- Myelophthisic anemias

Increased Loss or Destruction

I. Hemorrhage
- Acute blood loss anemia
- Chronic blood loss anemia

II. Hemolysis
  A. Intrinsic (intracorpuscular) abnormalities
    1. Hereditary
     (a). Membrane disorders
- Hereditary spherocytosis
- Hereditary elliptocytosis
- Hereditary stomatocytosis
- Acanthocytosis (abetalipoproteinemia)
     (b). Enzyme deficiency
      (i). Glycolytic (Embden-Myerhof) pathway
- Pyruvate kinase deficiency
      (ii). Hexose monophosphate shunt pathway
- G6PD deficiency
     (c). Structurally abnormal globin chain
- Sickle cell anemia
- Hemoglobin C disease
- Unstable hemoglobins
- Hemoglobins with abnormal oxygen affinity
- Methemoglobinemia
    2. Acquired
     (a). Membrane complement sensitivity
- Paroxysmal nocturnal hemoglobinuria

  B. Extrinsic (extracorpuscular) abnormalities
    1. Immune mediated
     (a). Isohemagglutinins
- Erythroblastosis fetalis
     (b). Autoantibodies
- Warm antibody–induced hemolysis
- Cold antibody autoimmune hemolytic anemia
     (c). Drug-induced immunologic injury to erythrocytes
    2. Mechanical trauma to erythrocytes
- Traumatic cardiac hemolytic anemia
- March hemoglobinuria
- Microangiopathic hemolytic anemia
    3. Hypersplenism (hyperactivity of mononuclear phagocyte system)
    4. Hemolytic anemia due to chemical or physical agents
    5. Hemolytic anemia due to infections

Multifactorial
- Alcohol-induced anemia

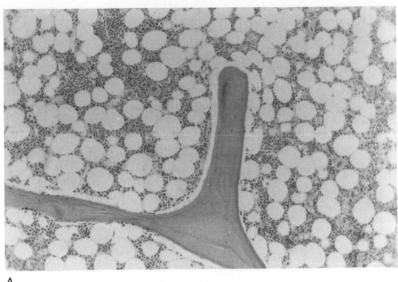

A

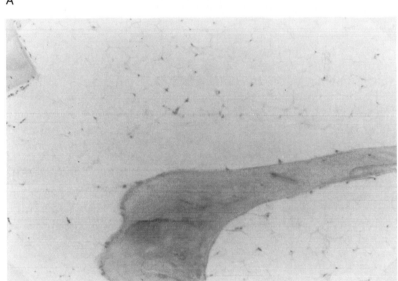

B

Figure 20-8. The bone marrow in aplastic anemia. *(A)* Normal bone marrow with a fat:cell ratio of 50:50. *(B)* Aplastic anemia. The marrow consists largely of fat cells and lacks normal hematopoietic activity.

mechanism of the anemia. For example, skin ulceration over the ankle malleoli is characteristic of sickle cell anemia. Concave or spoon-shaped fingernails—koilonychia—may rarely be observed in severe iron-deficiency anemia.

The pathophysiologic classification of the anemias is outlined in Table 20-11. This classification scheme is followed in the discussion of the specific anemias.

Aplastic Anemia

Aplastic anemia (aplastic pancytopenia) is a common hematopoietic precursor cell disorder, characterized by a decrease in all peripheral blood cell types (pancytopenia) and a hypocellular marrow (Fig. 20-8). A

cause is identified in only half of the cases. Possible causes include a variety of myelotoxic drugs and chemicals (e.g., chloramphenicol, benzene), ionizing radiation, certain viral infections (e.g., infectious hepatitis), and uncommonly, immunologically mediated injury to the bone marrow precursor cells. Fanconi's anemia is a rare familial form of aplastic anemia that occurs in the first decade of life and is associated with a variety of congenital malformations, including absent or hypoplastic thumbs and radii. Common laboratory findings in aplastic anemia include a normocytic, normochromic anemia, reticulocytopenia, granulocytopenia, and thrombocytopenia. The prognosis depends on the severity and duration of the bone marrow aplasia. Mortality is particularly high when aplastic anemia is associated

Table 20-12 The Myelodysplastic Syndromes: French-American-British (FAB) Classification

	REFRACTORY ANEMIA (RA)	REFRACTORY ANEMIA WITH RINGED SIDEROBLASTS (RARS)	REFRACTORY ANEMIA WITH EXCESS BLASTS (RAEB)	REFRACTORY ANEMIA WITH EXCESS BLASTS (RAEB) IN TRANSFORMATION	CHRONIC MYELOMONOCYTIC LEUKEMIA (CMML)
Peripheral Blood					
Hemoglobin	Decreased	Decreased	Decreased	Decreased	Variable
% myeloblasts	0–1	0–1	< 5	> 5	< 5
Monocytes	±	+	±	±	Increased > 1000/µl
Bone Marrow					
% myeloblasts	< 5	< 5	5–20	20–30	≤ 20 with monocytoid precursor cells
Ringed sideroblasts	±	> 15%	±	±	±

Variable peripheral blood granulocytopenia and thrombocytopenia and dyspoiesis of bone marrow and peripheral blood granulocytic and erythrocytic cells may be observed in the myelodysplastic syndromes.

with infectious hepatitis. Overall 5-year mortality for aplastic anemia is 70% in adults and 50% in children. Acute nonlymphocytic leukemia develops in 5% of the cases.

The Myelodysplastic Syndromes

The myelodysplastic syndromes comprise a heterogeneous group of disorders characterized by impaired function of the bone marrow pluripotential hematopoietic precursor cells and by peripheral blood abnormalities. The impaired precursor cell function is manifested as ineffective hematopoiesis or as increased intramedullary destruction of maturing hematopoietic cells. Peripheral blood abnormalities include cytopenias or any combination of anemia, granulocytopenia, thrombocytopenia, and abnormalities in morphologic appearance. Five subtypes of the myelodysplastic syndromes are recognized in the French-American-British classification (Table 20-12): refractory anemia, refractory anemia with ringed sideroblasts, refractory anemia with excess blasts, refractory anemia with excess blasts in transformation, and chronic myelomonocytic leukemia.

In the myelodysplastic syndromes, the cellularity of the bone marrow is normal or increased, and there may be prominent morphologic abnormalities of all three hematopoietic cell lines. Abnormalities of maturing erythroid cells include (1) a megaloblastoid appearance, particularly of the erythroid cell series, with large maturing erythroid cells showing loose chromatin, and (2) the presence of nucleated erythroid precursor cells with damaged, iron-laden mito-

chondria that encircle the cell nucleus (ringed sideroblasts). The mature granulocytes exhibit hyposegmentation of the nuclei with dense chromatin, called the acquired Pelger-Huet anomaly. In the peripheral blood neutropenia and monocytosis are common, and there may be thrombocytopenia, with large, atypically granulated platelets.

The clinical course of the myelodysplastic syndromes is unpredictable. As a result of the peripheral blood cytopenias, there may be complicating infections and bleeding. A progressively severe anemia may be observed, and leukemic transformation occurs in 5% to 10% of cases. Superimposed leukemia is most likely to occur when there is an abnormal morphologic appearance of multiple hematopoietic cell lines, severe peripheral blood cytopenias, and chromosomal abnormalities, the last of which are identified in approximately one-third of cases. The incidence of superimposed leukemia varies with the type of myelodysplastic syndrome. It is most common in refractory anemia with excess blasts in transformation, in which there is generally a rapid progression to acute leukemia.

Pure Red Cell Aplasia

Pure red cell aplasia is the result of an isolated failure of the erythroid precursor cells, with secondary anemia but without leukopenia or thrombocytopenia. Reticulocytopenia is characteristic. Pure red cell aplasia may present either as an acute and self-limited disorder or as several chronic hereditary and acquired disorders. The acute form of red cell aplasia frequently follows a parvovirus infection or a drug reaction. Spontaneous remission usually occurs following resolution of the viral illness or discontinuation of the offending drug. Pure red cell aplasia usually becomes clinically apparent only when there is simultaneous hemolysis or a shortened life span of the circulating erythrocytes. Without the normal bone marrow compensatory capacity, a life-threatening anemia rapidly develops. This is called the **aplastic crisis.**

The Diamond-Blackfan syndrome is a rare hereditary form of pure red cell aplasia, usually detected in the first year of life, in which defective erythroid precursor cells are insensitive to erythropoietin. Serum erythropoietin levels are generally increased. Bone marrow examination reveals a marked erythroid hypoplasia and normal granulocytopoiesis and megakaryocytopoiesis.

The chronic acquired form of pure red cell aplasia occurs usually in middle-aged adults, women being affected more than men. **Acquired red cell aplasia is associated with a mediastinal thymoma in half of the cases.** Serum antibodies with specificity for the erythroid precursor cells have been identified in half of the cases. Surgical removal of the thymoma, however, results in remission of the acquired pure red cell aplasia in only one-quarter of the cases.

Anemia of Chronic Renal Disease

A mild normocytic, normochromic anemia is commonly observed in association with chronic renal disease. The severity of the anemia is proportional to the degree of the uremia. The causes of the anemia in chronic renal disease reflect both a decreased rate of erythrocyte production and an accelerated peripheral loss of erythrocytes. Decreased bone marrow production of erythrocytes results from decreased production of erythropoietin by the damaged kidneys and from the suppression of marrow erythroid precursors by unidentified factors in the uremic serum. Blood loss due to gastrointestinal or gynecologic hemorrhage occurs in one-third to one-half of cases of chronic renal failure and may result in iron deficiency. The bleeding tendency is due to qualitative defects in platelet function or to abnormalities in vascular integrity that occur in uremia. The erythrocyte life span is also decreased, but the mechanism of hemolysis is incompletely understood. Finally, deficiencies in folic acid and iron may occur because of loss during hemodialysis. In chronic renal disease erythrocytes with regularly scalloped margins (burr cells) are characteristic.

Congenital Dyserythropoietic Anemias

The congenital dyserythropoietic anemias (CDA) are a group of rare, hereditary, refractory anemias. The pathogenesis of these anemias includes both ineffective erythropoiesis (increased intramedullary destruction of maturing erythroid cells) and dyserythropoiesis (abnormalities in differentiation and maturation). The erythroid cells exhibit abnormal morphologic features. Usually there is marked anisocytosis (variation in cell size) and poikilocytosis (variation in cell shape). Bizarre multinucleated erythrocytes may be identified. There are three types of CDA, the most common being type II, which is distinctive because the abnormal red cells may be lysed in sera at an acid pH. A common complication in the CDA is iron overload in tissues (hemosiderosis) caused by repeated transfusions.

Vitamin B₁₂ Deficiency (Megaloblastic Anemia)

The megaloblastic anemias are due to deficiency of either vitamin B_{12} or folic acid. Both types are characterized by abnormal DNA synthesis. In vitamin B_{12} deficiency the abnormal DNA synthesis is due to a coenzyme deficiency with consequent impaired conversion of deoxyuridylate (dUMP) to deoxythymidylate (dTMP). This results in a delay in nuclear maturation and an abnormality in cell division. The mitotic abnormality is particularly expressed in such rapidly dividing cells as erythroid, granulocytic, and megakaryocytic precursor cells. Because of the delay in nuclear maturation, the nuclear chromatin is loose rather than condensed, an abnormality that persists even in the more mature precursor cells. **In vitamin B_{12} and folic acid deficiency, the abnormal and delayed cell division results in a population of unusually large precursor cells, a distinctive morphologic alteration called megaloblastosis** (Fig. 20-9). Because of the abnormal cell maturation and division, there is ineffective hematopoiesis, with markedly increased intramedullary destruction of hematopoietic precursor cells. **Therefore, pancytopenia is characteristic of the megaloblastic anemias.**

In vitamin B_{12} deficiency the bone marrow is usually markedly hypercellular, and there is an increase in blast cells with dense, purple cytoplasm. The maturing erythroid cells exhibit loose chromatin, but cytoplasmic maturation is normal. In the granulocytic cell series, giant metamyelocytes and band neutrophils are present. The megakaryocytes exhibit nuclear hypersegmentation, with widely separated, or "exploded," nuclear lobes.

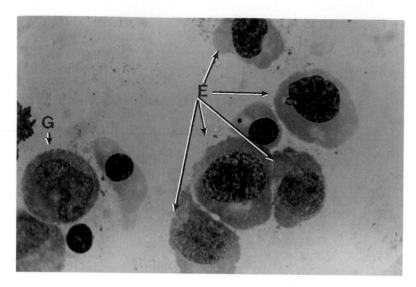

Figure 20-9. Bone marrow in megaloblastic anemia. Maturing erythroid *(E)* and granulocytic *(G)* precursor cells are large, and the chromatin is loose.

In the peripheral blood, large erythrocytes with an oval shape, called oval macrocytes, are identified. There is prominent poikilocytosis. Teardrop shaped erythrocytes are characteristic, and multilobed neutrophils, with five or more nuclear lobes, are seen. **This nuclear hypersegmentation of polymorphonuclear neutrophils is the first morphologic abnormality to appear in megaloblastic anemia and the last to disappear.** Characteristically, thrombocytopenia is accompanied by large platelets (megathrombocytes). Common laboratory findings include a decreased reticulocyte count because of the ineffective erythropoiesis and a decrease in the release of mature erythrocytes to the peripheral blood. LDH isoenzymes 1 and 2 are elevated because of ineffective erythropoiesis and hemolysis. Ineffective granulocytopoiesis leads to increased serum and urinary lysozyme.

Vitamin B_{12} is synthesized only by certain microorganisms. All animals depend ultimately on this microbiologic synthesis of the enzyme. Sources of vitamin B_{12} in the human diet include foods of animal origin, such as meat, seafood, liver, milk, and eggs.

The causes of B_{12} deficiency include dietary deficiency, defective absorption, increased requirements, and impaired utilization. Dietary deficiency is an exceedingly rare cause of B_{12} deficiency except in strict vegans—that is, persons who eat no food of animal origin, even milk and eggs. **Defective absorption in the gastrointestinal tract is the most common cause of B_{12} deficiency.** Absorption of vitamin B_{12} requires the initial complexing of B_{12} with intrinsic factor (IF), which is produced in the parietal cells of the gastric mucosa, and the presence of IF-B_{12} receptors in the mucosa of the terminal ileum (Fig. 20-10). **Defective absorption of vitamin B_{12} occurs in classic or addi-**sonian pernicious anemia because intrinsic factor is not produced by the gastric parietal cells. There is also a lack of secretion of gastric juice, gastric acid, and pepsin. This generalized deficiency of secretory function reflects an atrophy of the gastric mucosa, which is believed to be immunologically mediated. Antibodies to intrinsic factor are found in half of cases of pernicious anemia. Other autoantibodies, such as antiparietal cell and antithyroid antibodies, are also frequently identified. Vitamin B_{12} absorption also may be impaired in the postgastrectomy state and in a variety of disorders of the small bowel, such as regional enteritis and malignant lymphoma. In juvenile pernicious anemia, there is a congenital absence of intrinsic factor secretion in conjunction with normal gastric acid and gastric juice secretion. A deficiency of vitamin B_{12} may also result from competitive utilization within the small intestine. For example, deficiency may occur with infestation by the fish tapeworm diphyllobothrium latum or because of bacterial colonization in small intestinal blind loops or in diverticula. A rare cause of vitamin B_{12} deficiency is an increased requirement for the enzyme, such as occurs with certain metastatic tumors. In rare cases impaired utilization results from the lack of vitamin B_{12}-binding protein (transcobalamin II).

Because the daily requirement for vitamin B_{12} is only 1 μg and the total body stores are approximately 2 mg to 5 mg, it usually requires years for megaloblastic anemia to develop. Classic or addisonian pernicious anemia occurs most commonly in adults 40 to 80 years of age. Northern Europeans with a fair complexion are most commonly affected. In any vitamin B_{12} deficiency, a moderate to severe anemia is characteristic. A red, beefy tongue is common.

Combined system disease is a serious complication. Demyelination of the posterolateral columns of the spinal cord leads to peripheral neuropathy, spasticity, and ataxia. The pathogenesis of this demyelination is poorly understood. Personality changes, which may progress to "megaloblastic madness," may be observed.

Folic Acid Deficiency (Megaloblastic Anemia)

Folic acid deficiency is associated with a megaloblastic anemia that is similar to that caused by vitamin B$_{12}$ deficiency; however, the neurologic dis-

order of B$_{12}$ deficiency, combined system disease, is not observed in folic acid deficiency. In vitamin B$_{12}$ deficiency, administration of folic acid improves the hematologic status, but it does not halt the progression of the neurologic disorder. In megaloblastic anemia, therefore, a vitamin B$_{12}$ deficiency must first be excluded before folic acid is administered.

Folic acid functions as a coenzyme in a variety of one-carbon transfer reactions, acting either as a donor or as an acceptor. The consequence of folic acid deficiency is abnormal DNA synthesis. In the catabolism of histidine to glutamic acid, a deficiency of folic acid results in the accumulation of an intermediary product, formimino glutamic acid (FIGlu), which is excreted in the urine. The laboratory diagnosis of folic

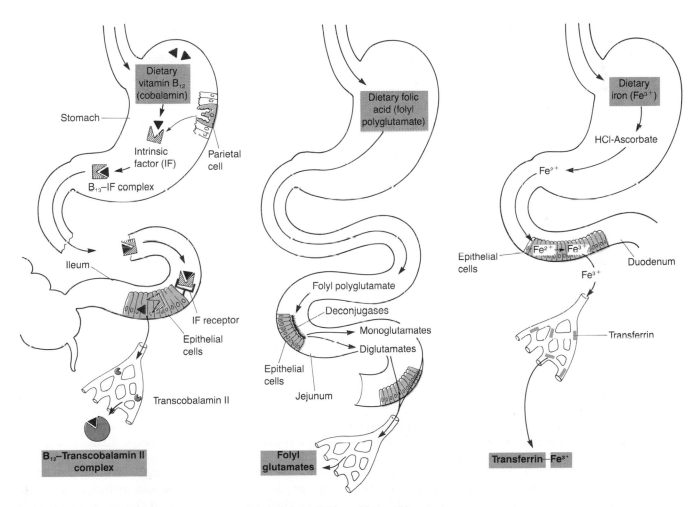

Figure 20-10. Absorption of vitamin B$_{12}$, folic acid, and iron. Absorption of vitamin B$_{12}$ requires initial complexing with intrinsic factor (IF), which is produced by the parietal cells of the gastric mucosa. Absorption then occurs in the terminal ileum where there are receptors for the IF-B$_{12}$ complex. Dietary folic acid is conjugated to polyglutamate. Absorption occurs in the jejunum following deconjugation in the intestinal lumen. Dietary ferric iron is reduced to ferrous iron in the stomach and absorbed principally in the duodenum.

acid deficiency is made by the demonstration of decreased levels of serum folic acid and is supported by the finding of increased urinary excretion of FIGlu after administration of a loading dose of histidine.

The principal sources of dietary folic acid are leafy vegetables, eggs, and meat products. Folic acid is heat labile, water soluble, and easily destroyed by extensive cooking. Dietary folic acid is conjugated to polyglutamate. Following deconjugation in the intestinal lumen, absorption of folic acid occurs in the jejunum (see Fig. 20-10).

The minimal daily requirement for folic acid is about 50 µg. Since total body stores are 2 mg to 5 mg, it takes 4 to 5 months for folic acid deficiency and megaloblastic anemia to develop. Deficient intake of folic acid is seen with **alcoholism**, in which a poor nutritional status is common; impaired intestinal absorption, such as occurs with **nontropical or tropical sprue;** administration of certain anticonvulsant drugs, such as **dilantin,** which impair the intestinal deconjugation of polyglutamate forms of folic acid; conditions associated with increased requirements for folic acid, such as **pregnancy** or the hyperactive hematopoiesis that occurs in **chronic hemolysis;** and impaired utilization, such as after treatment with **antineoplastic folic acid antagonists.**

Iron Deficiency

Iron, which is utilized principally in the production of hemoglobin, also functions as a cofactor with a variety of intracellular enzymes. An adequate dietary source provides approximately 20 mg of iron daily, of which 1 mg to 2 mg is absorbed, principally in the duodenum (see Fig. 20-10). The absorbed iron is equivalent to the 1 mg to 2 mg of iron that is lost daily in the desquamation of cells from the skin and gastrointestinal and genitourinary tracts.

Iron deficiency is the most common medical disorder worldwide. The causes of iron deficiency include inadequate dietary sources of iron, impaired intestinal absorption of iron, loss of iron due to hemorrhage or to intravascular hemolysis, and diversion of iron to the fetus during pregnancy and lactation. Dietary intake of iron is frequently inadequate in infants and in young children on unsupplemented iron-poor milk diets. Impaired iron absorption may occur in persons who have undergone surgical resection of portions of the upper gastrointestinal tract or who have a malabsorption syndrome. **Loss in the gastrointestinal tract is the most common cause of iron deficiency in the adult male and postmenopausal female. In women of reproductive age, iron de-**

ficiency usually is caused by loss in menses or during pregnancy. Iron is lost in the urine as hemosiderin in paroxysmal nocturnal hemoglobinuria and in traumatic or immunologically mediated intravascular hemolysis. Hemosiderinuria is detected by performance of the Prussian blue stain on a concentrated urine sediment.

In iron-deficiency anemia, **the bone marrow examination reveals a severe decrease in or absence of hemosiderin in macrophages and an absence of ferritin in developing normoblasts.** The normoblasts frequently have poorly hemoglobinized, or "ragged," cytoplasm. Hypochromic microcytic erythrocytes are seen on the peripheral blood smear. When the deficiency is severe, anisocytosis and poikilocytosis are prominent. The common laboratory findings include a decreased serum iron level and an increased total iron binding capacity, the latter being a quantitative measure of the transferrin level. Iron saturation, the proportion of transferrin bound to iron, is generally less than 10%, the normal value being about 30%. The serum ferritin level, which reflects total body iron stores, is decreased.

In iron-deficiency anemia, signs and symptoms are referable to the causal anatomic lesion, if any, such as a bleeding gastric ulcer; the anemia; and abnormal cellular function. Abnormal cellular function caused by a decrease in intracellular iron-containing enzymes is commonly expressed as epithelial changes, such as atrophic glossitis, angular stomatitis and, rarely, koilonychia (spoon-shaped fingernails). Pica, the craving to eat unusual substances, occurs in severe iron-deficiency anemia.

The Thalassemia Syndromes

The thalassemia syndromes are a heterogeneous group of genetic disorders that have in common a selective depression or absent synthesis of either the alpha (α) or the beta (β) chains of the normal hemoglobin A tetramer ($\alpha_2 \beta_2$). The specific thalassemia syndromes are defined by the globin chain affected. In the β-thalassemias, synthesis of the β-chain is defective, while in the α-thalassemias, there is an abnormal synthesis of the α-chain. **The pathophysiology of the thalassemias relates principally to the accumulation of excess globin chains, which precipitate and cause membrane damage. Ineffective erythropoiesis and chronic hemolysis result.** The severity of the anemia reflects both the erythroid cell destruction and the decreased erythrocyte hemoglobin content.

In the β-thalassemias, there may be either decreased (β^+) or absent (β°) synthesis of the β-chain. The genetic defects in β-thalassemia are heterogeneous but commonly relate to defective processing of messenger RNA. Heterozygous β-thalassemia (β-thalassemia minor) is the most common disorder. One β-globin gene is normal, but the second β-globin gene exhibits a variably impaired β-globin production. There is usually mild anemia. In the peripheral blood mild hypochromia, microcytosis, basophilic stippling of erythrocytes, and target cells are observed. The spleen is moderately enlarged. Hemoglobin A_1 ($\alpha_2\beta_2$) is slightly decreased, hemoglobin F ($\alpha_2\gamma_2$) is normal, and hemoglobin A_2 ($\alpha_2\delta_2$) is slightly increased (4–8%). Beta-thalassemia minor must be distinguished from iron-deficiency anemia. Iron should not be administered in β-thalassemia minor because it may cause iron overload.

Homozygous β-thalassemia (Cooley's anemia) is caused by a severe reduction in or absence of β-chain production. Hemoglobin electrophoresis reveals principally fetal hemoglobin ($\alpha_2\gamma_2$). Hemoglobin A_2 ($\alpha_2\delta_2$) is normal to moderately elevated. Splenomegaly and hepatomegaly reflect the massive sequestration and destruction of the damaged erythrocytes. There may be enlargement and distortion of facial and cranial bones because of the severe bone marrow erythroid hyperplasia. Pigment gallstones develop even in childhood because of chronic hemolysis and resulting hyperbilirubinemia. The peripheral blood erythrocytes are hypochromic and microcytic and show marked anisocytosis and poikilocytosis. Circulating nucleated red cells may be observed.

Alpha-thalassemias result from impaired α-chain synthesis. The defect appears to be a deletion of from one to all four α-globin genes found on the pair of chromosomes 16. Excess γ- and β-chains precipitate as hemoglobin Barts (γ_4) *in utero* and during the neonatal period and as hemoglobin H (β_4) in childhood and in adult life. A minor component of hemoglobin delta (δ_4) may be identified. The hemoglobin Barts, hemoglobin H, and δ-tetramers are more soluble and less toxic than the precipitated α-chains in the β-thalassemia syndromes. Red cell destruction is consequently generally less severe. However, the oxygen affinity of the tetramers is high, and the erythrocytes function poorly in the delivery of oxygen.

The clinical severity of the α-thalassemias reflects the number of α-genes deleted. In the silent carrier state, in which there is a deletion of one gene, the hematologic parameters are normal, and in infants up to 1% to 2% of the hemoglobin is hemoglobin Barts. In α-thalassemia trait, in which two genes are deleted, there is a mild hemolytic anemia and in infants up to 5% of the hemoglobin is hemoglobin Barts. In hemoglobin H disease, in which three genes are deleted, there is a moderate hemolytic anemia and hypochromia and microcytosis of erythrocytes; in the first year of life up to 25% hemoglobin Barts is identified. In adults the major hemoglobin is hemoglobin A, but a minor component of hemoglobin H is also found. If all four α-chains are deleted, death occurs either *in utero* or at the time of delivery. The predominance of the high-affinity hemoglobin Barts produces a severe impairment of oxygen delivery. There is massive hepatosplenomegaly as a result of compensatory extramedullary hematopoiesis, and generalized edema (hydrops fetalis) reflects severe heart failure.

Anemia of Chronic Disease

Mild to moderate anemia, with a hemoglobin of 9 g/dl to 10 g/dl, is common in infectious, inflammatory, and neoplastic disorders. The anemia, which is either normochromic or hypochromic, is caused by a slightly shortened erythrocyte life span, impaired release of storage iron from macrophages, an inadequate response of bone marrow erythroid precursors to erythropoietin, and inadequate elevation of erythropoietin in response to the anemia. Serum iron levels and total iron binding capacity are decreased, and iron saturation tends to be low (15–20%). Storage iron in bone marrow macrophages is increased, whereas sideroblast iron in developing erythroid cells is decreased.

Sideroblastic Anemia

Sideroblastic anemia is a disorder in which damage to the mitochondria of maturing erythroid cells produces a distinctive morphologic abnormality, the ringed sideroblast. There is an associated mild to moderate anemia because of the premature destruction of abnormally maturing erythroid cells in the bone marrow.

In the mitochondria of normally developing erythroblasts, iron is inserted into protoporphyrin to form heme. In the cytosol, heme then combines with globin to form hemoglobin. When heme production is impaired, iron in the form of ferritin accumulates in the mitochondria, causing damage to and even rupture of these organelles. In the developing normoblast, the mitochondria are situated in a perinuclear location. In sideroblastic anemia, the Prussian blue stain demonstrates the iron-laden mitochondria as a granular blue ring that encircles the cell nucleus.

This abnormal erythroid precursor cell is called the ringed sideroblast.

Sideroblastic anemia may occur as a hereditary disorder; as a secondary finding in a variety of hematologic, inflammatory, and neoplastic diseases; as a result of exposure to bone marrow toxins; and as an idiopathic acquired disorder. Hereditary sideroblastic anemia is rare and most commonly an X-linked recessive trait. As a result, young males are most commonly affected. Secondary ringed sideroblastic anemia occurs usually in adults in association with a variety of hemolytic anemias, hematologic and nonhematologic malignancies, and inflammatory conditions. Sideroblastic anemia has also been observed after the administration of antituberculous drugs and the antibiotic chloramphenicol. Marrow toxins such as alcohol and lead may be associated with sideroblastic anemia.

Idiopathic acquired sideroblastic anemia is seen in middle-aged and elderly people of either gender. About 10% of cases are associated with the subsequent development of acute nonlymphocytic leukemia. Therefore, idiopathic acquired sideroblastic anemia is included in the category of myelodysplastic syndromes. Bone marrow examination reveals erythroid hyperplasia with ringed sideroblasts. Occasionally there is a megaloblastic change, but serum B_{12} and folate levels are normal. In the peripheral blood there is a dimorphic population of microcytic hypochromic and normal erythrocytes.

Myelophthisic Anemias

The myelophthisic anemias are a consequence of bone marrow infiltrative disorders, most frequently metastatic carcinoma or malignant lymphoma. Leukemia, myelofibrosis, multiple myeloma, granulomatous inflammation, osteopetrosis, and lipid storage diseases also cause myelophthisic anemia. The pathogenesis of the myelophthisic anemia involves damage to the normal hematopoietic microarchitecture. Because of disruption of the sinus endothelial cells, hematopoietic precursor cells are released prematurely. On the peripheral blood smear the erythrocytes display prominent anisocytosis and poikilocytosis. Teardrop-shaped erythrocytes are numerous. There may be leukoerythroblastosis, with circulating immature granulocytes, erythroid cells, and giant platelets. Commonly there is a mild to moderate normocytic normochromic anemia. The diagnosis of a myelophthisic anemia is made by bone marrow biopsy. The course and prognosis are determined by the type of marrow infiltrative disorder.

Acute Blood Loss Anemia

In acute hemorrhage with consequent anemia, the clinical manifestations reflect both the rapidity and the volume of the blood loss. Following an acute hemorrhage, fluid shifts from the interstitial to the intravascular compartments in order to maintain the blood volume. This fluid shift accentuates the acute anemia due to hemorrhage because of a dilutional effect. The serum erythropoietin level rapidly increases and stimulates the pool of erythroid precursors. Since maturation and release of erythroid cells requires 2 to 5 days, the fluid shift and subsequent dilution cause the hemoglobin level to reach a nadir in 2 to 3 days. Thereafter, depending on the adequacy of the body iron stores, a gradual restoration of the red blood cell mass occurs. When bleeding occurs internally, such as into the body cavities, iron is recaptured and reutilized in the production of red blood cells.

Chronic Blood Loss Anemia

Chronic blood loss anemia is caused by iron deficiency and occurs only after the total body iron stores are depleted. The old clinical dictum is still valid: occult blood loss in a man or a postmenopausal woman requires that the diagnosis of intestinal tumor be excluded.

Hereditary Spherocytosis

Hereditary spherocytosis is an autosomal dominant disorder characterized by a distinctive spheroidal shape of the erythrocytes and hemolytic anemia. A defect in the cell membrane cytoskeleton leads to a low surface:volume ratio and dehydration of the red blood cells. The resulting spherocytes are incapable of the deformation required to traverse the splenic red pulp cords and are selectively destroyed at that site. Splenectomy is usually curative. Phagocytosis with premature destruction of erythrocytes in splenic macrophages is conspicuous, and enlargement of the spleen is usual. Macrophages and erythrocytes expand the red pulp cords, but the splenic sinusoids appear empty. Bone marrow examination reveals a marked erythroid hyperplasia. The common laboratory findings include a moderate normocytic hyperchromic anemia and a reticulocytosis. The erythrocyte osmotic fragility is increased.

Clinically, hereditary spherocytosis is manifested as the triad of jaundice, anemia, and splenomegaly. Because of increased bile pigment metabolism, pigment gallstones form even in pediatric patients. Intercurrent infections, especially with parvovirus, induce either temporary episodes of bone marrow failure (aplastic crises) or hyperfunction of the spleen, which leads to a hemolytic crisis.

Hereditary Elliptocytosis

Hereditary elliptocytosis is an autosomal dominant disorder characterized by circulating elliptical or oval-shaped erythrocytes. The pathogenesis again relates to a cytoskeletal defect in the erythrocyte membrane. Commonly, more than 75% of circulating erythrocytes are elliptical. Hemolysis is usually mild and may be only intermittent. In 10% to 15% of cases, moderate hemolysis occurs, and the peripheral blood smear shows signs of erythrocyte fragmentation. Elliptocyte destruction occurs principally in the spleen, and splenectomy is curative.

Hereditary Stomatocytosis

Hereditary stomatocytosis is an autosomal dominant disorder in which the erythrocyte membrane displays abnormal permeability to sodium and potassium ions. The structural basis for the membrane defect has not been defined. A gain in erythrocyte sodium leads to osmotic overhydration, in which case the cells exhibit a central, slitlike pallor. These distinctive erythrocytes are called stomatocytes. A decrease in erythrocyte sodium plus potassium produces underhydration, and central pooling of hemoglobin leads to the appearance of target cells. In hereditary stomatocytosis hemolysis is moderate and only partially corrected by splenectomy.

Abetalipoproteinemia (Acanthocytosis)

Abetalipoproteinemia, an autosomal recessive disorder that presents in the first 2 years of life, reflects the absence of the B protein of β-lipoprotein. Impaired fat absorption in the intestine results in a general decrease in plasma lipid levels, with a relative increase in the red cell membrane phospholipid sphingomyelin and a decrease in lecithin. Probably because of the increased sphingomyelin content, the red blood cells exhibit increased rigidity and decreased deformability, a situation that leads to irregularly spiculated erythrocytes. These spiculated red blood cells, called **acanthocytes,** are identical to the **spur cells** seen in liver disease. The clinical features of abetalipoproteinemia include diarrhea and steator-

rhea, due to the malabsorption of fat. Occasionally there is a mild hemolysis. The nonhematologic manifestations include a variety of neuromuscular abnormalities and degenerative changes in the retina, usually with retinitis pigmentosa.

Hereditary Nonspherocytic Hemolytic Anemia (Pyruvate Kinase Deficiency)

A mild chronic hemolytic anemia frequently occurs when there is a deficiency in or a kinetic abnormality of a variety of enzymes of the Embden-Meyerhof or glycolytic pathway. These heterogeneous disorders are collectively termed **hereditary nonspherocytic hemolytic anemias.** The most common mode of inheritance is autosomal recessive. The mechanism of the hemolysis is incompletely understood, but ATP depletion may be a common pathway in producing damage to the red blood cell membrane. Typically the erythrocytes show no distinctive morphologic abnormalities, although crenated erythrocytes are seen with severe enzyme deficiency and lack of ATP. Mild chronic hemolysis, anemia, jaundice, and splenomegaly are common. There is little or no improvement with splenectomy. The most common of the hereditary nonspherocytic hemolytic anemias, **pyruvate kinase deficiency,** is unusual in that a severe hemolysis of normal red blood cells may occur when there is a severe enzyme deficiency. In pyruvate kinase deficiency, splenectomy is associated with some improvement in the hemolysis, although the reticulocyte count may paradoxically increase.

Glucose-6-Phosphate Dehydrogenase Deficiency

Glucose-6-phosphate dehydrogenase (G6PD), an enzyme of the hexose monophosphate shunt pathway, maintains glutathione in the reduced form. **When G6PD is deficient, the erythrocytes are more susceptible to oxidant stresses.** With exposure to oxidants, such as some of the antimalarial drugs, oxidized denatured hemoglobin precipitates as **Heinz bodies,** which adhere to the red cell membrane. The abnormal red cells are phagocytosed and removed in the spleen.

G6PD deficiency comprises a heterogeneous group of X-linked recessive disorders. Most G6PD deficient males do not express clinical manifestations of their genetic trait. Fifteen percent of American blacks have the abnormal enzyme G6PD A, rather than the normal enzyme G6PD B. In this population hemolysis is generally mild because G6PD levels are nearly normal in the reticulocytes. In the Mediterranean type of G6PD deficiency, a severe enzyme deficiency may lead to life-threatening hemolysis. Severe, occasionally lethal, reactions precipitated by ingestion of the fava bean may occur in this Mediterranean variant of G6PD deficiency.

Sickle Cell Disease

In sickle cell disease, a single base mutation in DNA results in the substitution of valine for glutamic acid at the sixth position of the β-globin chain of hemoglobin. As a consequence of this point mutation, **aggregation and polymerization of globin chains occur under deoxygenated conditions, with the formation of rigid filamentous structures, or "tactoids."** These "tactoids" induce a characteristic deformity of the red blood cells, the sickled, or "hollyleaf," configuration. **Irreversibly sickled erythrocytes cannot traverse the red pulp cords of the spleen, and are there destroyed. Sickled erythrocytes occlude small blood vessels in any visceral organ and produce multifocal ischemic infarctions.**

Approximately 10% of American blacks are heterozygous for the sickle cell gene. One β^S- and one β^A-chain are synthesized. Hemoglobin S constitutes 30% to 40% and hemoglobin A 60% to 70% of the total. **The associated disorder is called sickle cell trait.** In sickle cell trait the peripheral blood count and the red blood cell life span are normal. Generally, there are no symptoms. Rarely, sickling may occur in the renal medulla owing to low oxygen tension, low pH, and high osmolarity, and the result may be ischemic infarction of the papillae. Sickling is rare but may occur in the lungs of persons with sickle cell trait who have a condition of low PO_2, such as pneumonia or atelectasis, or who are at a high altitude.

In homozygous sickle cell disease, only β^S-chains are synthesized. Hemoglobin S constitutes 80% to 95% of the total hemoglobin and hemoglobins F and A_2 constitute the residual minor components. The predominance of hemoglobin S leads to both **severe chronic hemolytic anemia and vaso-occlusive disease.** Hemoglobin levels may be reduced to 5 g/dl. Vaso-occlusion of small vessels by irreversibly sickled erythrocytes causes painful infarctions in any visceral organ, the so-called **sickle cell crisis,** and repeated splenic infarctions cause progressive fibrous scarring and eventual atrophy of the spleen. Commonly, by the time the affected person has reached adulthood, the spleen is reduced to a small, functionless fibrous

nodule, a process termed **autosplenectomy.** Ulceration of the skin in the region of the ankle malleoli, which results from occlusion of small dermal and subcutaneous vessels with consequent infarction, is characteristic of sickle cell disease.

The secondary complications of sickle cell disease reflect both chronic hemolysis and the vaso-occlusive episodes. Chronic hemolysis with hyperbilirubinemia predisposes to gallstones, which form in one-third of the cases. Iron overload, which is common, leads to disease of the heart, liver, and pancreas. The lack of normal splenic function predisposes to infections, salmonella osteomyelitis and pneumococcal pneumonia being especially characteristic. Intercurrent viral infections depress normal hematopoiesis, an effect that leads to a rapid fall in the hemoglobin level, in the presence of simultaneous hemolysis. This situation, labeled the **aplastic crisis,** may also be precipitated by a concurrent folic acid deficiency. In children intercurrent infections cause splenic hyperplasia, a massive splenic pooling of erythrocytes, and a rapid fall in the hemoglobin level. This potentially lethal complication is termed the **hyperhemolytic crisis.**

If the sickle gene is inherited with another abnormal globin gene or with a thalassemia gene, the clinical picture depends on the interaction of the two abnormal genes. **Hemoglobin S-C disease,** in which there is 50% hemoglobin S and 50% hemoglobin C, is associated with a severe hemolytic anemia. Painful crises and bone infarctions are common. **Infarction of the femoral head is especially characteristic of hemoglobin S-C disease.** Hemoglobin S-D disease, in which there is 50% hemoglobin S and 50% hemoglobin D, is asymptomatic, because the molecular interaction of hemoglobin D with hemoglobin S prevents the sickling of erythrocytes. The clinical features of hemoglobin S--thalassemia disease are variable, depending on the amounts of hemoglobins A and F, which protect from hemolysis. Hemoglobin S--thalassemia is usually a mild hemolytic disorder.

Hemoglobin C Disease

Hemoglobin C disease is an inherited hemoglobinopathy, due to a single base mutation in DNA, that results in the substitution of lysine for glutamic acid at the sixth position of the hemoglobin B globin chain. In homozygous hemoglobin C disease (hemoglobin C-C) the erythrocytes are dehydrated and rigid. They are susceptible to phagocytosis and removal in the spleen and, to a lesser extent, to fragmentation in the circulation. A mild anemia is characteristic. Enlargement of the spleen reflects the intrasplenic destruction of the abnormal erythrocytes. Although the hemolysis is mild, erythroid hyperplasia in the bone marrow does not maintain normal hemoglobin levels. A decreased oxygen affinity of erythrocytes in hemoglobin C disease increases the delivery of oxygen to the tissues, so that full compensation of hemoglobin levels is not necessary. **In homozygous hemoglobin C disease, prominent target cells are characteristic.** Occasionally, intraerythrocytic rhomboid hemoglobin C crystals are identified. Hemoglobin C trait (hemoglobin A-C) is an asymptomatic disorder. The red cell life span is normal.

Unstable Hemoglobins

Certain globin-chain amino acid substitutions or deletions affect the stability of hemoglobin. Amino acid substitutions involving the heme pocket of globin are particularly likely to induce instability. In some, such as **hemoglobin Köln,** heme tends to "fall out" of the heme pocket and is lost to the cell, and the globin becomes denatured. The abnormal, precipitated globin molecules adhere to the erythrocyte cell membrane as Heinz bodies, which are removed (pitted) from erythrocytes in the splenic red pulp. Mild chronic hemolysis, with splenomegaly and jaundice, is common. In a minority of cases there is a severe chronic hemolysis, or there are hemolytic episodes precipitated by oxidant drugs or by infections.

Hemoglobins with Abnormal Oxygen Affinity

Hemoglobins with amino acid substitutions at certain contact points between the globin chains may demonstrate an abnormally high affinity for the oxygen molecule. As a consequence these hemoglobins release oxygen poorly to the tissues, an effect that leads to tissue hypoxia. In turn, erythropoietin production, the hemoglobin level, and the red blood cell count are all augmented. The clinical disorder associated with high-oxygen-affinity hemoglobins is usually benign, although symptoms referable to the increased red cell mass may develop. **High-oxygen-affinity hemoglobins should be included in the differential diagnosis of erythrocytosis or polycythemia.**

Hemoglobins that have a low oxygen affinity release oxygen readily to the tissues, thereby leading to decreased erythropoietin production and a mild anemia. Cyanosis is visible because of the low hemoglobin oxygen saturation.

Hereditary Methemoglobinemia

In hereditary methemoglobinemia there is a substitution of tyrosine for one of the two histidines that bind to ferrous heme in the heme pocket of hemoglobin. This substitution predisposes to accelerated electron transfer, thus converting ferrous to ferric iron. Ferric iron combines with tyrosine to form an iron-phenolate complex, which prevents the reduction of ferric to ferrous iron. The consequence is markedly increased methemoglobin or hemoglobin with an oxidized heme moiety. Other than a striking cyanosis, there is no clinical disability.

Paroxysmal Nocturnal Hemoglobinuria

Paroxysmal nocturnal hemoglobinuria (PNH) is an acquired disorder of the common hematopoietic precursor cell. In PNH the erythrocytes, granulocytes, and platelets demonstrate an inordinate sensitivity to complement-mediated lysis. The disorder probably results from a defect in the clearance of complement from the cell membrane, owing to an absence of a decay-accelerating factor. The abnormal PNH cell clone frequently occurs in conjunction with a damaged bone marrow. The abnormality in the erythroid cell series is expressed either as intermittent episodes of acute hemolysis or as chronic hemolysis. The acute hemolytic episodes occur at night and are recognized by the passage of brown urine in the morning. Iron deficiency may result from the loss of hemoglobin. Because of complement-mediated platelet lysis, thrombocytopenia and secondary hemorrhages are complications. Venous thromboses, occasionally involving the hepatic veins (Budd-Chiari syndrome), are characteristic of PNH. This predisposition to thrombosis may reflect complement-mediated activation of platelets. Alternatively, ADP, which is released from damaged erythrocytes, may activate the circulating platelets.

Useful screening tests for PNH include the sucrose hemolysis test, which demonstrates an increased sensitivity of PNH erythrocytes to osmotic lysis, and the demonstration of hemosiderin pigment in the urine. The acid hemolysis (Ham) test is confirmatory for PNH. Most individuals affected by PNH ultimately succumb to a complication of the disorder. Rarely, death is due to superimposed acute nonlymphocytic leukemia or to aplastic anemia.

Warm-Antibody Autoimmune Hemolytic Anemia

Autoimmune hemolytic anemia is a heterogeneous group of disorders in which a shortened red cell survival is caused by an immune response against the autologous red blood cells. A positive Coombs' test confirms the presence of immunoglobulins on the erythrocyte membrane. Complement components are also identified on erythrocytes by the appropriate Coombs' reagents. **Warm-antibody autoimmune hemolytic anemia results from the production of antibodies, usually of the IgG class, which have maximum reactivity at 37°C** and which frequently exhibit specificity for Rh blood group determinants. **Warm antibodies cause 80% to 90% of cases of autoimmune hemolytic anemia.** Hemolysis occurs because of the coating of erythrocytes with anti-Rh antibody and complement components. Splenic macrophages have surface membrane receptors for the Fc portion of IgG and for the complement component C3b, and they therefore remove portions of the erythrocyte membrane. The result is the formation of spherocytes, which are ultimately destroyed by splenic macrophages.

Warm-antibody autoimmune hemolytic anemia occurs either as an idiopathic disorder or as a secondary disease in association with a variety of malignant or benign conditions. The lymphocytic lymphomas and chronic lymphocytic leukemia account for approximately half of all cases of secondary autoimmune hemolytic anemia. Secondary warm-antibody autoimmune hemolytic anemia may also occur in association with collagen vascular diseases (particularly systemic lupus erythematosus), viral infections, some solid tumors (e.g., carcinoma of the ovary), and certain inflammatory disorders (e.g., ulcerative colitis). The clinical course in warm-antibody autoimmune hemolytic anemia is intermittent and unpredictable. Anemia and jaundice are common clinical features. The usual causes of death are thromboembolic episodes, infections, and severe anemia. The prognosis in secondary autoimmune hemolytic anemia reflects the course of the associated disorder.

Cold-Antibody Autoimmune Hemolytic Anemia

Cold antibodies have maximal reactivity below 37°C and especially below 31°C. They usually are of the IgM class and generally have specificity for the I/i antigen complex. When blood is pooled in the extremities, IgM antibody fixes C3 to the erythrocyte membrane. Since IgM usually subsequently dissociates at 37°, only complement components are identified on the erythrocyte surface membranes by the appropriate Coombs' reagents. These complement-coated red blood cells are removed principally by hepatic Kupffer cells. This extravascular hemolysis may be associated with a mild chronic anemia.

Cold antibodies cause 10% to 20% of cases of autoimmune hemolytic anemia. This type of hemolytic anemia occurs as an idiopathic chronic disorder in elderly persons in whom features of a malignant lymphoma subsequently develop and as a secondary condition in young persons who have acute infections, such as mycoplasmal pneumonia or infectious mononucleosis.

Paroxysmal Cold Hemoglobinuria

In paroxysmal cold hemoglobinuria an IgG antibody with anti-P blood group specificity is induced during the course of certain infections. Historically, the disorder was associated with **syphilis,** and the antibody was called the **Donath-Landsteiner antibody.** Today, **paroxysmal cold hemoglobinuria usually follows a viral infection.** The IgG antibody fixes complement during exposure to the cold in the peripheral tissues. On rewarming, complement-induced lysis of erythrocytes takes place. The hemolysis in paroxysmal cold hemoglobinuria is generally self-limited and usually disappears after resolution of the precipitating infection. An idiopathic variant of cold hemoglobinuria, which is not associated with an infection, pursues a prolonged, but benign, course.

Drug-Mediated Immunologic Injury of Erythrocytes

Many drugs have been implicated in the production of immunologic injury of erythrocytes. There are three principal mechanisms of drug-mediated immunologic injury of erythrocytes: autoantibody induction, immune complex formation, and the hapten mechanism. In autoantibody induction a drug induces the formation of an autoantibody against a blood group determinant. The principal offender is the antihypertensive drug α-methyldopa. In 10% of those who take this medication the drug induces an IgG autoantibody directed against Rh blood group determinants, and in approximately 1% overt hemolytic anemia occurs. In the immune complex mechanism, a drug initially binds to a serum antibody, and the drug-antibody complex then reversibly binds to the erythrocyte. The erythrocyte is then destroyed by complement-mediated lysis. An example of this mechanism occurs with the anti-arrhythmic agent quinidine, which binds to an IgM antibody and forms quinidine-IgM complexes, which in turn bind to erythrocytes. In the hapten mechanism, a drug binds to an erythrocyte membrane protein, forming first a hapten. A serum antibody is then produced with specificity for this protein-drug complex. An example is the binding of penicillin to an erythrocyte membrane protein.

Drug-mediated immunologic destruction of erythrocytes is usually a benign process, with a good prognosis. In the hapten and autoantibody mechanism of drug-mediated immunologic injury of erythrocytes, a mild to moderate hemolysis is usually observed. However, severe hemolysis may occur in immune complex–mediated injury of erythrocytes.

Traumatic Cardiac Hemolytic Anemia

Shear-stress forces on circulating erythrocytes due to cardiac prostheses are associated with traumatic rupture of the red blood cell membrane and hemolytic anemia. Plastic prosthetic aortic valves are most commonly implicated. **Schistocytes** are commonly identified on the peripheral blood smear.

March Hemoglobinuria

March hemoglobinuria follows certain types of vigorous exercise, particularly walking long distances or running. Traumatic disruption of erythrocytes leads to hemoglobinemia and hemoglobinuria. The hemolysis is transitory, and recovery is usually complete.

Microangiopathic Hemolytic Anemia

A variety of disorders of the microvasculature are associated with intravascular fragmentation of erythrocytes, a condition termed **microangiopathic hemolytic anemia.** Disseminated intravascular coagulation plays a major role in the pathogenesis of most microvascular fragmentation syndromes.

Hypersplenism

Hypersplenism is defined as an increased functional activity of the mononuclear phagocytes of the spleen with increased sequestration and destruction of the peripheral elements of the blood. Variable anemia, leukopenia, and thrombocytopenia are noted. Because of the splenic hyperfunction, a bone marrow compensatory hyperplasia is common. Although the

Table 20-13 Alcohol-Induced Hematologic Abnormalities

Abnormalities of Erythrocytes

Hypoproliferative anemia
  Iron deficiency
  Folic acid deficiency
  Direct toxic effect on marrow normoblasts
    Vacuolated normoblasts
    Ringed sideroblasts
Acute blood loss anemia
  Esophageal varices
  Alcoholic gastritis
  Peptic ulcer
Hemolytic anemia
  Spur cell anemia
  Hypersplenism

Abnormalities of Leukocytes

Direct toxic effect
  Neutropenia
Functional defects of neutrophils

Abnormalities of Platelets

Thrombocytopenia
  Hypersplenism
  Folic acid deficiency
  Direct toxic effect on megakaryocytes

Abnormalities of Coagulation

Decreased hepatic synthesis of coagulation factors

increase in splenic phagocyte activity usually correlates with the increase in the size of the spleen, for poorly understood reasons hypersplenism is observed only in a minority of cases of splenomegaly.

Alcohol-Induced Anemia

Chronic alcohol abuse may be associated with abnormalities of the erythrocytes, leukocytes, and platelets. Blood coagulation may also be abnormal because of effects on both platelets and, when liver disease is present, the plasma protein coagulation factors. Cytoplasmic vacuolization of the bone marrow normoblasts due to the toxic effect of alcohol is a characteristic morphologic finding. The hematologic effects of alcohol are outlined in Table 20-13.

Erythrocytosis (Polycythemia)

Relative erythrocytosis is defined as an increase in the hemoglobin level consequent on a decrease in the plasma volume. The total red blood cell mass, as determined by ^{51}Cr labeling, is normal. The decreased plasma volume generally reflects fluid loss due to a variety of causes, such as water deprivation, diarrhea, diuresis, and extensive third-degree burns.

Relative erythrocytosis also occurs in an obscure and rare disorder called stress or "spurious" polycythemia **(Gaisbock's syndrome)**. Stress polycythemia afflicts obese, hypertensive, middle-aged men who are usually heavy smokers and who exhibit a decreased plasma volume. The mechanism is not understood.

Secondary erythrocytosis (polycythemia) refers to a true increase in the red blood cell mass, owing either to (1) appropriate increased production of erythropoietin, because of tissue hypoxia or increased production of androgens, or to (2) inappropriate erythropoietin production in the absence of tissue hypoxia or increased androgens. In the first category **(appropriate increased erythropoietin production)** are included arterial hypoxemia related to high-altitude low PO_2, pulmonary disease with impaired gas exchange, and cardiac disease with right-to-left shunts, as well as a variety of abnormal hemoglobins with high oxygen affinity that release oxygen poorly to the tissues. Tissue hypoxia then stimulates erythropoietin production. Increased androgen production in Cushing's disease or in the adrenogenital syndrome may cause increased erythropoietin production.

Inappropriate secondary erythrocytosis reflects secretion of erythropoietin in the absence of tissue hypoxia. Renal lesions such as cysts or hydronephrosis produce localized renal hypoxia by a pressure effect and consequently cause enhanced erythropoietin production. Erythrocytosis may occur in association with a variety of tumors, probably because of aberrant production of erythropoietin by tumor cells. Such erythropoietin-producing tumors include renal cell carcinoma, cerebellar hemangioblastoma, uterine leiomyomas, primary hepatocellular carcinoma, and adrenal adenomas. In inappropriate secondary erythrocytosis, correction of the renal abnormality or excision of the primary tumor generally results in a prompt return of the red blood cell mass to normal levels.

Benign Disorders of Polymorphonuclear Leukocytes

The polymorphonuclear leukocytes are a heterogeneous population of cells with distinctive morphologic features and cellular functions. They are called the polymorphonuclear leukocytes because of the complexity of their nuclear morphology. Three subtypes are defined by the staining of specific cytoplasmic granules: **the polymorphonuclear neutrophil, eosinophil,** and **basophil.** In adults, the polymorphonuclear neutrophil is the predominant leukocyte in the peripheral blood. Criteria for the adult white blood cell count are outlined in Table 20-9. In prepubertal children the lymphocyte is the predominant leukocyte in the peripheral blood.

The neutrophilic polymorphonuclear leukocyte, or neutrophil, is a phagocytic cell that is an important component of the first line of defense against a variety of invading microorganisms. Neutrophil cell kinetics are complex, and there is no sensitive indicator of bone marrow neutrophil production that is comparable to the erythroid reticulocyte. There is a large bone marrow neutrophil reserve, or storage pool, that is released by substances such as bacterial endotoxin or corticosteroids. There is also a peripheral blood pool of neutrophils that is marginated along the blood vessel walls and therefore not included in the total white blood cell count. The marginal pool comprises a cell population numerically equivalent to the circulating pool. The marginal pool is released to the circulating pool by epinephrine or by severe exercise. Because of this release, the white blood cell count may be increased up to twofold. **Neutrophils circulate in the peripheral blood briefly, with a half-life of only 6 hours.**

Neutrophilia

Neutrophilia is defined as an increase in the peripheral blood absolute neutrophil count to more than 7000 per microliter. Neutrophilia has many causes (Table 20-14). Kinetically, they relate to increased neutrophil mobilization from the bone marrow storage pool or the peripheral blood marginal pool; an increased bone marrow–effective granulocytopoiesis (i.e., a decreased destruction of maturing granulocyte precursor cells in the bone marrow); and an increased neutrophil survival time in the peripheral blood, owing either to immaturity of neutrophils, because of premature release from the bone marrow, or to diminished egress to the tissues.

A fleeting neutrophilia may occur within minutes because of an acute, stress-induced release of epinephrine, which transfers neutrophils from the marginal to the circulating neutrophil pools. This phenomenon is called "pseudoneutrophilia," because there is no absolute increase in the total blood granulocyte pool. **A sustained neutrophilia is caused by the release of granulocytes from the bone marrow storage pool in the presence of an acute inflammatory disorder or acute infection.**

Table 20-14 Principal Causes of Neutrophilic Leukocytosis

Infections (primarily bacterial)
Immunologic-inflammatory
   Rheumatoid arthritis
   Rheumatic fever
   Vasculitis
Tissue necrosis
   Infarction
   Trauma
   Burns
Neoplasia
Hemorrhage
Hemolysis
Metabolic disorders
   Acidosis
   Uremia
   Gout
Endocrinologic disorders
   Thyroid storm
   Glucocorticoids
Pregnancy
Toxins
Physical stimuli
   Cold
   Heat
   Stress
Emotional stress
Hereditary neutrophilia

Corticosteroids and endotoxins are also capable of mobilizing the bone marrow granulocyte storage pool. Chronic inflammation or infection, chronic blood loss, and malignant neoplasms increase effective granulocytopoiesis by augmenting the production of colony-stimulating factor neutrophil-monocyte (CSF-NM). A mild neutrophilia occurs in about 20% of women during the third trimester of pregnancy. Rare benign causes of neutrophilia include chronic idiopathic neutrophilia, in which neutrophil counts of 10,000 to 20,000 are typical, and hereditary neutrophilia. In the chronic myeloproliferative syndromes, which are malignant disorders of hematopoietic precursor cells, abnormalities in regulatory mechanisms of the bone marrow may result in chronic neutrophilia and the release of immature leukocytes to the peripheral blood.

In life-threatening infections there may be a pronounced neutrophilia, with circulating immature cells. This is termed a **leukemoid reaction,** since it may simulate the appearance of chronic leukemia. Clues to the benign, or reactive, nature of the process include the following: the cells in the peripheral blood are rarely less immature than myelocytes; leukocyte alkaline phosphatase activity is high; and neutrophils contain Döhle bodies (blue-staining cytoplasmic inclusions) and toxic granulation consisting of prominent azurophilic granules (Fig. 20-11).

Neutropenia

Neutropenia is defined as a decrease in the absolute neutrophil cell count in the peripheral blood to less than 1800 neutrophils per microliter. Neutropenia is due either to impaired bone marrow production of neutrophils or to increased peripheral destruction of neutrophils. Causes of impaired bone marrow production of neutrophils include toxic bone marrow suppression by drugs, alcohol, and irradiation; idiosyncratic reactions to drugs; aplastic anemia; ineffective granulocytopoiesis; infection; and hereditary disorders, the prototype of which is Kostmann's disease (infantile genetic agranulocytosis). The causes of excessive peripheral destruction of neutrophils include (1) antibody-mediated destruction of neutrophils—idiopathic, related to drugs, or in association with immunologic disorders such as systemic lupus erythematosus or Felty's syndrome—and (2) hypersplenism. In cyclic neutropenia, a genetic disorder with autosomal dominant inheritance, there is periodic failure of pluripotential bone marrow precursor cells, possibly owing to an abnormal bone marrow feedback mechanism. At 3-week intervals profound neutropenia, with secondary infections and fever, occurs. Cyclic neutropenia tends to become milder with time. The neutrophilic leukocyte response to a variety of stimuli may be attenuated or lost in persons with granulocytopenia induced by chemotherapy and in severely debilitated individuals, such as chronic alcoholics. In overwhelming sepsis, granulocytopoiesis may be suppressed, and neutropenia is an ominous prognostic sign. **Neutropenia is responsible for an increased susceptibility to infection,** which is proportional to the severity of the neutropenia. Infection is particularly common when the absolute neutrophil count is less than 500 per microliter.

Qualitative Disorders of Neutrophils

To provide a first line of protection against invading microorganisms, neutrophils must have normal chemotactic, phagocytic, and bactericidal capacities. Defects of each of these functions have been described.

Bactericidal function in the neutrophil is mediated predominantly by hydrogen peroxide (H_2O_2) and by the enzyme myeloperoxidase, which is delivered to cytoplasmic phagosomes by the degranulation of lysosomes. In **chronic granulomatous disease,** there is a defect in oxygen metabolism, with consequent im-

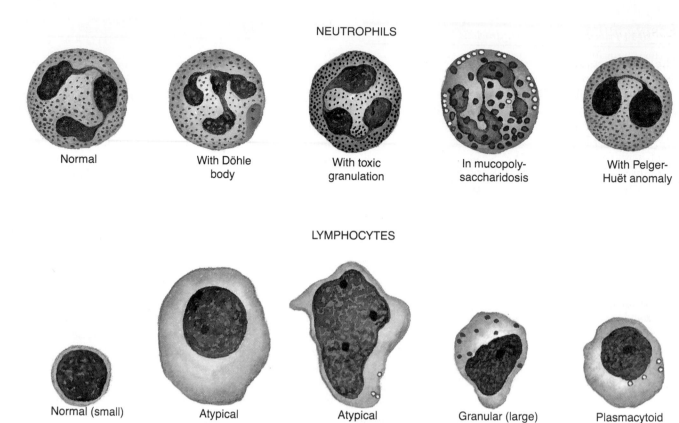

Figure 20-11. Abnormal leukocyte morphology. Abnormal neutrophils and lymphocytes are contrasted with normal cells. Döhle bodies are blue cytoplasmic inclusions that represent ribosome-associated endoplasmic reticulum. In toxic granulation there is prominent blue-black granulation in the cytoplasm. This represents persistence of prominent primary or azurophilic granules. Both Döhle bodies and toxic granulation are characteristic of benign or reactive processes. In the storage diseases or mucopolysaccharidoses, large blocklike cytoplasmic inclusions are seen. The Pelger-Huet anomaly consists of nuclear hyposegmentation, frequently with bilobed nuclei, and dense chromatin. Atypical lymphocytes are large, with deep blue to pale gray cytoplasm; they are seen in benign reactive processes. Large granular lymphocytes are medium to large lymphoid cells with some pink cytoplasmic granules. They are suppressor T-lymphocytes, some with natural killer function, and may be increased in benign or malignant disorders. Plasmacytoid lymphocytes have abundant blue cytoplasm and are seen in some reactive disorders.

paired production of bactericidal H_2O_2. As a result, bacteria multiply intracellularly. The common organisms involved in chronic granulomatous disease are *Staphylococcus aureus*, *Serratia marcescens*, and *Salmonella* species. Microscopically, both granulomatous inflammation and microabscesses, with necrosis and neutrophils, are observed.

Myeloperoxidase deficiency is an autosomal recessive disorder characterized by a lack of this bactericidal lysosomal enzyme. An unusual susceptibility to infection is not observed because a compensatory increase in intracellular hydrogen peroxide compensates for the enzyme deficiency.

The **Chediak-Higashi syndrome** is caused by a generalized defect in cell membrane formation. One consequence is impaired degranulation of neutrophils, with defective release of the lysosomal enzymes into cytoplasmic phagosomes. Giant cytoplasmic inclusions represent abnormal lysosomes in all the circulating leukocytes. Poor function of both neutrophils and lymphocytes leads to an increased susceptibility to infection.

Eosinophilia

The polymorphonuclear eosinophil differentiates in the bone marrow, subject to the inductive influence of an eosinophilopoietic factor produced by T-lymphocytes. The mature eosinophil is a distinctive cell with a bilobed nucleus and numerous large, refractile, red cytoplasmic granules. Eosinophils circulate briefly in the peripheral blood and migrate preferentially to the gastrointestinal and respiratory tracts and to the skin. Eosinophils respond to chemotactic substances produced by mast cells, including the eosinophil chemotactic factor of anaphylaxis and histamine. Because T-lymphocytes also produce eosinophilic chemotactic substances, eosinophils accumulate preferentially both in sites of mast cell degranulation and in sites of immune reactions. **Eosinophils function in the host immune defense against helminths and participate in some inflammatory reactions.** The causes of peripheral blood eosinophilia are outlined in Table 20-15.

Basophilia

The least numerous blood polymorphonuclear leukocyte, the basophil, differentiates in the bone marrow, circulates briefly in the peripheral blood, and then passes to the tissues, where its fate is uncertain. Basophils have a distinctive appearance, with abundant large, purple metachromatic granules, which frequently overlie and obscure the nucleus.

A number of cell mediators of the inflammatory response are contained in basophil granules, the most important being histamine. When contiguous IgE antibodies on the basophil plasma membrane are bridged by divalent or multivalent antigens for which the IgE antibodies have specificity, degranulation occurs, and histamine and other inflammatory media-

Table 20-15 Principal Causes of Eosinophilia

Allergic disorders
Skin diseases
Parasitic infestations
Malignant neoplasms
   Lymphoma
   Leukemia
   Myeloproliferative syndromes
   Epithelial malignancy
Collagen vascular disorders
   Polyarteritis nodosa
   Dermatomyositis
Idiopathic
   Hypereosinophilic syndromes

Table 20-16 Principal Causes of Basophilia

Allergy
Inflammation
   Juvenile rheumatoid arthritis
   Ulcerative colitis
Infection
   Viral
   Tuberculosis
Neoplasia
   Myeloproliferative syndromes
   Mastocytosis
   Basophilic leukemia
   Carcinoma
   Hodgkin's disease
Endocrinopathy
   Myxedema
   Estrogen administration

tors are released. Basophils play a prominent role, therefore, in immediate-type hypersensitivity reactions and probably also participate in certain cell-mediated hypersensitivity reactions.

The causes of basophilia are outlined in Table 20-16. A blood basophilia is most commonly observed in immediate type hypersensitivity reactions and in the chronic myeloproliferative syndromes.

Proliferative Disorders of Mast Cells

The mast cell, located in the connective tissues and probably derived from a hematopoietic precursor cell, is usually found near blood vessels. It exhibits a striking functional and some morphologic similarity to the circulating basophilic leukocyte. The mast cell is spindle-shaped or stellate and resembles the tissue histiocyte. The nucleus is round to elongate and centrally located, and the cytoplasm pink and finely granular (Fig. 20-12). The cytoplasmic granules are visualized by metachromatic stains, such as toluidine blue and Giemsa, and are positive with the chloroacetate esterase stain.

The mast cell granules contain histamine, heparin-like material, proteases, and acid hydrolases. The systemic symptoms in mast cell disease reflect degranulation of excess mast cells and include urticaria, flushing, pruritus, rhinorrhea, wheezing, headache, tachycardia, and hypotension. These symptoms are induced by histamine released from mast cells, either locally or systemically. Epistaxis and gastrointestinal bleeding result from the release of heparin-like material. Eosinophilia in peripheral blood or localized in

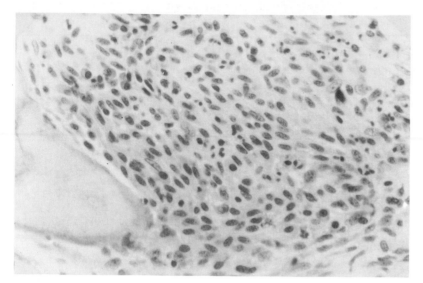

Figure 20-12. Bone marrow in mast cell disease. An infiltration of bland cells with centrally situated spindle-shaped nuclei and pale granular cytoplasm is seen.

tissue is caused by the release of eosinophilic chemotactic factor of anaphylaxis from mast cells.

Mast cell hyperplasia or reactive mastocytosis is observed both in tissues involved in hypersensitivity reactions and in lymph nodes that drain sites of malignant tumors. Infiltration of reactive mast cells is also prominent in certain lymphoproliferative disorders, in particular Waldenström's macroglobulinemia. Conspicuous mast cell hyperplasia in the bone marrow occurs in postmenopausal women with osteoporosis and in persons who have undergone antileukemic chemotherapy.

The spectrum of proliferative disorders of mast cells includes solitary mastocytoma, urticaria pigmentosa, systemic mast cell disease, and mast cell leukemia. **Solitary mastocytoma** is characterized by a single localized skin nodule, or at most several nodules, composed of a diffuse dermal infiltration of mast cells. The ventral aspect of the wrist is the more common site, and newborn infants are most commonly affected. The nodule tends to involute spontaneously, and only rarely is there progressive involvement of other skin sites. Systemic symptoms are absent. **Urticaria pigmentosa** affects children and, less commonly, young adults. Multiple cutaneous reddish macules and papules contain mast cells. Histamine release from mast cells, induced by a variety of stimuli (e.g., friction, heat, cold), causes local skin wheals or systemic symptoms. The disorder is generally restricted to the skin and systemic involvement is unusual. In most cases urticaria pigmentosa resolves at the time of puberty. **Systemic mastocytosis** occurs at any age, the peak incidence being in the sixth and seventh decades. The male:female ratio is

2:1. Mast cell infiltration is seen in the skin, bone marrow, spleen, lymph nodes, and liver. Osseous lesions occur in approximately two-thirds of the cases. The ribs, vertebrae, pelvis, skull, and proximal long bones are most commonly affected with both osteosclerotic and osteolytic lesions. On occasion marrow involvement with accompanying fibrosis leads to anemia, leukopenia, and thrombocytopenia. Mild hepatosplenomegaly and lymphadenopathy may be observed. **Mast cell leukemia** supervenes in 15% of cases of systemic mast cell disease, in which case the median survival is less than 2 years.

Proliferative disorders of mast cells must be distinguished from hairy cell leukemia, other types of acute and chronic leukemias, and the differentiated histiocytoses. In the presence of systemic symptoms, mast cell proliferative disorders must be distinguished from the carcinoid syndrome.

Benign Disorders of the Mononuclear Phagocyte System

Monocytosis

Monocytosis, an increase in the absolute blood monocyte count to above 800 per microliter, is associated with multiple disorders, including hematologic, immune, infectious, and inflammatory disorders (Table 20-17). Monocytosis is common in nonhematologic malignancies, such as carcinomas and sarcomas. Hematologic conditions, however, account for at least half of the disorders associated with monocytosis. Monocytosis is a common finding in the **hematopoietic dysplasias,** the so-called **preleukemic disorders.** Monocytes may be increased in the acute non-lymphocytic leukemias and in chronic myelogenous leukemia; in both they are a component of the neoplastic condition and may either be morphologically normal or exhibit atypical features. Monocytosis also occurs in a variety of neutropenic states. Finally, monocytosis is seen in association with the malignant lymphomas, Hodgkin's disease, and malignant histiocytosis.

Sinus Histiocytosis

The sinus histiocytes of the lymph nodes are derived from the cells that line the sinuses. The term *sinus histiocytosis* refers to an increase in these histiocytes or their functional counterparts, the phagocytic macrophages and the multinucleated giant cells, in the subcapsular and radiating sinuses of the lymph nodes. Expansion of the lymph node sinuses by benign nonphagocytic histiocytes and phagocytic macrophages is observed. The sinus histiocyte–macrophages have round or indented nuclei, which are eccentrically situated in an abundant pink cytoplasm. The chromatin is delicate, and the nucleoli are small (Fig. 20-13).

The cause of the sinus histiocytosis is often not determined, but it is a common finding in lymph nodes draining sites of cancer. The type of phagocytic debris identified in phagosomes may point to the cause. For example, mediastinal and scalene lymph nodes, which drain the pulmonary parenchyma,

often contain anthracotic (dust) pigment. In autoimmune hemolytic anemia, erythrocytes and hemosiderin pigment are identified in the macrophages. In the clinical staging of malignant neoplasms (e.g., the malignant lymphomas), radiopaque lipid contrast material, injected into the lymphatics of the lower extremities in lymphangiography, accumulates in the sinuses of the pelvic and abdominal lymph nodes. This material commonly elicits a histiocytic and macrophage reaction with multinucleated giant cells.

Sinus Histiocytosis with Massive Lymphadenopathy

Sinus histiocytosis with massive lymphadenopathy is a distinctive inflammatory disorder, with characteristic histologic and clinical features. Blacks in the first two decades of life are most commonly affected. Massive, bilateral, painless enlargement of the cervical lymph nodes, occasionally other lymph nodes, and even soft tissue sites is typical. In the lymph nodes the characteristic histologic features include capsular and pericapsular fibrosis, prominent sinus histiocytosis, and plasmacytosis of the medullary cords. In the sinus histiocytes cytoplasmic vacuoles that contain inflammatory cells, principally lymphocytes, are distinctive. This phenomenon, called **emperipolesis** (see Fig. 20-13), is not well understood. Although no causal agent has been identified, intermittent fever, neutrophilic leukocytosis, polyclonal hypergammaglobulinemia, and a high erythrocyte sedimentation rate suggest an infectious cause. The lymphadenopathy may persist for years before spontaneous resolution occurs, but affected persons usually remain in good health.

Dermatopathic Lymphadenopathy

In chronic dermatologic disorders drainage of lipid and melanin to the lymph nodes produces lymphadenopathy with a characteristic histologic appearance. Conspicuous paracortical and cortical hyperplasia of histiocytes and macrophages is observed. The cytoplasm of the macrophages either is pale and finely vacuolated, owing to the ingestion of lipid, or contains granular, brown melanin pigment (see Fig. 20-13).

Dermatopathic lymphadenopathy frequently occurs in association with mycosis fungoides, a dermatologic malignancy of T-helper lymphocytes.

Table 20-17 Principal Causes of Monocytosis

Hematologic disorders
  Preleukemia
  Myelogenous leukemia
    Acute
    Chronic
  Congenital and acquired neutropenia
  Malignant lymphoma
Immune and inflammatory disorders
  Collagen vascular diseases
  Inflammatory bowel disease
  Sarcoidosis
Infectious diseases
  Tuberculosis
  Subacute bacterial endocarditis
  Syphilis
  Protozoa
Epithelial malignancy

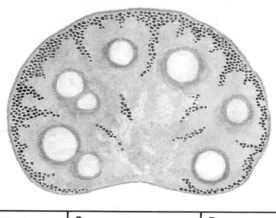

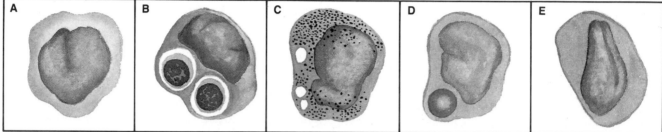

Figure 20-13. Mononuclear phagocyte system—benign disorders. In the lymph nodes, benign proliferations of mononuclear phagocytes first involve the nodal sinuses (*dots in lymph node cross section*) but may subsequently extend to involve the nodal stroma. In benign sinus histiocytosis, the nodal sinuses are expanded by bland histiocytes or phagocytic macrophages (*A*). In sinus histiocytosis with massive lymphadenopathy, the macrophages contain lymphocytes in cytoplasmic vacuoles (*B*). In dermatopathic lymphadenopathy, the macrophages contain cytoplasmic lipid and melanin pigment (*C*). In infection-induced hemophagocytic reticulosis, the macrophages contain phagocytosed red cells (*D*). In the differentiated histiocytoses the histiocytic-macrophages are bland, and a deep nuclear crease or fold is characteristic (*E*).

Infection-Induced Hemophagocytic Reticulosis

Infection-induced hemophagocytic reticulosis, a rare disorder that occurs in immunosuppressed individuals, is precipitated by a variety of infections. Hepatosplenomegaly, fever, and pancytopenia are typical clinical findings, and occasionally lymphadenopathy, skin rash and pulmonary infiltrates are observed. Proliferating benign histiocytes are identified in the spleen, lymph nodes, the hepatic sinusoids, and the bone marrow. A distinctive feature is prominent erythrophagocytosis by macrophages (see Fig. 20-13), but phagocytosis of neutrophils and platelets is also observed. The familial disorder, erythrophagocytic lymphohistiocytosis, probably represents the hemophagocytic syndrome in persons with a combined defect in both cellular and humoral immunity. Infection-induced hemophagocytic reticulosis clinically simulates the neoplastic proliferative disorder of mononuclear phagocytes, termed malignant histiocytosis. However, cytologic atypia of the histiocyte-macrophages is lacking.

Differentiated Histiocytoses

In the spectrum of disorders of the mononuclear phagocytes, the differentiated histiocytoses, a group of closely related proliferative conditions of histiocytes, occupy a central position between the benign immunoreactive hyperplasias and the neoplastic malignant histiocytosis. These maladies are of unknown cause and pathogenesis. Three syndromes that reflect the age of presentation and the extent of tissue and organ involvement are recognized: **acute disseminated histiocytosis (Letterer-Siwe disease), chronic disseminated histiocytosis (Hand-Schüller-Christian** disease), and **eosinophilic granuloma.** In the differentiated histiocytoses the extent and clinical aggressiveness of the disease correlate inversely with the age of the patient; the younger the patient, the more serious the prognosis.

Despite their clinical heterogeneity, these disorders have some common histopathologic features. Differentiated histiocytes are large cells with eccentric round or indented nuclei. Differentiated histiocytes display a deep nuclear crease, a feature that is unusual for histiocytes and macrophages (see Fig. 20-13). The abundant cytoplasm is pink and may be vacuolated, reflecting an increased lipid content. **The cell surface markers, which include Fc receptors, HLA-D/DR antigen, and OKT-6 (common thymic antigen), are identical to those of the epidermal Langerhans cell, an antigen-processing and -presenting cell that is included in the mononuclear phagocyte system.** By electron microscopy a cytoplasmic inclusion, **the X-body, Birbeck granule, or Langerhans cell granule,** is occasionally identified in differentiated histiocytes. The Birbeck granule is rod shaped or tubular with a dense core, a characteristic periodicity, and a bulbous end. **Because the Birbeck granule is found in epidermal Langerhans cells, it appears that the differentiated histiocytes may represent proliferative disorders of Langerhans cells;** the term **Langerhans cell granulomatosis** has therefore been applied to these disorders.

Acute disseminated histiocytosis (Letterer-Siwe disease) is an aggressive, sometimes fatal, systemic disorder in children usually less than 3 years of age. Frequently the clinical features suggest a malignant disease. Fever, generalized lymphadenopathy, hepatosplenomegaly, and failure to thrive are usual. Bone involvement, with cystic lesions of the skull, pelvis, and long bones, may be observed but are generally not prominent features. Involvement of the skin is common and is manifested by an eczematoid or seborrheic eruption, particularly of the scalp, face, and trunk. There may be purpura secondary to thrombocytopenia, caused either by extensive bone marrow replacement by histiocytes or by hypersplenism. Leukopenia and anemia may also be caused by extensive marrow replacement or hypersplenism. Interstitial pulmonary infiltration is common.

There may be extensive infiltration of differentiated histiocytes in virtually any organ or tissue, and the histiocytes may exhibit slight nuclear atypia. Phagocytosis is uncommon. Accompanying inflammatory cells, including eosinophils, are sparse. In the lymph nodes infiltration of differentiated histiocytes usually is identified first in the sinuses. Frequently there is extension to the lymph node stroma, and total effacement of the normal nodal architecture may ensue. In the liver infiltrating histiocytes are observed primarily in the sinusoids, whereas in the spleen they are observed primarily in the red pulp cords and sinuses.

Chronic disseminated histiocytosis (Hand-Schüller-Christian disease) occurs in children usually under the age of 5 years. Although multifocal involvement of organs is frequent, the course is usually benign. Lytic bone involvement, particularly of the bones of the skull, is characteristic. Destruction of the orbital bones, with extension into the orbit, may result in proptosis. Involvement of the hypothalamus or of the pituitary stalk may induce diabetes insipidus. The Hand-Schüller-Christian triad of defects in membranous bones, diabetes insipidus, and exophthalmos is seen in less than 15% of cases. Seborrhea with involvement of the scalp and ear canals is common. Generally, there is mild lymphadenopathy and hepatosplenomegaly. Histologically, there is infiltration of differentiated histiocytes, usually admixed with numerous inflammatory cells, principally eosinophils.

Eosinophilic granuloma is most commonly observed in adolescent males or in young adults. There is single (monostotic) or multifocal (polyostotic) involvement of bone. The ribs, skull, and femur are most commonly affected. Occasionally extraskeletal involvement in sites such as the lymph nodes, skin, and the lungs occurs. Differentiated histiocytes, with numerous eosinophils, infiltrate the tissues. The course in eosinophilic granuloma is benign.

Benign Disorders of Lymphoid Cells

Lymphoid Hyperplasia of Bone Marrow

Small lymphocytes constitute 10% to 20% of the nucleated cells of the bone marrow. The percentage of bone marrow lymphocytes, however, is age-dependent; from approximately 1 month to 2 years of age, up to 45% of bone marrow nucleated cells are lymphocytes. After 2 years of age, there is a gradual decline to the normal adult levels.

Lymphocytes are distributed interstitially in the hematopoietic tissues, but aggregates of lymphocytes, or "lymphoid nodules," are commonly observed in normal children and in elderly adults. At any age, the benign aggregates are small and well-delineated from the surrounding hematopoietic tissues. Small lymphocytes, with round hyperchromatic nuclei, are the predominant cell type in the lymphoid nodules. A few activated lymphocytes, transformed immunoblasts, plasma cells, and histiocyte-macrophages may be seen. Rarely, germinal center formation, indicative of a concurrent B-cell immunologic reaction, is present.

There is no precise definition as to what constitutes bone marrow lymphoid hyperplasia, or lymphocytosis. In bone marrow biopsy sections, lymphoid hyperplasia has been defined as 4 or more lymphoid aggregates in any low-power field (4X) or as the presence of a single lymphoid aggregate that measures at least 0.6 mm in greatest dimension. An adult with over 20% lymphocytes in either aspirate smears or biopsy sections should be considered to have a lymphocytosis. The differential diagnosis of bone marrow lymphocytosis includes an immunoreactive hyperplasia, such as that which occurs in viral infections or in tuberculosis, or an inflammatory disorder, such as a collagen vascular disease, or malignant lymphoproliferative disorder.

Plasma cells constitute 3% or less of the bone marrow nucleated cells and are linearly distributed along small blood vessels. A few plasma cells may be found at the margin of benign lymphoid nodules or scattered randomly in the hematopoietic stroma. The nucleus of the plasma cell is round, and the chromatin is marginated along the nuclear membrane in a distinctive distribution known as "clock face" chromatin. Nucleoli are generally not visualized. The nucleus is situated eccentrically in an abundant blue cytoplasm, and a paranuclear pale zone, representing the Golgi apparatus, is characteristic. Electron microscopy reveals abundant cisternae of rough endoplasmic reticulum and a prominent Golgi apparatus. These organelles reflect the function of the plasma cell, the production and external secretion of immunoglobulin. Immunoglobulin may accumulate in the cytoplasm and form an eosinophilic globule, termed the **Russell body.** Russell bodies are identified either in reactive disorders or in plasma cell neoplasia. Uncommonly, in neoplastic disorders of plasma cells, intranuclear invagination of protein-containing cytoplasm appears as intranuclear eosinophilic globules, called Dutcher bodies.

Reactive bone marrow plasmacytosis is characterized by a prominent perivascular cuff of plasma cells or an increase in irregularly distributed plasma cells. In reactive plasmacytosis, there is a conspicuous absence of cohesive sheets or clusters of plasma cells. Atypical cytologic features characteristic of neoplastic cells are lacking. Reactive bone marrow plasmacytosis occurs in a variety of disorders, including certain liver diseases, infectious diseases, and immunologic and inflammatory disorders. A marrow plasmacyto-

sis may occur as an immunologic response to epithelial malignancies, either localized or metastatic to the bone marrow. Bone marrow plasma cells may also be increased in amyloidosis.

Lymphocytosis

Peripheral blood lymphocytosis is defined as an absolute increase in the number of circulating lymphocytes. Since the lymphocyte count is higher in children than in adults, lymphocytosis is defined as an absolute lymphocyte count that exceeds 4000 per microliter in adults, 7000 per microliter in children, and 9000 per microliter in infants. **The most frequent cause of lymphocytosis is an acute or chronic viral or other infection (Table 20-18).** An absolute lymphocytosis is less commonly encountered than a relative lymphocytosis that reflects neutropenia. Thus, the absolute rather than relative blood neutrophil and lymphocyte counts should always be determined (see Table 20-9).

An evaluation of the morphologic features of circulating lymphocytes is important in determining the clinical significance of an absolute lymphocytosis. Normally, the blood lymphocytes are small to medium-sized and display coarse, clumped chromatin, small or indistinct nucleoli, and scant cytoplasm. Occasional large "transformed" lymphocytes with loose chromatin, distinct nucleoli, and abundant blue cytoplasm may be identified. There may also be a few medium-sized lymphocytes with prominent azurophilic granules—the large granular lymphocytes, which usually represent T cytotoxic-suppressor cells (see Fig. 20-11). **The morphologic hallmark of viral infections is the atypical lymphocyte, a term applied to a transformed lymphocyte in the blood.** The atypical lymphocyte characteristically has a round to irregular nucleus with relatively coarsely clumped chromatin, one to several distinct nucleoli, and abundant blue cytoplasm. Occasionally, atypical lymphocytes have moderate pale cytoplasm (see Fig. 20-11). A minority of atypical lymphocytes have sparse cytoplasm and fine chromatin, and these must be distinguished from the neoplastic blast cells of acute leukemia. The latter have uniformly finer chromatin and are clearly recognizable as belonging to a homogeneous population of abnormal cells; by contrast, atypical lymphocytes are a heterogeneous population of cells with a spectrum of cell sizes and morphologic features.

In infectious mononucleosis (Epstein-Barr virus infection), atypical lymphocytes usually constitute 20% or more of the peripheral blood nucleated cells. In cytomegalovirus and other virus infections, a mod-

Table 20-18 Principal Causes of Absolute Lymphocytosis

Acute infections
    Infectious mononucleosis
    Cytomegalovirus
    Bordetella pertussis
    Acute infectious lymphocytosis
    Toxoplasma gondii
Chronic infections
    Tuberculosis
    Brucellosis
Hematopoietic disorders
    Chronic lymphocytic leukemia
    Acute lymphocytic leukemia
    Prolymphocytic leukemia
    Hairy cell leukemia
Hypersensitivity reactions

erate atypical lymphocytosis is observed. *Toxoplasma gondii* infection, which is manifested by lymphadenopathy and circulating atypical lymphocytes, may mimic infectious mononucleosis. A moderate atypical lymphocytosis may be seen in brucellosis and in rickettsial infections. Finally, atypical lymphocytosis is encountered in inflammatory disorders, such as ulcerative colitis, and in immune reactions, such as hypersensitivity reactions and serum sickness.

Several unusual disorders are characterized by an increase in circulating normal small lymphocytes. Whooping cough (*Bordetella pertussis* infection) is associated with lymphocytosis, which may be due to release of a factor that inhibits the egress of small lymphocytes from the blood to the lymphoid tissues. In the childhood disorder **acute infectious lymphocytosis,** there is a marked increase in small T-lymphocytes, and the white blood cell count may be increased to 100,000 per microliter. Self-limited mild fever and diarrhea are typical, but a specific causal agent has not been identified. An increase in circulating small lymphocytes may also be observed in tuberculosis.

Chronic lymphocytic leukemia and the leukemic phase of some non-Hodgkin's malignant lymphomas must be distinguished from reactive lymphocytosis. Neoplasia may be suspected because of the clinical presentation and because of the uniformly abnormal cytologic features of the circulating cells. In some cases immunologic cell marker studies must be performed to establish a diagnosis of malignant disease.

Lymphocytopenia

Lymphocytopenia is an absolute blood lymphocyte count of less than 1500 per microliter in adults and less than 3000 per microliter in children. It is due to decreased production, to increased destruction, or to increased loss of lymphocytes. Decreased production of lymphocytes occurs in a number of congenital and acquired immunodeficiency syndromes. Decreased production of T-lymphocytes is also characteristic of advanced Hodgkin's disease. Irradiation, chemotherapeutic agents, antilymphocyte globulin, and ACTH or corticosteroid administration all lead to increased destruction of lymphocytes. Even localized radiotherapy may result in a significant lymphocytopenia. Corticosteroids have a poorly understood "lympholytic" effect. In Cushing's disease or in any stress-related increase in corticosteroid levels, there may be an associated lymphocytopenia. Abnormalities of the intestinal lymphatic system lead to an increased loss of lymphocytes. Damage to intestinal lymphatics, with loss of lymph into the lumen of the intestinal tract, may be accompanied by a significant depletion of lymphocytes. Associated disorders include the protein-losing enteropathies, acquired disorders of the small bowel, such as Whipple's disease, and any disorder associated with increased central venous pressure, such as right-sided heart failure and chronic constrictive pericarditis.

Peripheral Blood Plasmacytosis (Circulating Plasma Cells)

Plasma cells normally do not circulate in the peripheral blood. The most common cause of a blood plasmacytosis is plasma cell neoplasia. In multiple myeloma, the most common variant of plasma cell neoplasia, circulating plasma cells are usually identified only in the preterminal stages of the disease. Plasma cells may also occasionally be identified in the blood in various immunologic reactions and in viral infections. Sometimes atypical lymphocytes morphologically resemble plasma cells, in which case they are labeled **Turk cells** (see Fig. 20-11).

Reactive Hyperplasia of Lymph Nodes

A reactive hyperplasia of all or any combination of B cells, T cells, and mononuclear-phagocytic cells of the lymph nodes occurs in many infectious, inflammatory, and neoplastic diseases (Fig. 20-14). **Hyperplasia of the follicles and plasmacytosis of the medullary cords indicate immunoreactivity of B cells. Lymphoid hyperplasia of the deep cortex or paracortex (interfollicular hyperplasia) reflects immunoreactivity of T cells.** In benign reactive hyperplasia of lymph nodes, more than one immunologic compartment is frequently involved, a feature termed a "mixed pattern of reactivity."

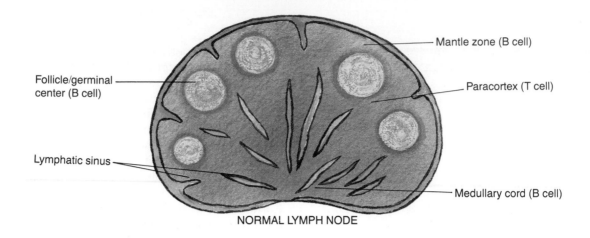

Follicle/germinal center (B cell)

Lymphatic sinus

Mantle zone (B cell)

Paracortex (T cell)

Medullary cord (B cell)

NORMAL LYMPH NODE

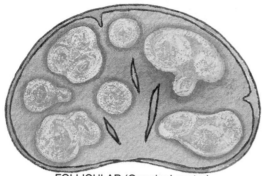

FOLLICULAR (Germinal center)

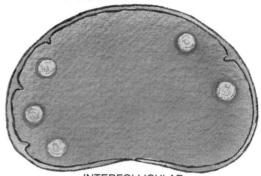

INTERFOLLICULAR

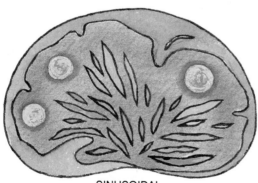

SINUSOIDAL

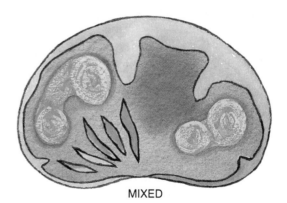

MIXED

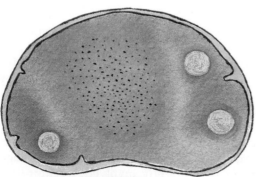

NECROTIZING

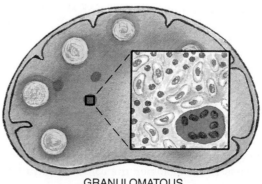

GRANULOMATOUS

The histologic appearance and degree of lymph node enlargement in benign reactive hyperplasia are influenced by the age of the patient (children exhibit a more pronounced lymphoid reactivity than adults), the immunologic competence of the host, and the specific infectious agent or type of inflammatory disorder.

The inguinal lymph nodes are frequently palpable in normal adults, and may measure up to several centimeters in greatest dimension. This nodal enlargement may persist unchanged for years, and in adults is generally of no clinical significance. Inguinal lymphadenopathy is usually a memento of previous infections, either of the lower extremities or of the groin region. The nodes show focal fibrosis and distortion of the normal architecture. Mild nonspecific paracortical lymphoid hyperplasia and partial fatty replacement are not unusual. Because these findings are common, biopsy of nodes other than the inguinal lymph nodes is generally preferred in the evaluation of a systemic disease. In children the cervical lymph nodes are frequently palpable because of previous infections. A moderate expansion of the paracortex and a mild follicular hyperplasia may be observed, but fibrosis is generally absent. **With the exception of such mild inguinal and cervical lymphadenopathy, enlargement of lymph nodes is not physiologic and suggests either a local or a systemic disease.**

The site of enlarged lymph nodes often provides a clue as to the likely cause. For example, the posterior auricular lymph nodes are commonly prominent in rubella infection, the occipital lymph nodes in scalp infections, the posterior cervical lymph nodes in toxoplasmosis, the axillary lymph nodes in infections of the upper extremities, and the inguinal lymph nodes in venereal infections and infections of the lower extremities. A generalized enlargement of the lymph nodes occurs in systemic infections, hyperthyroidism, drug reactions, collagen vascular diseases, and malignant lymphoproliferative disorders. Enlargement of a supraclavicular lymph node occasionally heralds metastatic carcinoma from the lung or from a primary abdominal malignancy.

Specific types of tissue reaction in the nonlymphoid tissues can also involve the lymph nodes. For example, in **acute suppurative lymphadenitis,** the lymph nodes draining a focus of acute bacterial infection commonly exhibit a rapid enlargement, with edema, infiltration of the sinuses and stroma by polymorphonuclear leukocytes, and a follicular hyperplasia. Such lymph nodes are tender because of acute distention of the lymph nodal capsule by edema, hyperemia, and infiltration of acute inflammatory cells. Suppuration may be complicated by abscess formation, and penetration of the infection to the skin may result in draining sinuses. With appropriate therapy, either complete resolution or residual fibrous scarring occurs.

Follicular Hyperplasia

Nonspecific Reactive Follicular Hyperplasia Nonspecific reactive follicular hyperplasia is characterized by prominent follicles in the lymph node cortex (Fig. 20-15). The follicles are enlarged and irregular and may be confluent. The activated follicular B-lymphocytes exhibit a spectrum of cell sizes and nuclear contours. A characteristic feature of benign follicles is the predominance of activated lymphoid cells toward one side of the follicle (the so-called polarized follicle.) In reactive follicles mitotic figures are numerous. Macrophages containing nuclear and cytoplasmic debris, so-called tingible bodies, are seen throughout such follicles (Fig. 20-15). **The presence of tingible body**

Figure 20-14. Lymph nodes—patterns of benign reactive hyperplasia. The patterns of benign reactive hyperplasia in lymph nodes are contrasted with the structure of a normal lymph node. Follicular hyperplasia with prominent enlarged and irregular benign follicles is characteristic of B-cell immunoreactivity. Interfollicular hyperplasia with expansion of the paracortex is characteristic of T-cell immunoreactivity. The sinusoidal pattern with expansion of sinuses by benign histiocyte-macrophages is characteristic of reactive proliferations of the mononuclear-phagocyte system. Mixed patterns of follicular, interfollicular, and sinusoidal hyperplasia are common in a variety of complex mixed immune reactions. In necrotizing lymphadenitis, variable necrosis of the lymph node architecture with residual cell debris is seen. In granulomatous inflammation, cohesive clusters of histiocytes with pink cytoplasm and occasional multinucleated giant cells are characteristic.

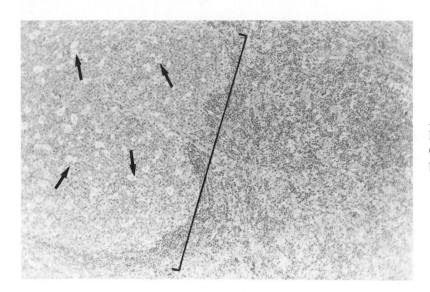

Figure 20-15.   Lymph node with reactive follicular hyperplasia. A prominent follicle *(bracket)* containing pale cytoplasmic macrophages *(arrows)* is seen.

macrophages is the hallmark of benign reactive follicular hyperplasia. Such macrophages are typically absent in the follicular lymphomas. Scattered large cells with vesicular nuclei and pale pink cytoplasm, **dendritic reticular cells,** are identified near the margin of the follicle. A perifollicular cuff of normal small lymphocytes is usually present and clearly demarcates the follicle from the surrounding interfollicular zone. A few immunoblasts and inflammatory cells may be located in the interfollicular zone, and an increase in medullary cord plasma cells is common. By definition, nonspecific reactive follicular hyperplasia is of unknown cause. Generally, a viral etiology is suspected. The course is typically benign, usually with rapid resolution of the lymphadenopathy.

Specific causes of follicular hyperplasia include rheumatoid arthritis, syphilis, toxoplasmosis, angiofollicular lymph node hyperplasia, and the acquired immunodeficiency syndrome (AIDS).

Rheumatoid Arthritis   The lymphadenopathy of rheumatoid arthritis is characterized by a conspicuous follicular hyperplasia, which involves the cortex and the paracortex and occasionally extends to involve the medulla. Interfollicular plasmacytosis is prominent.

Syphilis   In leutic or syphilitic lymphadenitis striking follicular hyperplasia and interfollicular plasmacytosis are also observed. In syphilis small clusters of epithelioid histiocytes, or sarcoid-like granulomas, are present together with fibrosis of the capsule and perinodal soft tissues. In the perinodal soft tissues, perivascular plasma cell infiltration is characteristic. The causal spirochetes may be identified with silver stains or with fluorescein-labeled antitreponemal antibody.

Toxoplasmosis   In toxoplasmosis lymphadenitis reactive follicles are prominent. Small clusters of interfollicular epithelioid histiocytes encroach upon, and are found within, the reactive follicles (Fig. 20-16). Frequently, the sinuses and perisinusal regions are expanded by B-lymphocytes with indented "monocytoid" nuclei (perisinusoidal hyperplasia). The combination of prominent follicles containing epithelioid histiocytes and perisinusoidal hyperplasia is highly suggestive of toxoplasmosis.

Angiofollicular Lymphoid Hyperplasia   Angiofollicular lymphoid hyperplasia (giant lymph node hyperplasia, Castleman's lesion) is an unusual inflammatory disorder of unknown etiology. Two distinct histologic subtypes are identified. The more common hyaline vascular type, comprising 90% of the angiofollicular lymphoid hyperplasias, usually presents as an asymptomatic mass, most frequently in the mediastinum. Other soft tissue sites may also be involved. Numerous small, follicle-like structures, frequently with radially penetrating capillaries, are seen. These capillaries extend from a highly vascular perifollicular tissue and may be sheathed in dense collagen. A perifollicular concentric layering of small lymphocytes (onion-skinning) is characteristic. In the less common plasma cell type, which constitutes 10% of all cases of angiofollicular lymphoid hyperplasia, large, more typical, reactive follicles with less prominent penetrating capillaries are present. There is a pronounced interfollicular plasmacytosis and prominent vascularity. Whereas hyaline vascular angiofollicular lymphoid hyperplasia is usually without systemic symptoms, the plasma cell variety is characterized by fever, polyclonal hypergammaglobulinemia, and anemia. These findings resolve with excision of the lesions. The cause of both types of angiofollicular lymphoid hyperplasia is unknown.

AIDS   In the persistent generalized lymphadenopathy of the AIDS-related complex, a florid follicular hyperplasia is characteristic. With progression to the full expression of AIDS, there is typically an involution of the exuberant follicular hyperplasia. Additionally, lymphoid cells in the paracortex are depleted. Superimposed infection is common, and special stains for microorganisms, including fungi and mycobacteria, should routinely be performed on all biopsy specimens. In AIDS there is a high incidence of superimposed Kaposi's sarcoma and high-grade, diffuse non-Hodgkin's lymphomas, including B cell immunoblastic lymphoma and Burkitt's lymphoma.

Interfollicular Hyperplasia

Nonspecific Reactive Interfollicular Hyperplasia   In nonspecific paracortical hyperplasia low-power microscopy reveals a mottled ("salt and pepper") appearance of the lymph node paracortex. At high power an admixture of small lymphocytes, activated lymphocytes (including immunoblasts), and scattered histiocytes is seen (Fig. 20-17). Typically, the postcapillary venules are prominent and have conspicuous endothelial lining cells. This benign immunoblastic reaction may be so florid that it completely effaces the normal lymph node architecture. Paracortical hyperplasia is seen in viral infections and in some immune reactions, but often no precise cause is found. However, there are occasionally histopathologic features that suggest a specific infectious agent.

Infectious Mononucleosis   In the lymphadenitis of infectious mononucleosis the immunoblastic reaction is usually severe and is accompanied by bizarre immunoblast variants, which may simulate or be indistinguishable from the Reed-Sternberg cells of Hodgkin's disease. A spectrum of noncohesive immunoblast variants may be observed "floating" in the lymph node sinuses.

Postvaccinial Lymphadenitis   In postvaccinial lymphadenitis bizarre immunoblast variants, indistinguishable from Reed-Sternberg cells, are also seen. Both infectious mononucleosis and postvaccinial lymphadenitis are distinguished from Hodgkin's disease by the presence of a spectrum of transforming lymphocytes and immunoblasts; in Hodgkin's disease the background cells consist of small, nonactivated lymphocytes.

Varicella-Herpes Zoster Lymphadenitis   In varicella-herpes zoster lymphadenitis, some endothelial cells may exhibit intranuclear eosinophilic inclusions (Cowdry type A inclusions), which are surrounded by a clear nuclear halo. Such inclusion-containing lymphoid cells are present in the typical cellular background of a viral lymphadenitis.

Measles Lymphadenitis   In measles lymphadenitis, multilobed or multinucleated cells with delicate nuclear chromatin (perikaryons) are present in the prodromal phase of the infection.

Cytomegalovirus Lymphadenitis   In cytomegalovirus lymphadenitis the nuclei of endothelial cells may contain very large eosinophilic, intranuclear inclusions, surrounded by a clear nuclear halo.

Histiocytic Necrotizing Lymphadenitis   Histiocytic necrotizing lymphadenitis (Kikuchi's disease), a disorder most common in young women, usually involves the cervical lymph nodes. The lesions typically show focal cortical and paracortical necrosis, with a prominent immunoblastic and histiocytic reaction (see Fig. 20-14). Despite the necrosis and abundant nuclear debris, granulocytes are lacking. Spontaneous resolution occurs in 3 to 4 months. A viral cause is suspected.

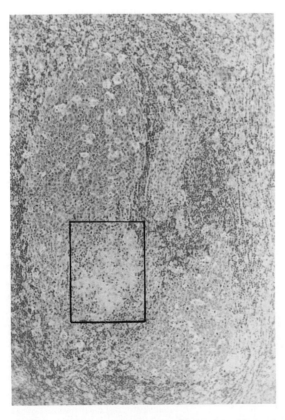

Figure 20-16.   Toxoplasmosis lymphadenitis. There is prominent follicular hyperplasia. Nests of epithelioid histiocytes encroach on the benign follicles *(box).*

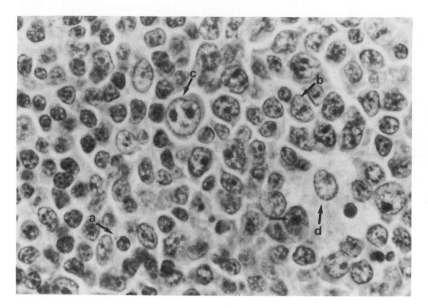

Figure 20-17. Lymph node with reactive interfollicular hyperplasia. A spectrum of lymphocytes undergoing transformation from a small lymphocyte (*a*) to a partially transformed lymphocyte (*b*) to a classic immunoblast (*c*) is seen in the T-dependent paracortex. One cytoplasmic histiocyte is seen (*d*).

Lymphadenopathy Associated With Systemic Lupus
In lymphadenopathy associated with systemic lupus erythematosus, there is a diffuse or paracortical lymphoid hyperplasia with immunoblastic reaction, plasmacytosis, and extensive necrosis. The lymphoid follicles tend to be inconspicuous. Arteriolitis, with fibrinoid necrosis of the vessel walls, is frequent. Extracellular, purple, amorphous deposits, which consist of altered DNA and are called "hematoxylin bodies," are diagnostic.

Angioimmunoblastic Lymphadenopathy Angioimmunoblastic lymphadenopathy comprises a spectrum of related disorders that are characterized by generalized lymphadenopathy, hepatosplenomegaly, and

a maculopapular rash. Middle-aged and elderly persons are most commonly affected. The common constitutional symptoms are fever, night sweats, and weight loss. Patients frequently have anemia, and the direct antiglobulin test (Coombs test) is often positive. Laboratory findings include polyclonal hypergammaglobulinemia and a peripheral blood eosinophilia. In approximately one-third of cases the disorder is precipitated by the administration of drugs. For example, the administration of diphenylhydantoin, an antiepileptic medication, may be associated with a condition that is indistinguishable from angioimmunoblastic lymphadenopathy. It has been speculated that these lymph node lesions rep-

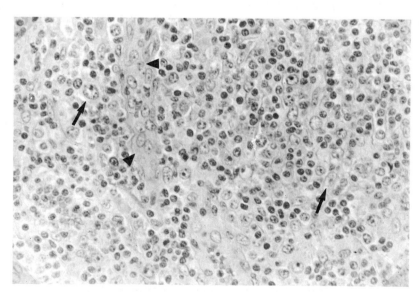

Figure 20-18. Angioimmunoblastic lymphadenopathy. A spectrum of lymphocytes undergoing transformation with scattered immunoblasts (*arrows*) is seen. Postcapillary venules are prominent and thick walled (*arrowheads*).

resent hyperimmune disorders involving an altered or abnormal immunologic reactivity. Indeed, a subtype of T-cell malignant lymphoma with a similar histopathologic appearance has been described. In angioimmunoblastic lymphadenopathy the involved lymph nodes exhibit a diffuse effacement of the normal architecture, although a few "burnt-out," or depleted, follicles may remain. Typically, there is a polymorphous cell infiltrate consisting of a wide spectrum of activated lymphocytes with immunoblasts, plasmacytoid immunoblasts, plasma cells, histiocytes, neutrophils, and eosinophils. The lymph node vasculature is prominent and thick walled (Fig. 20-18) and demonstrates an arborizing pattern. Deposition of an interstitial PAS-positive material, which represents either immunoglobulins secreted by B cells or the products of cell degeneration, is seen. A similar histologic picture is seen in involved skin, bone marrow, liver, and spleen. In one-third to one-half of cases, large transformed lymphoid cells appear in clusters and progressively obliterate the normal tissue architecture. The course and prognosis then are those of an aggressive large cell lymphoma. Even in the absence of malignant degeneration, the prognosis is poor because of progressive immune failure. Death usually is caused by superimposed infection.

Atypical Reactive Hyperplasia   In less than 5% of lymph node biopsies, atypical cytologic features of the lymphoid cells or atypical patterns of the nodal architecture are suggestive but not diagnostic of a malignant lymphoid neoplasm. In such cases the diagnosis of atypical reactive hyperplasia is appropriate. In one-third of the cases in which the diagnosis of atypical lymph node hyperplasia is made, a malignant lymphoma is subsequently diagnosed.

Extranodal Lymphoid Hyperplasia

Lymphocytes circulate in the vascular and lymphatic systems and preferentially home to the lymphopoietic organs. However, since they are recirculating cells, lymphocytes are found in almost any tissue, where they are available to participate in local immune reactions. Occasionally, prominent hyperplasia or benign reactive proliferation of these local tissue lymphocytes occurs. Although they are of unknown cause, such hyperplasias probably represent an exaggerated immune response, possibly on the part of defective lymphocytes to antigenic stimuli. The most common sites of such extranodal lymphoid hyperplasia include the lungs, stomach, soft tissues of the orbit, and skin (Table 20-19). Because they can pres-

Table 20-19 Extranodal Lymphoid Hyperplasia (Pseudolymphoma)

Focal Organ Involvement (Pseudolymphoma)

Lung
Stomach
Orbit
Skin

Diffuse Organ Involvement

Thyroid—Chronic lymphocytic thyroiditis
Salivary gland—Lymphoepithelial lesion
Small bowel—Nodular lymphoid hyperplasia

ent as mass lesions composed of lymphoid cells, both the clinical and the histologic findings suggest the diagnosis of malignant lymphoma. Therefore, benign extranodal lymphoid hyperplasia is termed **pseudolymphoma.**

Grossly, extranodal lymphoid hyperplasia presents as a white-gray firm mass that is well demarcated from the surrounding normal tissue. The mass may be large and measure up to 10 cm or more in greatest dimension. Microscopically, there is a polymorphous cell infiltrate, which consists of varying proportions of small lymphocytes, immunoblasts, plasma cells, eosinophils, histiocytes, and fibroblasts. The presence of scattered benign germinal centers is a characteristic feature.

Usually extranodal lymphoid hyperplasia follows a benign course, and excision is curative. Particularly with pulmonary extranodal lymphoid hyperplasia, there is a significant risk of progression to a non-Hodgkin's malignant lymphoma. There are instances when the histologic features might suggest early progression to a non-Hodgkin's lymphoma. In such instances, cell marker studies may determine whether the proliferation is polyclonal and therefore benign, or monoclonal and therefore malignant. Additionally, histologic examination of the regional lymph nodes may be useful in determining whether the lymphoid cell proliferation is benign or malignant. In extranodal lymphoid hyperplasia, the regional lymph nodes are normal or exhibit benign reactive hyperplasia. The finding of malignant lymphoma in the regional lymph nodes would suggest that the extranodal lesion is probably a malignant neoplasm.

In contrast to extranodal lymphoid hyperplasia, which presents as a localized mass, a more diffuse lymphoid cell infiltration may occur in the thyroid, the salivary glands, and the mucosa of the small bowel. In the thyroid the lesion is labeled chronic lymphocytic thyroiditis; in the salivary glands, a lymphoepithelial lesion; and in the small bowel, nodular lymphoid hyperplasia. In the thyroid and the salivary glands the lymphoid cell infiltration appears to be inflammatory, whereas in the mucosa of the small bowel it may represent an abnormal hyperplasia of immune cells.

Both in chronic lymphocytic thyroiditis and in lymphoepithelial lesions of the salivary glands, there is a significant risk of progression to a malignant lymphoma. In a small minority of cases of nodular lymphoid hyperplasia of the small bowel, there is progression to a malignant lymphoma.

Disorders of the Spleen

The spleen is an uncommon site of primary disease, but enlargement of the spleen is common, because the spleen is involved in reactions to systemic infections, participates in systemic immunologic-inflammatory disorders, enlarges in storage diseases, and is involved in generalized hematopoietic and, less consistently, lymphopoietic disorders. The causes of splenomegaly are outlined in Table 20-20.

Splenomegaly is sometimes associated with the syndrome of hypersplenism, a condition that reflects hyperplasia of splenic mononuclear phagocytes and

Table 20-20 Principal Causes of Splenomegaly

Infections
  Acute
  Subacute
  Chronic
Immunologic-inflammatory disorders
  Felty's syndrome
  Lupus erythematosus
  Sarcoidosis
  Amyloidosis
  Thyrotoxicosis
Hemolytic anemias
Pediatric immune thrombocytopenia
Splenic vein hypertension
  Cirrhosis
  Splenic and/or portal vein thrombosis or stenosis
  Right-sided cardiac failure
Primary or metastatic neoplasm
  Leukemia
  Lymphoma
  Hodgkin's disease
  Myeloproliferative syndromes
  Sarcoma
  Carcinoma
Storage diseases
  Gaucher's
  Niemann-Pick
  Mucopolysaccharidoses
Idiopathic
  Banti's disease

macrophage-mediated destruction of sequestered elements of the blood. Any combination of anemia, leukopenia, and thrombocytopenia results, and splenectomy is curative. The sporadic occurrence of hypersplenism in association with splenomegaly is poorly understood.

Congenital anomalies of the spleen are rare and include absence or **asplenia,** and multiple small spleens, or **polysplenia.** Both asplenia and polysplenia are often associated with other congenital anomalies. **Accessory spleens** are a common anomaly, occurring in 10% of normal individuals. Accessory spleens are usually small and spherical, measuring up to several centimeters in diameter, and are most frequently found near the tail of the pancreas or in the gastrosplenic ligament. Following splenectomy, accessory spleens can assume the role of the normal spleen; in certain hematologic disorders, such as hereditary spherocytosis, splenectomy may therefore be of no benefit.

Nonspecific acute reactive hyperplasia of the spleen (active hyperemia, nonspecific acute splenitis) occurs in response to a variety of acute systemic infections. The stimulus to splenic hyperplasia probably relates both to blood-borne bacteria and to the heterogeneous products of the inflammatory response. The spleen is modestly enlarged (up to 400 g) and hyperemic. Macrophages abound, and disintegrating bacteria may be identified in mononuclear phagocytes. An increase in neutrophils and plasma cells is also observed. Mild hyperplasia of the lymphoid white pulp is common.

Immunoreactive hyperplasia of splenic lymphoid tissue ("activated spleen") may be observed in a number of chronic immunologic-inflammatory disorders. Follicle or germinal center formation may be prominent, as in rheumatoid arthritis. Hyperplasia of mononuclear phagocytes and increased immunoblasts, plasma cells, and eosinophils are seen in the red pulp. Features characteristic of specific disorders may also be observed. For example, in **systemic lupus erythematosus** there may be fibrinoid necrosis of capsular and trabecular collagen and characteristic "onion-skin" thickening of penicilliary and central arterioles. In **infectious mononucleosis,** transformed lymphocytes (immunoblasts) prominently infiltrate the red pulp, while the white pulp may no longer be evident. Infiltration of the capsule, trabeculae, and blood vessels by lymphoid elements weakens the supporting structures of the spleen and accounts for a high incidence of splenic rupture. **Typhoid fever** is characterized by lymphoid infiltrates of the red pulp and hyperplasia of macrophages, often accompanied by prominent erythrophagocytosis. **Chronic malarial**

infection results in a huge spleen, with fibrous thickening of the capsule and trabeculae. Grossly, a slate-gray or black color reflects the presence of malarial pigment (hematin). Microscopically, myriads of macrophages contain malarial parasites and pigment.

Chronic passive congestion (fibrocongestive splenomegaly), caused by prolonged elevation of pressure in the splenic vein is most commonly seen as a complication of hepatic cirrhosis, in which case it reflects portal hypertension. Other causes of portal hypertension, such as thrombosis of the portal or splenic veins secondary to pylephlebitis or tumors, may lead to chronic passive congestion of the spleen. An increase in splenic vein pressure may also result from right-sided heart failure, due either to cor pulmonale or to tricuspid or pulmonary valve disease.

With chronic passive congestion, the enlarged spleen (500–1000 g) shows fibrosis of the capsule and the red pulp. The sinusoids are dilated and empty. Foci of old hemorrhage persist as **Gamna-Gandy bodies,** fibrotic nodules containing iron and calcium salts encrusted on collagenous and elastic fibers. There is atrophy of the white pulp. The clinical syndrome of hypersplenism is a potential complication.

Infarctions of the spleen result from occlusion of the splenic artery or one of its tributaries. The vascular occlusion is frequently due to emboli from the left heart, originating in mural thrombi or in vegetations on mitral or aortic valves damaged by endocarditis. Splenic infarctions may also result from local thrombosis caused by disorders such as sickle cell disease, polyarteritis nodosa, and the chronic myeloproliferative syndromes. Infarcts are usually wedge shaped, with their bases contiguous to the splenic capsule. Friction rubs may be audible, owing to a secondary fibrinous perisplenitis. With septic emboli, such as from a focus of bacterial endocarditis, suppuration and abscess formation may occur. Particularly after multiple infarcts, extensive fibrous scarring may result in atrophy of the spleen. Such "autosplenectomy" is especially characteristic of sickle cell disease.

Rupture of the spleen occurs most commonly as the result of blunt trauma. In the absence of trauma, an underlying predisposing disorder should be sought, since for practical purposes spontaneous rupture of a normal spleen does not occur. Diseases that predispose to rupture of the spleen include infectious mononucleosis, chronic malaria, typhoid fever, abscesses, and leukemia. Splenic rupture is a surgical emergency because of the potential for massive hemorrhage. Following rupture bits of splenic tissue may be seeded on the peritoneal surface, leading to the formation of splenic implants (splenosis).

Splenic cysts are rare. The parasite *Echinococcus granulosus* is the most common cause of splenic cysts, the rupture of which leads to secondary peritonitis. True benign epidermoid cysts, lined by normal squamous epithelium, are exceedingly rare. Pseudocysts, which are lined by a fibrous wall rather than a true epithelial lining, usually are a result of old hemorrhage and repair.

Primary tumors of the spleen are rare. The most common benign tumors are hemangiomas and lymphangiomas, which vary greatly in size, from minute foci to lesions that occupy most of the spleen. They are usually of the cavernous type; that is, they exhibit large, dilated, endothelium-lined spaces. In hemangiomas the spaces are occupied by erythrocytes, and in lymphangiomas by lymph. Other benign tumors, including chondromas, fibromas, and osteomas, are exceedingly rare. Primary malignant tumors of the spleen, which are also uncommon, include unusual primary splenic lymphomas, Hodgkin's disease, and hemangiosarcoma. The last, a highly malignant neoplasm of vascular endothelial cells, is aggressive and frequently metastasizes to the liver by way of the portal system.

In general, **the microenvironment of the spleen does not offer a favorable milieu for the implantation and growth of metastatic tumor cells.** Metastatic tumors to the spleen generally are observed only late in the course of most malignant neoplasms and are rare in the absence of extensive spread to other organ sites. The primary tumors that most commonly metastasize to the spleen are carcinomas of the lung, breast, stomach, colon, and prostate, and malignant melanoma.

Monoclonal Gammopathy of Unknown Significance

A homogeneous immunoglobulin molecule, a portion of an immunoglobulin molecule, or a single predominant kappa or lambda light chain, in the blood or urine is called a monoclonal gammopathy (M component). The abnormal protein is produced by a clone of B cells derived from a single aberrant B cell. Such a homogeneous protein is detected as a sharp peak, or "spike," in the serum or urine protein electrophoretic pattern (Fig. 20-19). By contrast, in benign or reactive processes a polyclonal immunoreactivity results in a polyclonal, or broad-based, increase in immunoglobulins.

In most persons in whom a monoclonal gammopathy is demonstrated, there is no evidence for an

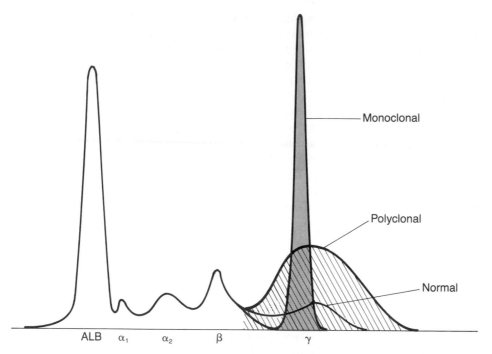

Figure 20-19. Serum protein electrophoretic patterns. Abnormal serum protein electrophoretic patterns are contrasted with a normal pattern. In polyclonal hyper-gammaglobulinemia, which is characteristic of benign reactive processes, there is a broad-based increase in immunoglobulins due to immunoglobulin secretion by a myriad discrete reactive plasma cells. In monoclonal gammopathy, which is characteristic of monoclonal gammopathy of unknown significance or plasma cell neoplasia, there is a narrow peak, or spike, due to the homogeneity of the immunoglobulin molecules secreted by a single clone of aberrant plasma cells.

associated malignant tumor or other disorder. In the bone marrow plasma cells are only slightly increased, and sheets of plasma cells, as seen in multiple myeloma, are not present. The incidence of monoclonal gammopathy of unknown significance increases from 1% at age 25 years to 3% at age 70 years to 10% at age 80 years. Despite the alternative label of "benign monoclonal gammopathy," 10% of affected individuals subsequently develop either plasma cell neoplasia or a B-cell malignant lymphoma. A minority of persons with monoclonal gammopathy have an associated disorder, such as an epithelial cancer or an infection. These associations are probably coincidental and may reflect an age-related increased incidence of all such disorders. **Monoclonal gammopathy of unknown significance is important, because it is common and must be distinguished from plasma cell neoplasia.** Clinical features, radiologic studies, and laboratory data must all be carefully considered in the differential diagnosis (Table 20-21).

The Chronic Myeloproliferative Syndromes

The chronic myeloproliferative syndromes are clonal disorders that arise from the neoplastic transformation of a single common hematopoietic precursor cell. Evidence for clonality and, by inference, for neoplasia is provided by analysis of glucose-6-phosphate dehydrogenase isoenzymes and by cytogenetic studies. These reveal the expression of only isoenzyme A or B of glucose-6-phosphate dehydrogenase or the presence of identical marker chromosomes in erythrocytic, granulocytic, and megakaryocytic precursor cells. By contrast, in benign or polyclonal proliferations, both isoenzymes A and B are expressed and marker chromosomes are absent.

Initially in the chronic myeloproliferative syndromes, the neoplastic common precursor cells retain their capacity for differentiation and maturation.

Thus, the bone marrow exhibits a trilineage hyperplasia (panhyperplasia), a generalized increase in erythrocytic, granulocytic, and megakaryocytic cell lines. Cohesive clusters of atypical megakaryocytes with hyperchromatic nuclei are the morphologic hallmark of the chronic myeloproliferative syndromes (Fig. 20-20).

Fibrosis of the bone marrow is common in the chronic myeloproliterative syndromes. Since the fibroblasts lack the restricted isoenzymes and the marker chromosomes, the proliferation of fibroblasts appears to be a reactive phenomenon. The fibroblast proliferation may be due to the secretion of a platelet-derived growth factor (PDGF) that induces fibroblasts to proliferate and produce collagen. The specific chronic myeloproliferative syndromes are defined by the predominant proliferating cell types. **Polycythemia vera** is characterized principally by erythroid cells, **chronic granulocytic leukemia** by granulocytes, and **primary hemorrhagic thrombocythemia** by megakaryocytes. In **myelofibrosis with myeloid metaplasia,** all the hematopoietic cell lines are proliferative and reactive fibrosis is prominent.

Polycythemia Vera

Polycythemia vera is a neoplastic disorder of the common hematopoietic precursor cell in which a pronounced increase in the production of erythroid cells is accompanied by a corresponding increase in the total red cell mass. The criteria for diagnosis of polycythemia vera are outlined in Table 20-22.

The cause of polycythemia vera is unknown, but it may relate to an abnormality of the erythroid committed-precursor cells. The erythroid precursors are

Table 20-21 Monoclonal Gammopathy of Unknown Significance Versus Plasma Cell Neoplasia

	MONOCLONAL GAMMOPATHY OF UNKNOWN SIGNIFICANCE	PLASMA CELL NEOPLASIA
Incidence	1% of young adult, > 3% elderly	0.003% annual incidence
Characteristic Protein Abnormality		
Typical monoclonal serum immunoglobulin concentration	IgG < 3 g IgM, IgA < 1.5 g	IgG > 3 g IgM, IgA > 1.5 g
Monoclonal light chain, urine (Bence-Jones proteinuria)	Absent, or present in very small amounts	Present in 80% (with or without serum-M component)
Stability monoclonal immunoglobulin over time	Stable	Tends to increase
Concentration, other immunoglobulins	Generally normal	Generally decreased
Pathology of Bone Marrow		
Marrow plasmacytosis	Normal, or mild increase (< 10%)	Generally > 15%
Plasma cells in clusters or sheets	Absent	Present
Plasma cell morphology	Normal	Atypical (nucleolated and nuclear-cytoplasmic asynchrony)
Clinical Findings		
Bone (radiologic)	Normal	Osteolytic lesion(s) or diffuse osteoporosis
Hypercalcemia	Absent	May be present
Anemia	Absent	May be present
Erythrocyte sedimentation rate	Normal	Frequently increased

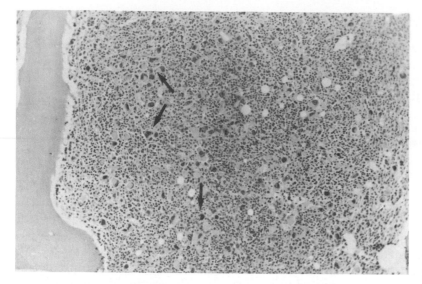

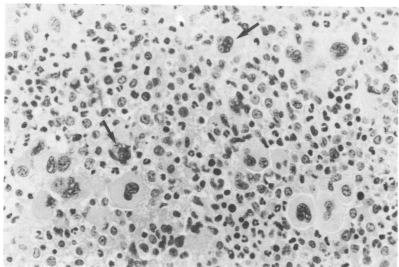

Figure 20-20. Bone marrow in chronic mye-loproliferative syndrome. The marrow is cellular, with hyperplasia of all hematopoietic elements. Megakaryocytes *(arrows)* are atypical and show hyperchromatic nuclei.

exquisitely sensitive to and, in turn, dependent on erythropoietin stimulation. However, in polycythemia vera these cells proliferate and form colonies in vitro even in the absence of erythropoietin. Although normal erythroid precursor cells are identified early in the course of polycythemia vera, the neoplastic cell clone has a proliferative advantage. With the passage of time the red blood cell mass increases, thereby shutting off erythropoietin production by the kidneys. Normal erythroid precursors are then gradually depleted because of the lack of erythropoietin stimulation.

The principal hematopathologic features of polycythemia vera are presented in Table 20-23. In addition to there being hyperplasia of the erythroid series, all hematopoietic cell lines are increased. Clusters of atypical megakaryocytes, the characteristic feature of

the chronic myeloproliferative syndromes, are often present. Bone marrow iron is depleted, owing both to diversion of storage iron to the developing erythrocytes and to blood loss from recurrent gastrointestinal hemorrhage. Bone marrow fibrosis is observed even early in the course of the disease, and in one-fifth of the cases, severe fibrosis with depletion of hematopoietic cells is a late complication.

In most cases of polycythemia vera, there is moderate enlargement of the spleen, which reflects expansion of the red pulp. The white pulp is atrophic (Fig. 20-21). The spleen is congested and commonly exhibits myeloid metaplasia (neoplastic extramedullary hematopoiesis), that is, islands of erythroid normoblasts, scattered megakaryocytes, and immature granulocytic cells. Myeloid metaplasia of the liver is observed principally in the hepatic sinusoids.

The common laboratory findings are shown in Table 20-24. They include a hemoglobin concentration of greater than 20 g/dl, a hematocrit of 60% or more, and a red blood cell count of 6 million to 10 million per microliter. Arterial oxygen saturation is normal, thereby excluding a cardiopulmonary cause for the erythrocytosis. The peripheral blood erythrocytes usually appear normal, but hypochromia and microcytosis may be observed in conjunction with superimposed iron deficiency. With progression of the disease, the erythrocytes may exhibit marked anisocytosis and poikilocytosis. Teardrop-shaped erythrocytes are seen when myeloid metaplasia develops in the spleen, owing to a lack of the normal conditioning of the red cell membrane. A leukocytosis of up to 25,000 per microliter occurs in two-thirds of cases. Uncommonly, the leukocyte count may be strikingly elevated, up to 100,000 per microliter, and circulating immature leukocytes may be identified. An increase in peripheral blood basophils is common and is characteristic of all the chronic myeloproliferative syndromes. The platelet count is moderately increased in half of the cases. The peripheral blood platelets are often abnormal, both morphologically (giant forms and abnormal granulation) and functionally. The leukocyte alkaline phosphatase score is often high. Because levels of this enzyme activity vary in the different chronic myeloproliferative syndromes, the score is useful in distinguishing these syndromes (see Table 20-24). In a quarter of the cases cytogenetic study reveals karyotypic abnormalities, such as aneuploidy or an extra C-group chromosome.

Polycythemia vera is typically a disorder of middle aged Caucasian men, the usual age at onset being 40 to 60 years. The clinical features are outlined in Table 20-25. The symptoms generally reflect the increased red blood cell mass, with secondary circulatory disturbances such as impaired blood flow, vascular stasis, and local tissue hypoxia. Almost any organ may be affected. Headache, dizziness, and visual disturbances result from impaired circulation in the central nervous system. Angina pectoris and intermittent claudication reflect poor circulation in the coronary and peripheral vascular systems, respectively. Hemorrhage and thrombosis occur in half of the cases and may involve the cerebral, coronary, and peripheral vascular systems. Gastric ulcers occasionally develop because of sludging of erythrocytes in gastric mucosal vessels and increased gastric acid secretion secondary to histamine release from basophils. Severe pruritus, also due to histamine release from basophils is associated with bathing in warm water.

The course of polycythemia vera is characterized by a protracted stable erythroid phase with polycythemia. However, 20% of cases ultimately progress to a "spent" phase, typified by progressive anemia, an enlarging spleen with prominent myeloid metaplasia, a peripheral blood leukoerythroblastic picture, and marrow fibrosis with depletion of hematopoietic cells. The prognosis is then very poor. In untreated polycythemia vera the risk of acute nonlymphocytic leukemia is 2% to 4%, and this risk is further increased by treatment with ^{32}P or alkylating agents. With treatment the median survival is about 13 years. The most common cause of death is thrombosis.

Chronic Myelogenous Leukemia

Chronic myelogenous leukemia is a neoplastic disorder of the common hematopoietic precursor cell in which the granulocytic cell series is predominantly affected. Typically, there is an accompanying proliferation of erythroid cells and of megakaryocytes. The fact that neoplastic cell markers are occasionally identified on lymphoid cells suggests that in some cases transformation of the pluripotential precursor cell has occurred.

Although the cause of chronic myelogenous leukemia is unknown, suggestive clues may be derived from epidemiologic associations, chromosomal studies, and some data obtained by the techniques of molecular biology. Agents that damage the bone marrow, exemplified by benzene, may be causal in a small minority of cases. The incidence of the disease is significantly augmented following excessive exposure to radiation, an observation made among sur-

---

Table 20-22 Criteria for the Diagnosis of Polycythemia Vera

Major (Category A)

A1	Increased RBC mass
	Male: ≥ 36 ml/kg
	Female: ≥ 32 ml/kg
A2	Normal arterial O$_2$ saturation (> 92%)
A3	Splenomegaly

Minor (Category B)

B1	Thrombocytosis: Platelets ≥ 400,000/μl
B2	Leukocytosis: WBC ≥ 12,000/μl (absence of fever or infection)
B3	Elevated LAP score: > 100 (absence of fever or infection)
B4	Elevated serum vitamin B$_{12}$ or unbound B$_{12}$
	Binding capacity: B$_{12}$ > 900 pg/ml; UB$_{12}$ BC > 2200 pg/ml

Diagnosis

1) All three parameters from Category A
   OR
2) A1 + A2 + any two parameters from Category B

Data obtained from Polycythemia Vera Study Group. (*RBC*, red blood cells; *WBC*, white blood cells; *LAP*, leukocyte alkaline phosphatase)

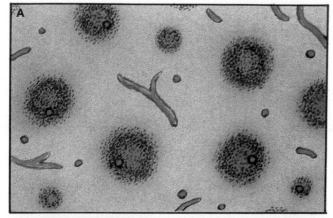

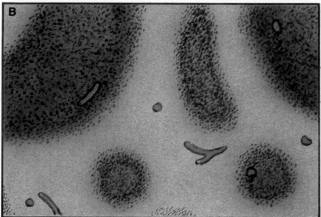

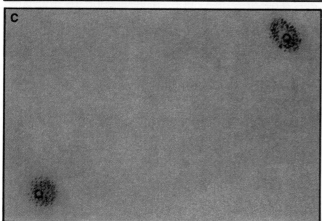

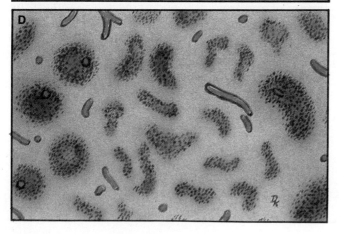

vivors of the nuclear explosions in Hiroshima and Nagasaki. After a latent period of approximately 3 years, this population suffered an increased incidence of chronic myelogenous leukemia, the peak being at 7 years. In Great Britain patients who were treated for ankylosing spondylitis with irradiation of the spine displayed an incidence of this form of leukemia about 13 times that of the general population.

Ninety percent of individuals with chronic myelogenous leukemia have an acquired chromosomal abnormality, the Philadelphia chromosome (Ph¹). This marker chromosome is identified in erythroid, granulocytic, and megakaryocytic cells and occasionally even in lymphoid cells. **Translocation of half of the long arm of chromosome 22, usually to chromosome 9, is demonstrated.** In approximately 5% of the cases translocation to other recipient chromosomes is detected. **The critical event appears to be the loss of a portion of the long arm of chromosome 22.** An oncogene, c-abelson (c-abl), is present at the breakpoint of chromosome 9 and is reciprocally translocated to chromosome 22.

The hematopathologic features of chronic myelogenous leukemia are outlined in Table 20-23. **In the bone marrow, there is trilineage hyperplasia with predominant proliferation of the granulocytic cell series, the myeloid:erythroid ratio varying from 10:1 to 50:1 (normal, 2:1 to 4.5:1).** Megakaryocytes are numerous, but the clustering and atypia of megakaryocytes characteristic of the chronic myeloproliferative syndromes may be lacking. Significant marrow fibrosis is distinctly uncommon.

Splenomegaly, occasionally massive (>1000 g), is seen in 90% of cases. The cut surface of the spleen exhibits a homogeneous expansion of the red pulp (see Fig. 20-21), but the white pulp is not visualized

Figure 20-21. Hematopoietic malignancy—patterns of splenic involvement. The patterns of splenic involvement in hematopoietic malignancies are contrasted with the architectural structure of the normal spleen (*A*). (*B*) In malignancies that primarily involve the lymphoid white pulp (Hodgkin's disease and non-Hodgkin's lymphomas), there is variable expansion of the white pulp with encroachment on the red pulp. (*C*) In malignancies that primarily involve the red pulp (acute non-lymphatic leukemia, myeloproliferative syndromes, malignant histiocytosis, hairy cell leukemia, plasma cell neoplasia, and mast cell disease), there is expansion of the red pulp with encroachment on, and ultimately obliteration of, the white pulp. (*D*) Some malignant disorders both expand the white pulp and initially infiltrate the red pulp (prolymphocytic leukemia, mycosis fungoides, small lymphocytic lymphoma–leukemia, and plasmacytoid lymphocytic lymphoma).

grossly. Microscopically, myeloid metaplasia of the sinuses, and less prominently of the cords, is identified. As the name of the disease indicates, proliferation of immature granulocytic cells is predominant. Islands of erythroid normoblasts and variable numbers of megakaryocytes are also observed. Moderate hepatomegaly is common, with or without myeloid metaplasia in the hepatic sinusoids.

The common laboratory findings in the myeloproliferative syndromes are shown in Table 20-24. Frequently there is a mild, normocytic normochromic anemia. Circulating erythrocytes are usually normal but may exhibit mild anisocytosis and poikilocytosis. **The peripheral blood white cell count is invariably elevated, typically exceeding 20,000 and often increased up to 200,000 per microliter. The entire spectrum of maturing granulocytic cells, from myeloblast to neutrophil, is observed. Myelocytes and neutrophils constitute the most numerous cell types.** Myeloblasts and promyelocytes together account for less than 10% of the peripheral blood leukocytes. Frequently, circulating basophils and eosinophils are increased in number. Blood monocytes may also be increased. Initially there is a moderate thrombocytosis in one-third of the cases. **The leukocyte alkaline phosphatase (LAP) score is typically markedly decreased in chronic myelogenous leukemia.** This low LAP score is useful in distinguishing the leukemia from a leukemoid reaction caused by infection, in which case the LAP is typically increased. However, a markedly decreased LAP score is not diagnostic of chronic myelogenous leukemia, since it may also be observed in such disorders as paroxysmal nocturnal hemoglobinuria, aplastic anemia, and hypophosphatasia. The LAP score increases when chronic myelogenous leukemia progresses to acute leukemia (blast crisis), an event that occurs in about 70% of cases.

In Western countries, chronic myelogenous leukemia constitutes 20% of all the leukemias. It is typically a disorder of middle-aged adults. The age at onset varies from 25 to 60 years, the median age being 45 years. A slight male predominance is observed. The clinical features are presented in Table 20-25. The symptoms relate either to a hypermetabolic state induced by the increased granulocytic cell turnover or to the prominent splenomegaly. Symptoms of hypermetabolism include malaise, weight loss, sweating, and fatigue. Symptoms referable to splenomegaly include early satiety with meals and abdominal discomfort in the left upper quadrant. Hemorrhagic manifestations are due to thrombocytopenia or to qualitative platelet abnormalities, and thrombosis is related to thrombocytosis.

In children and the elderly, the onset of chronic myelogenous leukemia in conjunction with the absence of the Ph[1] chromosome indicates a poor prognosis. The course of the disease is usually characterized by an initial stable, chronic phase, that persists for 2 to 8 years, with a mean of 3 years. Because only a subtle deficiency of granulocytic cell function is seen in the stable phase, with proper clinical management a normal life can be maintained.

In a minority of patients, an accelerated phase of the disease is heralded by an increasing or decreasing white blood cell count and frequently by a blood basophilia. Increasing splenomegaly and prominent symptoms of hypermetabolism provide evidence for disease progression. The accelerated phase is frequently a prelude to a terminal superimposed acute leukemia (blast crisis), the most common cause of death in chronic myelogenous leukemia. A loss of maturation capacity of the granulocytic cell series characterizes the blast crisis. Frequently, additional chromosomal abnormalities, including a second Ph[1] chromosome, are detected in this stage. The response of blast crisis to therapy is poor, and the median survival is only 2 to 3 months. Although the blasts are usually of myeloid origin, in one-quarter to one-third of the cases they originate from lymphoid elements. The median survival in lymphoid blast crisis is approximately 8 months.

Myelofibrosis with Myeloid Metaplasia

Myelofibrosis with myeloid metaplasia (MMM) is a neoplastic disorder of the common hematopoietic precursor cell. The bone marrow shows trilineage hyperplasia, with variable proliferative potential of the erythrocytic, granulocytic, and megakaryocytic cell lines. No single hematopoietic cell line is predominant. **A reactive marrow fibrosis (myelofibrosis) usually accompanies the neoplastic cell proliferation.** The fibroblasts in myelofibrosis with myeloid metaplasia lack neoplastic cell markers, and, as previously mentioned, the fibroblastic proliferation may be due to release of platelet-derived growth factor (PDGF) from the alpha granules of platelets and megakaryocytes. Abnormal secretion of PDGF by the expanded megakaryocyte cell clone in MMM may stimulate bone marrow fibroblasts to secrete the abundant collagen that is characteristic of this disorder.

In MMM there is prominent myeloid metaplasia in the sites of fetal extramedullary hematopoiesis, which include the spleen, the liver, and the lymph nodes. Myeloid metaplasia develops early and may even precede the development of myelofibrosis. Thus, myeloid metaplasia appears to represent an intrinsic expression of the neoplastic process and is

Table 20-23 The Myeloproliferative Syndromes: Hematopathologic Features

	POLYCYTHEMIA VERA	CHRONIC MYELOGENOUS LEUKEMIA	MYELOFIBROSIS WITH MYELOID METAPLASIA	IDIOPATHIC THROMBOCYTHEMIA
Bone Marrow				
Histopathology	Panhyperplasia (predominantly erythroid)	Panhyperplasia (predominantly granulocytic)	Panhyperplasia with fibrosis	Atypical megakaryocytes predominant
M:E ratio	≤ 2:1	10:1 to 50:1	2:1 to 5:1	Unevaluable
Marrow iron	↓ or absent	Normal or ↑	Normal or ↑	Normal to absent
Marrow fibrosis	15–20%	< 10%	90–100%	< 5%
Liver, Spleen				
Extramedullary hematopoiesis (myeloid metaplasia)	Moderate (predominantly erythroid)	Moderate to marked (predominantly granulocytic)	Moderate to marked	Slight (predominantly megakaryocytic)

Table 20-24 The Myeloproliferative Syndromes: Laboratory Features

	POLYCYTHEMIA VERA	CHRONIC MYELOGENOUS LEUKEMIA	MYELOFIBROSIS WITH MYELOID METAPLASIA	IDIOPATHIC THROMBOCYTHEMIA
Hemoglobin	> 20 g/dl	Mild anemia	Mild anemia	Mild anemia
RBC morphology	Slight aniso- and poikilocytosis	Slight aniso- and poikilocytosis	Immature erythrocytes and marked aniso- and poikilocytosis	Hypochromic microcytes
Granulocytes	Normal to mildly increased, may be a few immature forms	Moderate to markedly increased with spectrum of maturation Basophilia	Normal to moderately increased with some immature WBC	Normal to slightly increased
Platelets	Normal to moderately increased	Normal to moderately increased	Increased to decreased	Markedly increased with abnormal forms
Leukocyte alkaline phosphatase (LAP)	Normal to increased	Decreased to absent	Variable	Variable
Cytogenetics	Aneuploid (25%)	Philadelphia chromosome (Ph[1]) (90%)	Aneuploid (50%)	Aneuploid (25%)

(*RBC*, red blood cells; *WBC*, white blood cells)

Table 20-25 The Myeloproliferative Syndromes: Clinical Features

	POLYCYTHEMIA VERA	CHRONIC MYELOGENOUS LEUKEMIA	MYELOFIBROSIS WITH MYELOID METAPLASIA	IDIOPATHIC THROMBOCYTHEMIA
Male:female	1.2:1	3:2	1:1	1.2:1
Peak age range (years)	40–60	25–60	50–70	50–70
Clinical symptoms	Headache, dizziness, pruritus	Asymptomatic or LUQ discomfort, fatigability	Asymptomatic or LUQ discomfort, fatigability	Asymptomatic or LUQ discomfort
Clinical signs	Bleeding, thrombosis	Easy bruising, bleeding	Weight loss, gouty arthritis	Bleeding, thrombosis
Splenomegaly	75%	90%	100%	30% (slight)
Hepatomegaly	40%	50%	80%	40% (slight)
Leukemic conversion	1–3%	70% (blast crisis)	15–20%	Uncommon (incidence unknown)
Median survival (years)	13	3–4	3–4	Unknown

(*LUQ*, left upper quadrant)

not compensatory for marrow failure due to myelofibrosis. Myeloid metaplasia probably is the result of bone marrow precursor cells gaining access to the circulation and proliferating selectively in sites of fetal extramedullary hematopoiesis. The cause of MMM is unknown. In a minority of cases it may relate to prior bone marrow damage due to irradiation or exposure to benzene or unknown toxins. Polycythemia vera and chronic myelogenous leukemia may progress to a clinicopathologic appearance indistinguishable from that of MMM.

The hematopathologic features of MMM are listed in Table 20-23. **In the bone marrow, there is panhyperplasia of the hematopoietic cells, and clusters of atypical megakaryocytes with hyperchromatic nuclei are conspicuous.** Myelofibrosis involves particularly the central flat bones and the proximal long bones. Osteosclerosis (thickening of the bony trabeculae) may also be present. Early in the course of the disease, a cellular phase without accompanying myelofibrosis or osteosclerosis is common. This early cellular phase must be differentiated from chronic myelogenous leukemia.

The spleen in MMM is customarily massively enlarged, weighing up to 4000 g. It is firm and homogeneously red-purple, and the white pulp usually cannot be visualized (see Fig. 20-21). Microscopically, there is prominent myeloid metaplasia of the red pulp, especially of the sinusoids. Often the liver shows myeloid metaplasia of the hepatic sinusoids.

The common laboratory findings in MMM are listed in Table 20-24. Typically the blood shows a normocytic normochromic anemia and a leukoerythroblastic picture, with circulating immature erythroid and granulocytic cells and giant platelets. **Teardrop-shaped erythrocytes are particularly characteristic of MMM and serve as a diagnostic feature because they are inconspicuous in chronic myelogenous leukemia and polycythemia vera.** A mild leukocytosis of up to 20,000 per microliter is common. Alternatively, there may be leukopenia. A blood basophilia or eosinophilia may be observed. Platelet counts are variable but are usually normal to low. The LAP score is usually normal to increased, but in 20% of cases it is decreased. Chromosomal abnormalities, most commonly C-group trisomy, are found in half of the cases but are of no prognostic significance. **The Ph[1] chromosome is lacking, a finding which, together with the typically normal to high LAP score, is useful in distinguishing MMM from chronic myelogenous leukemia.**

The clinical features of MMM are presented in Table 20-25. The disorder occurs principally in middle-aged to elderly persons, with a median age of 60 years. There is no sex predominance. The course in MMM is usually characterized by progressive anemia, with gradually increasing transfusion requirements, and by progressive enlargement of the liver and spleen. The symptoms in MMM relate principally to the consequences of the anemia and to the splenomegaly. The median survival is 3 years. Infection, hemorrhage and thromboses—due to leukopenia and conditions that reflect qualitative platelet abnormalities or thrombocytosis—are the usual causes of death. In 15% to 20% of cases death is due to a superimposed acute nonlymphocytic leukemia.

Primary Hemorrhagic Thrombocythemia

Primary, or idiopathic, hemorrhagic thrombocythemia is a neoplastic disorder of the common hematopoietic precursor cell in which the megakaryocytic cell line is predominantly affected. Primary hemorrhagic thrombocythemia is the least common of the chronic myeloproliferative syndromes. The cause and pathogenesis of primary hemorrhagic thrombocythemia are not known. The hematopathologic features are outlined in Table 20-23. The bone marrow displays a pronounced megakaryocytic cell hyperplasia, with greatly increased platelet production. The neoplastic megakaryocytes exhibit atypical morphologic features, which include bizarrely lobulated and hyperchromatic nuclei. A mild erythroid and granulocytic cell hyperplasia may also be observed. Bone marrow iron is frequently decreased. Generally, marrow fibrosis is not seen. Modest splenomegaly and hepatomegaly are observed in one-third of cases. On cut surface, the red pulp is expanded (see Fig. 20-21). Histologically, myeloid metaplasia with predominance of proliferating megakaryocytes is noted, particularly in the sinusoids. Proliferating megakaryocytes may be numerous in the hepatic sinusoids.

The blood platelet count typically exceeds 1 million per microliter and may reach levels of 3 million per microliter or more. Circulating giant platelets (megathrombocytes), bizarrely shaped platelets, and megakaryocyte fragments are present. Qualitative platelet function abnormalities are common; for example, abnormalities of platelet aggregation occur in over 50% of cases. Generally, there is a mild neutrophilic leukocytosis of up to 20,000 per microliter without an increase in immature granulocytic cells. A mild iron-deficiency anemia is common and secondary to gastrointestinal blood loss. The LAP score is usually normal but may be increased or decreased. Cytogenetic study reveals aneuploidy in 25% of cases.

Primary hemorrhagic thrombocythemia occurs most commonly in persons 50 to 70 years of age. The symptoms relate most frequently to splenomegaly or to anemia, but hemorrhagic and thrombotic events are common. For poorly understood reasons, the increase in platelets more commonly predisposes to hemorrhage than to thrombosis. Bleeding into the gastrointestinal or genitourinary tract and in the skin occurs frequently. Thrombosis is seen in any organ. Thromboses in the spleen with consequent infarctions are especially important; they may result in splenic atrophy, in which case the decreased pooling capacity of the spleen is associated with a poor prognosis because of the loss of a sequestration site for the immensely increased blood platelet pool. Similarly, splenectomy may be associated with a catastrophic increase in blood platelets and is therefore contraindicated.

The natural history of primary hemorrhagic thrombocythemia is unclear, since there are few long-term studies of patients with this uncommon disorder. The median survival appears to be about 13 years, a duration similar to that associated with polycythemia vera. In a minority of cases progression to acute nonlymphocytic leukemia has been recorded, but its incidence is not known.

Primary hemorrhagic thrombocythemia must be distinguished from the reactive thrombocytosis that occurs in infections, inflammatory disorders, a variety of neoplasms, and iron deficiency. Thrombocytosis following hemorrhage, hemolysis, or splenectomy should also be ruled out. However, secondary causes of thrombocytosis rarely produce platelet counts in excess of 1 million per microliter. Moreover, in such cases the platelet counts return to normal levels with treatment or with resolution of the precipitating disorder.

Acute Myeloproliferative Syndromes: The Acute Nonlymphocytic Leukemias

The acute nonlymphocytic, or myelogenous, leukemias are a heterogeneous, but interrelated, group of neoplastic disorders of the hematopoietic precursor cells of the bone marrow. They are malignant proliferations that originate either from single multipotential precursor cells or from precursor cells with restricted lineage potential and thus exhibit trilineage, bilineage, or single-lineage descent.

In the acute nonlymphocytic leukemias (ANLL),

Table 20-26 Factors Predisposing to Acute Nonlymphocytic Leukemia

Genetic influences
  Sibling with leukemia
Down's syndrome
Syndromes with chromosome instability
  Bloom's syndrome
  Fanconi's anemia
  Ataxia telangiectasia
  Kostman's syndrome
Chemical exposure
  Benzene
Alkylating agent chemotherapy
Ionizing radiation
Myelodysplastic syndromes
Chronic myeloproliferative syndromes
Aplastic anemia
Paroxysmal nocturnal hemoglobinuria

the tumor cell generation time (time for one cell division) is prolonged compared with that of normal bone marrow blast cells. Thus, ANLL does not represent a disorder of rapidly proliferating neoplastic cells; rather, the pathophysiology involves a failure of maturation of the neoplastic cell clone. Because of this failure and the continued slow neoplastic cell proliferation, the bone marrow is gradually replaced by blast cells, with consequent encroachment on and loss of normal hematopoiesis. **The most important complications in ANLL, therefore, are progressive anemia, leukopenia, and thrombocytopenia.**

The cause of this form of leukemia is unknown. The risk factors for the development of ANLL include myelotoxic agents, certain chromosomal abnormalities, and several predisposing hematologic disorders (Table 20-26). The most common myelotoxic agents are ionizing radiation, benzene, and the antineoplastic alkylating agents. **In doses exceeding 100 rads, there is a linear relationship between radiation and the risk of ANLL.** The antineoplastic alkylating agents induce chromosomal breakage and are associated with a minor increase in incidence. **Downs' syndrome and the chromosomal instability syndromes are predisposing chromosomal abnormalities. In Downs' syndrome (trisomy 21) there is approximately a 15-fold increased risk of developing acute leukemia, principally acute lymphoblastic leukemia but in a minority of cases acute nonlymphocytic leukemia.** In the chromosomal instability syndromes, such as Bloom's syndrome, Fanconi's anemia, and ataxia telangiectasia, there is a small but significant increased risk of ANLL.

Hematologic disorders associated with an increased risk of ANLL include the chronic myeloproliferative syndromes, the myelodysplastic syndromes, aplastic anemia, and paroxysmal nocturnal hemoglobinuria. **Superimposed ANLL may constitute the terminal event in all of the chronic myeloproliferative syndromes, in particular chronic myelogenous leukemia, in which superimposed blast crisis occurs in approximately 70% of cases.** In the myelodysplastic syndromes, the incidence of superimposed acute leukemia is dependent on the subtype of myelodysplasia. In myelodysplastic syndromes in which abnormalities of all three cell lines are observed with accompanying pancytopenia, up to 50% of those affected are at risk of acute nonlymphocytic leukemia. In aplastic anemia and paroxysmal nocturnal hemoglobinuria, there is also an increased risk of ANLL. At least some acute leukemias are associated with transmissible RNA tumor viruses that show homologies with leukemogenic viruses of lower mammals. To date, however, only the Japanese type adult T cell leukemia-lymphoma, a lymphoid neoplasm, has been conclusively linked with a C-type RNA tumor virus, mainly the HTLV-1.

On Wright-Giemsa–stained smears of blood or bone marrow aspirates, the neoplastic blast cells in ANLL have delicate chromatin, frequently multiple nucleoli, and gray-blue cytoplasm. Pink-purple (azurophilic) granules represent primary lysomes. **Auer rods, an aberrant morphologic expression of the primary lysosomes, are azurophilic, rod shaped, cytoplasmic structures that are noted in up to 40% of the cases (Fig. 20-22).** The morphologic variants of ANLL, described by the French-American-British (FAB) task force on acute leukemia, are shown in Figure 20-23. In general, the FAB morphologic variants exhibit a similar clinical course. In acute promyelocytic leukemia the neoplastic blast cells have abundant azurophilic granules or Auer rods, both of which have tissue thromboplastin–like activity. Release of the granules, especially with therapy-associated cell lysis, may trigger the syndrome of disseminated intravascular coagulation. Acute monocytic leukemia, an aggressive variant of ANLL, is characterized by prominent infiltration of the skin, gums, and perirectal soft tissues, a high white blood cell count, and a poor response to therapy. Acute megakaryoblastic leukemia, a recently described variant now included as FAB M7 in the French-American-British classification of ANLL, presents either as a usual variant of ANLL or as a rare disorder known as acute myelofibrosis. The clinical syndrome of acute myelofibrosis includes pancytopenia, hyperplasia of all marrow elements, conspicuous fibrosis, and a rapid progression to an acute leukemia. The blast cells express the megakaryocyte cell markers Factor

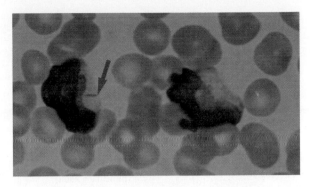

Figure 20-22. Acute nonlymphocytic leukemia. Two blast cells, one with a cytoplasmic Auer rod *(arrow)*, are identified on a Wright-Giemsa–stained peripheral blood smear.

VIII and platelet peroxidase. In acute myelofibrosis the lack of splenomegaly is useful in excluding the diagnosis of myelofibrosis with myeloid metaplasia. A rapidly fatal outcome is the rule.

The significance of the FAB classification lies in its precise grouping of variants of the nonlymphocytic and, as will be discussed, the lymphoblastic leukemias, thus aiding in their distinction. The differentiation of acute nonlymphocytic from acute lymphoblastic leukemias is important because of their markedly different prognoses and appropriate therapies. In addition to precise morphologic subclassification as defined by the FAB criteria, cytochemical studies are frequently required to distinguish acute nonlymphocytic from acute lymphoblastic leukemia (see Table 20-7; Fig. 20-24). Demonstration of the nuclear DNA-polymerizing enzyme terminal deoxynucleotidyl transferase (Tdt) identifies the acute leukemia as having a lymphoid rather than a nonlymphocytic phenotype; however, Tdt activity is also demonstrated in 2% to 5% of otherwise typical cases of ANLL (Table 20-27), so results must be interpreted cautiously.

Variable bone marrow replacement by blast cells is found in ANLL (Fig. 20-25). Although initially the leukemic blast cells are interspersed among the residual normal hematopoietic cells, progression to complete bone marrow replacement usually occurs (Fig. 20-26). Morphologic abnormalities of the residual maturing erythroid and granulocytic precursor cells, an abnormality termed "dyspoiesis," are often present. Dyspoiesis is distinctly uncommon in the acute lymphoblastic leukemias and therefore suggests that the leukemia has a nonlymphocytic origin. **A characteristic abnormality is an increase in small, single-lobed megakaryocytes.** Myelofibrosis may occur in any variant of ANLL.

MORPHOLOGY	CLASSIFICATION	NUCLEUS	NUCLEOLUS	CHROMATIN	CYTOPLASM
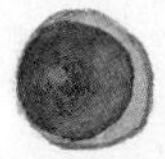	L1 ACUTE LYMPHOBLASTIC (principally pediatric)	Uniformly round, small	Single, indistinct	Slightly reticulated with perinucleolar clumping	Scant, blue
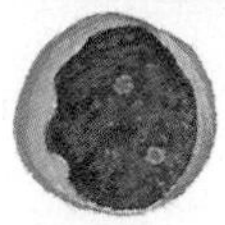	L2 LYMPHOBLASTIC (principally adult)	Irregular	Single to several, indistinct	Fine	Moderate, pale
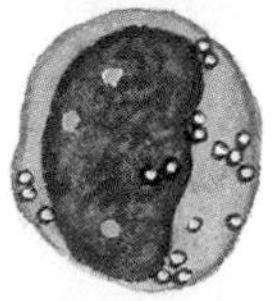	L3 BURKITT'S	Round to oval	Two to five	Coarse with clear parachromatin	Moderate, blue, vacuolated
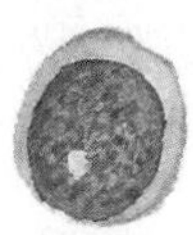	M1 MYELOBLASTIC (without maturation)	Round to oval	Single to multiple, distinct	Fine	Scant, nongranulated
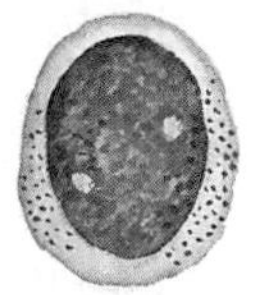	M2 MYELOBLASTIC (with maturation)	Round to oval	Single to multiple, distinct	Fine	Moderate azurophilic granules with or without Auer rods
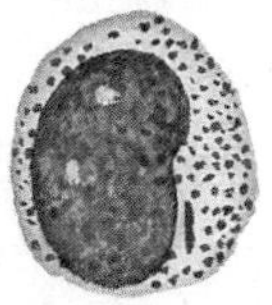	M3 PROMYELOCYTIC	Round to indented to lobed	Single to multiple (granules obscure)	Fine	Prominent azurophilic granules and/or Auer rods
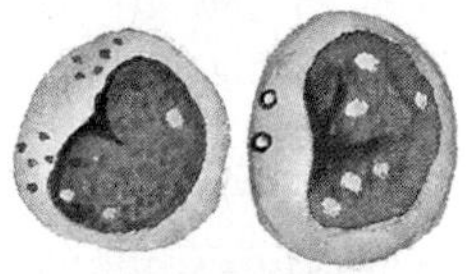	M4 MYELOMONOCYTIC (biphasic M1 and M5)	Round to indented, folded	Single to multiple, distinct	Fine	Moderate, blue to gray, may be granulated
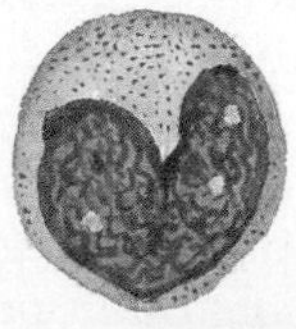	M5 MONOCYTIC	Round to indented, folded	Single to multiple, distinct	Variable, lacy or ropy	Scant to moderate, gray-blue, dustlike lavender granules
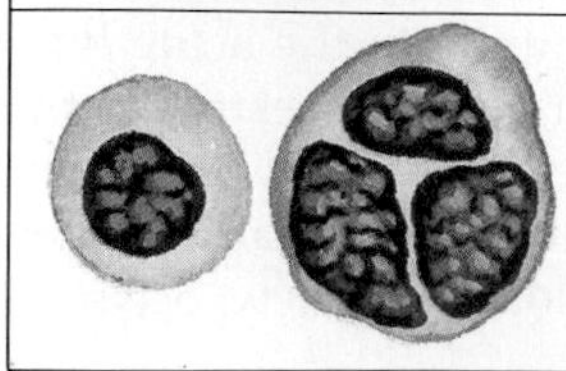	M6 ERYTHROLEUKEMIA	Single to bizarre multinucleated, multilobed	Single to multiple, distinct	Open "megaloblastoid"	Abundant, red to blue

Figure 20-23.   Acute leukemia—French-American-British classification.

Clinically, variable splenomegaly, hepatomegaly, and lymphadenopathy are observed. The initial leukemic cell infiltration involves the red pulp of the spleen (see Fig. 20-21), the sinusoids of the liver, and the paracortex of the lymph nodes (Fig. 20-27). Occasionally, within and outside of the bone marrow, there are discrete tumor masses composed of variable proportions of myeloblasts and promyelocytes. These tumors, termed **granulocytic sarcomas** or **chloromas**, commonly are located in the bones and the adjacent soft tissues of the orbit, the facial bones, the lymph nodes, and other soft tissue sites. Histologically, granulocytic sarcomas are difficult to distinguish from the large cell lymphomas or undifferentiated carcinomas. A positive chloroacetate esterase stain, the demonstration of lysozyme by the immuno-peroxidase technique, and the presence of azurophilic granules confirm the diagnosis of granulocytic sarcoma (Fig. 20-28).

The common laboratory findings in ANLL reflect the depletion of normal hematopoietic cell elements and the presence of blast cells. Frequently there is neutropenia with dyspoietic features of the residual maturing granulocytic cell series. The total white blood cell count may be decreased, normal, or increased up to 200,000 per microliter. Blast cells are generally predominant, particularly when the white blood cell count is increased. A moderate normocytic normochromic anemia is common. Basophilic stippling, circulating normoblasts, and other features of erythroid dyspoiesis may be observed. Thrombocytopenia is a common finding, although generally not as marked as in acute lymphoblastic leukemia. Serum and urinary lysozyme levels are elevated, particularly in acute monocytic leukemia, because monocyte cytoplasmic lysosomes contain abundant lysozyme. In acute promyelocytic leukemia (FAB M3) cytogenetic study reveals a characteristic translocation in approximately half of the cases (t15q + :17q-). Acute myeloid leukemia with maturation (FAB M2) frequently exhibits a characteristic translocation (t8q-:21q+). In radiation-induced or cytotoxic drug–induced acute leukemia, there may be loss of chromosome 5 or 7, or there may be trisomy 8.

ANLL constitutes 20% of all the leukemias, 85% of the acute leukemias in adults, and 15% to 20% of the acute leukemias in children. The clinical manifestations include fatigue due to anemia, infection because of granulocytopenia, and bleeding secondary to thrombocytopenia. The risk of infection correlates directly with the severity and duration of the granulocytopenia. Infection is common when the white blood cell count is less than 500 per microliter and

Table 20-27 Terminal Deoxynucleotidyl Transferase (Tdt) in Hematologic Disease

DISEASE	PERCENT POSITIVE
Acute lymphoblastic leukemia	80–90
Lymphoblastic lymphoma	90
Chronic granulocytic leukemia in blast crisis	30
Acute undifferentiated leukemia	60
Acute nonlymphocytic leukemia	2–5

Reaction	LYMPHOID	MYELOID	MONOCYTOID
PAS			
CAE			
SBB			
APh			
ANAE			
ANAE/NaF			

Figure 20-24. Acute leukemia—cytochemistry. (See Table 20-7 for key to abbreviations)

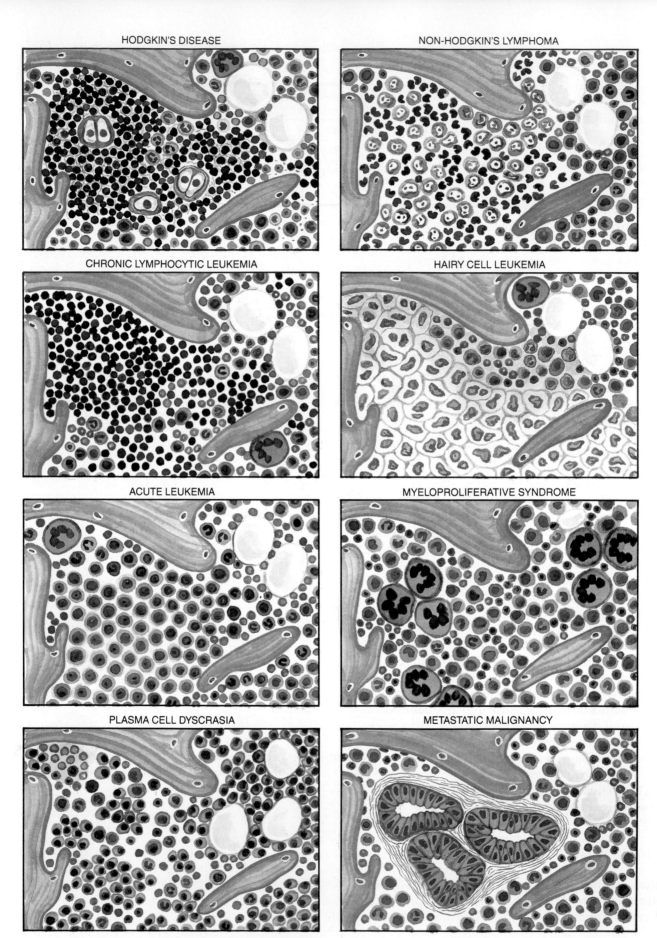

Figure 20-25. Bone marrow biopsy in hematologic disease.

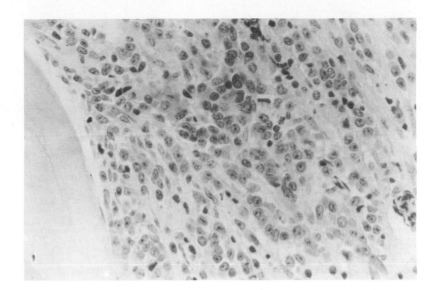

Figure 20-26 Acute nonlymphocytic leukemia. The bone marrow is diffusely hypercellular and consists largely of myeloblasts.

inevitable when the count is less than 200 per microliter. Similarly, the risk of bleeding correlates directly with the severity of the thrombocytopenia. With platelet counts of less than 20,000, and especially those of less than 5000 per microliter, there is a serious risk of gastrointestinal and central nervous system hemorrhage. Leukostasis or the occlusion of small blood vessels by blast cells occurs when the white blood cell count exceeds 100,000 per microliter. Blast cell infiltration of the leptomeninges produces the syndrome of leukemic meningitis. Arthralgias and bone pain are caused by expansion of the bone marrow spaces and by periosteal infiltration by leukemic blast cells. Hyperuricemia due to leukemic blast cell turnover predisposes to the complications of uric acid nephropathy and kidney stones.

The most common cause of death in ANLL is infection. Hemorrhage is a less frequent cause of death than in the past because of the efficacy of platelet transfusions. Leukostasis in patients with high blast cell counts may cause fatal brain hemorrhage.

Malignant Disorders of the Mononuclear Phagocyte System

Malignant Histiocytosis

Malignant histiocytosis is an aggressive and rapidly fatal systemic neoplasm of the histiocyte macrophages of the mononuclear phagocyte system. Malignant transformation of fixed tissue histiocytes and macrophages affects any organ in which the mononuclear phagocytes are normally found.

The cause is unknown, but a simultaneous onset in several family members has been described, suggesting an environmental or infectious agent. Malignant histiocytosis has also been described as a superimposed neoplasm in patients with previously diagnosed acute lymphoblastic leukemia. The pathophysiology of malignant histiocytosis relates to the systemic proliferation of functioning malignant histiocytes and the nonfunctioning precursor cells of these histiocytes. Typically, pancytopenia is caused by (1) phagocytosis by malignant histiocytes, which results in the destruction of erythrocytes, leukocytes, and platelets, and (2) replacement of the normal bone marrow hematopoietic tissues by the tumor cells. The physical findings include splenomegaly, hepatomegaly, mild lymphadenopathy, and papulonodular skin lesions.

Cytologically, malignant histiocytes exhibit bizarre and atypical morphologic features. The nuclei are single or multiple, are often eccentrically situated, and may be multilobed. The heterochromatin is irregularly clumped in a background of clear parachromatin, and the nucleoli are prominent. The pale to pink cytoplasm is abundant, particularly in the more mature histiocytes. The mitotic rate is high and abnormal configurations, such as tripolar or quadripolar forms may be observed. **Striking phagocytosis of erythrocytes, leukocytes, platelets, and nuclear and cytoplasmic debris is seen, particularly in the**

(Text continues on p. 1082)

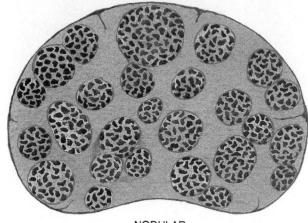

NODULAR

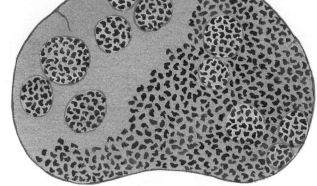

NODULAR AND DIFFUSE

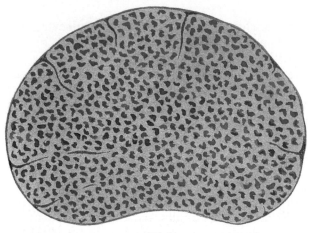

DIFFUSE

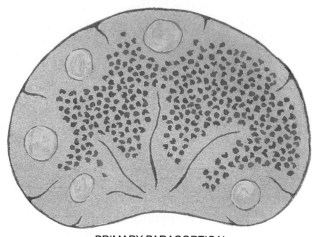

PRIMARY PARACORTICAL

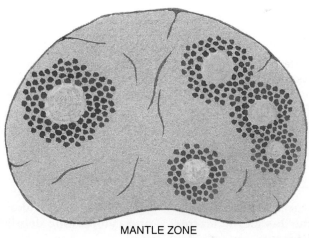

MANTLE ZONE

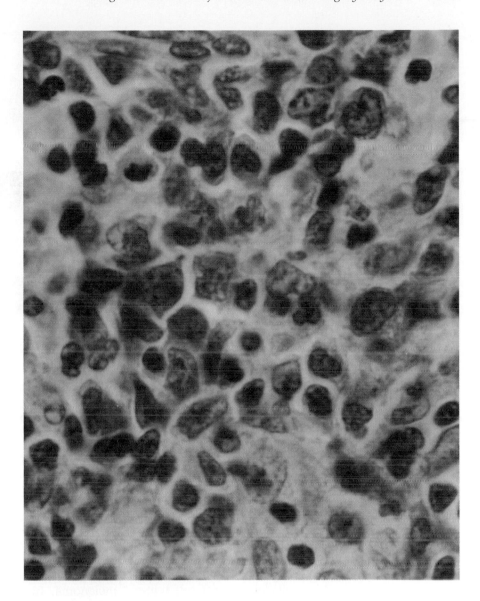

Figure 20-28. Granulocytic sarcoma (chloroma). A diffuse soft tissue infiltrate of the orbit contains primitive blast cells with round to lobulated nuclei. The napthol-AS-D chloroacetate esterase stain is focally positive (red).

Figure 20-27. The lymph node—patterns of involvement in leukemia and lymphoma. In the follicular lymphomas, there is replacement of the normal lymph node architecture by uniform nodular aggregates of neoplastic B-lymphocytes. In the follicular and diffuse lymphomas, there is variable replacement of the node architecture by neoplastic B-lymphocytes in both follicular and diffuse architectural patterns. In the diffuse lymphomas, there is partial to (frequently) total obliteration of the normal nodal architecture by neoplastic B- or T-lymphocytes. The architectural pattern is diffuse without proclivity to form follicles. With primary paracortical involvement, there is initial neoplastic cell infiltration of the T-cell–dependent paracortex. Involvement may progress to total effacement of the lymph node architecture. In mantle zone lymphomas, there is initial variable expansion of the B-cell cuff that surrounds normal germinal centers. Ultimately, there may be progression to total obliteration of the normal lymph node architecture.

MALIGNANT HISTIOCYTOSIS   "TRUE" HISTIOCYTIC LYMPHOMA

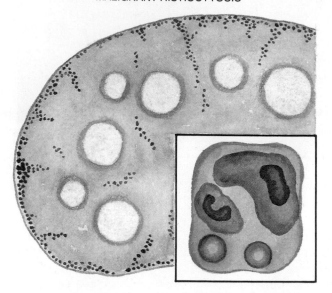

Figure 20-29. Malignant histiocytosis and "true" histiocytic lymphoma. The patterns of lymph node involvement in malignant disorders of the mononuclear phagocyte system are shown. In malignant histiocytosis there is initial involvement of the nodal sinuses, which are expanded by morphologically atypical malignant histiocytes. Neoplastic cell phagocytosis of erythrocytes and other formed elements of the blood may be observed. Ultimately, there may be progression to complete obliteration of the lymph node architecture. In "true" histiocytic lymphoma there is partial to total obliteration of the lymph node architecture by large, transformed cells that are morphologically indistinguishable from those of the large cell lymphomas.

more differentiated histiocytes (Fig. 20-29). Occasionally, bizarre binucleated or multinucleated cells with prominent nucleoli simulate the neoplastic Reed-Sternberg cells of Hodgkin's disease or the pleomorphic tumor giant cells of some T-cell lymphomas. A population of primitive cells with scant cytoplasm, so-called prohistiocytes, which resemble the blast cells of acute leukemia, may be identified. The malignant histiocytes usually exhibit cell markers characteristic of histiocyte macrophages. Lysozyme or muramidase levels may be elevated in the serum or urine. Detection of elevated lysozyme levels, produced by the malignant histiocytes, suggests the diagnosis of malignant histiocytosis.

Prominent sites of neoplastic histiocytic cell infiltration include the spleen, liver, lymph nodes, bone marrow, and skin. In the spleen the neoplastic histiocytic cells principally infiltrate the cords and sinusoids of the red pulp and eventually obliterate the white pulp (see Fig. 20-21). Erythrophagocytosis by the malignant histiocytes is best appreciated in the spleen. In the liver atypical neoplastic Kupffer cells are observed in the hepatic sinusoids. The subcap-

sular and radiating sinuses represent the sites of initial involvement of the lymph nodes (see Fig. 20-29).

Histologically, malignant histiocytosis must be distinguished from metastatic carcinoma and malignant melanoma, tumors that also commonly initially involve the sinuses of lymph nodes. Infiltration of the lymph node stroma by malignant histiocytes may occur secondarily, and the nodal architecture may ultimately be effaced. The histopathologic appearance may then be indistinguishable from that of the large cell lymphomas. A characteristic finding in the lymph nodes is prominent plasma cell infiltration of the medullary cords. In the skin the deep dermis typically shows perivascular and periadnexal infiltration.

Malignant histiocytosis may occur in persons of any age, but middle-aged and elderly men are most commonly affected. The presentation is usually dramatic, with a sudden onset characterized by fever, weight loss, and pancytopenia. The course is rapidly progressive, and the median survival is about 6 months. Death is usually caused by infection or, less commonly, hemorrhage. Infrequently, the course is more indolent, and the disease is initially localized to the spleen or other site, in which case the label "chronic malignant histiocytosis" is applied.

Malignant histiocytosis may be simulated by certain of the non-Hodgkin's lymphomas as well as by some benign reactive processes. For example, the clinical presentation may be similar in some malignant T-cell lymphomas in which the neoplastic T cells secrete a lymphokine that activates mononuclear phagocytes. The reactive proliferation of these benign, activated phagocytes may dominate the histologic appearance and obscure the underlying T-cell lymphoma; immunologic marker studies may then be required to identify the neoplastic T cells. Malignant histiocytosis must also be distinguished from the benign disorder infection-induced hemophagocytic reticulosis. In this disorder there is also prominent phagocytosis of the formed elements of the peripheral blood, but the phagocytic macrophages lack cellular atypia, and the course is self-limited.

"True" Histiocytic Lymphoma

In 5% or less of malignant neoplasms with the histologic appearance of a large cell lymphoma, neoplastic cell markers characteristic of mononuclear phagocytes are identified. Malignant tumors with these phenotypic markers are therefore not lymphomas or neoplasms of lymphoid cells, but rather true neoplasms of the mononuclear phagocyte system. Cytologically, **they are indistinguishable from some lymphomas of the large cell type** (see Fig. 20-29). In "true" histiocytic lymphoma, cytochemical stains performed on tissue imprints are generally positive for alpha-naphthyl acetate esterase sensitive to sodium fluoride inhibition and for alpha-naphthyl butyrate esterase. Immunohistochemical demonstration of lysozyme or alpha-1 anti-chymotrypsin on tissue sections confirms the cell origin of mononuclear phagocytes.

The Lymphocytic Leukemias

Chronic Lymphocytic Leukemia

Chronic lymphocytic leukemia is a malignant, clonal disorder of B-lymphocytes. The neoplastic cell is a **hypoproliferative, immunologically incompetent** small lymphocyte. The cell of origin may be the small memory B-lymphocyte, which in the lymph nodes is found in the medullary cords. **The disease distribution in chronic lymphocytic leukemia is leukemic,** **with primary involvement of the bone marrow and secondary release to the peripheral blood. The recirculating lymphocytes selectively infiltrate the lymph nodes, the spleen, and the liver. Therefore, as the disease progresses, lymphadenopathy, splenomegaly, and hepatomegaly develop.**

The cause is unknown, and there is no known association with ionizing radiation or with myelotoxic agents. Genetic influences may be important. **Of all the leukemias, chronic lymphocytic leukemia most conclusively demonstrates familial case clustering.** Additionally, the disease is rare in Japan and other Asian countries, and the incidence is still low, although slightly increased, among Asians who live in Western countries. **In Western countries chronic lymphocytic leukemia is the most common type of leukemia, comprising about one-quarter of all the leukemias** (Fig. 20-30).

There are possible hormonal and age-related influences in chronic lymphocytic leukemia. Male predominance is more accentuated in this disorder than in the other leukemias, with a male:female ratio of 2:1. The disease is observed most frequently in the elderly, the mean age at diagnosis being 60 years.

The pathophysiology is traced to the progressive accumulation of malignant lymphocytes in the bone marrow and in extramedullary tissue sites and to the secondary immunologic deficiency with hypogammaglobulinemia. Generalized lymphadenopathy is usual, but localized enlargement of lymph node groups is also common. The lymph nodes are soft and pale gray. The spleen is moderately enlarged and on cut surface exhibits a generalized enlargement of the white pulp with occasional prominent tumor nodules (Fig. 20-31). The liver is also moderately enlarged, but discrete tumor masses are usually not identified. The respiratory and gastrointestinal tracts, and less commonly the lungs, pleura, and other tissue sites, may be infiltrated. Cutaneous involvement appears as papulonodular lesions or as a more diffuse dermatitis.

In the bone marrow three distinctive microscopic patterns of lymphocytic infiltration are recognized: interstitial, nodular, and diffuse (see Fig. 20-25). The initial pattern of lymphocytic cell infiltration is often interstitial, with an increased population of lymphocytes irregularly distributed among normally maturing hematopoietic cells. The lymphocytes often cluster into cohesive nodular aggregates separated by normal hematopoietic stroma. Both the interstitial and the nodular patterns of tumor cell infiltration are associated with a favorable prognosis. Progression to a diffuse pattern of involvement, with obliteration of

(Text continues on p. 1086)

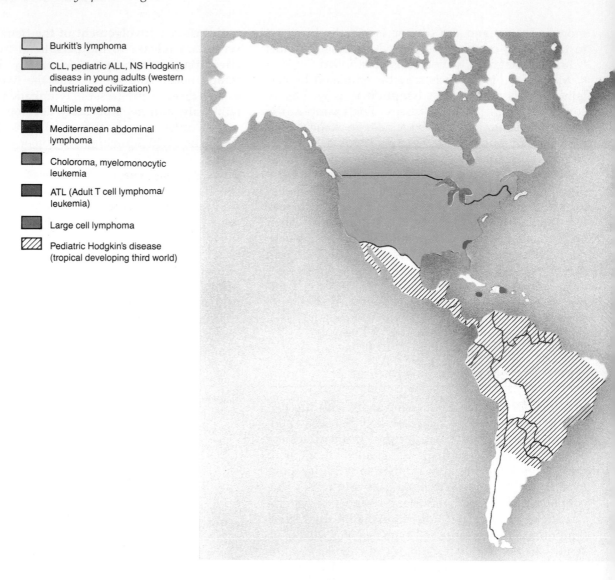

Burkitt's lymphoma

CLL, pediatric ALL, NS Hodgkin's disease in young adults (western industrialized civilization)

Multiple myeloma

Mediterranean abdominal lymphoma

Choloroma, myelomonocytic leukemia

ATL (Adult T cell lymphoma/ leukemia)

Large cell lymphoma

Pediatric Hodgkin's disease (tropical developing third world)

Figure 20-30.   Global epidemiology of lymphoma and leukemia. Burkitt's lymphoma is prominent in tropical equatorial Africa and in parts of New Guinea. In Western industrialized countries, including the United States and Western Europe, chronic lymphocytic leukemia, pediatric acute lymphoblastic leukemia, and nodular sclerosing Hodgkin's disease in young adults are common. Multiple myeloma is common in South Africa. Mediterranean abdominal lymphoma occurs commonly in the Eastern Mediterranean basin. Adult-type T-cell leukemia-lymphoma is common in the Southwestern islands of Japan, in certain Caribbean islands, and in the Southeastern United States. Acute myelomonocytic leukemia with chloromas is common in parts of Turkey. Large cell lymphomas are common in Japan, China, and Egypt. In tropical Third World countries, aggressive Hodgkin's disease is common in children.

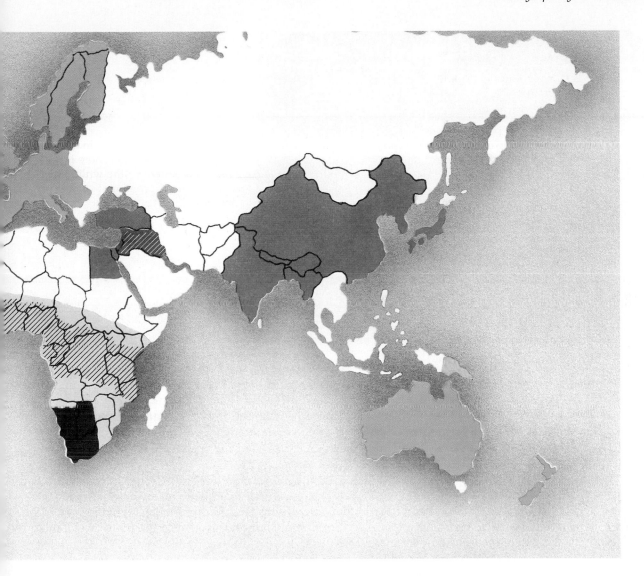

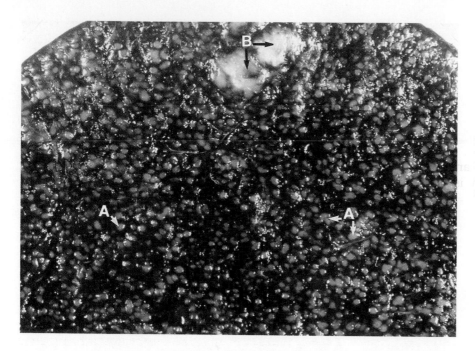

Figure 20-31. The spleen in chronic lymphocytic leukemia. There is diffuse enlargement of the white pulp *(A)*, with focal prominent tumor nodules *(B)*.

normal hematopoietic elements and fat cells, is associated with a poor prognosis. Regardless of the pattern of infiltration, when neoplastic lymphocytes replace more than half of the normal marrow elements, peripheral blood cytopenias are observed. The pattern of infiltration in involved soft tissues is always diffuse.

The neoplastic cells of chronic lymphocytic leukemia resemble normal small lymphocytes. The nuclei are round, the chromatin compact, the nucleoli inconspicuous, and the cytoplasm scant. Mitotic figures are rare, a finding that reflects the low proliferative potential of the neoplastic lymphocytes. Clusters of

partially transformed lymphoid cells, with round vesicular nuclei and more abundant cytoplasm, are common. Although they are characteristic of chronic lymphocytic leukemia in tissue sections, these clusters, called proliferation centers, have no prognostic significance.

In the blood the absolute lymphocyte count is elevated, exceeding 15,000 and occasionally 100,000 per microliter. The predominant circulating cell is a normal small lymphocyte, but often there is a variable size range, with admixed medium-sized lymphocytes (Fig. 20-32). Some tumor cells display large central nucleoli, in which case they are termed "prolympho-

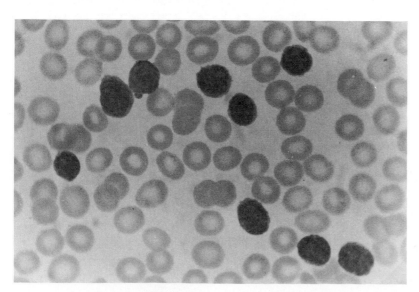

Figure 20-32. Chronic lymphocytic leukemia. Numerous small to medium-sized lymphocytes are seen in the peripheral blood smear.

cytes." Occasionally primitive lymphoblast-like cells are noted. The neoplastic lymphocytes are fragile and easily ruptured on preparation of the blood smear. The resultant amorphous, dark blue nuclear remnants, called "smudge cells," are characteristic of chronic lymphocytic leukemia.

The neoplastic B cells express limited surface membrane monoclonal immunoglobulin, usually IgM kappa. If the absolute peripheral blood lymphocyte count is only modestly increased and the diagnosis of chronic lymphocytic leukemia is in doubt, the demonstration of monoclonality or of light-chain restriction is accepted as evidence of B-cell neoplasia. The abnormal B cells form spontaneous rosettes with mouse red blood cells and may express Fc and complement receptors. Sometime during the clinical course, hypogammaglobulinemia is detected in half the cases. In 5% of cases a monoclonal serum immunoglobulin (paraprotein), usually IgM kappa, is detected. Trisomy of chromosome 12 has been reported in up to one-third of patients. A specific chromosomal translocation, t(11;14), may be identified.

The natural history of chronic lymphocytic leukemia is highly variable. Initially, there may be no associated symptoms, and the diagnosis is first suggested by examination of a routine peripheral blood smear or by the incidental detection of splenomegaly or lymphadenopathy. The Rai clinical staging system (Table 20-28), which is based on the extent of soft tissue involvement and the degree of compromise of bone marrow function at the time of diagnosis, has clinical utility in assessing prognosis. As the disease progresses, anemia may be caused by hypersplenism, bone marrow replacement, or autoimmune hemolytic anemia. Bleeding may result from thrombocytopenia owing to hypersplenism, marrow replacement, and immunologic destruction of platelets. Bacterial pneumonia and other infections are common, reflecting both hypogammaglobulinemia and neutropenia induced by the disease or by therapy. Occasionally there may be complicating viral infections, such as herpes zoster.

The median survival in chronic lymphocytic leukemia is 6 years, and the natural history is not altered by therapy. Infection is the leading cause of death.

In 5% of cases of chronic lymphocytic leukemia, there is a superimposed large cell lymphoma, the so-called **Richter's syndrome.** This syndrome probably represents a dedifferentiation or transformation of the malignant B cell clone, since the lymphoma cells express a surface membrane immunoglobulin identical to that expressed by the chronic lymphocytic leukemia neoplastic B cells. Richter's syndrome is an aggressive disorder that progresses rapidly; the median survival is less than 2 months. In less than 1% of cases, there is a superimposed acute lymphoblastic leukemia, that is, a blast crisis.

T-cell chronic lymphocytic leukemia is uncommon, constituting less than 5% of cases of chronic lymphocytic leukemia. It is characterized by a high peripheral blood white cell count, skin involvement, prominent splenomegaly, and a lack of lymphadenopathy. The cells are medium sized and have round or irregular nuclei, generally a single nucleolus, and moderately abundant blue cytoplasm, with azurophilic granules. The disease is aggressive, with a median survival of 6 months.

Prolymphocytic Leukemia

Prolymphocytic leukemia is an aggressive variant of chronic lymphocytic leukemia. The neoplastic cell, the prolymphocyte, is distinctive. It is medium sized, with a round nucleus in which the chromatin is reticulated. The most characteristic morphologic feature is the large central nucleolus. About 60% of cases are of B-cell origin, although T-cell (and, less commonly, null cell) prolymphocytic leukemias have been described.

Prolymphocytic leukemia is most common in middle-aged to elderly men, the male:female ratio being 2:1 to 3:1. Patients present with massive splenomegaly, a high white blood cell count, and a low platelet

Table 20-28 Chronic Lymphocytic Leukemia: Rai Clinical Staging System

STAGE	ABSOLUTE LYMPHOCYTOSIS ($\geq$ 15,000/μl)	ENLARGED NODES	HEPATOMEGALY/ SPLENOMEGALY	ANEMIA	THROMBOCYTOPENIA
0	+	−	−	−	−
I	+	+	−	−	−
II	+	±	+	−	−
III	+	±	±	+	−
IV	+	±	±	±	+

count. Lymph nodes are often modestly enlarged. Regardless of cell type, the prognosis is poor, and the median survival is less than 2 years.

Hairy Cell Leukemia

Hairy cell leukemia is a distinctive variant of chronic lymphocytic leukemia. The clinicopathologic features include circulating neoplastic cells with prominent cytoplasmic membrane filamentous processes, or "hairs"; prominent splenomegaly; pancytopenia; a marrow that is difficult to aspirate; and an indolent clinical course. Hairy cell leukemia, also called leukemic reticuloendotheliosis, constitutes only 2% of all the leukemias. The cell of origin appears to be a B-lymphocyte with aberrant morphologic and functional properties. The cause of hairy cell leukemia is unknown. The pathophysiology relates to (1) tumor cell infiltration of the spleen, with resulting splenomegaly and secondary hypersplenism, and (2) marrow infiltration, with replacement of normal hematopoietic elements.

The principal clinicopathologic finding is marked enlargement of the spleen, which occurs in 85% of cases. The parenchyma is a homogeneous dark red color, reflecting the expansion of the red pulp and obliteration of the white pulp (see Fig. 20-21). Mild hepatomegaly occurs in almost half the cases. Histologically, the spleen exhibits a diffuse infiltration of the red pulp cords and sinusoids by bland medium-sized lymphoid cells, with round to indented nuclei and poorly visualized cytoplasm. Mitotic figures are rare, since typically less than 1% of the cells are engaged in DNA synthesis. Spaces filled with red blood cells, so-called venous lakes, are lined by hairy cells. This finding probably reflects damage to the normal splenic sinusoidal wall by massive infiltration of hairy cells. Scattered reactive plasma cells may be identified. The white pulp is either inconspicuous or obliterated by the neoplastic cell infiltration. In the liver mild infiltration, primarily of the portal areas, is seen. Circulating hairy cells may also be observed in their traverse through the hepatic sinusoids. The lymph nodes reveal patchy involvement of the paracortex, cortex, and sinuses; eventually, the normal lymph node architecture is obliterated.

There is patchy to diffuse infiltration by hairy cells in the bone marrow. Biopsy sections of the marrow show a distinctive mosaic-like histologic pattern with bland round to indented lymphoid nuclei surrounded by a clear zone or halo representing the moderate cytoplasm and well-defined cytoplasmic margins (see Fig. 20-25). Mild, diffuse marrow fibro-

sis, with reticular fibers surrounding individual neoplastic cells, is common.

In smears of blood or marrow aspirates stained by the Wright-Giemsa method, hairy cells are 10 μ to 15 μ in diameter and show eccentric round, indented, or occasionally lobed nuclei, delicate chromatin, indistinct nucleoli, and a moderate amount of gray-blue cytoplasm. Occasionally azurophilic granules are observed in the cytoplasm. **The filamentous cytoplasmic membrane projections, for which this disorder is named, are usually well visualized on smears** (Fig. 20-33). Scanning electron microscopy reveals the projections to be surface membrane ruffles, a feature that is more characteristic of cells of the mononuclear phagocyte system. With transmission electron microscopy a specific cytoplasmic inclusion, the ribosomal lamellar complex, is identified in half of the cases; this structure is a hollow cylinder that has marginal parallel lamellae and interlamellar ribosome-like granules. On smears, ribosomal lamellar complexes appear as purple cytoplasmic rods.

In 90% of cases, a specific isoenzyme of acid phosphatase, number 5, is identified in the cytoplasm of the neoplastic cells. When the cytochemical stain for acid phosphatase is performed in the presence of inhibitory tartaric acid, there is little loss of activity. Such cells are said to have tartrate-resistant acid phosphatase (TRAP)-activity. With rare exceptions, such as an unusual disorder called **malignant lymphoma simulating hairy cell leukemia,** other lymphoproliferative disorders are TRAP-negative. Therefore, a positive TRAP stain in the appropriate clinicopathologic setting confirms the diagnosis of hairy cell leukemia.

Usually the hairy cells express B-cell markers. These include immunoglobulin heavy- and light-chain gene rearrangements and the presence of surface membrane immunoglobulin. However, immunologic and cytochemical markers indicative of monocyte differentiation may also be identified. These include nonspecific esterase activity sensitive to fluoride inhibition, phagocytosis of inert particles (latex beads), adherence to glass or plastic surfaces, and the frequent presence of avid Fc receptors. Rare T cell variants have been described in which the neoplastic cells form E rosettes with sheep erythrocytes. Thus, **hairy cell leukemia may constitute a neoplastic disorder of a pluripotential precursor cell that is principally committed to B-cell differentiation but that remains capable of expressing heterogeneous cell markers.**

The principal laboratory finding is pancytopenia, which reflects both the splenomegaly associated with secondary hypersplenism and the neoplastic cell re-

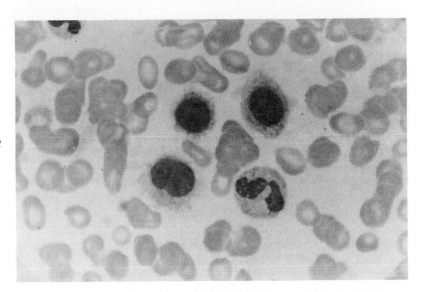

Figure 20-33. Hairy cell leukemia. Three typical hairy cells with fibrillar cytoplasmic margins are seen in the peripheral blood smear.

placement of bone marrow. In 10% of cases, leukocytosis, with a count above 11,000 per microliter, principally hairy cells, occurs late in the clinical course.

Hairy cell leukemia most commonly occurs in middle-aged to elderly men. The male:female ratio is 4:1, and the median age is 50 years. The onset is insidious, and the course is generally indolent and chronic. In 10% to 15% of cases, a more aggressive clinical course is characterized by progressive enlargement of the visceral organs and blood cytopenias. The most common cause of death is infection. Recurrent infectious episodes are frequent and reflect both neutropenia and monocytopenia, which occur in over 80% of cases. The infections may be caused either by common organisms, such as gram-negative bacteria, or by more unusual organisms, such as certain fungi and atypical mycobacteria. The median survival in hairy cell leukemia is 4 years, but a prolonged survival of over 10 years is not uncommon.

Acute Lymphoblastic Leukemia

Acute lymphoblastic leukemia is a malignant, clonal disorder of bone marrow lymphopoietic precursor cells. The cause is unknown. **Unlike acute nonlymphocytic (myelogenous) leukemia, there is no established association with ionizing radiation or with myelotoxic drugs or chemicals.** Acute lymphoblastic leukemia is rarely heralded by a prodromal myelodysplastic syndrome. Typically the onset is acute or subacute in a previously healthy child or, less commonly, in an adult. Certain observations suggest a genetic predisposition, at least in some cases: the incidence of leukemia, usually acute lymphoblastic leukemia, is increased 15-fold in Down's syndrome (trisomy 21), and if one identical twin develops acute lymphoblastic leukemia before the age of 6 years, there is a 20% chance that the other twin will also develop it.

The pathogenesis in acute lymphoblastic leukemia involves a progressive medullary and extramedullary accumulation of lymphoblasts that lack the potential for differentiation and maturation. **Of greatest clinical significance is inhibition by the expanding leukemic cell mass of the development of normal hematopoietic cell elements. Therefore, the clinical presentation is dominated by the untoward effects of progressive weakness and fatigue due to anemia, infection due to leukopenia, and bleeding due to thrombocytopenia.** There is prominent extramedullary soft tissue infiltration, frequently with generalized lymphadenopathy. Enlargement of the cervical lymph nodes is particularly common. Mild to moderate hepatosplenomegaly is also common. Before the era of modern therapy, involvement of the brain, particularly of the leptomeninges (leukemic meningitis), was common even early in the course of the disease. The leptomeninges were also a frequent site of relapse. The clinical presentation in leukemic meningitis frequently mimicked an acute bacterial meningitis, with headache, stiff neck, papilledema, confusion, nausea, and vomiting. The complication of leukemic meningitis is now usually prevented by routine prophylactic treatment of the craniospinal axis once the diagnosis of acute lymphoblastic leukemia has been made. However, late relapse may still occur in the leptomeninges. Bone pain is common, owing both to leukemic cell expansion of medullary spaces and to infiltration of the subperiosteum. There may be infiltration of the joint synovia and polyarthralgias that mimic rheumatic fever.

The involved lymph nodes are moderately enlarged and pale gray. The spleen is moderately enlarged, and the cut surface is pale red. The white pulp is not prominent. The liver is mildly enlarged and may display accentuation of the normal lobular markings. Microscopically, the normal marrow hematopoietic tissue is largely replaced (50–100%) by infiltrating blast cells (see Fig. 20-25). Mild fibrosis is observed in 15% of cases. The splenic red pulp is predominantly involved, but the white pulp may also be infiltrated. In the liver infiltration of both the sinusoids and the portal areas is usual. Initially, the paracortex or deep cortex of the lymph nodes is affected (see Fig. 20-27), but subsequently the normal nodal architecture may be completely effaced.

Acute lymphoblastic leukemia cells are morphologically and immunologically heterogeneous. FAB morphologic classification distinguishes three cell variants (see Fig. 20-23). L1 cells are small and have fine chromatin, indistinct nucleoli, and scant blue cytoplasm. **L1 cells are predominant in 85% of cases of childhood acute lymphoblastic leukemia and in approximately 35% of cases in adults.** L2 cells are moderate to large in size and exhibit finely reticulated chromatin, frequently irregular or cleaved nuclei, one to several nucleoli, and moderately abundant gray-blue cytoplasm. **L2 cells predominate in 65% of cases of adult acute lymphoblastic leukemia and in 10% of cases of the childhood disorder.** L3 cells are uniformly large, with round to oval nuclei, 2 to 5 small distinct nucleoli, coarsely reticulated chromatin, and a moderate amount of deeply basophilic and vacuolated cytoplasm. **L3 cells represent the leukemic or circulatory phase of Burkitt's lymphoma.** They are seen in less than 5% of cases of acute lymphoblastic leukemia, predominantly in children.

The immunologic classification recognizes B-cell, B-precursor, and T-cell variants of acute lymphoblastic leukemia. It is based on recognition of specific B- and T-cell markers as well as of a common acute lymphoblastic leukemia antigen (CALLA) (Table 20-29). The B-cell origin of most L3 cells (B ALL) is demonstrated by the presence of monoclonal surface membrane IgM. **In 80% of cases of acute lymphoblastic leukemia, an origin of neoplastic blast cells from early B-cell precursors is suggested by immunologic marker studies and by the demonstration of gene rearrangements of the immunoglobulin heavy and light chains. Fifteen percent to 20% of cases of acute lymphoblastic leukemia are of T-cell origin, as demonstrated by reactivity with monoclonal anti–T-cell antibodies and by rearrangement of the genes for the beta and gamma chains of the T-cell receptor.** T-cell acute lymphoblastic leukemia is morphologically classified in the FAB classification as either L1 or L2 acute lymphoblastic leukemia. A small minority of leukemias lack any distinguishing immunologic or other cell markers and are labelled null, or unclassified, leukemias.

A characteristic cytochemical finding in B-precursor and T-cell acute lymphoblastic leukemia is coarse (block positive) PAS cytoplasmic staining with the PAS reaction in over half of all cases. Focal cytoplasmic staining with acid phosphatase and alpha-naphthyl acetate esterase is observed in a majority of cases of T-cell ALL (see Fig. 20-24). **Ninety percent of T- and B-precursor cell acute lymphoblastic leukemias contain the nuclear DNA-polymerizing enzyme Tdt.** This marker is lacking only in the morphologically distinctive FAB L3 variant. Tdt is useful in distinguishing lymphoblastic from primitive nonlymphocytic or myelogenous leukemias, which are positive for Tdt only 2% to 5% of the time (see Table 20-27). **Demonstration of Tdt has important therapeutic and prognostic implications, because acute lymphoblastic leukemia has a much better prognosis than acute nonlymphocytic leukemia and responds to a less intensive chemotherapeutic regimen.**

The leukemic cells in most cases of acute lymphoblastic leukemia have an abnormal karyotype.

Table 20-29 Acute Lymphoblastic Leukemia (ALL): Immunologic Phenotypes

Subtypes	CALLA	TdT	Ia	Pan-T	Pan-B	C μ	SIg	Ig Gene Rearrangement
T ALL	−	+	−	+	−	−	−	−
B ALL	±	−	+	−	+	−	+	+
B Precursor ALL								
Pre-B	+	+	+	−	+	+	−	+
Non-Pre-B	+	+	+	−	+	−	−	+
Unclassified ALL	−	+	+	−	−	−	−	−

Aneuploidy, usually hyperdiploidy, and marker chromosomes, commonly involving the C and G groups, are the most frequent cytogenetic findings. The finding of hyperdiploidy is a favorable prognostic sign in acute lymphoblastic leukemia. The blast cells of 25% of adults and 5% of children with acute lymphoblastic leukemia have the Ph[1] chromosome. These cases may represent either presentation of chronic myelogenous leukemia in blast crisis or a different disorder. Ph[1]-positive acute lymphoblastic leukemia usually is an aggressive disorder and carries a poor prognosis. L3 (Burkitt's) leukemia is characterized by a translocation, involving the oncogene c-myc between chromosomes 2 and 8, 14 and 8, or 22 and 8. The specific translocation determines whether the neoplastic cells express surface membrane kappa or lambda light chains with the IgM heavy chain.

Acute lymphoblastic leukemia is predominantly a disease of childhood, 85% of all cases occuring in that age group. It is also the most common pediatric malignancy. In children the incidence peaks between 3 and 6 years. In this age group, most acute lymphoblastic leukemia is morphologically L1 and immunologically CALLA and Tdt positive **(B-precursor cell acute lymphoblastic leukemia).** Caucasian males are most commonly affected. L3 (Burkitt's) leukemia occurs in a slightly older age group, with a peak age range of 6 to 11 years. L3 acute lymphoblastic leukemia is further discussed in the section on non-Hodgkin's lymphomas.

The prognosis in the 3 to 6 year-old age group with L1 acute lymphoblastic leukemia has improved dramatically, and a cure can be anticipated in over half of cases. The prognosis in adult acute lymphoblastic leukemia is much less favorable. In acute lymphoblastic leukemia adverse risk factors include FAB L3 and T-cell subtypes of leukemia, the presence of the Ph[1] chromosome, a high blast cell count, the presence of a mediastinal mass, central nervous system involvement, and onset of disease either in infancy or in adulthood.

The Non-Hodgkin's Malignant Lymphomas

The non-Hodgkin's lymphomas are a clinically and pathologically diverse group of neoplastic disorders of lymphoid cells. The heterogeneity of the lymphomas reflects the potential for malignant transformation at any stage of B- or T-lymphocyte differentiation. The malignant lymphomas commonly first involve the lymph nodes or other lymphopoietic tissues. They have traditionally been called the non-Hodgkin's malignant lymphomas to distinguish them from Hodgkin's disease. This distinction may on occasion be difficult because of overlapping clinical and pathologic features. Clinical features helpful in distinguishing non-Hodgkin's lymphoma from Hodgkin's disease are shown in Table 20-30. Differences in preferential sites of initial involvement are outlined in Table 20-31.

The malignant lymphomas are characterized by the following: homogeneous neoplastic cell populations; a histologic pattern of tumor cell growth either as cohesive cellular aggregates, called the follicular, or nodular, pattern, or as diffuse infiltration; a prognosis determined principally by the histopathologic subtype; unpredictable spread of disease; frequent presentation as widespread or systemic disease; and pronounced clinical and pathologic differences between the malignant lymphomas of children and those of adults. In addition to the characteristic morphologic patterns, the demonstration of light-chain restriction, with the expression of only kappa or only lambda light chains, is confirmatory of monoclonality and hence of B-cell neoplasia (Fig. 20-34). The diagnosis of a T-cell lymphoma requires the demonstration of a homogeneous population of cytologically malignant lymphoid cells that express T-cell markers or rearrangement of the genes for either the beta or the gamma chains of the T-cell receptor.

Etiology

The cause of most non-Hodgkin's malignant lymphomas is unknown, but variations in global epidemiologic patterns provide suggestive clues (Table 20-32). Two uncommon clinicopathologic subtypes are associated with specific viruses. **There is a strong correlation between infection with the Epstein-Barr virus and endemic Burkitt's lymphoma in central equatorial Africa** (see Fig. 20-30). This association is less well established for the sporadic Burkitt's lymphomas that occur in the United States and elsewhere in nonendemic areas of the world. **A specific C-type retrovirus, the human T-cell leukemia/lymphoma virus (HTLV-I), is commonly associated with the adult T-cell leukemia/lymphoma that occurs in several geographically restricted areas of the world** (see Fig. 20-30). Evidence for HTLV-I infection either by serologic studies or by the demonstration of the HTLV-I viral genome in tumor cells is present in 90% to 100% of patients with adult type T-cell leukemia/lymphoma in endemic areas.

Table 20-30 Hodgkin's Disease Versus Non-Hodgkin's Malignant Lymphoma—Clinical Features

CLINICAL FEATURE	HODGKIN'S DISEASE	NON-HODGKIN'S MALIGNANT LYMPHOMA
Age range	Bimodal (15–34,> 50) (Western or type IV)	Increases with age (median, 50)
Sex incidence	Male:female, 1.5:1 (nodular sclerosis: male:female, 1:1)	Male:female, 1.5:1 (Mediterranean abdominal lymphoma: male:female, 1:1)
Pathologic stage at presentation	Frequently stage I or II (localized)	Generally stage III or IV (< 20% localized)
Constitutional symptoms at presentation	40%	15%
Pattern of spread	Predictable (to contiguous nodal groups)	Random
Leukemic conversion	Never	Variable (cell-type dependent)

Table 20-31 Hodgkin's Disease Versus Non-Hodgkin's Malignant Lymphoma—Preferential Sites of Involvement

SITE	HODGKIN'S DISEASE	NON-HODGKIN'S MALIGNANT LYMPHOMA
Initial involvement	Nodal (> 95%), extranodal (rare)	Nodal (80%), extranodal (20%)
Epitrochlear nodes	Rare	Occasional
Mesenteric nodes	Rare	Common
Mediastinal or hilar nodes	50%	20%
Pharyngeal lymphoid tissue (Waldeyer's ring)	Rare	Common
Spleen	Common	Common
Bone marrow	< 10%	Cell-type dependent: Small cleaved (50–70%) Large cell (5–10%)
Gastrointestinal tract	Rare	Diffuse (20%), follicular (< 10%)
Testicle	Rare	Common with lymphoblastic and large cell lymphoma
Central nervous system	Rare	Cell-type dependent: lymphoblastic (common), large cell (common after marrow involvement)
Skin	Rare	Common
Liver	Uncommon	Small cleaved (common), large cell (uncommon)

A number of disorders are associated with an increased risk for the development of B-cell large cell malignant lymphoma (Table 20-33). **Congenital and acquired immune deficiency states are associated with an increased risk for the development of large cell immunoblastic lymphomas.** The risk is increased when there is both immune deficiency and chronic antigenic stimulation. For example, renal and cardiac transplant recipients are clinically immunosuppressed in order to prevent allograft rejection and are simultaneously subjected to the chronic antigenic stimulation of the allograft. Such graft recipients are at risk for the development of large cell immunoblastic lymphomas of the central nervous system. The risk of secondary lymphoma is also increased in the collagen vascular diseases. The risk is greatest in Sjögren's syndrome, in which large cell immunoblastic lymphoma develops in up to 10% of cases. Irradiation does not appear to constitute a definite risk factor for the development of malignant lymphoma. Chemotherapy with alkylating agents carries a minor risk for the development of malignant lymphoma.

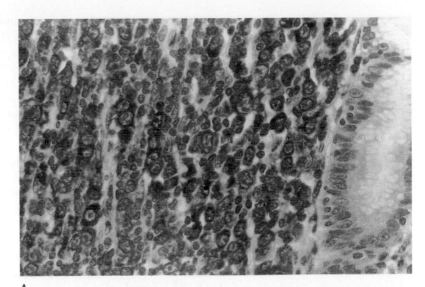

A

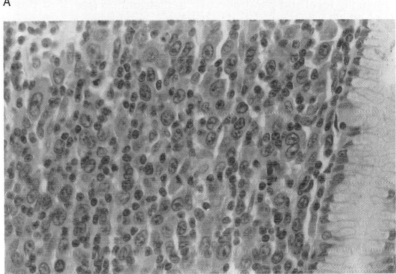

B

Figure 20-34. Plasmacytoid large cell lymphoma in the large bowel. *(A)* A positive immunohistochemical (peroxidase-antiperoxidase) stain for cytoplasmic kappa light chains. *(B)* A negative immunohistochemical stain for cytoplasmic lambda light chains.

General Features

In non-Hodgkin's malignant lymphomas, the involved lymph nodes are enlarged, soft, and pale gray, an appearance commonly described as "fish flesh." However, they may be firm if there is associated fibrosis. Fibrosis is most commonly observed in malignant lymphomas involving retroperitoneal, mediastinal, and inguinal sites. The presence of fibrosis does not influence the clinical course or the prognosis of the malignant lymphomas. Tumor necrosis is appreciated grossly as foci of opaque yellow softening. Characteristically, tumor necrosis is observed in the rapidly dividing large cell lymphomas and involves single cells rather than broad zones of tumor tissue.

Phagocytosis of nuclear and cytoplasmic debris by macrophages is conspicuous in the rapidly dividing lymphomas with cell necrosis, imparting the so-called **starry-sky** appearance on histologic sections.

In non-Hodgkin's lymphomas involving the spleen, there is primary involvement of the white pulp (see Fig. 20-21). Initially, the follicular centers are involved in B-cell lymphomas and the periarteriolar lymphoid sheath in T-cell lymphomas. There may be generalized expansion of the white pulp or discrete tumor masses. The liver may be grossly normal or variably enlarged, with accentuation of the normal lobular pattern. Uncommonly, tumor masses may be evident. Microscopically, the portal areas are first involved. In the bone marrow initial involvement

Table 20-32 Geographic Pathology of Lymphomas: Global Epidemiologic Patterns

Type I	Tropical countries with high prevalence of Burkitt's lymphoma
Type II	Tropical countries where Burkitt's lymphoma not prevalent but where there is high incidence of aggressive Hodgkin's disease in children
Type III	Tropical and subtropical countries with relatively high incidence of aggressive Hodgkin's disease in children and relatively high incidence of nodular sclerosing Hodgkin's disease in young adults
Type IV	Industrialized countries with low incidence of Hodgkin's disease in children and high incidence of nodular sclerosing Hodgkin's disease in young adults
Type V	Asian countries with low incidence of Hodgkin's disease and high incidence of large cell lymphoma

is usually focal and paratrabecular in distribution (see Fig. 20-25), but multifocal or diffuse involvement with marrow replacement may be observed. Radiologically, osteolytic or, less commonly, osteoblastic, lesions are identified.

Histologic examination reveals a monotonous lymphoid cell population that infiltrates and obliterates normal lymph nodal or other tissue architecture. Characteristically, the neoplastic cells exhibit uniformly atypical cytologic features. A spectrum of neoplastic cell size may be seen, but careful histologic examination usually reveals cytologic atypia of all of the infiltrating lymphoid cells. Only in small or well-differentiated lymphocytic lymphoma is cellular atypia lacking.

Microscopically, in 40% of the malignant lymphomas in adults, the initial tumor cell pattern is one of uniform aggregates of neoplastic cells, referred to as follicles or nodules (Fig. 20-35). All malignancies that exhibit a follicular pattern are of B-cell origin. A specific chromosomal translocation t(14;18) is present in 85% of the follicular lymphomas. Follicular

Table 20-33 Disorders Associated with Significantly Increased Risk of Secondary Malignant Lymphoma

Sjögren's syndrome
Renal and cardiac transplant
Acquired immunodeficiency syndrome (AIDS)
Congenital immune deficiency syndromes
    Chediak-Higashi
    Wiscott-Aldrich
    Ataxia telangiectasia
    IgA deficiency
    Severe combined immune deficiency
Alpha heavy-chain disease
Celiac disease
Hodgkin's disease posttreatment
X-linked lymphoproliferative disorder

lymphomas are generally indolent disorders and typically follow a chronic course. However, recurrent late relapses are common, and cure is exceptional. Follicular lymphomas progressively infiltrate the normal interfollicular tissues to become both follicular and diffuse. The final growth pattern is diffuse. Follicular lymphomas are most common in middle-aged to elderly adults, are uncommon in persons under the age of 30 years, and are exceedingly rare in children. The vast majority of malignant lymphomas in the pediatric age group are diffuse neoplasms that exhibit an aggressive clinical course and frequent leukemic distribution (Table 20-34). Follicular lymphomas must be distinguished from the benign or reactive follicular hyperplasias (Table 20-35).

In 60% of the malignant lymphomas in adults, the tumor is initially diffusely infiltrative, without a proclivity to form follicles or nodules. These diffuse lymphomas are of B- or T-cell origin. **With the exception of small lymphocytic lymphoma, diffuse lymphomas exhibit a more aggressive clinical course than the follicular lymphomas.** However, a clinical cure can now be anticipated in many of these more aggressive diffuse lymphomas. The patterns of neoplastic involvement of the lymph nodes by the non-Hodgkin's malignant lymphomas are shown in Figure 20-27.

Classification

Because the malignant lymphomas are pathologically diverse, a number of classification systems have been proposed to identify subtypes that have therapeutic and prognostic relevance. All of these nosologic systems require the identification of tumor cell types and tumor growth patterns. Three such classification systems (Table 20-36) are relevant to a current understanding of the malignant lymphomas: Rappaport, Lukes-Collins, and the International Working Formulation.

The Rappaport classification (1966) is based on morphologic evaluation of tumor cell size and morphologic appearance, and was formulated before the application of modern immunologic concepts to the study of the malignant lymphomas. Nevertheless, this classification is clinically relevant and prognostically significant and has been widely employed in clinical therapeutic trials. The major features of the Rappaport classification are as follows. First, if the nuclei of the tumor cells are smaller than the nuclei of benign histiocytes or vascular endothelial cells, the tumor is classified as lymphocytic lymphoma, well or poorly differentiated. Second, if the tumor cells are comparable in nuclear size to histiocytes or endoth-

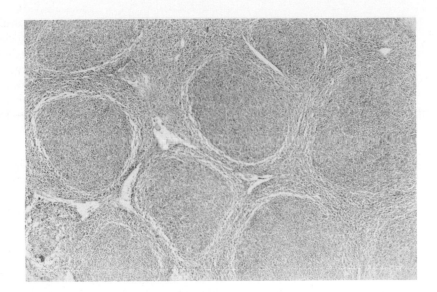

Figure 20-35. The lymph node in follicular lymphoma. The normal nodal architecture is replaced by homogeneous nodular aggregates of neoplastic B-lymphocytes.

elial cells, the neoplasm is labeled undifferentiated lymphoma, Burkitt's, or non-Burkitt's. Third, if the nuclei are still larger, the tumor is a histiocytic lymphoma. The term "histiocytic" was previously employed for aggressive large cell lymphomas because of a morphologic similarity between large neoplastic lymphoma cells and fixed tissue histiocytes. **Immunologic marker studies have subsequently clearly demonstrated that "histiocytic" lymphomas are in the majority of cases tumors of large transformed lymphocytes.**

The Lukes-Collins classification (1974) is based on a combined morphologic and functional or immunologic identification of B- and T-cell malignant lymphomas and tumors of true histiocytes. The small lymphocyte of the perifollicular or mantle zone is thought to give rise to the entity known as diffuse small lymphocytic lymphoma. All follicular lymphomas are thought to arise from the neoplastic trans-

formation of follicular center B cells. The type of follicular center cells and their corresponding lymphomas include small cleaved lymphocyte (small cleaved cell lymphoma), large cleaved lymphocyte (mixed small and large cell, or large cell, lymphoma), small noncleaved lymphocyte (Burkitt's and non-Burkitt's lymphoma), and large noncleaved lymphocyte (large cell lymphoma). A postfollicular large plasmacytoid cell in the interfollicular region of the lymph node is thought to give rise to a plasmacytoid large cell lymphoma, the so-called B immunoblastic sarcoma. Most diffuse lymphomas are also thought to arise from follicular center B cells and are cytologically identifiable because of retention of specific morphologic features. **Immunologic identification of B-cell malignant lymphomas is provided by the demonstration of monoclonal surface membrane immunoglobulin, usually IgM kappa, complement receptors, and Fc receptors.** Such B-cell markers are

Table 20-34 Non-Hodgkin's Malignant Lymphoma: Pediatric Versus Adult

	PEDIATRIC	ADULT
Sites of initial involvement	Commonly extranodal	Predominantly nodal
Histopathologic subtypes	Aggressive high-grade	Indolent to high-grade
Pattern of tumor cell growth	Diffuse, rarely follicular	Diffuse (60%), follicular (40%)
Leukemic conversion	Common	Occasional, cell-type dependent
Initial central nervous system involvement	Common	Common only with lymphoblastic lymphoma
Monoclonal gammopathy	Rare	Infrequent, cell-type dependent
Late relapse after 2 years	Rare	Common with follicular lymphomas

Table 20-35 Lymph Nodes—Reactive Follicular Hyperplasia Versus Follicular Lymphoma

REACTIVE FOLLICULAR HYPERPLASIA	FOLLICULAR LYMPHOMA
Follicles composed of spectrum of activated normal lymphoid cells	"Follicles" composed of uniformly atypical or spectrum of atypical neoplastic cells
Follicles with "starry sky" pattern due to presence of intrafollicular phagocytic macrophages and dendritic reticular cells	"Follicles" without "starry sky" pattern due to absence of phagocytic macrophages and dendritic reticular cells
Marked variation in size and shape of follicles	Minor variation in size and shape of follicles
Follicles sharply demarcated from surrounding lymph node tissue by cuff of normal lymphocytes	"Fading follicles" poorly demarcated from surrounding lymph node tissue
Follicles predominantly in cortex	"Follicles" closely apposed and evenly distributed in cortex and medulla
Preservation of normal lymph node architecture	Partial to complete effacement of normal lymph node architecture
Absent to moderate capsular and perinodal soft tissue infiltration in predominantly perivascular distribution	Frequent extensive capsular and perinodal soft tissue infiltration not selectively perivascular in distribution
Polyclonal B-cell population	Monoclonal B-cell population

present on the cells of follicular, and frequently diffuse, lymphomas that have the cytologic features of follicular center cells. In the Lukes-Collins classification, a minority of diffuse lymphomas are thought to be of T cell origin and to be morphologically identifiable because of a distinctive spectrum of abnormal cells with irregular or cerebriform nuclei.

Confirmation of T-cell origin is provided by the demonstration of the specific T-cell marker, the sheep cell (E) rosette. In the Lukes-Collins classification true histiocytic (mononuclear-phagocyte) cell markers Fc and complement receptors are identified on less than 5% of malignant tumors with morphologic features of a large cell lymphoma. The Lukes-Collins classification applies immunologic concepts to the understanding of the malignant lymphomas, but its therapeutic and prognostic relevance has not been fully assessed.

The International Working Formulation (1981) is based on an international pathologic review and clinical correlation of almost 1200 cases of malignant lymphoma. The Working Formulation compared six major lymphoma classifications and found that each defined three major subgroups: lymphomas with a low-grade (indolent) clinical course, an intermediate-grade clinical course, and a high-grade (aggressive) clinical course. The Working Formulation relates to

survival and provides a mode of translation between different classification systems. The schema of the Working Formulation is employed in the following discussion of the salient features of subtypes of the malignant lymphomas; corresponding terminology in the Rappaport and Lukes-Collins classifications is shown in Table 20-36. The cytologic features of each of the neoplastic cell subtypes, following the order of the Working Formulation, are illustrated in Figure 20-36. The preferential sites of involvement of the specific non-Hodgkin's malignant lymphomas and, for comparison, Hodgkin's disease are presented in Figure 20-37.

Low-Grade Non-Hodgkin's Malignant Lymphomas

In the Working Formulation low-grade non-Hodgkin's lymphomas are classified as **small lymphocytic, small lymphocytic plasmacytoid, follicular small cleaved,** and **follicular small cleaved and large cell.**

Small Lymphocytic Lymphoma

Small lymphocytic lymphoma is a diffuse B-cell lymphoma of morphologically normal but immunologically incompetent small lymphocytes. Most often it represents the tissue phase of chronic lymphocytic leukemia, but it does not invariably progress to a leukemic phase. The **tumor cell immunologic markers of small lymphocytic lymphomas are comparable to those of chronic lymphocytic leukemia.** These include weakly expressed monoclonal surface membrane immunoglobulin, usually IgM kappa, Fc and complement receptors, and pan B-cell antigens. A minority of small lymphocytic lymphomas express the common acute lymphoblastic leukemia antigen (CALLA). A specific chromosomal translocation t(11;14) is found in some cases of small lymphocytic lymphoma. **Histologically, the normal architecture of the lymph node is replaced by a monotonous population of morphologically normal small lymphoid cells with round hyperchromatic nuclei** (Fig. 20-38). Scattered pale clusters of larger, round lymphoid cells, called proliferation centers, are characteristic of small lymphocytic lymphoma. Mitotic figures are typically rare, and an increased mitotic rate (> 30 per 20 high-power fields) predicts a more aggressive clinical course. In the spleen the white pulp is uniformly expanded and spills over into the red pulp. In the liver the portal areas are first affected. The bone marrow shows involvement similar to that in chronic lymphocytic leukemia.

Table 20-36 Comparative Classification of Non-Hodgkin's Lymphoma

1981 NCI INTERNATIONAL WORKING FORMULATION (SURVIVAL)	1974(MODIFIED 1979) LUKES-COLLINS (MORPHOLOGIC-IMMUNOLOGIC)	1966 (MODIFIED 1976) RAPPAPORT (MORPHOLOGIC-CELL SIZE)
Low-Grade		
Small lymphocytic Consistent with chronic lymphocytic leukemia	Diffuse small lymphocytic	Diffuse well-differentiated lymphocytic
Plasmacytoid	Plasmacytoid lymphocytic	Well-differentiated lymphocytic with plasmacytoid differentiation
Follicular, predominantly small cleaved cell	Follicular small cleaved	Nodular poorly differentiated lymphocytic
Diffuse areas, sclerosis	Follicular and diffuse small cleaved	Nodular and diffuse poorly differentiated lymphocytic
Follicular, mixed small cleaved and large cell	Follicular small cleaved and large cell	Nodular mixed lymphocytic-histiocytic
Diffuse areas, sclerosis	Follicular and diffuse small cleaved and large cell	Nodular and diffuse, mixed lymphocytic histiocytic
Intermediate-Grade		
Follicular, predominantly large cell	Follicular, large cell	Nodular histiocytic
Diffuse areas sclerosis	Follicular and diffuse large cell	Nodular and diffuse histiocytic
Diffuse small cleaved cell sclerosis	Diffuse small cleaved	Diffuse poorly differentiated lymphocytic
Diffuse mixed small and large cell sclerosis, epithelioid component	Diffuse mixed small cleaved and large cell	Diffuse poorly differentiated lymphocytic-histiocytic
Diffuse large cell Cleaved cell	Diffuse large cleaved	Diffuse mixed lymphocytic-histiocytic or histiocytic
Noncleaved sclerosis	Diffuse large noncleaved	Diffuse histiocytic
High-Grade		

Large cell immunoblastic
    Plasmacytoid
    Clear cell
    Polymorphous
    Epithelioid cell component
	Immunoblastic sarcoma
	    B-cell type
	    T-cell type
	    B- or T-cell type
	    T-cell type
		Diffuse histiocytic

Lymphoblastic
    Convoluted
    Nonconvoluted
	Lymphoblastic, diffuse
	    Convoluted
		Diffuse lymphoblastic

Small noncleaved cell
    Burkitt's
    Follicular areas
	Small noncleaved
	    Burkitt's
		Diffuse undifferentiated
		    Burkitt's

	Burkitt's-like	non-Burkitt's

The clinical features of small lymphocytic lymphoma are similar to those of chronic lymphocytic leukemia. Generalized lymphadenopathy and hepatosplenomegaly are usual. The disease tends to be indolent. Middle-aged to elderly men are most commonly affected. Less than 5% of small lymphocytic lymphomas are of T-cell origin, and these are characterized by an aggressive course, with frequent leukemic distribution and extensive soft tissue involvement.

Small Lymphocytic Plasmacytoid Lymphoma

Small lymphocytic plasmacytoid lymphoma is a diffuse B-cell lymphoma of small lymphoid cells that exhibit variable plasmacytoid differentiation. The neoplastic cells usually secrete monoclonal IgM macroglobulin. Small lymphocytic plasmacytoid lymphoma usually represents the clinical entity commonly termed **Waldenström's macroglobulinemia.**

Generalized lymphadenopathy and hepatosplenomegaly are present, and involvement of the bone marrow is common. A leukemic phase with circulating tumor cells occurs in 10% to 15% of cases. The neoplastic cell population is heterogeneous, being composed of small lymphoid cells and plasmacytoid lymphoid cells that display eccentric lymphoid nuclei and abundant dark blue plasmacytoid cytoplasm. Histologic evidence for immunoglobulin production includes refractile eosinophilic globules of immunoglobulin in the nuclei (Dutcher bodies) and cytoplasm (Russell bodies).

(Text continues on p. 1100)

SMALL LYMPHOCYTIC
Nucleus: round
Chromatin: dense
Nucleolus: indistinct
Cytoplasm: scant, blue

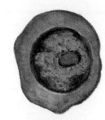

IMMUNOBLASTIC, B
Nucleus: round to oval
Chromatin: vesicular
Nucleolus: prominent
Cytoplasm: moderate, dense, blue

SMALL LYMPHOCYTIC, PLASMACYTOID
Nucleus: round, eccentric
Chromatin: dense
Nucleolus: variable
Cytoplasm: moderate, blue

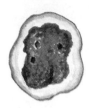

IMMUNOBLASTIC, T
Nucleus: round to irregular
Chromatin: variable
Nucleoli: variable
Cytoplasm: clear

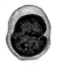

SMALL CLEAVED
Nucleus: indented
Chromatin: coarse
Nucleolus: small
Cytoplasm: scant

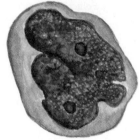

IMMUNOBLASTIC, POLYMORPHOUS
Nucleus: pleomorphic
Chromatin: variable
Nucleoli: variable
Cytoplasm: moderate

SMALL NONCLEAVED (BURKITT'S)
Nucleus: round to oval
Chromatin: coarsely reticulated
Nucleoli: small, 2-5
Cytoplasm: blue, vacuolated

LYMPHOBLASTIC, CONVOLUTED
Nucleus: irregular
Chromatin: delicate
Nucleolus: variable
Cytoplasm: blue, scant

LARGE CLEAVED
Nucleus: irregular, indented
Chromatin: delicate
Nucleoli: indistinct
Cytoplasm: scant, pale

LYMPHOBLASTIC, NONCONVOLUTED
Nucleus: round to oval
Chromatin: delicate
Nucleolus: variable
Cytoplasm: scant, blue

LARGE NONCLEAVED
Nucleus: round to oval
Chromatin: vesicular
Nucleoli: contiguous to membrane
Cytoplasm: moderate

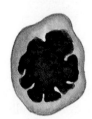

MYCOSIS FUNGOIDES
Nucleus: irregular, convoluted
Chromatin: dense
Nucleolus: indistinct
Cytoplasm: scant

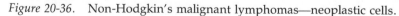

Figure 20-36.   Non-Hodgkin's malignant lymphomas—neoplastic cells.

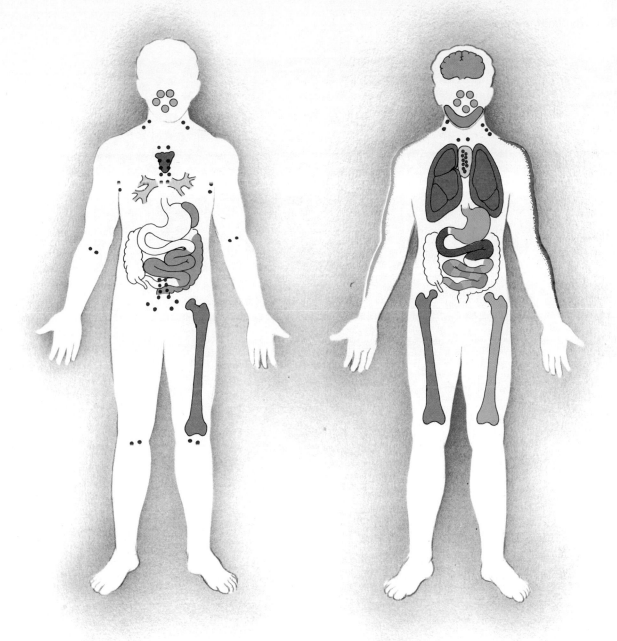

LYMPH NODES
SPLEEN (white pulp)
BONE MARROW
THYMUS
WALDEYER'S RING (lymphoid tissue of oronasopharynx)
GALT (gut-associated lymphoid tissue)
BALT (bronchial-associated lymphoid tissue)

HODGKIN'S DISEASE—lymph nodes
Lymphocyte predominant—high cervical
Mixed cellularity—left cervical
Nodular sclerosis—mediastinal and supraclavicular
SMALL LYMPHOCYTIC LYMPHOMA/LEUKEMIA—bone marrow
MEDITERRANEAN ABDOMINAL LYMPHOMA—proximal small bowel
BURKITT'S LYMPHOMA—maxilla, mandible, terminal ileum
EXTRANODAL LARGE CELL LYMPHOMA—stomach, terminal ileum, bone, skin, Waldeyer's ring
POST-TRANSPLANT IMMUNOBLASTIC SARCOMA (B cell)—central nervous system
T CELL LYMPHOMA—skin, pleura, lungs, nodes
LYMPHOBLASTIC LYMPHOMA—mediastinum

Figure 20-37. *(Left)* Normal immune system. *(Right)* Sites of preferential tumor involvement.

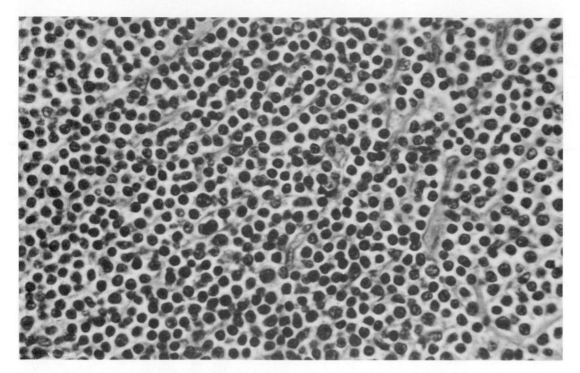

Figure 20-38. The lymph node in small lymphocytic lymphoma. Normal nodal architecture is replaced by a diffuse infiltration of normal-appearing small lymphocytes.

The clinical symptoms usually are due to increased serum viscosity secondary to the circulating IgM paraprotein of high molecular weight. When the serum viscosity exceeds 4.0 (normal, 1.4–1.8), circulatory disturbances, with symptoms referable particularly to the central or peripheral nervous systems may be observed. These include headache, dizziness, deafness, paresis, coma, and peripheral neuropathy. Small lymphocytic plasmacytoid lymphoma is associated with an average survival of 3 to 4 years. Occasionally, a superimposed large cell immunoblastic lymphoma, with identical immunologic cell markers, may usher in the terminal phase.

Rare B-cell tumors are associated with the secretion of an immunoglobulin heavy-chain molecule or portion of the heavy-chain molecule **(heavy-chain diseases)**. IgA heavy-chain disease, the most common, is endemic in certain Middle Eastern countries in the region of the eastern Mediterranean Sea (see Fig. 20-30). The disorder is observed predominantly in adults less than 30 years of age. There is no sex predominance. The pathogenesis seems to involve an inability to assemble a complete secretory IgA molecule. Appropriate immunologic responses to antigenic intestinal bacteria or parasites are therefore impaired. There is a compensatory hyperplastic re-

sponse of the defective plasma cells in the lamina propria of the duodenum and jejunum, a process that may be associated with a malabsorption syndrome, with diarrhea and steatorrhea. Additionally, the combined risk factors of immunodeficiency and chronic antigenic stimulation predispose to a high incidence of superimposed large cell immunoblastic lymphoma of the small bowel, the so-called **Mediterranean abdominal lymphoma.**

IgG heavy-chain disease is uncommon. In addition to generalized lymphadenopathy and hepatosplenomegaly, prominent involvement of Waldeyer's tonsillar ring, with secondary palatal edema, is typical. The neoplastic cell population is heterogeneous, consisting of lymphocytes, variably transformed lymphoid cells, and plasmacytoid cells. An aggressive clinical course is usual.

Follicular Small Cleaved Cell Lymphoma

Follicular small cleaved cell lymphoma, the most common variant of follicular lymphoma, is characterized by cohesive aggregates of small cleaved or notched and clefted lymphocytes. These cells, 10 μ to 15 μ in diameter, have small, hyperchromatic angulated nuclei, indistinct nucleoli, and scant or indistinguishable cytoplasm. Few mitoses are seen. The fact that up to 20% of the cells are large, transformed lymphoid cells suggests an incomplete block to transformation of follicular center cells.

Small cleaved cells exhibit prominent monoclonal surface membrane immunoglobulin, most commonly IgM kappa, complement receptors, and Fc receptors. Pan B-cell antigens are expressed, and in a minority of cases, the tumor cells also express CALLA.

Follicular small cleaved cell lymphoma is typically a disorder of middle and old age, the mean age at diagnosis being 50 years. Men and women are equally affected. Initially, lymphadenopathy and hepatosplenomegaly are observed. Early in the course there is usually widespread dissemination of disease, with hepatic and bone marrow involvement in at least 50% of cases. Frank leukemic dissemination occurs late in the course of the disease in 10% to 15% of cases. **The natural history of follicular small cleaved cell lymphoma is often characterized by progression to a follicular and diffuse, and finally to a diffuse, lymphoma, either of the small cleaved or, less frequently, of a mixed small cleaved and large cell type.** Late relapses are frequent, and cure is exceptional. The median survival is 7 to 9 years.

Follicular Small Cleaved and Large Cell Lymphoma

Follicular small cleaved and large cell lymphoma is similar in many respects to follicular small cleaved cell lymphoma, but the proportion of large lymphoid cells exceeds 20%. Histologically, a spectrum of neoplastic cell sizes is observed, with admixed small cleaved and transformed large lymphoid cells (Fig. 20-39). The median survival is similar to that associated with follicular small cleaved cell lymphoma, but early relapse is more common. Progression to a diffuse small cleaved and large cell lymphoma or to a diffuse large cell lymphoma may be observed.

Intermediate-Grade Non-Hodgkin's Malignant Lymphomas

Intermediate-grade malignant lymphomas are classified as: **follicular large cell, diffuse small cleaved cell, diffuse mixed small cleaved and large cell,** and **diffuse large cell, cleaved and non-cleaved.**

Follicular Large Cell Lymphoma

Follicular large cell lymphoma is a distinctly uncommon subtype of follicular lymphoma. The malignant follicles are composed predominantly of large neoplastic lymphoid cells. **Follicular large cell lymphoma is the only follicular lymphoma characterized by an aggressive clinical course.** The identification of accompanying diffuse areas suggests a biologic behavior similar to that of the diffuse large cell lymphomas. In follicular large cell lymphoma the residual neoplastic follicles are eventually obliterated and the disease progresses to a diffuse large cell lymphoma.

Diffuse Small Cleaved Cell Lymphoma

Diffuse small cleaved cell lymphoma is a B-cell lymphoma of follicular center cell origin in which there is a diffuse infiltration of small cleaved lymphocytes.

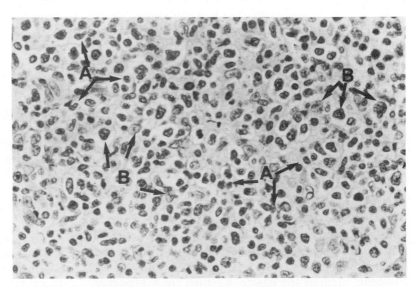

Figure 20-39. The lymph node in mixed small cleaved and large cell lymphoma. There is a variety in cell size, from small *(A)* to large *(B)* lymphocytes.

The age range of those affected is similar to that of adults with follicular lymphomas; however, the clinical course is more aggressive. Occasional T-cell lymphomas exhibit a diffuse infiltration of small, irregular lymphoid cells. An aggressive course is characteristic.

Diffuse Mixed Small and Large Cell Lymphoma

Diffuse mixed small and large cell lymphomas are of B- or T-cell type. In mixed small and large cell B-cell lymphomas, the neoplastic cells are of follicular center cell origin. Cytologically, they are identical to the malignant cells observed in follicular mixed small cleaved and large cell lymphomas. The disorder is usually widespread at the time of diagnosis, with disease in the bone marrow, liver, and other tissues. In mixed small and large cell lymphomas of the T-cell type, a spectrum of neoplastic cell size is also observed. **The contour of the tumor cell nuclear membranes is commonly irregular or cerebriform but may be round.** The cytoplasm is typically pale and clear. Tumor cells may be compartmentalized into small clusters or aggregates outlined by a delicate collagenous fibrosis. Postcapillary venules are frequently prominent. Admixed inflammatory cells and histiocytes are not unusual.

Immunologic studies may be required to establish that these tumors are of T-cell origin. Findings consistent with T-cell malignancy include marked predominance of helper or suppressor cell populations, expression of early T-cell markers such as T6 and T10, loss of mature or postthymic T-cell markers, and demonstration of gene rearrangements of the beta or gamma chains of the T-cell receptor.

Mixed small and large T-cell lymphomas are aggressive neoplasms manifested by generalized lymphadenopathy, particularly involving the retroperitoneal lymph node groups. Commonly, there is neoplastic involvement of such sites as the skin, lungs, pleura, palatine tonsils, bone marrow, and spleen.

Diffuse Large Cleaved Cell Lymphoma and Large Noncleaved Cell Lymphoma

Diffuse large cleaved cell lymphoma and diffuse large noncleaved cell lymphoma occur in persons of any age and can be manifested by either local or widespread systemic disease. The most common sites of origin are the lymph nodes or other lymphopoietic sites, but in 25% to 40% of cases an extranodal site of origin, such as the gastrointestinal tract (especially the stomach and distal small bowel), the thyroid gland, the bone, and the skin, is identified.

Histologically, there is diffuse infiltration by large transformed lymphoid cells with vesicular nuclei. The nuclear membrane contours may be either irregular (cleaved) or round (noncleaved) (Fig. 20-40). One to several nucleoli are noted. The tumor cell cytoplasm is scant to moderately abundant and pale to eosinophilic. Numerous mitoses are the rule.

More than half of all diffuse large cell lymphomas are of B-cell origin. The remainder are largely of T-cell origin, although in a minority of cases no identifying markers are observed. Surface immunoglobulin is frequently lacking in B-cell diffuse large cell lymphomas, in which case B-cell origin is confirmed by demonstration of specific B-cell antigens or by gene rearrangements of the immunoglobulin heavy and light chains.

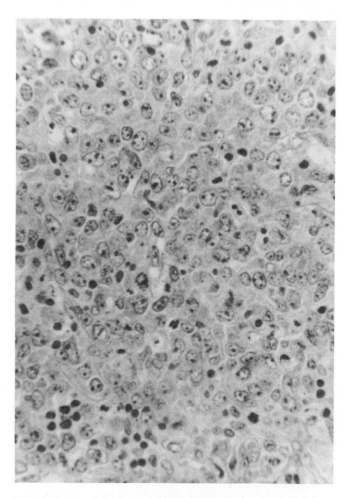

Figure 20-40.   The lymph node in large noncleaved cell lymphoma. The normal nodal architecture is replaced by a diffuse infiltration of transformed lymphoid cells with round vesicular nuclei.

Diffuse large cell lymphoma, cleaved or non-cleaved, is an aggressive neoplasm. Large cleaved cell lymphoma generally follows a more indolent course than does large noncleaved cell lymphoma. The clinical course in B-cell, T-cell, and null cell large cell lymphomas is similar. Cure can be anticipated in a majority of such neoplasms.

High-Grade Non-Hodgkin's Malignant Lymphomas

High-grade malignant lymphomas are classified as: **large cell immunoblastic, lymphoblastic,** and **small noncleaved cell (Burkitt's** and **Burkitt's-like lymphoma).**

Large Cell Immunoblastic Lymphoma

Large cell immunoblastic lymphoma is the most aggressive subtype of the large cell lymphomas. Subtypes of the immunoblastic lymphomas are described in the Working Formulation as plasmacytoid, clear cell, polymorphous, and epithelioid cell component.

The plasmacytoid variant is derived from B cells and is therefore termed **B immunoblastic lymphoma.** The neoplastic lymphoid cells exhibit nuclei with vesicular chromatin, a large central, eosinophilic nucleolus, and a moderate amount of dark blue plasmacytoid cytoplasm. **B immunoblastic lymphomas arise commonly in disordered immune states;** they include the lymphomas that arise in the central nervous system in renal allograft recipients, the lymphomas that complicate chronic lymphocytic thyroiditis and lymphoepithelial lesions of the salivary glands, the lymphomas that arise in one-third to one-half of the cases of immunoblastic lymphadenopathy, and the Mediterranean abdominal lymphoma, which may be superimposed on alpha heavy-chain disease of the proximal small bowel.

Variants of immunoblastic lymphoma defined as clear cell, polymorphous, and epithelioid cell component are generally of T-cell origin. **Clear cytoplasm is particularly characteristic of the T-cell malignant lymphomas.** Occasionally T-cell lymphomas exhibit bizarre or polymorphous cytologic features. Pleomorphic tumor cells, which morphologically simulate the Reed-Sternberg cells of Hodgkin's disease, may be identified. The distinction between non-Hodgkin's malignant lymphoma and Hodgkin's disease is based on the abnormal or neoplastic cytologic features of the background small lymphoid cells in T-cell lymphomas, as opposed to the background of normal small lymphocytes in Hodgkin's disease. Additionally, immunohistochemical staining for the granulocyte antigen Leu-M1 may be helpful in this distinction. Leu-M1 is commonly positive in Hodgkin's disease in a focal paranuclear and plasma membrane distribution. In T-cell lymphomas, staining for Leu-M1 is generally negative, although a minority of cases may exhibit positive staining frequently indistinguishable from that seen in Hodgkin's disease. The presence of benign epithelioid cell histiocytes, which are sufficiently numerous to partially obscure the underlying neoplastic lymphoid cell population, is a histologic feature that suggests a T-cell lymphoma.

Common clinical features of T-cell immunoblastic lymphomas include widespread (stage III–IV) disease, an aggressive clinical course, and frequent involvement of such anatomic sites as the skin, retroperitoneal lymph nodes, lungs, and pleura.

A distinctive T-cell malignancy, **the adult T-cell leukemia/lymphoma,** has recently been described. It is associated with a C-type retrovirus, the human T-cell leukemia/lymphoma virus (HTLV-1). **The disease is endemic in the islands of Southwestern Japan and in certain Caribbean islands** (see Fig. 20-30). There is also a higher than normal incidence of this disorder in the Southeastern United States. Morphologically, the neoplastic T cells display conspicuous nuclear membrane convolutions, which are best appreciated on peripheral blood smears. Both leukemic and lymphomatous distributions are seen, with involvement of the bone marrow, blood, lymph nodes, liver, spleen, and skin. Hypercalcemia secondary to bone lysis may be a complication. The bone destruction may reflect tumor cell secretion of an osteoclast-activating factor. **Adult T-cell leukemia/lymphoma is aggressive and is associated with a median survival of less than 1 year.**

Lymphoblastic Lymphoma

Lymphoblastic lymphoma is a diffuse malignant lymphoma, usually of mid-thymic or late thymic T-cell origin, that is closely related to the acute lymphoblastic leukemias. The neoplastic cell is a lymphoblast, 10 µ to 15 µ in diameter, that contains a round or convoluted nucleus. The chromatin is delicate, and one to several inconspicuous nucleoli are present. The cytoplasm is usually scant. The mitotic rate is extremely high. In 90% of cases the neoplastic cells express the nuclear DNA-polymerizing enzyme Tdt.

Lymphoblastic lymphoma is an aggressive disorder most commonly observed in adolescent and young adult males. In half of the cases a mediastinal mass is identified. Supradiaphragmatic lymphadenopathy is also common. The disease usually spreads rapidly to the bone marrow with a subsequent leukemic phase. The white blood cell count is high, frequently greater than 100,000 per microliter. Commonly, there is involvement of the central nervous system, with secondary leukemic meningitis.

Small Noncleaved Cell Lymphoma

Small noncleaved cell lymphomas include **Burkitt's lymphoma** and similar clinicopathologic disorders that lack the distinctive uniform morphologic features of Burkitt's lymphoma (Burkitt's-like lymphoma). **Initially described as a common malignant tumor of the jaw in young African children, Burkitt's lymphoma is endemic in tropical equatorial Africa and in certain areas of New Guinea** (see Fig. 20-30); it also occurs sporadically in other geographic locations. **Burkitt's lymphoma is an aggressive neoplasm of children that rarely occurs in adults.** In Africa the median age of onset is 7 years, and commonly the bones of the maxilla and mandible are initially involved; in Western countries the median age of onset is 9–11 years, and abdominal sites, including the terminal ileum, ovaries, and kidneys, are initially affected. The lymph nodes tend to be spared, both in endemic and in nonendemic areas. In the preterminal stage there may be leukemic distribution (FAB L3 or Burkitt's leukemia), with secondary involvement of the central nervous system.

Burkitt's lymphoma has a distinctive histologic and cytologic appearance; it is a diffuse lymphoma. Tumor cells in tissue sections are uniform and have round to oval nuclei, with coarsely reticulated chromatin, 2 to 5 small nucleoli, and a rim of dense cytoplasm, which frequently contains clear vacuoles. **Mitotic figures are numerous, a feature that demonstrates that Burkitt's lymphoma is one of the most rapidly dividing human neoplasms. Phagocytic macrophages containing nuclear and cytoplasmic debris impart the "starry sky" pattern. Burkitt's lymphoma is a B-cell tumor, and monoclonal surface membrane IgM usually is demonstrated.**

Burkitt's-like lymphoma is also a diffuse lymphoma, usually of the B-cell type, that arises either in lymph nodes or in extranodal sites. It occurs both in adults and in children. The size of the tumor cell nuclei approximates that of benign histiocytes, but there is greater variation in nuclear size and shape than in Burkitt's lymphoma. The chromatin is delicate, and one to several eosinophilic nucleoli are seen. The cytoplasm is scant and pale. Like Burkitt's lymphoma, non-Burkitt's lymphoma is clinically aggressive.

Miscellaneous Lymphomas

In the Working Formulation, several distinctive neoplastic disorders are included in a miscellaneous category. These include **mycosis fungoides** and **composite lymphoma.**

Mycosis fungoides is a cutaneous malignant disorder of mature or postthymic T-helper lymphocytes. The evolution of mycosis fungoides is typically indolent, and the disorder is initially manifested by a localized or generalized chronic erythematous or eczematous rash. In the early eczematous phase the histologic appearance is not diagnostic; focal perivascular and periadnexal lymphoid cell infiltrates in the superficial dermis are characteristic. **Over the course of months to years, the lesions progress to raised, flattened, indurated plaquelike papules and subsequently to fungating nodular tumor masses.** Both in the plaque and in the tumor stages a lymphoid bandlike dermal infiltrate lies contiguous to the epidermis. The infiltrate is composed of a spectrum of atypical lymphoid cells. Medium to large cell variants with hyperchromatic cerebriform nuclei are termed mycosis cells. Admixed inflammatory cells, including eosinophils and plasma cells, are present, particularly early in the course of the disease. Aggregates of atypical lymphoid cells in the epidermis, called **Darier-Pautrier's microabscesses, are characteristic but not diagnostic of mycosis fungoides.** Draining lymph nodes show dermatopathic lymphadenopathy and subsequently neoplastic cell infiltration, tumor first being observed in the T dependent paracortex (see Fig. 20-27). Subsequent involvement of such sites as the lungs, spleen, and liver is common.

The Sézary syndrome represents the leukemic phase of mycosis fungoides. A high white blood cell count reflects the presence of circulating neoplastic lymphoid cells with bizarre cerebriform nuclei (Fig. 20-41). Frequently a ring of perinuclear PAS-positive cytoplasmic vacuoles is demonstrated. Extensive skin involvement is prominent in the Sézary syndrome, with eczema or erythroderma.

Composite lymphoma is defined as the occurrence of two subtypes of non-Hodgkin's malignant lymphoma in the same anatomic site or the combination of contiguous Hodgkin's disease and a non-Hodgkin's malignant lymphoma. The most common example is combined follicular small cleaved and diffuse large noncleaved cell lymphomas. The prognosis in composite lymphomas is generally intermediate between that of the low-grade and that of the high-grade neoplastic cell components.

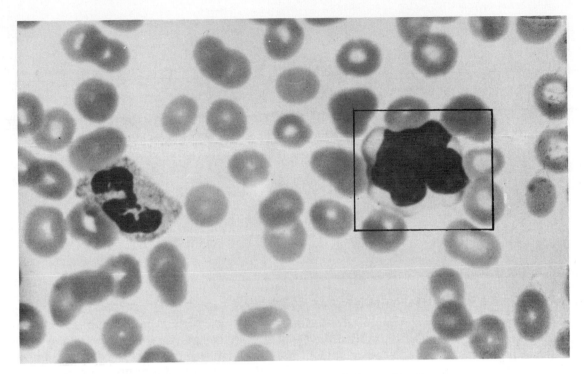

Figure 20-41. Sézary syndrome. A circulating neoplastic T-helper cell with prominent nuclear convolutions *(inset).*

Plasma Cell Neoplasia

Plasma cell neoplasia is a malignant, clonal disorder of the terminally differentiated B cell, namely the plasma cell. It is characterized by neoplastic plasma cell infiltration of the bone marrow and, less frequently, of the soft tissues. In most cases there is secretion either of a monoclonal immunoglobulin molecule or of a light chain. A serum or urine paraprotein is therefore generally detected.

There are three well-defined clinical presentations, but only one is common. Most plasma cell neoplasia occurs as multifocal disease of the bone marrow, in which case it is termed **multiple myeloma.** Uncommonly, a single destructive lesion of bone, **solitary myeloma,** is identified, but this tumor usually progresses to multiple myeloma. Localized plasma cell tumors of the soft tissues, called **extramedullary plasmacytomas,** are rare. They are located in the upper respiratory tract in 75% of cases (Fig. 20-42). Less commonly involved locations include the lower respiratory tract and other soft tissue sites. Extramedullary plasmacytomas usually do not progress to multiple myeloma.

The cause of multiple myeloma is unknown. A possible relationship to high-dose ionizing radiation has been suggested but not conclusively demonstrated. Chronic antigenic stimulation may be a predisposing factor. Intraperitoneal installation of mineral oil or solid plastic material induces a monoclonal plasmacytoma in mice. In humans rare cases of multiple myeloma have been associated with chronic infections, such as osteomyelitis, and with chronic inflammatory disorders, such as rheumatoid arthritis. In most cases no specific associations can be demonstrated. A genetic predisposition is suggested by an increased incidence of multiple myeloma and monoclonal gammopathy of unknown significance in family members of patients with myeloma, an increased frequency of the 4c complex of the HLA system in myeloma patients, and an increased incidence of multiple myeloma in blacks.

The pathophysiology in multiple myeloma relates to both progressive infiltration and destruction of bone by the malignant plasma cells and to the secondary effects of the serum or urine paraprotein.

The osseous tumors of multiple myeloma are red-gray, soft, gelatinous, and well demarcated from the contiguous normal bone. There may be mild enlargement of the lymph nodes, liver, and spleen, but the gross appearance is not distinctive.

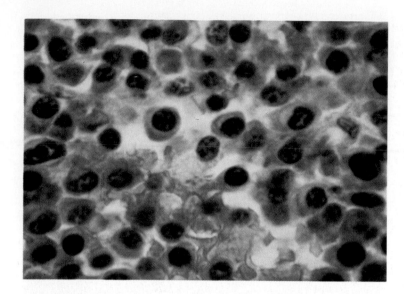

Figure 20-42. Extramedullary plasmacytoma. Infiltration of the larynx by neoplastic plasma cells, with eccentric hyperchromatic nuclei and abundant purple cytoplasm.

In histologic sections of bone marrow, **clusters or diffuse sheets of plasma cells are identified** (see Fig. 20-25). **Unlike reactive processes, neoplastic plasma cell infiltration is not selectively perivascular. A characteristic early histologic feature is the encircling of fat cells by plasma cells.** Ultimately both normal hematopoietic tissues and fat cells are replaced. Although neoplastic plasma cells may be indistinguishable from normal cells, they are more commonly immature and display atypical morphologic features. These include the presence of nucleoli, irregular chromatin distribution, binucleation or multinucleation, and a primitive blastlike appearance. Marrow osteoclast activity is increased, and numerous osteoclasts are located in resorption lacunae along the margins of bony trabeculae. This osteoclast proliferation may be a response to the secretion of osteoclast-activating factor by the neoplastic plasma cells. The bone resorption induced by the increased osteoclast activity may be responsible, at least in part, for the hypercalcemia that is a common complication of multiple myeloma.

In the spleen the disease involves principally the red pulp, with plasma cell infiltration of both the cords and the sinuses (see Fig. 20-21). The liver may show infiltration of the portal areas or, in the case of a leukemic phase, of the sinusoids. In the lymph nodes there may be initial patchy involvement of the medullary cords, which rarely progresses to extensive infiltration and obliteration of the normal nodal architecture.

Renal involvement (myeloma kidney) occurs in up to 80% of the cases. The kidneys may be normal in size, slightly enlarged, or contracted owing to the multiple damaging effects of hypercalciuria, hyper-

uricosuria, and acute or chronic pyelonephritis. Plasma cell infiltration of the kidneys, usually focal and interstitial, is common, but even extensive involvement may not affect renal function. Light chains are toxic to the renal tubular epithelium and are important in the genesis of the renal failure that is common in multiple myeloma. Frequently proteinaceous casts containing light chains and other proteins are found in the distal convoluted and collecting tubules. Morphologically, the casts are either homogeneous and finely granular or lamellar. They may induce destruction of the renal tubules, occasionally with an accompanying giant cell reaction or with proliferation of the tubular epithelium.

The diagnosis of multiple myeloma is made only after careful consideration of both the clinical and the pathologic findings (see Table 20-21). **The diagnosis requires the findings of sheets of plasma cells or a significant population of atypical plasma cells in the bone marrow, the presence (in the vast majority of cases) of a monoclonal paraprotein, and the radiologic demonstration (in the majority of cases) of lytic bone lesions (Fig. 20-43) or of diffuse osteoporosis.** Lytic bone lesions of the skull and other flat bones are a characteristic but not diagnostic radiologic finding in multiple myeloma.

The distribution of the serum and urine immunoglobulin abnormalities in multiple myeloma is shown in Table 20-37. In the majority of cases levels of the normal circulating immunoglobulins are depressed. A small serum or urine monoclonal protein can be identified in up to one-third of cases of solitary myeloma or of extramedullary plasmacytoma. These generally disappear following treatment of the isolated tumor.

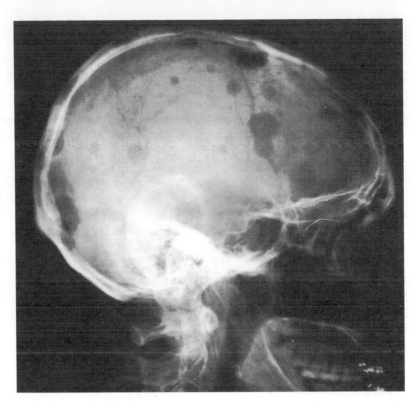

Figure 20-43. Multiple myeloma. A radiograph of the skull shows numerous "punched-out" radiolucent areas.

Common laboratory findings include a mild normocytic normochromic anemia and a mild neutropenia. A leukoerythroblastic reaction may be observed. Circulating plasma cells may be seen on the blood smear. Because of the increased serum immunoglobulin levels due to the paraprotein, there is typically a high erythrocyte sedimentation rate. Occasionally the peripheral blood smear exhibits rouleaux formation, described as a stacked coin appearance of erythrocytes. Serum calcium and uric acid levels are frequently elevated. Normal alkaline phosphatase levels attest to an absence of increased bone marrow osteoblast activity.

Multiple myeloma is usually a disease of the older age groups, the average age at diagnosis being 60 years. However, the disease may occur in young and middle-aged adults and has even been seen in teenagers. There is a slight male predominance. **The most common symptom is bone pain. Low back pain occurs in 70%, rib pain in 20%, and leg pain in 10% of the cases.** The bone pain may be intermittent and chronic, owing to slowly progressive plasma cell infiltration, or acute and severe, as in the case of pathologic fractures. Pathologic fractures most commonly involve the vertebrae, ribs, and long bones. Weakness and fatigue due to the normocytic normochromic anemia are also frequently encountered. Less commonly, there may be neurologic symptoms

due either to spinal cord compression or to infiltration of nerve trunks by neoplastic plasma cells. Nerve root symptoms may also be due to amyloid deposition. **Amyloidosis occurs in 10% to 15% of cases of multiple myeloma.**

Acute infections by gram-negative bacteria or by encapsulated gram-positive organisms, such as pneumococcus, streptococcus, and meningococcus, are common and often involve the lungs and genitourinary tract. The increased incidence of infection is caused by the decreased levels of normal serum immunoglobulins and by the neutropenia induced

Table 20-37 Multiple Myeloma: Distribution of Immunoglobulin Abnormalities

Immunoglobulin Abnormality	Percent
Serum monoclonal gammopathy	75
IgG	55–60
IgA	15–20
IgD	<1
IgE	Rare
IgM	Very rare
Urine light chain only (Bence-Jones protein)	20–25
Combined serum monoclonal gammopathy and urine light chain	70
Two or more serum monoclonal immunoglobulins	0.5
Nonsecretory	1

by therapy. The hyperviscosity syndrome, which reflects the high serum levels or unusual physicochemical properties of the paraprotein, is observed in 7% of cases. Rarely, the paraprotein has the properties of a cryoglobulin and reversibly precipitates in the colder portions of the extremities. Because of the cryoglobulin properties, Raynaud's phenomenon and purpura, which may progress to ulceration and gangrene of the distal fingers and toes, may occur. A bleeding diathesis, usually due to thrombocytopenia and rarely due to paraprotein complexing with clotting factors, may be observed.

The clinical course of multiple myeloma is frequently biphasic, with an initial chronic stable phase followed by an accelerated preterminal phase. The median survival in multiple myeloma is 30 months. The prognosis is worse if there is a large tumor cell burden, indicated by a hemoglobin level of less than 8.5 g/dl, a serum calcium level greater than 12 mg/dl, marked elevation of serum or urine paraproteins, and extensive lytic bone lesions.

A poor prognosis is also associated with the presence of a lambda light-chain paraprotein, since lambda light chains are particularly toxic to the renal tubular epithelium. A poor prognosis is also associated with those cases in which there is secretion of IgD heavy chain. This form of myeloma is aggressive and frequently associated with prominent extramedullary soft tissue involvement. The common causes of death in multiple myeloma are infection and renal failure. A small minority of patients succumb to superimposed acute nonlymphocytic leukemia, usually following chemotherapy with alkylating agents.

Hodgkin's Disease

Hodgkin's disease is a unique malignant disorder that commonly first involves the lymph nodes. Hodgkin's disease has traditionally been classified with the malignant lymphomas, but a number of unusual clinical and pathologic features distinguish Hodgkin's disease from the non-Hodgkin's malignant lymphomas and other malignant neoplasms. First, the clinicopathologic presentation frequently simulates an infectious process. Second, a significant proportion of tumor tissue commonly consists of benign host immune and inflammatory cells. Third, the classification of histopathologic subtypes is based on the type of host immune response rather than on the architectural or cytologic features of the neoplastic cells. Fourth, the origin of the neoplastic cell, the Reed-Sternberg cell, is controversial. Finally, Hodgkin's disease usually spreads predictably from involved nodes to adjacent nodal groups.

Etiology and Pathogenesis

The cause of Hodgkin's disease is unknown. An association with oncogenic viruses is suspected but not proved. Young adults with infectious mononucleosis (Epstein-Barr virus infection) have a threefold increased risk of developing Hodgkin's disease, but the viral genome has not been identified in tumor tissue. The possibility of horizontal transmission of an infectious agent has been suggested by reports of several self-limited "mini-epidemics" of Hodgkin's disease in children. Although this apparent case clustering has not been confirmed by broader epidemiologic studies, there may be a sevenfold increased risk in siblings, and the incidence is increased two- to threefold in family members of patients with Hodgkin's disease.

Global epidemiologic patterns suggest that age at first exposure to unidentified oncogenic agents may influence the incidence of specific histopathologic subtypes of Hodgkin's disease (see Table 20-32). In Western countries the incidence of indolent subtypes of Hodgkin's disease is higher than normal in young adults from small families and upper socioeconomic groups. Children younger than 10 years of age account for fewer than 10% of all cases of Hodgkin's disease. These observations suggest a delayed or decreased exposure to oncogenic agents. By contrast, in developing countries aggressive variants of Hodgkin's disease are common in childhood, and there is typically no peak of indolent disease in young adults. Early exposure to oncogenic agents is suggested in these cases.

The pathogenesis seems to involve a gradual malignant transformation of indigenous cells in lymph nodes or, less commonly, other tissues. The process of transformation appears to follow an orderly progression from normal to disordered cellular proliferation to overt neoplasia. Elucidation of the pathogenesis of Hodgkin's disease has been hindered by ignorance as to the origin of the Reed-Sternberg cell. In lymph nodes the T-dependent paracortex is first involved in Hodgkin's disease. Additionally, a deficiency in cell-mediated immunity is identified even early in the course of the disease. It has therefore been suggested that Reed-Sternberg cells evolve from transformed T cells. However, Reed-Sternberg cells lack specific T-cell markers. Both B-lymphocytes and cells of the mononuclear phagocyte system have been considered as possible precursors of Reed-Sternberg cells, but such an origin has not been confirmed by cell marker studies. More recent evidence has incriminated the antigen-processing and presenting cells—namely, the dendritic reticulum and interdigitating reticulum cells—as the possible culprits in Hodgkin's disease. These cells share certain common cell markers with Reed-Sternberg cells, including Fc and C_3b receptors and Ia antigen. Additionally, defects in antigen presentation to T cells because of neoplastic transformation of interdigitating reticulum cells could explain the abnormalities of delayed-type hypersensitivity detected even in newly diagnosed and untreated patients. However, despite such intriguing indirect evidence, the origin of Reed-Sternberg cells remains speculative.

Gross Pathology

Grossly, lymph nodes and other tissues involved by Hodgkin's disease are usually soft and pale gray, producing the so-called "fish flesh" appearance. Less commonly, firm, or "rubbery," tumor tissue reflects a variable degree of fibrosis. Focal necrosis may be visualized as areas of opaque yellow-gray discoloration. The lymph nodes may be matted together if tumor extends beyond the nodal capsules.

Routinely, the largest lymph node of a group of enlarged nodes should be removed for diagnostic biopsy. Smaller lymph nodes may exhibit only reactive changes and lack the histopathologic features diagnostic of Hodgkin's disease.

The spleen in Hodgkin's disease exhibits variable enlargement of the white pulp or a few dominant tumor nodules (Fig. 20-44). With early involvement (first in the T-dependent periarteriolar lymphoid sheath), there may be slight enlargement of one or several areas of the white pulp. Therefore, when Hodgkin's disease is suspected, the spleen should be carefully examined grossly at 2-mm to 3-mm intervals for detection of minute foci of involvement. In the liver the portal areas are first involved. Tumor nodules similar to those of metastatic carcinoma may be identified in the liver, usually late in the course of the disease.

Focal, multifocal, or diffuse infiltration of the bone marrow may be observed (see Fig. 20-25). Osteolytic or osteoblastic bone lesions are demonstrated radiographically.

Histopathology

Histopathologically, Hodgkin's disease exhibits a considerable heterogeneity of cell types, including classic Reed-Sternberg cells, variants of Reed-Sternberg cells that are characteristic of subtypes but not fully diagnostic of Hodgkin's disease, normal lymphocytes, and a spectrum of inflammatory cells. There may be delicate or dense fibrosis. **The diagnosis of Hodgkin's disease requires demonstration**

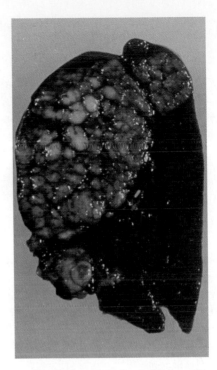

Figure 20-44. Hodgkin's disease involving the spleen. Several multinodular tumor masses partially replace the normal splenic parenchyma.

of the Reed-Sternberg cell, a distinctive tumor giant cell, in an environment of normal small lymphocytes and a heterogeneous population of benign inflammatory cells. Cells indistinguishable from Reed-Sternberg cells may be identified in other malignancies, such as carcinomas, sarcomas, and the non-Hodgkin's malignant lymphomas, and, rarely, in some reactive processes. In these disorders, however, Reed-Sternberg cells are not observed in the setting of normal small lymphocytes.

The classic Reed-Sternberg cell (Fig. 20-45) is binucleated and has large eosinophilic nucleoli centrally located in nuclei, which exhibit abundant clear parachromatin. Delicate threads of heterochromatin frequently extend from the nucleoli to a marginal rim of dense heterochromatin that accentuates the nuclear membranes. The cytoplasm is a pale pink. Multinucleated cells or cells with multilobed nuclei may be seen and are also considered diagnostic Reed-Sternberg cells. The identification of necrobiotic (mummified) Reed-Sternberg cells is characteristic of Hodgkin's disease.

Cytogenetic studies reveal an aneuploid, frequently hypotetraploid, neoplastic cell karyotype. No consistent chromosomal abnormalities are identified, but marker chromosomes indicative of monoclonality have been demonstrated, including additions to the long arm of chromosome 14 (14q +). The immuno-

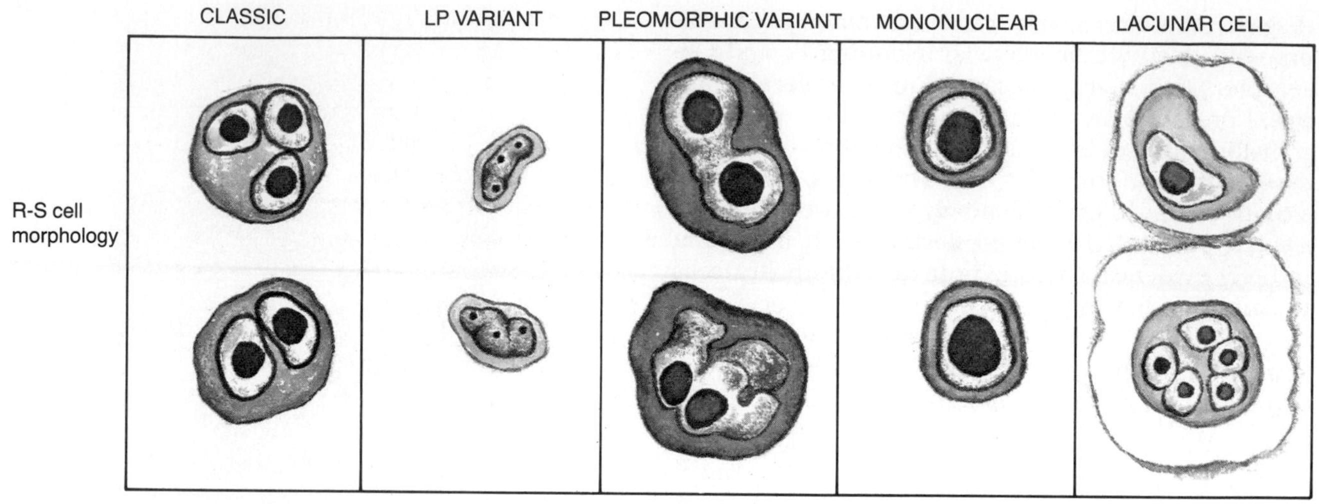

	CLASSIC	LP VARIANT	PLEOMORPHIC VARIANT	MONONUCLEAR	LACUNAR CELL
R-S cell morphology					

	CLASSIC	LP VARIANT	PLEOMORPHIC VARIANT	MONONUCLEAR	LACUNAR CELL
Nuclear Configuration	Binucleated to multinucleated to multilobulated	Single to multilobed	Single to multinucleated or multilobed	Single	Single to multilobed
Nucleoli	large (≥1/3 diameter of nucleus), eosinophilic	Small, punctate	Variable, prominent	large (≥1/3 diameter of nucleus), eosinophilic	Variable (generally <1/3 diameter of nucleus), eosinophilic
Chromatin	Clear parachromatin	Delicate	Variable, clear parachromatin to hyperchromatic	Abundant, clear parachromatin	delicate to clear parachromatin
Cytoplasm	Moderate to abundant, pale to pink	Scant, pale	Moderate to abundant, eosinophilic	Moderate, pale to pink	Abundant, pale[†]
Associated histologic subtype	Diagnostic in lymphocyte predominant, mixed cellularity, may be seen (diagnostic) in lymphocyte depleted, nodular sclerosis	Lymphocyte predominant (suggestive, not diagnostic)	Lymphocyte depleted[‡]	May be seen in any subtype	Nodular sclerosis[§]

[*] Mononuclear R-S cell variants are not diagnostic of Hodgkin's disease. However, these cells, in the appropriate environment, indicate involvement either in the staging work-up or in relapse

[†] Formalin fixation artifact: the cytoplasm of these cells may retract and the cell appears to lie in a clear space (lacuna or lake).

[‡] Pleomorphic large cell lymphoma of T-cell type must be ruled out

[§] Similar cells may occasionally be seen in mixed cellularity

Figure 20-45. Hodgkin's disease—Reed-Sternberg cells. Morphology of the classic Reed-Sternberg cell of Hodgkin's disease and variants of the Reed-Sternberg cell that are characteristic of Hodgkin's disease subtypes. Criteria for the identification of each cell type are shown in the accompanying table.

histochemical demonstration of focal paranuclear and plasma membrane staining for the granulocyte antigen Leu M1 is highly suggestive of, but not diagnostic for, Hodgkin's disease.

Cells with single nuclei and similar nuclear features are called mononuclear variants, or Hodgkin's cells (see Fig. 20-45). They may be seen in any subtype of the disease but are not diagnostic. Mononuclear variants may be difficult to distinguish from atypical reactive immunoblasts. Classic Reed-Sternberg cells may develop from the mononuclear variants by amitotic division, that is, nuclear replication without cell division. When rebiopsy is performed either for staging (establishing extent of disease) or for documentation of disease recurrence in a patient with a previously established diagnosis of Hodgkin's disease, the demonstration of mononuclear variants in the appropriate histopathologic setting of normal small lymphocytes and inflammatory cells is sufficient to confirm the diagnosis. Three additional Reed-Sternberg cell variants, the lymphocyte predominant, the pleomorphic, and the lacunar variant, are characteristic of several subtypes but are not fully diagnostic of Hodgkin's disease (see Fig. 20-45).

Four histopathologic subtypes of Hodgkin's disease are recognized, on the basis of specific cellular and stromal fibroblastic components of the host immune response (Fig. 20-46): **lymphocyte predominant (LP), mixed cellularity (MC), lymphocyte depleted (LD), and nodular sclerosis (NS). The subdivisions LP, MC, and LD are based on the ratio of normal lymphocytes to neoplastic Reed-Sternberg cells; NS is determined by the presence of distinctive Reed-Sternberg variants, the lacunar cells, and by the presence of dense, bandlike fibrosis.** The progression from lymphocyte predominant to mixed cellularity to lymphocyte depleted is characterized by decreasing numbers of normal small lymphocytes and by increasing numbers of Reed-Sternberg cells. Before the era of modern therapy, the histopathologic subtype represented an important prognostic indicator (LP>NS>MC>LD). With current therapy, the prognostic differences due to histopathologic subtype have largely evaporated.

The lymphocyte-predominant Reed-Sternberg cell variant is associated with the LP subtype of Hodgkin's disease. This variant, or "popcorn cell," has single or lobed nuclei, with delicate chromatin and small and inconspicuous nucleoli, and scant to moderate pale cytoplasm. There are no specific variants of the Reed-Sternberg cell that are characteristic of the mixed cellularity subtype. Classic binucleated or other diagnostic cells are usually numerous in mixed cellularity Hodgkin's disease. Pleomorphic variants

or classic binucleated Reed-Sternberg cells may predominate in the hypercellular or reticular variant of the lymphocyte-depleted subtype. Pleomorphic variants are bizarre multinucleated and/or multilobed cells with prominent nucleoli. In the hypocellular or diffuse fibrosis variant of lymphocyte-depleted Hodgkin's disease, there is usually marked depletion of both neoplastic Reed-Sternberg cells and immune and inflammatory cells. The tumor mass consists predominantly of a loose fibrillar proteinaceous material. The histopathologic expressions of both the reticular and the diffuse fibrosis variants of lymphocyte-depleted Hodgkin's disease are frequently identified in a single biopsy specimen.

Nodular sclerosis is a distinctive subtype of Hodgkin's disease characterized by dense, bandlike fibrosis and by a specific Reed-Sternberg cell variant, the lacunar cell. This cell has abundant pale cytoplasm and a lobulated nucleus, with eosinophilic nucleoli that are generally intermediate in size. The lacunar cell is so named because, in formalin-fixed tissue, the cytoplasm artifactually retracts toward the nucleus and the cell appears to lie in a lacuna, or lake. In the nodular sclerosis subtype, classic binucleated Reed-Sternberg cells may be difficult to identify among the clearly predominant lacunar cell variants. In nodular sclerosis, the fibrosis or sclerosis is prominent and initially involves the node capsule. Subsequently, bandlike fibrosis extends into the parenchyma to circumscribe nodules of lymphoid tissue. Characteristic lacunar cells are identified singly or in clusters in these lymphoid nodules. Uncommonly, lacunar cells and variants of lacunar cells may be numerous, occurring as extensive cohesive cellular infiltrates, the so-called syncytial variant of nodular sclerosis. This aggressive variant must be distinguished from carcinoma, melanoma, and other malignant disorders.

Clinical Features

Clinically, Hodgkin's disease is often characterized by a nontender enlarged lymph node or group of lymph nodes. The involved nodes may wax and wane in size before being removed for definitive diagnosis. **Central, or axial, lymph nodes are most commonly involved, particularly cervical (60% to 80% of cases) and mediastinal (50% to 60% of cases)** (Fig. 20-37). Left cervical lymph nodes are more commonly involved than are right cervical lymph nodes. Peripheral lymph node groups, such as the antecubital and popliteal, tend to be spared. Preferential sites of involvement are outlined in Table 20-31.

Figure 20-46.   Histopathologic subtypes of Hodgkin's disease. The characteristic histopathologic appearance of each of the principal subtypes of Hodgkin's disease is shown. The sequence from lymphocyte-predominant Hodgkin's disease to lymphocyte-depleted Hodgkin's disease is characterized by progressively fewer normal lymphocytes and by increasing numbers of Reed-Sternberg cells. The subtype of lymphocyte-depleted diffuse fibrosis is characterized by few lymphocytes, few Reed-Sternberg cells, and abundant loose fibrosis. The subtype nodular sclerosing Hodgkin's disease is distinctive because of dense, bandlike, collagenous fibrosis, which envelops cellular aggregates that contain lymphoid and inflammatory cells and the specific lacunar cell variants of the Reed-Sternberg cell. The specific criteria that define each of the Hodgkin's disease subtypes are outlined in the accompanying table.

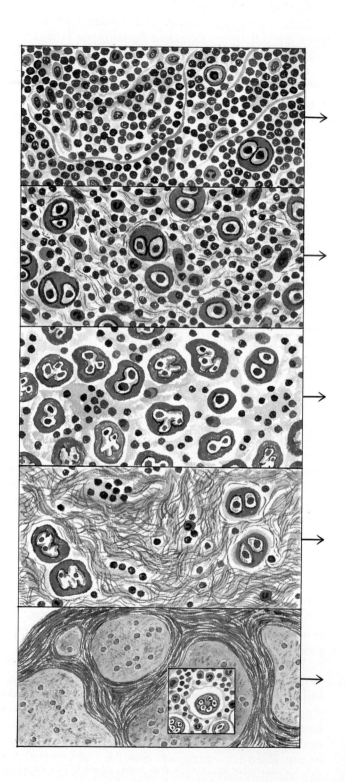

SUBTYPE	LYMPHOCYTE/REED-STERNBERG (R-S) CELL RELATIONSHIP			BACKGROUND ENVIRONMENT			LYMPH NODE INVOLVEMENT	
	NORMAL SMALL LYMPHOCYTES	REED-STERNBERG (R-S) CELL		MIXED INFLAMMATION (eosinophils, plasma cells, polys, histiocytes)	FIBROSIS	NECROSIS	PATTERN	EXTENT
		CLASSIC	VARIANT					
Lymphocyte predominant	Predominant*	Rare	Variable LP variants	Rare	Rare	Rare	Diffuse or vaguely nodular	Complete effacement
Mixed cellularity	Moderate	Variable (easily identified)	Mononuclear, lacunar, pleomorphic variants may be seen	Variable	Delicate	May be seen	Diffuse	Focal paracortical to complete effacement
Lymphocyte depleted, reticular	Scant	May be seen	Pleomorphic variant may be predominant	Scant	Delicate	May be seen	Diffuse	Complete effacement
Lymphocyte depleted, diffuse fibrosis	Scant	Rare	Rare pleomorphic variant	Scant	Abundant loose mesh-like	May be seen	Diffuse	Complete effacement
Nodular sclerosis	Predominant to scant	Rare to absent	Variable lacunar variant	Variable	Dense band-like	May be seen	Nodular (defined by collagenous fibrosis)**	Focal paracortical to complete effacement

*Benign histiocytes may constitute predominant population (histiocytic variant of lymphocyte-predominant Hodgkin's Disease).
**Vaguely nodular pattern without collagenous fibrosis (cellular phase nodular sclerosis) may be seen rarely.

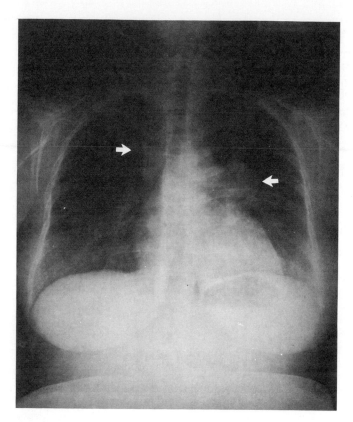

Figure 20-47. Hodgkin's disease—nodular sclerosis subtype. A radiograph of the chest shows enlarged hilar lymph nodes *(arrows).*

The spread of Hodgkin's disease appears to be by direct contiguity; that is, by direct spread between adjacent lymph node groups. There is an increased incidence of involvement of several associated anatomic sites. For example, there is often simultaneous involvement of the left supraclavicular and the abdominal periaortic lymph nodes, and of the right supraclavicular and the mediastinal lymph nodes. The spleen is involved at the time of diagnosis in one-third of cases. Hematogenous spread from the spleen is thought to be responsible for secondary hepatic and bone marrow involvement; the liver is rarely affected in the absence of splenic involvement.

In Western countries, nodular sclerosis accounts for 50% to 60% of cases of Hodgkin's disease, mixed cellularity for 30%, lymphocyte predominant for 5% to 10%, and lymphocyte depleted for 5% to 10%. The nodular sclerosis subtype commonly involves the lower cervical, supraclavicular, and mediastinal lymph nodes, particularly in young women. A mediastinal mass is common. Clinically, nodular sclerosis Hodgkin's disease is an indolent disorder, but late relapse is not uncommon. The mixed cellularity variety involves any lymph node group, but the left

cervical lymph nodes are most commonly affected. Any age group may be afflicted, but the disease is most common in middle-aged and elderly men. The lymphocyte-predominant type commonly involves the high cervical and less frequently involves the inguinal lymph nodes in men under the age of 35 years. This variety follows an indolent course and, before the era of modern therapy, was the only subtype associated with a good prognosis, even in the presence of widespread or systemic disease. Lymphocyte depleted is the most aggressive subtype of Hodgkin's disease. Visceral involvement, especially of the liver and bone marrow, is common at the time of diagnosis. Bulky lymphadenopathy may or may not be observed but is most common in the reticular subtype. In Western countries, lymphocyte depletion is most common in middle-aged and elderly men.

The salient clinical features of Hodgkin's disease are listed in Table 20-30. Fever, night sweats, and weight loss of 10% or more of baseline body weight within the 6 months before diagnosis are observed in one-third of cases. Patients with these symptoms are in the B group and have a worse prognosis than A-group patients, who lack these symptoms. Other distinctive symptoms include localized or generalized pruritus and alcohol-induced pain in involved sites.

All ages are affected in Hodgkin's disease. There is, however, a distinctive bimodal age peak, with an increased incidence between 15 and 34 years and a less well defined one over 50 years. The younger age peak principally reflects the increased incidence of nodular sclerosis Hodgkin's disease in young women. Overall there is a slight male predominance because of the higher incidence of Hodgkin's disease in middle-aged and elderly men.

The laboratory findings are generally nonspecific. They include a mild normocytic normochromic anemia of chronic disease and occasionally a moderate granulocytosis or eosinophilia. Lymphocytopenia (<1500 lymphocytes per microliter) may be observed late in the course of the disease. Elevation of the erythrocyte sedimentation rate correlates with disease activity.

The prognosis in Hodgkin's disease is principally dependent on the age of the patient and the extent of the disease or stage. In general, younger patients do better than older patients. In the assessment of the extent of disease, the comprehensive Ann Arbor staging system, which is based on clinical and pathologic findings, is employed (Table 20-38). **A more favorable prognosis is associated with a lower clinical stage (localized disease) and the absence of B symptoms.** The presence of noncaseating sarcoid-like granulomas in the bone marrow, liver, spleen, and

Table 20-38 Ann Arbor Staging System for Hodgkin's Disease

Stage I *A or B**	I	Involvement of a single lymph node region
		OR
	I_E	a single extralymphatic organ or site
Stage II *A or B**	II	Involvement of two or more lymph node regions on the same side of the diaphragm
		OR
	II_E	with localized contiguous involvement of an extralymphatic organ site
Stage III *A or B**	III	Involvement of lymph node regions on both sides of the diaphragm
		OR
	III_E	with localized contiguous involvement of an extralymphatic organ or site
		OR
	III_S	with involvement of spleen
		OR
	III_ES	both extralymphatic organ or site and spleen involvement
Stage IV *A or B**	IV	Diffuse or disseminated involvement of one or more extralymphatic organs with or without associated lymph node involvement

* *A*, asymptomatic; *B*, presence of constitutional symptoms (fever, night sweats, and weight loss exceeding 10% of baseline body weight)

lymph nodes in 10% to 15% of cases also carries a better prognosis. These granulomas may represent a host immune response to circulating tumor antigens or antigen-antibody complexes.

The therapy of Hodgkin's disease is increasingly effective, and in a majority of cases, clinical cure can be anticipated.

The complications of Hodgkin's disease include compromise of vital organs by progressive tumor growth, such as spinal cord compression and obstruction of ureters; infections due to defects in delayed-type hypersensitivity or to the immunosuppressive effects of therapy; direct toxicity of therapy, including pulmonary fibrosis, decreased thyroid function, and marrow suppression; and second cancers, due probably to the immunosuppressive and mutagenic effects of therapy (acute nonlymphocytic leukemia in less than 5% of cases and large cell malignant lymphoma in less than 1% of cases).

Bone Marrow: Metastatic Tumors

The bone marrow is a common site of metastatic tumors. The incidence of metastatic tumors is greater than that of primary bone tumors. In adults, carcinomas that arise in glandular or ductular epithelium are the most common cancers that metastasize to the bone marrow. **Carcinomas of the breast, lung, and prostate account for over 80% of the tumors that metastasize to the bone marrow.** In children, neuroblastomas and Ewing's tumor are the types of tumor that most commonly metastasize to the bone marrow. Sarcomas or tumors of mesodermal origin, with the exception of embryonal rhabdomyosarcoma of childhood, uncommonly metastasize to the bone marrow. Spread of malignant tumors to the bone marrow is usually by the hematogenous or blood-borne route. Occasionally, there may be direct spread from tumors that involve contiguous soft tissue sites.

The axial skeleton, including the cranium, vertebrae, ribs, and sacrum, is involved in 70% of cases of metastatic malignancy to bone. Neurologic symptoms are common, resulting from encroachment on and damage to the brain, spinal cord, and nerve roots. In 30% of cases of metastatic tumor, the appendicular skeleton, particularly the metaphyses of the proximal long bones, is first involved. Metastasis to the distal long bones below the elbows and knees is distinctly uncommon.

The microscopic diagnosis of metastatic cancer in the bone marrow is usually made without difficulty. Unlike the indigenous hematopoietic cells, which are loosely associated, metastatic tumor cells are generally cohesive and may exhibit a mosaic-like pattern. Metastatic tumor cells are generally also larger than the indigenous hematopoietic cells. Exceptions include tumor cells in the metastatic small cell anaplastic carcinomas and APUDomas, which may be similar in cell size to hematopoietic blast cells. Metastatic tumor cells often recapitulate the architectural patterns of the tissue of origin. The presence of glandular or ductular structures (see Fig. 20-25) or linear arrays of tumor cells, the so-called Indian filing, are features characteristic of metastatic carcinoma. The histopathologic features of metastatic thyroid and renal cell carcinomas and carcinomas of the large bowel are generally distinctive. Occasionally, however, metastatic renal cell carcinoma may simulate collections of benign foamy macrophages. Metastatic small cell or oat cell carcinoma of the lung and metastatic carcinoid tumor may be confused with malignant lymphoma.

Most metastatic tumors to the bone marrow cause osteolysis (destruction of the underlying bone). Such osteolytic metastases are particularly characteristic of metastatic thyroid, renal, and breast carcinomas. Metastatic tumors that induce new bone formation, termed osteoblastic metastases, are characteristic of metastatic prostatic carcinoma, carcinoid tumors, and some metastatic breast carcinomas. Frequently, mixed osteolytic and osteoblastic metastases are observed. A reactive fibrotic response in the marrow is especially characteristic of metastatic gastric and breast carcinomas.

Secondary, or reactive, changes in the bone marrow hematopoietic tissues adjacent to metastatic deposits include hyperplasias or hypoplasias of any or all of the hematopoietic cell lines. Megakaryocytic cell hyperplasia and eosinophilia are especially common. There may be a reactive marrow plasmacytosis, which on occasion requires distinction from plasma cell neoplasia.

Tumors metastatic to the bone marrow are frequently associated with peripheral blood neutrophilia and thrombocytopenia, and sometimes with moderate thrombocytosis. Indeed, an isolated peripheral blood thrombocytosis in the absence of other findings suggests the diagnosis of a metastatic malignant tumor. A normocytic normochromic anemia of chronic disease is common. A leukoerythroblastic reaction, with immature erythrocytes, leukocytes, and large platelets in the peripheral circulation, is an uncommon finding. Laboratory findings include an elevated serum acid phosphatase in metastatic carcinoma of the prostate gland and an elevated alkaline phosphatase in any osteoblastic bone metastasis. The increased serum alkaline phosphatase is due to hyperplasia of marrow osteoblasts involved in laying down new bone. Elevation of the serum alkaline phosphatase is a nonspecific finding, since it may also be increased with metastatic carcinoma to the liver. Identification of alkaline phosphatase isoenzymes is required to distinguish the specific bone and liver isoenzymes of alkaline phosphatase.

The principal clinical symptom in metastatic tumor to the bone marrow is the gradual onset of bone pain.

The pain is usually localized and generally worse at night. There may be pathologic fractures in sites of metastasis, usually involving the weight-bearing bones. The clinical syndrome is characterized by the sudden onset of severe pain in the site of the fracture.

Lymph Nodes: Metastatic Tumors

The regional lymph nodes that drain the sites of primary malignant tumors are commonly enlarged. This lymphadenopathy may be due either to benign reactive hyperplasia or to the presence of metastatic malignancy. Benign immunologic reactions to tumor-associated antigenic material may be expressed as follicular or interfollicular hyperplasia, sinus histiocytosis, and plasmacytosis. Sarcoid-like granulomas are occasionally observed. In certain tumors, such as carcinomas of the breast and stomach, interfollicular hyperplasia and sinus histocytosis have been associated with a favorable prognosis. By contrast, follicular hyperplasia and plasmacytosis have not been associated with an improved prognosis.

The regional lymph nodes are the most common site of initial metastatic spread of both carcinoma and malignant melanoma. Metastatic tumor cells first enter the lymph nodes by invading the tissue lymphatics, after which they are washed by lymph into the subcapsular sinus. Because they initially involve the lymph node sinuses, metastatic carcinoma or malignant melanoma cells can be confused with malignant histocytes or, if cytologically bland, with benign sinus histiocytes. Clues as to epithelial origin include cellular cohesion and characteristic architectural patterns, such as gland formation. Additionally, carcinoma cells rarely exhibit phagocytosis. Metastatic malignant melanoma may not demonstrate the cellular cohesion characteristic of metastatic carcinoma, but its characteristic cytologic features, including prominent eosinophilic nucleoli and cytoplasmic melanin pigment, often suggest the appropriate diagnosis.

Metastatic tumor cells fill and expand the subcapsular and radiating sinuses of lymph nodes before invading the stroma. The appearance of cohesive cells expanding the sinuses, with intervening residual normal lymphoid tissue, is characteristic of metastatic tumors. As the stroma is invaded, the margin of advancing tumor is well demarcated (pushing margins), a finding that is characteristic of metastatic tumors. Metastatic carcinoma often exhibits extensive areas of necrosis, in which case viable tumor cells may be identified only in a perivascular location.

The architectural patterns and cellular features of metastatic malignant tumors usually recapitulate those of the primary tumor, although variability in cellular differentiation is not infrequent. Occasionally the primary site cannot be identified on histopathologic grounds. The anatomic site of the involved lymph nodes is especially important in these cases. For example, the first site of metastasis is frequently the high cervical lymph nodes in many tumors of the head and neck; the right or left scalene lymph nodes in tumors of the thorax; the left supraclavicular and left scalene lymph nodes in abdominal cancers (especially carcinoma of the stomach); the axillary lymph nodes in breast cancer, malignant melanomas, and squamous cell carcinomas of the skin of the trunk and upper extremities; and the inguinal lymph nodes in tumors of the genitourinary system, the colorectum, and the skin of the lower extremities.

Sarcomas, which usually disseminate by the hematogenous route, are less likely to metastasize to the regional lymph nodes than are carcinomas or malignant melanomas. However, by either route, the regional or more distant lymph node groups may be sites of metastatic sarcoma. Of the sarcomas, lymph node involvement is most common with embryonal rhabdomyosarcoma of childhood. Synovial sarcoma and epithelioid sarcoma also occasionally metastasize to the lymph nodes.

Kaposi's sarcoma is a malignant tumor probably derived from vascular endothelial cells, and the tumor cells commonly are positive for Factor VIII antigen. Kaposi's sarcoma may involve the lymph nodes either as a primary malignant neoplasm or, more commonly, as a result of hematogenous spread from a cutaneous site. In either case, Kaposi's sarcoma is first identified in the lymph nodes in the region of the capsule as foci of proliferating, spindle-shaped, or elongate cells with accompanying vessel-like slits. Extravasated erythrocytes and deposition of hemosiderin or iron pigment are characteristic. The lymph node follicles may be prominent and contain hyalinized and thickened blood vessels. Rows of lymphocytes and increased interfollicular plasma cells surround the follicles. Thus, the histologic appearance mimics that of angiofollicular lymph node hyperplasia, and a possible relationship between these disorders has been postulated.

As with tumor metastatic to the bone marrow, immunologic cell marker studies are frequently useful in suggesting or confirming the diagnosis of metastatic carcinoma, malignant melanoma, and sarcoma in the lymph nodes.

Benign lymph node inclusions, such as müllerian glands in abdominal, pelvic, and inguinal lymph nodes, glandular and ductular elements of breast tissue in axillary lymph nodes, and nevoid elements in any peripheral lymph node group, must be distinguished from metastatic tumors. The location of such benign inclusions is typically the capsule and the trabeculae rather than the subcapsular and radiating sinuses. Additionally, in benign inclusions cytologic atypia and mitoses are absent.

SUGGESTED READING

BOOKS

DeVita VT, Hellman S, Rosenberg SA: Cancer, Principles & Practice of Oncology, Vol 2, 2nd ed. Philadelphia, JB Lippincott, 1985

Enriques P, Neiman RS: The Pathology of the Spleen: A Functional Approach. Chicago, American Society of Clinical Pathologists, 1976

Ioachim HL: Lymph Node Biopsy. Philadelphia, JB Lippincott, 1982

Jaffe ES: Major Problems in Pathology, Vol 16: Surgical Pathology of the Lymph Nodes and Related Organs. Philadelphia, WB Saunders, 1985

Kaplan HS: Hodgkin's Disease, 2nd ed. Cambridge, Harvard University Press, 1980

Rappaport H: Tumors of the hematopoietic system. In Atlas of Tumor Pathology, Section 3, Fascicle 8. Washington DC, Armed Forces Institute of Pathology, 1966

Rywlin A: Histopathology of the Bone Marrow. Boston, Little, Brown, 1976

Williams WJ et al: Hematology, 3rd ed. New York, McGraw-Hill, 1983

ARTICLES

Bennett JM, Catovsky D, Daniel MT et al: Proposals for the classification of the acute leukemias. Br J Haematol 33:451, 1976

Berard CW et al: Histopathological definition of Burkitt's tumor. Bull WHO 40:601–607, 1969

Dorfman RF, Warnke R: Lymphadenopathy simulating the malignant lymphomas. Hum Pathol 5:519–550, 1974

Jaffe ES et al: The pathologic spectrum of adult T-cell leukemia/lymphoma in the United States. Am J Surg Pathol 8:263–275, 1984

Lukes RJ: The immunologic approach to the pathology of malignant lymphomas. Am J Clin Pathol 72:657–669, 1979

Mann RB, Jaffe ES, Berard CW: Malignant lymphomas: A conceptual understanding of morphologic diversity. Am J Pathol 94:105–192, 1979

Nathwani BN: A critical analysis of the classification of Non-Hodgkin's lymphoma. Cancer 44:347–384, 1979

Rosenberg SA et al: National Cancer Institute–sponsored study of classification of non-Hodgkin's lymphomas: Summary and description of a working formulation for clinical usage. Cancer 49:2112–2135, 1982

21 The Endocrine System
Victor E. Gould and Sheldon C. Sommers

Pituitary Gland

Hypothalamus

Thyroid Gland

Parathyroid Glands

Adrenal Cortex

Adrenal Medulla and
Paraganglia

Thymus

Pineal Gland

Ectopic Hormones

Figure 21-1. The pituitary releases a variety of hormones that stimulate hormone secretion by other endocrine glands or act directly. Pituitary activity is modulated by releasing factors from the hypothalamus, which in turn responds to emotional and external stimuli. (*ACTH*, adrenocorticotropic hormone; *FSH*, follicle-stimulating hormone; *LH*, luteinizing hormone; *LTH*, luteotropic hormone [prolactin]; *STH*, somatotropin [growth hormone]; *TSH*, thyroid-stimulating hormone.)

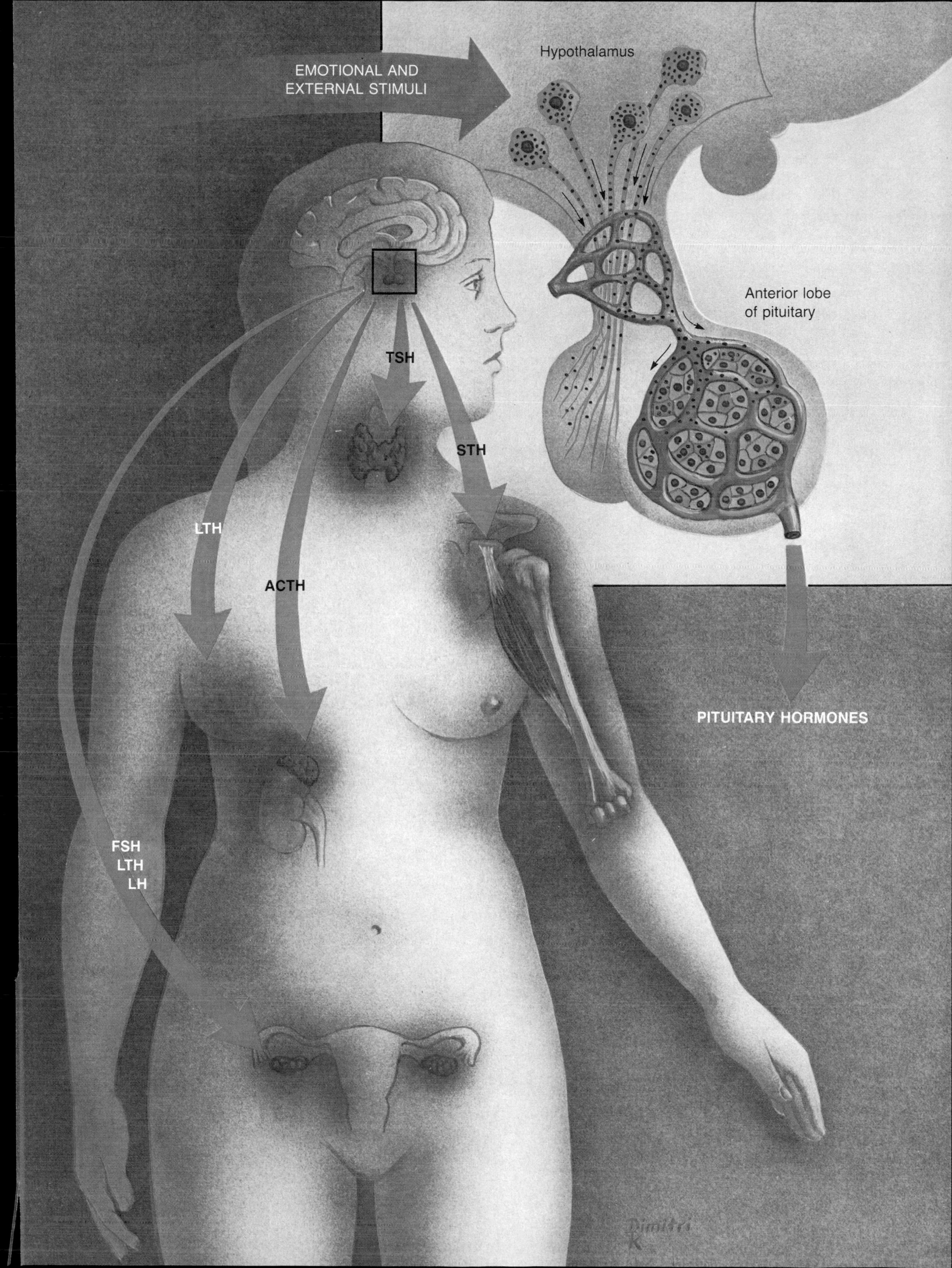
EMOTIONAL AND
EXTERNAL STIMULI
Hypothalamus
Anterior lobe
of pituitary
TSH
STH
LTH
ACTH
FSH
LTH
LH
PITUITARY HORMONES
Dimitri
K

Endocrine function refers to the transmission of a biological message by a chemical substance synthesized *in vivo* and acting on specific receptors. Chemical messengers that qualify as endocrine include amines, polypeptides, organic acids, and steroids. Widely distributed substances, such as glucose and cholesterol, are not regarded as endocrine messengers.

The notion that a given function in one part of the body can be mediated by the subtle release of a substance—a **hormone**—by a separate, and often distant, part of the body originated around the turn of the century. The notion of "ductless" (i.e., endocrine) glands implied that the chemical messenger entered the circulation, which carried it to the target organ. This original idea remains correct; however, subsequent discoveries have rendered it incomplete. We now recognize that important biologic messages are mediated by chemical modulators that do not enter the circulation, but rather travel short distances between secretory and target cells through the interstitial space. This mode of action is referred to as **paracrine.** Also, since the essence of the definition of endocrine activity involves the existence of a chemical intermediary, it follows that neuronal modulation of other cells—including other neurons—across synapses is essentially an endocrine function. Moreover, true neurons and paraneurons may also discharge their secretory products into the circulation; this function is referred to as **neuroendocrine.** Examples are provided by hypothalamic and posterior pituitary neurons, as well as by the adrenal medulla and paraganglia. These diverse forms of chemically mediated cell-to-cell communication are summarized in Figure 21-2.

Finally, chemical control substances need not necessarily travel from cell to cell, since there is evidence that certain cells are capable of producing materials destined to regulate some of their own activities. This mode of action is referred to as **autocrine.** An evolutionary example is the apparent production of an insulin-like material by unicellular organisms, including bacteria.

In addition to the well-known amino acids, amines, peptides, and steroids that belong to defined families of hormonal materials, other substances of varying chemical compositions are also regarded as having endocrine functions. These include the widely distributed prostaglandins, the functions of which relate to, for example, the central and peripheral nervous systems, circulation, respiration, reproduction, renal function, and coagulation. Also qualifying as hormones are thymus-produced thymosin and related materials; erythropoietin, mostly produced by the kidney and playing an important role in red blood cell maturation; kinins and related vasoactive substances; factors produced by B lymphocytes; nerve and epithelial growth factors; and a host of chemical messengers produced by mast cells, platelets, certain macrophages, and other cells.

The Dispersed Neuroendocrine System

Our knowledge has also expanded with regard to the distribution of many of the aforementioned chemical mediators in organs and cells that until very recently were not regarded as endocrine. It is now generally accepted that closely related, or even identical, transmitter substances, including certain amino acids, amines, and peptides ("common peptides"), are produced in the following:

- Neurons of the central nervous system,
- Peripheral nerves
- "Traditional" endocrine glands such as the pituitary
- Less clearly defined aggregates of endocrine cells, such as pancreatic islets and pulmonary neuroepithelial bodies
- A system of widely distributed cells located in numerous organs and tissues, including the gastrointestinal tract, the bronchopulmonary tree, and the skin

Cells that produce, store, and secrete the previously noted and related substances were originally classified together because of their capability to take up and decarboxylate relatively simple amine precursor substances, such as dihydroxyphenylalanine (DOPA) and 5-hydroxytryptamine (5-HT), thus producing biogenic amines. Given these "Amine Precursor Uptake and Decarboxylating" capabilities, such cells were designated by the acronym, **APUD cells,** and as a whole they were said to constitute the APUD system. It subsequently became evident that

Figure 21-2. Mechanisms of chemically mediated cell-to-cell communication. Biologic messages may be transmitted by mechanisms other than the classic endocrine pathway via the circulation. These include paracrine, synaptic, and neuroendocrine modes of communication.

ENDOCRINE
(e.g., insulin, ACTH,
parathyroid hormone)

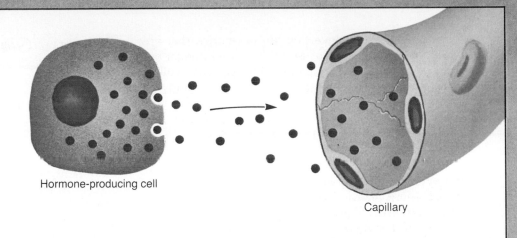

Hormone-producing cell

Capillary

PARACRINE
(e.g., somatostatin,
bombesin)

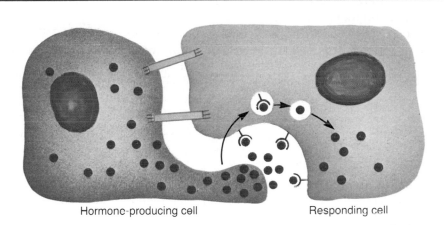

Hormone-producing cell

Responding cell

SYNAPTIC
(e.g., acetylcholine,
dopamine)

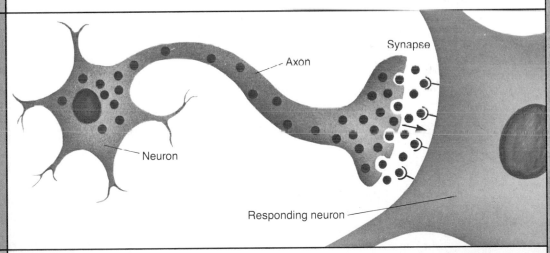

Synapse

Axon

Neuron

Responding neuron

NEUROENDOCRINE
(e.g., vasopressin,
epinephrine)

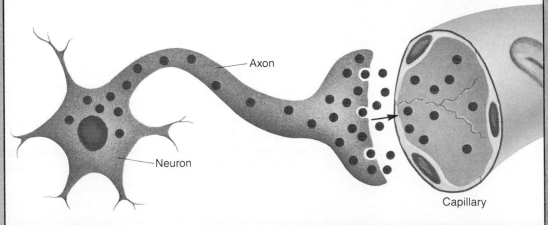

Axon

Neuron

Capillary

these cells also produce peptide hormones that are common to true neurons as well as to epithelial endocrine cells. Therefore, these cells are now collectively designated as neuroendocrine (NE), and the complex array of organs and tissues composed of or containing such cells is currently designated as the **Dispersed Neuroendocrine System (DNS).**

Neuroendocrine cells are readily characterized immunohistochemically by the demonstration of **neuron specific enolase,** a glycolytic enzyme common to all of these cells. Other significant markers are **chromogranin,** a protein of the secretory granule matrix, and **synaptophysin,** an integral membrane protein of neuronal presynaptic vesicles that is also present in epithelial neuroendocrine cells. Peptide hormones can also be shown immunohistochemically. By electron microscopy, neuroendocrine cells contain characteristic granules that consist of an electron-dense core, surrounded by a single membrane.

Hormone Function

The numerous types and wide distribution of hormone-producing cells do not account on a one-to-one basis for the larger number of chemical messengers that have been identified: We know in fact that many endocrine cells can synchronously secrete and store more than one hormone. It is also evident that the large and growing number of identified chemical messengers cannot account on a one-to-one basis for the much larger number of hormone-related functions. This discrepancy may be explained by the fact that a number of hormones are capable of conveying different messages and evoking diverse responses, depending on the site and the circumstances. For example, gastrin stimulates acid secretion by the stomach, and it acts as a growth factor during development and repair. Similarly, bombesin is a stimulator of gastrin release in the stomach, but in the bronchi it may modulate growth, development, and differentiation.

The significance of these hormonal materials extends beyond the physiology of the organs that produce them. Several of these peptide hormones, and likely others not yet identified, act as growth factors. For example, bombesin stimulates the growth of malignant tumors in experimental animals. The intriguing observation that bombesin is produced by certain rapidly growing human neoplasms, particularly neuroendocrine carcinomas of the lung, has led to the suspicion that bombesin may be an autocrine growth factor produced by certain tumors. The possibility exists that inhibition of such growth factors could curtail the growth of the tumor.

Pituitary Gland

Anatomy, Embryology, and Physiology

The pituitary gland, or hypophysis, has remarkable hormonal effects on growth, somatic and sexual development, reproductive functions, and metabolic regulation and lactation, as well as water conservation.

The anterior lobe (or adenohypophysis) is ectodermally derived, developing from Rathke's duct, which in embryos extends upward from the palatal region. Along its tract this craniopharyngeal duct leaves minute intrasphenoidal remnants of the anterior lobe, and in most adults its origin is perpetuated by microscopic squamous epithelial rests. These "Rathke" rests are considered the source of **craniopharyngioma,** a locally invasive solid and cystic neoplasm that closely resembles the tooth germ tumor called ameloblastoma.

The cell types comprising the anterior pituitary lobe as they appear in conventionally stained histologic sections are shown in Figure 21-3. Actually, anterior pituitary lobe cells are of four histologic types and six ultrastructural–immunohistochemical types, and produce seven important peptide hormones. These hormones control most of the major endocrine glands and endocrine responsive tissues. The hormones are listed here with their cell sources.

Growth hormone (somatotropic hormone) is produced by classic acidophilic cells; it stimulates the growth of many cells and tissues.

Prolactin (mammotropic hormone) is also produced by acidophils; it is essential to lactational secretion, and has over 80 additional metabolic activities.

Follicle stimulating hormone (FSH) is produced by classic strongly basophilic cells; it stimulates the formation of graafian follicles in the ovary.

Luteinizing hormone (LH) is produced by the same type of basophils as FSH; together these cells are called gonadotropic basophils or gonadotropes. LH induces ovulation and the formation of corpora lutea in the ovary.

Adrenocorticotropic hormone (corticotropin, ACTH) is secreted by a subset of basophils; it is the major hormone controlling adrenocortical secretion of cortisol and related glucocorticoid hormones.

Thyroid stimulating hormone (thyrotropin, TSH) is produced by pale basophilic or amphophilic

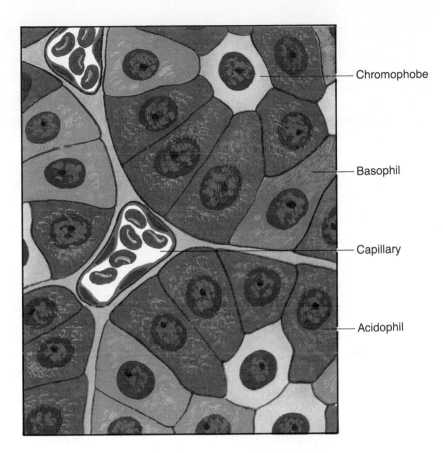

Chromophobe

Basophil

Capillary

Acidophil

Figure 21-3. Histology of the human anterior pituitary. The staining characteristics of the different cell types are those seen with hematoxylin and eosin. Note the intimate association of epithelial cells and blood capillaries.

cells; it controls the growth and function of thyroid follicular epithelial cells.

Melanocyte stimulating hormone (melanotropin, MSH), part of the molecule of ACTH prohormone, increases skin pigmentation. Some MSH also appears to be produced in the intermediate pituitary.

The posterior pituitary lobe (or neurohypophysis) is a downward projection of the central nervous system ectoderm, and is normally joined to the anterior lobe. There are two posterior lobe hormones: vasopressin and oxytocin. **Arginine vasopressin** (antidiuretic hormone, ADH), has the key function of promoting water resorption from the distal renal tubular fluid, thus conserving it for the body. Should any process sufficiently damage the posterior pituitary lobe or stalk, notable chronic water diuresis results, a disorder called **diabetes insipidus** (Fig. 21-4).

Diabetes insipidus can have many causes, including accidental or surgical trauma involving the pituitary stalk or posterior lobe, localized hemorrhagic or ischemic infarctions, infiltrates of histiocytic or granulomatous types, and neoplasms—either benign or metastatic cancers. These lesions interrupt the controls residing in the infundibular, supraoptic, and paraventricular regions of the hypothalamus, thus interfering with the neuronal secretions (see below, Hypothalamic–Pituitary Axis). The synthesis, storage, and release of vasopressin by the posterior pituitary cells are thus prevented, and diabetes insipidus ensues. It may be controlled by powdered posterior pituitary or arginine vasopressin administered as snuff.

Oxytocin is important in stimulating vigorous uterine muscle contractions during and after childbirth, although other factors also play a role.

Both the anterior and posterior pituitary are encapsulated within the bony sella turcica of the sphenoid bone. Between the anterior and posterior lobes in man lies the vestigial intermediate lobe, composed of a few colloid-filled follicles.

Congenital Anomalies

In severe congenital anomalies, such as anencephaly, proper connections among the pituitary stalk, posterior lobe, and anterior lobe are lacking. One result is a failure of the normal adrenocortical development,

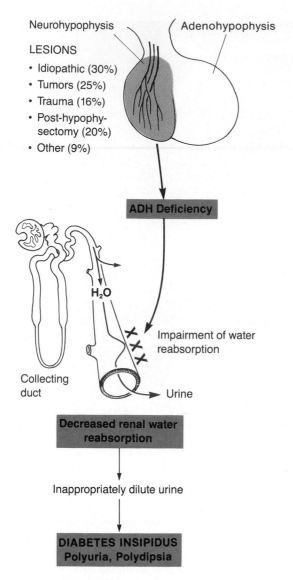

Figure 21-4.   The mechanism of diabetes insipidus.

groups in the hypothalamus secrete at least five factors that stimulate the anterior pituitary lobe: (1) growth hormone releasing factor (GRF), (2) gonadotropin releasing hormone (GnRH), (3) thyrotropin releasing hormone (TRH), (4) corticotropin releasing factor (CRF), and (5) melanotropin releasing hormone. There are three hypothalamic inhibitory hormones: prolactin inhibitory factor (PIF), growth hormone inhibitory factor (GHIF), and melanotropin inhibitory factor. These hypothalamic hormones are polypeptides, some of which have been synthesized. They are stored in and released from neuronal endocrine granules. These neurosecretory granules can be demonstrated by electron microscopy and by immunocytochemistry with the corresponding antibodies.

Secreted into the hypothalamic portal capillary network, the neuropeptides flow down through the collecting sinusoids in the pituitary stalk to be redistributed in the second portal capillary network of the anterior pituitary lobe, where their specific function is exerted.

The relation of the hypothalamus to the posterior pituitary is different. The posterior pituitary hormones are produced in the supraocular and paraventricular regions of the hypothalamus, by neurons that have axons that extend into the posterior pituitary lobe (see Fig. 21-1). The hormones are stored at the ends of the axons (in the posterior pituitary) and they are released into the general circulation upon the arrival of an action potential.

Hypothalamic–Pituitary Syndromes

Combined hypothalamic-pituitary syndromes are uncommon. **Laurence-Moon-Biedl syndrome** is of genetic origin, and comprises blindness due to retinitis pigmentosa, extra digits, pelvic girdle obesity, and failure of genital development with puberty. The specific hypothalamic abnormalities are uncertin. **McCune-Albright's syndrome** includes cutaneous café au lait spots, a bone disease (polyostotic fibrous dysplasia), and precocious puberty, principally in girls. This sporadic disease may be associated with a hypothalamic harmartoma, a nodule composed of excessive, misplaced neuron cell groups and nerve fibers centrally located in the hypothalamic tissues.

Other hypothalamic–pituitary syndromes are acquired. These include **Fröhlich's (or Babinski-Fröhlich) syndrome,** in which boys of pubertal age develop a girdle of obesity and feminine-type tapering limbs; the patients also fail to develop either primary or secondary sex characteristics. Any process that destroys enough anterior lobe tissue may be

secondary to insufficient ACTH stimulation. Cysts of developmental origin, arising from the third ventricle, the intermediate lobe, cystic Erdheim rests, or unidentified sites may become clinically evident in childhood or adult life because they expand and interfere with various pituitary or hypothalamic functions. Very rarely the pituitary gland is misplaced developmentally and forms a pedunculated mass hanging from the palate, a so-called epignathus tumor. Its removal results in total hypopituitarism.

Hypothalamic–Pituitary Axis

The hypothalamus, pituitary stalk, and pituitary gland constitute an integrated "neuroendocrine system," both anatomically and functionally. Neuron responsible. Such lesions include suprasellar cysts, infarction, inflammations—either nonspecific or specific (e.g., tuberculosis)—granulomatous or histiocytic infiltrates, and neoplasms (benign or malignant). Ordinary exogenous obesity and delayed puberty may sometimes give an appearance similar to that caused by hypopituitary dysfunction.

Hypopituitarism

In adults, severe panhypopituitarism may be caused by any process that destroys pituitary tissue, such as for example, ischemia, infection, or metastatic tumor. The disorder presents clinically as **Simmonds' disease** or "pituitary cachexia." The patient undergoes massive weight loss, and appears "skeletal," as if reduced to skin and bones. A psychiatric condition, anorexia nervosa, may simulate Simmonds' disease, but is not caused by a hypothalamic or pituitary lesion.

Sheehan's syndrome, a subcategory of Simmond's disease, is caused by shock-induced infarction of the pituitary in women who suffer a traumatic abortion or delivery, with considerable blood loss. Thereafter, they become amenorrheic and lack energy, muscle strength, and normal drive (Fig. 21-5). These patients are often regarded as neurotic, and are misdiagnosed until an alert physician tests any endocrine function—for example, that associated with thyroid or gonadal activity. Such functions are notably decreased, because *all* normal anterior lobe trophic functions are reduced. This particular variety of panhypopituitarism is caused by anterior pituitary hemorrhage and subtotal destruction, secondary to puerperal shock. Patients with Sheehan's syndrome appear normal or even obese (not emaciated), so that they escape a correct diagnosis for about 2 years after the original shock.

Some individuals with hypopituitarism are obese in youth and emaciated as older adults. This situation reflects complex hypothalamic–pituitary interactions and interrupted feedback controls from the anterior pituitary lobe, other endocrine glands, and target organs.

Precocious Puberty

Precocious puberty is most commonly constitutional, which means that the hypothalamic–pituitary time clock runs faster than normal. Another cause of precocious puberty is a centrally located protruding hypothalamic hamartoma, the size of the normal mamillary body.

Pituitary Tumors

Posterior Pituitary

Tumors of the posterior pituitary lobe are uncommon. Craniopharyngiomas originate in Erdheim's remnants or Rathke's embryonic duct, and as they grow they compress and damage adjacent structures. Hence, diabetes insipidus or other types of hypopituitarism may develop. These are slow-growing tumors, and patients occasionally survive for over 60 years. Craniopharyngiomas consist of anastomosing cords of epithelial cells that define irregular glandular spaces; keratin pearls are often formed (Fig. 21-6); calcifications may also occur.

Other posterior pituitary and hypothalamic neoplasms of histopathologic interest are granular cell tumors and the so-called pituicytomas. The former are composed of closely packed large pink-staining granular cells and are considered to be variants of Schwann cell tumors. Pituicytomas are astrocytic gliomas in the posterior lobe.

Anterior Pituitary

Adenomas

Pituitary adenomas are benign neoplasms of the anterior lobe. They are most common in men between the ages of 20 and 50 years. Small, apparently nonfunctioning pituitary adenomas are found incidentally in some 25% of adult autopsies. In inbred

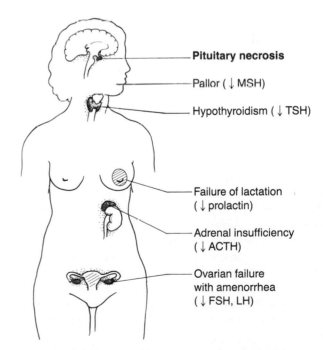

Figure 21-5. The major clinical manifestations of Sheehan's syndrome.

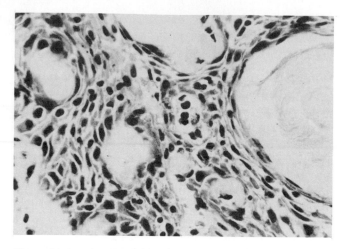

Figure 21-6. Craniopharyngioma of the posterior pituitary lobe. Anastomosing cell cords and glandlike spaces are apparent. The large space partly shown in the right field contains pale-staining material (keratin).

experimental animals pituitary tumors can be induced by endocrine imbalances, such as that following thyroidectomy. Probably man also has both genetic and endocrine dysfunctional factors that favor the development of pituitary adenomas. In the familial disorder known as multiple endocrine neoplasia (MEN) syndrome Type I, pituitary adenoma, adenomas of the thyroid gland, adrenal cortex, parathyroid gland, and sometimes the pancreatic islets coexist. These tumors may be clinically evident at the same time (synchronous) or be diagnosed sequentially, often with years elapsing (asynchronous).

A pituitary adenoma most commonly presents as an enlarging, space-occupying mass, without overt endocrine effects. It often produces lateral visual field abnormalities, including blindness, by pressure on the optic chiasm. Headaches are also characteristic. Rarely, pituitary adenomas are clinically silent until revealed by radiologic investigation.

Pituitary adenomas have classically been subdivided histologically according to the tinctorial properties of the neoplastic cells with conventional stains. Thus, pituitary tumors were classified as acidophil, basophil, or chromophobe. However, histochemical studies have demonstrated a lack of correlation between these properties and the type of hormone secretion. Therefore it is preferable to classify these tumors simply according to the hormones produced, although the surgical pathologist may for convenience use the older classification for descriptive purposes.

Chromophobe Adenomas   These tumors generally are over 1 cm in diameter, and consist of soft, pale tissue. Microscopically, there is a monotonous growth of small, regular cells with poorly stained cytoplasm, hence the old name, "chromophobe pituitary adenoma" (Fig. 21-7). **The majority of chromophobe adenomas contain prolactin.** The remainder include null cell and stem cell adenomas, which lack identifiable hormonal content or secretory granules.

After ionizing radiation or incomplete surgical removal, or without apparent cause, a chromophobe pituitary adenoma may grow aggressively outside the gland capsule or into the sphenoid bone. The cells are irregular, with aneuploid, enlarged, and bizarre nuclei. Such tumors are not considered pituitary carcinomas unless and until there is genuine invasion of the brain or basal blood vessels, or rarely, a metastasis. The same transition from benign pituitary adenoma to aggressive tumor to pituitary carcinoma develops in thyroidectomized mice.

Somatotropic Adenoma   Pituitary adenomas that secrete growth hormone produce dramatic bodily changes. If a somatotropic adenoma develops before adult growth is achieved, the individual becomes a **giant.** Most true giants, defined as over seven feet tall, have been found at autopsy to have had an acidophil pituitary adenoma. Sometimes the growth and pressure of a somatotropic adenoma so damages gonadotropic pituitary function that the individual eventually develops a eunuchoid habitus. The eunuchoid person is tall, exhibits elongated arms and legs, and suffers from deficient genital and secondary sex characteristics.

Should the somatotropic pituitary adenoma first develop after the long bone epiphyses have fused and the full adult height has been achieved, only

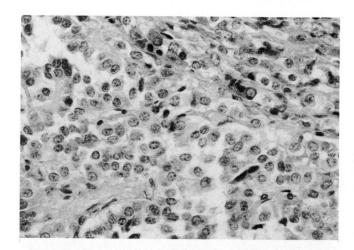

Figure 21-7. Chromophobe adenoma of the anterior pituitary. Compressed normal cells are evident at the upper right. The patient had no endocrine syndrome, but prolactin was shown by immunohistochemistry.

some bones still respond to excess growth hormone. These are, in particular, the bones of the hands, feet, mandible, and maxilla. The afflicted person develops coarse facial features with overgrowth of the mandible, mandibular and maxillary prognathism with spaces between the upper incisor teeth, a thickened nose, and enlarged, broad "spade-shaped" hands and feet. These osseous and associated soft tissue abnormalities are encompassed under the term **acromegaly** (Fig. 21-8). (Greek *acron*, extremities; *megalē*, great) The viscera are also hypertrophied. Although these persons are deformed to a greater or lesser degree, they are not necessarily handicapped.

The somatotropic pituitary adenoma is composed of sheets of acidophilic (pink) cells; thus, the old name "acidophil pituitary adenoma." Immunostains, and characteristic granule size identify the somatotropic adenoma. Since prolactin cells are also acidophilic, there are, as might be expected, adenomas that secrete both growth hormone and prolactin.

Oncocytoma Oncocytoma is another acidophilic pituitary adenoma, but, from the hormonal viewpoint, it is nonfunctional. Oncocyte is a generic term that pertains to the light-microscopic appearance of enlarged, eosinophilic (pink), and often granular epithelial cells that occur in older adults in the accessory bronchial glands, thyroid and parathyroid glands, pancreas, and elsewhere. These cells are packed with mitochondria that render the cytoplasm acidophilic, but usually show no notable secretory activity.

Among the various chromophobe and acidophil pituitary adenomas described, the most important microadenomas, defined as smaller than 1 cm, are prolactinomas. The **microprolactinoma** is a frequent cause of irregular menses, anovulation, and consequent infertility. The consistently elevated blood prolactin levels inhibit the surge in the secretion of pituitary luteinizing hormone necessary for ovulation. Treatment, either by transsphenoidal microsurgical removal or by pharmacologic inhibition with bromocriptine, may be effective in restoring fertility.

Basophil Adenomas **Basophil pituitary adenoma is the classic cause of Cushing's disease.** Excessive ACTH secretion induces adrenocortical hypersecretion of cortisol/cortisone. The hypercortisolemia in turn brings on the panoply of typical somatic, biochemical, and metabolic changes seen in Cushing's syndrome (Fig. 21-9). (See Adrenal Cortical Hyperfunction, under The Adrenal Cortex, below). The pituitary tumor is often small (Fig. 21-10), and its removal is curative.

Another type of basophil pituitary adenoma that secretes ACTH is iatrogenic. Some years after bilateral subtotal adrenalectomy for Cushing's syndrome, a space-occupying pituitary adenoma may develop.

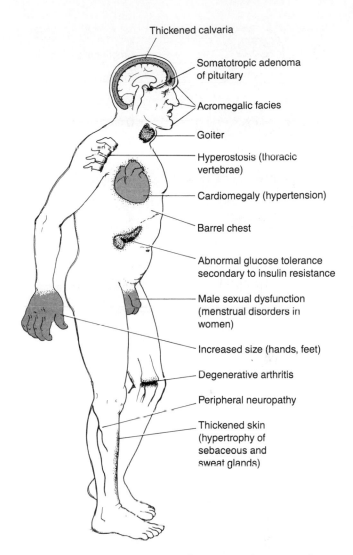

Thickened calvaria

Somatotropic adenoma of pituitary

Acromegalic facies

Goiter

Hyperostosis (thoracic vertebrae)

Cardiomegaly (hypertension)

Barrel chest

Abnormal glucose tolerance secondary to insulin resistance

Male sexual dysfunction (menstrual disorders in women)

Increased size (hands, feet)

Degenerative arthritis

Peripheral neuropathy

Thickened skin (hypertrophy of sebaceous and sweat glands)

Figure 21-8. The clinical manifestations of acromegaly.

In this situation the ACTH-cell pituitary adenoma is the cause of **Nelson's syndrome.**

A third type of ACTH adenoma is nonsecretory.

Rarely, faintly basophilic or chromophobic pituitary adenomas are composed of cells that exhibit gonadotropic or thyrotropic activity. As in the case of Nelson's syndrome, one suspects some antecedent deficiency in the feedback control exerted by the gonads or thyroid gland on the pituitary. Yet often there is no clearcut evidence of any such deficiency.

Anterior Pituitary Syndromes

Physiologic changes in the anterior pituitary lobe are associated with other endocrine alterations. Prolactin cells undergo hypertrophy and hyperplasia in the second half of pregnancy and lactation. These

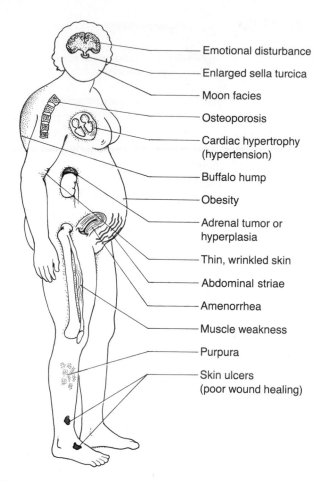

- Emotional disturbance
- Enlarged sella turcica
- Moon facies
- Osteoporosis
- Cardiac hypertrophy (hypertension)
- Buffalo hump
- Obesity
- Adrenal tumor or hyperplasia
- Thin, wrinkled skin
- Abdominal striae
- Amenorrhea
- Muscle weakness
- Purpura
- Skin ulcers (poor wound healing)

Figure 21-9. The major clinical aspects of Cushing's syndrome.

"Erdheim pregnancy cells" are responsible for the increased weight of the pituitary in pregnant women. Some women develop a coarsening of the facial features as a consequence of increased secretion of growth hormones. Pregnant women also occasionally suffer from hirsutism and focal increases in pigmentation, caused by increases in ACTH and MSH secretion.

Most dwarfs and midgets suffer from defects of constitutional origin. However, a few true pituitary dwarfs lack anterior lobe somatotropic cells that secrete growth hormone. African pygmies have normal growth hormone secretion, but their target tissues are relatively unresponsive.

Gonadotropic pituitary basophils in animals and humans undergo a notable vacuolar degeneration if the gonads are removed. These are the "pituitary castration cells."

Adrenalectomy and Addison's type of adrenocortical destruction lead to hypertrophy and hyperplasia of the weakly basophilic pituitary corticotropic cells. In a few patients this is a precursor state of Nelson's

corticotropic cell pituitary adenoma.

Corticotropic basophils in animals or humans who are exposed to elevated levels of corticosteroids, whether administered therapeutically or endogenously produced by adrenocortical hyperfunction, undergo a cobweb vacuolar degeneration and the loss of their basophilic cytoplasmic granules. These glassy appearing cells containing whorled intermediate filaments, called **hyaline basophils** or **Crooke's cells,** are a marker for hypercortisolemia and Cushing's syndrome. In Cushing's disease the basophil pituitary adenoma cells are autonomous and impervious to Crooke's cell degeneration. However, vacuolar changes may be noted in the uninvolved corticotropic basophils of the anterior lobe.

Hypothalamus

Anatomy and Physiology

The hypothalamus is a portion of the diencephalon that surrounds the third ventricle, and forms the inferior median surface of the brain between the mamillary bodies posteriorly and the optic chiasm anteriorly. From it, the dependent tuber cinereum and pituitary stalk connect with the posterior, intermediate, and anterior lobes of the pituitary. Nerves and a double portal vascular system connect the hypothalamus and pituitary. The first portal plexus is in the region of the median eminence and the second within the pituitary gland.

The hypothalamus is the master orchestrator of the endocrine system, since the hypothalamic peptide hormones stimulate or inhibit the release of the

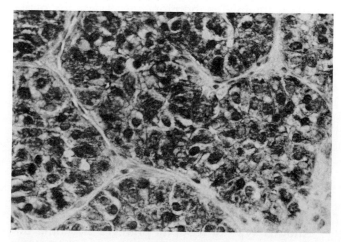

Figure 21-10. ACTH-producing pituitary adenoma immunostained with anti-ACTH antibody. The majority of neoplastic cells are stained.

major pituitary hormones, which in turn control other endocrine glands, and hence their target organs. It contains at least eight defined nuclei, which are collections of neuroendocrine cells that contain membrane-enclosed neurosecretory granules. The hypothalamus transduces neuronal electrochemical signals into endocrine secretions. Hypothalamic functions are pulsatile, and the frequency of discharge is different for different hormones; the intervals between discharges range from hourly to daily.

Remarkable progress is being made in the understanding of the interaction of hypothalamic functions with higher brain centers. Maps of the functional histology and histopathology of the hypothalamus resemble early drawings of new continents, with seaports identified and the hinterlands largely blank. Highlights of hypothalamic pathology include abnormalities in anencephalic fetuses and newborns, infantile failure to thrive (the so-called diencephalic syndrome), growth derangements, pubertal abnormalities, amenorrhea, menstrual irregularities, infertility, menopause, anorexia nervosa, obesity, aging, and the effects of primary or metastatic tumors. Much remains to be discovered.

Hypothalamic Syndromes

Anencephaly

In anencephaly, intrauterine growth of the fetus and placenta are retarded, and many anencephalic infants are born either prematurely or postmaturely. Excess amniotic fluid is often present, possibly reflecting intrauterine diabetes insipidus secondary to the interruption of hypothalamic control of vasopressin secretion. Deficiencies are found in hypothalamic growth hormone releasing factor (GRF), thyrotropin releasing hormone (TRH), and prolactin inhibiting factor (PIF). The fetal pituitary somatotropes remain small. On the other hand, the anterior pituitary responds to direct stimulation; the administration of vasopressin results in the secretion of growth hormone (GH) and thyrotropin (TSH).

Diencephalic Syndrome

Anorexia in infants, with resulting cachexia or emaciation, is classically associated with an anterior hypothalamic tumor (astrocytic glioma) or a hamartomatous malformation. Occasionally a fourth ventricle glioma has similar effects. Presumably GH secretion is inhibited by interference with the hypothalamic production of monoamine stimulators of GH release from the pituitary, such as the neurotransmitters dopamine, serotonin, and norepinephrine.

Growth Disorders

Dwarfism in children that is idiopathic or follows psychosocial deprivation is thought to reflect neurotransmitter dysfunction in the central nervous system. Possibly an increased β-adrenergic activity in the brain blocks the release of GH that would be expected after insulin-induced hypoglycemia. Other children, adolescents, and young adults with GH deficiency may have (a) hypothalamic dysfunction, with impaired synthesis or secretion of GRF, (b) isolated GH deficiency, (c) absent or low pituitary GH activity as a result of abnormal GH molecules or polymeric GH ("pituitary dwarfism, Type I"), or (d) unresponsiveness of the target organ to GH ("pituitary dwarfism, Type II"). African pygmies are thought to have the last defect.

Hypothalamic Causes of Gonadal Dysfunction

Pubertal Disorders

Delayed Puberty Progressive somatic growth, adrenogenital maturation, and circulating gonadotropins are prerequisites for normal menarche in pubertal girls. In general, a body weight of at least 70% of the ideal is required for normal pubertal maturation; a lower weight seems to inhibit the menarche. In malnourished children and in women who are thinner than two-thirds of their ideal body weight, plasma FSH levels may be normal but the 24 hour sleep–wake pattern of LH secretion is that of infants.

Precocious Puberty **Sexual precocity is usually, but not invariably, constitutional rather than pathologic.** Precocious puberty may arise as early as 20 months of age, in association with pubertal fluctuations of plasma FSH and LH. An inactive analog of LHRH can reverse the endocrine and bone growth changes, supporting the hypothesis that precocious puberty has a hypothalamic origin.

A midline hypothalamic hamartoma is the classic neoplastic cause of precocious puberty. Its neurons contain LHRH. As already mentioned, Albright's syndrome with precocious puberty is typically associated with a hypothalamic hamartoma. Suprasellar cysts and hypothalamic gliomas also may cause precocious puberty.

Amenorrhea and Related Disorders

Primary amenorrhea has many possible causes, among which hypothalamic dysfunction or lesions are infrequent. Ovarian absence (XO, Turner's syndrome) or dysgenesis (intersex gonads), congenital adrenal hyperplasia (adrenogenital syndrome), or even the rare so-called hypergonadotropic "resistant ovary syndrome" probably are more common. Isolated pituitary gonadotropin deficiency, a cause of primary amenorrhea, may be identified by the failure of the plasma prolactin level to rise after the injection of thyrotropin releasing hormone (TRH), a potent stimulator of prolactin secretion.

Secondary amenorrhea is often caused by increased circulating levels of prolactin. About one-third of cases are associated with a pituitary adenoma that secretes prolactin. In another third, unexplained prolactinemia is present for many years without evidence of a pituitary adenoma. Such patients are thought to have a functional disorder of the hypothalamic–pituitary axis.

Hyperprolactinemia has many causes besides hypothalamic disease, including hypothyroidism, chronic renal failure, and the administration of various therapeutic drugs and hormones.

Polycystic Ovary Syndromes

In polycystic ovary syndromes there is generally **an enhanced pituitary sensitivity to stimulation by LHRH.** An increased frequency or duration of hypothalamic LHRH secretion may be responsible, since LHRH induces its own receptors. Increased endogenous dopamine and endorphin secretions in the brain are thought to lead to a dissociation of the normal hypothalamic inhibitory mechanisms that control LHRH release. **Characteristically, the level of circulating LH is increased. The ovaries are enlarged and show multiple cysts, which are mostly luteinized owing to continuous and excessive gonadotropin secretion.**

Menstrual Cycle and Fertility

The integrated hypothalamic–pituitary–gonadal system is a morphologic and functional axis. In women who have enough pituitary FSH and LH secretion to stimulate maturation of ovarian graafian follicles, a midcycle pulse of LH secretion (the "LH spike") is essential to ovulation. In younger postpubertal women, ovulation is irregular, because the maturing hypothalamic–pituitary axis does not provide an LH spike every month. Consequently, the average fertility of women 13 to 15 years of age is less than that of older women.

In women older than age 40, fertility usually declines, because there is often a greater than normal secretion of pituitary LH during the preovulatory phase. The LH spike, if it occurs, is lower compared to the higher preovulatory levels of circulating LH. In animals, age-related changes in gonadotropin releasing hormone, and in FSH and LH cyclic secretion, may interfere with successful reproduction. Exceptionally, some women have had successful pregnancies at ages up to 57 years. Usually they have been grand multiparas.

Successful fertilization is a complex social, sexual, endocrine, and biological process, and many factors, including heredity, nutrition, and personal habits, may affect it. Clomiphene citrate is a gonadotropin-like medication that may induce single or multiple ovulations in infertile anovulatory women, who thereafter may experience multiple births far beyond the natural chance of occurrence.

Hypopituitarism in either sex prevents ovulation or spermatogenesis. Ordinarily, neither hypothalamic lesions nor functional disturbances are identified.

Menopause   Beyond 47 years of age most women cease to ovulate, and the menses stop, an event termed the menopause. The primordial ova disappear, and the ovaries become incapable of cyclic function and undergo atrophy. Hot flashes are a classic symptom of the menopause, whether natural or occurring after surgical removal of the ovaries. Abrupt skin vasodilation and attacks of sweating and a heat sensation occur, particularly involving the head and neck. Administration of estrogen ameliorates or prevents these attacks and some other postmenopausal manifestations, including osteoporosis.

Since pituitary gonadotropins are released in menopausal women, and the feedback effects of ovarian estrogens and progestogens on the hypothalamus cease, a hypothalamic–pituitary basis for hot flashes is suspected. We may recall that when males are given pulses of gonadotropin releasing hormone to induce puberty, they develop hot flashes. The vasomotor events may represent an effect of continued secretion of hypothalamic gonadotropin releasing hormone without estrogen feedback.

Male menopause has been described, but it is probably more a psychosocial than a biological entity.

Anorexia Nervosa

Anorexia nervosa is currently regarded as a predominantly psychiatric condition of adolescent girls who refuse to eat. Young women on diets, sometimes models, ballerinas, or schizophrenic women, and possibly male "obligatory runners," also may be afflicted. Amenorrhea and several endocrine dysfunctions are typical. As has been noted, FSH and LH responses to gonadotropin releasing hormone are depressed but return to normal with augmented body weight. Serum prolactin levels are increased. The normal diurnal variations in corticosteroid levels may disappear. Circulating concentrations of thyroid stimulating hormone (TSH) and the thyroid hormones T_3 and T_4 are decreased. Although gonadal dysfunctions predominate, other abnormalities occur, such as impaired thermoregulation and diabetes insipidus, with subnormal or erratic vasopressin secretion. **These changes are regarded as adaptive mechanisms in chronic starvation.** Indeed, in various wasting diseases the pituitary gonadotropes characteristically atrophy more than the other cell types, and the "low T_3 syndrome" occurs in diverse chronic diseases that also manifest an increased reverse T_3.

Hypothalamic astrocytic gliomas may also cause the anorexia nervosa syndrome.

Obesity

The obverse of anorexia nervosa, namely obesity, also has cultural, psychosocial, and psychosomatic aspects. Yet certain ancient fertility symbols were grossly obese female figures, an observation that indicates that it is no bar to human reproduction.

Women with refractory obesity have low plasma levels of growth hormone during oral glucose tolerance tests, but show normal GH and 11-hydroxycorticosteroid responses to insulin-induced hypoglycemia. Any hyperinsulinemia that accompanies obesity is considered secondary to it. Weight loss reduces the marginally elevated plasma prolactin levels, and GH levels remain normal. A hypothalamic origin for both obesity and amenorrhea in some women has been suspected. Some evidence indicates that elevated unbound plasma androgens may be characteristic of oligomenorrheic obese women, whether they are hirsute or not.

The relative unresponsiveness of obese individuals to internal cues of satiety could be of hypothalamic or higher origin, but the cause is unknown. The obesity that characteristically accompanies adolescent Fröhlich's or Laurence-Moon-Biedl types of hypothalamic–pituitary disorders clearly indicates that a relationship exists between obesity and some abnormal hypogonadotropic conditions. Similarly, the typical obesity of spayed or castrated animals and human eunuchs indicates a hypothalamic–pituitary relationship. It appears that the sluggishness among some obese individuals, while not evidence of hypothyroidism, is somewhat overcome either by weight loss or by exogenous thyroid hormone.

Some hypothalamic–pituitary–gonadotropic alterations in obesity appear to be epiphenomena rather than the cause of the obesity. Examples include the obesity of women with endometrial hyperplasia (or carcinoma) and polycystic ovaries, or estrogenic postmenopausal ovarian stromal alterations. Obesity provides abundant adipose tissue, in which the precursor hormone, androstenedione, is metabolized to estrogens, the hormones that continuously stimulate the endometrial and mammary target organs. **Hypothalamic–pituitary alterations in these situations are currently judged to be adaptive,** except possibly in rare chromosomally mosaic women with dysgenetic gonads.

Similarly, the obesity found in about 20% of patients with colorectal carcinoma is more likely to represent genetic endomorphy than hypothalamic–pituitary imbalance.

Hypothalamic Corticotropin and Thyrotropin Releasing Factors

Most instances of either excessive ACTH secretion or its deficiency are not ascribable to hypothalamic alterations. Both Cushing's disease, which is caused by a pituitary basophil adenoma, and Cushing's syndrome, which reflects increased glucocorticoid levels from any source, are explicable by pituitary–adrenocortical interactions. However, except for the ectopic ACTH syndrome associated with various carcinomas, the pathogenesis of Cushing's syndrome (with the exception of exogenous steroids), is not totally clear. A minority opinion is that hypothalamic corticotropin releasing factor may initiate the syndrome; the feedback effects of stress on the brain may alter the set point of a hypothalamic sensor that responds to changes in the plasma corticosteroid levels.

Hypothyroidism and hyperthyroidism are likewise largely explicable without implicating hypothalamic abnormalities. Nevertheless, the classic Cannon experiment, in which connecting the vagus nerve to the rabbit thyroid gland produces hyperthyroidism, and the considerable anecdotal information that stressful emotional situations may precede or trigger Graves' disease, attest to a possible autonomic and brain involvement in thyroid hyperfunctional states.

As well as the midline hypothalamic hamartoma responsible for precocious puberty, other small, posterolateral hypothalamic hamartomas are often found at autopsy. These tumors apparently lead to increased secretion of hypothalamic releasing factors, because they are associated with a higher incidence of hyperplasias of the pituitary anterior lobe, endocrine glands, and target organs. These posterolateral hypothalamic hamartomas resemble accessory hypothalamic tuberal nuclei, and are of unknown function.

Age Changes

Endocrine stimuli and target organ responses tend to decline with age. Ovarian failure, which initiates the menopause, conversely increases pituitary gonadotropin storage and secretion. Estrogen deficiency thus frees the hypothalamic–pituitary axis from feedback control.

Hypothalamic Tumors

To recapitulate, **a central hypothalamic hamartoma correlates with precocious puberty, and a posterolateral hamartoma is associated with pituitary–endocrine–target organ hyperplasias and neoplasms.** Sufficiently large pituitary adenomas, third ventricle cysts, craniopharyngiomas, and various granulomas or vascular lesions may press against the hypothalamus and interfere with its functions.

In children or adolescents, these diverse lesions affect growth, sexual maturation, and body weight. As discussed previously, dwarfism, eunuchoidism, Fröhlich's syndrome, Laurence-Moon-Biedl syndrome, Albright's syndrome, and diabetes insipidus may result. In adults, when tumors cause incomplete or complete hypopituitarism, Simmonds' pituitary cachexia or less dramatic symptoms may be present. Diabetes insipidus may be the chief clinical problem.

Emotional lability, insomnia, sexual hyperactivity, and either hyperbulemia or severe anorexia are common in hypothalamic disease.

The range of intrinsic hypothalamic lesions responsible for endocrine, physical, and psychic abnormalities is wide, as indicated in Table 21-1.

Thyroid Gland

Anatomy, Embryology, and Physiology

The thyroid gland is a bilobed endocrine organ situated below the thyroid cartilage anterior to the trachea. The thyroid mediates general metabolic activity. By six enzymatic processes, beginning with selective trapping of blood iodide within its parenchyma, the major active hormones triiodothyronine (T_3) and thyroxin (T_4) are produced for intrafollicular storage and secretion. There are thyroid hormone receptors in most tissue cells, and in hypermetabolic states a supranormal T_3 and T_4 attachment to tissues occurs, excepting only a few sites, such as the brain and spleen.

Embryologically, the thyroid anlage formed at the base of the tongue descends in the midline to reach its normal anatomic location. If it fails to descend, the entire functioning gland comprises a **lingual thyroid nodule.** Its removal results in total hypothyroidism. Nests of incompletely descended midline thyroid tissue may form **thyroglossal duct cysts** in adult life. Overdescent produces a mediastinal thyroid,

which if enlarged forms a **mediastinal goiter.** When trapped in the suprasternal notch, a mediastinal goiter may press on the trachea and compromise respiration.

Ectopic thyroid tissue is mostly a histopathologic curiosity in adjacent small lymph nodes. However, well-differentiated thyroid adenocarcinoma can be misdiagnosed as ectopic thyroid follicles, and vice versa.

Metabolic and Inflammatory Diseases

Nontoxic Nodular Goiter and Other Goiters

Goiter—or struma—means thyroid enlargement; a deficiency of iodine in the diet is its major cause. In areas far from salt water and seafood, which are rich sources of iodides, goiters are—or used to be—common. The Great Lakes area, Switzerland, south Austria (Styria), central Africa, and the Himalayas are such places. Iodized salt is an effective preventive dietary measure. This and similar public health mea-

Table 21-1. Hypothalamic Lesions

Hamartomas	Central
	Posterolateral
Neoplasms	Craniopharyngioma
	Astrocytoma
	Medulloblastoma
	Infundibuloma
	Pinealoma
	Ependymoma
	Ganglioneuroma
	Plasmacytoma
	Granular cell tumor
	Angioma
	Metastatic carcinoma
	Leukemia
Cysts	Choroid plexus
	Third ventricle
Inflammations	Viral encephalitis
	Epidemic encephalitis
	Smallpox
	Measles
	Varicella
Granulomas	Tuberculosis
	Sarcoidosis
	Histiocytosis X
Degenerations	Tuberous sclerosis
	Arteriosclerotic encephalomalacia
	Aneurysm
Trauma	Stalk section
	Foreign body

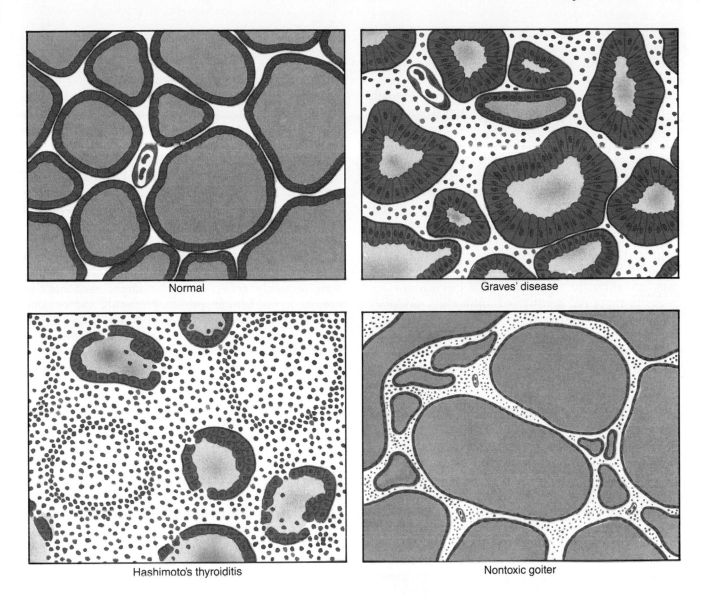

Normal

Graves' disease

Hashimoto's thyroiditis

Nontoxic goiter

Figure 21-11. Thyroid gland histology: Note the differences in size, architectural organization, and tinctorial affinities of the cells. *(A)* Normal. *(B)* Graves' disease. *(C)* Hashimoto's disease. Lymphoid infiltrates are evident. *(D)* Nontoxic goiter.

sures have contributed to the decrease of goiter in areas where it used to be common.

Endemic goiter due to iodine deficiency has various clinical and pathologic names, of which **nodular goiter** is the simplest. Other, synonymous terms are multinodular goiter, nontoxic nodular goiter, and adenomatous goiter. The normal adult thyroid weighs about 20 g to 35 g, whereas a nodular goiter may weigh 100 g or even 1000 g. It forms a palpable and often visible mass in the lower anterior neck. On removal the thyroid is grossly and microscopically nodular, and shows translucent gelatinous regions and foci of hemorrhage, fibrosis, and calcification. In iodine insufficiency the thyroid compensates for the

inability to produce small amounts of T_3 and T_4 by forming larger amounts of less effective hormones.

In iodine deficiency the thyroid tissue initially becomes vascular and hyperplastic. Subsequently, excessive amounts of colloid are stored in enlarged thyroid follicles, which form the nodules. A marker for nodular goiter is the presence of follicles larger than 2 mm in diameter. The follicular cells are low and flattened, in marked contrast to normal follicular cells (Fig. 21-11).

As nodules form and the thyroid enlarges, the local arterial and capillary networks become tortuous and stretched. The rupture of small vessels results in local hemorrhages, which are eventually organized into fibrous scars, in which calcific foci form. Hence the cut surface of a nodular goiter is a variegated tan, red, brown, and gray, and in places grates against the knife.

Conditions other than iodine deficiency eventually lead to similar nodular goiters. **Familial dyshormonogenesis,** a genetic deficiency of any one of the six enzymes that are required to synthesize and secrete T_3 and T_4, is associated with goiter, even in childhood and adolescence.

Congenital goiter most often reflects severe maternal iodine deficiency. The resulting lack of thyroid hormones leads to unopposed pituitary secretion of thyroid stimulating hormone (TSH), and a hyperstimulated fetal thyroid response.

Sporadic cretinism is associated with thyroid agenesis, an anomaly associated with intrauterine exposure to maternal antithyroid antibodies. **Endemic cretinism** occurs in remote, usually mountainous districts. Cretins with or without goiter suffer from the prenatal metabolic and developmental effects of nearly total maternal thyroid iodine insufficiency. They have large tongues, defective nervous system development, mental deficiency, neuromuscular abnormalities, and short stature. **Irreversible neurological damage is their most serious handicap.**

In developed countries neonatal thyroid deficiency may be clinically inapparent, and public health measures include required neonatal testing for increased levels of pituitary thyroid stimulating hormone (TSH). Most American states and all Canadian provinces have established mandatory testing programs to prevent neonatal hypothyroidism.

Increased TSH levels indicate an inadequate feedback control by thyroid T_3 and T_4. **If the diagnosis of neonatal hypothyroidism is missed, and replacement thyroid hormone is not given promptly, by age six months the infant will have irreversible mental deficiency.** Neonatal goiter may also be due to a block in any of the six enzymatic reactions previously mentioned.

Some mothers who receive antithyroid drug treatments during pregnancy, or considerable amounts of iodides, bromides, or radioactive iodine, bear offspring with goiter. Since these infantile thyroid enlargements formed in a few months, the hypertrophy is usually diffuse, rather than nodular. Either abundant colloid storage or very little is found, the latter associated with notable follicular epithelial hyperplasia. Such goiters usually involute as the infant grows and a normal metabolic balance is restored.

Adults with unrecognized and neglected recurrent hyperthyroidism eventually develop a nodular goiter. Foci of reddish thyroid hyperplasia may be evident on section of the enlarged gland. In some cases only the histopathologic signs of involution after previous epithelial overgrowth may be found. At this late stage those affected are ordinarily euthyroid.

Goitrogenic foods or medications cause a few nodular goiters. "Cabbage goiter" designates one food fad. Cyanates, isocyanates, resorcinols, cobalt, phenothiazines, and lithium are also goitrogenic substances.

About half of adults over the age of 40 years have one or two thyroid nodules, either palpable or impalpable. These nodules, like those in nodular goiters, are not neoplasms. They are foci of excessive colloid storage, with or without fibrosis. Since the thyroid gland containing such isolated nodules is of normal weight, it is not a goiter. Both nodular thyroid and the nodular adrenal cortex of middle-aged persons probably reflect irregular target responses to normal hypothalamic–pituitary stimuli. We emphasize this point because over 90% of solitary "cold" thyroid masses surgically removed because they may represent benign or malignant tumors prove to be simply the dominant nodule of a nodular thyroid gland.

Hyperthyroidism

Graves' disease, known in continental Europe as Basedow's disease, is the classic **primary hyperthyroidism.** The disorder is also termed **diffuse toxic goiter** and **primary thyroid hyperplasia.** In florid cases, Graves' disease is an arresting condition. The patient's eyes bulge, a condition called **exophthalmos,** and there is a symmetrical goiter. A local thyroid bruit of rushing blood is palpable or audible with a stethoscope. The skin is warm and sweaty, and there is a fine finger tremor. The afflicted person is jittery, anxious, and often hyperactive. Heat intolerance and hypomenorrhea or amenorrhea are the rule. Tachycardia, palpitations, and cardiomegaly are evident (Fig. 21-12). Older patients may present with a clinical picture of congestive heart failure, and may not show the overt signs and symptoms of florid hyperthyroidism. Women are especially affected, and, as in most thyroid diseases, predominate over men about 6:1.

Excessive thyroid hormonal activity is responsible for all these hypermetabolic effects, with the probable exception of the exophthalmos. Plasma T_3 and T_4 hormone levels and other biochemical markers of thyroid function are elevated. The condition waxes and wanes, if untreated. If there is a sudden, excessive thyroid hormonal discharge, a potentially lethal **"thyroid storm"** may develop, comprising a crisis of fever, abdominal pain, cardiorespiratory insufficiency, and shock.

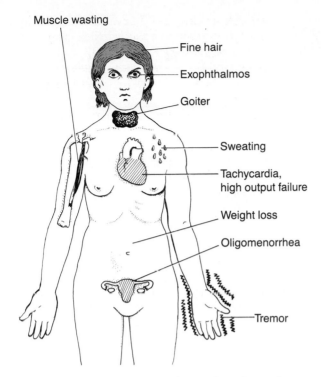

Muscle wasting

— Fine hair

— Exophthalmos

— Goiter

— Sweating

— Tachycardia, high output failure

— Weight loss

— Oligomenorrhea

—Tremor

Figure 21-12. The major clinical manifestations of Graves' disease.

At another extreme, old people develop **apathetic hyperthyroidism,** in which there are no dramatic symptoms or signs. The diagnosis is made only by measuring their metabolic derangements and levels of circulating thyroid hormones.

Autoimmunity is the common explanation of Graves' disease. One of the key phenomena in Graves' disease is presumed to be a genetically determined deficiency of antigen-specific suppressor T cells. Alternatively, antigen-specific helper T cells may be activated by Class II MHC antigens, which are present at the surface of thyroid follicular epithelial cells only under abnormal circumstances. In either case, subsets of B cells become activated and produce autoantibodies to TSH receptor antigens on the follicular cells. The TSH receptor autoantibodies are of two types—thyroid-growth immunoglobulins, which stimulate thyroid growth; and thyroid-stimulating immunoglobulins, which promote hypersecretion of thyroid hormones. In Graves' disease both types of antibodies are increased. These autoantibodies presumably bind to the follicular TSH receptors and mimic the effect of TSH. The several alternative pathways currently postulated to explain the pathogenesis of Graves' disease are outlined in Figure 21-13. These postulated mechanisms do not readily explain why Graves' disease appears only after several decades of life.

It has been suggested that HLA-DR3 immune-related genes are associated with the defect in the antigen-specific suppressor T cells. A number of initiating or triggering mechanisms have been suggested, ranging from viral or bacterial infections to recurrent episodes of severe physical or psychological stress. Once established, the autoimmune phenomena tend to be self-perpetuating. Contrary to traditional assumptions, the exophthalmos characteristic of Graves' disease is not the result of thyroid hormonal hyperactivity, but rather may have an autoimmune basis. The edematous orbital and periorbital fibroadipose tissues and muscles typically exhibit lymphocytic infiltrates. A circulating autoimmune antibody, presumably directed to an eye muscle tissue antigen, has been reported.

Although at present unfashionable, a certain skepticism persists regarding the ability of autoimmunity by itself to explain Graves' disease. The experimental model in rabbits, in which connecting the vagus nerve to the thyroid gland produced hyperthyroidism, should not be forgotten. Autoimmune reactions in Graves' disease, although present, do not necessarily represent the "cause" of the disease. Rather, as is the case in other diseases, autoimmune reactions could represent epiphenomena superimposed on other pathogenetic mechanisms.

The thyroid in Graves' disease is symmetrically enlarged, usually weighing 35 to 40 g, and has a thin translucent capsule covering firm, dark-red, glandular parenchyma. The tan translucence of the normal cut surface of the thyroid, attributable to stored colloid, is notably absent. Microscopically, colloid within the follicles is depleted or absent. If colloid remains, it is typically scalloped around the edges, as a result of increased proteolysis and subsequent reabsorption into the epithelium prior to hormone secretion. The follicular thyroid epithelium is normally regular and cuboidal, but in hyperthyroid states it becomes tall, cuboidal, or columnar (Fig. 21-14). Typically, intrafollicular folds or pleats of crowded thyroid epithelium are formed. As hyperthyroidism waxes and wanes the epithelium becomes, respectively, more and less hyperplastic, and the quantity of stored colloid is reduced and then increased. With recurrent hyperplasia, interstitial fibrosis develops. Even years later, when the patient with Graves' disease may be euthyroid, intrafollicular spurs of fibrous tissue remain as a souvenir of involuted follicular hyperplasia.

Ordinary iodine and antithyroid drugs alter the morphologic appearance of the thyroid in Graves' disease. Currently, the pathologist virtually never sees untreated Graves' disease; nevertheless an accurate diagnosis of the disease and assessment of the effects of therapy is possible.

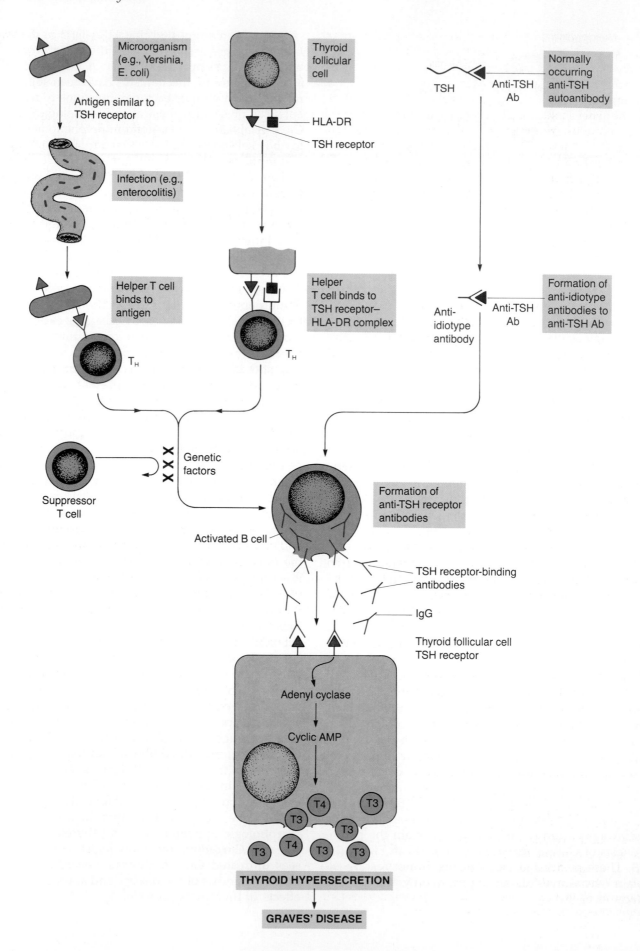

An exception to accurate cytological estimation of the severity of hyperthyroidism by morphometric analysis is seen in patients treated with certain antithyroid drugs, such as tapazole. Although the hypermetabolic state declines, the basic inhibitory effect of the drug is such that the histopathologic appearance remains frozen in the condition that obtained when drug therapy began. Iodine administration, on the other hand, decreases the height of the follicular epithelial cells, reduces vascularity, and increases colloid storage. The effects of radioiodine treatment of Graves' disease are considered below (see Hypothyroidism).

Less common causes of primary hyperthyroidism are hyperfunctioning thyroid adenoma and carcinoma. The rare hyperplastic or genuine toxic adenoma presents as a clinically "hot" nodule that concentrates a test dose of radioactive technetium and proves to be a benign follicular neoplasm. Similarly, a follicular adenocarcinoma may on occasion be hyperfunctional. An ovarian tumor largely composed of thyroid tissue—struma ovarii—usually resembles a nontoxic nodular goiter, but a few are hyperplastic and functional. The ovarian tumor concentrates radioactive iodine, and if a mistaken thyroidectomy is performed, the hyperthyroidism persists. Rarely, hyperthyroidism may be induced by the self-administration of, or injudicious treatment with, thyroid hormones.

Secondary hyperthyroidism affects some individuals with nodular goiter, a disorder termed **toxic multinodular goiter.** Usually the patient is elderly, the obvious goiter is longstanding, and the clinical presentation is less dramatic than in full-blown Graves' disease. A distinction between recurrent primary hyperplasia with eventual goiter formation and secondary hyperplasia arising in a nodular goiter is difficult.

Thyroiditis

Thyroiditis may be acute or chronic. Rarely, pharyngitis, tonsillitis, or cervical cellulitis spreads to the contiguous thyroid tissue, which may then exhibit acute inflammation with neutrophils.

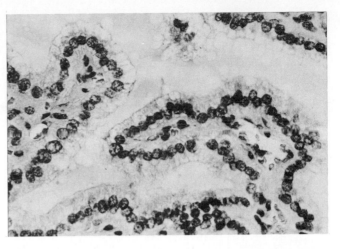

Figure 21-14. Graves' disease. Note the abnormal follicular architecture and the tall epithelial cells with vacuolated cytoplasm. Scalloping of pale-staining colloid is evident (compare with Fig. 21-11*B*).

Subacute thyroiditis is also called **granulomatous, pseudotuberculous,** or **de Quervain's thyroiditis.** It typically presents in a woman as a tender, enlarged, firm thyroid gland. Microscopically, many thyroid follicles are disrupted. There are nonspecific epithelioid cell granulomas and usually a prominent giant cell reaction to released colloid. This pattern should not be confused with that of tuberculosis, which sometimes affects the thyroid. The prognosis for functional recovery is good. The etiology of granulomatous thyroiditis is currently considered to be a viral infection of the thyroid gland, due to myxovirus, adenovirus, or other respiratory viruses.

Chronic thyroiditis is easy to define and difficult to subclassify pathologically. It shares with chronic inflammation elsewhere the presence of lymphocytes and plasma cells, which in this case appear in the thyroid connective tissue. Foci of lymphocytes and lymph follicles commonly accompany Graves' disease in younger people. These are considered to be attributes of the autoimmune state, and are not thought to represent ordinary chronic thyroiditis. Many thyroid gland specimens, whether removed

Figure 21-13. Possible mechanisms of the autoimmune pathogenesis of Graves' disease. The figure depicts three possible pathways by which B cells are activated to produce anti-TSH receptor antibodies. These antibodies, in turn, stimulate thyroid follicular cells to secrete T_3 and T_4. The mechanisms of B-cell activation may be indirect (*left* and *middle*)—that is, they may involve activation of helper T cells in conjunction with genetic factors that inhibit suppressor T cells. The two pathways illustrated differ with respect to mechanism of helper T cell activation. In the pathway shown on the right, anti-idiotype antibodies formed against anti-TSH antibodies cross react with the TSH receptor.

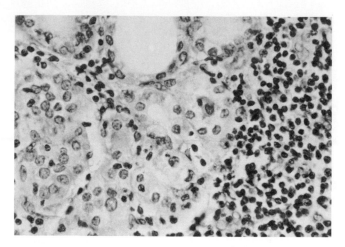

Figure 21-15. Hashimoto's disease. A dense lymphocytic infiltrate is evident on the right, and thyroid follicles can be recognized in the upper portion. The remaining epithelial cells are larger than normal and compactly arranged; their cytoplasm is granular and intensely pink (compare with Fig. 21-11C).

because of goiter or nodules thought to be neoplasms or obtained at autopsy, contain interstitial nests of plasma cells and lymphocytes. The follicular parenchyma appears largely intact and the individuals are euthyroid. Pathologically this banal and common condition is called **nonspecific chronic thyroiditis.** These "ordinary" forms of chronic thyroiditis are probably the end result of various viral infections or nonspecific toxic and degenerative changes, and have no apparent functional significance.

Hashimoto's disease, struma lymphomatosa, and **lymphadenoid goiter** are mellifluous names for the best known and clinically significant type of chronic thyroiditis. Characteristically, Hashimoto's disease develops in perimenopausal women; the patients present with an enlarged, hard thyroid gland, clinically believed to represent thyroid carcinoma. The major point of Hashimoto's original article was that not all large, hard, and microscopically cellular thyroid glands are cancerous.

Grossly, the thyroid gland in Hashimoto's struma is diffusely and uniformly enlarged and weighs from 60 g to 220 g. The capsule is thin, smooth, and intact, an unlikely feature if the lesion were a thyroid carcinoma or lymphoma of this size. Microscopically, in typical Hashimoto's disease it may not be easy at first to recognize the tissue as thyroid; it appears to be a lymph node. Further scrutiny reveals small, degenerated follicles containing minute droplets of colloid and scattered epithelial remnants of destroyed follicles. The tissue is overrun by sheets of lymphocytes,

with many lymph follicles that contain germinal centers. Few plasma cells are present.

The remaining thyroid epithelium characteristically has an eosinophilic, often granular, cytoplasm, and is arranged in cords, nests, and follicles. This metaplasia is often called "Hürthle cell" metaplasia. The cytoplasmic acidophilia is attributable to abundant mitochondria, as is the case with oncocytes, oxyphils, and oxyntic cells elsewhere (Fig. 21-15).

The pathogenesis of Hashimoto's disease, like that of Graves' disease, is thought to be based on autoimmune phenomena. The basic defect is a genetic deficiency in the antigen-specific suppressor T cells. In addition, antigen-specific helper T cells may be activated by recognizing the Class II MHC antigens expressed by the follicular epithelial cells. Thus, conditioned T cells may play a role in the injury and destruction of thyroid follicular epithelial cells and in the activation of B cells. The B cells, in turn, produce a number of autoantibodies against thyroid-related antigens. The most frequently demonstrated antibodies in patients with Hashimoto's disease are those against thyroid stimulating hormone (TSH) receptors and against thyroid microsomal fractions. Other antithyroid antibodies include those against thyroglobulin, against the nonthyroglobulin protein of the colloid material, and against the membrane of follicular cells.

TSH receptor autoantibodies are of two types—namely, those that promote glandular growth and those that stimulate hormonal hypersecretion. The pathogenesis of Hashimoto's struma may therefore be explained as an increase in the growth-stimulating antibodies without a parallel increase in those that stimulate hormone secretion. Alternatively, both types of autoantibodies may be increased, but a concomitant presence of blocking or anti–thyroid-stimulating antibodies would nullify the original antibody, thus "liberating" thyroid growth antibodies. Both situations—albeit hypothetically—would result in a goiter, without an associated increase in thyroid function.

It is important to distinguish nonspecific chronic thyroiditis from Hashimoto's disease. In nonspecific chronic thyroiditis, thyroid function is usually preserved, whereas Hashimoto's disease eventually destroys sufficient parenchyma to cause hypothyroidism. Therefore, subtotal thyroidectomy is not a desirable treatment for Hashimoto's disease. Therapy with thyroid hormone sometimes seems to rest the remaining thyroid parenchyma, and even may enable its functional recovery.

Riedel's struma is a rare form of chronic thyroiditis. It is also called ligneous thyroiditis, meaning hard as wood. At surgery a dense white scar involves part of the gland, the thyroid capsule, and the adjacent connective tissues and muscles. The original thyroid gland may be difficult to distinguish grossly, and even microscopically (Fig. 21-16). Like Hashimoto, Riedel, a German surgeon, emphasized that not all hard thyroid masses are cancer. Sometimes mediastinal or retroperitoneal fibrosis, or fibrosclerosis of other sites, may accompany Riedel's struma. The cause is unknown, but immune-related phenomena have been implicated.

Hypothyroidism

Hypothyroidism refers to a decrease in thyroid function. It has numerous causes and the severity of the syndrome may vary greatly. Degenerations, depositions, or infiltrations may adversely affect thyroid function. Aging is associated with mild thyroid atrophy and microscopic oxalate crystal deposition. The most extreme forms of thyroid atrophy and degeneration lead to **myxedema,** the most severe hypothyroid state. Patients who suffer from myxedema are sluggish, irritable, and display dry skin, loss of lateral eyebrow hairs, pasty swollen faces, an enlarged tongue, intolerance to cold, and excessive (anovulatory) menstrual bleeding in premenopausal women (Fig. 21-17). The individual with myxedema, aside from hypometabolic activity, suffers from disordered bowel and kidney functions, and may slip into myxedema coma. Thyroid hormone supplementation is curative. The term "myxedema" actually refers to hard edema of subcutaneous tissue. Paradoxically, localized pretibial myxedema occasionally accompanies hyperthyroidism.

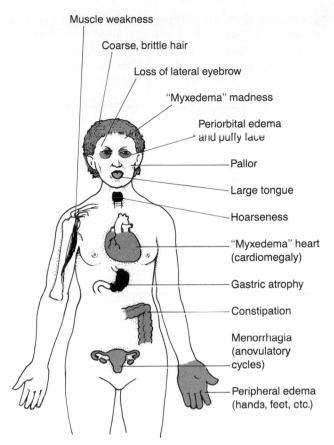

Figure 21-17. The dominant clinical manifestations of hypothyroidism.

The thyroid gland in myxedema may weigh as little as 6 g and consist largely of connective tissue and blood vessels. Microscopically, only isolated minute thyroid follicles with colloid droplets remain in a fibrofatty stroma. Of course, pituitary insufficiency may cause secondary hypothyroidism, but the cause of primary myxedema is not always readily diagnosable.

It has been suggested that most dysfunctional thyroid diseases have an autoimmune pathogenesis. This spectrum of dysfunctional stages may begin with Graves' primary hyperthyroidism, progress to Hashimoto's chronic thyroiditis, and end as subtotal atrophy with myxedema. Alternatively, it may begin with Hashimoto's disease and end with myxedema. This hypothesis, while attractive, is not invariably supported by clinical observations. Moreover, thyroid diseases seem to be too complex to be explained by a single, unifying pathogenetic mechanism.

Ionizing radiation, either external x-irradiation or radioisotopic iodine, damages thyroid tissue and leads to follicular epithelial necrosis and sloughing into follicles. Subsequently, epithelial regeneration

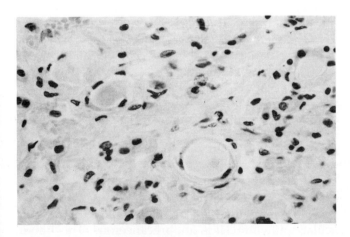

Figure 21-16. Riedel's struma. The thyroid is barely recognizable as such; a few isolated follicles are still noted. Densely fibrotic stroma predominates.

occurs, together with atypism of follicular cells, particularly nuclear aneuploidy. Hyaline interstitial fibrosis and vascular sclerosis and telangiectasia are also noted. These changes may be the eventual endpoint of the radioiodine treatment of Graves' disease; not surprisingly, hypothyroidism is noted in half or more of these patients.

Among the rarer causes of hypothyroidism is amyloid deposition localized to the thyroid. Metastatic or primary carcinomas, malignant lymphomas, or melanomas only rarely cause hypothyroidism.

Thyroid Tumors

Thyroid neoplasms are almost all either adenomas or carcinomas. A few primary or metastatic malignant lymphomas, sarcomas, and miscellaneous rare neoplasms also affect the thyroid gland.

Thyroid Adenoma

Thyroid adenomas are classified as follicular, papillary, or atypical.

Follicular Adenomas   Follicular adenoma is the prototypical endocrine adenoma. Recall that only 10% or less of clinical solitary thyroid nodules prove to be genuine adenomas. Why make a distinction? The reason is that a true adenoma is a benign clonal neoplasm, with small but clear cancerous potential, while a thyroid nodule is not.

The typical follicular adenoma ordinarily presents as a "cold" thyroid nodule—that is, one that does not take up radioiodine. When removed it is entirely encapsulated, and on transection the compressed tissue everts. The adenoma is tan, usually 2 to 3 cm in

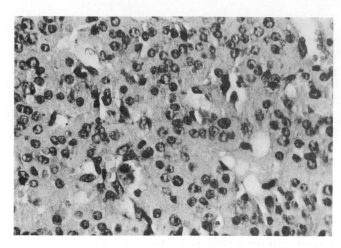

Figure 21-19.   Hürthle cell adenoma of the thyroid. Note the solid architecture; no follicles are recognized. The cytoplasm is granular and intensely pink.

diameter and may have a central scar or degenerative cysts. The follicles are small and uniform, and show limited colloid storage (Fig. 21-18). These are the so-called fetal follicles, and an old name for this adenoma is thyroid "fetal adenoma." Less commonly one sees solid cords of embryonal-type epithelium, admixed with follicles of small or ordinary size; an adenoma may also comprise variable proportions of oncocytes or Hürthle cells—a Hürthle cell adenoma (Fig. 21-19). Current classifications lump all these varieties under the designation of follicular thyroid adenoma. In summary, a genuine follicular thyroid adenoma is entirely encapsulated, contains a compressed solid growth, is morphologically uniform, and differs from the surrounding thyroid tissue. Furthermore, except in inbred racial isolates and after irradiation, most adenomas are solitary.

Papillary Adenoma   Papillary thyroid adenoma is morphologically unusual as well as uncommon. There is a fibrous shell around a cystic tumor, which is filled with dark red fluid. Macroscopically the cyst lining has small, granular, gray, papillary projections. Microscopically these papillae are covered by uniform, cuboidal, follicular-type epithelium, with fibrovascular cores. **Complete encapsulation is the exception, and hence most or all papillary adenomas may in fact be papillary carcinomas.** Removal, nonetheless, is curative.

Atypical Adenoma   Atypical adenoma refers to a solid encapsulated growth of closely packed, uniform spindle cells, which are unlike ordinary thyroid follicular epithelium. It is not precancerous. This tumor may represent an adenoma composed of parafollicular or C-cells, which are discussed later with medullary thyroid carcinoma.

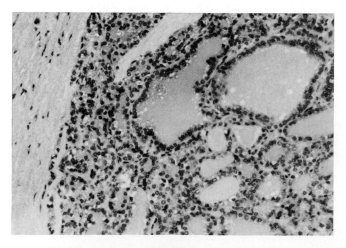

Figure 21-18.   Follicular adenoma of the thyroid. A dense capsule is evident on the left. The size and shape of the follicles and solid areas are notably irregular.

Thyroid Carcinoma

Thyroid carcinomas occur in three distinguishable varieties: microscopically recognized, grossly evident, and clinically obvious. Histologically these correspond to well, moderately, and poorly differentiated carcinomas. The prognosis varies with the differentiation, the well-differentiated tumors having the most favorable prognosis and the poorly differentiated ones the least.

Papillary Carcinoma **Papillary carcinoma is the most common thyroid cancer,** and is not unusual in the young age group. It may form a visible and palpable thyroid nodule, or first become evident as a lymph node metastasis in the lateral neck (Fig. 21-20). Unless one believes all papillary thyroid tumors to be malignant, the definitive diagnosis is only made microscopically. **If a papillary tumor is incompletely encapsulated and has spread into the adjacent thyroid tissue, or if it is multifocal without a dominant mass, it is almost certainly carcinoma.** Papillary thyroid carcinoma is recognized by (1) epithelium piled up on the surfaces of papillae, (2) empty, ground glass, "Orphan Annie eye" nuclei, and (3) laminated masses of calcareous material (so-called "psammoma bodies") in half the cases (Fig. 21-21). Psammoma bodies, even when found alone in thyroid tissue, strongly suggest a nearby papillary carcinoma. Also, the ground glass nuclei observed in almost any variety of differentiated thyroid carcinoma are now considered to indicate its papillary nature.

Papillary thyroid carcinoma typically invades lymphatics and spreads to the regional cervical lymph nodes. Sometimes the primary carcinoma is small, about 2 mm, and the involved lymph nodes are large. In these different clinical presentations, papillary thyroid carcinoma ordinarily grows sluggishly. With local surgical excision alone, the 5-year survival is now over 90%, and the 10-year survival rate is over 85%.

Therapeutic irradiation to the face, neck, and upper chest regions was given several decades ago for various benign conditions, such as presumed thymic enlargement, chronic tonsillitis, and acne. Such treatment included the thyroid in the field of radiation. This practice, now totally abandoned, often involved infants and children, who subsequently displayed a higher than usual incidence of papillary thyroid carcinomas. In addition, nodular thyroid regeneration, goiter, and single or multiple benign adenomas may develop after irradiation. These radiation-related thyroid diseases, however, are not usually associated with hypothyroidism.

Follicular Carcinoma Another important form of thyroid carcinoma is the **adenoma with invasion** (synonyms include malignant adenoma, adenoma with capsular invasion, angioinvasive adenoma). Multiple microscopic sections of what clinically and grossly appears to be a follicular adenoma show histologic foci of epithelium, either invading veins or penetrating the fibrous capsule (Fig. 21-22). The large majority are cured by local tumor excision, but metastasis or local recurrence are seen in about 15%. Metastases to the lungs, bones, and other sites may occur many years after removal of the thyroid lesion. Other diagnostic terms for this condition include encapsulated follicular carcinoma, and carcinoma arising in follicular adenoma. Of major importance for the physician is the understanding that metastases are uncommon, and radical intervention is not appropriate.

Among the histologic subtypes of thyroid follicular adenoma, those with embryonal or solid, trabecular growth patterns are the most likely to invade (about 25%), while invasion in the fetal microfollicular type adenoma is uncommon (about 10%). Hürthle cell carcinomas may or may not originate in corresponding adenomas, but in any case seem to have a higher propensity for aggressive behavior than their counterparts.

Follicular thyroid carcinoma is the prototype of the moderately differentiated, grossly identifiable carcinoma. It forms a hard thyroid mass that, on section, appears as a granular, pale gray-white, stellate invasive tissue, resembling many other visceral carcinomas. The neoplastic follicles are formed by cells with abnormally enlarged, crowded, and misshapen nuclei (Fig. 21-23). These follicles closely abut, with scanty intervening stroma; the tumor invades the adjacent thyroid tissue, the thyroid gland capsule, and blood vessels.

Follicular thyroid carcinoma typically spreads via the bloodstream and metastasizes to the lungs and bones (see Fig. 21-20). After its extirpation about 40% have five-year survival without disease, **only half the survival rates for papillary carcinoma or invasive adenoma.** Some follicular carcinomas localize radioiodine and can, therefore, be controlled by therapeutic doses.

Medullary Carcinoma **Medullary thyroid carcinoma** is different from all other thyroid carcinomas because of its cellular differentiation, its endocrine activities, and its morphologic appearance.

Medullary thyroid carcinoma forms bulky, soft, gray tumors, sometimes bilaterally. Despite its ominous gross and microscopic appearance, it ordinarily grows slowly. The 5-year survival rate, usually with residual tumor present, is about 40%, a figure similar to that of follicular carcinoma. It readily metastasizes

PAPILLARY CARCINOMA

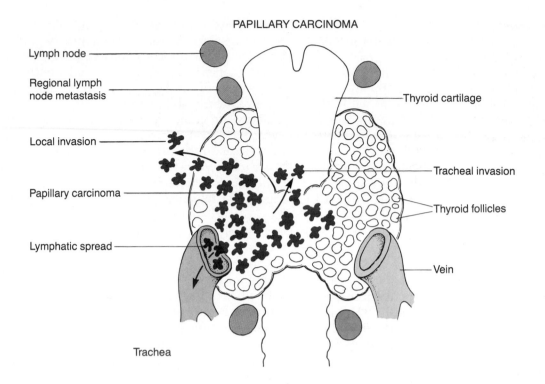

FOLLICULAR CARCINOMA

MEDULLARY CARCINOMA

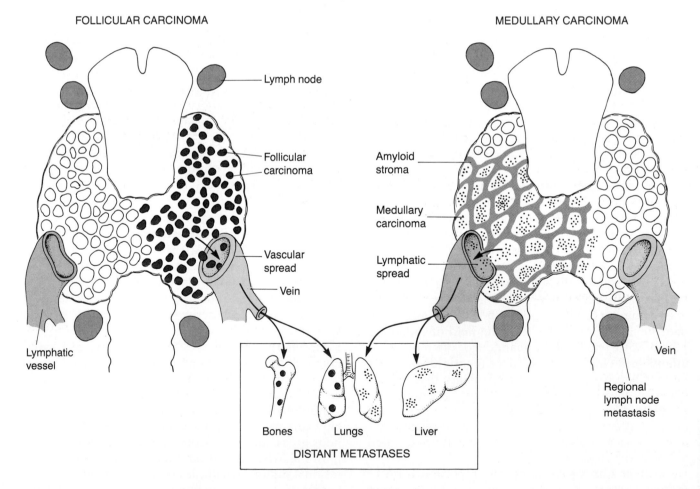

DISTANT METASTASES

via lymphatic channels to regional lymph nodes, but may also invade blood vessels and metastasize to the liver, lungs, and bones (see Fig. 21-20).

Medullary carcinoma does not resemble normal thyroid tissue, for it is composed of pale, cuboidal, and often spindle-shaped cells. In sections stained with hematoxylin and eosin the compact masses of tumor cells are surrounded by abundant, uniformly pink or violet stroma that represents amyloid (Fig. 21-24). Other histologic patterns resemble carcinoid tumors, or show ribbon-like islet cell tumors, or may even include a few follicles or glands with mucus. Because of the characteristic stromal change, the diagnostic term often employed is "medullary carcinoma with amyloid stroma." Spread and metastasis of medullary thyroid carcinoma resemble the pattern of follicular carcinoma.

Immunohistochemical studies of medullary carcinoma show not only calcitonin, but also serotonin, somatostatin, and bombesin, a situation similar to that in normal C-cells. The interstitial and follicle-lining C-cells are normally so inconspicuous in the adult thyroid as to escape identification, unless immunostains for calcitonin are utilized. Calcitonin antagonizes the hypercalcemic effect of parathyroid hormone, but hypocalcemia due to excessive calcitoninemia is extremely rare.

Ultrastructurally there are several different types of cytoplasmic neurosecretory granules. The medullary carcinoma cells are argyrophilic with the Grimelius or equivalent silver stains. Further, ectopic hormones such as ACTH are sometimes present. Hence medullary thyroid carcinoma may cause the carcinoid syndrome or Cushing's syndrome. **These characteristics mark C-cells as a component of the dispersed neuroendocrine system, and medullary thyroid carcinomas as neuroendocrine carcinomas.**

Familial medullary thyroid carcinoma is part of a genetic condition associated with pheochromocytoma, often bilateral, and parathyroid hyperplasia or adenoma. This combination is designated as multiple endocrine neoplasia (MEN) Type IIa. MEN Type IIb is a related condition, which has multiple mucosal neuromas, especially of the lips and tongue, but in which the parathyroid hyperplasia or adenoma is apparently atypical or absent. Children in such families, who had subtotal thyroidectomies as a prophylactic measure to forestall medullary carcinoma development, showed diffuse or nodular C-cell hy-

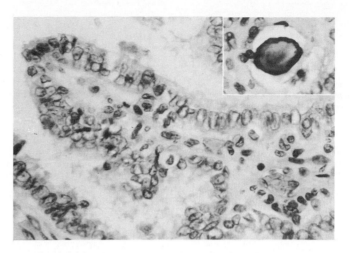

Figure 21-21. Papillary carcinoma of the thyroid. A papilla projects toward the upper left, and vesicular "Orphan Annie" nuclei are evident. *(Inset)* Typical psammoma body.

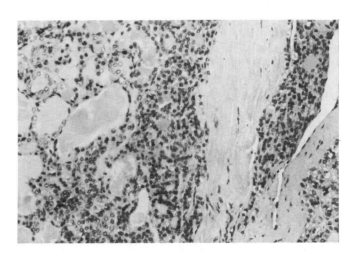

Figure 21-22. Angioinvasive follicular thyroid adenoma. Follicles and solid areas can be seen. The thick fibrous capsule has been penetrated by tumor (lower right). A large vein, part of whose lumen is seen, has also been invaded by tumor.

perplasia bilaterally. These increased C-cell populations correlated with elevated levels of circulating calcitonin. Similarly, some family members have diffuse or nodular adrenal medullary hyperplasia, presumably predisposing them to the development of a pheochromocytoma.

Figure 21-20. Principal gross characteristics and patterns of growth and metastases of papillary, follicular, and medullary carcinomas of the thyroid gland.

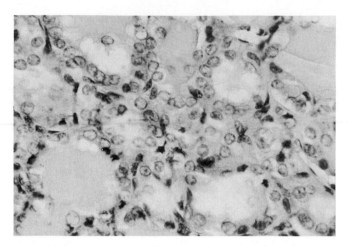

Figure 21-23. Follicular thyroid carcinoma. Well-formed, uniform, and closely packed follicles are evident. The nuclei are larger than normal and irregularly shaped.

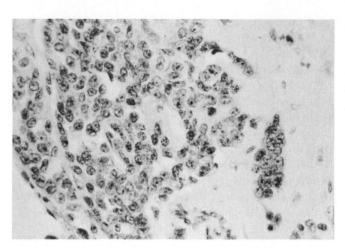

Figure 21-24. Medullary thyroid carcinoma. A solid arrangement of rather small cells (compare with Figs. 21-21, 21-23, and 21-25 at identical magnification) is surrounded by solid stroma containing abundant amyloid.

Undifferentiated Carcinoma Undifferentiated thyroid carcinomas are usually clinically obvious and rapidly lethal. The fast growing, hard neck mass is composed of dense, granular grayish tissue. These aggressive cancers typically occur in older women; they often develop in a preexistent goiter, with or without associated, better differentiated carcinomas.

Microscopically, the best known pattern is a bizarre cellular proliferation of spindle and giant cells, with polyploid nuclei, many mitoses, tumor necrosis, and stromal fibrosis. The diagnosis is spindle and giant cell thyroid carcinoma (Fig. 21-25).

Less common types of undifferentiated thyroid carcinoma are small cell anaplastic carcinoma, which vaguely resembles a breast carcinoma, and small cell diffuse carcinoma. These highly malignant tumors compress and destroy local structures; dysphagia and dyspnea due to tracheal compression or invasion are frequent. Most patients die within a few months after diagnosis.

As mentioned above, some cases of undifferentiated thyroid carcinoma have a long history, beginning with goiters in youth. Others have preceding papillary or follicular carcinoma, and end 20 or more years later with a spindle and giant cell thyroid carcinoma.

Other than ionizing radiation, especially before age 20 years, no carcinogenic factor for the human thyroid gland has been clearly identified. Countries with endemic goiter supposedly have a higher incidence of thyroid cancer, but there are more thyroidectomies as well. Subclinical minute papillary thyroid carcinomas have been found in serial sections

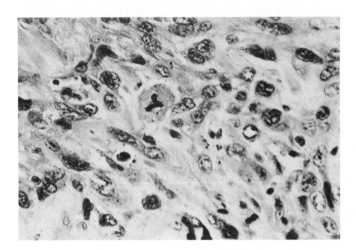

Figure 21-25. Undifferentiated spindle and giant cell carcinoma of the thyroid. A tripolar mitosis can be seen slightly left and above center.

of over 25% of random Japanese autopsies and 17% of autopsies in young Finns. Nevertheless, there is no convincing evidence that such findings are clinically significant.

Thyroid Lymphomas

Malignant lymphomas of the thyroid, though uncommon, appear to be increasing in frequency. They usually are of the large cell or mixed large cell and lymphocytic types. If restricted to the thyroid gland, malignant lymphoma has a reasonable prognosis, similar to that of gastric or retrobulbar malignant lymphomas.

Parathyroid Glands

Anatomy, Embryology, and Physiology

The four parathyroid glands are derivatives of branchial clefts III and IV. Occasionally five, and rarely up to eight, are seen. Normally they are found on the posterior thyroid surface, the lowest two (from branchial cleft III) adjacent to the inferior thyroid arteries. The upper two glands are adherent to the upper posterolateral third of each thyroid lobe. A parathyroid gland may be entirely intrathyroid or intrathymic, or may be located between the trachea and esophagus, or in other ectopic locations. Hence surgical identification and removal of a functioning parathyroid tumor may be difficult.

Each gland is the size and color of a grain of saffron-cooked rice. Half is normally adipose tissue and half chief cells. The overall weight per gland is 31 to 59 mg and the net parenchymal weight per gland 20 to 40 mg. The total net parenchymal parathyroid weight is 80 to 150 mg. Loose fibroconnective tissues, and particularly fat, are irregularly distributed in the parenchyma (Fig. 21-26). An adipose hamartoma may form a palpable cervical mass, with the parathyroid chief cells scattered through the fatty connective tissue.

The parathyroid glands are not under anterior pituitary control, but are most directly influenced by circulating ionized calcium and magnesium concentrations. This situation is similar to that in the adrenal zona glomerulosa, in which secretion of aldosterone responds to alterations in sodium levels. Parathyroid hormone concentrations in the blood control the levels of circulating calcium ions. The prohormone formed in the gland undergoes proteolysis and the molecule is further cleaved to provide the functional secretory polypeptide. The active parathyroid hormone (PTH) has a short circulating half-life. Magnesium, a cation closely related to calcium, acts as a brake on parathyroid hormone secretion. Consequently, in magnesium deficiency, increased parathyroid hormone secretion is evident.

Hypoparathyroidism

Hypoparathyroidism most often occurs after thyroidectomy, when three or four glands are either removed or have their vasculature damaged. The result is a prompt fall in the blood calcium level, with clinical tetany. The jaw locks, several tendon reflexes become exaggerated, and striated muscles twitch or cramp. Calcium infusion temporarily relieves the condition.

Hypoparathyroidism less commonly is an infantile condition, due either to gland agenesis or congenital hypoplasia, and is characterized by tetany or convulsions and a failure to thrive. Sometimes it is familial; other cases are sporadic. A pediatric syndrome of hypoparathyroidism, Addison's adrenocortical deficiency, and chronic candidal fungus infection is intriguing. Occasionally hypoparathyroid adults have excessive calcium deposits in the spine, joints, or cerebral basal ganglia. Lifetime therapy with parathyroid hormone and vitamin D, or subcutaneous transplantation of fetal human parathyroid tissue, restores the calcium balance.

Pseudohypoparathyroidism designates a group of conditions that exhibit target organ resistance or insensitivity to parathyroid hormone (PTH). The blood calcium level is low; phosphate levels and alkaline phosphatase activity are high. Kidney resistance to injected PTH is shown by failure to increase urinary excretion of cyclic AMP and phosphate and deficient renal calcium reabsorption. Pseudohypoparathyroidism (Type I) may or may not be accompanied by overt bone disease, but bone biopsy does show the osteolytic effects of excessive PTH. Some patients display short metacarpals or metatarsals, short stature, cataracts, subcutaneous calcifications, or mental deficiency—the so-called **Albright hereditary osteodystrophy somatotype.** Usually the activity of G-protein in fibroblast, platelet, and erythrocyte membranes is decreased. This protein binds guanine nucleotides and functions to couple PTH hormone receptors to the catalytic unit of the adenylate cyclase complex.

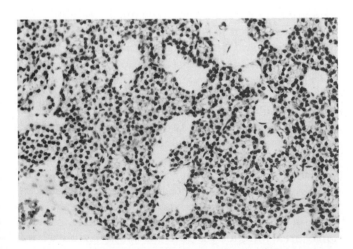

Figure 21-26. Normal parathyroid of a human adult. Observe the mingled solid epithelial nests and adipose tissue.

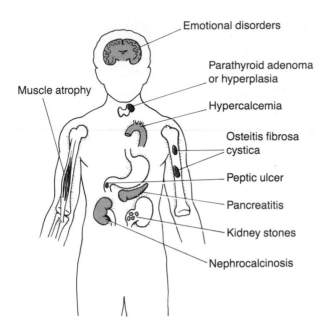

Muscle atrophy

Emotional disorders

Parathyroid adenoma or hyperplasia

Hypercalcemia

Osteitis fibrosa cystica

Peptic ulcer

Pancreatitis

Kidney stones

Nephrocalcinosis

Figure 21-27.   The major clinical features of hyperparathyroidism.

Thus, patients with Type I pseudohypoparathyroidism are resistant not only to PTH, but also to thyrotropin (TSH), glucagon, and the gonadotropins, FSH and LH. Variable expressions of this PTH resistance may correlate with variations in cell cyclic AMP concentrations. Patients without bone disease sometimes suffer from vitamin D_3 deficiency. However, if circulating vitamin D levels are normal the individual is normocalcemic.

Pseudopseudohypoparathyroidism reads like a typographic error. The term refers to rare cases in which the Albright's somatotype described above is associated with nail abnormalities, skull and dental anomalies, and a prominent forehead. In addition to these inherited anomalies there are abnormalities of the parathyroids, PTH, or PTH receptors.

In pseudopseudohypoparathyroidism (Type II pseudohypoparathyroidism) there is a marked rise in the urine cyclic AMP level after PTH is given, but the serum calcium does not rise, and renal phosphate reabsorption remains excessive. Apparently the intracellular cyclic AMP message is not received or is improperly transduced. G-protein activity is normal.

Hyperparathyroidism

Hyperparathyroidism, (i.e., parathyroid hyperfunction) most often is due to a parathyroid adenoma that secretes PTH. In its originally recognized, most florid state, hyperparathyroidism is clinically characterized by rubbery, deformed long bones, attributable to excessive calcium reabsorption. The bone lesions are called either brown tumors, because the fibrous tissue is pigmented by hemosiderin, or osteitis fibrosa cystica, a term that describes the radiologic appearance and locally cystic bones. The blood calcium level is elevated, because calcium is mobilized from bones. Deposition of calcium in the kidneys can result in kidney stones, secondary renal infections, and even renal failure. Calcium deposition may occur in other sites, such as the lungs and soft tissues. Clinical manifestations associated with hyperparathyroidism also include hypertension, pancreatitis, and peptic ulcers (Fig. 21-27). The pathogenesis of these problems and their direct or indirect relationship to hyperparathyroidism, remain obscure.

In the past, calcium kidney stones attracted attention to excessive parathyroid function. Nowadays, routine blood screening tests show hypercalcemia in about 3% of those examined, and from this group only a few patients with otherwise subclinical clearcut hyperparathyroidism are identified. In the remainder with isolated hypercalcemia, the need for any treatment is uncertain. Malnutrition, with osteomalacia, avitaminosis D, hypothyroidism, or magnesium deficiency, may mask hyperparathyroidism.

The diagnostic criteria for hyperparathyroidism are significant hypercalcemia, low blood phosphate, and high alkaline phosphatase activity. Dental X-rays show absence of the lamina dura, which is a fine calcified line around tooth roots. Radiological changes in the digital bones, characterized by subperiosteal resorption, are regarded as virtually pathognomonic of hyperparathyroidism, although similar cystic changes may be noted in other bones (Fig. 21-28).

Parathyroid Adenoma

Primary hyperparathyroidism is due to a single parathyroid adenoma in about 80% of cases, two adenomas in 5%, and diffuse parathyroid hyperplasia in 15%. Functioning parathyroid carcinoma may account for 1% or 2%. The size and weight of the responsible parathyroid adenoma are correlated with the severity of the hypercalcemia.

Hyperparathyroid crisis is a life-threatening emergency caused by an unrecognized or neglected, usually rather large, parathyroid adenoma. Palpation of the neck may set off the crisis. The blood calcium level rises above 15 mg/dl, and muscular weakness, lethargy, and acute brain, cardiovascular, or gastrointestinal symptoms may appear. The blood phosphate falls, urea nitrogen rises, renal failure follows, and about 60% of the patients die.

Exacerbation of an unrecognized chronic hyperparathyroidism is the usual circumstance. Emergency operation is lifesaving. Surgical neck exploration, with removal of the abnormal parathyroid(s), is the curative procedure for primary hyperparathyroidism. Pathologists are given, for intraoperative frozen-section examination, small tissue specimens that the surgeon suspects as the likely parathyroid tumor. Often, at first small lymph nodes or thyroid nodules are mistaken for parathyroid tissue. Then, after search, an elongated, typically mustard-colored, thinly encapsulated soft mass is removed. Microscopic examination reveals a solid parathyroid cell growth, partly surrounded by a rim of unaltered parathyroid gland, half of which is adipose tissue. Reduced intracellular fat indicates hyperfunctional parathyroid cells, either adenomatous or hyperplastic. The most common diagnosis is parathyroid chief cell adenoma (Fig. 21-29).

Parathyroid parenchymal cell types, normally and abnormally, are predominantly chief cells, but transitional forms, and pale, water-clear cells are present in adenomas and in hyperplasias. Oxyphil parathyroid cells are found in middle-aged or older individuals, and may form small nodules, more commonly in women. These acidophilic cells are rich in mitochondria, and are usually nonfunctional. However, a

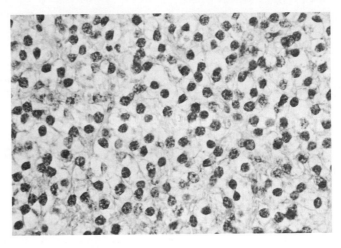

Figure 21-29. Parathyroid adenoma. Solidly arranged epithelial cells with pale cytoplasm are evident.

number of hyperfunctioning parathyroid oxyphil adenomas have been identified. A few tumors with considerable adiposity are designated as lipoadenomas.

Parathyroid adenomas may undergo infarctive, hemorrhagic, and cystic degeneration. Lymphocytic and plasma cellular infiltrates may be seen. Sometimes the hyperparathyroid state spontaneously remits.

The pathogenesis of parathyroid adenoma generally is unknown. Hyperplasias do not evolve into adenomas. Genetic factors may be present, since parathyroid adenoma (or hyperplasia) is a typical feature of both multiple endocrine neoplasia (MEN) syndromes Types I and IIa, but not of MEN IIb. Familial parathyroid adenoma, alone or with papillary thyroid carcinoma, forms another syndrome. Ionizing radiation clearly is a cause of parathyroid adenoma. Prolonged thiazide diuretic therapy may also be a cause. Claims are advanced that high-phosphate diets may initiate parathyroid hyperplasia, and that a few functioning parathyroid adenomas develop in longstanding primary or secondary hyperplasias.

Parathyroid Hyperplasia

Primary parathyroid hyperplasia, as already noted, is a less common cause of primary hyperparathyroidism. Because of claims that parathyroid adenomas are polyclonal and really represent the dominant nodule of a general parathyroid hyperplasia, some surgeons, after removing an adenoma, will biopsy one additional parathyroid gland to prove it is histologically normal.

Primary parathyroid hyperplasia involves all four glands. These are grossly enlarged and tan, and are

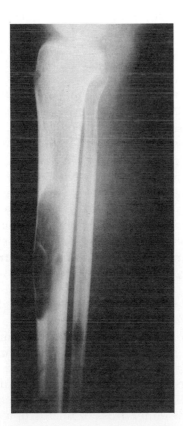

Figure 21-28. Radiograph depicting the tibia and fibula of a patient with severe hyperparathyroidism. Several cystic areas corresponding to "brown tumors" are noted.

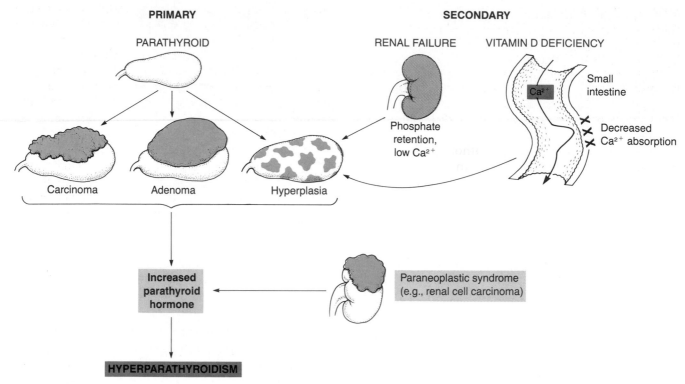

Figure 21-30.   Major pathogenetic pathways leading to clinical primary and secondary hyperparathyroidism.

composed of nearly solid chief cell parenchyma, with little residual adipose tissue. At one time, primary hyperplasia of clear cell type predominated; these appeared grossly as brownish parathyroid glands, the superior pair often being more enlarged than the inferior pair. For unknown reasons clear cell hyperplasia is now less frequently observed.

Secondary parathyroid hyperplasia is commonplace at autopsy. It is encountered in patients with renal diseases and renal insufficiency, in whom these conditions result in important bone lesions. The inadequate renal conservation of calcium lowers blood calcium levels and causes the parathyroids to increase their PTH secretion, a sequence that results in increased calcium resorption from bones.

The hyperplastic parathyroids are enlarged twofold or more, and parathyroid cells replace part or most of the adipose tissue normally present. Chief, transitional, or water-clear cells may predominate, the hypersecretion of PTH increasing in that order.

Parathyroid hyperfunction, either primary or secondary, predisposes to metastatic calcification in the lungs, kidneys (nephrocalcinosis or stones), meninges, synovial membranes, and sometimes other tissues. As mentioned, pancreatitis with calcification, hypertension, and peptic ulcers complicate some

cases. A diagrammatic outline of the various forms of primary and secondary hyperparathyroidism is presented in Figure 21-30.

Tertiary hyperparathyroidism, sometimes called autonomous parathyroid hyperplasia, is a complication of chronic renal failure treated by bilateral nephrectomy followed by long-term hemodialysis. Many such patients have normal calcium homeostasis, but some show persistent hypercalcemia. Surgical exploration often yields two to four irregularly enlarged glands with nodular parathyroid hyperplasia. Some nodules consist of chief cells; adjacent nodules are composed of water-clear or oxyphil cells. They are functionally autonomous, in that endocrine control of hypercalcemia is not achieved without their extirpation.

Parathyroid Carcinoma

Parathyroid carcinoma is very uncommon. Some cases are nonfunctional. A neck mass that is difficult to distinguish from a clear cell or small cell thyroid carcinoma possesses ultrastructural features of parathyroid cells. A few hyperfunctioning parathyroid tumors show either gross or microscopic penetration of the gland capsule, with invasion of the adjacent connective tissues or striated muscle. Occasional mitoses raise the suspicion of parathyroid carcinoma. Local invasion alone does not invariably prove that a parathyroid tumor is malignant. (This is also true of tumors of the anterior pituitary and pancreatic islets, and perhaps thyroid adenomas.)

Incomplete resection of the parathyroid adenoma is undesirable because the hyperparathyroid state may persist thereafter for many years. Also, local recurrences of adenomas may involve the adjacent tissues, with questionable "malignant" invasion. In parathyroid carcinoma, with or without previous surgery, multiple metastases in the lungs, soft tissues, and bones may accompany the clinical onset or a recurrence of hyperparathyroidism.

Microscopically, some parathyroid carcinomas are cytologically overtly malignant neoplasms, with lymphatic and blood vessel invasion. Others have a bland growth pattern and monotonous cellularity. The prognosis is generally poor. Occasional atypical or giant nuclei in a parathyroid adenoma are not a sign of cancer; again, this is also true of pituitary and adrenocortical adenomas.

Hypercalcemia

Hypercalcemia may have numerous causes other than hyperparathyroidism. These include hypervitaminosis D, milk–alkali overuse in individuals

Table 21-2. Some Causes of Hypercalcemia

Primary hyperparathyroidism, adenoma, hyperplasia, or parathyroid carcinoma
Secondary hyperparathyroidism, chronic renal disease
Disuse atrophy, bones
Familial hypocalciuria
Granulomas due to silicone implants
Metastatic cancer, bones
Munchausen syndrome, surreptitious calcium ingestion
Sarcoidosis
Thyrotoxicosis
Vitamin D intoxication

Table 21-3. Some Causes of Hypercalcemia with Cancer

Bone destruction
Colony-stimulating factors for granulocytes
Osteoclast activating factor
Parathyroid hormone, ectopic
Parathyroid adenoma
Parathyroid hormone receptor interacting factor
Prostaglandin E_2
Transforming growth factors for fibroblasts
Tumor peptide stimulating renal adenylate cyclase
Calcitriol (1α,25-dihydroxyvitamin D_3)

treating their own peptic ulcers, excessive calcium ingestion, familial hypocalciuria, and metastatic cancers that destroy bones and mobilize their calcium (Table 21-2). In the absence of any of these conditions and without renal failure, hypercalcemia may accompany a variety of cancers, particularly renal, lung, or breast carcinomas, and lymphoma or leukemia. The parathyroid glands and circulating PTH are typically normal. In a few cancer cases ectopic PTH has been demonstrated both in the blood and tumor tissue. A number of other tumor products have been implicated, including the E prostaglandins, osteoclast-activating factor, and at least three other biologically identified factors (Table 21-3). Proper biochemical studies can successfully distinguish hypercalcemia related to cancer from primary hyperparathyroidism.

The Adrenal Cortex

Anatomy

The adrenal gland (also called suprarenal gland) is actually two organs in one; it comprises the cortex, derived from the mesoderm, and the medulla, derived from the neuroectoderm. The adrenal glands are necessary to maintain life; cortical aldosterone maintains salt and water balance, and cortisol and cortisone are important hormonal controls of glucose metabolism.

The adrenal cortex is zonate. From the capsule inward it consists of the zona glomerulosa, a site of aldosterone synthesis, the zona fasciculata, where cortisol is formed, and the zona reticularis, the source of adrenal androgenic and estrogenic hormones.

Congenital Anomalies

Various anomalies in the number, location, or fusion of adrenal glands are clinically unimportant. One adrenal gland was found inside the skull. Hepatoadrenal or adrenorenal fusion is usually unilateral. Small accessory adrenocortical foci are commonplace adjacent to the adrenal capsule, or rarely, elsewhere in the retroperitoneum, pelvic connective tissues, and gonads.

Congenital adrenal hyperplasia comprises important inborn functional deficiencies of adrenocortical steroidogenesis. One of five enzymes required for the formation of intermediate steroids from cholesterol is lacking or defective. **All these defects are autosomal recessive, and in all those affected in a given family the same enzyme deficiency is present.**

In desmolase deficiency the cortical cells are rich in cholesterol, but no further steroid synthesis is achieved, so that extrauterine life is brief.

Of the five congenital enzyme deficiencies the absence of 21-hydroxylase is the most common. No step in cortisol synthesis beyond 17-α-hydroxyprogesterone is completed. **The affected infants or children are susceptible to lethal shock after trivial trauma or respiratory infections.** Side reactions encourage an excessive androgenic steroid synthesis, and at birth affected females have external genitalia that resemble a penis and scrotum, owing to clitoral and labial hypertrophy. Congenital adrenal hyperplasia is the most common cause of female pseudohermaphroditism, in which a genetic female appears male at birth, and may be so reared. When comparable endocrine abnormalities appear later in life the condition is termed the adrenogenital syndrome.

Some patients with 21-hydroxylase deficiency also manifest aldosterone deficiency. Salt and water balance is imperfect, with salt being lost into the urine. Although handicapped in growth, and in physical and mental development, and with precocious external genital development in boys and partial virilization in girls, such individuals may live to become adults, if they are supplemented with the appropriate corticosteroids.

Adrenocortical hormone deficiency in infants may develop if bilateral hemorrhages complicate the normal postnatal involution of the innermost fetal cortical zone. *In utero* the fetal cortical zone contributes estrogens and androgens to the fetal–placental unit, a process that acts to increase maternal circulating estrogen levels in late pregnancy.

Adrenal Cortical Insufficiency

Chronic adrenocortical insufficiency has the classical name of **Addison's disease.** In times past, destructive bilateral adrenal tuberculosis was the usual cause. Now autoimmune destruction of the adrenal cortex is the most common cause, and infiltrates of lymphocytes and macrophages populate the residual connective tissue. Patients with Addison's disease suffer from muscle weakness, asthenia, low blood pressure, low serum sodium, and a tendency to suffer shock after minor infections or injuries. Their skin and mucous membranes are pigmented brown through the effects of melanocyte stimulating hormone (MSH) that has been liberated from the feedback control provided by cortisol and related corticosteroids. Replacement therapy with adrenocortical steroids maintains such individuals in reasonable health.

Cortisone-type hormones inhibit normal inflammatory reactions and granuloma formation. For example, tuberculosis or histoplasmosis of the adrenal glands cause more caseation or nonspecific necrosis, and fewer well-developed granulomas, than these infections usually induce in other tissues.

Systemic viral infections, especially herpesvirus or cytomegalovirus, tend to damage the adrenals, and their viral inclusion bodies are evident in cortical cell nuclei. Numerous other infections and toxic states produce foci of adrenocortical necrosis. Such conditions rarely result in adrenocortical insufficiency.

Depositions may replace the adrenal cortex focally or diffusely, and sometimes cause functional deficiency. Amyloid is one such deposit, metastatic cancer is another. Addison's disease due to any type of deposition is uncommon. In the elderly, foci of ordinary adipose cells may replace parts of the adrenal cortex; that is possibly a sign of sluggish function, but not of true insufficiency.

The adrenal glands are resistant to ionizing radiation damage, but inner zone fibrosis may result.

Adrenocortical atrophy is, as might be expected, a result of long continued therapy with adrenocortical steroids for arthritis, connective tissue and muscle diseases, asthma, or other disorders. The adrenal glands shrink from the normal weight of 6 grams each to 3 grams or less. Should the corticosteroid therapy be abruptly discontinued, a temporarily serious deficiency state of Addisonian type may develop. It is, therefore, desirable to taper the corticosteroid dose gradually.

In children and some adults the most dramatically **acute adrenocortical destruction** is known as the **Waterhouse-Friderichsen syndrome.** This often lethal condition is characterized by sudden shock, loss of plasma electrolyte balance, skin petechiae and purpura, all caused by massive bilateral adrenal hemorrhage and necrosis. Most commonly, meningococcal septicemia is responsible, but gram-positive cocci may be found. Although the mechanism is not entirely understood, it probably is a form of endotoxic shock reaction analogous to the Shwartzman phenomenon. In the truly acute Waterhouse-Friderichsen syndrome, shock kills the patient before cortical hormone deficiency can develop. Should the patient survive the acute phase with significant destruction of the adrenal cortex, an Addisonian-type cortical insufficiency syndrome ensues.

In stressful circumstances that follow a major injury, burn, operation, sepsis, or toxic condition, the stored adrenocortical lipid and hormone contents are rapidly mobilized and discharged into the bloodstream. In chronic illness the steroids are secreted as fast as they are formed, and there is little intracellular lipid storage. Hence, bright-yellow, lipid-rich adrenocortical tissue is an indicator of sudden death without preexisting chronic disease. Conversely, autopsies performed on chronically ill patients yield adrenal glands that are less yellow than their normal counterparts; these glands are said to be "lipid depleted." In the acute reaction to stress, after about 16 hours not only is most of the adrenocortical lipid gone, but portions of the cellular cords may undergo necrosis. Subsequently, as the cortex regenerates, between 16 and 36 hours after the shocking event, the zona fasciculata cells, where the reactive changes are most severe, form hollow cords with empty centers. This "tubular degeneration" is a marker for a recent serious event. After 36 hours, the usual solid adrenocortical structure and some lipid content are usually restored.

Adrenal Cortical Hyperfunction

Hyperfunction, hypertrophy, and hyperplasia of the adrenal cortex follow appropriate stimulation. The zona glomerulosa, site of aldosterone synthesis, is normally discontinuous (in humans). If chronically stimulated, as by the salt and water imbalance associated with liver cirrhosis and ascites, the cells of the zona glomerulosa become enlarged and form a continuous subcapsular zone. This is designated as **adrenocortical hyperplasia of secondary hyperaldosteronism.** The glands are not measurably enlarged because the outermost cortical zone contributes less than 8% of the adrenal weight.

Hypertrophy and hyperplasia of the zona fasciculata constitute the major adrenal reactions to chronic illness. The zona fasciculata comprises about 75% of the gland mass, so that its changes are often evident both grossly and microscopically. The glands reach weights of 10 to 12 grams each, compared to the normal 6 grams. The cortical cells become enlarged, and the mitochondria and the rough and smooth endoplasmic reticulum are increased, changes which indicate accelerated glucocorticoid synthesis.

Cells of the zona reticularis are enlarged and their numbers increased in **adrenal virilism.** This uncommon condition affects some perimenopausal women, often but not invariably of Mediterranean ethnic origin. These patients develop male hair patterns in the facial, limb, chest, and pubic areas. It has been speculated that declining ovarian function at the menopause releases pituitary gonadotropins to stimulate adrenal androgen secretion.

Specific adrenocortical hyperfunctional states also may involve any one or two of the three cortical zones. The most important of these hyperfunctional states is **Cushing's syndrome.** These patients, unlike those with Cushing's disease, do not have a definable pituitary adenoma. However, many have irregular aggregates of corticotropin-producing cells called pituitary microadenomas. In a small subset of patients, not even microadenomas can be found, an observation that has led to the suggestion that the hypothalamus may be the site of the functional derangement. The variants in which ACTH hypersecretion stems from the pituitary have been termed "pituitary Cushing's syndrome" and account for two-thirds of the cases.

When excess ACTH is produced by an extrapituitary neoplasm, the condition is termed **ectopic Cushing's, or ectopic ACTH syndrome.** The tumors most frequently implicated are neuroendocrine carcinomas of the lung, thymus, and pancreatic islets. In rare cases, cancers producing ACTH-releasing factor (CRF) have also been reported.

The direct hormonal effects of Cushing's syndrome are due to hypercortisolism; thus Cushing's syndrome can also be based on functional adenomas, carcinomas, or unilateral hyperplasia of the adrenal cortex (Fig. 21-31).

Patients with Cushing's syndrome typically present with (a) a rounded, moon-shaped face, (b) obesity around the shoulder girdle, called a buffalo-hump, (c) thin skin that may stretch and show red striae over the abdomen, (d) osteoporosis, (e) plethoric features reflecting erythrocythemia, (f) a diabetic type of glucose tolerance test, and (g) psychological disturbances (see Fig. 21-9). These changes are common side effects of prolonged treatment with large doses of corticosteroids. Indeed, **iatrogenic Cushing's syndrome is, by far, the most common variety seen today.**

Typically, the adrenal glands in spontaneous Cushing's syndrome are both enlarged to 8 to 12 g and display hyperplasia of the zona fasciculata. A few glands are of normal size but these also have enlargement of the outer zona fasciculata, due to swollen, lipid-rich cortical cells that contain increased steroidogenic organelles. Subtotal adrenalectomy relieves the somatic, metabolic, and endocrine abnormalities. Three-quarters of cases of spontaneous Cushing's syndrome are due to this type of bilateral adrenocortical hyperplasia, which in turn, may be either primary or secondary to pituitary lesions.

Some patients with Cushing's syndrome are partly virilized women or, rarely, feminized men. The bilateral adrenocortical hyperplasia in such individuals involves the zona reticularis as well as the fasciculata.

In middle age the adrenal cortices often become nodular, without a significant change in weight or

PITUITARY

PARANEOPLASTIC SYNDROME

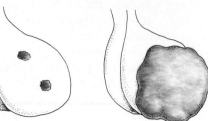

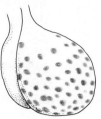

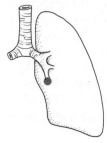

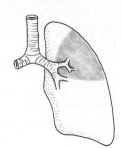

Basophilic
microadenomas

Basophilic or
chromophobe adenoma

Basophilic
hyperplasia

Carcinoid tumor
(e.g., bronchial)

Small (oat) cell
carcinoma of lung

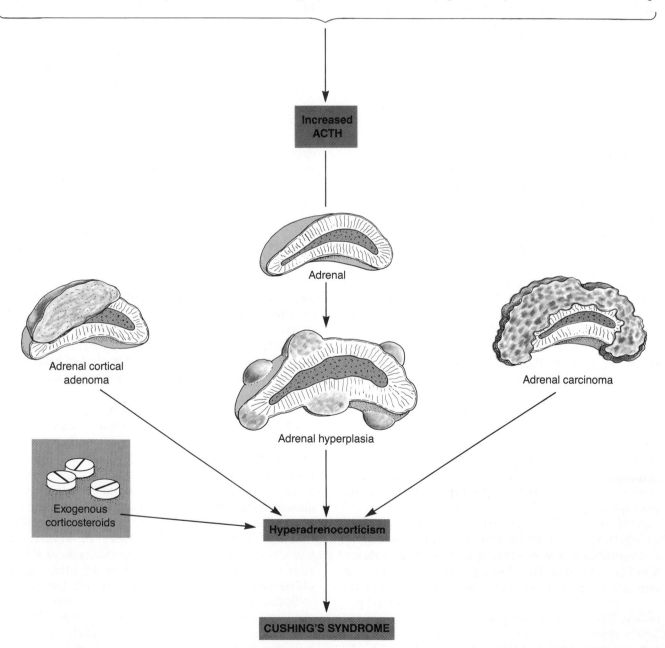

Increased ACTH

Adrenal

Adrenal cortical
adenoma

Adrenal carcinoma

Adrenal hyperplasia

Exogenous
corticosteroids

Hyperadrenocorticism

CUSHING'S SYNDROME

associated functional abnormalities. This nodularity also affects the thyroid gland, and is believed to be due to irregular responses of target organs to normal pituitary stimuli. True adrenocortical hyperplasia may be similarly nodular.

Neoplasms

Adrenocortical Adenomas

Adrenocortical adenoma is a frequent incidental finding at autopsy, most commonly in diabetics, older women, and the obese. The adenoma is a bright yellow, spheroidal mass of some 2 cm in diameter, compressing the adjacent uninvolved adrenal gland and sometimes possessing a partial fibrous capsule. Microscopically, the enlarged adenoma cells, which have a lipid-rich cytoplasm, are arranged in nodules and cords (Fig. 21-32). Since there is no overt endocrine disease, and the uninvolved and contralateral adrenal glands appear unaltered, the adenoma is considered nonfunctional.

Cushing's syndrome due to adrenal adenoma is clinically indistinguishable from that due to bilateral hyperplasia of the zona fasciculata. In children, adenoma is a more common cause than hyperplasia, and there is a rare type with nodular adrenocortical dysplasia. Pathologically, the nontumorous adrenal cortices are narrowed, and their cells are atrophic, because the adenoma overproduces cortisol type steroids, which in turn, inhibit pituitary ACTH secretion.

Few virilizing or feminizing adrenal adenomas are known, and these endocrine dysfunctional states more frequently result from adrenocortical carcinomas.

Aldosteronoma Aldosteronoma is functionally the most notable type of adrenocortical adenoma. It is usually small, 0.9 to 2.0 cm in size. The sectioned aldosteronoma is more orange than yellow, and histologically resembles other adrenocortical adenomas. Ultrastructurally, the mitochondria in some cases have plate-like, stacked cristae, typical of the normal zona glomerulosa. Others have tubulovesicular mitochondrial plicae of the zona fasciculata type, since in man this zone may also produce aldosterone.

Conn's syndrome, characterized by **hypertension, low plasma potassium, high sodium, alkalosis, and edema,** is relieved by the removal of an aldoste-

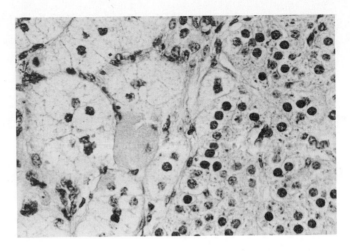

Figure 21-32. Adrenal cortical adenoma without clinical manifestations. Small, normal cortical cells are evident on the right, and notably larger adenoma cells can be seen on the left.

ronoma. Curiously, typical primary hyperaldosteronism in Conn's syndrome is closely imitated by pseudoprimary aldosteronism, a condition in which no adrenal adenoma is found, and for which subtotal adrenalectomy to relieve hypertension is not curative. Even the adrenocortical histologic alterations in pseudoprimary aldosteronism are disputed.

Other Benign Tumors

Various incidental benign neoplasms may involve the adrenal gland. Among them myelolipoma, a mixture of mature adipose tissue and hematopoietic marrow, is notable for its occasional large size. Hemangioma, neurofibroma, schwannoma, and leiomyoma occur here as in other soft tissues.

Adrenal Carcinoma

Adrenal carcinomas are usually first recognized as upper abdominal masses that are beyond clinical control. **At least half are clinically nonfunctional.** The diagnostic criteria of adrenocortical carcinoma include large tumor size, capsular and vascular tumor invasion, hemorrhage and necrosis within the mass, and occasional local or distant metastases. Microscopically, cytologic atypicality and abundant mitoses are common; other cases show only moderate cellular pleomorphism, but are similarly malignant (Fig. 21-33). The diagnosis of adrenocortical carcinomas is

Figure 21-31. The pathogenetic pathways of Cushing's syndrome.

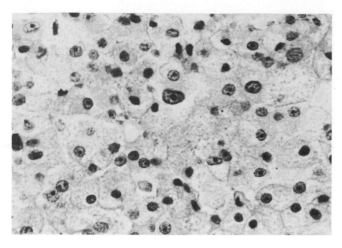

Figure 21-33. Adrenal cortical carcinoma in a virilized woman. Note the lack of distinct architecture, the irregularity of size and shape of the cells, and the occasional large and dark nuclei. Compare with Figure 21-32, which is at identical magnification.

often difficult by light microscopy. The tumors may be identified by electron microscopy, which reveals mitochondria typical of steroidogenic cells and abundant profiles of endoplasmic reticulum.

Slightly less than half the adrenal carcinomas have clinically evident endocrine effects. Cushing's syndrome, virilization, feminization, and hyperaldosteronism occur in decreasing order of frequency. If the tumor is extirpated, the syndrome resolves, unless the carcinoma recurs.

Metastatic Cancer

Metastatic cancer to the adrenal glands commonly originates from carcinomas of the lung or breast or from malignant melanoma. The glands may be unilaterally or bilaterally massively enlarged, up to 20 to 45 grams each, and largely replaced by carcinoma, with necrosis and hemorrhage. Usually, enough adrenocortical parenchyma and function remain so that Addison's disease does not develop, particularly in view of the limited survival of these patients.

The Adrenal Medulla and Paraganglia

Most abnormalities of clinical interest in the adrenal medulla are neoplasms: neuroblastoma in infants and pheochromocytoma in children and adults. It should be remembered that most medullary tissue is in the head of each adrenal gland, the parts closest to the spine. Sections from the more lateral adrenal body and tail may lack any medulla.

Vascular Lesions and Hyperplasias

Vascular lesions, particularly venous thrombosis or hemorrhage, may cause both medullary and cortical adrenal necrosis. As the innermost fetal adrenocortical zone involutes in the weeks after birth, excessive hemorrhage sometimes destroys both glands, and death from adrenocortical insufficiency may ensue. Acute or chronic adrenal medullary inflammation is practically unknown. Groups of plasma cells and lymphocytes around adrenal medullary veins represent a part of the perirenal chronic phlebitis that characteristically accompanies chronic pyelonephritis.

Adrenal medullary hyperplasia is rare and must be confirmed morphometrically, not simply established by gross and microscopic visual examination. Adrenal medullary hyperplasia is sometimes found in clinically unaffected family members of the multiple endocrine neoplasia (MEN) syndrome Type II, and may be a forerunner or contralateral manifestation of pheochromocytoma formation.

Neoplasms

Pheochromocytoma

Pheochromocytoma, also referred to as a type of chromaffin paraganglioma, is the most important neoplasm of the adrenal medulla in adults or older children. "Chromaffin" refers to the dark brown color that typically develops when fresh pheochromocytoma tissue is dipped in chromate solutions. The color test involves epinephrine (adrenalin), a major hormone product of such tumors. Norepinephrine (noradrenalin) does not provide a chromaffin reaction, and hence the test is considered to have a negative result if the tumor produces only norepinephrine. The normal adrenal medulla in childhood chiefly contains norepinephrine, while epinephrine predominates in adults. The majority of pheochromocytomas produce norepinephrine as well as epinephrine, although the former usually predominates.

Clinical presentations of pheochromocytoma are of four types:

1. episodic hypertension, with accompanying headache, psychic disturbances, or sweating;
2. persistent hypertension;
3. multiple endocrine neoplasia, Type IIa and Type IIb;
4. silent asymptomatic pheochromocytoma.

Multiple endocrine neoplasia (MEN) Type IIa, is a familial syndrome, with unilateral or bilateral adrenal

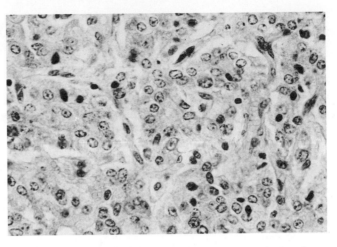

Figure 21-35. Adrenal pheochromocytoma with the classic syndrome of paroxysmal hypertension. The tumor cells are arranged in solid clusters, and mild pleomorphism is evident.

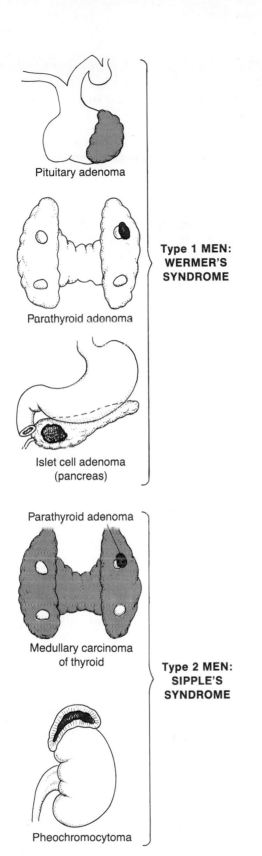

Pituitary adenoma

Parathyroid adenoma

Islet cell adenoma (pancreas)

Type 1 MEN: WERMER'S SYNDROME

Parathyroid adenoma

Medullary carcinoma of thyroid

Pheochromocytoma

Type 2 MEN: SIPPLE'S SYNDROME

Figure 21-34. The major forms of MEN (multiple endocrine neoplasia) syndromes.

tumors, thyroid medullary carcinoma, and parathyroid hyperplasia or adenoma (Fig. 21-34). In MEN Type IIb, there are mucosal neuromas, particularly affecting the lips and tongue, but the parathyroid adenoma or hyperplasia appears to be atypical or altogether absent.

A pheochromocytoma may be silent and then first manifest as extreme or lethal hypertension during an unrelated surgical procedure, such as a breast biopsy or hernia repair. A sudden massive infusion of epinephrine and norepinephrine is responsible, and the cause may be revealed only by a forensic autopsy.

Pheochromocytoma is diagnosed by finding increased urinary levels of catecholamine (epinephrine or norepinephrine) metabolites, particularly vanillylmandelic acid (VMA), metanephrine, and conjugated catecholamines. Plasma and platelet catecholamines likewise are elevated.

Most pheochromocytomas are encapsulated, spongy, reddish masses, with prominent central scars and enlarged vascular spaces. As noted, the tissue typically turns dark brown after exposure to potassium chromate and similar fixative solutions. The tumor cells are of widely variable size and shape, forming twisted cords or rounded clusters. They contain cytoplasmic basophilic granules, some rendered brown by the chromaffin reaction. The nuclei are large and irregular, an appearance similar to that of cancer (Fig. 21-35). However, **only a few pheochromocytomas are malignant,** as defined by the development of metastases. This is one of a small number of neoplasms in which **histologic atypicality is not an accurate indicator of biologic behavior.**

The cytoplasmic granules represent, for the most part, packaged catecholamines. Ultrastructurally, the norepinephrine granules are characteristic; they display a wide clear halo between the single delimiting membrane and the often eccentric osmiophilic core (Fig. 21-36). Granules containing epinephrine lack the halo and resemble other neuroendocrine (APUD) secretory granules. The granules are large, often measuring 300 nm or more in diameter. Smaller granules measuring 80 to 250 nm in diameter may also be found. The latter indicate that pheochromocytomas may also produce and store other peptide hormones, including calcitonin, bombesin, VIP, and ACTH, which occasionally are associated with clinical syndromes (Fig. 21-37).

If a pheochromocytoma should recur or metastasize after surgery, hypertension again develops. Removal of the metastasis alleviates the condition. The metastasis resembles the original pheochromocytoma, without any overtly malignant architectural or cytologic alterations.

Neuroblastoma

Neuroblastoma is a common neoplasm in children. Approximately two thirds of neuroblastomas are found in children under 5 years of age, but they may be encountered in older children, adolescents, and young adults. They may occasionally be congenital, and have been found even in premature stillborns. The overwhelming majority of neuroblastomas occur "sporadically." There have been a few reports of increased incidence of neuroblastomas developing in certain families. In the latter cases, neuroblastomas

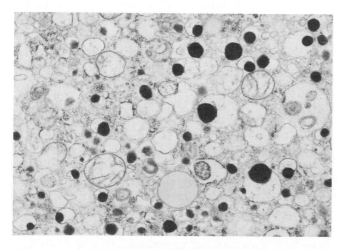

Figure 21-36.   Pheochromocytoma; same case as Figure 21-35. An electron micrograph depicts numerous, large neurosecretory granules with eccentric dense cores characteristic of norepinephrine.

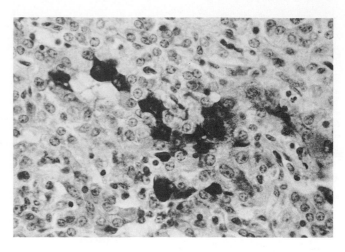

Figure 21-37.   Pheochromocytoma; same case as Figures 21-35 and 21-36. Immunostaining with anti-VIP antibody is responsible for the very dark cytoplasm seen in a few cells.

may be multiple and may arise in sites other than the adrenal medulla.

The adrenal medulla is the most frequent site of origin of neuroblastomas. However, they may develop anywhere in the retroperitoneal space, particularly in the upper portion. Neuroblastomas are not rare in the posterior mediastinum; they also arise within or around the brain, particularly in the posterior fossa, and the neck.

Depending on how early in their growth they are discovered, neuroblastomas may range from minute, barely discernible nodules to masses readily palpable through the abdominal wall. They are round, irregularly lobulated masses that may weigh 50 g to 150 g or more. They are soft and friable, and upon sectioning they may fall apart. In the case of small neuroblastomas, a yellow rim of compressed adrenal cortex may be noted. The cut surface ranges from gray to dark-red and hemorrhagic. Large tumors may show extensive central necrosis, scarring, and focal calcifications. The last are significant because they may be noted in abdominal radiographs, and constitute an important clinical diagnostic point.

The cells are small and are often compared with lymphocytes, although they are slightly larger. Characteristically, neuroblastoma cells range from round to fusiform; their nuclei are very dark and the cytoplasm is scanty. Mitoses are frequent. The neoplastic cells are arranged in ill-defined sheets which show areas of necrosis. The classic microscopic rosettes are defined by a rim of dark tumor cells in a circumferential arrangement around a central pale circle (Fig. 21-38). By electron microscopy, the rosettes consist of complex tangles of cytoplasmic processes, which show arrays of microtubules and small neurosecretory granules.

Neuroblastomas readily infiltrate the surrounding structures and metastasize to regional lymph nodes and hematogenously to the liver, lungs, bones, and other sites. Occasionally metastases may be found earlier than the primary tumor. Hutchison's neuroblastoma refers to extensive metastases to the skull, orbital bones, and soft tissues, resulting in exophthalmos. Occasional neuroblastomas may present with extensive and diffuse involvement of bones. In these cases the neoplastic cells replace the marrow and should be differentiated from Ewing's sarcoma and from lymphomas and leukemias.

Neuroblastomas secrete variable amounts of dopamine and catecholamines. **The overwhelming majority of patients with neuroblastoma excrete catecholamines and some of their metabolites in the urine.** Among the latter vanillylmandelic acid (VMA) and homovanillic acid are significant because their determination aids in the diagnosis and in monitoring the response to therapy. Occasionally neuroblastomas may secrete peptides. In addition, a neuroblastoma antigen, carcinoembryonic antigen (CEA), and poorly defined immune complexes have been described. It has been suggested that immune mechanisms may play a role in the rare, but well-documented, cases of total spontaneous regression of neuroblastomas.

Although neuroblastomas are malignant tumors, their clinical course, evolution, and response to therapy vary greatly. They tend to be clinically less aggressive in young infants. Also intriguing is their reported maturation to a more differentiated and clinically less aggressive, indeed benign, neoplasm, the ganglioneuroma. Maturation of neuroblastomas has been reported "spontaneously" and also following various forms of therapy. Mixed forms, for example, ganglioneuroblastomas, also occur.

In general, the presence of mature elements (i.e., ganglion cells) correlates with an improved prognosis. Nevertheless, the majority of neuroblastomas discovered over the age of 1 year already have demonstrable metastases at the time of the initial diagnosis. Combined forms of therapy, including surgery, radiotherapy, and chemotherapy, have dramatically improved the prognosis when metastatic disease (beyond regional lymph nodes) is not present.

Paragangliomas

Pheochromocytomas that develop in paraganglia other than the adrenal medulla are best designated as paragangliomas. The organs of Zuckerkandl comprise a retroperitoneal cluster of paraganglia, that usually involute during infancy, which are located along the abdominal aorta down to its bifurcation. This organ, the posterior mediastinum, and the urinary bladder may develop such tumors. Bladder paraganglioma may manifest with a peculiar syndrome of headaches and paroxysmal hypertension upon urination. Compared to pheochromocytomas, paragangliomas are more often malignant.

Paragangliomas may also arise in the base of the skull, in the neck, in vagal or aortic bodies, or in any organ that contains paraganglionic tissue, such as the larynx and small intestine. They arise in such paraganglia as the glomus jugulare, the carotid body, and other named and unnamed vasoreceptor bodies.

The carotid body tumor is a prototypic paraganglioma. Usually it forms a palpable mass in the neck, closely surrounding or enveloping the carotid vessels. When the tumor is removed, the tissue is soft and pale yellow. Larger tumors may be extensively hemorrhagic.

Microscopically, paragangliomas are indistinguishable from pheochromocytomas. The growth pattern is characteristically solid, and there are cell aggregates (Zellballen) in a richly vascular stroma. The individual cells are large, and show abundant, eosinophilic, and often granular cytoplasm. The nuclei range from vacuolated to dark and atypical. Moderate pleomorphism is frequent, but mitoses are rare. As with pheochromocytomas, **the presence of cytologic atypia in paragangliomas does not necessarily indicate malignancy.** Although most paragangliomas do not metastasize, they tend to recur or spread locally, and metastasize more frequently than adrenal pheo-

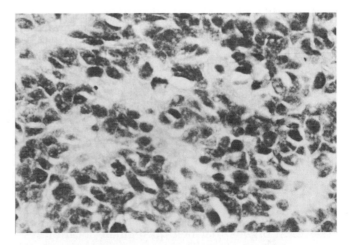

Figure 21-38. Neuroblastoma of the adrenal gland. Round to slightly spindle-shaped cells define irregular, round spaces with faintly fibrillar contents (rosettes).

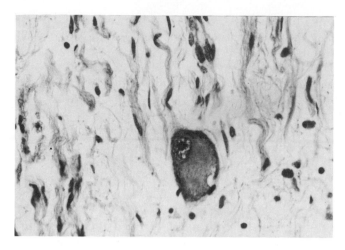

Figure 21-39. Ganglioneuroma of posterior mediastinum. A single, large, mature ganglion cell, small spindle cells, and abundant stroma are seen.

chromocytomas. Occasional paragangliomas may develop metastases 10 to 30 years after removal of the primary tumor.

Paragangliomas contain typical neurosecretory granules and small amounts of extractable catecholamines. In exceptional cases, paragangliomas secrete sufficient amounts of norepinephrine to produce hypertension. Many paragangliomas also contain ectopic peptide hormones, such as ACTH, VIP, calcitonin, somatostatin, and serotonin. Clinical manifestations associated with such materials are rare.

Ganglioneuromas

Ganglioneuromas appear grossly as well encapsulated tumors, with myxoid, glistening, cut surfaces. Microscopically, they show exquisitely differentiated, mature ganglion cells, associated with scanty spindle cells in a loose and abundant stroma (Fig. 21-39). The cytoplasmic processes of the ganglion cells contain neurosecretory granules. Typical neuroendocrine substances, such as neuron-specific enolase and certain peptide hormones, are readily demonstrated.

There are close embryogenetic, structural, and functional relationships among the group of neoplasms comprising neuroblastomas, ganglioneuromas, pheochromocytomas, and paragangliomas of all sites. All are regarded as neural crest neoplasms, with close anatomic relations to blood vessels. They arise from organs that help to regulate local or systemic vascular and chemical homeostasis. Also, these tumors may be regarded as a spectrum of neuroendocrine neoplasms that possess the capability of

producing neuropeptide hormones. This property explains, for instance, the occasional cases of ganglioneuroma producing vasoactive intestinal polypeptide, associated with watery diarrhea syndrome.

Thymus

Anatomy, Embryology, and Physiology

Embryologically, the thymus derives from the third pair of pharyngeal pouches. Inconstantly, the fourth pair of pharyngeal pouches also contribute to the formation of the thymus. Since the fourth pair also contribute to the formation of the lower parathyroids, parathyroid tissue may be found in the mediastinum near to or within the thymus; conversely, thymic tissue may also be found in the neck.

The thymus is irregularly pyramidal with its base located inferiorly and its two lobes fused in the midline. Its fibrous capsule extends into the parenchyma, forming septa which delimit lobules. The thymus is largest in relation to total body size and weight at birth, at which time it averages about 25 g. It continues to grow until puberty, and then may weigh 45 g. Each lobule has a peripheral, dark cortex that contains predominantly lymphoid cells, which normally lack follicular arrangement. The pale, central medulla includes the epithelial component. The epithelial cells, in addition to their main cytoplasmic masses, possess abundant cytoplasmic extensions that intertwine and form a complex network. Bundles of tonofilaments and desmosomes are prominent. Concentric aggregates of epithelial cells with focal keratinization are present in the medullary zone. These structures are termed Hassall's corpuscles.

The thymus is a complex organ which has a lymphoid and an epithelial component. It has been traditionally classified as an endocrine organ, although its precise role long remained obscure. More recently, the thymus has emerged as the key site for the differentiation of T lymphocytes. "Uncommitted" lymphocytes have their surface proteins rearranged or otherwise modified as a result of their interaction with the thymic epithelial cells. It appears that cell-to-cell contact and secretion of "thymic lymphopoietic factors" are required for lymphocyte processing. Various polypeptides of thymic origin have been described—thymosin, thymopoietin, thymin. Whether these materials are truly distinct, or constitute variants of a single indispensable factor, is not yet clear. Regardless, it now appears evident that thymic secretory products are indispensable for the development and maintenance of an immunologically competent T lymphocyte system. To a lesser extent the thymus also has a role in immunosurveillance and immunologic tolerance.

Since the lymphopoietic substances are secreted into the blood and act as true hormones by fulfilling their function at a distance from the site of their production, the thymus is an endocrine organ in the traditional sense. Moreover, the thymus also has a small population of neuroendocrine cells, the physiologic role of which remains undetermined, although they help to explain the occurrence of neuroendocrine tumors in this organ. The thymus also exhibits a complement of myoid cells, which have many structural and functional features similar to those of striated muscle cells, but are nevertheless regarded as epithelial cells. Myoid cells may play a significant role in the autoimmune pathogenesis of myasthenia gravis.

Agenesis and Hypoplasia

Pathologic alterations of the thymus are not frequent, but they range from totally asymptomatic tumors to lesions that have profound local and systemic consequences. Agenesis or congenital hypoplasia of the thymus may be found in the newborn or in young infants, and is associated with combined immunodeficiency disorders, telangiectatic ataxia, reticular dysgenesis, and Nezelof's or DiGeorge's syndrome. In DiGeorge's syndrome, the thymus disorder is accompanied by parathyroid agenesis. In all these instances the thymus may be "represented" by scattered groups of lymphocytes in fibrous tissue.

With advancing age, the thymus normally atrophies and is progressively replaced by fibroadipose tissue, although its components may still be identified microscopically. Thymic atrophy in young people is caused by ionizing radiation, severe malnutrition, or prolonged administration of glucorticoid or cytotoxic therapy.

Hyperplasia

A diagnosis of thymic hyperplasia cannot be made exclusively on the basis of increased weight of the gland, given the wide range of normal weights in all age groups. Thus, **the most reliable criterion of thymic hyperplasia is the presence of lymphoid follicular structures** (Fig. 21-40).

Thymic follicular hyperplasia may be found in association with a spectrum of chronic inflammatory and immunologic disorders, as well as with myas-

thenia gravis. The follicles tend to occupy and distort the medullary zones. Interestingly, the total weight of the gland may be within the normal range, although it is usually increased. It has been speculated that in some instances of myasthenia gravis the activated B lymphocytes of the hyperplastic follicles may play a role in the development of antibodies to the acetylcholine receptors of the neuromuscular junctions. Thymic follicular hyperplasia may also be found in numerous other diseases in which autoimmunity plays a role, such as Graves' disease, some instances of Addison's disease and numerous "connective tissue diseases", including systemic lupus erythematosus, scleroderma, and rheumatoid arthritis. Rarely, thymic follicular hyperplasia is found incidentally at autopsy in patients who had no clinical manifestation.

Tumors

The term **thymoma** is currently applied to tumors of the thymus in which the thymic epithelial cells are regarded as neoplastic. Whether scarce or prominent, the lymphocytic elements are not considered neoplastic. Thymomas, while uncommon, are significant neoplasms of the anterior mediastinum, together with dysgerminomas, true teratomas, and ectopic thyroid tumors. Notably, some are associated with other diseases, including myasthenia gravis, various types of hematocytopenias, other tumors, and a variety of immune disorders.

The vast majority of thymomas (80% to 95%) are clinically benign. Benign thymomas are irregularly

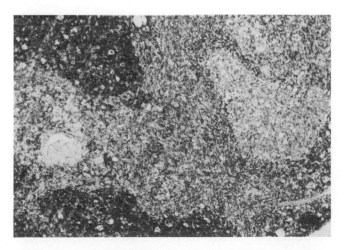

Figure 21-40. Hyperplasia of the thymus. The dark areas are closely packed lymphocytes. A lymphoid follicular structure is evident on the right. A pale, small Hassall's corpuscle is noted on the left.

shaped masses which range from a few centimeters to 15 cm or more in major diameter. They are encapsulated, firm, and gray to yellow. Fibrous tissue septa divide the tumors into lobules. Large tumors show foci of hemorrhage and necrosis, and cysts are frequent. The epithelial cells of thymomas may be obvious or may be obscured by the dominating non-neoplastic lymphocytes. In such cases, ultrastructural or immunohistochemical studies for cytokeratin or other epithelial markers will uncover the epithelial cells (Fig. 21-41). The epithelial cells are round or fusiform (spindle cell thymoma). The epithelial variant (round cells) tends to be associated with myasthenia gravis, whereas the spindle cell type is commonly seen with hypogammaglobulinemia or erythroid aplasia. The most characteristic microscopic pattern is one of irregular sheets of epithelial cells. Squamous features are frequent, while glands, basaloid clear cells, and other patterns are uncommon.

The neoplastic, i.e., epithelial, thymomas are invariably accompanied by a complement of T lymphocytes, which are larger than usual and have prominent vesicular nuclei, features suggestive of activation. Mitotic activity of the non-neoplastic lymphocytic component of thymomas generally exceeds that of the neoplastic epithelial cells. The dominant lymphoid component of occasional thymomas may result in an erroneous diagnosis of lymphoma.

Malignant thymomas are carcinomas of the thymus, which occur principally in middle age, without sex or ethnic predilection. They are diagnosed by marked cellular and nuclear atypism and a brisk mitotic activity of the neoplastic epithelial cells. More often than not, however, the diagnosis of malignant thymomas is based on macroscopic criteria, particularly invasion of the surrounding structures including the lung, pericardium, and large vessels. The demonstration of microscopic penetration of the capsule, and lymphatic and vascular invasion, is important.

Surprisingly, many thymomas are incidentally found as the result of chest radiographs obtained for unrelated reasons. A number of thymomas are found as a result of studies initiated because of systemic diseases, with which they may be associated, while the rest are encountered because of the local disorders associated with the physical presence of the tumors, such as cough, dyspnea, dysphagia, and vascular compression.

Neuroendocrine tumors of the thymus may be carcinoids (benign) or carcinomas (malignant). Since these tumors are composed of epithelial cells they may be viewed as thymomas, and their malignant variants as thymic carcinomas. Thymic carcinoids are morphologically similar to those occurring in the bronchi and other sites, showing well-defined cellular cords, nests, and ribbons separated by delicate fibrovascular septa. Neurosecretory granules are common and neuropeptide hormones and other related markers are demonstrable (Fig. 21-42). Neuroendocrine carcinomas of the thymus are composed of intermediate size or small oat cells; cellular atypicality is prominent and mitotic activity brisk. A significant proportion of these neuroendocrine neoplasms is associated with hormonal syndromes, particularly Cushing's syndrome.

Miscellaneous tumors in the thymus or anterior mediastinum include seminomas or dysgerminomas, choriocarcinomas, and teratomas. The evolution of these neoplasms is similar to that of their counterparts in more frequent sites, but may be aggravated by their intimate association with surrounding vital structures. Similarly, primary thymic lymphomas occur, as does Hodgkin's disease, which is often of the nodular sclerosing type.

Tumors consisting of admixtures of thymic and adipose tissues have been termed thymolipomas. Non-neoplastic tumors include thymic and mesothelial cysts, and enteric-type cysts.

Pineal Gland

Anatomy, Embryology, and Physiology

The pineal gland, or epiphysis cerebri, is but 5 to 7 mm in maximal diameter and weighs barely 100 to 180 mg. Shaped like a minute pine cone, it is located below the posterior edge of the corpus callosum and

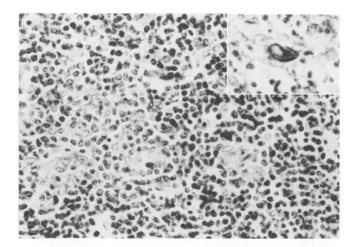

Figure 21-41. Thymoma. The picture is dominated by small, dark-staining lymphocytes. However, larger and paler epithelial cells represent the neoplasm. The inset *(upper right)* shows one of these epithelial cells immunostained with antibody against keratin.

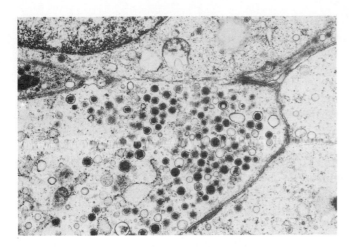

Figure 21-42. Neuroendocrine carcinoma of the thymus with production of ACTH and associated Cushing's syndrome. An electron micrograph shows several adjacent cytoplasmic processes, one of which contains numerous neurosecretory granules. (Compare these small granules with those in Fig. 21-36 at identical magnification).

between the superior colliculi. It develops as an outpouch of the posterior segment of the roof of the third ventricle, to which it remains linked by a stalk. The stalk is not a vestigial structure; it is rich in nerve fibers and seemingly arises from the brain. The significance of these fibers is unclear, and their connection with pineal cells remains controversial. Most of the pineal is wrapped in pia mater, from which connective tissue septa originate; the septa penetrate the gland and divide it into lobules.

Microscopically, most of the pineal gland is composed of cords and clusters of cells termed pinealocytes. As in paraganglia, interlacing cytoplasmic processes and neurosecretory granules are seen. A second cell type is similar to brain astrocytes. It is not clear whether these cells are simply glial or whether they represent an anatomically and functionally distinct cell class.

The pineal gland produces a number of neurotransmitter substances, among which the most abundant and readily demonstrable is **melatonin.** Although in lower animals melatonin has a significant depigmenting effect, such an action has not been shown in mammals. However, in higher mammals and humans melatonin induces sleep and increases brain serotonin. Melatonin is found in the blood, cerebrospinal fluid, and urine. Since the levels are distinctly higher at night, it has been suggested that melatonin may function as a sleep inducer.

Serotonin and several peptides are also produced by the pineal. Significant among the peptides is arginine vasotocin, a hormone which has been shown to have important antigonadotropic activity in ani-

mals. Melatonin may act as a releasing factor for arginine vasotocin.

About the time of puberty, calcifications in the pineal gland can be shown in autopsy specimens or by various radiologic techniques. Focal cystic changes may also be seen, but these alterations do not seem to have clinical manifestations.

Neoplasms

Tumors of the pineal gland are rare, and represent less than 1% of brain tumors. The most frequent neoplasms are apparently not derived from pineal parenchymal cells or their precursors, but from germ cells. Germinomas, or dysgerminomas, account for about 60% of pineal tumors. They are morphologically indistinguishable from, and thought to be equivalent to, testicular seminomas, ovarian dysgerminomas, and their counterparts in other sites. As in those tumors, the germinoma is comprised of large round cells, with pale cytoplasm and vesicular nuclei, organized in cords and clusters. Fibrovascular septa often contain infiltrates of mature lymphocytes (Fig. 21-43).

Other variants of germ cell neoplasms in the pineal gland are embryonal carcinomas, choriocarcinomas, and teratomas, tumors which are similar to their counterparts in other sites.

Pinealomas presumably arise from the pinealocyte. These rare tumors are of two types, pineoblastomas and pineocytomas. **Pineoblastomas** occur in the young. Soft masses, often showing hemorrhagic and necrotic areas, invade and infiltrate the surrounding structures. Microscopically, they consist of

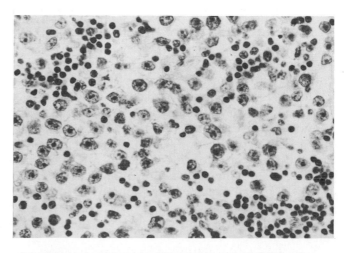

Figure 21-43. Dysgerminoma of the pineal gland. The large neoplastic cells, with poorly defined cytoplasm and nuclei that show prominent nucleoli, contrast with the smaller non-neoplastic lymphocytes.

small oval cells, with dark nuclei and scanty cytoplasm. Mitoses are generally numerous. Many features of these tumors are highly reminiscent of primitive medulloblastomas and neuroblastomas, but identifiable rosettes are rare. These tumors are very aggressive.

Pineocytomas represent the better differentiated counterpart of the pineoblastomas. They are most frequent in an older age group, and tend to be clinically less aggressive than pineoblastomas. Pineocytomas are well delineated; they impinge upon surrounding tissues but do not invade them. Pineocytomas often show a dual neuronal and glial differentiation, somewhat reminiscent of primitive neural neoplasms in other sites. Some pineocytomas may be indistinguishable from well-differentiated astrocytomas, whereas others are more distinctly neuroblastic and display prominent rosettes.

Regardless of histologic type, tumors of the pineal gland present with signs and symptoms related to their impact on the surrounding structures, including headaches and visual and behavioral anomalies. Destruction of the pineal, neoplastic or otherwise, in children is frequently associated with precocious puberty, the pathogenesis of which is thought to be based on the decreased or absent gonadotropic suppression normally exerted by melatonin. This syndrome occurs predominantly in boys. The prognosis of pineal tumors is poor in the case of the poorly differentiated types, but is also guarded in pineal tumors with a high degree of differentiation. Even non-neoplastic pineal cysts, because of the difficulties involved in their removal, pose a great threat to life.

Ectopic Hormones

Traditional and Current Concepts

The concept of "ectopic hormones" arose as it became evident that occasional neoplasms developing in "nonendocrine" organs are associated with significant endocrine syndromes. The notion of ectopic hormones is particularly pertinent in relation to the dispersed neuroendocrine system, since the materials that are presumed to be ectopically produced are generally neuroamines or neuropeptides. We should also remember that peptide hormones comprise groups that are closely related biochemically, and may indeed derive from common precursor molecules.

According to the traditional concept, a carcinoma of the lung which produced ACTH, and was associated with Cushing's syndrome, was regarded as a typical example of ectopic hormone production, because the tumor developed in an organ presumed to be nonendocrine. A somewhat different example was that of a carcinoma of the islet cells of the pancreas which produced gastrin, and was associated with recurrent peptic ulcers, i.e., Zollinger-Ellison syndrome. In this instance, the tumor arose in an organ known to have an endocrine cell component. However, it produced a peptide that was presumably not normal at that particular site, and gastrin production in that sense was viewed as ectopic, although the endocrine cells were indigenous to the site.

The development of the concept of a dispersed neuroendocrine system has seriously challenged older notions. It is becoming increasingly apparent that cells with the capability of producing endocrine products are far more widespread than previously assumed. Until very recently, the lung could hardly be regarded as an endocrine organ. But we now know that the bronchi include a significant population of solitary neuroendocrine cells and aggregates, termed neuroepithelial bodies. Although the amounts of hormones produced and their precise physiologic significance are not entirely clear, cells that produce serotonin, bombesin, calcitonin, and leucine enkephalin are found in normal bronchial epithelium. Therefore, the demonstration of elevated levels of calcitonin in association with a neuroendocrine carcinoma of the lung should no longer be regarded as an "ectopic" marker, since neither the presence of endocrine cells nor their production of calcitonin can be said to be foreign to the lung. On the other hand, we may still regard ACTH production by a small cell neuroendocrine lung carcinoma as ectopic. Whereas the lung may be rightly viewed as an endocrine organ, ACTH production is currently not regarded as indigenous to the normal lung. The same may be said when islet cell neoplasms produce hormonal material such as gastrin or vasoactive intestinal peptide (VIP).

Overproduction of the aforementioned hormonal materials—ectopic or eutopic—is not necessarily associated with malignant neoplasms. Examples to the contrary are provided by benign carcinoids and similarly benign ganglioneuromas that may be associated with overproduction of various hormones and significant endocrine syndromes. A further interesting observation is that endocrine populations that undergo severe hyperplasia may also overproduce hormones, as indicated by the occasional case of Zollinger-Ellison syndrome that is caused by diffuse hyperplasia of gastrin-producing cells in the stomach mucosa.

It is now generally accepted that many neuroendocrine cells are capable of synchronous production of more than one hormone. This physiologic capability is retained by benign and malignant neoplasms, and is occasionally shown by tumors associated with more than one hormonal activity, e.g., overproduction of gastrin and ACTH. Sometimes, we may also observe that a neuroendocrine neoplasm which was not associated with an endocrine syndrome upon first diagnosis may develop one later. Switching from one hormonal syndrome to another has also been observed.

Clinical Implications and Outlook

Until recently, many malignant tumors that did not reveal obvious differentiation by conventional light microscopy were regarded as "undifferentiated." However, the application of modern methods, such as electron microscopy and immunohistochemistry, has demonstrated that many of these tumors indeed have endocrine characteristics. Nevertheless, the majority of these endocrine tumors produce seemingly imperfect or immature molecules, or fragments with limited or no biological activity. They may, in fact, produce mature hormonal products, but only in small amounts. As a result, despite their endocrine character, the majority of these tumors are not demonstrably associated with overt hormonal syndromes.

We may, therefore, rightly question the clinical significance of many of these observations. Simply stated, these findings are important because the hormonal or related substances produced by many of these neoplasms are readily demonstrable in the tumors themselves, in the serum, or in the urine, and thus constitute valuable markers for the diagnosis and clinical monitoring of these tumors. Examples are the demonstration of catecholamine metabolites in the urine of patients with neuroblastomas, and the finding of calcitonin, bombesin, or neuron-specific enolase in patients with neuroendocrine carcinomas of the lung, despite the fact that the majority of these tumors are silent from the hormonal standpoint.

We may reasonably expect that the diagnostic and even the therapeutic significance of these markers will increase as our understanding of them improves. Newer markers and better methods for their demonstration may emerge in the future.

SUGGESTED READING

HYPOPHYSIS AND HYPOTHALAMUS

Ezrin C, Kovacs K, Horvath E: Pathology of the Adenohypophysis. In Bloodworth JMB (ed): Endocrine Pathology, 2nd ed, pp 101–132. Baltimore, Williams and Wilkins, 1982

Scheithauer BW: Pathology of the Pituitary and Sellar Region. Pathol Annu 20 (II): 67–155, 1985

Sheehan HL, Kovacs K: Neurohypophysis and Hypothalamus. In Bloodworth JMB (ed): Endocrine Pathology, 2nd ed, pp 455–499. Baltimore, Williams and Wilkins, 1982

THE THYROID GLAND

Rose NE: The Thyroid as Source and Target of Autoimmunity. Lab Invest 52: 117–119, 1985

Sommers SC: The Thyroid Gland. In Bloodworth JMB (ed): Endocrine Pathology, 2nd ed, pp 155–203. Baltimore, Williams and Wilkins, 1982

Strakosch CR, Wenzel BE, Row VV, Volpe R: Immunology of Autoimmune Thyroid Diseases. N Engl J Med 307: 1499–1507, 1982

THE PARATHYROID GLANDS

Golden A, Kerwin DM: The Parathyroid Glands. In Bloodworth JMB (ed): Endocrine Pathology, 2nd ed, pp 205–220. Baltimore, Williams and Wilkins, 1982

Grimelius L, Åkerstrlüm G, Johansson H, Bergström R: Anatomy and Histopathology of Human Parathyroids. Pathol Annu 16 (II): 1–24, 1981

THE ADRENAL CORTEX

Symington T: The Adrenal Cortex. In Bloodworth JMB (ed): Endocrine Pathology, 2nd ed, pp 419–471. Baltimore, Williams and Wilkins, 1982

Van Couter E, Refetoff S: Evidence of Two Subtypes of Cushing's Disease Based on the Analysis of Secretion. N Engl J Med 312: 1343–1349, 1985

ADRENAL MEDULLA AND PARAGANGLIA

Gould VE, Sommers SC: Adrenal Medulla and Paraganglia. In Bloodworth JMB (ed): Endocrine Pathology, 2nd ed, pp 473–511. Baltimore, Williams and Wilkins, 1982

THE THYMUS

Arya S, Gilbert EF, Hong R, Bloodworth JMB: The Thymus. In Bloodworth JMB (ed): Endocrine Pathology, 2nd ed, pp 767–832. Baltimore, Williams and Wilkins, 1982

Rosai J: Tumors and Tumor-like Conditions of the Thymus. In Ackerman's Surgical Pathology, 6th ed, pp 304–316. St Louis, C V Mosby, 1981

THE PINEAL GLAND

Moskowitz MA, Wurtman RJ: New Approaches to the Study of the Human Pineal Organ. In Bloodworth JMB (ed): Endocrine Pathology, 2nd ed, pp 133–154. Baltimore, Williams and Wilkins, 1982

22 Diabetes

John E. Craighead

Type I Diabetes Mellitus

Type II Diabetes Mellitus

Complications of Diabetes

Figure 22-1. Capillary lesion in Type II diabetes mellitus. An electron micrograph of a capillary in the muscle of a 56-year-old woman shows a thickened basement membrane, a characteristic late lesion in this disease.

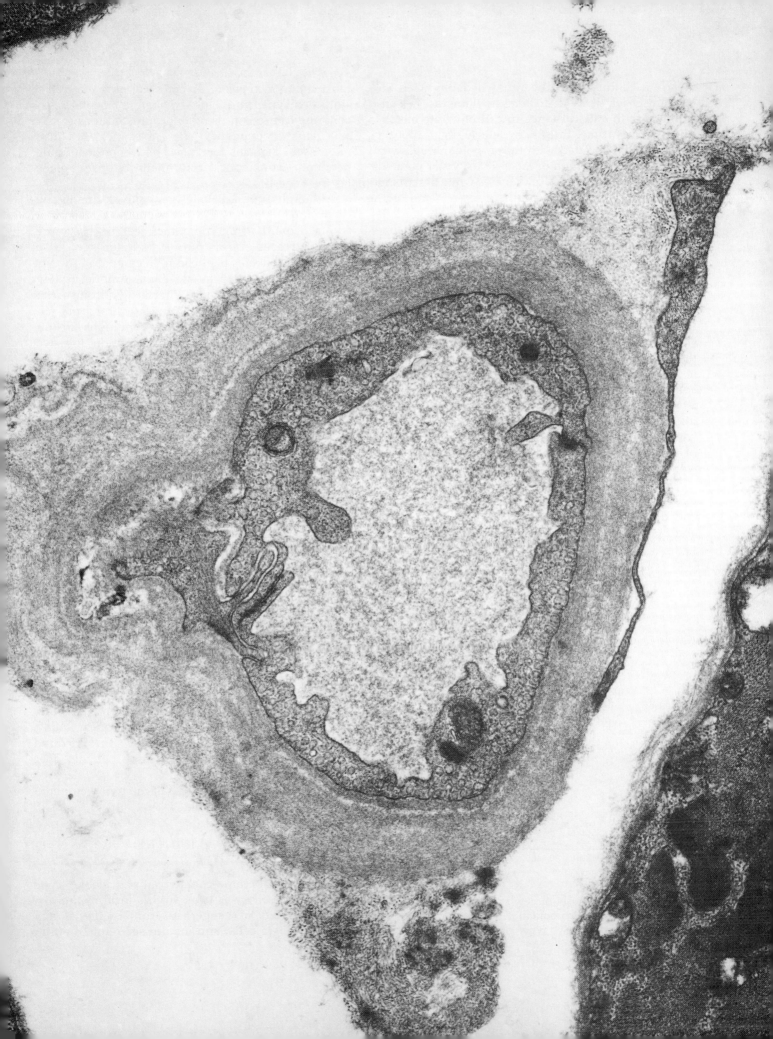

Nearly a century ago, the renowned physician Sir William Osler defined diabetes mellitus as "a **syndrome due to a disturbance in carbohydrate metabolism from various causes**, in which sugar appears in the urine associated with thirst, polyuria, wasting and imperfect oxidation of fats." Thus, Osler pointed out the diverse etiologies of diabetes while describing the salient clinical features of the disease. Years later, a noted specialist defined the disease as "a **genetically determined** disorder of carbohydrate metabolism . . . with **specific microvascular complications** and **accelerated atherogenesis**." In this definition, the heritable predisposition to diabetes and the secondary effects of the disease were stressed. Finally, in the 1970s, a governmental commission concluded that diabetes is "a **complex metabolic derangement**, characterized by either **relative** or **absolute insulin deficiency**."

Despite our increase in understanding since Osler's time, it remains difficult to define diabetes satisfactorily. A recent survey of physicians specializing in diabetes revealed that the experts employed widely divergent diagnostic criteria. More than half of the patients considered to be abnormal by some were classified as normal by others.

The terms used by physicians to refer to the different types of diabetes are confusing. Various names and descriptors were in vogue for periods of time and then discarded. Yet the legacies persist. The two most common types of diabetes are now referred to simply as Type I and Type II diabetes. Yet, physicians continue to use confusing and outdated terms, such as "insulin-dependent," "ketosis-prone," or "juvenile onset" diabetes for Type I and "non-insulin dependent, "nonketotic," and "maturity-onset" diabetes for Type II.

Although Type I diabetes generally occurs in children and teenagers, it occasionally develops in adults. Type II also is sometimes seen in the young, but most cases appear during the later decades of life. Type I diabetes is uncommon compared to Type II; the latter affects 5 to 10 million Americans (Fig. 22-2). There are also rare clinical syndromes that cause either frank hyperglycemia or abnormal glucose metabolism. Because these conditions are uncommon and have a genetic predisposition, they will not be considered in detail here, but information can be found in the classification of the National Diabetes Data Group (see Suggested Reading).

The currently accepted criteria for the diagnosis of diabetes define pragmatically a disease that exhibits enormous variability in its biochemical and clinical features. If a patient has typical symptoms and markedly elevated concentrations of blood glucose, the diagnosis is obvious. But when symptoms are vague and the **fasting** blood glucose is normal or only slightly elevated, the question is more difficult to resolve. Under these circumstances, physicians often "challenge" the patient's metabolism by giving a large amount of glucose by mouth or by vein—the so-called **glucose tolerance test**. If blood glucose concentrations increase excessively and remain elevated for an inordinate time, the findings are consistent with diabetes.

Some patients have impaired glucose metabolism but are not frankly diabetic. A few of these individuals develop classic diabetes later in life. In the past, such patients were considered to have "chemical," "latent," "borderline," "subclinical," or "asymptomatic" diabetes. These terms rarely appear today, and their use is discouraged because the impaired glucose metabolism in most of these patients does not progress to diabetes.

We will now consider in detail the two major clinical types of diabetes (Table 22-1).

Type I Diabetes Mellitus

Before insulin became commercially available, Type I diabetes usually was fatal. **In this form of the disease, the islets of Langerhans contain few if any functional beta cells, and insulin secretion is either**

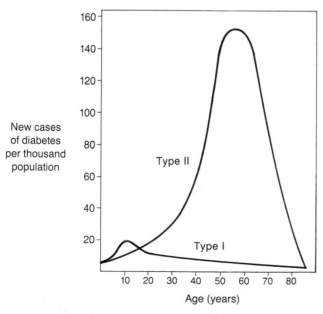

Figure 22-2. Age of onset of new cases of Types I and II diabetes in a large clinic population. Note the relative number of cases of the two types of diabetes.

Table 22-1. Comparison of Type I and Type II Diabetes

	TYPE I	TYPE II
Age at onset	usually before 20	usually after 30
Type of onset	abrupt; often severe	gradual; usually subtle
Usual body weight	normal	overweight
Genetics—parents or siblings with diabetes	<20%	~60%
Monozygotic twins	50% concordant	90% concordant
HLA associations	yes	no
Islet cell antibodies	yes	no
Islet lesions		
EARLY	inflammation	—
LATE	atrophy and fibrosis	fibrosis, amyloid
Beta cells	markedly reduced	normal or slightly reduced
Blood insulin	markedly reduced	elevated or normal
Clinical management	insulin and diet	diet; occasionally drugs or insulin

substantially reduced or nonexistent. As a result, body fat is metabolized as a source of energy, and ketone bodies (acetoacetic acid and β-hydroxybutyric acid) are released into the blood. Systemic metabolic acidosis develops as a result. Hyperglycemia and glucosuria produce fluid and electrolyte imbalances that can ultimately lead to coma and death (Fig. 22-3). Diabetes is often first identified when the patient is hospitalized because of metabolic acidosis, dehydration, and electrolyte imbalance. These events may occur unexpectedly and precipitously, and are life-threatening emergencies. More often, however, patients with Type I diabetes experience vague symptoms for weeks or months before diagnosis. Prominent among these are an increase in urine output (polyuria) caused by glucosuria and the resulting thirst (polydipsia). Many patients have an insatiable appetite (polyphagia), but nonetheless lose weight because of defective carbohydrate metabolism and wasted calories. Often the appearance of diabetes coincides with the metabolic stresses of an acute illness, such as an infection.

Type I diabetes usually develops during childhood, the peak incidence being at puberty. For this reason, until a few years ago, Type I diabetes was familiarly known as juvenile diabetes. However, we now know that some cases develop during the first years of life, and a few after maturation. Fewer than 20% of Type I diabetics have a parent or sibling with the disease. Many investigators argue that inherit-

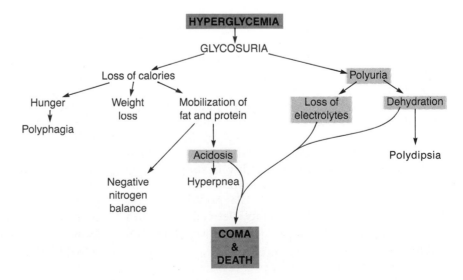

Figure 22-3. Symptoms and signs of acute diabetes mellitus.

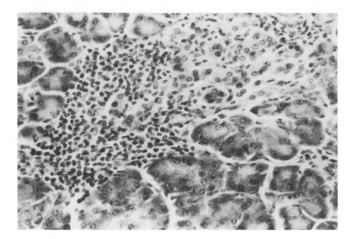

Figure 22-4. Type I diabetes. Mononuclear inflammatory cell infiltrate in and around an islet of Langerhans. Such inflammation is found in the pancreas of many Type I diabetics at the time of diagnosis.

ance of this form of diabetes is autosomal recessive with variable penetrance, but this claim is not universally accepted. Insight into the genetics of this disorder has grown out of studies of identical (monozygotic) twin pairs in which one or both twins were diabetic. Interestingly, both twins were affected in only about half of the families. This observation suggests that **environmental factors contribute to the causation of the disease, possibly superimposed on a heritable predisposition.**

Additional genetic evidence comes from studies of the antigens of the major histocompatibility complex. Certain Class I (A, B, and C loci) and Class II (DR locus) antigens are unusually common in patients with Type I diabetes; many patients possess DR-3 and DR-4 Class II antigens. It now appears that the gene or genes influencing the development of diabetes are located close to the DR locus. Because coding for immunologic responsivity is also situated near the DR locus on the sixth chromosome, a role for immune mechanisms in the causation of Type I diabetes has been postulated.

The concept of an **autoimmune pathogenesis** is appealing, because Type I diabetics who die shortly after the onset of disease display an infiltrate of mononuclear cells in and around the islets of Langerhans (Fig. 22-4). This possibility is supported by the observation that serum antibodies to islet cells are present in almost all newly diagnosed diabetics. Many of these patients develop islet cell antibodies months or years before the appearance of clinical symptoms.

Although serum antibodies might play a role in the causation of diabetes, other immune mechanisms could be involved. Considerable evidence now points to cellular immunity, perhaps resulting from the action of cytolytic T cells on the beta cells. The finding that pancreatic islets transplanted from a healthy to a diabetic monozygotic twin have been met by transplant rejection strengthens theories of immune pathogenesis of Type I diabetes. Some diabetic patients have now been successfully treated with cyclosporin, a drug that alters cellular immunity. This finding offers hope that Type I diabetes can be aborted at the outset by immunosuppressive treatment.

What triggers the immunologic injury to the islets of Langerhans? Are diabetics genetically programmed to develop an aberrant immunologic response, or do insults to the islets from environmental agents initiate the autoimmune process? Recently, viruses and chemicals have been implicated as causative factors in at least some cases of Type I diabetes. For example, the disease develops occasionally after mumps, and group B Coxsackie viruses have been shown to infect the islets and cause acute-onset diabetes. Children and young adults who were infected *in utero* with rubella virus also occasionally develop diabetes, presumably as a result of viral injury of the pancreas. The role of chemicals in the initiation of Type I diabetes is more problematic. Some nitrosamines, such as streptozotocin, exhibit specific affinity for beta cells and cause diabetes in experimental animals. Recently, inadvertent consumption of a rodenticide, Vacor, was found to cause diabetes in man, even though the agent had no effect on islet function in animals. Although environmental factors are important, and probably play a causative role in some patients, the etiology in most cases of Type I diabetes is still obscure.

Type II Diabetes Mellitus

Type II diabetes usually develops in the adult, and its prevalence increases with advancing age. Indeed, almost 10% of persons over 65 years of age are affected. Four out of every five patients with Type II diabetes are overweight (Fig. 22-5).

The pathogenesis of Types I and II diabetes differ in most respects. **Genetic influences are a key factor in the occurrence of Type II diabetes;** about 60% of patients have either a parent or a sibling with this type of diabetes. When one member of a monozygotic twin pair has the disease, almost invariably the second twin is also affected. However, an association

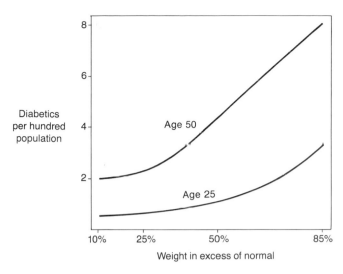

Figure 22-5. Occurrence of diabetes in relation to body weight in young and older adults of both sexes.

with genes of the major histocompatability complex similar to that occurring in Type I diabetes is not found. Despite the high familial prevalence of the disease, the mode of inheritance remains to be defined, probably because this form of diabetes has several etiologies masquerading as a single clinical syndrome. In addition, **constitutional factors, such as obesity and exercise, influence the expression of the condition** and thus confuse genetic analyses.

Two pathogenetic factors appear to be critical to the development of Type II diabetes. First, in many but not all hyperglycemic patients **insulin release by the beta cells is impaired.** Second, **tissue sensitivity to insulin is reduced in major organs**, with the exception of the brain. There also appear to be changes in the function of intracellular mediators of insulin action. Thus, uptake and metabolism of glucose are altered. A variety of microscopic lesions are found in the islets of Langerhans of many, but not all, patients with Type II diabetes. These changes occasionally are found in the general population and are not diagnostic. In the islets of some patients, fibrous tissue accumulates, sometimes with sufficient prominence to obliterate the islets. In other patients, one sees a hyaline material that has many of the properties of amyloid (Fig. 22-6). This material is composed of polypeptide chains of the insulin molecule, a finding that suggests that secretion of insulin by beta cells is defective.

In view of these observations, can we conclude that production of insulin by beta cells in the islets of Langerhans is reduced? Probably not, according to the incomplete evidence currently available. **Type II diabetics have either normal or only slightly reduced amounts of insulin in the pancreas.** Moreover, the islet lesions appear to develop late in the course of the disease and generally are found in older patients.

Metabolic studies provide further insight into the pathogenesis of Type II diabetes. **Deficient insulin release occurs during the early response of the beta cell to glucose stimulation, a defect most prominent in those with severe hyperglycemia.** Although recognition of glucose by the beta cell is impaired, the blood insulin concentration of many Type II diabetics is actually increased. This paradoxical finding is now attributed to a reduction in the number of functional insulin receptors in the plasma membranes of cells that utilize insulin. Thus, **patients with Type II diabetes are hyperglycemic, but their cells are relatively deficient in insulin receptors, and so they metabolize glucose inefficiently despite normal or elevated levels of insulin in the blood** (Fig. 22-7).

The insulin receptor comprises two linked glycoprotein subunits, a beta component that attracts and binds insulin and an alpha component that serves as a transmembrane protein kinase. However, information on the functional properties of these receptors in diabetes is limited. For example, the number of receptors on cells remains low when blood insulin concentrations are high, even though receptors turn over rapidly. Since receptor activity improves when blood insulin concentrations return to normal, insulin

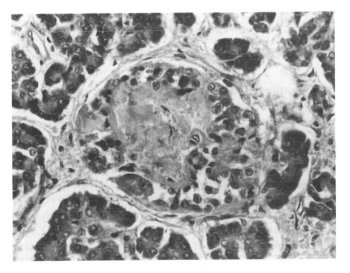

Figure 22-6. Type II diabetes. Hyalinization and fibrosis of a pancreatic islet in an elderly patient are prominent.

Amyloid, a generic term that refers to a group of diverse extracellular protein deposits, is associated with many different diseases. Amyloid deposits have common morphologic properties, stain with specific dyes, and have a characteristic appearance under polarized light. Though varying in amino acid sequence, all amyloid proteins are folded in such a way as to share common ultrastructural and physical properties.

Although disorders associated with amyloid deposition have been known for more than 300 years, it was not until Virchow's time in the mid-19th century that attempts were made to define the nature of the tissue deposits by their staining properties.

Amyloid stained blue with iodine, which was then in use for demonstrating cellulose or starch. The positive reaction not only led to the coining of the term "amyloid" (applied by Virchow and meaning starchlike), but also incorrectly suggested its fundamental nature. Starch is not a constituent of amyloid. A different complex carbohydrate is responsible for its iodine staining properties.

Amyloid deposits are composed of at least three constituents:

1. A fibrillary protein, the nature of which varies with the underlying disease. The tertiary structure of this protein and the manner in which it interacts with fellow molecules are responsible for the morphologic, structural, and some staining characteristics of amyloid. Furthermore, it is the particular nature of this fibrillary protein that is now the determining factor in the classification of amyloid.
2. Stacks of a pentagonal, doughnut-shaped protein, called the amyloid component or AP. All types of amyloid, with only one exception, possess this amyloid P component. AP is identical to, and is derived from, a normal circulating serum protein termed serum amyloid P component, or SAP.
3. A complex carbohydrate (a glycosaminoglycan—in most cases, heparan sulfate). This molecule is probably responsible for the iodine-staining properties of amyloid.

It is important to emphasize that not all amyloids are the same. The protein responsible for the fibrillary characteristics varies significantly. In amyloid associated with multiple myeloma, the fibrillary component is a product of immunoglobulin light chains produced by the myeloma cells. In amyloid associated with inflammatory diseases, the fibrillary component is derived from the amino-terminal two-thirds of an acute phase protein. This protein is produced by the liver and is unrelated to immunoglobulins. In these two cases, amyloid is deposited systemically. In other situations, amyloid is deposited locally in isolated organs. Amyloid in medullary carcinoma of the thyroid is restricted to the tumor deposits, and its fibrillary component is derived from a polypeptide hormone. In the pancreatic islets of Langerhans, amyloid associated with an islet cell tumor or diabetes mellitus is a peptide related to calcitonin.

Clearly the nature of the deposits varies widely, and the conditions under which they occur are disparate. However, a century of usage has entrenched the term "amyloidosis" as connoting a single disease. This notion has been replaced by the concept that amyloidosis, in a generic sense, should be used only to designate a group of diseases in which there are proteinaceous tissue deposits with common morphologic, structural, and staining properties, but with variable protein composition.

General Features of Amyloid Deposits

Staining Properties

The staining properties and general appearance of amyloid are governed primarily by its protein nature. Because of their compact nature, the amyloids have few structural features visible by light microscopy. With routine stains, they are amorphous, glassy, and almost cartilage-like, characteristics that are responsible for their so-called hyaline appearance.

Although the amyloids stain no differently than many other proteins when using hematoxylin and eosins, the specific nature and underlying organization of the amyloid proteins, as well as that of associated molecules (glycosaminoglycans and the amyloid P component), allow amyloid to be stained in specific ways.

All amyloids stain red with the Congo red dye (Fig. 23-2A). When the sections stained with Congo red are viewed under polarized light, the deposits exhibit a red–green birefringence (Fig. 23-2B). The fibrillary deposits organized in one plane have one color and those organized perpendicularly to the first have the other color. Rotation of the prism changes the orientation of the polarized light and results in a reversal of the colors. Congo red is the stain most commonly used for the diagnosis of amyloidosis.

Staining with thioflavin T, though not entirely specific for amyloid, allows the amyloid to fluoresce when viewed in ultraviolet light. The presence of

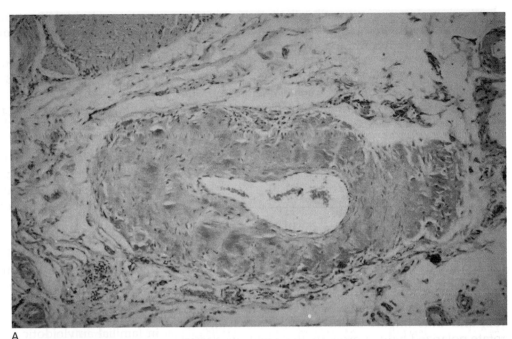

A

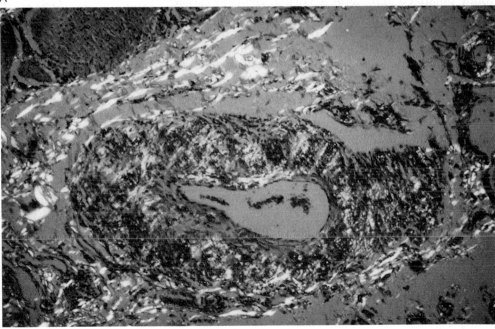

B

Figure 23-2.   AL amyloid involving the wall of an artery, stained with Congo red. The appearance under ordinary light (*A*) and polarized light (*B*) is shown. Note the red–green birefringence of the amyloid. Collagen has a silvery appearance.

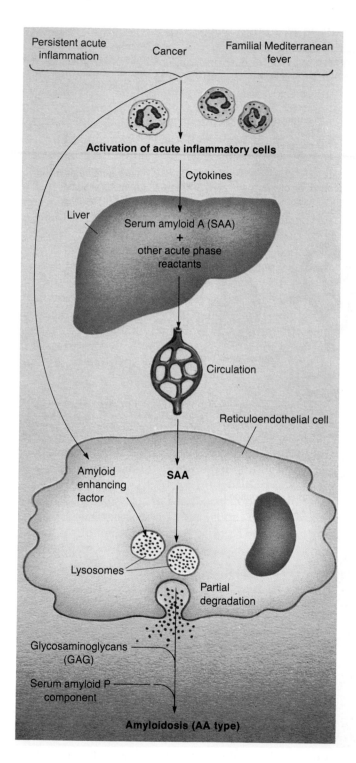

Figure 23–4. The mechanism of AA amyloid deposition. A variety of diseases are associated with the activation of polymorphonuclear leukocytes, which in turn leads to the release of acute phase reactants, including SAA, by the liver. These disorders also are accompanied by the appearance of amyloid enhancing factor. SAA, in the presence of amyloid enhancing factor, is partially degraded by reticuloendothelial cells, and the released product complexed with GAG and SAP is deposited as AA amyloid.

does not occur without the concomitant presence of AEF. AEF is a naturally occurring glycoprotein, the concentration of which increases markedly during inflammation, that alters the metabolic processing of SAA. **Thus, during inflammation at least two coincident processes are apparently necessary for AA amyloid deposition. The first is the pathway that generates the amyloid precursor; the second is the pathway that generates AEF.** Even these two processes, however, are not sufficient for amyloid deposition. Animals that receive interleukin-1 in the absence of a full blown inflammatory process have elevated levels of SAA. Yet if AEF is passively transferred to such animals, they fail to deposit the AA protein. At least one further process stemming from acute inflammation is necessary for AA amyloid deposition, but its nature has not been identified.

In both AA and AL amyloid deposition, partial degradation of a protein by a phagocytic cell occurs. It is the distribution of these cells that seems to determine the anatomic distribution of the AL and AA forms of amyloid.

Deposition of Amyloids Associated with Prealbumin

Familial amyloidotic polyneuropathy is inherited in an autosomal dominant fashion. Heterozygous individuals express both genes, with both the variant and normal prealbumins present in the serum. Apparently the entire molecule of A prealbumin is deposited, rather than a fragment. **In contrast to the AL and AA amyloids, a proteolytic mechanism is not involved in the pathogenesis of familial amyloidotic polyneuropathy.**

Additional genetic variants of prealbumin have been associated with familial forms of amyloidosis of the polyneuropathic form. Different mutations involving the same protein, but at different locations, give rise to similar clinical entities. As in the AL and AA forms of amyloidosis, tissue glycosaminoglycans and serum amyloid P are deposited in association with the prealbumin.

Deposition of Other Amyloids

There is a lack of information about mechanisms involved in the deposition of other forms of amyloid. Procalcitonin, which is associated with medullary carcinoma of the thyroid, is a fragment of a larger molecule, a finding implying that a proteolytic step is involved in the genesis of this amyloid. Morpho-

logically, the close association of this form of amyloid with tumor cells that contain many lysosomes suggests that the proteolytic mechanism operates at a local site.

An Underlying Mechanism?

Given the diverse nature of amyloid proteins and their markedly different amino acid sequences, it is surprising that they fold in similar ways, thereby giving rise to constant ultrastructural characteristics and staining properties. However, there are several features in most of these amyloids that suggest that common processes are involved in their deposition. In many situations, a proteolytic process is involved in cleaving a protein fragment from a larger molecule (although in the case of prealbumin this may not be true). **It may well be that proteolysis is the common mechanism for providing protein fragments.** In virtually all amyloids, highly charged glycosaminoglycans and serum amyloid P component are present in close association with the amyloid deposits. The protein fragments interact with the highly charged glycosaminoglycan molecules and SAP, a process that forces them to fold as fibrils, which in turn interact as β-pleated sheets. Thus, the basic fibril is probably not formed simply as a result of the primary structure of the protein fragment; it is most likely influenced significantly by the manner in which the protein fragment interacts with additional components. The common secondary and tertiary organization of the proteins then results in common structural and staining properties.

Features of Amyloid Deposits in Different Tissues

In addition to the common structural features of the amyloid deposits themselves, there are several features of the deposits that are related to the tissues in which they are laid down. **Because amyloid is deposited along stromal networks, the deposits take on the architectural framework of the organs involved.** The morphologic differences in amyloid deposition from one organ to the next simply relfect the differing stromal organization of each tissue. For example, in the medulla of the kidney, amyloid is laid down in a longitudinal fashion, parallel to the tubules and vasa recta. In the glomerulus (Figs. 23-5 and 23-6), amyloid is deposited in a pattern determined by the lobular architecture of the glomerulus itself. Splenic amyloid may be deposited in one of two

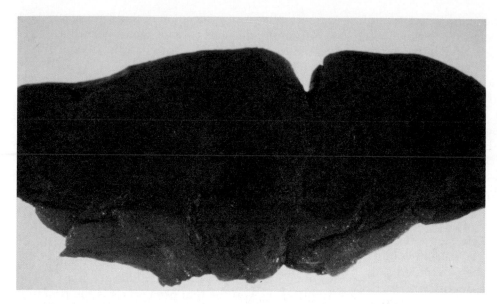

Figure 23-5. Kidney containing AA amyloid stained with the iodine reaction originally used to identify amyloid. Note the staining of the glomeruli in the cortex.

patterns. It may be associated primarily with the stroma of the red pulp or, alternatively, with the stroma of the white pulp. On a cut surface, the former has a diffusely pale and waxy appearance, the so-called **lardaceous spleen.** The cut surface of the latter shows multiple pale foci scattered throughout the spleen, the so-called **sago spleen.** Deposits in the liver follow the arteries of the portal triads, or are laid down along central veins and radiate into the parenchyma along the liver plates.

Amyloid adds interstitial material to sites of deposition, a process that increases the size of affected organs. This increase may be counterbalanced by the deposition of amyloid in vessels (Fig. 23-7), an effect that may impair circulation and lead to organ atrophy. Affected organs may, therefore, increase or decrease in size. The compact protein deposits are essentially avascular, a property that makes organs paler and adds a firmness to their consistency.

The fibrils when first deposited are usually in close association with subendothelial basement membranes (Fig. 23-8). **Regardless of whether amyloid is laid down in a systemic or local fashion, the deposits tend to occur between parenchymal cells and their blood supply. Extension of these deposits eventually entraps the parenchymal cells, interferes with their nutrition, and leads to their strangulation and atrophy (Fig. 23-9).**

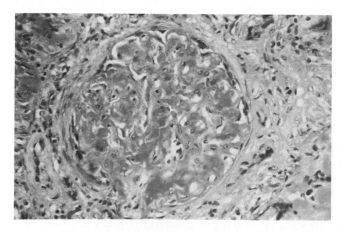

Figure 23-6. The microscopic appearance of AA amyloid from the glomeruli of the specimen in Figure 23-5. Note the lobular pattern of the deposit and the involvement of the afferent arteriole.

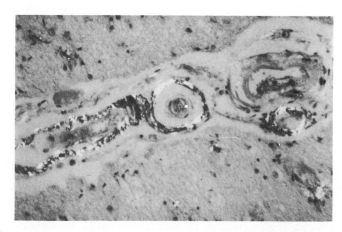

Figure 23-7. Cerebrovascular amyloid from a case of Alzheimer's disease.

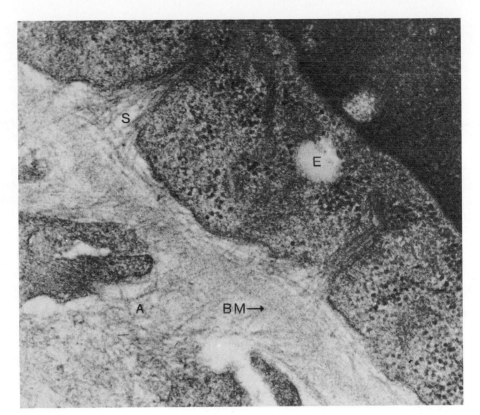

Figure 23-8. Electron micrograph of glomerular amyloid (*A*) illustrating its location relative to the basement membrane (*BM*). Amyloid spicules (*S*) extend into the cytoplasm of the glomerular epithelial cells (*E*).

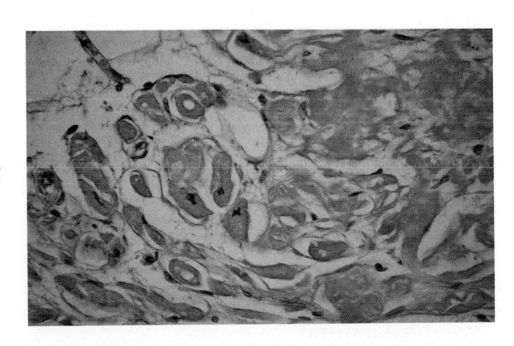

Figure 23-9. Myocardial amyloid (AL type), showing the encroachment upon and strangulation of individual myocardial fibers.

Clinical Features of Amyloidosis

The symptomatology of amyloidosis is governed by both the underlying disease and the type of protein deposited. **No single set of symptoms points unequivocally to amyloidosis as a diagnosis.** In fact, amyloidosis may be found as a completely unexpected disorder, with no clinical manifestations. Renal and cardiac complications are common in several varieties of amyloidosis. Patients with multiple myeloma, chronic long-standing inflammatory disorders, or familial Mediterranean fever who develop the nephrotic syndrome should be suspected of having amyloidosis. Proteinuria, particularly in patients with multiple myeloma or plasma cell dyscrasias, may be overlooked if the patients are already excreting a Bence-Jones protein. Progressive glomerular obliteration may ultimately lead to renal failure and uremia.

Amyloid involvement of the myocardium should be suspected in systemic forms of amyloidosis, in which congestive failure or cardiomegaly is associated with low voltage on the electrocardiogram. Entrapment of the conduction system may lead to arrhythmias, which in turn can result in sudden death. Not only does congestive failure secondary to cardiac amyloidosis respond poorly to digitalis therapy, but amyloid fibrils sequester and concentrate digoxin, thus precipitating digitalis toxicity and fatal arrhythmias. Sufficient amyloid deposition within the myocardium also impairs ventricular distensibility and filling, an effect that appears clinically as a restrictive form of cardiomyopathy. Similarly, it can masquerade as a restrictive type of pericarditis.

Gastrointestinal ganglia, smooth muscle vasculature, and submucosa all may be involved by amyloid. Deposits in these locations alter gastrointestinal motility and absorption. Patients may complain of either constipation or diarrhea, occasionally in association with malabsorption. Enlargement of the tongue and interference with its motor function may be of sufficient degree to affect speech and swallowing.

The familial polyneuropathic forms of amyloid usually present with paresthesias and loss of temperature and pain sensation of the extremities.

In all systemic forms of amyloidosis, the patient's course is usually unremitting and ultimately fatal. Patients with myeloma and AL amyloidosis generally die within 1 to 2 years, from either the malignancy or the cardiac and renal complications of amyloidosis. Patients with AA amyloidosis secondary to long-standing inflammatory disease have a more protracted course, but death usually occurs within 5 years of the diagnosis, usually from cardiac or renal failure. Patients with deposition of A prealbumin of the familial type have an extended course of from 15 to 25 years. Symptoms may begin at any age, but are usually postpubertal, with death most common in the fifth and sixth decades.

For the most part, amyloid is a stable, static protein deposit. However, successful treatment of the underlying condition, such as multiple myeloma or an inflammatory disorder, may on rare occasion lead to the resorption and resolution of these deposits. Treatment directed specifically at resorption is not available.

Diagnosis of Amyloidosis

Even when one suspects amyloidosis, the diagnosis ultimately rests on its histologic demonstration in biopsy specimens. Amyloid is readily demonstrated in gingival and rectal biopsy specimens and in abdominal subcutaneous fat. Amyloid is commonly demonstrated in renal biopsy tissue taken as part of a general investigation of impaired renal function.

Individuals who carry the genes for familial amyloidotic polyneuropathy can be identified by demonstrating the substitution of methionine for valine in A prealbumin. Since virtually all patients with this gene ultimately develop symptoms, the detection of carriers is valuable in genetic counselling.

SUGGESTED READING

Axelrad MA, Kisilevsky R, Wilmer J, Chen SJ, Skinner M: Further characterization of amyloid-enhancing factor. Lab Invest 47:139, 1982

Durie BGM, Persky B, Soehnlen BJ, Grogan TM, Salmon SE: Amyloid production in human myeloma stem-cell culture with morphologic evidence of amyloid secretion by associated macrophages. N Engl J Med 307:1689, 1982

Glenner GG: Amyloid deposits and amyloidosis: The B-fibrilloses (Parts I & II). N Engl J Med 302:1283 & 302:1333, 1980

Glenner GG, Costa PP, deFreitas AF (eds): Amyloidosis: Proceedings of the Third Symposium of Amyloidosis, Povoa de Varzim, Portugal. Amsterdam, Excerpta Medica, 1980

Kang J, Lemaire HG, Unterbeck A, Salbaum JM, et al: The precursor of amyloid A4 protein resembles a cell-surface receptor. Nature 325:733, 1987

Kisilevsky R: From arthritis to Alzheimer's disease: current concepts on the pathogenesis of amyloidosis. Can J Physiol Pharm 65:1085, 1987

Kisilevsky R, Boudreau L: The kinetics of amyloid deposition. I. The effects of amyloid-enhancing factor and splenectomy. Lab Invest 48:60, 1983

Parmelee DC, Tinani K, Ericsson LH, Eriksen N, Benditt EP, Walsh KA: Amino acid sequence of amyloid-related apoprotein (apoSAA$_1$) from human high-density lipoprotein. Biochemistry 21:3298, 1982

Pitkanen P, Westermark P, Cornwell GG: Senile systemic amyloidosis. Am J Pathol 117:391, 1984

Saraiva MJM, Birken S, Costa PP, Goodman DS: Amyloid fibril protein in familial amyloidotic polyneuropathy, Portuguese type. Definition of molecular abnormality in transthyretin (prealbumin). J Clin Invest 74:104, 1984

Saraiva MJM, Costa P, Goodman DS: Studies on plasma transthyretin (prealbumin) in familial amyloidotic polyneuropathy, Portuguese type. J Lab Clin Med 102:590, 1983

Sletten K, Westermark P, Natvig JB: Characterization of amyloid fibril proteins from medullary carcinoma of the thyroid. J Exp Med 143:993, 1976

24

The Skin

Wallace H. Clark, Jr.

The Skin: The Cosmetic
Organ of the Creature of
Adornment

Anatomic and Physiologic
Considerations

The Patterns of Cutaneous
Disease

Diseases Primarily Affecting
the Epidermis

Diseases Primarily Affecting
the Basement Membrane
Zone: Pathology of the
Dermal-Epidermal Interface

Inflammatory Diseases of the
Superficial and Deep Vascular
Bed

Disorders Manifested
Primarily by Alterations of
the Dermal Connective Tissue

Inflammatory Disorders of
the Panniculus

Disorders of the
Pilosebaceous Unit

Primary Neoplasms of the
Skin

Figure 24-1. The dermis and its vasculature. The fact that the dermis is divided into two distinct anatomic regions is of importance in studying cutaneous pathology. The papillary dermis, with its vascular plexus, and the epidermis usually react together in most diseases that are primarily limited to the skin. The reticular dermis and subcutis are altered in association with systemic diseases that are manifested in the skin. *DSUP*, deep superficial venular plexus; *SAP*, superficial arterial plexus; *USVP*, upper superficial venular plexus.

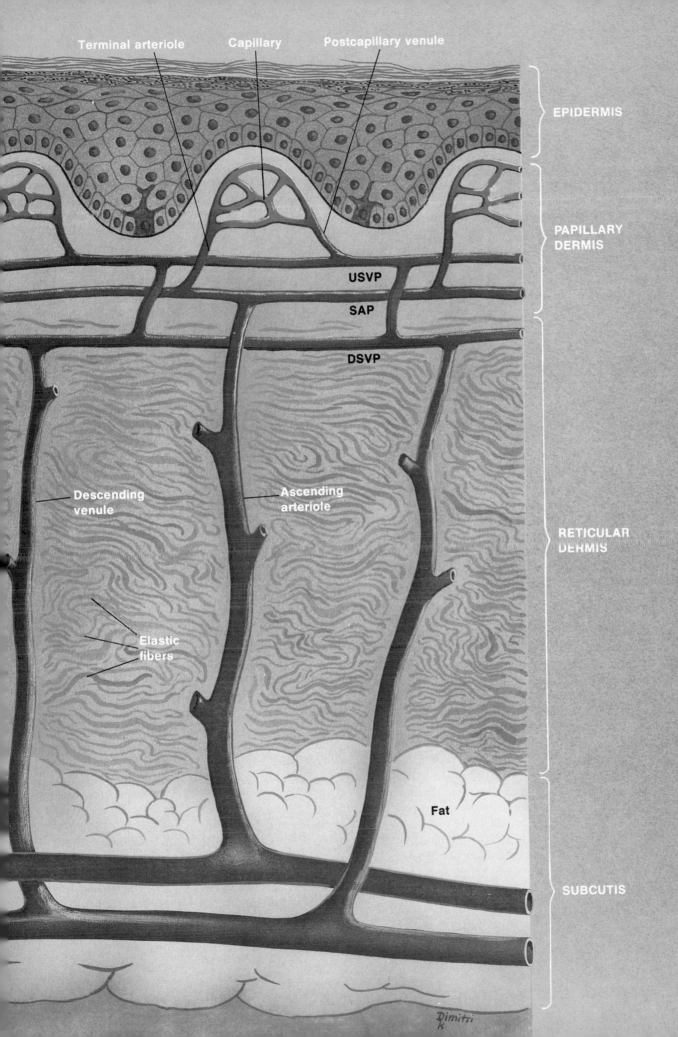

Terminal arteriole   Capillary   Postcapillary venule

EPIDERMIS

PAPILLARY DERMIS

USVP

SAP

DSVP

Descending venule

Ascending arteriole

Elastic fibers

RETICULAR DERMIS

Fat

SUBCUTIS

Dimitri K

The skin is a particularly favorable organ for studying the principles of pathology, including pathogenesis and even morbid anatomy. Except for diseases of highly specialized tissues—for instance, those of the alveolus or the glomerulus, or the demyelinating diseases of the central nervous system—all classes of disease are seen in the skin. On the other hand, some diseases—the dyshesive, blistering ones quickly come to mind—are manifested only in the skin, except for some involvement of the mucous membranes. The skin has many functions, but one of its most important functions—the cosmetic packaging of the individual organism—may not even be alluded to in standard medical texts.

The Cosmetic Organ of the Creature of Adornment

Except for the first of living things and the late-arriving but currently fashionable evolutionary product *Homo sapiens,* all creatures, save a worm or two, have a beautiful, fascinating or interesting integument, as a minimum gift of Nature's hand. From the Precambrian epoch to the Cambrian explosion of life—through the flood of time stamped with names struggling to comprehend that very flood: Ordovician, Devonian, Permian, Jurassic, to our current Quaternary way-station—only the ameba and man have a boring integument. Divest yourself of your adornments, all of them, and stand before a mirror. Look. Better still, imagine one or two hundred diverse kinds of *Home sapiens,* caged, zoo-like, also stripped of their adornments and paints. Standing there, contentedly munching their hors d'oeuvres and sipping their martinis, willingly available for careful inspection. Where does your eye go? The genitalia, the buttocks, the breasts, the eyes, the mouth, the nose, the hair, even the hands and feet, and surely, the whole package. The skin? No. Its color perhaps registered in passing. One could even note the warmth of a rich, ebony-black or deep red-brown. Basically, however, the whole package is dull because of a pedestrian integument. Now disperse your disrobed self and your brothers throughout a complete zoo—Noah's Zoo—and see how you fare in competition with the compellingly attractive coats of the kingdom of living things. How would you like to be between a magnificent Siberian tiger (*Panthera tigris*), and, arguably, the most beautiful of all birds, Blythe's Tragopan (*Tragopan satyra*)? This rarely seen inhabitant of the Himalayan hillsides is brilliantly red, sequined with small white spots delineated from the red by a black halo. Some of the sequins are held together by golden threads. The face is blue and the chapeau black and red. Even were you to be arrayed with less spectacular creatures such as the pileated woodpecker or spotted skunk, the unadorned skin of *Homo sapiens* is, by comparison, a scenic disaster.

Man, having certain advantages over the ameba, uses another derivative of his neuroectoderm, the central nervous system, to correct his native cutaneous decorative flaws. And does he correct the flaws! Down through the relentless march of years from early Pleistocene to the ubiquitous cosmetic counters of this very day in Holocene time, *H. sapiens* has painted his skin; draped strands and bits of metal over its narrow places and outcroppings; punched holes in it; covered it with metal and stones of all descriptions; made it lighter if it was dark and darker if it was light; cut the hair, let the hair grow, colored the hair, abandoned the hair, and covered the skin with cloth, leather and fur of unending variety and color. *Now,* take your decorated self back to Noah's Zoo (take your drink and melted brie with you) and stand with some pride between the common peacock and the giant panda. Your conspecifics will now give you notice and you him. Much of your daily time is spent looking at the decorations *H. sapiens* uses and in formulating your own integumentary modifications. The skin is the way we present ourselves to ourselves and to each other. The skin is the cosmetic organ. Man spends much of his time, creativity, and money in altering the drabness of his integument. The decorative act is a common behavioral thread firmly linking creatures of diverse cultures into a common cosmetic union. Man is a creature of adornment.

Considering the imperatives of appearance in human relationships, it is not surprising that an alteration in the appearance of the skin may be the single most important feature of cutaneous disease. Many cutaneous diseases have minor symptomatology, while others have none at all. Few are life-threatening and many are self-limited. (There are notable exceptions to this statement.) However, even the self-limited, asymptomatic cutaneous diseases are of great concern to the patient. For example, the symptoms of acne are minor, but the disease can totally change a life. Vitiligo, a completely asymptomatic, progressive, mottled depigmentary disorder, commonly converts a normal human being into a recluse. Loss of some unneeded scalp hair has generated an industry of significant size.

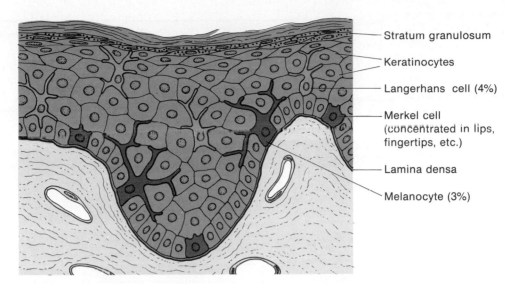

Figure 24-2. Normal epidermis and the epidermal immigrant cells. The keratinocytes form the multilayered epidermis, protecting against water loss and bacterial invasion. The melanocytes, forming some 3 percent of the cells of the epidermis, provide color, as well as protection against ultraviolet radiation. The Langerhans cells, which are slightly more numerous than melanocytes, are the cellular manifestation of the skin's function as an immunologic organ. The Merkel cells are markers of one of the tactile functions of the skin. They are confined to special sites, such as the lips.

Anatomic and Physiologic Considerations

The functions of the skin not related to appearance are compellingly related to survival. The skin serves a protective barrier function: microorganisms find it almost impossible to traverse the epidermis and water loss is inhibited. The skin is also vital in regulating temperature and in protecting against ultraviolet light radiation. A wide variety of sensory receptors communicate details related to the immediate environment. The skin is an important part of the immune system. This list is hardly complete, and many of the skin's functions are related to specialized cutaneous cells, special structural organizations, and highly distinctive organelles typical of many cutaneous cells.

The Epidermis and the Keratinocytic Cellular System

Basically, the human epidermis is a multilayered sheet of keratin-synthesizing cells. From the lowermost basal layer to the outermost shedding cells of the stratum corneum, there is a progressive change in form (Fig. 24-2). The cylindrical basal cells are stem cells that replicate. The nonviable, superficial, cornified cells are flattened plates, the long axes of which are parallel to the surface of the skin. The layering of keratinocytes is not without order, since there is an intrinsic stacking architecture related to (a) the rate of proliferation, (b) the order of desquamation, and (c) the regulation of water loss. **Keratinocytes** synthesize a sulfur-poor filamentous protein, the **tonofibril,** which is directly related to the keratin molecule of the stratum corneum. In addition to various specialized attachment zones, the keratinocytes are distinguished by two structural products. The **keratohyaline granule,** the defining hallmark of the stratum granulosum, is a histidine-rich protein whose function is not well understood and whose chemical composition is not precisely defined. It does, however, clearly contribute to the stratum corneum, forming the electron-dense, amorphous matrix of the cornified cells. The **Odland bodies** (keratinosome, membrane-coating granules) are the only known, structurally distinctive, secretory product of the epidermis (Fig. 24-3). They are formed in the outer spinous and granular layers and discharge their uniquely lamellated contents into the intercellular space, there form-

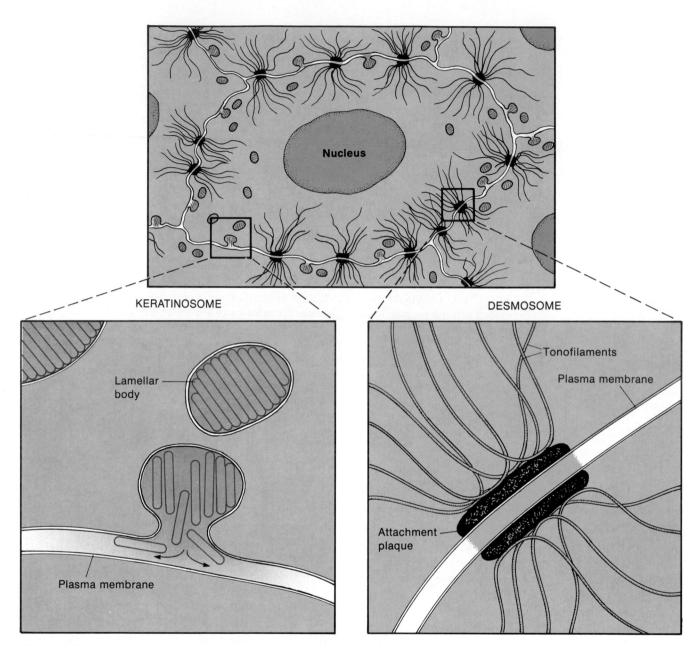

KERATINOSOME

Lamellar body

Plasma membrane

DESMOSOME

Tonofilaments

Plasma membrane

Attachment plaque

Figure 24-3. The keratinocyte, keratinosome, and desmosome. The keratinocyte cytoplasm is dominated by delicate keratin fibrils, the tonofilaments. These form a part of the cytoskeleton of the cell, and loop within the attachment plaque of the desmosome. The lamellar body of the keratinocyte extrudes its contents into the intercellular space. The material probably has a role in cellular cohesion.

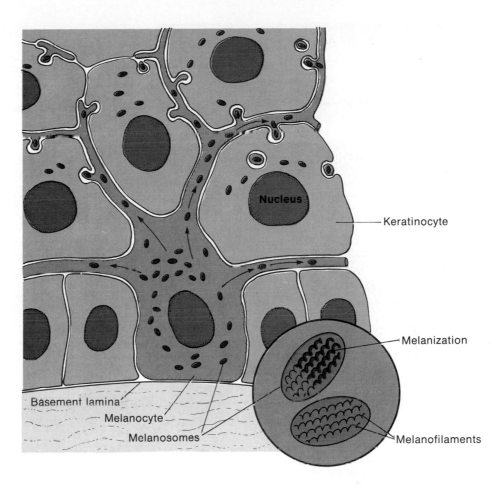

Figure 24-4. The melanocyte supplies approximately 36 keratinocytes with melanin granules by way of complex dendritic cytoplasmic extensions. The melanin granules are transferred to keratinocytes and come to lie in a supranuclear cap, a site suggestive of the protective function of these pigment granules. Pigment is actually formed in the melanocytes within distinctive organelles—the melanosomes—which are the parents of the pigment granule. Pigment is synthesized on small filaments within this organelle (see inset).

ing lamellar masses that parallel cytomembranes. The Odland body and its discharged lamellated products are related to the epidermal barrier function that is most clearly manifested in the outer granular layer. They may also be involved in cholesterol synthesis and storage, and may possibly induce the conversion of vitamin D3 by ultraviolet light. An increase in Odland bodies and their intercellular products in some ichthyoses may play a role in the abnormal retention of the stratum corneum.

The Epidermal Immigrant Cells

The epidermis harbors immigrant cells of neuroectodermal or mesenchymal origin. These cells do not synthesize keratin and have their own highly distinctive phenotypic organelles. All appear in varying numbers and at varying levels of the epidermal strata as cells with a clear perikaryon. Two of the cells, **melanocytes** and **Langerhans** cells, are dendritic; the third, the **Merkel cell,** is associated with a terminal neuraxon. (see Fig. 24-2).

The Melanocytes

The melanocytes, which are dendritic cells that are largely responsible for the color of human skin, originate in the neural crest. After a mesenchymal migratory pathway, they come to lie in the epidermis from the eighth embryonic week forward, and are the first immigrant cells to arrive in the epidermis. Melanin synthesis begins in these cells by the fourth month of pregnancy, and the transfer of the synthesized pigment granules occurs by the sixth month. This is the beginning of the constitutive (native) color of the individual. In postembryonic life, the melanocytes come to lie in the basal layer of the epidermis, tending to hang down, as a teardrop, into the papillary dermis; however, they are separated from it by the basement membrane zone. Through their dendrites, the cells acquire a relation to some 36 keratinocytes. This cellular complex has come to be known as an **epidermal–melanin unit** (Fig. 24-4).

Melanin is synthesized in a complex organelle called the **melanosome** (Fig. 24-4). This organelle is bounded by a membrane and has a highly character-

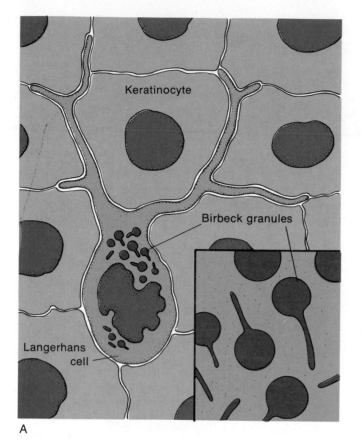

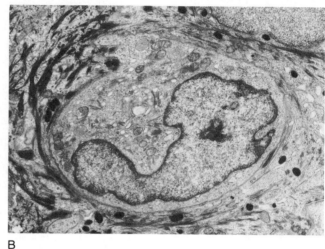

A   B

Figure 24-5.   The dendritic Langerhans cell can recognize and process antigens. The unique, racquet-shaped organelles (*A*) may be related to antigen presentation by the cell. (*B*) An electron micrograph of the Langerhans cell shows the distinctive linear bars with a central dark line which represent the racquet-shaped handles of Birbeck granules. A few profiles show a bulbous end, representing the "paddle" of the racquet. Most of the distinctive organelles are within or near the large nuclear indentation.

istic internal structure on electron microscopy. When melanin synthesis is active, the internal structure is characterized by a filamentous appearance. The filaments (melanofilaments) have a distinctive periodicity—in the range of 9 nm—and are arranged in a parallel array along the long axis of the dirigible-shaped organelle. In some profiles, the melanofilaments seem to be cross-linked coincident with their periodic structure, a feature which results in a highly distinctive striated appearance. With melanization (a tyrosinase-dependent process), the orderly internal structure is progressively obliterated, and the organelle then presents as an electron-opaque granule. This granule is responsible for protection from ultraviolet light and provides the diverse coloration of man and much of the animal kingdom. Interestingly, the black cloud that obscures the retreat of the squid is secreted by a gland that synthesizes massive quan-

tities of melanin. The color of the skin is based largely on the number, size, and packaging of melanosomes in cells other than the one where they are formed, and is not primarily dependent on variations in the final chemical structure of melanin. Chemically, there are two basic melanins—namely, eumelanin (the brown-black insoluble melanin) and phenomelanin (the yellow-red melanin that is soluble in dilute alkali). Melanins accomplished their protective and decorative functions by moving from the modulating environment, where they are synthesized, to other cells, where they assume a static array. When transferred to keratinocytes, they form a supranuclear cap that acts as a shield against ultraviolet radiation. In hair and epidermal keratinocytes, they are packaged in such a fashion that they variably absorb and reflect visible light, thereby forming the integumentary colors.

Langerhans Cells

The next immigrants to the epidermis (and dermis)—the Langerhans cells—arrive in embryonic skin in the last month of the first trimester of pregnancy, following the melanocytes by some 4 to 5 weeks. With the arrival of these HLA-DR–positive cells, the skin acquires a new dimension. It can recognize and process antigens and, consequently, becomes a part of the immune system. Uncommon in the dermis, these cells are distributed throughout the nucleated layers of the epidermis, where they constitute some 4 percent of the nucleated epidermal cells. In routine light microscopic preparations, Langerhans cells are difficult to see. The cytoplasm, in relation to that of a keratinocyte, is translucent, and is formed of a perikaryon and blunt dendrites. The plasma membranes do not form specialized zones with the opposed keratinocytes. In electron micrographs, the cytoplasm contains a moderate number of specialized organelles, the **Birbeck granules.** In two dimensions, they appear to be racquet-shaped, but three-dimensional reconstruction has shown them to be cup-shaped (Fig. 24-5). The function of these unique organelles is, unfortunately, unknown, although it is possible that their function is related to that of Langerhans cells as antigen-presenting cells. In the proliferating Langerhans cells of the histiocytoses, granules are attached to the plasma membrane and are in direct communication with the extracellular space. Further, they have a fuzzy coat of clathrin, a feature of "coated pits," suggesting that they may be related to receptor-mediated endocytosis and, in turn, to antigen processing and recognition. In this respect, Langerhans cells have specific receptor sites for the Fc fragment of IgG and for the C3B component of complement.

Merkel Cells

Merkel cells become residents of the basal layer at the beginning of the second trimester of pregnancy. They are not ubiquitous immigrants to all areas of the epidermis, but are found in special regions, such as the lips, oral cavity, or external root sheath of the hair follicles, in the glabrous skin of the digits, or as a part of certain tactile discs. Merkel cells project short, blunt, cytoplasmic fingers into adjacent keratinocytes and, in contrast to other immigrant cells, are attached to adjacent keratinocytes by desmosomes. This fact suggests that they may be ectodermal in origin rather than neuroectodermal. Along with the other immigrant cells to the skin, Merkel cells have a distinctive phenotypic organelle, a membrane-bound, dense-cored granule that is 100 nm or

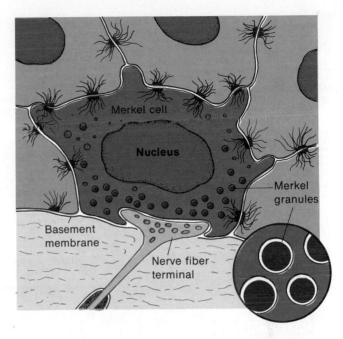

Figure 24-6. The Merkel cell, which differs from other immigrant cells, forms desmosomes with keratinocytes, and is attached to a small nerve plate (nerve fiber terminal). The membrane-delimited, dense cored granule is distinctive (see inset).

larger in width (Fig. 24-6). At its base, the tactile Merkel cell is opposed to a small nerve plate, connected by a short, nonmyelinated axon to a myelinated axon. This complex structure functions as a tactile mechanoreceptor.

The Basement Membrane Zone

The basement membrane zone, which serves as an interface between the epidermis and dermis, is as diverse in function as it is complex in structure (Fig. 24-7). It is responsible for epidermal–dermal adherence, and probably serves as a selective macromolecular filter. It is also the major site of immune reactant localization in cutaneous disease. Neoplastic cells must acquire certain properties to be able to traverse the basement membrane zone. If these properties are not acquired by neoplasms arising in the epidermis, these tumors would remain *in situ* indefinitely, and invasion and metastasis would not occur. The basement membrane zone includes:

- The innermost part of the basal keratinocytes, especially the tonofilaments that attach to the inner face of the hemidesmosome
- The hemidesmosome itself, with its subdesmosomal dense plate

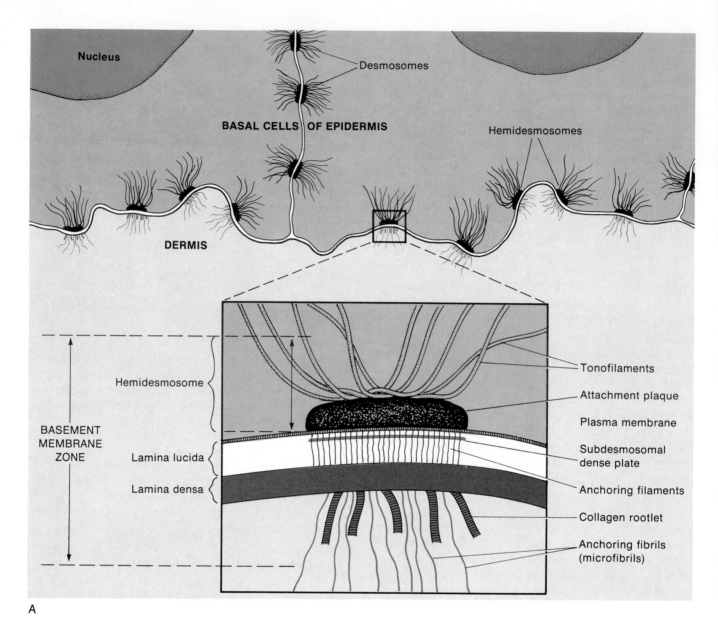

A

Figure 24-7.   The dermal-epidermal interface and the basement membrane zone. (*A*) This epithelial-mesenchymal interface is the site of the basement membrane zone, a complex structure that is mostly synthesized by the basal cells of the epidermis. Each of its complex structures, from tonofilaments and attachment plaques of basal cells to collagen rootlets and microfibrils, attached to the inner face of the lamina densa, is a site of change in specific diseases.

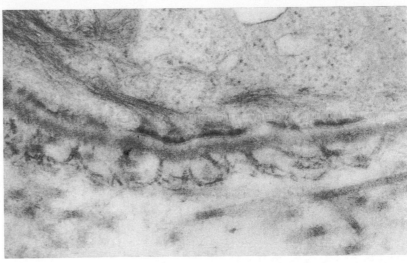

Figure 24-7 (continued). (B) An electron micrograph shows the hemidesmosomal attachment plaques with their inserting tonofilaments (near the center of the micrograph). The subdesmosomal dense plates, the lamina lucida, the lamina densa, and the subjacent collagen rootlets are well demonstrated. Compare this with the illustration in *A*.

B

- That portion of the plasma membrane of basal cells that faces the dermis
- The anchoring filaments that extend from the subdesmosomal dense plates across the lamina lucida and insert into the lamina densa
- The lamina lucida, an electron lucent layer, where adherence proteins, such as laminin, are located
- The lamina densa, basically composed of type IV collagen
- Anchoring fibrils, which are collagen rootlets that extend from the inner face of the lamina densa for a short distance into the papillary dermis.
- Microfibrils, which are delicate, long, elastic fibrils that blend with the underlying elastic fibrillary system of the skin.

It is of interest that all of the structures of the basement membrane zone are elaborated by the epidermis, except for the anchoring fibrils and microfibrils.

The Dermis

The organization of the collagen and elastic tissue of the dermis is a distinctive feature of human skin. Except for swine, it is not duplicated in the skin of other animals. Swine, also in common with man, enjoy lying in the sun, tan in response to the sun, and will drink beer in large quantities. Immediately deep to the epidermis, there is a narrow zone where collagen is disposed in unit fibrils. This zone, the papillary dermis, is pale pink on hematoxylin and eosin staining, and has little structure when viewed with the light microscope (see Fig. 24-1). Its delicate connective tissue extends as a narrow sheath about blood vessels, nerves, and skin appendages. The entire network of this collagen is termed the adventitial dermis. The majority of dermal collagen is organized into coarse bundles that form the reticular dermis (see Fig. 24-1). Each bundle is associated with elastic tissue fibers that are demonstrated only with special stains. It is particularly important to differentiate between the papillary dermis (and its ramifications as the adventitial dermis) and the reticular dermis. As a rule, the papillary dermis is altered in conjunction with epidermal disease and disorders that affect the superficial venular bed. **The three structures—the epidermis, papillary dermis, and superficial capillary-venular bed—react conjointly and influence each other in complex ways.** Primary skin diseases with few or no systemic manifestations involve these superficial cutaneous structures.

Psoriasis and lichen planus are classical forms of such skin diseases. The reticular dermis and subcutis (also formally designated as a cutaneous structure) are less common sites of pathologic change and, when diseased, are usually manifestations of systemic disease. Scleroderma (progressive systemic sclerosis) and erythema nodosum exemplify this principle of cutaneous pathology.

Mast Cells

Mast cells are normally present about the venules of the skin and provide for the immediate release of vasoactive and chemotactic substances. The cells play a vital role in inflammation of all types (their function

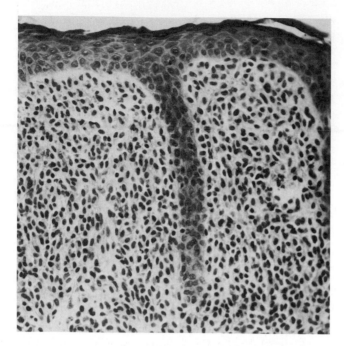

Figure 24-8. Urticaria pigmentosa. All the uniform cells filling the papillary dermis are mast cells.

is discussed in the sections on urticaria and angioedema). Occasionally they proliferate in clusters as a specific disease entity termed **urticaria pigmentosa** (Fig. 24-8).

Cutaneous Vasculature

As the skin receives about 10 times the amount of blood needed for its nutrition, the skin's vasculature and its circulating blood play a complex role in organismal life quite beyond nutrition. Temperature regulation is an example and, in this regard, the skin is of great importance. Many aspects of cutaneous inflammation involve the superficial cutaneous vascular unit. An ascending arteriole arises from arterial structures in the subcutis and directly crosses much of the reticular dermis (see Fig. 24-1). In the outer part of the reticular dermis, in conjunction with other similar ascending arteries, a superficial arteriolar plexus is formed. From this plexus, a terminal arteriole extends into each dermal papilla, where an arterial capillary is formed. The arterial capillary makes a U-turn and becomes a venous capillary and a postcapillary venule before forming a complex venular plexus in the reticular dermis, immediately deep to the papillary dermis. **The venular end of this vascular structure is extensively involved in the mediation of the cutaneous inflammatory response.**

The lymphatics of the skin form a complex and random network, beginning as lymphatic capillaries near the epidermis. A superficial lymphatic plexus may then be formed, from which lymphatic channels drain to regional lymph nodes. The lymphatic channels are involved in metastasis of cutaneous cancers, especially malignant melanoma.

The Skin Appendages

Hair Follicles, the Hair Cycle, and Alopecia

The large hairs of the scalp and the bearded areas of the male grow in a cyclical fashion. The growing hair has a bulb of epithelial and mesenchymal tissue firmly embedded within the subcutis. A cross section of this bulb reveals a cap of actively dividing, keratin-synthesizing cells, which become arrayed in layers that join at the top of the bulb to form the cylindrical hair shaft. As the differentiating hairs form the roof of the epithelial bulb, they interact with an island of melanocytes; these melanocytes contribute melanin to the passing keratinocytes, a process which results in hair color. The colored keratinocytes lose their nuclei as they form the final cylindrical hair shaft. Curly hair is formed from an angulated bulb. In a healthy scalp with a normal complement of hair, about 90 percent of hairs are in the *anagen phase,* the actively growing hair phase just described. These growing hairs have a mosaic distribution and are interspersed with hairs showing no evidence of growth, termed **telogen hairs,** and those that are in the process of ceasing growth, called **catagen hairs.** Catagen hairs still have a hair shaft, but it ends in the lower reticular dermis as a slightly widened structure, similar to a club. This shaft is surrounded by a rim of nucleated keratinocytes, but the hair bulb with dividing keratinocytes and the prominent mesenchymal papillae are no longer present. A strikingly thickened and widened lamina densa surrounds the catagen hair. As the telogen phase (resting follicle) is reached, the end of the hair retreats to the level of the arrectores pilorum as a rule. The hair shaft is missing, leaving but a rudiment of the original follicle. From its attenuated tip, however, one may see a delicate, vascularized mesenchymal tract, the telogen tract. At the top of this tract, the early anagen hair forms again, and with growth, follows the delicate pathway through the reticular dermis into the fat, there forming a mature anagen follicle and a new hair simultaneously.

Two phenomena permit one to appreciate alopecia—one that has doubtless afflicted man from antiquity and the other of recent iatrogenic origin. Common alopecia, which affects both men (male pattern baldness) and women (female pattern), results from a complex and poorly understood interaction of heritable and hormonal factors. If a male who is genetically destined to become bald is castrated before puberty, he will not lose his scalp hair and he will fail to grow a beard. If, as an adult, he is given testosterone, he will lose his scalp hair and will grow a beard. This loss of scalp hair, both in this unusual circumstance and in common baldness, results in **the replacement of a telogen hair follicle with a vellus hair follicle,** the parent of the delicate fuzz on the cheeks of women and on the upper cheeks of men.

Growing hair is the site of active mitosis, and many systemic diseases cause cessation of mitoses in this location. When the malady has passed, regrowth occurs. If a person is subjected to a potent antimitotic regimen, such as chemotherapy for advanced cancer, the hair reacts protectively, as in the lower mammals. Hair follicles stop growth and modulate to a telogen phase, a sequence in which hair is lost. With cessation of therapy, hair regrows. Almost any kind of follicular inflammation can induce the telogen phase, and if fibrosis ensues and involves the telogen tract (the regrowth pathway), permanent loss of that follicle results.

Vellus hair probably plays some role in touch perception in many mammals, but in man, this pale, short hair has no major function. Microscopically, it is a diminutive anagen hair, with a small active bulb high in the reticular dermis, along with small sebaceous glands.

The third kind of hair follicle is the **sebaceous follicle.** It develops with puberty and is clinically important because it is affected by acne. This type of follicle has a minute vellus hair at its base. However, instead of the small sebaceous glands of the vellus hair, it has large sebaceous glands that dwarf the vellus hair and fill the follicular canal with sebum.

The Patterns of Cutaneous Disease

Cutaneous diseases are presented in this chapter according to how they affect the primary anatomic structures of the epidermis. For example, if the stratum corneum is greatly thickened without significant alteration of the remaining epidermis or dermis, the pathologic process will involve flawed cornification, one of the hallmarks of the ichthyoses. If the epidermal cells stick poorly and intraepidermal blisters form, the disease is one of the epidermal dyshesive (flawed cellular cohesion) disorders. Disease of the subcutaneous fat is often suggestive of specific systemic granulomatous inflammation elsewhere in the

body. Thus, in making a diagnosis by microscopic criteria, it is important to locate the affected structures, observe the pathologic changes, and evaluate the pathogenesis. Because a comprehensive treatment of skin pathology is not feasible in this text, the following discussion will focus on diseases that illustrate important mechanisms of lesional pathogenesis. For instance, the increase in the incidence of malignant melanoma is greater than that for any other form of human cancer, and it clearly illustrates certain pathogenetic principles in neoplasia. It is, therefore, covered in some detail. The formation of blisters, an important feature of many cutaneous diseases, is a process largely limited to the skin. Consequently, the diverse mechanisms leading to blisters are thoroughly reviewed.

Diseases Primarily Affecting the Epidermis

Heritable Disorders Associated With Excessive Cornification

Ichthyoses

Definition and Clinical Features
The ichthyosiform dermatoses comprise a heterogeneous, heritable group of disorders that show a striking thickening of the stratum corneum. This thickening is usually disproportionate to the thickening of the deeper nucleated epidermal layers. In severe forms of ichthyosis, such as lamellar ichthyosis, excessive cornified material presents clinically as coarse, fishlike scales over the cutaneous surfaces, hence the name applied to this group of diseases. There are four major ichthyoses, namely ichthyosis vulgaris, sex-linked (X-linked) ichthyosis, lamellar ichthyosis, and epidermolytic hyperkeratosis (congenital ichthyosiform erythroderma). Several rare forms of ichthyosis are associated with other abnormalities, such as abnormal lipid metabolism, neurologic disorders, and bone diseases.

Pathology

General Considerations   As already noted, in contrast with most other skin disorders, **all ichthyoses** (with the possible exception of lamellar ichthyosis) **show a stratum corneum that is disproportionately thick in comparison to the thickness of the nucleated epidermal layers.** Virtually any diseases characterized by thickening of the nucleated epidermal layers also exhibit hyperkeratosis. For example, chronic

Table 24-1 A Comparison of the Major Ichthyoses

	MODE OF INHERITANCE	PRESENT AT BIRTH	PATHOGENETIC MECHANISM	HISTOLOGY
Ichthyosis vulgaris	Autosomal dominant	No; onset in childhood	Normal epidermal turnover. A retention keratosis due to a delay in a dissolution of adhesive mechanism in stratum corneum.	Hyperkeratosis, loosely woven; disproportionately thick in relationship to a relatively thin stratum spinosum. Thin granular layer with abnormal keratohyaline granules.
Sex-linked ichthyosis	X-linked recessive	Yes; onset may be in infancy	Normal epidermal turnover. Constitutional absence of steroid sulfatase and arylsulfatase-C. A retention keratosis due to a failure to break down cholesterol sulfate, an important compound in corneal cohesion.	Compact, disproportionately thick stratum corneum. Normal granular layer. Stratum spinosum only slightly thick.
Epidermolytic hyperkeratosis (bullous congenital ichthyosiform erythroderma)	Autosomal dominant	Yes	Increased germinative cell hyperplasia and decreased transit through the epidermis. Increased number of keratinosomes and increase of intercellular substance.	Tonofilaments aggregate at the cell periphery and show a distorted association with desmosomes. This may lead to "acanthosis" and vesicle formation. Entire skin is rarely involved.
Lamellar ichthyosis (nonbullous congenital ichthyosiform erythroderma)	Autosomal dominant	Yes	Same as for epidermolytic hyperkeratosis	Moderate hyperkeratosis; normal or thickened granular layer. Moderate epidermal hyperplasia. May be psoriasiform with parakeratosis. Entire skin and nails are involved.

scratching or rubbing of normal skin causes a thickened epidermis and dermal changes, a condition known as **lichen simplex chronicus.** In this ailment, both the nucleated epidermal layers and the compacted stratum corneum are likely to be three times their normal thickness. By contrast, in ichthyosis, the stratum corneum may be four or five times thicker than normal, but it commonly overlies a disproportionately thin, nucleated epidermis.

Ichthyosis Vulgaris and Epidermolytic Hyperkeratosis Ichthyosis vulgaris and epidermolytic hyperkeratosis are compared with the other major ichthyotic disorders in Table 24-1. **Ichthyosis vulgaris** is the prototype of disproportionate corneal thickening. The stratum corneum is loose and has a basket-weave appearance which differs little from the normal, except in amount. The granular layer is greatly diminished, and often seems absent (Fig. 24-9). On electron microscopy, the keratohyaline granules are small and spongelike, an appearance indicative of defective synthesis. The basal and spinous layers seem entirely normal. Thus, **the primary defect in ichthyosis vulgaris is in the granular and cornified layers,** the epidermal zones responsible for the final stage of keratinization and cornification. A synonym for **epidermolytic hyperkeratosis** is bullous congenital ichthyosiform erythroderma. Both of these names connote **epidermal lysis** and, consequently, the potential for the formation of **vesicles and bullae.** The stratum spinosum does, indeed, show a faulty tonofilament structure that readily explains the tendency for vesiculation. The spinous keratinocytes present thick, eosinophilic tonofilaments that whorl around the nucleus in a concentric fashion (Fig. 24-10). The cytoplasm displays a clear zone peripheral to the perinuclear tonofilaments, but at the periphery of the cell, these filaments again become condensed. Electron microscopy reveals a faulty insertion of tonofilaments into desmosomes. This flaw, together with other abnormalities in tonofilament structure, may be responsible for cell lysis and the formation of vesicles. The stratum corneum is again, disproportionately thick (Fig. 24-11).

Pathogenesis

Three general defects seem to be involved in the excessive epidermal cornification of the ichthyoses: increased cohesiveness of the cells of the stratum corneum (retention keratosis), possibly related to altered lipid metabolism; abnormal keratinization, expressed as impaired tonofilament formation and keratohyaline synthesis, and excessive cornification; and increased germinative cell hyperplasia and decreased transit time of keratinocytes across the epidermis. Increased corneal cohesiveness is characteristic of ichthyosis vulgaris, but there are no clues as to the reason for this phenomenon. Two mechanisms for abnormal retention of cornified cells are likely in X-linked ichthyosis and lamellar ichthyosis. In X-linked ichthyosis, there is a constitutional absence of steroid sulfatase and arylsulfatase-C, enzymes that degrade cholesterol sulfate in the epidermis. The resulting increase in cholesterol sulfate is directly related to increased cohesiveness and retention keratosis. La-

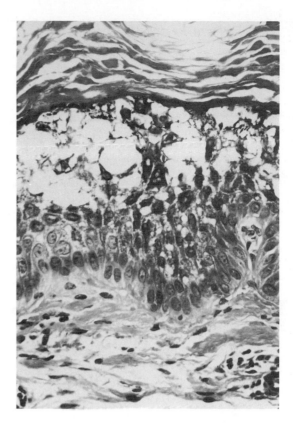

Figure 24-10.   Epidermolytic hyperkeratosis. The cells of the stratum spinosum, immediately above the basal layer, show clumping of their tonofilaments. As a result, their cytoplasm is relatively clear, with small fibrils. In the outer spinous layers, the clumped fibrils are further compacted, and whorl about the nucleus, resulting in cells with a dark cytoplasm. These cells separate from each other to produce epidermolysis.

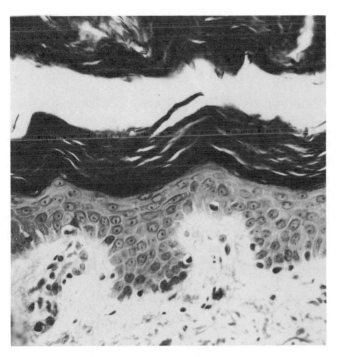

Figure 24-9.   Ichthyosis vulgaris. There is disproportionate thickening of the stratum corneum in relationship to the normal thickness of the nucleated epidermal layers. The stratum granulosum is absent.

mellar ichthyosis is typified by an increased number of keratinosomes, and an increased amount of intercellular substance. Excessive keratinosomes and intercellular substance are thought to be related to increased cohesiveness of the horny layer, and consequently, to retention keratosis. A clinical and histologic state similar to ichthyosis vulgaris may occasionally be associated with other diseases or may follow the use of drugs that affect cholesterol metabolism. The lymphomas, especially Hodgkin's disease, may be associated with ichthyosis. However, other types of neoplasms, systemic granulomatous disorders, and connective tissue disease also may have an ichthyotic cutaneous manifestation. It is possible that the drugs that produce ichthyotic changes by interfering with cholesterol metabolism act through pathways similar to those involved in some of the rare ichthyoses. In these uncommon keratotic diseases, cutaneous changes are apparently due to abnormal-

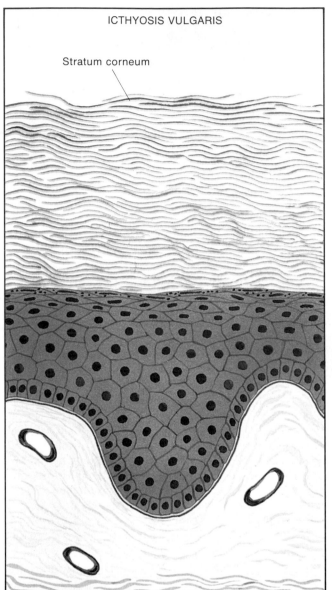

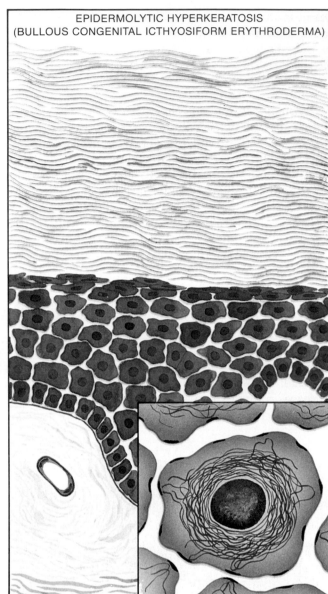

Figure 24-11.   Both diseases (*A*) ichthyosis vulgaris and (*B*) epidermolytic hyper-keratosis (bullous congenital ichthyosiform erythroderma) are characterized by thickening of the stratum corneum relative to the nucleated layers. Epidermolytic hyperkeratosis is characterized by abnormal keratin synthesis that is manifested by whorled keratin filaments about the nucleus and diminished cohesiveness of the keratinocytes (*inset*).

ities in lipid metabolism—for instance, phytanic acid storage disease (Refsum's disease).

Darier's Disease (Keratosis Follicularis)

Definition and Clinical Features

Darier's disease, an inherited autosomal dominant disorder, is pathogenetically related to the ichthyoses in that it is a disorder of keratinization. However, the lesions of Darier's disease are focal keratoses, rather than the generalized scales of the ichthyoses. The chest, nasolabial folds, back, scalp, forehead, ears, and groin exhibit multiple lesions. These first appear late in childhood or in adolescence as skin-colored papules that later become crusted. The affected area exhibits numerous warty elevations that are 2 to 4 mm in diameter.

Pathology

Microscopically, the warty papule shows a cleft above the basal layer. Above and to the side of the cleft, **dyskeratotic cells** with eosinophilic cytoplasm are defined by keratin fibrils that whorl about the nucleus (Fig. 24-12). The roof of the cleft is formed by a cone of compact keratotic material. In the stratum spi-

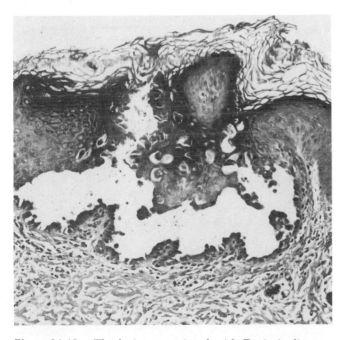

Figure 24-12. The lesion associated with Darier's disease is a suprabasal cleft caused by focal dyskeratosis of keratinocytes. It is not a true vesicle, as most true vesicles contain inflammatory cells, which are noticeably absent here. The dyskeratosis is further evidenced by the cells in the cornified material (above the cleft) that are surrounded by clear lacunae.

nosum, some of these cells, called **corps ronds,** have pyknotic nuclei, whereas the eosinophilic, seedlike remains of dyskeratotic cells in the stratum corneum are called **corps grains.**

Psoriasis: Epidermal-Dermal Disease Characterized by Persistent Epidermal Hyperplasia

Definition and Clinical Features

Psoriasis is a chronic, frequently familial, worldwide disease that affects 1 to 2 percent of the population. **In its classical form it is characterized by large, erythematous, scaly plaques commonly observed on the extensor-dorsal cutaneous surfaces.** The severity of the disease varies from annoying scaly lesions over the elbows to a serious debilitating disorder, involving most of the skin, which at times may be associated with arthritis. A single lesion of psoriasis may be a small focus of scaly erythema or an enormous confluent plaque covering much of the trunk. A typical plaque is 4 to 5 cm in diameter, is sharply demarcated at its margin, and has a surface of silvery scales. When the scales are detached, pinpoint foci of bleeding dot the underlying glossy erythematous surface. Diseases that tend to simulate psoriasis clinically, such as seborrheic dermatitis, are said to be **psoriasiform.** Diseases characterized histologically by epidermal hyperplasia and preservation and exaggeration of the rete papillae pattern are also termed psoriasiform.

Pathology

A psoriasiform appearance is one of the common patterns of cutaneous pathology. For example, seborrheic dermatitis (severe dandruff with associated scaly erythema of the nasolabial fold and midline of the chest), reaction to chronic trauma (lichen simplex chronicus), and cutaneous T-cell lymphoma (mycosis fungoides) all may exhibit a psoriasiform epidermal change. Psoriasis, which by definition is the prototype of the psoriasiform disorders, is a disease of intermittent activity and variable presentation. These variations are related to the degree of influence of heritable factors, as well as to the amount of neutrophilic chemotactic factors produced in a given lesion or patient. Familial psoriasis is usually severe. In some variations of the disease, neutrophilic pustules dominate the pathologic process. The most distinctive pathologic changes are seen at the periphery of a classical psoriatic plaque. **The epidermis is thickened and shows both hyperkeratosis and parakeratosis.** Parakeratosis may present as circumscribed, ellipsoid foci, or it may be diffuse, in which case the

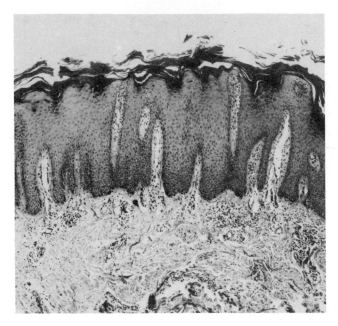

Figure 24-13. In psoriasis, the rete ridges are uniformly elongated. The dermal papillae are elongated, and some present prominent, elongated venules.

granular layer is diminished or absent. The nucleated layers of the epidermis are thickened several-fold in the rete, and frequently are thinner over the dermal papillae (Fig. 24-13). The papillae, in turn, are elongated and appear as sections of cones, with their apices toward the dermis. In chronic lesions, the papillae may appear as bulbous clubs with short handles (Fig. 24-14). The rete ridges of the epidermis have a profile reciprocal to that of the dermal papillae, and the skin shows interlocked mesenchymal and epithelial clubs with alternating reversed polarity (see Fig. 24-14). The capillaries of the papillae are dilated and tortuous. Electron micrographs show the capillaries to be venule-like; neutrophils may emerge at their tips and migrate into the epidermis above the apices of the papillae. The acute inflammatory cells may become localized in the epidermal spinous layer, or in small collections in the stratum corneum and be associated with circumscribed areas of parakeratosis (Fig. 24-15). The dermis, below the papillae, exhibits a varying number of mononuclear inflammatory cells, which are mostly lymphocytes, about the superficial vascular plexus. There is little extension of the inflammatory process into the subjacent reticular dermis.

Etiology and Pathogenesis

In psoriasis, the entire skin—both that with lesions and that without—is abnormal. About one third of affected patients have a family history of the disease. The more severe the disease, the greater is the likelihood of a familial background. A variety of inductive stimuli, such as physical injury, infection, and photosensitivity, may produce characteristic lesions in clinically normal skin. The pathogenesis of the psoriatic plaques may be appreciated by contrasting the effect of chronic cutaneous trauma in persons with and without psoriasis. Chronic trauma (for instance, that caused by rubbing) of the skin of a normal person produces a tough, scaly, cutaneous plaque that is psoriasiform both clinically and histologically. However, with cessation of the trauma, the lesion disappears. In the psoriatic patient, even less severe trauma produces a distinctive psoriatic plaque that may persist for years after the initial injury. Although there is no universally accepted explanation for this unique response to injury, evidence suggests that a **deregulation of epidermal proliferation and an abnormality in the microcirculation of the dermis are responsible** (Fig. 24-16). This abnormal proliferation is probably related to defective epidermal cell surface receptors. For example, the beta-adrenergic receptors are thought to be defective in psoriasis. The faulty surface receptors are associated with a decrease in the activity of adenylate cyclase which, in turn,

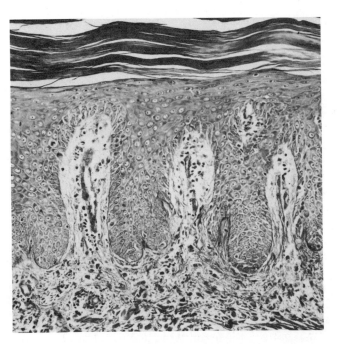

Figure 24-14. Psoriasis with clubbed papillae and prominent venules. The papillae and venules present an interlocking pattern of alternately reversed "clubs." The prominent venules are part of the venulization of capillaries that is of histogenetic importance in psoriasis.

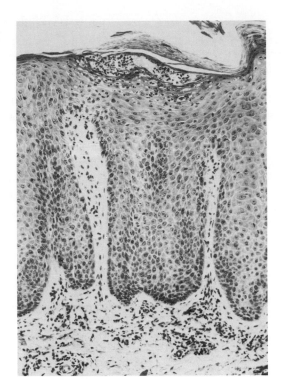

Figure 24-15. Intraepidermal neutrophils are a manifestation of the transepidermal migration of these cells in psoriasis. They emerge from the venulized capillaries at the tips of the dermal papillae and migrate to the location illustrated here. In time, they extend into the stratum corneum, which commonly is parakeratotic, as shown in this micrograph.

diminishes cAMP (cyclic 3',5' adenosine monophosphate) in the lower proliferative compartment of the epidermis. The decrease in cAMP alters cutaneous responses to trauma in complex ways that are not fully understood, but there appears to be a growth factor effect and induction of neutrophilic inflammation. The growth factor effect operates through an increase in cAMP-regulated proteinases and augmented polyamines of low molecular weight. The induction of neutrophilic inflammation follows an increase in phospholipase A_2, which enhances the production of arachidonic acid. This, in turn, through its lipoxygenase metabolites—notably, leukotriene B4 (LTB-4)—has a potent chemotactic effect (see Fig. 24-16). The capillary loops of the dermal papillae become venular, showing multiple layers of basal lamina material, wide lumina, and bridged fenestrations between endothelial cells. This vascular change, which is associated with a striking increase in neutrophilic chemotactic factors, causes extrusion of many neutrophils at the tips of the dermal papillae, after which

the inflammatory cells migrate through the epidermis. This unusual pattern of neutrophilic inflammation is responsible for the dense collections of neutrophils in the stratum corneum, as well as for the scattering of neutrophils throughout the epidermis. Thus, psoriasis involves latent defects in the epidermis and dermis that contribute to a fully developed psoriatic plaque. The complex pathogenetic mechanisms likely to be operative in psoriasis are depicted in Figure 24-16.

Quite recently severe intractable psoriasis has been observed in some patients with AIDS. The pathogenetic mechanism responsible for psoriasis in these immunocompromised patients is not known, but could be related to an imbalance in the T-cell system.

Dyshesive Disorders

Pemphigus

Definition and Clinical Features
The term pemphigus, derived from the Greek *pemphix*, meaning bubble, defines a blistering disease. All blistering diseases were once classified as pemphigus. **Pemphigus vulgaris is but one of a group of diseases characterized by blister formation secondary to diminished cohesiveness (dyshesion) of epidermal cells. This dyshesion is related to the reaction of autoantibodies to surface antigens on the cells of stratified squamous epithelia.** Pemphigus vulgaris, a severe dyshesive disorder usually fatal without corticosteroid therapy, is the prototype for this group of blistering diseases. The characteristic lesion of pemphigus vulgaris is a large, easily ruptured blister that leaves extensive denuded or crusted areas. The lesions are most common on the scalp and mucous membranes, and in the periumbilical and intertriginous areas. Without treatment, the disease is progressive, and much of the epidermis may become denuded.

Pathology
The blister in pemphigus vulgaris forms because of the separation of the stratum spinosum and outer epidermal layers from the basal layer. This suprabasal dyshesion results in a blister that has the intact basal layer as a floor and the remaining epidermis as a roof (Figs. 24-17 and 24-18). The vesicle contains a moderate number of lymphocytes, macrophages, eosinophils, neutrophils, and distinctive, rounded keratinocytes that shed into the vesicle during the process of dyshesion. These keratinocytes are called **acantholytic cells,** a term that implies "lysis of a

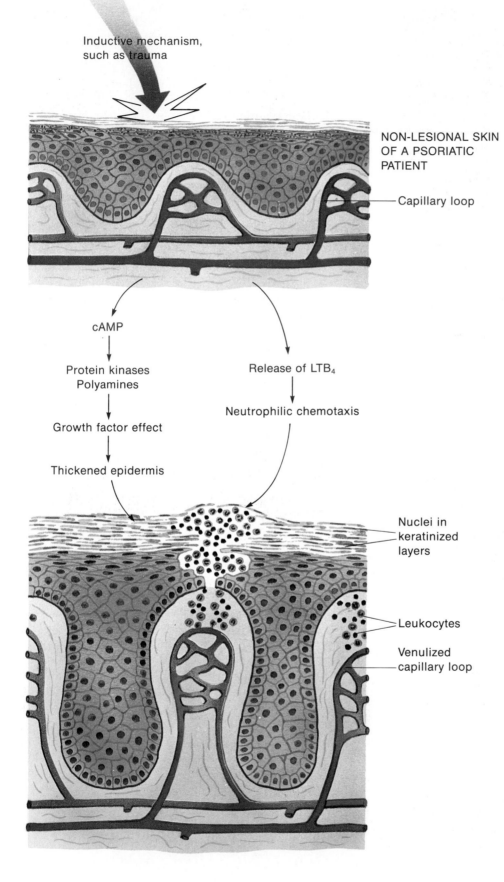

Inductive mechanism,
such as trauma

NON-LESIONAL SKIN
OF A PSORIATIC
PATIENT

Capillary loop

cAMP

Protein kinases
Polyamines

Release of LTB$_4$

Growth factor effect

Neutrophilic chemotaxis

Thickened epidermis

Nuclei in
keratinized
layers

Leukocytes

Venulized
capillary loop

Figure 24-16. Pathogenetic mechanisms in psoriasis. The drawing depicts the deregulation of epidermal growth, venulization of the capillary loop, and a unique form of neutrophilic inflammation. The altered epidermal growth is thought to be caused by defective epidermal cell surface receptors. This results in a decrease in cAMP, together with the effects indicated. The decrease in cAMP is also likely to be related to the increased production of arachidic acid which, in turn, leads to activation of LTB-4. This potent neutrophilic chemotactic agent acts on a venulized capillary loop. Neutrophils then emerge from the tips of the capillary loop at the apex of the dermal papilla, rather than from the postcapillary venule, as is the rule in most inflammatory skin diseases.

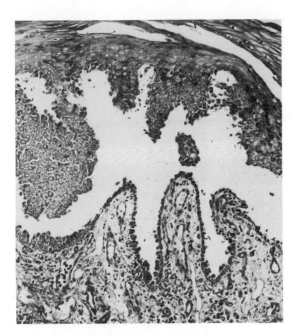

Figure 24-17. Suprabasal dyshesion in pemphigus vulgaris. A classic suprabasal vesicle is evident.

spine." These keratinocytes had a fancied resemblance to a spiny leafed plant of the genus acanthus. Before the fine structure of the epidermis was clarified, it was thought that a fine fibril of keratin coursed from epidermal cell to epidermal cell through the desmosome, forming a small spine, or spike, as it left the cell. Pemphigus vulgaris was thus thought to develop by dissolution of this spine—hence, the name acantholysis. It is now known that the flawed cohesiveness of the epidermal cells that is characteristic of this disorder is due to the action of proteases on many of the epidermal cohesive forces, and does not simply reflect "dissolution of the spine." Consequently, the term dyshesion aptly describes the "flawed sticking" of the epidermal cells in this disease. The dyshesion may extend along the adnexa, and is not always strictly suprabasal. The subjacent dermis shows a moderate infiltrate of lymphocytes, macrophages, eosinophils, and neutrophils, predominantly about the capillary venular bed. Occasionally, eosinophils are numerous.

Etiology and Pathogenesis
There are specific circulating autoantibodies in pemphigus, as well as *in vivo*-bound IgG in the intercellular substance of the epidermis and other stratified squamous epithelia. Electron microscopy suggests that the antibody reacts with a component of the outer layer of the epidermal plasma membrane. The

circulating antibodies in patients with pemphigus vulgaris react with an epidermal surface antigen that is not species-specific, and is found in other mammals and birds. It is not known whether the autoantibody reflects an alteration of the immune system (as in a breakdown of immune tolerance) or a change in the antigen, rendering it "non-self." Pemphigus may be associated with other autoimmune diseases, such as myasthenia gravis and lupus erythematous, and may also be seen with benign thymomas. The clinical activity of the disease correlates with the titer of pemphigus autoantibodies. The autoantibodies are related to the dyshesion, and the purified antibodies can induce dyshesion in animal skin. Moreover, antibodies produced in rabbits in response to the administration of purified antigen cause lesions similar to pemphigus in the skin of the newborn mouse.

By what mechanism does antigen-antibody union at the cell surface diminish epidermal cohesiveness and lead to vesicle formation? The function and precise nature of the antigen in pemphigus is unknown. If it is related to cell-to-cell adhesion, an antibody to pemphigus antigen could directly induce dyshesion. However, present evidence suggests that the binding

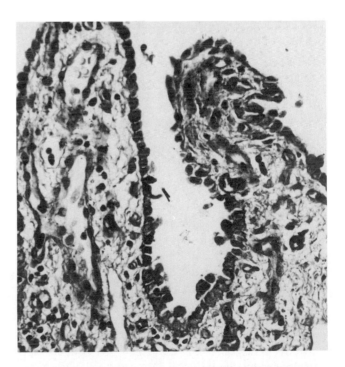

Figure 24-18. Higher power magnification of the suprabasal dyshesion in pemphigus vulgaris. The crisply delineated basal cells, slightly separated from each other and completely separated from the stratum spinosum, are still firmly attached to the basement membrane zone.

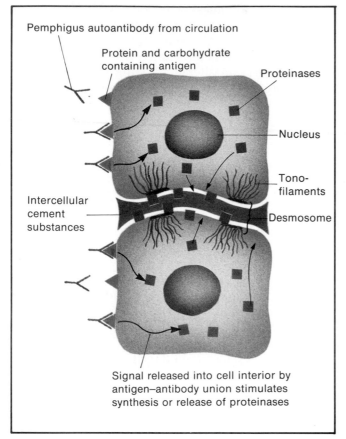

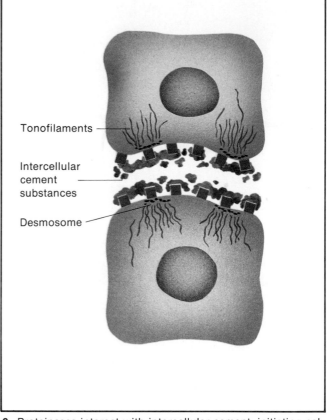

1. Antigen–antibody union activates intracellular proteinases.

2. Proteinases interact with intercellular cement, initiating cellular dyshesion (acantholysis).

Figure 24-19. The pathogenetic mechanisms of suprabasal dyshesion in pemphigus vulgaris. A circulating autoantibody of unknown origin reacts with an antigen on the outer leaflet of the plasma membrane of epidermal cells, especially in the basilar regions. (*1*) Antigen-antibody union results in release of a proteinase (plasmin). (*2*) The proteinase interacts with intercellular cement, initiating dyshesion.

of antibody to this antigen causes an increase in synthesis of plasminogen activator and, hence, activation of plasmin. This proteolytic enzyme acts on the intercellular substance and is probably the dominant factor in dyshesion. Cytopathologic processes within the cell may also contribute to dyshesion. Internalization of the antigen-antibody complex, disappearance of attachment plaques, and perinuclear tonofilament retraction all may act in concert with proteinases to cause dyshesion and vesiculation (Fig. 24-19).

Related Diseases
Other diseases caused by dyshesion that have a pathogenetic mechanism similar to that of pemphigus vulgaris include pemphigus vegetans, pemphigus foliaceus, Brazilian pemphigus foliaceus, and pemphigus erythematosus. The specific antigen of pemphigus foliaceus and Brazilian pemphigus, called desmoglein I, is in the desmosomes of the outer spinous and granular layers. Consequently, autoantibodies to desmoglein I cause dyshesion in the outer spinous and granular epidermal layers (Fig. 24-20). These differences between the various forms of pemphigus are outlined in Table 24-2. Other maladies may simulate the histologic appearance of pemphigus vulgaris—notably, familial benign chronic pemphigus and transient acantholytic dermatosis—but none of these histologic stimulants show IgG antibodies reacting with epidermal antigen.

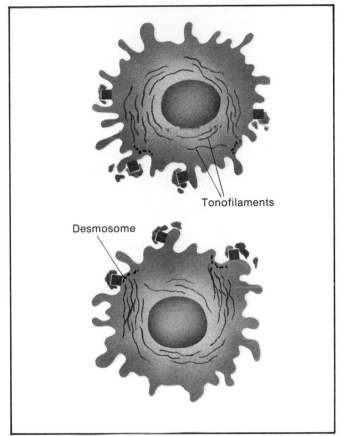

3. Complete dyshesion (acantholysis). Acantholytic cells separate, round up, and form micropapillary projections on the cell surface. Desmosomes deteriorate and tonofilaments clump about nucleus.

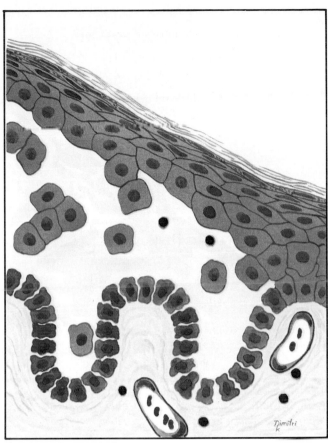

4. Intraepidermal bulla

Figure 24-19 (continued). *(3)* Desmosomes deteriorate, tonofilaments clump about the nucleus, the cells round up, and separation is complete. *(4)* A vesicle, which is usually suprabasal, forms.

Diseases Primarily Affecting the Basement Membrane Zone: Pathology of the Dermal-Epidermal Interface

Blister Formation Due to Dermal-Epidermal Separation

Epidermolysis Bullosa

Definition and Clinical Features

The term epidermolysis bullosa embraces a heterogeneous group of disorders, loosely held together by being hereditary and by a tendency to form blisters at sites of minor trauma. The diseases vary from a minor annoyance to a widespread, life-threatening, blistering disease. Although as many as 16 varieties of epidermolysis bullosa have been recorded, only a few representative examples of this class of disease will be discussed. An appreciation of the clinical significance of these blistering diseases requires an understanding of the exact structure within the dermal-epidermal interface where separation occurs, the clinical presentation of the disease, and the type of inheritance. Although a few apparently specific biochemical abnormalities have been described in some of the variants of epidermolysis bullosa, these have not been easily or definitively related to pathogensis.

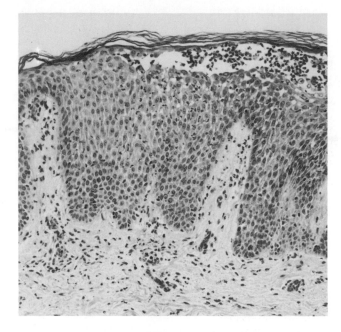

Figure 24-20. Dyshesion in the outer spinous layer in pemphigus foliaceus. Compare the distinctive site of separation, illustrated here, with that in pemphigus vulgaris (see Figure 24-18). The offending antigen in pemphigus foliaceus is in the outer spinous layers; thus, separation occurs at this site.

Table 24-2 Diseases of the Pemphigus Group
Reactive Antibodies of the IgG Type to Antigen on the Plasma Membrane of
Stratified Squamous Epithelia or to Desmosomal Antigen

	CLINICAL FEATURES	PATHOLOGY
Pemphigus vulgaris	Flaccid, easily ruptured bullae commonly involving the scalp, periumbilical region, intertriginous areas, and mucous membranes. Commonly occurs during fourth and fifth decades of life. Occurs predominantly in people of Jewish origin and other Mediterranean peoples. Frequently fatal if untreated.	Suprabasal vesicle with a sparse infiltrate of lymphocytes, macrophages, and eosinophils.
Pemphigus vegetans	A variant of pemphigus vulgaris, but healing in intertriginous areas is characterized by complex papillary epidermal hyperplasia, resulting in verrucous or vegetating lesions.	The same as for pemphigus vulgaris with superimposed extensive epidermal hyperplasia. Eosinophils may be numerous, and may be disposed in the nests in the epidermis.
Pemphigus foliaceous	Bullae occur early on, but may not be present. The disease may be eczematoid, with shallow erosions, scales, and crusting. The scalp, face, throat, back, and abdomen are commonly involved, but mucous membrane involvement is uncommon. Not fatal if untreated. Question of slight predominance in Jews.	Dyshesion is in the spinous layer. Granular cells may peel apart; appearance is of shedding granular cells one by one. Variable number of inflammatory cells. Neutrophils may be numerous with formation of subcorneal pustules. Antibody is in desmosomes of the outer epidermal layers.
Brazilian pemphigus foliaceous	Clinically and immunologically identical to pemphigus foliaceous. Occurs in two rural areas of south central Brazil as a common endemic disease. Two-thirds of patients are women. Common in children and young adults.	Same as for pemphigus foliaceous
Pemphigus erythematosus	Similar to pemphigus foliaceous, but dominated by a lupus-like area on the butterfly area of the face. Immunologically, patients have pemphigus antibodies *and* the autonuclear antibodies and immune complex deposits of lupus.	Same as for pemphigus foliaceous

Table 24-3 Classification of Epidermolysis Bullosa (Selected Variants)

CLASS	SITE OF BLISTER FORMATION	NAME OF VARIANT	HEALING RESIDUUM	HEREDITY
Epidermolytic	Within the basal keratino-cytic layer	Localized epidermolysis bullosa simplex	None	Autosomal dominant
		Generalized epidermolysis bullosa simplex	None	Autosomal dominant
Junctional	Lamina lucida	Epidermolysis bullosa letalis	None or atrophic scars	Autosomal recessive
		Generalized atrophic benign epidermolysis bullosa	Atrophic scars	Autosomal recessive
Dermolytic	Immediately deep to the lamina densa	Dystrophic epidermolysis bullosa (hyperplastic variant)	Hyperplastic scars Nails deformed	Autosomal dominant
		Dystrophic epidermolysis bullosa	Scars Teeth and nails deformed	Autosomal recessive

Thus, the classification is anatomic, and is based upon the site of blister formation in the basement membrane zone:

Epidermolytic epidermolysis bullosa—Blister formation occurs as a result of disruption of the integrity of the keratinocytic basal cells.

Junctional epidermolysis bullosa—Blisters form within the lamina lucida.

Dermolytic epidermolysis bullosa—Blisters are located immediately deep to the lamina densa and are apparently related to flaws of the anchoring fibrils.

Accompanying each of these primary forms of epidermolysis bullosa are clinical presentations that are either innocuous or severe. Junctional or dermolytic blisters may be associated with abnormalities of the nails and teeth. As a rule, healing proceeds differently in the various classes of epidermolysis bullosa. The epidermolytic forms (so-called simplex) heal without scarring; the junctional form heals without scarring, or with residual flat, shiny areas (atrophic lesions); and the dermolytic form heals with scarring (dystrophic lesions). All forms of epidermolytic disease are autosomal dominant, whereas all varieties of junctional epidermolysis bullosa are autosomal recessive. Dermolytic disease may be either dominant or recessive, the latter being more severe. This classification is outlined in Table 24-3.

Pathology

In cases of epidermolysis bullosa, a cursory inspection with low-power magnification of hematoxylin and eosin preparations shows a subepidermal vesicle with few inflammatory cells in the dermis. The proper classification of vesiculation in epidermolysis bullosa requires periodic acid-Schiff (PAS) staining of paraffin and plastic embedded materials and, occasionally, low-power electron microscopy. These methods, applied to the study of early vesicles or to sites of deliberate minor trauma prior to vesiculation, demonstrate the different mechanisms of blister formation that underlie each of the three major categories of epidermolysis bullosa (Fig. 24-21).

Epidermolytic Epidermolysis Bullosa In epidermolytic epidermolysis bullosa, intracellular edema below the nuclei of the basal keratinocytes precedes vacuolization in this area, eventual disruption of the basal cell plasma membranes, and the formation of an intraepidermal vesicle. The roof of the vesicle is an almost intact epidermis with a fragmented basal layer, whereas its floor shows bits of basal cell cytoplasm attached to the lamina densa, which is seen as a well-preserved pink line at the base of the vesicle. Inflammatory cells are sparse.

Junctional Epidermolysis Bullosa The roof of the vesicle formed in junctional epidermolysis bullosa is preserved epidermis, and the plasma membranes of the basal cells remain intact. The floor of the vesicle is an intact lamina densa, as in epidermolysis bullosa, but the attached fragments of basal cell cytoplasm are lacking. The split that initiates the blister occurs within the lamina lucida. Both lesional and non-lesional skin show fewer hemidesmosomes, which have poorly developed attachment plaques and subbasal dense plates.

Dermolytic Epidermolysis Bullosa The roof of the

EPIDERMOLYTIC

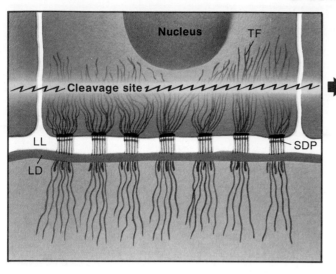
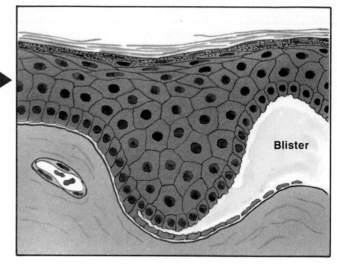

JUNCTIONAL

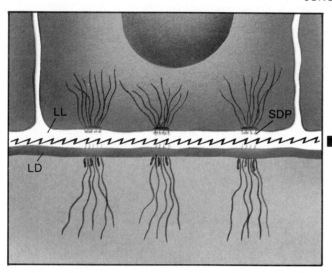
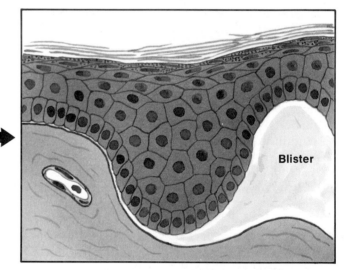

DERMOLYTIC

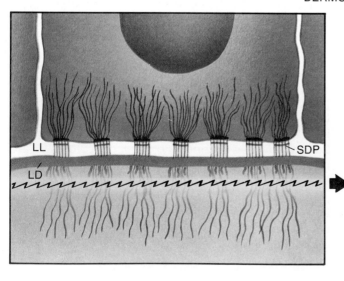
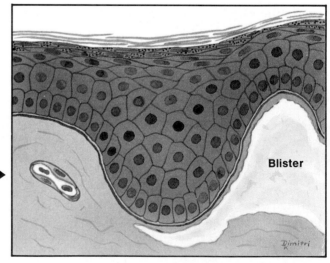

vesicle seen in dermolytic epidermolysis bullosa is normal epidermis with an attached, intact lamina lucida and lamina densa. The base of the vesicle is formed by the outer part of the papillary dermis. Electron microscopy reveals rudimentary anchoring fibrils which are decreased in number. Such changes are present in lesional and non-lesional skin in the severe, autosomal recessive form of the disease.

Pathogenesis

In general, the pathogenesis of epidermolysis bullosa cannot be explained by the heritable biochemical defects that have been described in a few forms of the illness. For example, although gelatinase activity in cultured fibroblasts is greatly decreased in a generalized form of epidermolytic epidermolysis bullosa, it does not explain the basal cell cytolysis. Increased degradation of chondroitin sulfate in the skin has been reported in one form of dermolytic epidermolysis bullosa, but this does not explain the abnormality in anchoring fibrils. Although the pathogenesis of dermolytic epidermolysis bullosa remains vague, some clues are emerging, based on the following observations:

- Anchoring fibrils are diminished in number. When skin from recessive dermolytic epidermolysis bullosa is grafted onto a chorioallantoic membrane, anchoring fibrils do not form.
- The fibroblasts of dermolytic epidermolysis bullosa synthesize excessive collagenase.
- A noncollagenous component of the lamina densa has been shown to be defective.

In summary, **the dermolytic forms of epidermolysis bullosa involve extensive flaws in the dermal component of the basement membrane zone, including malformation of anchoring fibrils, excessive breakdown of collagen, and a defect in a critical structural protein of the lamina densa.**

Bullous Pemphigoid

Definition and Clinical Features

Bullous pemphigoid is a blistering disease with clinical similarities to pemphigus vulgaris, hence the name "pemphigoid." The disease has a predilection for the later decades of life, but has no significant racial or sexual prevalence. The blisters are large and tense, and may appear on normal-appearing skin or on an erythematous base. The medial thighs and flexor aspect of the forearm are commonly affected, but the groin, axilla, and other cutaneous sites may also develop blisters. The disease is self-limited but chronic, and the patient's general health is usually unaffected. The course of the disease is greatly shortened by systemic steroids.

Pathology

The blisters of pemphigoid are subepidermal, with the roof of the blister being formed by an intact epidermis, and the base by the lamina densa of the basement membrane zone (Figs. 24-22 and 24-23). The blister contains fibrin, lymphocytes, neutrophils, and eosinophils, with the last usually appearing as the dominant cell form. Vesicles that contain only sparse eosinophils are designated as cell-poor bullous pemphigoid. Even before becoming erythematous, the normal skin around the lesions of pemphigoid shows mast cell migration from the venule toward the epidermis. With the onset of erythema, eosinophils appear in the upper dermis and are occasionally arranged in a linear array at the basement membrane zone. By electron microscopy, the first site of dermal-epidermal separation is in the lamina lucida, and is associated with disruption of anchoring filaments.

Etiology and Pathogenesis

The cause of bullous pemphigoid is unknown. It is thought to be an autoimmune disease, and is characterized by circulating IgG antibodies to a normal

---

Figure 24-21. Three distinct mechanisms of blister formation in epidermolysis bullosa. Electron microscopic images are on the left, whereas light microscopic images are depicted on the right. **Epidermolytic epidermolysis bullosa** is caused by disintegration of the lowermost regions of the epidermal basal cells. The bottom portions of the basal cells cleave, and the remainder of the epidermis lifts away. Small fragments of basal cells remain attached to the basement membrane zone. **Junctional epidermolysis bullosa** is characterized by cleavage in the lamina lucida. **Dermolytic epidermolysis bullosa** is associated with rudimentary and fragmented anchoring fibrils. The entire basement membrane zone and epidermis split away from the dermis in relationship to these flawed anchoring fibrils. *LL,* lamina lucida; *LD,* lamina densa; *SDP,* subdesmosomal dense plate.

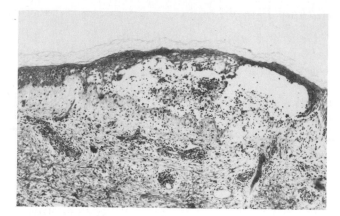

Figure 24-22.   Subepidermal vesicle in bullous pemphigoid. Inflammatory cells are prominent in the vesicle and in the dermis.

glycoprotein of the lamina lucida in or near the basal keratinocyte hemidesmosome. This glycoprotein, known as BP-antigen, together with laminin and anchoring filaments, contributes to dermal-epidermal adherence. Most cases of pemphigoid display a linear deposit of IgG and C3 in the lamina lucida of the basement membrane zone. The BP-antigen–antibody complex in the lamina lucida may injure the basal cell plasma membrane through the formation of C5b-C9 membrane attack complex, and this damage might interfere with the elaboration of adherence factors by

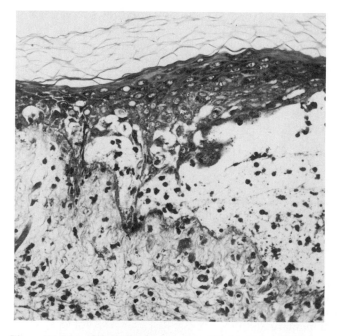

Figure 24-23.   The subepidermal vesicle is above the lamina densa (*arrows*) in bullous pemphigoid.

basal cells. Of greater importance is the production of the anaphylatoxins C3a and C5a following activation of complement. In turn, these anaphylatoxins cause degranulation of mast cells and the release of factors that are chemotactic for eosinophils, neutrophils, and lymphocytes. The eosinophilic granules contain tissue-damaging substances, including eosinophil peroxidase and major basic protein. These, together with proteases of neutrophilic and mast cell origin, cause dermal-epidermal separation, primarily within the lamina lucida (Fig. 24-24). Protease inhibitors, such as alpha$_2$–macroglobulin, block dermal-epidermal separation in normal skin cultured with pemphigoid blister fluid. Although a dense inflammatory infiltrate eventually causes extensive destruction of the entire basement membrane zone, the primary site of dermal-epidermal change in pemphigoid remains within the lamina lucida, the site of antigen-antibody union.

Dermatitis Herpetiformis

Definition and Clinical Features

Dermatitis herpetiformis is an intriguing disease characterized by urticaria-like plaques, which may develop small vesicles, over the extensor surfaces of the body. The lesions are especially prominent over the elbows, knees, and buttocks. The intensely pruritic vesicles may become grouped in a fashion similar to herpes. Because they are so pruritic, emerging vesicles may be rubbed until broken, and a patient may first present with crusted lesions only, and no intact vesicles. Although the disease is of varying severity and is characterized by remissions, it is disturbingly chronic. The healing lesions often leave scars. **The ailment is related to gluten sensitivity in patients of the HLA-B8/DRW3 haplotype; most of these patients also have a gluten sensitivity enteropathy.** The cutaneous lesions are related to deposits of granular IgA at the dermal-epidermal interface, mainly at the tips of the dermal papillae.

Pathology

The pathologic changes associated with dermatitis herpetiformis are best appreciated by studying sequential biopsies over a 72-hour period after cessation of therapy. Dapsone or sulfapyridine completely control the signs and symptoms of the disease, probably by inhibiting the inflammatory cascade and neutrophilic lysosomal functions. Twenty-four hours after cessation of therapy, however, patients develop erythematous, urticarial plaques about the elbows and knees. In these lesions, concomitant with the emergence of a delicate perivenular lymphocytic infiltrate,

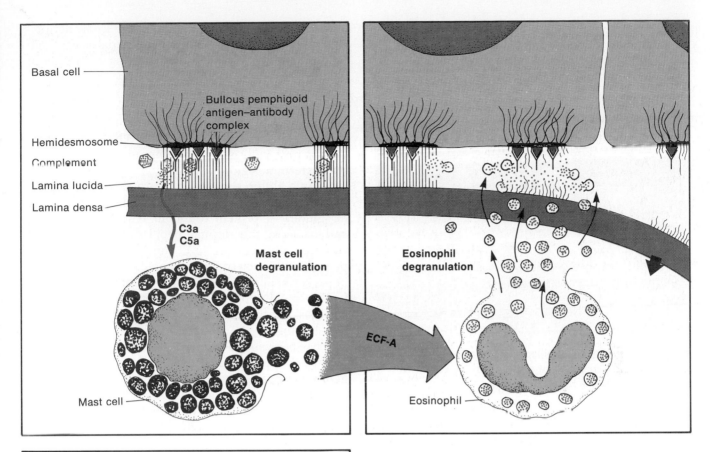

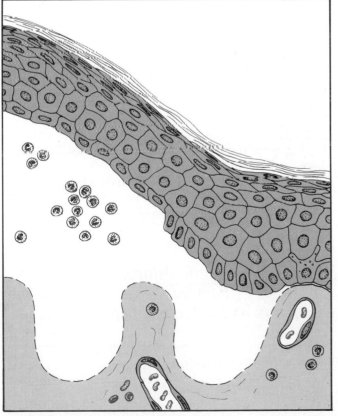

Figure 24-24. Pathogenetic mechanisms of blister formation in bullous pemphigoid. A circulating antibody to an apparently normal glycoprotein—BP antigen—in the lamina lucida precipitates the pathogenetic events in bullous pemphigoid. *A*, Antigen-antibody union activates complement, and the anaphylatoxins C3a and C5a are produced. These degranulate mast cells, resulting in release of eosinophilic chemotactic factor. *B* and *C*, the tissue-damaging substances of eosinophilic granules cause vesicle formation at the lamina lucida, with some breakdown of the lamina densa (ECF-A—Eosinophil chemotactic factor-A).

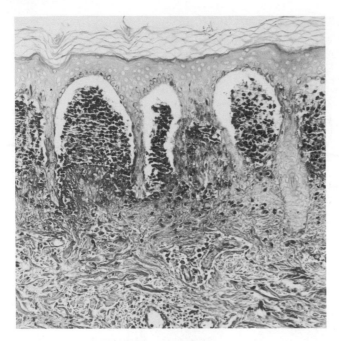

Figure 24-25.   Dermal papillary abscesses with early dermal-epidermal separation at that site are essentially unique to dermatitis herpetiformis.

a row of neutrophils appears immediately deep to the lamina densa. Within 36 hours, **the neutrophils aggregate in clusters of 10 to 25 at the tips of the dermal papillae, to create a highly distinctive, essentially diagnostic histologic picture.** There are two related mechanisms of dermal-epidermal separation. In one, associated with the sheetlike spread of a layer or two of neutrophils at the dermal-epidermal interface, the entire epidermis detaches from the papillary dermis, carrying the basement membrane zone with it (Fig. 24-25). The roof of such a vesicle contains the intact lamina densa, whereas the floor is made up of papillary dermis with a prominent neutrophilic infiltrate. In striking contrast to bullous pemphigoid, eosinophils are uncommon early in the course of dermatitis herpetiformis. When an increased number of neutrophils rapidly accumulate at the tips of dermal papillae, the release of large amounts of neutrophilic lysosomal enzymes in the outer portion of the dermal papillae results in **the uncoupling of the epidermis from the dermis at the tips of dermal papillae, disruption of the basement membrane zone in the outer part of the papillae, and tearing of the epidermis across the adjacent rete ridges. In the resulting vesicle, the roof has alternating tears across its epidermal covering, whereas the floor shows residual epidermal pegs alternating with the basal half of dermal papillae.** Regardless of the kind of vesicle formed, eosinophils appear late within the dermal

infiltrate and extend deeply into the reticular dermis, deeper than in other vesiculobullous diseases. Such an extension is responsible for scarring at the site of some vesicles.

Etiology and Pathogenesis

The patients with dermatitis herpetiformis are, for the most part, of the HLA-B8/DRW3 haplotype. This locus is physically close to the immune response gene that determines gluten sensitivity, and most patients develop a gluten sensitivity enteropathy, although it may be only minimally expressed. There is a receptor for gluten—a protein found in wheat, barley, rye, and oats—in the dermal papillae of human skin. Granular deposits of IgA immune complexes are present at the tips of dermal papillae, and are greater in perilesional skin than in non-lesional skin. Importantly, a gluten-free diet controls the disease, whereas reintroduction of dietary gluten provokes new lesions.

It has been suggested that patients of the B8/DRW3 haplotype express two genes. One is responsible for gluten sensitivity enteropathy, while the other controls dimeric IgA antibody formation in response to partially digested forms of gluten and other dietary proteins that pass through a defective mucosal epithelial barrier that has been damaged by gluten sensitivity. The resultant IgA immune complexes are deposited in the skin at gluten receptor sites, where they accumulate at locations, such as the elbow, that frequently sustain trauma.

IgA immune complexes are inefficient in complement activation, and only a few neutrophils are attracted to the site. However, the neutrophils elaborate the leukotrienes, which attract more neutrophils. Through their lysosomal enzymes, the epidermis is cleaved from the dermis. The immune complexes are deposited deep to the lamina densa in intimate relation to the collagen rootlets (microfibrils) which, along with anchoring fibrils, are important in the attachment of the lamina densa to the subjacent papillary dermis (Fig. 24-26).

Basal Keratinocytic Injury, Excessive Synthesis of Lamina Densa, and Immune Reactants at the Basement Membrane Zone

Lupus Erythematosus

Definition and Clinical Features

Systemic lupus erythematosus, the paradigm of human immune complex disease, is characterized by an excess of a variety of autoantibodies. The nature of the antibodies and their antigenic targets vary from patient to patient, as well as at different times in the same patient. The type of the immune complex and its site of deposition are responsible for the extremely variable symptoms and course of lupus. The organ systems involved include the kidney, the central nervous system, the joints and muscles, the hematopoietic system, the pleura, the lungs, the heart, the gastrointestinal tract, and the skin. Although cutaneous involvement may be severe and cosmetically devastating, it is not life-threatening. However, the nature and pattern of immune reactants in the skin serve as an excellent guide to the likelihood of systemic disease. The various forms of cutaneous lupus erythematosus have been classified as chronic (discoid), subacute, or acute. Chronic cutaneous lupus erythematosus is usually a disease of the skin alone. Subacute cutaneous lupus may be accompanied by involvement of the musculoskeletal system, but severe disease of other organs is uncommon. By contrast, acute cutaneous lupus is associated with serious involvement of a variety of organ systems, especially progressive renal disease.

The lesions of chronic cutaneous lupus erythematosus are generally above the neck—on the face, scalp, and ears. The lesions begin as slightly elevated, violaceous papules that have a rough scale of keratin on the surface. As they enlarge, the lesions assume a disklike appearance, with a hyperkeratotic margin and a depigmented center. This form of the disease is not associated with involvement of other organs. These cutaneous lesions may culminate in disfiguring scars.

Subacute cutaneous lupus erythematosus, a disease of young and middle-aged Caucasian women, differs from chronic cutaneous lupus erythematosus in a number of ways. The lesions are seen in the "V" area of the upper chest, upper back, and extensor surface of the arms, a distribution that suggests that light may have a role in the pathogenesis of this form of the disease. Indeed, photosensitivity is common. The early lesions are scaly erythematous papules, but they enlarge into psoriasiform or annular lesions which, in turn, may fuse. Significant scarring does not occur.

The most serious form of lupus—namely, acute systemic lupus erythematosus—may be associated with inconspicuous and transient acute cutaneous lesions. Frequently, the only manifestation is the **classic butterfly rash**—a delicate erythema of the malar area of the face that may pass in a few hours or a few days. Occasionally, the upper chest or extremities may be involved.

Pathology

There is an inverse relationship between the prominence of skin pathology and the extent of systemic pathology in lupus erythematosus. Chronic cutaneous lupus erythematosus (discoid lupus erythematosus) presents distinctive and diagnostic histologic changes, but is rarely associated with systemic pathology. The nucleated epidermal layers are modestly thickened or somewhat thin, but hyperkeratosis and plugging of hair follicles are prominent. The rete papillary pattern of the dermal epidermal interface is partially effaced (Fig. 24-27). Unique changes are seen in the basal cells and the basement membrane zone. The basal cells are vacuolated, and fibrillary bodies, which provide evidence of the death of keratinocytes (see the discussion of lichen planus that follows), are noted. The lamina densa is greatly thickened and reduplicated. On PAS staining, multiple layers of lamina densa are found to extend into the subjacent dermis. The excessive quantity of lamina densa, a product of the basal cells, reflects a response of basal cells to damage. **The vacuolated basal cells, the fibrillary bodies, and the alterations of the lamina densa all indicate one essential pathogenetic characteristic of lupus-induced skin disease—namely, injury to basal keratinocytes** (Figs. 24-28 and 24-29). A variety of immune complexes are present in the basement membrane zone. These are located predominantly deep to the lamina densa, but are also seen on the lamina densa and within the lamina lucida; a haphazard array is to be expected in a disease involving numerous, diverse antigens.

This pattern may be contrasted with that of bullous pemphigoid, in which there is but a single offending antigen precisely localized to the lamina lucida. In lupus, the basal keratinocytic layer and basement membrane zone also show a diffuse, only moderately dense, lymphocytic infiltrate that focally penetrates the basal layer. Deeper in the dermis, the lymphocytic infiltrate may be the most prominent feature of discoid lupus erythematosus. In this area, there are dense patches of mature lymphocytes that are positive for T4 and T8 cell markers. The cells are commonly disposed about the skin appendages. Resolving lesions may show fewer lymphocytes, but the lamina densa remains remarkably thickened, and there may be fibrosis of the papillary dermis.

The more severe the systemic lesions of lupus, the more subtle is the cutaneous pathology. For example, in subacute cutaneous lupus erythematosus, edema of the papillary dermis, thickening of the lamina densa, and prominent vacuolar degeneration of the basal layer are noted. There are some lymphocytes in the basement membrane zone, but deeper, dense

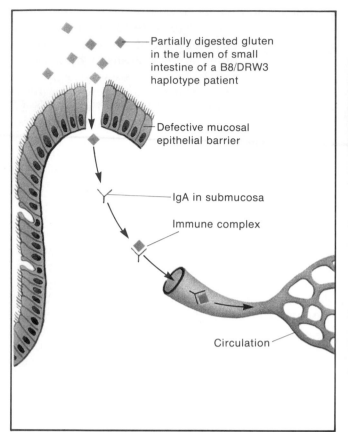

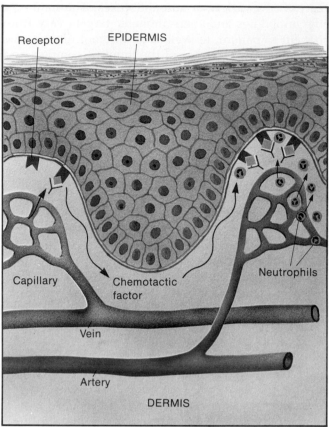

1. Formation of immune complexes in submucosa of small intestine. Passage of immune complexes into circulation.

2. Receptor–immune complex union releases neutrophil chemotactic factor. Neutrophils migrate to the tips of the papillae.

Figure 24-26. The pathogenesis of the cutaneous lesions in dermatitis herpetiformis. The disease is initiated in the small intestine and is expressed in the skin because of a gluten receptor immediately deep to the lamina densa.

patches of lymphocytes are not observed. By contrast, in acute cutaneous lupus erythematosus, in which progressive renal involvement is common, the earliest malar blush may show only edema of the papillary dermis. More commonly, the changes are similar to those in the subacute form of lupus, and are diagnostic. It follows then, that **the essential cutaneous pathology of lupus is seen in the basal keratinocytic layer, the basement membrane zone, and the papillary dermis.**

Etiology and Pathogenesis
As already noted, lupus erythematosus is characterized by a large number of different autoantibodies and the presence of immune complexes in the basement membrane zone of the kidney and the skin. Included among the antibodies are those against na-

tive (double-stranded) DNA, single-stranded DNA, small nuclear and cytoplasmic ribonuclear proteins, IgG, lymphocytes, and platelets. Antibodies against double-stranded DNA are not only diagnostic of systemic lupus, but also predict a high probability of renal involvement. On the other hand, antibodies against one of the small cytoplasmic ribonuclear proteins (Ross-A) is also indicative of systemic lupus erythematosus, but is associated with only a low incidence of renal involvement and a high incidence of photosensitivity. Although an impressive case can be made for the pathogenetic significance of immune complexes in renal diseases, they are not likely to be responsible for the production of cutaneous lesions. In this respect, immune complexes are present in both lesional and non-lesional skin in systemic lupus, so the deposition of immune reactants along the

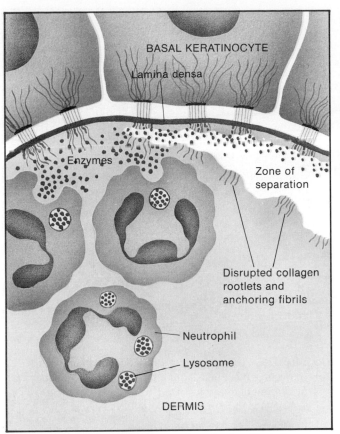

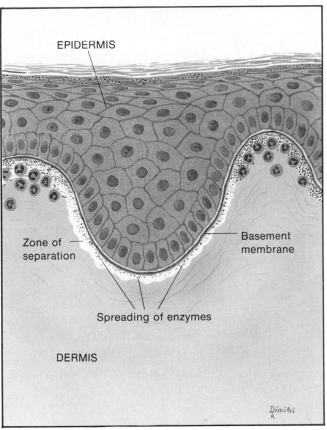

3. Dissolution of basal rootlets and anchoring fibrils by enzymes released by neutrophils. Early dermo-epidermal separation.

4. Concentration of neutrophils at the tips of the papillae. Spreading of enzymes along basement membrane. Lifting away of lamina densa.

basement membrane zone of "normal" skin (positive lupus band test) is important in the diagnosis of systemic lupus erythematosus.

The mechanisms underlying the pathology of the skin lesions of lupus are complex. First, epidermal injury seems to be caused by exogenous agents, such as ultraviolet light, and cell-mediated immune reactions similar to those in graft-versus-host disease. The manifestations of epidermal injury include vacuolization of basal cells with some diminution in epidermal thickness and hyperkeratosis, release of DNA and other nuclear and cytoplasmic antigen into the circulation, and deposition of DNA and other antigenic determinants in the basement membrane zone (lamina densa and immediately subjacent dermis) (Fig. 24-30). The deposition of circulating immune complexes in the kidney and skin is accompanied by

the local formation of immune complexes in the basal laminae of the two organs (see Fig. 24-30). **Thus, epidermal injury, local immune complex formation, and deposition of circulating complexes all seem to act in concert in the pathogenesis of cutaneous lupus.**

The course of the disease is clearly influenced by genetic and hormonal influences. Two HLA-DR antigens—DR2 and DR3—are more common in systemic lupus erythematosus. Commensurate with the dominance of this disease in women is the demonstration of altered estrogen metabolism in lupus patients of both sexes, who produce compounds, such as 16-α-hydroxyestrone, that have potent estrogenic activity. The underlying mechanisms of autoantibody production in lupus is the focus of much research effort. Presumably, B-cells frequently produce anti-

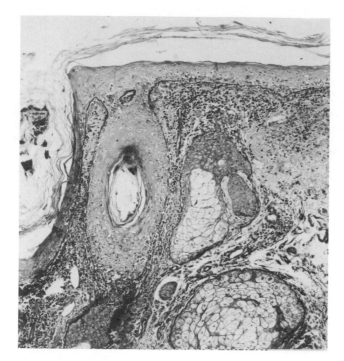

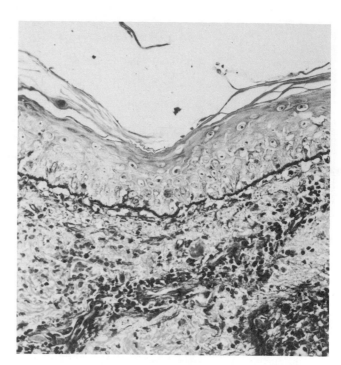

Figure 24-27. In lupus erythematosus, the lamina densa (the dark line separating the epidermis from the dermis) is thickened, and there is plugging of the hair follicle with keratin.

Figure 24-28. In this case of lupus erythematosus, the prominently thickened lamina densa with sublaminar vacuolization is evident.

bodies to circulating DNA and other antigens of exogenous or endogenous origin, but in normal individuals, such production is controlled by the action of suppressor T-cells. Antilymphocyte antibodies, or even a deficiency of suppressor T-cells, may impair this response. In concert with this possible flaw in T-cell suppressor activity, polyclonal B-cell hyperactivity in systemic lupus may then overwhelm the suppressor T-cell system.

Basal Keratinocytic Injury with a Lymphocytic Infiltrate Obscuring the Dermal-Epidermal Interface— Lichenoid Tissue Reactions and Diseases

Lichen Planus

Definition and Clinical Features
Disorders involving lichenoid tissue reactions are named because of a fancied or actual resemblance to certain lichens that form a scaly growth on rocks or tree trunks. Microscopically, lichen planus is distinguished by a **dense, bandlike infiltrate of lympho-**

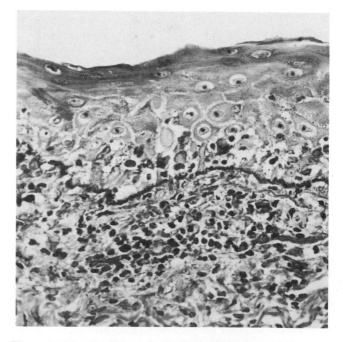

Figure 24-29. In this case of lupus erythematosus, the basal lamina is again prominently thickened. In this instance, the basal cells are vacuolated and poorly preserved, which is evidence of damage to these cells.

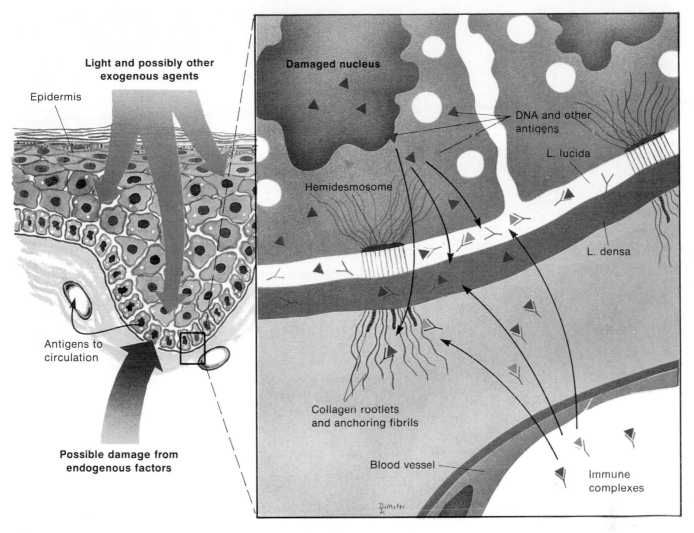

Figure 24-30.   In lupus erythematosus, there is epidermal generation of a variety of autoantibodies, as well as deposition of diverse immune complexes in and about the basement membrane zone. The epidermis is damaged by light, other exogenous agents, and endogenous mechanisms, especially cell-mediated immune reactions. Such injury releases a large number of antigens into the circulation, some of which return as immune complexes. Immune complexes are also formed in the skin, and the complexes are deposited throughout the basement membrane zone.

cytes and macrophages at the dermal-epidermal interface, which is frequently obscured by the infiltrate. This infiltrate is so characteristic that the term **lichenoid** is used to describe other diseases that have a similar histologic appearance. Lichen planus is characterized by violaceous, flat-topped papules that usually appear on the flexor surface of the wrists. White patches or streaks may also be present on the oral mucous membranes. The lesions may be pruritic and chronic, lasting one or more years.

Pathology

The prototypic disorder of the group is lichen planus itself. The lesions of this disease present with compact hyperkeratosis, with little or no parakeratosis. The stratum granulosum is thickened, frequently in distinctive, focal, wedge-shaped pattern. The base of the wedge abuts against the stratum corneum. The stratum spinosum is variably thickened. **The distinctive pathology is at the dermal-epidermal interface.** The basal layer is no longer a distinctive row of cu-

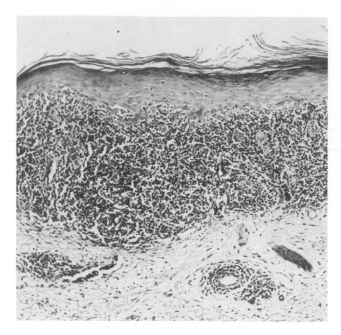

Figure 24-31. In lichen planus, there is a prominent bandlike lymphocytic infiltrate.

boidal cells, but is replaced by flattened or polygonal keratinocytes. The normal, gently undulating, interface, which passes from the dermal papilla to the rounded profile of the rete ridge, is replaced by papillae that are densely infiltrated with lymphocytes and macrophages and separated by sharply pointed (saw-toothed), inwardly projecting wedges of keratinocytes. The entire interface is obscured by the infiltrate of lymphocytes, macrophages, and melanophages (Fig. 24-31). Commonly admixed with the infiltrate (in the epidermis or dermis) are circular, fibrillary, eosinophilic bodies that are 15 to 20 μ in diameter (Figs. 24-32 and 24-33). These structures, which are variously termed colloid, Civatte, Sabouraud, or fibrillary bodies, are, in all likelihood, a manifestation of the focal death of keratinocytes. The fibrils within the bodies are similar to keratin filaments when studied by electron microscopy and with monoclonal antibodies. Histochemical studies of the fibrillary bodies have shown sulfhydryl cross-linking similar to that of the horny layer. An increased number of epidermal Langerhans cells is seen in early lichen planus. The lichenoid reactions that simulate lichen planus are more likely to show parakeratosis and eosinophils.

Etiology and Pathogenesis

The etiology of classic lichen planus is unknown, even though the disease is occasionally familial and,

at times, is associated with an increased incidence of glucose intolerance. The disease sometimes accompanies a variety of disorders thought to be autoimmune—for instance, lupus erythematosus, thymoma, myasthenia gravis, and ulcerative colitis. Drugs, such as gold, chlorothiazide, and chloroquine, may induce lichenoid reactions. External agents, such as color developer, may also evoke a lichenoid response. Finally, lichen planus-like lesions are commonly observed in the early stages of chronic graft-versus-host disease. These varied observations suggest that complex immunologic mechanisms are responsible for lichen planus. The morphologic manifestations of the disease—especially the fibrillary bodies that are thought to result from keratinocytic destruction and the increased epidermal cell turnover indicated by epidermal cell kinetic studies—provide evidence that the lesions are the result of cell destruction followed by reactive epidermal proliferation.

It has been suggested that idiopathic lichen planus is similar in pathogenesis to graft-versus-host disease. An unknown agent injures the epidermal cells, thereby altering their antigenic structure (Fig. 24-34). The altered antigen is then presented by epidermal and dermal Langerhans cells to T-cells which, in turn, stimulate B-cells. Lymphokines produced by T-helper cells lead to macrophage-mediated epidermal cell

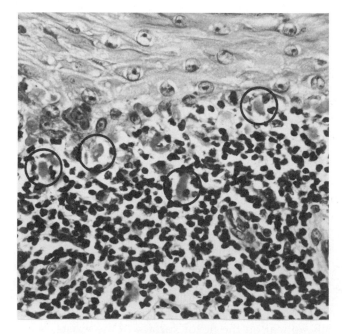

Figure 24-32. Lichen planus is often associated with a thickened granular layer, fibrillary bodies, and lymphocytic infiltrate. The pale grey, irregular bodies (*circled*) at the dermal-epidermal interface are fibrillary bodies.

damage, whereas the antibodies formed by the B-cells are deposited in the skin, especially within the eosinophilic fibrillary bodies. Excessive reactive proliferation of the epidermis in response to immune-mediated damage is manifested by a brisk lymphocytic response and results in the distinctive pathology of lichen planus.

Inflammatory Diseases of the Superficial and Deep Vascular Bed

Disorders Without Significant Epidermal Involvement

Urticaria and Angioedema (Neutrophilic, Eosinophilic Infiltrate)

Definition and Clinical Features

Urticaria, or hives, present as raised, pale, well-delimited, almost plaquelike, pruritic areas on the skin that appear and disappear within a few hours. **Hives represent edema of the superficial portions of the dermis.** When the edema involves the deeper dermis or subcutaneous fat, the resulting egglike swelling is prominent, and is termed **angioedema.** These rapidly developing disorders may simply be annoying or may be part of a life-threatening allergic reaction. All such reactions are related to a rapid and dramatic increase in permeability of the venule, because of the action of an array of vasoactive compounds. The activity of the vasoactive agents may be triggered by an IgE-dependent sensitivity to specific antigens, complement activation along the classical pathway, the direct action of certain compounds on mast cells, or by unknown mechanisms. Dermatographism, a linear hive with a rich pink flare, is an exaggerated IgE-dependent response to brisk stroking found in about 4 percent of the population. One may write on the skin of individuals affected by dermatographism, thereby creating a hive in the form of a legible word. This section is concerned with urticaria, angioedema, and similar reactions that are IgE-dependent.

Pathology

In urticaria, the model for IgE-dependent reactions, the collagen fibers and fibrils are pushed apart and are separated by clear areas where excess fluid occupies space *in vivo*. This separation of fibers gives rise to pale staining with eosin in the outer dermis. The lymphatics are dilated and the venules show margination of neutrophils and eosinophils, associ-

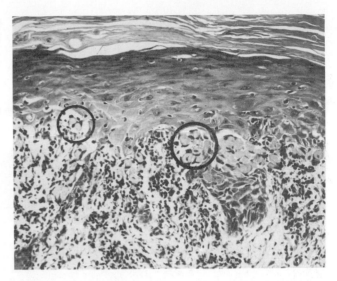

Figure 24-33. Fibrillary bodies (*circled*) in lichenoid actinic keratosis are a manifestation of altered keratinocytes in a neoplastic system; cells are no longer recognized as "self."

ated with a cuff of a few lymphocytes. Perivenular mast cell degranulation is important. When the urticarial lesion persists for 24 hours (an urticarial plaque reaction), the number of lymphocytes and eosinophils is greatly increased, whereas the number of neutrophils is diminished.

Etiology and Pathogenesis

The majority of cases of urticaria are IgE-dependent, and the final pathway of this abnormal reaction is an **exaggerated venular permeability due to degranulation of mast cells,** of which there are approximately 7,000 to 12,000/mm³ of normal skin. An almost unending list of materials may react with IgE antibodies at the mast cell surface, and this urticarial mechanism may occur in both atopic and nonatopic patients. Atopic patients have an intensely pruritic skin eruption, a family history of similar eruptions, and a personal or family history of allergies, such as allergic rhinitis and asthma. The study of these patients is important in understanding the pathogenesis of this disorder as they commonly exhibit an elevation of circulating IgE. Although IgE antibodies circulate in only small amounts, their Fc fragment has an affinity for the mast cell plasma membrane that is 10,000 to 20,000 times that of other immunoglobulin isotypes. Following exposure to a sensitizing antigen, IgE molecules attach to the plasma membrane. Antigen couples with two adjacent IgE molecules and, following such union, degranulation occurs at many sites on a given cell. Initially, the venule reacts by increased

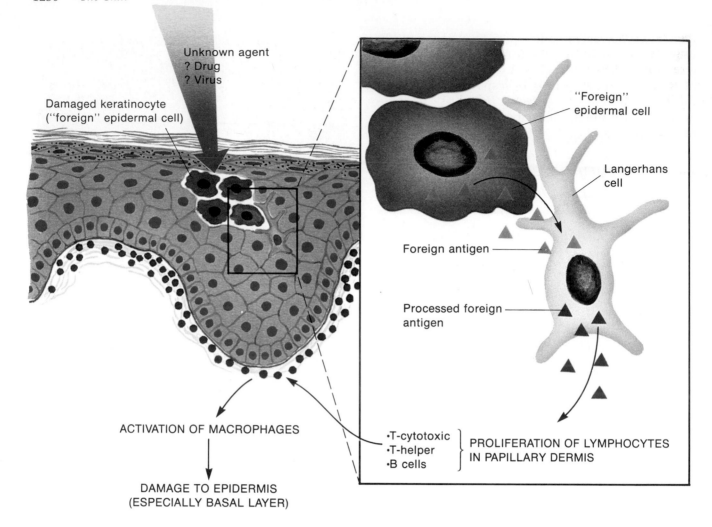

Unknown agent
? Drug
? Virus

Damaged keratinocyte
("foreign" epidermal cell)

"Foreign"
epidermal cell

Langerhans
cell

Foreign antigen

Processed foreign
antigen

ACTIVATION OF MACROPHAGES

• T-cytotoxic
• T-helper
• B cells

PROLIFERATION OF LYMPHOCYTES
IN PAPILLARY DERMIS

DAMAGE TO EPIDERMIS
(ESPECIALLY BASAL LAYER)

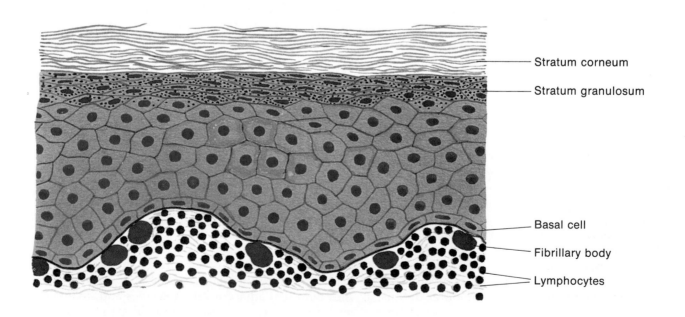

Stratum corneum

Stratum granulosum

Basal cell

Fibrillary body

Lymphocytes

permeability to fluid, with consequent rapidly forming edema. If the reaction persists, inflammatory cells are attracted to the area and a persistent urticarial plaque (lasting for more than 24 hours) is the result. Such plaques may occasionally show true venulitis.

Cutaneous Necrotizing Venulitis (Neutrophilic and Eosinophilic with Venular Damage)

Definition and Clinical Features

All inflammatory diseases are characterized by transvascular (usually across a venule) migration of white blood cells of all kinds. Some diseases are distinguished by the accumulation of inflammatory cells within the walls of blood vessels and by evidence of partial destruction of the vessel wall, frequently manifested by fibrin deposition. Diseases with such vascular reactions are called vasculitis, and are classified by the type of vessel involved and by the dominant inflammatory cell. Arteries, veins, and venules may be affected, but commonly, only one type of vessel is affected in a given disorder. In polyarteritis nodosa, small arteries are affected, but venules are spared. This discussion focuses on cutaneous vasculitis, which has variously been termed allergic cutaneous vasculitis, leukocytoclastic vasculitis, hypersensitivity angiitis, and cutaneous necrotizing venulitis. The last name is the most accurately descriptive.

Clinically, cutaneous necrotizing venulitis is distinguished by the purpuric papule, a red, palpable lesion that is 2 to 4 mm in width and that does not blanch under pressure. Multiple lesions characteristically appear in crops on the lower extremities or at sites of pressure. The lesions are confined to the skin in an otherwise healthy person, or may involve small blood vessels in the joints, gastrointestinal tract, or kidney. In about half of the cases, the cause of vasculitis is unknown. In the other half, the vascular disorder is either secondary to an infectious disease, is an allergic reaction to a drug, or is associated with

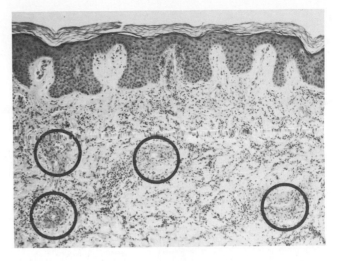

Figure 24-35. Cutaneous necrotizing venulitis. Damaged venules may be seen to the left, in the center, and in the lower right portion of the photograph (*circled*).

a chronic disease, such as systemic lupus erythematosus.

Pathology

Vasculitis is defined as inflammatory cells within the wall of the vessel, associated with at least partial disruption of the anatomic integrity of the vessel wall. The venule is virtually obliterated by a neutrophilic infiltrate (Fig. 24-35). The endothelial cells and mesenchymal wall are hard to visualize. The damage to the vessel is manifested by fibrin deposition and extravasation of erythrocytes (Fig. 24-36). Many of the neutrophils are also damaged, resulting in dust-like nuclear remnants, a process known as leukocytoclasia (Fig. 24-37). The collagen between affected venules is infiltrated by neutrophils, eosinophils, and leukocytoclastic cellular remnants.

Pathogenesis

The available evidence indicates that necrotizing cutaneous venulitis is an immune complex disease.

Figure 24-34. Pathogenetic mechanisms in lichen planus. Lichen planus is apparently initiated by epidermal damage. This damage causes some epidermal cells to be treated as "foreign." The antigens of such cells are processed by Langerhans cells. The processed antigen induces lymphocytic proliferation and macrophage activation. The macrophages, along with T-cytotoxic lymphocytes, injure the epidermal basal cells, resulting in a reactive epidermal proliferation and the formation of fibrillary bodies.

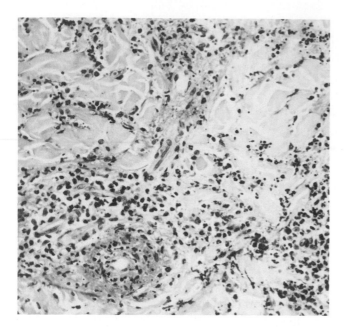

Figure 24-36.   In cutaneous necrotizing venulitis, there is prominent venular damage and leukocytoclasia (neutrophilic fragmentation).

Circulating immune complexes are deposited in the venular walls, probably at the sites of injury, or where circulation is slow, such as in the lower extremity. The elaborated anaphylatoxins C3a and C5a attract neutrophils which degranulate with release of lysosomal enzymes, resulting in endothelial damage and fibrin deposition (Fig. 24-38). Cutaneous necrotizing venulitis may be either primary (that is, occurring without a known precipitating event) or associated with a specific infectious agent (such as hepatitis B virus), or it may represent a secondary process in a wide variety of chronic illnesses, such as rheumatoid arthritis, systemic lupus erythematosus, and ulcerative colitis.

Disorders with Varied Epidermal Reactions and Dermal Alterations Dominated by Lymphocytes

Allergic Contact Dermatitis (Poison Ivy): A Lymphocytic Dermatitis with Epidermal and Dermal Edema

Definition and Clinical Features

More than 50 percent of the population of the United States is sensitive to the toxicodendrons (a term denoting "toxic tree"), which are members of the Rhus genus of plants. The common offenders are *R. radi-cans* (poison ivy), *R. quericifolium* (poison oak), and *R. vernix* (poison sumac). These plant dermatitides are so common that the resultant disease is synonymous with the offending plant. The patient states "I have poison ivy," and he comes to the physician for relief, not diagnosis. The ailment is self-limited and serves as the archetype for the study of delayed hypersensitivity in man, defined as an immunologically specific, mononuclear, inflammatory response that reaches its peak 24 to 48 hours after antigenic challenge in a sensitive subject. When a person comes into contact with poison ivy for the first time, it may not even be noted. Some five to seven days later, the site of contact becomes intensely pruritic, after which erythema and small vesicles develop rapidly. Over the ensuing few days, the area enlarges, becomes fiery red, presents numerous vesicles, and exudes a large amount of clear, proteinaceous fluid. During this evolution, pruritus is intense. The entire process lasts about 3 weeks. Exudation gradually subsides, and the whole area is covered by an irregular crust, which eventually falls off. Pruritus diminishes and healing occurs without scarring. When such a patient again comes into contact with poison ivy, the entire process is greatly accelerated. Within 24 to 48 hours, the lesions appear, spread rapidly, and produce the same clinical appearance. However, the reaction is usually more intense. Again, the lesions clear within about 3 weeks.

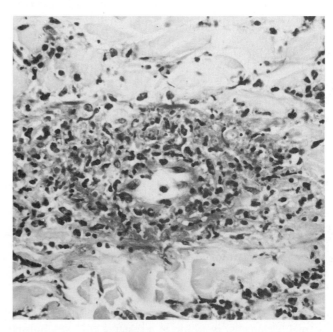

Figure 24-37.   A damaged venule with fibrin deposition and leukocytoclasia is evident in this case of cutaneous necrotizing venulitis.

Pathology

Biopsies of affected areas during the initial 24 hours following exposure show numerous lymphocytes and macrophages about the superficial venular bed, some of which extend into the epidermis. The epidermal cells are partially pulled apart, yielding a spongelike appearance (spongiosis). The stratum corneum contains some coagulated eosinophilic material. Later biopsies show an exaggeration of this process, with numerous mononuclear inflammatory cells, severe spongiosis of the epidermis, vesicles containing lymphocytes and macrophages, and large amounts of eosinophilic material in the stratum corneum (Fig. 24-39). At this time, eosinophils also infiltrate. This histologic appearance is typical for allergic contact dermatitis.

Etiology and Pathogenesis

The offending plant contains low-molecular-weight compounds called haptens. These are not active in sensitization unless they combine with a carrier protein. This happens, in all likelihood, at the cell membrane of the Langerhans cell. Formation of the hapten-carrier complex requires about 1 hour, after which it is processed as an antigen by the Langerhans cell, which is HLA-DR–positive. The processed antigen is then presented to a T cell, which becomes sensitized.* The now-sensitized lymphocytes ("peripheral sensitization") are transported to the regional lymph nodes, where they induce paracortical (T-cell) hyperplasia. The proliferating and sensitized T-cells return to the original site of contact via the bloodstream (Fig. 24-40). Emergence from the venule is, in all likelihood, dependent on mast cells. The vasoactive substances released from mast cells produce increased permeability of the venules, thereby permitting the transudation of large quantities of protein, lymphocytes, and macrophages into the perivenular tissue and subsequently, into the epidermis (Fig. 24-41). Mast cell degranulation also attracts the eosinophils, which are a part of the inflammatory response. In the perivenular bed of the skin, as well as in the epidermis, a further amplification of the lymphocytic response occurs through the interaction of the Langerhans cells, macrophages, and epidermal keratinocytes, all of which release interleukin-1. Interleukin-1 activates helper T-cells at the site, producing interleukin-2 which, acting as a growth factor, expands the lymphocyte population. These and other lymphokines activate macrophages, which partici-

* If the site of initial contact is excised in an experimental animal within 24 hours, sensitization does not occur.

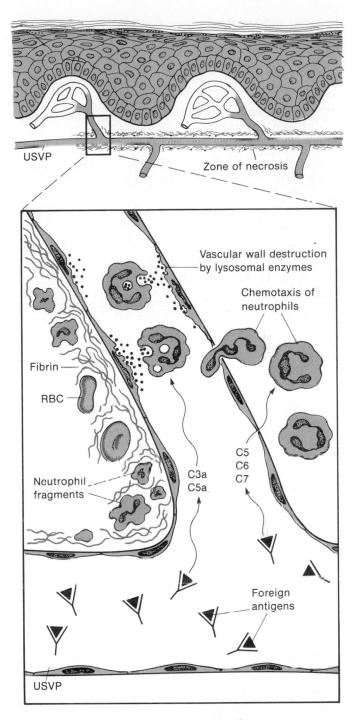

Figure 24-38. Pathogenesis of venular damage in cutaneous necrotizing venulitis. The site of the venular pathology is indicated in the upper diagram. Circulating immune complexes activate complement. There is neutrophilic chemotaxis (C3a and C5a) and neutrophilic destruction. Venular damage occurs with extravasation of erythrocytes, fibrin deposition, and leukocytoclasia. RBC, red blood cell; DSVP, deep superficial venular plexus.

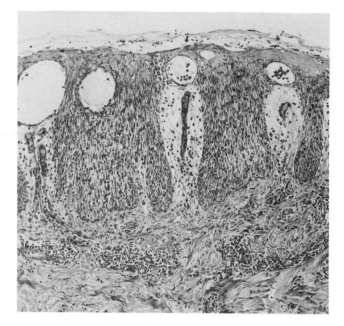

Figure 24-39. Epidermal spongiosis and dermal edema in allergic contact dermatitis secondary to poison ivy. The epidermal vesicles are termed spongiotic vesicles.

pate in the effector arm of the immunologically specific inflammatory process.

Disorders Manifested Primarily by Alterations of the Dermal Connective Tissue

Sclerosis of the Reticular Dermis

Progressive Systemic Sclerosis: Scleroderma

Definition and Clinical Features

Scleroderma is defined by progressive sclerosis and tightening of the skin. Its initial manifestation is frequently on the distal portion of the upper extremities and on the face about the mouth. Progression of the disease results in widespread thickening of the skin, with dense fibrosis and a striking decrease in cutaneous motility. A similar disease that involves only patchy circumscribed areas of the skin is designated **morphea.** Scleroderma is characterized by varying structural and functional involvement of internal organs, including the kidneys, lungs, heart, esophagus, and small intestine. It is an excellent example of how disorders of the reticular dermis accompany diseases of internal organs.

Pathology

The initial manifestations of scleroderma are in the lower reticular dermis, but eventually, the entire reticular dermis and even the papillary dermis become involved. There is a diminution of interbundle space in the reticular dermis and a tendency for the collagen bundles to be ill-defined and parallel to each other. A patchy lymphocytic infiltrate with a few plasma cells is common, and may also be present in the underlying subcutaneous tissue. Sweat ducts are entrapped in the thickened fibrous tissue, and hair follicles are completely lost (Fig. 24-42). Vascular disease often accompanies scleroderma, particularly in the gastrointestinal tract and kidney. In the kidney, the vascular lesions are responsible for the severe hypertension commonly seen in patients with scleroderma.

Etiology and Pathogenesis

The cause of progressive systemic sclerosis is unknown. The presence of a variety of autoantibodies, which is somewhat reminiscent of the multiple autoantibodies of lupus erythematosus, suggests that some form of autoimmunity is involved in the pathogenesis of scleroderma. In this regard, chronic graft-versus-host disease is characterized by diffuse sclerosis that simulates scleroderma, at least in its cutaneous manifestations. There is some evidence that the patient with scleroderma forms antibodies to the centromere, as well as a distinctive antibody, referred to as SCL-70 antibody. There is also evidence of lymphokine production by T-cells, which induces collagen synthesis and probably, fibroblast proliferation. Macrophage activation may act through interleukin-1 and fibronectin to induce fibroblast recruitment by chemotaxis and proliferation. Mast cells are also increased in diffuse scleroderma, and may be related to the fibrosis.

Alteration of Elastic Tissue

Pseudoxanthoma Elasticum

A single example of a hereditary disorder of connective tissue—pseudoxanthoma elasticum—is presented to show the complex interrelationship between connective tissue disease of the reticular dermis and systemic connective tissue syndromes. This disease may be inherited in recessive or dominant forms.

Definition and Clinical Features

In areas where the skin is folded, such as the axillary folds, about the neck, or in the inguinal area, the

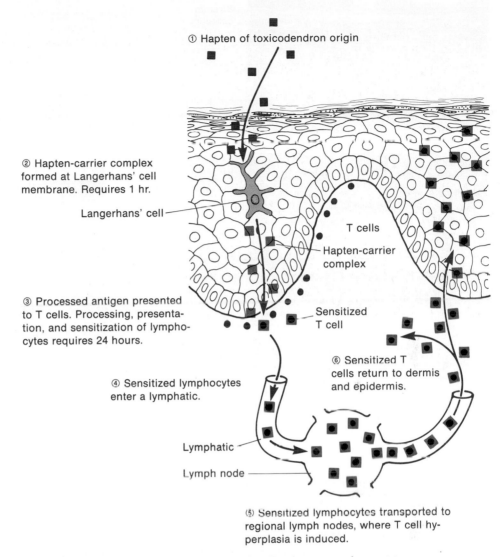

① Hapten of toxicodendron origin

② Hapten-carrier complex formed at Langerhans' cell membrane. Requires 1 hr.

Langerhans' cell

T cells

Hapten-carrier complex

③ Processed antigen presented to T cells. Processing, presentation, and sensitization of lymphocytes requires 24 hours.

Sensitized T cell

⑥ Sensitized T cells return to dermis and epidermis.

④ Sensitized lymphocytes enter a lymphatic.

Lymphatic

Lymph node

⑤ Sensitized lymphocytes transported to regional lymph nodes, where T cell hyperplasia is induced.

Figure 24-40. Pathogenetic mechanisms in allergic contact dermatitis.

skin of patients with pseudoxanthoma elasticum is thickened, pebbled, and yellowish-orange. The lesions have a fancied resemblance to xanthomas—and thus the name. Elastic tissue in other organs of the body is significantly altered, as in the fundus of the eye, where it appears as broad streaks ("angioid streaks") that radiate from the optic disc. In addition, lesions in the walls of coronary arteries may lead to vascular insufficiency of the myocardium. Elastic tissue disease of the renal vessels causes hypertension, whereas in the gastrointestinal tract, it leads to hemorrhage.

Pathology

As in the systemic tissues, elastic fibers in the skin are fragmented early. They are deeply basophilic,

even in routine preparations, owing to the deposition of calcium about the altered connective tissue fragments (Fig. 24-43). The damaged areas also frequently display an inflammatory response dominated by foreign body giant cells.

Etiology and Pathogenesis

Even though the heritable pattern of this disease has been elucidated in considerable detail, the basic biochemical defect is unknown.

Granulomatous Inflammation

Sarcoidosis

The cutaneous manifestations of sarcoidosis are characterized by asymptomatic involvement of the dermis

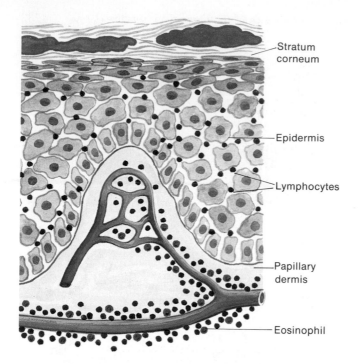

Stratum corneum

Epidermis

Lymphocytes

Papillary dermis

Eosinophil

Figure 24-41. Allergic contact dermatitis. The superficial venule bed is infiltrated by eosinophils, lymphocytes, and macrophages. Spongiosis of the epidermal cells is present. The stratum corneum contains coagulated eosinophilic material.

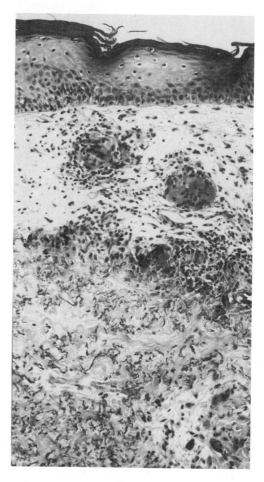

Figure 24-43. Pseudoxanthoma elasticum is characterized by clumped, fragmented, elastic fibers.

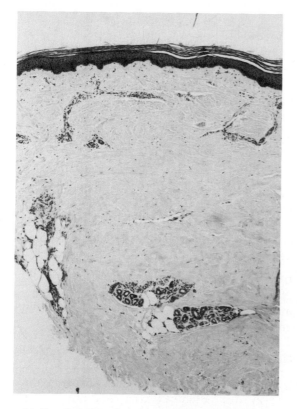

Figure 24-42. In scleroderma, the dermis is sclerotic and displays entrapped eccrine ducts.

and subcutaneous tissue. Some lesions may be annular, and those that involve the subcutaneous tissue present as irregular nodules.

Definition and Clinical Features

Sarcoidosis is of unknown etiology and commonly affects both the skin and the lungs. The disease may be unusually widespread and the cutaneous lesions so prominent as to simulate a diffusely infiltrative neoplasm. There may also be involvement of the lymph nodes, spleen, and eyes. The illness may be indolent and not debilitating, but may be a symptomatic, severe disorder.

Pathology

The lesions of sarcoidosis are of the classic epithelioid cell tubercle type (Fig. 24-44). Caseation necrosis is minimal or absent. A few lymphocytes may be present about the periphery of the tubercle. This prototypic example of granulomatous inflammation occurs both in the dermis and in the subcutaneous tissue.

Etiology and Pathogenesis

The etiology of sarcoidosis is unknown. For some years, it has been thought to be an abnormal reaction to an unknown antigen, possibly of infectious origin. According to this theory, activated T-helper cells stimulate macrophages to proliferate and to form the nodular configurations characteristic of the disease. These macrophages fuse to form the giant cells characteristic of the epithelioid cell granulomas. The activated macrophages of the granulomas release lymphokines, which further stimulate T-helper cells, as well as induce tissue fibrosis. The presence of an excess number of T4 helper cells, both in pulmonary and cutaneous infiltrates, suggests that these cells, reacting in an abnormal fashion, perpetuate the persistent granulomatous inflammation in both the lung and skin.

Inflammatory Disorders of the Panniculus

Predominantly Septal Panniculitis

Erythema Nodosum

A number of ailments are manifested by inflammation, of one sort or another, in subcutaneous tissue. These disorders are classified according to involvement of the subcutaneous septa, the lobule, or the subcutaneous blood vessels. One of the most common of these disorders—erythema nodosum—is seen in patients who have some other systemic disease, commonly one characterized by granulomatous inflammation. Erythema nodosum may also be an abnormal immune response to a drug.

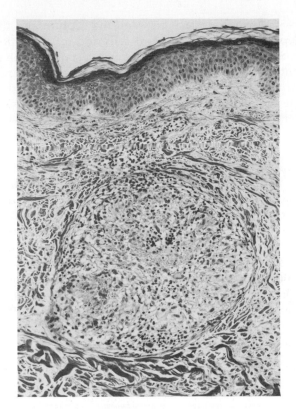

Figure 24-44. Sarcoidosis. A single dermal granuloma is seen.

Definition and Clinical Features

Erythema nodosum classically presents acutely on the anterior portion of the lower limbs of women as **dome-shaped, exquisitely tender, elevated, erythematous nodules.** These lesions come to resemble bruises and finally, less tender, firm nodules that may disappear in time, only to be followed by other evolving nodose lesions. Many affected patients prove to have sarcoidosis, tuberculosis, or deep fungus infections, such as histoplasmosis.

Pathology

Early in the course of the malady, the lesions are in the fibrous septa of the subcutaneous tissue, where a neutrophilic inflammation associated with the extravasation of erythrocytes is seen. In chronic lesions, the septa are widened, and show focal giant cell inflammation about small areas of altered collagen, as well as an ill-defined lymphocytic infiltrate (Fig.

24-45). At the interface between the septum and the surrounding fat lobule, giant cells and inflammation extend into the lobule. Secondary vascular involvement is occasionally noted. The histologic appearance is not absolutely diagnostic, and careful clinicopathologic correlation is often required to classify a lesion as erythema nodosum.

Etiology and Pathogenesis

Erythema nodosum occurs so commonly in association with a variety of infectious diseases that it may be accepted as an altered immune response. However, the precise mechanisms underlying its development have not been elucidated. The characteristic early neutrophilic inflammation suggests that it is a response to the activation of complement and the resulting neutrophilic chemotaxis. The subsequent chronic inflammation is probably secondary to fibroplasia in the septa, breakdown of fat at the interface of septa and lobule, and a foreign body giant cell response to degraded fat.

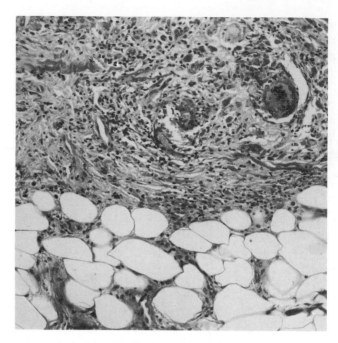

Figure 24-45. Erythema nodosum. A septal panniculitis with foreign body giant cells is evident.

Disorders of the Pilosebaceous Unit

Neutrophilic Inflammation and the Sebaceous Follicle

Acne

Definition and Clinical Features

Acne is an inflammatory disorder of the sebaceous follicle that is related to hormonally-induced, excessive production of sebum; abnormal cornification of portions of the follicular epithelium; and a response to the anaerobic diphtheroid, *Propionibacterium acnes*. The disease is usually manifested in adolescence, and can be both cosmetically disfiguring and psychologically debilitating.

Pathology

Fully evolved acne lesions show intense neutrophilic inflammation surrounding a ruptured sebaceous follicle. Numerous macrophages accumulate as a response to the rupture of the sebaceous follicle.

Etiology and Pathogenesis

The sebaceous follicle contains a vellus hair and prominent sebaceous glands. The change in an individual's hormonal status at puberty leads to production of sebum in the follicle and altered cornification in the follicular infundibulum. These two effects produce early dilatation of the follicular canal. Another round of excessive sebum production is as-

sociated with the desquamation of cells and the accretion of keratinous debris, a situation which provides a rich environment for the proliferation of *P. acnes*. These combined changes lead to the formation of a **comedone** which is a distended, plugged follicle. Hydrolytic enzymes released by neutrophils attack the wall of the follicle, permitting the escape of sebum, keratin, and bacteria into the perifollicular tissue, where they stimulate further acute inflammation (Fig. 24-46). The development of an allergy to *P. acnes* intensifies the inflammatory response. Patients with acne react much more intensely to injections of *P. acnes* than do normal subjects. **The combination of various hormonal factors, changes in the follicular epithelium, excessive sebum production, proliferation of *P. acnes*, and eventual rupture of the follicles constitutes the basic pathogenesis of acne.**

Primary Neoplasms of the Skin

Etiology and Pathogenesis

Neoplasia in the skin is an important paradigm for the understanding of cancer in general, particularly since it is known that the most important carcinogenic agent in most cutaneous cancers is ultraviolet light. The lesions of cutaneous neoplasia are on the body surface, where their development and evolution are readily observed. The pathology of most of the developmental stages of specific skin neoplasms is known, and the ready availability of lesions has permitted *in vitro* studies of cells derived from the tumors to be correlated with the observed biologic progression of the clinical disease. Furthermore, strong support for the somatic mutation theory of carcinogenesis comes from the study of xeroderma pigmentosum, a human disease characterized by an inherited sensitivity to cellular injury induced by ultraviolet light.

The Etiologic Role of Ultraviolet Light

The following contrasting histories are presented to provide a background for understanding the induction and progression of human epidermal keratinocytic neoplasia.

White Skin A boy of Scotch-German ancestry is born in the Southern part of the United States. He has brown hair and brown eyes, and develops a moderate number of freckles over the face and arms between the sixth and seventeenth year. He has somewhat fewer freckles over the exposed surfaces of the trunk and lower extremities. He does not tan well in the sun and is easily burned. By age 30, there is loss of cutaneous elasticity, and by age 35, a few foci of hyperkeratosis have appeared on the backs of the hands and forehead. At age 40, a small, pearly-white papule from the left cheek is removed and diagnosed as basal cell carcinoma. At age 50, a rapidly growing keratotic lesion from the right wrist is resected, and the diagnosis of keratoacanthoma is made. At age 56, one of the keratotic lesions on the left hand gradually becomes prominent because of persistent, thick, keratotic material. When it is removed at age 58, it proves to be a squamous cell carcinoma. By age 65, the backs of the hands present numerous keratoses, the intervening skin is atrophic, and telangiectasia is prominent. Cutaneous elasticity is essentially lost.

Black Skin A black male child, also born in the South, has rich brown skin and dark brown eyes. By age 65, there is a modest loss of cutaneous elasticity, but no keratoses or carcinomas have ever developed. His skin, except for a few wrinkles, is not remarkably different from its appearance as a young adult.

An Albino A brother of the black child, born 4 years after his birth, has pink-white skin at birth, gray irides, and white hair. The diagnosis of tyrosinase-negative, oculocutaneous albinism is established. By age 14, he has developed four squamous cell carcinomas, one basal cell carcinoma, and numerous keratoses. He is legally blind by the age of 16 years,

and has lost much cutaneous elasticity by the age of 30.

Xeroderma Pigmentosum A black male child, the third offspring of a couple of West African descent, is born with skin and eyes similar to that of his older siblings. At the age of 8 months, his color becomes somewhat mottled, and later he begins to freckle. Over the ensuing years, areas of the skin become even lighter, and by the age of 11 years, his face and hands are speckled. He dislikes the sun and avoids direct sunlight when possible. At age 18, keratoses appear on his forehead and the backs of his hands. One, on the cheek, slowly becomes more prominent than the rest, and upon removal, the tumor is diagnosed as squamous cell carcinoma. Over the ensuing years, he develops squamous cell carcinoma of the conjunctiva and three basal cell carcinomas of the skin. At age 41, a malignant melanoma arises on his forearm. During these years, appropriate studies establish a diagnosis of xeroderma pigmentosum ("pigmented dry skin"), complementation group A.

Discussion The preceding histories reflect much of the biology of cutaneous neoplasia and illustrate some of the fundamental principles of carcinogenesis. People who do not tan well and who are exposed to a great deal of ultraviolet light are those who are commonly affected by cutaneous carcinoma. The keratinocytes of such patients are damaged by ultraviolet light, but the cells repair much of the damage to DNA; thus, cutaneous cancer develops relatively late in life. In black persons, little ultraviolet light is delivered to the keratinocytic target because it is absorbed by melanin pigment. Thus, normal blacks do not develop cutaneous squamous or basal cell carcinomas. However, when the melanin shield which protects the nucleus of the keratinocyte is absent, as in inherited albinism, unimpeded ultraviolet light damages the DNA. DNA repair mechanisms are then overwhelmed, and cutaneous carcinoma is likely to occur early in life. Patients with xeroderma pigmentosum have a risk for basal and squamous cell carcinomas that is increased a thousand-fold, and they are also at a greatly increased risk for developing melanoma. Moreover, skin cancers appear at a median age of 8 years, some 50 years earlier than in the population at large, despite a normal amount of pigment. It is now known that **xeroderma pigmentosum is an inherited disorder in which defective ultraviolet endonuclease activity compromises DNA repair.** A rare form of the disease, called the variant form, is associated with a defect in the postreplication repair of DNA. The inability to repair DNA damage produced by ultraviolet light is responsible for the high incidence of skin cancer.

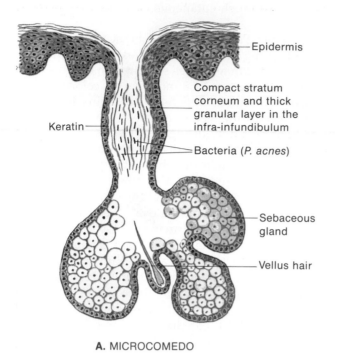

Epidermis

Compact stratum corneum and thick granular layer in the infra-infundibulum

Keratin

Bacteria (*P. acnes*)

Sebaceous gland

Vellus hair

A. MICROCOMEDO

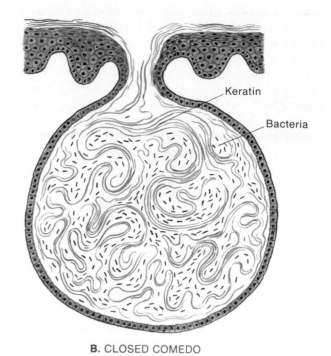

Keratin

Bacteria

B. CLOSED COMEDO

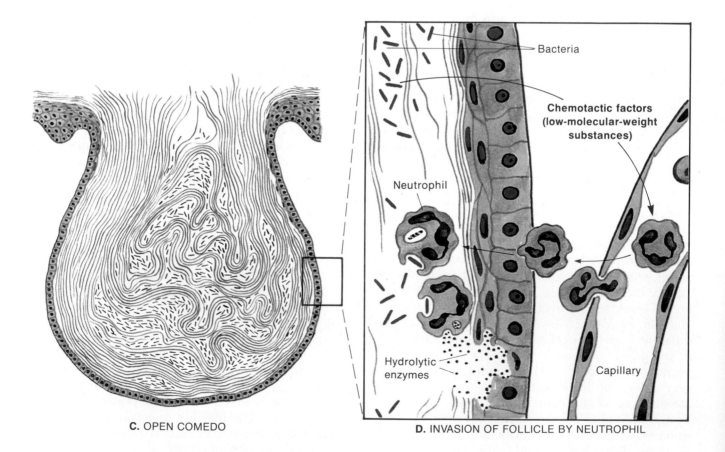

Bacteria

Chemotactic factors (low-molecular-weight substances)

Neutrophil

Hydrolytic enzymes

Capillary

C. OPEN COMEDO

D. INVASION OF FOLLICLE BY NEUTROPHIL

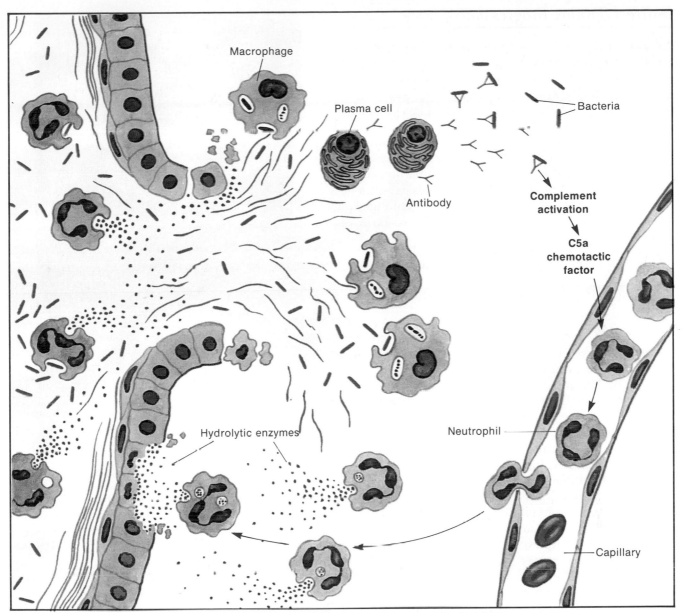

E. INFLAMMATION AND RUPTURE OF SEBACEOUS FOLLICLE

Figure 24-46. Pathogenesis of follicular distention, rupture, and inflammation in acne. Acne is a disease of the follicular canal of a sebaceous follicle. A compact stratum corneum and a thickened granular layer in the infrainfundibulum are the beginning of the formation of a comedone. Microcomedones (*A*) and closed (*B*) and open (*C*) comedones form. Excessive sebum secretion occurs, and the bacterium, *P. acnes*, proliferates. The organism produces chemotactic factors, and neutrophils enter the intact comedone. Neutrophilic enzymes are released, and the comedone ruptures, inducing a cycle of chemotaxis and intense neutrophilic inflammation (*D* and *E*).

Indirect Tumor Progression

An animal responds to a specific carcinogen not, as a rule, by developing cancer, but rather by developing a series of benign, proliferative lesions. Thus, cancer is actually a rare event, occurring after one half or more of the life span of the animal has passed. Enshrouded within this paradox is another basic principle of neoplastic development—namely, tumor progression. The principle of tumor progression is elegantly illustrated by the events of human melanocytic neoplasia. As in keratinocytic neoplasia, ultraviolet light may be causally related to malignant melanoma. Yet, exposure to light begins at birth, whereas malignant melanoma appears at a median age of 50 years. What of the intervening years?

Common Acquired Melanocytic Nevi (Moles)

Most people, regardless of their native skin color, who are exposed to a significant amount of light in the first 15 years of life, develop 10 to 50 moles on their skin. The moles do not ordinarily develop in areas protected from light, such as the breasts of women. A notable exception to the light induction of melanocytic nevi occurs in the red-haired, blue-eyed person with milk-white skin. These individuals are exquisitely sensitive to light and form freckles, but they do not exhibit a significant number of melanocytic nevi. Although there is an unequivocal causal relationship between ultraviolet light and melanocytic nevi (and malignant melanoma), the relationship is clearly complex; some light-sensitive skins form few nevi, whereas some dark skins develop many moles. Melanocytic nevi begin to appear between the first and second year of life and continue to emerge for the first two decades of life. The advent of significant numbers of moles beyond the twentieth year is regarded as abnormal. A mole is first recognized as a small tan dot that does not exceed 0.1 to 0.2 cm in diameter. Over a period of 3 to 4 years, the dot enlarges as a uniformly colored, tan to brown area. During this period of enlargement, the outline of the melanocytic nevus is regular and either circular or oval. When the nevus is 4 to 5 mm in diameter, it is flat or slightly elevated and stops enlarging at the periphery. When peripheral enlargement ceases, the uniformly colored, rich brown mole becomes sharply demarcated from the surrounding normal skin. Over the next 10 years, the lesion begins to elevate and color is slightly diminished. Gradually, the mole becomes a tan skin tag. For one to two decades, it

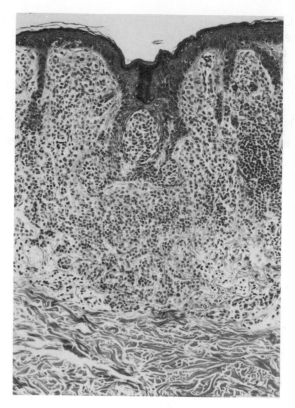

Figure 24-47. The melanocytes that form a compound nevus are within the epidermis and dermis.

gradually flattens and the skin may return to a normal appearance. Most people experience a gradual decrease in the number of moles through the years, as reflected in the statement, "We come into this world without moles, and we leave without moles."

Histologic Changes

There are precise histologic developments that parallel the foregoing description of the evolution of a normal mole. At the very beginning, an increased number of melanocytes in the basal epidermal layer is associated with hyperpigmentation. Subsequently, the melanocytes form nests at the tips of rete ridges, and melanocytes migrate into the dermis, where they form a cellular lesion. These small cells are circular and bear a superficial resemblance to a lymphocyte. With further passage of time, as the lesion becomes clearly elevated, the dermal component differentiates, and the cells evolve along the lines of Schwann cells, forming small structures similar to nerve endings. Gradually, this differentiation encompasses the entire dermal component of the lesion, and the core of a 20-year-old nevus may be composed of a delicate neuromesenchyme. This stage is followed by fibrosis, flattening, and eventual disappearance of the nevus.

Classification

The foregoing description of the histologic changes that the common acquired melanocytic nevus undergoes has given rise to a classification system that does not denote separate entities, but rather change with time in one entity. When the cells are limited to the basal layer of the epidermis, the lesion is called **lentigo.** At the stage of nest formation by melanocytes in the epidermis, the term **junctional nevus** is used. When nests of melanocytes are seen in both the epidermis and dermis, the lesion is labeled a **compound nevus** (Fig. 24-47). After intraepidermal melanocytic growth has ceased, the lesion is identified as a **dermal nevus** (Fig. 24-48). When the dermal component has differentiated into a delicate neuromesenchyme, the lesion is indistinguishable from a small skin tag. The appearance of a population of cells focally that grows for a while and differentiates is commonly seen in most neoplastic systems. Experimentally, most carcinogens produce a series of focal, benign, proliferative lesions that differentiate and disappear in time. In this respect, the evolution of hepatic nodules, discussed in Chapter 5, is analogous to that of the melanocytic nevus.

Dysplastic Nevi

Occasionally, common acquired nevi do not follow the normal pattern of growth, differentiation, and disappearance just described. Their evolution is flawed, and their differentiation aberrant. One or several moles in a patient with dysplastic nevi show focal areas of eccentric melanocytic growth, and become larger and more irregular. The peripheral irregular area is flat (macular) and extends asymmetrically from the parent mole. Initially, in these areas, the growth of melanocytes in the basal region of the epidermis appears no different from that which occurs at the beginning of the development of a common mole. It is abnormal in pattern, not in cytologic features. With the passage of time, melanocytes with large atypical nuclei that have some similarities to cancer cells appear. The combination of an abnormal growth pattern and cytologic abnormality of melanocytes (melanocytic nuclear atypia) defines a **dysplastic nevus** (Figs. 24-49 through 24-52). These areas of dysplasia are usually associated with a subjacent lymphocytic infiltrate. More than half of the malignant melanomas of the superficial spreading type have a mole precursor, the majority of which show melanocytic dysplasia, or have dysplastic nevi away from the site of the primary melanoma.

Malignant Melanoma of the Superficial Spreading Type

There are four common forms of malignant melanoma and several uncommon forms of the disease. Only the common forms are discussed here, with emphasis on the most frequently encountered variety—namely, superficial spreading melanoma—because it clearly illustrates tumor progression within an established cancer.

The incidence of malignant melanoma of the superficial spreading type is increasing at a rate greater than that of any other form of human cancer. It is estimated that 1 percent of children born today will develop malignant melanoma. The early stages of the disease are curable and clinically distinctive. Consequently, expeditious diagnosis is of great importance. The cells during the early stages of superficial spreading melanoma, though invasive, do not exhibit metastatic potential, a property reserved for the later stages of tumor progression.

Clinical and Histologic Appearance in the Radial Growth Phase (Before Competence for Metastasis Develops)

Except for the smallest lesions (those that are less than 6 mm in diameter), superficial spreading mela-

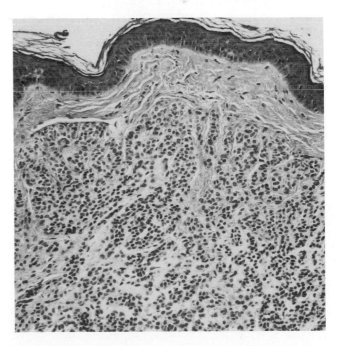

Figure 24-48. The cells of the dermal nevus are entirely confined to the dermis.

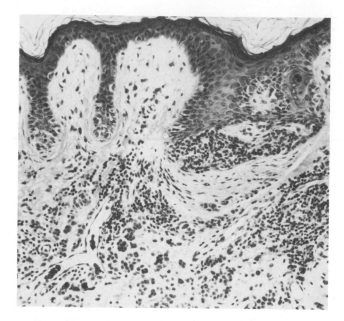

Figure 24-49.   Compound nevus with melanocytic dysplasia. The epidermal melanocytic component, the dermal component, lamellar fibroplasia, dermal nevus cells, and a lymphocytic infiltrate are illustrated.

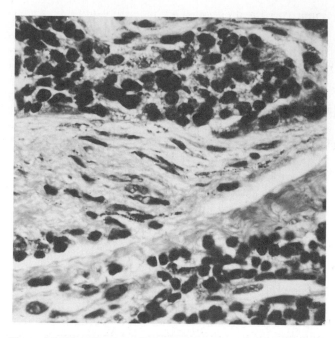

Figure 24-50.   The lamellar fibroplasia in a compound nevus with melanocytic dysplasia is shown at higher magnification.

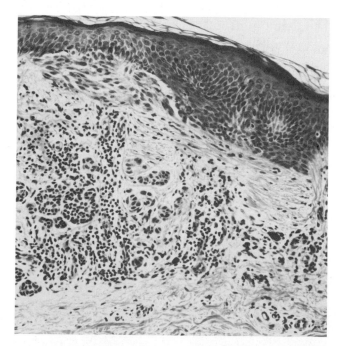

Figure 24-51.   An ellipsoid nest of atypical melanocytes is shown immediately below the epidermis in this compound nevus with melanocytic dysplasia.

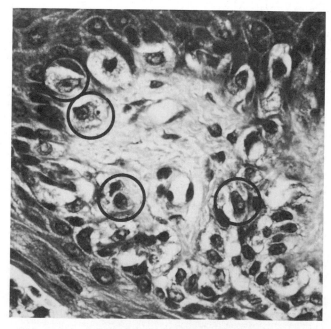

Figure 24-52.   The large, epithelioid melanocytes with atypia that are characteristic of a compound nevus with melanocytic dysplasia are shown (circled).

noma can be diagnosed in its radial growth phase with considerable accuracy merely by clinical inspection, and it may be distinguished from a nevus, even an abnormal one. However, the clinical diagnosis must be confirmed by excisional biopsy.

Initially, the lesions usually have a diameter of 10 mm or more and have a slightly elevated and palpable border. The neoplasm is variably and haphazardly colored. Some parts are unusually black or dark brown, while lighter brown shades are mingled with pink and light blue tints. On the other hand, the entire lesion may be uniformly dark brown (Fig. 24-53).

On microscopic examination, large, epithelioid melanocytes are dispersed in nests and as individual cells throughout the entire thickness of the epidermis (Fig. 24-54). They invade the dermis, but are confined to the papillary zone. Here, the disposition of the cells is highly characteristic of the radial growth phase. The cells are arranged in small nests or as individual cells. No nest of cells has a growth preference over the surrounding cells (see Fig. 24-54). As a rule, the cells of the radial growth phase are associated with a brisk lymphocytic response. The cells of the radial growth phase grow in all directions: upward in the epidermis, peripherally in the epidermis, downward from the epidermis into the dermis, and peripherally in the papillary dermis. The net clinical enlargement of these lesions is at the periphery, along the radii of an imperfect circle—thus the

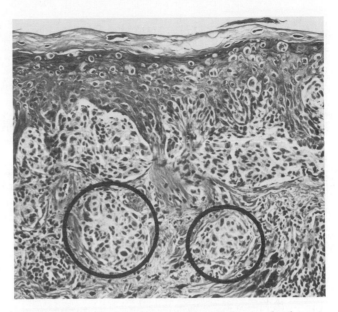

Figure 24-54. The histology of the radial growth phase in malignant melanoma of the superficial spreading type. Tumor cells grow at all levels of the epidermis, including the granular layer. Tumor cells are present in the papillary dermis (*circled*) but no nest has preferential growth over any other nest.

name radial growth phase. It is critical that this phase be recognized by clinicians and pathologists because **tumors having the characteristics of the radial growth phase have not been observed to metastasize.** As will be discussed later, most tumors in the radial growth phase are said to be invasive to anatomic level II.

Clinical and Histologic Appearance in the Vertical Growth Phase: The Acquisition of Competence for Metastasis

After a variable time (usually 1 to 2 years), the character of the growth of cells in the dermis changes focally. Foci of new cells appear in the dermis and the primary tumor possesses metastatic potential. The cells grow as spheroidal nodules (in a manner similar to the growth of metastatic nodules), expanding more rapidly than the rest of the tumor in the surrounding papillary dermis (Fig. 24-55). The net direction of growth tends to be perpendicular to that of the radial growth phase—hence, the term **vertical growth phase** (Figs. 24-56 through 24-59). The characteristics of the vertical growth phase are as follows:

- The cells tend to differ in appearance from those of the radial growth phase. For example, they may contain little or no pigment, whereas cells in the radial growth phase are melanotic.

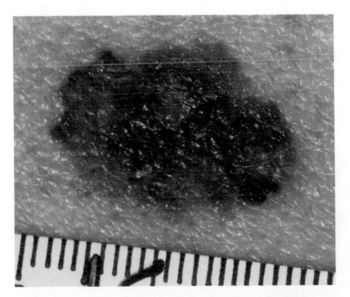

Figure 24-53. The clinical appearance of the radial growth phase in malignant melanoma of the superficial spreading type. The larger diameter is 1.8 cm.

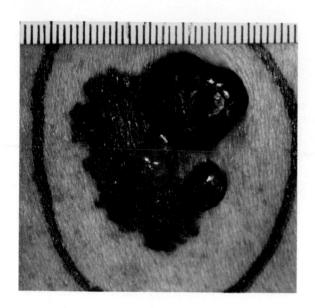

Figure 24-55.   Clinically, the radial growth phase in malignant melanoma of the superficial spreading type is represented by the relatively flat, dark, brown-black portion of the tumor. There are three areas in this lesion that are characteristic of the vertical growth phase. All are nodular in configuration; two have a pink coloration, and the largest is a rich, ebony black.

- The cellular aggregate that characterizes the vertical growth phase is larger than the clusters of cells that form the intraepidermal and invasive components of the radial growth phase. The dominant site of tumor growth is shifted from the epidermis to the dermis.
- Tumors that extend into the lower half of the reticular dermis are, by definition, in the vertical growth phase.
- The cellular immune response of the host is frequently absent at the base of the vertical growth phase.

Although malignant melanoma was once regarded as a particularly malignant tumor, its reputation is no longer deserved. The prognosis is excellent if the lesion is recognized before it enters the vertical growth phase. **When the vertical growth phase produces a lesion that is more than 4.0 mm in thickness, however, 75 to 80 percent of affected patients will die of metastatic disease,** a figure to be contrasted with the negligible mortality in the radial growth phase. With proper awareness on the part of physicians and the general public, the mortality from melanoma should be less than 5 percent.

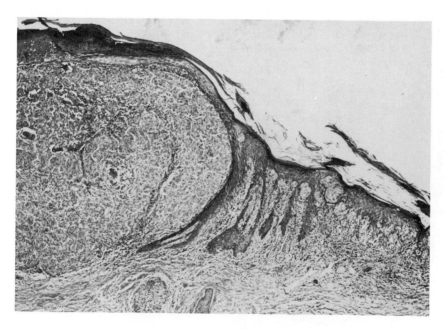

Figure 24-56.   The histologic appearance of the vertical growth phase in malignant melanoma of the superficial spreading type is manifested by the distinct spheroidal nodule of tumor cells—a focus of cells that clearly has a growth advantage over that in the radial growth phase.

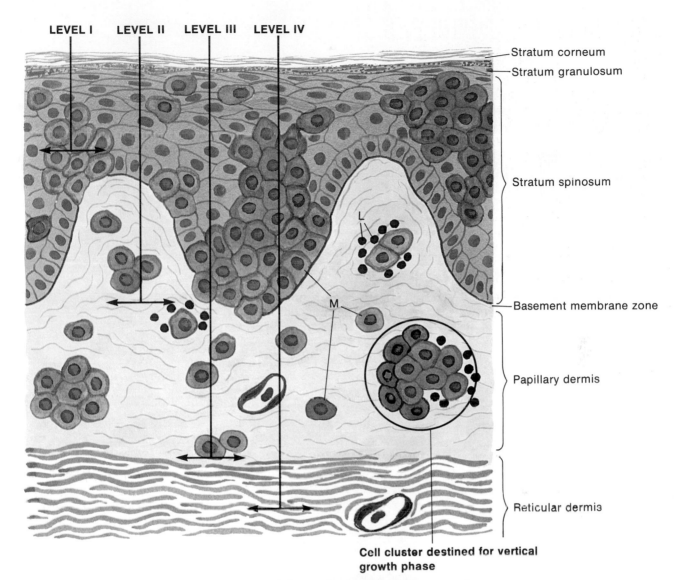

LEVEL I   LEVEL II   LEVEL III   LEVEL IV

Stratum corneum
Stratum granulosum
Stratum spinosum
L
M
Basement membrane zone
Papillary dermis
Reticular dermis

Cell cluster destined for vertical growth phase

Figure 24-57.   Schematic depiction of the radial growth phase in malignant melanoma of the superficial spreading type. In the **radial growth phase,** cells grow in the epidermis and are present in the dermis. They grow in all directions: outward, peripherally, and downward. However, the net direction of growth is peripheral—along the radii of an imperfect circle. Growth, as manifested by mitotic activity, is largely in the epidermis. No cells in the dermis seem to have a growth preference over others. The nest depicted here will be shown as it evolves into the **vertical growth phase** in Figs. 24-58 and 24-59. The anatomic landmarks of the levels of invasion are shown. Level III is not simply the occasional impingement of a tumor cell against the reticular dermis, but indicates a collection of cells that fills and widens the papillary dermis and broadly abuts the reticular dermis. Level III invasion is usually a manifestation of the vertical growth phase. Level IV invasion should be designated only when tumor cells clearly permeate between otherwise unaltered collagen bundles of the reticular dermis.

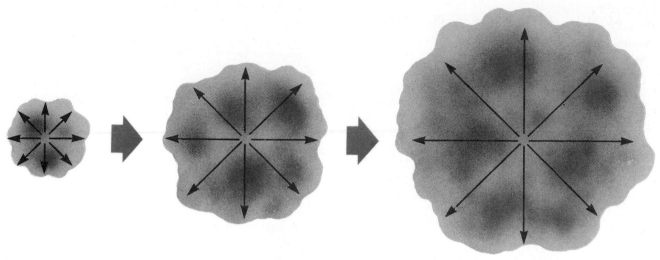

Figure 24-58. Development and evolution of the vertical growth phase in malignant melanoma of the superficial spreading type. A cell (clonal event?) or a nest of cells in the dermis of the radial growth phase will, in time, develop a growth preference over other cells in the tumor. In this phase, the focus of growth shifts from the epidermis to the dermis. The cells frequently expand in a balloon-like fashion, as illustrated. In other instances, they may form a plaque.

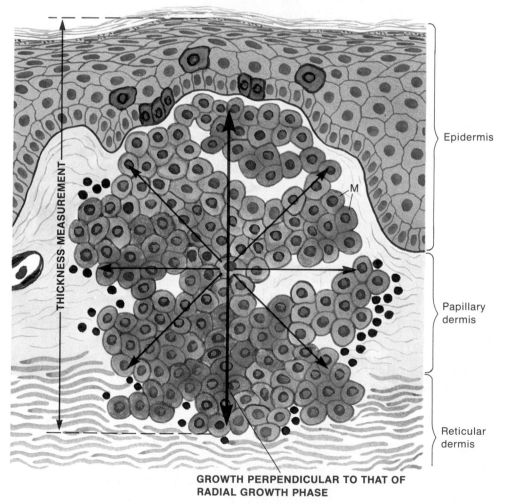

Epidermis

Papillary dermis

Reticular dermis

THICKNESS MEASUREMENT

M

GROWTH PERPENDICULAR TO THAT OF RADIAL GROWTH PHASE

Figure 24-59. Schematic depiction of the evolved vertical growth phase in malignant melanoma of the superficial spreading type with an indication of how thickness is measured. In this illustration, the vertical growth phase has extended into the reticular dermis. However, small nodules of tumor cells that clearly have a growth preference over other tumor cells may be a manifestation of the vertical growth phase. Thickness measurements (*arrows*) are taken from the outermost granular layer across the tumor in its thickest part.

Metastatic Melanoma

Metastatic melanoma, the final stage in tumor progression, arises from the cells of the vertical growth phase. Initial metastases in malignant melanoma usually involve the regional lymph nodes, but metastases via the bloodstream are also common. When bloodstream metastases do occur, they are unusually widespread in comparison with other neoplasms; virtually every organ system may be involved.

From the foregoing, one may answer the question previously posed, "What of the intervening years?" They are filled with a distinctive series of proliferative lesions, each of which has characteristic properties. In this melanocytic neoplastic system, that series of proliferative lesions proceeds as follows:

1. The common acquired melanocytic nevus (the ordinary mole)
2. A melanocytic nevus with a focus of flawed differentiation, called aberrant differentiation
3. A melanocytic nevus with aberrant differentiation and focal nuclear cytologic atypia of melanocytes, the combination being termed a dysplastic nevus
4. The radial growth phase of a primary melanoma
5. The vertical growth phase of a primary melanoma
6. Metastatic melanoma

Importantly, progression from one step to the next is not obligatory. In fact, it is rare in the first three steps, but common in the last three steps.

In vivo–In vitro Correlations in Tumor Progression

Growth regulation at the level of the cell or at the level of the organism is complex, and is controlled by multiple, diverse factors. One would not expect such a complex mechanism to become deregulated or dysregulated in a single cell generation or in a single lesional step. Each lesion that represents a given step in tumor progression has a predictable and characteristic behavior that is reflected, to some extent, in the characteristics of the cells from that lesion, grown in tissue culture. Cells from all the foregoing lesions of tumor progression may be grown in tissue culture.

The lesions of the first three steps do not show evidence of autonomous growth *in vivo* and, even though the cells grow in culture, permanent cell lines cannot be established. Further, while the cells are growing for several generations, they are nontumorigenic in animals. Most of these cells are diploid, but occasional random chromosomal abnormalities are seen in cells derived from dysplastic nevi. Autonomous growth *in vivo* is seen with the onset of the radial growth phase. However, it should be recalled that melanomas in the radial growth phase rarely give rise to metastases. Permanent cell lines may be established, but with great difficulty, and such cell lines are not usually tumorigenic in animals. Nevertheless, they show nonrandom chromosomal abnormalities at chromosome 6. The onset of the vertical growth phase marks the acquisition of competence for metastasis by a primary tumor. Metastases are postulated to come from the cells of the vertical growth phase. Cells cultured from the vertical growth phase and from metastases readily form permanent cell lines. Nonrandom chromosomal abnormalities are commonly seen at chromosomes 1, 6, and 7, and the cell lines are routinely tumorigenic in animals.

Direct Tumor Progression in Malignant Melanoma

Malignant Melanoma of the Nodular Type

Even though a cancer generally acquires its properties in a stepwise fashion, occasional cancers may arise that have all of their characteristics expressed in the initial lesion. Nodular malignant melanoma illustrates this form of tumor progression. These lesions, which fortunately are the rarest form of melanoma in man, appear as circumscribed, elevated nodules that tend to be spheroidal initially—that is, they do not develop through a radial growth phase (Fig. 24-60). Histologically, the tumor is composed of one or more nodules of cells that clearly grow in an expansile (balloon like) fashion in the dermis (Figs.

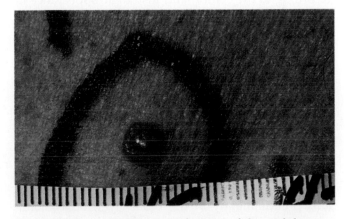

Figure 24-60. In malignant melanoma of the nodular type, the primary focus of growth of this 0.5-cm lesion is in the dermis.

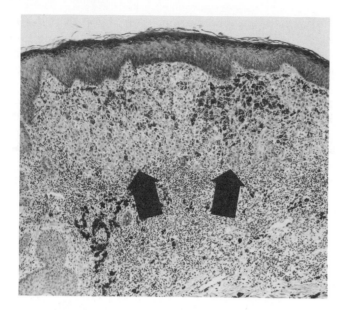

Figure 24-61.   The histology of the dermal growth in malignant melanoma of the nodular type is shown. Intraepidermal growth is essentially absent. Arrows point to deep margin of the tumor.

24-61 and 24-62). The tumor is in the vertical growth phase from the outset. The prognosis is dependent, in part, upon the thickness of the spheroidal nodule when the tumor is removed.

Other Examples of Indirect Tumor Progression in Malignant Melanoma

The other two common forms of malignant melanoma, which occur much less frequently than does the superficial spreading type, also evolve through radial and vertical growth phases. They are classified according to the clinical and histologic appearance of the radial growth phase.

Lentigo Maligna Melanoma

Lentigo maligna melanoma, which occurs almost exclusively in fair, usually elderly Caucasians, affects the exposed surfaces of the body and is probably related to ultraviolet light exposure. In its radial growth phase, it is a flat, irregular, brown to black lesion that may cover a large part of the face or back of the hand prior to the onset of the vertical growth phase (Fig. 24-63). The cells of the radial growth are seen predominantly in the basal layer, occasionally forming small nests that "hang down" into the papillary dermis (Fig. 24-64). Invasion is not as prominent or as extensive in the radial growth phase of

lentigo maligna melanoma as it is in superficial spreading melanoma. Cells of the radial growth phase, especially those disposed in nests, are of variable size. The subjacent dermis shows a modest lymphocytic infiltrate and, almost invariably, advanced solar degeneration of the elastic tissue. In the vertical growth phase (Fig. 24-65), the cells tend to be spindle-shaped. Occasionally, cells of this phase synthesize connective tissue and form a firm plaque; this condition is called **desmoplastic melanoma.** Cells of the vertical growth phase may also grow along small nerves, forming a **neurotropic vertical growth phase.**

Acral Lentiginous Melanoma

Acral lentiginous melanoma is the most common form of melanoma in dark-skinned people. The tumor is essentially limited to the palms, soles, and subungual regions. Although rare, a similar tumor affects the mucous membranes, and is termed **mucosal lentiginous melanoma.** In the radial growth phase, acral lentiginous melanoma forms an irregular, brown to black, flat area which covers a large part of the palm or sole or arises under a nail, usually the large toe or thumb (Fig. 24-66). Microscopically, the

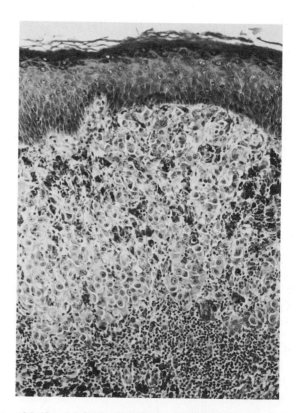

Figure 24-62.   Malignant melanoma of the nodular type. Melanoma cells in the dermis with host response are shown at a higher magnification.

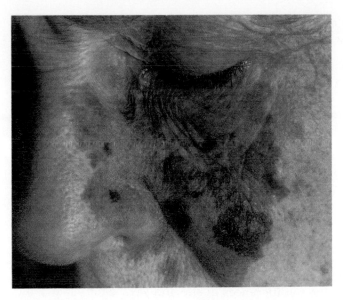

Figure 24-63. The radial growth phase in malignant melanoma of the lentigo maligna type.

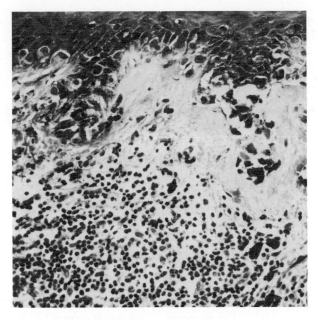

Figure 24-64. The histology of the radial growth phase in malignant melanoma of the lentigo maligna type. The growth is largely at the dermal-epidermal interface. Nests of melanocytes form, "hanging down" into the papillary dermis. Invasion of the dermis and upward growth in the epidermis are much less prominent than in malignant melanoma of the superficial spreading type.

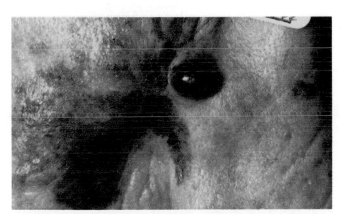

Figure 24-65. The clinical appearance of the radial and vertical growth phase in malignant melanoma of the lentigo maligna type. The lesion is 1 cm in diameter.

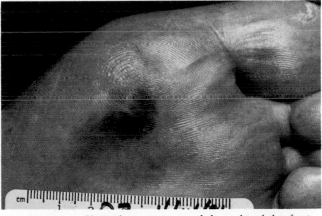

Figure 24-66. Clinical appearance of the sole of the foot in a patient with malignant melanoma of the acral lentiginous type (radial growth phase).

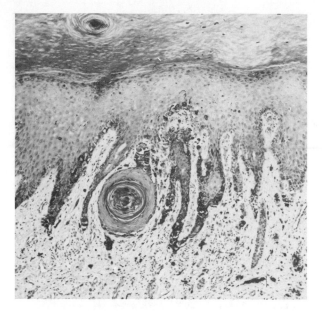

Figure 24-67. The histology of the radial growth phase in malignant melanoma of the acral lentiginous type. The tumor cells are largely in the basal layer, giving it a dark appearance at this magnification.

cells are, for the most part, confined to the basal layer, and maintain long dendrites (Figs. 24-67 and 24-68). Frequently, a brisk lichenoid lymphocytic response is present. As the vertical growth phase approaches, cells may grow upward in the epidermis and become more epithelioid. The vertical growth phase (Fig. 24-69) is similar to that of lentigo maligna melanoma, and spindle cells are common (Fig. 24-70). Neurotropism is also occasionally seen.

Prognostic Indicators in Malignant Melanoma (Derived from the Study of Primary Melanomas

Radial and Vertical Growth Phases

It has already been noted that malignant melanomas should first be divided into those that are in the radial growth phase and those that are in the vertical growth phase, and that patients with tumors that are entirely within the radial growth phase are not expected to have a recurrence or develop metastasis following complete excision of the lesion. In excising a melanoma that is in a radial growth phase, it is a common practice to include a radius of normal skin about 1 cm around the lesion. Those tumors that are in the vertical growth phase generally require exci-

sions with a radius of 2.5 cm or more around the original lesion.

Tumor Thickness in the Vertical Growth Phase

The best single prognostic indicator in malignant melanoma is the thickness of the tumor in the vertical growth phase. Tumor thickness is measured from the outermost layer of the stratum granulosum to the deepest penetration of the tumor in the dermis. Those tumors in a vertical growth phase that are less than 0.75 mm in thickness have a survival of 90 to 95 percent; those 0.76 mm to 1.69 mm a survival of 70 to 90 percent; those 1.70 mm to 3.60 mm a survival of 40 to 85 percent; and those greater than 3.61 mm a survival of 20 to 70 percent. The wide ranges are due to differences in site and sex.

Levels of Invasion

The level of tumor invasion refers to the degree of tumor penetration within the important anatomic layers of the skin. **Level I** tumors are *in situ*—that is, they are entirely above the basement membrane zone. **Level II** is the designation for those tumors in which the invasive cells are present only in the pap-

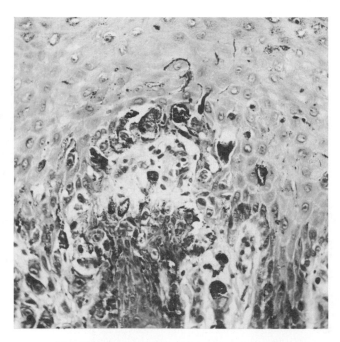

Figure 24-68. Large melanocytes with prominent dendrites, which are characteristic of malignant melanoma of the acral lentiginous type, are present in the basal region of the epidermis.

illary dermis, and generally coincides with the radial growth phase. **Level III** tumors are those that have entered the vertical growth phase and that impinge upon the reticular dermis, forming small expansile nodules that widen the papillary dermis. **Level IV** invasion denotes clear permeation of tumor cells between the collagen bundles of the reticular dermis. **Level V** invasion refers to tumors that extend into the fat. These levels of invasion are also predictors of the likelihood of metastasis from malignant melanoma, although they are not as accurate in this regard as is tumor thickness. Determining the level of invasion does, however, provide additional prognostic information for tumors that are thicker than 1.70 mm.

Site

In general, melanomas on the extremities have a better prognosis than do those on the head, neck, or trunk. However, acral lentiginous tumors of the sole of the foot or the subungual region are not necessarily associated with this better prognosis.

Sex

For every site and thickness, women have a better prognosis than men. For example, tumors that are 0.76 mm to 1.69 mm on the trunk of women are associated with a survival of about 86 percent, but in

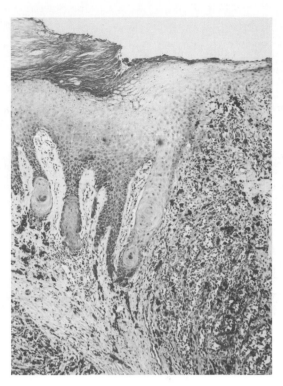

Figure 24-70. Histologic depiction of the vertical growth phase (right side of photograph) in malignant melanoma of the acral lentiginous type.

men the survival is only 71 percent, site and thickness being the same.

Lymphocytic Response

The evaluation of the interaction of lymphocytes and tumor cells in the vertical growth phase is of considerable prognostic importance. The response is stated to be **infiltrative** when the lymphocytes actually infiltrate and disrupt the tumor, frequently forming rosettes about the tumor cells (Fig. 24-71). When this infiltrative host response is not present, or when there is no host response at all, the prognosis is much poorer.

Mitotic Rate

In the vertical growth phase, if the number of mitoses per square millimeter is 0, the patient has a much improved prognosis. An intermediate mitotic rate of 1 to 6/mm^2 is associated with a somewhat poorer prognosis, whereas a mitotic rate greater than 6.1/mm^2 is indicative of an extremely poor prognosis. There are other adverse prognostic attributes, such as regression and satellitosis.

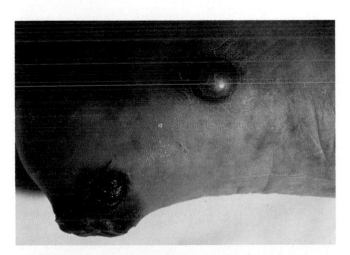

Figure 24-69. Clinical presentation of malignant melanoma of the acral lentiginous type (radial and vertical growth phases). The lesion on the heel is the primary tumor. The flat portion represents the radial growth phase, whereas the elevated portion is indicative of the vertical growth phase. The dark nodular lesion on the instep is a metastasis.

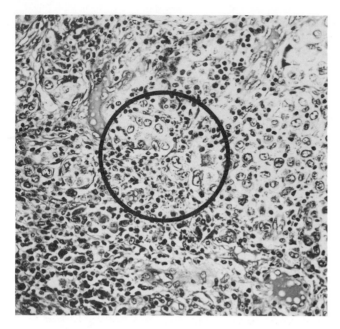

Figure 24-71. The vertical growth phase in this case of malignant melanoma of the superficial spreading type shows the characteristics of an infiltrative host response (*circled*).

Other Benign Tumors of Melanocytic Origin

Congenital Melanocytic Nevi

Approximately 1 percent of children are born with some form of pigmented lesions on their skin. Sometimes, these lesions are as inconspicuous as an area of pale tan hyperpigmentation. Rarely, the trunk or an extremity may be covered by a large, pigmented lesion that is cosmetically deforming. Such areas show a striking increase in intraepidermal and dermal melanocytes that extend deeply into the subcutaneous tissue. These large congenital melanocytic nevi can develop into malignant melanomas. Affected children should be followed carefully, and their families should be instructed in proper techniques for examining the lesions. Some physicians attempt to remove these large lesions, but in many instances, the size of these nevi makes surgical removal impossible.

Spitz Tumors (Epithelioid Cell Nevi)

Spitz tumors occur in children and, with somewhat less frequency, in adults. The greatest problem presented by these tumors is overdiagnosis as a malignant melanoma. The Spitz tumor, which presents as

an elevated, spheroid, pink, smooth nodule, grows rapidly, increasing in diameter to approximately 3 to 5 mm within 6 months. This lesion is composed of large, epithelioid melanocytes that extend into the epidermis and often extend well into the dermis (Fig. 24-72). The cells are so atypical that a false diagnosis of melanoma may be made. In a child, therefore, one should be compellingly certain that a lesion is truly malignant before making a diagnosis of malignant melanoma. True malignant melanoma is exquisitely rare in childhood.

Keratinocytic Neoplasia

Benign Keratinocytic Neoplasms (Including Those of Viral Etiology)

Seborrheic Keratosis

Although seborrheic keratosis is one of the most common keratoses of man, its etiology is unknown. It generally presents in the later years of life, and tends to be familial. The lesion is a scaly, frequently pigmented, elevated lesion the scales of which are easily rubbed off by hand. Microscopically, the lesions seem

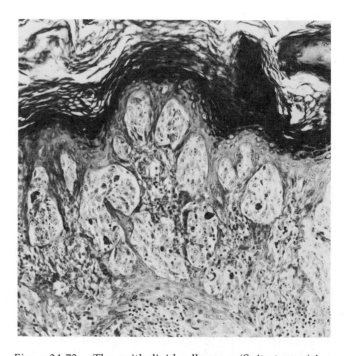

Figure 24-72. The epithelioid cell nevus (Spitz tumor) is composed of large melanocytes with prominent nuclei. The cells are disposed in nests. Even though the cells are large and, at first glance, suggestive of melanoma, they are much more uniform than the cells of most melanomas.

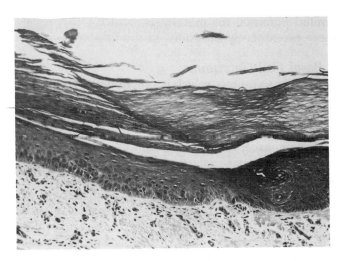

Figure 24-73. Actinic keratosis is shown on the left. Parakeratosis and loss of polarity are evident. The lesion is separated from the relatively normal epidermis by a diagonal line, which is a common histologic appearance.

to be tacked onto the skin, and are composed of broad anastomosing cords of mature, stratified, squamous epithelium, associated with small cysts of keratin called **horn cysts.** These lesions are innocuous, but represent a cosmetic nuisance.

Verruca Vulgaris

A number of interesting papillary hyperplasias of the epidermis are induced by viruses. Some of these are venereally transmitted (for example, condyloma acuminatum), whereas others are apparently spontaneous in origin. **An example of a viral papilloma is the common wart, termed verruca vulgaris.** It is characterized by pale, delicate, pointed spines that represent a circumscribed area of epidermal hyperplasia. Microscopically, there is marked hyperkeratosis and hyperplasia of mature stratified squamous epithelium. Early lesions show distinct, eosinophilic, intranuclear, and intracytoplasmic inclusions that are diagnostic of the viral infection.

Actinic Keratosis (From the Sun's Rays)

The sequence of events that relates hyperplasia of the keratinocytic epithelium to squamous cell carcinoma is analogous to that described for malignant melanoma, and is similar to the development of squamous carcinoma in other sites (for instance, the cervix or bronchus). Actinic keratosis ("from the sun's rays") is an atypical hyperplasia of keratinocytes, and is analogous to a dysplastic nevus. It presents in solar damaged skin as a circumscribed area of hyperkeratosis, commonly on the backs of the hands or the face. Microscopically, the stratum corneum is no longer loose and basket-weaved, but is replaced by a dense parakeratotic material (a result of the retention of nuclei in the stratum corneum). The underlying basal cells show significant atypia (Fig. 24-73). With passage of time, these lesions may evolve into squamous cell carcinoma *in situ,* and finally into invasive squamous cell carcinoma. However, as in the case of dysplastic nevi, the lesions are generally stable or may even regress.

Malignant Keratinocytic Neoplasms

Squamous Cell Carcinoma

The end stage of keratinocytic tumor progression, except for metastasis, is squamous cell carcinoma. These lesions characteristically arise on the backs of the hands or the face. An area of localized hyperkeratosis, which is usually actinic, produces increasing amounts of keratin. Microscopic examination reveals atypical keratinocytic hyperplasia involving all of the epidermal layers (Fig. 24-74). However, of far greater importance is the extension of atypical keratinocytes into the underlying connective tissue as an invasive squamous cell carcinoma. These tumors have only a

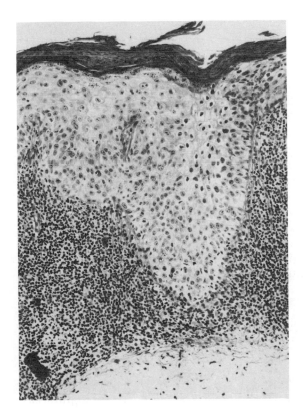

Figure 24-74. In this case of squamous cell carcinoma *in situ,* the entire epidermis is replaced by atypical keratinocytes. A brisk lymphocytic response is evident.

25

The Head and Neck

Károly Balogh

Oral Cavity

Salivary Glands

Nose and Paranasal Sinuses

Nasopharynx

Ear

Figure 25-1. Anatomy of the ear. (*A*) The relationships of the external, middle, and inner ear. Note the tympanic membrane, the ossicles of the middle ear, the location of the eustachian tube, and the proximity of the meninges and the brain. (*B*) Diagrammatic visualization of the tympanic membrane and the ossicles. The arrow indicates the normal position of the stapes in the oval window. A cross section of the cochlea demonstrates the relationship of the cochlear duct (carrying endolymph) to the scala tympani and scala vestibuli (filled with perilymph).

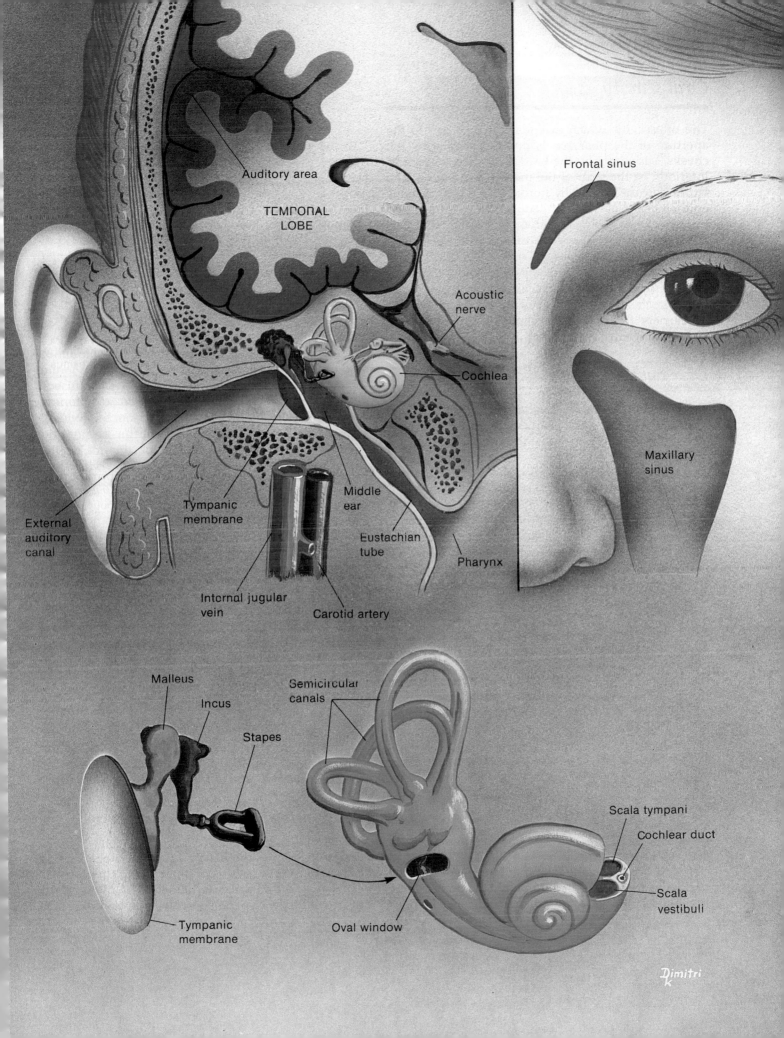

Auditory area

TEMPORAL LOBE

Frontal sinus

Acoustic nerve

Cochlea

Maxillary sinus

Tympanic membrane

Middle ear

External auditory canal

Eustachian tube

Pharynx

Internal jugular vein

Carotid artery

Malleus

Incus

Stapes

Semicircular canals

Scala tympani

Cochlear duct

Scala vestibuli

Tympanic membrane

Oval window

Dimitri
K

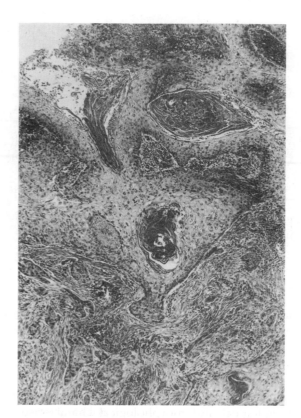

Figure 25-9. Squamous cell carcinoma of tongue. Nests and sheets of epithelial cells have invaded the stroma. This well-differentiated tumor shows marked keratinization.

Grading and Metastases   Variations in differentiation in squamous cell carcinoma have led to a system of grading tumors. Accordingly, a grade I carcinoma is well-differentiated and is frequently keratinizing (Fig. 25-9). At the other end of the spectrum, grade IV carcinomas are so poorly differentiated that their origin is difficult to detect microscopically. In general, the less differentiated a tumor, the faster it grows and spreads. Metastases from oral carcinoma occur mainly in the submandibular, superficial, and deep cervical lymph nodes. Lymph node involvement at the time of diagnosis carries a poor prognosis. More than half of patients who die of squamous carcinoma of the head and neck have distant, blood-borne metastases, most commonly in the lungs, liver, and bones. In establishing therapy, clinical staging is also useful. The TNM system (T, primary tumor; N, regional lymph nodes; M, distant metastases) is commonly employed.

Malignant Melanoma

As a primary tumor, malignant melanoma is rare in the oral mucosa, where its features are similar to those in the skin. It occurs in middle-aged or elderly individuals and is twice as common in men as in women. The tumor is highly malignant and carries a poor prognosis.

Sarcomas

Since all connective tissue elements are present in the soft tissues of the oral cavity, sarcomas arise in this site, albeit rarely. Fibrosarcomas, liposarcomas, angiosarcomas, neurogenic sarcomas, leiomyosarcomas, rhabdomyosarcomas, and synovial sarcomas do not differ from similar tumors elsewhere.

Locally aggressive fibrous lesions in the oral soft tissues include nodular fasciitis, aggressive fibromatosis, fibrous histiocytoma, and proliferative myositis. These lesions do not metastasize and must not be confused with sarcomas.

Kaposi's Sarcoma   In its classic form, Kaposi's sarcoma is a slowly progressive cutaneous neoplasm of the elderly that rarely metastasizes to the oral cavity. This tumor has attained wide publicity due to its notorious association with AIDS. The newly recognized, epidemic type of Kaposi's sarcoma in AIDS frequently involves the mucous membranes, including those of the oral cavity (Fig. 25-10). Early in the course of AIDS, sometimes among its first complications, the characteristic purple to brown-red, mucocutaneous nodules of Kaposi's sarcoma appear. Their size and number grow and they may bleed, although they seldom become bulky. The tumor is not life-threatening and the patients invariably die of other complications of AIDS.

Metastatic Carcinomas and Sarcomas

Metastases to the oral soft tissues are exceptionally rare and most are diagnosed incidentally. The most common sources are primary carcinomas of the breasts, lungs, and kidneys, and malignant melanomas.

Malignant Lymphomas and Hodgkin's Disease

Malignant lymphomas and Hodgkin's disease occasionally involve the oral cavity, either as an initial manifestation of the disease or in the course of its spread from other body sites. Some non-Hodgkin's lymphomas may remain localized and can be successfully treated, thereby suggesting a primary malignant lymphoma of the oral cavity. Similar situations have been observed with plasmacytomas.

Burkitt's lymphoma was originally described as a childhood tumor of the jaws in equatorial Africa. It is now thought to be related to infection with the Epstein-Barr virus. A rare, sporadic (American) form of Burkitt's tumor involves the jaws in only 5% of cases and is not associated with the Epstein-Barr virus.

Diseases of the Lips

The lips, covered externally by skin and internally by mucous membrane, contain skeletal muscle, areolar tissue, fat, numerous small mucous glands, blood vessels, lymphatics, and nerves. These anatomic structures are affected by a variety of degenerative, inflammatory, and proliferative processes. Some of these processes, particularly those expressed in the skin and oral mucous membranes, are systemic; others reflect localized disease (Fig. 25-11, 25-12).

Diseases of the Tongue

The tongue is a muscular structure situated in the floor of the mouth and invested by mucous membrane. The mucosa of the base of the tongue contains numerous lymphoid follicles, which constitute the lingual tonsils and are a part of Waldeyer's ring. The tongue consists mainly of striated muscle. Between the muscle bundles are minor salivary glands, adipose tissue, blood vessels, lymphatics, and nerves.

Macroglossia

All of the components of the tongue may be involved by various localized or systemic diseases, some of which can lead to enlargement of the tongue, that is, **macroglossia.** If present at birth, macroglossia is usu-

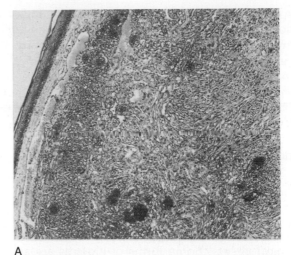

A

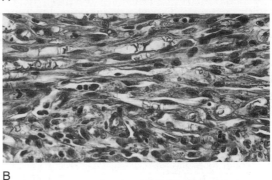

B

Figure 25-10. Kaposi's sarcoma. (*A*) The nasopharynx in a patient with AIDS contains a vascular lesion that extends close to the mucosal epithelium. Intervening bundles of cells and foci of hemorrhage are distinctive. (*B*) Thin-walled vessels and endothelial-lined spaces are seen among spindle cells.

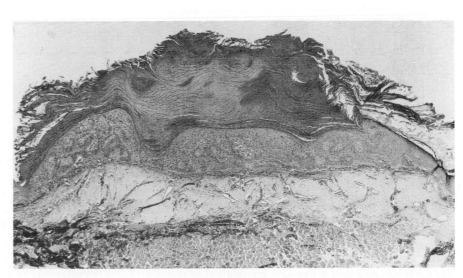

Figure 25-11. Solar cheilitis. A lesion analogous to a solar keratosis is present in the vermilion border of the lower lip. Hyperkeratosis and epithelial hyperplasia and dysplasia are evident. This lesion may develop into squamous cell carcinoma.

ally due to diffuse lymphangioma or hemangioma, although rarely enlargement is caused by congenital neurofibromatosis or true muscular hypertrophy. An enlarged tongue that protrudes from the mouth is seen in congenital hypothyroidism, Hurler's syndrome, glycogen storage disease type II (Pompe's disease), Beckwith-Wiedemann syndrome, and trisomy 21 syndrome. Secondary or acquired macroglossia is due to amyloidosis, acromegaly, and infiltration or lymphatic obstruction by tumors.

Glossitis

Inflammation of the tongue, called glossitis, is caused by various microorganisms, physical effects, or chemical agents. Some forms of glossitis are associated with systemic diseases or vitamin deficiencies.

In **pernicious anemia** the tongue is often inflamed and "beefy red." The gradual atrophy of the papillae results in a smooth or "bald" tongue (Hunter's glossitis). The changes rapidly disappear after treatment with vitamin B_{12}.

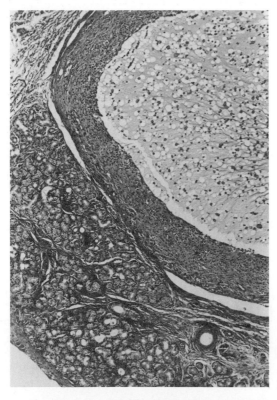

Figure 25-12.   Mucocele of lower lip. This cystic lesion is associated with the minor salivary glands and is probably caused by trauma that permits escape of mucus. The cyst has a fibrous wall and is lined by granulation tissue. The lumen is filled with mucus that contains numerous macrophages.

In **riboflavin (vitamin B_2) deficiency** a similar glossitis is characterized by atrophy of the filiform papillae. At the angles of the mouth maceration and fissuring, termed **cheilosis,** occur.

In **pellagra, the syndrome caused by niacin (nicotinic acid) deficiency,** the oral mucosa becomes fiery red and painful, and the epithelium of the tongue desquamates. A similar process affects the gums; an acute necrotizing and ulcerative gingivostomatitis is often superimposed.

The oral lesions of **pyridoxine (vitamin B_6) deficiency** bear a striking resemblance to the stomatitis of pellagra.

Diseases of the Teeth and Periodontal Tissues

The teeth and their attachments, together with the jawbones in which they are anchored, function as an apparatus. Developmental disturbances of the oral structures and jaws may be manifestations of hereditary syndromes or anomalies caused by a variety of insults during pregnancy.

Dental Caries

One of the oldest and most prevalent chronic diseases of the calcified tissues of the teeth is caries. It affects persons of both sexes and every age group throughout the world, and its incidence has increased with modern civilization.

Although the important etiologic factor seems to be a diet of processed foods, the cause of dental caries is not clear, and several theories have been proposed. The most often cited is the **acidogenic theory,** which is over 100 years old. This theory is supported by experiments demonstrating that acids, chiefly lactic acid, produced by microorganisms through the fermentation of sugars and cooked starches, decalcify enamel and dentin in vitro. Among the numerous microorganisms, the presence of *Bacillus acidophilus* was thought to be of critical importance. Experiments on germ-free hamsters have shown that oral inoculation of pure cultures of certain streptococci isolated from hamster caries induce lesions of teeth that closely resemble those seen in the conventional animals. Acid is held in place by the **dental plaque,** which is a bacterial colony on the surface of the tooth.

The **proteolytic theory,** also more than 100 years old, emphasizes the important role of the organic constituents of teeth in the development of caries. Proteolysis by invading microorganisms produces acid in both enamel and dentin. It has been pointed out that bacteria that produce acid from carbohydrate also degrade protein. The **proteolysis—chelation hypothesis** holds that the products of the initial proteolysis form soluble chelates with the mineralized components of enamel, thereby decalcifying it.

None of these theories is entirely satisfactory. The mere presence of microorganisms on a tooth surface is clearly insufficient to produce caries in all instances. Indirect factors which contribute to the development of caries include the chemical composition, morphologic characteristics, and position of the teeth. The composition of saliva, its pH, viscosity, quantity, and antibacterial properties also seem to play a role in the production of caries.

Dietary Factors

There is a consensus that one of the most important factors in the development of caries is a high carbohydrate intake. Raw and unrefined foods contain a great deal of roughage that cleanses the teeth and necessitates more mastication, which further contributes to the cleansing of the teeth. By contrast, soft and refined foods tend to stick to the teeth and also require less chewing. Deficient intake of vitamin D, calcium, and phosphorus has been claimed to contribute to dental caries, but it is difficult to draw definite conclusions. Of great practical significance is the fact that the presence of fluoride in the drinking water protects against dental caries. Fluoride is incorporated into the crystal lattice structure of enamel where it forms fluoroapatite, a less acid-soluble compound than the apatite of enamel. The fluoridation of drinking water in many communities has been followed by a dramatic reduction in the incidence of dental caries in children, whose teeth were formed while they drank fluoride-containing water.

Calcium

There is no relation between pregnancy or lactation, both of which drain calcium stores, and caries. In this connection it is noteworthy that, unlike the situation in bone, there is no mechanism for the physiologic mobilization of calcium from teeth.

Pathology

Microscopically, caries begin with the disintegration of the enamel prisms after decalcification of the interprismatic substance, events which lead to the accumulation of debris and microorganisms (Fig. 25-13, 14). When the process reaches the dentinoenamel junction, it spreads laterally and also penetrates the dentin along the dentinal tubules. Calcification of the dentinal tubules may seal them off, thereby barring further penetration by microorganisms. However, decalcification of dentin usually continues and leads to a focal coalescence of the destroyed dentinal tubules. Damage of dentin stimulates the odontoblasts which line the wall of the pulp chamber, to form secondary dentin. Unfortunately this reparative process usually does not prevent the microorganisms of the oral flora from reaching the dental pulp and causing pulpitis.

Diseases of the Pulp and Periapical Tissues

The dental pulp consists of delicate connective tissue enclosed within the calcified walls of dentin. The pulp chamber is lined by odontoblasts and has a minute apical foramen, through which blood vessels, lymphatics, and small nerves penetrate.

Pulpitis

Inflammation of the dental pulp, known as **pulpitis,** is usually due to invasion by oral bacteria in dental caries. In **acute pulpitis,** pain is caused by the increase in pressure of the pulp chamber by edema and exudate. Increased pressure in the pulp chamber also facilitates the spread of inflammation. A large open cavity may prevent an increase in pressure. Acute pulpitis may be accompanied by the formation of a small pulp abscess, and several small abscesses may lead to necrosis of the entire pulp.

Chronic pulpitis may be the outcome of a subsiding acute inflammation, or may be a chronic inflammation from its onset.

Acute or chronic pulpitis, if untreated, ultimately results in complete necrosis of the dental pulp. Another consequence of untreated pulpitis is the spread of infection through the root canals into the periapical region. The most common sequel of pulpitis is the formation of chronically inflamed periapical granulation tissue, termed **periapical granuloma** (Fig. 25-15). The inflammatory tissue gradually becomes surrounded by a fibrous capsule, and when the tooth is extracted, the encapsulated granuloma is found attached to the root. Histologic examination of periapical granulomas reveals the presence of stratified squamous epithelium, which may be derived from a periodontal pocket, or from oral epithelium lining a fistula. Since this epithelium proliferates, a cavity lined by stratified squamous epithelium forms in this inflammatory tissue, and is labelled an **apical periodontal cyst.** A **periapical abscess** develops as a result of pulpitis, either directly or after the formation of periapical granulomas and cysts. This abscess, if not contained, rapidly extends to the adjacent bone, where it produces osteomyelitis. Bacteriologic cultures in all stages of pulpitis and periapical infection

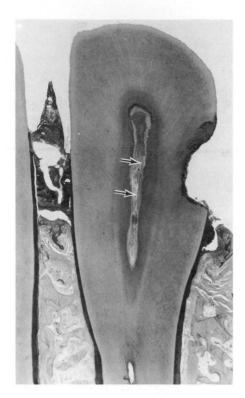

Figure 25-13. Dental caries. A large cavity close to the gingival margin is illustrated. Arrows point to the band of secondary dentin that lines the pulp chamber. This newly formed dentin is opposite the area of tooth destruction and was produced by the stimulated odontoblasts.

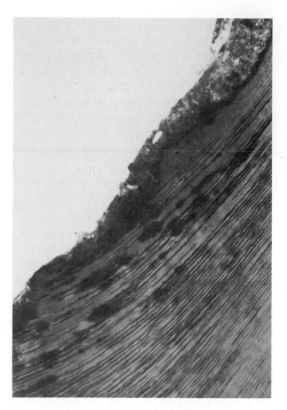

Figure 25-14. Dental caries. A deposit of debris covers the surface. Bacterial colonies (*black*) have extended into dentinal canals.

grow *Staphylococcus aureus, Staphylococcus albus,* various streptococci, or mixed organisms.

Osteomyelitis

Osteomyelitis of the jawbones, like that of other bones, may become localized or propagate within the bone. It may break through the cortical bone and spread in various tissue spaces of the head and neck, causing cellulitis (phlegmon) or abscesses. The purulent exudate may discharge into the surface of the mucous membranes or skin and create fistulas. In advanced cases the infection follows the line of gravity in the tissue planes and ultimately reaches the mediastinum. These grave complications of dental infection were often lethal in the days before antibiotics.

Diseases of the Periodontal Tissues

The gingiva is that part of the oral mucosa which surrounds the teeth and ends in a thin edge (free gingiva) closely adherent to the teeth. The periodontal ligament is composed of collagen fibers that hold the tooth in position by suspending it in the socket (alveolus) of the jawbones. Many mucocutaneous disorders affect the gums, among which are the most frequent infections of the oral mucosa. Other important diseases encompass several vitamin deficiencies.

Scurvy, due to vitamin C deficiency, is not only of historical interest, but is, in less dramatic forms, still encountered, particularly in poor, neglected, or ignorant individuals. Scurvy frequently affects the marginal and interdental gingiva, which becomes swollen and bright red and readily bleeds and ulcerates. Hemorrhage into the periodontal membrane causes loosening and loss of teeth.

A number of hematologic disorders affect the oral tissues, but some strike the gums with particular frequency. **Agranulocytosis** causes necrotizing ulcers anywhere in the oral and pharyngeal mucosa, but involvement of the gingiva is particularly common. **Infectious mononucleosis** is frequently accompanied by oral symptoms. Acute gingivitis and stomatitis, with exudate and ulceration, are among its common manifestations.

Acute and chronic **leukemias** of all types cause oral lesions. The most common involvement of oral tissues is seen in acute monocytic leukemia of the histiocytic type, in which 80% of the patients exhibit gingivitis, gingival hyperplasia, petechiae, hemorrhage, and ulceration. These may be early manifestations of the leukemic process and can suggest the correct diagnosis to the alert dentist or physician. Necrosis and ulceration of the gingiva lead to severe superimposed infection which may cause loss of teeth and alveolar bone.

Purpura, a purplish discoloration of the mucous membranes and skin caused by spontaneous, multifocal extravasation of blood, is seen in a wide variety of diseases and may affect the oral tissues.

Hemorrhage from various sites in the oral cavity is associated with various hemorrhagic diatheses, including hemophilia, hypofibrinogenemia, macroglobulinemia, anticoagulation, and deficiencies of vitamins C and K.

Gingivitis and Periodontal Disease

Although acute inflammation of the gum is not common, chronic gingivitis is one of the most widespread disorders. Local factors which cause gingivitis include microorganisms, calculus, food impaction, tooth malposition or defects, irritating restorations or prostheses, topical drugs, and chemicals. The most important and most frequent causes of chronic gingivitis are microorganisms alone or in combination with one of the listed physical or chemical irritants.

Often the inflammation starts as a marginal gingivitis and, if untreated, progresses to severe chronic periodontitis (Fig. 25-16). This disease usually occurs in adults, particularly in individuals with poor oral hygiene. Chronic inflammation weakens and destroys the periodontium, causing loosening and eventual loss of teeth. **Chronic periodontitis causes loss of more teeth in the adult than does any other disease, including caries.**

Odontogenic Cysts and Tumors

The mandible and maxilla, similar to other bones, are affected by both generalized and localized forms of skeletal diseases. They are, however, unique in that they provide an abode for the teeth. Besides the inflammatory processes of dental origin described above, a variety of odontogenic cysts and tumors arises in the jawbones and the adjacent soft tissues, the pathogenesis of which can be understood on the basis of dental histogenesis (Fig. 25-17).

Odontogenic cysts have been classified according to the stage of odontogenesis during which they originate. The most common is the **radicular, or apical periodontal, cyst,** which involves the apex of an erupted tooth, usually following an infection of the dental pulp. The cyst is lined by stratified squamous epithelium derived from the epithelial rests of Malassez.

Dentigerous cysts are associated with the crown of an impacted, embedded, or unerupted tooth, most often with the mandibular and maxillary third molars. The cyst forms after the crown of the tooth has completely developed, and fluid accumulates between the crown and the overlying enamel epithelium (see Fig. 25-17). Dentigerous cysts are usually unilocular and are lined by a thin layer of stratified squamous epithelium. Pressure by an enlarging cyst can cause marked resorption of bone and adjacent teeth. Among the potential complications of a dentigerous cyst are recurrence after incomplete removal, development of an ameloblastoma from the cyst lin-

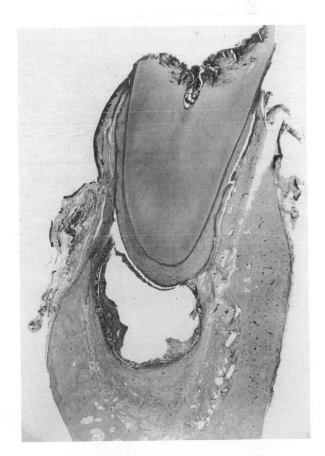

Figure 25-15. Advanced caries with periapical granuloma. The crown of the tooth has been destroyed by caries. Chronic infection of the pulp has led to chronic inflammation and the development of periapical granulation tissue.

ing or from epithelial rests of Malassez and development of squamous cell carcinoma.

Ameloblastoma is a tumor of the jaws, although rare cases have been reported in other sites (long bones, sella turcica). The origin of the tumor is not clear, but it clearly derives from odontogenic epithelium, most likely from cell rests of the enamel organ.

The large majority of ameloblastomas arise in the mandible, and most of these occur in the ramus or molar area. Ameloblastomas in the maxilla are also most common in the molar area, but they can also involve the maxillary antrum or floor of the nasal cavity. The tumor tends to grow slowly as a central lesion of bone. Radiographs, particularly of advanced tumors, show a multilocular cystlike appearance, with a smooth periphery, expansion of the bone, and thinning of the cortex. Microscopically, the ameloblastoma resembles the enamel organ in its various stages of differentiation; a single tumor may show various histologic patterns. Accordingly, the tumor cells resemble ameloblasts at the periphery of the epithelial nests or cords, where columnar cells are oriented perpendicularly to the basement membrane (Fig. 25-18). The centers of these cell nests consist of loosely arranged, larger polyhedral cells that resemble the stellate reticulum of the developing tooth. Frequently the complete breakdown of these looser areas results in the formation of microcysts.

The prognosis of ameloblastomas is favorable. Incompletely excised tumors recur, but malignant transformation is exceedingly rare.

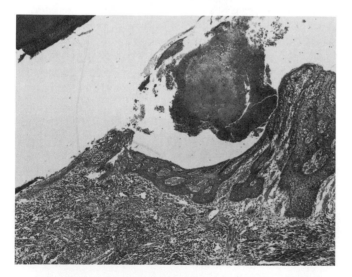

Figure 25-16. Hyperplastic chronic gingivitis. A labiolingual section shows marked hyperplasia of the epithelium and extensive chronic inflammation of the underlying tissues. Calculus can be seen in the pocket. The tooth separated from the gums during processing of the tissue.

Other Odontogenic Tumors

Several rare odontogenic neoplasms are characterized by the simultaneous occurrence of an ameloblastoma and proliferation of mesenchymal tissue. These true mixed tumors include **ameloblastic fibroma, ameloblastic fibrosarcoma** and **ameloblastic hemangioma.** An **odontoma** is a mixed tumor in which the epithelial and mesenchymal components are completely differentiated, that is, enamel and dentin are seen.

Salivary Glands

The minor and major salivary glands develop as buds of the oral ectoderm. Fully developed, they are tubuloalveolar structures that secrete saliva. The minor salivary glands are widespread, being present under the mucosa of the lips, cheeks, palate, and tongue. The major salivary glands are paired organs, secreting serous (parotid) or mixed serous and mucous (submandibular and sublingual) saliva.

Xerostomia

Xerostomia (decreased salivary flow) results from many causes. Diseases that involve the major glands and produce xerostomia include epidemic parotitis, Sjögren's syndrome, sarcoidosis, radiation-induced atrophy (Fig. 25-19), and drug sensitivity (antihistamines, tricyclic antidepressants, hypotensive drugs, phenothiazines).

Sialorrhea

Sialorrhea (increased salivary flow) is associated with many conditions, for example acute inflammation of the oral cavity, as in aphthous stomatitis, and Parkinson's disease, rabies, mental retardation, nausea, and pregnancy.

Enlargement

Enlargement of the major salivary glands, if unilateral, is due to inflammation, cysts, or neoplasms. Bilateral enlargement is caused by inflammation (mumps, Sjögren's syndrome), granulomatous disease (sarcoidosis), or diffuse neoplastic involvement (leukemia or malignant lymphoma).

Sialolithiasis

Salivary stones (calculi) are usually found in the ducts of a major gland, most commonly in the submandib-

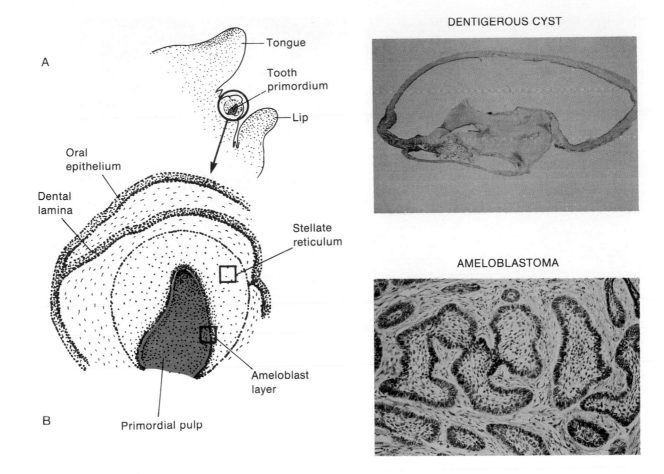

Figure 25-17. Development of dental and odontogenic tumors. Diagrammatic representation of the normal development of a tooth and the mode of formation of a dentigerous cyst and ameloblastoma. (*A*) Sagittal section of the lower jaw of a human embryo at 14 weeks, through the primordium of the lower central incisor. (*B*) Higher power representation of the circled area in *A*. The enamel organ at this stage is a double-walled sac, composed of an outer convex wall and an inner concave wall. Between the two are looser ectodermal cells (stellate reticulum). The stellate reticulum gives rise to dentigerous cysts, while the ameloblasts may form an ameloblastoma.

ular gland. The etiology of this disorder is unknown, although in some instances stones have been found around a foreign body. The most important consequence of stone formation is obstruction of the duct, often followed by inflammation distal to the occlusion.

Inflammation

Acute suppurative parotitis is caused by the ascent of bacteria (usually *Staphylococcus aureus*) from the oral cavity when the salivary flow is reduced. It is most frequently seen in debilitated or postoperative patients.

Acute and chronic inflammation of the major salivary glands is often associated with stricture or obstruction of the ducts by calculi (sialoliths). The stagnant secretions serve as a medium for retrograde bacterial invasion.

Epidemic parotitis (mumps) is an acute viral disease of the parotid glands that spreads with infected saliva. The submandibular and sublingual salivary glands may also be involved. In addition to involvement of the salivary glands, viral-induced pancreatitis and orchitis are common. Microscopically, the

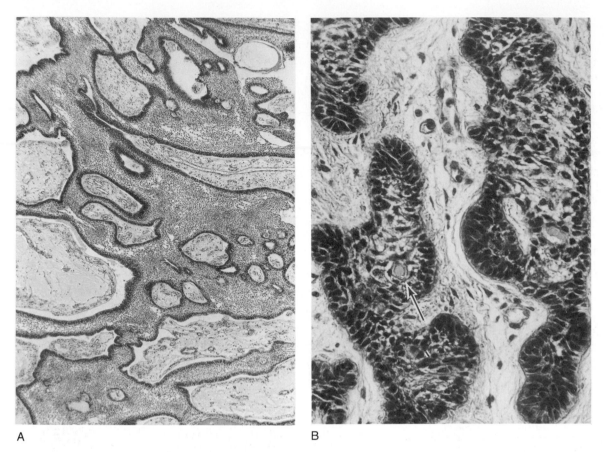

A   B

Figure 25-18.   Ameloblastoma. (*A*) A common histologic pattern is characterized by confluent islands of epithelium. The peripheral cells form a band that separates the tumor from the stroma. (*B*) A higher magnification of *A* shows tumor nests with central areas of stellate cells and squamous cells. The arrow indicates focal keratinization. The peripheral layer of cuboidal cells rests on a basement membrane.

salivary glands are densely infiltrated by lymphocytes and histiocytes; the infiltration is accompanied by degenerative changes and necrosis of the epithelial cells.

Sjögren's Syndrome

Sjögren's syndrome is a chronic inflammatory disease which is probably of autoimmune etiology. It is characterized by a set of inflammatory changes consisting of keratoconjunctivitis sicca, pharyngolaryngitis sicca, rhinitis sicca, rheumatoid arthritis, enlargement of the parotid gland (and sometimes, submandibular salivary gland) and xerostomia. Sjögren's syndrome may be accompanied by other presumably autoimmune disorders, such as primary biliary cirrhosis, chronic active (lupoid) hepatitis,

dermatomyositis, systemic lupus erythematosus, scleroderma, polyarteritis nodosa, Waldenström's macroglobulinemia, and Hashimoto's thyroiditis. The overwhelming majority of the patients are postmenopausal women.

The following features of Sjögren's syndrome favor an autoimmune etiology:

- Hypergammaglobulinemia
- Autoantibodies to the cytoplasm of salivary duct epithelium in more than 50% of cases
- Rheumatoid factor in more than 75% of cases
- Rheumatoid arthritis associated with more than 50% of cases
- Antithyroglobulin antibodies and antinuclear factor in many cases
- Common association with other connective tissue diseases

Pathology

The involved salivary glands are, unilaterally or bilaterally, enlarged. Sialograms reveal punctate, globular, or cavitary dilatation of the major ducts (sialectasis). Histologically, an initial periductal round cell infiltrate gradually extends to the acini until the glands are completely replaced by a sea of lymphocytes, immunoblasts, germinal centers, and plasma cells. Proliferating myoepithelial cells surround remnants of the damaged ducts and form so-called "epimyoepithelial islands" (Fig. 25-20). The irreversible destruction of the glandular acini causes marked dryness of the mucous membranes, and the rate of flow of saliva is below normal. Similar changes can be seen in the lacrimal glands and in the minor salivary glands. Focal lymphocytic sialadenitis is demonstrated in labial biopsies in 70% of patients with Sjögren's syndrome (Fig. 25-21).

Mikulicz's disease is a symmetrical enlargement of the salivary and lacrimal glands caused by a benign lymphoepithelial process characteristic of Sjögren's syndrome. At one time symmetrical enlargement of the salivary and lacrimal glands due to a specific disease, such as leukemic infiltrates, malignant lymphoma, amyloidosis, tuberculosis, and sarcoidosis, was labeled Mikulicz's syndrome. The use of this term in such situations is not warranted, since it does not indicate the etiology of the disease.

Sarcoidosis

Sarcoidosis, a chronic granulomatous inflammatory disorder of unknown etiology, may involve the salivary glands unilaterally or bilaterally. **Heerfordt's syndrome (uveoparotid fever)** is a triad that consists of parotid enlargement, uveitis, and facial nerve paralysis, due to involvement by sarcoidosis.

Tumors of Major and Minor Salivary Glands

Several classifications of salivary gland tumors have been based on histogenesis, but today the most widely used classifications combine histological and clinical features.

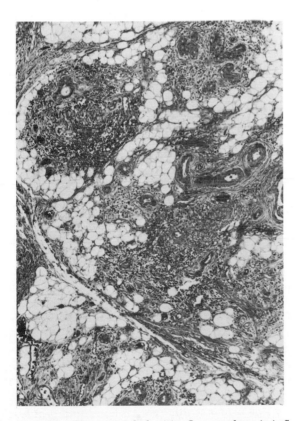

Figure 25-19. Chronic sialadenitis. Severe chronic inflammation and marked atrophy of submandibular gland are present after irradiation of adjacent oral cancer. The atrophic acini have been replaced by fat tissue.

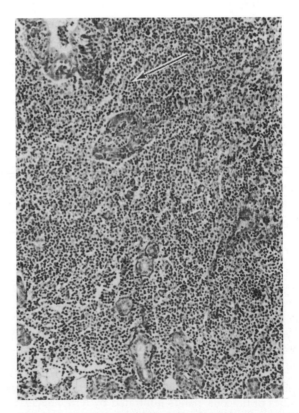

Figure 25-20. Sjögren's syndrome. A massive lymphoid infiltrate (*arrow*) and epimyoepithelial islands in the parotid gland are shown. Marked acinar atrophy caused xerostomia.

Pleomorphic Adenoma (Mixed Tumor)

This is the most common tumor of the salivary glands, and is now considered of epithelial origin, hence the label "adenoma." About 70% of all tumors of the major salivary glands and about 50% of those in the minor ones, are pleomorphic adenomas. The tumor is about nine times more frequent in the parotid than in the submandibular salivary gland, and usually arises in the superficial lobe of the parotid gland. It occurs most frequently in middle-aged persons and shows a female preponderance. Pleomorphic adenoma presents as a slowly growing, painless, movable, firm mass which has a smooth surface. Those which arise in the deep portion may grow between the ramus of the mandible and the styloid process and stylomandibular ligament into the parapharyngeal space, presenting as swellings of the lateral pharyngeal or tonsillar region.

Pleomorphic adenomas are characterized microscopically by a mixture of epithelial tissue intermingled with myxoid, mucoid, or chondroid areas (Fig. 25-22). The epithelial component consists of two cell types, ductal and myoepithelial. The cells lining the ducts form tubules or small cystic structures and contain clear fluid or eosinophilic, PAS-positive material. Around the duct epithelial cells are the smaller myoepithelial cells, which form well-defined sheaths, cords, or nests (Fig. 25-23). Often the myoepithelial cells are separated by acellular ground substance that resembles cartilaginous, myxoid, or mucoid material. This ground substance appears to be the product of the myoepithelial cells.

Pleomorphic adenomas have a fibrous capsule, and as they grow the surrounding fibrous tissue condenses around them. The tumors become larger and tend to protrude focally into the adjacent tissues, thus becoming nodular (Fig. 25-24). At surgery these protuberances can be missed if the tumor is not carefully dissected so as to leave an intact capsule and an adequate margin of surrounding glandular parenchyma. Tumor implanted during surgery, or nodules left behind, continue to grow as recurrences in the scar tissue of the previous operation. When the recurrent tumor is removed, the facial nerve may have to be sacrificed. It is difficult to dissect the branches of this nerve because they are embedded in dense scar tissue and are surrounded by irregular small

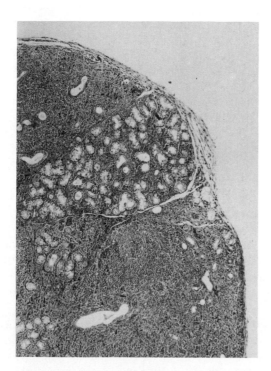

Figure 25-21. Sjögren's syndrome. A lip biopsy shows lobules of mucous glands infiltrated by lymphocytes and plasma cells. Slightly dilated ducts without acini indicate glandular atrophy.

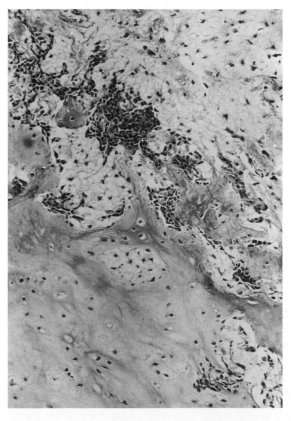

Figure 25-22. Pleomorphic adenoma of the parotid gland. Myoepithelial cells spread out into (*top*) myxoid and (*bottom*) chondroid areas.

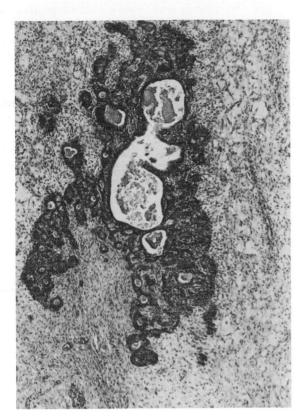

Figure 25-23. Pleomorphic adenoma of the parotid gland. Many myoepithelial cells have a fusiform appearance and are partly dispersed in a mucoid background. Nests of dark myoepithelial cells surround dilated ducts that contain eosinophilic material.

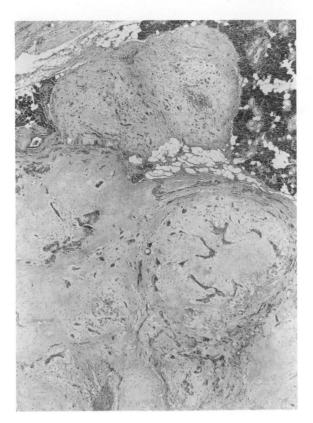

Figure 25-24. Pleomorphic adenoma of the parotid gland. The tumor contains characteristic myxoid and chondroid portions. The tumor is partly encapsulated, but a nodule protruding into the parotid gland lacks a capsule. If such nodules are not included in the resection, the tumor will recur.

nodules of non-encapsulated tumor. It is important to remember that recurrence of the tumor represents local growth and does not reflect metastatic disease.

Monomorphic Adenomas

About 5% to 10% of benign epithelial tumors of the salivary glands consist of epithelium arranged in a regular, usually glandular, pattern without a mesenchyme-like component. The most common tumor in this group is **adenolymphoma,** or **Warthin's tumor,** which occurs almost exclusively in the parotid gland. Adenolymphoma is the only tumor of the salivary glands which is more common in men than in women. It can be bilateral, or multifocal within the same gland, but is, with exceedingly rare exceptions, benign.

Adenolymphomas generally arise after the age of 30 years, with the majority arising after age 50. The tumors are composed of glandular spaces, which tend to become cystic and show papillary projections. The cysts are lined by characteristic eosinophilic epithelial cells (oncocytes) and are embedded in lymphoid tissue with germinal centers (Fig. 25-25). The histogenesis of this peculiar tumor has been much debated. Lymph nodes, which are normally found in the parotid gland and in its immediate vicinity, usually contain a few ducts or small islands of salivary gland tissue. It has been suggested that adenolymphomas arise from the proliferation of these salivary gland inclusions.

Oncocytes are benign epithelial cells that are swollen with mitochondria that impart a granular appearance to the cytoplasm. (Fig. 25-26). Oncocytes can be found scattered or in small clusters among the epithelial cells of various normal organs. For unknown reasons they begin to appear in early adulthood and their number increases with age. Their function is unknown. In addition to adenolymphomas, these cells form **oncocytomas** (oxyphilic adenomas), solid tumors composed of nests or cords of benign oncocytes. Most of these rare tumors occur in the parotid glands of elderly persons.

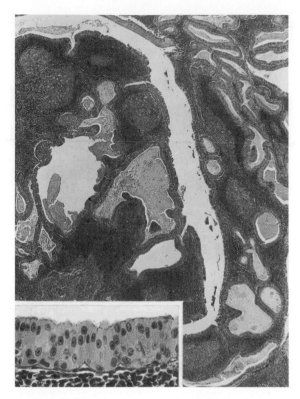

Figure 25-25.   Adenolymphoma (Warthin's tumor) of the parotid gland. A compact portion of the tumor shows a papillary adenomatous arrangement in follicular lymphoid tissue. The cystic spaces and ductlike structures are lined by oncocytes. (*Inset*) Oncocytes have finely granular cytoplasm.

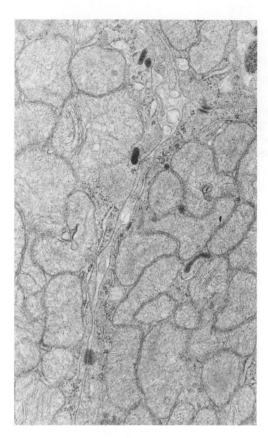

Figure 25-26.   Oncocytoma of the parotid gland. An electron micrograph of oncocytes shows cytoplasm packed with mitochondria.

Mucoepidermoid Carcinoma

Mucoepidermoid carcinomas are composed of malignant squamous cells, mucus-secreting cells, and cells of an intermediate type. These tumors probably originate from ductal epithelium, which has a considerable potential for metaplasia. They account for 5% to 10% of major salivary gland tumors and 10% of those in the minor salivary glands. Within the major salivary glands 90% arise in the parotid gland. In the minor salivary glands they develop most frequently in the palate. Most tumors occur in adults and do not show a sex predilection. Mucoepidermoid carcinomas grow slowly and present as a firm painless mass. Microscopically, well-differentiated mucoepidermoid carcinomas form irregular duct-like and cystic spaces that are lined by squamous or mucus-secreting cells (Fig. 25-27). Poorly differentiated tumors contain few mucus-secreting cells and resemble squamous cell carcinomas. Even well-differentiated tumors can metastasize, but the 5-year survival is better than 90%, regardless of the primary site. Poorly differentiated mucoepidermoid tumors, however, have a much lower survival rate (20% to 40%).

Adenoid Cystic Carcinoma (Cylindroma)

Adenoid cystic carcinomas constitute about 5% of all tumors of the major salivary glands and about 20% of all tumors of the minor salivary glands. Of all adenoid cystic carcinomas, a third arise in the major salivary glands and two-thirds in the minor ones. These tumors occur not only in the oral cavity, but also develop in the lacrimal glands, nasopharynx, nasal cavity, paranasal sinuses, and lower respiratory tract. They are most common between 40 and 60 years of age. The tumor grows slowly, but invades adjacent tissues. It is notorious for its predilection to infiltrate the perineural spaces and is therefore frequently painful.

Histologically, adenoid cystic carcinomas present varying patterns of cellular arrangement (Fig. 25-28). The tumor cells are small, have scant cytoplasm, and grow in solid sheets or as small groups, strands, or columns. Within these structures, the tumor cells interconnect to enclose cystic spaces, resulting in a cribriform (sieve-like) arrangement. The tumors probably originate from the intercalated ducts. The myoepithelial cells produce the homogeneous material that is deposited around the cell groups and that gives them the characteristic cylindromatous appearance (Fig. 25-29). **Although adenoid cystic carcinomas grow slowly and do not metastasize for many years, their long term prognosis is poor, because of frequent nerve involvement or local recurrence.** A particularly unfavorable sign is facial nerve paralysis, and most patients with this complication die within five years.

Carcinoma in Pleomorphic Adenoma (Malignant Mixed Tumor)

On rare occasions, carcinomas arise in pleomorphic adenomas. A pleomorphic adenoma which has been present for many years may begin to grow rapidly or become painful. Histologic examination reveals an unequivocal carcinoma in a readily recognizable pleomorphic adenoma. These carcinomas are usually adenocarcinomas, but mucoepidermoid or adenoid cystic carcinomas may also develop in pleomorphic adenomas. These tumors metastasize to the same sites (vertebrae, lungs) and are microscopically similar to the usual carcinomas of salivary gland origin.

Rare forms of salivary gland carcinomas include **adenocarcinoma, squamous cell carcinoma,** and **undifferentiated carcinoma.**

Connective Tissue Tumors

Hemangioma is the most common connective tissue tumor of the salivary glands and usually occurs in young children. The tumor is a hamartoma, rather than a neoplasm, and is frequently present at birth or becomes evident during infancy. Histologically, the glandular tissue is partly replaced by numerous vascular channels, mostly of capillary size.

Other benign mesenchymal tumors in the salivary glands are lymphangioma, neurilemoma, neurofibroma, lipoma, and leiomyoma. The malignant counterparts have also been reported.

Intraparotid lymph nodes may be involved in a variety of inflammatory, reactive, or proliferative processes, including malignant lymphoma. They may also become enlarged by leukemic infiltrates. Rarely, intraparotid lymph nodes harbor metastatic tumor, particularly malignant melanoma from primary sites in the face or scalp.

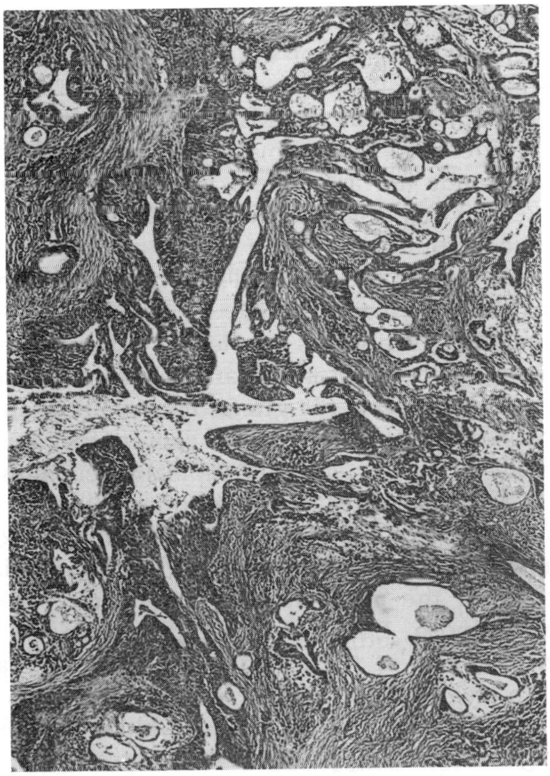

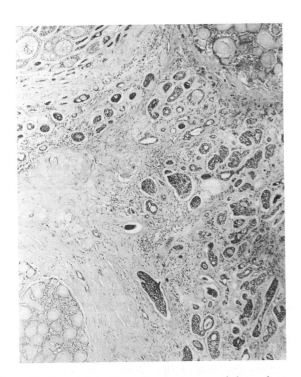

Figure 25-28. Adenoid cystic carcinoma of the palate. The tumor shows a cribriform arrangement, duct-like structures, and small groups of cells in a dense stroma.

Figure 25-27. Mucoepidermoid carcinoma of a minor salivary gland. This tumor invades the fibrous stroma and forms irregular duct-like and cystic spaces. The cysts, lined by squamous and mucus-secreting cells, contain mucus.

Table 25-2 Causes of Perforation of the Nasal Septum

Trauma
Specific infections (tuberculosis, syphilis, leprosy)
Wegener's granulomatosis
Lupus erythematosus
Chronic exposure to dust (containing arsenic, chromium, copper, etc.)
Cocaine abuse
Malignant tumors

Allergic Rhinitis   A large number of allergens is constantly present in our environment, and sensitivity to any one of them can cause allergic rhinitis. Often called **hay fever,** allergic rhinitis may be acute and seasonal, or chronic and perennial. The typical clinical and microscopic finding is **edema of the nasal mucosa,** especially of the inferior turbinates. Mucosal edema is a consequence of increased capillary permeability, mediated by vasodilator substances. The few plasma cells of the nasal mucosa normally produce IgE. After the antigen combines with IgE, the release of histamine and other vasoactive mediators leads to edema. Microscopic examination of the nasal secretions or mucosa reveals numerous eosinophils.

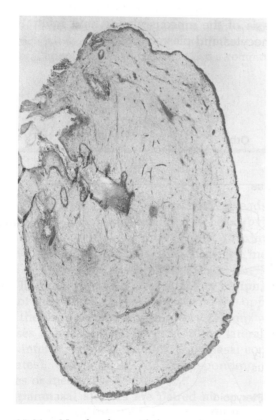

Figure 25-31.   Nasal polyp with loose edematous stroma.

Polyps

Allergic Polyps   If an allergic reaction is recurrent, fluid accumulates in the mucosa of the nose and paranasal sinuses, causing chronic mucosal swelling and enlargement of the turbinates. Eventually, mucosal edema may lead to localized bulging that grows to form polyps (Fig. 25-31). The polyps are usually multiple and appear as smooth, pale, movable, rounded tumors. They may be sessile or pedunculated, although the stalk is often not well seen. Polyps protrude into the airway and cause symptoms of nasal obstruction or, in the case of the paranasal sinuses, changes visible radiographically.

Nonallergic Polyps   These lesions arise in cases of chronic rhinitis and chronic sinusitis and are not related to allergic diseases of the nose. In most respects they are similar to allergic polyps, but show a hyaline condensation of the basement membrane under the ciliated respiratory epithelium, often associated with goblet cell hyperplasia. There is a variable infiltrate of neutrophils, lymphocytes, and plasma cells in the superficial tissues (Fig. 25-32).

Sinusitis

Acute sinusitis is caused predominantly by the extension of inflammation from the nasal mucosa. Maxillary sinusitis may also be due to odontogenic infections, when inflammation from the roots of the first and second molar teeth extends through the thin bony plate that separates them from the floor of the maxillary sinus. **Chronic sinusitis** is a sequel of acute inflammation, either as a result of incomplete resolution of the infection or because of recurrent acute complications. Any condition (inflammation, neoplasm, foreign body) that interferes with drainage or aeration of a sinus renders it liable to infection. If the ostium of a sinus is blocked, the secretion or exudate accumulates behind the obstruction.

The accumulation of mucous secretions in a nasal sinus leads to the formation of a **mucocele**; a collection of purulent exudate results in **empyema** (Fig. 25-33). Mucoceles occur most often in the anterior compartments ("cells") of the ethmoid sinus and in the frontal sinus. They develop slowly and by pressure cause resorption of bone (pressure atrophy). Mucoceles of the anterior ethmoid or frontal sinuses may be large enough to displace the contents of the orbit. Infection of a mucocele results in a **pyocele**, a sinus filled with mucopurulent exudate. Suppurative inflammation of the frontal sinus may extend to bone and cause **osteomyelitis**. The infection may also penetrate the bone and spread to the frontal and diploic venous system, thereby producing **septic thrombo-**

phlebitis. Osteomyelitis may also spread rapidly between the outer and inner tables of the skull. If this process is slow, osteonecrosis and formation of a sequestrum may ensue. Infection of the walls of a nasal sinus may spread through Volkmann's canals to the periosteum, producing periostitis and a subperiosteal abscess. If these occur on the orbital side of the bone, **orbital cellulitis** or an **orbital abscess** forms. The skin overlying the infection is often markedly edematous, and subcutaneous cellulitis or a subcutaneous abscess may also develop.

Another life-threatening complication of sinusitis is the **spread of septic (or aseptic) thrombophlebitis to the cavernous venous sinus** via the superior ophthalmic veins. Further intracranial complications include epidural, subdural, and cerebral abscesses, and purulent leptomeningitis. These consequences may develop without extensive destruction of the bone, since the infection can spread via the lymphatics or veins. Before the days of chemotherapy these dreaded complications often led to death within a few days. With proper treatment, they are today uncommon.

Tuberculosis

A tuberculous granulomatous infection of the nose is almost always secondary to tuberculosis of the lungs, from where the tubercle bacilli spread by droplet infection. Tuberculosis of the facial skin, called **lupus vulgaris,** may spread to the nasal vestibule and then to the nasal mucosa. **Granulomatous tuberculosis of the nasal mucosa** usually originates on the anterior nasal septum. Unlike syphilis it seldom destroys the bony or cartilaginous septum, and therefore does not cause collapse of the nose (saddle nose). However, if the tuberculous lesion in the vestibule heals, scar formation and retraction may cause a deformity that narrows or even occludes the nostrils. Tuberculous infection may spread into the paranasal sinuses or along the nasolacrimal duct to cause tuberculous dacryocystitis and conjunctivitis.

Syphilis

Although a primary chancre in the nose is rare, the mucosal lesions of secondary syphilis are commonly observed in the nose and nasopharynx. In tertiary syphilis the inflammatory process may involve large portions of the nasal mucosa, the underlying cartilage, and bone. The gumma, a necrotizing granuloma, is usually perichondrial or periosteal, and therefore destroys nasal cartilage and bone. The nasal bridge collapses and the so-called **saddle nose** of syphilis develops. Destruction of bony walls of the nose may also lead to perforation of the nasal septum, hard palate, wall of the orbit, or maxillary sinus.

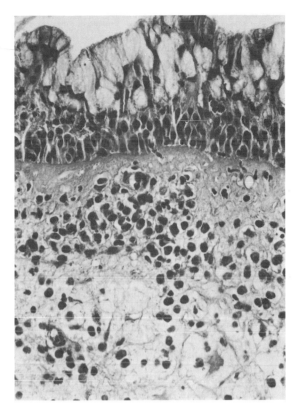

Figure 25-32. Nasal polyp. The ciliated respiratory epithelium has been replaced by goblet cells. The basement membrane is thickened, and the edematous submucosa is infiltrated by lymphocytes and plasma cells.

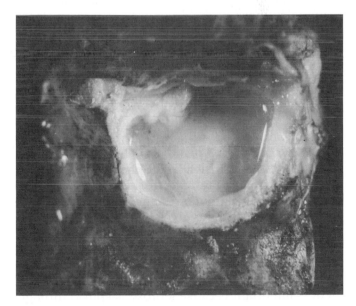

Figure 25-33. Empyema of the maxillary sinus (*sagittal section*). Infection followed chronic obstruction of the orifice caused by adenocarcinoma of the nasal mucosa.

26 Bones and Joints

Alan L. Schiller

Bone

Bone as an Organ

Bone as a Tissue

The Cells of Bone

Bone Formation and Growth

Disorders of Growth and Maturation of the Skeleton

Fracture

Osteonecrosis

Reactive Bone Formation

Infections

Metabolic Bone Disease

Paget's Disease of Bone

Neoplasms of Bone

Fibrous Dysplasia

Joints

Classification of Synovial Joints and Their Movements

Osteoarthritis

Rheumatoid Arthritis

Gout, Calcium Pyrophosphate and Apatite Deposition Disease (Chondrocalcinosis and Pseudogout)

Hemophilia, Hemochromatosis, and Ochronosis

Tumors and Tumor-Like Lesions Involving Joints

Soft Tissue Tumors

Figure 26-1. Anatomy of bone. A schematic representation of cortical and trabecular bone is presented. The longitudinal section on the left shows the vasculature entering the periosteum via the periosteal perforating arteries, and coursing through the bone perpendicular to the long axis in Volkmann's canals. The vessels that proceed longitudinally, or parallel to the long axis, are located in Haversian canals. Each artery is accompanied by a vein. Within the cortex, osteocytes reside in lacunae, and their cell processes extend into the canaliculi. The cross sectional view (*right*) illustrates the various types of lamellar bone in the cortex. Circumferential lamellar bone is located adjacent to the periosteum and borders the marrow space. Concentric lamellar bone surrounds the central haversian canals to form an osteon. Each layer of the concentric lamellar bone displays a change in the pitch of the collagen fibers, such that each layer has a different arrangement of collagen. The marrow space is filled with fat, and its trabecular bone is contiguous with the cortex. The interstitial lamellar bone occupies the space between osteons. Multinucleated osteoclasts are present, and palisaded osteoblasts surround the bone surfaces. The perforating arteries from the periosteum and the nutrient artery from the marrow space communicate within the cortex via haversian and Volkmann's canals.

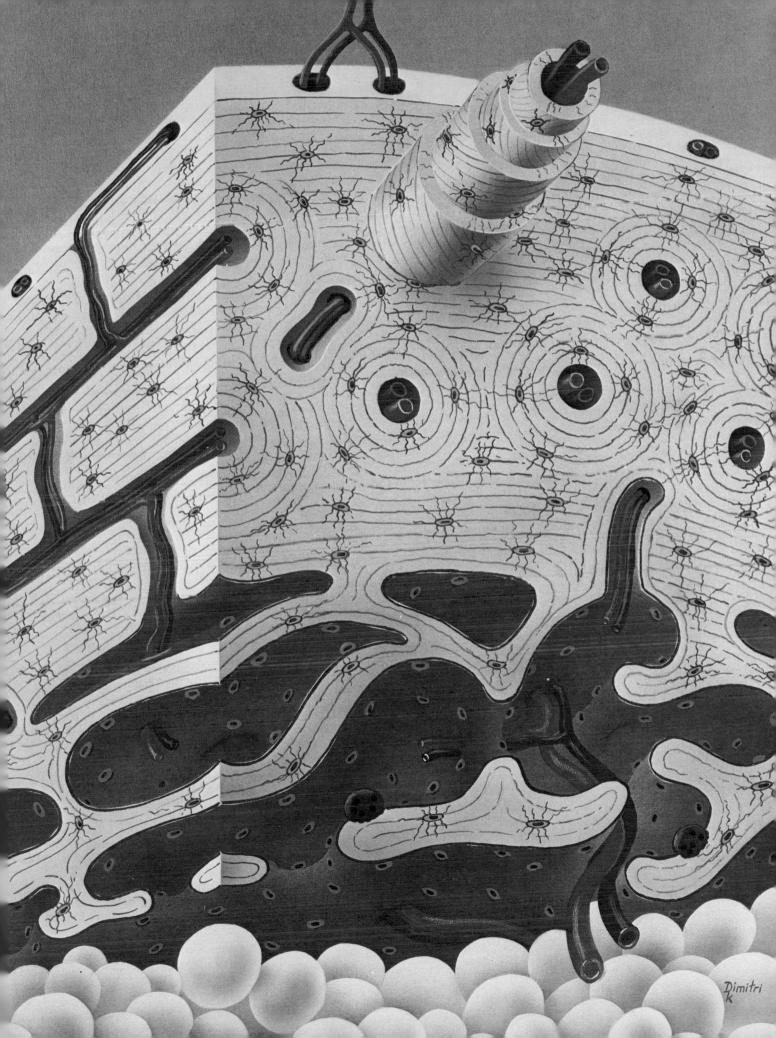

Bone

The functions of bone are classified as **mechanical, mineral storage,** and **hematopoietic.** Its mechanical functions include protection for the brain, spinal cord, and the viscera of the chest, and rigid internal support for the limbs. Bone is the principal reservoir for calcium and also stores other ions, such as phosphate, sodium, and magnesium. The bones also serve as hosts for the hematopoietic bone marrow.

The **mechanical properties** of bone are related to its specific type of construction and internal architecture. Although extremely light, bone has high tensile strength. This combination of strength and light weight is a result of its hollow tubular shape, layering of bone tissue, and internal buttressing of the matrix.

The term **bone** can refer to both an organ and a tissue. The "organ" is composed of bone tissue, cartilage, fat, marrow elements, vessels, nerves, and fibrous tissue, whereas bone "tissue" is described in microscopic terms and is defined by the relationship of its collagen and mineral structure to the bone cells.

Bone as an Organ

Macroscopically two types of bone are recognized. **Cortical bone,** which is dense, compact bone, is the outer shell that defines the shape of the bone as an organ. **Coarse cancellous bone** (also termed spongy, trabecular, or marrow bone) is generally found at the ends of long bones and internal to the cortical bone. All bones have both cancellous and cortical bone (Fig. 26-1) but proportions differ. The body, or shaft, of a long tubular bone, such as the femur, is composed of cortical bone, and the marrow is composed principally of fat. Toward the ends of the femur, the cortex becomes thin, and coarse cancellous bone becomes the predominant structure. By contrast, the skull is formed by outer and inner tables of compact bone, with only a little cancellous bone within the marrow space, called the "diploë." Both cortical and cancellous bone are composed of matrix and bone cells **(osteocytes).** The **extracellular matrix** consists of collagen fibers embedded in a ground substance. The inorganic mineral salts that give bone its hardness are deposited on the collagen fibers of the matrix.

The gross configuration of a typical long tubular bone is important in understanding bone disease. The anatomic structures of this bone are defined in relation to a transverse cartilage plate that is present in the growing child, and that is termed the **epiphyseal cartilage plate,** the **growth plate,** or the **physis** (Fig. 26-2). Thus, the three terms *epiphysis, metaphysis,* and *diaphysis* are defined in relation to the physis. The **epiphysis** is the area of the bone that is above or closest to the joint side of the epiphyseal cartilage plate. The **metaphysis** includes the nonjoint side of the epiphyseal cartilage plate, where the bone tends to have a fluted or funnel shape and contains coarse cancellous bone. The **diaphysis,** which corresponds to the body or shaft of the bone, is the zone between the two epiphyseal plates in a long tubular bone. The metaphysis blends into the diaphysis and generally corresponds to the area where the coarse cancellous bone dissipates. Because the metaphysis contributes to major longitudinal growth, it is the site of most active cellular processes within bone, including cell division and vascular invasion. It is, therefore, the area of bone that is particularly important in a discussion of hematogenous infections, tumors, and malformations and dysplasias of the skeleton.

Two additional terms are essential to an understanding of the organization of bone: **endochondral ossification** and **intramembranous ossification.** The process by which bone tissue replaces cartilage is called endochondral ossification. When bone tissue supplants membranous or fibrous tissue, the designation intramembranous ossification is applied. All bones in the body are formed by at least some intramembranous ossification, but the bulk of the skeleton is derived from endochrondral ossification. Some bones—for instance, the calvaria of the skull—are forged purely by intramembranous ossification. Microscopically, it cannot be determined whether bone formation occurred as a result of replacement of cartilage or fibrous tissue. Since bone tumors tend to recapitulate their embryologic origins, it is not surprising that cartilaginous tumors of the frontal bone have not been seen, since the calvaria of the skull do not originate from cartilage.

The Bone Marrow

The marrow is found in the space bounded by the cortical bone, called the marrow, or endosteal space. It is supported by a delicate connective tissue framework that enmeshes the marrow cells and the blood vessels. Three types of marrow may be seen by the naked eye: **red, yellow,** and **gray or white** marrow. **Gray or white marrow is always a pathologic tissue in a nongrowing adult bone or in areas removed from the epiphyseal cartilaginous plate in a child.** The colors of the marrow are useful in determining pathologic changes; yellow or red marrow may also be pathologic, depending on the age of the patient and the site of the marrow. The red marrow, which corresponds to hematopoietic tissue, is found in vir-

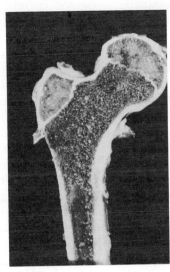
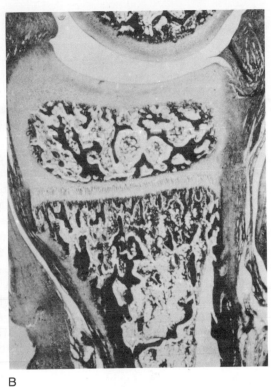

Figure 26-2. Anatomy of a long bone. (*A*) A gross specimen of the proximal femur illustrates the various anatomic parts of a long bone. The epiphyses of the femoral head and the greater trochanter are separated from the metaphysis by their respective epiphyseal plates. The cortex and medullary space are well visualized. The trabecular bone of the medullary cavity disappears in the diaphysis. (*B*) A section of a growing long bone illustrates the epiphysis, epiphyseal growth plate, metaphysis, and proximal portion of the diaphysis. The articular cartilage at this stage is contiguous with the cartilage anlage of the developing epiphysis. Coarse cancellous bone comprises the trabeculae of the marrow space.

A   B

tually all bones at the time of birth. As growth proceeds, at about the time of adolescence, the red marrow becomes confined to the axial skeletal bones, which include the skull, vertebrae, sternum, ribs, scapulae, clavicles, pelvis, and the proximal humerus and femur. Yellow marrow, which corresponds microscopically to fat tissue, is found in the bones of the limbs. Thus, the presence of red marrow in the diaphysis of the femur in, for example, a 55-year-old man is abnormal and may reflect underlying disease, such as leukemia. Likewise, yellow marrow in a vertebral body at any age is also abnormal, and should be investigated.

The Blood Supply of a Bone

The long tubular bones are supplied with blood from two sources. The first is the **nutrient artery,** which enters the bone through a nutrient foramen and supplies the marrow space and the internal one third to one half of the cortex. The second source comprises small, straight **perforating arteries** from the periosteal vessels lying on the external surface of the periosteum, the fibrous capsule of the bone. The two layers of the periosteum include an internal layer called the **cambium** layer, which is directly applied to the surface of the bone, and the outer layer, called the **fibrous layer,** which is directly contiguous with

soft tissue planes and fascia. The perforating arteries anastomose within the cortex, with branches from the nutrient arteries coming from the marrow space. Within the cortex, those vessels that run perpendicular to the long axis of the cortex are called **Volkmann's** canals; those vessels that course parallel to the long axis are called **haversian** canals. Each artery has its paired vein and, perhaps, free nerve endings. Drainage of the veins proceeds either from the cortex to the periosteal veins or into the marrow space and out the nutrient veins.

Bone as a Tissue

Bone tissue is composed of cells (10% by weight), a mineralized phase (hydroxyapatite crystals, representing 60% of the total tissue), and organic matrix (30%). Thus, with the exception of the cells, bone is a **biphasic** structure comprising an organic and an inorganic matrix.

The mineralized matrix consists of a poorly crystalline hydroxyapatite structure, $Ca_{10}(PO_4)_6(OH)_2$. Because of its net negative charge, this material can neutralize substantial amounts of acid. The hydroxyl component can be substituted by a fluoride ion, but this reduces the acid solubility of the compound. Other important ions in bone are carbonate, citrate, fluoride, chloride, sodium, magnesium, potassium, and strontium. The mechanism by which hydroxyapatite is combined with the organic matrix, the cellular control of such nucleation, and the internal organization of the crystal are the objects of extensive experimental work.

The organic matrix consists of 88% type I collagen, negligible amounts of type V collagen, 10% other proteins, and 1% to 2% lipid and glycosaminoglycans. **Thus, type I collagen essentially defines the organic matrix.** Yet, studies of the minor proteins are of great interest because these components may be related to bone morphogenesis and mineral crystallization. For instance, **osteocalcin,** produced by the osteoblast, may function as a binding factor for calcium and as a stimulus for the attraction of monocytes to the site of bone remodeling, where an osteoclast eventually forms. This compound may be measured accurately, and requires vitamins K, C, and D as cofactors. Other compounds, such as **osteonectin,** which is also made by the osteoblast, are present in platelets and may help bind collagen to calcium hydroxyapatite. Phosphoproteins that contain phosphoserine may also facilitate the nucleation of the mineral crystal. Factors that increase the concentrations of calcium or phosphate ions, and thereby increase nucleation sites, may also be involved. Other factors presumably oppose the action of inhibitors that prevent calcification. Inhibitors, such as **pyrophosphate,** which function by covering the crystal and stopping its growth, may require removal before bone can be mineralized. The same is probably true for the epiphyseal cartilaginous plate, where the **proteoglycans** tend to remain intact in the nongrowing area of the epiphyseal plate, but are fragmented in the areas where calcification of the cartilage is taking place.

Wolff's Law

Since bone is a dynamic system, it is not surprising that its shape is determined by its function. According to Wolff's law, **bone responds to stress in such a way that its shape is altered by mechanical forces from muscle, disease processes, or developmental abnormalities.** The orthopaedist and orthodontist harness Wolff's law to the advantage of the patient. For instance, the repositioning of teeth in the jaw by the use of orthodontic braces is based on the principle of exerting stress on one portion of the tooth root, thereby eliciting bone resorption; on the opposite surface of the tooth, bone deposition takes place. As a result, the teeth migrate within the jaw bones. Similar principles are employed by the orthopaedist

in the treatment of fractures with appliances such as a brace or cast. The mechanism by which Wolff's law is mediated—or, in other words, how mechanical stress is translated into morphologic expression—is unknown. An attractive view holds that piezoelectric currents exist in bone tissue. It is known that an electric current is generated when a macerated or dried piece of bone is simply bent or deformed. These electrical signals may exert an influence on osteocytes and osteoblastic and osteoclastic cells, stimulating bone deposition or bone resorption in a localized area and thereby allow the remodeling of bone. For example, a negative charge attracts osteoblasts, whereas a positive one attracts osteoclasts. However, the process is not a simple one; osteoblasts may be found in regions of osteoclastic activity, possibly because they release factors, such as osteocalcin, that aid in the formation of osteoclasts and remove surface osteoid seams to uncover the bone surface matrix, thereby exposing this matrix to the action of osteoclasts.

The Cells of Bone

There are four types of cells related to bone tissue, each of which has specific functions.

Osteoprogenitor Cell   **The osteoprogenitor cell is a ubiquitous cell found in the marrow, periosteum, and all the supporting structures within the marrow cavity.** This cell is not readily recognized by microscopy because it resides in tissue as a small, nonspecific, stellate or spindle-shaped cell. In response to an appropriate signal, this stem cell gives rise to other cells in the marrow.

Osteoblasts   **The osteoblast, which arises from the osteoprogenitor cell, is the protein-synthesizing cell that makes bone tissue.** It is a large mononuclear and polygonal cell, with a nucleus that is polarized opposite to the area of bone surface. It has a complex cytoplasm containing a prominent Golgi apparatus, mitochondria with calcium-containing granules, and abundant endoplasmic reticulum. Cytoplasmic processes that extend into the osteoid are in contact with cells embedded within the matrix, called **osteocytes.** It is thought that, when the osteoblast is inactive, it may flatten out on the surface of bone tissue. The osteoblast contains alkaline phosphatase, manufactures osteocalcin, and has a parathyroid hormone receptor that stimulates the production of cyclic adenosine monophosphate (cAMP). Collagenase in the osteoblasts may be used to disperse the osteoid on the surface of bone, thereby exposing calcified bone to osteoclastic activity.

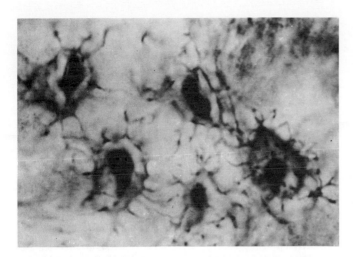

Figure 26-3. Osteocytes. Osteocytes represent trapped osteoblasts embedded in a bony matrix. They are located in lacunae, and their cytoplasm extends into bony canals, called canaliculi. The connections between the processes of the osteocytes make the bone a viable communication network.

Osteocytes **The osteocyte is an osteoblast that becomes entrapped in the bone matrix.** It is similar in structure to an osteoblast, except that over a period of time, it loses its capacity for protein synthesis, and the Golgi apparatus and endoplasmic reticulum become inconspicuous. The hallmark of the osteocyte is a cell that is completely embedded in matrix and isolated in a lacuna (Fig. 26-3). The osteocyte has numerous processes that extend through bony canals, called canaliculi, to communicate with processes from other osteocytes and eventually reach the marrow space. These cytoplasmic processes contain actin filaments and exhibit tight gap junctions with processes from other osteocytes.

As noted earlier, **the osteocyte may be the main mediator of Wolff's Law** because its surface volume is conspicuously increased by its cytoplasmic processes, which may detect electrical signals generated by small deformations of the bone matrix. Presumably, the cells transfer these signals from one osteocyte to the next, a system that eventually culminates in attracting either an osteoblast or an osteoclast to the bone surface for remodeling. Furthermore, the osteocyte deposits and resorbs small amounts of bone matrix (in a process called osteocytic osteolysis) about its lacuna, and thus may play a major role in calcium homeostasis.

Osteoclasts **The osteoclast—the cell that resorbs bone—is derived from circulating monocytes within the bloodstream and, possibly, from the tissue-fixed stem cells.** It is a multinucleated cell that contains many lysosomes and lysosomal enzymes. These cells, which produce tartrate-resistant acid phosphatase and carbonic anhydrase, are found on the surface of bones in a small depression, termed a **Howship's lacuna.** The active portion of the osteoclast is its ruffled border, which is composed of many invaginations of the cytoplasmic membrane and which increases the surface area of the cell several-fold. Adjacent to the ruffled border is a cytoplasmic area, known as the clear zone, which contains no organelles. This clear zone may function as a "sucker" that (1) allows the osteoclast to fasten to the bone, (2) isolates the area within it from the extracellular environment, and (3) permits appropriate enzymatic activity for degradation of the bone. Although the machinery of an osteoclast is superbly suited for bone resorption, it functions only if the matrix is mineralized. Any bone that contains osteoid or unmineralized cartilage is actually protected from osteoclastic activity. In rickets, because the epiphyseal cartilage plate does not calcify normally, it grows without osteoclastic resorption and becomes very thick.

Microscopic Organization of Bone Tissue

Microscopic examination reveals two types of bone tissue: lamellar bone and woven bone (Fig. 26-4). Both types of tissue may be mineralized or unmineralized, with the latter being termed osteoid.

Woven bone is defined by three characteristics: (1) an irregular arrangement of type I collagen fibers—hence, the term "woven," (2) numerous osteocytes in the matrix, and (3) variation in the size and shape of the osteocytes. **Lamellar bone** (see Fig. 26-4) is also defined by three characteristics: (1) a parallel arrangement of type I collagen fibers, (2) few osteocytes in the matrix, and (3) uniform osteocytes in lacunae parallel to the long axis of the collagen fibers. The occurrence of lamellar or woven bone is related to the rates and sites of bone deposition. **The more rapidly deposited tissue is woven bone, which is haphazardly arranged and of low tensile strength, but which serves as a temporary scaffolding for support.** It is not surprising that woven bone is found in the developing fetus, in areas surrounding tumors and infections, and as part of a healing fracture.

Lamellar bone, which is slowly produced and highly organized, is the strongest of all bone tissues and is the type of bone that forms the adult skeleton. Anything other than lamellar bone in the skeleton is abnormal. Thus, the presence of woven bone in the adult skeleton always represents a pathologic condition, and provides a clue that reactive tissue has been produced in response to some stress in the

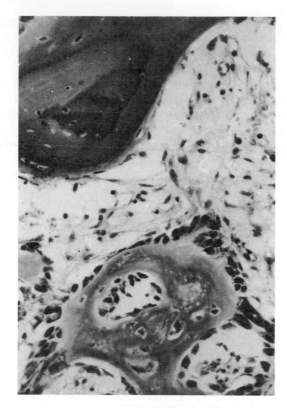

Figure 26-4. Woven and lamellar bone. Woven bone (*bottom*) is characterized by a random distribution of collagen fibers, numerous osteocytes, and variation in the size of the osteocytes. In this photograph, osteoblastic palisading about the woven bone spicule is prominent. The lamellar bone at the top of the photo shows a parallel arrangement of the collagen fibers, few osteocytes, and little variation in the size and shape of the osteocytes. The intervening marrow is composed of loose fibrous tissue.

bone. The presence of woven bone may signal tumor, infection, fracture, or a response to a necrotic focus.

Four types of lamellar bones are found. **Circumferential bone** forms the outer periosteal and inner endosteal lamellar plates of the cortex. **Concentric lamellar bone** is arranged around the haversian canal. In two dimensions, the concentric lamellar bone and its haversian artery and vein constitute the **osteon** (Fig. 26-1). In three dimensions, the osteons compose the **Haversian system**. These cylinders of bone around the haversian canal run parallel to the long axis of the cortex and are the strongest bone made. **Interstitial lamellar bone** represents remnants of circumferential lamellar bone or concentric lamellar bone which are wedged between the existing osteons. These three types of lamellar bone are found in the cortex (Fig. 26-5). The osteons form only if there is appropriate stress. For example, a paralyzed limb in a child has no haversian systems, but rather, a cortex composed exclusively of circumferential lamellar bone. The fourth kind of lamellar bone, called **trabecular lamellar bone,** forms the coarse cancellous bone of the medullary cavity. It exhibits plates of lamellar bone perforated by the marrow spaces.

A few points related to the presence of woven or lamellar bone deserve emphasis.

Slowly manufactured bone tends to be lamellar, whereas rapidly deposited bone is woven. Therefore, a persistent stress, such as that produced by a slowly growing tumor or an indolent infection, may actually be walled off by pathologic lamellar bone, whereas a rapidly growing tumor or virulent infection may stimulate woven bone formation.

Woven bone is the product of most bone-forming tumors. In contrast, lamellar bone is rarely found in bone-forming tumors.

The presence of a fragment of haversian bone and interstitial lamellar bone in a small biopsy specimen indicates the presence of cortical tissue. Importantly, by itself, the presence of such tissue does not exclude the presence of a medullary lesion—unless the biopsy sample contains both coarse cancellous tissue, which is indicative of marrow location, and marrow tissue itself, the biopsy is inadequate and must be repeated.

The presence of woven bone in an adult indicates that there is some pathologic process in the region, since woven bone is never present in the normal adult skeleton.

Bone Formation and Growth

Two terms related to the growth of bone tissue are important. **Appositional growth** refers to an increase in the mass of the matrix that stems from deposition of new matrix on the surface by adjacent surface cells. **Interstitial growth** implies that the matrix is increased from within by cell proliferation within the matrix. **Bone tissue only grows by appositional growth,** whereas virtually all other tissues, especially cartilage, increase by both forms of growth.

Most of the skeleton develops from cartilage models, called anlagen, that are present during fetal development. Thus, **bone as an organ is first represented by the tissue cartilage,** which is eventually resorbed and replaced with bone by a process termed **endochondral ossification.** The development of bone can be explained by using a limb as an example. By 5 weeks gestation, a thin layer of mesenchymal cells

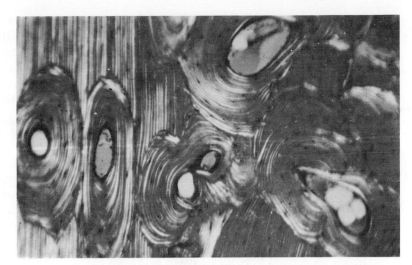

Figure 26-5. Cortical lamellar bone. Under partially polarized light, the concentric lamellar bone is arranged around the empty space where a haversian canal traverses. The black dots represent osteocyte lacunae.

forms between the ectoderm and entoderm of the limb bud. These cells condense into a core of hyaline cartilage. This cartilaginous anlage becomes the precursor of the future long bone of that limb. By definition, the fibrous capsule of the cartilage anlage is called a **perichondrium.** The width of the cartilaginous anlage is increased by appositional growth of chondroblasts, which deposit cartilage matrix on the internal surface of the perichondrium. At the same time, the anlage increases in length by a combination of appositional and interstitial growth of the chondrocytes. At this stage, the long "bone" is really composed of cartilage.

Bone Tissue

The first true bone tissue is laid down in the mid portion of the bone, the future diaphysis, by intramembranous bone formation at the site of the perichondrium. At this genetically determined site, the vascular bed increases, and the perichondrium begins to lay down woven bone on the surface of the cartilage core. This circumferential sleeve of woven bone is the **primary center of ossification,** since it is the first bone tissue to be formed. At the same time, the increased vascularity on the surface of the bone stimulates the chondrocytes within the cartilaginous anlage to form proliferating columns of chondrocytes, which eventually undergo focal calcification. This is the signal for osteoclastic resorption and invasion of vessels into the cartilaginous mass. Thus, the earliest endochondral ossification occurs after the cartilage is hollowed out from the center of the anlage. This "cavitation" of the cartilaginous core forms the future marrow space. The progressive hollowing

of the diaphysis is termed **cylinderization.** The swollen, hypertrophied chondrocytes within the central cartilage core begin to die, and capillary invasion becomes more extensive. The surfaces of the isolated, calcified cartilage cores become enveloped by woven bone laid down by osteoblasts, which arrive there via the pleuripotential mesenchymal tissue that enters with the capillaries. This cartilage core, surrounded by woven bone, is called **primary spongiosum** or **primary trabeculum.** It is the first bone formed after the replacement of cartilage in the process of endochondral ossification. As this process continues the cavitation extends along the future diaphysis toward each end of the bone. Meanwhile, the bone enlarges in width by appositional bone growth from the ever-increasing periosteal sleeve, which makes additional woven bone for the future cortex. The chondrocytes renew themselves by interstitial growth to keep pace with the ever-enlarging cavitation of the future marrow cavity.

The cartilaginous ends of the future bone undergo the same sequence of events, termed the **endochondral sequence.** Resting, or reserve, cartilage is stimulated to become columns of proliferating cartilage, which then become hypertrophied chondrocytes and eventually, calcified cartilage. Capillaries and osteoblasts invade, after which the deposition of primary spongiosum takes place. The **secondary center of ossification** (Fig. 26-6), or epiphyseal center of ossification, occurs at the ends of the bone when cartilage is resorbed. The centrifugal enlargement of the secondary ossification is called **hemispherization,** and occurs simultaneously with the longitudinal development of the marrow cavity of the diaphysis. Eventually, as the ends of the bone expand during hemispherization, and cylinderization occurs in the future

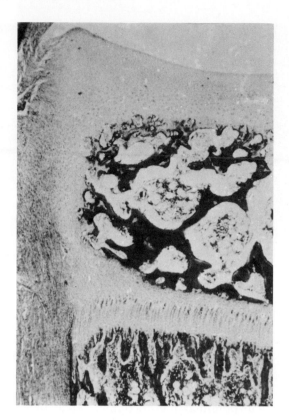

Figure 26-6.   Secondary ossification. The secondary center of ossification is located at the epiphysis of this developing tubular bone. The cartilage at the top represents a combination of the true articular cartilage and the remnant of the cartilage anlage deep to it. The cartilage below is the epiphyseal growth plate. At this stage, the trabecular bone of the epiphysis is transversely applied to the epiphyseal plate, thereby sealing it off, so that it grows toward the metaphysis. The marrow space in the epiphysis already has hematopoietic tissue.

diaphysis, a zone of cartilage is trapped between the end of the bone and the diaphysis. This cartilage is destined to be the physis or the **epiphyseal cartilage plate,** also termed the **growth plate** (Fig. 26-7). **The epiphyseal plate is a layer of modified cartilage between the diaphysis and the epiphysis,** and its structure is essentially unchanged from early fetal life to skeletal maturity. **It is this structure that controls the longitudinal growth of bones and that ultimately determines the height of the individual.**

The chondrocytes of the epiphyseal plate are arranged in vertical rows that, in three dimensions, are really spirals. When viewed longitudinally, the growth plate, proceeding from the epiphysis to the metaphysis, is divided into zones (Fig. 26-8). The **reserve zone** or **resting zone** is supplied by the epiphyseal arteries, and has small chondrocytes and very little matrix. An additional peripheral zone, known as the **zone of Ranvier,** lies directly under the perichondrium. The next zone is the **proliferative zone,** where active proliferation of chondrocytes occurs both longitudinally transversely, although the main growth thrust is in the longitudinal direction. In a very active growth plate, the proliferative zones can form more than half the thickness of the epiphyseal plate. The **hypertrophy zone** is characterized by a substantial increase in the size of the chondrocytes. In this zone, the oxygen tension is low; the chondrocytes contain glycogen and employ anaerobic pathways, and the matrix has abundant proteoglycan aggregates. The intercellular matrix is prominent, and chondrocytes are surrounded by a dense zone, called the **territorial matrix.** The **zone of calcification** is the zone closest to the metaphysis, where the matrix becomes mineralized. In this area, calcium hydroxy-

Figure 26-7.   Anatomy of the epiphyseal plate. (*A*) Normal growing epiphyseal plate. The epiphysis is separated from the epiphyseal plate by transverse plates of bone that seal the plate so that it grows only toward the metaphysis. The various zones of cartilage are illustrated. As the calcified cartilage migrates toward the metaphysis, the chondrocytes die, and the lacunae are empty. At the interface of the epiphyseal plate and the metaphysis, osteoclasts bore into the calcified cartilage, accompanied by a capillary loop from the metaphyseal vessels. Osteoblasts follow the osteoclasts and lay down osteoid on the cartilage core, thereby forming the primary spongiosum, or primary trabeculae. (*B*) Normal closure. The epiphyseal cartilage has ceased to grow and metaphyseal vessels penetrate the cartilage plate. Transverse bars of bone separate the plate from the metaphysis.

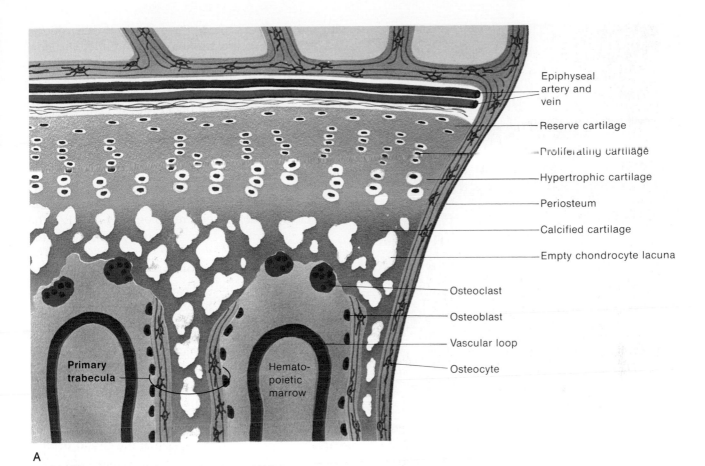

Epiphyseal artery and vein

Reserve cartilage

Proliferating cartilage

Hypertrophic cartilage

Periosteum

Calcified cartilage

Empty chondrocyte lacuna

Osteoclast

Osteoblast

Vascular loop

Osteocyte

Primary trabecula

Hemato-poietic marrow

A

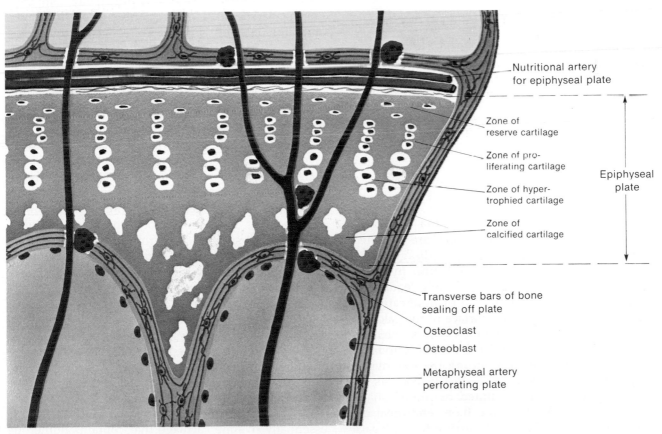

Nutritional artery for epiphyseal plate

Zone of reserve cartilage

Zone of pro-liferating cartilage

Zone of hyper-trophied cartilage

Zone of calcified cartilage

Epiphyseal plate

Transverse bars of bone sealing off plate

Osteoclast

Osteoblast

Metaphyseal artery perforating plate

B

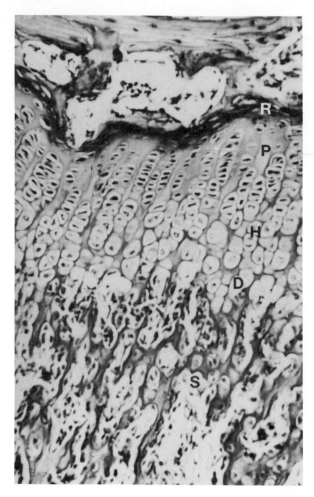

Figure 26-8. The normal epiphyseal plate. The epiphyseal side of the plate seals off the cartilage with transverse bars of lamellar bone. The nourishment for the epiphyseal plate is supplied by vessels that lie between the epiphyseal bone and the resting zone of the epiphyseal cartilage plate. *R,* resting cartilage; *P,* proliferating cartilage; *H,* hypertrophied cartilage; *D,* degenerating calcified cartilage; *S,* primary spongiosum of new woven bone laid down on the cores of cartilage.

apatite accumulates in the mitochondria and eventually in the matrix. Glycogen stores are depleted within chondrocytes, proteoglycans disaggregate, and the mitochondria release calcium hydroxyapatite crystals into the matrix, thereby leading to mineralized cartilage. In the **zone of ossification**, a coating of bone is laid on the surface of the calcified cartilage. The formation of the metaphysis, which is called **funnelization,** occurs at the **ring of Ranvier,** a periosteal cuff of bone surrounding the epiphyseal cartilage. Here, a wave of periosteal osteoclasts resorbs the cortex, so that a fluted or funnel shape begins to appear. At the same time, endosteal osteoblastic bone deposition is occurring to keep pace

with and to offset some of the osteoclastic resorption. The net result is the funnel or fluted shape of the bone.

Obliteration of the epiphyseal plate (Fig. 26-7B) normally occurs at a specific age for each location. In general, the epiphyseal plates cease growing and close earlier in girls than boys. The renewal of chondrocytes slows down and ultimately ceases. The metaphyseal vessels continue to permeate the plate, and endochondral ossification is therefore promoted. The entire plate is eventually replaced by bone. In some individuals a transverse bony plate representing the site of closure can be seen radiologically.

Cartilage

In contrast to bone tissue, **cartilage does not contain blood vessels, nerves, or lymphatics.** It is capable of both appositional and interstitial growth, and may be focally calcified to provide some internal strength in the appropriate areas. Like bone, cartilage may be viewed as an organic and inorganic biphasic material. The inorganic phase is composed of calcium hydroxyapatite crystals, equivalent to those found in bone matrix. However, the organic matrix is vastly different from that of bone. Essentially, cartilage is hyperhydrated, with water comprising some 80% of its weight. The remaining 20% is principally composed of two macromolecular substances, type II collagen and proteoglycan. Trace amounts of neutral lipids, phospholipids, lysozyme, and possibly, glycoproteins are found. The water content is extremely important in the function of articular cartilage, because it enhances the resilience and lubrication of the joint. The proteoglycans are complex macromolecules composed of a central linear protein core to which are attached long side arms of polysaccharides, called glycosaminoglycans. These polysaccharides are polyanionic because of the regular presence of carboxyl groups and sulfates along the molecules. Cartilage glycosaminoglycans comprise three long-chained, unbranched, repeating, polydimeric saccharides, chondroitin-4-sulfate, chondroitin-6-sulfate, and keratan sulfate. The chondroitin sulfates are the most abundant, accounting for 55% to 90% of the cartilage matrix, depending on the age of the tissue.

There are three types of cartilage. **Hyaline cartilage** is the prototypic cartilage, comprising the articular cartilage of the joints, the cartilaginous anlage of developing bones, the epiphyseal plates, the costochondral cartilages, the cartilages of the trachea, bronchi, and larynx, and the nasal cartilages. It is the most common cartilage in tumors, in a fracture callus, and in areas of relative avascularity. **Fibrocartilage** is essentially hyaline cartilage that contains numerous type I collagen fibers for tensile and structural strength. It is found in the anulus fibrosus of the intervertebral disc, tendinous and ligamentous insertions, menisci, the symphysis pubis, and insertions of joint capsules. Fibrocartilage may also occur in a fracture callus and in some cartilage-forming tumors. **Elastic cartilage** is hyaline cartilage that contains elastin. This yellow cartilage is found in the pinna of the ears, in the epiglottis, and in the arytenoid cartilages of the larynx.

The chondrocytes are derived from a primitive mesenchymal cell that is similar to the precursor of the bone cells. The chondroblast gives rise to the chondrocyte, and the cell that destroys calcified cartilage is called a chondroclast. Since this last cell is identical to the osteoclast, the term osteoclast is preferred. In contrast to bone, the chondrocyte is capable of division; thus, the cartilage matrix can grow by both interstitial and appositional growth. In general, the presence of high oxygen tension and vascular invasion is inimical to cartilage growth; therefore, it undergoes endochondral ossification in the presence of high oxygen tension. It is intriguing to speculate that inhibitors secreted by chondrocytes in the various zones of the endochondral sequence may prevent vascular invasion and mineralization; when these inhibitors are removed, vascular invasion and calcification take place. The isolation of these inhibitors is actively being pursued by researchers.

Disorders of Growth and Maturation of the Skeleton

The abnormalities of growth and maturation are classified in four ways: (1) as systemic or local disorders; (2) in relation to etiology, (3) in relation to a specific anatomic site (e.g., the epiphyseal plate) and its disorders, (4) in terms of specific tissue defects.

Delayed or Disorganized Cartilage Maturation

Cretinism

Cretinism, which results from maternal iodine deficiency, has profound effects on the skeleton, including severe dwarfism and delayed appearance of the deciduous teeth. The fontanels of the skull do not close, and there is a delay in closure of the epiphyses, as well as radiologic stippling of the epiphyses. **The histopathology is related to a defect in cartilage maturation.** The chondrocytes do not follow the orderly progression of the endochondral sequence. Instead,

the maturation of the hypertrophied zone is retarded, and the zone of proliferative cartilage is narrow. Therefore, endochondral ossification does not proceed appropriately, and metaphyseal transverse bars of bone seal off the epiphyseal plate from further capillary invasion. Although the epiphyseal plates may remain open, the failure of endochondral ossification produces severe dwarfism. The malshaped epiphyses seen on radiography reflect the incomplete penetration of the secondary centers of ossification of the epiphysis.

Morquio's Syndrome

Morquio's syndrome (Morquio's epiphyseal-metaphyseal dysplasia) is an inherited autosomal recessive disease. It is a mucopolysaccharidosis characterized by dental defects, mental retardation, corneal opacities, and increased urinary excretion of keratin sulfate. Mucopolysaccharides accumulate in the chondrocytes, a process that ultimately interferes with the normal endochondral sequence (Fig. 26-9). The net result is a disorganized epiphyseal plate, which is also sealed off by transverse bars of bone so that capillary penetration does not occur. The consequence is dwarfism. Cretinism and Morquio's syndrome, although of different etiologies, both produce dwarfism by altering the epiphyseal plate and preventing endochondral ossification.

Disorders of the Epiphyseal Plate

Achondroplasia

Achondroplasia, a genetic disease in which the specific defect is unknown, is one of the most common types of dwarfism. The epiphyseal plate is greatly thinned, and the zone of proliferative cartilage is either absent or extensively attenuated (Fig. 26-10). The zone of provisional calcification, if present, undergoes endochondral ossification, but at a greatly reduced rate. A transverse bar of bone often seals off the epiphyseal plate, thus preventing extensive bone formation and causing dwarfism. Interestingly, the secondary centers of ossification and the articular cartilage seem to be normal. Because intramembranous ossification is undisturbed, the periosteum functions normally, and bones often become very short and thick. For the same reasons, the head of affected patients appears unusually large, compared to the bones formed from cartilage of the face. The spine is of normal length, but the limbs are abnormally short. These patients have normal mentation and a normal life span. However, in some cases severe kyphoscoliosis and its complications develop.

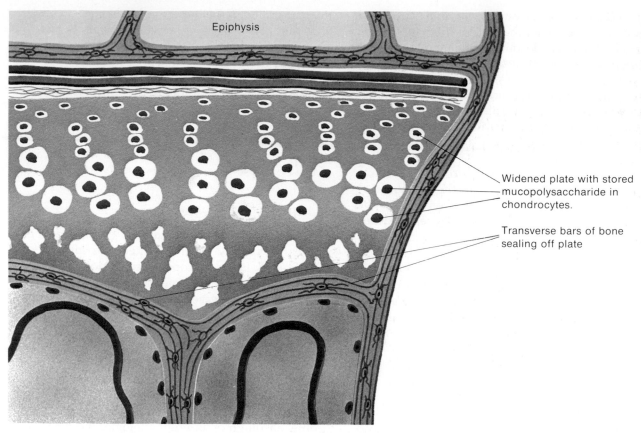

Epiphysis

Widened plate with stored mucopolysaccharide in chondrocytes.

Transverse bars of bone sealing off plate

Figure 26-9.   The epiphyseal plate in the mucopolysaccharidoses. These disorders are characterized by disorganized and abbreviated columns of swollen chondrocytes that are engorged with mucopolysaccharides. There is interference with the normal endochondral sequence, and the epiphyseal plate is sealed off by transverse bars of bone from the metaphysis. Dwarfism results from the lack of vascular penetration into the epiphyseal plate. Such penetration normally sustains new bone formation, thereby allowing continued lengthening of the bone.

Hemihypertrophy   Hemihypertrophy refers to a number of conditions that may stimulate the epiphyseal plate in one limb to undergo rapid and prolonged endochondral ossification. As a consequence, the limb is much longer than the contralateral one. An infection in the metaphyseal area may stimulate the epiphyseal plate to grow rapidly. Arteriovenous malformations may also cause the epiphyseal plate to grow faster than its opposite counterpart. Fractures and tumors near the epiphyseal plate may produce the same result.

Scurvy (Vitamin C Deficiency)

Today, scurvy is a rare disease, and is seen only in patients with other nutritional deficiencies, such as rickets. The disease was well known in antiquity, and was a perennial scourge of sailors until the publica-

tion in 1757 of James Lind's *Treatise of Scurvy,* which advocated the use of lime juice as an antiscorbutic. Vitamin C (ascorbic acid) is a water-soluble compound that is easily absorbed in the small intestine and stored in various organs, particularly the adrenal gland. Humans, monkeys, and guinea pigs cannot synthesize adequate supplies of this vitamin, as other animals do, and therefore must seek exogenous sources of vitamin C. Vitamin C is found in potatoes, green vegetables, and fruits, and can also be readily synthesized. Today, cases of scurvy usually occur only in inmates of poorly maintained mental asylums and in the third world countries, where starvation is a major problem.

Vitamin C is essential for the synthesis and proper structure of collagen. Therefore, wound healing and bone growth are impaired in patients with scurvy. Furthermore, the basement membrane of capillaries

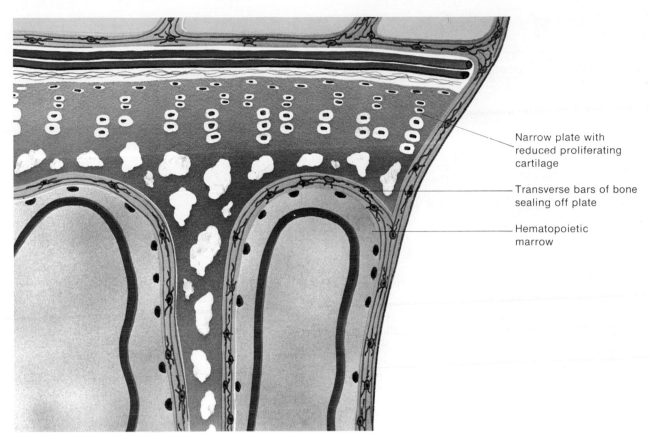

Narrow plate with
reduced proliferating
cartilage

Transverse bars of bone
sealing off plate

Hematopoietic
marrow

Figure 26-10. The epiphyseal plate of an achondroplastic dwarf. In achondroplasia, the epiphyseal plate is reduced in thickness, and the zones of proliferating cartilage are attenuated. Osteoclastic activity is inconspicuous, and the interface between the plate and the metaphysis is often sealed by transverse bars of bone that prevent further endochondral ossification. As a result, the bones are shortened.

is also damaged by this disease, and widespread capillary bleeding is common in affected patients. Children with scurvy are anorexic, irritable, and poor thrivers, do not gain weight, and have visible bone deformities, similar to those associated with rickets. In adults, weakness, bleeding gums, and skin hemorrhages are common. Bone deformities are not seen in adults, but subperiosteal bleeding may occur, leading to joint and muscle pain.

The pathologic skeletal changes of scurvy reflect the lack of osteoblastic function. Because the osteoblasts cannot produce collagen, woven bone is not formed. At the epiphyseal plate, the chondrocytes continue to grow. The zone of calcified cartilage may actually become more prominent, since it is more heavily calcified. Osteoclasts resorb this zone, but the primary spongiosum does not form properly, and there is irregular vascular perforation of the cartilage plate (Fig. 26-11). Fractures and capillary bleeding occur, leading to further disorganization in the metaphysis—hence, the German term *Trümmerfeld,* or "field of ruin," for this subepiphyseal plate area. The subperiosteal bleeding may be severe, leading to diminution of the cortex and appositional growth and osteoporosis. Sometimes, dislocation of the epiphyseal plate also occurs.

Asymmetric Cartilage Growth

Asymmetric cartilage growth, such as occurs in patients with knock-knees and bowed legs, develops when one part of the epiphyseal plate—a medial or a lateral side—grows faster than the other. The most common cause is probably hereditary, but mechanical forces, such as trauma near the plate, may stimulate one side of the plate to grow faster or in an asym-

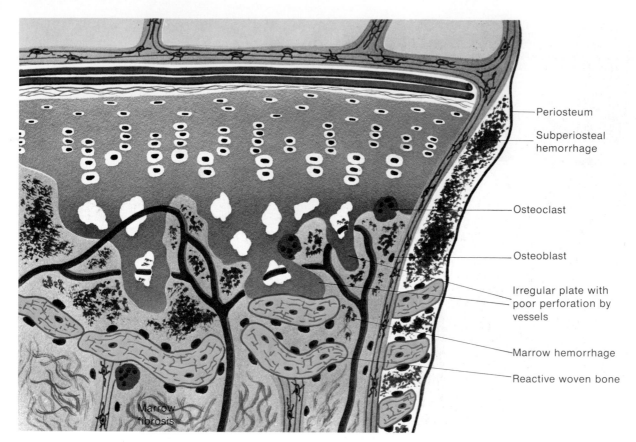

Periosteum

Subperiosteal hemorrhage

Osteoclast

Osteoblast

Irregular plate with poor perforation by vessels

Marrow hemorrhage

Reactive woven bone

Marrow fibrosis

Figure 26-11.   The epiphyseal plate in scurvy. Defective collagen formation leads to capillary fragility and periosteal hemorrhage. Osteoclasts do not perforate the plate in a regular fashion. There is often extensive hemorrhage in this region. Microfractures cause secondary microcalluses; reactive bone is, therefore, seen in this region.

metric fashion. To correct such a condition in a child, the growth of this portion of the plate is retarded by a surgically implanted staple or a brace or cast, thus allowing the opposite side of the plate to grow. In an adult, since the epiphyseal plates have already closed, surgical osteotomy (fracture) is employed. Aside from the cosmetic appearance, these conditions may require correction to prevent future incongruity, eventual loss of articular cartilage, and joint destruction.

Scoliosis

Scoliosis is an abnormal lateral curvature of the spine, usually affecting adolescent girls. Kyphosis is an abnormal anteroposterior curvature. The cause is asymmetric cartilage growth of the end plates of vertebral bodies, which correspond to the epiphyseal plates of the long tubular bone. This asymmetric growth produces severe curvatures of the spine. A vertebral body grows in length (height) from epiphyseal-like

cartilage which corresponds to the end plates, and which is peripheral to the anulus fibrosus of the intervertebral disc. As in any standard tubular bone, the vertebral bodies increase in width by appositional bone growth from the periosteum. **In scoliosis, for unknown reasons, one portion of the end plate grows faster, thereby producing a lateral curvature of the spine.** Applying Wolff's law, the treatment is appropriate stress on the vertebral body, through the use of braces or internal fixation, to straighten the spine. If the scoliotic spine remains in a severe S-shaped curve, it causes impairment of lung expansion, cardiac abnormalities, and joint problems, particularly involving the hip.

Osteochondroma

An osteochondroma is frequently classified as a neoplasm, but it is actually an abnormality that arises from a defect at the ring of Ranvier of the epiphyseal plate. The ring of Ranvier guides the growth of the

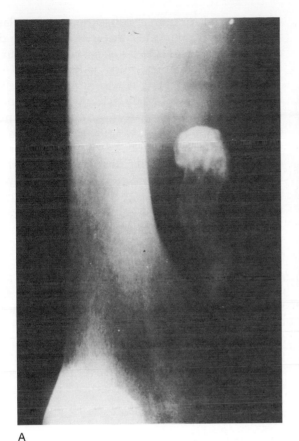

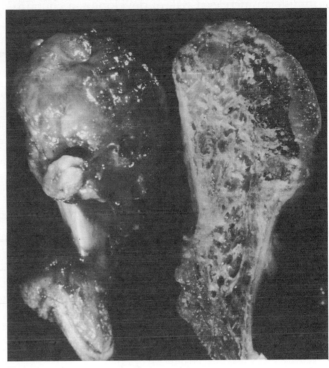

A

B

Figure 26-12. Osteochondroma. (*A*) A radiograph of an osteochondroma growing at the distal end of the femur shows a lesion that is directly contiguous with the marrow space. The osteochondroma grows away from the joint and is capped by radiodense, calcified cartilage. (*B*) The gross specimen of the resected osteochondroma shows the cap of calcified cartilage, the coarse cancellous bone, and the communication with the medullary cavity of the femur.

epiphyseal cartilage toward the metaphysis. If the ring of Ranvier is absent or defective, epiphyseal cartilage grows laterally into the soft tissue. Vessels originating in the marrow cavity of the bone extend into this cartilage mass. If this process continues, a cartilage-capped, bony, stalked osteochondroma results, which is in direct continuity with the marrow cavity of the parent bone (Fig. 26-12). These lesions tend to grow away from the joint. The pathognomonic radiologic appearance is that of a cartilage mass with direct continuity to the parent bone and without an underlying cortex. This appearance is evidence that no cortex formed between the cartilage mass and the bone in the embryologic stage. On histologic examination, a cartilage-capped, bony mass is surrounded by a surface fibrous membrane, which actually represents the perichondrium. Active endochondral ossification deep to the cartilage cap allows the bony protuberance to lengthen.

There are two forms of this disease. The most common is a **solitary osteochondroma,** which may have to be removed if it is cosmetically displeasing or presses on an artery or nerve. A second form of the disease, termed **hereditary multiple osteochondromatosis,** is inherited as an autosomal dominant disorder, and is characterized by multiple osteochondromas. This multiple form is not rare. It occurs predominantly in men, and although it is transmitted as a mendelian dominant disorder, an unaffected female from an afflicted family may also transmit the disorder. In severe cases, dwarfism may result because of the displacement of the longitudinal growth laterally as an osteochondroma. Metacarpals may be shortened, and pronation and supination may develop if these lesions occur in the forearm and interfere with the function of the wrist. Further orthopaedic difficulties may be caused by unequal leg length and joint function because of the encroaching osteochondromas. On histologic and gross examination, the multiple form is identical to that of the solitary osteochondroma. Especially in the multiple form, there is a long-term increased risk of developing a chondrosarcoma in the cartilage cap, but this is a rare event. The enlargement of a known osteochondroma is worthy of investigation, although it may be attributable to adjacent trauma, or to pregnancy and lactation in a woman.

Modeling Abnormalities

Another way of conceptualizing some of the peculiar developmental abnormalities, or so-called dysplasias, of bone is to observe the dynamic processes of funnelization and cylinderization.

Pyle's Disease

Pyle's disease is a disorder in which funnelization does not take place. Patients with this disease have bones with a flask shape rather than a tubular or flared shape.

Osteopetrosis

Osteopetrosis, or marble bone disease of Albers-Schönberg, is a rare disorder characterized by abnormally dense bone. The autosomal recessive form is a severe, sometimes fatal disease affecting infants and children. The death of infants with this severe variant is attributable to marked anemia, cranial nerve entrapment, hydrocephalus, and infections. A more benign form, which is transmitted as an autosomal dominant trait and presents in adulthood or adolescence, is associated with mild anemia or no symptoms at all. The defect involves defective bone remodeling and, more specifically, the function of osteoclasts. Hypofunction of the osteoclasts results in the retention of the primary spongiosum with its cartilage cores, lack of funnelization of the metaphysis, and a thickened cortex. The result is short, blocklike, radiodense bones—hence, the term marble bone disease (Fig. 26-13). Although these bones are extremely radiopaque, they are basically weak because the bone structure is intrinsically disorganized and Wolff's law is not operative. Although mineralized cartilage is extremely radiodense, it is weak and friable; therefore, these bones fracture easily. Since the primary spongiosum remains, the marrow cavity is severely attenuated. As a consequence, the hematopoietic marrow is deficient, a condition which results in severe anemia and death. Cranial nerve involvement is secondary to the lack of enlargement

of the neural foramina. Subsequent strangulation of nerves leads to blindness and deafness. The disease occurs in waves, with osteoclasts functioning adequately at some times, and inadequately at others. Thus, radiographs may reveal normal, as well as osteopetrotic, areas. To compensate for the encroachment on the marrow space, extramedullary hematopoiesis occurs in the liver, spleen, and lymph nodes, with resulting enlargement of these structures. The cause of osteopetrosis is not known, and the only treatment currently employed is bone marrow transplantation, which may give rise to a new clone of functional osteoclasts.

Progressive Diaphyseal Dysplasia

A disorder in which cylinderization does not proceed appropriately has been termed progressive diaphyseal dysplasia (Camurati-Engelmann disease). In this condition, there is a symmetrical thickening in and an increased diameter of the diaphyses of long bones, particularly of the femur, tibia, fibula, radius, and ulna. Patients experience pain over the affected areas, fatigue, muscle wasting, atrophy, and gait abnormalities.

Delayed Maturation

Osteogenesis Imperfecta

Osteogenesis imperfecta refers to a group of heritable disorders of the connective tissues, which tend to affect the skeleton, joints, ears, ligaments, teeth, sclerae, and skin. The basic disorder is the defective synthesis of collagen. There are at least four types of osteogenesis imperfecta, each with a different mode of inheritance and clinical features.

Osteogenesis Imperfecta Type I
Type I osteogenesis imperfecta, inherited as an autosomal dominant disorder, is a common form of the disease. It is characterized by multiple fractures after birth, blue sclerae, and hearing abnormalities. In some cases, abnormalities of the teeth are conspicuous. The initial fractures usually occur after the infant begins to sit and walk. There may be hundreds of fractures a year with minor movement or trauma. On radiologic examination, the bones are extremely thin, delicate, and abnormally curved (Fig. 26-14). When a fracture occurs, the fracture callus may be so extensive as to resemble a tumor. As a child grows, the fractures tend to decrease in severity and frequency, and stature is generally unaffected. The sclerae are very thin, with the blue color being attributable to

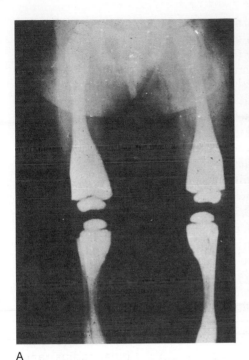
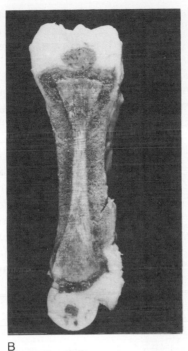
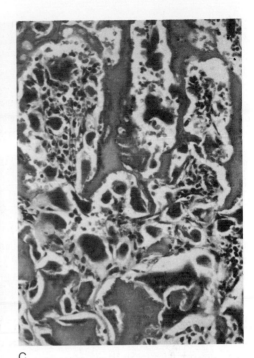

A   B   C

Figure 26-13. Osteopetrosis. (*A*) A radiograph of a child shows markedly dense bones of the lower extremities secondary to the preservation and retention of primary trabeculae, along with their calcified cores of cartilage. This increased density gives rise to the term "marble bone disease." The bones are also misshapen. (*B*) A gross specimen of the femur shows the original femur in the center, with virtually no marrow space remaining. The new bone deposited on the surface of the original femur accommodates the marrow space, which has been crowded out by osteopetrosis. The developing secondary centers of ossification at both ends of the specimen are also deficient in normal marrow elements. (*C*) A photomicrograph illustrates the preservation of the primary trabeculae, together with their cores of calcified cartilage and osteoclasts. Although the osteoclasts are more numerous than normal, they do not function appropriately.

the underlying choroid. The progressive hearing loss, which develops to total deafness in adulthood, is secondary to fusion of the ossicles. The joint laxity associated with the condition may eventually lead to kyphoscoliosis and flat feet. Because of hypoplasia of the dentine and pulp, the teeth are misshapen and bluish-yellow.

Osteogenesis Imperfecta Type II

Also a common form of this disorder, type II osteogenesis imperfecta is a lethal, perinatal disease. In some families, it is inherited as an autosomal recessive disorder, although it also occurs sporadically. Those affected are stillborn or die within a few days. These infants are, in a sense, crushed to death. They exhibit markedly short stature and severe deformities of the limbs, and almost all of the bones sustain fractures during delivery or during uterine contractions in labor. As in type I, the sclerae are blue.

Osteogenesis Imperfecta Type III

Osteogenesis imperfecta type III, the progressive, deforming type of this disease, is characterized by many bone fractures, growth retardation, and severe skeletal deformities, and seems to be inherited as an autosomal recessive disorder. The fractures are present at birth, but the bones seem to be less fragile than in the type II form. These patients may eventually develop severe shortening of their stature because of progressive bone fractures and severe kyphoscoliosis. Although the sclerae may be blue at birth, they become white shortly thereafter. Abnormalities of the teeth are common.

Osteogenesis Imperfecta Type IV

Type IV osteogenesis imperfecta, which is inherited as an autosomal dominant disorder, is similar to type I, except that the sclerae are normal. It seems to be a heterogeneous condition, and there may or may

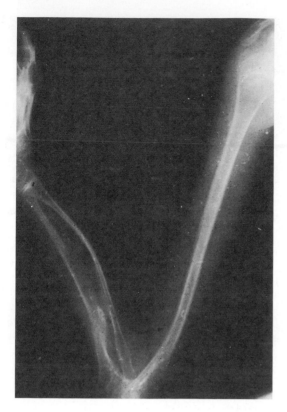

Figure 26-14. Osteogenesis imperfecta. A radiograph illustrates the markedly thin and attenuated humerus and bones of the forearm. There is a fracture callus in the proximal ulna.

not be dental disease. In this disorder, abnormal cross linkages of collagen are thought to result in thin, delicate, and weak collagen fibrils. This inappropriate collagen does not allow the bone cortex to mature, so at birth, patients have a cortex resembling that of a fetus. The cortex is composed of woven bone and small areas of lamellar bone. Over a period of years, the cortex matures, but this may not occur until adolescence or even later. In any event, the occurrence of fractures tends to decrease over a long period of time. These patients are vigorously treated with orthopaedic devices, including rods inserted into the medullary cavities, to prevent the dwarfing effect of multiple fractures.

Enchondromatosis (Ollier's Disease)

Although enchondromatosis is not specifically a disease of delayed maturation of bone, it is a condition wherein residual hyaline cartilage, anlage cartilage, or cartilage from the epiphyseal plate does not undergo endochondral ossification and remains in the bones. As a consequence, the bones show multiple,

tumor-like masses of abnormally arranged hyaline cartilage, with zones of proliferative and hypertrophied cartilage (Fig. 26-15). These masses tend to be located in the metaphyses; as the growth plates continue to proliferate, they settle in the diaphysis of adolescents and adults. This disease is asymmetrical and may cause bone deformities. These cartilage masses are all called **enchondromas,** and to some investigators, they represent true neoplasms. These cartilage nodules exhibit a strong tendency to undergo malignant change into a chondrosarcoma in adult life. Therefore, a patient with this condition who experiences increasing pain or an increasingly significant abnormality at one site should be evaluated to rule out an underlying sarcoma.

The presence of multiple enchondromas and cavernous hemangiomas of the skin is termed **Maffucci's syndrome.** This condition is thought to have an even higher predilection for malignant change, with chon-

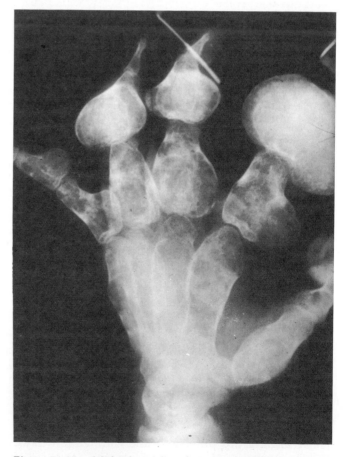

Figure 26-15. Multiple enchondromatosis (Ollier's disease). A radiograph of the hand shows bulbous swellings that represent cartilage masses composed of hyaline cartilage, which is sometimes admixed with more primitive myxoid cartilage.

drosarcoma developing in as many as 50% of all patients. There is also a solitary form of enchondroma that has the same histologic features (perhaps less atypical) as the chondrocytes in the multiple form, and also principally affects the hands and feet. This solitary form is less likely to undergo malignant change. It is noteworthy that **all chondrosarcomas of the skeletal system probably arise from a pre-existing cartilage rest or an enchondroma.**

Fracture

The most common bone lesion is a fracture, which is essentially defined as a discontinuity of the bone. If the applied force is axial, the resulting fracture is caused by compression of the bone. A torsional force results in a spiral fracture, and combined tension and compression shear forces cause angulation and displacement of the fractured ends. A force powerful enough to fracture a bone also injures the adjacent soft tissues. There is often extensive muscle necrosis, hemorrhage because of shearing of capillary beds and larger vessels of the soft tissues, tearing of tendinous insertions and ligamentous attachments, and even nerve damage, caused by stretching or direct tearing of the nerve.

Fracture Healing

In the repair of a bone fracture, **anything other than the formation of bone tissue at the fracture site represents incomplete healing.** The healing of a fracture is divided into three phases: the inflammatory phase, the reparative phase, and the remodeling phase (Fig. 26-16). The duration of each phase depends on the patient's age, the site of fracture, the patient's overall health and nutritional status, and the degree of soft tissue injury. Furthermore, local factors, such as vascular supply and mechanical forces at the site, also play a role in healing. Again, it must be emphasized that **the scar of bone is bone;** anything less is considered nonhealing.

The Inflammatory Phase

In the first 1 to 2 days after a fracture, there is extensive tearing of the periosteum. The resultant rupture of blood vessels in the periosteum and adjacent soft tissue leads to extensive hemorrhage. In addition, muscle and other soft tissues undergo necrosis and hemorrhage. There is also extensive necrosis of bone at the fracture site because of the disruption of large vessels in the bone and the interruption of the cortical vessels (i.e., the Volkmann and haversian canals). **The hallmark of dead bone is the absence of osteocytes and empty bone lacunae.**

In about 2 to 5 days, the hemorrhgae forms a large clot, with formation of fibrin. This is a relatively avascular area that must be resorbed so that the fracture can heal. Peripheral to this blood clot, which may extend deeply into the soft tissues and the medullary cavity of the bone, neovascularization begins to occur. There is dilatation of adjacent vessels, transudation and exudation of fluids into the soft tissue and marrow, and the standard inflammatory response of leukocytes, macrophages, and mononuclear cells at the peripheral portion of the clot. By the end of the first week, most of the clot is organized by invasion of blood vessels and early fibrosis.

By the end of the first week the earliest bone (invariably woven) has formed. This corresponds to the "scar" of bone. Since bone formation requires a good blood supply, the woven bone spicules begin to form at the periphery of the clot, where vascularization is greatest. Pleuripotential mesenchymal cells from the soft tissue and within the bone marrow give rise to the osteoblasts, which synthesize the woven bone. In most fractures, cartilage is also found in relatively avascular tissue, and is eventually resorbed by endochondral ossification. The granulation tissue containing bone cartilage is termed a **callus.** Woven bone also forms inside the marrow cavity at the periphery of the blood clot because vascular tissue is also present in this location. At this time, the actual fracture site has not undergone remodeling, since it is basically avascular.

The Reparative Phase

The reparative phase begins after the first week and extends for months, depending on the degree of movement and the fixation of the fracture. By this time, the acute inflammatory cells seen in the first week have dissipated. The reparative process involves modulation of such pleuripotential cells as fibroblasts and chondrocytes. Extensive neovascularization introduces mononuclear cells that form osteoclasts. The repair process proceeds from the most peripheral portion toward the fracture site, and accomplishes two objectives: (1) it organizes and resorbs the blood clot, and more importantly, (2) it furnishes neovascularization for the construction of callus that will eventually bridge the fracture site. Osteoclasts extend from the haversian canals and bore into the cortex toward the fracture site in a process called a **cutting cone.** The cutting cone tun-

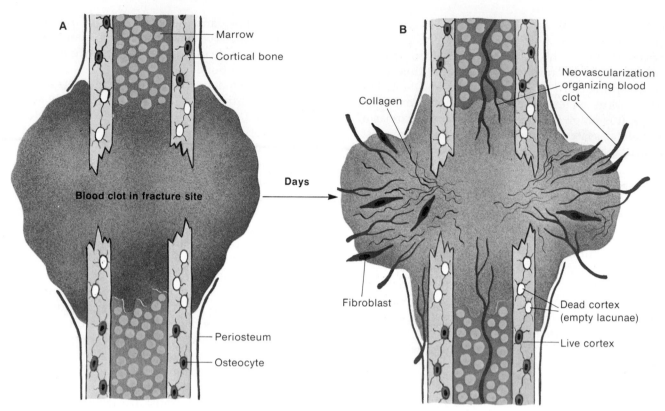

Figure 26-16. Healing of a fracture. (*A*) Soon after a fracture is sustained, an extensive blood clot forms in the subperiosteal and soft tissue, as well as in the marrow cavity. The bone at the fracture site is jagged. (*B*) The inflammatory phase of fracture healing is characterized by neovascularization and beginning organization of the blood clot. Because the osteocytes in the fracture site are dead, the lacunae are empty. The osteocytes of the cortex are necrotic well beyond the fracture site, owing to the traumatic interruption of the perforating arteries from the periosteum.

nels into the cortex by way of an army of osteoclasts, followed by a wave of osteoblasts. A new vessel accompanies the cutting cone, supplying nutrients to these cells and providing more pleuripotential and mononuclear cells for cell renewal. At the same time, the external callus, which is found on the surface of the bone and is formed from the periosteum and the soft tissue mesenchymal cells, continues to grow toward the fracture site. Simultaneously, an endosteal, or internal, callus forms within the medullary cavity and also grows toward the fracture site. At this time, if the cortical cutting cones reach the fracture site, the ends of the fractured bone begin to appear beveled and smooth, as the site is remodeled by osteoclasts. The same is true of the endosteal surface of the cortex, as the internal callus works its way to the fracture site. Where there are large areas of cartilage, neovascularization invades the calcified cartilage, and the endochondral sequence duplicates the normal formation of bone at the epiphyseal plate.

The Remodeling Phase

After the bone ends have been sealed by ingrowth of callus (generally, several weeks after the fracture occurs), remodeling begins. In the remodeling phase, the bone is reorganized, so that the original cortex is restored. Occasionally, the bone is strong enough to qualify as a clinically healed fracture, but biologically, the fracture may not be truly healed and may continue to undergo remodeling for years. For instance, the callus of rib fractures remains almost throughout life, because the continual movement of the ribs, caused by breathing, shears blood vessels and preserves extensive cartilage callus. In a child in whom the epiphyseal plates are still open, the normal mod-

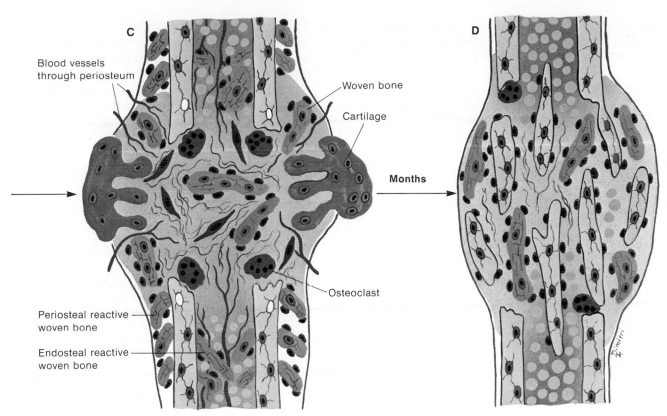

Figure 26-16 (continued). (*C*) The reparative phase of fracture healing is characterized by the formation of a callus of cartilage and woven bone near the fracture site. The jagged edges of the original cortex have been remodeled and eroded by osteoclasts. The marrow space has been revascularized and contains reactive woven bone, as does the periosteal area. (*D*) In the remodeling phase, during which the cortex is revitalized, the reactive bone may be lamellar or woven. The new bone is organized along stress lines and mechanical forces. Extensive osteoclastic and osteoblastic cellular activity is maintained.

eling process of growing bone overtakes the callus, so that a fracture may not be recognizable as such when adulthood is reached. Similarly, in a child, the angulation of a bone at its fracture site may be corrected by a normal modeling process. If the fracture is near the epiphyseal plate, differential growth rates of the epiphyseal plate also correct the angulation. In an adult, however, since the plates are closed, angulation often requires correction with external or internal devices.

Special Considerations

There are unusual nuances to fracture healing that deserve mention. If a fracture does not result in bone displacement and soft tissue injury (for example, in the case of a drill hole in the bone cortex or a controlled fracture, or osteotomy, created with a fine saw

under orthopaedic supervision), there is almost no soft tissue reaction and callus formation because the bone is rigidly fixed. In such instances, the fracture callus grows directly into the fracture site by a process called **primary healing.** Under these circumstances, there is rapid restitution of the cortex, including restoration of the haversian systems. Similarly, if a fracture site is held in rigid alignment by metal screws and plates, there is also little external callus. The cortical cutting cones will then be prominent, and will heal the fracture site quickly.

If a fracture site does not heal, the condition is termed **nonunion.** Causes of nonunion include interposition of soft tissue at the fracture site, excessive motion, infection, poor blood supply, and other factors previously mentioned. Continued movement at the unhealed fracture site leads to **pseudarthrosis,** a condition in which joint tissue is formed. Pleuripotential tissue cells become synovial cells, which secrete synovial fluid and form a "joint." In such cases, the fracture never heals and must be removed surgically.

Prospective treatment modalities for fractures, other than mechanical devices, are being sought. Some investigators are using electric currents to promote bone healing. Others are adding osteocalcin and other bone proteins to the fracture site to stimulate more rapid repair. These methods are still investigational.

Stress Fractures (Fatigue or March Fractures)

A stress fracture occurs when the bone cortex does not have an adequate supply of osteons, which form only when stress is applied to the cortex. If the ill-prepared cortex (e.g., in the 5th metatarsal) undergoes repeated stress, such as jogging, skiing, or ballet dancing, the bone produces cutting cones in an attempt to implant osteons. If the stress continues, periosteal and endosteal calluses develop to strengthen the bone while active remodeling takes place. An actual fracture occurs as the last event, if the stresses are continually applied during remodeling. The clinical signs of a stress fracture include pain and swelling in the region of exuberant remodeling and adjacent neovascularization. When the actual fracture occurs, the pain becomes more severe. Thus, at the site of a stress fracture, callus forms **before** the fracture occurs. In the early stages of this condition, prior to the actual fracture, the radiologic appearance may resemble that of tumor, as the cortex is riddled with cutting cones for remodeling, which is also the case with an invasive tumor.

Osteonecrosis (Avascular and Aseptic Necrosis)

Osteonecrosis refers to the death of bone and marrow in the absence of infection. Causes of osteonecrosis include the following:

- Trauma, including fractures and surgery
- Emboli producing focal bone infarction
- Systemic diseases, such as polycythemia, lupus erythematosus, Gaucher's disease, sickle cell disease, and gout, all of which may produce focal necrosis
- Radiation, either internal or external, which kills osteocytes and produces bone necrosis

- Steroid administration, which produces focal bone necrosis through unknown mechanisms
- Specific focal bone necrosis at various sites—for instance, in the head of the femur, where it is called **Legg-Calvé-Perthes** disease, or in the navicular bone, where it is called **Köhler's disease.**
- Osteochondritis dissecans, a condition in which a piece of articular cartilage and subchondral bone breaks off into a joint. It is thought that a focal area of bone necrosis occurs and eventually detaches. The etiology of this condition is unknown.
- Autografts and allografts.
- Thrombosis of local vessels secondary to the pressure of adjacent tumors or other space-occupying lesions
- Idiopathic factors, as in the high incidence of osteonecrosis of the head and the femur (Fig. 26-17) in alcoholics.

It is important to recognize that necrotic bone heals differently in the cortex and in the underlying coarse cancellous bone. **Necrotic coarse cancellous bone** heals by a process called "creeping substitution," whereby the necrotic marrow is replaced by invading, or "creeping," neovascular tissue, which provides the pleuripotential cells needed for bone remodeling. The necrotic bony trabeculae may be resorbed directly by osteoclastic activity, but more commonly, they are surrounded by new woven or lamellar bone generated by the osteoblastic activity of the granulation tissue. Eventually, the "sandwich," composed of necrotic bone in the center and the surrounding viable bone, is remodeled by osteoclastic activity, and new bone is laid down through intramembranous bone formation. By contrast, **necrotic cortical bone** is healed by a cutting cone. The cutting cone, as discussed earlier, forms via the pre-existing vascular channels in the cortex. The appropriate signals reach this vascular channel and stimulate neovascularization by the surrounding pleuripotential mesenchymal tissue. Osteoclasts are formed by fusion of the circulating monocytes, and make their way into the dense compact cortical bone, with osteoblasts trailing behind. As a result, tunnels bore their way into the necrotic cortex, leading to new bone formation. This is a slow process, and the bone is often laid down *de novo* as lamellar bone.

In Legg-Calvé-Perthes disease, which involves the femoral head in children, or in idiopathic osteonecrosis, which occurs in a similar location in adults, a collapse of the femoral head may lead to joint incongruity and eventual severe osteoarthritis. The col-

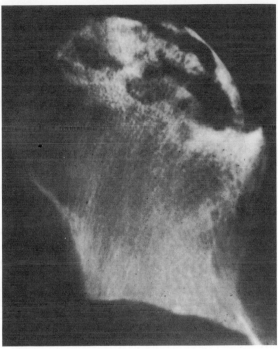

A

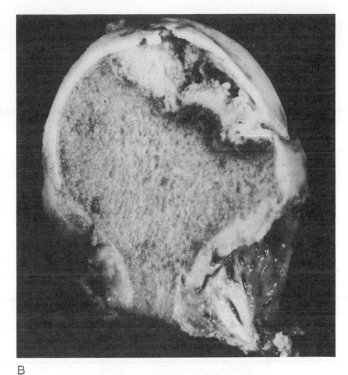

B

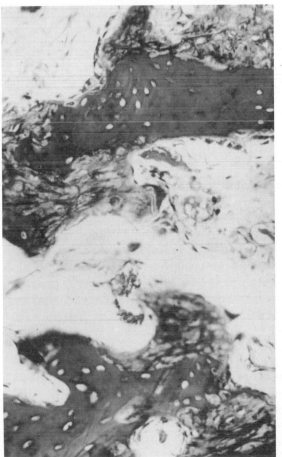

C

Figure 26-17.   Osteonecrosis of the femoral head. (A) A radiograph of the resected femoral head shows a subchondral bone plate fracture as a translucent semilunar space. The necrotic area deep to the fracture is more radiodense because of the collapse of pre-existing bone, the calcification of fatty marrow, and the ingrowth of new bone (creeping substitution). The interface between preserved coarse cancellous bone and the necrotic zone is sharply demarcated. (B) In the specimen shown in A, the necrotic zone is a white area deep to the articular cartilage, with some cystic areas of hemorrhage. The interface between the necrotic zone and the preserved marrow is dark because of neovascularization and repair tissue. The crack in the subchondral bone plate extends through the articular cartilage. (C) A photomicrograph shows that the necrotic lamellar bone contains empty osteocyte lacunae surrounded by viable woven bone. The marrow is loosely fibrotic, and osteoblasts and osteoclasts are seen.

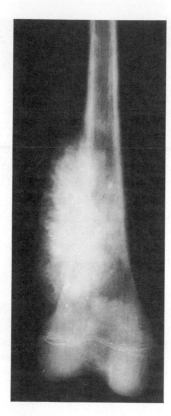

Figure 26-18. Osteosarcoma. A radiograph of the re-sected femur shows a sunburst pattern of hyperdense new bone in the distal diaphysis and metaphysis. This radiodensity is due to woven bone produced by the sarcoma. The epiphyseal plate is represented as a transverse lucent line that separates the metaphysis from the epiphysis. The radiating radiodense bone extends beyond the periosteum into the soft tissues, obscuring the underlying bone architecture.

lapse of the subchondral bone occurs as a result of several mechanisms:

- Necrotic bone, which does not respond to stress and does not obey Wolff's law, may sustain fatigue fractures and compaction over a long period of time.
- The portion peripheral to the necrotic bone may undergo neovascularization. On radiologic examination, there is a relatively lucent area surrounding the necrotic zone which allows for displacement of the necrotic zone downward.
- The rigid articular cartilage and subchondral bone may actually crack as the subchondral necrotic zone collapses, producing a fracture.

A radiograph of such an area often shows the necrotic zone as radiodense, because of the compaction of the pre-existing dead bone, the addition of new bone through creeping substitution, and the formation of calcium soaps that arise as a result of the necrosis of the marrow fat. Since this necrotic zone tends to be wedged-shaped, it may be that a focal vascular insufficiency has occurred, but this has not been confirmed.

Reactive Bone Formation

Reactive bone is formed in response to stress on bone or soft tissue. Conditions such as tumors, infections, trauma, or generalized or focal disease can stimulate bone formation. The periosteum may respond with a so-called **sunburst pattern** (Fig. 26-18), as seen with certain tumors, or a progressive layering of the periosteum, which produces an **onion skin pattern** of the cortex. The endosteal or the marrow surface may produce new bone, so that on radiologic studies, the cortex appears to be thickened and the coarse cancellous bone appears to be more dense. Importantly, the reactive bone may be woven or lamellar, depending on the rates of deposition of the reactive bone. For example, reactive bone around an indolent infection, such as a chronic osteomyelitis, may be laid down *de novo* as lamellar bone from the periosteum because the bone, as an organ, has time to respond to the persistent stress. Similarly, a benign tumor may also stimulate a lamellar bone reaction. By contrast, a rapidly growing tumor may stimulate woven bone formation as a response to the rapid growth of the tumor cells. **Invariably, reactive bone is of the intramembranous type, as it is usually derived from the periosteum or the endosteal tissue of the marrow.**

A point of distinction should be made between reactive bone formation and heterotopic calcification. The latter is simply deposition of acellular mineral in soft tissue. **Heterotopic bone formation** or **reactive bone formation** refers directly to the production of woven or lamellar bone, which may or may not be mineralized. Radiologically, these entities are usually distinctive. Heterotopic **ossification** often has a spicular or trabeculated pattern, whereas heterotopic **calcification** has an irregular, splotchy, and amorphous appearance. Heterotopic calcification tends to occur in necrotic soft tissue or in cartilage, and is usually more dense than bone on radiography. **Metastatic calcification** occurs in conditions in which there is an increase in calcium–phosphorus product. Thus, hypercalcemic states or hyperphosphatemic conditions predispose soft tissues to calcification. **Dystrophic calcification** is seen focally in soft tissues related to tumors, degenerative disease, such as arteriosclerosis, and trauma. Furthermore, loss of neurologic function, as seen in quadriplegia and hemiplegia, predispose the affected parts to soft tissue calcification.

Myositis Ossificans

Myositis ossificans, a common condition related to heterotopic or reactive bone formation affects young people. It often mimics a malignant neoplasm, but is entirely benign. The lesion occurs as a result of blunt trauma to the muscle and soft tissues, usually of the lower limb. Peripheral neovascularization of the resulting hematoma leads to early spicular bone formation in the soft tissue within a week or so. Because these lesions often occur near a bone, such as the femur or tibia, on radiography they may mimic a malignant bone-forming tumor (Fig. 26-19). Histologically, woven bone is formed within the granulation tissue. In a young lesion, the cells of the woven bone and surrounding soft tissue are pleomorphic and show abundant mitoses, a histologic appearance that also resembles that of a malignant tumor. The key feature distinguishing this lesion from a neoplasm is that **the woven bone is well formed peripherally, whereas it is immature or not formed at all in the center of the lesion.** This growth pattern reflects the ingrowth of neovascular tissue from the peripheral portion into the center of the damaged area. The reason for this peripheral formation of bone is not understood, but it is well known that the closer the trauma is to the periosteum, the more likely it is that the healing tissue will contain reactive bone. Occasionally, myositis ossificans, especially in the late stages, contains cartilage and even lamellar bone, so that in a well-formed lesion, it may mimic a sesamoid bone in the soft tissue. In this late stage, it is not difficult to distinguish this reactive lesion from a malignant tumor, which never forms such well-delineated bone. The phenomenon of peripheral maturity with central immaturity is called the **zonation effect,** and clearly indicates a reactive process. A neoplasm has an opposite zonation effect, since the most mature tissue of the tumor is located centrally.

Infections

Osteomyelitis

Osteomyelitis is an inflammation of bone caused by a pyogenic organism. Despite the common use of antibiotics, osteomyelitis is still a major diagnostic and therapeutic problem. The most common pathogens are staphylococcus species, but other organisms, such as *Escherichia coli* and *Neisseria gonorrhea, Haemophilus influenzae,* and salmonella species, are also seen.

Pathogenesis and Clinical Presentation

The organisms are introduced either through the **hematogenous** route or by **direct introduction** of the organisms into the bone in areas of trauma.

Infection by direct penetration or extension of bacteria is now the most common cause of osteomyelitis in the United States. Bacterial organisms are introduced directly into the bone by penetrating wounds, fractures, or surgery. Staphylococci and streptococci are still commonly incriminated, but there are now many other organisms that produce such infections. *Staphylococcus aureus* is the most common organism involved following elective surgical procedures without preoperative antibiotics. When preoperative antibiotics are administered, *S. epidermidis* is the organism most frequently isolated. Anaerobic organisms are isolated in 25% of postoperative infections when preoperative antibiotics are used. Rarely, a gram-negative organism may seed a hip following a urologic or gastrointestinal surgical procedure.

In **hematogenous osteomyelitis,** the organisms reach the bone from a focus elsewhere in the body. Often, the focus itself—for instance, a skin pustule or infected teeth and gums—poses little threat. Some researchers suggest that the mere brushing of teeth creates a temporary bacteremia, which may allow organisms to reach the bone. **The most common sites affected by hematogenous osteomyelitis are the ends of the long bones, such as the knee, ankle, and hip.** Hematogenous osteomyelitis principally affects boys 5 to 15 years of age, but it may be seen in slightly older age groups as well. Drug addicts may also develop hematogenous osteomyelitis from infected needles.

Hematogenous osteomyelitis primarily affects the metaphyseal area because of the unique vascular supply in this region (Fig. 26-20). Normally, arterioles enter the calcified portion of the epiphyseal plate, form a loop, and then drain into the medullary cavity without establishing a capillary bed. This loop system permits slowing and sludging of blood flow, thereby allowing bacteria time to penetrate the walls of the blood vessels and establish an infective focus within the marrow. If the organism is virulent and continues to proliferate, it creates increased pressure on the

(Text continues on p. 1332)

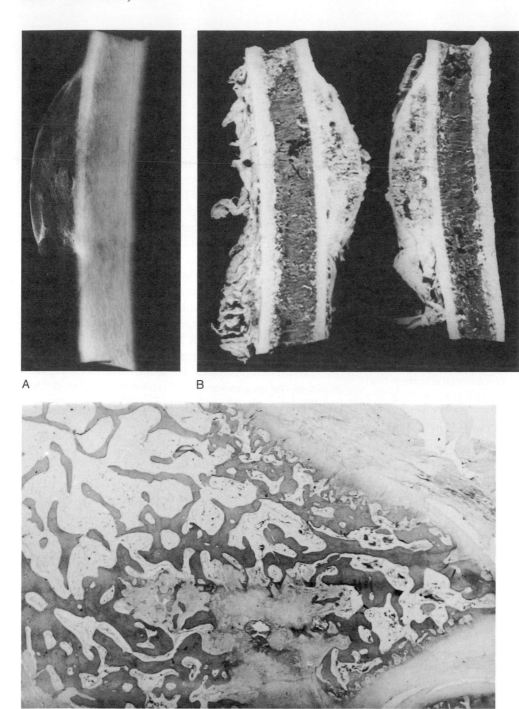

A

B

C

Figure 26-19.   Myositis ossificans. (*A*) A radiograph of the middiaphyseal region of a long bone shows a surface excrescence of bone that represents long-standing myositis ossificans. The lesion is composed of distinct bony trabeculae and cortical bone. (*B*) The gross specimen illustrated in *A*. The presence of marrow in the zone of myositis ossificans indicates a long-standing lesion. (*C*) A photomicrograph reveals mature bone on the periphery of the lesion and immature bone in the center. The peripheral bone is lamellar, and the center contains woven bone surrounded by fibrous tissue. The more peripheral bone is surrounded by fatty marrow. The entire lesion is surrounded by fibrosis or compressed, atrophic, skeletal muscle. The diagnostic features of peripheral maturation and central immaturity of the bone indicate that myositis ossificans is a repair reaction to soft tissue damage rather than a neoplastic process.

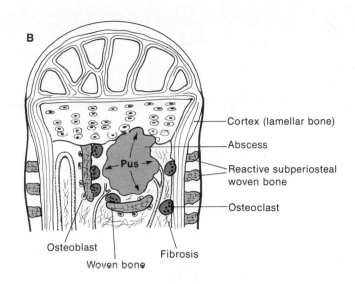

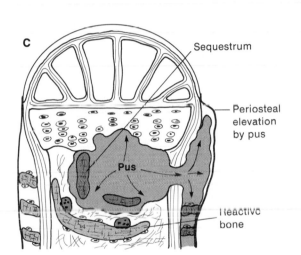

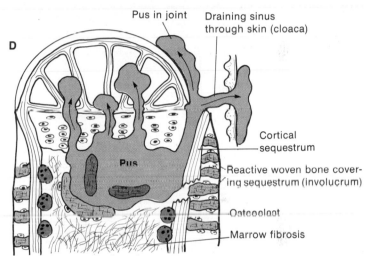

Figure 26-20. Pathogenesis of hematogenous osteomyelitis. (*A*) The epiphysis, metaphysis, and epiphyseal plate are normal. A small, septic microabscess is forming at the capillary loop. (*B*) The expansion of the septic focus stimulates resorption of adjacent bony trabeculae. Woven bone begins to surround this focus. The abscess expands into the cartilage and stimulates reactive bone formation by the periosteum. (*C*) The abscess, which continues to expand through the cortex into the subperiosteal tissue, shears off the perforating arteries that supply the cortex with blood, thereby leading to necrosis of the cortex. (*D*) The extension of this process into the joint space, the epiphysis, and the skin produces a draining sinus. The necrotic bone is called a sequestrum. The viable bone surrounding a sequestrum is termed the involucrum.

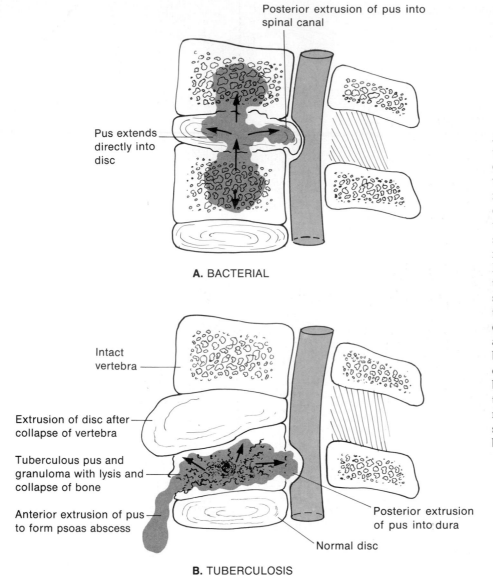

Posterior extrusion of pus into
spinal canal

Pus extends
directly into
disc

A. BACTERIAL

Intact
vertebra

Extrusion of disc after
collapse of vertebra

Tuberculous pus and
granuloma with lysis and
collapse of bone

Anterior extrusion of pus
to form psoas abscess

Posterior extrusion
of pus into dura

Normal disc

B. TUBERCULOSIS

Figure 26-21. Osteomyelitis of the vertebral body. (*A*) Bacterial osteomyelitis expands from one vertebral body to the next by direct invasion of the intervertebral disc, and may actually push posteriorly into the spinal canal. The sequence of events in the marrow cavity is similar to that in a long bone. (*B*) In tuberculous osteomyelitis, the bone is destroyed by resorption of bony trabeculae, which results in mechanical collapse of the vertebrae and extrusion of the intervertebral disc. Tuberculous organisms cannot penetrate the intervertebral disc directly; rather, they extend from one vertebra to the next after mechanical forces destroy and extrude the intervertebral disc.

adjacent thin-walled vessels because they lie in a closed space—namely, the marrow cavity of bone. Such pressure further compromises the vascular supply in this region and produces bone necrosis. The necrotic areas coalesce into an avascular zone, thereby allowing further bacterial proliferation.

If the infection is not contained, pus and bacteria extend into the endosteal vascular channels that supply the cortex and spread throughout the Volkmann and haversian canals of the cortex. Eventually, pus forms underneath the periosteum, shearing off the perforating arteries of the periosteum and further devitalizing the cortex. The pus flows between the periosteum and the cortex, isolating more bone from its blood supply, and may even invade the joint. Eventually, the pus penetrates the periosteum and the skin to form a draining sinus. The hole formed in the bone during this process is termed a **cloaca.** A fragment of necrotic bone, called a **sequestrum,** is often embedded in the pus.

Periosteal new bone formation and reactive bone formation in the marrow tend to wall off the infection. At the same time, osteoclastic activity resorbs bone. If the infection is virulent, this attempt to contain it is overwhelmed, and the infection races through the bone with virtually no bone formation but extensive bone necrosis.

The bone generally has several options for repair.

Marrow cells may modulate into osteoblasts and osteoclasts in an attempt to wall off the infection. Alternatively, a **Brodie's abscess** may form, consisting of reactive bone from the periostum and the endosteum that contained the infection. The third option occurs when periosteal new bone formation is extensive. In such cases the reactive new bone forms a sheath around the necrotic sequestrum, giving rise to an **involucrum.** This may be at a microscopic level, or the entire cortex may represent an involucrum. An involucrum that involves an entire bone may exist for several years before a patient seeks medical attention. In very young children (1 year old or younger), the adjacent joint is often involved by osteomyelitis because the periosteum is not firmly adherent to the cortex, and only a few perforating arteries supply the cortex. From the age of 1 year to puberty, subperiosteal abscesses are common. In adults, spread to adjacent joints may also occur. A sinus tract that extends from the cloaca to the skin may become epithelialized by skin epidermis that grows into the sinus tract. When this occurs, the sinus tract invariably remains open, continually draining pus, necrotic bone, and bacteria.

Occasionally, osteomyelitis involves vertebral bodies (Fig. 26-21). The intervertebral disc is not a barrier for bacterial osteomyelitis, particularly for staphylococcal infection. Infections travel from one vertebra to the next by directly invading and traversing the intervertebral disc. Some researchers consider that the intervertebral disc is the primary source of infection—so-called discitis. The disc expands with pus and is eventually destroyed as the pus bores into the adjacent vertebral bodies. Fifty percent or more of the cases of **vertebral osteomyelitis** are caused by *Staphylococcus aureus.* Twenty percent are caused by *E. coli* and other enteric organisms, many of which originate from the urinary tract. Salmonella is also seen in the vertebral bodies, as are brucella species. The predisposing factors are intravenous drug abuse, upper urinary tract infections, urologic procedures, and hematogenous spread of organisms from other sites. Back pain, with point tenderness over the area of infection, is associated with low-grade fever and an elevated sedimentation rate.

Occasionally, a paravertebral abscess draining the bone may "point" and emerge in the groin or elsewhere. The complications of vertebral osteomyelitis include vertebral collapse with paravertebral abscesses; spinal epidural abscesses, with cord compression from the abscess or from displaced fragments of the infected bone; and compression fractures of the vertebral body, leading to neurologic deficits.

Complications

The complications of osteomyelitis include the following:

- **Septicemia** may occur in infants secondary to bone infection. It is unusual for osteomyelitis to occur secondary to septicemia.
- **Acute bacterial arthritis** may arise as a result of osteomyelitis in children and in adults, and represents a medical emergency. Direct digestion of cartilage by inflammatory cells destroys the articular cartilage and leads to osteoarthritis. Rapid intervention to prevent this complication is mandatory.
- **Pathologic fractures** may occur as a result of osteomyelitis. These fractures heal poorly because of the infected tissue, and may require surgical drainage.
- **Squamous cell carcinoma** develops in the bone or in the sinus tract of long-standing chronic osteomyelitis, often years after the initial infection. Squamous tissue arises from the epithelialization of the sinus tract, and may eventually undergo carcinomatous change.
- **Amyloidosis** was a common complication of chronic osteomyelitis in the preantibiotic era, and patients often would die from cardiac and renal disease. Currently, it is extremely rare in industrialized countries.
- **Chronic osteomyelitis,** especially that involving the entire bone, is incurable because antibiotic therapy does not eradicate all the organisms. In this condition, necrotic bone or sequestra function as foreign bodies in avascular areas, and antibiotics cannot reach the bacteria. Therefore, chronic osteomyelitis is treated symptomatically with surgery or antibiotics for the duration of the patient's life.

Treatment

The treatment of osteomyelitis depends on the stage of the infection. Early osteomyelitis is treated by administration of intravenous antibiotics for a period of 6 or more weeks. Surgery may be used to drain and decompress the infection within the bone, or to drain abscesses that do not respond to antibiotic therapy. As already mentioned, in long-standing, chronic osteomyelitis, antibiotics alone are not curative, and high-dose antibiotic therapy with extensive surgical debridement of necrotic bone is often required.

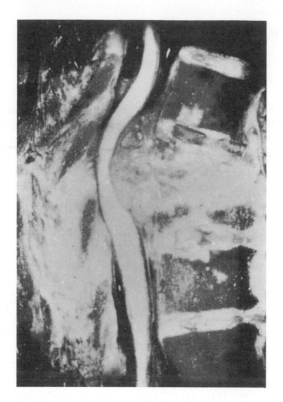

Figure 26-22. Tuberculous spondylitis (Pott's disease). A vertebral body is replaced by tuberculous tissue that extends anteriorly into the soft tissues and posteriorly into the spinal canal, where it compresses the spinal cord. The infection has extended into the adjacent vertebral bodies because the intervertebral disc has been extruded anteriorly.

Tuberculosis

Tuberculosis of bone is invariably secondary to a primary focus elsewhere in the body—the lungs or lymph nodes in the human type, or the gut or tonsils in the rare bovine type. The mycobacteria spread to the bone hematogenously; only rarely is there direct spread into the rib, spine, or sternum from a lung or lymph node.

Tuberculous Spondylitis (Pott's Disease)

Tuberculous spondylitis, inflammation of the spine, a feared complication of childhood tuberculosis, affects the vertebral bodies, sparing the lamina and spines and adjacent vertebrae (Fig. 26-21, Fig. 26-22). With antibiotic treatment, Pott's disease is rare. The thoracic vertebrae are usually affected, especially T11, with the lumbar and cervical vertebrae being less commonly involved.

The pathologic process is similar to that in other sites. The tuberculous granulomas first produce ca-

seous necrosis of the bone marrow, an effect that leads to slow resorption of bony trabeculae, and occasionally, to cystic spaces in the bone. Because there is little or no reactive bone, **collapse of the affected vertebra is usual,** after which kyphosis and scoliosis ensue. The intervertebral disc is crushed and destroyed by the compression fracture rather than by invasion of organisms. If the infection ruptures into the soft tissue anteriorly, pus and necrotic debris drain along the spinal ligaments and form a **cold abscess,** a term that signifies that acute inflammation is sparse or nonexistent. A **psoas abscess** forms near the lower lumbar vertebrae and dissects along the pelvis, to emerge through the skin of the inguinal region as a draining sinus. Such a process may occur without any prior symptoms, and may be the first manifestation of tuberculous spondylitis. Paraplegia in Pott's disease is secondary to vascular insufficiency of the spinal nerves, rather than to direct pressure.

Arthritis

In tuberculous arthritis, the focus of tuberculosis, again reflecting hematogenous spread, begins in the joint capsule, synovium, or intracapsular portion of

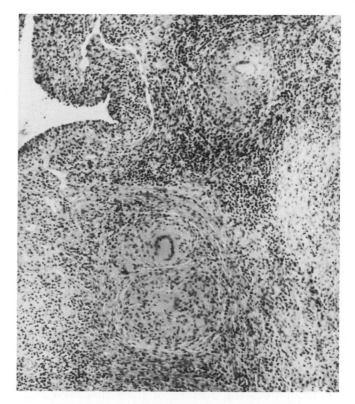

Figure 26-23. Tuberculous arthritis. The chronically inflamed synovium is filled with granulomas that contain Langhans-type giant cells.

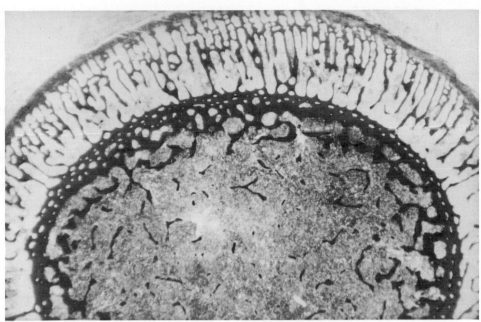

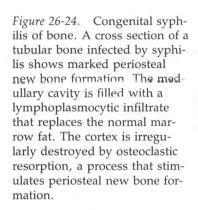

Figure 26-24. Congenital syphilis of bone. A cross section of a tubular bone infected by syphilis shows marked periosteal new bone formation. The medullary cavity is filled with a lymphoplasmocytic infiltrate that replaces the normal marrow fat. The cortex is irregularly destroyed by osteoclastic resorption, a process that stimulates periosteal new bone formation.

the bone. Tuberculosis induces proliferation of granulomas in synovial tissue (Fig. 26-23). This tissue then becomes edematous and papillary, and may fill the entire joint space. There is also massive destruction of the articular cartilage from undermining granulation tissue in the bone. The destroyed joint is replaced by osseous tissue, the result being bony ankylosis.

Osteomyelitis of the Long Bones

Osteomyelitis of the long bones is the least common bone manifestation of tuberculosis. Tuberculous osteomyelitis in a long bone occurs near the joint, and produces a simultaneous arthritis. For unknown reasons, the greater trochanter of the femur is a common site for this disease.

Syphilis

Syphilis (lues), which is caused by the spirochete *Treponema pallidum,* causes a slowly progressive, chronic, inflammatory disease of bone that is characterized by granulomas, necrosis, and marked reactive bone formation. It may be acquired through sexual contact, or it may be passed through the placenta from mother to the fetus. The bone changes in syphilis depend on the age of the patient, the endosteal and periosteal changes, and the presence or absence of gummas.

Congenital Syphilis

Congenital syphilis may appear as early as the fifth month of gestation, and is fully developed at birth. In this disease, the spirochetes are ubiquitous and are present in the epiphysis and periosteum, where they produce osteochondritis (epiphysitis) and periostitis, respectively (Fig. 26-24). If the disease is severe, the epiphysis may become dislocated, leaving the child with a functionless limb (pseudoparalysis of Parrot). The knee is most often affected. The epiphyseal plate is irregularly widened and is discolored yellow. The zone of calcified cartilage is destroyed, and the marrow spaces are filled by a sea of lymphocytes, plasma cells, and spirochetes. Because the periosteum is stimulated to produce reactive new bone, the thickness of the cortex may actually be doubled. The inflammatory infiltrate permeates the cortex through the Volkmann and haversian canals, and settles in the elevated periosteum. Ultimately, the affected bones become short and deformed.

Acquired Syphilis

Acquired syphilis in adults usually produces lesions early in the tertiary stage, 2 to 5 years after inoculation of the organisms. Periostitis is predominant because the epiphyseal plates have already closed. The bones most commonly affected are the tibia, nose, palate, and skull. The tibial lesions often produce a marked periostitis with deposition of new bone on

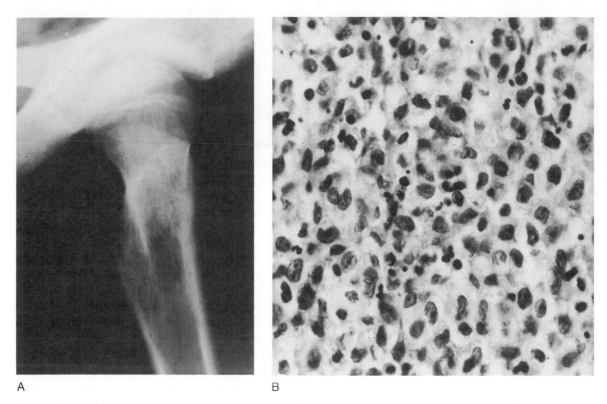

A   B

Figure 26-25.   Histiocytosis. (*A*) A radiograph of the proximal femur shows a well-defined lucency in the subtrochanteric proximal diaphysis. (*B*) A photomicrograph of the femur in *A* reveals sheets of histiocytes and scattered polymorphonuclear leukocytes and eosinophils.

the medial and anterior aspects of the shaft, a process that leads to the "saber shin" deformity. The skull is also increased in thickness because of periosteal stimulation.

The formation of gummas is most common during the tertiary stage of the disease. A **gumma** (so named because of gray, viscid, necrotic tissue that resembles gum arabic) is a granulomatous reaction with associated necrosis. The adjacent bone is slowly replaced by fibrous marrow. Ultimately, perforations occur through the cortex. The markedly irregular, thickened periosteal surfaces, which are perforated by pits and serpiginous ulcerations, are characteristic of syphilis. There may be collapse and total lysis of small bones, such as the nasal and palatal bones, producing the classic "saddle nose" defect—namely, perforation, destruction, and collapse of the nasal septum.

Histiocytosis

Histiocytosis, formerly called histiocytosis X, is a disease of unknown etiology in which cholesterol-laden macrophages collect in the bones and soft tissues

(Fig. 26-25). The complex of histiocytosis comprises three nosologic entities: a localized form labeled **eosinophilic granuloma;** a disseminated variant called **Hand-Schüller-Christian** disease; and a severe generalized disease termed **Letterer-Siwe disease.** Histiocytosis occurs predominantly in infants and young adults, but it may also affect middle-aged adults. Eosinophilic granuloma and Hand-Schüller-Christian disease may be asymptomatic, but in Letterer-Siwe disease, the course may be fulminant and fatal.

The histologic appearance of the bone in all three diseases is identical, and is characterized by collections of large macrophages that contain cholesterol. By electron microscopy these cells have a microtubular structure that is similar to that of the Langerhans cells of the skin (Fig. 26-26). Numerous, scattered eosinophils are located throughout the lesion, occasionally forming a collection called an "eosinophilic abscess." Multinucleated giant cells of the foreign body, or Touton, type are often seen in the lesion, as are chronic inflammatory cells. **The diagnostic feature of this lesion is the peculiar macrophage with its lobulated nucleus.** Lesions may occur in any portion of the body, including bones, skin, brain, lungs, lymph nodes, liver, and spleen. Although cholesterol deposition is prominent in the macrophages, there is no defined abnormality related to cholesterol metabolism, and these patients exhibit neither hypercholesterolemia nor peripheral eosinophilia. No specific enzyme defect or causative organism has been found.

The radiologic findings in all three diseases are identical. The lesions may occur in the metaphysis or diaphysis of a long bone, or in a flat bone, especially in the skull. They are visualized as punched-out, lytic defects, with virtually no reactive bone. Such a lesion may lead to a fracture and periosteal callus formation.

Clinical Presentation

Eosinophilic Granuloma

Clinically, eosinophilic granuloma presents as a self-limited disease, with one or two lytic lesions in the bone. These lesions may cause mild pain or may be an incidental finding in a routine chest radiograph. The disease is usually manifested in the first two decades of life, but it occasionally affects older people. Lesions in the lower thoracic or upper lumbar vertebrae may lead to focal collapse and pathologic fracture.

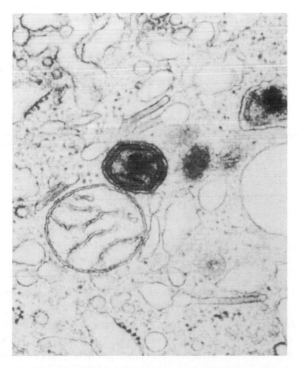

Figure 26-26 Histiocytosis. An electron micrograph of a histiocyte demonstrates microtubular structures, some of which look like tennis rackets. These structures have been termed Birbeck bodies, a finding that is diagnostic for histiocytosis.

Eosinophilic granuloma may be difficult to distinguish from osteomyelitis because a macrophage background may be present in chronic osteomyelitis. However, the macrophages in eosinophilic granuloma usually produce S100 protein, whereas the macrophages in osteomyelitis do not. Furthermore, the characteristic infolding of the macrophage nuclei strongly suggests eosinophilic granuloma. Hodgkin's lymphoma is associated with malignant histiocytes and the classic Reed-Sternberg cells, which are not present in eosinophilic granuloma.

Hand-Schüller-Christian Disease

Hand-Schüller-Christian disease also occurs in young individuals, but is much more widespread than eosinophilic granuloma, and is accompanied by symptoms related to the affected organ systems. Some patients are abnormally short, and their weight is reduced. Infiltration of the stalk of the hypothalamus leads to diabetes insipidus. A lesion may infiltrate the retro-orbital space, producing exophthalmos. Lytic lesions in the jaw bone yield a radiologic impression of floating teeth. Twenty percent of patients have lymphadenopathy and lung infiltrates. Crusty, red, and weepy skin lesions occur at the hairline, the extensor surfaces of the extremities, the abdomen, and occasionally on the soles of the feet. Deafness occurs when the external auditory canal and mastoid air cells are involved. About 30% of affected patients demonstrate liver and spleen involvement, and 40% have bone lesions, half of which involve the skull. Therefore, the classic triad of Hand-Schüller-Christian disease—namely, **lytic lesions of the skull, diabetes insipidus,** and **exophthalmos**—occurs in only one third of patients.

Letterer-Siwe Disease

Letterer-Siwe disease is an aggressive systemic disease that usually occurs in children under the age of 2 years. Affected children fail to thrive and become cachectic. Multiple organ involvement culminates in massive hepatosplenomegaly, lymphadenopathy, anemia, leukopenia, and thrombocytopenia. Widely scattered skin lesions, often hemorrhagic, are usual. The bone lesions are not prominent, but progressive marrow replacement and pulmonary infiltration occasionally cause death.

Treatment

Eosinophilic granuloma is a self-limited disease, and most of the lesions disappear if left alone. A lytic lesion in bone may have to be curetted and packed with bone chips. Sometimes, the biopsy itself is enough to stimulate repair of the lytic lesion. The collapsed vertebra may actually reconstitute itself over a period of time. Hand-Schüller-Christian disease may require radiation therapy for some bone and retro-orbital lesions. Diabetes insipidus seems to be irreversible, despite irradiation of the pituitary region. Powerful drugs, such as steroids, cyclophosphamide, and tumoricidal agents may also be used to treat Hand-Schüller-Christian disease. Similarly aggressive therapy for Letterer-Siwe disease may improve the prognosis.

Metabolic Bone Disease

The term metabolic disease refers to a number of skeletal disorders that are generalized; that is, they involve **all** the bones of the skeleton. **In metabolic bone disease, there are no normal areas of bone tissue in the skeleton.** A disease such as Paget's disease, which is discussed in a later section, is not considered a metabolic bone disease because although it may be widespread, foci of normal bone tissue are also present.

Calcium Metabolism

Some general principles related to calcium metabolism should be mentioned. The normal adult body contains 20 to 25 grams of calcium per kilogram of fat-free tissue, a total of 1000 to 1500 grams. Ninety-nine percent of this body calcium is present in bone, and the other 1% is found in the blood and cells. Of the 1 to 2 grams of calcium in the extracellular fluid, 50% is bound to protein, and the remaining 50% is found as free calcium ions. **Thus, the skeleton is the major reservoir for calcium when needed; the calcium is liberated from it only by bone resorption.**

The homeostatic mechanisms that control metabolism of calcium and phosphorus operate under three basic constraints.

- The salt of calcium, $CaHPO_4$, is not freely soluble in water. At the pH of body fluids, the concentrations of calcium and phosphate ions in the serum actually exceed the critical solubility product. They are presumed to be held in solution by an elaborate inhibitor system. This metastability allows the deposition of hydroxyapatite during bone formation with a minimal expenditure of energy.
- The blood calcium concentration is exquisitely tuned. Reduced levels of calcium in the blood produce irritability and contractile and conduc-

tive abnormalities of smooth and skeletal muscle (expressed as tetany), convulsions, and even death. Conversely, increases in the concentration of calcium produce muscle weakness, somnolence, and ventricular fibrillation.

Calcium cannot enter cells without a transport system. The transport of calcium across a mucosal cell of the intestine, through the renal tubular cell, or across a bone cell membrane involves the action of the active form of vitamin D and parathyroid hormone, and is inhibited by an increase in the concentration of cytosolic phosphate. For example, the absorptive intestinal cell (duodenum and proximal jejunum) has receptors for parathyroid hormone. Circulating parathyroid hormone increases in response to a decrease in serum calcium. The parathyroid hormone binds to the receptor of the intestinal cell, thereby activating an intracellular mechanism by which ATP is converted to cAMP through the action of adenyl cyclase. This cAMP renders the cell membrane more permeable to ionic calcium and also induces the mitochondria to release calcium. Both of these actions increase the intracellular concentration of calcium, but do not promote Ca^{2+} transport to the extracellular space. The active form of vitamin D (1,25-dihydroxyvitamin D) promotes the transcription of a messenger RNA which, in turn, codes for the synthesis of a calcium-binding or transport factor. This protein transports calcium across the cell membrane into the pericellular space and the extracellular fluid. Thus, parathyroid hormone and vitamin D, although they work independently, are synergistic. An increased concentration of parathyroid hormone leads indirectly to an increased rate of synthesis of 1,25-dihydroxyvitamin D from 25-hydroxyvitamin D. On the other hand, the action of the active form of vitamin D is essential to the action of PTH.

Phosphate Metabolism

The role of phosphate in this system is less well understood than that of calcium. If the cytosolic concentration of phosphate increases—as, for instance, in chronic renal failure—the calcium transport system is turned off, and at the level of the renal tubule, there is a decrease in synthesis of 1,25-dihydroxyvitamin D. This action presumably prevents the critical solubility product for calcium and phosphorus from being exceeded. High levels of phosphate inhibit the absorption of phosphate from the gastrointestinal tract, the resorption of calcium from the renal tubules, and probably, the resorption of bone. However, high levels of phosphate do not protect the bones from osteoclastic resorption when there is an excessive concentration of parathyroid hormone, as occurs in hyperparathyroidism.

In summary, the role of **parathyroid hormone** in calcium homeostasis is critical. The parathyroid hormone acts at all levels to increase serum calcium. In the intestine, its principal effect is to control the efficiency of calcium absorption by promoting the hydroxylation of 1,25-dihydroxyvitamin D in the kidney. In the kidney, parathyroid hormone regulates calcium loss. It is also the principal hormone directing both bone resorption and phosphate excretion. If there is a net deficit of calcium in the diet, parathyroid hormone induces a net transfer of calcium from bone to the extracellular fluid. The resorption of bone to liberate calcium and phosphate protects against a drop in the extracellular fluid calcium level to a serious or lethally low value. However, it does not affect parathyroid hormone action at the level of the intestine and kidney. The action of **vitamin D** is synergistic with that of parathyroid hormone on the bone, and is the most important direct influence on calcium absorption.

Phosphate absorption in the intestine is less important than calcium absorption, since phosphate is virtually ubiquitous in all foods. Phosphate is released together with calcium when bone is resorbed by osteoclasts. Calcium concentrations can abruptly increase or decrease, whereas changes in phosphate concentration are less dramatic. Abnormalities related to vitamin D levels are characterized by low concentrations of both calcium and phosphorus. By contrast, low serum calcium and high phosphorus levels indicate parathyroid-hormone–related abnormalities. The major source of control for calcium then becomes the gut, whereas for phosphorus, it is the kidney.

It is helpful to bear in mind that vitamin D controls calcium ion homeostasis day by day, whereas parathyroid hormone controls it minute by minute. The main actions of parathyroid hormone include: (1) stimulation of the production of 1,25-dihydroxyvitamin D; (2) an increased transfer of calcium from bone into the extracellular fluid; (3) an increase in the renal tubular resorption of calcium; and (4) a decrease in tubular phosphate resorption, and thus a promotion in the excretion of phosphate. Decreases in the concentration of 1,25-dihydroxyvitamin D lead to the following: (1) increased secretion of parathyroid hormone, (2) increased size of the parathyroid glands,

(3) decreased urinary calcium levels, (4) decreased levels of calcium in the extracellular fluid, and (5) nonresorption of bone. The effect on phosphate is a decrease in its extracellular concentration and an increase in its urine concentration.

As previously noted, hormones regulate the rate and duration of skeletal growth. However, other factors, such as inadequate thyroid function, may delay growth and retard maturation. A decreased amount of growth hormone brought about by somatomedin produces dwarfism, and a deficiency of sex hormones also retards growth and maturation. Another important point is related to remodeling of bone. As indicated earlier, bone formation and bone resorption are "coupled." The signals for the respective cells to act—whether they be mechanical, electrical, or chemical—are not well understood, and at present, there are no drugs that selectively "uncouple" bone formation from resorption.

Remodeling of Bone

The remodeling of bone, a continuous process that persists even in adults, is accomplished by resorption and building of haversian systems, as well as of trabecular bone. A number of techniques, including microradiography, radioisotopic studies, and the fluorescence of tetracyclines, are used to study this remodeling process.

Tetracycline binds to newly incorporated mineralized sites shortly after it is administered. A bone biopsy taken some time after the administration of tetracycline reveals fluorescence if mineralization has taken place during that time interval. A **bone deposition surface** is a smooth, sharp surface of bone that shows uptake of tetracycline, and may be of low mineral density. **Active bone-forming surfaces** are covered by prominent osteoblasts. **Osteoid seams** result from a time lag between the deposition of collagen and the appearance of the calcium salt. In general, adults make 1 μm of bone a day, but it requires about 10 days to mineralize this new bone; therefore, the thickness of osteoid seams should not exceed 12 μm. Osteoclastic **bone resorptive surfaces** are the irregular configurations that represent the Howship's lacunae. In general, bone resorption precedes formation but does not persist as long as bone formation. In adults, about 10% to 15% of the trabecular bone surfaces are covered with osteoid, and about 4% have active resorptive surfaces. Interestingly, kinetic studies indicate that approximately **18% of the total skeletal calcium may normally be removed and deposited over a period of a year.**

General Classification

The classification of metabolic bone disease is based on the relationship of the mineral phase to the matrix of bone, and the relative rates of formation and resorption of bone (Fig. 26-27).

Low Ratio of Mineral to Matrix Phase
The rate of resorption may be low to high, depending on the disorder.

Osteomalacia—Rickets   The histologic features of osteomalacia and rickets are characterized by an increased thickness of osteoid and by an increased area of bone surface covered by osteoid.

Normal Ratio of Mineral to Matrix Phase, When the Rate of Bone Resorption Exceeds That of Bone Formation

Osteitis Fibrosa   In osteitis fibrosa, which is often caused by hyperparathyroidism, bone destruction exceeds formation. However, bone formation is also augmented in an attempt to repair the bone lesions. Histologic, examination reveals numerous osteoclasts resorbing the bone, and adjacent marrow fat is replaced by fibrosis. Extensive hemorrhage in the area is also prominent.

Osteoporosis   Resorption of bone occurs at a greater rate than bone formation in osteoporosis. The rate of bone formation is usually normal, or may actually be decreased, depending on the cause. The bone marrow remains normal, and little or no osteoblastic activity is seen.

Normal Ratio of Mineral to Matrix Phase, When the Rate of Bone Formation Exceeds That of Bone Resorption

Hypoparathyroidism   Hypoparathyroidism is the sole example of disease in the presence of a normal mineral-to-matrix ratio when the rate of bone formation proceeds at a faster pace than bone resorption. The histopathology in this condition is normal, since the kinetic changes are not striking.

Low Ratio of Mineral to Matrix Phase, When the Rate of Bone Formation Exceeds That of Bone Resorption

Osteopetrosis   As previously noted, the rate of resorption of bone is low in osteopetrosis, but the bone formed may be poorly mineralized. Even though the bone mass is increased, the bone that is formed displays osteomalacia. Characteristically, preserved calcified cartilage is surrounded by poorly mineralized woven or lamellar bone, because the primary spongiosum is not properly resorbed by osteoclastic activity and persists into adult life. The osteoclasts may be more numerous than normal, but apparently do not function.

The Healing Phase of Osteitis Fibrosa.   If a parathyroid adenoma or other hyperfunctioning parathyroid tissue is removed, bone resorption ceases, but bone formation continues at an increased rate. Histologically, this situation presents as excessive osteoblastic activity and minimal osteoclastic activity. Osteoid is prominent. Although the osteons and trabeculae are being restored at a rapid rate, there is a time lag before mineralization takes place.

Figure 26-27.   Metabolic bone diseases. (*A*) Normal trabecular bone and fatty marrow. The trabecular bone is lamellar and contains evenly distributed osteocytes. (*B*) Osteoporosis. The lamellar bone exhibits discontinuous, thin trabeculae. (*C*) Osteomalacia. The trabeculae of the lamellar bone have abnormal amounts of nonmineralized bone (osteoid). These osteoid seams are thickened, and cover a larger than normal area of the trabecular bone surface. (*D*) Primary hyperparathyroidism. The lamellar bone trabeculae are actively resorbed by numerous osteoclasts that bore into each trabecula. The appearance of osteoclasts dissecting into the trabeculae, a process termed dissecting osteitis, is diagnostic of hyperparathyroidism. Osteoblastic activity is also pronounced. The marrow is replaced by fibrous tissue adjacent to the trabeculae. (*E*) Secondary hyperparathyroidism. The morphologic appearance is similar to that of primary hyperparathyroidism, except that prominent osteoid covers the trabeculae. Osteoclasts do not resorb osteoid, and wherever an osteoid seam is lacking, osteoclasts bore into the trabeculae. Osteoblastic activity, in association with osteoclasts, is again prominent.

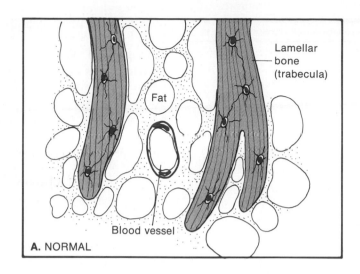

A. NORMAL

Lamellar bone (trabecula)

Fat

Blood vessel

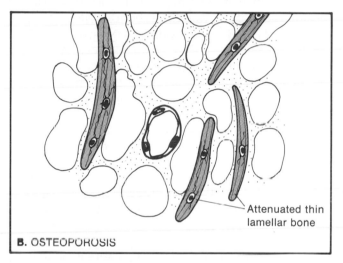

B. OSTEOPOROSIS

Attenuated thin lamellar bone

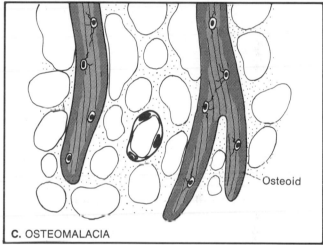

C. OSTEOMALACIA

Osteoid

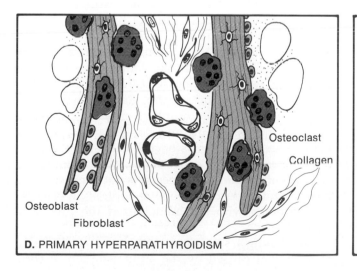

D. PRIMARY HYPERPARATHYROIDISM

Osteoclast

Collagen

Osteoblast

Fibroblast

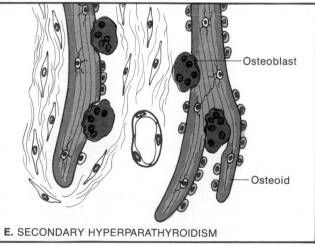

E. SECONDARY HYPERPARATHYROIDISM

Osteoblast

Osteoid

Table 26-1 Classification of Osteoporosis

Primary

    Postmenopausal osteoporosis
    Involutional osteoporosis
    Idiopathic osteoporosis (juvenile, adult)

Secondary

    Primary biliary cirrhosis
    Rheumatoid arthritis
    Chronic pulmonary disease
    Endocrine causes
        Hyperthyroidism
        Cushing's syndrome (endogenous or exogenous)
        Diabetes
        Lactation and pregnancy
        Hypogonadism
        Hyperparathyroidism
    Nutritional causes
        Intestinal malabsorption
        Protein malnutrition
        Scurvy
        Calcium deficiency (?)
    Immobilization
    Drugs
        Anticonvulsants
        Heparin
    Heritable disorders of the connective tissue
        Osteogenesis imperfecta
        Menkes' syndrome
        Homocystinuria
        Adult hypophosphatasia
    Neoplasms
        Multiple myeloma
        Myelomonocytic leukemia
        Systemic mastocytosis
        Waldenström's macroglobulinemia

Osteoporosis

Osteoporosis refers to a **group of diseases** of many etiologies (Table 26-1) which have as their **common denominator a reduction in the bone mass to a level below that required for normal bone support.** Although reduced in mass, the bones are normal with respect to mineralization. Histologically, there is a decrease in the thickness of the cortex and the number and size of trabeculae of the coarse cancellous bone. By contrast, the osteoid seams are of normal width (see Fig. 26-27). The trabecular bone loses its continuous arrangement, so that it is no longer a sheet. Rather, isolated struts are seen microscopically as minute, cigar-shaped fragments of bone. Therefore, the major problem in this disease is that the **rate of bone resorption exceeds that of bone formation.**

Increased osteoclastic activity, decreased osteoblastic activity, and combinations of both are observed in the various forms of osteoporosis (see Table 26-1). Thus, low, normal, or high rates of bone turn-over may occur in osteoporosis, depending on the type.

In general, after the age of 40 or 50 years, the skeletal mass begins to decrease at a faster rate in women than in men, and at different rates in various parts of the skeleton. For example, the rate of bone loss is greater in the metacarpals, the femoral neck, and the vertebral bodies than in the midshaft of the femur, the tibia, or the skull. The degree of bone loss may be striking, amounting to as much as a 30% to 50% reduction in skeletal mass, compared to that at age 30 to 40 years. In elderly patients, the rate of resorption is high, whereas the rate of bone formation remains in the normal range. In the normal process of remodeling, most of the resorption tends to occur at the cortical and endosteal surfaces. In osteoporosis, this may be exaggerated, and bone loss also includes the coarse cancellous bone and the endosteal surface of the cortex. Cortical cutting cones resorb bone and produce a thin, hollowed cortex.

The cause for this age-associated decrease in bone mass and increase in osteoclastic resorption, which is especially common in elderly women after menopause, is unknown. The disease is not as common in American blacks as in whites. It is thought that blacks have an initially larger skeleton than whites, so that adequate bone still remains after the age of 40 years and older. Other parameters that have not been implicated as a cause of osteoporosis are parathyroid hormone, calcium intake in the diet, and adrenal cortical function, all of which remain normal in osteoporotic patients. The roles of prostaglandins and osteoclast-activating factors have yet to be studied in these patients. The possibility that excessive acid intake, particularly in the form of high-protein diets, leads to resorption of bone as an attempt to buffer the extra acid has been promulgated as a possible cause. Likewise, the anticoagulant heparin has been associated with osteoporosis, since heparin potentiates bone resorption *in vitro*. Patients with osteoporosis have increased numbers of mast cells (which synthesize heparin) in their bone marrow, and patients with systemic mastocytosis also have areas of lysis. Since, as Wolff's law states, bone responds to all kinds of mechanical forces, it is not surprising that immobilization leads to bone resorption; in osteoporotic patients who are immobilized the process is aggravated.

In Cushing's syndrome, either the spontaneous form or that caused by the administration of corticosteroids, there may be deficient bone production, as well as an increased rate of bone resorption. An increased rate of bone resorption seems also to be the mechanism in hyperthyroidism, even though the rate is only slightly higher than normal. Thus, **the combination of decreased osteoblastic activity and increased osteoclastic activity is responsible for the striking changes seen in osteoporosis.**

Epidemiology of Osteoporosis

Osteoporosis is the most common metabolic bone disease in the United States. Fifteen percent of white women older than 65 years of age have significant osteoporosis. Thirty percent of those women 75 years of age or older have suffered fractures secondary to osteoporosis. **These fractures usually occur in the proximal humerus, lower forearm, hip, spine, and pelvis.** A typical patient with osteoporosis is a thin, sedentary, postmenopausal, white woman of Northern European descent who smokes and has breastfed several children. Her diet is usually deficient in calcium and vitamin D, and she has little sun exposure. Black women and obese women are less likely to develop the disease.

There may be two subsets of osteoporosis after the age of 50 years. Type I osteoporosis affects a small subset of women, aged 51 to 65 years, with predominantly vertebral or wrist fractures that involve mostly trabecular bone. Type II osteoporosis presents in women and men older than 75 years of age who sustain fractures of the hips, humerus, or tibia. In these subsets, it is thought that the net decrease in trabecular or cortical bone is due to decreased bone formation.

The Idiopathic variety of osteoporosis, which affects postmenopausal women, usually becomes recognizable 10 years after the onset of menopause. Since these patients are predisposed to vertebral fracture, compression fractures and shortening of the spine are common.

Diagnosis

The diagnosis of osteoporosis is primarily made on the basis of the radiologic finding of thin cortices, a condition labelled **osteopenia** (meaning "little bone"). Radiologists use this term because they are unable to distinguish between loss of bone with normal mineralization (osteoporosis), and osteoid with incomplete mineralization (osteomalacia). The radiographic features of osteoporosis include the loss of coarse cancellous bone and the presence of thin, hollowed cortices (Fig 26-28). The skull is usually spared. In vertebral body fractures, the vertebra is deformed, with anterior wedging and total collapse of the structure. If the vertebral body is not fractured, there is a general outline of the end plates, both craniad and

caudad, with virtually all the coarse, cancellous bone being absent. It is significant that the laboratory findings, including serum calcium and phosphorus levels, are basically normal.

Treatment

There is no cure for osteoporosis, despite the fact that virtually every mode of therapy has been tried. Agents such as estrogens, androgens, and calcium supplements have been used to decrease resorption and stimulate bone formation. Fluorides have also been administered in an attempt to increase bone formation. At best, these therapeutic strategies may retard the loss of bone, but they do not definitively increase bone mass. Currently, increased calcium supplementation and the administration of high doses of vitamin D are in vogue. Since there are many causes of osteoporosis, some of which may be malignant (for instance, multiple myeloma, lymphoma, leukemia, and carcinoma), appropriate tests should be done to rule out these conditions prior to initiation of treatment.

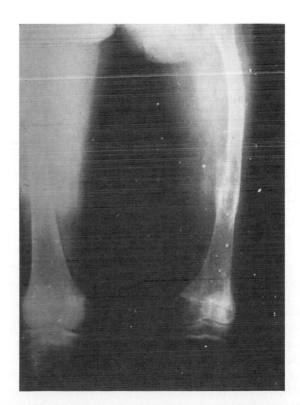

Figure 26-28. Disuse osteoporosis. A radiograph shows thin cortices, attenuated trabeculae, and associated soft tissue atrophy in a previously fractured left femur.

Osteomalacia

Osteomalacia ("soft bones") refers to a group of diseases in which there is a failure to form the normal inorganic calcium phosphate phase in relation to the organic matrix of bone. This defective mineralization results in exaggeration of the osteoid seams, both in the thickness and in the proportion of trabecular surface covered (see Fig. 26-27). The term **rickets** means osteomalacia of the growing skeleton, a disorder that involves not only bone but also cartilage. The mechanisms underlying osteomalacia are related to the type of disease producing it. Causes include **deficiency of dietary or endogenous vitamin D (see Ch. 8), intestinal malabsorption, acquired or hereditary renal disorders, and miscellaneous factors.**

The clinical diagnosis of osteomalacia is often difficult. Patients usually have nonspecific complaints, such as muscle weakness or diffuse aches and pains. In mild forms of the disease, only slowly progressive changes in bone are seen, and many patients are totally asymptomatic for years. In advanced cases, poorly localized bone pain and tenderness are common, especially in the spine, pelvis, and proximal parts of the extremities. Muscular weakness and hypotonia lead to a waddling gait; in severe cases, patients may not be able to walk at all.

As already noted, osteomalacia is also a cause of the **osteopenic** x-ray pattern. The only findings may be compression fractures and a decrease in bone thickness, as seen in osteoporosis. However, some specific findings may be seen in osteomalacia, including the **pseudofractures of Milkman-Looser syndrome.** These represent radiolucent transverse defects, and are most common on the concave side of a long bone, the medial side of the neck of the femur, the ischial and pubic rami, the ribs, and the scapula. Histologically, these areas of pseudofracture display abundant osteoid and at times, may function as stress points for fracture. In most cases, these areas do not evoke formation of callus and do not extend through the entire diameter of the bone.

Rickets

Clinical Presentation

Children with rickets are apathetic and irritable. They have a short attention span and are content to be sedentary, assuming a Buddha-like posture. They are short and exhibit characteristic changes of bone and teeth. Flattening of the skull, prominent frontal bones ("frontal bossing"), and prominent suture lines are typical. The teeth show delayed dentition, with severe dental caries and enamel defects. The chest has the classic rachitic "rosary" appearance, which is pro-duced by the enlargement of the costal cartilages and indentations of the lower ribs at the insertion of the diaphragm. The sternum is marked by pectus carinatum, or "pigeon breast," which is an outward curvature. The overall musculature is weak, and abdominal weakness leads to a pot belly. The limbs are shortened and deformed, with severe bowing of the arms and forearm and frequent fractures. The femoral head may dislocate from the epiphyseal plate (slipped capital femoral epiphysis).

Radiologic and Histologic Findings

Because rickets affects children, there are extensive changes at the epiphyseal plate (Fig. 26-29). The epiphyseal plate is not adequately mineralized, and the calcified cartilage and the zones of hypertrophy and proliferative cartilage continue to grow, because osteoclastic activity does not resorb the cartilage growth plate. As a consequence the epiphyseal plate is conspicuously thickened, irregular, and lobulated. Endochondral ossification proceeds very slowly and preferentially at the peripheral portions of the metaphysis. The net result is a flared and cup-shaped epiphysis. The largest part of the primary spongiosum is composed of lamellar or woven bone, which importantly is unmineralized.

On histologic examination, the epiphyseal plate exhibits striking changes. Although the resting zone is relatively normal, the zones of proliferating cartilage are greatly distorted. The ordered progression of spiral-forming chondrocytes is lost, and is replaced by a disorderly profusion of cells separated by small amounts of matrix. The resulting lobulated masses of proliferating and hypertrophied cartilage are associated with an increasing width of the epiphyseal plate, which may be 5 to 15 times the normal width. The zone of provisional calcification is poorly defined, and only a minimal amount of primary spongiosum is formed. Masses of proliferating cartilage extend into the metaphyseal region, without any apparent vascular invasion, and with little osteoclastic activity.

Pathogenesis

Rickets in the United States is rare, but it is sometimes encountered in children who have abnormal diets as a result of food fads, in premature infants, and in patients hospitalized in mental institutions. In the industrialized countries, osteomalacia is more often caused by diseases that are associated with intestinal malabsorption than by poor nutrition. For instance, in obstructive jaundice, the lack of bile salts in the intestine precludes adequate absorption of lipids and lipid-soluble substances, among which is the fat-soluble vitamin D. Calcium absorption from the gut is also impaired. Furthermore, with sufficient

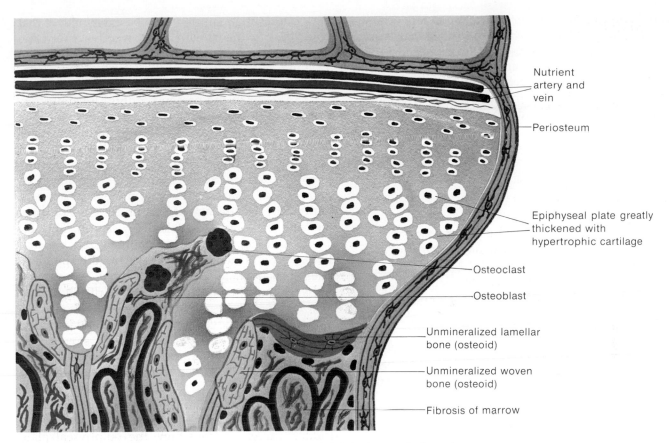

Nutrient artery and vein

Periosteum

Epiphyseal plate greatly thickened with hypertrophic cartilage

Osteoclast

Osteoblast

Unmineralized lamellar bone (osteoid)

Unmineralized woven bone (osteoid)

Fibrosis of marrow

Figure 26-29. The epiphyseal plate in rickets. The epiphyseal plate is thickened and disorganized, with a large zone of hypertrophic cartilage cells. There is irregular perforation of the cartilage plate by osteoclasts because there is little calcified cartilage. The woven bone on the surface of some of the primary trabeculae is unmineralized and therefore easily fractured. Such microfractures often lead to hemorrhage at the interface between the plate and the metaphysis.

liver damage, the hydroxylation of vitamin D is also reduced. The absorption of vitamin D and calcium is also decreased in gluten-sensitive enteropathy, Crohn's disease, sarcoidosis, and tuberculosis. In dietary vitamin D deficiency, the serum levels of calcium and phosphorus are both low owing to decreased intestinal absorption, particularly of calcium. **A low serum calcium level stimulates the parathyroid glands, thus producing secondary hyperparathyroidism.**

Vitamin D-Resistant Rickets
Vitamin D–resistant rickets, or osteomalacia, may be acquired or genetic. The disease is characterized by an abnormally high urinary excretion of phosphate, glucose, amino acids, water, bicarbonate, and some unusual substances, such as ketone bodies and glycine. There may be deposition of cystine crystals in the liver, bone marrow, and anterior chamber of the eye (Lignac-Fanconi syndrome), or pure renal tubular acidosis (Butler-Albright syndrome).

There are four distinct causes of vitamin D–resistant rickets: phosphate diabetes, in which there is a failure of the resorptive mechanisms for phosphate; failure of production of 1,25-dihydroxyvitamin D, which causes so-called vitamin D–dependent rickets, end organ insensitivity to 1,25-dihydroxyvitamin D; and renal tubular acidosis.

In patients with **phosphate diabetes,** the defect is in the renal tubule, where there is a failure to reabsorb phosphate from the glomerular infiltrate. Although other resorptive defects may exist, such as for glucose and amino acids, the main cause of the rickets is probably the hyperphosphaturia and the profound hypophosphatemia. The serum calcium level is normal.

Renal tubular acidosis caused by an acquired or genetic error in the renal handling of fixed base or bicarbonate. In one form of the disease, the kidney is unable to establish a hydrogen ion gradient and, therefore, excretes fixed base, including sodium and calcium, in the urine. In another form, the tubule fails to reabsorb bicarbonate, a defect that also causes a loss of these ions. In either case, the net result is the development of a syndrome of renal tubular acidosis that is characterized by hyperchloremic, hyponatremic, and hypokalemic acidosis, with alkaline urine. In addition, impaired reabsorption of phosphate accentuates the metabolic bone disease.

Renal Osteodystrophy

Chronic renal failure affects virtually every organ system, and the skeletal system is no exception. Diseases such as osteoporosis, osteomyelitis, or gout are associated with chronic renal failure. Furthermore, the use of corticosteroids in the treatment of renal failure accentuates osteoporosis, and may even produce osteonecrosis. Renal dialysis also exacerbates osteomalacia. However, a distinct syndrome in which bone is directly affected by renal failure is termed **renal osteodystrophy.**

Pathogenesis

The pathogenesis of renal osteodystrophy is essentially similar to that of osteomalacia, with **secondary hyperparathyroidism exerting its influence by way of osteoclastic resorption on the bone** (see Fig. 26-27). The pathophysiology of renal osteodystrophy may be summarized as follows:

1. Damage to the glomerulus causes retention of phosphate, thereby producing hyperphosphatemia.
2. Tubular injury leads to a reduction in 1,25-dihydroxyvitamin D.
3. Intestinal calcium absorption is, in turn, decreased, leading to profound hypocalcemia.
4. Hypocalcemia stimulates the elaboration of parathyroid hormone and, within a short time, there is marked secondary hyperparathyroidism, with clear cell hyperplasia of all four glands.
5. This increased amount of parathyroid hormone does not effectively promote intestinal calcium absorption or renal tubular resorption of calcium because of the absence of vitamin D and the increased level of phosphate. Therefore, the principle action of parathyroid hormone is resorption of skeletal calcium.

An interesting feature, yet to be explained, is that about 20% of patients with renal osteodystrophy also show increased bone formation, most frequently in the spine, but sometimes in the long bones as well.

In chronic renal insufficiency, mineralization defects can occur in the presence of high serum phosphorus and low or normal calcium. Such cases suggest the involvement of inhibitors of mineralization. Aluminum, which can contaminate dialysis media, can inhibit mineralization and therefore promote osteomalacia. Alternatively, the metabolic acidosis of chronic renal failure may inhibit mineralization as a result of the substitution of H^+ for Ca^{2+} in hydroxyapatite.

On microscopic examination, trabecular bone in affected areas is increased and haphazardly arranged. In terminal patients with chronic renal disease who are hyperphosphatemic, metastatic calcification may occur at various sites, including the eyes, skin, muscular coats of arteries and arterioles, and periarticular soft tissues.

Thus, the four components of renal osteodystrophy are osteomalacia, secondary hyperparathyroidism, osteosclerosis (new bone), and ectopic calcification or ossification. Acidosis and hypoalbuminemia are accompanied by low serum calcium and elevated inorganic phosphate levels. The alkaline phosphatase and parathyroid hormone levels are increased, but the concentrations of 1,25-dihydroxyvitamin D are also decreased. The urinary calcium level is low, whereas fecal calcium is increased.

Treatment

The management of renal osteodystrophy involves not only the treatment of the primary disorder of renal failure by dialysis or kidney transplantation, but also the control of phosphate levels by appropriate drug therapy and infusions. Occasionally, parathyroidectomy is necessary to control hyperparathyroidism, and the administration of vitamin D may also be necessary.

Primary Hyperparathyroidism

Primary hyperparathyroidism, the oversecretion of parathyroid hormone, is prominently associated with bone disease. The disorder may be caused by one or more adenomas (90% of cases), hyperplasia of all four glands (10% of cases), or more rarely, by parathyroid carcinoma. Since parathyroid hormone promotes excretion of phosphate in the urine, low serum phosphate and high serum calcium levels are characteristic.

Clinical Presentation

The symptoms related to this abnormality of calcium ion homeostasis has been summarized as "stones, bones, moans, and groans." The "stones" refer to kidney stones, and the "bones" to the usual skeletal changes. The "moans" relate to psychiatric depression and other abnormalities associated with hypercalcemia, while the "groans" characterize the gastrointestinal irregularities associated with a high serum calcium level.

Radiographic Appearance

The skeletal disease of hyperparathyroidism is also called **von Recklinghausen's disease.** On radiologic examination, there is a generalized decalcification of the entire skeleton, and the weakened bones are associated with deformities such as platybasia, biconcave vertebrae, and bowing of the long bones, and with fractures. Similar deformities are also seen in osteomalacia and, less frequently, in osteoporosis. A distinctive radiologic peculiarity, referred to as **subperiosteal bone resorption,** is seen in the subperiosteal outer surface of the cortex. This occurs on the outer table of the skull, the tufts of the terminal digits, and the shafts of the metacarpals, and results in mottled bone cortex, with an irregular frayed surface. Resorption around the tooth sockets causes the lamina dura of the teeth to disappear.

In addition to the generalized osteopenia seen on radiography, there are multiple, localized, lytic lesions that represent hemorrhagic cysts or masses of fibrous tissue, called **brown tumors** (Fig. 26-30). These eccentric and well-demarcated lesions are separated from the soft tissue by a periosteal shell of bone. The lesions may be multiple or solitary. **It is important to remember that these focal, tumor-like, lytic lesions always occur in the context of an abnormal skeleton produced by the hyperparathyroidism.** If a single lesion is examined without considering the rest of the skeleton, it may be mistaken for a primary neoplasm of bone. Conversely, multiple lytic lesions of bone may indicate hyperparathyroidism, in which case a search should be made for chemical abnormalities, such as those of calcium, phosphorus, and parathyroid hormone. The changes of secondary hyperparathyroidism of renal osteodystrophy usually resemble those of osteomalacia. The differential diagnosis of hyperparathyroidism includes other causes of hypercalcemia, such as osteolytic metastases, steroid therapy, sarcoidosis, vitamin D intoxication, and rarely, multiple myeloma.

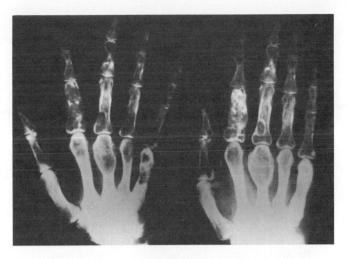

Figure 26-30. Primary hyperparathyroidism. A radiograph of the hands reveals bulbous swellings ("brown tumors") and numerous cavities, both representing bone resorption.

Histopathologic Changes

The histopathology of primary hyperparathyroidism that culminates in osteitis fibrosa cystica may be classified into three stages.

In the early stage of the disease, osteoclasts are stimulated by the elevated parathyroid hormone levels to resorb bone. From the subperiosteal and endosteal surfaces, osteoclasts bore their way into the cortex as cutting cones, a process that accounts for the radiologic finding of subperiosteal resorption. The pattern of osteoclasts boring into the trabecular bone is termed **dissecting osteitis** (see Fig. 26-27) because each trabeculum is continually hollowed out by osteoclastic activity. At the same time, the endosteal marrow modulates into fibrous tissue and additional osteoclasts that also penetrate bone. Adjacent, then, to the zone of dissecting osteitis is a loose, fibrous marrow closely tied to the surface of bone where the osteoclasts are active. Although osteoblastic activity may be seen, it is not as prominent as the osteoclastic activity.

In the second stage of hyperparathyroidism, the trabecular bone is ultimately resorbed, and the marrow is replaced by loose fibrosis, hemosiderin-laden macrophages, areas of hemorrhage from microfractures, and reactive woven bone. This combination of features constitutes the **osteitis fibrosa** portion of the complex.

As the disease progresses and hemorrhage progressively increases, cystic degeneration ultimately occurs, leading to **osteitis fibrosa cystica,** the third and final stage of the disease. The areas of fibrosis

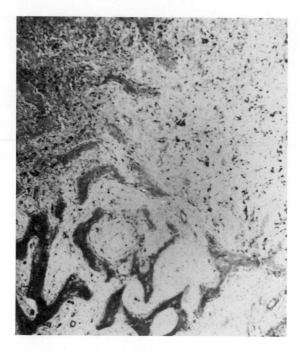

Figure 26-31.   Primary hyperparathyroidism. A photomicrograph of a "brown tumor" shows reactive woven bone, numerous macrophages filled with hemosiderin, fibrosis, and foci of hemorrhage.

with reactive woven bone and hemosiderin-laden macrophages often display many giant cells of the foreign body type, as well as osteoclasts, an appearance that has been termed a **brown tumor** (Fig. 26-31). This is not a true tumor, but rather a repair reaction as an end stage of hyperparathyroidism. An important diagnostic point is that brown tumors always present in the setting of a diffuse skeletal abnormality. A brown tumor does not occur if the adjacent skeleton is normal, since it represents the ultimate loss of bone caused by excess parathyroid hormone secretion.

In **secondary hyperparathyroidism,** the histopathology is that of osteomalacia with superimposed osteoclastic activity, usually dissecting osteitis. The latter process represents the parathyroid component. As mentioned earlier, osteoclastic activity is retarded by unmineralized bone. Therefore, when seen in secondary hyperparathyroidism osteoclasts are found only on mineralized bone surfaces.

Treatment

The treatment for primary hyperparathyroidism is to remove the parathyroid adenoma, thereby arresting the skeletal process. A gradual waxing of osteoblasts correlates with a waning of osteoclastic activity, so that the cortical cutting cones fill with osteoblastic

activity and fibrosis, and there is a restoration of the coarse cancellous bone of the marrow cavity. Although this healing activity may take months or years to complete, the lesions are usually reversible over a long period of time. In the cases in which parathyroid hyperplasia is the cause of the disease three and one-half glands are usually removed. The remaining fragment ensures that the patient does not develop severe hypocalcemia and tetany.

Gaucher's Disease

Gaucher's disease is a hereditary metabolic disease affecting the bones in which histiocytes contain increased amounts of a lipid called **glucocerebroside.** The affected macrophages exhibit a characteristic infolding of their cytoplasm, and are termed **Gaucher cells.** The disease is caused by a relative deficiency in the activity of lysosomal glucocerebrosidase needed for the hydrolysis of glucosylceramide to glucose and ceramide. A low concentration of this enzyme in the cells of the peripheral blood, bone marrow, or amniotic fluid is diagnostic for the disease, and identifies carriers. The gene for glucocerebrosidase has been mapped to chromosome 1q, and the expression of the gene has been accomplished in bacteria. All forms of Gaucher's disease are transmitted as autosomal recessive traits. There are essentially three types of the disease. **Type I,** the most common form of the disease, is also referred to as the **non-neuronopathic phenotype.** This type has a high prevalence in Ashkenazy (Eastern European) Jews, in whom the carrier frequency is estimated to be as high as 1 in 12. **Type II** Gaucher's disease, also referred to as the **acute neuronopathic type,** is much less common and has no ethnic predilection. **Type III,** or the **subacute neuronopathic form,** is uncommon, and has been seen worldwide in various ethnic groups.

Clinical Features

Type I Gaucher's disease is not only the most common disorder of this complex, but is actually the most common hereditary lipidosis. The patient may present with symptoms related to the hematopoietic system, even though there may be no other symptoms referable to the skin or other organs. The skin and conjunctivae often exhibit a yellowish-brown to gray, flaky, macular rash. Recent studies indicate that this pigmentation is caused either by hemosiderin or by melanin, and is not directly related to the accumulation of the glucocerebroside. The conjunctivae show asymptomatic, pinguecula-like lesions, which start at the outer or inner canthus, and which may be present even in childhood. The presenting symptom in most patients is usually related to splenomegaly, and, in rare cases, to splenic rupture. Infarcts in the spleen may produce sudden abdominal pain. Hepatomegaly is also common. The hematopoietic system generally bears the brunt of the disease process. Affected patients experience easy fatigability and generalized weakness, and are frequently pale. Pancytopenia may be caused by hypersplenism, and may be corrected by splenectomy. However, in some patients, late in the course of the disease, marrow failure again occurs.

Most patients with Gaucher's disease have hematocrit values of less than 30 and platelet counts of less than 100,000/μl. The sedimentation rate is often elevated. A significantly increased bleeding time is one of the most consistent abnormalities in Gaucher's disease, and is accompanied by a bleeding diathesis. Thus, epistaxes, conjunctival hemorrhages, petechiae and ecchymoses of the skin, and bleeding gums are common. The activity of tartrate–resistant acid phosphatase in the serum is usually elevated. Examination of the bone marrow reveals the presence of Gaucher's cells, a finding that confirms the diagnosis. Patients with Gaucher's disease, particularly those over 50 years of age, have a higher than normal incidence of myeloma and amyloidosis. Abnormal immunoglobulins in the blood often create difficulties in diagnosis, and a bone marrow biopsy may be the only way to distinguish among these various diseases.

Virtually all patients with Gaucher's disease have some abnormality of the skeleton that is related to the excessive storage of glucosylceramide in the macrophages of the marrow space. **The following bone changes occur: failure of remodeling, localized and diffuse bone loss, corticomedullary osteonecrosis, Gaucher's crisis, fractures, and osteomyelitis.** It is an interesting fact that the severity of the bone disease does not correlate well with any individual factors, such as the extent of visceral involvement, the extent of bone marrow depression, the degree of enzyme deficiency, or the concentration of circulating glucosylceramide.

The most common and least troublesome skeletal abnormality is the **failure of remodeling** of the distal femur, proximal tibia, and at times, other bones. In about 80% of affected patients, the distal femur and proximal tibia are involved bilaterally. There is an absence of appropriate flaring, and therefore, funnelization and cylinderization are abnormal (Fig. 26-32). The resulting bone has an "Erlenmeyer flask shape," similar to that seen in other modeling deformities, such as Pyle's disease and osteopetrosis.

Diffuse and localized bone loss is manifested radiologically as localized lytic lesions, cortical thinning, and loss of coarse cancellous bone. Bone loss is usually most severe in the axial skeleton and the proximal appendicular skeleton. On histologic examination, areas of new bone formation are found to contain marrow packed with Gaucher cells. These patients are generally asymptomatic until a fracture or osteonecrosis occurs. The **osteosclerotic lesions** represent increased bone formation in the medullary cavity of the long bones and pelvis. Reactive new bone forms in areas that have undergone osteonecrosis, as evidenced by the presence in these zones of dead bone, fat necrosis, and calcification of fat. Occasionally, osteosclerotic lesions are present in the flat bones of the skull.

Corticomedullary osteonecrosis, the most disabling of the skeletal problems associated with Gaucher's disease, affects the femoral head or proximal humerus or, less commonly, a femoral or tibial condyle, talus, or capitulum. It may involve the shaft of long bones, as well. Osteonecrosis occurs most commonly in young patients between the ages of 8 and 35 years. It is bilateral in more than 50% of the patients, and is often multifocal. The pathogenesis of this lesion is not clear; one suggestion is that it involves an occlusion of a vessel leading to the femoral or humeral head.

Gaucher's crisis, which occurs in only a few patients with the disease, is intensely painful and disabling. Although the cause is unknown, the crisis seems to result from an acute infarction of a large segment of bone (usually the spine, pelvis, or femoral heads). The lesion may even be multifocal in one or several bones. In many cases, Gaucher's crisis occurs after an acute viral illness. The patients present with sudden, severe, and progressive pain, which is localized to an anatomic focus. Fever, tenderness in the area of the bone, and soft tissue swelling are characteristic. An elevated white blood count and erythrocyte sedimentation rate may confuse the issue, leading to an erroneous diagnosis of osteomyelitis. Interestingly enough, x-ray studies are generally normal, although late in the course of the disease, lysis of bone, endosteal and periosteal new bone formation, and increased marrow calcification suggest an infarction. Gaucher's crisis lasts for 2 or more weeks and then gradually improves. The **pathologic fractures** that occur in Gaucher's disease may be compression fractures of the vertebrae or fractures of the long bones and even the pelvis.

Patients with Gaucher's disease seems to be unusually prone to infections of the bones and joints. **Hematogenous osteomyelitis** and **septic arthritis** oc-

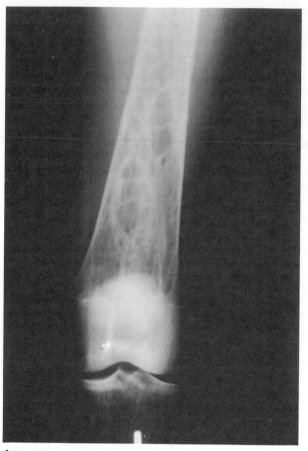

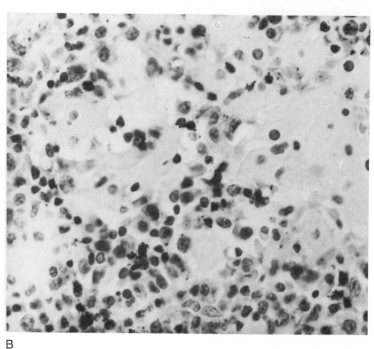

A

B

Figure 26-32.   Gaucher's disease. (*A*) A radiograph of the distal femur displays the characteristic lack of funnelization of the metaphysis that produces a carafe-shaped bone. Numerous radiolucencies, a thin cortex, and osteoporotic trabeculae are seen. (*B*) The normal hematopoietic marrow is infiltrated by large histiocytes that have small nuclei and abundant cytoplasm.

cur in these individuals, and the incidence of post-operative wound infection is also high. There does not appear to be any associated immunodeficiency, and the most common agents are coliform or anaerobic organisms. It may be that bacteria are deposited in areas of bone infarction, or perhaps the phagocytic cells filled with glucocerebroside are incompetent and cannot respond to the invading bacteria.

Therapeutic Considerations

The management of patients with Gaucher's disease is, for the most part, symptomatic, and many of the orthopaedic complications are treated conservatively. Surgical operations are avoided, if possible, since the risk of infection is high. Unfortunately, many of the cases of acute osteomyelitis proceed to chronic disease, and patients may have draining sinuses for

years. At times, despite all therapy, amputations are required to control the disease locally.

Pathology

The classic appearance of the **Gaucher cell** is specific for this disease (see Fig. 26-32). This cell is a large macrophage with a folded cytoplasmic membrane, which is represented in smears as linear striations within the cytoplasm that resemble **folded cigarette paper.** Electon micrographs show that the folds in the cytoplasmic membranes are microtubules filled with glucocerebroside. The nucleus is small. The Gaucher cell always has excess iron, and is positive on testing with the periodic acid Schiff (PAS) stain. The cells lie in sheets, and by crowding out the normal marrow elements, simulate a neoplasm. Alternatively, they may spread individually through the marrow and insinuate between existing cellular elements.

Paget's Disease of Bone

Paget's disease is common, and some manifestation of the disorder is found in 3% to 4% of all autopsies in elderly individuals. On radiographic examination, about 4% of aged persons exhibit some changes that are characteristic of Paget's disease. The disease is seen in both sexes, and generally affects persons older than 60 years of age. Paget's disease has an unusual worldwide distribution, generally afflicting populations of the British Isles and following their migrations throughout the world. English peoples living in areas of the United States, Australia, New Zealand and Canada have a high incidence of the disease. Furthermore, Northern Europeans tend to have more Paget's disease than Southern Europeans. The white populations of Africa and the European populations of South America have a higher incidence than the native populations. It is striking that the disease is almost nonexistent in Asia and in native populations of Africa and South America.

Paget's disease is not considered a metabolic bone disease because there are always areas of normal bone in the skeleton. The disease, which may be monostotic or polyostotic, is of unknown etiology. Interestingly, when James Paget first described this disease over 100 years ago, he called it **osteitis deformans,** implying that it was an infection of bone. Since that time, virtually every type of disease process, including a neoplasm, has been proposed as the cause. Recently, inclusions consistent with the structure of a virus have been demonstrated in the osteoclasts of Paget's disease. This, along with epidemiologic evidence, suggests the possibility of a slow-acting virus which, in the appropriate genetic setting, is triggered by an unknown stimulus (Fig. 26-33).

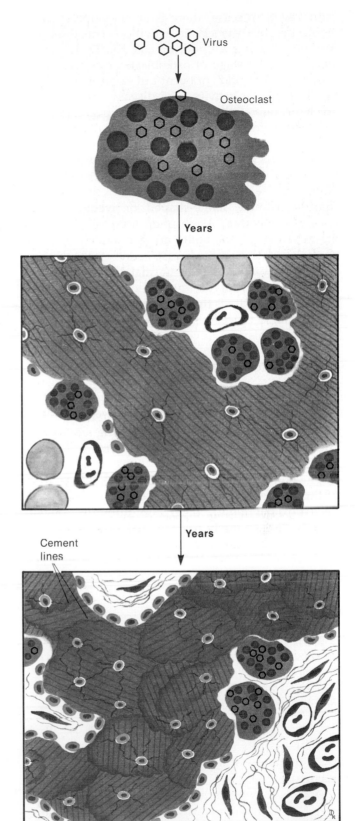

Figure 26-33. Hypothetical viral etiology of Paget's disease of bone. A virus infects osteoclastic progenitors or osteoclasts and stimulates osteoclastic activity, thereby leading to excessive resorption of bone. Over a period of years, the bone develops a characteristic mosaic pattern, produced by chaotically juxtaposed units of lamellar bone that form irregular cement lines. The adjacent marrow is often fibrotic, and there is a mixture of osteoclasts and osteoblasts on the surface of the bone.

In Paget's disease, there is an uncoupling of osteoblastic and osteoclastic activities. The disease is triphasic, having a "hot" or osteoclastic resorptive stage, a mixed stage of osteoblastic and osteoclastic activity, and a "cold" or burnt-out stage characterized by little cellular activity. The disease need not progress through all three stages, and in polyostotic disease, different foci may be in different stages.

The radiologic appearance of the disease correlates with the histopathologic stage of the disease (Fig. 26-34). For example, if the disease is in the lytic, or "hot," phase, the bone shows a characteristic, sharply defined, **flame-shaped** or **wedged-shaped lysis of the cortex,** which often mimics a tumor. In the mixed stage, the bones are generally larger than normal; in fact, Paget's disease is one of two diseases that produces **larger than normal bones,** the other being fibrous dysplasia (discussed later). The cortex in the mixed phase is thickened, and the accentuation of the coarse cancellous bone makes the bone look heavy and enlarged. Involvement of vertebral bodies leads to a "picture frame" appearance, as the cortices and end plates become greatly exaggerated in comparison to the coarse cancellous bone of the vertebral body. Although the bone is abnormal, it responds to Wolff's law, so that the distorted coarse cancellous bone and cortex still tend to align along stress lines. The pelvis is often thickened in the area of the acetabulum.

The bones involved in this disease tend to be those of the axial skeleton, including the spine, skull, pelvis, proximal femur, tibia, and humerus. Solitary Paget's disease rarely involves the humerus, but in polyostotic disease, lesions involving this bone are common.

Focal Manifestations

The most common focal symptom of Paget's disease is pain, although its cause is not clear. The pain may be related to microfractures, the stimulation of free nerve endings by dilated blood vesels adjacent to the bones, or weight bearing in weaker bones. The skull may exhibit localized lysis, generally in the frontal and parietal bones, which is termed **osteoporosis circumscripta.** Alternatively, there may be thickening of the outer and inner tables, which is most pronounced in the frontal and occipital bones. The skull becomes very heavy and may collapse over the C1 vertebra, thereby producing **platybasia,** with compression of the neurologic structures in the posterior fossa and spinal cord. Hearing loss is caused by involvement of the ossicles and bony impingement on the eighth cranial nerve at the foramen. On rare occasions, optic atrophy may occur. Occasionally patients feel lightheaded, a symptom thought to be due to so-called **pagetic steal,** in which blood is shunted from the internal carotid system to the bone, rather than to the brain. The jaws may be grossly affected and misshapen, and the teeth may fall out. Often, the facial bones increase in size, producing the so-called **leontiasis ossea,** the "lion-like" face. This deformity is particularly likely to result when the maxillary bones are affected. Involvement of the pelvis leads to hip problems. The loss of subchondral bone compliance causes a loss of articular cartilage and, therefore, osteoarthritis.

Fractures in Paget's disease are common, the bones snapping transversely like a piece of chalk. There may also be incomplete fractures without displacement—the so-called **infractions.** With extensive Paget's disease, the blood flow to bone and subcutaneous tissue is remarkably increased, and the cardiac output is also increased. High-output cardiac failure is thus a potential complication of the disorder.

Sarcomatous change in a focus of Paget's disease occurs in less than 1% of all cases. Such a change is usually found in the femur, humerus, or pelvis—for unknown reasons, the skull and vertebrae (which are the bones most commonly involved in Paget's disease) rarely undergo sarcomatous change. The sar-

Figure 26-34. Paget's disease of bone. (*A*) A radiograph of the spine demonstrates a sclerotic and enlarged vertebral body (*arrow*) in which the trabeculae and the cortex are coarsened and thickened. Paget's disease is one of the few diseases that can enlarge a bone. (*B*) The lytic phase of Paget's disease is illustrated in this radiograph. A sharply defined, lucent lesion has thinned the cortex. (*C*) A radiograph of the skull shows the thickening and distortion of the bone by osteoblastic and osteolytic foci. (*D*) A gross specimen of bone from the skull demonstrates marked thickening of the outer and inner tables, which narrows the diploë (hematopoietic marrow).

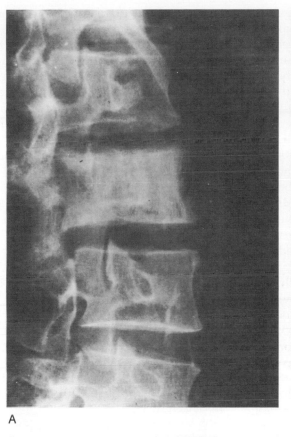

A

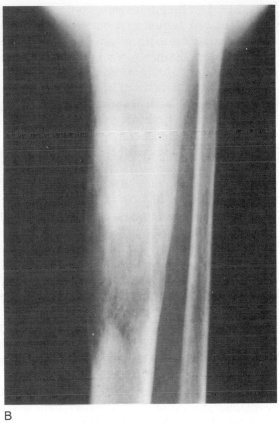

B

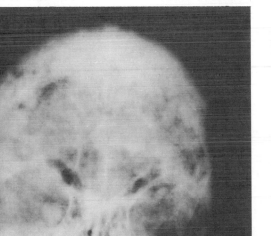

C

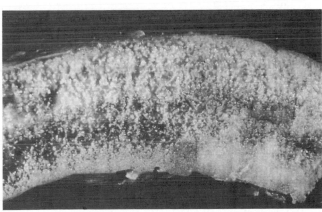

D

coma may be fibrogenic, osteogenic, or cartilaginous. The **giant cell tumor** that occurs in Paget's disease seems not to be a neoplasm, but rather a reactive phenomenon, similar to that seen in hyperparathyroidism as the "brown tumor." The lesion is thought to represent an overshoot of osteoclastic activity and associated fibroblastic response. Radiotherapy of the giant cell tumor is curative in many cases.

Although hypercalcemia is rare in Paget's disease, it does occur if the patient is immobilized. The serum calcium and phosphorus levels are normal, but the turnover rate of bone is increased by more than 20-fold. The collagen structure of bone in Paget's disease is entirely normal, but because of the accelerated bone turnover, collagen breakdown products are elevated in the serum and urine, especially hydroxyproline and hydroxylysine. Hydroxyproline excretion may reach 1000 mg per day (normally, less than 35 to 40 mg of hydroxyproline is excreted per day). The serum alkaline phosphatase level is enormously increased, and correlates with osteoblastic activity. The alkaline phosphatase levels are disproportionately high with skull involvement, but tend to be low when the pelvis is affected. A sudden elevation of the activity of serum alkaline phosphatase may reflect sarcomatous change within a lesion.

Histologic Features

The diagnostic feature of Paget's disease is the abnormal arrangement of lamellar bone, in which islands of irregular bone formation resembling pieces of a jigsaw puzzle are separated by prominent "cement lines" (Fig. 26-35). The result is a **mosaic pattern** in the bone, which can be seen particularly well under polarized light. In the cortex of an affected bone, the osteons tend to be destroyed, and concentric lamellae are incomplete. Although the changes in lamellar bone are diagnostic, it is not uncommon to see woven bone as part of the pathologic process. In this situation, the woven bone is a reactive phenomenon, as in a microcallus, and represents a temporary bridge between islands of the mosaic bone of Paget's disease.

The osteoclast of Paget's disease is characteristic, and to some, is diagnostic. The osteoclast is very large, possessing more than 12 nuclei, each of which is hyperchromatic. The osteoclast thus appears as a large cell with dark, smeared nuclei. These cells are the ones that exhibit the virus-like particles seen on electron microscopy, although the osteoclast precursor cells do not contain such particles. Even in the "hot" phase, in which osteoclasts predominate, there is always some osteoblastic activity, presumably to counteract the osteoclastic bone resorption. The marrow is fibrotic and sometimes contains scattered inflammatory cells. In the lytic, or "hot," phase, the mosaic pattern may not be prominent, but in the mixed and "cold" phases of the disease, mosaic patterns are abundant. The marrow space contains large, dilated vessels, but there are no arteriovenous shunts. In areas of fracture, callus tends to obscure the characteristic changes of Paget's disease. Similarly, a neoplasm may invade the bone and blot out the underlying disease.

Treatment

Fortunately, most patients with Paget's disease are asymptomatic, and therefore require no specific treatment. Fractures, osteoarthritis, and other orthopaedic complications are treated symptomatically. Several drugs may be used for the treatment of Paget's disease because they are directed at abnormal osteoclast function. These include calcitonin, diphosphonates and mithramycin. Porcine, salmon, and human calcitonins are used to prevent osteoclastic activity in the Paget's focus. Diphosphonates depress bone resorption, but unfortunately they also increase the amount of osteoid, which may increase the patient's susceptibility to pathologic fractures in areas of osteomalacia. Mithramycin is administered to suppress osteoclastic activity, but this very toxic drug should only be used with great care. Sodium fluorides have also been used to stimulate bone formation, but with indifferent results. At present, there is no cure for Paget's disease.

Neoplasms of Bone

Bone tumors are uncommon, but are nevertheless important neoplasms, particularly in young people. A primary bone tumor may arise from any one of the cellular elements of bone. Most neoplasms of bone occur near the metaphyseal area, and over 80% of primary tumors occur in either the distal femur or the proximal tibia (Fig. 26-36). In the growing child these areas are characterized by conspicuous growth activity and are, therefore, more likely to develop a tumor.

Benign Tumors

Solitary Bone Cyst

The solitary bone cyst is a benign, fluid-filled, usually unilocular lesion found in children or adolescents. There is a male predilection of 3:1 over females.

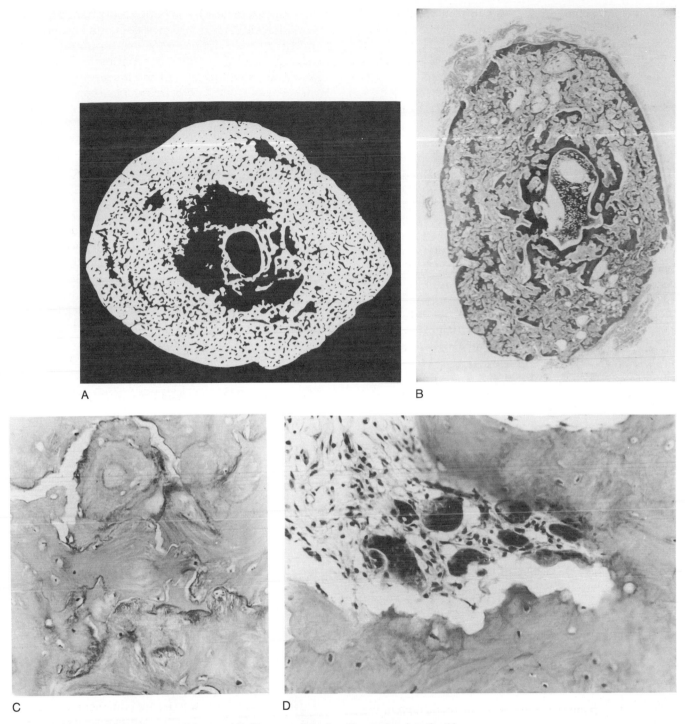

Figure 26-35.   Paget's disease of bone. (*A*) Cross-sectional radiograph of a rib. The cortex is markedly thickened, and the marrow space is narrowed. (*B*) A histologic section of the specimen in *A*. (*C*) The characteristic mosaic pattern of lamellar bone units fastened together in a random fashion is evident. The mosaic pattern is produced by the interfaces of the units of lamellar bone, termed cement lines. Artifactual cracks along the cement lines separate the units of lamellar bone. (*D*) The osteoclasts in Paget's disease have numerous hyperchromatic nuclei.

BENIGN TUMORS

EPIPHYSIS

Chondroblastoma,.
Giant cell tumor

METAPHYSIS

Osteoblastoma
Osteochondroma
Non-ossifying fibroma
Osteoid osteoma
Chondromyxoid fibroma
Giant cell tumor

DIAPHYSIS

Enchondroma
Fibrous dysplasia

MALIGNANT TUMORS

DIAPHYSIS

Ewing's sarcoma
Chondrosarcoma

METAPHYSIS

Osteosarcoma
Juxtacortical osteosarcoma

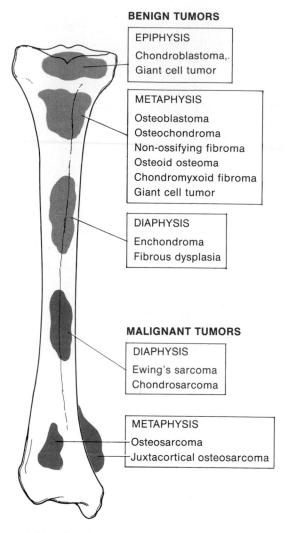

Figure 26-36.   Location of primary bone tumors in long tubular bones.

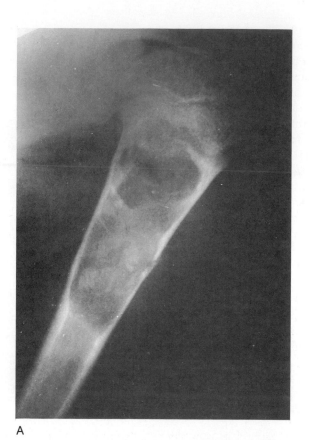

A

Figure 26-37.   Solitary bone cyst. (*A*) A radiograph of the proximal humerus of a child (note the epiphyseal plate) shows a large, well-demarcated, lytic, epiphyseal and diaphyseal lesion. The cortex is thinned, but there is no cortical distortion or malformation of the shape of the bone. (*B*) A low power microscopic view of the lining of the cyst shows it to be composed of a thin fibrous membrane.

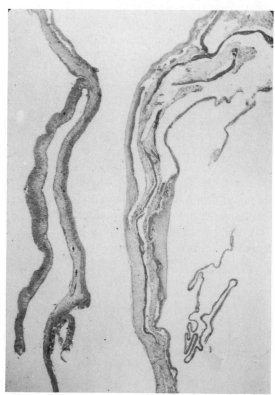

B

About 65% to 75% of all solitary bone cysts occur in the upper humerus or femur, often in the metaphysis adjacent to the epiphyseal plate. The lesion seems to be not a true neoplasm but rather a disturbance of bone growth with superimposed trauma. Secondary organization of a hematoma or some abnormality of the metaphyseal vessels causes serum accumulations. This "tumor" grows by expansion of the fluid cavity and the resulting pressure causes resorption of bone, mediated by osteoclasts of the surrounding bone. The process is slow, so that as the endosteal surface of the cortex is destroyed, a thin periosteal shell of new bone is laid down. This process results in a thin, ballooned, lytic bone lesion that is particularly susceptible to pathologic fracture (Fig. 26-37).

The cyst is lined by fibrous tissue, a few giant cells, hemosiderin-laden macrophages, chronic inflammatory cells, and reactive bone. Osteoclasts, seen in the advancing front of the cyst, enable the expansion of the lesion. Curettage and the deposition of bone chips are curative.

Osteoid Osteoma

Osteoid osteoma, a small, painful lesion that is often about 1 cm in diameter, occurs in persons ranging in age from 5 to 24 years. It occurs more commonly in males than in females, with a ratio of 3:1. The pain is diaphyseal and intracortical, and principally affects the lower extremity, including the small bones of the foot. The severity of the pain is out of proportion to the size of the lesion.

Osteoid osteoma is characterized by a dense, vascular center of woven bone and osteoid (Fig. 26-38), which may be partially mineralized and is seen radiographically as a radiolucent nidus surrounded by very dense, reactive bone. If the nidus is calcified, the lesion resembles a target on radiography, having a dense center, a thin, peripheral, radiolucent zone, and a very dense outer zone of bone. Surgical excision is usually curative.

Osteoblastoma

Osteoblastoma is an uncommon tumor that is histologically similar to osteoid osteoma, but is larger. It does not stimulate a bone reaction, but rather appears as a purely lytic lesion, with only a thin shell of surrounding bone. Osteoblastoma occurs in persons between the ages of 10 and 35 years, with no sex predilection, and mainly affects the spine (spines, bodies, arches) and long bones (metaphyses and shaft) of the limbs (Fig. 26-39).

Chondroblastoma

Chondroblastoma is an uncommon cellular tumor (representing 2% of bone tumors) that is found almost exclusively in the epiphyses of large bones, especially the upper femur, tibia, and humerus. It is more common in males than in females (2:1), and about 90% of cases occur in persons between the ages of 5 and 25 years. The tumor grows slowly, and on radiologic examination displays an eccentric lytic appearance with sharply defined borders (Fig. 26-40).

A chondroblastoma consists of primitive chondroblasts arranged as cellular masses of sharply delineated, round to polyhedral cells with large nuclei. Often, calcific granules and reticular fibers lie between the cells, together with foci of calcification and mineralized cartilage of varying degrees of maturity. This histologic appearance accounts for the mottled pattern seen on radiographs in at least 50% of the cases of chondroblastoma. The tumor expands by stimulating osteoclastic resorption. In fact, these tumors may perforate the cortex, although they remain confined by the periosteum.

Malignant Tumors

Osteosarcoma (Osteogenic Sarcoma)

Osteosarcoma is the most common primary malignant bone tumor, representing one-fifth of all malignant bone tumors. It is a highly malignant lesion that often requires amputation for treatment, and is associated with a poor prognosis (the 5-year survival rate ranges from 10% to 60%). The tumor most commonly occurs in persons between the ages of 10 and 20 years, and it affects males more often than females. It is often found around the knee—that is, the lower femur, upper tibia, or fibula—but any metaphyseal area of a long bone may be affected. The hands, feet, skull, and jaw are less common sites for this disease, but they are affected more frequently in patients older than 24 years of age. The serum alkaline phosphatase level is elevated in about 50% of patients and may decrease after amputation, only to rise again with a recurrence or metastasis. Radiologic evidence of bone destruction and bone formation is characteristic, with the latter representing tumor bone. Often, the periosteum is elevated by reactive bone adjacent to the tumor, a pattern that appears

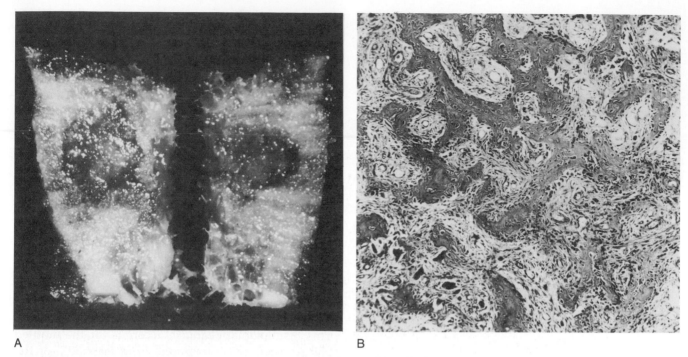

A   B

Figure 26-38.   (*A*) A gross specimen of an osteoid osteoma shows the nidus, which is less than 1 cm in diameter, as a small hemorrhagic area. (*B*) A photomicrograph of the nidus reveals irregular trabeculae of woven bone surrounded by osteoblasts, osteoclasts, and fibrovascular marrow.

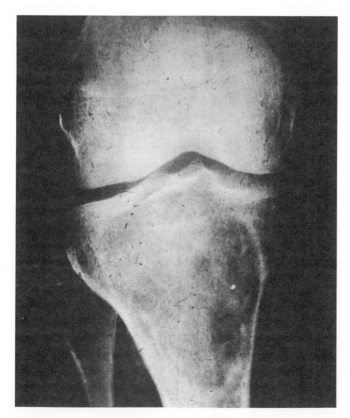

Figure 26-39.   Osteoblastoma. A radiograph of the proximal tibia shows a large lytic lesion, surrounded by reactive bone (margination), that extends from the metaphysis into the epiphysis. Innumerable bone spicules produced by the tumor are represented as hazy densities.

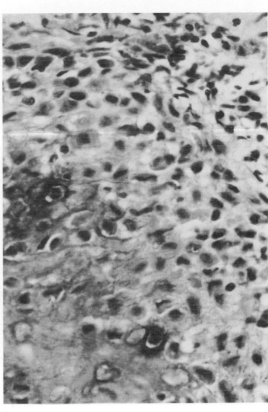

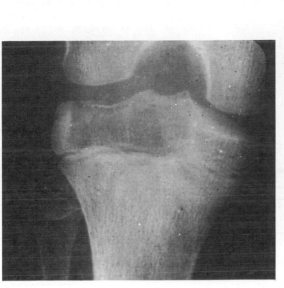

A   B

Figure 26-40. Chondroblastoma. (*A*) A radiograph of the knee shows a well-delineated lucency that involves almost the entire epiphysis and extends to the epiphyseal plate. (*B*) The histologic appearance of a chondroblastoma is defined by
plump, round cells (chondroblasts) surrounded by a mineralized matrix.

on radiographic studies as a triangular area between
the cortex and the periosteal bone (Codman's
triangle).

Histologic examination reveals malignant mesenchymal cells that modulate into malignant osteoblasts, producing osteoid and tumor bone (Fig.
26-41). This almost wholly woven bone is laid down
haphazardly, and is not aligned along stress lines.
Thus, it is the tumor bone that gives the radiologic
"sunburst" appearance (see Fig. 26-28). Often, foci
of malignant cartilage cells or malignant giant cells
are intermixed with the stromal tumor. In areas of
lysis, osteoclasts are found at the advancing front of
the tumor. The tumor spreads via the bloodstream to
the lungs (over 90% of patients who die from this
disease have lung metastases) and, less commonly,
to other bones (14%).

Juxtacortical osteosarcoma, a rare variant of osteosarcoma, occurs on the periosteal surface of the bone,
especially the lower posterior metaphysis of the femur (in 72% of cases). Unlike the usual osteosarcoma,

most patients are older than 25 years of age, and the
tumor is more common in women. Juxtacortical osteosarcoma spares the deep cortex and medulla of
the bone and grows external to the shaft (Fig. 26-42).
Usually, no Codman's triangle is evident. Amputation is the treatment of choice, and the prognosis is
good, with a 5-year survival over 80%.

Chondrosarcoma

Chondrosarcoma arises *de novo* in a pre-existing cartilaginous rest or in a benign tumor. It usually presents within the bone rather than as a juxtacortical
lesion. It is the second most common primary malignant bone tumor, occurs more commonly in men
than in women (2:1), and is most frequently seen in
the fourth to sixth decades (average age of 45 years).
The tumor is often a lobulated mass in the pelvic
bones, but may be seen in the long bones, ribs, spine,
scapula and sacrum.

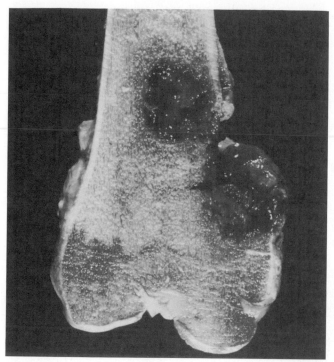
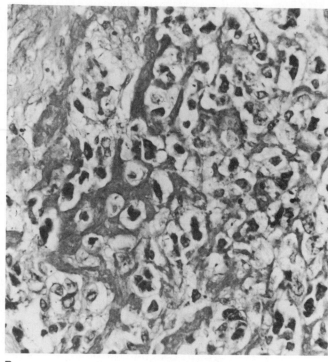

A   B

Figure 26-41.   Osteosarcoma. (*A*) The distal femur contains a tumor composed of hemorrhagic tissue. The dense white tissue that fills the metaphyseal marrow represents new bone formation. (*B*) A photomicrograph of the tumor in *A* shows malignant osteocytes and woven bone matrix.

Histologically, chondrosarcomas are composed of malignant cartilage cells in various stages of maturity. Occasionally, a well-differentiated chondrosarcoma would be difficult to diagnose were it not for its large size. Zones of calcification are often conspicuous, and are seen on radiography as splotches or bulky masses (Fig. 26-43). The tumor expands by osteoclastic stimulation and often breaks through the cortex. Most tumors grow slowly, but hematogenous metastases to the lungs are common. Amputation is often necessary, and the 5-year survival rates varies between 45% and 75%.

Giant Cell Tumor

Giant cell tumors are locally aggressive lesions with the capacity to metastasize, especially if manipulated surgically. They are thought to arise from primitive stromal cells with the capacity to modulate into osteoclasts. Indeed, the giant cell tumor is often a lytic lesion that grows slowly enough to allow a periosteal reaction. Thus, the tumor is usually surrounded by a thin, bony shell and expands the bone. Often, it

has a multiloculated or "soap bubble" appearance, representing the outpouchings of the bone (Fig. 26-44). The tumor usually occurs in the third and fourth decades, predominantly in women. In the long bones, it invariably involves the metaphysis after the epiphysis is closed, but it often extends into the epiphysis. It may also be found in the pelvis and sacrum. The mononuclear "stromal" cells are plump and oval, with large nuclei and scanty cytoplasm. Large osteoclastic giant cells, some with more than 100 nuclei, are scattered throughout the richly vascularized tumor.

Amputation may be necessary for treatment if an en bloc excision cannot be performed; otherwise, recurrences are inevitable. In older patients, giant cell tumors may also arise secondary to Paget's disease or irradiation.

Ewing's Sarcoma

Ewing's sarcoma, which at one time was the most deadly primary bone tumor, has been thought to arise from primitive marrow elements or immature

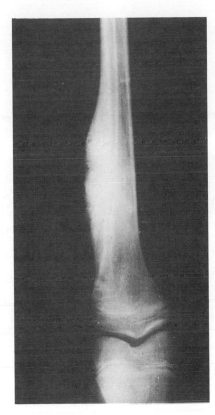

Figure 26-42. Juxtacortical osteosarcoma. A radiograph of the tibia shows a large bony excrescence on the lateral cortex of the proximal diaphysis. The medullary cavity is spared.

mesenchymal cells. Newer evidence suggests a neural histogenesis for this tumor. Fortunately, Ewing's sarcoma is relatively uncommon, representing only about 4% to 5% of all bone tumors.

Ewing's sarcoma is primarily a tumor of the long bones, especially the humerus, tibia, and femur, where it occurs as a midshaft or metaphyseal lesion. However, it may occur in any bone of the body, including those in the hands and feet. It is a tumor of childhood and adolescence, with two-thirds of the cases occurring in patients younger than 20 years of age. Males are affected more often than females (2:1). The onion skin pattern that is seen on radiologic examination represents a circumferential layer of reactive periosteal bone associated with a lytic lesion involving the medulla and endosteal surface of the cortex. The tumor cells are found in sheets that permeate all the bony interstices, including the haversian canals, and that extend along the shaft in both directions.

On histologic examination, the cells resemble primitive lymphocytes, and are visualized as small, closely packed cells with little cytoplasm; they are two to three times larger than a lymphocyte (Fig. 26-45). There is little or no interstitial stroma, and mitoses occur infrequently. Ewing's sarcoma metastasizes to many organs, including the lungs and brain. Other bones, especially the skull, are common sites for metastases (45–75% of cases). With irradiation and chemotherapy, the 5-year survival rate is approximately 50%.

Multiple Myeloma

Multiple myeloma, a malignant tumor of plasma cells, may be either local or diffuse. It occurs most often in older patients (average age, 64 years) and affects men twice as commonly as women. Multiple myeloma is characterized by overproduction of immunoglobulins in more than 90% of patients with disseminated disease. Bence Jones protein may be seen in 50% of cases. The hematologic aspects of multiple myeloma are discussed in detail in Chapter 20. The lesions are almost exclusively lytic, although rare examples of radiodense bone lesions have been reported. The bones most frequently involved are the skull, spine, ribs, pelvis, and femur (Fig. 26-46). Pathologic fractures are common. On microscopic examination, the sheets of plasma cells show varying degrees of maturity, but the prognosis does not correlate with the histologic appearance. Amyloid deposits, in both skeletal and extraskeletal sites, are seen in at least 10% of patients. Despite irradiation and chemotherapy, the prognosis is poor (the median survival time is 32 months). Solitary myeloma has a better prognosis, with a 60% 5-year survival. The cause of death is usually infection or kidney failure.

Metastatic Tumors

The most common malignant tumor of bone is metastatic cancer, with carcinomas comprising the vast majority of lesions. Specifically, tumors of the breast, prostate, lung, thyroid, and kidney frequently spread to bone. Tumor cells usually arrive in the bone via the bloodstream; in the case of spinal metastases, they are transported particularly by the vertebral veins. It is estimated that skeletal metastases are found in at least 85% of cancer cases that have run their full clinical course. The vertebral column is, by far, the most commonly affected bony structure. Some tumors (cancers of the thyroid, gastrointestinal tract, and kidney, and neuroblastoma) produce mostly lytic lesions by stimulating osteoclasts. A few

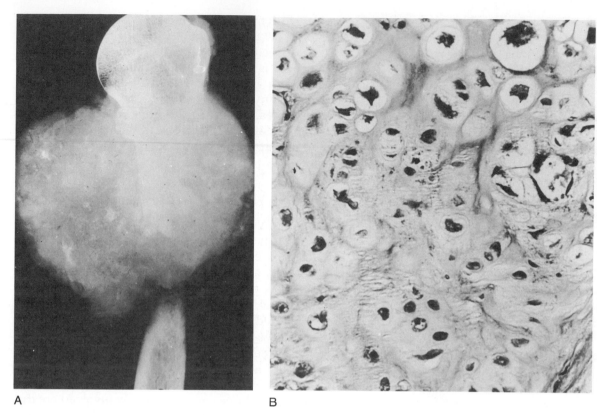

A   B

Figure 26-43.   Chondrosarcoma. (*A*) A radiograph of the resected proximal humerus reveals a bulky, destructive, mineralized lesion in the diaphysis. There is extensive bone destruction and extension of the tumor into the soft tissue. (*B*) A photomicrograph of *A* reveals a hypercellular tumor composed of malignant chondrocytes embedded in a sparse matrix.

tumors (prostate, breast, lung, and stomach cancers) stimulate osteogenic components to make bone; these appear on radiographic studies as dense, osteoblastic foci (Fig. 26-47). However, most foci of metastatic cancer have mixtures of both lytic and blastic elements. It is important to remember that the cancer itself does not resorb or make bone, but instead stimulates, by unknown mechanisms, the mesenchymal elements of the marrow.

Fibrous Dysplasia

Fibrous dysplasia is a condition characterized by a disorganized mixture of fibrous and osseous elements in the interior of affected bones. The disorder probably represents a peculiar developmental abnormality of the skeleton rather than a neoplasm, although it is neither familial nor hereditary. It occurs in children or adults, and may involve a single bone (monostotic) or many bones (polyostotic). The skeletal lesions may be associated with skin pigmentation and endocrine dysfunction, in which case the term Albright's syndrome is applied.

Monostotic fibrous dysplasia is the most common form of the disease and is most often seen in the 2nd and 3rd decades. The bones that are commonly involved are the proximal femur, tibia, ribs, and facial bones, but any bone may be involved. The disease may be asymptomatic, or it may lead to a pathologic fracture. Persons of either sex may have monostotic fibrous dysplasia.

In **polyostotic fibrous dysplasia** (osteitis fibrosa disseminata) more than one bone is involved; 25% of patients exhibit disease in more than half of the skeleton, including the facial bones. Symptoms usually present in childhood, and almost all patients suffer from pathologic fractures, limb deformities, or limb length discrepancies. Polyostotic fibrous dysplasia is

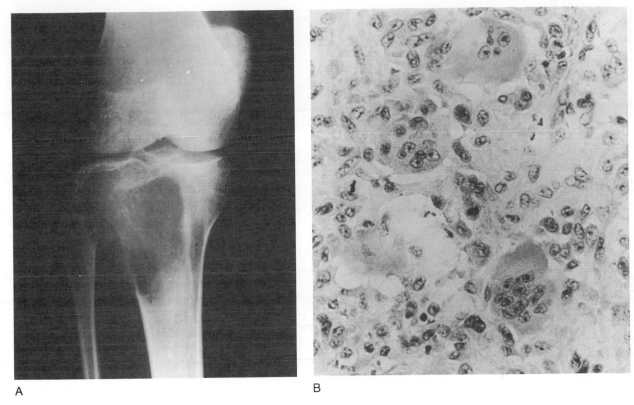

A   B

Figure 26-44.   Giant cell tumor of bone. (*A*) A radiograph of the proximal tibia shows an eccentric lytic lesion, with virtually no new bone formation. The tumor extends to the subchondral bone plate and breaks through cortex into the soft tissue. (*B*) A photomicrograph shows osteoclast-type giant cells and plump, oval, mononuclear cells. The nuclei of both types of cells are identical.

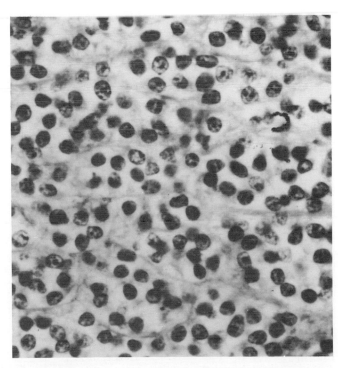

Figure 26-45.   Ewing's sarcoma. Small, round cells, with glycogen-filled clear cytoplasm, are uniformly distributed.

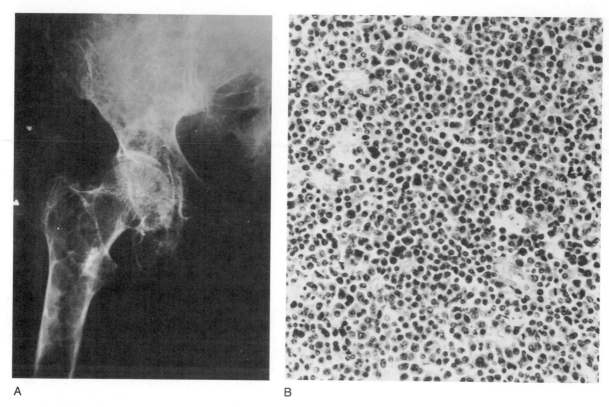

A   B

Figure 26-46. Multiple myeloma. (*A*) A radiograph of the right pelvis and proximal femur reveals large, lucent areas, as well as a diffuse osteoporotic pattern that particularly involves the pelvis. (*B*) A photomicrograph of *A* shows sheets of plasma cells, some of which are binucleated or pleomorphic.

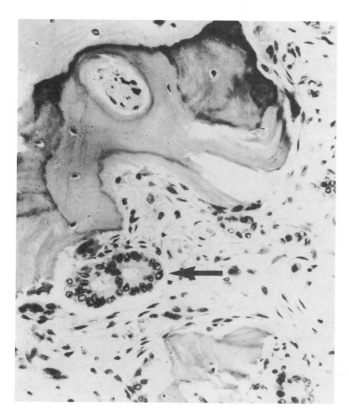

Figure 26-47. Metastatic adenocarcinoma to bone. The neoplastic glands (*arrow*) have stimulated new woven bone formation. The marrow has been replaced by loose fibrosis. This focus is an osteoblastic metastasis.

more common in females. Sometimes the disease becomes quiescent at puberty, whereas pregnancy may stimulate the growth of lesions.

The endocrine dysfunctions of Albright's syndrome may include acromegaly, Cushing's syndrome, hyperthyroidism, and vitamin-D-resistant rickets. However, the most common endocrine abnormality is precocious puberty in females (males rarely have Albright's syndrome). As a result, premature closing of the epiphyseal plates may occur, leading to shortness. The most frequent extraskeletal manifestations of this form of fibrous dysplasia are the characteristic skin lesions. These are pigmented macules (café au lait spots) with indented ("coast of Maine") borders that do not cross the midline of the body and are usually located on the buttocks (Fig. 48A), and back, and over the sacrum. These skin "freckles" have a tendency to overlie the skeletal lesions.

The radiographic features of fibrous dysplasia are distinctive. The bone lesion has a lucent ground-glass appearance with well-marginated borders and a thin cortex. The bone may be ballooned, deformed, or enlarged, and involvement may be focal, or it may encompass the entire bone (Fig. 26-48B).

All the forms of fibrous dysplasia have an identical histologic pattern—benign fibroblastic tissue arranged in a loose, whorled pattern. Irregularly arranged, purposeless, woven bone spicules that lack osteoblastic rimming are embedded in the fibrous tissue. In about 10% of cases, irregular islands of hyaline cartilage are also present. Occasionally, cystic degeneration occurs, with hemosiderin-laden macrophages, hemorrhage, and osteoclast-type giant cells congregated about the cyst (Fig. 26-48C). Rarely, malignant degeneration into sarcoma (osteosarcoma, chondrosarcoma, or fibrosarcoma) has been reported, but most of these cases involved previous irradiation. Treatment consists of curettage, repair of fractures, and prevention of deformities.

Joints

A joint or an articulation is a union between two or more bones, whose construction varies with the function of that joint. There are two types of joints: (1) a **synovial** or **diarthrodial joint,** which is a movable joint that is lined by a synovial membrane; and (2) a **synarthrosis,** which is a joint that has little movement. Synarthroses are further divided into four subclassifications:

- **Symphyses** are articulations joined by fibrocartilaginous tissue and firm ligaments that allow for little movement. Examples are the symphysis pubis and the ends of vertebral joints.
- **Synchondroses,** which are found at the articulated ends of bones, have articular cartilage, but there is no synovium or significant joint cavity. An example of such a joint is the sternal manubrial joint.
- **Syndesmoses** connect bones by fibrous tissue without any cartilaginous elements. Examples are the distal tibiofibular articulation and the cranial sutures.
- **Synostoses** are pathologic bony bridges between bones, as seen in ankylosis of the spine.

Joint disease is one of the oldest diseases known, having been found in the fossil bones of dinosaurs. Fifteen to 30% of the population of the United States over the age of 50 years will develop some form of clinically significant joint disease. The most important disease affecting the joints is arthritis. The two most common forms of this disease—namely, osteoarthritis and rheumatoid arthritis, will be discussed to emphasize the different pathophysiologic mechanisms involved. Diseases caused by the deposition of crystals, especially gout, will also be examined.

Classification of Synovial Joints and Their Movements

The synovial joints (or diarthrodial joints) are classified according to the type of movement they permit. A **uniaxial joint** allows movement around only one axis. In a hinge joint, such as the elbow, the axis is transverse across the articular surfaces, permitting both flexion and extension. In a pivot joint, such as radioulnar joint, the axis is longitudinal along the shaft of the bone, and the motion is rotational. A **biaxial joint** allows movement around two axes. In the condyloid joint of the wrist, where the articular surfaces are oval, one axis is along the long diameter and the other is along the short diameter of the articular surfaces. This joint permits four-way movement—namely, flexion, extension, abduction, and adduction. In a saddle joint, such as the carpometacarpal joint of the thumb, the joint surfaces allow for movement as in a condyloid joint. **Polyaxial joints** permit movement in virtually any axis. In a ball-and-socket joint, such as is found in the shoulder and hip, all movements, including rotation, are possible. The plane joint, represented by the patella, allows the articular surfaces to glide over one another, the surfaces being essentially flat.

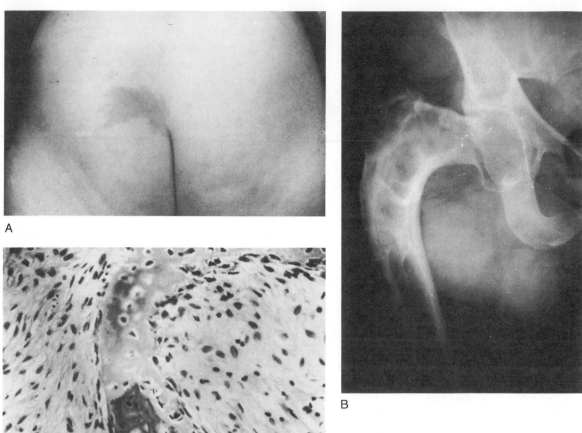

A

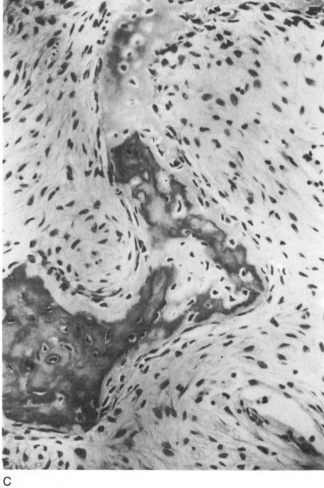

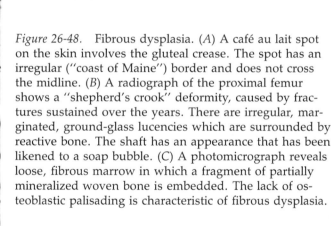

B

C

Figure 26-48. Fibrous dysplasia. (*A*) A café au lait spot on the skin involves the gluteal crease. The spot has an irregular ("coast of Maine") border and does not cross the midline. (*B*) A radiograph of the proximal femur shows a "shepherd's crook" deformity, caused by fractures sustained over the years. There are irregular, marginated, ground-glass lucencies which are surrounded by reactive bone. The shaft has an appearance that has been likened to a soap bubble. (*C*) A photomicrograph reveals loose, fibrous marrow in which a fragment of partially mineralized woven bone is embedded. The lack of osteoblastic palisading is characteristic of fibrous dysplasia.

The most important principle in the understanding of joint function is the concept of **unit load.** The unit load is the compressive force in kilograms per cubic centimeter of articular cartilage. The size of the joint is irrelevant, as is the load on the joint itself. However, the unit load is fairly constant over the hip, knee, and ankle, generally ranging from 20 to 26 kg/cm^3 along the articular surfaces. If the load exceeds these values, the articular cartilage is injured. A number of mechanisms protect the joint from exceeding the unit load. The adjacent muscles are the major shock-absorbing structures that protect the joint. In addition, deformation, even to the extent of microscopic fractures of the coarse cancellous bone also helps to protect the joint. Moreover, the joint incongruity allows for increasing contact area with increasing load. With these mechanisms in mind, it is not surprising that the thickest articular cartilage is generally about 6 mm thick. But 90% or more of the absorption of energy across the knee joint is by active muscle contraction, and 10% or less is by secondary mechanisms, such as absorption of force by the coarse cancellous bone of the knee joint. Thus, virtually any structure is sacrificed, even to the point of a bone fracture, to protect the articular cartilage from forces that would exceed the critical unit load, thereby killing the irreplaceable articular cartilage. In diarthrodial joints, there may be intra-articular structures, such as ligaments and menisci. The menisci generally allow for two planes of motion, such as flexion and rotation.

Vascular and Nerve Supply

There is a rich arterial and venous supply to the joints, including arteriovenous connections that communicate with the vessels of the periosteum. Large arteries supply the synovium near the joint capsule, giving off many branches that ultimately communicate with the subsynovial tissue. Precapillary arterioles play a major role in controlling the circulation of the synovial lining. A large surface area in the synovial capillary bed, which is located only a few cell layers deep to the joint cavity, allows for trans-synovial exchange of substances and the common phenomena of effusion and hemarthrosis. If the joint is subjected to heat, blood flow increases through the synovial capillaries. Exercise, immobilization, and even joint effusions may reduce blood flow into the synovium.

There is a dual nerve supply to each joint. Specific articular nerves arise from adjacent peripheral nerves and enter the capsule, and articular branches arise from related muscle nerves. The body senses the position of the joint by nerve endings in the muscles, as well as in the joint capsule.

Development of Diarthrodial Joints

In discussing the formation of diarthrodial joints, two basic principles should be stressed. The first is that the appendicular skeleton develops proximal to the distal skeleton. This means that the proximal structures are developed before the distal ones; for example, the shoulder joint develops before the elbow joint. The second principle maintains that development progresses in a cranial to caudal manner. This means that the upper limb develops approximately 24 hours or more before the lower limb. These principles are important in understanding certain developmental abnormalities. Thus, it is unusual to find developmental abnormalities of the humerus and femur in the same patient, because injurious agents act during discrete time intervals.

The upper limb bud appears when the embryo is 26 days of age, and is completely formed 4 weeks later. The limb bud is covered by ectodermal tissue, and by 31 days, the tip of the upper limb bud has a well-defined, ridgelike area called the **apical ectodermal ridge.** This structure is necessary for the sequential development of the limb elements, and it stimulates the underlying mesoderm to proceed in a proximal to distal direction. If the apical ectodermal ridge is removed, mesodermal proliferation is discontinued. The mesodermal tissue condenses to form a blastema soon after the limb bud appears. In the region of the future bone, the blastema differentiates to form cartilage. The space between two adjacent bones destined to become the future joint is termed the **interzone.**

The synovial tissue arises from the periphery of the interzone. Joint capsules, interarticular ligaments, menisci, tendons, and all other joint structures develop from this synovial mesenchyme. Vascular penetration takes place in this tissue, and the synovium soon becomes a rich capillary network, bringing to this area extra blastema cells, such as mast cells and macrophages. The macrophages, which secrete acid phosphatase and other esterases, play a major role in cavitation. **Cavitation** is a process by which vascular tissue is removed from the interzone region, thereby creating a future joint cavity (Fig. 26-49). Administration of corticosteroids at this time arrests joint development. The joint becomes fused, leading to syndactyly of the hands. **Cleft palate** results when the two palatine bones grow toward the midline and

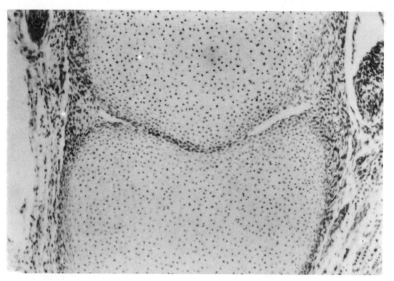

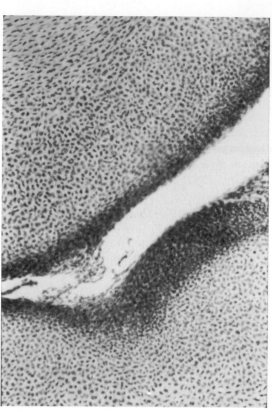

A   B

Figure 26-49.   Development of a diarthrodial joint. (*A*) The earliest development
of the joint is characterized by cavitation at the interzone between two masses of
hyaline cartilage. The adjacent tissue, of mesodermal origin, gives rise to the joint
capsule, muscles, and synovium. (*B*) A high-power view of the interzone. The
condensation of hyaline cartilage cells, destined to be the true articular cartilage, is
evident.

the intervening tissue is not resorbed. **Syndactyly,**
which is a fused or web-shaped hand, occurs because
the tissue between the digits is not removed. Movement also plays a major role in the formation of a
joint. A lack of movement retards joint development
and may result in a rare but extremely crippling disease termed **arthrogryposis,** which is characterized
by joint fusion. This condition may be produced experimentally by administering curare to chick embryos, thereby paralyzing movement.

Structures of the Synovial Joint

The Synovium

Synovial joints are partially lined on their internal
aspects by the synovium. In a synovial joint, only
the articular cartilage surfaces are devoid of syno-

vium. The recesses and internal aspects of the capsule, as well as the areas around the intra-articular
structures, such as the menisci and ligaments, all
show synovial lining tissue. The synovial lining is
not a true membrane, as there is no basement membrane separating the synovial lining cells from the
subsynovial tissue. Neither are there tight gap junctions or desmosomes between the synovial cells. The
synovium is composed of one to three layers of synovial lining cells and is made up of two types of cells,
recognizable only by electron microscopy. **Type A
cells** are macrophages that contain lysosomal enzymes and dense bodies. The secretory **B cells** produce hyaluronic acid. The synovial cell membranes
are disposed in villi and microvilli, an arrangement
that creates an enormous surface area. It is estimated
that, in the knee alone, there are 100 m^2 of synovial
lining. The subsynovial tissue is a loose, vascularized

areolar tissue. In some locations, the synovium is closely applied to the dense connective tissue of the joint capsule. On the other hand, if the synovial tissue lines a fat pad—for example, that of the knee—then the subsynovial tissue is composed mostly of adipose tissue.

The synovium controls diffusion in and out of the joint; ingestion of debris; secretion of hyaluronate, immunoglobulins, and lysosomal enzymes; and lubrication of the joints by secretion of glycoproteins. The clear, sticky, viscous synovial fluid, which is present in small amounts not exceeding 1 to 4 ml, is the chief source of nourishment for chondrocytes of the articular cartilage that lack a blood supply. The synovial fluid is an ultrafiltrate that functions as a molecular sieve. It does not contain fibrinogen and therefore has no clotting capacity. It does not normally contain alpha-2 macroglobulin, but in disease states, this protein may accumulate in the synovial fluid. Hyaluronate, a very large molecule, has a great affinity for water because of its high number of negative charges. The function of hyaluronate may be disturbed if the charges are altered. For example, when a hemophiliac bleeds into a joint, the positive iron charges bind to and neutralize the negative charges. In another disease, ochronosis, homogenistic acid also binds to the negative charges of the hyaluronate, thereby altering its molecular charge. As a result, the synovium becomes a leaky sieve, and fibrinogen, alpha-2 macroglobulin, and other foreign substances gain entrance to the joint cavity. The analysis of synovial fluid is often important in the diagnosis of joint disease.

Articular Cartilage

The hyaline cartilage that covers the articular ends of the bones does not participate in endochondral ossification, and is well suited for its dual role in absorbing shocks and lubricating the surface of the movable joint. On gross examination, the articular cartilage is glistening, smooth, white, and semi-ridged, and has a thickness that generally does not exceed 6 mm.

Histologic Characteristics

Although the articular surface appears smooth on gross examination, scanning electron microscopy reveals gentle waves and pits that correspond to the underlying lacunae of the surface chondrocytes. There are five histologic zones in the articular cartilage (Fig. 26-50).

Tangential or Gliding Zone   The tangential or gliding zone is the region closest to the articular surface, where the chondrocytes are elongated, flattened, and parallel to the long axis of the surface. Within this zone, a condensation of type II collagen fibers forms the so-called "skin" of the articular cartilage.

Transitional Zone   The next, slightly deeper zone is called the transitional zone. The chondrocytes in this zone are larger, more ovoid, and more randomly distributed than in the tangential zone. The standard hyaline cartilage matrix is present, and there seems to be a random distribution of collagen fibers. However, electron microscopy reveals that the fibers are arranged transverse to the articular surface.

Radial Zone   The next deeper zone is the radial

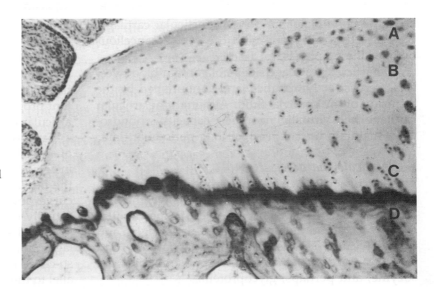

Figure 26-50. The zones of normal articular cartilage. *A*, tangential zone; *B*, transitional zone, *C*, radial zone; *D*, calcified zone, separated from the radial zone by the prominent tide mark. The articular cartilage is supported by a layer of subchondral bone plate.

Pathology

The earliest histologic changes of osteoarthritis involve the loss of proteoglycans from the surface of the articular cartilage, manifested as a decrease in metachromatic staining. At the same time, empty lacunae in the articular cartilage indicate the death of chondrocytes (Fig. 26-51). The viable chondrocytes becomes large, aggregate into groups or **clones,** and are surrounded by basophilic-staining matrix, called the **territorial matrix.** The disease may arrest at this stage for many years before it proceeds to the next stage, which is characterized by **fibrillation,** the development of surface cracks parallel to the long axis of the articular surface. These fibrillations also may persist for many years before further progression occurs. As these cracks propagate, synovial fluid begins to flow into the defects. The cracks are progressively oriented more vertically, tending to parallel the long axis of the collagen fibrils in the arcades of Benninghoff. In so doing, synovial fluid works its way deeper into the articular cartilage along the crack. Eventually, pieces of articular cartilage break off and lodge in the synovium, there inducing mild inflammation and a foreign body giant cell reaction. The result is a hyperemic and hypertrophied synovium.

As the crack extends down toward the tide mark and eventually crosses it, neovascularization from the epiphysis and subchondral bone extends into the area of the crack, inducing subchondral osteoclastic bone resorption. Adjacent osteoblastic activity also occurs, and the net result is a thickening of the subchondral bone plate in the area of the crack. As neovascularization progressively extends into the area of the crack, mesenchymal cells invade, and fibrocartilage forms as a poor substitute for the articular hyaline cartilage. These fibrocartilaginous plugs may persist, or they may be swept into the joint. The subchondral bone becomes exposed and burnished as it grinds against the opposite joint surface, which

is undergoing the same process. These thick, shiny, and smooth areas of subchondral bone are referred to as **eburnated** ("ivory-like") bone (Figs. 26-52 and 26-53). In some areas, the eburnated bone eventually cracks, allowing synovial fluid to extend from the joint surface into the subchondral bone marrow, where it eventually leads to a **subchondral bone cyst.** These cysts increase in size as synovial fluid is forced into the space but cannot exit. Eventually, there is bone resorption by osteoclasts and an attempt to wall off the area by osteoblastic activity. The net result is a subchondral bone cyst filled with synovial fluid, with a well-marginated, reactive bone wall.

An **osteophyte** may be found (usually, in the lateral portions of the joint) when the mesenchymal tissue of the synovium modulates into osteoblasts and chondroblasts, cells that form a mass of cartilage and bone. On gross examination, these osteophytes are pearly, grayish-bone nodules appearing on the peripheral portion of the joint surface. These osteophytes, or bony spurs, also occur at the lateral portions of the intervertebral discs, extending from the adjacent vertebral bodies and producing the "lipping" pattern seen on radiologic studies as osteoarthritis of the spine. In the fingers, osteophytes at the distal interphalangeal joints are termed **Heberden's nodes.**

Biochemical Abnormalities

The biochemical changes of osteoarthritis primarily involve proteoglycans. There is a decrease in proteoglycan content and aggregation, as well as a decrease in the chain length of the glycosaminoglycans. Compared to the levels in normal articular cartilage, keratan sulfate is decreased and chondroitin sulfate is increased. There is also a decline in the glucosamine concentration, but there is no change in the concentration of galactosamine. The collagen fibers are thicker than normal, and the arcades of Benninghoff

Figure 26-51.   Histogenesis of osteoarthritis. The death of chondrocytes leads to a crack in the articular cartilage that is followed by an influx of synovial fluid and further loss and degeneration of cartilage. As a result of this process, cartilage is gradually worn away. Below the tide mark, new vessels grow in from the epiphysis, and fibrocartilage is deposited. The fibrocartilage plug is not mechanically sufficient and may be worn away, thereby exposing the subchondral bone plate, which becomes thickened and eburnated. If there is a crack in this region, synovial fluid leaks into the marrow space and produces a subchondral bone cyst. Focal regrowth of the articular surface leads to the formation of osteophytes.

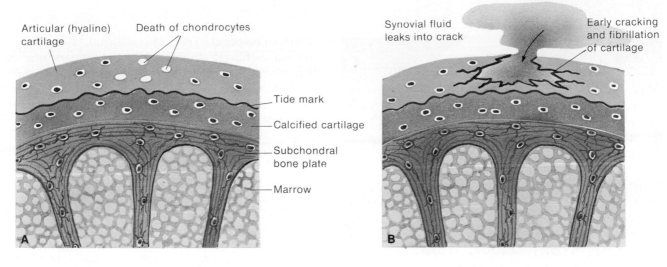

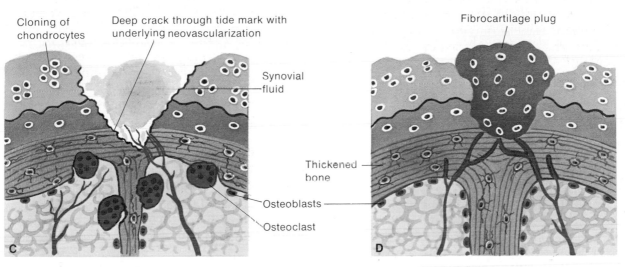

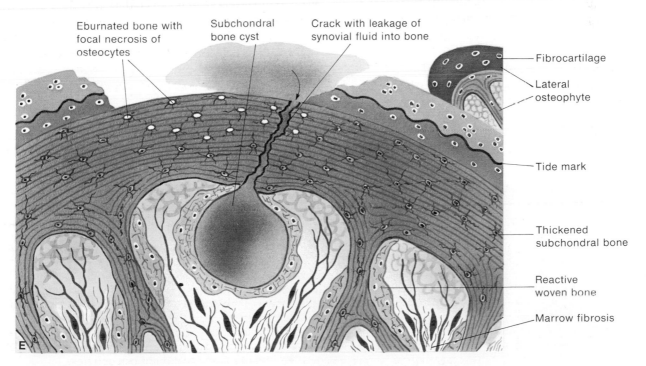

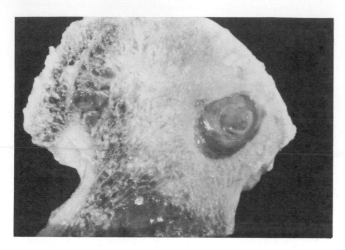

Figure 26-52.   Osteoarthritis. The femoral head is flattened, with loss of articular cartilage and an eburnated subchondral bone plate. A subchondral bone cyst, surrounded by new bone, is evident.

it fails to respond to reparative stimuli. In contrast to normal cartilage, chondrocytes in osteoarthritic cartilage begin to replicate and form clones of chondrocytes. However, over a long period of time and with the advance of osteoarthritic changes, cell metabolism gradually diminishes, as does cell replication. Acid cathepsin, which exerts a proteolytic action on the protein cores of the matrix macromolecules, is increased in osteoarthritic cartilage. Collagenase, which is not present in normal cartilage, is also found in osteoarthritic cartilage. Recent evidence indicates that ascorbic acid and vitamin E inhibit proteoglycan degradation in osteoarthritic cartilage.

At present, there is no specific treatment for arresting the osteoarthritic process. Therapy is directed at specific orthopaedic conditions and, when appropriate, may include joint replacement, exercise, weight loss, and other supportive measures.

Rheumatoid Arthritis

Rheumatoid arthritis is a systemic, chronic, inflammatory disease that involves the joints. Its onset usually occurs in the third or fourth decade, but it may occur at any age. The joints that are commonly affected are those of the extremities, which are usually afflicted at the same time and often in a symmetrical pattern. The course of the disease is variable, and is often punctuated with remissions and exacerbations. The broad spectrum of clinical manifestations ranges from barely discernible and mild forms to severe, destructive, and mutilating disease.

are disrupted. The water content of osteoarthritic cartilage is increased. It is thought that the reduction in proteoglycans allows more water to be bound to the collagen fibers. Thus, osteoarthritic cartilage, or any cartilage that is fibrillated, tends to swell more than normal cartilage.

In the early stages of osteoarthritis, synthesis of matrix by chondrocytes is augmented, presumably as a reparative reaction. As the osteoarthritis progresses, protein synthesis eventually tends to decrease, suggesting that the cell reaches a point where

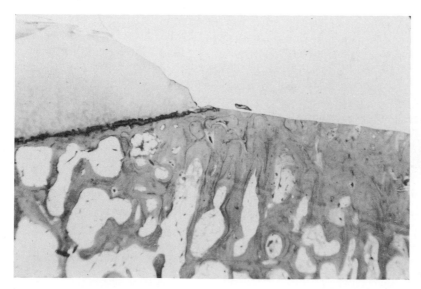

Figure 26-53.   Osteoarthritis. The articular cartilage has been lost (*right*). Remnants of the articular cartilage are evident on the left. The thickened subchondral bone corresponds to the eburnated bone seen on gross inspection.

The diagnosis is based primarily on the clinical course, rather than the histopathology, because there is no one specific finding that is diagnostic of rheumatoid arthritis. Rheumatoid factor is usually present in the serum, but some patients are persistently seronegative. Furthermore, rheumatoid factor is not specific for rheumatoid arthritis. It is now thought that classic rheumatoid arthritis probably comprises a heterogeneous group of disorders; patients who are persistently seronegative for rheumatoid factor may have disease of a different etiology than do those who are seropositive. As well as the classic form of rheumatoid arthritis in which joint manifestations are predominant, rheumatoid-like diseases exist that are associated with underlying maladies such as inflammatory bowel disease and cirrhosis.

Rheumatoid arthritis and its variants are characterized histologically by a progressive proliferation of the synovium, which eventually destroys the articular cartilage and leads to severe osteoarthritis as the final common pathway of joint destruction.

Classification and Incidence

Clinically, rheumatoid arthritis is considered to be a disease without a specific biologic marker. The diagnosis is based primarily on a number of criteria, and the incidence varies depending upon which criteria are employed. Rheumatoid arthritis affects less than 1% of the adult population; its incidence is greater in women than in men (with a ratio of 3:1). A genetic origin for the disease is suggested by the association of the haplotype HLA-DW4 and a related B-cell alloantigen, HLA-DRW4, with severe seropositive rheumatoid arthritis in white patients.

Pathogenesis

The cause of rheumatoid arthritis is unknown. Infectious bacteria or viruses have never been detected in the joints of patients with rheumatoid arthritis, although in animal models, some bacterial wall fragments have produced a chronic synovitis. It is thought that immunologic mechanisms play an important role in the pathogenesis of the disease. Lymphocytes and plasma cells, which are increased in number in the synovium, produce immunoglobulins, mainly of the IgG class. Deposits of immunoglobulins and complement components are present in the articular cartilage and the synovium. Although it has not yet been demonstrated that a virus can cause rheumatoid arthritis, structures resembling viruses have been reported early in the course of the disease.

It has been suggested that the Epstein-Barr virus may play a role in this disease, especially considering the high incidence of precipitating antibodies to an antigen that is produced following infection with this virus. Moreover, the Epstein-Barr virus is a polyclonal B-cell activator that stimulates production of rheumatoid factor. Synovial cells cultured from rheumatic joints exhibit a decreased response to glucocorticoids, and also demonstrate increased production of hyaluronate. These cells release a peptide ("connective-tissue–activating peptide") that may influence the function of other cells, producing increased amounts of prostaglandins, particularly PGE_2. Increased serum levels of immunoglobulins IgM, IgA, and IgG, may also be found in patients with rheumatoid arthritis.

Rheumatoid factor actually represents multiple antibodies, principally IgM, directed against the Fc fragment of IgG in humans and several animals. Rheumatoid factors of the IgM class are detected by latex fixation, bentonite flocculation, and sensitized sheep red blood cell agglutination. **Up to 80% of patients with classic rheumatoid arthritis are positive for rheumatoid factor, depending on the test used.** In a few cases, negative tests or low titers of rheumatoid factors are obtained because circulating IgG inhibits rheumatoid factor activity. In rare cases, rheumatoid factors may be absent in the serum but detectable in synovial fluid. Significant titers of rheumatoid factor are found in patients with related disease, such as systemic lupus erythematosus, progressive systemic sclerosis, and dermatomyositis. Rheumatoid factor also may occur in a wide variety of nonrheumatic disorders, including pulmonary fibrosis, cirrhosis, sarcoidosis, Waldenström's macroglobulinemia, tuberculosis, kala-azar, lepromatous leprosy, and viral hepatitis. Rheumatoid factor tests may be positive in patients who were recently vaccinated against smallpox, and in those who have received skin grafts or who suffer from subacute bacterial endocarditis. Healthy, elderly people, particularly women, may also test positive for rheumatoid factor. Interestingly, although patients with classic rheumatoid arthritis may be seronegative, the presence of high titer rheumatoid factor is frequently associated with severe and unremitting disease, many systemic complications, and a grave prognosis. In addition to IgM, rheumatoid factors may also be IgG and IgA. The presence of IgG may be associated with the development of systemic complications, such as necrotizing vasculitis. In addition IgG immune complexes may be found in the synovial fluid.

In summary, a pathogenetic theory maintains that, initially, in a joint or elsewhere, an unknown agent, possibly a virus, stimulates the formation of antibodies (immunoglobulins). These immunoglobulins act as new antigens, triggering the production of anti-idiotype antibodies (the rheumatoid factor). Immune complexes, which contain rheumatoid factors, are phagocytosed by leukocytes, which release lysosomal enzymes and other products. Similarly, mononuclear phagocytes within the synovium may also phagocytose the immune complexes, as rheumatoid factor and other immunoglobulins are made locally, as well as in distinct lymphoid tissue. This hypothesis is supported by the demonstration of immune complexes (IgG rheumatoid factor with IgG) and complement components in synovium, synovial fluid, and extra-articular lesions. Furthermore, patients with seropositive rheumatoid arthritis have lower levels of complement in their synovial fluid than do patients who have seronegative rheumatoid arthritis; the latter have complement levels that are comparable to those seen in noninflammatory joint diseases, such as osteoarthritis.

It has also been postulated that cell-mediated immunity contributes to rheumatoid arthritis. Abundant T-lymphocytes in the rheumatoid synovium are frequently Ia positive ("activated") and of the helper type. They are frequently in close contact with HLA-DR–positive cells, which are either macrophages or so-called dendritic Ia-positive cells that do not demonstrate antigens of the monocyte lineage. The T-cells may act as helper cells and may also function in other immune capacities. Furthermore, T-cells may directly or indirectly interact with macrophages through the production of soluble products that inhibit migration and division. Such substances have been found in rheumatoid synovial fluid and in supernatants from rheumatoid tissue explants. It has further been observed that interleukin I can stimulate the production of collagenase and prostaglandins in cultured synovial cells. Patients with rheumatoid arthritis demonstrate a reactivity of T-lymphocytes with collagen types I and III. In therapeutic trials drainage of the thoracic duct, which primarily contains T-cells, improved the condition of patients with rheumatoid arthritis. A related observation is the fact that irradiation of lymphoid tissue may also improve the clinical condition of patients.

Pathology

The early synovial changes of rheumatoid arthritis are edema and the accumulation of plasma cells, lymphocytes, and macrophages (Fig. 26-54). There is a concomitant increase in vascularity, and exudation of fibrin in the joint space. Conspicuous fibrin deposition may result in small fibrin nodules that float in the joint, termed **rice bodies.** The synovial lining cells, which are normally one to three layers thick, undergo hyperplasia and form layers 8 to 10 cells thick. Multinucleated giant cells are often found among the synovial cells. **The net result is a synovial lining thrown into the numerous villi and frondlike folds that fill the peripheral recesses of the joint.** As the synovium undergoes hyperplasia and hypertrophy, it creeps over the surface of the articular cartilage and adjacent structures. This inflammatory synovium, now containing mast cells, is termed a **pannus** ("cloak"). The pannus proceeds to cover the articular cartilage and isolate it from its nutritional synovial fluid. Lymphocytes aggregate into masses and eventually develop a follicular center, an appearance termed an **Allison-Ghormley body** (Fig. 26-55).

The **synovial fluid** contains abundant polymorphonuclear leukocytes, although they are rarely present in the **synovial tissue.** As the disease waxes and wanes over the years, the degree of acute inflammation also correlates with the varying activity of the rheumatoid process. The pannus may also burrow deep to the subchondral bone plate, where it erodes

Figure 26-54. Histogenesis of rheumatoid arthritis. A virus or an unknown stress stimulates the synovial cells to proliferate. The influx of lymphocytes, plasma cells, and mast cells, together with neovascularization and edema, leads to hypertrophy and hyperplasia of the synovium. Lymphoid nodules are prominent. The proliferating synovium extends into the joint space, burrows into the bone beneath the articular cartilage, and covers the cartilage as a pannus. The articular cartilage is eventually destroyed by direct resorption or deprivation of its nutrient synovial fluid. The synovial tissue continues to proliferate in the subchondral region, as well as in the joint. Eventually, the joint is destroyed and becomes fused, a condition termed ankylosis.

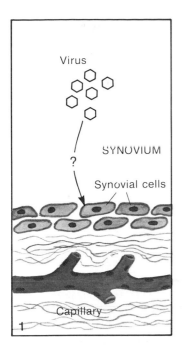

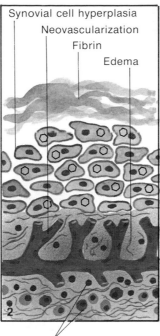

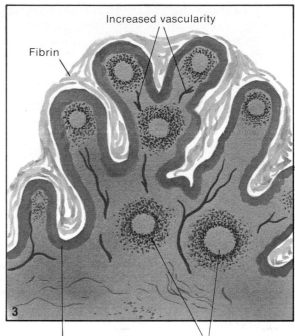

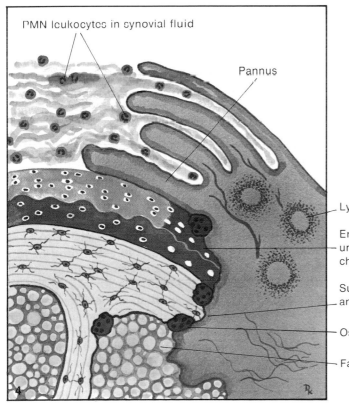

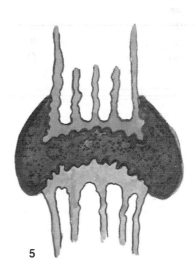

Destruction of joint by fibrosis and loss of articular cartilage, with periarticular bone loss

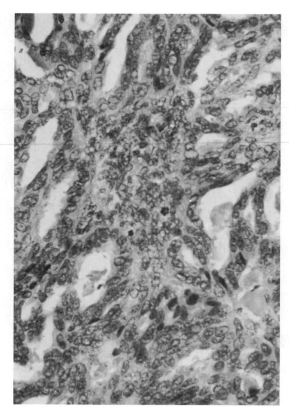

Figure 26-71. Synovial sarcoma. Irregular spaces are lined by plump, synovial-like, neoplastic cells. The intervening tissue contains neoplastic cells with similar nuclei. There are no basement membranes separating the joint-like spaces from the more spindle-shaped interstitial tumor cells. This pattern is typical of a biphasic synovial sarcoma.

the center of the clusters leads to the "alveolar" pattern. Malignant rhabdomyoblasts, identifiable by their cross striations, occur less commonly in the alveolar variant than in embryonal rhabdomyosarcoma, being present in only 25% of cases.

Pleomorphic rhabdomyosarcoma, the least common form of rhabdomyosarcoma, is found in the skeletal muscles of older persons. This tumor differs from the other types of rhabdomyosarcoma in the pleomorphism of its irregularly arranged cells. Large, granular, and eosinophilic rhabdomyoblasts are common, although cross striations are virtually nonexistent.

The previously dismal prognosis associated with most rhabdomyosarcomas has improved in the last 20 years as a result of the introduction of combined therapeutic modalities, including surgery, radiotherapy, and chemotherapy. Today, more than 80 percent of patients with localized or regional disease are cured.

Kaposi's Sarcoma

A lesion worthy of special attention is Kaposi's sarcoma, a skin tumor of endothelial cell origin that is typified by irregular bundles of spindle-shaped cells with vascular, slitlike spaces. These spaces are lined by atypical endothelial cells, and contain extravasated erythrocytes. Hemosiderin-laden macrophages are scattered throughout the tumor.

The disease was first described in the 19th century, and was seen in two forms. One occurred among elderly, white people, many of whom had another disease that impaired the immune system. This neoplasm was indolent, but was often followed by another malignant disease, usually a lymphoproliferative disorder. A more aggressive variant of Kaposi's sarcoma commonly occurred in African blacks. The high incidence of this tumor in patients with acquired immunodeficiency syndrome (AIDS) supports the previous theory of a viral etiology in Kaposi's sarcoma. In these patients, the cytomegalovirus has been suggested to play a role.

Synovial Sarcoma

As previously discussed, synovial sarcoma should be considered a soft tissue tumor. The lesion is classically described as having a **biphasic pattern** that forms microscopic spaces in a sarcomatous spindle cell background (Fig. 26-71). These slit-like spaces are filled with fluid similar to hyaluronic acid. If these spaces are not present, a diagnosis of **monophasic sarcoma** may be established, but it is difficult to differentiate such a tumor from fibrosarcoma. Synovial sarcoma often appears to be well circumscribed in the deep tissues of the limbs, a characteristic that may lead to a falsely benign diagnosis. In such cases, the surgeon may "shell out" the lesion, leaving behind small wisps of malignant tumor. The recurrence rate of this tumor is high, and metastases occur in over 60% of cases. The 5-year survival rate is about 50%, and those who die have extensive lung metastases.

SUGGESTED READING

BOOKS

Aviota LV, Crane SM (eds.): Metabolic Bone Disease. New York, Academic Press, 1978

Collins DH: Pathology of Bone. London, Butterworth & Co, 1966

Enzinger FM, Weiss SW: Soft Tissue Tumors. St. Louis, CV Mosby, 1983

Evarts CM (ed.): Surgery of the Musculoskeletal System. New York, Churchill Livingstone, 1983

Kelley WN, Harris ED, Jr, Ruddy S, Sledge CB: Textbook of Rheumatology, 2nd ed. Philadelphia, WB Saunders, 1985

Rodman GP, Shumacher HR (eds.): Primer in the Rheumatic Diseases, 8th ed. Atlanta, GA, Arthritis Foundation, 1983

Spjut HJ, Dorfman HD, Fechner RE, Ackerman LV: Tumors of Bone and Cartilage, Fascicle 5. Armed Forces Institute of Pathology, Washington, DC, 1971

REVIEW ARTICLES

Enneking F, Spanier SS, Goodman MA: A system for the superficial staging of musculoskeletal sarcoma. Clin Orthop 153:106, 1980

Glimcher MJ: On the Form and Function of Bone: from Molecules to Organs. Wolff's Law Revisited. In Veis A (ed.): Chemistry and Biology of Mineralized Connective Tissue. New York, Elsevier-North Holland, 1981

Kane SM: Heberden Oration 1980: Aspects of the cell biology of the rheumatoid lesion. Ann Rheum Dis 40:433–448, 1981

Seminars on Paget's Disease of Bone. Arthritis Rheum 23:1073–1171, 1980

Schiller AL: Diagnosis of borderline cartilage lesions of bone. Semin Diagn Pathol 2:42–61, 1985

Sledge CB: Structure, development, and function of joints. Orthop Clin North Am 6:619–629, 1975

27

Skeletal Muscle

Vernon W. Armbrustmacher

Normal Muscle

Enzyme Histochemical Stains

Muscle Biopsy

Noninflammatory Myopathies

Inflammatory Myopathies

Metabolic Diseases

Denervation

Figure 27-1. Anatomy of skeletal muscle. The composite drawing demonstrates the morphologic features of striated muscle from grossly visible to macromolecular levels. In the upper left, a portion of a muscle is contained by a distinct outer connective tissue layer, called the epimysium or fascia. Fascicles are groups of muscle fibers separated by connective tissue septa called perimysium. Within the fascicle, individual muscle fibers (myofibers) are closely packed and are surrounded by an intricate array of microvasculature and a barely perceptible network of connective tissue called the endomysium. The enlarged fascicle also shows scattered, flattened cells (*green*), called satellite cells, lying on the surface of the fiber. Each muscle fiber is covered by a basement membrane (*orange*) and packed with bundles of myofilaments called myofibrils. The endoplasmic reticulum (sarcoplasmic reticulum) forms an extensive, complex tubular network with periodic dilatations (cisternae) around each myofibril. The cisternae are closely apposed to the transverse tubules, which are derived from the cell membrane (sarcolemma) and form a transverse network, which resembles chicken wire, around each myofibril, giving extensive communication between the internal and external environments. The cross striations of striated muscle are created by the arrangement of the myofilaments of the myofibril. The dark A-band results from the thick myosin filaments and the thinner, partially overlapping actin filaments. In the middle portion of the myosin filaments, where the actin does not overlap, there is a lighter band called the H-zone or H-band. In the middle of the H-band, the center of each myosin filament thickens, forming intermolecular bridging with the adjacent myosin filament and giving rise to the M-line. The finer actin filaments are anchored on the dark Z-disc of the lighter I-band. With contraction, the myosin filaments pull the actin filaments, causing the H-zone to disappear, the A-band to widen, and the I-band to shrink. The mitochondria are scattered throughout the sarcoplasm among the myofibrils. In the final enlargement, the myosin filament is covered with myosin heads that attach to receptor sites on the surrounding actin filaments. The movement of these heads, with attachment and detachment, pulls the actin filaments, ratchet fashion, past the myosin filament.

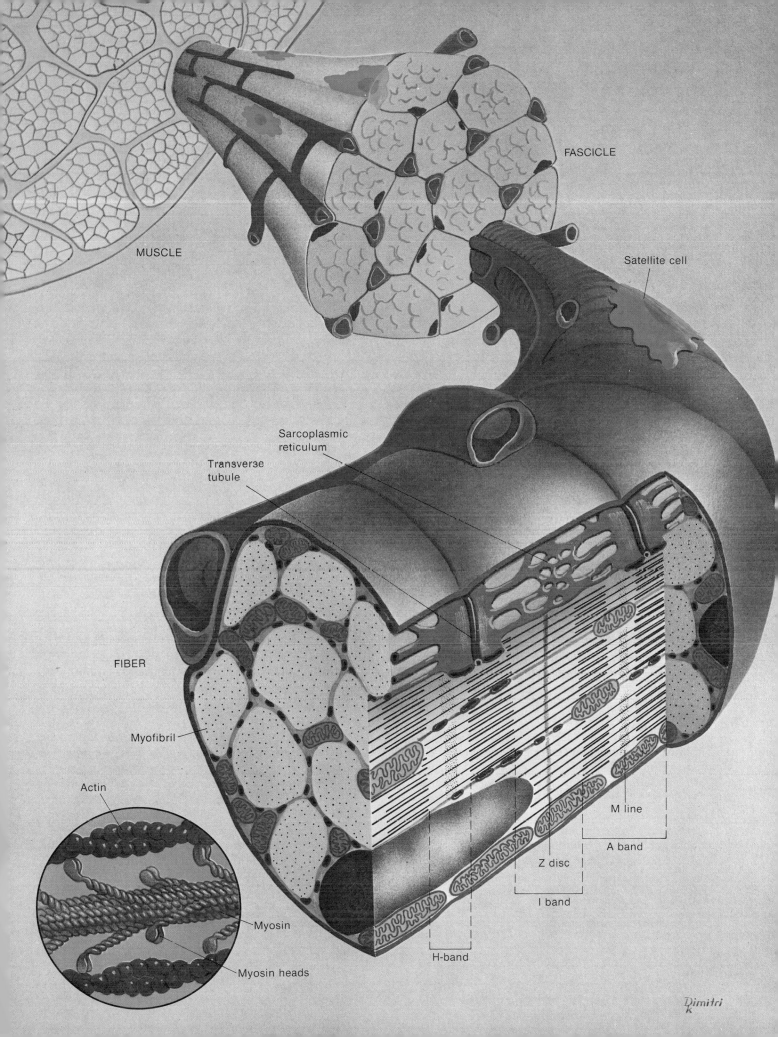

MUSCLE

FASCICLE

Satellite cell

Sarcoplasmic
reticulum

Transverse
tubule

FIBER

Myofibril

Actin

Myosin

Myosin heads

H-band

Z disc

I band

M line

A band

Dimitri
K

Normal Muscle

The myoblast, a primitive cell committed to developing into skeletal muscle, is postmitotic, contains myosin and actin filaments within its cytoplasm, and contains nicotinic receptor sites for acetylcholine on the surface membrane. The myoblast develops the capacity to fuse with other myoblasts to form the multinucleated myotube. This structure soon assumes a cylindrical configuration, with rapid accumulation of myofibrils, composed of, among other proteins, myosin and actin. The myosin and actin become arrayed in a specific pattern, causing the cross-banded pattern seen in striated muscle (see Fig. 27-1). The nuclei of the myotube, situated in the center of the cell, are large and vesicular with a prominent nucleolus. The myotube does not mature completely until it is innervated by the terminus of a lower motor neuron. Prior to innervation the sarcolemma of the myotube contains diffusely distributed nicotinic receptor protein for acetylcholine. When innervation occurs the diffuse nicotinic receptor protein (now designated extrajunctional receptor) disappears from the sarcolemma, except at the developing motor endplate, where it becomes highly concentrated. Possibly, the restriction of this extrajunctional receptor to the motor endplate prevents innervation of a fiber by more than one nerve terminal. Although one muscle fiber is innervated by only one nerve ending, a given motor neuron may innervate numerous muscle fibers. The lower motor neuron and the fibers that it innervates are referred to as the motor unit. The size of a motor unit varies from five to six fibers in the intrinsic muscles of the hand up to 2000 fibers in the belly of the quadriceps femoris muscle. The extraocular muscles are exceptional in that they may have more than one motor endplate per muscle fiber.

Only after innervation has occurred can the muscle fiber progress to maturity. It becomes packed with myofibrils, each myofibril being a cable of myofilaments, and the nuclei arrange themselves in a regular pattern in a subsarcolemmal position. The myofibrils are surrounded by an elaborate membranous network called sarcoplasmic reticulum, which has irregular dilatations (cisternae) that are juxtaposed to a transverse tubular network, which is derived from the sarcolemma itself. This tubular network is transversely arranged across the fiber like chicken wire, each ring wrapping around an individual myofibril. (See Fig. 27-1.) This allows an electrical stimulus proceeding along the surface of the muscle fiber to become diffusely and rapidly internalized by way of the lumen of the transverse tubular system. The electrical signal is translated to a chemical signal between the transverse tubule and the cisternae of the sarcoplasmic reticulum. The chemical signal consists of the release of calcium ion diffusely throughout the sarcoplasm. The chemical signal activates the chemical process that results in muscle contraction.

The functional unit of the myofibril, and therefore of the muscle fiber, is the sarcomere. A single sarcomere extends from one Z-band to the next. The Z-band is a distinct electron-dense band that anchors the thin actin filaments that extend from the Z-disc in hexagonal clusters. The actin filaments surround each thick myosin filament, giving the appearance of a thick dark band, which is designated an A-band. In the midportion of the A-band where the actin filaments end, there is a relatively pale zone called the H-zone. At the midline of the A-band, a zone of intermolecular bridging and thickening of the myosin filaments forms a thin, slightly darker electron-dense band, designated the M-line. Movement occurs by the sliding of the actin filaments past the myosin filaments (see Fig. 27-1).

Another important aspect of maturation which occurs only after innervation is the development of a characteristic metabolic profile for different muscle fibers. It is obvious that not all muscle tissue is the same. Some muscles have a deep red color, while others have a paler or white color. It has been recognized that if a nerve to a dark (red) muscle is stimulated, the resulting contraction is slower and more prolonged than when a nerve to a white muscle is stimulated, the latter stimulation eliciting a faster, shorter, and more powerful contraction. For this reason red muscles have been classified as "slow twitch," while white muscles are labeled as "fast twitch." The red (slow-twitch) fibers tend to have more oxygen-storing red pigment (myoglobin), and more numerous mitochondria. The mitochondrial enzymes of the Krebs cycle, which are responsible for aerobic oxidation, are all present in greater amounts in the red, slow-twitch muscle than in the white, fast-twitch muscle. Glycogen, phosphorylase, and other enzymes in the Embden-Meyerhof pathway, which produces energy by anaerobic glycolysis, are present in high concentrations in white muscle. In the clinical pathologic literature, it has become customary to classify the two types of muscle fibers as either Type I or Type II, Type I corresponding to red muscle and Type II to white muscle. Type I and II fibers are best identified with the alkaline adenosine triphosphatase (ATPase) reaction, which gives a crisp distinction between the two fiber types. Type II fibers stain darkly and Type I are almost unstained (Fig. 27-2A). These staining characteristics are maintained even in the presence of the advanced pathologic alterations due to neuromuscular disease.

It is important to understand that the lower motor neuron determines the fiber type. Although fiber typing does not develop until the muscle is innervated, this process is also reversible. That is, reinnervation of a muscle of one type from the nerve endings of another type causes the muscle to reverse its histochemical profile. It is not clear exactly how the lower motor neuron causes this profound change to occur in muscle fibers, but it is apparent that the rate of discharge or discharge pattern is important. Since the nerve is responsible for determining the fiber type, it follows that all the muscle fibers in a given motor unit are of the same type. When looking at a cross section of human muscle that has been stained with the alkaline ATPase reaction, one sees a random intermixture of fiber types (Fig. 27-2A), because the motor units interdigitate extensively with each other.

There are no muscles that are completely of one type. However, the proportion of fiber types varies from muscle to muscle. For example, the soleus is predominately (up to 80%) Type I. The pattern of fiber types in a given muscle varies between individuals, a difference which is apparently genetically determined. There is some evidence that changing the use of a muscle over a long period through intensive training may change the pattern of muscle fiber types, although this concept is controversial.

Functionally, Type I muscles have the greater capacity for long, sustained contractions, which they can generate without fatigue. A good example of Type I function is seen in a postural muscle, such as the soleus. By contrast, a typical Type II muscle is suitable for rapid, short, powerful contractions. Type II fibers react to training with hypertrophy. Androgenic steroids cause hypertrophy of Type II fibers, and disuse results in their selective atrophy. Type I fibers change very little in size, with or without exercise, but conditioning of these fibers results in increases in those enzymes necessary for aerobic glycolysis.

Enzyme Histochemical Stains

Application of enzyme histochemical reactions is very helpful in the interpretation of pathologic changes in muscle biopsies. The alkaline ATPase reaction, the most important stain for identifying the fiber types, can be reversed by preincubating the sections in an acid buffer, which causes the Type I fibers to become dark and the Type II fibers to be white. This is referred to as the "reverse ATPase reaction".

Another important stain is the nonspecific esterase reaction, in which the Type I fibers are slightly darker than the Type II fibers. This reaction is important in identifying denervation atrophy, since many of the atrophic denervated fibers are selectively stained, whether they are Type I or Type II fibers (Fig. 27-3). Histiocytes are also intensively stained, as are motor endplates, due to their acetylcholine esterase activity. Lipofuscin granules are dark, and in some cases of myotonic dystrophy, there are irregular areas of dark staining in some fibers. A dark rim of staining is normally present around the perimeter of fibers as they insert into the collagen of a tendon.

The reaction product in the nicotinamide adenine dinucleotide–tetrazolium reductase (NADH–TR) reaction, the reduced tetrazolium (formazan), is a dark precipitate that has an affinity for lipid membranes. Therefore, the staining pattern reflects mainly the distribution of the sarcoplasmic reticulum and the mitochondria. Myofibrils are visible as unstained areas. Since Type I fibers have more mitochondria they appear darker with this stain. The fiber type distinction is not as clear as with the ATPase reaction, and many fibers of intermediate density are present. In addition, the fiber type identity is often not maintained in pathologic situations. Fibers that are atrophic due to denervation are often excessively dark, whether they were originally Type I or Type II fibers. The value of this stain is its reflection of the architecture of the membranous organelles. Abnormal collections of mitochondria (as in "ragged red" fibers, Fig. 27-4) and sarcoplasmic masses (aggregates of membranous material in degenerating fiber) are darkly stained. Target fibers characteristic of denervation are best recognized with this stain (Fig. 27-5).

Normally, muscle fibers are unstained with the alkaline phosphatase technique. Small blood vessels (probably arterioles) appear black. However, regenerating fibers are selectively stained. Cases of inflammatory myopathy often exhibit abnormal staining of the perifascicular connective tissue, which may be a helpful sign of the inflammatory nature of the disease (Fig. 27-6).

The PAS stain is helpful for demonstrating the basement membrane of muscle fibers and capillaries. Within the fiber most of the PAS-positive material seen is glycogen, a finely granular material distributed around the myofibrils throughout the fiber. The PAS stain is helpful in the diagnosis of glycogen-storage diseases.

(Text continues on p. 1400)

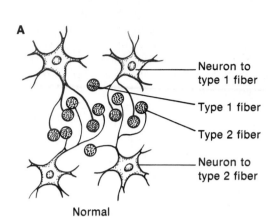

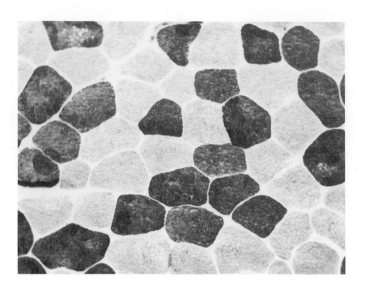

Figure 27-2. Denervation/reinnervation.

(*A*) **Normal.** Two neurons (*red*), representing Type I neurons, each innervate a number of muscle fibers, causing them to be Type I fibers (*red*). These fibers are intermixed with Type II fibers (*black*), innervated by Type II neurons. The photomicrograph shows the normal intermixed distribution of Type I (*light*) and Type II (*dark*) muscle fibers as demonstrated by staining for ATPase.

(*B*) **Denervation.** With early (mild) denervation, portions of the axonal tree degenerate, resulting in angular atrophy of scattered Type I and Type II muscle fibers. In the photomicrograph, a modified Gomori trichrome stain shows a single angular atrophic muscle fiber. With more advanced (severe) denervation, entire lower motor neurons or numerous axonal processes degenerate, causing groups of angular atrophic fibers to appear. In the photomicrograph, a hematoxylin and eosin stain shows groups of angular atrophic Type I and Type II muscle fibers.

(*C*) **Reinnervation.** As neurons degenerate, surviving neurons grow more nerve endings and reinnervate all or some of the denervated fibers, depending on the magnitude of the denervating process. These reinnervated fibers become Type I or Type II, depending on the type of neuron that reinnervates them. This process results in fewer, but larger, motor units and the appearance of clusters of fibers of one type adjacent to clusters of the other type, a pattern called type grouping. In the photomicrograph, a stain for ATPase demonstrates type grouping. (Compare with the normal pattern illustrated in the photomicrograph in *A*.) Depending on the tempo of the denervating process, there may or may not be other evidence of denervation (e.g., target fibers, scattered angular atrophic fibers or group atrophy). This field would appear normal if it were stained with hematoxylin and eosin.

B DENERVATION

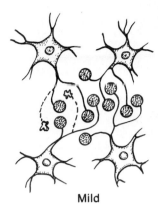

Mild

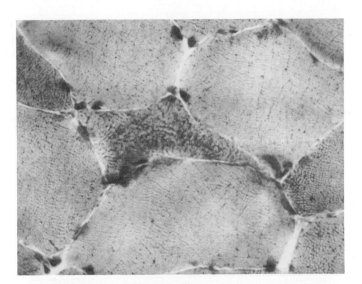

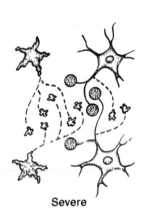

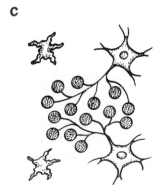

Severe

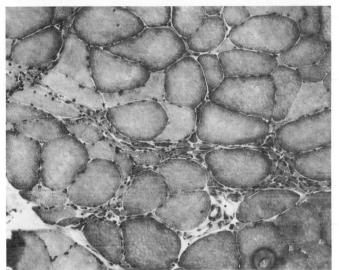

C

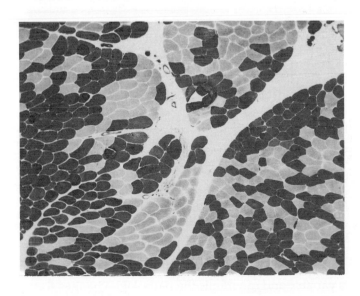

REINNERVATION WITH "TYPE GROUPING"

Mild

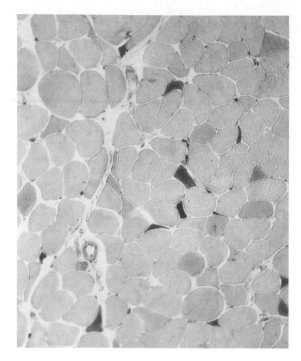

Figure 27-3. Denervation atrophy. A cross section of striated muscle treated with a nonspecific esterase stain shows scattered angular atrophic fibers that are excessively stained, a feature typical of denervation atrophy.

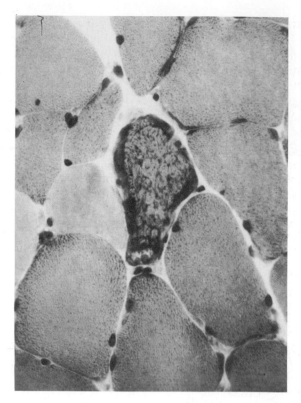

Figure 27-4. Mitochondrial myopathy. A cross section of striated muscle treated with a modified Gomori trichrome stain shows a single fiber containing abundant, coarse, granular, brilliant red material—a so-called "ragged red fiber." Electron microscopy reveals that the red material consists of aggregates of pleomorphic mitochondria.

Muscle Biopsy

Most neuromuscular diseases are generalized, and therefore the pathologic changes can be demonstrated in biopsy specimens from almost any muscle. It is advantageous to limit the biopsy to the same muscle from case to case because the normal pattern, which varies considerably from muscle to muscle, is more constant. Biopsies from either the quadriceps femoris or the biceps brachii are suitable for biopsy in most neuromuscular diseases. However, some conditions are more focal, and judgment must be exercised accordingly. Biopsy from minimally, but definitely, involved muscle is desired because the earliest changes are the most informative for understanding the pathophysiology of the disease. The surgeon should also avoid the site of a tendon insertion because the histology of a normal myotendinous area is variable and can mimic the pathologic changes seen in some neuromuscular diseases.

Noninflammatory Myopathies

Muscular Dystrophy

The term muscular dystrophy was developed in the middle of the nineteenth century, as recognition was given to the fact that diseases characterized by progressive weakness of the voluntary muscles could be due either to involvement of the nervous system or to primary degeneration of muscles. The term muscular dystrophy was applied to the latter group, which was frequently found to be hereditary, or at least familial, and relentlessly progressive. Morphologic study of muscle tissue from these patients, obtained with a "muscle harpoon," showed degeneration of muscle fibers, with regenerative activity, progressive fibrosis, and infiltration of the muscle with fatty tissue (Fig. 27-7). No inflammation was recognized.

In subsequent years many variants of this type of

muscle disease were described, and a classification of hereditary, progressive, noninflammatory degenerative conditions of muscle has been developed. In none of these conditions is the exact metabolic defect defined. Application of new techniques in the study of neuromuscular disease has led to the reevaluation and reclassification of some of these entities. In general, many of these conditions show similar pathologic alterations, that is, evidence of a chronic, active, noninflammatory myopathic process. The identification of a specific disease is a clinical decision that must be based on the family history, clinical symptoms, physical findings, laboratory data, and histologic changes.

Progressive Muscular Dystrophy (Duchenne Muscular Dystrophy)

Duchenne muscular dystrophy, the most clearly defined noninflammatory myopathy, is a severe, progressive, sex-linked, recessively inherited condition. Boys with Duchenne muscular dystrophy have markedly elevated serum creatine kinase from birth and morphologically abnormal muscle, even *in utero*. The clinical weakness is not detectable during the first year and usually becomes evident during the third or fourth year. The weakness is noted mainly around the pelvic and shoulder girdles (proximal muscle weakness) and is relentlessly progressive.

The patients are usually wheelchair-bound by the age of 10 years and bedridden by the age of 15. The most common causes of death are complications of respiratory insufficiency caused by the muscular weakness, or cardiac arrhythmia due to myocardial involvement. The patients have a striking tendency to form contractures when immobilized for a short period of time, even as a result of such minor trauma as a muscle biopsy. For this reason biopsies should be done only if necessary to establish the diagnosis, and biopsy samples should be taken from the quadriceps muscle rather than the gastrocnemius muscle. The weak muscles eventually become atrophic and are replaced by fibrofatty tissue. Eventually, a "pseudohypertrophy" of the calf muscles develops.

Occasional cases that are indistinguishable from Duchenne muscular dystrophy but occur in girls may represent a genetically different disease, a nonrandom inactivation of the X chromosome, or Turner's Syndrome (XO) with a Duchenne-dystrophy-carrying chromosome.

The earliest pathologic changes in the muscle tissue consist of scattered foci of degenerating and regenerating muscle fibers, together with scattered,

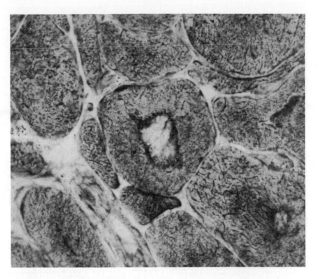

Figure 27-5. Target fiber. A cross section of striated muscle treated with an NADH–TR stain demonstrates a "target fiber," a characteristic feature of some cases of denervation. Since the stain is selectively fixed to membranous organelles, the centers of the target fibers appear devoid of mitochondrial and sarcoplasmic reticulum. The myofibrils may or may not be intact. Target fibers are seen in 20% or less of cases of denervation.

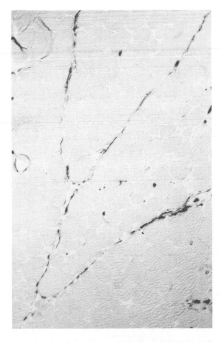

Figure 27-6. Polymyositis. A cross section of skeletal muscle treated with an alkaline phosphatase stain shows the normally unstained fibers. The staining of the perifascicular connective tissue is not normal, however, and is often seen in inflammatory myopathies.

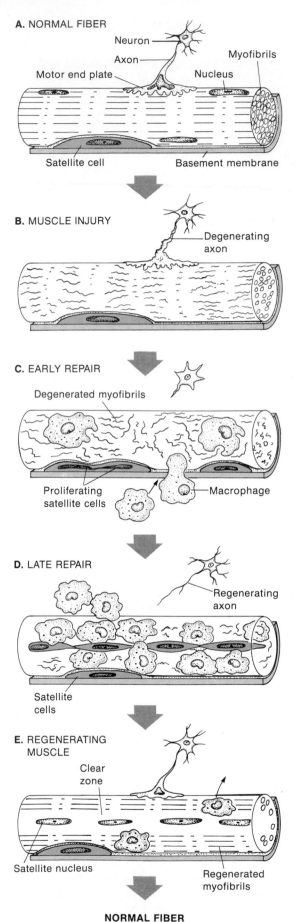

A. NORMAL FIBER

Neuron
Axon
Myofibrils
Motor end plate
Nucleus
Satellite cell
Basement membrane

B. MUSCLE INJURY

Degenerating axon

C. EARLY REPAIR

Degenerated myofibrils
Proliferating satellite cells
Macrophage

D. LATE REPAIR

Regenerating axon
Satellite cells

E. REGENERATING MUSCLE

Clear zone
Satellite nucleus
Regenerated myofibrils

NORMAL FIBER

Figure 27-7. Degeneration/regeneration.

(*A*) A normal muscle fiber, communicating with the lower motor neuron via the motor endplate, contains subsarcolemmal nuclei, is packed with myofibrils, and is covered by a basement membrane. Scattered satellite cells are situated on the surface of the sarcolemma, but inside the basement membrane. These are dormant myoblasts, capable of proliferating and differentiating into muscle fibers. They constitute 3% to 5% of the nuclei seen in a cross section of skeletal muscle.

(*B*) In types of injury to the muscle fiber that preserve the integrity of the basement membrane (such as alcoholic rhabdomyolysis, Duchenne muscular dystrophy, or polymyositis) the sarcoplasmic structures begin to disintegrate and the terminus of the motor endplate breaks down.

(*C*) The damaged fiber attracts circulating macrophages, which penetrate the basement membrane and begin to digest and engulf the sarcoplasmic contents (myophagocytosis). In the meantime, regenerative processes begin with the activation and proliferation of the satellite cells, which, in contrast to the macrophages, are confined by the intact cylinder of basement membrane.

(*D*) At a later stage, myophagocytosis is prominent, satellite cells have proliferated and are beginning to fuse, protein synthesis has begun, and the damaged axon terminus is beginning to regenerate.

(*E*) Regeneration is prominent. The nuclei of the regenerating fiber are immature (large, vesicular with nucleoli) and centrally located. Myofibrils are developing, mostly at the periphery, and the ribosome-rich sarcoplasm appears basophilic with a hematoxylin and eosin stain. The motor endplate has reformed at its original site. This fiber will process to complete maturity, reconstituted as in *A*.

large, hyalinized dark fibers, which are overly contracted and in an early stage of degeneration (Fig. 27-8). Breakdown of the sarcolemma, which probably accounts for the early striking elevation of serum creatine kinase in these patients, is one of the earliest ultrastructural changes noted. Myophagocytosis, the infiltration of histiocytes into degenerating muscle fibers, is almost invariable but does not reflect an inflammatory process. There is a brisk regenerative response to the degeneration. These regenerating fibers, which are alkaline phosphatase positive, have more basophilic sarcoplasm, as seen with the hematoxylin and eosin stain, and have large vesicular nuclei with prominent nucleoli (see Fig. 27-8).

Another typical change of Duchenne dystrophy is endomysial fibrosis, which develops early and becomes prominent with time. The process consists of constant focal degeneration of muscle fibers, with a prolonged effort at repair and regeneration, together with progressive fibrosis. The degenerative process eventually outstrips the regenerative capacity of the muscle. As a consequence there is a progressively decreasing number of muscle fibers and increasing amounts of fibrofatty connective tissue. The end stage is characterized by an almost complete loss of skeletal muscle fibers, but an interesting sparing of the muscle spindle fibers. The muscle spindle is surrounded by a capsule that creates a blood–spindle barrier similar to the blood–brain barrier. The sparing of the spindle fibers and the predominantly left ventricular, subendocardial involvement in the heart raise the possibility that a noxious circulating factor mediates the damage selectively to striated muscle cells. A search for such a circulating factor has been unsuccessful.

Enzyme histochemical studies of skeletal muscle demonstrate that both fiber types are equally affected, and there is no excess staining of the endomysial connective tissue with the alkaline phosphatase reaction, such as is seen in primary inflammatory myopathies.

Carrier Detection

Since Duchenne muscular dystrophy is inherited as an X-linked recessive disease, there is considerable interest in attempting to identify women who might be carriers. At present the best method of detecting carriers is multiple determination of serum creatine kinase levels. Biopsy of putative carriers adds little information. In the best of hands no more than 70%–80% of carriers can be detected, so that a woman who is a potential carrier cannot be assured that she is not

a carrier. There is considerable variability in expression of the carrier state, probably because of variations in the random inactivation of the X chromosome (the Lyon hypothesis). In addition, there is a high spontaneous mutation rate (30% of cases), which indicates that the woman would have no expression of the condition, since she would not be heterozygous.

The gene for Duchenne muscular dystrophy has now been identified. After it has been sequenced and cloned, the detection of the carrier state and an understanding of the pathogenesis of the disease should be facilitated.

Other Forms of Muscular Dystrophy

Many other forms of muscular dystrophy have been described. With improved techniques, reevaluation of many of these conditions has resulted in reclassification of the diseases into chronic forms of lower motor neuron disease or a variety of other metabolic conditions. Therefore, it has been recommended that some of these conditions be designated syndromes, rather than diseases.

Congenital Myopathies

Occasionally a newborn infant manifests generalized hypotonia, with decreased deep tendon reflexes and muscle bulk. Many of these children have a difficult perinatal period because of the weakness of respirations and consequent pulmonary complications. Some have a "malignant" hypotonia, which is progressive and results in death within the first twelve months of life. Werdnig-Hoffmann disease and infantile acid maltase deficiency (Pompe's disease) are examples. In other cases, the weakness is severe, but apparently not progressive.

Some of these hypotonic patients never become ambulatory and develop severe secondary skeletal complications, such as kyphoscoliosis, due to the hypotonia and debility. Careful study may reveal a mild form of nonprogressive lower motor neuron disease, sometimes designated Kugelberg-Welander disease or spinal muscular atrophy. Other hypotonic patients may have one of the metabolic diseases (see below).

Finally, some hypotonic patients have a "benign" course. Although the hypotonia persists throughout their lives, it is not progressive and they become ambulatory and live a normal life span, somewhat complicated by secondary skeletal complications of the hypotonia. It is this group of patients that is

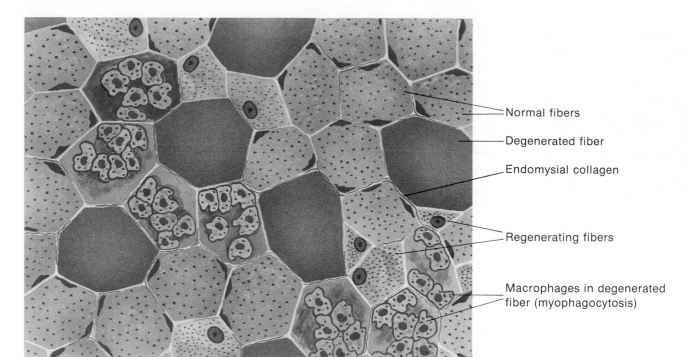

Normal fibers

Degenerated fiber

Endomysial collagen

Regenerating fibers

Macrophages in degenerated fiber (myophagocytosis)

Figure 27-8. Duchenne muscular dystrophy. The pathologic changes seen in skeletal muscle as stained with the modified Gomori trichrome stain are illustrated. Some fibers are slightly larger and darker than normal. These represent overcontracted segments of sarcoplasm situated between degenerated segments. Some fibers are packed with phagocytes (myophagocytosis) clearing out degenerated sarcoplasm. Some fibers are smaller than normal and have granular sarcoplasm. These fibers have enlarged, vesicular nuclei with prominent nucleoli and represent regenerating fibers. Developing endomysial fibrosis is represented by the deposition of collagen around individual muscle fibers. The changes are those of a chronic, active noninflammatory myopathy.

subsumed in the category of "congenital myopathies."

Morphologic study of the muscle of some patients with congenital myopathy reveals three distinct groups of conditions, although variations in presentation often make the exact diagnosis difficult. The three groups are central core disease, nemaline (rod) myopathy, and central nuclear myopathy. (See Fig. 27-9.)

Some generalizations can be made about these three conditions. In addition to presenting with congenital hypotonia, decreased deep tendon reflexes, decreased muscle bulk, and delayed motor milestones, the morphologic abnormality expressed in the muscle biopsy in all three conditions is confined to the Type I (red) fibers. Furthermore, these patients have an abnormal predominance of Type I fibers or, perhaps more accurately, a failure of Type II (white) fibers to develop. The skeletal muscle does not show signs of active degeneration, and the patients do not ordinarily have elevated levels of serum creatine kinase.

Central Core Disease

Central core disease can be sporadic, autosomal recessive, or autosomal dominant. It is characterized by congenital hypotonia, with proximal muscle weakness, decreased deep tendon reflexes, and delayed motor development. A typical patient does become ambulatory, although the muscle strength never develops to a normal level.

Muscle biopsy typically reveals a striking predominance of Type I fibers. In many or all of the Type I fibers there is a central zone of degeneration that is best seen with the NADH tetrazolium reductase reaction. This is referred to as a central core abnormality and is characterized by loss of membranous organelles, with or without disorganization of the myofibrillar architecture. This central core runs the entire length of the fiber. It is difficult to see with the hematoxylin and eosin stain, but can often be demonstrated with a PAS reaction (Fig. 27-9B). Electron microscopic study reveals that membranous organelles are absent in the central portion of the core but condense around its margin. The ultrastructure of the fiber is otherwise unremarkable. The myofibrils may show considerable disorganization or may be intact.

The central core anomaly bears a striking resemblance to the target fibers (see Fig. 27-5) seen in active denervating conditions. However, no evidence of active denervation is seen in patients with central core disease. The motor endplates are architecturally unremarkable, and no extrajunctional nicotinic acetylcholine receptors are present in the muscle membrane.

Rod (Nemaline) Myopathy

This myopathy was initially named "nemaline" myopathy because the inclusions within the muscle fiber were interpreted as a tangled, threadlike mass. Since then it has been determined that the inclusions are clusters of rod-shaped inclusions, and the term rod myopathy has become established.

This entity probably includes a heterogeneous group of diseases that have in common the accumulation of rodlike inclusions within the sarcoplasm of skeletal muscle. The classic congenital form is characterized by congenital hypotonia and a clinical course of delayed motor milestones of variable clinical severity, with associated secondary skeletal changes, such as kyphoscoliosis. In some cases there is severe involvement of muscles of the face, pharynx and neck. Later-onset (childhood and adult) forms have been noted, and these tend to be associated with some muscle degeneration, elevations of serum creatine kinase levels, and a slowly progressive course. Many patients originally designated as having limb girdle muscular dystrophy have eventually been found to have rod myopathy.

The pathologic findings on muscle biopsy consist of a variable predominance of Type I fibers and the accumulation of rod-shaped structures within the sarcoplasm of the skeletal muscle. These inclusions, found mostly in the Type I fibers, are brilliant red when stained with the modified Gomori trichrome stain (Fig. 27-9C) and may or may not be visible with a standard hematoxylin and eosin stain. The rods are almost always positive with a phosphotungstic acid hematoxylin (PTAH) reaction and are negative with the ATPase and NADH tetrazolium reductase stains. Ultrastructural studies demonstrate that the inclusions are indeed rod-shaped and can be seen to arise from the Z-band, which they resemble ultrastructurally. The etiology of the condition is unknown.

It should be pointed out that rods have been described in a variety of neuromuscular diseases, including denervation atrophy, muscular dystrophy, and inflammatory myopathies. They can be produced experimentally in tenotomy preparations, in which the peripheral nerve is intact. In rod myopathy, however, they constitute the predominant pathologic change.

Central Nuclear Myopathy (Myotubular Myopathy)

Central nuclear myopathy is also clinically and genetically heterogeneous. It has been recognized as an autosomal recessive, autosomal dominant, and X-linked recessive condition. In the X-linked recessively inherited condition the newborn infant is strikingly weak and hypotonic and may die of respiratory insufficiency during the neonatal period. The autosomal dominant form tends to be of later onset and is associated with modestly elevated serum creatine kinase levels. It has a slowly progressive course and, like rod myopathy, resembles the so-called limb girdle muscular dystrophy syndrome. In some patients, there is striking involvement of the facial and extraocular musculature.

Biopsy specimens from patients with central nuclear myopathy are variable, but are characterized by Type I predominance; many of the Type I fibers are small and round, with a single central nucleus (Fig. 27-9D). In this respect they resemble the myotubular stage in the embryogenesis of skeletal muscle. For this reason considerable interest has been generated in the relationship of the lower motor neuron to the muscle fiber, since it is recognized that the trophic influence of the lower motor neuron is necessary for subsequent maturation of the fiber. Studies of the lower motor neuron, including the motor endplate, have failed to demonstrate any abnormality in these patients. The later onset forms of myotubular myopathy are characterized morphologically by more mature muscle fibers (i.e., the fibers are larger and have more numerous myofibrils). The single central nucleus also appears more mature.

Patients have been described with a Type I predominance of muscle fibers in which the Type I fibers are smaller and more round than normal, but do not contain a single central nucleus. This condition has been designated as "congenital fiber type disproportion," but some authors feel that it represents a variant of central nuclear myopathy.

Inflammatory Myopathies

Inflammatory myopathies are easily recognized, the hallmark being an unequivocal inflammatory infiltrate within the skeletal muscle. In this category we do not include conditions caused by known infectious agents, but rather those in which the muscle tissue itself is the primary target of the inflammatory reaction. This targeting may be highly specific, as in polymyositis, or generalized, as in some of the diffuse collagen vascular diseases.

Figure 27-9.   Congenital myopathies.
(*A*) **Normal.** A microscopic field of a frozen section of normal skeletal muscle stained with the modified Gomori trichrome (MGT) stain is depicted. The nuclei are purple, the membranous organelles (mitochondria and sarcoplasmic reticulum) are red, myofibrils are light green, and perifascicular collagen is light green. The fibers are of uniform size and somewhat polygonal.
(*B*) **Central core myopathy** (MGT stain). Many fibers are slightly smaller than normal and contain a round central core that is devoid of membranous organelles, which form a condensed ring around the core. Staining for ATPase would identify the fibers with cores as Type I. The cores run the length of the muscle fiber. "Core fibers" resemble target fibers (see Fig. 27-5), although, as yet, no neuropathic process has been demonstrated in central core disease.
(*C*) **Rod myopathy** (MGT stain). Many fibers are slightly smaller than normal and contain brilliant red granules. The abnormal fibers would all be identified as Type I with an ATPase stain. Electron microscopy would reveal the granules to be clusters of electron-dense, rod-shaped structures that arise from the Z-band.
(*D*) **Central nuclear myopathy** (MGT stain). Many fibers are smaller and rounder than normal. Some contain a round central pole zone, while others contain a single, central nucleus. Again, ATPase staining would identify the abnormal fibers as Type I. These fibers resemble the myotube stage of the embryogenesis of skeletal muscle.

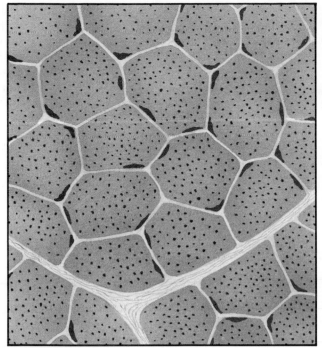

A. NORMAL

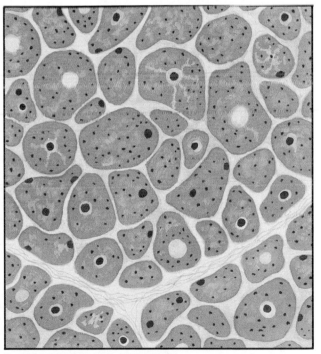

B. CENTRAL CORE DISEASE

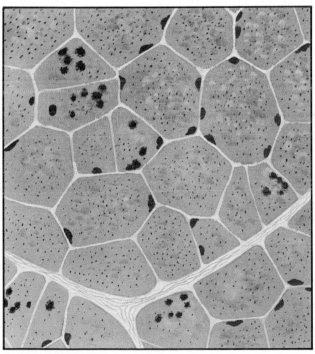

C. ROD MYOPATHY

D. CENTRONUCLEAR MYOPATHY

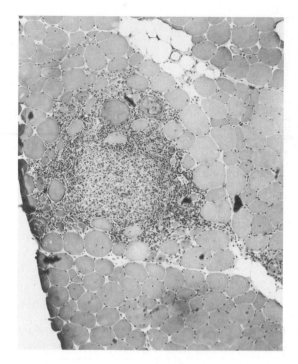

Figure 27-10. Polymyositis. With hematoxylin and eosin staining a cross section of skeletal muscle shows a focus of mononuclear inflammation within a muscle fascicle. At the perimeter of the inflammatory focus there is a zone of degenerating and regenerating fibers. A biopsy could easily miss the focus of inflammation but would probably show the scattered degenerating and regenerating fibers.

Polymyositis/Dermatomyositis

Polymyositis, an inflammatory myopathy of unknown etiology, is characterized by an inflammatory reaction of mononuclear cells (lymphocytes and histiocytes) confined to the striated muscle. Cardiac muscle is not involved. The onset of the disease is usually subacute and often follows a "viral syndrome" by several days or weeks. Untreated, the disease is characterized by exacerbations and remissions, with progressive weakness and, ultimately, a high mortality rate. The patients present with muscular pain, and proximal muscle weakness, often accompanied by difficulty in swallowing. Most often seen in young adult women, the disease also occurs in young children and older patients. Rarely, the disease is insidious and only slowly progressive, in which case it may be difficult to distinguish from a chronic form of muscular dystrophy. At the other extreme, the disease may be fulminant and resemble an episode of acute rhabdomyolysis.

Patients with polymyositis respond dramatically to corticosteroid therapy. However, as the patient is being tapered from the steroids, remissions may occur, in which case the corticosteroid therapy must be reinstituted. These patients have a moderate to markedly elevated serum creatine kinase level, together with an elevated erythrocyte sedimentation rate. In addition to the skeletal muscle symptoms and signs, some develop an erythematous skin rash, in which case the disease is designated dermatomyositis. Whether or not there is skin involvement, the disease typically responds to corticosteroid therapy. When dermatomyositis or polymyositis occurs in a middle-aged man, there is an associated increased risk of an epithelial cancer, most commonly carcinoma of the lung.

Biopsy of skeletal muscle in patients with polymyositis ordinarily demonstrates the inflammatory nature of the myopathy (Fig. 27-10). Scattered degenerating and regenerating muscle fibers are surrounded by a focal or diffuse mononuclear infiltrate that occurs in the endomysium and the interstitium, as well as around blood vessels. However, because of the focal nature of the inflammatory infiltrate, a given biopsy may show degenerating and regenerating fibers, but no evidence of inflammation. Thus the apparent absence of inflammation does not rule out an inflammatory myopathy.

Another morphologic feature that reveals the inflammatory nature of polymyositis is a pattern recognized as "perifascicular atrophy." In these biopsy specimens the periphery of a fascicle or group of fascicles shows degeneration and regeneration. Even in the absence of an inflammatory infiltrate, this pattern strongly suggests polymyositis.

A third helpful finding in a biopsy without definite inflammation is the presence of an abnormal staining of the endomysial connective tissue with the alkaline phosphatase reaction, which also selectively demonstrates regenerating muscle fibers.

The presence of eosinophils in the inflammatory infiltrate may be associated with the extremely rare eosinophilic polymyositis, but is more often associated with a parasitic infestation, typically *Trichinella spiralis*. So-called eosinophilic polymyositis probably represents a manifestation of "hypereosinophilic syndrome," a diffuse inflammatory condition that affects many organs, responds poorly to corticosteroids, and has a poor prognosis.

Occasionally, one sees a granulomatous inflammatory infiltrate in skeletal muscle. The most common cause is sarcoidosis, in which condition the granulomas infiltrate the endomysium, but do not destroy the muscle fibers. These patients also do not have elevated serum creatine kinase. In the analysis of granulomas, special stains for fungal and acid fast organisms should be used and serial sections to search for parasites should be carried out. A rare primary granulomatous polymyositis has been reported, which seems to respond to corticosteroid therapy.

Metabolic Diseases

The skeletal muscle tissue is dramatically affected by a variety of generalized diseases, such as Cushing's disease, Addison's disease, hypothyroidism, hyperthyroidism, and conditions associated with hepatic or renal failure. In the following disorders, however, a primary abnormality in the metabolism of skeletal muscle results in the abnormal function of the muscle.

Glycogen Storage Diseases (Glycogenoses)

The glycogen storage diseases are inherited metabolic disorders characterized by an interference in the ability to metabolize glycogen. A genetic mutation affecting the function of any of the enzymes associated with glycogen synthesis or breakdown could theoretically cause a glycogenosis. There are in excess of a dozen known glycogenoses caused by abnormalities of different enzymes involved in glycogen metabolism. An enzyme can have many different genetic lesions, which can cause variations in the manifestations associated with deficiency of a given enzyme activity.

For the purpose of this discussion we identify five conditions that significantly affect the function of skeletal muscle. When these conditions were described initially, they were often identified according to the individual who recognized the abnormality (Pompe's disease, McArdle's disease). Later, as the specific enzyme deficiency was identified, the disorder was classified according to the deficient enzyme (acid maltase deficiency, myophosphorylase deficiency). However, it is now recognized that different genetic mutations can affect the same enzyme and lead to different clinical syndromes. For example, this results in the recognition of infantile acid maltase deficiency and adult-onset acid maltase deficiency.

Another nomenclature attaches a Roman numeral to the enzyme deficiency. For instance, Pompe's disease (acid maltase deficiency, infantile acid maltase deficiency) is also known as Type II glycogenosis.

Type II Glycogenosis (Acid Maltase Deficiency, Alpha-1,4- Glucosidase Deficiency, Pompe's Disease)

Various genetic mutations affect the acid maltase activity of muscle and lead to distinctly different clinical syndromes. The first acid maltase deficiency to be recognized, described by Pompe, is the most severe form and occurs in the neonatal or early infantile stage. These patients have severe hypotonia and areflexia, and clinically resemble patients with Werdnig-Hoffmann disease (discussed later, under "Denervation"). Sometimes the patients have an enlarged tongue and cardiomegaly and, in fact, cardiac failure is a common cause of death, usually within the first year or two of life. The serum creatine kinase level is only slightly to moderately elevated. Many tissues are affected, but the most significant involvement is in skeletal and cardiac muscle, the central nervous system, and the liver.

In all forms of glycogenosis due to acid maltase deficiency the morphologic changes are distinctive and almost pathognomonic. Acid maltase is a lysosomal enzyme that participates in the degradation of glycogen. When the enzyme is deficient, glycogen is not broken down, accumulates within lysosomes, and remains membrane-bound. The muscle in Pompe's disease displays massive accumulation of membrane-bound glycogen and apparent lysis of the myofilaments and other sarcoplasmic organelles. Surprisingly, there is very little regeneration, and apparently inactive satellite cells are seen on the surface of muscle fibers which have been almost completely destroyed by the disease process.

The late infantile, juvenile, and adult-onset forms of the disease are milder and the morphologic changes are more subtle. By light microscopy, only small, rounded, empty vacuoles are noted, which are PAS positive and disappear on predigestion with diastase (Fig. 27-11). Ultrastructurally scattered small membrane-bound vacuoles filled with glycogen granules are found. The diagnosis should be confirmed with an assay of the muscle for acid maltase activity.

Many patients with the later onset form of the disease have a mild but relentlessly progressive myopathy, which in the past was often mistaken for limb girdle muscular dystrophy.

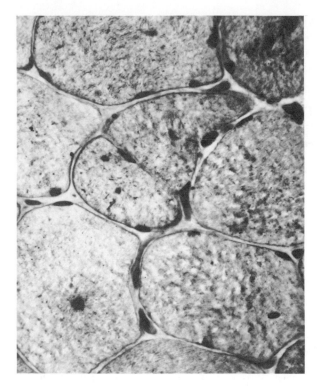

Figure 27-11. Acid maltase deficiency—adult onset. A cross section of skeletal muscle treated with a PAS stain shows dark-stained granules in the cytoplasm. These disappear on predigestion with diastase, proving that they are glycogen. The reason they are present as coarse granules is that they are membrane-bound, a hallmark of acid maltase deficiency.

Type III Glycogenosis (Debranching Enzyme Deficiency, Cori's Disease, Forbes' Disease, Limit Dextrinosis, Amylo-1,6-Glucosidase Deficiency)

Type III glycogenosis is an extremely rare glycogenosis that may affect children or adults and is inherited as an autosomal recessive trait. Hepatomegaly and growth retardation are usual. The muscle involvement and symptoms are variable, and the most severe and consistent involvement is related to liver dysfunction. These patients are unable to hydrolyze glycogen beyond the 1,4-glycosidic linkages, owing to the absence of a debranching enzyme which cleaves the 1,6-glycosidic bonds. Glycogen without surface 1,4-glycosidic chains is referred to as "limit dextrin."

Electron microscopy reveals masses of glycogen granules free in the sarcoplasm, an appearance similar to that in other forms of glycogenosis. A definitive diagnosis rests on the biochemical demonstration of the absence of debranching enzyme activity.

Type V Glycogenosis (McArdle's Disease, Myophosphorylase Deficiency)

Type V glycogenosis, a more common metabolic myopathy, is usually not progressive and is usually not severely debilitating. The absence of myophosphorylase causes muscle cramps with exercise. If the patients avoid strenuous exercise, the disease does not seriously interfere with their lives. However, persistence in exercise may lead to massive rhabdomyolysis and severe metabolic consequences. The absence of myophosphorylase activity renders the skeletal muscle glycogen inaccessible for energy production during periods of physical exertion.

These patients are unable to produce lactate during ischemic exercise, a defect that is the basis of a metabolic test for the condition. The muscle biopsy may appear completely normal, except for the complete absence of phosphorylase activity. However, there is usually some evidence of abnormal accumulation of glycogen granules within the sarcoplasm, predominantly within the subsarcolemmal area (Fig. 27-12). The diagnosis can be specifically made histochemically or biochemically by the absence of myophosphorylase activity.

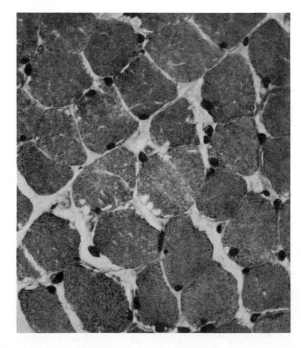

Figure 27-12. McArdle's disease (myophosphorylase deficiency). A cross section of skeletal muscle treated with hematoxylin and eosin shows that some fibers have subsarcolemmal vacuoles that appear empty. Electron microscopy, however, demonstrates that they consist of masses of glycogen granules, non-membrane-bound, in the sarcoplasm.

Type VII Glycogenosis (Tarui's Disease, Phosphofructokinase Deficiency)

Phosphofructokinase deficiency is less common than McArdle's disease, but causes an identical clinical syndrome. Phosphofructokinase is a key enzyme in the Embden-Myerhof pathway that catalyzes the conversion of fructose-6-phosphate to fructose-1,6-diphosphate. In muscle this enzyme is composed of two identical subunits (MM), whereas in erythrocytes it consists of two nonidentical subunits (MR), each under separate genetic control. As a result, a genetic lack of the muscle subunit results in a complete absence of phosphofructokinase activity in muscle, but only a 50% decrease in activity in erythrocytes.

These patients often have a slight anemia or low-grade hemolysis (decreased erythrocyte survival, elevated reticulocyte count).

The morphologic findings are identical to those in McArdle's disease, except that these patients have phosphorylase activity. Confirmation of the diagnosis is made by quantitative biochemical assay of phosphofructokinase activity in skeletal muscle.

Lipid Myopathies

Occasionally, the muscle biopsy specimen from patients with exercise intolerance or muscle weakness exhibits an accumulation of neutral lipid vacuoles. When the number of mitochondria is also increased, the cases are referred to as mitochondrial myopathies (see Fig. 27-4). Such conditions are probably caused by a variety of metabolic conditions affecting lipid metabolism.

Carnitine Palmityl Transferase Deficiency

Patients with carnitine palmityl transferase deficiency are unable to metabolize long-chain fatty acids because of an inability to transport these lipids into the mitochondria for beta oxidation. After prolonged exercise, these individuals characteristically have muscular pain, which may progress to severe rhabdomyolysis. Prolonged fasting can produce the same symptoms. Biopsy specimens show no microscopic abnormalities. The diagnosis depends on the biochemical assay for carnitine palmityl transferase activity.

Carnitine Deficiency

Carnitine, which is synthesized in the liver and is present in large quantities in skeletal muscle, is necessary for the transport of long-chain fatty acids into the mitochondria. Patients with muscle carnitine deficiency have progressive proximal muscle weakness and atrophy and often show signs of denervation and peripheral neuropathy.

The absence of carnitine leads to massive accumulation of lipids outside the mitochondria. The activity of carnitine palmityl transferase activity is normal, but carnitine levels are diminished. Sometimes oral carnitine therapy, with or without associated corticosteroid therapy, may alleviate the symptoms.

Rhabdomyolysis

Rhabdomyolysis refers to a diffuse destruction or lysis of skeletal muscle fibers. It is analogous to hemolytic anemia and has many causes, only some of which are known. Rhabdomyolysis may be acute, subacute, or chronic. When acute, the sarcoplasmic contents are poured into the circulation, an event which may result in myoglobinuria and acute renal failure. During acute rhabdomyolysis the muscles are swollen and tender, and there is profound weakness. Occasionally, an episode may complicate or follow an episode of "flu".

Some patients develop rhabdomyolysis with apparently mild exercise and probably have some form of ill-defined metabolic myopathy. After recovery a subsequent biopsy may reveal muscle that is morphologically normal.

Rhabdomyolysis may also complicate heat stroke and malignant hyperthermia after the administration of a triggering anesthetic agent, such as halothane. Alcohol intoxication is occasionally associated with either acute or chronic rhabdomyolysis.

The pathologic changes are classified as a noninflammatory myopathy, with varying degrees of degeneration and regeneration of muscle fibers. Clusters of macrophages are seen in and around muscle fibers, but these are not accompanied by lymphocytes or other inflammatory cells (see Fig. 27-7).

Myoadenylate Deaminase Deficiency

A staining technique that can be applied to gels used for electrophoretic separations or to frozen sections of skeletal muscle has been developed for the demonstration of the enzyme adenosine monophosphate deaminase (AMP-DA). This enzyme is present in large quantities in skeletal muscle, particularly in the Type II fibers. It is an important enzyme in the regulation of the purine nucleotide cycle that helps to maintain the ATP/ADP ratio during exercise.

A group of patients who suffer from mild proximal

muscle weakness and exercise intolerance has been found to have complete absence of AMP-DA activity. It is a common, autosomal recessive condition, being seen in 1% to 2% of all muscle biopsy specimens. There is a question as to whether this represents a separate disease entity, a malady that is unmasked by other neuromuscular diseases, or simply a genetic curiosity.

Periodic Paralysis

Periodic paralysis, a disease characterized by abrupt onsets of complete paralysis, is associated with abnormalities in potassium metabolism. Although there are three clinically and genetically distinct syndromes, the pathologic changes and the therapy (carbonic anhydrase inhibitors) for all three are similar. The three conditions are hyperkalemic, hypokalemic, and normokalemic periodic paralysis.

Biopsy specimens from patients with periodic paralysis appear completely normal between attacks, although occasionally, large, central vacuoles containing PAS-positive material are seen. Electron microscopic examination reveals that these vacuoles are composed of markedly dilated sarcoplasmic reticulum. In some cases a distinct subpopulation of fibers (Type IIB) contains large numbers of tubular aggregates, which are derived from the tubular network of the sarcoplasmic reticulum.

Denervation

Despite the application of enzyme histochemical studies to skeletal muscle biopsy samples, it is still occasionally difficult to distinguish myopathic changes from those caused by denervation of muscle, particularly when the disease is chronic. The pathologic changes, although they may be severe, tend to show a mixture of "neuropathic" and "myopathic" features. However, in most cases a careful analysis of the muscle biopsy specimen, using enzyme histochemical techniques, will resolve the problem.

It should be remembered that the pathology of denervation reflects lesions of the lower motor neuron. Lesions of the upper motor neuron, as seen in multiple sclerosis or cerebral vascular stroke, result in paralysis and atrophy. Yet the lower motor neuron is intact and the pathologic changes are those of a nonspecific diffuse atrophy rather than of denervation atrophy.

A muscle biopsy is a highly sensitive test for detecting a lesion of the lower motor neuron, but the pattern of denervation does not identify the cause of the lower motor neuron lesion. It is, therefore, difficult to distinguish between a disease such as amyotrophic lateral sclerosis and a peripheral neuropathy due to diabetes. The morphologic changes can, however, indicate whether denervation is present, and if so, whether it is chronic, or possibly relapsing. When a skeletal muscle fiber becomes separated from contact with its lower motor neuron, it invariably becomes progressively more atrophic, owing to progressive loss of myofibrils and myofilaments. On cross section the atrophic fiber has a characteristic angular atrophic configuration, being compressed by surrounding normal muscle fibers (see Fig. 27-2B). If the fiber is not reinnervated, the atrophy progresses to complete loss of myofibrils and myofilaments, and the nuclei condense into aggregates. In longitudinal section, the end-stage of atrophy consists of an aggregate of nuclei connected by a thin strand of sarcoplasm to another aggregate of nuclei. On cross section these nuclei are seen as pyknotic nuclear clumps. A section between clusters of nuclei may fail to demonstrate that a muscle fiber was even present.

The early phase of denervating disease is characterized by irregularly scattered angular atrophic fibers. As the disease progresses, these angular atrophic fibers are seen in groups, at first in small clusters of several fibers and later in progressively larger groups (see Fig. 27-2B) . Angular atrophic fibers which are denervated are excessively dark when stained with the nonspecific esterase (see Fig. 27-3) and the NADH tetrazolium reductase reactions, in contrast to a case involving nonspecific atrophy due to disuse or wasting. With the ATPase reaction, the clusters of angular atrophic fibers which are excessively dark-stained are found to be a mixture of Type I and Type II fibers. In virtually all of the known denervating conditions there is no selective denervation of one type of motor neuron.

Another abnormality occasionally present in a denervating condition is the "target fiber" (see Fig. 27-5), seen in 20% or less of cases. This change is apparently transient, occurring during or shortly after the process of denervation, and indicating that the denervating process is active. A central pallor of the muscle fiber is surrounded by a condensed zone which in turn is surrounded by a normal zone of sarcoplasm. Target fibers are difficult to see with the hematoxylin and eosin stain, but they can usually be detected with the PAS reaction. Because the earliest target change consists of clearing of the central portion of the fiber of its membranous organelles, these fibers are always demonstrable with an NADH tetrazolium reductase reaction (see Fig. 27-5).

With every episode of denervation there is an effort at reinnervation. In a slowly progressive denervating process reinnervation may actually keep pace with denervation. New sprouting nerve endings make synaptic contact with the muscle fiber at the site of the previous motor endplate. Shortly after denervation the muscle fiber becomes covered with the nicotinic receptor for acetylcholine (extrajunctional receptor), a situation similar to that in the myotubular phase of embryogenesis. With reinnervation the extrajunctional receptor again disappears from the sarcolemma, except at the point of synaptic contact. In a chronic denervating condition, in which reinnervation is at least partially able to keep pace with denervation, progressively fewer motor units are seen, but each motor unit becomes larger. Thus, there is a tendency for a given lower motor neuron to take over the innervation of a given field of fibers, and a group of fibers of one type is seen adjacent to fibers of another type. **This pattern is designated type grouping and is pathognomonic of denervation followed by reinnervation** (see Fig. 27-2C).

Patients with striking type grouping often have symptoms of muscle cramping in addition to progressive muscular weakness. After a single episode of denervation, such as occurs with poliomyelitis, there is often a remarkable recovery of strength, owing to reinnervation. Years later a pattern of type grouping with scattered pyknotic nuclear clumps is conspicuous. In such a case there are no angular atrophic fibers, which are excessively dark with esterase, or target fibers, which are associated with active denervation.

Occasionally a biopsy specimen reveals an abnormal prominence of one fiber type over the other. This situation is designated **type predominance** and may involve either Type I or Type II fibers. The explanation for this is often not clear, but frequently there is also evidence of denervation. It could be that type predominance is a form of reinnervation in which reinnervation favors one type of lower motor neuron over another. It is not uncommon to see occasional muscle fibers undergoing degeneration or regeneration in neuropathic conditions. In these patients a modest elevation in serum creatine kinase reflects mild muscle degeneration, a consistent finding in patients who have amyotrophic lateral sclerosis.

One denervating condition which can often be specifically identified is Werdnig-Hoffmann disease, or infantile spinal muscular atrophy. This autosomal, recessively inherited condition results in extreme weakness at birth. The disease is progressive and

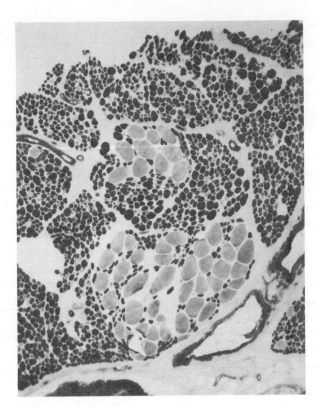

Figure 27-13. Werdnig-Hoffmann disease (infantile spinal muscular atrophy). This cross section of skeletal muscle stained for ATPase is from an infant with severe hypotonia. It shows normal fascicles of Type I and Type II fibers, groups of extremely atrophic, rounded Type I and Type II fibers, and clusters of markedly hypertrophied fibers, all of which are Type I. These are typical features of Werdnig-Hoffman disease.

severe, and these infants seldom live beyond the first year of life. The denervation seems to have already occurred *in utero* after the establishment of the motor units. The histologic pattern is virtually pathognomonic (Fig. 27-13). Groups of minute, rounded, atrophic fibers are still identifiable with the ATPase reaction as being either Type I or Type II. In addition there are fascicles of normal muscle fibers and, almost invariably, striking clusters of markedly hypertrophied fibers, all of which are Type I.

There are rarer forms of spinal muscular atrophy of varying degrees of severity, some of which are nonprogressive. These later onset forms have been designated Kugelberg-Welander disease and may be autosomal recessive, autosomal dominant, or sex-linked recessive. Previously, these patients have often been designated as having a limb-girdle muscular dystrophy. The presence of type grouping and other evidence of denervation helps to identify these patients.

Type II Atrophy

A commonly misinterpreted pathologic pattern in muscle biopsy specimens is atrophy due to disuse, wasting, upper motor neuron disease, and corticosteroid toxicity. This diffuse, nonspecific atrophy is manifested histologically by a selective angular atrophy of Type II fibers. Using the routine hematoxylin and eosin stain, it is sometimes impossible to distinguish this pattern of atrophy from that of denervation (Fig. 27-14). However, with the ATPase reaction all of the angular atrophic fibers are Type II, and virtually all of the Type II fibers are angular and atrophic (Fig. 27-15). Furthermore, these angular atrophic fibers do not stain excessively with the nonspecific esterase reaction or the NADH tetrazolium reductase reaction. Type II atrophy is a common condition which is often an epiphenomenon of a more chronic problem.

The so-called steroid myopathy is characterized histologically by Type II atrophy. This is an important distinction to make, since oftentimes patients with polymyositis, which is an inflammatory myopathy, are treated with large doses of corticosteroids. If the patient suffers an episode of worsening weakness, the physician must decide whether this represents a recurrence of the polymyositis and requires an increase in the dose of corticosteroids, or whether it is a manifestation of corticosteroid toxicity, in which case a decrease in the dosage is indicated. If the increased weakness is due to corticosteroid toxicity, the patient does not demonstrate an increase in the serum creatine kinase and histologically has selective atrophy of Type II fibers in the absence of muscle fiber degeneration and inflammation. Fiber degeneration and inflammation would be expected if the inflammatory myopathy is recurring, a process that would be reflected in an elevation of the serum creatine kinase.

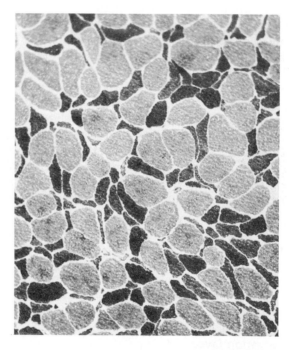

Figure 27-15. Type II fiber atrophy. The angular atrophic fibers here stained for ATPase were not excessively stained with the esterase stain and are virtually all Type II fibers. Denervating conditions do not involve only Type II fibers. Selective atrophy of Type II fibers is associated with wasting, chronic inactivity (disuse atrophy), and corticosteroid toxicity and is often mistaken for denervation atrophy.

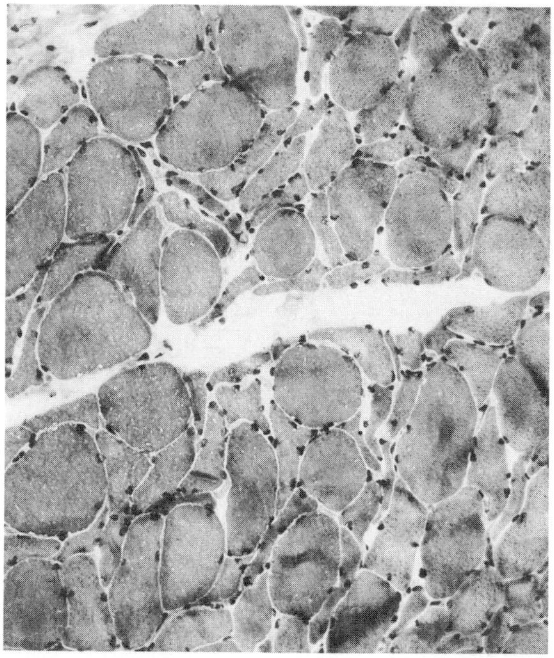

Figure 27-14. Type II fiber atrophy. This cross section of striated muscle treated with a modified Gomori stain is from a man who had suffered an unexplained 30-pound weight loss and proximal muscle weakness. He was found to have a malignant tumor. The numerous angular atrophic fibers suggest denervation. (See Fig. 27-2).

SUGGESTED READING

BOOKS

Dubowitz V: Muscle Biopsy, A Practical Approach, 2nd ed. Bailliere Tindall, 1985

Mastaglia FL, Walton J: Skeletal Muscle Pathology. Edinburgh: Churchill Livingstone, 1982

Vinken PS, Bruyn GW: Handbook of Clinical Neurology. In Ringel S (ed): Vol. 40–41, Diseases of Muscle, Part I. Amsterdam, Elsevier North Holland, 1979

Walton J: Disorders of Voluntary Muscle. 4th ed. Edinburgh, Churchill Livingstone, 1981

REVIEW ARTICLES

Callen JP: Dermatomyositis. Neurol Clin 5:379, 1987

Moser H: Duchenne muscular dystrophy: pathogenetic aspects and genetic prevention. Hum Genet 66:17, 1984

Temple JK, Dunn DW, Blitzer MG, et al: The "muscular variant" of Pompe disease: Clinical, biochemical, and histologic characteristics. Am J Med Genet 21: 597, 1985

ORIGINAL ARTICLES

Bodrug SE, Ray PN, Gonzalez IL, et al: Molecular analysis of a constitutional X-autosome translocation in a female with muscular dystrophy. Science 237:1620, 1987

Burr IM, Asayama K, Fenichel GM: Superoxide dismutases, glutathione peroxidase, and catalase in neuromuscular disease. Muscle Nerve 10:150, 1987

Darras BT, Harper JF, Francke U: Prenatal diagnosis and detection of carriers with DNA probes in Duchenne's muscular dystrophy. N Engl J Med 316:985, 1987

Hoffman EP, Monaco AP, Feener, CC, et al: Conservation of the Duchenne muscular dystrophy gene in mice and humans. Science 238:347, 1987

28 The Nervous System

F. Stephen Vogel and Thomas W. Bouldin

The Central Nervous System

Trauma
Circulatory Disorders
Inflammatory Diseases
Congenital Malformations

Demyelinating Diseases
Neoplasia
Metabolic Disorders
Degenerative Diseases

The Peripheral Nervous System

General Pathology
Peripheral Neuropathies
Nerve Trauma
Tumors

Figure 28-1. The brain. The anatomic structures of the brain are well visualized by magnetic resonance imaging.

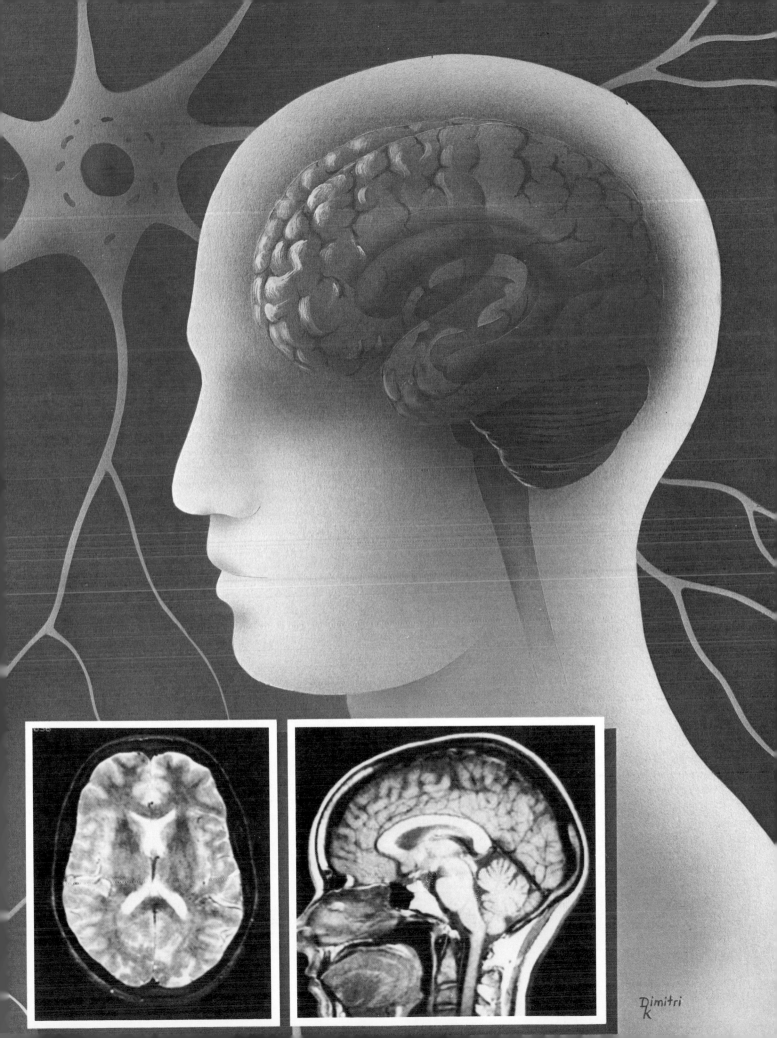

Dimitri
K

The Central Nervous System

F. Stephen Vogel

The nervous system evolved phylogenetically over many millions of years, yet its functional capacity for cognition was an abrupt and remarkable acquisition. It is this aptitude that permits us to inquire into the nature of the disorders of this enormously complex biologic system.

The functional properties of the nervous system are topographically localized. Not surprisingly, the diseases that affect the organ are also geographically distributed, and thus, their topographies serve to individualize them and to facilitate their recognition. For example, among the degenerative disorders, Huntington's disease is characterized by selective involvement of the caudate nuclei; parkinsonism targets the substantia nigra; and amyotrophic lateral sclerosis singles out the motor neurons of the spinal cord, brain stem, and cerebrum. Similarly, inflammatory lesions have preferred locations: poliomyelitis involves the anterior horn cells of the spinal cord and the motor nuclei of the brain stem, herpes simplex localizes preferentially in the temporal lobes of the cerebrum, and rabies seeks out the medulla. Hypertension is responsible for spontaneous hemorrhage, which predictably occurs in the deep nuclear regions of the cerebrum. Spontaneous hemorrhage occurs less frequently in the pons and cerebellum, and almost never elsewhere. Multiple sclerosis creates plaques of demyelination, which are focal lesions that are widely scattered throughout the cerebrum, brain stem, and spinal cord. Nevertheless, they exhibit a predilection for the visual system and the paraventricular areas, with a total avoidance of the myelin of the peripheral nerves. Although the expressions of neoplasia are numerous, they, too, are patterned. For example, the gliomas of childhood affect the brain stem and cerebellum, whereas those in the adult predominantly involve the cerebrum. Thus, an understanding of neurologic diseases not only encompasses morphology and pathogenesis, but also embodies the topographic distribution that individualizes each disease process.

Generally, disorders of the nervous system progress with a characteristic tempo. For example, among the inflammatory processes, the suppurative meningitides—such as those caused by meningococcus, pneumococcus, or streptococcus—without treatment progress to death within days. By contrast, the tempo of tuberculous meningitis is cast in weeks, that of cryptococcal meningitis evolves over a period of months, and that of leutic meningovascular disease spans decades. Poliomyelitis and amyotrophic lateral sclerosis share the symptoms of weakness because each involves the motor neurons. However, poliomyelitis runs its course in days, whereas the course of amyotrophic lateral sclerosis progresses over a number of years. Cerebral hemorrhage is an abrupt process. Within hours, it creates a mass which, by transtentorial herniation, commonly attains sufficient size to threaten life. On the other hand, an abscess expands during an interval of days or weeks, but it also ultimately attains a size that initiates the same lethal mechanism—namely, transtentorial herniation. In the case of neoplasia, transtentorial herniation is also a frequent terminal event. When the tumor is well differentiated the symptomatology prior to herniation may persist for many years, but when the lesion is anaplastic the clinical course is abbreviated.

Unlike diseases of other organs, neurologic disorders generally assail the nervous system throughout the entire lifespan. Nevertheless, within this spectrum an individual disease process commonly manifests a predilection for a select age group. For example, inborn errors of metabolism, such as Tay-Sachs disease, the leukodystrophies, and several species of neoplasms, are encountered largely in childhood. Multiple sclerosis tends to occur in young adults, with the onset rarely occurring before puberty or after the age of 40 years. Huntington's disease and amyotrophic lateral sclerosis typically strike the youthful and middle-aged adult. Parkinsonism, a disorder that shares many cytologic features with Huntington's disease and amyotrophic lateral sclerosis, is rarely manifested clinically before the late decades of life. Alzheimer's disease and cerebrovascular disease are maladies of the aging biologic system. Advanced

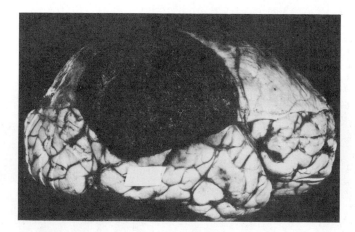

Figure 28-2.   Epidural hematoma. A fracture of the temporoparietal bone transected the right middle meningeal artery, permitting blood (under arterial pressure) to create a discoid hematoma between the skull and the dura. The patient died of transtentorial herniation.

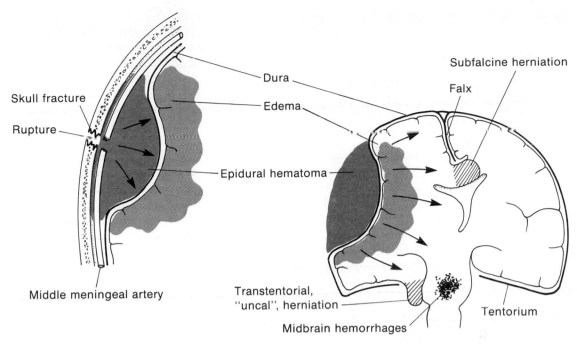

Figure 28-3. Development of an epidural hematoma. Transection of a branch of the middle meningeal artery by the sharp edge of a fracture initiates bleeding under arterial pressure. This bleeding slowly dissects the dura from the calvarium and produces an expanding hematoma. After an asymptomatic interval of several hours, transtentorial herniation becomes life-threatening.

age is also associated with the highest incidence of neoplasia.

A differential diagnosis is thus based on answers to three cardinal questions: Where is the lesion? How long has it been present? Is the age of the patient relevant?

Trauma

Epidural Hematoma

The intracranial dura, securely bound to the inner aspect of the calvarium, is analogous to the periosteum. The two middle meningeal arteries that occupy the theoretical space between the dura and the calvarium are grooved into the inner table of the bone and are fixed securely by the underlying dura. Branches of the middle meningeal artery splay across the temporoparietal area, generally as three major tributaries. The temporal bone is the thinnest bone of the skull, with the exception of the orbital surfaces of the frontal bone. Transection of one or several of the branches of the middle meningeal artery is frequently a consequence of a regional skull fracture. Skull fractures may also traverse a dural sinus, initi-

ating less forceful venous bleeding into the epidural space. Nevertheless, **the classic epidural hematoma results from a fracture of the temporoparietal bone, with severance of a branch of the middle meningeal artery.** These anatomic characteristics explain why a seemingly minor blow to the side of the head, with a consequent fracture of the skull, may result in a potentially lethal epidural hematoma (Figs. 28-2 and 28-3).

It is important, at this point, to distinguish between the phenomenon of concussion and other injuries. Consciousness is a positive neurologic activity that is dependent upon the intactness and function of specific neurons—namely, those of the reticular formation of the brain stem. By definition, concussion is the transient loss of consciousness secondary to trauma. It is exemplified in the boxing ring, generally as the consequence of a blow that deflects the head upward and posteriorly, often with a rotatory component. These motions impart a quick torque upon the brain stem, an effect that presumably causes functional paralysis of the neurons of the reticular formation. It is a fallacious clinical notion that a patient not rendered unconscious by a blow to the head poses little cause for concern. As defined above, the initiation of an epidural hematoma is predicated upon a skull fracture, which, in turn, results from trauma to the side of the head. As the falx precludes displacement of the cerebral hemispheres laterally, a blow to the temporoparietal area does not stress the anatomy of the brain stem. Therefore, the absence of a loss of consciousness in a patient with suspected epidural hematoma has little clinical relevance.

Transection of one or several branches of the middle meningeal artery permits the escape of blood under arterial pressure, with a pulsating cadence that slowly deflects the dura from the calvarium. The firm adhesiveness of the dura to the calvarium is slowly but progressively overcome by this relentless arterial force, which eventually creates a true epidural compartment engorged with blood. The hematoma enlarges relentlessly. During an early interval of several hours the cutaneous abrasion may be associated with regional pain and tenderness, but the intracranial events characteristically are asymptomatic. The firm adherence of the dura to the calvarium generally dictates that this asymptomatic interval lasts 4 to 8 hours. The subsequent and meaningful symptomatology, which generally is manifested after the hematoma has attained a volume of 30 to 50 ml, is a reflection of the space-occupying nature of the lesion. Central to the subsequent events is the fact that the supratentorial compartment has a fixed volume; thus, the introduction of a space-occupying mass necessitates the displacement of an equal volume from this compartment.

During the asymptomatic interval, the earliest volumetric adjustment is accomplished by the displacement of cerebrospinal fluid. This fluid, which is derived from the subarachnoid space and from the intravascular chambers, is dispelled through the aperture in the tentorium. Normally, the supratentorial compartment contains about 60 ml of cerebrospinal fluid. However, because the chambers of the lateral and third ventricles and the estuaries of the subarachnoid space are not fully compressible, less than 60 ml of volume can be accommodated. Accommodation of the progressively enlarging hematoma thus necessitates additional space. When the increased intracranial pressure exceeds the intravenous pressure, the veins (represented principally by large venous sinuses) are compressed, and transiently yield space. This collapse of the venous conduits impedes arterial flow and creates circulatory stagnation, thereby causing cerebral ischemia and hypoxia. The initiation of the Cushing reflex is a protective response designed to enhance cerebral circulation and to increase cerebral oxygenation. The heart rate slows so as to increase ventricular filling, and ventricular contraction

becomes more forceful. Blood pressure, particularly the systolic pressure, is elevated while the heart rate is slowed. During this interval of global cerebral hypoxia, the patient manifests diffuse cortical impairment, evidenced by confusion and disorientation.

The hematoma attains a volume of approximately 60 ml within an interval of 6 to 10 hours. Once compensatory mechanisms have been exhausted, the brain shifts laterally away from the side of the lesion. The medial aspect of the temporal lobe on the same side as the hematoma is compressed against the midbrain and displaced downward through the horseshoe-shaped opening of the tentorium. This extremely important phenomenon, termed **transtentorial herniation,** compresses the tissues of the uncus of the hippocampus against the midbrain and also against contiguous structures, such as the third nerve. Thus, the ocular motor nerve is forced against the edge of the tentorium, an effect that causes palsy of the third nerve. The pupil on the side of the lesion generally becomes fixed and dilated. The herniated uncus also compresses the vasculature of the midbrain—most importantly, the mesencephalic veins (great veins of Rosenthal). This creates venous stagnation in the midbrain. Stagnation and hypoxia impair neuronal function, notably that of the reticular formation, and this is expressed clinically as a decline in the level of consciousness. Shortly thereafter, stagnation causes hemorrhage and necrosis, after which the regional injury to the reticular formation becomes irreversible. Death of the injured patient is then imminent or, if supratentorial pressure is relieved, unconsciousness is permanent. Epidural hematomas are invariably progressive; when not recognized and evacuated, they are lethal, usually within 24 to 48 hours (Fig. 28-4).

Subdural Hematoma

The cerebral hemispheres, composed of approximately 90% liquid, submerged in cerebrospinal fluid, and tethered loosely by blood vessels and cranial nerves, are free to float in an anteroposterior direction. The venous drainage from the cerebral hemispheres flows upward through veins in the pia. These veins first reach the parasagittal region; then, leaving the pia, they cross the subarachnoid space, penetrate the arachnoid, traverse the theoretical subdural space, breach the dura, and enter the dural sinus. Significantly, the arachnoid is intimately applied to the undersurface of the dura, being held in close apposition by the underlying layer of noncom-

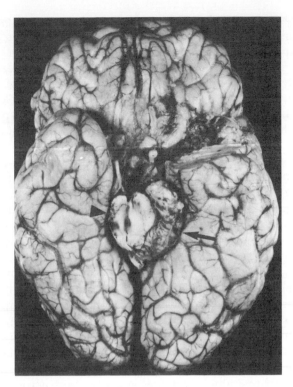

Figure 28-4. Transtentorial herniation. An expanding lesion above the tentorium in the left cerebral hemisphere caused a left-to-right shift of midline structures, notably of the midbrain, and initiated downward displacement of a ridge of neural tissue, the uncus of the hippocampus, through the aperture of the tentorium (*arrow*). Compression of the venous drainage from the midbrain resulted in secondary midbrain hemorrhages. As a terminal event, the shift of the brain stem brought the right cerebral peduncle into forceful contact with the edge of the tentorium, causing laceration of the posterior aspect of the right cerebral peduncles, a lesion referred to as Kernohan's notch (*arrowhead*).

pressible spinal fluid. The arachnoid is secured to the cerebral hemispheres, whereas the dura is bound to the calvarium. The arachnoid is unattached to the dura, yet intimately subjacent to it, an apposition analogous to two pages of a book. The gelatinous consistency of the cerebral tissues permits the energy of trauma to disfigure the cerebrum and to initiate shock waves that pass through the hemispheres like ripples through gelatin. In concert, these anatomic features are targeted by trauma applied in the sagittal plane. It is in this way that subdural hematomas are initiated (Fig. 28-5).

The cerebral hemispheres are displaced in an anteroposterior direction when the frontal or occipital portion of the moving head strikes a fixed object.

Alternatively, the forehead or posterior portion of the stationary head may be struck by a blunt object. It is not surprising that **subdural hematomas occur most frequently when the moving head strikes a fixed object,** a circumstance in which movement is already inherent both in the brain and the skull. The abrupt arrest of movement of the skull forcefully brings the moving cerebral hemispheres against the inner aspect of the occipital or frontal bone. The soft cerebral tissues compact and then recoil, a response that generates shock waves. The motions of the skull and the brain are thereafter asynchronous. Since the dura is adherent to the skull and the arachnoid is attached to the cerebrum, the interface between these two disparately moving membranes localizes a shearing phenomenon to the subdural space. **This motion cleaves the cortical veins as they pass through the theoretical subdural compartment.** Thus, with rare exceptions, the bleeding is venous in origin. The liberated blood enters a compartment that is readily expansile, unlike the restricted epidural space. Fortunately, because the bleeding is venous in origin, in most instances it stops spontaneously after an accumulation of 25 to 50 ml. The hematoma compresses the severed veins and initiates thrombosis.

The nature of the lesion is defined by the characteristics and the vulnerability of the normal anatomy.

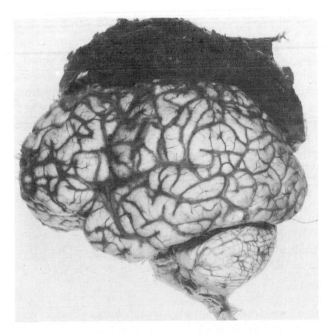

Figure 28-5. Subdural hematoma. A recent subdural hematoma is exposed by upward deflection of the dura. Note the absence of blood in the subarachnoid space. The patient died of transtentorial herniation.

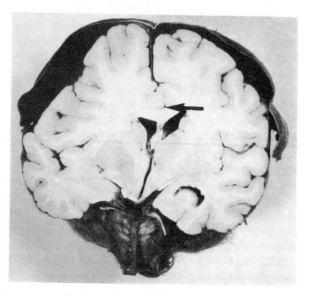

Figure 28-6. Subdural hematoma. A coronal section of the brain reveals large, bilateral, subdural compartments filled with blood. The subdural hematoma on the left is larger, and has caused a shift of the ventricular system from left to right. Note the flattened contour of the left cerebral convexity, the disfigurement and displacement of the ventricles, and the subfalcine herniation of the cingulate gyrus (*arrow*).

The magnitude of the force required to produce such a lesion is similarly defined; namely, it is one that is sufficient to displace the cerebral hemispheres in the anteroposterior direction. A backward fall, without intervention, propels the skull at a rate of about 20 miles per hour against the floor. The skull stops instantaneously, and for a moment the brain continues its downward movement. This is then followed by the impact of the brain against the skull and subsequent recoil. A similar condition is created when a moving head strikes a windshield in a head-on automobile collision. As brain structures are bilateral and symmetric, and the force is directed sagittally, it is not surprising that **subdural hematomas are frequently bilateral.**

A hematoma that is not enlarging and that is too small to cause symptoms or transtentorial herniation nevertheless initiates important tissue responses. The surface of contact between the hematoma and the inferior aspect of the dura becomes the site of granulation tissue formation, which proceeds for days. This layer of granulation tissue, which is rich in capillaries and fibroblasts, is referred to as the "outer membrane." From it, migratory fibroblasts enter the subjacent hematoma. These cells travel downward and knit a fibrous membrane across the deep, or inner, aspect of the blood clot. Approximately 2

weeks pass before this "inner membrane" is grossly visible. Unlike the outer membrane, this delicate encapsulating inner membrane lacks blood vessels.

The hematoma, which is static in size and generally asymptomatic, has three potential routes of evolution: **reabsorption,** as occurs regularly when blood is introduced experimentally into the subdural space of most laboratory animals; **maintenance of the status quo** with the potential for calcification; or **enlargement.** Expansion of the hematoma and the onset of symptoms is most often the result of rebleeding from the outer membrane. The granulation tissue, analogous to a wet scab, is extremely vulnerable to minor trauma, even the mild pressure exerted by an underlying cerebral hemisphere that has been set in motion by shaking the head. Rebleeding creates a new hematoma that lies subjacent to the outer membrane. With time, it becomes compartmentalized from the original hematoma by the development of a second inner membrane. Such episodes of sporadic rebleeding expand the lesion periodically and at unpredictable time intervals. Alternatively, it has been postulated that lysis of the original hematoma creates a hyperosmotic state that attracts fluid across the inner membrane, thus enlarging the lesion. This phenomenon seems to be of lesser consequence than rebleeding, as the appearance of a subdural hematoma at surgery or postmortem examination resembles dense, clotted blood, undiluted by clear fluid (Fig. 28-6).

As has been mentioned, enlargement of a subdural hematoma may occur unpredictably during an interval after the initial trauma. However, since the outer membrane, as well as the hematoma, may be reabsorbed, this interval probably does not exceed 6 months.

The symptoms of a subdural hematoma are protean. Stretching of the meninges may cause headaches. Pressure on the motor cortex may produce contralateral weakness. Irritation of the cortex may initiate seizures. Diffuse, often bilateral, subdural hematomas may impair cognitive function, an effect that may be manifested as dementia and that is often misinterpreted as senility. One or several rebleeds may enlarge the mass sufficiently to cause transtentorial herniation and death (Fig. 28-7).

Subarachnoid Hemorrhage

Unless the dura has physically been breached by a depressed skull fracture, this dense fibrous membrane is an invulnerable barrier to the diffusion of blood from the epidural compartment. Remarkably, during the genesis of a subdural hematoma, sever-

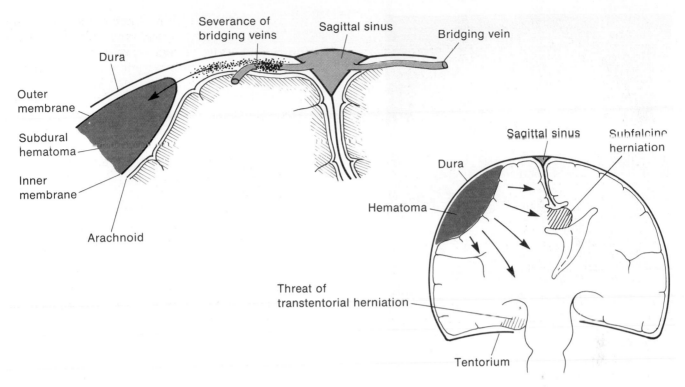

Figure 28-7. Development of a subdural hematoma. With head trauma, the dura moves with the skull and the arachnoid moves with the cerebrum. As a result, the bridging veins are sheared as they cross between the dura and the arachnoid. Venous bleeding creates a hematoma in the expansile subdural space. Subsequent transtentorial herniation is life-threatening.

ance of the cortical bridging veins is so precisely localized to the subdural space that blood is compartmentalized away from the cerebrospinal fluid. Throughout the evolution of a subdural hematoma, the diaphanous arachnoid generally preserves its continuity, its integrity, and its individuality. It is not incorporated into the inner membrane nor, for unexplained reasons, does it participate in this contiguous fibroblastic proliferation. Thus, the absence of blood in the cerebrospinal fluid does not negate the presence of a subdural hematoma.

On rare occasions, a severe rotatory force causes a traumatic dissecting aneurysm, particularly of the internal carotid arteries. These aneurysms may subsequently rupture into the subarachnoid space. Trauma can also cause the rupture of a coincidental vascular defect—notably, a saccular aneurysm. However, such events are extremely rare. Therefore, the presence of blood in the cerebrospinal fluid of a patient who has sustained head trauma usually denotes a cerebral contusion or laceration that has torn the pia, permitting blood from the contused cortex to gain entry into the cerebrospinal fluid.

Cerebral Contusion

The flotation of the cerebral hemispheres in the anteroposterior direction and the soft, gelatinous quality of cerebral tissues are predisposing factors for bruising or laceration of the cortex by force applied to the head. The inner aspect of the occipital bone has a smooth, curved contour, whereas the bony concavities of the frontal and middle fossa are corrugated. Cerebral contusions, like subdural hematomas, are generally the result of energetic anteroposterior displacement when the moving head strikes a fixed object. Logically, the magnitude of the contusion parallels the velocity of the motion and the abruptness of deceleration. Stumbling over a curb and sustaining an uninhibited forward fall can cause contusions of the polar tips of the frontal or temporal lobes. When the contusion occurs immediately internal to the point of surface impact, the lesion is referred to as a coup contusion. When the occipital area strikes the ground in a backward fall, the resultant abrasions are situated on the opposite sides of the brain in the frontal or temporal cortex, and

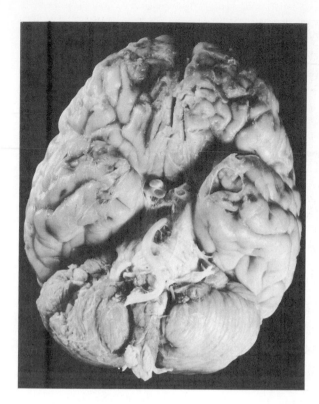

Figure 28-8. Cerebral contusion. The orbital surfaces of both frontal lobes and the tips of both temporal lobes are the sites of superficial lesions caused by the forceful impact of the soft cortical tissues against the rough surfaces of the base of the skull. The initial hemorrhage and edema have regressed, and the injured cortical tissue has been removed by the action of macrophages.

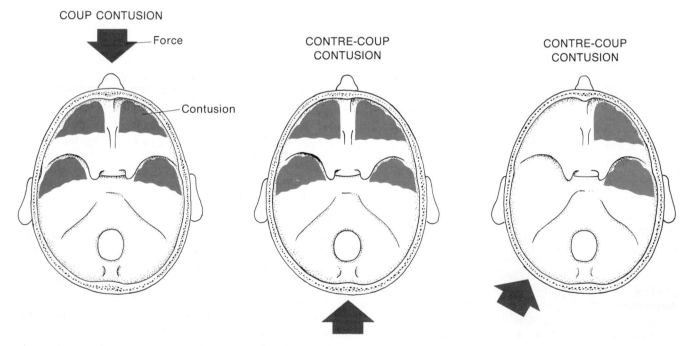

Figure 28-9.   Mechanisms of cerebral contusion. The cerebral hemispheres float in the cerebrospinal fluid. Rapid deceleration or, less commonly, acceleration of the skull causes the cortex to impact forcefully into the anterior and middle fossa. The position of a contusion is determined by the direction of the force and the intracranial anatomy.

the lesion is designated a contrecoup contusion (Figs. 28-8 and 28-9).

The distant position of contrecoup lesions underscores the significant determinants that are established by the anatomy—notably, the broad, smooth contour of the occipital bone against which the cerebrum first impacts; the gelatinous quality of the cerebral tissues that causes recoil and initiates disparate motion between the cerebrum and the skull; and the irregular, cobbled surface of the frontal and middle fossa against which the frontal and temporal poles impact. If the force is minimal, the contusion is limited to the gray cortex and is restricted to the apex of one or several gyri. Greater forces destroy larger expanses of the cortex, creating deeper cavitary lesions that extend into the white matter, or that lacerate the cortex and initiate cortical or subcortical hemorrhages. Large lesions are associated with considerable edema which, together with hemorrhage, forms a mass lesion that threatens life by transtentorial herniation (Fig. 28-10).

Contusions are permanent. Bruised, necrotic tissue is promptly phagocytized by macrophages and is transported into the blood stream. Mild, regional, astrocytic proliferation forms a regional scar, and the lesion persists as a telltale crater.

The injury may be only microscopic. Axons may be fractured and retracted into spheroids, a process accompanied by a loss of myelin. These changes are typically present in the parasagittal white matter and are often accompanied by multiple small hemorrhages. They are attributed to the shearing phenomenon that occurs during forceful rotatory acceleration and deceleration. These forces create laminar planes of parenchymal displacement. The parasagittal cortex is anchored by its attachment to the arachnoid villi (pacchionian granulations), whereas the lateral aspect of the cerebral hemispheres have greater freedom of motion. These shearing lesions commonly occur as a result of an automobile accident. Typically, the patient is rendered comatose and the computerized tomography (CT) scan discloses cerebral edema without hemorrhage.

Penetrating Head Wounds

Objects such as bullets and knives may enter the cranium and traverse the brain at variable velocities. In the absence of direct injury to the vital medullary centers, the immediate threat to life is hemorrhage (Fig. 28-11). Bleeding creates a space-occupying mass which, when present in or about the cerebrum, may

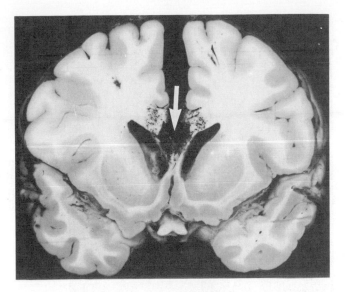

Figure 28-10.   Contusion and laceration. Deceleration of the moving head, with forceful upward displacement, caused transection of the corpus callosum (*arrow*) by the stationary edge of the falx.

lead to transtentorial herniation. When the hemorrhage occurs in the cerebellum, the immediate threat is herniation of the cerebellar tonsils into the foramen magnum and compression of the medulla.

Velocity contributes a blast effect to a projectile. Thus, a high- or intermediate-caliber bullet, as it traverses the brain, disrupts tissues not only by its own mass but also by a centrifugal blast that enlarges the diameter of the cylinder of disruption. A high-velocity military bullet can cause immediate death through an explosive increase in intracranial pressure. This pressure forcefully herniates the cerebellar tonsils into the foramen magnum and compresses the medulla, thereby causing immediate cardiac or respiratory paralysis (Fig. 28-12).

When **hemorrhage** has been less than lethal, or when it is controlled by surgery, a second complication arises from the introduction of microorganisms by the projectile. **Infection** is usually anticipated clinically, and is generally controlled by antibiotics. The onset of **seizures** is a tertiary manifestation that may appear 6 to 12 months after sustaining a penetrating wound. Collagen is displaced into the brain from the scalp or dura and subsequently proliferates to form a dense scar. Because a collagen scar is more contractile than a glial one, it causes greater distortion of neurons. The precise mechanism by which the scar produces the neuronal activation that causes seizures remains obscure.

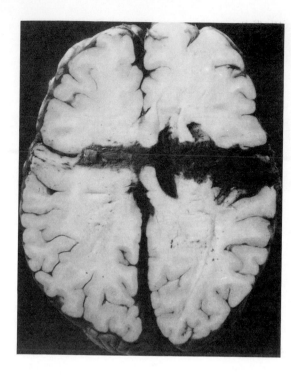

Figure 28-11. Penetrating head wound. A 22-caliber bullet entered the cranial compartment on the right. Its course through the cerebral hemispheres was attended by considerable hemorrhage. Note the petechiae in the area of the shock wave beyond the point of penetration of the bullet.

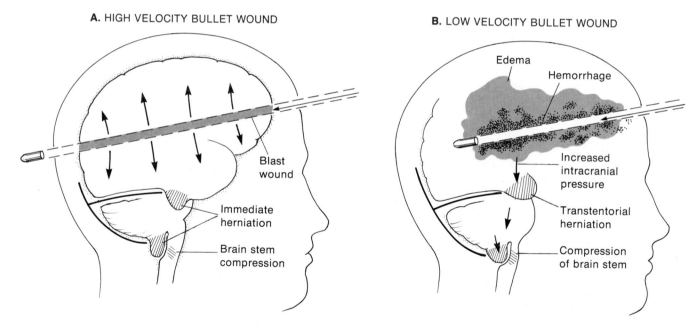

Figure 28-12. Consequences of high- and low-velocity bullet wounds. (*A*) The "blast effect" of a high-velocity projectile causes an immediate elevation in supratentorial pressure and results in death because of impaction of the cerebellum and medulla into the foramen magnum. (*B*) A low-velocity projectile elevates the pressure at a more gradual rate through hemorrhage and edema.

Spinal Cord Injuries

The bodies of the vertebrae are separated by intervertebral discs, and are stabilized in normal alignment by two longitudinal ligaments, as well as by the posterior bony processes. The anterior spinal ligament adheres to the ventral surface of the vertebral bodies, whereas the posterior spinal ligament is affixed to the posterior surface of this column of bony cubes. It should be recalled that the dura hangs free from the foramen magnum, once it has left the cranial compartment. There is, therefore, a slender spinal epidural space that contains a vestment of connective tissue. The angulation of the bony vertebral column brings the spinal cord forcefully into contact with bone or, alternatively, interferes with the regional circulation. Thus, a **hyperextension injury** occurs when the forehead is struck and is driven posteriorly, as in the impact of a dive into shallow water. This posterior displacement tears the anterior spinal ligament and permits a sharp, posterior angulation of the spinal canal. At the point of angulation, the posterior aspect of the spinal cord is brought into forceful contact with the posterior process of the stationary vertebral body that is, the vertebra that lies immediately caudal to the angulation (Fig. 28-13).

Hyperflexion injuries result when the head or shoulders are struck from behind by an object of considerable weight, or when the falling body strikes the ground in a flexed position. The head is driven forcefully forward and caudal. The anatomy of the vertebrae is again vulnerable, particularly in the cervical region. The force causes one vertebral body to impact on the underlying one. This frequently causes a fracture of a lip of the underlying vertebral body, with forward slippage of the underlying one and downward displacement. This disfigurement of the spinal canal results in sharp angulation of the spinal cord. The ventral surface of the angulated cord forcefully contacts the posterosuperior edge of the stable, underlying vertebral body.

A consequence of spinal injury is hemorrhage into the central core of the cord, a condition termed **hematomyelia**. Intramedullary hemorrhage is invariably accompanied by edema and softening, a combination designated **myelomalacia**. Severe trauma may cause transection of the spinal cord (Fig. 28-14).

Circulatory Disorders

The primitive neuroectoderm is initially, but very transiently, nourished by an infusion of ambient fluid and substrates. By the eighth week of fetal development, vessels that have formed within the neural tissues anastomose with the carotid and vertebral basilar arteries. Thereafter, the functional and structural integrity of the brain is critically dependent upon the systemic circulation.

The consequences of abnormal angiogenesis are immediately expressed in disordered neural development by the evolution of such entities as anencephaly, hydroanencephaly, and hemiatrophy, among others. Alternatively, abnormal angiogenesis induces a focal lesion, such as an arteriovenous (AV) malformation. This entity may remain clinically latent for several decades, eventually expressing its presence symptomatically through hemorrhage or seizures. Abnormal development of the cerebral vasculature also leaves the angles of bifurcation defective in their musculature. Through an interval of years, these deficiencies evolve into aneurysms, designated as berry, medial defect, or saccular aneurysms. These aneurysms are associated with an ever-increasing risk of rupture and consequent subarachnoid hemorrhage.

Ischemia and Infarction

Occlusive cerebrovascular disease may be classified into five categories, in accordance with the caliber and nature of the involved vessel. These categories are (1) large, extracranial and intracranial vessels, such as the carotid, vertebral, and basilar arteries; (2) arteries of the circle of Willis and their immediate branches; (3) parenchymal arteries and arterioles; (4) capillaries; and (5) large veins and dural sinuses.

Large Extracranial and Intracranial Vessels

The progressive character of atherosclerosis dictates that, in the course of time, the circulation to the brain will become compromised and the incidence of lesions, such as infarcts and hemorrhages, will increase. A recent infarct of the brain transforms the cerebral tissue into putty-like material, and the necrotic tissue is ultimately phagocytized by macrophages (Figs. 28-15 and 28-16).

Unlike infarcts of the heart and kidneys, **cerebral infarcts are not repaired by fibroblasts.** As an early response, capillaries proliferate at the margin of the lesion and become numerous by the fifth day. In accord with the size of the lesion, but generally within a period of months, the necrotic area is excavated by phagocytosis, and the lesion becomes a **permanent cyst.** During this interval, neovascularity regresses. If the initial area of the infarction is large,

(Text continues on p. 1431)

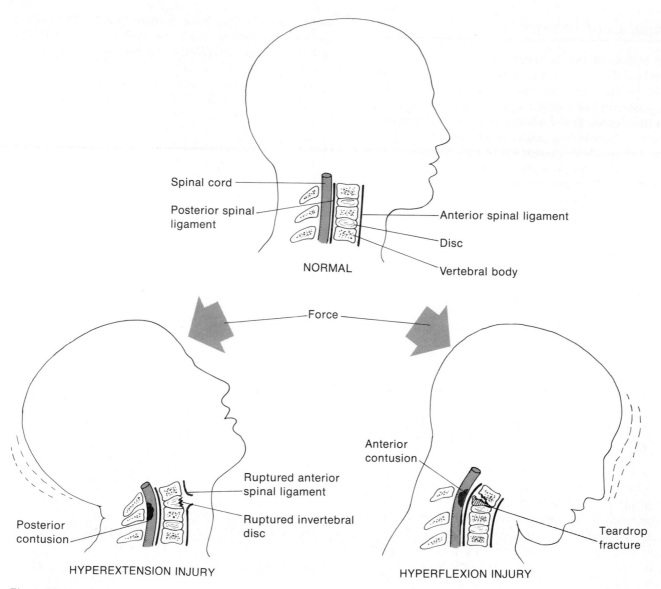

Figure 28-13. Spinal injury. Numerous angles of force can be applied to the highly vulnerable cervical spine. Posterior (hyperextension) and anterior (hyperflexion) injuries are the most common. Hyperextension injury causes rupture of the anterior spinal ligament and permits excessive posterior angulation. Hyperflexion injury causes compression, frequently associated with a "teardrop" fracture of a vertebral body, and produces excessive forward angulation of the cord.

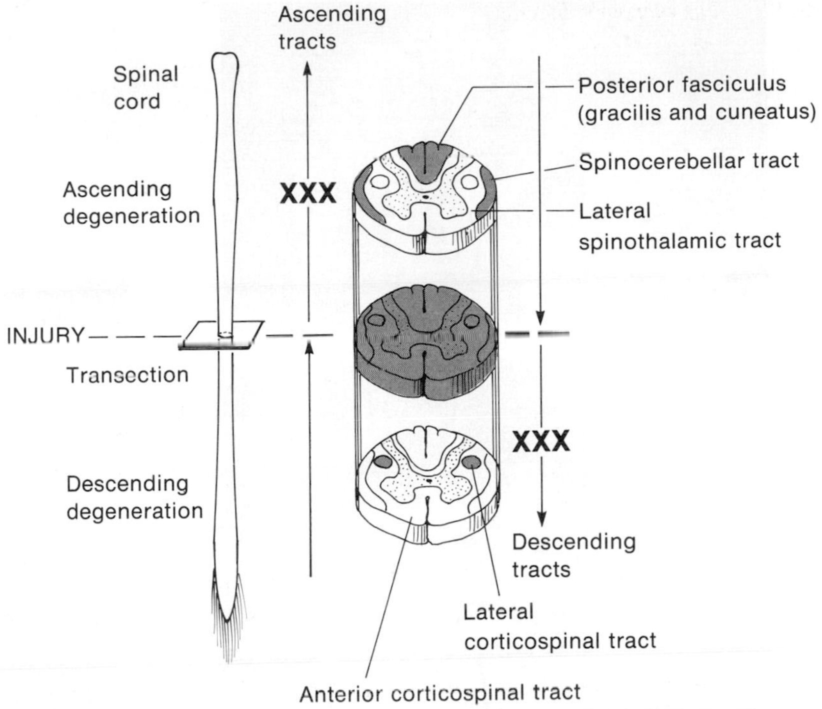

The following labels appear on the diagram at the top of the page:

Ascending tracts

Spinal cord

Ascending degeneration

XXX

Posterior fasciculus (gracilis and cuneatus)

Spinocerebellar tract

Lateral spinothalamic tract

INJURY —

Transection

Descending degeneration

XXX

Descending tracts

Lateral corticospinal tract

Anterior corticospinal tract

Figure 28-14. The consequences of spinal cord transection. Transection of an axon initiates distal wallerian degeneration. Thus, descending pathways degenerate below a transecting spinal cord injury, whereas ascending tracts degenerate above the level of injury.

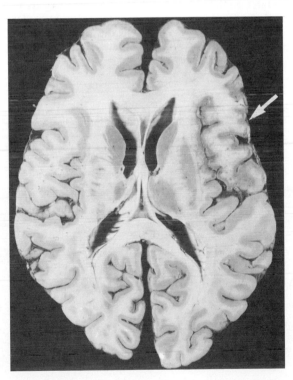

Figure 28-15. Ischemic cerebral infarct. A horizontal section of the cerebral hemisphere shows an area of ischemic necrosis (*arrow*) of about 5 days duration in the distribution of the left middle cerebral artery distal to the trifurcation. Note the preservation of the lenticulate nuclei, structures supplied by the striate branches from the middle cerebral artery. The occlusion resulted from thrombosis in situ initiated by severe atherosclerosis.

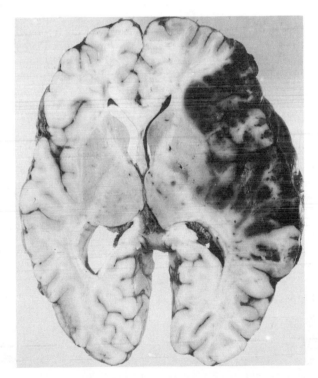

Figure 28-16. Hemorrhagic cerebral infarct. The trifurcation of the left middle cerebral artery was occluded by an embolus of thrombotic material from a mural thrombus in the heart. The hemorrhage and edema in the left hemisphere caused left-to-right displacement of the ventricular system. Death resulted from transtentorial herniation.

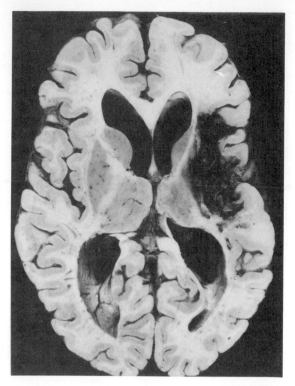

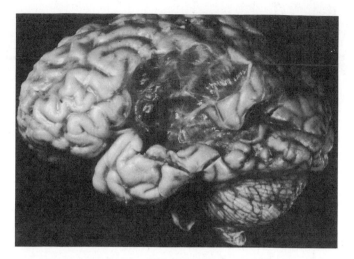

Figure 28-17. Remote cerebral infarct. An occlusion of the left middle cerebral artery at the trifurcation caused infarction in the left hemisphere in the region supplied by the distal branches of this major vessel. Note that the left caudate nucleus is preserved, as it is supplied predominantly by the anterior cerebral artery. The thalamus, which receives its circulation principally from the posterior cerebral artery, also remains intact. Over a period of months, macrophages removed the necrotic tissue and established a permanent cystic lesion.

Figure 28-18. Remote cerebral infarct. A surface view of the infarct depicted in Figure 28-17 defines the areas of cortical involvement and provides an explanation for the patient's aphasia, facial weakness, and hemiparesis. The cystic nature of the lesion is evident.

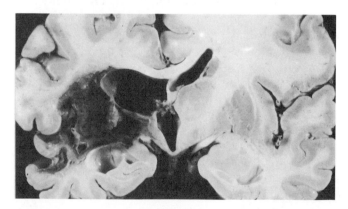

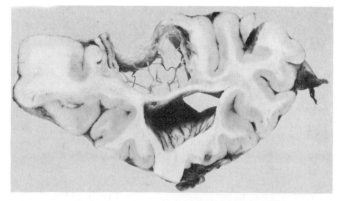

Figure 28-19. Remote cerebral infarct. A coronal section reveals a cystic area of infarction in the distribution of the striate branches of the left middle cerebral artery. The loss of tissue has resulted in compensatory dilatation of the left lateral ventricle and, to a lesser degree, the third ventricle. Note that the ependymal membrane remains intact, as it receives nutrition from the cerebrospinal fluid.

Figure 28-20. Remote cerebral infarct. A cystic area of infarction is frequently traversed by atretic blood vessels. The lesion is covered by a slender membrane formed of astrocytes that are nourished by cerebrospinal fluid. This membrane is not present above an area of contusion. Note again the preservation of the ependymal membrane.

the residual cyst is customarily bridged by a cobweb of atretic blood vessels. Because the cyst is filled with fluid, cerebral infarcts have been referred to as examples of liquefactive necrosis. However, the fluid is derived from seepage, and is not the end product of necrosis. Thus, it is more accurate to speak of cerebral infarctions as examples of coagulative, rather than liquefactive, necrosis (Figs. 28-17 through 28-20).

Cerebral infarcts are either hemorrhagic or bland. This overly simplistic description admits of only two extreme possibilities. However, in general, **infarcts that are caused by embolization are the sites of varying degrees of hemorrhage, whereas those initiated by thrombotic occlusion in situ are largely ischemic and, therefore, bland.** The differences are attributable to the tempo of the injury. An embolus occludes vascular flow abruptly, after which the ischemic region undergoes necrosis. The collateral blood vessels that traverse the area of infarction also become necrotic and leak blood into the area of infarction. Occlusion by thrombosis in situ progresses more slowly, and the collateral vessels also thrombose, thus guarding against secondary hemorrhage.

As previously discussed, specific neurologic functions are located within defined anatomic regions and, in turn, anatomic areas have defined relationships to the cerebral vasculature. It is, therefore, not surprising that distinctive neurologic deficits or syndromes are produced by cerebral infarcts, and that these are related to the occlusion of specific vessels. For example, the lengthy, slender, striate arteries that originate in the proximal trunk of the middle cerebral artery are commonly occluded by atherosclerosis and thrombosis. The resultant infarct often transects the internal capsule, producing hemiparesis or hemiplegia. Similarly, the trifurcation of the middle cerebral artery, a point of major step-down in vascular caliber, is not only a natural place for the lodgment of emboli, but it is also a common location for artherosclerosis that disposes to thrombosis in situ. Occlusions at this trifurcation deprive the parietal cortex of circulation and produce motor and sensory deficits, which may be accompanied by aphasias when the dominant hemisphere is involved (Fig. 28-21).

Frequent sites of atherosclerosis are the large vessels in the neck, most notably the common carotid artery at its bifurcation—that is, the point of origin of the external and internal branches. A thorough physical examination of an elderly patient includes the application of a stethoscope to this region (specifically, beneath the angle of the jaw) to listen for a bruit. Occlusion or severe stenosis of the internal carotid artery affects the ipsilateral hemisphere proportional to the degree of collateral circulation

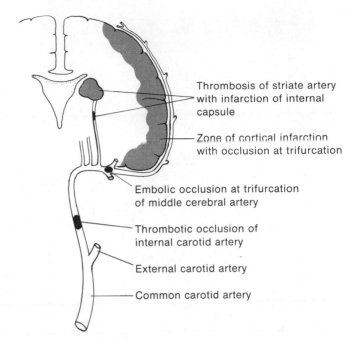

Figure 28-21. Distribution of cerebral infarcts. The normal geographic distribution of the cerebral vasculature defines the pattern and size of infarcts, and consequently, their symptomatology. Occlusion at the trifurcation initiates cortical infarction, with motor and sensory loss and often, aphasia. Occlusion of a striate branch transects the internal capsule and causes a motor deficit.

Labels in figure:
Thrombosis of striate artery with infarction of internal capsule
Zone of cortical infarction with occlusion at trifurcation
Embolic occlusion at trifurcation of middle cerebral artery
Thrombotic occlusion of internal carotid artery
External carotid artery
Common carotid artery

through the anterior and posterior communicating arteries. Most often, it initiates infarction in the distribution of the middle cerebral artery, with a less intense insult to the ipsilateral frontal lobe. The latter area is partially spared because of circulation through the anterior communicating artery.

Circle of Willis and Its Branches

The significance of an occlusion of a vessel of the circle of Willis depends on the normality—or the degree of deviation therefrom—in the developmental configuration of the circle. Thus, a large anterior communicating artery may provide circulation to a frontal lobe, the arterial supply of which has been compromised by occlusion of the ipsilateral internal carotid artery. **Among the immediate branches of the circle of Willis, the middle cerebral artery is most often occluded by emboli, as well as by atherosclerosis and thromboses.** As has been mentioned, because the trifurcation represents a major step-down in vascular caliber, it is the predominant site of occlusion by embolized thrombotic material derived from a mural thrombus in the heart. Characteristically, these

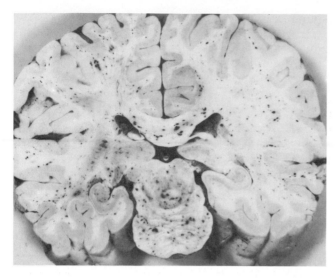

Figure 28-22. Fat embolization. Droplets of fat liberated from the bone marrow at the site of a fracture of the femoral bone passed through the pulmonary vascular bed and lodged in the cerebral capillaries. The white matter is more vulnerable to the ischemia of partial occlusion by a fat droplet because the white matter contains fewer capillaries than does the gray matter. Diapedesis of red cells and petechiae result when the endothelial integrity is compromised. Thus, petechiae are restricted to the white matter, although fat droplets are also present in the capillaries of the gray matter.

emboli have diameters of 5 mm or greater, fitting snugly behind the trifurcation or entering and occluding a branch of the middle cerebral artery.

Parenchymal Arteries and Arterioles

The parenchymal arteries and arterioles are small in caliber and are not disposed to atheromatous deposition. However, they are often affected by hypertension, and become stenotic because of fibromuscular hyperplasia. The integrity of their walls is further compromised by the deposition of lipid and hyalin material, a transformation that is spoken of as lipohyalinosis. **The weakening of the wall leads to aneurysm formation of the Charcot-Bouchard variety.** These small, fusiform aneurysms, which are located on the trunk of a vessel rather than at a bifurcation, are disposed to rupture and hemorrhage. Alternatively, as a result of hypertension, fibromuscular proliferation impinges on the caliber of these arteries and leads to microinfarction. The microinfarcts, like the hemorrhages, are small. They are conventionally referred to as lacunae or **lacunar infarcts.** When multiple, these minute infarcts impair cognition and create the entity referred to as multiple infarct dementia.

Cerebral Capillaries

The capillary bed is the site of occlusion by small emboli, notably those of fat and air. Droplets of fat are carried downstream through the gradient of the cerebral vessels until the caliber of the embolus exceeds that of the tributaries beyond a bifurcation. When they lodge, their semifluid consistency creates a major, but not absolute, barrier to blood flow. The distant capillary endothelium becomes hypoxic and permeable, and petechiae develop. Typically, these petechiae are restricted to the white matter, because the greater density of capillaries in the gray cortex provides regional nutritional support and endothelial integrity is adequately preserved (Fig. 28-22). Similarly, the introduction of air into the vascular system liberates a multitude of bubbles. Each bubble divides as it encounters a constricting bifurcation, until the surface tension of the bubble exceeds the forces applied by vascular flow. Upon lodgment, a bubble of air acts in a manner comparable to that of a droplet of fat, depriving the distant capillary endothelium of oxygenation. This again results in the formation of

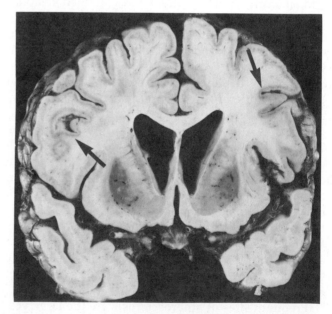

Figure 28-23. Laminar necrosis. Global ischemia initiates laminar necrosis in the terminal regions of the short penetrating arteries that enter the gray mantle from the overlying pia. These slender vessels branch and terminate near the gray-white junction. The lesion appears as a linear discoloration in the deeper zones of the cortex (*arrows*). Note that the necrosis is most conspicuous bilaterally in the parasagittal areas. These regions mark the interface between the anterior and middle cerebral arteries, the so-called watershed areas.

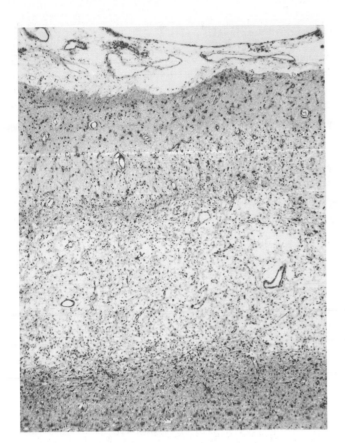

Figure 28-24. Laminar necrosis. A photomicrograph shows a horizontal band of ischemic necrosis that occupies the third to fifth neuronal cell layers. Neurons have disappeared from the overlying gray mantle and have been replaced by astrocytes. Macrophages and capillary proliferation mark the zone of cystic necrosis. There is astrogliosis and wallerian degeneration in the underlying white matter.

petechiae, typically less restricted to the white matter than in the case of fat embolization.

Cerebral Veins

The cerebral veins empty into large conduits called the venous sinuses. Among these, the sagittal sinus occupies a position of prominence, as it accommodates the venous drainage from the superior portions of the cerebral hemispheres. Blood flows sluggishly in these aqueducts, the walls of which are irregularly contoured with estuaries. One would expect that thrombosis would be common, but it is, fortunately, rare. **Venous sinus thrombosis** is, however, a serious complication of **systemic dehydration,** as occurs in the adult with chronic alcoholism or in the infant with gastrointestinal fluid loss; **phlebitis,** as might result from regional mastoiditis or from bacteremia;

obstruction by a neoplasm, notably a meningioma; and **red blood cell sickling** in sickle cell disease. Venous obstruction causes stagnation upstream. Thus, abrupt thrombosis of the sagittal sinus frequently results in bilateral hemorrhagic infarctions of the frontal regions of the cerebral hemispheres. A more indolent mechanism of occlusion, such as occurs with invasion by a meningioma, permits the recruitment of collateral circulation through the inferior sagittal sinus.

Global Ischemia

Global ischemia or hypoxia, as results from cardiac arrest (ischemia) or from near-drowning (hypoxia), imparts a generalized, or global, insult to the brain. The character of the injury reflects the topography of the cerebral blood vessels and the gradient in sensitivity of individual species of neurons to oxygen deprivation and to lactic acid intoxication. Global ischemia is characterized by laminar necrosis, whereas hypoxia leads to selective destruction of the cerebellar Purkinje cells and the neurons of Sommer's section of the hippocampus (Figs. 28-23 through 28-25).

The topography of the cerebral vasculature is primarily responsible for two lesions: **watershed infarcts** and **laminar necrosis.** The major cerebral vessels—notably the anterior, middle, and posterior cerebral arteries—provide overlapping collateral circulation where they interface with the distribution of a contiguous vessel. Thus, the anterior cerebral arteries supply the cortex on the medial aspects of both cerebral hemispheres and also interface with the distribution of the middle cerebral arteries in the para-

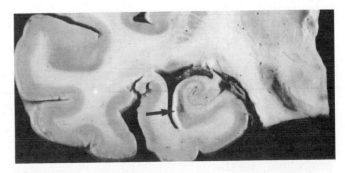

Figure 28-25. Ischemic necrosis of Sommer's sector. A coronal section through the hippocampus reveals a darkened area of necrosis in the region of Sommer's sector (*arrow*). The lesion exemplifies the unusual sensitivity of these neurons to ischemia.

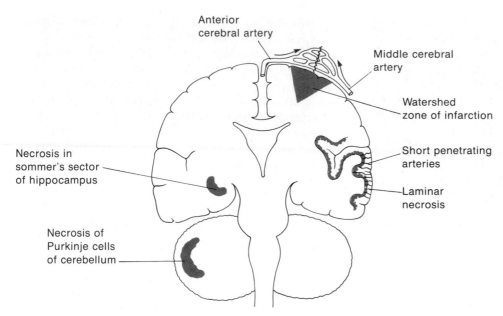

Figure 28-26. Consequences of global ischemia. A global insult induces lesions that reflect the vascular architecture (watershed infarcts, laminar necrosis) and the sensitivity of individual neuronal systems (pyramidal cells of Sommer s section, Purkinje cells).

sagittal cortex. A precipitous decline in circulatory flow, as occurs during cardiac arrest, abruptly diminishes the circulation in the terminal branches of both the anterior and middle cerebral arteries, and thus inflicts a dual insult to the zones of collateral circulation, or "watershed" areas (Fig. 28-26).

Similarly, laminar necrosis is an injury whose pattern reflects the topography of the normal cerebral vasculature. The cerebral gray matter receives its major blood supply through the "short penetrators" that originate at right angles from larger vessels in the pia. Having this origin, they form a cascade as they penetrate into the gray matter. They branch frequently and finally construct a rich plexus of capillaries deep in the gray matter, notably in the fourth to sixth neuronal cell layers. An abrupt loss of circulatory pressure selectively diminishes flow through this terminal capillary plexus. The necrotic zone is laminar in configuration, parallel to the surface of the cortex, and the necrosis is understandably most severe in the deep layers of the gray cortex.

Selective neuronal sensitivity to hypoxia is expressed most dramatically in the Purkinje cells of the cerebellum and the pyramidal neurons of Sommer's sector in the hippocampus. Presumably, these neurons have unusual metabolic requirements for oxygen, or an inordinate sensitivity to lactic acid.

The lesions of ischemia and hypoxia are intimately related. Thus, in a patient who has experienced car-

diac arrest and global ischemia, or who has been deprived of oxygen by near-drowning or by entrapment in a burning building, and who survives for several days (the period required for the morphologic lesions to become evident), the brain can be expected to show one or a variety of changes. These include laminar necrosis, watershed infarcts, a marked loss of Purkinje cells, or necrosis of Sommer's sector.

Aneurysms

Fluid under pressure exploits weaknesses of the arterial wall and may produce focal dilatations, or aneurysms. Such weaknesses may be the result of developmental defects, which give rise to berry, saccular, or medial defect aneurysms; atherosclerosis; hypertensive lipohyalinosis, the harbinger of Charcot-Bouchard aneurysms; bacterial inflammation, the forerunner of mycotic aneurysms; or trauma, which is rarely the instigator of a dissecting aneurysm.

Intracranially, atherosclerosis adheres to the same general principles that govern its deposition and evolution elsewhere. Thus, it preferentially localizes in the major vessels—namely, the vertebral, basilar, and internal carotid arteries. The degree of involvement tapers in the smaller branches.

The evolution of atherosclerosis in the brain, as in other organs, is rooted in the genesis of the atheromatous plaque. Chapter 10 deals more fully with the complexity of this process; here we merely take note that the plaque narrows the lumen by its own mass and serves as a potential site of intimal disruption and thrombus formation. Fibrous replacement of the muscularis and the destruction of the internal elastic membrane weaken the wall and permit aneurysmal dilatation. Characteristically, atherosclerotic aneurysms are fusiform. As an aneurysm acquires girth, the vessel also becomes elongated. Thus, an atherosclerotic aneurysm of the basilar artery moves laterally into the cerebellar pontine angle, where it constitutes a mass that compresses cranial nerves and produces neurologic deficits. The major clinical complication of a cerebral atherosclerotic aneurysm is thrombosis, not rupture. Thus, pontine infarctions are the anticipated sequelae of atherosclerotic aneurysms of the basilar artery (Fig. 28-27).

The terms saccular and berry aneurysm are synonymous with medial defect aneurysm. The lesion originates during embryonic development. A vessel that bifurcates creates a crotch, which, together with the parent artery, creates a Y-shaped configuration.

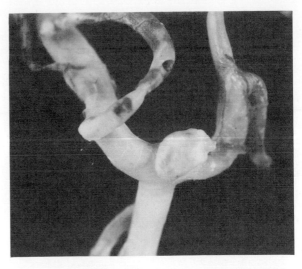

Figure 28-28. Saccular aneurysm. A small spherical outpouching occurred at the bifurcation of the middle cerebral artery in the crotch of two branches. This is the point of impact of the circulatory stream. The apical wall of the aneurysm consists only of adventitial fibrous tissue; it lacks a muscularis, and the internal elastic membrane has disintegrated.

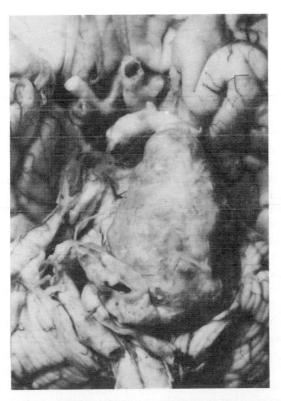

Figure 28-27. Atherosclerotic aneurysm. Atherosclerosis weakens the wall of the major cerebral vessels—notably, the basilar and carotid arteries—and aneurysms may result. In this photograph, the basilar artery is greatly dilated. A redundancy in length permitted the mass lesion to shift from the midline into the left cerebellopontine angle.

The muscularis of the parent vessel, and that of the two branches, are individually circumferential. These muscular coats may fail to interdigitate adequately in the notch. Thus, a point of congenital muscular weakness is created, bridged only by endothelium, internal elastic membrane, and a slender coating of adventitia. The point of the angle is also the site of impact of the bloodstream from the parent vessel. Time and trauma exploit the weakness. When the internal elastic membrane degenerates or fragments, the endothelium yields. A saccular aneurysm evolves, with its apical portion precariously formed only of adventitia. Rupture of a berry aneurysm causes life-threatening subarachnoid hemorrhage, associated with a 35% mortality during the initial bleed (Figure 28-28).

For reasons not understood, **more than 90% of saccular aneurysms occur at branch points in the carotid system.** They are about equally distributed at the unions of the anterior cerebral and anterior communicating arteries, the internal carotid–posterior communicating–anterior cerebral–anterior choroidal artery complex, and at the trifurcation of the middle cerebral artery.

Enlargement of a saccular aneurysm may constitute a mass that is of sufficient size to compress cranial nerves and produce palsies, or to impinge on parenchymal structures and induce neurologic symptoms. Palsies of cranial nerves III, IV, and VI, or seizures initiated by the compression of the medial

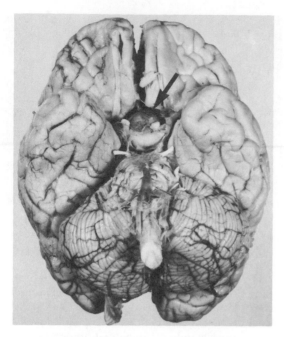

Figure 28-29. Saccular aneurysm. A saccular aneurysm (*arrow*) originated in the union between the left anterior cerebral and anterior communicating arteries. Its mass compressed the optic chiasm, impairing vision.

aspect of the temporal lobe are the most common manifestations of a giant saccular aneurysm on the internal carotid complex (Figs. 28-29 through 28-31).

Mycotic aneurysms result from the embolization of thrombotic material, usually from an infected cardiac valve, which contains microorganisms. The embolus, composed of fibrin and platelets and populated by bacteria, is characteristically smaller than those derived from an endocardial mural thrombus. Typically, it flows through the carotid circulation and lodges in a branch of the middle cerebral artery. Being small, it enters the arteries of the pia and lodges at the origin of a short, penetrating vessel. The bacteria proliferate, inducing inflammation and diminishing the integrity of the arterial wall. The compromised vessel yields to an aneurysm, which may rupture and present as an intracerebral or subarachnoid hemorrhage. Alternatively, microorganisms are released from the bed of inflammation and produce a cerebral abscess or suppurative meningitis.

Vascular Malformations

There are four major categories of vascular anomalies: **arteriovenous malformations, cavernous angiomas, telangiectasias,** and **venous angiomas.** The arterio-venous malformation is the most common, and it has the greatest clinical significance. The lesion evolves during embryonic development from disordered angiogenesis that is secondary to focal absence of a capillary bed, thus permitting direct communication between cerebral arteries and veins (Fig. 28-32). The resultant conglomeration of abnormal vessels usually involves a region of the cerebral cortex and the contiguous underlying white matter. The involved area enlarges as a result of the gradual recruitment of tributary vessels. Symptoms usually appear in the second or third decades, and include seizure disorders and cerebral hemorrhages. Cavernous angiomas, formed of large vascular spaces compartmentalized by prominent fibrous walls, are considerably less common. Rupture is uncommon, and cavernous angiomas usually remain asymptomatic. A telangiectasia is a focal aggregate of uniformly small vessels with intervening parenchyma. These lesions may initiate seizures, but they rarely rupture. A venous angioma consists of enlarged veins, which are usually few in number and are distributed randomly in a focus of parenchyma. The lesion is generally asymptomatic.

Hemorrhages

Hemorrhages that occur in the brain independent of trauma are referred to as spontaneous, but most are secondary to a vascular anomaly or are the consequence of long-standing hypertension. **The common sites of hypertensive hemorrhage are the basal ganglia-thalamus (65%), the pons (15%), and the cerebellum (8%).** Interestingly, although the frequency is notably increased by the presence of hypertension, the topographic pattern is not altered by the absence of this major contributory factor.

Long-standing hypertension is associated with the occurrence of Charcot-Bouchard aneurysms, which are fusiform, segmental dilatations along the course of small arteries and arterioles. They are unrelated to branch points, and thus differ in configuration and position from berry aneurysms. The aneurysmal site is marked by lipohyalinosis, lipid deposition within the media, and hyalin replacement of the muscularis. Lipohyalinosis, usually accompanied by Charcot-Bouchard aneurysm, occurs in a geographic distribution that closely corresponds to the pattern of spontaneous hemorrhages. This fact argues for a relationship between hypertension, lipohyalinosis, and Charcot-Bouchard aneurysms on the one hand, and spontaneous cerebral hemorrhages on the other.

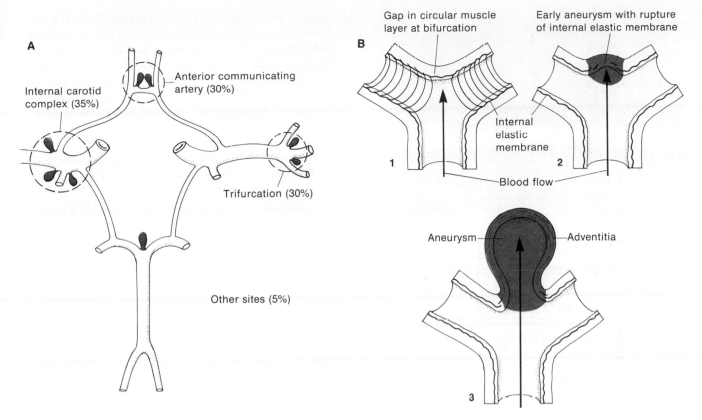

Figure 28-30. Saccular aneurysm. (*A*) The incidence of saccular aneurysms (berry aneurysms), which preferentially involve the carotid tributaries, is depicted. (*B*) Their pathogenesis is illustrated. The lesion evolves as a result of blood acting on an early embryonic defect.

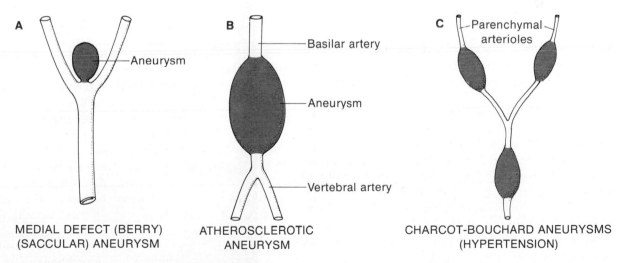

Figure 28-31. Types of aneurysms. The etiology of an aneurysm (congenital, atherosclerotic, hypertensive) defines its location, size, and shape.

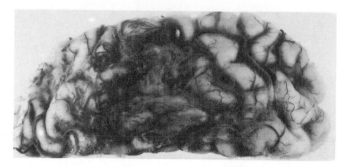

Figure 28-32.   Arteriovenous malformation. An arteriovenous malformation results from altered embryonic angiogenesis, wherein veins communicate directly with arteries without intervening capillaries. This lesion, which involves the right cerebral hemisphere, is viewed from above. Its presence initiated seizures, a common symptom of arteriovenous malformations.

Most hypertensive cerebral hemorrhages begin in the region of the external capsule—that is, peripheral to the basal ganglia and thalamus. The onset of symptoms is abrupt, and is dominated by weakness. When hemorrhage is progressive (and it usually is), the time span during the appearance of symptoms is a period of hours or several days. During this interval, the hematoma may attain a size that is sufficient to cause death by transtentorial herniation or rupture into a lateral ventricle. The latter event initiates massive intraventricular hemorrhage (Fig. 28-33).

Intraventricular hemorrhage rapidly distends the entire ventricular system with blood. At postmortem examination, the forward edge of this column of blood expands the fourth ventricle but rarely emerges from the foramina of Magendie and Luschka. This indicates that the rush of blood through the ventricular system causes death by distention of the fourth ventricle, with compression of the vital centers in the medulla.

A **spontaneous hemorrhage in the pons** is, similarly, a catastrophic event. Loss of consciousness reflects damage to the reticular formation, an injury that overshadows all other specific cranial nerve deficits. The hematoma generally originates in the midpons, and thus is more caudal than hemorrhages induced by transtentorial herniation. Pontine hemorrhage encroaches upon the vital medullary centers. Patients rarely survive; death frequently occurs before arrival at the hospital (Fig. 28-34).

The symptomatology of a **cerebellar hemorrhage** is also dynamic. The patient abruptly experiences ataxia, usually accompanied by a severe occipital headache and vomiting. The expanding hematoma threatens life acutely through compression of the medulla—either directly or secondarily—as a conse-

quence of cerebellar tonsilar herniation into the foramen magnum. The lack of localized functional representation in the cerebellum generally permits surgical evacuation of the lesion without serious neurologic deficits, and thus contrasts favorably with the almost universally disappointing surgical results of drainage or resection of cerebral hematomas (Fig. 28-35).

Cerebral hemorrhages also have other causes. Among these are leakage from an arteriovenous malformation; erosion of a vessel by a primary or secondary neoplasm; a bleeding diathesis, as exemplified by thrombocytopenic purpura; endothelial injury by microorganisms, notably rickettsia; and embolic infarction with consequent hemorrhage into the area of necrosis. The locations of hypertensive hemorrhage are shown in Figure 28-36.

Cerebrospinal Fluid Dynamics

Phylogenetic development has ingeniously evolved an accessory circulatory system, and has individualized it to the needs of the brain and spinal cord. This body of fluid flows passively and leisurely from its

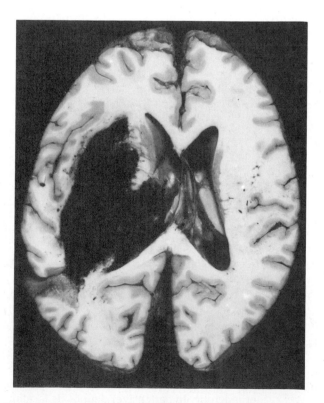

Figure 28-33.   Cerebral hemorrhage. The basal ganglia-thalamus is the most frequent site of hypertensive hemorrhage. Note the contouring of the hematoma on the left by the external capsule. Blood has dissected through the thalamus into the left lateral ventricle.

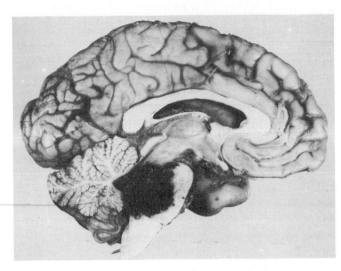

Figure 28-34. Pontine hemorrhage. The pons is the second most common site of hypertensive hemorrhages. Characteristically, bleeding begins in the tegmentum and ruptures through the floor of the fourth ventricle. Note that blood has not passed through the foramen of Magendie into the subarachnoid space.

intraventricular origin to its site of reabsorption—principally, the sagittal sinus by way of the arachnoid villi. Its flow transports metabolites, thereby providing nutrition for the ependymal membrane, which remains intact even when it is subjacent to a massive cerebral infarct. The cerebrospinal fluid also serves as a sump of metabolic waste; most importantly, however, its fluid properties create a protective jacket for the brain and spinal cord. Consequently, the cerebral hemispheres float within the calvarium.

The cerebrospinal fluid is present in a volume of 120 to 150 ml and is formed principally by the choroid plexus in estimated amounts of 500 ml per day. A small volume of fluid is formed near the surface of the brain and reaches the subarachnoid compartment through the Virchow-Robin spaces. In striking contrast to the renal glomeruli, the choroid plexus is not marked for obsolescence, either by disease or by the ravages of time and atherosclerosis. Age disfigures the delicate anatomy of the choroid by the deposition of fibrous tissue, cholesterol, and calcium, but its filtration capacity is maintained, and no disease state is characterized by a dearth of spinal fluid.

The choroid plexus stretches as a cord along the roof of the third ventricle, bifurcates, and passes through each foramen of Monro. It then angles sharply posterior to lie on the floor of the lateral ventricles, curves gently downward to enter the temporal horn of each ventricular chamber, and expands appreciably in this curvature to form a bulbous mass, the glomus. Thus, the choroid plexus is not present in the frontal or occipital poles of the lateral ventricles, nor does it enter the aqueduct of Sylvius.

During embryonic development, the cerebellum rotates upon its transverse axis, and the pia is carried onto the posterior surface of the fourth ventricle, where it comes into contact with ependyma. Through the combined participation of these two structures, the tela choroidea is formed from the pia, and the cuboidal epithelium of the choroid is contributed by the ependyma. Thus, the posterior aspect of the fourth ventricle is covered by choroid plexus that extends laterally through the foramen of Luschka into the immediate subarachnoid space of the cerebello-pontine angle. Analogously, the inward rotation of the cerebral hemispheres contributes pia to the formation of the choroid plexus, which ultimately resides in the third and lateral ventricles.

Obstruction to the flow of cerebrospinal fluid results in hydrocephalus. When the obstruction is within the ventricular chambers, the hydrocephalus is designated as **noncommunicating.** By contrast, an impediment in the subarachnoid space creates **communicating** hydrocephalus (Fig. 28-37).

Flow through a ventricular chamber or a foramen may be obstructed by a congenital malformation, a neoplasm, inflammation, or hemorrhage. As will be discussed later, **the aqueduct of Sylvius is the most common location of an obstructive congenital malformation.** Some neoplasms, notably papillomas or carcinomas of the choroid plexus, and ependymomas arise within the ventricular chambers. Obstruction with hydrocephalus and increased intracranial pressure predominate in the production of the clinical

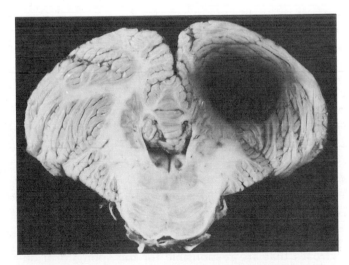

Figure 28-35. Cerebellar hemorrhage. The cerebellum is the third major area of hypertensive hemorrhage. The expanding lesion may displace the cerebellum forcefully through the foramen magnum to compress the medulla.

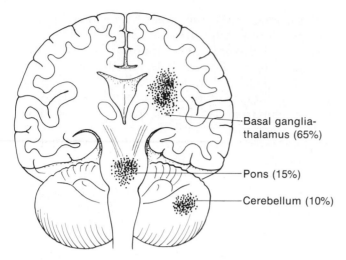

Figure 28-36.   The distribution of hypertensive hemorrhages. The location and relative incidence of hypertensive hemorrhages is in accord with the distribution of Charcot-Bouchard aneuryms.

symptomatology. Interestingly, in addition to physical obstruction, neoplasms of the choroid plexus form excessive volumes of spinal fluid. Tumors of the parenchyma, notably gliomas, compress the aqueduct or a ventricular chamber, causing hydrocephalus behind the point of obstruction. The ependyma is sensitive to viral infections, particularly during embryonic development; thus, ependymitis is possibly a cause of congenital aqueductal stenosis. Inflammation of the meninges produces fibrosis and may obstruct cerebrospinal fluid flow, thereby inducing communicating hydrocephalus.

Inflammatory Diseases

A consideration of intracranial and intraspinal infections must recognize the biologic properties of a wide variety of infectious agents. It must acknowledge the anatomic distribution of lesions and the nature of diverse tissue responses. Ultimately, it must interrelate the geographic patterns and the time intervals of tissue injury with the clinical symptomatology. The list of offending organisms is long, and includes **bacteria,** the majority of which initiate suppurative responses, whereas a few are responsible for granulomatous diseases; **conventional viruses,** but also an occasional renegade, notably the so-called **slow viruses** that are responsible for the spongiform degeneration associated with kuru, scrapie, and Creutzfeldt-Jakob disease; **fungi;** and **spirochetes,**

Rickettsia, and **protozoa,** as well as a host of **parasites.**

It is important to recall that **most species of organisms localize in preferred intracranial and intraspinal sites.** Thus, poliomyelitis is individualized by its selectivity for the motor neurons of the spinal cord and bulbar area, herpes simplex encephalitis by its localization in the temporal lobes, and progressive multifocal leukoencephalopathy by its preferred involvement of the parasagittal white matter. **Bacteria generally localize in the leptomeninges and induce meningitis.** However, the same organism can, on occasion, lodge in the parenchyma, producing a cerebritis which is prone to progress to abscess formation. On rare occasions, these same organisms enter the subdural compartment and clandestinely induce subdural empyema. Some fungi are rigidly opportunistic; most benefit by an incompetency of the immune system of the host. Some, such as *Cryptococcus neoformans,* grow indolently in the leptomeninges. Others, such as *Aspergillus fumigatus,* aggressively induce cerebral abscesses and occasionally initiate leptomeningitis.

Spirochetes gain access to the nervous system through the bloodstream. The treponema may as-

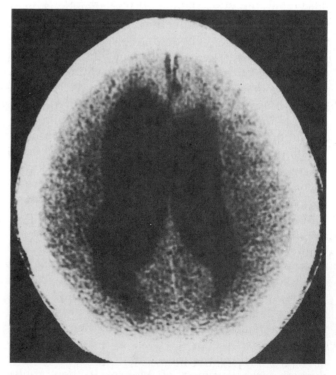

Figure 28-37.   Hydrocephalus. In this computed tomography (CT) scan of the brain, the ventricular system is remarkably dilated, even though the brain is contained within the limiting confines of the cranial compartment.

sume a prolonged residency in neural tissues, where they propagate and induce highly distinctive, chronic tissue reactions that are responsible for the clinical manifestations of dementia paralytica. On other occasions, the spirochete selects the meninges, where it initiates fibrosis and an obliterative endarteritis, thereby creating meningovascular syphilis. Rickettsial infections, such as Rocky Mountain spotted fever, target endothelial cells. When the endothelial cells of the brain are injured by this microorganism, petechiae and cerebral edema result, and the global nature of this process induces a serious encephalopathy. *Toxoplasma gondii* pits its low virulence against the natural resistance of adult humans and generally is unable to induce an active infection. Yet, through transplacental transmission, it gains access to the fetal brain, exploits its susceptibility, and induces subependymal necrosis and calcification in the basal ganglia and thalamus (Fig. 28-38). This protozoan also recognizes the susceptibility of the immunocompromised adult, and therefore constitutes a significant source of infection in patients with acquired immunodeficiency syndrome (AIDS).

Clearly, the anatomic location of the infection, the character of the tissue response, and the age and nature of the patient are all cardinal factors in an understanding and recognition of an intracranial infection.

Meningitis

The term **leptomeningitis** denotes an inflammatory process that is localized to the interfacing surfaces of the pia and arachnoid, the encasement for the cerebrospinal fluid. Thus, the characteristics of the inflammation are portrayed in the composition of this fluid, notably in its cellular constituency, its protein and sugar contents, its electrolyte composition, and its serologic reactivities.

Pachymeningitis is inflammation of the dura. It is usually the consequence of focal, contiguous inflammation, such as chronic sinusitis or mastoiditis. The dura is a substantial barrier, and the inflammation is usually restricted to its outer surface.

With few exceptions, all forms of meningitis are initiated by microorganisms, with bacteria being the principal offender. Among these, suppurative organisms predominate. In the neonate, in whom resistance to gram-negative bacteria has not yet developed fully, *Escherichia coli* is the prime offender. *Hemophilus influenzae* plagues the early years of life, whereas pneumococcus, meningococcus, and the tubercle bacillus predominate thereafter. **Because most organ-**

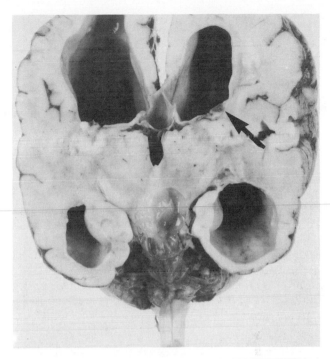

Figure 28-38. Toxoplasmosis of the brain. *Toxoplasma gondii* crosses the placental barrier and manifests a strong tropism for the paraventricular areas of the cerebral hemispheres. This region contains the germinal mantle, an area of high cellularity and high metabolic activity. The inflammation initiates necrosis that typically calcifies (*arrow*). The proximity of the lesion to the third ventricle often induces hydrocephalus. The organisms may become encysted, and the active infection may abate.

isms initiate a purulent or suppurative response, the presence of polymorphonuclear leukocytes in the spinal fluid is the most definitive index of meningitis. Yet, lymphocytes are the hallmark of tuberculosis, and this is also true of the viral meningitides, as well as chronic infections, such as those attributable to *Cryptococcus neoformans*.

Gross examination of the brain discloses an exudate of leukocytes and fibrin that imparts opacity to the arachnoid and, when extreme, a creamy appearance to this membrane. The intensity of the exudate may be so slight as to be equivocal to the naked eye, whereas at other times, it is sufficiently marked to form white cords along the vessels that traverse the sulci, particularly those in the parasagittal areas and those in proximity to the Sylvian fissure. A purulent exudate is most prominent over the convexity of the cerebral hemispheres, but it also extends about the base of the brain where the interpeduncular fossa generally constitutes a reservoir. Since the intracranial and intraspinal subarachnoid spaces are in con-

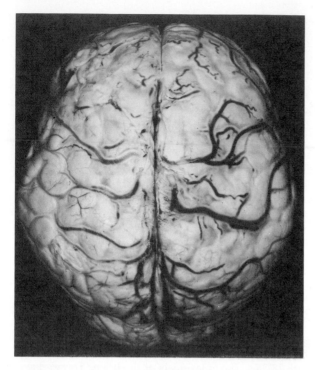

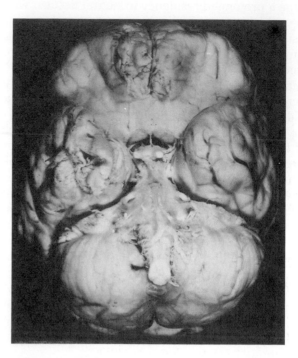

Figure 28-39.   Purulent meningitis. An exudate is most prominent over the convexities, which is characteristic of purulent meningitis. The presence of pneumococci in the fluid-filled compartment of the subarachnoid space caused an outpouring of leukocytes.

Figure 28-40.   Purulent meningitis. Purulent meningitis also involves the base of the brain, typically with an accumulation of exudate in the cisternae.

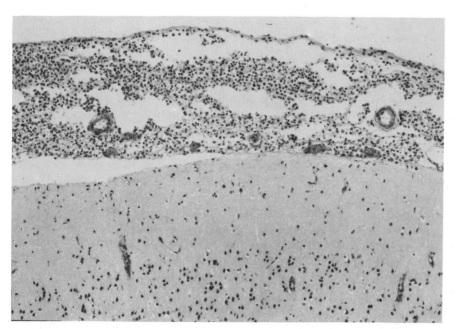

Figure 28-41.   Purulent meningitis. A photomicrograph demonstrates an exudate composed of neutrophils and fibrin in the subarachnoid space; this represents a response to bacterial infection of the cerebrospinal fluid. The pia is a delicate membrane, but it serves as a remarkable barrier to the passage of leukocytes into the underlying cerebral tissue.

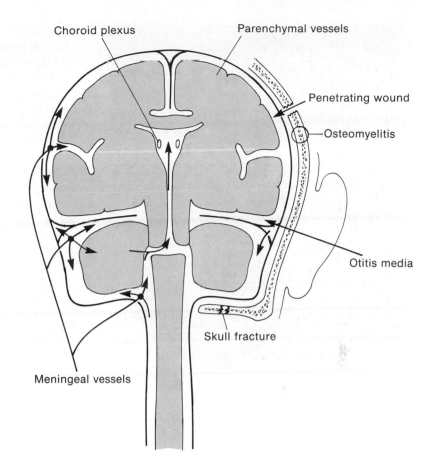

Choroid plexus

Parenchymal vessels

Penetrating wound

Osteomyelitis

Otitis media

Skull fracture

Meningeal vessels

Figure 28-42. Routes of entry of infectious organisms into the cranial cavity.

tinuity, the exudate passes freely between these conjoined compartments. The pia, although structurally diaphanous, is a remarkably efficient barrier against the spread of infection and generally precludes involvement of the underlying brain. Thus, cerebral abscesses are rare as a complication of meningitis. The effectiveness of this barrier is further underscored when one recalls that the pia forms conical sleeves about each vessel as it penetrates through the surface of the brain. These slender, perivascular compartments, termed the Virchow-Robin spaces, are in direct continuity with the subarachnoid space. They may harbor leukocytes and microorganisms, but rarely do they provide a portal of entry for infection into the parenchyma (Figs. 28-39 through 28-41).

Most organisms reach the intracranial compartment by way of the bloodstream. It is not clear, however, by what means they exit from the vascular channels. Blood-borne bacteria may lodge in the pial blood vessels, produce an arteritis, escape into the spinal fluid, and interact with the meningeal surfaces to induce meningitis. Alternatively, they may gain entry into the cerebrospinal fluid by way of the choroid plexus. At postmortem examination of patients with tuberculous meningitis, granulomas are frequently encountered in the choroid plexus. However, this

defines an end-stage characteristic and does not necessarily constitute an initial event. Tubercle bacilli may also lodge in parenchymal capillaries, as is true of pyogenic organisms that produce abscesses. These tubercle bacilli might then initiate a tuberculoma which secondarily erodes into the subarachnoid space. Perhaps all of these potential portals—namely, pial blood vessels, the choroid plexus, and the parenchymal capillaries—are functional portals on occasion. Enlightenment may come from studying the Rhesus monkey, an animal that is highly susceptible to tuberculosis and greatly disposed to hematogenous dissemination, yet rarely develops tuberculous meningitis. This situation implies that there is a single portal of entry from the bloodstream, as it seems unlikely that numerous portals would all be patent in humans and all be closed in the monkey. The routes of entry of microorganisms into the cranial cavity are summarized in Figure 28-42.

Bacterial Meningitis

Many organisms are capable of initiating acute, purulent inflammation in the meninges or the brain. As has been mentioned, the list is headed by *E. coli* and *H. influenzae* in the neonate and child, and by pneu-

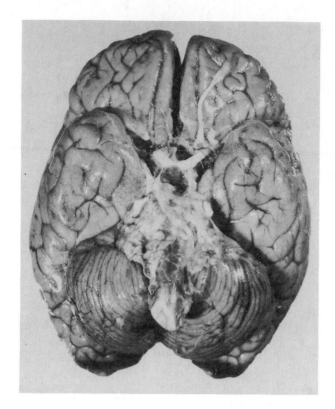

Figure 28-43. Tuberculous meningitis. Tuberculous meningitis involves the base of the brain. Granulomatous lesions are scattered in the leptomeninges of the pons, in the interpeduncular fossa, and in the Sylvian fissure.

mococcus, meningococcus, staphylococcus, and streptococcus at older ages. Of note is the unusually high incidence of pneumonococcal meningitis, which is often recurrent in patients with a history of basilar skull fracture.

The cross-placental transfer of maternal IgG imparts protection to the neonate against many bacteria. However, IgM, which is required to neutralize *E. coli* and similar gram-negative organisms, is not normally transported across the placental barrier. Meningitis induced by gram-negative organisms quickly produces a dense, purulent exudate, and is often lethal in infancy.

Hemophilus influenzae is also a gram-negative organism. However, environmental exposure is somewhat delayed, and the incidence of meningitis is maximal between 3 months and 3 years. This organism evokes a dense, leukocytic exudate that is rich in fibrin. Loculation of this exudate creates a barrier against chemotherapy.

The meningococcus frequents the human nasopharynx. Its airborne transmission in crowded environments causes epidemic meningitis, a serious problem in military barracks. The initial phase of the

infection is a bacteremia manifested as fever, malaise, and a petechial skin rash. During this interval, an intravascular coagulopathy may be associated with lethal adrenal hemorrhages **(Waterhouse-Friderichsen syndrome).** Untreated bacteremia often initiates an acute fulminant meningitis.

Tuberculous Meningitis and Tuberculomas

The granulomatous expression of tuberculosis in the meninges is analogous to that in visceral sites. Individual tubercules are structured about areas of caseous necrosis, with epithelioid cells, Langerhans giant cells, and lymphocytes. Inadequately treated tuberculous meningitis expresses two further attributes—namely, a propensity for scar formation and a tendency to involve blood vessels. Meningeal fibrosis is responsible for the sequelae of communicating hydrocephalus, whereas involvement of vessels leads to parenchymal infarcts. These infarcts are most often found in the distribution of the striate arteries, as tuberculosis has a strong predilection for the base of the brain and particularly for the Sylvian fissure. Untreated tuberculous meningitis is uniformly fatal within 2 to 4 weeks (Fig. 28-43).

Parenchymal involvement by tuberculosis produces a solitary mass which, typically, is a spherical lesion with a central area of caseous necrosis surrounded by granulomatous tissue. In the early era of neurosurgery, these tuberculomas accounted for 10% or more of intracranial "tumors" (Fig. 28-44).

Tuberculosis of the spinal column (Pott's disease)

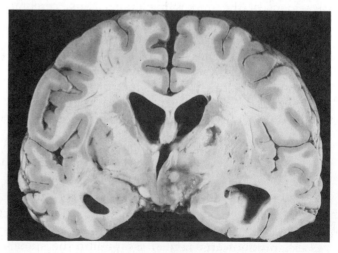

Figure 28-44. Tuberculoma. A tuberculoma present in the right hypothalamus produced a mass lesion that disfigures the third ventricle. It impaired circulation through the striate arteries and caused an infarct in the right internal capsule.

produces an epidural mass of granulomatous tissue. Frequently, it causes destruction and angulation of the spine, and carries the risk of spinal cord compression.

Cryptococcal Meningitis

Cryptococcal meningitis is an indolent form of infection wherein the virulence of the causative agent marginally exceeds the resistance of the host. Thus, on rare occasions, the organism establishes a progressive meningitis in a noncompromised host. However, in most instances, it acts opportunistically, producing meningitis in an immunosuppressed host, the progression of which takes place within a period of months. The organism customarily enters the human host by the inhalation of contaminated particulates. Birds are a major reservoir for *Cryptococcus neoformans*, and their excreta is a vehicle of disease transmittal to humans. The inhaled organisms initiate a transient or progressive pneumonitis, after which they enter the bloodstream and the intracranial compartment. The tissue response in the meninges is typically sparse. To the naked eye, it appears as discrete white nodules that are approximately 1 mm in diameter. The lesions are widely disseminated in the meninges, ependyma, and choroid plexus. Although the organisms may abound, particularly in the Virchow-Robin spaces, the tissue response is meager. It features an occasional multinucleated giant cell, sometimes with phagocytized organisms, accompanied by scant epithelioid cells and a scattering of lymphocytes. The organisms are encapsulated spheres that are 5 to 15 μ in diameter. They have an external gelatinous capsule and reproduce by budding. When a drop of contaminated spinal fluid is mixed with India ink, microscopic examination shows a clear halo about the encapsulated organism. Importantly, this capsule sheds antigens, and the detection of these in the spinal fluid by the latex cryptococcal antigen test is of immediate diagnostic significance.

Syphilitic Meningitis and Related Lesions

Syphilis attests to the potential chronicity of intracranial infections. The spirochete *Treponema pallidum* enters the bloodstream from a primary lesion, the chancre. Interestingly, its rate of multiplication in this location is intense. Dark-field preparations obtained several weeks after a few organisms have entered the dermis and subcutaneous tissue typically disclose the chancre to be teeming with spirochetes. The onset of secondary syphilis is indicated externally by the ap-

pearance of a maculopapular rash on the skin and mucous membranes, and internally by a few lymphocytes and plasma cells and an elevated protein level in the spinal fluid. This is also the period when the blood-borne spirochetes come to reside, at least transiently, in the meninges. As will be discussed later, spirochetes can also infect the cerebral tissues during this interval. The organisms do not survive for long in the meninges. They cannot be demonstrated histologically in cases of meningovascular syphilis, and characteristically, the serologic tests of the spinal fluid yield negative results. Nevertheless, on occasion, the transitory presence of the spirochete initiates a fibroblastic response in the meninges that is accompanied by a **proliferative, obliterative endarteritis** of the subjacent cortical arterioles. **Plasma cells are the hallmarks of syphilis.** They abound in the chancre and are present about the vasa vasorum of the aorta in luetic aortitis. Similarly, they are the inflammatory cells that prominently cuff the cortical arterioles in meningovascular syphilis. Obliterative endarteritis induces multiple, small, cortical infarcts.

Tabes dorsalis is commonly portrayed as a degeneration of the posterior fasciculi of the spinal cord, but the initial lesion is a variant of chronic luetic meningitis (Fig. 28-45). The dorsal nerve roots that approach the spinal cord proximal to the dorsal root ganglia are met by a conical sleeve of arachnoid. This sleeve is filled with cerebrospinal fluid, and may be the site of chronic luetic inflammation. With time, the inflammatory response generates fibrous tissue that constricts the nerve root and causes wallerian degeneration. The axons that course cephalad in the posterior fasciculus do not synapse with intramedullary neurons, as do the axons of all other ascending pathways in the cord. Rather, they are direct extensions of axons from the posterior roots. Therefore, **wallerian degeneration** that is initiated in the dorsal spinal nerve roots extends directly into the posterior fasciculi. This is the most readily visualized morphologic lesion of tabes dorsalis (Fig. 28-46).

The spirochetes that lodge in the cerebral parenchyma may be clinically latent for one or several decades. Ostensibly, they replicate sluggishly but escape eradication, being shielded from the immune system by the blood–brain barrier. Their presence can be demonstrated in histologic sections taken several decades later. The spirochetes induce a focal loss of cortical neurons; a disfigurement in the topography of the residual nerve cells, producing a "wind-blown appearance;" a marked astrogliosis; a conversion of microglia into elongated forms encrusted with iron, termed rod cells; and a nodular ependymitis. These morphologic alterations are accompanied by marked

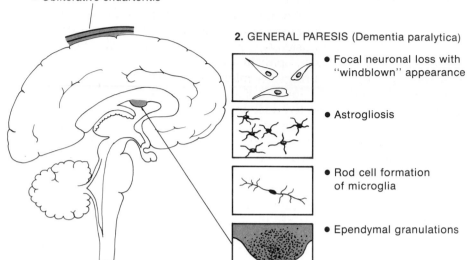

1. MENINGOVASCULAR SYPHILIS
- Thickened meninges
- Obliterative endarteritis

2. GENERAL PARESIS (Dementia paralytica)

- Focal neuronal loss with "windblown" appearance

- Astrogliosis

- Rod cell formation of microglia

- Ependymal granulations

Figure 28-45.   Involvement of the central nervous system in syphilis.

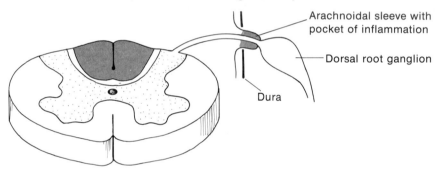

3. TABES DORSALIS (Posterior column degeneration)

Arachnoidal sleeve with pocket of inflammation

Dorsal root ganglion

Dura

decrements in cognitive function, referred to as dementia paralytica.

In summary, inflammation of the meninges may last only a few days or it may span a few decades. There are deficiencies in our knowledge about the onset, pathogenesis, and course of these categories of disease. As the etiologic agents of the meningitides generally reach the meninges through the bloodstream, it is fortunate that meningitis is rare, compared to the frequency of bacteremia.

We are also ignorant of the mechanism by which meningitis kills. For example, a healthy adult may contract meningococcal meningitis and die with only a meager outpouring of leukocytes in the leptomeninges. It has been suggested that toxins are absorbed by the brain stem and paralyze the cardiac and respiratory centers.

Abscess Formation

The cerebral gray matter and the immediately subjacent white matter are vascularized by a rich plexus of branching capillaries that constitute the terminal vasculature of arteries. These arteries, referred to as "short penetrators," form a cascade of branches originating at right angles from arteries in the pia and coursing perpendicularly through the cerebral cortex. The arteries branch frequently and form the richest capillary bed in the brain. Therefore, it is not surprising that microorganisms carried by the bloodstream lodge preferentially in this location. In the cortex, they replicate and generate a colony that stimulates inflammation. As a result, the vascular bed becomes permeable, and the escape of fluid produces regional edema, which is soon permeated by leukocytes. The term **cerebritis** is applied to this transient phase of inflammation. Typically, within several days, the leukocytic component intensifies, and lytic enzymes produce **liquefactive necrosis.** The lesion then becomes an abscess.

Astrocytes are inadequate to restrain such a suppurative process because of its strong propensity for tissue destruction and its rapid expansion. Because of these properties, an abscess threatens life, either by **transtentorial herniation** or by **rupture into a ventricle.** Thus, although astrocytes are usually the designated cell for cerebral repair, in this unique situation, they yield the role of containment to fibroblasts. The fibroblasts knit a capsule about regions of liquefactive necrosis. As a physical barrier, the capsule becomes a defined structure within a week or so, after which time it progressively thickens. In a subordinate role, astrocytes multiply at the peripheral margin of the lesion—that is, outside the fibrous capsule. However, the contribution of astrocytes to encapsulation is minimal. If the abscess is not excised, or if the infection is not totally restrained by antibiotic therapy, pressure builds within the abscess cavity. Edema develops in the underlying white matter, an area that is already vulnerable because of the normal paucity of blood vessels. This region is further disposed to ischemia because the abscess compresses the deep penetrating vessels that course perpendicularly from the pia into the depths of the white matter. Thus, the region below an abscess is susceptible

to the growth of microorganisms that escape from the primary abscess. Frequently, a secondary abscess forms subjacent to the primary lesion. Through the evolution of one or several generations of contiguous abscesses, the inflammatory process is carried inward to threaten intraventricular rupture. Purulent material liberated into the ventricle passes through the chambers and across the absorptive ependymal surfaces, and hence through the foramina of Magendie and Luschka into the meninges. The event is promptly fatal, presumably because of the absorption of toxic products. Alternatively, the expansion of an abscess may threaten life through transtentorial herniation (Fig. 28-47 through 28-49).

Viral Infections

Poliomyelitis, rabies, herpes simplex encephalitis, von Economo's encephalitis, subacute sclerosing panencephalitis, progressive multifocal leukoencephalopathy, the putative "slow" viral infections, and AIDS constitute prototypes of a heterogeneous and large category of infections (Fig. 28-50).

Viral infections are prone to localize in specific areas of the nervous system. Thus, poliomyelitis selects the motor neurons of the spinal cord and bulbar area. Rabies assails the brain stem. Herpes simplex targets the temporal lobes. von Economo's encephalitis acquired the synonym "sleeping sickness" because the inflammation localizes in the midbrain and hypothalamus. In this region, it also produces postencephalitic parkinsonism through its destruction of the substantia nigra. Subacute sclerosing panencephalitis and progressive multifocal leukoencephalopathy afflict the cerebral hemispheres; the former generally occurs in childhood, whereas the latter generally affects immunocompromised patients. The "slow viruses" (scrapie, kuru, and Creutzfeldt-Jakob disease) elicit a histologic response, termed **spongiform degeneration,** and originate a symptom complex that combines dementia and ataxia through global involvement of the cerebral and cerebellar cortices. The incidence, distribution, and significance of the viral encephalopathy of AIDS remain unclear.

The mechanism of viral tropism is largely obscure. There are specific binding sites for the poliovirus on the plasma membranes of specific motor neurons. Thus, the injection of poliovirus into the occipital lobes of a monkey fails to elicit reactivity at the injection site. Rather, the virus "seeks out" the motor neurons, to which it binds and into which it penetrates. It is less clear why other viral encephalitides are distributed regionally. For example, why does the

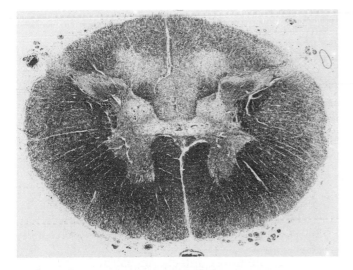

Figure 28-46. Tabes dorsalis. A myelin preparation shows the loss of axonal cylinders in the posterior column. The lesion is an expression of wallerian degeneration that results from constriction of the dorsal spinal roots proximal to the dorsal root ganglia. Axons that do not synapse in the spinal cord degenerate in a cephalad direction in the posterior fasciculus.

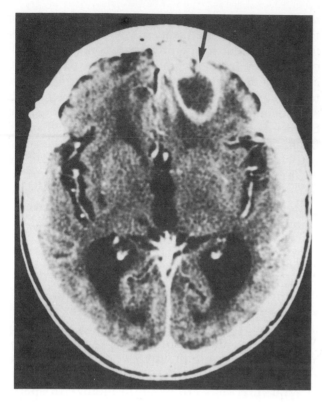

Figure 28-47. Cerebral abscess. A CT scan of the brain shows the variable tissue densities of an abscess (*arrow*) (a liquefied center, an encapsulating zone, and surrounding edema). This configuration may create a "ring lesion."

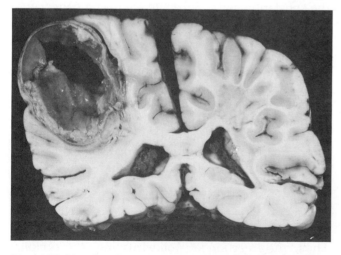

Figure 28-48. Cerebral abscess. An abscess of the left cerebral hemisphere is encapsulated by dense fibrous tissue. The center of the abscess is liquid; the wall is coated with a purulent exudate, fibrin, and necrotic tissue debris. The patient died of transtentorial herniation.

herpes simplex virus preferentially involve the temporal lobes? Because this virus resides latently in the gasserian ganglia, it has been suggested that the proximity of these ganglia to the temporal lobes is responsible for the geographic distribution of herpetic encephalitis. However, the validity of this concept requires confirmation.

The mobility of viruses within the neural tissues, and specifically within axons, is clearly exemplified in the pathogenesis of the herpetic "cold sore." It is also dramatically evident from studies of rabies. Intra-axonal transmission of the viral particles of rabies has been demonstrated to occur in peripheral nerves, from the site of the bite to the spinal cord or brain stem. Transmission also occurs centrifugally as, for example, from the cranial nerves to the salivary glands.

Perivascular cuffs of lymphocytes, principally in small arteries and arterioles, are the classic, but not universal, hallmark of viral infections of the central nervous system. A more precise diagnostic feature is the formation of inclusion bodies (Fig. 28-51), although this morphologic expression is by no means a consistent finding. Inclusion bodies are not present in some classic infections, such as poliomyelitis, nor are they features of atypical infections, such as Creutzfeldt-Jakob disease. The inclusions of **herpes simplex** and **herpes zoster** are small, intranuclear, and eosinophilic, but their morphologic appearance does not distinguish one from the other. By contrast, the cytoplasmic **Negri body** is unequivocal evidence of **rabies encephalitis.** The inclusions of **progressive multifocal leukoencephalopathy,** caused by a papovavirus ("JC virus"), are intranuclear, distinctively within oligodendroglial cells, typically associated with mild nucleomegaly, and of a "ground glass" appearance. They transform the size and chromatin composition of the entire nucleus within the formation of a discrete body. The inclusions of **subacute sclerosing panencephalitis** are intranuclear, frequently basophilic, and characteristically discrete, with a prominent halo. The inclusions of an infection by the **cytomegalovirus** are present both in the nucleus and cytoplasm, but are most conspicuous in the nucleus, where they are discrete, associated with nucleomegaly, and surrounded by a halo. The cytomegalovirus commonly infects an astrocyte, which is typically enlarged; when appropriately stained, it is shown to harbor small, inconspicuous, cytoplasmic inclusions. Thus, inclusions add significant direction and security to a diagnosis but, except in the case of rabies, are rarely pathognomonic.

As a further adjunct to diagnosis, viral particles

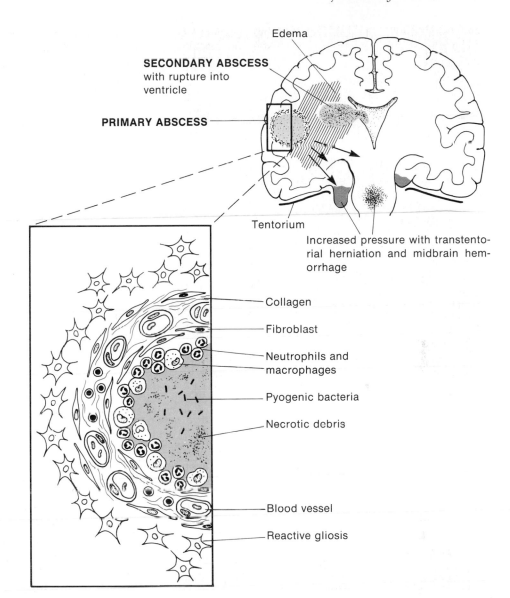

Edema

SECONDARY ABSCESS
with rupture into
ventricle

PRIMARY ABSCESS

Tentorium

Increased pressure with transtentorial herniation and midbrain hemorrhage

Collagen

Fibroblast

Neutrophils and macrophages

Pyogenic bacteria

Necrotic debris

Blood vessel

Reactive gliosis

Figure 28-49. Brain abscess and its complications. A cerebral abscess may cause death through the production of secondary abscesses with intraventricular rupture; alternatively, death may result from transtentorial herniation.

may be visualized by electron microscopy; again, the usefulness of this technique varies with the etiologic agent. Intranuclear viral particles abound in progressive multifocal leukoencephalopathy, and they are generally visible in herpes simplex. Nevertheless, exhaustive searches for the "slow virus" agent have so far been unsuccessful, although protein particles that do not contain nucleotides (termed "prions") have been claimed to be infectious. The utilization of immunohistochemical techniques in the demonstration of specific proteins is an important adjunct to the identification of viral infections.

The onset of most viral encephalitides is abrupt. The more specific neurologic deficits—for example, the paralysis of poliomyelitis, the somnolence of von

Economo's encephalitis, and the difficulty in swallowing (and thus the fear of drinking, or hydrophobia) of rabies—reflect the geographic localization of the lesions. Although most encephalitides run a brief course, the tempo of the diseases is variable. For example, the clinical course of subacute sclerosing panencephalitis may extend over many years. It is likely that the same would be true for progressive multifocal leukoencephalopathy were this infection not present in a host already ravaged by a primary major illness. The herpes simplex virus, as mentioned above, resides latently in the gasserian ganglion for decades, and there is suggestive evidence that it can do likewise in the brain. Creutzfeldt-Jakob disease not only has a prolonged latent incubation

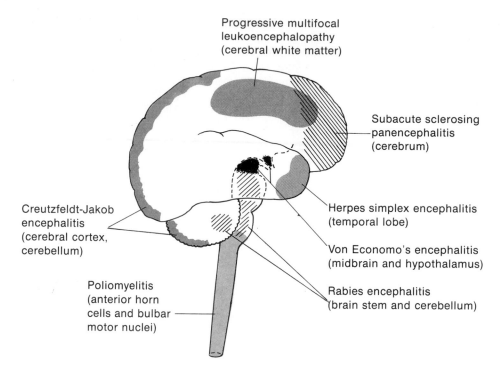

Progressive multifocal leukoencephalopathy (cerebral white matter)

Subacute sclerosing panencephalitis (cerebrum)

Creutzfeldt-Jakob encephalitis (cerebral cortex, cerebellum)

Herpes simplex encephalitis (temporal lobe)

Von Economo's encephalitis (midbrain and hypothalamus)

Poliomyelitis (anterior horn cells and bulbar motor nuclei)

Rabies encephalitis (brain stem and cerebellum)

Figure 28-50. Distribution of the lesions of viral encephalitides.

period, but its active phase can also be indolent. Thus, there are unresolved concerns about the potential role of viral infections in the genesis of chronic disorders, such as epilepsy and multiple sclerosis. Clearly, the full scope of viral infections of the nervous system—their tempos, tissue reactions, and clinical expressions—extends far beyond our current knowledge.

Poliomyelitis (Infantile Paralysis)

Generically, **the term poliomyelitis refers to inflammation of the gray matter of the spinal cord.** However, in common usage, it implies an inflammation by one of three strains of poliovirus (Brunhilde, Lancing, or Leon). The organism belongs to the enterovirus group, which also contains the coxsackievirus and echovirus. On occasion, the latter two viruses induce inflammation predominantly in the gray matter of the spinal cord, and thus can mimic poliomyelitis clinically.

Historical evidence suggests that poliomyelitis has occurred in epidemic form since antiquity. The recent medical triumph over this disease depended upon prior observations. In 1908, Landsteiner transmitted the infection to monkeys by an intraperitoneal inoculation of contaminated spinal fluid. Three years later, he reported that the virus replicates in the tonsils and intestinal tract of humans, and that these reservoirs of infection produce viremia. The next year, Flexner provided evidence of the capacity for host immunoresistance. About a half century later, the development and application of a vaccine eliminated epidemics of poliomyelitis. The polio virus binds to receptor sites on motor neurons, enters these cells, and produces injury and death of the cells (Fig. 28-52). An influx of fluid into the cytoplasmic compartment of an infected cell disperses the Nissl substance (rough endoplasmic reticulum) and displaces the nucleus peripherally. These structural events are collectively termed **chromatolysis.** Thereafter, the dead neuron appears contracted, and is phagocytosed by macrophages. This process is referred to as **neuronophagia.** These events produce inflammation that transiently features polymorphonuclear leukocytes; however, these cells soon yield to lymphocytes. The inflammation is centered in the anterior horns of the spinal cord and in the medulla. Inflammatory cells surround parenchymal blood vessels and involve the meninges to a lesser degree. The motor cortex usually does not exhibit frank inflammation, but may contain **glial nodules.** These are focal collections of small, round cells that are thought to represent microglia or lymphocytes. Interestingly, glial nodules are hallmarks of several types of inflammation, including those caused by viruses (e.g., poliomyelitis, herpes simplex); by Rickettsia (Rocky Mountain spotted fever); and by protozoa (toxoplasmosis) (Fig. 28-53).

Importantly, in poliomyelitis, the immunologic response of the host sterilizes the tissues within several weeks, thereby halting the progression of clinical disease and limiting the duration of the inflammation.

Rabies

Rabies has been recognized throughout recorded time. In humans it is a lethal encephalitis. Carnivores, such as the dog, wolf, fox, and skunk, are the principal reservoirs, but the infection extends to bats and to some domesticated animals, such as cattle, goats, and swine. The infectious agent is transmitted to humans through contaminated saliva introduced into the wound of a bite. The virus enters a peripheral nerve and is transported by centripetal axoplasmic flow to the spinal cord and brain. The latent interval varies in proportion to the distance of transport, being as short as 10 days or as long as 3 months. Centrifugal intra-axonal transport of the virus contaminates visceral organs, particularly the salivary glands, which in turn contaminate the saliva.

Although it is not understood why the virus seeks out the brain stem, this pattern of localization initiates the classic symptoms of difficulty in swallowing and the painful spasms of the throat that justify the term **hydrophobia**. The clinical symptoms—namely, irritability, agitation, seizures, and delirium—also reflect a **general encephalopathy**. The spinal fluid is altered in accord with the "typical viral response:" a modest pleocytosis by lymphocytes, a moderate elevation of protein content (50 to 100 mg/ml), and an unaltered glucose level and spinal fluid pressure. The illness progresses to death within one to several weeks.

Lymphocytes aggregate about the small arteries and veins in the brain stem. Scattered neurons show chromatolysis and neuronophagia. Glial nodules attest to the infectious nature of the process. The geographic distribution of the inflammation, centered in the brain stem with spillage into the cerebellum and hypothalamus, strongly suggests rabies. The presence of **Negri bodies** validates the diagnosis. Negri bodies are discrete, intracytoplasmic, deeply eosinophilic inclusions that measure several microns in diameter (See Fig. 28-51). They occur in neurons of the brain stem, particularly those in the hippocampus, and in the Purkinje cells of the cerebellum.

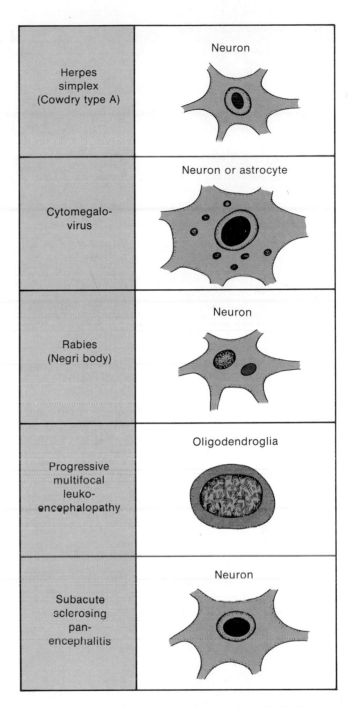

Figure 28-51. Inclusion bodies in viral encephalitides.

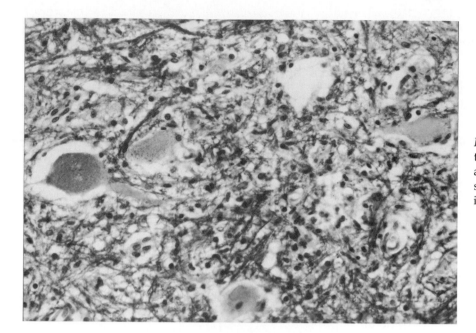

Figure 28-52.   Poliomyelitis. A photomicrograph shows variable degeneration of the anterior horn cells of the spinal cord. The neuropil is diffusely infiltrated by mononuclear cells.

Herpes Simplex Encephalitis and Related Infections

An important genus of pathogenic viruses includes herpes simplex (type I and II), the varicella-zoster virus, cytomegalovirus, Epstein-Barr virus, and the simian B virus.

Type I herpes virus is largely responsible for the

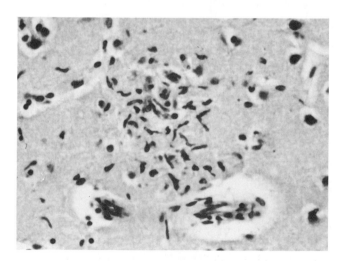

Figure 28-53.   Glial nodule. A photomicrograph shows elongated nuclei, presumably microglial cells, unassociated with necrosis. A glial nodule is a hallmark of inflammation, and may occur in viral rickettsial and protozoan infections.

"cold sore." This vesicular cutaneous lesion is connected anatomically with the gasserian ganglion through its mandibular nerve trunk. The virus resides latently within the gasserian ganglion, where it proliferates during periods of stress, and is transmitted centrifugally through the nerve trunk to the lip. Similarly, type II herpesvirus initiates a vesicular lesion on the genital labia of women and is coupled with a latent infection in the pelvic ganglia.

At the present time, herpes encephalitis constitutes the most important viral infection of the human nervous system. In adults, the encephalitis is caused principally by the type I virus, and curiously is localized predominantly in one or both temporal lobes. The reason for this geographic preference is uncertain, but as mentioned previously, it is thought to result from intra-axonal spread of the virions from the gasserian ganglion to the overlying brain through meningeal nerve fibers. However, this explanation is weakened by the occurrence of encephalitis in individuals who lack a history of cold sores, and also by the frequently concurrent onset of bitemporal lobe involvement.

Typically, herpes encephalitis is a fulminant infection. The temporal lobes become swollen, hemorrhagic, and necrotic. The exudate is predominantly lymphocytic and perithelial, an appearance consistent with inflammation initiated by a virus (Fig. 28-54). However, because the small arteries and arterioles characteristically become necrotic and filled with fibrin thrombi, the parenchyma becomes hemorrhagic and edematous. Intranuclear inclusions occur

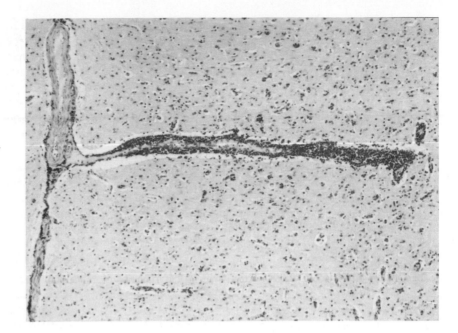

Figure 28-54.   Herpes simplex encephalitis. A photomicrograph illustrates perivascular lymphocytic cuffing, a feature shared by most viral encephalitides.

predominantly in neurons, but also involve astrocytes and oligodendrocytes (Fig. 28-55). They are weakly eosinophilic, occupy less than half the volume of a nucleus, and are usually surrounded by an inconspicuous halo. The detection of viral proteins by immunohistochemical techniques is diagnostic.

In neonates, encephalitis is induced predominantly by type II herpesvirus, as an acquired infection from the birth canal. At this age, the neural tissues are extremely vulnerable, and the infection promptly causes extensive necrosis in the cerebrum and cerebellum.

The pattern of **herpes zoster–varicella viral infection** is anatomically analogous to the gasserian ganglion/cold sore complex of herpes simplex. **The vesicular cutaneous eruption of "shingles" occurs in the distribution of a dermatome, the dorsal root ganglion of which harbors the virus.** Rarely does this infection spread to the central nervous system.

The **cytomegalovirus** induces encephalitis *in utero* as a crossplacental infection and also initiates encephalitic lesions in the adult brain of immunocompromised hosts. Characteristically, the lesions in the embryonic nervous system predominantly occur in the periventricular areas, and are characterized by necrosis and calcification. Because of their proximity to the third ventricle and the aqueduct, they are prone to induce hydrocephalus.

The simian B virus contaminates the saliva of lower primates and is transmitted to humans through a bite wound. The ensuing encephalitis and myelitis are fulminant.

Encephalitis Lethargica (von Economo's Encephalitis)

Unlike the lengthy historical accounts of poliomyelitis and rabies, the agent of encephalitis lethargica induced a single, severe epidemic which began in the winter of 1916, lasted for about 5 years, and was concurrent with the influenza epidemic. Although the infectious agent was neither isolated nor identified, the characteristics of the inflammation testified unequivocally to its viral nature. It featured perivascular cuffs of lymphocytes in the region of the midbrain and hypothalamus. As the name implies, the dominant symptom was somnolence which, on occasion, persisted for weeks. In a few patients, the period of lethargy was followed by the onset of parkinsonism, a symptom complex of hyperkinesia, involuntary movements, athetosis, and tremors. These symptoms reflected injury to the substantia nigra. Other patients developed parkinsonism (postencephalitic parkinsonism) a decade or so later. This occurrence gave rise to the theory that subclinical injury to the substantia nigra during an acute encephalitic episode compromises the longevity of the neurons. This theory suggested that many neurons of the substantia nigra are killed during an acute episode, but that enough remain to preserve clinical function. Subsequently, as neurons are progressively lost with aging, clinical insufficiency of the substantia nigra—that is, parkinsonism—would become apparent.

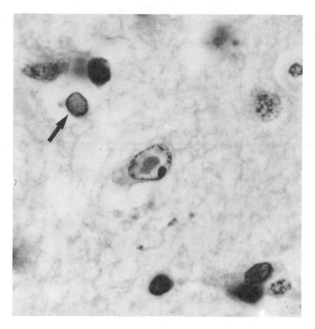

Figure 28-55.   Herpes simplex encephalitis. A photomicrograph shows the inclusion bodies of herpes simplex encephalitis. They are intranuclear and may be discrete, with a halo, as depicted in the neuron in the center of the field, or they may occupy the entire nucleus, as is shown in an astrocyte (*arrow*).

Interestingly, it is thought that the infectious agent of encephalitis lethargica manifested only a transitory pathogenic relationship to humans. Although brief epidemics of encephalitis, such as the "Saint Louis encephalitis" of 1933, have been ascribed by some investigators to the same agent, such a recurrence remains uncertain.

Subacute Sclerosing Panencephalitis

The morphologic and clinical characteristics of an encephalitis are expressions of the pathogenicity of the virus, as well as the defense mechanisms of the host. Subacute sclerosing panencephalitis serves to emphasize that a major alteration in one of these areas significantly modifies the nature and course of the disease.

The entity now known as subacute sclerosing panencephalitis was first recognized by Dawson in 1933 and was descriptively termed "subacute inclusion body encephalitis" (or "Dawson's inclusion body encephalitis"). A decade later, principally through the observations of van Bogaert, it was recognized that this encephalitis primarily affects children, but also occurs in adults; that its course is characteristically

protracted, but may be as brief as several months; and that the inflammation centers in the cerebral gray matter, but may also involve the white matter.

The classic, protracted disease insidiously disturbs cognitive function, alters personality and behavior, produces motor sensory deficits, and ultimately leads to stupor and death over a period of several years. The spinal fluid is minimally altered, but typically displays an elevated titer against the measles virus. The inflammation is highlighted by the presence of prominent, haloed, intranuclear inclusions within neurons; a marked astrogliosis; a patchy loss of myelin; and the customary perivascular cuffs of lymphocytes and macrophages.

The etiology of subacute sclerosing panencephalitis remained uncertain until 1969, when it was demonstrated that an agent having the general properties of the measles virus proliferated in cells maintained in co-culture with infected tissues of the host. The protracted course of the infection in the human central nervous system is thought to result from a defect in the cycle of measles virus replication and release in the infected neuron. As a consequence, the virus is not released from the cell, and viral products accumulate intracellularly, creating inclusions and causing neuronal dysfunction and cell death.

Progressive Multifocal Leukoencephalopathy

Progressive multifocal leukoencephalopathy exemplifies many fundamental characteristics of neurotropic viruses, including opportunism; selectivity for

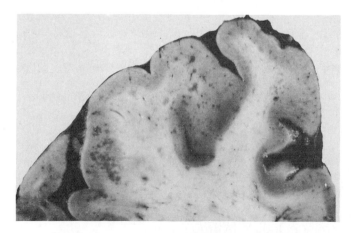

Figure 28-56.   Progressive multifocal leukoencephalopathy. Focal demyelinating lesions are widespread in the cerebral hemispheres, with a preference for the gray-white junction.

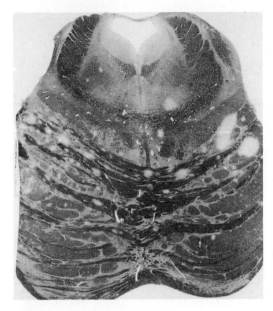

Figure 28-57. Progressive multifocal leukoencephalopathy. A myelin stain of the pons reveals numerous demyelinating lesions.

an individual cell species—in this instance, for oligodendrocytes; the capacity to induce demyelination through interference in the normal functional relationship of oligodendrocytes to the metabolism of myelin; and oncogenicity. The latter two characteristics have broad implications for major disease processes, namely for demyelinating states, such as multiple sclerosis, and neoplasia in the nervous system.

The causative agent of progressive multifocal leukoencephalopathy is a papovavirus bearing the name **JC virus,** in accord with the initials of the first human source of the identified virus. The agent is closely related to the simian oncogenic SV40 virus. The human nervous system becomes vulnerable through immunosuppression. Thus, with few exceptions, the encephalitis is a terminal complication in patients with cancer or lupus erythematosus, in recipients of organ transplants, and particularly, in patients with AIDS.

Characteristically, the lesions appear as discrete foci of demyelination near the gray-white junction in the cerebral hemispheres (Fig. 28-56). Nevertheless, in most instances, they are also widely disseminated through the cerebrum and brain stem (Fig. 28-57). A typical lesion is spherical, measuring several millimeters in diameter; exhibits a central area that is largely devoid of myelin but contains axons; is sparsely populated by oligodendrocytes; displays no necrosis, although it is infiltrated by macrophages;

and is distinguished by the presence of pleomorphic astrocytes, which appear to be anaplastic. The diagnosis is established on the basis of a peripheral area of demyelination in the presence of enlarged oligodendrocytes, which are homogeneously dense and hyperchromatic, and which contain intranuclear inclusions that lack a halo and have a ground-glass appearance (see Fig. 28-51; Fig. 28-58). Electron microscopy discloses intranuclear, crystalline arrays of spherical virions that are 35 to 40 nm in diameter. The nuclei of the pleomorphic astrocytes are often multiple and irregular, and possess dense chromatin material. This anaplastic morphologic appearance is compatible with the development of astrocytomas in a few cases.

The characteristic morphologic features of the acute viral encephalitides are summarized in Figure 28-59.

Slow Viral Infections

The category of infectious diseases caused by "slow viruses," and its relationship to certain degenerative disorders of the human central nervous system remain enigmatic. An awareness of this possible relationship dates from 1956, when a medical officer in New Guinea provided an account of individuals in an isolated tribe whose illness was characterized by trembling. The disease, known as **kuru,** takes its

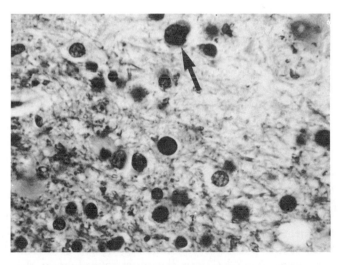

Figure 28-58. Progressive multifocal leukoencephalopathy. A photomicrograph of the marginal areas of demyelination shows enlarged oligodendroglial cells, with nuclei that have a ground-glass, hyperchromatic appearance. A pleomorphic astrocyte shows an enlarged irregular nucleus (*arrow*).

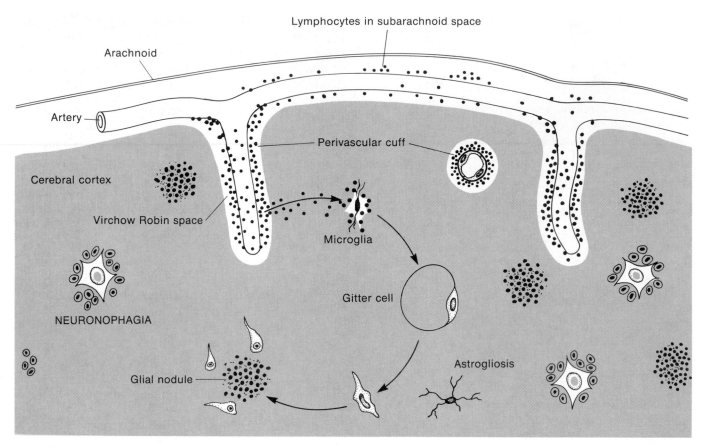

Figure 28-59.   The lesions of viral encephalitis.

name from the word "trembling" in the Fore language of this tribe.

The morphologic lesions of kuru are limited to the central nervous system and are descriptively represented by the term **spongiform degeneration.** Their morphologic appearance is analogous to that of scrapie, a disease of sheep that had been studied extensively, principally in England and Iceland, and that had been shown to be transmissible by the inoculation of infected tissue. Curiously, such inoculation was followed by a prolonged latent period of a year or more. Subsequently, infected tissues from patients with kuru were inoculated into chimpanzees, and the disease was successfully transmitted.

As the term spongiform degeneration connotes, the cardinal feature of Creutzfeldt-Jakob disease and kuru is the presence of small aggregates of microcysts (Fig. 28-60). These are most prevalent in the cortical gray matter, but also involve the deeper nuclei of the basal ganglia and hypothalamus and, importantly, the cerebellum. The involvement of the cerebellum adds ataxia to the predominant symptom of dementia and distinguishes Creutzfeldt-Jakob dis-

ease clinically from Alzheimer's disease. Within the areas of spongiform degeneration, neurons disappear, and astrogliosis becomes prominent. The corticospinal pathways degenerate. Of singular interest is the absence of inflammatory cells, a factor that accounts for the fact that Creutzfeldt-Jakob disease was mistakenly classified as a degenerative disorder for many years.

Acquired Immunodeficiency Syndrome (AIDS)

Approximately 50% of patients with AIDS manifest an encephalopathy. Of these patients, half were found at postmortem examination to exhibit a recognizable infection of the central nervous system (such as toxoplasmosis, cytomegalovirus, progressive multifocal leukoencephalopathy, or herpes simplex encephalitis) or a neoplasm (e.g., primary lymphoma or Kaposi's sarcoma). **Recent evidence indicates that the AIDS virus possesses neurotropic properties.** Particularly in childhood cases of AIDS, scattered

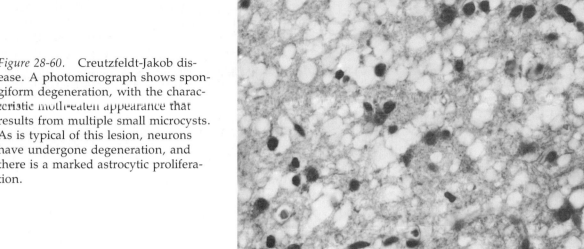

Figure 28-60. Creutzfeldt-Jakob disease. A photomicrograph shows spongiform degeneration, with the characteristic moth-eaten appearance that results from multiple small microcysts. As is typical of this lesion, neurons have undergone degeneration, and there is a marked astrocytic proliferation.

perivascular cuffs of lymphocytes and distinctive, solitary, multinucleated glia attest to a response to infection by the virus.

Congenital Malformations

As in all organs, each individual morphologic event during the development of the central nervous system is the cornerstone for those that follow. Accordingly, it is logical to conclude that a specific congenital malformation may have many causes, all sharing a common, time-related target. For example, anencephaly can be induced experimentally in a number of ways, including induction of maternal anoxia or exposure to ionizing radiation, provided that the event occurs at precisely the same interval in the biologic sequence of development. For instance, in the gestational rat, anoxia or ionizing irradiation early in the eighth day induces anencephaly in the offspring. The same treatment applied a few hours later fails to induce anencephaly, but rather results in a cleft palate.

Anencephaly

The incidence of anencephaly is second only to that of spina bifida with meningomyelocele among lethal malformations of the nervous system. It occurs with a frequency of approximately 0.5 to 2.0 per thousand births, with a modest female predominance. Anen-

cephalic fetuses are either stillborn or die within the first few days of life. This entity is discussed at some length because it exemplifies the nature of the conundrums that confront the student of developmental anomalies.

Anencephaly is characterized by an absence of the cranial vault; the cerebral hemispheres are represented by a discoid mass of highly vascularized, poorly differentiated, neural tissue, the so-called **cerebrovasculosa** (Fig. 28-61). This diminutive mass lies upon the flattened base of the skull, behind two well-formed and normally positioned eyes that mark the anterior margin of disturbed organogenesis. A well-differentiated retina attests to the differentiation and preservation of this particular neuroectoderm. Short segments of the optic nerve extend posteriorly. The posterior aspect of the malformation is a transitional zone, which varies from case to case. On occasion, it permits recognition of midbrain structures, but most often, the entire brain stem and cerebellum are rudimentary. The upper spinal cord is generally hypoplastic and deformed. A rachischisis may involve the cervical area, appearing as a dysraphic bony defect of the posterior spinal column (see Chapter 6).

Typically, the discoid mass, which represents a residuum of the underdeveloped cerebral hemispheres, contains discrete islands of immature neural and glial tissue. It also contains cavities that are partially lined by ependyma and that occasionally contain choroid plexus. However, the discoid mass is composed predominantly of variably sized vascular channels that are lined by endothelium, but that are

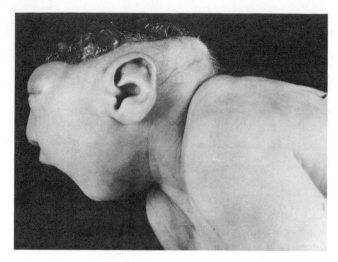

Figure 28-61. Anencephaly. The absence of a calvarium has exposed a discoid mass of highly vascularized tissue, in which there are rudimentary neuroectodermal structures. Characteristically, the lesion of anencephaly involves the cerebral hemispheres; thus, it is usually bounded anteriorly by normally formed eyes and posteriorly by the brain stem.

largely devoid of muscularis. Beneath this discoid mass, but sharing a common origin with the brain, are cranial nerves and intraosseous ganglia.

The concurrence of anencephaly with other dysraphic states, such as spina bifida, suggests a shared pathogenetic mechanism, wherein failure of closure of the anterior neuropore is believed to be the primary event. This concept is supported by the occurrence of anterior dysraphic states among aborted early human embryos. However, the morphologic attributes of anencephaly cast doubt on the validity of this concept. For example, the presence of well-formed eyes attests to the prior existence of properly formed optic cups. These, in turn, arise as out-pouches of the lateral walls of the diencephalon at a time that postdates the expected closure of the neural tube during the fourth week. Thus, the presence and proper positioning of the eyes suggests a normal alignment of the lateral walls of the diencephalon during the formation of the optic cups. Similarly, the maturation and preservation of the retina affirm the absence of significant intrinsic deficiencies in the neuroectodermal potential for differentiation. The presence of the choroid plexus implies that the pia has been brought into physical contact with the ependyma through infolding of the neural tube, events that also postdate the closure of the anterior neuropore. In the formation of the choroid plexus, the pia contributes the tela, or membranous portion of the choroid, whereas ependymal differentiation provides the cuboidal epithelium. These structural features

date the cerebral injury at, or slightly after, the sixth week of gestation.

Importantly, among the many events that occur about the sixth week is the normal incorporation of the cerebrum into the systemic circulation. By the sixth to seventh week of fetal development, the carotid and vertebral arteries have united to form the circle of Willis. This becomes the hub for vessels that establish union with the intrinsic parenchymal vasculature, an event that integrates the developing cerebrum into the systemic circulation. Because the intrinsic blood pressure of a vessel is the determinant for smooth muscle proliferation, the scant muscularis in the vessels of the cerebrovasculosa attests to the lack of intrinsic pressure and suggests that these channels represent the "unused" parenchymal vascular bed that failed to unite with the systemic circulation. Accordingly, it is of interest that the eyes are not dependent upon the internal carotid circula-

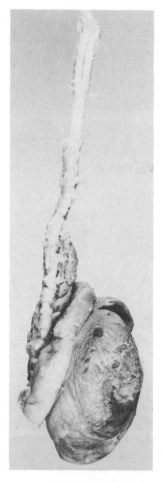

Figure 28-62. Spina bifida with meningomyelocele. The illustration shows a cystic lesion that protrudes above a discoid mass of skin and subcutaneous tissue in which the underlying lumbosacral segment of the spinal cord is enmeshed.

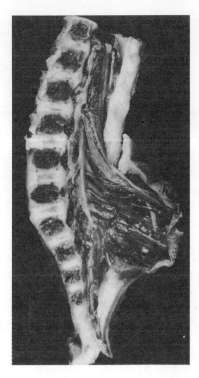

Figure 28-63. Spina bifida with meningomyelocele. A sagittal section of the spine reveals displaced nerve roots of the cauda equina entering the meningomyelocele.

tissue. Characteristically, the spinal cord appears as a flattened, ribbon-like structure, suggesting lack of closure of the neural tube. The term **meningomyelocele** is applied to this entity (Figs. 28-62 and 28-63). The extreme defect converts the spinal column into a gaping canal, often without a recognizable spinal cord. This lesion is termed a **rachischisis.**

Spina bifida is induced readily in rats and chicks by certain chemicals, such as trypan blue, or by hypervitaminosis A. A favored concept suggests that spina bifida results from a failure of closure of the neural tube. However, since the minor lesion of spina bifida occulta involves only the bone, the validity of this concept has been questioned.

The spectrum of neurologic deficits is similarly scaled, ranging from an absence of symptoms in spina bifida occulta to lower limb paresis or paralysis, sensory loss, and rectal and vesical incontinence with meningomyelocele. Importantly, the appearance of such a lesion implies the possibility of other malformations. In the case of meningomyelocele, Arnold-Chiari malformation, hydrocephalus, polymicrogyria, and hydromyelia may also be present. The last is a segmental dilatation of the central canal of the spinal cord, usually in the thoracic segment, and is generally asymptomatic (Fig. 28-64).

tion alone, having acquired a dual blood supply that includes the external carotid vessels. Clearly, more evidence is needed to determine whether the involution of the cerebrum is a consequence of such a disturbance in angiogenesis, or alternatively, whether it represents a dysraphic state that results from a lack of closure of the neuropore.

Spina Bifida

A dysraphic state refers to a defective closure in the dorsal aspects of the vertebral column. Spina bifida is a dysraphic state that occurs most commonly in the lumbosacral region. When the defect is restricted to the vertebral arches, the entity is termed **spina bifida occulta.** Generally, this condition is asymptomatic, although its presence is frequently marked by a dimple or small tuft of hair. A more extensive bony and soft tissue defect, known as a **meningocele,** permits protrusion of the meninges as a fluid-filled sac. The lateral aspects of the sac are characteristically covered by skin, whereas the apex is usually ulcerated. More extensive defects expose the spinal canal and cause the nerve roots, particularly those of the cauda equina, to be entrapped in subcutaneous scar

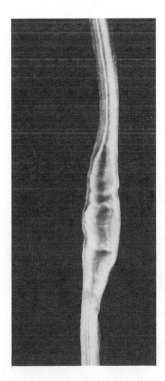

Figure 28-64. Hydromyelia. The spinal cord demonstrates cystic dilatation of the central canal. Hydromyelia is distinguished from syringomyelia, in which the cystic lesion primarily involves the parenchyma.

Arnold-Chiari Malformation

The Arnold-Chiari malformation is usually associated with a lumbosacral meningomyelocele and involves structures in the posterior fossa and the upper cervical cord. The brain stem and cerebellum are compacted into a shallow, bowl-shaped, posterior fossa, with a low-positioned tentorium. A cardinal sign of the deformity is herniation of the caudal aspect of the cerebellar vermis through an enlarged foramen magnum (Figs. 28-65 through 28-67).

This cerebellar tissue protrudes as a tongue upon the dorsal aspect of the cervical cord, often reaching the level of C3-C5. The herniated tissue shows pressure atrophy. Purkinje and granular cells are depleted, and the tongue of the cerebellum is usually bound in position by thickened meninges. The brain stem is also displaced caudally. Typically, the displacement is more exaggerated dorsally then ventrally; thus, landmarks, such as the obex of the fourth ventricle, are appreciably more caudal than are ven-

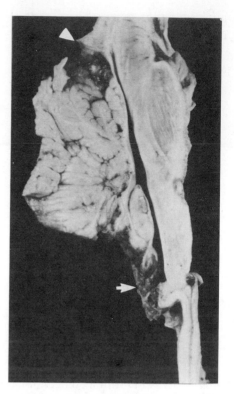

Figure 28-66.   Arnold-Chiari malformation. A sagittal section of the brain stem illustrates the features enumerated in Figure 28-65. A tongue of tonsillar tissue extends downward over the dorsum of the cervical cord (*arrow*). Note the sharp beak of the posterior colliculus (*arrowhead*).

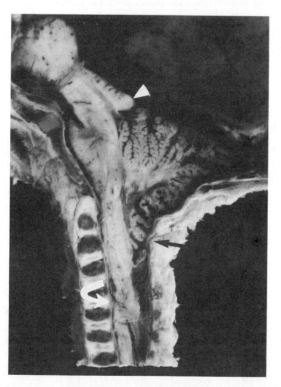

Figure 28-65.   Arnold-Chiari malformation. The cerebellar tonsils are herniated below the level of the foramen magnum (*arrow*). The excessive downward displacement of the dorsal portion of the cord causes the obex of the fourth ventricle to occupy a position below the foramen magnum. The beaking of the inferior colliculus of the quadrigeminal plate (*arrowhead*) and the S-shaped angulation of the upper cervical cord (*curved arrow*) are seen.

tral structures, such as the inferior olives. As viewed from a lateral aspect, the lower medulla is sharply angulated in its midsegment, thereby creating a dorsal protrusion. The foramina of Magendie and Luschka are compressed by the bony ridge of the foramen magnum. The cerebellum is typically flattened and resembles a clam; it has a discoid, rather than an ovoid, contour. Frequently, the quadrigeminal plate is also deformed by a beak-shaped, dorsal protrusion of the inferior colliculus.

One theory of pathogenesis maintains that a meningomyelocele causes fixation of the lower end of the spinal cord and that the growth that elongates the vertebral column creates downward traction on the medulla. This theory is challenged both by the curvature of the medulla and by the beaking of the quadrigeminal plate. Another theory proposes that the downward thrust is initiated by increased intracranial pressure of hydrocephalus. Still another focuses upon the restricted size of the posterior fossa, viewing the bony defect of the skull as the primary event, with the extrusion of the cerebellar tissue through the foramen magnum as a consequence.

Consideration of the Arnold-Chiari malformation is important in the clinical management of a patient with meningomyelocele. It is also a cause of hydrocephalus, through obstruction of the foramina of Magendie and Luschka.

Congenital Hydrocephalus

The excessive accumulation of cerebrospinal fluid intracranially is termed hydrocephalus. The entity is classified as **noncommunicating** when the blockage is situated within the ventricular system, and is considered to be **communicating** when the obstruction is positioned distal to the foramina of Magendie and Luschka. The conical herniation of the cerebellar tonsils into the foramen magnum in the Arnold-Chiari malformation compromises the outflow from the fourth ventricle. Alternatively, as an accompaniment of the Arnold-Chiari malformation, the obstruction may be at the level of the aqueduct of Sylvius.

The most frequent solitary malformation responsible for congenital hydrocephalus is an obstruction

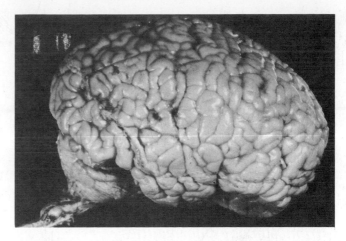

Figure 28-68. Polymicrogyria with Arnold-Chiari malformation. The surface of the brain exhibits an excessive number of small, irregularly sized and randomly distributed gyral folds.

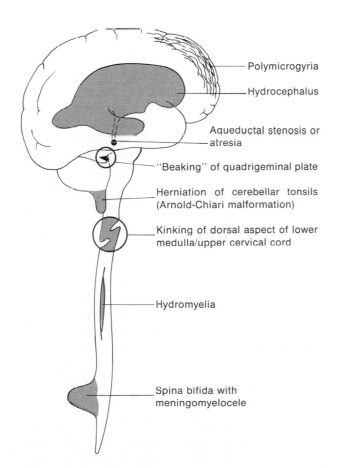

Polymicrogyria

Hydrocephalus

Aqueductal stenosis or atresia

"Beaking" of quadrigeminal plate

Herniation of cerebellar tonsils (Arnold-Chiari malformation)

Kinking of dorsal aspect of lower medulla/upper cervical cord

Hydromyelia

Spina bifida with meningomyelocele

Figure 28-67. Arnold-Chiari and associated malformations.

in the continuity of the aqueduct. Histologic examination usually reveals multiple, small, ependymal-lined canals that lack directional orientation, caliber, and continuity. In some instances, the single aqueduct or the clustered, aborted canals are surrounded by astrogliosis, in which case the condition is thought to represent an inflammatory ependymitis, probably attributable to an intrauterine viral infection. This concept is supported by experimental studies in pregnant rats inoculated with myxoviruses. In this context, aqueductal atresia or stenosis is classified as congenital. With only rare exceptions, communicating hydrocephalus is acquired, and results predominantly from meningitis.

Polymicrogyria

A significant number of infants with meningomyelocele and the Arnold-Chiari malformation not only develop hydrocephalus, but also show abnormalities in gyral topography. Abnormalities of the cerebral gyri cause numerous deviations from normal and are regularly associated with mental retardation. These deviations include a spectrum of entities, such as **polymicrogyria,** a term descriptive of the presence of small and excessive gyri (Fig. 28-68); **pachygyria,** a condition in which the gyri are too few and too broad; and **lissencephaly,** a disorder in which the cortical surface is smooth or only lightly furrowed. Such malformations arise from disturbances in neuronal migration, a highly patterned event of the first trimester of embryonic development. The primitive neurons move centrifugally from the germinal mantle to populate the cortex. Their population densities and positions in the cortex are determining factors in the redundancy of the cortical mantle which, in turn, initiates the infolding that creates sulci.

A focal disturbance in neuronal migration also leads to nodular collections of ectopic neurons, usually in the white matter, which are termed **heterotopias.** Their functional significance lies in the likelihood of mental retardation and seizures. Importantly, migrational disturbances of neurons have also been associated with maternal alcoholism.

Congenital Defects Associated with Chromosomal Abnormalities

Derangements of the larger autosomes (1 through 12) are incompatible with sustained intrauterine life, and affected fetuses are spontaneously aborted. Structural and functional abnormalities attributable to gross chromosomal derangements are best exemplified by the trisomies of groups 13–15 and 21.

Trisomy 13–15 has an incidence of approximately 1 per 5,000 births, with a modest female predominance. The deformities involve the brain, facial features, and extremities. Holoprosencephaly, arhinencephaly, microphthalmia, cyclopia, low-set ears, harelip, and cleft palate dominate the complex. The extremities exhibit polydactyly and rocker-bottom feet.

Holoprosencephaly refers to a microcephalic brain that features an absence of the interhemispheric fissure (Fig. 28-69). The noncleaved cerebral hemispheres are horseshoe-shaped with an uncleaved frontal pole, across which the gyri have an irregular,

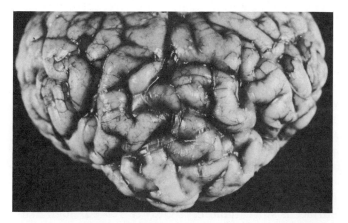

Figure 28-69.   Holoprosencephaly. A view from the frontal aspect of the brain shows horizontally positioned gyri without the cleavage of the interhemispheric fissure. This malformation is commonly associated with trisomy 13.

horizontal orientation. Behind this lens-shaped cortex, there is a common ventricular chamber created by the lateral displacement of the posterior portions of the cerebral hemispheres. A velum, the meninges, covers this ventricle. The base of the common ventricular chamber is formed by the bilobed structures of the caudate nuclei and thalami. Holoprosencephaly is rarely compatible with life beyond a few weeks or months. The absence of the olfactory tracts and bulbs, either associated with holoprosencephaly or as a solitary malformation, is designated **arhinencephaly.**

The corpus callosum is regularly absent in holoprosencephaly, but its absence can also be a solitary lesion. The **absence of the corpus callosum** is a remarkably latent maldevelopment, notably without significant impairment of interhemispheric functional coordination. Occasionally, however, this malformation is associated with seizures. The corpus callosum physically tethers the hemispheres; its absence permits the lateral ventricles to be displaced outward and upward. Radiographic documentation of this position is diagnostic, and provides meaningful information in the case of congenital absence of the corpus callosum associated with seizures.

Down's syndrome is an expression of several chromosomal abnormalities, each of which involves chromosome 21, and is predominantly associated with duplication and the formation of a trisomy. Translocation is responsible for about 5% of cases, whereas variable expressions of mosaicism are even more rare. Functional deficiencies in cognition exceed the minor gross and cytologic abnormalities. However, the weight of the brain is moderately reduced, and the organ is shortened in its anteroposterior dimension. There is a simple gyral pattern, with disproportionately slender superior temporal gyri. On histologic examination, the cytoarchitecture of the cortex so closely approximates that of normal cortex that it is generally indistinguishable from it. Of interest is the nearly absolute propensity for this chromosomal abnormality to predispose patients to the **precocious development of the histologic features of Alzheimer's disease.** Typically, these lesions occur before the middle of the fourth decade of life.

Demyelinating Diseases

The category of demyelinating diseases becomes meaningful when the definition is restricted to those disorders in which myelin is lost selectively while other neural structures are preserved. In this context, the leukodystrophies, multiple sclerosis, central pontine myelinolysis, and perhaps progressive multifocal leukoencephalopathy are appropriately viewed as demyelinating states. By contrast, the coagulative necrosis of an infarct, the liquefactive necrosis of an abscess, the traumatic injury of a contusion, and the secondary demyelination of wallerian degeneration serve only as reminders that myelin has a delicate tissue structure and is vulnerable to many injuries. Importantly, the restricted definition permits a search for mechanisms of a highly selective tissue reaction, as well as causative agents that are uniquely directed to the vulnerability of this membranous structure.

The Leukodystrophies

Although the prefix "leuko" refers specifically to the white matter, the conditions classified as the leukodystrophies comprise a heterogeneous group of disorders. Nevertheless, they share a profound disturbance in the formation and preservation of myelin.

Metachromatic leukodystrophy is the most common and also the best understood disorder among a group of entities that include Krabbe's disease, Alexander's disease, and **adrenoleukodystrophy**. Metachromasia is a phenomenon wherein a dye undergoes a predictable color transformation through its reactions with tissue, for example from blue to purple. Metachromasia lends its name to an autosomal recessive disorder of the central and peripheral myelin. Metachomatic leukodystrophy occurs predominantly in infancy, but also has a rare juvenile or adult form. The course is progressive and the disease is always fatal, usually within several years. Postmortem examination discloses a diffuse, confluent loss of myelin that is most advanced in the cerebrum. The degradation of myelin is attributed to an inborn error of metabolism in which the enzyme arylsulfatase-A, although present, is enzymatically inactive. The functional inadequacy of this enzyme leads to the breakdown of myelin and the accumulation of sulfatide-rich lipids, which exhibit a metachromatic reaction to staining with toluidine blue. These products enter the bloodstream, accumulate in the kidneys, and are excreted in the urine. Histologically, the cerebral hemispheres feature a diffuse loss of myelin, with preservation of the subcortical arcuate fibers, prominent astrogliosis, and the pathognomonic accumulation of small globules of metachromatic material, principally in the white matter. The involvement of the peripheral nerves is less severe.

Krabbe's disease also appears in the early months of life, and progresses to death within a year or two. The symptomatology reflects a diffuse involvement of the nervous system, with severe motor, sensory, and cognitive impairments. The disorder, an autosomal recessive trait caused by a deficiency of galactocerebroside, β-galactosidase, is expressed histologically by the presence of perivascular aggregates of globoid cells. These cells have an epithelial quality and are often multinucleated, so that they mimic a foreign body reaction. The loss of myelin is diffuse, but marbled areas of partial and total demyelination are present. Both central and peripheral myelin are involved. Astrogliosis is typically severe.

The degradation of myelin into lipid products was the basis for the identification of a childhood condition that was initially referred to as sudanophilic leukodystrophy or **Schilder's disease.** It is now appreciated that most of these cases represent an X-linked recessive entity, termed **adrenoleukodystrophy,** which conjoins an inborn metabolic error of lipids in the adrenals and a disturbance in the preservation of myelin. Again, the clinical signs, which are variably motor, sensory, or cognitive, develop in the first decade of life and progress insidiously for about a year. The central nervous system and, to a lesser degree, the peripheral nervous system, are depleted of myelin. The adrenals are characteristically atrophic, and electron microscopy reveals pathognomonic, cytoplasmic, membrane-bound, curvilinear inclusions, or clefts, in the cortical cells of the adrenal.

It is remarkable that an entity as morphologically distinctive as **Alexander's disease,** although still rare, was not described until the mid-1900s. The degeneration of myelin—in this instance, its lack of formation—suggests an inborn error of metabolism. The histologic appearance of the central nervous system is strikingly abnormal because of the presence of innumerable **Rosenthal fibers.** These irregular, beaded formations of lipoproteins are deposited in the subpial mantle of the cerebrum, in the molecular cortex of the cerebellum, in the periphery of the spinal cord, and in the outer margins of the optic and olfactory nerves. Less intense depositions surround the blood vessels. The content of myelin in the white matter is strikingly deficient. Small Rosenthal fibers are present in glial processes, presumably during their formative development. Larger fibers consist of extracellular accumulations, which are irregular, but are generally elongated or spiral. They stain in a manner similar to that of myelin.

The primitive glial cells originate in the germinal mantle and migrate centrifugally into the hemispheres, where they normally align with axons for the purpose of myelination. It has been suggested that, in Alexander's disease, they fail to establish this critical structural alignment and, as a consequence, continue to migrate outward until they encounter a barrier, such as a blood vessel or the pia. It is presumed that these cells then elaborate lipoproteins in this ectopic position, and that these deposits understandably have the staining characteristics of myelin, but not the membranous configuration that is normally acquired through an anatomic relationship with an axon. Interestingly, in Alexander's disease, the myelin is well preserved in the peripheral nerves.

Multiple Sclerosis

There are few diseases about which knowledge is so lacking and yet are so common and have such an array of distinctive clinical and pathologic characteristics as multiple sclerosis. Classically, multiple sclerosis has its clinical onset during the third or fourth decades of life. The disease is marked thereafter by indolent periods, punctuated by abrupt and brief episodes of clinical progression. The disease has a protracted course of 5 to 20 years or more. Each exacerbation is the expression of additional focal plaques of demyelination. The visual system is particularly vulnerable, whereas the peripheral nerves are uniformly spared.

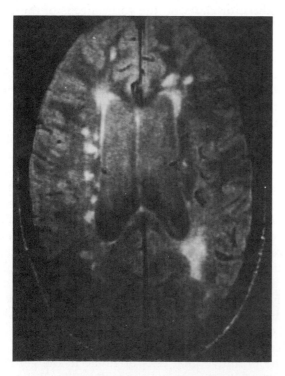

Figure 28-70.   Multiple sclerosis. A magnetic resonance imaging scan of the brain demonstrates multiple sclerotic plaques and shows their preference for the periventricular areas.

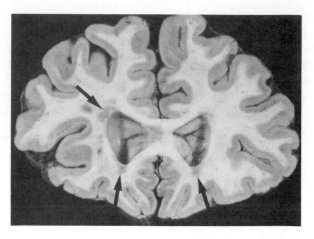

Figure 28-71.   Multiple sclerosis. Multiple sclerotic plaques appear gray as a result of the loss of white myelin (*arrows*). Note the sharply demarcated, rather smoothly contoured plaques in the white matter of the left frontal lobe. The predilection for the paraventricular regions is seen in the four quadrants of the anterior horns of the lateral ventricles. There is also a zone of demyelination in the genu of the corpus callosum.

The plaque is the hallmark of multiple sclerosis. Characteristically, plaques of variable size, rarely more than 2 cm in diameter, accumulate in great numbers. They are remarkably discrete and frequently possess smoothly rounded edges. Usually situated in the white matter, the plaques occasionally breach the gray-white junction, and rarely are seated entirely in the gray cortex (Figs. 28-70 and 28-71). As previously mentioned, the lesions exhibit a preference for the optic nerves and chiasm, and almost always localize in the periventricular white matter of the corona radiata. Otherwise, their distribution is highly random, and they indiscriminately involve the cerebrum, cerebellum, brain stem, and spinal cord.

The evolving plaque is marked by a selective loss of myelin in a region of axonal preservation, a few lymphocytes that cluster about small veins and arteries, an influx of macrophages, and considerable edema (Fig. 28-72). When neurons are encompassed by the boundaries of a plaque, the neuronal cell bodies are remarkably spared. The number of oligodendrocytes is moderately diminished, but they show no distinctive structural alterations. As the lesion ages, the plaque becomes more discrete and edema regresses. This serves to emphasize the focal nature of the tissue injury, its selectivity for myelin, and its severity, as demyelination is typically total within the area of the plaque. Rarely, a plaque is traversed by a few myelinated fibers, in which case the lesion is referred to as a shadow plaque. The discrete appear-

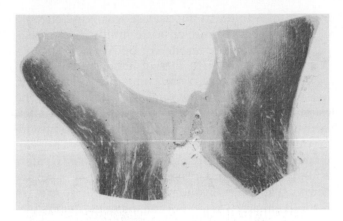

Figure 28-72. Multiple sclerosis. A horizontal section through a demyelinated plaque in the optic chiasm depicts the lack of wallerian degeneration and underscores the preservation of axonal cylinders.

ance of the plaque indicates that an axon that approaches the area of tissue injury loses its myelin sheath abruptly, in precisely the same physical relationship to the plaque as that of all other neighboring axons, although some may be motor and others sensory (Fig. 28-73). The denuded axons traverse the plaque and in unison again acquire myelin on the contralateral edge of the lesion. The aging plaque acquires astrocytes and, with time, the tissue becomes dense with glial processes that presumably impair the structural integrity of the axons. Oligodendroglia are lost without evidence of abortive attempts at remyelination. Plaques rarely exhibit frank necrosis.

There have been many theories about the etiology and pathogenesis of multiple sclerosis. These theo-

ries have sought clues from the clinical nature of the disease, its relapsing and remitting course, the predilection of the disease for young adults, the heightened incidence of the disorder in the northern latitudes, its possible genetic predisposition, and the characteristic tissue reaction. Yet, the theories that have postulated immunologic insults; specific etiologic agents, such as viruses, and vascular insults have provided few insights into the genesis of the disease. The acceptance of such theories has waxed and waned, a pattern similar to the disease itself. At the moment, a viral etiology is a particularly popular theory. This proposed etiology gained favor when it was demonstrated that the papovavirus (JC virus) of progressive multifocal leukoencephalopathy can selectively induce demyelination. In this circumstance, the virus replicates in the nuclei of the oligodendrocytes, where it produces intranuclear inclusions and presumably interferes with the capability of these cells to sustain myelin. There are no visible inclusion bodies in the oligodendrocytes of a plaque of multiple sclerosis, nor has an infectious agent been visualized or isolated. However, a viral etiology for multiple sclerosis which, by necessity, implies a chronic, relapsing infectious process, is made tenable by the occurrence of a similarly persistent infection by the herpes simplex virus in the gasserian ganglion, with periodic exacerbations during periods of stress. Indeed, the human nervous system has long been known to be colonized chronically by *Treponema pallidum* throughout the many years of latency before the clinical expression of dementia paralytica. Similarly, the protozoon *Toxoplasma gondii*, in its encapsulated form, can reside unobtrusively in the human brain.

Figure 28-73. Multiple sclerosis. A photomicrograph shows that the myelinated axons that approach the zone of demyelination (*top*) lose their myelin in parallel positions. The myelinated axon that runs tangential to the plaque (horizontal axon) reflects injury in several "beaded" enlargements.

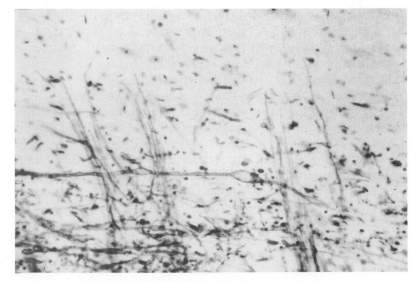

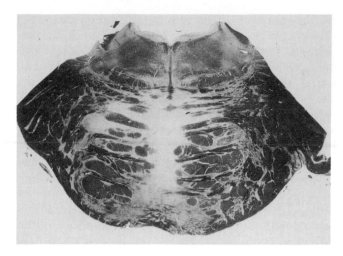

Figure 28-74. Central pontine myelinolysis. The crossed fibers of the pons have lost myelin in the region of the central raphe. As this early lesion progresses, it will widen laterally.

Although there are no good models of multiple sclerosis in lower animals, interesting parallels may be drawn with the focal demyelination that occurs in human central pontine myelinolysis.

Perivenous Encephalomyelitis

Historically, perivenous encephalomyelitis, also termed postvaccinial or postinfectious encephalomyelitis, occurred after immunization against rabies, smallpox, and typhoid-paratyphoid. With changes in manufacturing methods, the eradication of smallpox, and immunization against measles, such episodes have virtually disappeared. Today, perivenous encephalomyelitis primarily follows upper respiratory infections or viral exanthems, such as measles. It may also occur spontaneously without any clinically apparent preceding illness. This acute demyelinating disease is thought to result from sensitization to myelin basic protein (MBP), one of the principal constituents of myelin. An experimental analogue of this disease, called experimental allergic encephalomyelitis, can be produced in mice by immunization with MBP.

The onset of perivenous encephalomyelitis is abrupt, and in severe cases, headache and delirium proceed to coma and even death. Seizures and a flaccid paralysis of the limbs may complicate the disease course. The cerebrospinal fluid contains increased protein and lymphocytes. Without a history of immunization or a preceding viral infection, it is difficult to distinguish the disease from viral encephalitis, Reye's syndrome, or acute multiple sclerosis.

The histologic appearance of perivenular encephalomyelitis is similar to that of acute multiple sclerosis, except for more conspicuous demyelination in the subpial zone and meningeal inflammation. The lesions are most intense in the cerebral white matter, particularly in the periventricular areas, although minor inflammation of the gray matter occurs. The lymphocytes and macrophages form minute clusters around venules, and plasma cells may also be numerous, especially in the Virchow-Robin spaces. In the inflammatory regions, conspicuous demyelination is present, and there is an intense microglial response in the damage area. Hypertrophic astrocytes are distributed within and around the lesions. The resulting morphologic appearance resembles a string of beads along the course of the venule.

Experimental allergic encephalomyelitis, induced by immunization with MBP, is mediated by T-cells. The T-cells attract macrophages, which are the effector cells that destroy myelin. T-cells from animals with experimental allergic encephalomyelitis can be used to transfer the disease to untreated recipients.

Central Pontine Myelinolysis

Discrete areas of selective demyelination were first observed as solitary lesions in the pons of chronic alcoholics who entered the hospital with severe electrolyte disturbances. The lesions resembled those of

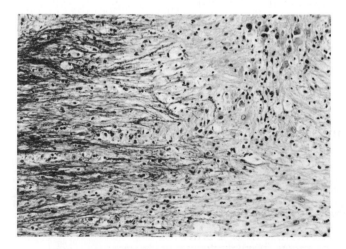

Figure 28-75. Central pontine myelinolysis. A photomicrograph shows a myelinated tract as it approaches the zone of demyelination (*right*). The neurons within the area of demyelination are preserved, emphasizing the selectivity of the injury for myelin.

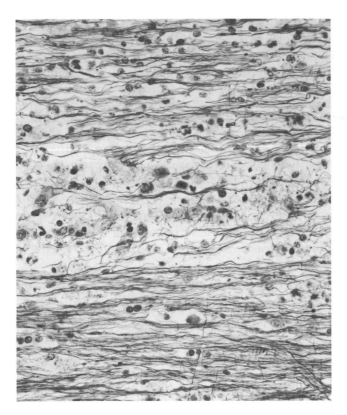

Figure 28-76. Central pontine myelinolysis. A photomicrograph demonstrates that the zone of demyelination retains axons that are splayed by an influx of macrophages.

multiple sclerosis in their selectivity for myelin, in their discrete appearance, and in their abrupt onset. However, they differed from the lesions of multiple sclerosis in their unique localization and rigid conformity to the midline of the upper pons. Additional experience has made it clear that **the electrolyte abnormality is of primary significance, and that chronic alcoholism is merely the setting for its occurrence.** It is now thought that the rapid correction of hyponatremia is instrumental in the initiation of the selective demyelination that characterizes central pontine myelinolysis (Figs. 28-74 through 28-76).

Neoplasia

Deviation and Behavior

Neoplastic lesions in the cranial cavity can be classified according to five fundamental origins: (1) the neuroectoderm (principally, gliomas), (2) mesenchymal structures (notably, meningiomas and schwannomas), (3) tissues and cells that have been ectopically displaced intracranially during embryonic development (craniopharyngiomas, dermoid and epidermoid cysts, lipomas, and dysgerminomas), (4) retained embryonal structures, and (5) metastases. Intracranial tumors constitute approximately 2% of "malignant" neoplasms, but their frequent occurrence in childhood weighs heavily upon their clinical importance. About 60% of primary intracranial neoplasms are gliomas, slightly less than 20% are meningiomas, and all others account for the remainder (Fig. 28-77).

Tumors of neuroectodermal origin are predominantly glial. They are derived from astrocytes, oligodendroglia, or ependyma, and are designated accordingly as **astrocytomas, oligodendrogliomas,** and **ependymomas.** Within each of these three cell species, there is a spectrum or gradient of anaplasia. Thus, the astrocytic gliomas are conventionally subclassified in a three-tiered fashion as astrocytoma, anaplastic astrocytoma, and glioblastoma multiforme. These terms are used to signify increasing degrees of anaplasia. In accord with the degree of anaplasia, tumors of oligodendroglial and ependymal origins are conventionally designated as oligodendrogliomas or anaplastic oligodendrogliomas and, by analogy, either ependymomas or anaplastic ependymomas.

The descriptive terms "benign" and "malignant" require qualification when these intracranial tumors, particularly the gliomas, are contrasted with tumors in other body sites. For example, even the cytologically well-differentiated astrocytoma infiltrates freely through the surrounding brain tissue and has a poorly defined margin. The term benign is frequently applied to this lesion because its growth is indolent, despite the fact that its expansion and infiltration ultimately cause death in 5 to 10 years. Conventionally, anaplastic astrocytoma and glioblastoma multiforme are designated as malignant neoplasms. These lesions grow rapidly, infiltrate without restraint, and are rapidly fatal. Yet, unlike malignant tumors elsewhere in the body, these anaplastic gliomas rarely metastasize.

Infrequently, the neuroectoderm gives rise to a neoplasm of neuronal heritage. These neoplasms occur most often in childhood, and the cellular composition is usually primitive. An important example is the medulloblastoma that arises in the cerebellum, generally in the first decade of life. This tumor is usually situated in the vermis; its growth is rapid, and regional infiltration is extensive. It has been emphasized that the neuroectodermal tumors, even

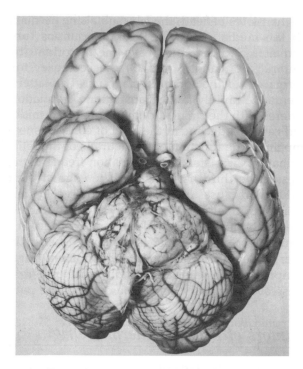

Figure 28-78.   Astrocytoma of the brain stem. The expansile nature of an astrocytoma is shown by the enlargement of the pons, particularly laterally, but also ventrally, where it encircles the basilar artery. Pontine gliomas involve the cranial nerve nuclei and interfere with the long tracts that pass through the pons. The tumor may also obstruct the flow of cerebrospinal fluid, producing hydrocephalus.

proximately 10% of cases, the tumor becomes more anaplastic, and life expectancy is shortened.

An **anaplastic astrocytoma** is distinguished from the usual astrocytoma by a greater degree of cellularity, by cellular pleomorphism, and by the features of anaplasia. Its topographic distribution parallels that of the better-differentiated astrocytoma. The growth of an anaplastic astrocytoma is accelerated, and life expectancy is reduced to about three years.

Glioblastoma multiforme, the extreme expression of anaplasia among the glial neoplasms, accounts for 40% of all primary intracranial tumors. Most glioblastomas have constituent cells with recognizable astrocytic properties, but they generally display marked cellular pleomorphism, frequent mitoses, regional zones of necrosis, and endothelial proliferation. Endothelial proliferation is a manifestation of induced cellular hyperplasia. A similar hyperplasia of fibroblasts, also initiated by the presence of neoplastic cells in proximity to the dura and vascular adventitia, may lead to malignant transformation.

The sarcomatous growth intermingles fibrosarcoma with the glioma, in which case, the entity is designated a **gliosarcoma.**

Characteristically, the glioblastoma infiltrates extensively, frequently crossing the corpus callosum and producing a bilateral lesion likened to a butterfly in its gross configuration and mottled red and yellow color (Fig. 28-80). These colors are imparted by multiple areas of recent (red) and remote (yellow) hemorrhage and necrosis. The cardinal histologic features of a glioblastoma multiforme are dense cellularity, with variable degrees of cellular pleomorphism, often accompanied by multinucleation; serpentine areas of necrosis surrounded by zones of increased tumor cell density ("palisading"); and endothelial cell proliferation that creates clusters of small vessels, referred to as **glomeruloid formations** (Fig. 28-81).

The clinical course of this neoplasm rarely exceeds a year and a half. Glioblastoma multiforme predominates in the latter decades of life, and has a frequency twice that of the astrocytomas.

Oligodendroglioma, in accord with the cell of origin, arises in the white matter, predominantly in the cerebral hemispheres of adults. Although the lesion is infiltrative, its slow growth permits survival for 5 to 10 years. The oligodendroglioma displays the small, rounded nuclei of oligodendrocytes. The tumor is pleomorphic and of variable cell density. Calcospherites, often detected on radiologic examination, appear as grains of sand scattered randomly throughout the lesion; usually, however, they are most prominent at its periphery. The slow growth of this neoplasm is reflected in an absence of mitotic figures. Necrosis is an uncommon feature. Seizures are often the first symptom.

Ependymoma, a lesion that occurs most commonly in the fourth ventricle, is accompanied by symptoms that are predominantly caused by obstruction and hydrocephalus (Fig. 28-82). Together with astrocytomas, the ependymoma is the second most common intramedullary tumor of the spinal cord. It arises from the central canal or the filum terminale, and generally presents at the lumbosacral level. This differs from the preference of astrocytomas for the cervicothoracic level of the spinal cord. An ependymoma rarely involves the lateral or third ventricles. Normal ependymal cells have an epithelial appearance. Similarly, the tumor cells of an ependymoma characteristically possess ovoid nuclei, with coarse chromatin material and well-defined plasma membranes. The tumor cells form clefts, or they may be arranged around blood vessels, creating a mantle of glial processes about the adventitia in which nuclei

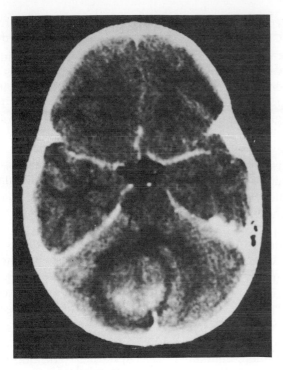

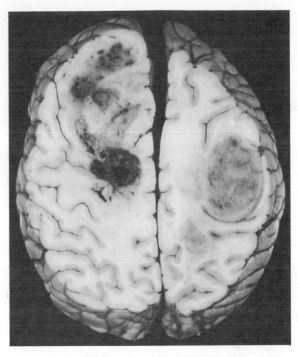

Figure 28-79.   Astrocytoma of the cerebellum. An astrocytoma in the right cerebellar hemisphere appears in a CT scan as a spherical area of increased density, surrounded by a halo of decreased density (edema).

Figure 28-80.   Glioblastoma multiforme. This extremely anaplastic tumor of the astrocytic series is represented by a necrotic, hemorrhagic lesion that has crossed the corpus callosum and has spread throughout both hemispheres.

Figure 28-81.   Glioblastoma multiforme. The characteristic microscopic features of this anaplastic tumor include prominent cellularity, areas of necrosis around which nuclei are palisaded, and the presence of numerous blood vessels that show endothelial proliferation.

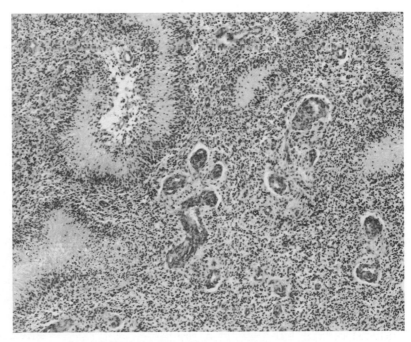

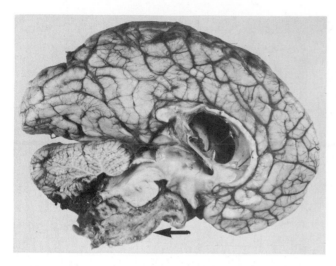

Figure 28-82.   Ependymoma. This tumor (*arrow*) originated in the fourth ventricle and spread outward over the base of the brain. The obstruction to the flow of cerebrospinal fluid caused dilatation of the aqueduct of Sylvius, enlargement of the third ventricle, dilatation of the foramen of Monro, and a marked expansion of the lateral ventricles. The symptomatology associated with ependymoma of the fourth ventricle often reflects increased intracranial pressure.

are absent. The tumor generally grows slowly, but it can seed in the subarachnoid space.

Medulloblastoma, the most common intracranial neuroblastic tumor, arises exclusively in the cerebellum and has its highest frequency in the first decade of life. The progenitor cell is of neuronal origin and is derived from the transient, external, granular cell layer of the cerebellum. The lesion infiltrates aggressively and frequently disseminates throughout the spinal fluid. The neuroblastic quality of the cells is occasionally expressed in a rosette formation, a distinctive feature of embryonic and neoplastic neuroblasts. The tumor cells feature crowded, hyperchromatic, round-to-oval nuclei, with scant cytoplasm and no structural pattern. The tumor, in accord with embryonic neuroblasts, is highly sensitive to ionizing radiation.

Ganglioglioma is a rare lesion comprised of mature and immature neurons in a stroma of glia. Generally a discrete lesion in the cerebrum, it expresses itself clinically by producing seizures during the first two decades of life. The neuronal constituents are represented by small, rounded nuclei of neuroblasts; intermediate forms; large nuclei with prominent nucleoli; and well-defined cytoplasm of ganglionic cells. The matrix is contributed by astrocytes.

Tumors of Mesenchymal Origin

Meningiomas account for almost 20% of all primary intracranial neoplasms, having a maximum frequency in the fourth to fifth decades, but with a significant incidence in young adults, as well. They originate in the arachnoid villi and produce a globoid or discoid ("meningioma en plaque") mass (Fig. 28-83). Because they occur in diverse locations, they cause a variety of symptoms. The propensity for the tumor to invade contiguous bone permits a confident radiographic diagnosis. The superficial position of meningiomas in relation to the brain and spinal cord, coupled with neural displacement rather than infiltration, permits total surgical excision (Fig. 28-84). However, particularly with lesions at the base of the brain, invasion of the bone may limit complete resection, and recurrence is common.

The histologic hallmark of meningiomas is the whorled pattern of "meningothelial" cells in association with psammoma bodies (Fig. 28-85). The latter are small, laminated calcospherites. Although the meningothelial appearance is distinctive, it is often obscured by a predominantly fibroblastic proliferation. Other meningiomas exhibit prominent blood vessels (angioblastic meningioma), some have a pap-

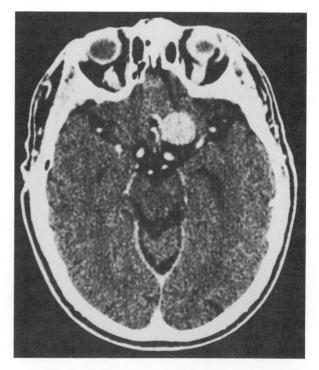

Figure 28-83.   Meningioma. On a CT scan meningiomas appear as discrete lesions.

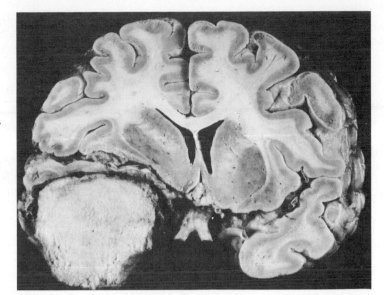

Figure 28-84. Meningioma. This globoid tumor, which underlies the temporal lobe, compresses but does not infiltrate this portion of the brain. The presence of the meningioma "irritated" the cortex, initiating a seizure disorder.

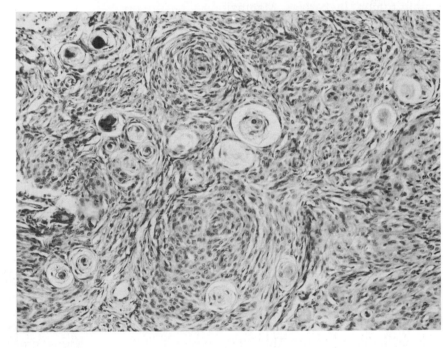

Figure 28-85. Meningioma. A photomicrograph shows the classic features of a meningioma. Whorls of uniform, round nuclei are interspersed with dark psamoma bodies. The general absence of mitotic activity and necrosis attests to the slow growth of this neoplasm.

illary appearance (papillary meningioma), and a rare lesion features microcystic formations (microcystic meningioma).

The indolent growth of meningiomas creates a symptomatic interval that often spans years. Because the lesion displaces rather than infiltrates the brain, seizures, rather than neurologic deficits, frequently characterize the clinical presentation. This is particularly true of parasagittal meningiomas and those located over the convexity of the hemispheres. In other locations, meningiomas compress functional structures. For instance, those in the olfactory groove produce anosmia, those in the suprasellar region cause visual deficits, those in the cerebellopontine angle are associated with cranial nerve palsies, and those in the spinal column produce spinal nerve root and cord dysfunctions. Because meningiomas are intimately related to meninges that are innervated with pain fibers, headaches are common. Infiltration of the calvarium may create a tumor mass on the external table of the skull, historically recognized as a "brain tumor" by barbers. Meningiomas that are not completely excised recur, but the symptom-free interval is variable. The typical meningioma has an average estimated doubling time of about 2 years.

Schwannoma (neurilemoma, perineural fibroblastoma, neurinoma) is derived from Schwann cells, a cell species that produces collagen as well as myelin. Accordingly, schwannomas have a dense mesenchymal appearance. Histologically, they feature spindle cells in fascicles and occasionally, in parallel, picketed, and regimented patterns termed Verocay bodies. Fortunately, malignant transformation is a rare event among Schwann-cell tumors, and nuclear pleomorphism, particularly when isolated to an occasional cell, does not indicate an accelerated growth.

Intracranial schwannomas are largely restricted to the eighth nerve, and are often referred to as acoustic neurinomas. Interestingly, the new growth invariably begins where the stromal matrix undergoes transition from oligodendrocytes to Schwann cells. This junction corresponds anatomically to the position of the internal auditory meatus. Thus, the occurrence of the lesion not only initiates tinnitus and deafness, but also expands the bony meatus, an effect that is useful for radiographic diagnosis. Growth causes the lesion to protrude into the cerebellopontine angle, where compression initiates cranial nerve palsies. Schwannomas also arise on spinal nerve roots. On occasion, they are entirely within the spinal canal; at other times, they span a bony foramen with a dumbbell configuration. Together with meningiomas, Schwann-cell tumors constitute the greatest propor-

tion of intradural-extramedullary neoplasms. Tumors of Schwann cell origin also occur on peripheral nerves as schwannomas or neurofibromas.

Tumors Derived from Ectopic Tissues

Craniopharyngiomas arise from epithelium derived from Rathke's pouch, a derivative of the embryonic nasopharynx that migrates cephalad and gives origin to the anterior lobe of the pituitary. It is thought that remnants of this epithelium are positioned above the sella turcica, where they may generate cystic and solid lesions, termed craniopharyngiomas (Fig. 28-86). Some cystic craniopharyngiomas are lined by squamous epithelium, whereas others, referred to as adamantinomas, are solid and have a dense histologic pattern that resembles lesions of dentiginous origin. Craniopharyngiomas generally become symptomatic in the first two decades of life, creating visual deficits and causing headaches.

Dermoid and epidermoid cysts represent cutaneous structures that may be displaced into the bone of the skull and occasionally into the intracranial compartment. These displaced squamous cells proliferate and develop into a cyst whose inwardly oriented epithelium desquamates keratotic debris. A cystic mass is created, the content of which, when viewed through the thin capsule, resembles "mother of pearl." The intracranial lesions are prone to occur in the posterior fossa or about the sella turcica.

Lipomas arise from rudiments of adipose tissue that have been carried inward as the brain infolded embryologically. Not surprisingly, therefore, lipomas are positioned either along the superior aspect of the corpus callosum, across the dorsum of the quadrigeminal plate, or down the dorsal sagittal plane of the spinal cord to the level of the cauda equina. They enlarge slowly, if at all, but may enmesh cranial or spinal nerves, interfering· with nerve conduction. Histologically, lipomas mimic normal fat cells. Most lipomas are encountered incidentally at postmortem examination.

Dysgerminomas comprise a spectrum of lesions derived from displaced germ cells. Among the circulating embryonic germ cells intended entirely for the gonads, an occasional renegade cell may lodge intracranially. Tumors derived therefrom show a strong preference for the pineal area or the region of the infundibulum above the sella turcica: Subsequent neoplastic growth permits a number of phenotypic morphologic expressions that parallel gonadal neoplasms—namely, seminomas, choriocarcinomas, em-

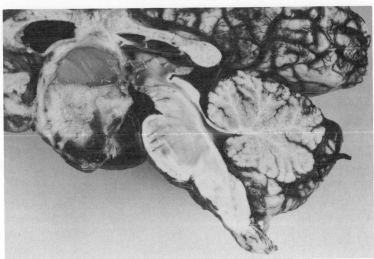

Figure 28-86. Craniopharyngioma. This cystic tumor, which originates from rudiments of Rathke's pouch in the suprasellar area, has a fibrous capsule that adheres to the undersurface of the corpus callosum. The lower portion of the cyst contains cellular debris; a coagulum of protein-rich fluid occupies the upper part of the cyst. Obstruction of the third ventricle is reflected in the dilatation of the lateral ventricles.

bryonal carcinomas, entodermal sinus tumors, and teratoid tumors. As a family, these lesions greatly exceed the incidence of true neoplasms of the pineal gland, or **pinealomas.**

True pineal tumors express histologic characteristics of the phylogenetic past. They resemble neoplasms of the retina and, on occasion, form prominent rosettes.

Destruction of the pineal by a dysgerminoma in childhood may produce precocious puberty, particularly in boys. A mass in the pineal area compresses the superior colliculus and restricts ocular motion. It also compresses the aqueduct of Sylvius and causes hydrocephalus.

Hemangioblastomas originate principally in the cerebellum, without a well-defined cell of origin. These tumors are highly vascularized and feature endothelial-lined canals interspersed with plump cells that do not generate factor VIII. In about 20% of cases, these cells secrete erythropoietin and induce polycythemia. Although this lesion is encountered predominantly in the cerebellum, a few lesions arise in the spinal cord and, rarely, above the tentorium. A few case studies have disclosed a hereditary pattern. When the lesions are restricted to the cerebellum, the term **Lindau's syndrome** is applied. When the cerebellar lesion coexists with one in the retina, the term **von Hippel-Lindau syndrome** is used.

Lymphomas may originate as primary lesions in the brain, in a manner analogous to their occurrence in the stomach, small bowel, and testes. In the brain, these tumors often arise deep in the cerebral hemispheres, and they are often bilateral in a periventricular position. The histologic diagnosis is suggested by the tendency of lymphocytes and larger histiocytic forms to encircle blood vessels and, particularly, to occupy their walls. The constituent cells are generally identified as B-lymphocytes. Interestingly, the lesion has a close, but not absolute, relationship with immunosuppression, and is recognized as a complication of AIDS.

Metastatic Tumors

Metastatic tumors are the most common neoplasms of the central nervous system. They reach the intracranial compartment through the bloodstream, generally in patients with advanced cancer. It is not clear why tumors of different organs or different cell types exhibit differences in the incidence of intracranial metastases. In this respect, a patient with disseminated malignant melanoma has greater than a 50% likelihood of acquiring intracranial metastases, whereas the incidence of cerebral metastases in patients with carcinoma of the breast and lung is about 35%, and that in carcinoma of the kidney or bowel is 5%. All sarcomas and certain carcinomas, such as those of the prostate, liver, and adrenals, rarely metastasize to the brain. Most metastatic lesions seed to the gray-white junction, a reflection of the rich capillary bed in this area.

A metastasis contrasts with a primary glioma in its discrete appearance, globoid shape, and its halo of edema. Metastases to the leptomeninges permit tumor cells to grow in the cerebrospinal fluid, suspended as in tissue culture. This entity is termed carcinomatosis of the meninges.

A. CENTRAL NERVOUS SYSTEM

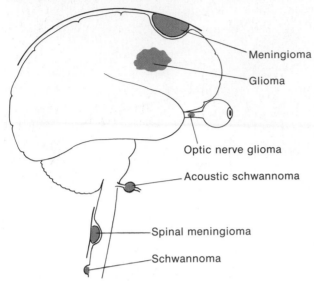

Meningioma

Glioma

Optic nerve glioma

Acoustic schwannoma

Spinal meningioma

Schwannoma

B. PERIPHERAL NERVOUS SYSTEM

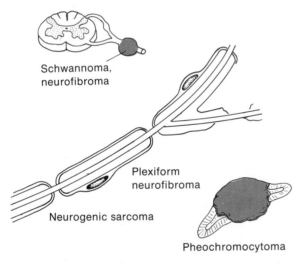

Schwannoma, neurofibroma

Plexiform neurofibroma

Neurogenic sarcoma

Pheochromocytoma

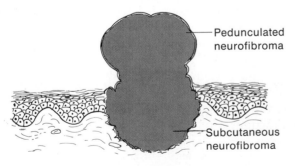

Pedunculated neurofibroma

Subcutaneous neurofibroma

Figure 28-87. Tumors associated with von Recklinghausen's disease.

Tumors Derived from Embryonic Structures

Colloid cysts (paraphyseal cyst, third ventricular cyst) are distinctive for their anterior, midline location in the segmental portion of the third ventricle. This site causes the mass to occlude the foramina of Monro, elevate and compress the fornix, and press upon the lateral wall of the third ventricle. This anatomic relationship creates hydrocephalus, alterations in personality, weakness of the lower legs, and loss of bladder control. The pyramidal fibers to the legs pass medially in the internal capsule subjacent to the ependyma, and the same is true for the pathway that originates in the cingulate gyrus to control the bladder. The colloid cyst is lined by cuboidal epithelium. The lesion enlarges slowly, usually over decades, because of the accumulation of desquamated and secretory products. The origin of the colloid cyst remains in doubt, but it is conjectured that it arises from the paraphysis, a sense organ of lower vertebrates that may remain as a vestigial structure in man.

Genetic Contributions to Intracranial Neoplasms

Three genetically expressed entities deserve consideration. They include von Recklinghausen's disease, tuberous sclerosis, and Lindau's disease.

von Recklinghausen's disease (neurofibromatosis) is inherited as an autosomal dominant disorder, with a high degree of penetrance. In addition, a high mutation rate accounts for cases without a familial history. Its genetic contribution to the incidence of intracranial neoplasia is complex, and involves the peripheral and central nervous systems. There is a high incidence of neurofibromas and schwannomas of the peripheral nerves. In addition, there is a high incidence of meningiomas, acoustic and spinal schwannomas, and gliomas (Fig. 28-87).

Tuberous sclerosis (Bourneville's disease) is transmitted as a mendelian dominant disorder, with frequent examples of formes frustes. In this entity, disordered migration and arrested maturation of the neuroectoderm result in "tubers" of the cerebral cortex and the appearance of subependymal astrocytic nodules. The "tubers" are discrete, firm, cortical areas composed of bizarre cells that possess both neuronal and glial features. The subependymal nodules have been likened to candle drippings, and provide the substrate for the highly characteristic gemistocytic astrocytomas (Fig. 28-88). The gemistocytic astrocyte is a plump, swollen cell. In addition to the intracranial neuroectodermal lesions, the syndrome includes angiofibromas of the face (adenoma sebaceum), rhabdomyomas of the heart, and mixed mesenchymal tumors of the kidney (angiomyolipomas).

As has been mentioned previously, some hemangioblastomas of the cerebellum display a hereditary pattern (**Lindau's** syndrome). An identical tumor may occur in the retina (**von Hippel-Lindau** syndrome). In addition, a hemangioblastoma may be associated with cysts in the kidneys and pancreas.

Metabolic Disorders

Cellular and tissue metabolism may be altered genetically and the derangements expressed neonatally in certain entities, such as Tay-Sachs disease, Hurler's syndrome, Hunter's syndrome, Gaucher's disease, and Niemann-Pick disease (see Ch. 6). Alternatively, genetic disruptions may be expressed predominantly as functional disorders, as exemplified by phenylketonuria or cretinism. Extraneuronal metabolism may also be altered by genes that exert adverse secondary influences on the nervous system, a relationship that characterizes Wilson's disease. Furthermore, normal metabolism can also be modified by nutritional deficiencies, as in Wernicke-Korsakoff's syndrome (thiamine deficiency) and posterior combined degeneration of the spinal cord (vitamin B_{12} deficiency).

Numerous exogenous toxins alter the metabolism of the nervous system; many modify function, and some alter structure. Alcohol is a prominent example among many that include lead, mercury, and tin. Importantly, because neurons do not replicate in the adult, their metabolism may be altered during the passage of time, perhaps through the accumulation of exogenously or endogenously induced errors. Parkinsonism, amyotrophic lateral sclerosis, Huntington's disease, and Alzheimer's disease are possible examples.

Neuronal Storage Diseases

Tay-Sachs disease (amaurotic familial idiocy) is the morphologic and functional expression of an autosomal recessive genetic disorder. A deficiency of hexosaminidase A permits the accumulation of a ganglioside within the neurons of the central and

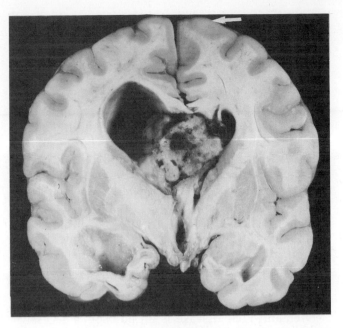

Figure 28-88. Tuberous sclerosis with secondary neoplasia. A neoplasm occupies the midline between the two cerebral hemispheres, creating a bosselated mass that histologically is composed of large, gemistocytic astrocytes. This neoplasm originated from subependymal "candle drippings," a stigmata of tuberous sclerosis. A cortical tuber (*arrow*) is present in the right parasagittal region of the gray cortex, where the definition of the gray mantle is obscured.

peripheral nervous systems. Retinal involvement increases the transparency of the macula, resulting in a cherry-red spot (see Ch. 29). The infant appears normal at birth, but shows a delay in motor development by the age of 6 months. Thereafter, the child deteriorates to a state of flaccid weakness, blindness, mental inactivity, and ultimately death, generally by the end of the second year. The brain becomes heavier, and on histologic examination, shows the universal presence of lipid droplets within the cytoplasm of distended nerve cells, both in the central and peripheral nervous systems. Electron microscopy reveals the lipid to be largely within lysosomes, in the form of whorled myelin figures. The neural tissues respond with a diffuse astrogliosis.

Hurler's syndrome reflects a hereditary disturbance in glycosaminoglycan metabolism that results in the intraneuronal accumulation of mucopolysaccharides. The clinical variants of this syndrome are distinguished by the involvement of visceral organs and the nervous system. Typically, Hurler's syndrome is expressed in infancy or early childhood by dwarfism, corneal opacities, skeletal deformities, and hepatosplenomegaly. The intraneuronal storage distends the cytoplasmic compartment, and astrocytes respond with proliferation.

Gaucher's disease results from an autosomal recessive genetic disorder involving a deficiency of glucocerebroside β-glucosidase. As a result, glucocerebroside accumulates, principally in the reticuloendothelial system. The central nervous system is most severely involved in the infantile type (type II) of Gaucher's disease, in which intraneuronal storage is not as conspicuous as neuronal loss, which is accompanied by severe, diffuse astrogliosis. These infants fail to thrive, and die at an early age. The accumulation of glucocerebroside is minimal, even though glucocerebrosidase activity in the tissue is virtually absent, a situation that suggests a complex disturbance in cerebral metabolism and neuronal maturation.

Niemann-Pick disease is an autosomal recessive disorder characterized by intraneuronal storage of sphingomyelin that results from a deficiency of sphingomyelinase. The clinical symptoms occur early, and the disease is marked by failure of the infant to develop and thrive. The reticuloendothelial system is targeted for storage, but symptoms may predominantly affect the nervous system during infancy. The brain becomes atrophic and shows marked astrogliosis. Retinal degeneration may produce a cherry-red spot similar to that which occurs in Tay-Sachs disease.

Impaired Neuronal Metabolism

Phenylketonuria is an autosomal recessive disorder that is clinically manifested in homozygotes as an enzymatic deficiency in phenylalanine hydroxylase (see Ch. 6). This abnormality results in the excessive accumulation of phenylalanine in the blood and tissues because of a block in the conversion of phenylalanine to tyrosine. Symptoms of the disease include mental retardation, seizures, and retarded physical development, and generally become apparent in the early months of life. Patients who are not treated with a rigid diet rarely obtain an IQ of greater than 50. This entity exemplifies an inborn metabolic error that seriously impairs cognitive function without consistent alterations in neuronal cytoarchitecture. Occasionally, the brain is underweight and deficient in myelination.

Cretinism is a consequence of maternal iodine deficiency, with a resulting lack of thyroxin (see Ch. 21). Severe hypothyroidism in infancy alters the func-

tional capacity of the central nervous system. As with phenylketonuria, this disorder is reversible—in this instance, by the administration of thyroxin. When the deficiency persists beyond a few months, the disease becomes irreversible. Interestingly, even in this dysfunctional state, the brain achieves a near-normal weight, has appropriate neuronal cytoarchitecture, and is well myelinated. However, the patient is typically stunted in growth and severely handicapped intellectually.

Wilson's disease is an autosomal recessive disorder of copper metabolism (see Ch. 14). Copper accumulates in toxic amounts in the liver and the brain, especially the putamen—hence, the term **hepatolenticular degeneration.** The cerebral intoxication is generally manifested in the second decade by athetoid movements. Before, during, or after the appearance of neurologic symptoms, an insidiously developing cirrhosis of the liver may present as hepatic failure.

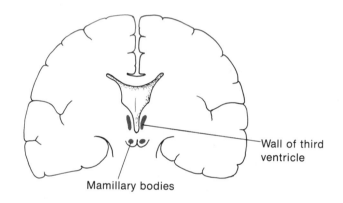

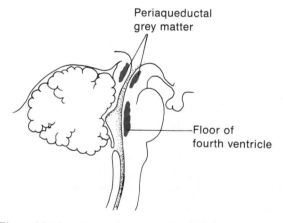

Figure 28-89. Wernicke's encephalopathy. The geographic distribution of "ring hemorrhages" in Wernicke's encephalopathy include the mamillary bodies, the wall of the third ventricle, the periaqueductal gray matter, and the floor of the fourth ventricle.

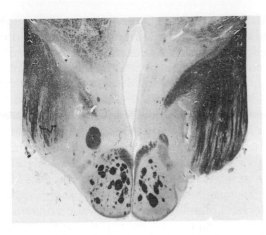

Figure 28-90. Wernicke's encephalopathy. A coronal section through the hypothalamus, the third ventricle, and mamillary bodies discloses clusters of "ring hemorrhages" in the mamillary bodies.

The deposition of copper in the limbus of the cornea produces a visible golden-brown band, the Kayser-Fleischer ring. Although the functional disturbances of the nervous system greatly exceed the morphologic alterations, on gross examination, the lenticulate nuclei may show a light golden discoloration. In 25% of the cases, small cysts or clefts are evident to the naked eye, either in the region of the putamen or in the lower margins of the cortical gray mantle. Histologically, a scant loss of neurons and a mild gliosis in the lenticulate nuclei present a sharp contrast to the severe chorioathetoid movement disorder that characterizes the clinical disease.

Deficiencies of Dietary Intake and Nutrient Utilization

Wernicke's syndrome results from a deficiency of thiamine (vitamin B_1) (see Ch. 8). **In the industrialized world, the disease is most commonly associated with chronic alcoholism.** Typically, the onset of symptoms is precipitous, and the symptoms reflect lesions in the hypothalamus and mamillary bodies, in the periaqueductal regions of the midbrain, and in the tegmentum of the pons (Fig. 28-89). These lesions are manifested clinically by a disturbance in thermal regulation, altered consciousness, ophthalmoplegia, and nystagmus. The condition may progress rapidly to death, but is promptly reversible with the administration of thiamine. The acute tissue response features petechiae about small capillaries. Neurons and myelin are remarkably spared. The petechiae vary geographically from case to case, but regularly involve the mamillary bodies (Fig. 28-90), hypothalamus, periaqueductal gray matter, and the floor of the fourth ventricle. The prior occurrence of petechiae is permanently marked by the presence of brown hemosiderin. The mamillary bodies become atrophic.

Wernicke-Korsakoff's syndrome refers to a clinical state of disordered memory for recent events, which is often compensated for by confabulation, in the setting of chronic alcoholism. The histologic changes, when present, are distinguishable from those of Wernicke's syndrome and are represented by chromatolysis and degeneration of neurons in the medial dorsal nucleus of the thalamus. Thus, although Wernicke's syndrome and Korsakoff's psychosis occur concurrently in the setting of chronic alcoholism, their causes are seemingly different. Indeed, Korsakoff's psychosis is now thought to be nonspecific and to occur in conditions other than alcoholism.

Alcoholism creates a complex problem that embraces both nutrition and intoxication (see Ch. 8). Four cerebral conditions warrant consideration: cortical atrophy, atrophy of the superior aspect of the vermis of the cerebellum, Wernicke's syndrome, and central pontine myelinolysis (Fig. 28-91). The intimacy of the association of alcoholism with cortical atrophy is still debated, but it does not appear to be absolute, nor is the role of toxicity versus malnutrition defined. The same lack of precise etiology prevails with regard to the atrophy of the Purkinje and

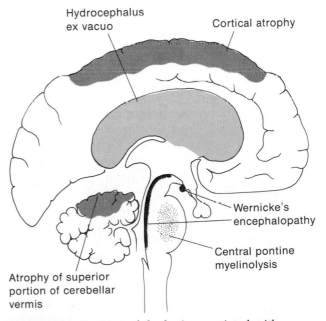

Figure 28-91. Lesions of the brain associated with chronic alcoholism.

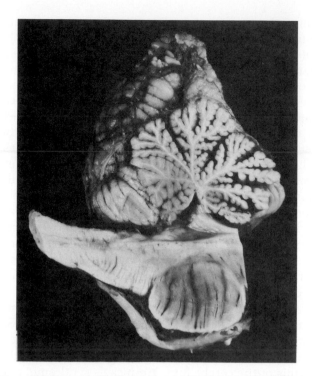

Figure 28-92. Alcoholism. The cerebellum shows atrophy of the superior portion of the vermis. The open, fernlike appearance is indicative of a loss of parenchyma which accentuates the individual folia.

granular cells of the cerebellum (Fig. 28-92). This alteration is, perhaps, the most common corollary of chronic alcoholism, and is ostensibly the cause of the truncal ataxia that persists during periods of sobriety. As noted previously, the fourth lesion, central pontine myelinolysis, is presumably an iatrogenic complication related to the rapid correction of hyponatremia.

Hepatic encephalopathy is an expression of liver failure, evidenced as delirium, seizures, and coma. In general, the clinical symptoms greatly exceed their morphologic corollaries in the brain. The latter are restricted to a response by astrocytes, termed **Alzheimer type II change,** wherein the nuclei enlarge moderately and the chromatin material is marginated to the nuclear membrane. These changes are generally more prominent in the thalamus.

Subacute combined degeneration (posterolateral combined degeneration) results precipitously from a deficiency of vitamin B$_{12}$, most often in association with pernicious anemia treated only with folic acid. The lesion begins as a symmetric loss of myelin and axons in the midthoracic or lower thoracic level of the spinal cord, and extends caudally and cephalad, producing an edematous, spongiform appearance in the posterolateral areas. A burning sensation in the soles of the feet ushers in a rapidly progressive, only partially reversible, neurologic deficit. Although astrogliosis is typically mild in the acute lesion, with time, the area of degeneration loses its spongiform appearance, and the cord becomes atrophic. Historically, subacute combined degeneration was intimately associated with pernicious anemia. Today, its occurrence complicates rare cases of extensive gastric resection, as well as other malabsorption syndromes. Because vitamin B$_{12}$ is not synthesized by humans, some extreme vegetarians, who eschew even animal products, such as milk and eggs, have developed subacute combined degeneration after many years on the restricted diet.

Degenerative Diseases

The heterogeneous group of degenerative diseases places under a common heading several entities, such as parkinsonism, Huntington's disease, amyotrophic lateral sclerosis, and spinocerebellar degenerations (Fig. 28-93). These disorders involve individual neuronal species, select systems or anatomic regions, or alternatively, may affect the nervous system diffusely, as in the case of Alzheimer's disease and Pick's disease.

Parkinsonism

Parkinsonism (paralysis agitans) is a neuronal disorder that primarily involves the substantia nigra. The neurons in this location are unable to maintain a normal functional state and ultimately die. The clinical expression of tremors at rest, muscular rigidity, and emotional lability are usually evidenced in the sixth to eighth decade of life. Thus, the focus is upon an intraneuronal metabolic state that is involved in the transmission and reception of information within the extrapyramidal system. These neurons exert their action principally by secreting dopamine and, in the early period of metabolic impairment, substitution therapy using L-dopa is functionally beneficial. However, this mode of therapy does not rectify the defective metabolic state and, with the passage of several years, neuronal viability is lost and therapy becomes ineffective.

Gross examination of the brain typically reveals a loss of pigment in the substantia nigra and locus ceruleus (Fig. 28-94). Microscopic examination reveals a depletion of pigmented neurons in these areas. Transient, small deposits of melanin result from the death of neurons. Some residual nerve cells are atrophic, and a few contain spherical, eosino-

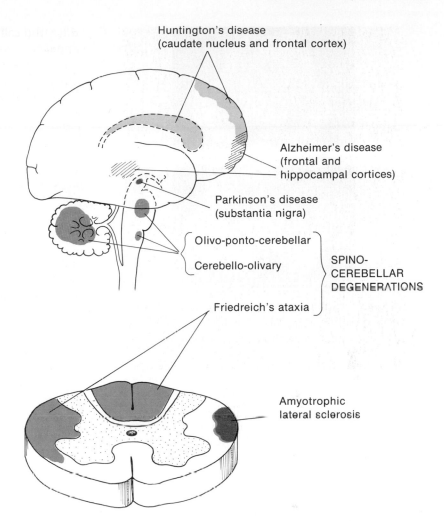

Huntington's disease
(caudate nucleus and frontal cortex)

Alzheimer's disease
(frontal and
hippocampal cortices)

Parkinson's disease
(substantia nigra)

Olivo-ponto-cerebellar

Cerebello-olivary

SPINO-
CEREBELLAR
DEGENERATIONS

Friedreich's ataxia

Amyotrophic
lateral sclerosis

Figure 28-93. Distribution of degenerative diseases of the central nervous system.

philc, cytoplasmic inclusions termed **Lewy bodies**. As viewed by electron microscopy, these are dense accumulations of filaments. The degenerative effect of parkinsonism extends beyond the substantia nigra throughout the dopaminergic nigrostriatal pathways. Secondary degenerative changes are present in the striatum, particularly the putamen.

The basis of parkinsonism secondary to von Economo's encephalitis (encephalitis lethargica) has been discussed. Interestingly, the residual pigmented neurons associated with this form of postencephalitic parkinsonism exhibit neurofibrillary tangles rather than Lewy bodies.

Huntington's Disease

Huntington's disease is an autosomal dominant, hereditary disorder in which the expression of an abnormal gene alters the metabolism of a specific neu-

ronal cell species and initiates a progressive functional deficiency that terminates in cell death. The abnormal gene resides on the short arm of chromosome 4. Remarkably, the clinical expression of this gene abnormality is clinically dormant, and the patients remain asymptomatic through the first three to five decades of life. The primary disorder concerns the extrapyramidal system, and initial symptoms usually include an athetoid movement disorder. Subsequent involvement of the cortex leads to a loss of cognitive function, often accompanied by paranoia and delusions. Death occurs a decade or so later, and postmortem examination shows marked, symmetrical atrophy of the caudate nuclei, with lesser involvement of the putamen (Fig. 28-95). The frontal cortex is symmetrically atrophic. The neuronal population of the caudate and putamen, particularly the small neurons, is greatly depleted. This degenerative process is accompanied by a moderate astroglial response. The cortical neurons are similarly, but less

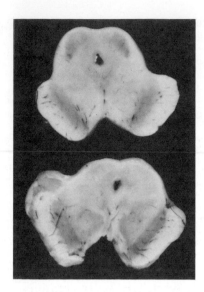

Figure 28-94. Parkinsonism. Transverse sections of the midbrain show a marked loss of melanin pigmentation in the substantia nigra, reflecting a loss of neurons in that area.

severely, depleted. Biochemical assays at the termination of the disease show a marked decrease in gamma-aminobutyric acid (GABA) and in glutamic acid decarboxylase. There is also a marked increase in iron content.

Amyotrophic Lateral Sclerosis

Amyotrophic lateral sclerosis reiterates the common theme of a precocious dysfunction of a select system of neurons that is followed by neuronal death, presumably as an expression of disordered intraneuronal metabolism. This disease relates specifically to motor neurons—that is, the anterior horn cells of the spinal cord; the motor nuclei of the brain stem, particularly the hypoglossal nuclei; and the upper motor neurons of the cerebral cortex. The structural counterpart of the agonal events prior to neuronal death is reflected in the "dying back phenomenon." This process is best visualized in the retrograde degeneration of the lateral pyramidal pathways in the spinal cord. The axons of this system originate from the cell bodies of the upper motor neurons in the cerebral cortex. These neurons lose their metabolic potential and become unable to sustain the structural integrity of the distal portions of their axons. Thus, initially, the lateral columns degenerate at the lumbosacral level. Thereafter, the degeneration progresses retrograde or cephalad, but a gradient of severity persists. With

time, the cell body itself undergoes atrophy and disappears.

Spinocerebellar Degeneration

Spinocerebellar degeneration represents a category of disease that contains numerous heterogeneous entities. However, they are unified by three features: a broad but system-based geographic topography, a genetic influence, and a precocious loss of neurons and tracts in the cerebellum, brain stem, and spinal cord. The symptomatology reflects the topography of the lesions. Thus, patients display ataxia and intention tremor with involvement of the cerebellum; rigidity and tremor with degeneration of the brain stem; and loss of deep tendon reflexes, vibratory sense, and pain sensation with involvement of the spinal cord. Because there is a greater anatomic and clinical uniformity among familial cases than among random ones, case reports have generally focused upon an individual family, and the researcher's name has frequently individualized that series. For example, an inherited form of cerebello-olivary degeneration is designated cerebello-olivary degeneration of Holmes, which is distinguished from sporadic cerebello-olivary degeneration of Marie. In turn, these cases share many anatomic features with olivopontocerebellar degeneration of Menzel. A similar complexity of entities pertains to the spinal cord, but in this location, Friedreich's ataxia predominates. Thus,

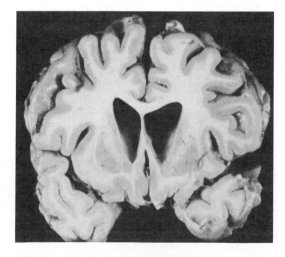

Figure 28-95. Huntington's chorea. Selective degeneration of the caudate nuclei bilaterally has straightened the normal concave contour of the lateral walls of the lateral ventricles, and has brought the ependyma in close proximity to the internal capsules. There is a moderate degree of cortical atrophy.

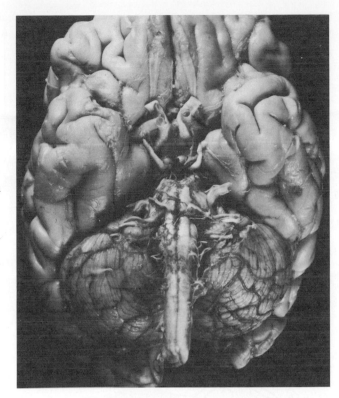

Figure 28-96.   Spinocerebellar degeneration. Degeneration of the pons is conspicuous in this case of olivopontocerebellar degeneration.

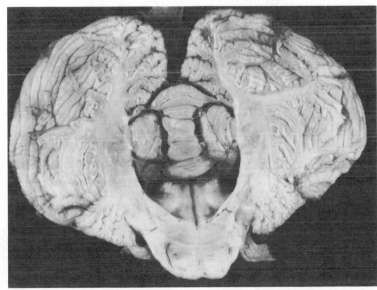

Figure 28-97.   Spinocerebellar degeneration. The small size of the pons compared to that of the fifth cranial nerve emphasizes the pontine atrophy. The enlargement of the fourth ventricle reflects severe loss of substance in the middle cerebellar peduncles.

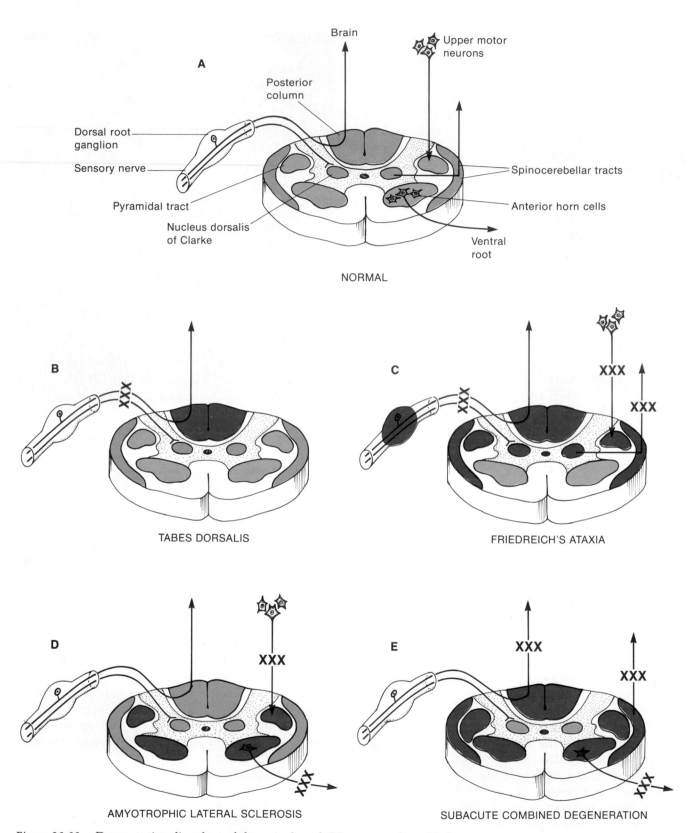

Figure 28-98.   Degenerative disorders of the spinal cord. Many ascending (*blue*) and descending (*green*) pathways traverse the spinal cord. The four diseases illustrated produce differing patterns of disruption (*red*) of these pathways depending on the location of the primary pathologic process.

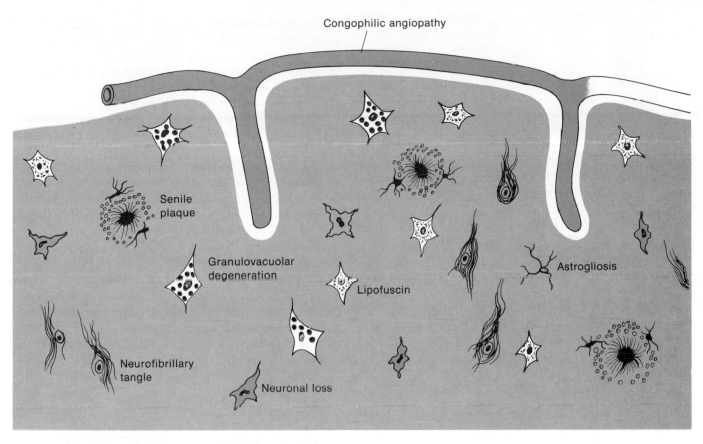

Figure 28-99.   Microscopic lesions of Alzheimer's disease.

it would appear that small anatomic subunits of the cerebellopontine spinal system degenerate precociously as a result of different abnormal genes (Figs. 28-96 and 28-97).

Cerebello-olivary degeneration of Holmes is an autosomal inherited disorder that is commonly expressed clinically during the second and third decades of life. Progressive cerebellar ataxia predominates, but brain stem involvement often causes dysphagia and nystagmus. There is precocious loss of Purkinje cells and a varying degree of loss of neurons of the inferior olives.

Friedreich's ataxia is an autosomal dominant disorder that involves the spinal cord (Fig. 28-98). The symptoms of this disorder first appear during the first and second decades of life, and the course is insidiously progressive for 10 years or more. The classic lesion features degeneration of the posterior columns, the corticospinal pathways, and the spinocerebellar tracts. Interestingly, but for reasons not understood, a chronic, interstitial cardiomyopathy develops. Cardiac hypertrophy and fibrosis may lead to heart failure.

Alzheimer's disease is characterized by the formation of senile (neuritic) plaques, neurofibrillary tangles, and granulovacuolar degeneration (Fig. 28-99). These structural changes are most likely responsible for the dementia that affects about two-thirds of persons who are institutionalized because of impaired cognitive function. The morphologic alterations are also present, but to a lesser degree, in the cerebrum of a large number of elderly individuals with symptoms as minor as forgetfulness. Indeed, the "disease process" is seemingly as inescapable in the aging human brain as is systemic atherosclerosis.

The term Alzheimer's disease was originally restricted to patients in whom the typical morphologic features and dementia occurred prior to the age of 65 years. "Presenile dementia" was the designation given the disorder affecting the middle-aged population, whereas an analogous clinical and morphologic state in the later decades of life was termed "senile dementia." Currently, the term Alzheimer's disease is employed generically for all ages and identifies a specific morphologic corollary of dementia. Alzheimer's disease is clearly distinguishable from

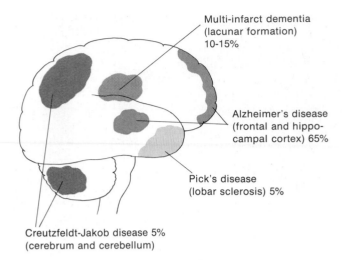

Figure 28-100. Diseases associated with dementia.

other disorders associated with dementia, such as Creutzfeldt-Jakob disease, Huntington's disease, multi-infarct dementia, and Pick's disease (Fig. 28-100).

During the course of Alzheimer's disease, neurons and neuritic processes are lost, the gyri narrow, the sulci widen, and cortical atrophy becomes apparent (Fig. 28-101). The brain weight is reduced by about 200 g in an interval of 3 to 8 years. The atrophy is bilateral and symmetric and principally involves the cortex of the frontal lobes and hippocampus (Fig. 28-102). The most conspicuous histologic lesion, the **senile or neuritic plaque,** is a focal, discrete area that is several hundred microns in diameter. Within these small, spherical regions, electron microscopy discloses segmental enlargement of the neuritic processes and stagnation of axoplasmic flow, as evidenced by the accumulation of mitochrondria and lysosomes. The segmental dilatation of dendritic processes as they traverse a region of tissue injury is somewhat analogous to the regional loss of myelin as axons traverse a plaque of multiple sclerosis. On light microscopy, the maturing neuritic plaque is argentophilic and contains abundant glial processes and deposits that stain positively for amyloid. Ultrastructurally, the characteristic fibrillar structure of amyloid is also observed.

The second member of the morphologic triad, **neurofibrillary tangles,** are helical filaments within neurons that are formed in such abundance as to engorge the perikaryon (Fig. 28-103). These filaments have the same protein composition and diameter (10 nm)

as normal neurofilaments and neurotubules. However, they are present in great excess and are abnormally paired into helical complexes. The third constituent of the morphologic triad is **granulovacuolar degeneration,** which is largely restricted to the pyramidal cells of the hippocampus. The term is used to describe multiple, small, cytoplasmic vacuoles, each of which contains one or several dark granules (Fig. 28-104).

The cause of Alzheimer's disease remains obscure. At present, there are two prominent theories regarding the pathogenetic mechanisms for Alzheimer's disease, but both fall short of accounting for all of the features of the disorder. One hypothesis incriminates aluminum as a toxic cause of Alzheimer's disease. However, the presence of low and inconsistent levels of the metal in some affected individuals raises the question of whether its presence represents the cause of the disease or an epiphenomenon that reflects chelation. Another theory creates an analogy to parkinsonism, wherein Meynert's nucleus serves as the counterpart of the substantia nigra. According to this concept, a deficiency of cholinergic com-

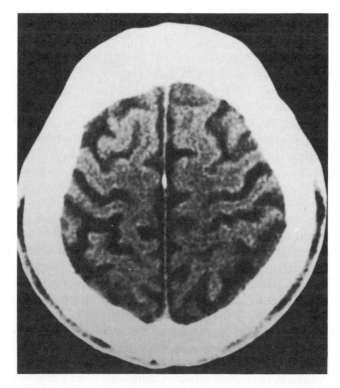

Figure 28-101. Alzheimer's disease. A CT scan reveals widening of the sulci and narrowing of the gyri, evidence of cortical atrophy.

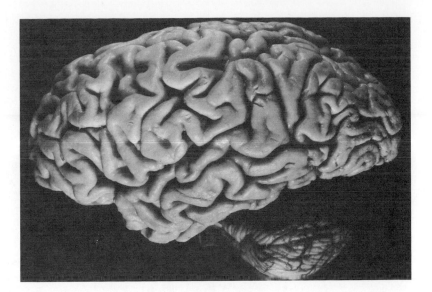

Figure 28-102. Alzheimer's disease. The cortex of the frontal, temporal, and parietal areas of the brain are atrophic.

pounds, rather than of dopamine, is involved. This hypothesis relies upon biochemical determinations performed at the termination of a chronic disease, when primary events may be obscured by a multitude of epiphenomena.

As mentioned previously, there is a predictable and precocious development of neuritic plaques, neurofibrillary tangles, and granulovacuolar degeneration in persons with Down's syndrome. This provides a natural human model with which to seek biochemical events that antedate the morphologic expressions of the disease. Recent evidence suggests that an amyloid protein, derived from a larger precursor protein, may play a role in the pathogenesis of Alzheimer's disease. The gene for this amyloid β-protein, an important component of the amyloid plaques of Alzheimer's disease and Down's syndrome (trisomy 21), has been localized to chromosome 21. Importantly, the gene responsible for the hereditary form of Alzheimer's disease has also been localized to the same region of chromosome 21. Taken together, these data suggest that Alzheimer's disease may result from an abnormality in the gene that codes for amyloid β-protein or the processing of its precursor protein.

The prevalence of severe dementia in the United States is estimated to exceed 1.3 million cases. As indicated earlier, Alzheimer's disease is the predominant cause of this severe dementia. Other entities, such as Creutzfeldt-Jakob disease, Huntington's disease and multiple infarct dementia, have been discussed previously. Pick's disease is extremely rare in

the United States, but its incidence is significant in European countries, and its morphologic appearance is highly distinctive.

Pick's disease (lobar sclerosis) is expressed clinically as dementia that is essentially indistinguishable from that of Alzheimer's disease. The disease becomes symptomatic in midadulthood and progresses relentlessly over a period of 3 to 5 years. Some examples of Pick's disease cluster in a single family, but the case distributions do not conform to a hereditary pattern. Women are affected by the disease more often than men.

The brain in Pick's disease is atrophic, but unlike Alzheimer's disease, the atrophy is typically localized in a frontal or a temporal lobe, and it may attain extreme proportions (Fig. 28-105). Histologically, the involved cortex is markedly depleted of neurons, and their absence is accentuated by a marked astrogliosis (Fig. 28-106). Many residual neurons have a "ballooned" cytoplasm, and in some, there is one or several faintly eosinophilic inclusions, termed **Pick bodies,** whose presence is validated by their intense argentophilia (Fig. 28-107). These bodies are formed of densely aggregated neurofilaments. Thus, a quantitative and qualitative disturbance in neurofilament formation characterizes a number of neuropathologic states, such as a tangle formation in Alzheimer's disease, the Lewy body in parkinsonism, the Pick body, and the nonpaired neurofilamentous accumulations in progressive supranuclear palsy (Steele-Richardson-Olszewski syndrome).

(Text continues on p. 1490)

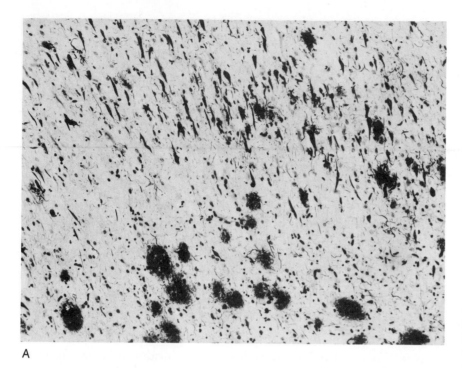

A

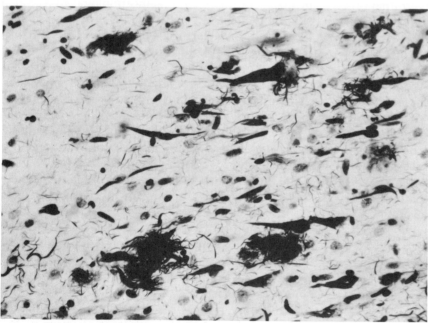

B

Figure 28-103. Alzheimer's disease. (A) A photomicrograph of the hippocampal cortex demonstrates extensive neurofibrillary degeneration of many neurons. There are numerous senile plaques, the presence of which is made apparent by their argentophilia. (B) High-power view of A.

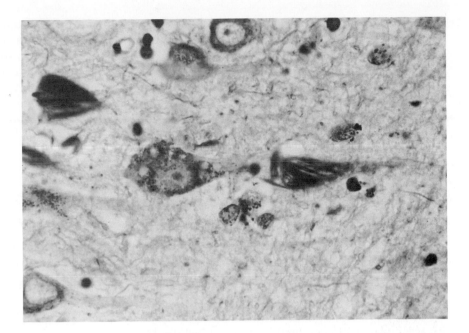

Figure 28-104. Alzheimer's disease. The neurofibrillary tangles are also argentophilic. Note that the neuron with granulovacuolar degeneration (*center*) does not show neurofibrillary degeneration.

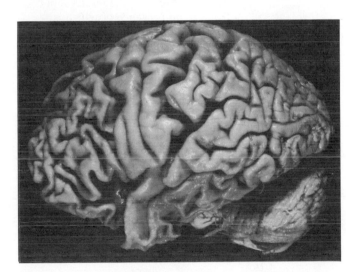

Figure 28-105. Pick's disease. Atrophy is extreme in the temporal lobe, pronounced in the frontal region, and moderate in the parietal area.

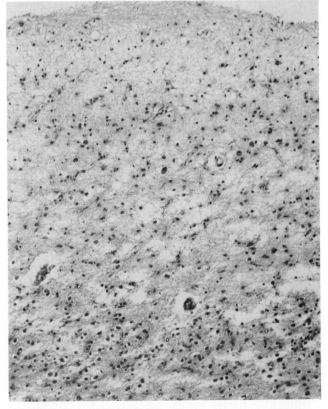

Figure 28-106. Pick's disease. A photomicrograph shows advanced neuronal depopulation and marked astrogliosis.

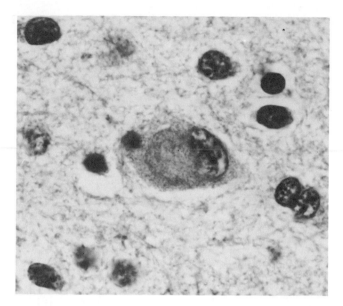

Figure 28-107.   Pick's disease. The Pick body is a spherical accumulation of neurofibrillary material that displaces the nucleus.

of unmyelinated fibers measures 0.4 to 2.4 μm. Myelin is an elaboration of the Schwann cell's plasmalemma and is necessary for saltatory nerve conduction. Schwann cells ensheath both the myelinated and the unmyelinated fibers. The axon determines whether the ensheathing Schwann cell differentiates into a myelin-forming cell. Myelin sheath thickness, internodal length (i.e., the distance between two nodes of Ranvier), and conduction velocity are proportional to the axonal diameter.

General Pathology

Peripheral nerve fibers display only a limited number of reactions to injury. The major types of nerve fiber damage are axonal degeneration and segmental de-

The Peripheral Nervous System

Thomas W. Bouldin

The peripheral nervous system is external to the brain and spinal cord and includes the cranial nerves, dorsal and ventral spinal roots, spinal nerves and their continuations, and ganglia. Peripheral nerves carry somatic motor, somatic sensory, visceral sensory, and autonomic fibers. The somatic motor and preganglionic autonomic fibers arise from neuronal cell bodies within the central nervous system. The sensory and postganglionic autonomic fibers arise from neuronal cell bodies within ganglia located on cranial nerves, dorsal roots, and autonomic nerves. The neurons and satellite cells of the ganglia and all of the Schwann cells are derived from the neural crest. The peripheral nerves, but not their ganglia, have a blood–nerve barrier analogous to the blood–brain barrier. Endoneurial connective tissue surrounds the individual nerve fibers, which are bundled into fascicles by the perineurial connective tissue. Epineurial connective tissue binds the fascicles together and contains the nutrient arteries.

Peripheral nerve fibers are either myelinated or unmyelinated (Fig. 28-108). Myelinated fibers range from 1 to 20 μm in diameter, whereas the diameter

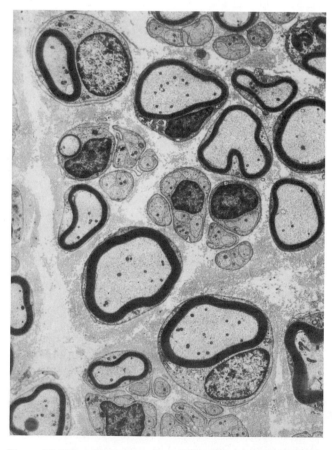

Figure 28-108.   Structure of peripheral nerve. An electron micrograph of a peripheral nerve shows myelinated fibers interspersed with groups of unmyelinated fibers. Note that, in contrast to myelinated axons, several unmyelinated axons may share a Schwann cell.

myelination. The peripheral nervous system differs from the central nervous system in its capacity for axonal regeneration and segmental remyelination.

Axonal Degeneration

Degeneration (necrosis) of the axon occurs in many neuropathies and reflects significant injury of the neuronal cell body or its axon. Axonal degeneration is quickly followed by breakdown of the myelin sheath and Schwann-cell proliferation. The myelin debris is cleared by Schwann cells and macrophages. In many neuropathies, axonal degeneration is initially restricted to the distal ends of the larger, longer fibers (Fig. 28-109). Peripheral neuropathies exhibiting this selective degeneration of distal axons are known as **dying-back neuropathies (distal axonopathies)** and typically present as distal ("glove-and-stocking") neuropathies. The basis for the selective vulnerability of the distal axon in these neuropathies is unknown. Axonal degeneration may also be secondary to degeneration of the neuronal cell body, as occurs in poliomyelitis.

Neuropathies characterized by selective degeneration of the neuronal soma are referred to as **neuronopathies,** and are much less common than distal axonopathies. The axonal degeneration that occurs in a nerve distal to a transection or crush of the nerve is termed **wallerian degeneration.**

Segmental Demyelination

The loss of myelin from one or more internodes (segments) along a myelinated fiber is common in many neuropathies and reflects Schwann-cell dysfunction (Fig. 28-109). This Schwann-cell dysfunction may be caused by direct injury of the Schwann cell/myelin sheath, or it may be secondary to underlying axonal abnormalities **(secondary demyelination).** The myelin debris is cleared by Schwann cells and macrophages. Degeneration of the internodal myelin sheath is followed sequentially by Schwann-cell proliferation, remyelination of the demyelinated segments, and recovery of function. The remyelinated internodes have shortened internodal lengths. Repeated episodes of segmental demyelination and remyelination of peripheral nerves, as occurs in chronic demyelinating neuropathies, lead to the accumulation of supernumerary Schwann cells around axons **(onion-bulb formation)** and nerve enlargement (hypertrophy). (Fig. 28-110). Neuropathies characterized

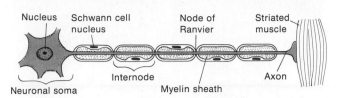

A. INTACT MYELINATED FIBER

Nucleus Schwann cell nucleus Node of Ranvier Striated muscle Neuronal soma Internode Myelin sheath Axon

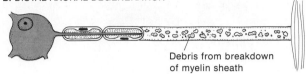

B. DISTAL AXONAL DEGENERATION

Debris from breakdown of myelin sheath

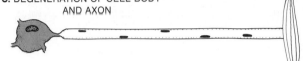

C. DEGENERATION OF CELL BODY AND AXON

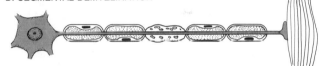

D. SEGMENTAL DEMYELINATION

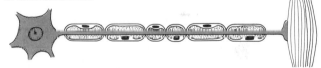

E. REMYELINATION

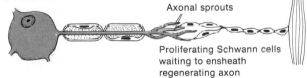

F. REGENERATING AXON

Axonal sprouts

Proliferating Schwann cells waiting to ensheath regenerating axon

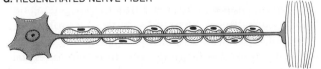

G. REGENERATED NERVE FIBER

Figure 28-109. Axonal degeneration and regeneration after peripheral nerve injury.

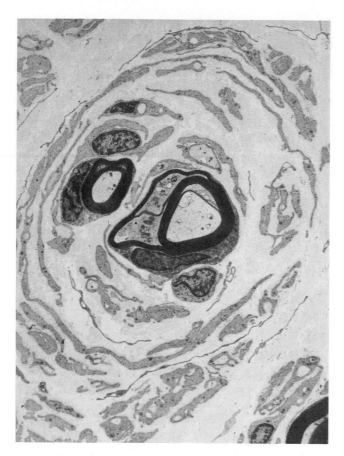

Figure 28-110.   Onion-bulb formation in peripheral nerve. An electron micrograph shows multiple layers of flattened Schwann cell processes encircling two myelinated axons. Onion bulb formations are common in certain hereditary neuropathies and in chronic inflammatory demyelinating neuropathy.

by conspicuous onion-bulb formation and nerve hypertrophy are known as **hypertrophic neuropathies.**

Peripheral Neuropathies

The major clinical manifestations of peripheral neuropathy are muscle weakness, muscle atrophy, alterations of sensation, and autonomic dysfunction. Motor, sensory, and autonomic functions may be equally or preferentially affected. The clinical manifestations may have an acute (within days), subacute (within weeks), or chronic (within months or years) evolution. They may be localized to one nerve (mononeuropathy) or several individual nerves (mononeuropathy multiplex), or they may be diffuse and symmetric (polyneuropathy). On pathologic exami-

nation, a neuropathy may show mainly axonal degeneration (axonal neuropathy), mainly segmental demyelination (demyelinating neuropathy), or a mixture of axonal degeneration and segmental demyelination. The etiologic classification of peripheral neuropathies is presented in Table 28-1.

Inflammatory Demyelinating Neuropathy

Acquired inflammatory demyelinating neuropathy usually presents as an acutely evolving, predominantly motor polyneuropathy (**Landry-Guillain-Barré syndrome**). Occasional patients have a chronic course of disease characterized by multiple relapses or a slow, continuous progression (**chronic inflammatory polyneuropathy**). Severe cases are associated with respiratory embarrassment. Resolution of the neuropathy commences 2 to 4 weeks after onset, and most patients make a good recovery. The pathogenesis of the demyelination is unknown, but current evidence suggests that it may be immunologically mediated. The neuropathy may be sporadic, may follow immunization, surgery, or viral and mycoplasmal infections, or it may complicate cancer.

The neuropathy may involve all levels of the peripheral nervous system, including spinal roots, ganglia, craniospinal nerves, and autonomic nerves, with the distribution of the lesions varying from case to case. The involved regions show endoneurial infiltrates of lymphocytes and macrophages, segmental demyelination, and relative sparing of axons. The lymphoid infiltrates are often perivascular, but there is no true vasculitis. Macrophages are frequently found adjacent to degenerating myelin sheaths and have been observed to strip off and phagocytose the superficial myelin lamellae (macrophage-mediated demyelination). The chronic form of the disease may show numerous onion-bulb formations owing to the recurring episodes of demyelination and remyelination. Lumbar puncture characteristically reveals an increase in the protein level of the cerebrospinal fluid, but only slight pleocytosis. The elevated protein level is attributable to the inflammation of the spinal roots.

Diabetic Neuropathy

Diabetes mellitus, a major cause of neuropathy, is associated with distal sensory or sensorimotor polyneuropathy, autonomic neuropathy, mononeuropathy, or mononeuropathy multiplex. Symmetric polyneuropathy is characterized by a mixture of segmental demyelination and axonal degeneration. The

Table 28-1 Etiologic Classification of Neuropathies

Autoimmune
   Inflammatory demyelinating neuropathy

Metabolic
   Diabetic polyneuropathy
   Uremic neuropathy
   Hypothyroid neuropathy
   Hepatic neuropathy
   Porphyric neuropathy

Nutritional
   Alcoholic neuropathy
   Beriberi neuropathy
   Neuropathy related to Vitamin B12 deficiency
   Neuropathy related to Vitamin E deficiency
   Neuropathy related to the postgastrectomy state
   Neuropathy related to celiac disease

Ischemic
   Vasculitic neuropathy
   Neuropathy of peripheral vascular disease
   Some diabetic mononeuropathies

Toxic See Table 28-2
Paraneoplastic
Amyloid
Paraproteinemic
Inherited See Table 28-3
Infectious
   Herpes zoster
   Leprosy
   Diphtheria (toxin)
   Acquired immune deficiency syndrome (AIDS)

Sarcoid
Radiation-induced
Cryptogenic

axonal degeneration may involve fibers of all sizes or may preferentially involve the small myelinated fibers and the unmyelinated fibers. There may also be neuronal loss in the dorsal root ganglia and anterior horns. The segmental demyelination and axonal degeneration are presumed to have a metabolic basis, but the pathogenesis is unknown. Although the pathogenesis of the diabetic mononeuropathies is not well defined, it has been suggested that many are caused by focal nerve ischemia secondary to arteriosclerosis.

Uremic Neuropathy

A distal sensorimotor polyneuropathy may complicate chronic renal failure. It is characterized pathologically by both distal axonal degeneration and seg-

mental demyelination. The pathogenesis of the nerve fiber damage is not known, but recent studies suggest that the segmental demyelination is a consequence of the underlying axonal abnormalities, rather than a result of a primary metabolic derangement of the Schwann cell. The neuropathy usually resolves after successful renal transplantation.

Alcoholic Neuropathy

The distal sensorimotor polyneuropathy associated with alcohol abuse is generally attributed to concomitant nutritional deficiencies, rather than to a direct toxic effect of alcohol on the peripheral nerves. Peripheral nerves show loss of nerve fibers secondary to axonal degeneration of the dying-back type.

Vasculitic Neuropathy

Systemic vasculitis involves the nutrient arteries of nerves and produces nerve ischemia. Ischemic neuropathy typically presents as a mononeuropathy or mononeuropathy multiplex, and is characterized pathologically by axonal degeneration and a lesser degree of demyelination. Vasculitic neuropathy has been associated with periarteritis nodosa, allergic granulomatosis, hypersensitivity angiitis, rheumatoid arthritis, systemic lupus erythematosus, progressive systemic sclerosis, Sjögren's syndrome, Wegener's granulomatosis, temporal arteritis, and cryoglobulinemia.

Table 28-2 Agents Associated with Toxic Neuropathy

Drugs	Environmental Agents
Amiodarone	Acrylamide
Amytriptyline	Arsenic
Chloramphenicol	Buckthorn toxin
Dapsone	Carbon disulfide
Disulfiram	Chlordecane
Glutethimide	2,4-Dichlorophenoxyacetic
Gold	acid (2,4-D)
Hydralazine	Dimethylaminopropionitrile
Isoniazid	Diphtheria toxin
Lithium	*n*-Hexane
Metronidazole	Methyl-*n*-butyl ketone
Misonidazole	Lead
Nitrofurantoin	Methyl bromide
Perhexiline	Organophosphates
Platinum	Polybrominated biphenyls
Pyridoxine (Vitamin B$_6$)	Thallium
Vincristine	Trichloroethylene

Toxic Neuropathies

Many drugs and toxic agents produce peripheral neuropathy (Table 28-2). Most toxic neuropathies are characterized by axonal degeneration, usually of the dying-back type. Buckthorn and diphtheria toxins are notable for producing demyelinating neuropathies. Because diphtheria toxin does not cross the blood–nerve barrier, the demyelination in diphtheritic neuropathy is limited to the barrier-deficient ganglia and contiguous regions of the spinal roots and nerves.

Paraneoplastic Neuropathies

The remote effects of cancer on the nervous system include an encephalomyelitis, necrotizing myelopathy, cerebellar degeneration, several types of peripheral neuropathy, and the Eaton-Lambert syndrome. The pathogenetic mechanisms responsible for these paraneoplastic diseases are unknown. Remarkably, the onset of a paraneoplastic disorder may precede recognition of the cancer in some cases. The paraneoplastic neuropathies are of several clinicopathologic types: a distal sensorimotor polyneuropathy showing axonal degeneration and a variable amount of segmental demyelination, a subacute sensory polyneuropathy secondary to dorsal root ganglionitis, a subacute motor polyneuropathy caused by the loss of anterior horn cells, and an acute or chronic inflammatory demyelinating polyneuropathy of the Landry-Guillain-Barré type. The dorsal root ganglionitis is characterized microscopically by neuronal loss and chronic inflammatory infiltrates, and is often accompanied by similar changes in the central nervous system (paraneoplastic encephalomyelitis).

Amyloid Neuropathy

A distal sensorimotor polyneuropathy, often with prominent autonomic dysfunction, complicates hereditary systemic amyloidosis or the acquired form of systemic amyloidosis that is associated with plasma cell dyscrasias (primary amyloidosis, multiple myeloma, Waldenström's macroglobulinemia). The neuropathy is characterized pathologically by deposition of amyloid in peripheral nerves, dorsal root ganglia, and autonomic ganglia. The interstitial amyloid deposits are both endoneurial and epineurial, and frequently involve the walls of blood vessels. The deposition of amyloid is accompanied by loss of myelinated and unmyelinated fibers, and segmental

demyelination. Postulated mechanisms for the nerve fiber damage include direct mechanical injury of nerve fibers and ganglion cells by the amyloid deposits or nerve ischemia secondary to amyloid infiltration of the vasa nervorum.

A chronic entrapment neuropathy of the median nerve at the wrist (**carpal tunnel syndrome**) is another complication of systemic amyloidosis. The nerve entrapment is secondary to amyloid infiltration of the flexor retinaculum.

Paraproteinemic Neuropathies

Plasma cell dyscrasias may be associated with a paraneoplastic sensorimotor neuropathy, an amyloid neuropathy, or a chronic demyelinating neuropathy. The chronic demyelinating neuropathy has been associated with benign IgM monoclonal gammopathies, and is characterized pathologically by extensive segmental demyelination, a variable number of onion-bulb formations, axonal loss, and deposition of the monoclonal paraprotein on the myelin sheaths. It has been shown that the IgM paraprotein binds to myelin-associated glycoprotein. The role of paraproteins in the pathogenesis of nerve fiber damage is currently an area of intense investigation.

Hereditary Neuropathies

Peripheral neuropathy is a manifestation of a number of inherited diseases. Among these inherited diseases are several in which peripheral neuropathy is the major clinical manifestation. These hereditary neuropathies show relatively selective involvement of lower motor neurons, primary sensory neurons, or both lower motor and primary sensory neurons. This selective involvement of different neuronal populations is reflected in the clinical presentation of these hereditary diseases as motor neuropathies, sensory neuropathies, or sensorimotor neuropathies, respectively. The biochemical abnormalities for most of these hereditary neuropathies are unknown; thus, current classifications are based on mode of inheritance, clinical presentation, and pathologic features (Table 28-3).

Cryptogenic Neuropathies

A significant number of patients have peripheral neuropathies for which no etiology is apparent, despite careful and extensive investigations. Pathologically,

Table 28-3 Hereditary Neuropathies

DISEASE	INHERITANCE	CLINICAL PRESENTATION	PATHOLOGY
HMSN type I (Peroneal muscular atrophy; Charcot-Marie-Tooth disease)	AD	Distal sensorimotor neuropathy; onset after first decade; slow progression; palpably enlarged nerves, severe slowing of nerve conduction	Extensive demyelination with numerous onion bulbs and nerve hypertrophy; distal axonal degeneration
HMSN type II (Peroneal muscular atrophy; Charcot-Marie-Tooth disease)	AD	Similar to HMSN type I except no nerve hypertrophy and less slowing of nerve conduction	Distal axonal degeneration
Dejerine-Sottas disease (HMSN type III)	AR	Distal sensorimotor neuropathy; onset in infancy; palpably enlarged nerves; severe slowing of nerve conduction	Extensive demyelination with numerous onion bulbs and nerve hypertrophy; distal axonal degeneration
Refsum's disease (HMSN type IV)	AR	Distal sensorimotor neuropathy; pigmentary retinopathy; enlarged nerves; accumulation of phytanic acid in serum	Extensive demyelination with onion bulbs and nerve hypertrophy; distal axonal degeneration
HSN type I	AD	Distal sensory neuropathy; onset in adolescence; sensory loss leads to mutilation of feet	Axonal degeneration
HSN type II	AR	Similar to HSN type I except earlier onset and mutilation of hands and feet	Axonal degeneration
Werdnig-Hoffman disease (acute infantile spinal muscular atrophy)	AR	Motor neuropathy; onset in infancy; proximal muscle weakness; progressive and fatal	Axonal degeneration with chromatolysis and loss of lower motor neurons

HMSN, hereditary motor and sensory neuropathy; HSN, hereditary sensory neuropathy; AD, autosomal dominant; AR, autosomal recessive.

these cryptogenic neuropathies are often chronic axonal neuropathies.

Nerve Trauma

Traumatic Neuroma

Shortly after the transection of a peripheral nerve, regenerating axonal sprouts arise from the distal ends of the intact axons in the proximal nerve stump. If the severed ends of the proximal and distal nerve stumps are closely approximated, the regenerating axonal sprouts may find and reinnervate the distal stump. The regenerating axons advance in the distal stump at a rate of about 1 mm per day. In many instances, however, the severed ends of the nerve are not closely approximated, and there is considerable scar tissue between the proximal and distal stumps. This scar tissue and the wide gap between the proximal and distal stumps prevent the regenerating sprouts from successfully reinnervating the distal stump. In this situation, the axonal sprouts ensheathed by Schwann cells grow haphazardly into the scar tissue at the end of the proximal stump to form a painful swelling known as a traumatic or amputation neuroma.

Plantar Neuroma (Morton's Neuroma)

Plantar neuroma, a painful, sausage-shaped swelling of the plantar digital nerve between the second and third or third and fourth metatarsal bones, is probably caused by repeated nerve compression. The swelling is not a true neuroma, as it is secondary to endoneurial, perineural, and epineural fibrosis, rather than a mass of regenerating axons. The fibrotic nerve also shows nerve fiber loss and areas of myxoid degeneration.

Tumors

Primary tumors of the peripheral nervous system are of neuronal or nerve sheath origin. The neuronal tumors (for instance, neuroblastoma and ganglioneuroma) usually arise from the adrenal medulla or sympathetic ganglia. The common nerve sheath tumors are schwannoma and neurofibroma.

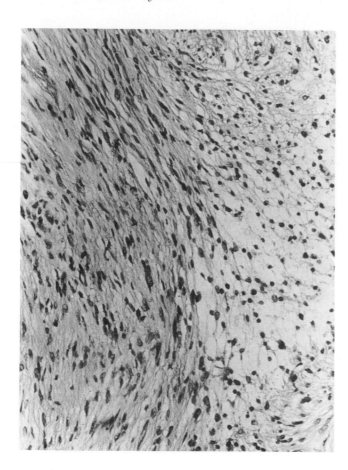

Figure 28-111.   Schwannoma. A photomicrograph shows the characteristically abrupt transition between the compact Antoni type A cellular pattern (*left*) and the spongy Antoni type B cellular pattern (*right*).

Schwannoma (Neurilemoma)

Schwannoma, a benign, slowly growing neoplasm of Schwann cells, may arise in any nerve. The tumor is oval and well demarcated, and varies in diameter from a few millimeters to several centimeters. The nerve of origin, if sufficiently large, may be identifiable. The cut surfaces of the schwannoma are firm and tan to gray, and often show foci of hemorrhage, necrosis, xanthomatous change, and cystic degeneration. Microscopically, the proliferating Schwann cells form two distinctive histologic patterns (Fig. 28-111). One pattern, termed **Antoni type A,** is characterized by interwoven fascicles of spindle cells with elongated nuclei, eosinophilic cytoplasm, and indistinct cytoplasmic borders. The nuclei may palisade in areas to form structures known as **Verocay bodies.** The second histologic pattern, termed **Antoni type B,** is characterized by spindle or oval cells with indistinct cytoplasm in a loose, vacuolated background. Degenerative changes in schwannomas are common, and include collections of foam cells, recent or old hemorrhage, foci of fibrosis, and hyalinized blood

vessels. Scattered atypical nuclei are frequently encountered in schwannomas, but mitotic figures are uncommon.

Schwannomas may arise from cranial nerves, spinal roots, or peripheral nerves, and most often present in adults. Intracranial schwannomas are most common, accounting for 8% of all intracranial tumors. With rare exceptions, the intracranial schwannomas arise from the eighth cranial nerve **(acoustic schwannoma)** within the internal auditory canal or at the meatus, and cause unilateral hearing loss and tinnitus. The slowly growing tumor enlarges the meatus, extends medially into the subarachnoid space of the cerebellopontine angle (cerebellopontine-angle tumor), and compresses the fifth and seventh cranial nerves, brain stem, and cerebellum. The posterior fossa mass may also lead to increased intracranial pressure, hydrocephalus, and tonsillar herniation. Most acoustic schwannomas are unilateral and are unassociated with neurofibromatosis. Bilateral acoustic schwannomas are a defining feature of the central type of neurofibromatosis.

Intraspinal schwannomas arise most often from

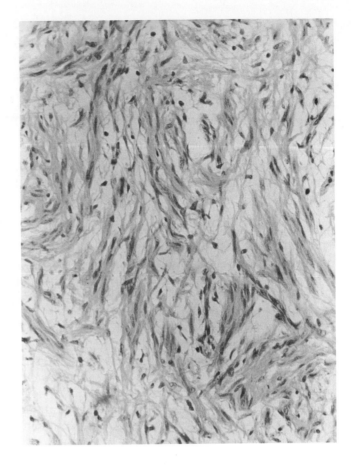

Figure 28-112. Neurofibroma. A photomicrograph shows that the proliferating Schwann cells form small strands that course haphazardly through a myxoid background matrix.

the dorsal (sensory) spinal roots. They typically present as intradural, extramedullary tumors producing radicular (root) pain and spinal cord compression. These tumors occasionally extend through the intervertebral foramen and acquire an hourglass shape (dumbbell tumor). Intraspinal and peripheral schwannomas are usually solitary and unassociated with neurofibromatosis.

Neurofibroma

The Schwann cell is the principal constituent of neurofibroma, which may be more hamartomatous than neoplastic. A distinction between neurofibroma and schwannoma is warranted because of the close association of neurofibroma with von Recklinghausen's neurofibromatosis and its potential for sarcomatous degeneration. On gross examination, the neurofibroma involves the large nerves, appearing as a poorly circumscribed, fusiform enlargement of the nerve. The diffuse, intrafascicular growth of the tumor within multiple nerve fascicles may so enlarge

the nerve's fascicles that they appear grossly as the cords of a nerve plexus (plexiform neurofibroma). The neurofibroma may involve long segments of the nerve, making complete surgical excision impossible. When neurofibromas arise from small nerves, the nerve of origin may not be apparent. Cutaneous neurofibromas arise from dermal nerves and present as soft, nodular, or pedunculated skin tumors.

The cut surfaces of a neurofibroma are soft and light gray, and the enlarged nerve fascicles of the plexiform neurofibroma may be prominent. Microscopically, the neurofibroma arising in large nerves is characterized by an endoneurial proliferation of spindle cells with elongated nuclei, eosinophilic cytoplasm, and indistinct cell borders. The spindle cells often aggregate to form tiny strands coursing haphazardly through the tumor (Fig. 28-112). Interspersed among the spindle cells are wavy bands of collagen, an extracellular myxoid matrix, and residual nerve fibers. The coursing of nerve fibers through the neurofibroma contrasts with the pattern in schwannoma, in which nerve fibers are pushed peripherally into the tumor capsule. When arising from small nerves, the neurofibroma usually extends beyond the nerve and diffusely infiltrates the surrounding tissue. A small but clinically significant proportion of neurofibromas exhibits sarcomatous transformation, with foci of malignant schwannoma. The presence of increased cellularity and mitotic figures heralds the malignant transformation.

Neurofibromas are solitary or multiple, arise on any nerve, and are found in children or adults. Most commonly, they involve the skin, major nerve plexuses, large deep nerve trunks, retroperitoneum, and gastrointestinal tract. Most **solitary cutaneous neurofibromas** occur outside the context of neurofibromatosis, and these tumors do not have the potential of their deeper counterparts for sarcomatous degeneration. **The presence of multiple neurofibromas is diagnostic of neurofibromatosis.** The occurrence of one large plexiform neurofibroma or of bilateral acoustic schwannomas is also considered to be evidence of neurofibromatosis. Other potential manifestations of neurofibromatosis include multiple tan skin macules (café-au-lait spots), gliomas, meningiomas, hamartomas and heterotopias of the central nervous system, hydrocephalus, mental retardation, pigmented iris nodules (Lisch nodules), skeletal abnormalities, pheochromocytomas, and other endocrine tumors.

Malignant Schwannoma (Neurofibrosarcoma)

The histogenesis of malignant schwannoma, a poorly differentiated, spindle cell sarcoma of the peripheral nerve, is uncertain. The tumor may arise *de novo* or from malignant transformation of a neurofibroma. The malignant schwannoma rarely arises from malignant transformation of a schwannoma. **About half of these sarcomas are found in patients with neurofibromatosis.** There is an increased incidence of malignant schwannomas in areas of previous irradiation. The neoplasm presents grossly as an unencapsulated, fusiform enlargement of a nerve. Microscopically, the neoplasm resembles fibrosarcoma. The tumor is prone to local recurrence and blood-borne metastases, and has a worse prognosis in the context of neurofibromatosis. Malignant schwannomas most often occur in adults.

SUGGESTED READING

BOOKS

Burger PC, Vogel FS: Surgical Pathology of the Nervous System and Its Coverings, 2nd ed. New York, John Wiley and Sons, 1982

Davis RL, Robertson DM: Textbook of Neuropathology. Baltimore, Williams and Wilkins, 1985

Greenfield JG: Neuropathology. London, Edward Arnold, 1985

Russell D, Rubinstein L: Pathology of Tumors of the Nervous System, 4th ed. Baltimore, Williams and Wilkins, 1977

Schochet SS, McCormick WE: Neuropathology Case Studies, 3rd ed. New Hyde Park, NY, Medical Examination Publishing Co, 1984

Vogel FS: An Introduction to Disease. Chicago, Field, Rich & Assoc, 1985

REVIEW ARTICLES

Burger PC, Vogel FS: Cerebrovascular disease. Am J Pathol 92:253, 1978

Burger PC, Vogel FS: Degenerative and demyelinating diseases. Am J Pathol 99:479, 1980

Chervenak FA, Isaacson G, Mahoney MJ: Advances in the diagnosis of fetal defects. N Engl J Med 315:305–308, 1986

Gusella JF, Tanzi RE, Anderson MA, Hobbs W, Gibbons K, Rashtchian R, Gilliam TC, Wallace MR, Wexler NS, and Conneally PM: DNA markers for nervous system diseases. Science 225:1320–1326, 1984

Mozar HN, Bal DG, Howard JT: Perspectives on the etiology of Alzheimer's disease. JAMA 257:1503, 1987

Poser CM: Pathogenesis of multiple sclerosis: A critical reappraisal. Acta Neuropathol 71:1, 1986

Prusiner SB, DeArmond SJ: Prions causing nervous system degeneration. Lab Invest 56:349, 1987

ORIGINAL ARTICLES

Gajdusek DC, Zigas V: Degenerative disease of the central nervous system in New Guinea. The epidemic occurrence of "kuru" in the native population. N Engl J Med 257:974, 1957

Gajdusek DC, Gibbs CJ Jr, Alpers M: Experimental transmission of a kuru-like syndrome to chimpanzees. Nature 209:794, 1966

Goldgaber D, Lerman MI, McBride OW, Saffiotti U, Gajdusek DC: Characterization and chromosomal localization of a cDNA encoding brain amyloid of Alzheimer's disease. Science 235:877, 1987

Gusella JF, Wexler N, Conneally PM, Naylor SL, Anderson MA, Tamzi RE, Watkins PC, Ottina K, Wallace MR, Sakaguchi AY, Young AB, Shoulson I, Bonilla E, Martin JB: A polymorphic DNA marker genetically linked to Huntington's disease. Nature 306:234, 1983

Hirano A, Malamud N, Kurland LT: Parkinsonism-dementia complex: An epidemic disease on the island of Guam. II. Pathological features. Brain 84:662, 1961

Hockberg FH, Miller G, Schooley RT, Hirsch MS, Feorino P, Heule W: Central nervous system lymphoma related to Epstein-Barr virus. N Engl J Med 309:745–748, 1983

Kristensson K, Zeller ND, Dubois-Dalcq ME, Lazzarin RA: Expression of myelin basic protein gene in the developing rat brain as revealed by *in situ* hybridization. J Histochem Cytochem 34:467–473, 1986

Sima AAF, Finkelstein SD, McLachlan DR: Multiple malignant astrocytomas in patients with spontaneous progressive multifocal leukoencephalopathy. Ann Neurol 14:183, 1983

ZuRhein GM, Chou SM: Particles resembling papovavirus in human cerebral demyelinating disease. Science 148:1477, 1965

29 The Eye

Gordon K. Klintworth

Infections, Inflammation, and
Immunologic Disorders

Neoplasms

Physical and Chemical
Injuries to the Eye

Developmental Anomalies
and Genetically Determined
Disorders

Vascular Disorders

The Eye in Systemic Disease

Common Disorders of
Specific Ocular Tissues

Figure 29-1. The retinal basis of vision. The retina, the specialized tissue which responds to light, contains neurons arranged in distinct layers. In the vertebrate retina, light passes through the entire eye before reaching the photoreceptors (rods and cones). The outer segment of each photoreceptor is its light sensitive region. The rod outer segment contains a dense stack of disc membranes in which the photoprotein, rhodopsin, is embedded. In the dark a current normally flows through this cell ("dark current"). In the presence of light the circulating dark current is reduced by the closure of Na⁺-selective ion channels in the plasma membrane. Cyclic guanosine 3',5'-monophosphate (cGMP) seems to be involved in the light response.

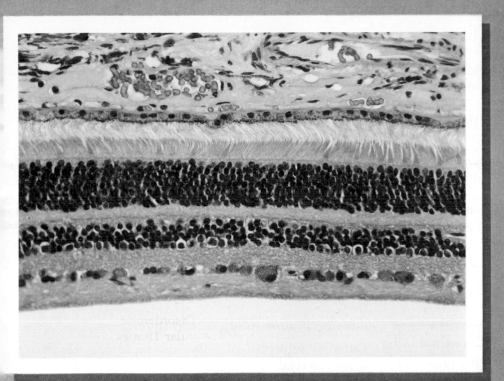

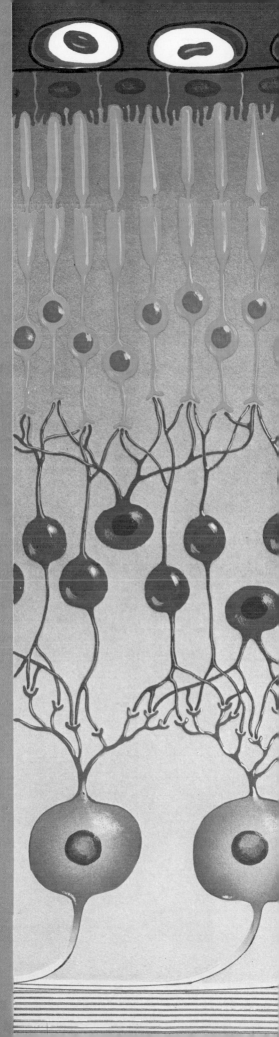

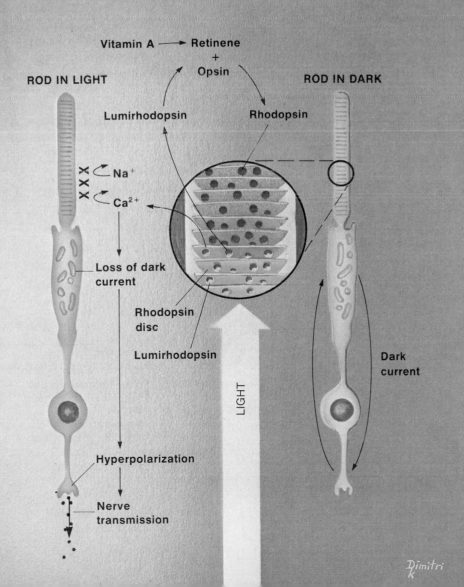

Vitamin A $\longrightarrow$ Retinene
$+$
Opsin

ROD IN LIGHT

ROD IN DARK

Lumirhodopsin

Rhodopsin

$\times \times \times$ ⟲ Na$^+$
$\times \times \times$ ⟲ Ca^{2+}

Loss of dark
current

Rhodopsin
disc

Lumirhodopsin

Dark
current

LIGHT

Hyperpolarization

Nerve
transmission

Dimitri
K

Largely because of its superficial location, the eye is exposed to a myriad of microorganisms, antigens, and toxic chemicals, as well as to solar radiation and adverse climatic conditions. The unprotected position of the eye also makes it vulnerable to a host of injuries. Disorders of the eye are common and many of its afflictions result in loss of sight. While the reactions of the eye to injurious agents are basically identical to those in other parts of the body, a mass of jargon in ophthalmic nomenclature has evolved, making ophthalmic pathology virtually an exercise in a foreign language.

Infections, Inflammation, and Immunologic Disorders

Microorganisms lodging on the surface of the eye frequently cause conjunctivitis, keratitis, or corneal ulcers, and sometimes, as with *Mycobacterium tuberculosis*, enter the body by way of the ocular mucous membranes to cause systemic disease. The eye may also become infected by hematogenous spread from a focus of infection elsewhere. Ocular infections also occasionally complicate surgical procedures, such as cataract extractions, corneal grafts, and the installation of ocular lenses. Adenoviruses and other pathogens may be introduced into the eye by physicians using infected eyedrops or a contaminated tonometer (an instrument used to measure intraocular pressure). Numerous pathogens affect the ocular tissues, but only a few representative infections will be discussed.

The Conjunctiva

At some stage in life everyone suffers from conjunctivitis. This commonest of eye diseases is characterized by hyperemic conjunctival blood vessels ("pink eye"). The inflammatory exudate that accumulates in the conjunctival sac commonly crusts, causing the eyelids to stick together in the morning. The conjunctival discharge may be purulent, fibrinous, serous, or hemorrhagic, and contains inflammatory cells that vary with the etiologic agent. In keeping with the seasonal nature of many allergens, allergic conjunctivitis sometimes occurs only during a particular time of the year.

Trachoma and Related Infections

Different serotypes of *Chlamydia trachomatis* cause ocular, genital, and systemic infections (trachoma, inclusion conjunctivitis, and lymphogranuloma venereum) in millions of individuals.

About five hundred million people are afflicted by trachoma (Fig. 29-2), an acute, infectious, cicatrizing keratoconjunctivitis due to *Chlamydia trachomatis* (serotypes A, B, and C) and the commonly associated bacteria. **This is the commonest cause of blindness in the world and is especially prevalent in Asia, the Middle East, and parts of Africa. In the United States it is almost restricted to the American Indian population in the southwestern region of the country.** Trachoma is not very contagious, but overcrowding and poor hygienic conditions favor its transmission by fingers, fomites, and flies. Spontaneous

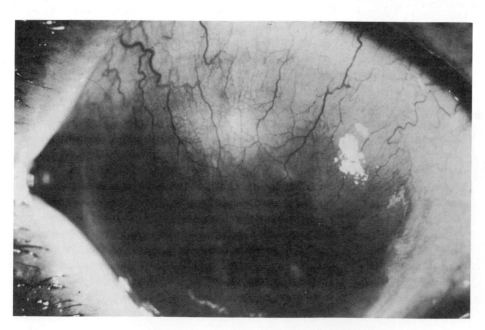

Figure 29-2. Trachoma. A clinical photograph of the cornea of a patient with severe trachoma shows an extensive fibrovascular opacity (pannus) in the superior cornea.

healing is common in children, but in adults the disease progresses more rapidly and rarely heals in the absence of treatment.

Trachoma is virtually always bilateral and involves the upper half of the conjunctiva more extensively than the lower. The cellular infiltrate is predominantly lymphocytic, and conjunctival lymph follicles with necrotic germinal centers are characteristic. Eventually lymphocytes and blood vessels invade the superior portion of the cornea between its epithelium and Bowman's zone (trachomatous pannus), and scarring of the conjunctiva and eyelids distorts the lids. On microscopic examination the desquamated conjunctival epithelium exhibits glycogen-rich intracytoplasmic inclusion bodies and large macrophages containing nuclear fragments (Leber cells).

Chlamydia is responsible for a purulent conjunctivitis (inclusion blennorrhea) that develops in the newborn who becomes infected during natural birth. The infection is also acquired by swimming in nonchlorinated pools ("swimming pool conjunctivitis"), or from discharges of lesions of the conjunctiva, urethra, or cervix uteri. In adults and older children, chlamydia causes a chronic follicular conjunctivitis with focal lymphoid hyperplasia (inclusion conjunctivitis) and intracytoplasmic inclusion bodies indistinguishable from those of trachoma. In contrast to trachoma, however, the lower tarsal conjunctiva is involved, scarring and necrosis do not develop, and keratitis is rare and mild.

Ophthalmia Neonatorum

Neisseria gonorrhoeae causes a severe, acute conjunctivitis with a copious purulent discharge, especially in the newborn. The infection, a common cause of blindness in some parts of the world, is complicated by corneal ulceration, perforation and scarring, and panophthalmitis. The infant usually becomes infected while passing through the birth canal of an infected mother. Aside from gonorrhea, ophthalmia neonatorum has other causes, including other pyogenic bacteria, *Chlamydia trachomatis* (serotypes D to K, also known as *Chlamydia oculogenitalis)*, and even the silver nitrate administered to the conjunctiva of newborns to prevent gonococcal conjunctivitis.

The Cornea

Herpes simplex

Herpesvirus has a predilection for the corneal epithelium, but it can invade the corneal stroma and occasionally other ocular tissues. Primary infection by herpes simplex type I usually causes subclinical or undiagnosed localized ocular lesions in childhood,

these often being accompanied by regional lymphadenopathy, systemic infection, and fever. Herpes simplex type II, which can produce widespread infection of the cornea and retina, rarely causes ocular infection, except in the neonate who becomes infected during natural birth from a mother harboring genital herpes. Most corneal lesions due to herpesvirus are asymptomatic plaques of diseased epithelial cells that contain replicating virus. These usually heal without ulceration, but an acute unilateral follicular conjunctivitis may occur. Corneal ulcers appear after the serum antibodies become elevated.

A high rate of recurrence at one site characterizes secondary herpes infection (reactivation disease). The herpes simplex virus commonly causes multiple, minute, discrete, intraepithelial ulcers (superficial punctate keratopathy). While some of these lesions heal, others enlarge and eventually coalesce to form linear or branching fissures (dendritic ulcers, from Greek *dendron*, a tree). The epithelium between the fissures desquamates, causing sharply demarcated, irregular geographic ulcers. The corneal ulcers are readily seen in the patient after the cornea has been stained with fluorescein. The affected epithelial cells, which may become multinucleated, contain eosinophilic, intranuclear inclusion bodies (Lipschütz bodies).

Recurrence of corneal ulcers due to herpes simplex may be precipitated by ultraviolet light, trauma, menstruation, emotional and physical stress, exposure to light or sunlight, vaccination, and other factors. These recurrences occur despite high titers of circulating, highly stable, neutralizing antibodies and specific cell-mediated immunity.

Herpes simplex is thought to reside in the trigeminal ganglion, and recurrent infection follows extension of the virus down the nerves. In contrast to primary infection by herpes simplex, reactivation disease is characterized by ulceration and a more severe inflammatory reaction, while fever and lymphadenopathy are not seen.

The lesions of the corneal stroma in herpes simplex vary. Typically, a central disc-shaped corneal opacity develops beneath the epithelium, due to edema and a minimal inflammatory cell infiltrate (disciform keratitis). The corneal stroma may become markedly thinned and Descemet's membrane may bulge into it (descemetocele). Corneal perforation can also occur.

Onchocerciasis

The nematode *Onchocerca volvulus*, which is transmitted by bites of infected black flies *(Simulium sp.)* is by far the most important helminthic infection of the eye. This parasite is estimated to account for blindness in at least half a million individuals in endemic regions of Africa and Latin America. Five to six years after the appearance of subcutaneous nodules (cercomas), the living microfilaria that are released from fertilized adult female onchocerca migrate into the superficial cornea, bulbar conjunctiva, aqueous humor, and other ocular tissues. Following the demise of intracorneal microfilaria, an inflammatory response causes corneal opacification and visual impairment ("river blindness"). Less frequently, endophthalmitis, retinal lesions, and optic atrophy occur.

Uvea

Inflammation of the iris and ciliary body typically causes a red eye, sensitivity to bright light (photophobia), moderate pain, blurred vision, a pericorneal halo, dilated deep ciliary vessels (ciliary flush) and slight constriction of the pupil (miosis). Leukocytes aggregate on the posterior surface of the cornea as small clusters (keratic precipitates), or if abundant, they settle to the bottom of the anterior chamber (hypopyon). The increased protein content in the anterior chamber is evident clinically with the slit-lamp because of the reflection of the light beam (flare). As a sequel to iritis, adhesions develop between the iris and the lens (posterior synechiae) or between the peripheral iris and the anterior chamber angle (peripheral anterior synechiae), thereby causing glaucoma.

Sympathetic Ophthalmitis (Sympathetic Ophthalmia)

An important complication of a perforating ocular injury and prolapse of uveal tissue is a progressive, bilateral, diffuse, granulomatous inflammation of the uvea. This uveitis, which also rarely follows evisceration and intraocular melanomas, develops in the originally injured eye ("exciting eye") after a latent period of at least 10 days (usually 4–8 weeks, sometimes many years). The uninjured eye ("sympathizing eye") becomes affected at the same time or shortly thereafter. Vitiligo and graying of the eyelashes sometimes accompanies the uveitis. Nodules containing reactive retinal pigment epithelium, epithelioid cells, and macrophages commonly appear between Bruch's membrane and the retinal pigment epithelium (Dalen-Fuchs nodules).

It is widely believed that the condition is an autoimmune reaction to sensitization by uveal isoantigens. Because melanin granules are frequently found within macrophages in sympathetic ophthalmia, they were once suspected of containing the offending antigen, but evidence for this is weak. In recent years experimental studies have suggested that the offending antigen resides in the photoreceptors of the retina ("S-antigen").

Another immunologically evoked ocular granulomatous response sometimes occurs around or within the lens (or its remains) in an eye with a traumatized or cataractous lens, or after the surgical removal of a cataractous lens (phacoanaphylactic endophthalmitis). A similar reaction may occur spontaneously in the contralateral eye months or years later. This autoimmune reaction to unique lens proteins, which are normally sequestered throughout life from the immune system, can be provoked experimentally by immunization with autologous lens material.

Eyelids

Inflammation of the eyelids (blepharitis) is common and sometimes presents as an acute, red, tender inflammatory mass in the eyelid (sty, hordeolum). Acute inflammation of the meibomian glands (internal hordeolum) and acute folliculitis of the glands of Zeis (external hordeolum) are common. Chronic, foreign-body, granulomatous inflammation centered around the meibomian or Zeis glands produces a painless swelling in the eyelid (chalazion).

Orbit

The term "inflammatory pseudotumor of the orbit" is applied to an idiopathic chronic inflammatory reaction associated with a variable degree of fibrosis. It is a common cause of proptosis and partial immobility of the eyeball.

Neoplasms

The eye and the structures around it contain a wide variety of cell types and, as one might expect, benign and malignant neoplasms arise from them (Table 29-1). However, the frequency with which the different cell types become neoplastic varies immensely. **Intraocular neoplasms arise mostly from immature retinal neurons (retinoblastoma) and uveal melanocytes (melanoma).** Although the retinal pigment epithelium often undergoes reactive proliferation, it seldom becomes neoplastic. No bona fide neoplasm of the human lens epithelium has been documented.

Melanoma

While melanomas, **the most common primary intraocular malignancy,** may arise from melanocytes in any part of the eye, the choroid is the most common site. Choroidal melanomas are usually circumscribed and invade Bruch's membrane, causing a collar stud or mushroom-shaped mass (Fig. 29-3). By contrast, some are flat (diffuse melanoma) and either cause a gradual visual deterioration over many years or do not become apparent until extraocular or distant dissemination has occurred. Orange lipofuscin pigment is evident over the surface of some choroidal melanomas. Based on the microscopic appearance of uveal melanomas, they have been subdivided into different types (spindle A, spindle B, fascicular, necrotic, mixed, and epithelioid types). Melanomas of the ciliary body and iris may extend circumferentially around the globe ("ring melanoma"). Melanomas in the iris present clinically one to two decades earlier than those in the choroid and ciliary body, perhaps because they are more easily seen. Aside from hematogenous spread, uveal melanomas disseminate by traversing the sclera to enter the orbital tissues, usually at sites where blood vessels and nerves pass through the sclera. Unlike melanomas of the skin, those of the uvea do not exhibit lymphatic spread, because the eye lacks lymphatics. Intraocular melanomas secondarily cause hemorrhage, cataract, glaucoma, retinal detachment, and inflammation. Each of these manifestations may mask the basic pathologic disorder.

Occasionally one or more irregular areas of pigmentation appears spontaneously in a nonpigmented portion of the conjunctiva of one eye at about 40 to 50 years of age. This condition, designated primary acquired melanosis, is analogous to the lentigo-maligna variety of melanoma in the skin and may regress spontaneously or evolve into a malignant melanoma. Other malignant melanomas of the conjunctiva are preceded by a nevus, or have no overt antecedent lesion. Others represent an extension of an intraocular melanoma.

Retinoblastoma

Retinoblastoma, the most common intraocular, potentially fatal, neoplasm of childhood (Fig. 29-4), is estimated to affect 1:20,000–34,000 live births. It arises from the retina and most frequently presents within the first two years of life, and sometimes even at birth. The presenting signs include a white pupil (leukocoria), squint (strabismus), poor vision, spontaneous hyphema or a red, painful eye, often with

Table 29-1 Primary Neoplasms of the Eye and its Adnexa

Intraocular Neoplasms

Retinoblastoma
Medulloepithelioma
Teratoid medulloepithelioma
Glioneuroma
Adenomas and adenocarcinomas of ciliary epithelium
Melanoma
Leiomyoma
Neurofibroma
Schwannoma
Lymphoma

Neoplasms of Eyelid and Lacrimal Drainage Apparatus

BENIGN

Squamous papilloma
Seborrheic keratosis
Inverted folliculoma (inverted follicular keratosis)
Calcifying epithelioma of Malherbe
Adenoma of sebaceous glands (Meibomian glands)
Adenoma of Krause's accessory lacrimal gland
Adenoma of sweat glands, and apocrine glands (Moll's glands)
Keratoacanthoma
Papilloma of lacrimal sac
Leiomyoma
Trichoepithelioma
Neurofibroma
Schwannoma

MALIGNANT

Basal cell carcinoma
Squamous cell carcinoma
Sebaceous carcinoma (Meibomian gland carcinoma)
Malignant melanoma
Lymphoma
Adenocarcinoma of sweat gland
Extramammary Paget's disease
Adenoacanthoma

Neoplasms of Conjunctiva

Dysplasia	"Primary Acquired Melanosis"
Intraepithelial carcinoma	Melanoma
(carcinoma-in-situ)	Oncocytoma
Squamous cell carcinoma	Neurofibroma
Lymphoma	

Neoplasms of Orbit

Neoplasms of lacrimal gland:	Mucoepidermoid carcinoma
Mixed tumors	Oncocytoma
Adenocystic carcinoma	
Neoplasms of optic nerve:	
Meningioma	Astrocytoma

OTHER ORBITAL TUMORS:

Benign

Hemangiopericytoma	Chondroma
Fibrous histiocytoma	Leiomyoma
Schwannoma	Aneurysmal bone cyst
Lipoma	Fibrous dysplasia
Osteoma	Fibrous xanthoma
Fibroma	Myxoma
Hemangioendothelioma	

Malignant

Rhabdomyosarcoma	Malignant hemangioendothelioma
Malignant lymphomas	Malignant hemangiopericytoma
Plasma cell myeloma	Malignant fibrous histiocytoma
Neurofibrosarcoma	Chondrosarcoma
Liposarcoma	Kaposi's sarcoma
Osteogenic sarcoma	

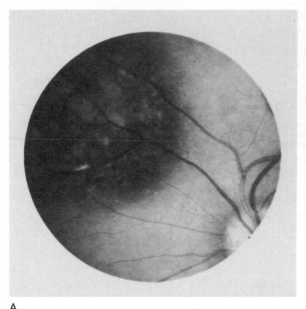
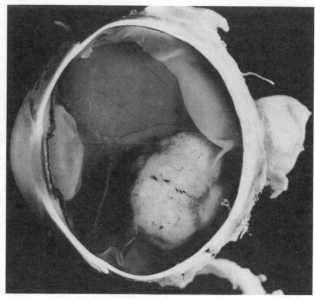

A   B

Figure 29-3. Malignant melanoma. (*A*) A malignant melanoma of the choroid is apparent as a dark mass visible beneath the retinal blood vessels. (*B*) A mushroom-shaped melanoma of the choroid is present in this eye. Choroidal melanomas commonly invade through Bruch's membrane and result in this appearance.

secondary glaucoma. Light entering the eye reflects a yellowish color similar to that from the tapetum of a cat ("cat's eye reflex"). While most retinoblastomas are unilateral, up to 25% of the sporadic cases and most inherited retinoblastomas are bilateral.

Most retinoblastomas (about 95%) occur sporadically, but some (6% to 8%) are inherited and recent evidence suggests that the retinoblastoma (R*b*) susceptibility gene, located on the long arm of chromosome 13 (13q14), is actually recessive, and not dominant as once thought. The R*b* gene, which has been sequenced, is located on chromosome 13 in close proximity to the gene for esterase D. The oncogene N-*myc* is amplified 10 to 200 fold in some retinoblastomas and may play a cardinal role in the tumorigenesis of retinoblastoma. A recent hypothesis suggests that the R*b* gene normally regulates a set of proto-oncogenes, and that when both alleles of this gene are lost or inactivated, the structural transforming gene (which may be an oncogene) is expressed. Even survivors of sporadic retinoblastoma sometimes transmit the tumor to their offspring in an apparent "autosomal dominant" manner. These offspring are especially prone to bilateral tumors. There is a high incidence of retinoblastoma in individuals with a deletion of chromosome 13.

Some retinoblastomas grow towards the vitreous humor and can be seen clinically with an ophthal-moscope (endophytic retinoblastoma). Others grow between the sensory retina and the retinal pigment epithelium, thereby detaching the retina (exophytic retinoblastoma). Other retinoblastomas are both endophytic and exophytic. The retina often contains several distinct foci of tumor in the same eye, some of which represent distinct points of origin, while others reflect tumor implantations from intravitreal dissemination.

This cream-colored tumor usually contains scattered, chalky white, calcified flecks within yellow necrotic zones. The amount of calcification within retinoblastomas is often sufficient to be detected radiologically. Retinoblastomas are intensely cellular and display several morphologic patterns. In some instances, densely packed, round neoplastic cells with hyperchromatic nuclei, scant cytoplasm, and abundant mitoses are randomly distributed. In other tumors the cells are commonly arranged radially around a central cavity (Flexner-Wintersteiner rosettes), as they differentiate towards photoreceptors. In some retinoblastomas the cellular arrangement resembles the fleur-de-lis (fleurette). Viable tumor cells align themselves around blood vessels, while necrotic areas with calcification are seen a short distance from the vascularized regions.

Retinoblastomas disseminate by several routes. They commonly extend into the optic nerve, from

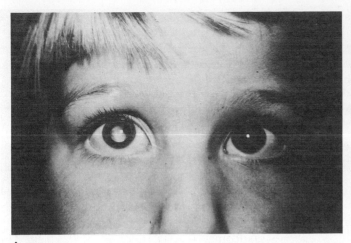
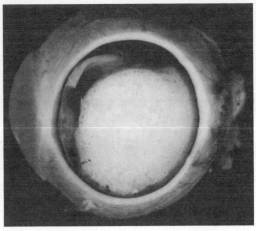

A

B

Figure 29-4. Retinoblastoma. (*A*) The white pupil (leukocoria) in the right eye is the result of an intraocular retinoblastoma. (*B*) This surgically excised eye is almost filled by a cream-colored intraocular retinoblastoma with white calcified flecks.

where they spread intracranially. They also invade blood vessels, especially in the highly vascular choroid, before metastasizing hematogenously throughout the body. The bone marrow is a common site of blood-borne metastases, but surprisingly the lung is rarely involved. Retinoblastomas are almost always fatal if left untreated. However, with early diagnosis and modern therapy, survival is high (about 90%). On rare occasions, spontaneous regression occurs for reasons that remain unknown. Individuals with retinoblastomas have an increased susceptibility to other potentially fatal neoplasms, including osteogenic sarcoma, Ewing's sarcoma and pinealoblastoma.

Some features of retinoblastomas are compared with similar attributes of melanomas in Table 29-2.

Metastatic Intraocular and Orbital Neoplasms

Metastatic neoplasms in the eye are more common than those that arise within the ocular tissues. Sometimes the ocular metastasis is the presenting clinical manifestation of the cancer, but most cases are only diagnosed after death. Most intraocular metastases involve the posterior choroid, and while any malignant tumor may, in theory, metastasize to the ocular tissues, leukemia, carcinoma of the breast, and carcinoma of the lung account for most cases. Neuroblastoma frequently metastasizes to the orbit in in-fancy and childhood. Malignant neoplasms of the eyelid, conjunctiva, paranasal sinuses, nose, nasopharynx, and intracranial cavity may invade the orbit.

Physical and Chemical Injuries to the Eye

Trauma to the eye commonly causes ecchymosis of the highly vascular eyelids ("black eye"), and when this occurs other parts of the eye may also be injured. Superficial disruptions of the corneal epithelium follow traumatic abrasions, prolonged wearing of a contact lens, foreign bodies on the eye, exposure to ultraviolet light, and chemical exposure. Blunt trauma increases the intraorbital pressure momentarily, causing the bones in the floor of the orbit to fracture into the maxillary sinus ("blowout fracture"). The inferior rectus muscle may become entrapped in the fracture, thereby causing the eye to sink into the orbit (enophthalmos).

An infinite variety of foreign materials commonly injure the eye. While small particles commonly lodge in the superficial ocular tissues, some penetrate into or through the eye. The patient may not even be aware of the intraocular foreign body, if it reaches the eye at high velocity, as with industrial machinery. A foreign particle may damage the eye during entry or because of secondary infection following the introduction of organisms. Some foreign bodies provoke a prominent acute inflammatory or granulomatous reaction, others, such as those containing iron, cause retinal degeneration and even discoloration of the ocular tissues (siderosis bulbi), effects which may not occur for several years. Other complications of ocular injuries include cataracts, retinal detachment, and glaucoma.

The eye is commonly injured by a variety of household and industrial chemicals that enter it accidentally or maliciously. The damage created depends upon the nature of the chemical.

Developmental Anomalies and Genetically Determined Disorders

Anomalous development of the eye results in a variety of malformations that involve the entire globe or specific parts of it. The causes of many of these developmental anomalies are unknown, but some are genetically determined or due to chromosomal abnormalities, viruses, or drugs. Some genetically determined diseases of the eye have been linked to specific chromosomes, such as the X chromosome, which carries the genes for ocular albinism, retinitis pigmentosa, retinoschisis, choroideremia, Norrie's disease, and red–green color blindness (protanopia or deuteranopia). The genes that specify the protein

moieties ("opsins") of the three different color-sensitive pigments in the human retina have been isolated and characterized. The mutant genes responsible for color blindness have been sequenced and cloned.

Vascular Disorders

Hyperemia

Hyperemic conjunctival blood vessels (called conjunctival injection by ophthalmologists) occur in conjunctivitis, certain corneal diseases, iridocyclitis, and glaucoma.

In conjunctivitis, irrespective of cause, a diffuse hyperemia of the conjunctival vessels occurs, the engorged vessels tapering towards the corneoscleral limbus.

Another variety of conjunctival hyperemia is associated with iritis and corneal epithelial defects. In this condition (called ciliary flush by ophthalmologists), finer vessels radiate for a short distance from the limbus.

Hemorrhage

Conjunctiva   Conjunctival hemorrhage may follow blunt trauma, anoxia, or severe bouts of coughing,

Table 29-2 Comparison Between Melanoma and Retinoblastoma

	MELANOMA	RETINOBLASTOMA
Inheritance	Rare	Some 5-8%
Cell of Origin	Melanocytes and related precursors	Retinal neurons
Age	Most after 50 years Rare before puberty	Infancy
Location	Choroid (most) Ciliary body Iris Conjunctiva Eyelid (rare)	Retina
Race	Mostly Caucasian Uncommon in blacks Rare in Orientals	No predisposition
Sex	No sex predisposition	No sex predisposition
Bilaterality	Rare	Common (30%)
Color	Variable Gray to black	Creamy with chalky white flecks
Spread		
Hematogenous	Yes	Yes
Via optic nerve	Rare and only in blind glaucomatous eye	Common
Transcleral	Common	Uncommon

or it may occur spontaneously, often first noted on arising after sleep. Conjunctival hemorrhages do not extend into the cornea because of the barrier imposed by the close apposition of the corneal epithelium to the underlying substantia propria.

Retina Retinal hemorrhages are a feature of many disorders, including hypertension, diabetes mellitus, and central retinal vein occlusion. The appearance varies with the location. Hemorrhage in the nerve fiber layer spreads between axons and causes a flame-shaped appearance on funduscopy, while deep retinal hemorrhages tend to be round. When located between the retinal pigment and Bruch's membrane, blood appears as a dark mass and clinically resembles a melanoma.

Choroid After accidental or surgical perforation of the globe, choroidal hemorrhages may detach the choroid and displace the retina, vitreous humor, and lens through the wound.

Vitreous and Anterior Chamber When blood is present in the vitreous humor and anterior chamber, it gravitates to the most dependent part.

Retinal Occlusovascular Disease

Vascular occlusion results from thrombosis, embolism, stenosis (as in atherosclerosis), vascular compression, intravascular sludging or coagulation, and vasoconstriction (for instance in hypertensive retinopathy and migraine). Thrombosis of the ocular vessels may accompany disease of these vessels, as in giant cell arteritis.

Certain disorders of the heart, and of major vessels such as the carotid arteries, predispose to emboli that lodge in the retina (see Table 29-3) and are evident on funduscopic examination at points of vascular bifurcation. The detection of fat, air, and other emboli within the retina may aid in the clinical diagnosis of embolization. A frequent site of embolic obstruction of the central retinal artery is that portion of the sclera which is perforated for the passage of the optic nerve (lamina cribrosa), where the arterial lumen is narrower than in the orbital portion of the artery.

The effect of vascular occlusion depends upon the size of the vessel involved, the degree of resultant ischemia, and the nature of the embolus. Small emboli often do not interfere with retinal function, while septic emboli may cause foci of ocular infection. Ischemia of any cause deprives the retina of oxygen and other essential metabolites and frequently results in the appearance of white fluffy patches that resemble cotton ("cotton-wool patches") on ophthalmoscopic examination. These spots, which are generally round and seldom wider than the optic disc, consist of aggregates of varicose swollen axons in the nerve fiber layer of the retina. The affected axons contain numerous degenerated mitochondria and other dense bodies related to the lysosomal system that accumulate because of impaired axoplasmic flow. Histologically, cross sections of the individual swollen axons resemble cells ("cytoid bodies"). Cotton-wool spots are reversible if the circulation is restored in time.

Central Retinal Artery Occlusion

The neurons of the retina (Fig. 29-5), like those in the rest of the nervous system, are extremely susceptible to hypoxia. Central retinal artery occlusions (Figs. 29-6 and 29-7) may follow thrombosis of the retinal artery, as in atherosclerosis or giant cell arteritis, or emboli of various types. Intracellular edema, manifested by retinal pallor, is prominent, especially in the macula where the ganglion cells are most numerous. The vascularized choroid beneath the center of the macula (foveola) stands out in sharp contrast as a prominent "cherry red spot". The lack of retinal circulation reduces the retinal arterioles to delicate threads (Fig. 29-7).

Permanent blindness follows central retinal artery obstruction, unless the ischemia is of short duration. Unilateral blurred vision, lasting a few minutes (amaurosis fugax), occurs with small retinal emboli. Hemorrhage is not a feature, inasmuch as the blood is not under increased pressure and simply drains away.

Central Retinal Vein Occlusion

Following central retinal vein occlusion flame-shaped hemorrhages develop in the nerve fiber layer of the retina, especially around the optic disc, as a result of the high intravascular pressure that dilates the veins and collateral vessels (Fig. 29-8). Edema of the optic disc and retina occur because of an impaired absorption of interstitial fluid. Vision is generally poor, but may recover surprisingly well, considering the severity of the funduscopic changes. An intractable closed angle glaucoma, with severe pain and repeated hemorrhages, commonly ensues 2 to 3 months after central retinal vein occlusion ("100 day glaucoma", "thrombotic glaucoma"), owing to neovascularization of the iris and adhesions between the iris and the anterior chamber angle (peripheral anterior synechiae).

Table 29-4 summarizes certain attributes of central retinal artery and central retinal vein occlusion.

(Text continues on p. 1514)

Table 29-3 Systemic Disease with Ocular Involvement

OCULAR TISSUE	OCULAR ABNORMALITIES	DISEASE
Choroid	Hemangioma	Sturge-Weber syndrome
Conjunctiva	Bitot's spot	Vitamin A deficiency
	Crystals	Cystinosis
	Dry eyes	Avitaminosis A
		Benign mucous membrane pemphigoid
		Familial dysautonomia (Riley-Day syndome)
		Giant cell arteritis
		Polyarteritis nodosa
		Psoriatic arthritis
		Rheumatoid arthritis
		Sjögren's syndrome
		Systemic lupus erythematosus
		Systemic sclerosis
		Stevens-Johnson syndrome
	Granulomatous inflammation	Sarcoidosis
	Telangiectasia	Ataxia telangiectasia (Louis-Bar syndrome)
Cornea	Amyloid deposits	Inherited amyloid neuropathy type IV (Meretoja)
	Arcus lipoides (arcus senilis)	Hyperlipoproteinemia type II
		Hyperlipoproteinemia type III (occasionally)
		Hyperlipoproteinemia type IV
	Band keratopathy	Hyperparathyroidism
		Marie-Strümpell disease
		Sarcoidosis
		Severe renal disease
		Still's disease
		Vitamin D toxication
	Clouding/opacification	Familial lecithin cholesteral acyltransferase deficiency
		Familial high-density lipoprotein deficiency (Tangier disease)
		Metachromatic leukodystrophy variant
		Mucolipidosis type III
		Mucopolysaccharidoses (some types)
	Crystals	Benign monoclonal hypergammopathies
		Cystinosis
		Multiple myeloma
	Dry cornea	(See under conjunctiva, dry eyes)
	Kayser-Fleischer ring	Hepatolenticular degeneration (Wilson's disease)
	Thick corneal nerves	Multiple endocrine neoplasia syndrome type II B
	Ulcers (dendritic)	Tyrosinemia
	Verticillate lines	Fabry's disease
Eyelid	Epicanthic folds	de Lange syndrome
		Deletion of short arm of chromosome 5 (5p−)
		Deletion of long arm of chromosome 13 (13q−)
		Deletion of short arm of chomosome 18 (18p−)
		Down's syndrome
		Ehlers-Danlos syndrome
		Klinefelter's syndrome (45X and mosaic variants)
		Marinesco-Sjögren syndrome
		Rubinstein-Taybi syndrome
		Turner's syndrome (XXY, XXXY, XXXXY)
	Xanthomas/xanthelasmas	Hyperlipoproteinemia type I, II and V
		Hyperlipoproteinemia type III (occasionally)
Iris	Aniridia	Nephroblastoma (Wilms' tumor)
	Blue color	Various forms of oculocutaneous albinism
	Heterochromia iridis	Waardenburg-Klein syndrome
	Neovascularization	Carotid cavernous fistula
		Carotid ischemia
		Diabetes mellitus
Lacrimal gland	Granulomatous inflammation	Sarcoidosis
Lens	Cataract	Alport's syndrome
		Cretinism
		Diabetes mellitus
		Down's syndrome
		Fabry's disease
		Galactosemia

Table 29-3 Systemic Disease with Ocular Involvement (Continued)

OCULAR TISSUE	OCULAR ABNORMALITIES	DISEASE
Lens (cont.)	Cataract (cont.)	Sturge-Weber syndrome
		Hidrotic ectodermal dysplasia (Marshall type)
		Hypocalcemia
		Incontinentia pigmenti
		Laurence-Moon-Biedl syndrome
		Mannosidosis
		Marinesco-Sjögren's syndrome
		Myotonic dystrophy
		Norrie's disease
		Pierre Robin syndrome
		Rothmund-Thomson syndrome
		Rubella (congenital)
		Trisomy 13
	Dislocated/subluxation	Ehlers-Danlos syndrome
		Homocystinuria
		Marfan's syndrome
Miscellaneous	Glaucoma	Lowe's oculocerebrorenal syndrome
		Sturge-Weber syndrome
	Photophobia	Chédiak-Higashi syndrome
		Oculocutaneous albinism (various types)
	Progressive myopia	Stickler's progressive arthro-ophthalmopathy
Muscles	Strabismus	Gaucher's disease type II (infantile, acute neuronopathic)
Optic nerve	Optic atrophy	Globoid cell leukodystrophy (Krabbe's disease)
		GM_2 gangliosidosis type III
		Neuronal ceroid lipofuscinosis type I (infantile, Hagberg-Haltia-Santavuori)
Orbit	Proptosis	Hyperthyroidism
Retina	Angioid streaks	Paget's disease of bone
		Pseudoxanthoma elasticum
	Astrocytic hamartomas	Tuberous sclerosis
	Cherry red spot at macula	GM_1 gangliosidosis type I
		GM_2 gangliosidosis type II (Tay-Sachs)
		GM_2 gangliosidosis type II (Sandhoff)
		Mucolipidosis type I
		Niemann-Pick disease
	Cotton-wool spots	Collagen disease
		Diabetes mellitus
		Malignant hypertension
		Pernicious anemia
	Degeneration	Farber's disease
		Hyperornithinemia (chorioretinal gyrate atrophy)
		Neuronal ceroid-lipofuscinosis type I (infantile, Hagberg-Haltia-Santavuori)
		Niemann-Pick disease
		Sulfatide lipidosis (metachromatic leukodystrophy)
		X-linked copper malabsorption syndrome (Menke's disease)
		(See also pigmentary retinopathy, below)
	Emboli	Atrial myxoma
		Bacterial endocarditis
		Calcified cardiac valves
		Cardiac mural thrombi
		Ulcerated atheromatous plaques
	(of fat)	Fractures of long bones
	(of air)	Sudden barometric decompression
	(of air)	Surgical procedures or accidental injuries to neck or thorax
	(of talc)	Intravenous drug addiction
	Hemangioblastoma	Von Hippel-Lindau disease
	Lipemia retinalis	Hyperlipoproteinemia types I and V
		Young diabetes with marked acidosis
	Microaneurysms	Aortic arch syndrome
		Diabetes mellitus
		Macroglobulinemia

(Continued)

Table 29-3 Systemic Disease with Ocular Involvement (Continued)

OCULAR TISSUE	OCULAR ABNORMALITIES	DISEASE
Retina (cont.)	Neovascularization	Diabetes mellitus
		Retinopathy of prematurity
		Sickle cell disease
	Occlusovascular disease	Aortic arch syndrome (Takayasu's disease, pulseless disease)
		Atherosclerosis
		Diabetes mellitus
		Disseminated intravascular coagulation
		Giant cell arteritis
		Sickle cell disease
	Pigmentary retinopathy	Cystinosis
		Abetalipoproteinemia (Bassen-Kornzweig syndrome)
		Neuronal ceroid lipofuscinosis
		Type II Late infantile (Janský-Bielschowsky)
		Type III Juvenile (Spielmeyer-Sjögren-Batten)
		Niemann-Pick disease
		Phytanic acid storage disease (Refsum's syndrome)
		Cockayne's syndrome
		Congenital ichthyosis
		Drugs
		chloroquine
		quinacrine hydrochloride (Atabrine)
		Chlorpromazine
		Hallervorden-Spatz syndrome
		Hallgren's syndrome
		Kearns-Sayre syndrome
		Laurence-Moon-Biedl syndrome
		Pelizaeus-Merzbacher syndrome
		Usher's syndrome
		Vitamin A deficiency
		Mucopolysaccharidoses
		Type I-H (Hurler)
		Type I-S (Scheie)
		Type II (Hunter)
		Type IIIA and IIIB (Sanfilippo)
		Postinflammatory and degenerative conditions
		Behçet's disease
		Cytomegalovirus
		Measles
		Onchocerciasis
		Rubella
		Smallpox vaccination
		Syphilis
		Toxoplasmosis
		Typhoid fever
	Retinal detachment	Norrie's disease
	Retinopathy	Diabetes mellitus
		Hypertension
		Sickle cell hemoglobin C disease
Sclera	Pigmentation	
	brown/black	Alkaptonuria (ochronosis)
	blue	de Lange syndrome
	blue	Ehlers-Danlos syndrome
	blue	Osteogenesis imperfecta
	yellow	Jaundice
	yellow	Liver disease
Vitreous humor	Amyloid deposits	Inherited amyloid neuropathy type II (Rukavinas)

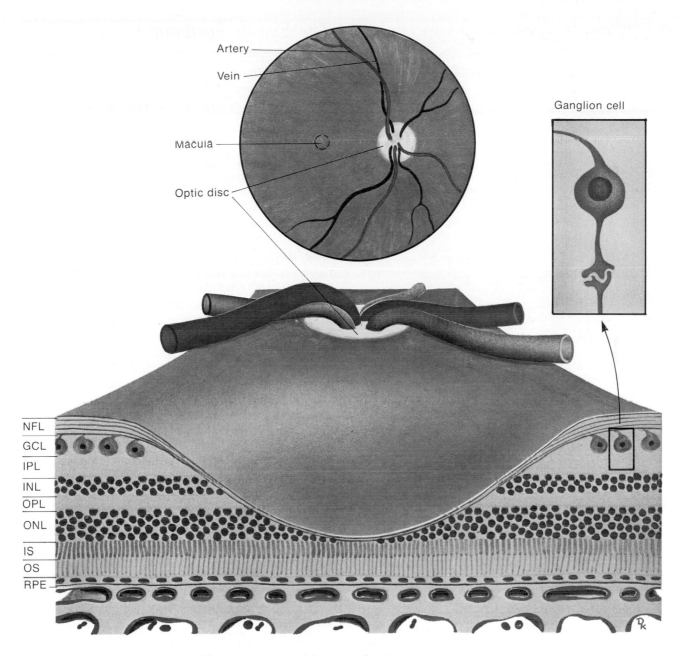

Artery

Vein

Macula

Optic disc

Ganglion cell

NFL
GCL
IPL
INL
OPL
ONL
IS
OS
RPE

Figure 29-5. The normal retina. The constituents of the normal retina are arranged in distinct layers. These include the nerve fiber layer *(NFL)*, ganglion cell layer *(GCL)*, inner plexiform layer *(IPL)*, inner nuclear layer *(INL)*, outer plexiform layer *(OPL)*, outer nuclear layer *(ONL)*, inner segments *(IS)* and outer segments *(OS)* of the photoreceptors, and the retinal pigment epithelium *(RPE)*. The axons from the ganglion cells enter the nerve fiber layer and converge toward the optic disc. The inner retina contains arteries and veins. The retina is thinnest at the center of the macula, where bare photoreceptors rest upon the retinal pigment epithelium. While only one cell thick in most of the retina, the ganglion cell layer is multilayered at the macula.

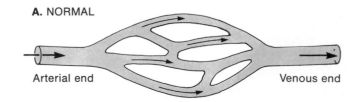

A. NORMAL

Arterial end   Venous end

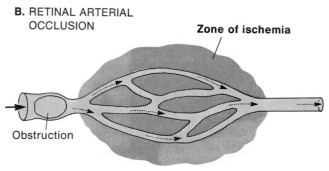

**B. RETINAL ARTERIAL
OCCLUSION**

Zone of ischemia

Obstruction

Neuronal functional impairment → Visual loss

Edema → Pallor

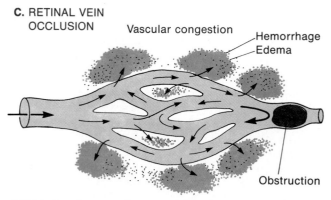

**C. RETINAL VEIN
OCCLUSION**

Vascular congestion

Hemorrhage
Edema

Obstruction

Mild ischemia; normal neuronal function

Figure 29-6.   Occlusion of the retinal artery and vein. (*A*) In the retina, as in other parts of the body blood normally flows through a capillary network. When the retinal arteries become occluded, as with an embolus, a zone of retinal ischemia ensues. This is accompanied by impaired neuronal function and visual loss, and the ischemic retina becomes pale (*B*). Because the intravascular pressure within the ischemic tissue is low, hemorrhage is inconspicuous. On the other hand, with retinal vein occlusion (C) vascular congestion, hemorrhage, and edema are prominent, while ischemia is mild and neuronal function may remain intact.

The Eye in Systemic Disease

The eye is involved in numerous systemic diseases (Table 29-3), and the recognition of ocular abnormalities aids in the diagnosis of many conditions.

Hypertensive Vascular Disease

Elevated systemic blood pressure commonly affects the retina, causing changes that can readily be seen with the ophthalmoscope and which relate to the severity of the hypertension (Figs. 29-9 and 29-10). Features of hypertensive retinopathy include (a) variable degrees of arteriolar narrowing, (b) hemorrhages in the retinal nerve fiber layer ("flame-shaped hemorrhages"), (c) exudates, including some that fan out around the center of the macula ("macular star"), (d) fluffy white bodies in the superficial retina ("cotton wool spots"), and (e) microaneurysms. In cases of severe hypertension, the retinal arterioles are much narrower than normal, and edema of the optic nerve head ensues. Arteriolosclerosis accompanies long standing hypertension and commonly affects the retinal and choroidal vessels. The thickened retinal arterioles become attenuated, increasingly tortuous, and of irregular caliber.

At sites where the arterioles cross veins, the veins may appear kinked (arteriovenous nicking), but the venous diameter is not narrower distal to the compression, an appearance which indicates that the kinked appearance of veins is not due to compression by a taut sclerotic artery. Instead it reflects sclerosis within the venous walls, because retinal arteries and veins share a common adventitia at sites of arteriovenous crossings.

The abnormal retinal arterioles appear clinically as parallel white lines at sites of vascular crossings (arterial sheathing). The narrowed lumen of the retinal vessels decreases the visibility of the blood column and makes them first appear orange on ophthalmoscopic examination ("copper wiring"). However, eventually as the blood column becomes completely obscured, light reflected from the sclerotic vessels appears as threads of silver wire ("silver wiring").

Hypertensive retinopathy has been classified according to severity in Grades 1 through 4, with the higher numbers having more serious changes and a poorer prognosis. Small superficial or deep retinal hemorrhages often accompany retinal arteriolosclerosis. In malignant hypertension, a necrotizing arteriolitis, with fibrinoid necrosis and thrombosis of the precapillary retinal arterioles, occurs.

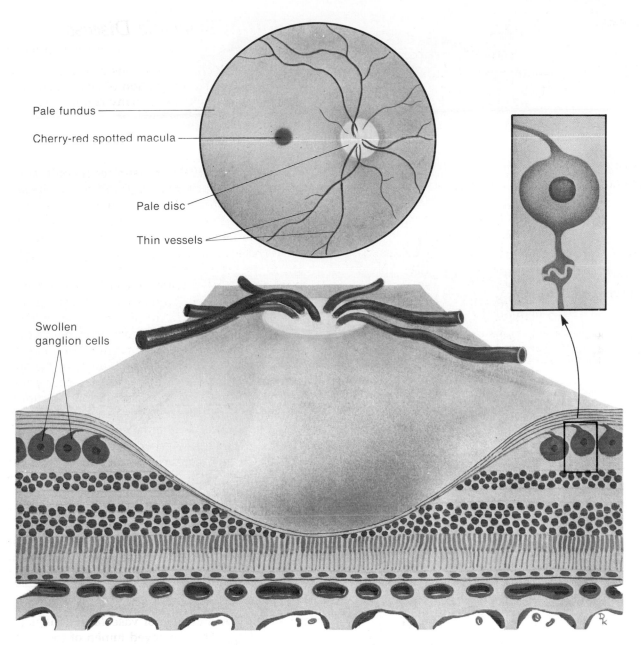

Figure 29-7. Central retinal artery occlusion. When the central retinal artery becomes occluded, as with an embolus, the entire retina becomes edematous and pale and the decreased blood flow makes the retinal vessels less visible on funduscopic examination. The macula becomes cherry-red in color, owing to the prominent, but normal, underlying vasculature of the choroid.

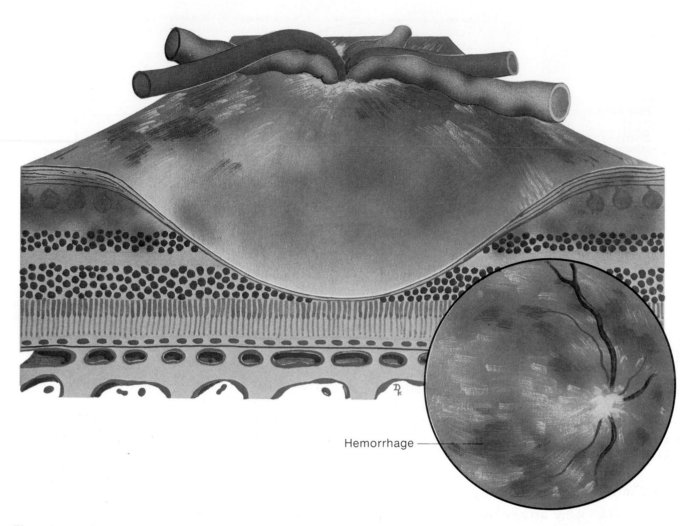

Hemorrhage

Figure 29-8.   Central retinal vein occlusion. In contrast to central retinal artery occlusion, central retinal vein occlusion produces considerable vascular engorgement and retinal hemorrhage as a consequence of the elevated intravascular pressure.

Table 29-4 Comparison Between Central Retinal Vein and Central Retinal Artery Occlusions

	CENTRAL RETINAL VEIN OCCLUSION	CENTRAL RETINAL ARTERY OCCLUSION
Incidence	More common	Less common
Intravascular pressure	High	Low
Metabolites	Impaired drainage	
Funduscopic features		
Hemorrhage	Marked	Not a feature
	Flame shaped	
Cherry red spot	Absent	Present
Cotton-wool spot	Occasionally	Uncommon*
Veins	Engorged and tortuous	Collapsed
Retinal arterioles	Prominent	Delicate threads
Vision	Poor	Poor
Recovery	Good	Poor
Onset	Gradual	Sudden
Ischemia	Less prominent	Prominent
Sequelae		
Glaucoma	Common	Uncommon
Iris neovascularization	Common	Uncommon

* Sometimes seen in patients with ischemia (e.g., carotid artery stenosis) preceding central retinal artery occlusion

Diabetes Mellitus

The eye is frequently involved in diabetes mellitus, and ocular symptoms, which occur in 20% to 40% of diabetics at the clinical onset of the disease, may be a presenting manifestation of this common cause of blindness.

Diabetic Retinopathy

Diabetic retinopathy usually follows 10 to 20 years after the onset of diabetes, and its prevalence increases with the duration of the disease (75% to 90% of patients have retinal changes after 25 years of diabetes; see Figs. 29 11 to 29 13). The incidence of diabetic retinopathy is increasing because of the improved life expectancy of treated diabetics. Diabetic retinopathy under the age of 10 is rare, and most cases are over the age of 50 years. Women are not only more prone to diabetes than men, but also develop diabetic retinopathy more frequently. The retinopathy does not seem to be closely related to the severity of the diabetes nor to the cause of it, but similar to other delayed lesions in diabetes mellitus, the retinopathy is an outcome of vascular disease. Diabetic retinal microangiography correlates directly with diabetic glomerulosclerosis.

Retinal ischemia, which can account for most features of diabetic retinopathy, including the cotton-wool spots, capillary closure, microaneurysms, and retinal neovascularization, may result from narrowing or occlusion of retinal arterioles (as from arteriolosclerosis or platelet and lipid thrombi), or from atheromatosis of the central retinal or ophthalmic arteries. The progression of diabetic retinopathy is retarded by treating the retina in multiple sites by laser photocoagulation.

The retinopathy of diabetes is characterized by nonproliferative and proliferative stages. Nonproliferative diabetic retinopathy exhibits venous engorgement, small hemorrhages ("dot and blot hemorrhages"), capillary microaneurysms, and exudates. These lesions usually do not impair vision, unless associated with macular edema. The retinopathy begins at the posterior pole, but eventually may involve the entire retina.

The first discernible clinical abnormality in nonproliferative diabetic retinopathy is engorged retinal veins, with localized sausage-shaped distension, coils, and loops. This is followed by small hemorrhages in the same area, mostly in the inner nuclear and outer plexiform layers. With time, "waxy" exudates accumulate, chiefly in the vicinity of the microaneurysms. The retinopathy of the elderly diabetic frequently displays numerous exudates (exudative diabetic retinopathy), while this is not a feature in juvenile diabetics. Because of the hyperlipoproteinemia of diabetics, the exudates are rich in lipid, and hence appear yellowish ("waxy" exudates).

Capillary microaneurysms appear in areas of poor retinal vascular perfusion and are best seen in the living eye by taking numerous sequential photographs of the retinal fundus after an intravenous injection of fluorescein (fluorescein angiograph). Capillary microaneurysms can also be seen in flat preparations of the retina.

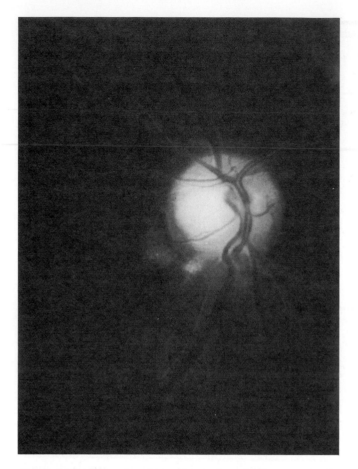

Figure 29-9.   Hypertensive retinopathy. A photograph of the ocular fundus in a patient with chronic hypertension shows silver wiring of the retinal arteries and venous dilatation.

After many years the retinopathy becomes proliferative; delicate new blood vessels grow with fibrous and glial tissue toward the vitreous humor. Neovascularization of the retina is a prominent feature of diabetic retinopathy and of other conditions caused by retinal ischemia. Chronic hypoxia is presumed to provoke the secretion of a diffusible angiogenic factor by retinal cells. Tortuous new vessels first appear on the surface of the retina and optic nerve head and then grow into the vitreous cavity. The newly formed friable vessels bleed easily, and the resultant vitreal hemorrhage obscures vision by impairing the ability of light to reach the retinal photoreceptors. The neovascularization is associated with a proliferation and migration of astrocytes, which grow around the new vessels to form delicate white veils (gliosis). The proliferating, preretinal, fibrovascular, gliotic tissue contracts, often causing retinal detachment and blindness.

In young diabetics with marked acidosis the retinal vessels are light pink to yellowish because of hyperlipidemia (lipemia retinalis).

Frequently, features of hypertensive and arteriolosclerotic retinopathy are associated with diabetic retinopathy. Usually both eyes are affected simultaneously and more or less equally.

In diabetes mellitus blindness results when the macula is involved in the retinopathy, but it also follows vitreous hemorrhage, retinal detachment, and glaucoma. **Diabetic retinopathy now equals glaucoma as a leading cause of irreversible blindness in the United States.** Once blindness ensues it heralds an ominous future for the patient, since the average life expectancy is then less than 6 years, and only one-fifth of blind diabetics survive 10 years.

Thickened Basement Membranes

In patients with diabetes the basal lamina of the retinal capillaries and of the pigmented epithelium of the ciliary body is frequently duplicated and consid-

Figure 29-10.   Hypertensive retinopathy. Various abnormalities develop within the retina in hypertension. The commonly associated arteriolosclerosis affects the appearance of the retinal microvasculature. Light reflected from the thickened arteriolar walls mimics silver or copper wire. Blood flow through the retinal venules is not well visualized at the sites of arteriolar–venular crossings. This effect is due to a thickening of the venular wall rather than to an impediment to blood flow caused by compression; the column of blood proximal to the compression is not wider than the part distal to the crossing. Impaired axoplasmic flow within the nerve fiber layer, secondary to ischemia, results in swollen axons with cytoplasmic bodies. Such structures resemble cotton on funduscopy ("cotton-wool spots"). Hemorrhages are common in the retina, and exudates frequently form a star around the macula.

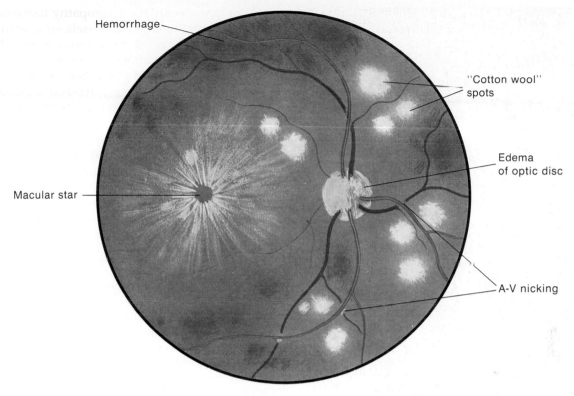

Hemorrhage

"Cotton wool" spots

Edema of optic disc

Macular star

A-V nicking

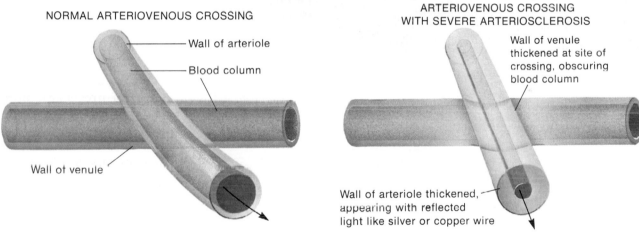

NORMAL ARTERIOVENOUS CROSSING

Wall of arteriole

Blood column

Wall of venule

ARTERIOVENOUS CROSSING
WITH SEVERE ARTERIOSCLEROSIS

Wall of venule thickened at site of crossing, obscuring blood column

Wall of arteriole thickened, appearing with reflected light like silver or copper wire

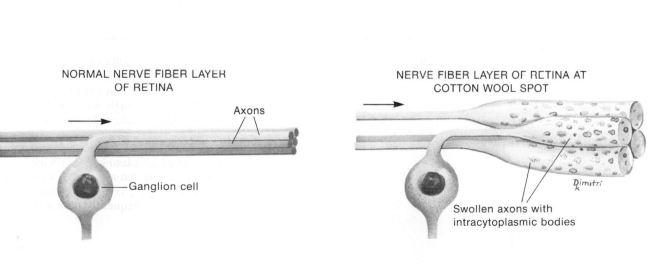

NORMAL NERVE FIBER LAYER
OF RETINA

Axons

Ganglion cell

NERVE FIBER LAYER OF RETINA AT
COTTON WOOL SPOT

Swollen axons with intracytoplasmic bodies

Dimitri
k

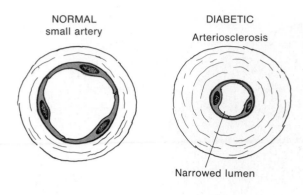

NORMAL
small artery

DIABETIC
Arteriosclerosis

Narrowed lumen

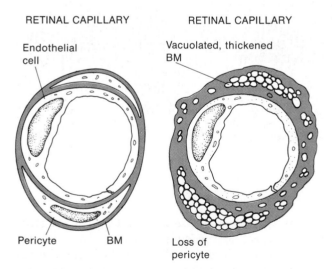

Endothelial Cell/
Pericyte ratio 1:1

Endothelial cell nucleus

Pericyte nucleus

Endothelial Cell/
Pericyte ratio > 1:1

Obliterated region of
capillary network

Pericytes
lost

Microaneurysm

RETINAL CAPILLARY

Endothelial
cell

Pericyte   BM

RETINAL CAPILLARY

Vacuolated, thickened
BM

Loss of
pericyte

Figure 29-11.   Diabetic retinopathy. In diabetic retinopathy the microvasculature is abnormal. Arteriosclerosis narrows the lumen of the small arteries. Pericytes are lost and the endothelial cell:pericyte ratio is greater than 1. Capillary microaneurysms are prominent, and portions of the capillary network become acellular and show no blood flow. The basement membrane of the retinal capillaries is thickened and vacuolated.

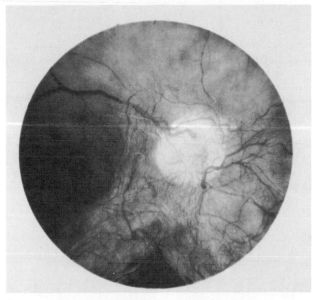

Figure 29-12. Diabetic retinopathy. (*A*) An extensive network of newly formed blood vessels extends into the vitreous cavity from the region of the optic disc in a patient with advanced diabetic retinopathy. (*B*) Numerous microaneurysms are present in this flat preparation of a diabetic retina.

A

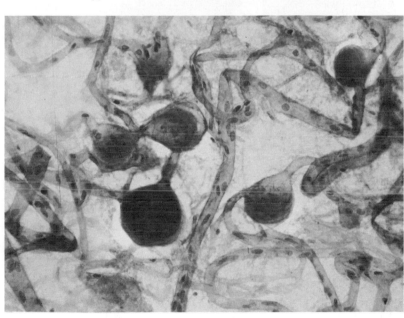

B

erably thicker than normal. The thickened basement membrane is identical to that in the kidney and other locations in diabetics.

Diabetic Iridopathy

In diabetics with severe retinopathy, a fibrovascular layer frequently grows along the anterior surface of the iris and in the anterior chamber angle. Because such iris neovascularization ("rubeosis iridis") is a feature of several conditions associated with retinal ischemia, it is believed to be due to an angiogenic factor produced by the ischemic retina. The fibrovascular membrane leads to adhesions between the iris and the cornea (peripheral anterior synechiae) and between the iris and lens (posterior synechiae), while traction by the fibrovascular membrane pulls the iris pigment epithelium around the pupillary margin (ectropion uveae). The friable new vessels on the iris bleed easily and cause hyphema.

Similar to diabetic retinopathy, and usually involving both eyes, iris neovascularization is clinically im-

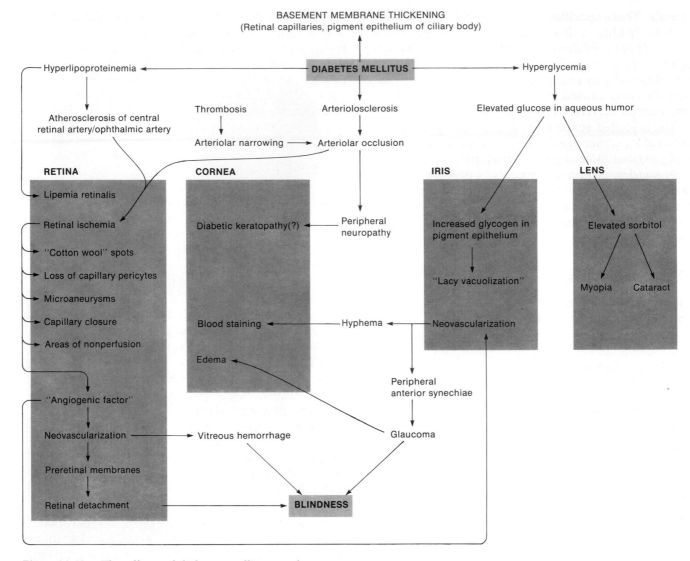

Figure 29-13.   The effects of diabetes mellitus on the eye.

portant because it frequently culminates in a blind painful eye due to a secondary glaucoma ("neovascular glaucoma").

The elevated aqueous sugar level that accompanies hyperglycemia leads to glycogen storage in the pigmented epithelium of the iris, a phenomenon analogous to that produced in the renal tubules by glycosuria (Armanni-Epstein phenomenon). When tissue sections of diabetic eyes are processed in the usual manner, the pigment epithelium of the iris sometimes contains numerous vacuoles that impart a lacy appearance. The vacuoles result from the loss of glycogen in the preparation of tissue sections. The glycogen storage within the pigment epithelium of the iris is thought to account for the scattering of the iris pigment that is observed clinically in diabetic irises.

Diabetes and the Lens

In juvenile diabetics (15 to 25 years old) and, exceptionally, in diabetic infants, a blanket of white needle-shaped opacities collects in both crystalline lenses immediately beneath the anterior and posterior lens capsule. These opacities, which resemble snowflakes, coalesce within a few weeks in adolescents, and within days in children, until the whole lens becomes opaque. This "snowflake" cataract can be produced experimentally in young animals and results from an osmotic effect caused by an accumulation of sorbitol (the alcohol derived from glucose).

The so-called senile cataracts occur in elderly diabetics at an earlier age than in the general population and progress more rapidly to maturity.

A sudden temporary myopia, caused by an increase in the refractive power of the lens, may be the presenting manifestation of diabetes. The increased sorbitol content of the lens causes imbibition of water and an enlargement of the lens.

Other Ophthalmic Manifestations

Diabetics are at increased risk for inflammation of the anterior segment of the eye, phycomycosis (mucormycosis) of the orbit, and primary open-angle glaucoma. Diabetics are also prone to unequal, irregular-shaped pupils that react to accommodation, but not to light (Argyll Robertson pupil). Cranial nerve palsies, especially of the oculomotor nerve, are seen. Some individuals with longstanding diabetes develop a keratopathy that is characterized by recurrent epithelial erosions, and that is believed to be due to an impaired corneal innervation.

Retinopathy of Prematurity (Retrolental Fibroplasia)

In the United States and in some other countries during and after World War II, the retinopathy of prematurity (Fig. 29-14) was the leading cause of blindness in infants. This bilateral, iatrogenic ocular disorder is almost restricted to premature infants and is caused by the administration of high concentrations of oxygen. When a premature infant is exposed to excessive amounts of oxygen, as in an incubator, the developing retinal blood vessels become obliterated and the peripheral retina, which is normally avascular until the end of fetal life, does not vascularize. The more mature the retina, the less the vaso-obliterative effect of hyperoxia. When the infant eventually returns to ambient air, an intense proliferation of vascular endothelium and glial cells begins at the junction of the avascular and vascularized portions of the retina. This becomes apparent 5 to 10 weeks after removal from the incubator, and, as previously discussed (see "Diabetic Retinopathy"), is thought to result from the liberation of an angiogenic factor produced by the avascular peripheral retina that is now ischemic. This angiogenic factor is also thought to account for the neovascularization of the iris that sometimes accompanies the retinal angiogenesis in the retinopathy of prematurity. In approximately 25% of cases the retinopathy progresses to a cicatricial phase, characterized by retinal detachment and a retrolental, fibrovascular mass.

Thyroid Disease

Forward protrusion of the eyeball from the orbit, termed exophthalmos, is most frequently due to Graves' disease and may precede or succeed other manifestations of the thyroid dysfunction. While usually bilateral, one side may be involved earlier or more extensively than the other. Other ocular manifestations of hyperthyroidism include retraction of the upper eyelid (due to increased sympathetic tone), and a characteristic stare or apparent proptosis, owing to exposure of the conjunctiva above the corneoscleral limbus.

Exophthalmos due to thyroid disease usually occurs in early adult life, especially in women, who are affected more often than men (about 4:1). It may be severe and progressive, particularly in middle life, when the exophthalmos no longer correlates well with the state of the thyroid function. This dysthyroid exophthalmos may be associated with lid edema, chemosis (edema of the conjunctiva), and limited ocular motility. Sequelae of severe exophthalmos include several potentially blinding complications, namely corneal exposure with subsequent ulceration, secondary glaucoma, and optic nerve compression. Thyroidectomy enhances the severity and the incidence of dysthyroid-induced exophthalmos.

Dysthyroid exophthalmos results from an increase in the volume of orbital tissue, produced largely by (a) an increase in orbital water, imbibed because of the osmotic pressure of glycosaminoglycans, and (b) enlarged extraocular muscles that are infiltrated with lymphocytes and other mononuclear cells.

The pathogenesis of dysthyroid exophthalmos remains uncertain, but patients with Graves' disease appear to develop autoimmunity to thyroglobulin. Since normal orbital tissue contains thyroglobulin, or an antigenically related molecule, an autoimmune reaction involving sensitized lymphocytes presumably takes place on the surface of extraocular muscles and in other thyroglobulin-containing orbital tissues. The serum of most individuals with Graves' disease contains stimulating autoantibodies which are directed against the receptor for thyroid-stimulating

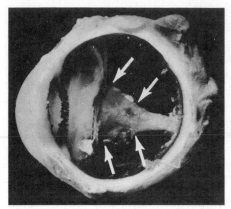

A

Figure 29-14. Retinopathy of prematurity. (*A*) A horizontal section through an eye with advanced retinopathy of prematurity (retrolental fibroplasia) shows a totally detached retina adherent to a fibrovascular mass (*arrows*) behind the lens. (*B*) A histologic section of the retina at an early stage in the retinopathy of prematurity shows pronounced vascularization of the inner retina.

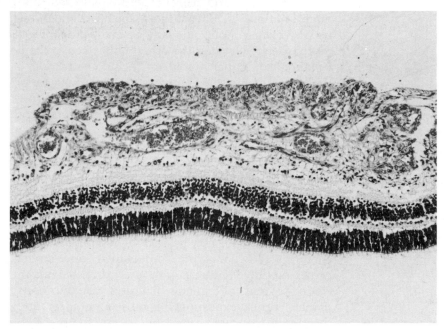

B

hormone on the thyroid cell surface, but these thyroid-stimulating immunoglobulins do not seem to be the cause of dysthyroid exophthalmos. Thyroglobulin–antithyroglobulin complexes bind to membranes of extraocular muscle better than to membranes of other tissues. There they may trigger an orbital autoimmune reaction that damages the extraocular muscles, thus eliciting inflammation and proptosis.

Exophthalmos-producing substances have been identified in pituitary extracts, sera of patients with Graves' disease, and in digests of thyroid-stimulating hormone, but the significance of these substances in the pathogenesis of dysthyroid exophthalmos remains uncertain.

Sarcoidosis

Ocular involvement occurs in at least one-fourth to one-third of patients with sarcoidosis and is often the presenting clinical manifestation. While any of the ocular and orbital tissues may be involved, this granulomatous disease has a predilection for the anterior segment of the eye. Ocular involvement is usually bilateral and most often takes the form of a granulomatous uveitis. Other ocular manifestations include band keratopathy, cataracts, retinal vascularization, vitreous hemorrhage, and bilateral enlargement of the lacrimal and salivary glands (Mikulicz's syndrome).

Common Disorders of Specific Ocular Tissues

Conjunctiva

Dry Eye Syndrome

Basal tear production is diminished in certain ocular or systemic diseases (see Table 29-3), but may also be decreased for no apparent reason, especially in older women, sometimes during the menopause. Dry eyes associated with xerostomia and a systemic immune disorder (Sjögren's syndrome) usually affects middle-aged women and is associated with atrophy of the lacrimal and salivary glands and of other mucosal glands, and with infiltration by lymphocytes and plasma cells. Frequent findings in the blood of patients with Sjögren's syndrome include hypergammaglobulinemia, rheumatoid factor, antinuclear antibodies, and autoantibodies to salivary duct cytoplasm, gastric parietal cells, and thyroglobulin. Affected individuals often develop malignant lymphomas.

Pinguecula and Pterygium

The commonest conjunctival lump, the pinguecula, is most often located nasal to the corneoscleral limbus. Despite its yellowish appearance the lesion does not contain fat, but consists of sun-damaged connective tissue identical to that in similarly injured skin ("actinic elastosis").

Another common conjunctival lesion, the pterygium, consists of a triangular fold of vascularized conjunctiva that grows horizontally onto the cornea in the shape of an insect wing.

Cornea

Arcus Lipoides

A white ring due to lipid deposition occurs in the peripheral cornea with aging (arcus senilis). While not necessarily associated with elevated serum lipids, the same reaction accompanies certain hyperlipoproteinemias, (Table 29-3) and its presence alerts the astute clinician to the systemic disorder.

Band Keratopathy

Calcium phosphate may deposit in a horizontal band across the superficial central cornea in hypercalcemia. However, this so-called calcific band keratopathy most often occurs in the absence of an elevated serum calcium, as in chronic uveitis and other ocular disorders.

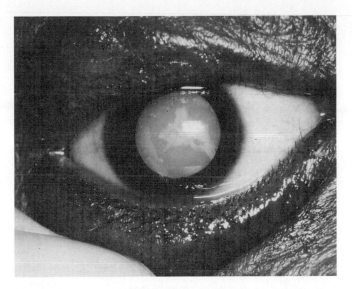

Figure 29-15. Cataract. The white appearance of the pupil in this eye is due to complete opacification of the lens ("mature cataract").

Lens

Cataracts

Some ophthalmologists call any opacity in the lens a cataract, while others restrict the term to lens opacities that impair vision (Fig. 29-15). Cataracts, a major cause of visual impairment and blindness throughout the world, are the outcome of numerous conditions. Cataracts can be caused by disorders of carbohydrate metabolism that result in monosaccharide excesses, or they can be caused by deficiencies in riboflavin or tryptophan. Numerous cataracts are the result of genetic disorders. Others result from toxins, drugs, or physical agents. Examples of toxins or drugs which may cause cataracts are dinitrophenol, naphthalene, ergot, phospholine iodide (topical), corticosteroids (systemic), and phenothiazines. Physical agents can be heat, some categories of electromagnetic radiation (ultraviolet light, microwaves), trauma, intraocular surgery, ultrasound, or electric shock.

Ocular diseases which may result in cataracts include uveitis, intraocular neoplasms, glaucoma, retinitis pigmentosa, and sensory retinal detachment. Cataracts are also associated with rubella virus, aging, some skin diseases (atopic dermatitis, scleroderma), and various systemic diseases (see Table 29-3).

Fortunately cataractous lenses can be surgically removed, and an optical device can be provided to permit the focusing of light on the retina (spectacles, contact lenses, implantation of intraocular lenses).

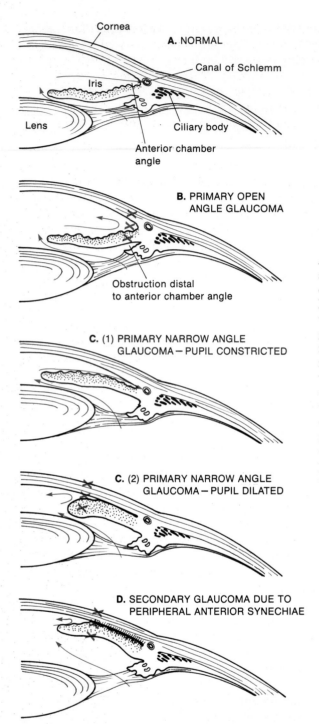

A. NORMAL

Cornea

Canal of Schlemm

Iris

Lens

Ciliary body

Anterior chamber
angle

**B. PRIMARY OPEN
ANGLE GLAUCOMA**

Obstruction distal
to anterior chamber angle

**C. (1) PRIMARY NARROW ANGLE
GLAUCOMA – PUPIL CONSTRICTED**

**C. (2) PRIMARY NARROW ANGLE
GLAUCOMA – PUPIL DILATED**

**D. SECONDARY GLAUCOMA DUE TO
PERIPHERAL ANTERIOR SYNECHIAE**

Figure 29-16. Pathogenesis of glaucoma. The anterior segment of the eye is affected differently in various forms of glaucoma. (*A*) shows the structure of the normal eye. In primary open-angle glaucoma (*B*) the obstruction to the aqueous outflow is distal to the anterior chamber angle, and the anterior segment resembles that of the normal eye. In primary narrow-angle glaucoma (*C*) the anterior chamber angle is open, but narrower than normal when the pupil is constricted (*C1*). When the pupil becomes dilated in such an eye the thickened iris obstructs the anterior chamber angle (*C2*) thereby causing an increase in intraocular pressure. The anterior chamber angle can become obstructed by a variety of pathologic processes, including an adhesion between the iris and the posterior surface of the cornea (peripheral anterior synechia) (*D*).

The most common cataract in the United States is associated with aging (senile cataract). In such cataracts, clefts appear between the lens fibers, and degenerated lens material accumulates in these spaces (Morgagnian corpuscles, incipient cataract). The degenerated lens material exerts an osmotic pressure, causing the cataractous lens to increase in volume by imbibing water. Such a swollen lens may obstruct the pupil and cause glaucoma ("phakomorphic glaucoma"). After the entire lens degenerates ("mature cataract"), its volume diminishes because lenticular debris escapes into the aqueous humor through a degenerated lens capsule ("hypermature cataract"). After becoming engulfed by macrophages the extruded lenticular material may obstruct the aqueous outflow and produce glaucoma ("phakolytic glaucoma"). The compressed lens fibers in the center of the lens normally harden with aging (simple nuclear sclerotic cataract) and may become brown or black. If the peripheral portion of the lens (lens cortex) becomes liquified (Morgagnian cataract), the sclerotic nucleus may sink with gravity within the lens.

Presbyopia

At the equator of the crystalline lens, the cuboidal subcapsular cells differentiate into elongated lens fibers throughout life. Once formed, these lens fibers persist indefinitely, and older fibers become displaced into the center of the lens, causing it to enlarge with age. After this has occurred for many years, the lens loses its elasticity, an effect which interferes with its normal tendency to become spherical, thereby diminishing the power of accommodation (presbyopia).

Aqueous Humor

Glaucoma

After being produced by the ciliary body, the aqueous humor enters the posterior chamber (the space between the iris and the zonules) before passing through the pupil to enter the anterior chamber (between the iris and the cornea). From that site it drains into veins by way of the trabecular meshwork and Schlemm's canal (Fig. 29-16). A delicate balance between the production and drainage of the aqueous humor maintains intraocular pressure within its physiologic range (10–20 mm Hg). In certain pathologic states aqueous humor accumulates within the eye, and the intraocular pressure, which is measured by determining the force required to indent or flatten the cornea, becomes elevated, producing temporary or permanent impairment of vision and damage to the optic nerve. When this occurs, usually when the intraocular pressure is above 20 mm Hg, the term glaucoma is applied. Vision becomes impaired because of degenerative changes in the retina and optic nerve head (a result of ocular hypertension and resultant ischemia), and because of corneal edema and opacification.

Causes of Glaucoma

Glaucoma almost always follows a congenital or acquired lesion of the anterior segment of the eye that mechanically obstructs the aqueous drainage. The obstruction may be located between the iris and lens, in the angle of the anterior chamber, in the trabecular meshwork, in Schlemm's canal, or in the venous drainage of the eye. Glaucoma resulting from a hypersecretion of aqueous humor is extremely rare, if it occurs at all.

Glaucoma may develop in a person with no apparent underlying eye disease (primary glaucomas), or it may follow a known antecedent or concomitant ocular disorder (secondary glaucomas).

Types of Glaucoma

Congenital Glaucoma (infantile glaucoma, buphthalmos)   By tradition the term congenital glaucoma refers to glaucoma caused by an obstruction of the aqueous drainage by developmental anomalies, even though the intraocular pressure may not become elevated until early infancy or childhood. Most cases of congenital glaucoma are males (60% to 70%), and an X-linked recessive mode of inheritance is common. The developmental anomaly usually involves both eyes and, while often limited to the angle of the anterior chamber, may be accompanied by a variety of other ocular malformations. Congenital glaucoma is often associated with a deep anterior chamber, corneal cloudiness, sensitivity to bright lights (photophobia), excessive tearing, and enlarged eyes (buphthalmos).

Primary Glaucomas   Primary glaucomas are of two types, namely open-angle glaucoma and closed-angle (narrow-angle) glaucoma.

Primary Open-Angle Glaucoma   **Primary open-angle glaucoma, the commonest type of glaucoma and a major blinding disorder in the United States, is estimated to affect 1% to 3% of the population over the age of 40 years and occurs principally in the sixth decade.** The intraocular pressure becomes elevated insidiously and asymptomatically, and while almost always bilateral, one eye may be affected more severely than the other. With time, damage to the retina and optic nerve causes an irreversible loss of peripheral vision. The angle of the anterior chamber is open and appears normal, but an increased resistance to the outflow of the aqueous humor is present within the vicinity of Schlemm's canal. Individuals with diabetes mellitus and myopia appear to have an increased risk of primary open-angle glaucoma.

Primary Closed-Angle Glaucoma   Primary narrow-angle glaucoma occurs, especially after the age of 40 years, in individuals who possess an abnormally narrow angle, in which the peripheral iris is displaced anteriorly towards the trabecular meshwork. When the pupil is constricted (miotic), the iris remains stretched, so that the chamber angle is not occluded. However, when the pupil dilates (mydriasis), the iris obstructs the anterior chamber angle, thereby impairing aqueous drainage and resulting in sudden episodes of intraocular hypertension. This is accompanied by ocular pain, and halos or rings are seen around lights. In such individuals the intraocular pressure may also become elevated if the pupil becomes blocked, for example by a swollen lens, and aqueous humor accumulates in the posterior chamber. Primary-closed angle glaucoma affects both eyes, but it may become apparent in one eye 2 to 5 years before it becomes apparent in the other. The intraocular pressure is normal between attacks, but after many episodes adhesions form between the iris and the trabecular meshwork and cornea (peripheral anterior synechiae) and accentuate the block to the outflow of the aqueous humor.

Secondary Glaucomas   The causes of secondary glaucoma are many, and the anterior chamber angles may be open or closed. Because the underlying disorder is usually limited to one eye, secondary glaucomas are usually unilateral.

"Low Tension Glaucoma"   The characteristic visual field defect and all of the ophthalmoscopic features of chronic simple (open-angle) glaucoma often occur in the elderly without an elevation in intraocular pressure. While some eyes might be hypersensitive to normal intraocular pressure, most cases of this "low tension glaucoma" probably represent an infarction of the optic nerve head.

Effects of Elevated Intraocular Pressure

Individuals vary in their ability to tolerate an elevated intraocular pressure. Some do not develop a visual field loss or optic atrophy after having an intraocular pressure of three standard deviations above the mean (24 mm Hg) for many years.

Prolonged ocular hypertension has several effects on the eye:

- In adults it leads to a characteristic cupped excavation of the optic disc (glaucomatous cupping), accompanied by a nasal displacement of the retinal blood vessels. In infants cupping of the optic disc tends to be less prominent.
- The cornea or sclera bulges at weak points, such as sites of scars in the outer coat of the eye.
- Optic atrophy, with a loss of axons, gliosis, and thickening of the pial septa, follows the retinal degeneration and damage to the nerve fibers at the optic disc.
- The ganglion cell layer of the retina degenerates, thereby impairing vision. The outer retina, which derives its nutrition from the underlying choroid, remains intact.
- When the intraocular pressure becomes elevated before the age of 3 years, the pliable eye sometimes enlarges extensively and may resemble an ox eye (buphthalmos). After the first few years of life, a rigid sclera prevents glaucomatous eyes from enlarging under the elevated pressure.

Retina

Retinal Detachment

During development the space between the sensory retina and the retinal pigment epithelium is obliterated when these two layers become apposed. However, the sensory retina readily separates from the retinal pigment epithelium when fluid (liquid vitreous humor, hemorrhage, or exudate) accumulates within the potential space between these structures.

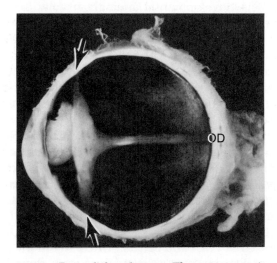

Figure 29-17.   Retinal detachment. The sensory retina is completely detached from the retinal pigment epithelium in this eye. It remains attached at the optic disc (*OD*) and at the boundary of the retina and ciliary body (ora serrata, *arrows*).

Such a separation is designated a retinal detachment (Fig. 29-17), and three varieties of this common cause of blindness are recognized, namely rhegmatogenous, tractional, and exudative.

Rhegmatogenous retinal detachment, the commonest form of retinal detachment, is associated with a retinal tear and often degenerative changes in the vitreous or peripheral retina. Full thickness holes in the retina are usually not complicated by retinal detachment, unless liquid vitreous humor gains access to the potential space between the retina and the retinal pigment epithelium, and even then some vitreoretinal traction seems to be necessary for retinal detachment to occur. Retinal detachment follows intraocular hemorrhage (as after trauma) and is a potential complication of cataract extractions and several other ocular operations.

In tractional retinal detachment, the retina is detached by being pulled toward the center of the eye by adherent vitreoretinal adhesions, as occurs in proliferative diabetic retinopathy and the retinopathy of prematurity, and after intraocular infection.

An accumulation of fluid in the potential space between the sensory retina and the retinal pigment epithelium causes an "exudative retinal detachment" in disorders such as choroiditis, choroidal hemangioma, and choroidal melanomas.

Factors predisposing to retinal detachment include retinal holes (due to trauma or certain retinal degenerations), vitreous traction, diminished pressure on the retina (as after vitreous loss), and weakening of the fixation of the retina. The photoreceptors and retinal pigment epithelium normally function as a unit. After they separate in a retinal detachment, oxygen and nutrients that normally reach the outer retina from the choroid need to diffuse a greater distance, a situation which causes the photoreceptors to degenerate and cyst-like extracellular spaces to appear within the retina.

Retinitis Pigmentosa

The misnomer "retinitis pigmentosa" is a generic term that comprises a variety of bilateral, progressive, degenerative retinopathies that are characterized by pigment accumulation within the retina and loss of retinal photoreceptors (rods and cones). This noninflammatory reaction presumably results from multiple genetic abnormalities. While often an isolated ocular disorder, with autosomal dominant, autosomal recessive, or X-linked recessive modes of inheritance, the pigmentary retinopathies are associated with many neurologic and systemic disorders (see Table 29-3).

The clinical manifestations of these cases, including the appearance and distribution of the retinal pigmentation, vary with the cause of the retinopathy. The familial cases usually present in childhood with night blindness due to the loss of rods in the peripheral retina. As the condition progresses, contraction of the visual fields eventually leads to blindness. Retinal pigment epithelium migrates into the sensory retina, and melanin, which appears within slender processes of spidery cells, accumulates mainly around small branching retinal blood vessels (especially in the equatorial portion of the retina) like spicules of bone. A gradual attenuation of the retinal blood vessels ensues, and the optic nerve head acquires a characteristic waxy pallor.

Macular Degeneration

At the center of the macula where visual acuity is greatest there is a high concentration of cones resting on the retinal pigment epithelium. Surrounding this foveola the retina has a multilayered concentration of ganglion cells. With aging, in certain drug toxicities (for example chloroquine), and in several inherited disorders, the macula degenerates, and central vision is impaired. Perhaps the most common cause of reduced vision in the elderly in the United States is senile or involutional macular degeneration, which is sometimes associated with bleeding into the subretinal space (hemorrhagic macular degeneration).

Cherry Red Spot at the Macula

In lysosomal storage diseases (see Table 29-3), including GM_2-gangliosidosis type II (Tay-Sachs disease), a myriad of intracytoplasmic lysosomal inclusions within the multilayered ganglion cell layer of the macula imparts a striking pallor to the affected retina. As a result the central foveola appears bright red ("cherry red spot") because of the underlying choroidal vasculature (Fig. 29-18).

Following a central retinal artery occlusion, a cherry red spot also occurs at the macula, but for a different reason. Edema causes the entire retina to appear pale, a condition which highlights the subfoveolar vascular choroid.

Angioid Streaks

In a variety of systemic conditions (see Table 29-3), Bruch's membrane fractures spontaneously, thereby causing characteristic irregular lines that radiate beneath the retina from the optic nerve head (angioid streaks).

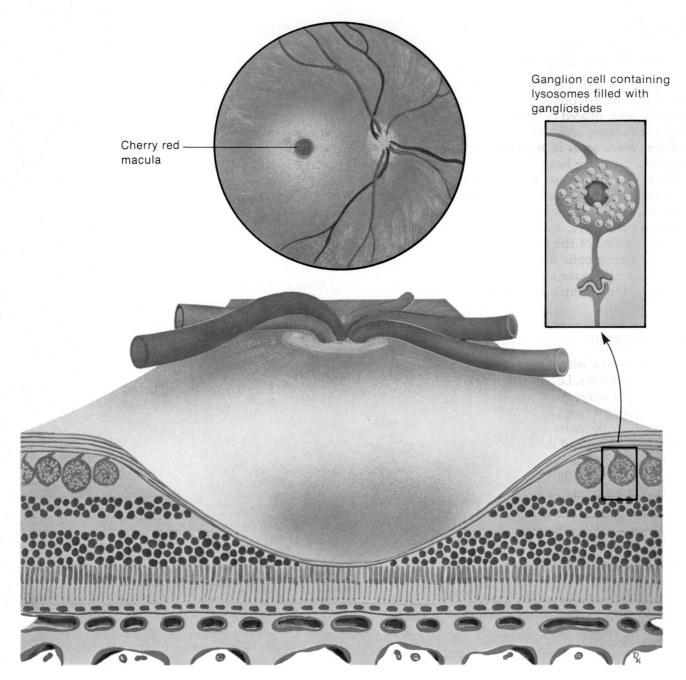

Cherry red macula

Ganglion cell containing lysosomes filled with gangliosides

Figure 29-18. Cherry-red macula. A cherry-red spot appears at the macula in several lysosomal storage diseases that are characterized by intracytoplasmic accumulations within the retinal ganglion cells, such as GM$_2$ gangliosidosis type II (Tay-Sachs disease). The macula develops this appearance because the pallor created by the deposits within the multilayered ganglion cells enhances the visibility of the underlying normal choroidal vasculature.

Optic Nerve

Edema of Optic Disc (Papilledema)

Edema of the optic nerve head is characterized clinically by a swollen optic disc which displays blurred margins and dilated vessels. Frequently, hemorrhages, exudates, and "cotton wool" spots are seen, and concentric folds of the choroid and retina may surround the nerve head.

Optic disc edema can result from various causes, the most important of which is increased intracranial pressure. Other causes are obstruction to the venous drainage of the eye, such as may occur with compressive lesions of the orbit, an infarct of the optic nerve (ischemic optic neuropathy), inflammation of the optic nerve close to the eyeball (optic neuritis, papillitis), and multiple sclerosis.

Optic Atrophy

The nerve axons within the optic nerve may be lost in many conditions. Longstanding papilledema, optic neuritis, optic nerve compression, glaucoma, and retinal degeneration are all possible causes. Optic atrophy can also be caused by some drugs, examples being ethambutol and isoniazid.

The optic disc is usually flat and pale in optic atrophy, but when this disorder follows glaucoma the disc is excavated (glaucomatous cupping).

Eyelid

Xanthelasma

In this disorder, yellow plaques of lipid-containing macrophages appear, usually involving the nasal aspect of the eyelids. It is seen more often in older individuals.

Miscellaneous Disorders

Proptosis

Numerous conditions cause an abnormal forward protrusion of the eyeball. The most common cause is thyroid disease, followed by orbital hemangiomas and lymphomas. Other orbital conditions can cause proptosis: various inflammatory lesions, developmental anomalies, vascular problems, and neoplasms all contribute some cases. Proptosis can also result from lesions of the paranasal sinuses and intracranial lesions.

Myopia

Myopia affects more than 70 million individuals in the United States, causing them to wear glasses or contact lenses or to undergo a controversial operation called a radial keratotomy.

In this refractive ocular abnormality, light from the visualized object focuses at a point in front of the retina because of a longer than usual anteroposterior diameter of the eye. Myopia usually begins in youth and varies in severity. A mild form (stationary or simple myopia) is generally nonprogressive after the cessation of body growth, while a genetically determined "progressive myopia" is more severe.

SUGGESTED READING

Garner A and Klintworth GK (eds): Pathobiology of Ocular Disease: A Dynamic Approach, 2 vols. New York, Marcel Dekker, 1982

Klintworth GK and Landers MB III: The Eye: Structure and Function in Disease. Baltimore, William and Wilkins, 1976

Spencer WH (ed): Ophthalmic Pathology: An Atlas and Textbook, 3rd ed, 3 vols, Philadelphia, WB Saunders, 1985

Yanoff M and Fine BS: Ocular Pathology: A Text and Atlas, 2nd ed, New York, Harper and Row, 1982

Acknowledgments

The editors are grateful for the valuable assistance of Lawrence S. Friedman and Shmuel Eidelman in the preparation of the chapters on the gastrointestinal tract and the liver. We thank the following for providing us with important photographs: Henry D. Applemann, Jules L. Dienstag, Michael A. Gerber, Ali Z. Hameli, Victor H. Nassar, Giuseppe G. Pietra, Si-Chun Ming, Fiorenzo Paronetto, M. James Phillips, Hans Popper, Heidrun Rotterdam, Mateo Russo, and John H. Yardley.

Hugh Bonner is grateful for the assistance of Regina Cohen and Hugh Bonner III. Wallace H. Clark acknowledges the assistance of Carol Blumenthal, William Witmer, Patricia Clark, and William Ju. Daniel Conner and Dean Gibson thank the following: Douglas J. Wear, Isaac S. Banks, J. Kevin Baird, Charles K. English, Ronald C. Neafie, Yvonne Koch, Christopher R. Lissner, Abe M. Macher, Wayne M. Meyers, Ann Marie Nelson, Meade Pimsler, and Jorge L Ribas. John E. Craighead thanks Joseph R. Williamson for an electron micrograph. Ivan Damjanov thanks Olaf H. Iversen for contributing photographs to his chapter. Gordon K. Klintworth thanks James S. Tiedeman for supplying a photograph for his chapter. Dante Scarpelli is grateful to the following individuals for contributing photographs to his chapter: Hartmann H.R. Friederici, Mary Jumbelis, Yashpal S. Kanwar, Robert J. Marder, Janardan K. Reddy, I. Sanford Roth, Donald F. Steiner, Robert Vogelzang, and Heidejiro Yokoo.

Specific acknowledgment is made for permission to use the following material:

Chapter 1, Figure 33. DeBusk FL: The Hutchinson-Gilford progeria syndrome. J Pediat 80, (4): 706, 1972

Chapter 4, Figure 11. Photograph from Armed Forces Institute of Pathology.

Chapter 9. All photographs from Armed Forces Institute of Pathology.

Chapter 11, Table 6. Reimer K, Jennings RB: Myocardial ischemia, hypoxia, and infarction. In Fozzard HA, Haber E, Katz AM, et al (eds): The Heart and Cardiovascular System. New York, Raven Press, 1986.

Chapter 11, Figure 3. Hackel DB: Delayed complications of myocardial infarction. Cardiovasc Rev Rep 3(9): 1353, 1982

Chapter 11, Figures 14 and 15. Hackel DB: The coronary arteries in acute myocardial infarction. Circulation 68 (suppl 1): 1, 1983

Chapter 11, Figure 30. Hackel DB: Diseases of the pericardium. In Edwards J (ed): Clinical-Pathologic Correlations, I. Cardiovasc Clin 4(2): 147, 1972. By permission FA Davis Company

Chapter 13, Figure 12. Photograph from Armed Forces Institute of Pathology.

Chapter 13, Figure 55. Appelman HD: Epithelial neoplasia of the appendix. In Norris TH (ed): Pathology of the Colon, Small Intestine, and Anus. New York, Churchill Livingstone, 1983

Chapter 16, Figure 1. Galtone VH, Evan AP: Quantitative renal vascular casting in nephrology research. Scan Elect Micros 1:256, 1986

Chapter 16, Figures 2, 3, 10, 12, 13, 15, 17, 19–24, 26, 29, 31, 34, 36, 38, 41, 42, 44, 50, 52, 53, 59, and 62. Spargo, BH, Seymour AE, Ordonez NG: Renal Biopsy Pathology with Diagnostic and Therapeutic Implications. New York, John Wiley & Sons, 1980

Chapter 16, Figures 46, 47, and 61. Peterson, ROP: Urologic Pathology, Philadelphia, JB Lippincott, 1987

Chapter 16, Figure 48. Heptinstall R: Pathology of the Kidney, 3rd ed. Boston, Little Brown, 1983

Chapter 17, all photographs. Peterson ROP: Urologic Pathology, Philadelphia, JB Lippincott, 1987

Chapter 29, Figure 2. Darougar S, Treharne JD: Chlamydial infections. In Garner A, Klintworth GK: Pathobiology of Ocular Disease. A Dynamic Approach. New York, Marcel Dekker, 1982

Chapter 29, Figures 3B, 4B, 14B, 15, and 17. Klintworth GK, Landers MD III: The Eye: Structure and Function in Disease. Baltimore, Williams & Wilkins, 1976

Index

Page numbers in boldface represent major discussions; t and f following page numbers indicate tables and figures, respectively.

AA amyloid protein, 1185, 1186–1189, 1188f
A-band, of muscle, 1396
Abdominal angina, 672
Abetalipoproteinemia, 1043, 678–679
ABO incompatibility, maternal-fetal, 246
Abortion, spontaneous, 985
Abrasion, 307
Abruptio placentae, 283f
Abscess:
  of Bartholin's gland, 950
  of bone, staphylococcal, 383
  of brain, 1446–1447, 1448f–1449f
    amebic, 416–417
    in drug addiction, 287, 289f
  of breast, 383, 997
  Brodie's, 1333
  cold, 1334
  crypt, 698
  liquefactive necrosis in, 15, 16f
  of liver:
    amebic, 416
    cholangitic, 788, 788f
  of lung, 552–553, 552f–553f
  mechanism of formation of, 36
  in melioidosis, 370–371
  periapical, 1271
  pericholecystic, 804
  peritonsillar, 1292
  psoas, 1334
  pylephlebitic, 788
Acanthocytosis, 1043
Acantholytic cells, 1211–1213
Acanthosis nigricans, 188
Acetaldehyde, tissue injury induced by, 287
Acetaminophen, hepatocellular necrosis due to, 26–27
Achalasia:
  esophageal cancer due to, 639
  of esophagus, 633, 633f–634f
Achondroplasia, 1315–1316, 1317f
Achrondroplastic dwarfism, 224
Acid maltase deficiency, 1409, 1410f
Acidophilic bodies, 747–748, 747f
Acinus:
  anatomy of, 545–546
  normal, 594f
Acne, 1238, 1240f–1241f
Acoustic schwannoma, 1496
Acoustic trauma, 1302

Acquired immunodeficiency syndrome. See AIDS
Acral lentiginous melanoma, 1250–1252, 1251f–1253f
Acrania, 203
Acrodermatitis enterohepatica, 325
Acromegaly, 1127, 1127f
ACTH production, in cancer, 185
ACTH syndrome, ectopic, 1151, 1152f
Actinic keratosis, 1255, 1255f
Actinomycosis, 392–393, 393f
  cervicofacial, 1264–1265
  of female genital tract, 948–949
  of lung, 573
Addison's disease, 1150
Adenocarcinoma:
  of breast, 146, 146f
  of cervix, 959–961
  of colon and rectum, 151, 151f, 709–712. See also Colorectal cancer
  of endometrium, 965–967, 966f, 967t
  of esophagus, 640
  of gallbladder, 806, 806f
  of lung, 556, 557f
  of ovary, 977
  of pancreas, 279, 279f
  of prostate, 932–937
  of small intestine, 682
  of stomach, 144
  of thyroid, 146, 146f
  of urinary bladder, 908
  of vagina, 248
Adenoid cystic carcinoma, of lung, 559
Adenoids, 1292
Adenolymphocele, 433
Adenolymphoma, of salivary glands, 1279, 1280f
Adenoma, 143
  of adrenal cortex, 1153, 1153f
  of colon, villous, 704–705, 704f
  of gallbladder, 806
  of liver, 292, 792–793, 792f
  of nipple, 1004
  of parathyroid glands, 1146–1147, 1147f
  of pituitary, 1125–1127
  renal cell, 889
  of salivary glands, 1278–1279, 1278f–1279f
  of small intestine, 681
  of thyroid, 143, 144f, 1140

Adenomatoid tumor, of testicular tunic, 924
Adenomatous polyp, 143
Adenomyoma, of gallbladder, 806
Adenomyosis, 963
Adenosarcoma:
  müllerian, 968
  of uterus, 968
Adenosine deaminase deficiency, 124
Adenosis, of vagina, 953–954, 953f
Adenovirus:
  in bronchiolitis, 550
  in carcinogenesis, 173
  in diarrhea, 343
  in pneumonia, 344
Adherence protein defect, 57t
Adipose tumors, 1390, 1390f–1391f
ADP, endothelial cell metabolism of, 473
Adrenal cortex, 1149–1154
  adenoma of, 1153, 1153f
  anatomy of, 1149
  atrophy of, 1150
  carcinoma of, 1153–1154, 1154f
  congenital anomalies of, 1149–1150
  congenital hyperplasia of, 1149–1150
  hormonal deficiency in, 1150
  hyperfunction of, 1150–1153
  insufficiency of, 1150
  metastatic cancer of, 1154
Adrenal glands, in shock, 273
Adrenal medulla, 1154–1158
  neuroblastoma of, 1156–1157
  pheochromocytoma of, 1154–1156
  vascular lesions and hyperplasias of, 1154
Adrenal virilism, 1151
Adrenocorticotropic hormone, 1122
Adrenoleukodystrophy, 1463
Adult T-cell leukemia/lymphoma, 1103
AE amyloid protein, 1185
Aflatoxin B1, 162f, 163
African trypanosomiasis, 404f, 405–406
Agammaglobulinemia, Bruton's, 122–123, 124f
Agenesis, in morphogenesis, 201
Aging:
  atrophy in, 9
  cellular, 29–33
  endocrine responses in, 1131–1132
  nonerosive gastritis due to, 645

Aging:
  physiologic capacity, decline in, 30, 31f
  structural changes in, 30, 31f
Agranulocytosis, gingiva in, 1272
Agricultural chemicals, 296
AIDS, **124–129**, 126t, 127f–128f
  classification of, 126t
  conditions associated with, 125, 127f
  cryptosporidiosis in, 419
  encephalopathy in, 1456–1457
  Kaposi's sarcoma in, 494–495, 1257,
    1257f–1258f
  laboratory features of, 126, 129
  lymphadenitis in, 1061
  opportunistic infections in, 450–451,
    450t
  pathogenesis of, 128f
  Pneumocystis carinii in, 414
  psoriasis in, 1211
Air embolism, 268, 620
Airflow:
  central obstruction of, 585–593
  chronic obstruction of, 583–598
Air pollution, as respiratory irritant, 551
Airspace enlargement, 593, 593t
Alagille's syndrome, 792
AL amyloid protein, 1184–1185, 1186, 1187f
Albinism, 219, 231–232, 232f
Albright's syndrome, 1124, 1145
Alcoholic liver disease, 284, 284f–285f,
    751–760
  cirrhosis in, 760, 761f
  epidemiology of, 752, 754f
  fatty liver in, 754–758, 756f–757f
  hepatocellular carcinoma and, 795
Alcoholism, **282–287**
  blood in, 286, 1047, 1047t
  brain lesions in, 286, 1479–1480, 1479f–
    1480f
  cancer and, 286
  cardiomyopathy in, 285, 539
  complications of, 284f
  definition of, 283
  endocrine system in, 285, 738
  fetal effects of, 206
  gastrointestinal tract in, 285–286
  heart in, 285, 539
  immune system in, 286
  liver in, 284, 284f–285f, **751–760**. *See also*
    Alcoholic liver disease
  neuropathy in, 1493
  pancreas in, 284–285, 814, 816
  rhabdomyolysis in, 285
  skeletal muscle in, 285
  tissue injury in, 286–287
  tolerance in, 283–284
Aldosteronoma, 1153
Alexander's disease, 1463
Alkaptonuria, 232
Allergic bronchopulmonary aspergillosis,
    422–423, 550–551
Allergic contact dermatitis, 1232–1233,
    1234f–1236f
Allergic purpura, 1027
Allison-Ghormley body, 1376, 1378f
Alopecia, 1204–1205
Alpha cell, pancreatic, 822–823, 822f
Alpha cell tumors, 825, 826
Alport's syndrome, 869
Altitude-related illness, 304–306. *See also*
    High-altitude sickness

Aluminum intoxication, 300
Alveolar-arterial capillary block syndrome,
    607
Alveolar macrophage, 547, 547f
Alveolar rhabdomyosarcoma, 1391–1392
Alveoli:
  anatomy of, 542f–543f, 546
  filling defects of, idiopathic, 581–583
  injury to:
    diffuse, 552, 577–581
      drug-induced, 581
      environmental causes of, 580
      iatrogenic causes of, 580–581
    with intact basement membrane, 93
    with ruptured basement membrane,
      93–94
  lipoproteinosis of, 581, 582f
  type I cells of, 546
  type II cells of, 546
Alveolitis:
  extrinsic allergic, 612, 613f–614f
  fibrosing, 609
  toxic, in drug reaction, 290
Alzheimer's disease, **1485–1487**, 1485f–
    1489f
  amyloid deposits in, 1184
  cause of, 1486–1487
  genetic theory of, 1487
  granulovacuolar degeneration in, 1486,
    1489f
  neurofibrillary tangles in, 1486, 1488f
  senile plaque in, 1486, 1488f
Alzheimer type II change, 1480
Amebiasis, 414–417, 415f–416f
  of liver, 788–789, 789f
Amebic colitis, 414–417, 415f–416f
Amebic meningoencephalitis, 417
Ameboma, 416
Ameloblastoma, of jaw, 1274, 1276f
Amenorrhea:
  hypothalamus in, 1129–1130
  in obesity, 316
American trypanosomiasis, 402, 402f
Ames test, 160, 164, 165f
Amine, aromatic, 163
Amino acid metabolism, inborn errors of,
    230–232, 232f
γ-Aminobutyric acid, 736
Aminotransferase, 739
Ammonia:
  in hepatic encephalopathy, 735
  as respiratory irritant, 551
Amniocentesis, 236
Amniotic fluid aspiration, 238, 238f
Amniotic fluid embolism, 268, 620
Amniotic membrane, premature rupture
    of, 283f
Ampulla of Vater, carcinoma of, 806
Amygdalin, 296–297
Amylo–1,6-glucosidase deficiency, 1410
Amyloid enhancing factor, 1186
Amyloid neuropathy, 1493t, 1494
Amyloidosis, **1178–1193**
  AA amyloid in, 1185, 1186–1189, 1188f
  AE amyloid in, 1185
  AL amyloid in, 1184–1185, 1186, 1187f
  in cancer, 188
  classification of, 1183t
    clinical, 1182–1184
    by protein type, 1184–1185
  clinical features of, 1192

Amyloidosis:
  deposits in, 1179f
    constituents of, 1180
    definition of, 1182
    mechanisms of, 1185–1189
    staining properties of, 1180–1182,
      1181f
    structure of, 1182
    types of, 1182
    underlying mechanism of, 1189
    in various tissues, 1189–1190, 1190f–
      1191f
  diagnosis of, 1192
  familial, 1183–1184
  of heart, 538f, 539
  isolated, 1184
  of kidney, 848–850, 849f–850f, 1189,
    1190f
  of lung, 576
  paraproteinemia in, 868
  prealbumin in, 1185, 1189
  primary, 1182–1183
  of renal pelvis and ureter, 893
  secondary, 1183
  of urinary bladder, 903
Amyloidotic polyneuropathy, familial,
    1184
Amyotrophic lateral sclerosis, 1482
Anagen hairs, 1204
Anal canal:
  carcinoma of, 712–713
  fibrous polyp of, 702
  imperforate anus, 688
  malformation of, 688
  malignant melanoma of, 713
  sphincter, 686
  tag, 702
  varices of, in portal hypertension, 780
Analgesics, renal damage due to, 874
Anaphylactic syndrome, 105
Anaphylatoxins, biologic activity of, 45,
    46f
Anaphylaxis, in drug reaction, 293
Anaplasia, 147, 148f, 156
Ancylostoma duodenale, 436, 437f
Ancylostomiasis, 436, 437f
Andersen's disease, 227f
Anemia, **1030–1047**
  in abetalipoproteinemia, 1043
  alcohol-induced, 1047, 1047t
  aplastic, 290, 1035–1036
  aplastic crisis in, 1037
  blood loss, 1042
  in cancer, 187
  characteristic morphologic features of,
    1032f–1033f
  in chronic disease, 1041
  in chronic renal disease, 1037
  clinical symptoms of, 1034–1035
  Cooley's, 1041
  dyserythropoietic, congenital, 1037
  erythrocyte indices in, 1031
  Fanconi's, 1035
  in G6PD deficiency, 1043–1044
  in hemoglobin C disease, 1044–1045
  hemoglobin Kohn and, 1045
  hemolytic:
    cold-antibody autoimmune, 1046
    in drug reaction, 290
    hereditary nonspherocytic, 1043
    microangiopathic, 880, 1047

Anemia:
    traumatic cardiac, 1047
    warm-antibody autoimmune, 1046
  in hereditary elliptocytosis, 1043
  in hereditary methemoglobinemia, 1045
  in hereditary spherocytosis, 1042–1043
  in hereditary stomatocytosis, 1043
  iron deficiency, 1040
  ischemic heart disease and, 518
  in lead poisoning, 297–298
  megaloblastic:
    in alcoholism, 286
    in drug reaction, 290
    folic acid deficiency in, 1039–1040
    vitamin B$_{12}$ deficiency in, 1037–1039,
       1038f–1039f
  morphologic classification of, 1031–1034,
       1031t
  myelodysplastic, 1036, 1036t
  myelophthisic, 1042
  of neonate, congenital, 245
  normal blood values and, 1030, 1031t
  in paroxysmal cold hemoglobinuria,
       1046
  in paroxysmal nocturnal hemoglobinu-
       ria, 1045
  pathophysiologic classification of, 1030–
       1031, 1031t, 1034t
  pernicious, 1038
    glossitis in, 1270
    nonerosive gastritis with, 645–647
  pyridoxine-responsive, 322
  red cell aplasia in, 1036–1037
  refractory, 1036t
    with excess blasts, 1036t
    with ringed sideroblasts, 1036t
  secondary hemochromatosis in, 769
  in sickle cell disease, 220, 884, 1044
  sideroblastic, 1041–1042
  thalassemia in, 1040–1041
Anencephaly, 203–205, 204f, 1129, 1457–
       1459, 1458f
Aneuploidy, autosomal, 213, 213t
Aneurysm, 455, **488–491**
  aortic, smoking and, 277
  atherosclerotic, 489–490
    of basilar artery, 1435, 1435f
  cerebral artery, 490
  Charcot-Bouchard, 1436, 1437f
  dissecting, 490–491, 490f
    coronary artery involvement in, 518
  gross appearance of, 489
  location of, 488–489, 488f
  luetic, 489, 489f
  mycotic, 490, 1436
  saccular or berry, 490, 1435, 1435f
  syphilitic, 489, 489f
  types of, 1437f
  ventricular, true and false, 523–524, 525f
Angina:
  abdominal, 672
  intestinal, 672
  preinfarction, 515
  Prinzmetal's, 515, 516
  unstable, 515
  variant, 515
  Vincent's, 1292
Angina pectoris, 471, 515
Angiodysplasia, colon in, 701
Angioedema, 1229–1230

Angiofibroma, juvenile, of nasopharynx,
       1292–1293, 1293
Angiogenesis, 455
Angiogenesis factor, 77, 455
  in wound healing, 79, 82f
Angioid streaks, ocular, 1529
Angioimmunoblastic lymphadenopathy,
       1062
Angiolipoma, 1390
Angioma, 493, 1257
Angiomyolipoma, of kidney, 887–888
Angiosarcoma, 1391
  of liver, 494
Angiostrongyliasis, 438
Angiostrongylus cantonensis, 438
Angiotensin-converting enzyme, 43
Aniline dyes, 639
Anisakiasis, 439–440
Anitschkow cells, 527, 527f
Ankylosing spondylitis, 1381, 1381f
Anlagen, 1310–1311
Anoplura, 448
Anorectal disorders. *See* Anal canal
Anorexia, in cancer, 185
Anorexia nervosa, 1130–1131
Anovulatory bleeding, 962
Anterior chamber, hemorrhage of, 1509
Anthracosilicosis, 604
Anthracosis, 13
Anthrax, 358
  gastrointestinal, 358
  pulmonary, 358
Antibody:
  anticentromere, 136
  anti-HAV, 740
  antinuclear. *See* Antinuclear antibody
  cytotropic, 105
  heterophile, 338
Antibody-dependent, cell-mediated cyto
       toxicity, 107–109
Anti-D immunoglobulin, 246
Anti-diuretic hormone, inappropriate pro-
       duction of, 185
Antigen:
  carcinoembryonic, 151
  factor VIII-related, 151
  human leukocyte (HLA), 102, 131–132
  prostate-specific, 151
  tumor-associated, 183
Antiglomerular basement membrane dis-
       ease, 582, 857, 858f–859f
Antinuclear antibody:
  in mixed connective tissue disease, 138
  in scleroderma, 136
  in Sjögren's disease, 135
  in systemic lupus erythematosus, 131,
       132
Antioxidant defense mechanisms, 21f
α$_1$-Antiprotease, 55
Antiribonucleoprotein antibody:
  in mixed connective tissue disease, 138
  in polymyositis/dermatomyositis, 137
α$_1$-Antitrypsin deficiency, 595
  cirrhosis in, 774–775, 775f
  peptic ulcer disease in, 653
Ants, 448–449
Anus. *See* Anal canal
Aorta:
  aneurysm of, smoking and, 277
  coarctation of, 512, 513f

Aorta:
  dissecting aneurysm of:
    abdominal, 490f
    coronary artery involvement in, 518
  function of, 253
  infantile (tubular) coarctation of, 512,
       513f
  in Marfan's syndrome, 222
  postductal (adult) coarctation of, 512,
       513f
  tubular hypoplastic, 512
Aortic arch:
  derivatives of, 510f
  right, 509
Aortic stenosis, 513–514
  subvalvular, 513
  supravalvular, 513
  valvular, 513
Aortic stenosis syndrome, supravalvular,
       513
Aortic valve, in bacterial endocarditis,
       534, 535f
Aortitis, luetic, 355, 355f, 456, 489, 489f,
       518, 540
Aortopulmonary window, 509
Apatite arthropathy, 1385
Apgar score, 240t
Aphthous stomatitis, 1263
Aphthous ulcer, 386
Aplasia, in morphogenesis, 201
Aplastic crisis, 1037, 1044
Apolipoproteins, 467t
Apoptosis, 15
Appendices epiploicae, 686
Appendicitis, 714–715
  acute, 714–715, 715f
  chronic, 715
  tuberculous, 715
Appendix, **714–717**
  mucocele of, 715–716, 715f
  tumors of, 716
  vermiform, 686
Appropriate for gestational age infant, 238
APUD system, 824–825, 1120
Aqueous humor, common disorders of,
       1527–1528
Arachidonic acid metabolism, 47–48, 48f
Arachnids, 447–448
Arachnodactyly, in Marfan's syndrome,
       222, 222f
Arboviruses, 332
Arcus lipoides, 1525
Argentaffin cells, 641
Argentine hemorrhagic fever, 331
Arginine vasopressin:
  inappropriate production of, in cancer,
       185
  production of, 1123
Arginine vasotocin, 1161
Argyrophil cells, gastric, 641
Arhinencephaly, 1462
Arias-Stella reaction, 961
Armanni-Epstein phenomenon, 1522
Arnold-Chiari malformation, 1460–1461,
       1460f–1461f
Arrhythmia:
  in drug reaction, 290
  in myocardial infarction, 523
Arsenic, 299
Arteriohepatic dysplasia, 792

Arterioles, 457
  in hypertension, 480, 480f
  vasoconstriction or vasodilatation, 37
Arteriolosclerosis, 481, 481f
  benign, 481
  in diabetes mellitus, 1174
  hyaline, 481
  malignant, 481
  onion-skin appearance in, 481, 481f
Arteriosclerosis, 481
  benign, 481
  malignant, 481
Arteriovenous malformation, 1390–1391
  in brain, 1436, 1438f
Arteritis:
  coronary, 518
  giant cell, 483–484, 484f
  temporal, 483–484, 484f
Artery(ies). *See also individual types, e.g.*
      Coronary artery
  elastic, 455
  embolism of, 267–268, 268f
  endoreplication of smooth muscle cells
      of, 455, 457f
  fibrinoid necrosis in, 16, 18f
  muscular, 456, 457, 480, 480f
  resistance, 457
  structure of, 455–459, 457f
  total occlusion of, 256
  transposition of, 511–512, 512f
Arthritis:
  gouty, 1382, 1384, 1384f
  rheumatoid, **1374–1381**. *See also* Rheu-
      matoid arthritis
  septic, staphylococcal, 383
  tuberculous, 1334–1335, 1334f
Arthrogryposis, 1368
Arthropathy:
  apatite, 1385
  in hemochromatosis, 771
Arthropod disease, **447–449**, 447t
Arthus reaction, 111–113, 112f
Arytenoid cartilage, 544
Asbestos, in carcinogenesis, 168–169
Asbestos bodies, 604, 604f, 605
Asbestos bronchiolitis, 604
Asbestosis, 604
Asbestos pneumoconiosis, 601f, 604–605,
      604f
Ascariasis, 439, 439f
  of liver, 789
Ascaris lumbricoides, 439, 439f
Aschoff body, 527, 527f
Ascites, 265
  in portal hypertension, 781–782, 781f
Ascorbic acid deficiency, 322–323, 323f
Asherman's syndrome, 963
Ash-Upmark kidney, 837
Aspergilloma, 422
Aspergillosis, 422–423
  acute, 422
  allergic bronchopulmonary, 422–423,
      550–551
  of lung, 574, 575f
  of nose, 1287
  rhinocerebral, 1287
Aspergillus fumigatus, 422
Aspergillus niger, 422
Aspiration, amniotic fluid, 238, 238f
Aspirin:
  platelet effects of, 1029

Aspirin:
  Reye's syndrome and, 784
Asplenia, 1064
Asplenia syndrome, 510
Asterixis, 735
Asteroid body, 427, 427f
Asthma, **587–591**
  antigen-induced, 587, 589
  in drug reaction, 290, 291f, 587
  exercise-induced, 589
  hidden, 589
  hypersensitivity reaction in, 590
  occupation-related substances in, 587
  pathogenesis of, 587–589, 588f, 590
  pathology of, 589–590, 590f
  pollution-related, 587
  status asthmaticus in, 589, 590f
  viral respiratory infection in, 587
Asthmatic bronchitis, 589
Astrocytes, in hepatic encephalopathy,
      736
Astrocytoma, 1469–1470, 1470f–1471f
  anaplastic, 1470
  fibrillary, 1469
  juvenile pilocytic, 1469
Atelectasis, 551–552
Atheroma, 463–465, 464f
Atherosclerosis, **459–471**
  aneurysm in, 489–490, 1435, 1435f
  of brain, 1434–1435, 1435f
  characteristic lesion of, 463–465, 464f
  complicated lesions of, 465
  of coronary artery, 476, 476f, 516, 517f
  in diabetes mellitus, 1172–1174
  encrustation hypothesis of, 460
  fatty streak of, 461–462, 464f
  genetic factors in, 470–471
  in hypertension, 481
  initial lesion of, 461–463, 464f
  insudation hypothesis of, 460
  intimal cell mass hypothesis of, 461, 463
  mechanisms of lesion progression in,
      465–466, 465f–467f
  monoclonal hypothesis of, 461
  in muscular arteries, 456
  obesity and, 315
  pathology of, 460–461
  reaction to injury hypothesis of, 460–
      461
  risk factors for, 466
  sites of, 477f
  smoking and, 277
  unifying hypothesis of, 461, 462f
  viruses and, 471
ATPase reaction, for muscle, 1397
Atresia, in morphogenesis, 201
Atrial natriuretic factor, 259–261, 478
Atrial septal defect, 506–507, 508f
  ostium primum, 507
  ostium secundum, 507
Atrioventricular canal, persistent com-
      mon, 507
Atrioventricularis communis, 507
Atrioventricular node, congenital polycys-
      tic tumors of, 541
Atrioventricular septal defect, 507
Atrophie blanche, 486
Atrophy, **6–9**
Auer rods, 1075, 1075f
Autoantibodies:
  nucleolar, in scleroderma, 136

Autoantibodies:
  in primary biliary cirrhosis, 763
  regulated production of, 129
  in type II hypersensitivity reactions,
      109, 109f
Autocrine activity, 1120
Autoimmune disease, **129–138**. *See also in-
      dividual diseases*
  hepatitis, 738–751
  hypersensitivity reactions in, 130–131,
      131t
  mechanisms of, 129–130, 130t
  mixed connective tissue disease, 138
  polymyositis/dermatomyositis, 137–138
  primary biliary cirrhosis as, 763–764
  progressive systemic sclerosis, 136–137
  Sjögren's, 135–136
  systemic lupus erythematosus, 131–135
  thyroiditis, 1137–1139
  tissue injury in, 130–131, 131t
  type I diabetes, 1116–1168
Autonomic nerve dysfunction, in diabetes
      mellitus, 1175
Autosomal dominant inheritance, 220, 220f
Autosomal recessive inheritance, 224, 224f
Autosplenectomy, 1044
Axial regeneration, 68
Axonal degeneration, 1491, 1491f
Axonal regeneration, 94
Axonopathy, distal, 1491, 1491f
Azo dyes, in carcinogenesis, 163

Babesiosis, 413
Babinski-Fröhlich's syndrome, 1124
Backwash ileitis, 686, 697
Bacteremia:
  in AIDS, 450
  in tuberculosis, 571
Bacteria:
  complement system activation by, 46
  opsonization of, 46
Bacterial diseases, **358–392**. *See also indi-
      vidual types*
Bacterial endotoxin, in septic shock, 269–
      270
Bacterial infection, filamentous, 392–394,
      393f
Balanoposthitis, 938
Balantidiasis, 418
Balantidium coli, 418
Baldness, male pattern, 1204–1205
Bancroftian filariasis, 431–432
Band keratopathy, 1525
Bantu siderosis, 769
Barr body, 217, 233
Barrett's epithelium, 635
Bartholin's gland:
  abscess of, 950
  cyst of, 950
Bartonella bacilliformis, 379–380
Bartonellosis, 379–380
Basal cell carcinoma, 144
  of skin, 1256, 1256f
Basal cell epithelioma, 144
Basedow's disease, 1134–1137
Basement membrane, 72–73, 72f, 73t
  alveolar, in wound healing, 93–94
  capillary, in diabetes mellitus, 486–487,
      487f, 1174

Basement membrane:
  composition of, 73, 73t
  of epidermis, 1201–1203, 1202f–1203f
  function of, 73
  glomerular, 72, 72f, 834–836, 835f–837f
    anatomy of, 834, 835f
    disease of, 857, 858f–859f
  retinal capillary, 1518–1521
  of skin, diseases of, 1215–1229
  in tumor invasion, 153–155, 154f
Basilar artery, atherosclerotic aneurysm
    of, 1435, 1435f
Basophilia, 1051, 1051t
Basophils:
  function of, 40–42
  hyaline, 1128
B cell differentiation factor, 100t
B cell growth factor, 100t
B cells, 100–101
  in autoimmune disease, 130
  ontogeny of, cell markers for, 1023t
  in systemic lupus erythematosus, 132
Bedbugs, 448
Bees, 448–449
Beetles, 448
Behçet's disease, 486
Bejel, 356–357
Benzene, 295–296
Berger's disease, 862, 863t
Beriberi, 319
Beriberi heart disease, 537
Bernard-Soulier syndrome, 1029
Berry aneurysm, 490, 1435, 1435f–1436f
Berylliosis, 605
Beta cell, pancreatic, 822f, 823
Beta cell tumors, 826f–827f, 827
Bezoar, 662, 662f
Bile:
  impairment of flow of, 732–734, 820. See
      also Cholestasis
  secretion of, 725
  white, 767
Bile acid:
  in intestinal absorption, 672
  in malabsorption, 672–673
Bile duct:
  carcinoma of, 169, 796–797, 797f, 806
  common, 724
  congenital dilatation of, 800f, 801
  microhamartoma of, 794
Bile infarct, 734, 735f
Bile lake, 734, 735f, 767
Bile peritonitis, 720, 804
Bilharziasis, 440–441, 440f
Biliary atresia, of neonate, 791–792
Biliary cirrhosis, primary, 760–764. See also
      Cirrhosis, primary biliary
Biliary colic, 801
Biliary concretions, 767, 767f
Biliary nephrosis, 737
Biliary obstruction, extrahepatic, 766–767,
      766f–767f
Bilirubin, 727
Bilirubin metabolism, 727–732
  decreased conjugation in, 728–730
  decreased transport of conjugated bili-
      rubin in, 730–732
  decreased uptake in, 728
  normal, 727
  overproduction, 727, 728, 729f
Birbeck granules, 1200f, 1201

Birth defects, 198, 198f
Birth injury, 246–247
Birth weight, maternal smoking and, 280–
    281, 282f
Bittner milk factor, 170
Bittner virus, 170
BK virus, 171
Black lung, 13, 595
Blackwater fever, 409
Black widow spider, 447
Bladder. See Urinary bladder
Blast cells, 1017, 1022
Blastema, 68
Blastoma, 248
  of lung, 559
Blastomere:
  exogenous toxins and, 200–201
  incomplete separation of, 201
Blastomyces dermatitidis, 423, 423f, 574
Blastomycosis, 420f–421f, 423, 423f
  of lung, 574
Bleeding time, 1026t
Blennorrhea, inclusion, 1503
Bleomycin, alveolar damage due to, 581
Blepharitis, 1504
Blister beetles, 448
Blood, 1014–1117. *See also individual compo-
    nents*
  cellular components of, 38f
  fecal occult, 712
  normal CBC values for, 1030, 1031t
Blood flow:
  regulation of, 253
  velocity of, vascular cross-section and,
      458f
Blood group A, in carcinoma of stomach,
    657
Blood group O, in peptic ulcer disease,
    650
Blood group system, Rh, 243, 245
Blood islands, embryonic, 455, 456f
Blood pressure. *See also* Hypertension
  ischemic heart disease due to decrease
      in, 518
  oxygen demand and, 518
  structural autoregulation of, 480f
Blood vessels. *See individual types;* Vascu-
      lature
Blood volume, effective vs total, 258–259
Blowout fracture, 1507
Blue bloater, 598
Blue-domed cyst, 999, 1002f
Boerhaave's syndrome, 637
Boils, 382
Bolivian hemorrhagic fever, 331
Bombesin, 1122
Bone, 1304–1365
  abscess of, staphylococcal, 383
  anatomy of, 1305f
  blood supply of, 1307
  calcium metabolism in, 1338
  cells of, 1308–1310
  circumferential, 1310
  coarse cancellous, 1306
  concentric lamellar, 1310
  cortical, 1306
  cortical lamellar, 1310, 1311f
  cyst, solitary, 1354–1357, 1356f
  disorders of growth and maturation of,
      1315–1323
  embryonic formation of, 1310–1311

Bone:
  fibrous dysplasia of, 1362–1365, 1366f
  formation and growth of, 1310–1315
  fracture of, 1323–1326
  functions of, 1306
  in Gaucher's disease, 1349, 1350f
  histiocytosis of, 1336–1338
  infections of, 1329–1338
  interstitial lamellar, 1310
  lamellar, 1309, 1310f
  lead poisoning signs in, 297
  metabolic disease of, 1340–1350, 1341f
  microscopic organization of, 1309–1310,
      1310f–1311f
  mineralized matrix of, 1307–1308
  modeling abnormalities of, 1320
  neoplasms of, **1354–1362**
    benign, 1354–1357
    malignant, 1357–1361
    metastatic, 1361–1362
  as organ, 1306–1307
  organic matrix of, 1308
  phosphate metabolism in, 1338–1339
  reactive formation of, 1328–1329
  remodeling of, 1339
  resorption of, subperiosteal, 1347
  subchondral cyst of, 1372, 1374f
  syphilis of, 1335–1336, 1335f
  as tissue, 1307–1308
  trabecular lamellar, 1310
  tuberculosis of, 1334–1335, 1334f
  Wolff's law of, 1308
  woven, 1309, 1310f
Bone marrow:
  in acute lymphoblastic leukemia, 1078f,
      1090
  anatomy of, 1306–1307
  in chronic lymphocytic leukemia, 1078f,
      1083–1086
  examination of, 1017–1018, 1017t–1018t
  function of, 1016–1017
  grey or white, 1306–1307
  in hairy cell leukemia, 1078f, 1088
  in hematologic disease, 1078f
  lymphoid hyperplasia of, 1055–1056
  metastatic tumors of, 1114–1115
  in multiple myeloma, 1078f, 1106
  in myeloproliferative syndrome, 1067,
      1068f
  normal adult, 1017t
  plasmacytosis in, 1056
  red, 1016, 1306–1307
  structure of, 1016
  in visceral leishmaniasis, 408, 408f
  yellow, 1016, 1306–1307
Bone marrow embolism, 620
Bone plate, subchondral, 1370
Botryomycosis, 383
Botulism, 374f–375f, 376
Bourneville's disease, 1476–1477, 1477f
Bowenoid papulosis, 938–939
Bowen's disease, 938–939
Box-jellies, 450
Bradykinin, 42–43, 44f
Brain:
  abscess of, 1446–1447, 1448f–1449f
    amebic, 416–417
    in drug addiction, 287, 289f
  in alcoholism, 286
  in amebic meningoencephalitis, 417
  anatomy of, 1417f

Brain:
  arteriovenous malformations of, 1436, 1438f
  atherosclerosis of, 1434–1435, 1435f
  in blastomycosis, 423f
  cavernous angioma of, 1436
  cryptococcosis in, 426
  cysticercosis of, 446–447, 447f
  edema of, 261
  global ischemia vs hypoxia of, 1432f–1434f, 1433
  in Hartmannella-acanthameba meningoencephalitis, 417–418
  hypertensive hemorrhage of, 1436–1438, 1438f
  infarct of, 257, 1427–1431, 1429f–1431f
  liquefactive necrosis of, 15
  in malaria, 409, 411f–412f
  in premature infant, 239
  in shock, 273
  spongiform degeneration of, 1456, 1457f
  subacute combined degeneration of, 1480
  in toxoplasmosis, 413, 413f, 1441, 1441f
  tumor of, 1467–1477. *See also* Central nervous system, neoplasia of
Brain capillaries, permeability of, 459
Brain stem, astrocytoma of, 1470f
Branchial cleft cyst, 1262, 1262f, 1263f
Brazilian pemphigus foliaceous, 1216t
Breast, **990–1013**
  abscess of, 383, 997
  adenocarcinoma of, scirrhous, 146, 146f
  anatomy of, 991f–995f, 992–996
  carcinoma of, **1004–1011**. *See also* Breast cancer
  congenital anomalies of, 996
  cystic atrophy of, 995
  duct ectasia of, 997
  elastosis of, 995
  embryology of, 991f, 992
  fat necrosis of, 997–998
  fibroadenoma of, 1000, 1003f
  fibrocystic disease of, 998–999, 1000f–1002f
    adenosis in, 999, 1001f
    apocrine metaplasia in, 998–999, 1001f
    blue-domed cysts in, 999, 1002f
    carcinoma risks in, 999, 1004t
    ductal epithelial hyperplasia in, 999, 1001f
    etiology of, 999–1000
    histology of, 999, 1002f
    lobular hyperplasia in, 999, 1001f
    morphology of, 998–999, 1000f–1002f
    sclerosing adenosis in, 999, 1001f
  intraductal papilloma of, 1004
  juvenile hypertrophy of, 996
  juvenile papillomatosis of, 999
  lactating adenoma of, 1000
  in lactation, 995
  lymphatic drainage of, 996
  malignant lymphoma of, 1012
  in menopause, 995
  menstrual effects on, 992–995
  morphology of, 992–996
    female, 992–995, 993f–995f
    male, 996
  neonatal hypertrophy of, 996
  nipple of, 996
  non-neoplastic disease of, 996–998

Breast:
  parenchyma of, 992
  peau d'orange skin of, 1010, 1011
  phyllodes tumor of, 1011–1012, 1012f
  in pregnancy, 995
  at puberty, 992
  radiation effects on, 998
  supernumerary, 996
  tubular adenoma of, 1000
Breast cancer, **1004–1011**
  carcinoma in situ, 1005–1007, 1006f
  classification of, 1005t
  comedocarcinoma, 1005–1007
  epidemiology of, 1004–1005
  geographic and ethnic factors in, 193
  histologic prognostic features of, 1010–1011, 1010t
  inflammatory, 1010
  intraductal, 1005, 1006f
  invasive, 1007–1009, 1007f–1009f, 1007t
  lobular carcinoma, 1005, 1006f
  in male, 1010
  metaplastic, 1010
  metastasis from, 1011
  morphology of, 1005–1010
  mucinous, 1009
  risk factors for, 1004, 1004t
  scirrhous carcinoma, 1007, 1007f
  signet ring, 1009
  staging of, 1010–1011
  treatment of, 1011
  tubular, 1009–1010
  well-differentiated, 1009–1010
Brenner tumor, 977
Brill-Zinsser disease, 350
Brodie's abscess, 1333
Bromobenzene, hepatocellular necrosis due to, 26–27
Bronchi:
  anatomy of, 542f–543f, 545
  atresia of, 550
  fungal infections of, 550–551
  gaseous irritants of, 551
  obstruction and aspiration in, 551–553
  viral infections of, 550
Bronchial epithelium, squamous metaplasia of, 11, 13f
Bronchiectasis, 591–593, 592f
  cylindrical, 592
  post-infective, 592
  saccular, 592
  varicose, 592, 592f
Bronchioloalveolar tumors, 557–559
Bronchioles:
  anatomy of, 542f–543f, 545
  terminal, 545
Bronchiolitis, 550, 591
  asbestos and, 604
  mild chronic airflow obstruction in, 591
  rheumatoid arthritis and, 591
  severe chronic airflow obstruction in, 591
  toxic gases causing, 591
Bronchiolitis obliterans, 610
Bronchitis:
  asthmatic, 589
  chronic, 585–587, 586f
Bronchoalveolar tumor, intravascular, 627
Bronchocentric granulomatosis, of lung, 615
Bronchogenic carcinoma. *See* Lung cancer

Bronchogenic cyst, 563
Bronchopleural fistula, 568, 615–616
Bronchopneumonia, 566, 568f
Bronchopulmonary aspergillosis, allergic, 422–423, 550–551
Bronchopulmonary dysplasia, 243
Bronchopulmonary foregut malformation, 631
Bronchovascular bundle, 546
Bronze diabetes, 771
Brown recluse spider, 447–448
Brown tumors, 1146, 1147f, 1347, 1347f, 1348, 1348f
Brucellosis, 371–372
Brugia malayi, 431–432
Brunner's glands, 663
Brunn's buds, 894
Brunn's nests, 894
Bruton's agammaglobulinemia, 122–123, 124f
Bruton's X-linked infantile hypogammaglobulinemia, 122–123, 124f
Budd-Chiari syndrome, 778–779, 779f
Buerger's disease, 278, 485–486, 485f
Bullous congenital ichthyosiform erythroderma, 1206–1207, 1206t, 1207f–1208f
Bullous pemphigoid, 1219–1220, 1220f–1221f
  blister formation in, 1221f
  definition and clinical features of, 1219
  etiology and pathogenesis of, 1219–1220, 1221f
  pathology of, 1219, 1220f
Bundle of His, 500
Bundle of Kent, 500
Burkitt's lymphoma, 248, 1084f–1085f, 1104
  chromosomal translocation in, 175, 177f
  Epstein-Barr virus in, 171, 339f
  geographic and ethnic factors in, 194
  maxilla and mandible in, 340f
  in migrant populations, 194
  of oral cavity, 1268–1269
Burns, 303–304, 304f
  electrical, 304, 305f
  staphylococcal infection of, 383
Buruli ulcer, 401
Butler-Albright syndrome, 1345
Butterfly rash, 132, 1223
Byler's disease, 731–732

C1 esterase inhibitor, 46
C1 INA deficiency, 46
C2 deficiency, 46
C3a:
  biologic activity of, 45, 46f
  formation of, 44, 45
  regulation of, 46
C4a, biologic activity of, 45, 46f
C4b binding protein, 46
C5a:
  biologic activity of, 45, 46f
  formation of, 44, 45
  regulation of, 46
Cachectin, 185
Cachexia, in cancer, 185
Cadmium, 299

Calcification, 27–29
dystrophic, 27–29, 1328–1329
heterotopic, 1328
of lung, 577
metastatic, 29, 1328
in stone formation, 29
zone of, 1312–1314
Calcium:
concentration gradient of, 16
dental caries and, 1271
deposits, in coagulative necrosis, 16–17, 19f
intracellular:
in inflammatory cell activation, 49
in ischemia, 19–20
metabolism of, 1338
Calcium pyrophosphate deposition disease, 1385
California encephalitis, 332–333
Call-Exner bodies, 977–978, 978f
Calymmatobacterium granulomatis, 380, 380f, 945
cAMP:
in inflammatory cell modulation, 52–54, 52f
in tumor growth, 159
Campylobacter enteritis, 369–370
Campylobacter fetus, 370
Campylobacter gastroenteritis, 667–668
Camurati-Engelmann disease, 1320
Cancer. *See also individual types;* Carcinogenesis; Tumor, malignant
in alcoholism, 286
amyloidosis in, 188
anorexia and weight loss in, 185
causes of, **159–181**. *See also* Carcinogenesis
cutaneous syndromes in, 188
dysplasia and, 12–13
endocrine syndromes due to, 185–186
epidemiology of, 140f, **190–195**
age as factor in, 190, 192f
criteria in, 190
ethnic factors in, 192–194
geographic factors in, 192–194
in migrant populations, 194–195
in United States, 190, 191f–192f, 192t
excessive iron storage and, 14
fever in, 185
gastrointestinal syndromes in, 187
genetic basis of, 173
grading and staging of, 156–157, 156f
hematologic syndromes in, 187
heredity and, 188–190, 189t
host effects of, **184–188**
hypercoagulability in, 187
neurologic syndromes in, 186–187
in oral contraceptive use, 292
due to radiation, 310–314
renal syndromes in, 188
smoking and, 278–279, 278f–279f
Cancer cell, biochemistry of, 157
Cancrum oris, 381, 382f
Candida albicans, 424–425
Candidiasis, 424–425
of bronchi, 551
of endocardium, 424–425
of esophagus, 636
of lung, 575
mucocutaneous, 123, 424

Candidiasis:
of nose, 1286
of oral cavity, 424, 1265
of skin, 424
of small intestine, 669
systemic, 424
of vagina, 424, 949
Canker sores, 1263
Canthariasis, 448
Capillaria hepatica, 434
Capillaria philippinensis, 434
Capillariasis, 434
Capillaries, 457
basement membrane of, in diabetes mellitus, 486–487, 487f, 1174
of brain, 459
endothelium of, 457–459
fenestrated, 459
of heart, 250f
permeability of, 459
proliferation of, in wound healing, 79, 82f
Capillary hemangioma, 493, 1390, 1391f
Capillary lymphangioma, 495
Caplan's syndrome, 603
Caput medusae, in portal hypertension, 780
Carbon monoxide poisoning, 518
Carbon tetrachloride, 295
hepatocellular necrosis due to, 25–26, 27f
Carboxypeptidase N, 43
Carbuncles, 382, 383
Carcinoembryonic antigen, 151
in carcinoma of stomach, 661
in colorectal cancer, 712
Carcinogenesis, **159–181**
altered differentiation in, 180–181
chemical, **160–167**
factors influencing, 163–164
initiation and promotion of, 160, 161f
metabolic activation in, 160–163, 162f
multiple steps in, 164–167, 166f
mutagenicity assay (Ames test) in, 164, 165f
chromosomal alterations and, 175–177
chromosomal translocations in, 212
physical, 167–169
asbestos in, 168–169
foreign body in, 169
ultraviolet radiation in, 167–168
x-irradiation in, 167, 314
viral, **169–175**
adenoviruses in, 173
DNA viruses in, 170–173, 172f
hepatitis B virus in, 171–173
herpesviruses in, 171, 339f
historical overview of, 169–170
papillomaviruses in, 170–171
polyomaviruses in, 171
poxviruses in, 173
RNA viruses (retroviruses) in, 173–175, 174f
Carcinoid heart disease, 537–538
Carcinoid syndrome, 684
Carcinoid tumor:
of colon, 712
of lung, 559, 560f
of pancreas, 828
of small intestine, 683–684, 685f
of stomach, 661

Carcinoma. *See also individual types, e.g.,* Squamous cell carcinoma
of adrenal cortex, 1153–1154
of ampulla of Vater, 806
of anal canal, 712–713
basal cell, 144, 1256, 1256f
of bile duct, 169, 796–797, 797f, 806
of breast, **1004–1011**. *See also* Breast cancer
bronchogenic. *See* Lung cancer
of cervix:
herpes simplex type 2 and, 171
human papillomavirus, 957–958
in situ, 957–959, 958f, 959t
verrucous, 959
cholangiocellular, 441
cholangiohepatocellular, 797
of colon and rectum. *See* Colorectal cancer
electron microscopy in, 149, 149f
of endometrium, 316, 965
epidermoid. *See* Squamous cell carcinoma
of esophagus, **637–640**, 639f. *See also* Esophagus, carcinoma of
geographic and ethnic factors in, 193
due to smoking, 278–279
of gallbladder, 806, 806f
of larynx, 278
of liver, **794–796**, 796f. *See also* Hepatocellular carcinoma
of lung. *See* Lung cancer
of nasal cavity and paranasal sinuses, 1289, 1290f
of nasopharynx, 1293–1294, 1294f
Epstein-Barr virus in, 171, 339f
geographic and ethnic factors in, 193
of oral cavity, 278
in situ, 1267
of ovary, 975–977, 977t
of pancreas, exocrine, 819–821
of parathyroid, 1148–1149
of penis, verrucous, 939
of prostate, 193, 937
renal cell, 888–889, 888f–889f
of renal pelvis, 889, 895–896
of salivary glands, 1280–1282
of skin, 193, 1256, 1256f
of stomach, **656–661**. *See also* Stomach, carcinoma of
of testicle, 193, 919, 919f
of thyroid, 1141–1144
transitional cell, 144
of ureter, 895–896, 896f
of urethra, male, 911
of urinary bladder:
geographic and ethnic factors in, 193–194
in situ, 905, 906f
papillary transitional cell, 905–907, 907f
due to parasitic infestation, 169
due to smoking, 279
of vulva:
in situ, 951, 951t
verrucous, 952
Carcinomatosis, of peritoneum, 151, 152f, 977
Carcinosarcoma, 144
of lung, 559
Cardiac cirrhosis, 254, 503, 531, 787

Cardiac fibrosis, of liver, 787
Cardiac glands, 641
Cardiac output, 252
    ischemic heart disease due to, 518
    oxygen demand and, 518
Cardiogenic shock, 269, 523
Cardiomyopathy, 539
    alcoholic, 285, 539
    in Chagas's disease, 403
    congestive, 539
    hypertrophic, 539
    restrictive, 539
Cardiospasm, 632
Caries, dental, 1270–1271, 1272f
Carnitine deficiency, 1411
Carnitine palmityl transferase deficiency, 1411
Caroli's disease, 800f, 801
Carotid artery aneurysm, 1435, 1435f, 1436f
Carotid body tumor, 1157
Carpal tunnel syndrome, 1493t, 1494
Cartilage:
    articular, 1369–1371, 1369f
        calcified zone of, 1369f, 1370
        chemical characteristics of, 1370–1371
        histologic characteristics of, 1369–1370, 1369f
        radial zone of, 1369–1370, 1369f
        tangential or gliding zone of, 1369, 1369f
        transitional zone of, 1369, 1369f
    asymmetric growth of, 1317–1318
    delayed or disorganized maturation of, 1315
    elastic, 1314–1315
    growth and development of, 1314–1315
    hyaline, 1314
Caruncle, of urethra, 910, 910f
Caseous necrosis, 16, 17f
Castleman's lesion, 1060–1061
Catagen hairs, 1204–1205
Cataract, 1525–1527, 1525f
    due to radiation injury, 310
    senile, 1523, 1527
    snowflake, 1523
    sunflower, in Wilson's disease, 773
    in TORCH complex, 208
Cathartic colon, 713
Cathepsin G, 54, 55
Cat scratch disease, 392, 392f
Cavernous angioma, 1436
Cavernous hemangioma, 493, 1390
Cavernous lymphangioma, 495
Cavernous venous sinus, thrombophlebitis of, 1285
Ceelin's disease, 583
Celiac compression syndrome, 672
Celiac disease, 675–678, 676f–677f
    cereal proteins in, 675–676, 676f
    clinical features of, 677
    dermatitis herpetiformis and, 677
    epidemiology of, 675
    etiology and pathogenesis of, 675–677, 676f
    genetic and immunologic factors in, 676–677
    pathology of, 677–678, 677f
Cell cycle, 75, 76f
Cell injury, 2–33
    atrophy in, 6–9

Cell injury:
    chemical, 25–27, 27f
    chronic adaptation in, 6, 8f
    coagulative necrosis in, 15–27. *See also* Necrosis, coagulative
    dysplasia in, 12–13
    hydropic swelling as, 5, 5f–6f
    hyperplasia in, 10–11, 12f
    hypertrophy in, 9, 9f–11f
    ionizing radiation causing, 22–24, 25f, 307–308
    irreversible, **14–27**
    ischemic, 17–20
    metaplasia in, 11–12, 13f
    oxygen radicals causing, 20–22, 21f–24f
    persistent, 8–9
    in persistent stress, 5–6, 8f
    responses to, 4–5
    reversible, **5**
    ultrastructural changes in, 5, 6f–7f
    viruses in, 24–25, 26f
Cells. *See also individual cell types*
    labile, 75, 76f
    nutrient delivery and waste elimination in, 252
    permanent, 77
    proliferation of, 75–77
    stable, 76–77
    stem, 75–76
Cell-to-cell communication, 1120, 1121f
Cellular aging, 29–33
    developmental-genetic theories of, 32
    error theory of, 31–32
    functional and structural changes in, 30, 31f
    genetics and, 32f–33f, 33
    immunologic theory of, 32
    intrinsic mutagenesis theory of, 32
    lipid peroxidation in, 32–33
    neuroendocrine theories of, 32
    random event (stochastic) theories of, 31–32
    somatic mutation theory of, 31
Cellular atypia, 147
Cellular oncogene, 158, 159
Cellular space, 252
Cellular storage, 13–14
Centipedes, 449
Central core disease, 1405, 1407f
Central nervous system, **1418–1487**
    age group in diseases of, 1418
    in cancer, 186
    circulatory disorders of, 1427–1440
    congenital malformations of, 1457–1462
    degenerative disorders of, 1480–1490
    demyelinating diseases of, 1462–1467
    inflammatory disorders of, 1440–1457
    metabolic disorders of, 1477–1480
    neoplasia of, **1467–1477**
        deviation and behavior of, 1467–1468
        distribution of, 1467, 1468f
        from ectopic tissues, 1474–1475
        from embryonic structures, 1476
        genetic contributions to, 1476–1477
        location of, 1468–1469
        of mesenchymal origin, 1472–1474
        metastatic, 1475
        of neuroectodermal origin, 1468–1472
        symptoms of, 1469
        terminology of, 1467
    in radiation, 308, 309f

Central nervous system:
    tempo of diseases of, 1418
    topographic distribution of disease of, 1418
    trauma to, 1419–1427
    viral infections of, 1447–1450, 1450f
    wound healing in, 94
Central nuclear myopathy, 1406, 1407f
Cerebello-olivary degeneration of Holmes, 1485
Cerebellum:
    astrocytoma of, 1470f
    degeneration of, alcoholic, 286
    hemorrhage of, 1438, 1439f
Cerebral arteries, aneurysm of, 490
Cerebral capillaries, fat embolization of, 1432–1433, 1432f
Cerebral contusion, 1423–1425, 1424f
Cerebral edema, 261, 306
Cerebral infarct, 257, 259f, 1427–1431, 1429f–1431f
Cerebritis, 1446
Cerebrospinal fluid, 1438–1440, 1440f
Cerebrovascular disease, **1427–1434**
    of cerebral capillaries, 1432–1433, 1432f
    of cerebral veins, 1432f–1433f, 1433–1434
    of circle of Willis and branches, 1431–1432
    of large extracranial and intracranial vessels, 1427–1431, 1429f–1431f
    of parenchymal arteries and arterioles, 1432
Cerebrovasculosa, 1457, 1458f
Cervical lymph node hyperplasia, 1059
Cervicitis, 956
Cervix, **955–961**
    adenocarcinoma of, 959–961
    anatomy of, 955–956
    carcinoma of:
        herpes simplex type 2 and, 171
        human papillomavirus, 957–958
    connective tumors of, 957
    dysplasia and carcinoma in situ of, 957–959, 958f, 959t
    inflammatory disease of, 956
    intraepithelial neoplasia of, 957–959, 958f, 959t
    leiomyoma of, 957
    microglandular hyperplasia of, 956–957
    polyp of, 956
    squamous cell carcinoma of, 959, 959t, 960f
        geographic and ethnic factors in, 193
        microinvasive, 959
    transformation zone of, 956
    verrucous carcinoma of, 959
Cestode disease, **444–447**
Chagas' disease, 402–405, 402f–403f
    acute, 402f–403f, 403
    chronic, 403–405
    congenital, 403
Chagoma, 403
Chalazion, 1504
Chancre, syphilitic, 354
Chancroid, 365, 945
Charcot-Bouchard aneurysm, 1436, 1437f
Charcot-Leyden crystals, 589
Charcot-Marie-Tooth disease, 1495t
Charcot's joints, 356
Chediak-Higashi syndrome, 1015
Cheilitis, solar, 1269f

Cheilosis, 321, 321f
Chemicals, **293–300**
  accidental exposure to, 294–295
  agricultural, 296
  aromatic halogenated hydrocarbons, 296
  arsenic, 299
  cadmium, 299
  cyanide, 296–297
  iron, 299–300
  lead, 297–298, 298f
  mercury, 298–299
  metals, 297–300
  nickel, 299
  responses to, 294–300
  toxicity of, 293–294
  toxic vs hypersensitivity responses of, 294
  volatile organic solvents and vapors, 295–296
Chemodectoma, of middle ear, 1299, 1299f
Chemotactic factors, 48–50, 50f
Cherry red macula, 1529, 1530f
Chickenpox. *See* Varicella
Chief cells, 641
Chikungunya hemorrhagic fever, 330
Chilopoda, 449
Chlamydial infections, **346–349**
  genital, 348–349, 947
  inclusion conjunctivitis, 347
  lymphogranuloma venereum, 347–348, 348f
  psittacosis, 346–347
  trachoma, 347
Chlamydia trachomatis pneumonia, 566
Chloasma, in oral contraceptive use, 291
Chlorine, as respiratory irritant, 551
Chloroform, 295
Chloroma, in leukemia, 1077, 1081f
Chocolate cyst, 989
Cholangiocarcinoma, 796–797, 797f
Cholangiocellular carcinoma, 441
Cholangiohepatocellular carcinoma, 797
Cholangitis:
  ascending, 788
  chronic destructive, in primary biliary cirrhosis, 762, 763f
  sclerosing, primary, 805
Cholecystenteric fistula, 804
Cholecystitis:
  acalculous, 805
  acute, 804–805
  chronic, 805
  gangrenous, 804
Choledochal cyst, 800f, 801
Choledochal diverticulum, 800f, 801
Choledochocele, 800f, 801
Choledocholithiasis, 804
Cholelithiasis, **801–804**
  cholesterol stones in, 801–803, 802f
    pathogenesis of, 801–802, 802f
    risk factors in, 803
  clinical course of, 803–804
  complications of, 804
  in oral contraceptive use, 291
  pigment stones in, 803
Cholera, 366, 367f
  diarrhea in, 675
  pancreatic, 828
Cholestasis, **732–734**
  benign recurrent, 731

Cholestasis:
  canalicular properties in, 733
  cellular mechanisms of, 732–734
  chronic, 734
  definition of, 732
  extrahepatic, 732
  familial fatal intrahepatic, 731–732
  feathery degeneration in, 734
  intrahepatic, 732, 736f
  lobular distribution of, 732–733, 733f
  morphology of, 734
  in toxic necrosis of liver, 784–785
Cholestatic hepatitis, 748
Cholesteatoma, in otitis media, 1299
Cholesterol:
  in ischemic heart disease, 526
  transport pathways of, 467–470, 468f–469f
Cholesterol granuloma, in otitis media, 1297
Cholesterolosis, of gallbladder, 805
Chondroblastoma, 143, 1357, 1359f
Chondrocalcinosis, 1385
Chondrocytes, 1315
Chondroma, 143, 143f
Chondromalacia, of knee, 1371
Chondromatosis, synovial, 1386, 1387f
Chondrosarcoma, 144, 145f, 1359–1360, 1362f
Chordoma, of nasopharynx, 1294, 1295f
Chorioadenoma destruens, 987
Chorioamnionitis, 985
Choriocarcinoma, 981
  geographic and ethnic factors in, 193
  of testis, 918
Chorionic villus biopsy, 236
Choristoma, 143, 248
Choroid, in systemic disease, 1510t
Choroidoretinitis, in TORCH complex, 208
Choroid plexus, 1439
Chromogranin, 149
Chromomycosis, 428–429, 429f
Chromosomal alterations:
  anaphase lag as, 213
  autosomal aneuploidies as, 213
  autosomal monosomy as, 213
  autosomal trisomy as, 213–214
  in Burkitt's lymphoma, 175, 177f
  in carcinogenesis, 175–177, 177f
  causes of, 213–214
  central nervous system defects in, 1462
  deletion as, 212
  incidence of, 214t
  inversion as, 212
  isochromosomes as, 212
  mosaicism as, 214
  nomenclature of, 214
  nondisjunction as, 213
  numerical, 213–214, 213t
  reciprocal translocations in, 212
  rings as, 212
  Robertsonian translocations in, 212
  structural, 210–212, 211f
Chromosome:
  acrocentric, 210–211f
  banding of, 210
  metacentric, 210, 211f
  normal, 210
  Philadelphia, 175–177
  submetacentric, 210–211f

Chronic obstructive lung disease, 279, 280f
Churg-Strauss syndrome, 615
Chylothorax, 616
Cicatrization, 89
Cigarette smoking, **276–282**
  cancer due to, 278–279, 278f–279f
  cardiovascular disease due to, 277–278, 277f
  disease associated with, 275f
  in emphysema, 598, 599f
  in esophageal cancer, 638
  ischemic heart disease and, 526
  lung cancer and, 554
  morbidity and mortality statistics of, 276, 276f
  non-neoplastic disease due to, 279–280, 280f
  oxygen deprivation in, 518
  in pancreatic carcinoma, 820
  peptic ulcer disease due to, 279–280, 649–650
  in women, 280–282, 281f–283f
Circle of Willis, occlusion of, 1431–1432
Cirrhosis, **764–776**
  alcoholic, 284, 284f. *See also* Alcoholic liver disease
  in α₁-antitrypsin deficiency, 774–775, 775f
  cardiac, 254, 503, 531, 787
  in chronic active hepatitis, 751, 752f
  in cystic fibrosis, 774
  in duodenal ulcer disease, 651–652
  edema in, 261
  etiology of, 766, 766t
  in extrahepatic biliary obstruction, 766–767, 766f–767f
  in galactosemia, 775–776
  in glycogen storage disease, 775
  in hemochromatosis, **767–771**
  in hepatocellular carcinoma, 795
  in hepatolenticular degeneration, 772–774
  in hereditary fructose intolerance, 776
  Indian childhood, 776
  Laennec's, 764
  macronodular, 764–766, 765f
  mechanism of, 89, 92f
  micronodular, 761f, 764
  mixed, 764
  morphology of, 761f, 764–766, 765f
  in peptic ulcer disease, 651–652
  in portal hypertension, 777
  posthepatitic, 766
  primary biliary, **760–764**
    basic lesion of, 760
    clinical features of, 762
    complications of, 762
    duct lesion in, 762, 763f
    end-stage cirrhosis in, 762–763
    immunopathogenesis of, 763–764
    pathology of, 762–763, 763f
    scarring in, 762
  in tyrosinemia, 776
  in Wilson's disease, 772–774
Claudication, intermittent, 471
Clear cell adenocarcinoma:
  of ovary, 977
  of vagina, 248
Cleft palate, 235–236, 236f, 1367–1368
Cloaca, 1332

Clonorchiasis, 441, 443f
Clonorchis sinensis, 789–790
Clostridial disease, **372–377**, 374f–375f
  botulism, 376–377
  food poisoning, 373
  myonecrosis (gas gangrene), 373–374
  necrotizing enteritis, 373
  tetanus, 374–376
Clostridium difficile, 689
Clostridium perfringens, 373, 374f–375f, 668
"Cloudy swelling," cellular, 5
Coagulation, 474–476, 474f, 474f, 475t, **1024–
    1030**. *See also* Hemostasis
  in coronary artery occlusion, 476
  disseminated intravascular, 487–488,
      1028–1029, 1028f
    in cancer, 187
    in hepatorenal syndrome, 737
  extrinsic pathway of, 474, 474f, 1025–
      1026, 1025f
    in hepatorenal syndrome, 737–738
  intrinsic pathway of, 474, 474f, 1025–
      1026, 1025f
  screening tests of, 1026t
Coagulation cascade, 1025–1026, 1025f
Coagulation factors, disorders of, 1029–
    1030
Coagulative necrosis, 15–27. *See also under*
    Necrosis, coagulative
Coal pneumoconiosis, 601f, 603–604
Cobalt poisoning, 300
Coccidioides immitis, 420f–421f, 425–426,
    425f, 573
Coccidioidomycosis, 420f–421f, 425–426,
    425f, 573–574
Coccidiosis, 418–419
$^{14}CO_2$-cholyl-glycine breath test, 675
Codon, 219
Coin lesions, 395, 561–562, 562f
Cold abscess, 1334
Cold sore, 336, 337f
Coleoptera, 448
Colic, lead, 297
Colitis:
  amebic, 414–417, 415f–416f
  ischemic, 700–701
  ulcerative, **694–700**
    appendicitis in, 715
    clinical features of, 695–697
    colon cancer and, 698
    colorectal cancer and, 710
    crypt abscess in, 698
    differential diagnosis of, 700
    epidemiology of, 695
    epithelial dysplasia in, 698–699, 699f
    etiology and pathogenesis of, 695
    extraintestinal manifestations of, 696f,
        697
    inflammatory polyps in, 698, 699f
    microscopic features of, 698, 699f
    mild, 697
    moderate, 697
    pathology of, 697–698, 698f–699f
    severe or fulminant, 697
    treatment of, 700
Collagen, **69–72**
  assembly of, 67f, 71
  biosynthesis of, 67f, 70–71
  catabolism of, 71
  composition and distribution of, 69, 69t
  genetic types of, 69–70, 69t, 70f

Collagen:
  gross structure of, in various organs,
      220
  metabolism of, heritable diseases of,
      220–223, 221f
  morphology and function of, 71–72
  secretion of, 67f
  in wound healing, 79
Collagenase:
  actions of, 71
  synthesis and secretion of, 71
  type IV, tumor production of, 155
  in wound healing, 79
Collagen bundles, 71
Collagen fibers, 71
Collagen fibrils, 71
Collagen type I, 69
Collagen type II, 69, 1370–1371
Collagen type III, 69
Collagen type IV, 70, 73, 73t
Collagen type V, 70
Collagen type VI, 70
Collateral blood vessels, of coronary ar-
      tery, 516–518
Colloid cyst, intracranial, 1476
Colon, **686–714**
  adenocarcinoma of, 151, 151f
  anatomy of, 686–687
  in angiodysplasia, 701
  bacterial flora of, 666
  benign tumors of, 702–709
  bleeding in, 716f
  carcinoid tumor of, 712
  carcinoma of. *See* Colorectal cancer
  cathartic, 713
  congenital disorders of, 687–688
  diverticulosis of, 689–691, 691f
  endometriosis of, 713
  histologic anatomy of, 686
  infarct of, 257–258
  infections of, 688–689. *See also* Colitis
  lymphoma of, 712
  obstruction of, 717f
  polyps of, **702–709**
    adenomatous, 702f–705f, 703–706
      benign vs malignant, 703–704, 703f
      carcinoma in situ in, 704
      colorectal cancer and, 705–706
      histogenesis of, 705, 705f
      inherited syndrome of, 706, 706f
      tubular, 702f–703f, 703–704
    hyperplastic, 707–708, 707f
    inflammatory, 708
    juvenile, 708, 708f
    lymphoid, 708
    metaplastic, 707–708, 707f
    retention, 708, 708f
    tubulovillous, 704
    villous, 704–705, 704f
  regions of, 686
  in shigellosis, 368
  in shock, 273
  stercoral ulcer of, 713–714
  trichuriasis of, 436, 436f
  vascular disease of, 700–702
Colony stimulating factor, 63, 100t
Colorectal cancer, **709–712**
  adenocarcinoma, 710–711, 710f
  adenomatous polyps and, 705–706
  clinical features of, 712
  Crohn's disease and, 710

Colorectal cancer:
  direct spread of, 711–712
  Dukes' classification of, 711, 711f
  geographic and ethnic factors in, 193
  pathogenesis of, 709
  pathology of, 710–712, 711f
  risk factors in, 709–710
  ulcerating, 710, 710f
  ulcerative colitis and, 698–699, 710
Comedocarcinoma, 146
Commensalism, 328
Complement system, **43–46**
  alternative pathway of, 44–45, 45t
  anaphylatoxins of, 45, 46f
  bacterial activation of, 46
  classical pathway of, 43–44, 45t
  deficiencies of, 46
  regulation of, 45–46
  in type II hypersensitivity reactions,
      106–107, 108f
Complete blood count, 1030, 1031t
Compound nevus, 1242f, 1243
Concussion, 1419
Conducting system, of heart, 500–502, 500t
Condyloma acuminatum:
  of female genital tract, 947–948
  of penis, 938, 938f
Condyloma lata, 354, 947
Congestive heart failure. *See* Heart failure,
      congestive
Conjunctiva:
  common disorders of, 1525
  hemorrhage of, 1508–1509
  hyperemia or injection of, 1508
  in systemic disease, 1510t
Conjunctivitis, 347, 1502–1503
Connective tissue, heritable diseases of,
      220–223
Connective-tissue-activating peptide, 1375
Conn's syndrome, 1153
Contact dermatitis, allergic, 1232–1233,
      1234f–1236f
Contraceptives, oral. *See* Oral contracep-
      tives
Contractures, 77, 89
Contrecoup contusion, 1424f, 1425
Contusion, 306–307
Cooley's anemia, 1041
Copper:
  deficiency of, 325
  metabolism of, in Wilson's disease, 772
Cori's disease, 227f, 1410
Cornea, 1503–1504
  common disorders of, 1525
  herpes simplex infection of, 1503
  onchocerciasis of, 1503–1504
  in systemic disease, 1510t
  vascularization of, 321, 321f
Coronary arteritis, 518
Coronary artery:
  anatomy of, 496f–497f, 498, 499f–500f
  anomalous origin of, 518
  atherosclerosis of, 476, 476f, 516, 517f
  collateral blood vessels of, 516–518
  in dissecting aneurysm, 518
  left anterior descending, 498, 499f
    intramural, 518
  left circumflex, 498, 499f
  occlusion of:
    left ventricular infarct due to, 498,
        499f

Coronary artery:
    pathogenesis of, 476–477, 476f, 516,
      517f
    pulmonary artery origin of, 514
    right, 498, 499f
    spasm of, 516
Coronary sinus defect, 507
Coronavirus, human respiratory, 345
Cor pulmonale, 533, 621
Corpus callosum, absence of, 1462
Corpus luteum, 961
Corpus luteum cyst, 973
Corticomedullary osteonecrosis, 1349
Corticosteroids:
    mechanism of action of, 47–48
    wound healing and, 88
Corticotropin, 1122
Corticotropinoma, 830
Corynebacterium diphtheriae, 377
Cotton wool spots, retinal, 481, 1509
Councilman bodies:
    in acute viral hepatitis, 747–748, 747f
    in yellow fever, 330, 330f
Courvoisier's sign, 819
Cowdry type A intranuclear inclusion, 334
Coxiella burnetii infection, 566
Coxsackievirus, 345
C particles, enzymes of, 55
Craniopharyngioma, 1122
Craniorachischisis, 203
Cranium, routes of entry for microorga-
    nisms in, 1443, 1443f
Creola bodies, 589
CREST variant scleroderma, 136
Cretinism, 1134
    bone formation in, 1315
    central nervous system in, 1478
Creutzfeldt-Jakob disease, 1456, 1457f
Cricoid cartilage, 544
Crigler-Najjar disease, 728–730
    type I, 728–730
    type II, 730
Crimean hemorrhagic fever, 330–331
Crohn's disease, 672, **692–694**, 694f
    adenocarcinoma of small intestine and,
      682
    appendicitis in, 715
    colorectal cancer and, 710
    epidemiology of, 692
    etiology and pathogenesis of, 692–693
    granulomas in, 693–694
    pathology in, 693–694
Crooke's cells, 1128
Croup, 548
Cryoglobulinemia, paraproteinemia in,
    869
Cryotherapy, gastritis due to, 648
Crypt abscess, 698
Cryptococcoma, of lung, 426
Cryptococcosis, 420f–421f, 426–427, 574
Cryptococcus neoformans, 420f–421f, 426–
    427, 574, 1445
Cryptorchidism, 912–913, 912f–914f
Cryptosporidiosis, 419
Crypts of Lieberkuhn, 686
Curling's ulcer, 643
Curschmann's spirals, 589
Cushing's syndrome, 1127, 1128f
    in cancer, 185
    osteoporosis in, 1342–1343
    paraneoplastic, 559–560

Cushing's syndrome:
    purpura in, 1026
Cushing's ulcer, 643
Cutaneous disorders. *See under* Skin
Cyanide, 296–297, 518
Cyclophosphamide, cystitis due to, 903
Cylinderization, 1311
Cylindroma, 1256, 1256f
Cyst:
    apical periodontal, 1271
    Bartholin's gland, 950
    blue-domed, 999, 1002f
    of bone, 1354–1357, 1356f
    bronchogenic, 563
    chocolate, 989
    choledochal, 800f, 801
    colloid, 1476
    dentigerous, 1273, 1275f
    enteric, 665
    gas, gastrointestinal, 684–686
    of liver, 794
    mesenteric, 720
    odontogenic, 1273–1274, 1275f
    omental, 720
    of ovary, 973–974, 974f
    of pancreas, 811
    pilonidal, 688
    of seminal vesicles, 927
    of spleen, 1065
    of subchondral bone, 1372, 1374f
    of vulva, 950
    of wolffian ducts, 953
Cystadenoma, of exocrine pancreas, 816,
    819
Cysticercosis, 446–447, 447f
Cysticercus, racemose, 447
Cystic fibrosis, 225–226, 225f–226f
    bronchiectasis in, 592
    cirrhosis in, 774
    meconium ileus in, 666
    Pseudomonas aeruginosa pneumonia in,
      569
Cystic hydatid disease, 790
Cystic lymphangioma, 495
Cystitis, **900–904**
    chronic interstitial, 901
    in cyclophosphamide therapy, 903
    eosinophilic, 901
    honeymoon, 870
    iatrogenic, 903
    polypoid, 900–901
    radiation-induced, 903
Cystitis cystica, 900
Cystitis glandularis, 11, 900
Cystosarcoma phyllodes, 1011–1012, 1012f
Cytogenetics. *See* Chromosomal altera-
    tions
Cytokeratin, 149
Cytomegalic inclusion disease, 337–338,
    948
Cytomegalovirus infection:
    in AIDS, 124, 451
    in carcinogenesis, 171
    in encephalitis, 1453
    inclusion bodies of, 1448, 1451f
    lymphadenitis in, 1061
    in pneumonia, 345, 563
    in TORCH complex, 206–208, 206f, 207t,
      208f
Cytoplasm, in coagulative necrosis, 14f–
    15f, 15

Cytoskeleton, ischemia effects on, 19
Cytotrophoblast, 981

Dane particle, 741, 742f
Darier-Pautrier's microabscesses, 1104
Darier's disease, 1209, 1209f
Death, sudden:
    in ischemic heart disease, 515
    in pulmonary embolism, 618
Debranching enzyme deficiency, 1410
Dedifferentiation, 68, 180
Deformation, morphologic, 203
Dehiscence, wound, 88
Dehydration, pathology of, 265
Dejerine-Sottas disease, 1495t
Delta cell, pancreatic, 822f, 823
Delta cell tumor, 827–828
Dementia, diseases associated with, 1486f
Demyelination, segmental, 1491–1492,
    1491f–1492f
Dendritic reticular cells, 1018, 1020
Dengue fever, 330
Dengue hemorrhagic fever, 330
Dental caries, 1270–1271, 1272f
Dentigerous cyst, 1273, 1275f
de Quervain's thyroiditis, 1137
Dermal-epidermal disease, **1215–1229**
    basal keratinocytic injury:
      lamina densa synthesis, immune
        reactants in, 1222–1226
      lymphocytic infiltrate in, 1226–1229
    blister formation due to, 1215–1222
    with persistent epidermal hyperplasia,
      1209–1211, 1210f–1212f
Dermal eruptions, in bartonellosis, 379–
    380
Dermal nevus, 1243, 1243f
Dermatitis:
    allergic contact, 1232–1233, 1234f–1236f
    in niacin deficiency, 320, 320f
    onchocercal, 433
    seborrheic, in riboflavin deficiency, 321,
      321f
Dermatitis herpetiformis, 1220–1222
    celiac disease and, 677
    definition and clinical features of, 1220
    etiology and pathogenesis of, 1222,
      1224f–1225f
    pathology of, 1220–1222, 1222f
Dermatographism, 1229
Dermatomyositis, 1408–1409, 1408f
Dermatopathic lymphadenopathy, 1053
Dermatophytosis, 431
Dermis, 1203
    connective tissue diseases of, 1234–1237
    papillary, 1203
    reticular, sclerosis of, 1234, 1236f
Dermoid cyst, 979
    intracranial, 1474
Desmin, 150
Desmoid tumors, 1389
Desmoplakin, 150
Desmoplasia, 155
Developmental association, 203
Developmental sequence anomaly, 202
Developmental syndrome, 202–203
Diabetes insipidus, 1123, 1124f

Diabetes mellitus, **1164–1176**
  arteriolosclerosis in, 1174
  atherosclerosis in, 1172–1174
  bronze, 771
  capillary basement membrane thicken-
      ing in, 486–487, 487f, 1174
  complications of, 1171–1176, 1173f
  diagnostic criteria for, 1166
  gestational, 1176
  glomerulonephritis in, 867
  glomerulosclerosis in, 487, 847–848,
      848f–849f, 1174–1175, 1175f
  in hemochromatosis, 771
  infection in, 1175–1176
  iridopathy in, 1521–1522
  lens in, 1522–1523
  neuropathy in, 1492–1493
  in pancreatic carcinoma, 820
  peripheral sensory and autonomic
      nerve dysfunction in, 1175
  pregnancy and, 1176
  renal failure in, 1174
  retinal capillary basement membrane in,
      1518–1521
  retinal capillary microaneurysms in, 487
  retinopathy in, 1174f, 1175, 1517–1518,
      1520f–1522f
  type I, 1166–1168
    age of onset of, 1166, 1166f
    autoimmune pathogenesis of, 1168
    clinical symptoms of, 1167, 1167f
    environmental factors in, 1168
    genetic inheritance of, 1167–1168
    type II vs, 1167t
  type II, 1168–1171
    age of onset of, 1166, 1166f
    capillary lesion in, 1165
    insulin metabolism in, 1169, 1170f
    islet cell hyalinization and fibrosis in,
        1169, 1169f
    obesity and, 315, 1169f, 1170–1171,
        1172f
    pathogenesis of, 1168–1169
    type I vs, 1167t
  wound healing in, 88
Dialysis, peritoneal, peritonitis due to,
    718–720
Dialysis encephalopathy, 300
Diamond-Blackfan syndrome, 1037
Diaphragmatic hernia, congenital, 642
Diaphyseal dysplasia, progressive, 1320
Diaphysis, 1306, 1307f
Diarrhea, **666–668**
  adenovirus, 343
  in AIDS, 450
  bacterial, 666–668
  Campylobacter, 667–668
  in cholera, 366, 367f, 675
  Clostridium perfringens, 668
  in disaccharide deficiency, 675
  E. coli, 369, 667
  in food poisoning, 668
  invasive bacteria in, 667–668
  in malabsorption, 675
  in nontyphoidal salmonellosis, 667
  Norwalk-like viral, 342–343
  Norwalk virus in, 668
  in pseudomembranous colitis, 689
  rotaviral, 342, 668
  in shigellosis, 667
  Staphylococcus aureus, 668

Diarrhea:
  toxigenic, 666–667
  traveler's, 369, 667
  in typhoid fever, 667
  Yersinia in, 667
Diencephalic syndrome, 1129
Diet:
  in carcinoma of stomach, 657
  chemical carcinogenesis and, 164
  in colorectal cancer, 709
  in diverticulosis, 690
  esophageal cancer due to, 639
  in pancreatic carcinoma, 820–821
Diethylstilbestrol:
  tumor in offspring due to, 248, 292
  vaginal adenosis due to, 953–954, 953f–
      954f
Differentiation, 247
Diffusion, 252
DiGeorge syndrome, 123
  partial, 123, 124f
Diphtheria, 377–378, 378f
  oral cavity in, 1264
Diplopoda, 449
Diptera, 449
Dirofilariasis, 433
  of lung, 433, 576
  subcutaneous, 433
Disaccharide deficiency, 675
Dispersed neuroendocrine system, 1120–
    1122
Dissecting aneurysm, 490–491, 490f
  coronary artery involvement with, 518
Disseminated intravascular coagulation:
  in cancer, 187
  in hepatorenal syndrome, 737
Diverticular disease, 690
Diverticulitis, 690
Diverticulosis, 689–691, 691f
  clinical symptoms of, 690–691, 691f
  epidemiology of, 690
  etiology of, 690
  pathology of, 690–691, 691f
Diverticulum:
  choledochal, 800f, 801
  of esophagus, 632
  Meckel's, 665–666, 665f
  of renal pelvis, 892
  of stomach, 662
  of ureter, 892
  of urethra, 909
  of urinary bladder, 897–899
  Zenker's, 632
Division failures, in morphogenesis, 201
DNA viruses, in carcinogenesis, 170–173,
    172f
Döhle bodies, 1027
Donovan bodies, 380, 380f
Double monsters, 201
Double outlet right ventricle, 511
Doubling time, tumor, 157
Down's syndrome, 214–215, 215t, 216f
  central nervous system in, 1462
  lung in, 593
Dracunculiasis, 434
Dressler's syndrome, 524
Driving pressure, 252
Drug abuse, 287–288, 288f–289f
Drug reactions, **288–293**
  blood in, 290

Drug reactions:
  female reproductive tract in, 291–292,
      292f
  gastrointestinal tract in, 289
  heart in, 290
  immunologic response in, 293
  kidney in, 290
  liver in, 289
  lungs in, 290, 291f
  metabolic effects of, 290
  musculoskeletal system in, 292–293
  nervous system in, 289–290
  skin in, 290
  thrombocytopenia in, 1028
Dry eye syndrome, 1525
D1 tumors, 828
Dubin-Johnson syndrome, 730–731, 731f
Duchenne muscular dystrophy, 234, 234f,
    1401–1403, 1404f
Duct ectasia, of breast, 997
Ducts of Luschka, 800
Ductus arteriosus:
  embryologic development of, 507
  patent, 243, 507–509
  prostaglandin effects on, 509
Duodenum:
  anatomy of, 663
  blood and lymphatic supply of, 663
  peptic ulcer disease of, **648–655**. *See also*
      Peptic ulcer disease
Dwarfism, 1129
  achondroplastic, 224
Dysentery, shigellosis, 368
Dysgerminoma, 978–979
  intracranial, 1474–1475
  of pineal gland, 1161, 1161f
Dyshormonogenesis, familial, 1134
Dyskinesia, tardive, 289
Dyslipoproteinemia, 470t
Dysphagia, 632
Dysplasia, 12–13
  in morphogenesis, 201
Dysraphic anomalies, 201
Dystopia, in morphogenesis, 202

Ear, **1295–1302**
  anatomy of, 1261f
  cauliflower, 1296
  external, 1295–1296
    anatomy of, 1295
    neoplasms of, 1296
  inner, 1300–1302
    anatomy and function of, 1300
    neoplasms of, 1302
  keloid of, 1296
  middle, 1296–1299
    anatomy of, 1296–1297
    otitis media of, 1297–1299. *See also*
        Otitis media
    tumors of, 1299, 1299f
  polyps of, 1296
  relapsing polychondritis of, 1296, 1296f
Eastern equine encephalitis, 332
Eaton-Lambert syndrome, 186
Ebola virus disease, 331–332
Ebstein's malformation, 514
Ecchymosis, 253
Echinococcosis, 444–446, 445f
  of liver, 790

Echinococcus granulosus, 444–446, 445f
Echinococcus multilocularis, 445–446
Echinococcus vogeli, 446
Echovirus, 345
Eclampsia, 983, 984f
Ectopia, in morphogenesis, 201
Ectopic ACTH syndrome, 830, 1151, 1152f
Ectopic hormones, 1162–1163
Ectopic hypercalcemia syndrome, 830
Ectopic pregnancy, 971–972, 972f
Edema, **258–263**
   capillaries in formation of, 459
   cerebral, 261, 306
   in cirrhosis of liver, 261
   effects and causes of, 258–259, 261t, 262f
   generalized, salt metabolism and, 258–259
   granulocytic, 261
   in high-altitude sickness, 305
   hydrocephalic, 261
   hydrostatic, 263f
   inflammatory, 263f
   local, 258
   mechanism of, 37, 459
   in nephrotic syndrome, 261
   oncotic, 263f
   of optic disc, 1531
   pitting, 261
   pulmonary, 261–263, 624–626, 625f–626f. *See also* Pulmonary edema
   traumatic, 263f
Effusion:
   definition of, 37
   peritoneal, 265
   pleural, 263–265, 616
Ehlers-Danlos syndrome, 222–223
Eisenmenger's complex, 506
Elastase, 54, 55
Elastic fibers, morphology and function of, 73–74
Elastin, 74
Electrical burns, 304, 305f
Electrolytes. *See* Fluid and electrolyte disorders
Electrophoresis, serum protein, 119, 120f
Elephantiasis, 431–432, 492
Elliptocytosis, hereditary, 1043
Embolism, **265–268**, 267f, 471, 472. *See also* Thromboembolism
   air, 268, 620
   amniotic fluid, 268, 620
   arterial, 267–268, 268f
   bone marrow, 620
   fat, 268, 619–620
      of cerebral capillaries, 1432–1433, 1432f
   of lung, 265–267, 266f, **618–621**, 619f
      consequences of, 618–619
      without infarction, 619
      infarction in, 618–619
      multiple recurrent, 619
      pulmonary hypertension due to, 622
      sources of, 618
   paradoxical, 267–268
   saddle, 618, 619f
   schistosomiasis, 620
   talc, 620
   tumor, 620
Embryo, preimplantation, exogenous toxins and, 200–201

Embryoma, 248
Embryonal cell carcinoma, 919, 919f, 979
Embryonal rhabdomyosarcoma, 1391
Emperipolesis, 1053
Emphysema, **593–598**
   centrilobular, 594f, 595
   cigarette smoking in, 279, 280f, 598, 599f
   clinical features of, 595–598, 596f–597f
   coal pneumoconiosis in, 595
   definition of, 593
   etiology and pathogenesis of, 598, 599f
   familial, 595
   panacinar, 594f, 595
   panacinar with centrilobular, 595
   pink puffer and blue bloater, 598
   proteolysis-antiproteolysis theory of, 598, 599f
   proximal acinar (centriacinar), 593–595, 594f
   pulmonary hypertension and, 623
   types of, 594f
Empyema, 616
   of gallbladder, 804
   in pneumococcal pneumonia, 568
   in sinusitis, 1284, 1285f
Encephalitis, viral, 1447–1450, 1450f
   arbovirus, 332
   cytomegalovirus, 1453
   herpes simplex, 1452–1453, 1453f–1454f
   simian B virus, 1453
   in TORCH complex, 208
   toxoplasmosis, 413, 413f, 450–451
   von Economo's, 1453–1454
Encephalitis lethargica, 1453–1454
Encephalomyelitis, perivenous, 1466
Encephalopathy:
   dialysis, 300
   hepatic, 735–737, 1480
   high-altitude, 306
   lead, 297
   portal-systemic, 735
   Wernicke's, 286, 1478f, 1479
Enchondromas, 143, 1322
Enchondromatosis, 1322–1323, 1322f
Endocardial cushion defect, 507
Endocardial fibroelastosis, 514–515
Endocarditis:
   bacterial, 533–534, 534t, 535f
      acute, 534t
      in drug addiction, 287, 288f
      glomerulonephritis in, 867
      staphylococcal, 384
      streptococcal, 388
      subacute, 534t
   candidal, 424–425
   Libman-Sacks, 134, 532
   marantic, 534–535
   nonbacterial thrombotic, 187, 534–535
   rheumatic, 528, 528f
   in systemic lupus erythematosus, 134
Endocervical polyp, 956
Endochondral ossification, 1306
Endochondral sequence, 1311
Endocrine cells:
   of small intestine, 664
   of stomach, 641
Endocrine system, **1118–1163**. *See also* individual organs
Endodermal heterotopia, congenital, 541
Endolymphatic stromal myosis, 967

Endometriosis, 987–989, 988f
   of colon, 713
   of rectum, 713
   of ureter, 893
   of urinary bladder, 903–904
Endometritis:
   acute, 962
   chronic, 962
   tuberculous, 962
Endometrium, **961–970**
   adenoacanthoma of, 965
   adenocarcinoma of, 316, 965–967, 966f, 967t
   adenosquamous carcinoma of, 965
   anatomy of, 961
   clear cell adenocarcinoma of, 966
   contraceptive steroidal effects on, 963
   estrogen effects on, 962
   hyperplasia of, 964–965, 965f
   during menstrual cycle, 961
   physically induced lesions of, 963
   polyps of, 963, 965f
   in pregnancy, 961
   secretory carcinoma of, 965
   serous adenocarcinoma of, 966
   stromal sarcoma of, 967–968, 968f
   stromatosis of, 967
Endomysial fibrosis, 1403
Endophlebitis, in hepatitis, 748
Endoplasmic reticulum:
   dilated cisternae of, 5, 6f
   proliferation of, 9, 9f
Endoreplication, of smooth muscle cells, 455, 457f
Endothelial sarcoma, sclerosing, 627
Endothelium:
   antithrombotic activity of, 473
   in atherosclerosis, 466, 466f–467f
   of blood vessels, 455t
   capillary, 457–459
   cellular, of blood vessels, 454–455, 454f, 455t
   denuding injury of, 473
   prothrombotic activity of, 473–474
   in thrombus formation, 472–474, 473f
Endotoxin, bacterial, in septic shock, 269–270
Entactin, in basement membrane, 73, 73t
Entamoeba histolytica, 414–417, 415f–416f
Enteric cysts, 665
Enteritis:
   necrotizing, 373, 374f–375f
   radiation, 680
   salmonella, 667. *See also under* Diarrhea
Enterobiasis, 438–439
Enterobius vermicularis, 438–439
Enterochromaffin cells:
   gastric, 641
   pancreatic, 823
Enterochromaffin cell tumors, of pancreas, 828
Enterocolitis:
   necrotizing, 243
   pseudomembranous, 689
   radiation and, 702
   Yersinia, 667. *See also under* Diarrhea
Enteropathy, protein-losing, 187, 679–680
α-Enterotoxin, 373
β-Enterotoxin, 373
Entodermal sinus tumor, 979
   of vagina, 955

Environmental chemicals, **293–300**. *See also*
    Chemicals
Environmental pathology, 276
Eosinophil chemotactic factor, 106
Eosinophilia, 63, 1050, 1050t
    in cancer, 187
    tropical, 432, 575, 583
Eosinophilic bodies, 747–748, 747f
Eosinophilic granuloma, 1055
    of bone, 1337
    of lung, 610–612, 611f
Eosinophilic pneumonia, 575, 583, 584f
Eosinophilic polymyositis, 1408
Eosinophils:
    in chronic inflammation, 59
    morphology and function of, 61f
    oxygen radical production by, 57
Ependymoma, 1470, 1472f
Epidermal growth factor, 158
Epidermal hyperplasia, 11, 12f
Epidermal-melanin unit, 1199, 1199f
Epidermis, 1197–1203
    basement membrane zone of, 1201–
        1203, 1202f–1203f
    diseases of, **1205–1214**. *See also individual*
        diseases
        dyshesive, 1211–1214
        excessive cornification in, 1205–1211
    immigrant cells of, 1197f, 1199
    normal, 1197, 1197f
Epidermodysplasia verruciformis, 170
Epidermoid carcinoma. *See* Squamous cell
        carcinoma
Epidermoid cyst, intracranial, 1474
Epidermolysis bullosa, **1215–1219**
    blister formation in, 1218f
    definition and clinical features of, 1215–
        1217
    dermolytic, 1217, 1217t
    epidermolytic, 1217, 1217t
    esophagus in, 636–637
    junctional, 1217, 1217t
    pathogenesis of, 1219
    pathology of, 1217–1219
Epidermolytic hyperkeratosis, 1206–1207,
        1206t, 1207f–1208f
Epididymis, **924–926**
    inflammatory disease of, 924–926
    papillary cystadenoma of, 926, 926f
Epididymitis, 924–926
Epidural hematoma, 1419–1420, 1419f–
        1421f
Epiglottic cartilage, 544
Epiglottis, 544–545
Epiglottitis, 548
    H. influenzae, 364
Epiphyseal plate, 1312, 1313f, 1314f
    in achondroplasia, 1315, 1317f
    disorders of, 1315–1320
    hemihypertrophy of, 1316
    in mucopolysaccharidoses, 1316f
    obliteration of, 1314
    in rickets, 1344, 1345f
    in scurvy, 1318f
Epiphysis, 1306, 1307f
Epispadias, 909
Epistaxis, 1282–1283
Epithelial cell disease, nephrotic, 841–842,
        842f–843f
Epithelioid cell nevi, 1254, 1254f
Epithelioid cells, 60–61, 62f, 102

Epithelioma, 143
    basal cell, 144
Epstein-Barr virus:
    in Burkitt's lymphoma, 171, 339f
    in carcinogenesis, 171, 339f
    in infectious mononucleosis, 338–340,
        339f
    in nasopharyngeal carcinoma, 171, 339f
Erdheim pregnancy cells, 1128
Erosions, repair of, 78
Error theory of aging, 31–32
Erucism, 448
Erysipelas, 386
Erythema gyratum repans, 188
Erythema nodosum, 1237–1238, 1238f
    in drug reaction, 290
    streptococcal, 388
Erythroblastic island, 1017
Erythroblastosis fetalis:
    clinical presentation in, 245
    diagnosis of, 246
    immunoprophylaxis in, 246
    pathogenesis of, 244f, 245
Erythrocytosis, 187, 1047–1048
Erythroderma, bullous congenital ich-
        thyosiform, 1206–1207, 1206t,
        1207f–1208f
Erythrogenic toxin, 385
Erythroid cell series, maturation of, 1022
Erythroid pronormoblast, 1022
Erythroplasia of Queyrat, 938–939
Erythropoietin, 77
Escherichia coli infection, 368–369
    enteroadhesive, 369
    enteroinvasive, 369, 667
    enterotoxigenic, 369
Escherichia coli pneumonia, 569
Esophageal sphincter, lower, 630, 635
Esophageal varices:
    bleeding, 780
    in portal hypertension, 779–780
Esophagitis, **635–637**
    candidial, 636
    chemical, 636
    esophageal cancer due to, 639
    herpetic, 636
    infectious, 636
    physical agents causing, 637
    reflux, 635–636
    in systemic illness, 636–637
Esophagus, **630–640**
    achalasia of, 633, 633f–634f
    adenocarcinoma of, 640
    in alcoholism, 285
    anatomy of, 630, 631f
    atresia of, 630–631
    Barrett's epithelium of, 635
    carcinoma of, **637–640**, 639f
        clinical features of, 639–640
        etiology of, 638–639
        geographic and ethnic factors in, 192
        geographic distribution of, 637–638
        pathology of, 640
        due to smoking, 278–279
    congenital disorders of, 630–631
    diverticula of, 632
        epiphrenic, 632
        intramural, 632
        pulsion, 632
        traction, 632
    in epidermolysis bullosa, 636–637

Esophagus:
    in graft-vs-host disease, 637
    lacerations of, 637
    motor disorders of, 632–633
    nasogastric tube trauma to, 637
    nonneoplastic disorders of, 638f
    in pemphigoid, 637
    perforation of, 637
    in peripheral neuropathy, 633
    radiation injury of, 637
    scleroderma of, 633
    stenosis of, congenital, 631
    stricture of, due to reflux, 635
    ulcer of, 635
    varices of, 491
    webs of, 631–632, 631f
Espundia, 1287
Esterase reaction, nonspecific, for muscle,
        1397, 1400f
Esthesioneuroblastoma, 1468
Estrogen:
    endometrial effects of, 962
    metabolism of, smoking effects on, 280,
        281f
    prostate and, 928–929
Ethanol:
    metabolism of, 752–754, 755f
    tissue injury induced by, 286–287
Ethinyl estradiol, side effects of, 291
Ethylene glycol, 295
Eumelanin, 1200
Eumycetoma, 422
Euploidy, 213, 213t
Ewing's sarcoma, 1360–1361, 1363f
Exophthalmos, dysthyroid, 1134, 1523–
        1524
Exstrophy, of urinary bladder, 897, 898f
Extracellular matrix, **68–75**
    basement membranes in, 72–73, 72f, 73t
    collagen in, 69–72, 69t, 70f
    components of, 69
    elastic fibers in, 73–74
    fibronectin in, 74
    functions of, 68–69
    proteoglycans in, 74–75, 75f
Exudate, 616
    definition of, 37
    transudate vs, 503t
Eye, **1500–1531**
    developmental and genetic anomalies
        of, 1508
    disorders of specific tissues of, 1525–
        1531
    infections, inflammations, immunologic
        disorders of, 1502–1504
    neoplasms of, 1504–1507
    in onchocerciasis, 433
    physical and chemical injury to, 1507–
        1508
    in systemic disease, 1510t–1512t, 1514–
        1524
    vascular disorders of, 1508–1509
Eyelid:
    common disorders of, 1531
    inflammation of, 1504
    in systemic disease, 1510t

Fabry's disease, 228f, 538
Facial cleft, 1262

Factor H, actions of, 46
Factor VIII-related antigen, 151
Factor XII:
    activation of, 42, 43f
    vasoactive mediator production by, 42–43, 43f
Fallopian tube, 970–972
    anatomy of, 970
    infections of, 970–971
    neoplasms of, 972
    pathophysiology of, 970
Familial Mediterranean fever, 720
Familial paroxysmal polyserositis, 720
Familial polyposis coli, 706, 706f
Fanconi's anemia, 1035
Fanconi's pancytopenia, 1027
Fanconi's syndrome, 298
Farber's lipogranulomatosis, 228f
Fasciitis, nodular, 146, 147f, 1389, 1389f
Fasciola hepatica, 444, 789–790
Fascioliasis, 444
Fasciolopsiasis, 444
Fasciolopsis buski, 444
Fat, tumors of, 1390, 1390f–1391f
Fat embolism, 268, 619–620
    of cerebral capillaries, 1432–1433, 1432f
Fatigue fracture, 1326
Fat necrosis, 15–16, 16f
Fatty-acid binding protein, 727
Fatty liver:
    alcoholic, 754–760
        pathogenesis of, 756–758, 757f
        ultrastructural changes in, 754–756, 756f
    morphology in, 13
    of pregnancy, 784
    in Reye's syndrome, 784
    toxic, 783–784
        macrovesicular steatosis in, 783
        microvesicular steatosis in, 783f, 784
        due to phospholipidosis, 784
Fatty streak, of atherosclerosis, 461–462, 464f
Fecal occult blood test, 712
Female genital tract. *See also individual anatomic parts*
    embryology of, 944–945
    infectious diseases of, 944t, 945–949
Feminization, in hepatorenal syndrome, 738
Femoral head, osteonecrosis of, 1326, 1327f
Fenton reaction, 57t
Ferritin, 14, 768
Ferruginous bodies, 168
Fertility, hypothalamus in, 1130
Fetal alcohol syndrome, 206
Fetal hydantoin syndrome, 205–206
Fetal tobacco syndrome, 280–282, 282f
α-Fetoprotein, 151
    in hepatocellular carcinoma, 795
    in testicular germ cell tumors, 918
Fetor hepaticus, 735
Fetus:
    drug withdrawal syndrome in, 288
    effects of maternal smoking on, 280–282, 282f–283f
    heart of, 506, 507
    lungs of, 238–239
    pulmonary circulation in, 240
    radiation effects on, 308–309

Fetus in fetu, 201
Fever, 303. *See also individual type, e.g., Yellow fever*
    in cancer, 185
    mechanism of, 62–63
    oxygen demand and, 518
Fever blister, 336, 337f
Fibrinoid necrosis, 16, 18f, 113, 481
Fibrinolysis, 474–476, 475f
Fibrinous exudate, 37
Fibroadenoma, of breast, 1000, 1003f
Fibroblast activating factor, 100t
Fibroblasts:
    morphology and function of, 77, 78f
    proliferation of, 78–79
Fibrocartilage, 1314–1315
Fibrocystic breast disease, 998–999, 1000f–1002f. *See also Breast, fibrocystic disease of*
Fibroelastoma, papillary, of heart, 541
Fibroelastosis, endocardial, 514–515
Fibroepithelial polyps, of renal pelvis and ureter, 894
Fibroma:
    of oral cavity, 1266
    of ovary, 978
Fibromatosis, 1389
Fibronectin:
    morphology and function of, 74
    in phagocytic cell adherence, 58
    in wound healing, 79
Fibrosarcoma, 144, 1389–1390, 1390f
Fibrosis, 67–93
    in heart, in wound healing, 93f, 94
    onion skin, of liver, 767
    pipestem, 441, 443f
    retroperitoneal, 720
Fibrous cap, atherosclerotic, 463–465, 464f
Fibrous dysplasia, 1362–1365, 1366f
    monostotic, 1362
    polyostotic, 1362
Fibrous histiocytoma, malignant, 1390
Filariasis:
    bancroftian, 431–432
    Malayan, 431–432
Filtration, 252
Fire ants, 449
Fleas, 449
Flies, true, 449
Flora, of colon, 666
Flow cytometry, 119, 121f–122f, 122
Fluid and electrolyte disorders, 258–265
    edema in, 258–263, 261t, 262f
    fluid in body cavities in, 263–265, 264f
    fluid loss or overload in, 265
Fluidization, of plasma membrane, 287
Foam cells, 463, 464f
Folic acid deficiency, 322, 1039–1040
Follicle cyst, 973
Follicle stimulating hormone, 1122
Follicular hyperkeratosis, 318, 318f
Follicular hyperplasia, 62
Food poisoning, 668
    salmonella, 373, 374f–375f
    staphylococcal, 384
Foot:
    immersion, 302
    mycetoma of, 421–422, 421f
Foramen ovale, 507, 508f
Forbes' disease, 1410

Foreign body:
    in carcinogenesis, 169
    tracheal, 549
Foreign body giant cell, 61, 62f
Fossa ovalis, 507, 508f
Fracture, **1323–1326**
    healing of, 1323–1326, 1324f–1325f
        callus in, 1323
        cutting cone in, 1323–1324
        inflammatory phase of, 1323
        primary, 1325
        remodeling phase of, 1324–1325
        reparative phase of, 1323–1324
    nonunion of, 1325
    stress (march, fatigue), 1326
    types of, 1323
Francisella tularensis, 363
Friedländer's bacillus pneumonia, 378–379
Friedreich's ataxia, 1484f, 1485
Fröhlich's syndrome, 1124
Frostbite, 302
Fructose intolerance, hereditary, cirrhosis in, 776
Functional demand, reduced, 6–8
Fungal disease, **421–431**. *See also individual types*
Fungus balls, 422, 550
Funnelization, 1314
Furuncles, 382

Gaisböck's syndrome, 1048
Galactocele, 998
Galactosemia, cirrhosis in, 775–776
Gallbladder, **799–806**. *See also under Biliary*
    anatomy of, 799–800
    benign tumors of, 806
    carcinoma of, 806, 806f
    cholesterolosis of, 805
    congenital anomalies of, 800–801, 800f
    empyema of, 804
    hydrops of, 804
    porcelain, 804
    strawberry, 805
Gallstone ileus, 804
Gallstones, **801–804**. *See also Cholelithiasis*
Gamna-Gandy bodies, 255, 780, 1065
Ganglioglioma, 1472
Ganglioneuroma, 1158, 1158f
Gangliosidosis:
    heart in, 538, 538f
    metabolic disturbance in, 228t
Gangrene:
    gas, 373–374, 374f–375f
    of lung, 569
Gangrenous cholecystitis, 804
Gangrenous stomatitis, 382f
Gardnerella infection, 945
Gardner's syndrome, 706–707
Gas cyst, gastrointestinal, 684–686
Gasoline, 295
Gastric cancer. *See Stomach, carcinoma of*
Gastric glands, 641
    endocrine cells of, 641
    mucous neck cells of, 641
    parietal (oxyntic) cells of, 641
    zymogen or chief cells of, 641
Gastric outlet obstruction, in peptic ulcer disease, 655
Gastric rugae, 640, 641f

Gastric ulcer, nonerosive gastritis with, 645
Gastrinoma, of pancreas, 828–830
Gastritis, **642–648**
    atrophic, 644–645
    in drug reactions, 289
    eosinophilic, 648
    erosive (acute), 642–643
        causes of, 642–643
        pathogenesis of, 643
        pathology of, 643
    giant hypertrophic, 647–648, 647f
    granulomatous, idiopathic, 648
    miscellaneous causes of, 648
    nonerosive (chronic), 644–647
        achlorhydria in, 644
        antral, 644
        atrophic, 644, 645f
        fundal, 644
        intestinal metaplasia in, 644–645, 646f
        pathogenesis and consequences of, 645–647
        pathology of, 644, 645f–646f
        postgastrectomy, 645
        pseudopyloric metaplasia in, 645
        stomach cancer and, 647
        superficial, 644
Gastroenteritis:
    Campylobacter, 369–370, 667–668. *See also under* Diarrhea
    S. enteritidis, 359
    shigellosis, 368
    staphylococcal, 384
    vibrio, 368
    viral, 342–343, 668
Gastroenteropancreatic system, 825
Gastroesophageal reflux, 635–636
    in hiatal hernia, 635
Gastrointestinal tract, **628–721**. *See also individual anatomic parts*
    in alcoholism, 285–286
    anthrax of, 358
    bleeding in, 284, 285f, 716f
    in drug reactions, 289
    lymphoid tissue in, 1020
    obstruction of, 717f
    in radiation, 308, 309f
    zygomycosis of, 430
Gaucher cell, 1349f, 1350
Gaucher's crisis, 1349
Gaucher's disease, 229–230, 230f, 538, **1348–1350**, 1350f
    bone in, 1349, 1350f
    central nervous system in, 1478
    clinical features of, 1348–1350, 1350f
    pathology in, 1349f, 1350
    secondary, 1348–1350, 1350f
    therapy in, 1350
    types of, 1348
Gay bowel syndrome, 689
G cell hyperfunction, 650
Gelatinase, 55
Gene amplification, 177
Genes, Mendelian inheritance of, 218
Genetic abnormalities, **218–234**
    autosomal dominant, 220–224, 220f
    autosomal recessive, 224–232, 224f
    biochemical basis of, 218–220
    prenatal diagnosis of, 236
    due to radiation, 309
    sex-linked, 232–234, 233f

Genetic factors:
    in atherosclerosis, 470–471
    in carcinoma of stomach, 657
    in celiac disease, 676–677
    in hemochromatosis, 768–769
    in peptic ulcer disease, 650
    in Wilson's disease, 772
Genital tract:
    chlamydial infection of, 348–349
    female. *See also individual anatomic parts*
        embryology of, 944–945
        infectious diseases of, 944t, 945–949
    herpes infection of, 336–337, 337f
Geographic pathology, 276
German measles, 341
Germ cell tumors, 978–981, 979f
Germinoma, of pineal gland, 1161, 1161f
Gestation, multiple, 983–985
Gestational diabetes, 1176
Gestational trophoblastic disease, 986–987
Ghon complex, 395
Giant cell arteritis, 483–484, 484f
Giant cell granuloma, peripheral, of oral cavity, 1266, 1266f
Giant cell hepatitis, 791, 791f
Giant cells, 102
    foreign body, 61, 62f
    Langhans', 61, 63f
    multinucleated, 61
    Warthin-Finkeldey, 341, 341f
Giant cell tumor:
    of bone, 1360, 1363f
    multinucleated, 147, 148f
    in Paget's disease, 1354
    of tendon sheath, 1387
Giant platelet syndrome, 1029
Giardia lamblia, 418
Giardiasis, 418
Gilbert's syndrome, 730
Gingival disease, 1272–1273
Gingivitis, 1273, 1274f
    acute necrotizing ulcerative, 1264
Glanders, 371
Glands of Lieberkuhn, 686
Glanzmann's thromboasthenia, 1029
Glaucoma, 1526f, 1527–1528
    closed-angle, 1528
    congenital, 1527
    effects of, 1528
    low tension, 1528
    open-angle, 1527–1528
    phakolytic, 1527
    phakomorphic, 1527
    secondary, 1528
Glial fibrillary acidic protein, 150
Glial filament protein, 150
Glial nodules, 1450, 1452f
Glioblastoma multiforme, 1470, 1471f
Gliosarcoma, 1470
Gliosis, 94
Glomangioma, 493–494
Glomerular basement membrane, 72, 72f
    anatomy of, 834–836, 835f–837f
    anti-glomerular basement membrane disease of, 857, 858f–859f
Glomerular capillaries, 834, 836f
Glomeruloid formation, 1470, 1471f
Glomerulonephritis, **850–864**
    acute, streptococcal, 388
    acute (postinfectious), 852–855, 853f–855f

Glomerulonephritis:
    in bacterial endocarditis, 867
    cell-mediated processes in, 852
    cellular proliferation in, 851
    circulating immune complexes in, 851–852
    complement activation in, 852
    crescentic, 855–857, 856f, 857t
        differential diagnosis of, 857t
        idiopathic, 857, 857t
    in diabetes mellitus, 867
    exudative, 851
    focal, 859–865, 863f–864f, 863t
    focal embolic, in bacterial endocarditis, 534
    hereditary, 869
    in situ immune complex formation in, 852
    intracapillary deposits in, 851
    membranoproliferative, 858–859, 860f–862f
        dense deposit, 859
        mesangial interpositioning in, 859
        with subendothelial deposits, 859, 860f
        type I, 859, 860f
        type II, 859
        type III, 859
    mesangial deposits in, 851
    in paraproteinemia, 867–869, 868f
    pathogenetic mechanisms of, 851–852
    patterns of injury in, 851
    poststreptococcal, 857t
    rapidly progressive, 836, 855
    subendothelial deposits in, 851
    subepithelial deposits in, 851
    in systemic lupus erythematosus, 133–134, 133f–134f, 865–867, 865f–866f. *See also Lupus nephritis*
Glomerulosclerosis, 93
    in diabetes mellitus, 487, 847–848, 848f, 1174–1175, 1175f
    diffuse, 847
    focal segmental, nephrotic, 842–845, 844f
    kappa light-chain, 868
    nodular, 847
Glomerulus:
    anatomy of, 834, 834f–836f
    hyalinosis of, 843
    inflammatory lesions of, 850–864. *See also Glomerulonephritis*
    noninflammatory lesions of, 841–850
    in polyarteritis nodosa, 483
Glomus bodies, 493–494
Glossitis, 1270
Glottic tumor, 548
Glottis, 545
Glucagon:
    physiologic actions of, 825t
    synthesis of, 822f, 823
Glucagonoma, 825, 826
Glucose homeostasis, liver in, 726
Glucose–6-phosphate dehydrogenase deficiency, 1043–1044
α-1,4-Glucosidase deficiency, 1409, 1410f
β-Glucuronidase deficiency syndrome, 231f
Gluten, in celiac disease, 675–676, 676f
Gluten-sensitive enteropathy B-cell antigen, 676

Glycogen, catabolism of, 227f
Glycogenoses, 226–229, 227f
    biochemical basis of, 219
    type II, 1409, 1410f
    type III, 1410
    type V, 1410, 1410f
    type VII, 1411
Glycogen storage disease, 1409–1411
    cirrhosis in, 775
    heart in, 538, 538f
Glycoproteins, in phagocytic cell adherence, 58
Glycosaminoglycans, 74
Goblet cells, of small intestine, 664
Goiter, 1132–1134
    congenital, 1134
    diffuse toxic, 1134–1137
    lymphadenoid, 1138
    nodular, 1133
    toxic multinodular, 1137
Gonadal dysgenesis, 913–915
Gonadoblastoma, of testis, 921–922
Gonadotropic syndromes, in cancer, 186
Gonococcal infection, 389–391, 390f–391f
Gonorrhea, 389–391, 390f–391f, 945–946
Goodpasture's disease, 109, 110f, 857
Goodpasture's syndrome, 582, 852
Gout, **1381–1384**
    acute arthritic, 1382, 1384, 1384f
    classification of, 1381
    clinical features of, 1382–1383, 1382f
    epidemiology and etiology of, 1381–1382
    kidney in, 1382–1383
    pathology of, 1383–1384, 1383f–1384f
    primary, 1381
    saturnine, 1383
    secondary, 1381
    tophi of, 1382, 1382f
    treatment of, 1384
Graft-vs-host disease, 119
    esophagus in, 637
Granular cell tumor:
    of pituitary, 1125
    of vagina, 954
Granulation tissue, 58, 58f, 79, 82f
Granulocyte, 1017, 1022
Granulocyte count, in cancer, 187
Granulocytic edema, 261
Granulocytic sarcoma, in leukemia, 1077, 1081f
Granuloma:
    cholesterol, in otitis media, 1297
    in Crohn's disease, 693–694
    eosinophilic, 1055
        of bone, 1337
        of lung, 610–612, 611f
    in extrahepatic biliary obstruction, 767
    formation of, 60 61, 62f
    lethal midline, of face, 1288, 1289f
    periapical, 1271, 1273f
    peripheral giant cell, of oral cavity, 1266, 1266f
    pyogenic:
        of nose, 1282
        of vulva, 950
    in sarcoidosis, 607, 607f
    spermatic, 926
    swimming pool, 401–402
    in tuberculosis, 397f
Granuloma inguinale, 380, 380f, 945

Granulomatosis:
    bronchocentric, of lung, 615
    lymphomatoid, 615
    necrotizing sarcoidal, 615
    Wegener's, 484, 485f
        of kidney, 880
        of lung, 614
Granulomatous disease, chronic, neutrophils in, 1049–1050
Granulomatous inflammation, 59–62, 62f–63f
Granulosa cell tumors, 977–978, 978f
Graves' disease, 1134–1137
    autoantibodies in, 109, 109f
    autoimmune pathogenesis of, 1135, 1136f
    clinical manifestations of, 1134, 1135f
    ocular manifestations of, 1523–1524
    thyroid architecture in, 1135, 1137f
Gray, 307
Great arteries, transposition of, 511–512, 512f
Growth, intrauterine, retardation of, 238
Growth disorders, 1129
Growth factor:
    oncogene interaction with, 175, 176f
    tumor cells and, 158–159
Growth hormone:
    deficiency of, 1129
    production of, 1122
Growth plate. *See* Epiphyseal plate, 1312, 1313f, 1314f
Guarnieri's bodies, 334
Gum, inflammatory hyperplasia of, 1266
Gumma, 356, 356f, 1336
Gynecologic pathology, **942–989**. *See also individual types*
Gynecomastia, 10, 996–997, 997f

Haber-Weiss reaction, 22, 57t
Hageman factor:
    activation of, 42, 43f
    vasoactive mediator production by, 42–43, 43f
Hair:
    anagen, 1204
    catagen, 1204–1205
    telogen, 1204–1205
    vellus, 1205
Hairballs, 662, 662f
Hair cycle, 1204–1205
Hair follicles, 1204–1205
Halothane hepatitis, 785
Hamartoma, 143, 145f, 247–248, 493
    of lung, 561, 562f
Hand-Schüller-Christian disease, 1054–1055, 1337
Hansen's disease, 397–401, 398f–400f
Hartmannella-acanthameba group, 417–418
Hashimoto's disease, 1138–1139, 1138f
Haustra, 686
Haversian canals, 1307
HBV antigen, localization of, 748
Head:
    in birth injury, 246–247
    penetrating wounds of, 1425, 1426f

Head and neck, **1260–1303**. *See also individual anatomic parts*
Healing. *See* Wound healing
Heart, 252–253
    in alcoholism, 285
    in amyloidosis, 538f, 539
    capillary system of, 250f
    conducting system of, 500–502, 500t
    fetal, development of, 506, 507
    functional anatomy of, 498–502
    in gangliosidosis, 538, 538f
    in glycogen storage disease, 538, 538f
    in hyperthyroidism, 537
    hypoplastic left, syndrome of, 513
    in hypothyroidism, 537
    in mucopolysaccharidosis, 538, 538f
    myocyte of, 498–500, 501f
    in myxedema, 537
    normal vs failing, 504, 505f
    in polyarteritis nodosa, 532
    pulmonary hypertension and, 623
    in rheumatoid arthritis, 532
    sarcomere of, 498–500, 501f
    in scleroderma, 532
    in shock, 271
    in sphingolipidosis, 538, 538f
    in systemic lupus erythematosus, 531–532
    in thiamine deficiency, 320
    in toxoplasmosis, 412, 412f
    tumors of, 540–541
    work of, calculation of, 502, 502f
    wound healing in, 93f, 94
Heart block, complete, congenital, 514
Heart disease:
    carcinoid, 537–538
    congenital, **504–515**. *See also individual types*
        classification of, 505–506, 506t
        etiology of, 505
        incidence of, 504
    hypertensive, 532 533, 533f
    ischemic, **515–527**. *See also* Ischemic heart disease
    luetic, 540
    rheumatic, **527–531**. *See also* Rheumatic heart disease
    thiamine deficiency (beriberi), 537
    thyrotoxic, 537
Heart failure, **502–504**
    backward, 502
    causes of, 503–504
    congestive, 259–261
        biochemical characteristics of, 504, 505f
        in drug reaction, 290
        in hemochromatosis, 771
        liver in, 786–787, 786f
    effects of, 502–503, 503f, 503t
    forward, 502
Heart failure cells, 254
Heart rate:
    ischemic heart disease due to increase in, 518
    oxygen demand and, 518
Heavy-chain disease, 1100
Heberden's nodes, 1372
Hebra nose, 378
Heerfordt's syndrome, 1277
Heimlich maneuver, 549
Heinz bodies, 1043

Helminthic infection, of liver, 789–790
Hemangioblastoma, intracranial, 1475
Hemangioendothelioma, infantile, of
    liver, 794
Hemangioma, 493–494, 1390, 1391f
    capillary, 493, 1390, 1391f
    cavernous, 493, 1390, 1391f
    juvenile or strawberry, 493
    of liver, 794
    of oral cavity, 1266–1267
    pulmonary, 626
    of salivary glands, 1281–1282
    of vulva, 950
Hemangiomatous syndrome, multiple,
    493
Hemangiopericytoma, 494
Hemangiosarcoma, 494
    of liver, 786, 797–798
Hematocephalus, neonatal, 242–243, 243f
Hematoma, 253, 307
    epidural, 1419–1420, 1419f–1421f
    retroplacental, 983
    subdural, 1420–1422, 1421f–1423f
Hematomyelia, 1427
Hematopoietic system, 1016–1019
    bone marrow of, 1016–1018, 1017t–1018t
    cellular differentiation and maturation
        in, 1015f, 1017t
    embryologic development of, 1016
    in radiation, 308, 309f
Hematoxylin bodies, in lupus nephritis,
    865
Hemihypertrophy, of epiphyseal plate,
    1316
Hemiptera, 448
Hemispherization, 1311
Hemochromatosis, 14, **767–771**
    arthropathy in, 771
    complications of, 768f
    congestive heart failure in, 771
    definition of, 767
    diabetes mellitus in, 771
    genetic inheritance of, 768–769
    joints in, 1386
    laboratory diagnosis of, 771
    liver in, 769–771, 770f
    pathology of, 769–771, 770f
    primary, 768–769
    secondary, 769
    skin in, 771
    testicular atrophy in, 771
    treatment of, 771
Hemodynamic disorders, of perfusion,
    253–258
Hemoglobin:
    high oxygen affinity, 1045
    normal concentration of, 1030, 1031t
Hemoglobin C disease, 1044–1045
Hemoglobin Kohn, 1045
Hemoglobin S-C disease, 1044
Hemoglobin S-D disease, 1044
Hemoglobin S-thalassemia disease, 1044
Hemoglobinuria:
    march, 1047
    paroxysmal cold, 1046
    paroxysmal nocturnal, 1045
Hemoglobinuric nephrosis, 409
Hemolytic anemia, in drug reaction, 290
Hemolytic uremic syndrome, 880–881,
    881f, 1029
Hemophagocytic reticulosis, 1054

Hemophilia, 233–234
    joints in, 1385–1386, 1386f
Hemophilia A, 1029–1030
Hemophilia B, 1030
Hemophilus ducreyi, 945
Hemophilus influenzae infection, 363–364
    in meningitis, 1444
Hemorrhage, 253–254
    anterior chamber, 1509
    of brain, 1438, 1439f
        hypertensive, 1436–1438, 1438f–1440f
    gastrointestinal, 716f
        in alcoholism, 284, 285f
    intraocular, 1508–1509
    intraventricular, 1438
    of lung, 581–583
    in peptic ulcer disease, 654
    in periventricular germinal matrix, neo-
        natal, 242–243, 243f
    pontine, 1438, 1439f
    of retina, in high-altitude sickness, 305
Hemorrhagic fever, viral, 329–332
Hemorrhagic thrombocytopenia, primary,
    1072t, 1073–1074
Hemorrhoids, 491, 701–702
Hemosiderin, 14, 768
Hemosiderosis, 14
Hemostasis, 471, 474–476, **1024–1030**. See
    also Coagulation
    disorders of, 1026–1030
        blood vessels in, 1026–1027
        characteristics of, 1026
        coagulation factors in, 1029–1030
        platelet disorders in, 1027–1029
    normal, 1025–1026
    primary, 1025
    screening tests of, 1026t
Hemothorax, 616
Henoch-Schönlein nephritis, 862–863
Heparan sulfate, 473
Heparan sulfate proteoglycan, in base-
    ment membrane, 73, 73t
Hepar lobatum, 356, 790
Hepatic duct, common, 724
Hepatic encephalopathy, 735–737, 1480
    morphology of, 736–737
    pathogenesis of, 735
Hepatic failure, 734–738
    complications of, 737f
    encephalopathy in, 735–737
    jaundice in, 735
Hepatic fibrosis, congenital, 840
Hepatic necrosis, confluent, 748–749, 749f
Hepatic porphyria, in drug reaction, 290
Hepatic vein, thrombosis of, in portal hy-
    pertension, 779, 779f
Hepatic veno-occlusive disease, 779
Hepatitis, **738–751**
    acute viral, 738–746
        hepatocytes in, 747–748, 747f
        lobular disarray in, 748
        morphology of, 753f
        pathology of, 747–748, 747f
    alcoholic, 757f, 758f–760f, 759–760
        central hyaline sclerosis in, 759, 760f
        hepatocellular necrosis in, 758f, 759
        portal tracts in, 759–760
    autoimmune, 746
    cholestatic, 748
    chronic, 746–747, 750–751
        active, 750–751, 751f–753f

Hepatitis:
    persistent, 750, 750f–751f, 753f
    in drug reactions, 289
    fulminant, 749
    giant cell, 791, 791f
    halothane, 785
    infectious agents causing, 739t
    lupoid, 746
    neonatal, 790–791, 790t, 791f
    subacute, 749
    in toxic liver necrosis, 785
    type A, 739–741, 739f–740f
        clinical features of, 739–740, 740f
        comparative features of, 754t
        epidemiology of, 740–741
        virus in, 739, 739f
    type B, 741–745, 742f–745f
        acute, self-limited, 741–744
        antigen localization in, 748
        in carcinogenesis, 171–173
        chronic, 746–747
        chronic carrier state in, 744
        clinical features of, 741, 743f
        comparative features of, 754t
        epidemiology of, 745–746
        hepatocellular carcinoma and, 794–
            795
        indirectly cytopathic, 24–25, 26f
        outcomes of infection with, 745f
        vaccine for, 745
        virus in, 741, 742f
    type D, 745–746
    type non-A, non-B, 746
        chronic, 747
        comparative features of, 754t
Hepatoblastoma, 797
Hepatocarcinogenesis, in rat, 164–167, 166f
Hepatocellular carcinoma, **794–796**, 796f
    cirrhosis and, 795
    fibrolamellar, 796
    geographic and ethnic factors in, 193
    in hemochromatosis, 771
    hepatitis B and, 173, 794–795
    in migrant populations, 194
    pleomorphism in, 796
    pseudoglandular, 796
    trabecular, 796, 796f
Hepatocellular nodules, 167, 751, 752f
Hepatocyte:
    anatomy of, 725–726
    in fatty liver, 754–756, 756f
    feathery degeneration in, 734, 767
    functions of, 726–727
    ground glass, 750, 751f
    hydropic swelling in, 5f–6f
    hypertrophy of, 9, 9f–10f
    necrosis of:
        in acute viral hepatitis, 747–748, 747f
        in alcoholic hepatitis, 758f, 759
    ribosome disaggregation in, 5, 7f
    toxic centrilobular necrosis of, 782f, 783
    triglyceride accumulation in, 13
Hepatolenticular degeneration, 772–774.
    See also Wilson's disease
    central nervous system in, 1478–1479
Hepatorenal syndrome, **737–738**
    coagulation in, 737–738
    endocrine complications of, 738
    feminization in, 738
    hypoalbuminemia in, 738
    pulmonary complications of, 738

Hepatotoxins, metabolism of, 25–27, 27f
Hermaphroditism, 915
Hernia:
  diaphragmatic, congenital, 642
  hiatal, 633–635, 634f
    paraesophageal, 633–635
    sliding, 633
  incisional, 88
Heroin nephropathy, 287
Herpes simplex:
  in atherosclerosis, 471
  in carcinogenesis, 171
  in corneal infection, 1503
  in encephalitis, 1452–1453, 1453f–1454f
  in esophageal infection, 636
  inclusion bodies of, 1448, 1451f
  infections with, **334–340**
  in pneumonia, 344–345
  in stomatitis, 1265
  in TORCH complex, 206–208, 206f, 207t
Herpes simplex type 1 infection, 335–336, 337f
Herpes simplex type 2 infection, 336–337, 337f
  in cervical carcinoma, 171, 957
  of female genital tract, 948
Herpes zoster, 335
  inclusion bodies of, 1448, 1451f
  in lymphadenitis, 1061
Heterophile antibody, in infectious mononucleosis, 338
Heterotopia, 248
  in morphogenesis, 201
  neuronal, 1462
Heyman nephritis, 845
Hiatal hernia, 633–635, 634f
  paraesophageal, 633–635
  sliding, 633
Hidradenoma, of vulva, 950
High-altitude sickness, 304–306
  deterioration in, 306
  flatus in, 305
  mountain sickness, 306
  pulmonary edema and cerebral edema in, 306
  retinal hemorrhage in, 305
  systemic edema in, 305
Hirschsprung's disease, 687–688, 687t–688f
Histamine:
  mast cell release of, 41
  platelet release of, 40
  in type I hypersensitivity reaction, 106
Histiocytic lymphoma, true, 1082f, 1083
Histiocytic necrotizing lymphadenitis, 1061
Histiocytoma, malignant fibrous, 1390
Histiocytosis:
  acute disseminated, 1054–1055
  of bone, 1336–1338
    clinical presentation in, 1337
    histology in, 1336, 1336f–1337f
    treatment of, 1337–1338
  chronic disseminated, 1054–1055
  malignant, 1079–1083
    cytologic abnormalities in, 1079–1082, 1082f
    spleen in, 1070f, 1082
  of sinus, 62, 1053
    with massive lymphadenopathy, 1053
Histoplasma capsulatum, 427–428, 428f, 573

Histoplasmosis, 427–428, 428f
  of lung, 573
  of small intestine, 669
HIV infection. *See* AIDS
HLA (human leukocyte antigen), 102
  in systemic lupus erythematosus, 131–132
Hodgkin's cells, 1110, 1110f
Hodgkin's disease, **1108–1114**
  Ann Arbor staging system for, 1115t
  clinical features of, 1092t, 1111–1114
  etiology and pathogenesis of, 1108–1109
  gross pathology in, 1109, 1109f
  histopathology of, 1109–1111, 1110f
  Hodgkin's cells in, 1110, 1110f
  in migrant populations, 195
  nodular sclerosis in, 1111, 1114f
  non-Hodgkin's lymphoma vs, 1092t, 1108
  of oral cavity, 1268
  prognosis in, 1114
  Reed-Sternberg cell in, 1109–1110, 1110f
  sites of involvement of, 1092t
  spread of, 1111
  subtypes of, 1110, 1112f–1113f
Hofbauer cells, 245
Holoprosencephaly, 1462, 1462f
Honeycomb lung, 608, 608f
Hookworm infection, 436, 437f
Hordeolum, 1504
Horder's spots, 346
Hormones:
  ectopic, 1162–1163
  function of, 1122
  hypertrophic response to, 9
Hornets, 448–449
Horseshoe kidney, 837
Howship's lacuna, 1309
Human chorionic gonadotropin, as tumor marker, 151
Human pancreatic polypeptide, 825t
Hunner's ulcer, 901
Hunter's syndrome, 231f
Huntington's disease, 1481–1482
Hurler's syndrome:
  central nervous system in, 1477–1478
  metabolic disturbance in, 231f
  pathogenesis, 230
Hutchinson's teeth, 209, 356
Hutchinson's triad, 209
Hyaline, 29
Hyaline arteriolosclerosis, 481
Hyaline basophils, 1128
Hyaline membranes, in respiratory distress syndrome, 242, 242f
Hyalinosis, of glomerulus, 843
Hydantoin, fetal effects of, 205–206
Hydatid disease, 444–446, 445f
Hydatidiform mole, 986–987
  complete, 986–987
  invasive, 987
  partial, 987
Hydrocarbon:
  aromatic halogenated, 296
  polycyclic, in carcinogenesis, 162
Hydrocele, 922–924, 925f
Hydrocephalic edema, 261
Hydrocephalus, 1439, 1440f
  congenital, 1461
Hydrogen peroxide:
  formation of, 57t
  production of, 20, 21f

Hydromyelia, 1459, 1459f
Hydronephrosis, 885–886
Hydropic swelling:
  mechanism of, 5, 5f
  ultrastructural changes in, 5, 6f
Hydrops fetalis, 245, 245f
Hydrosalpinx, 948
Hydrostatic pressure gradient, 252
Hydrothorax, 616
21-Hydroxylase deficiency, 1150
Hydroxyl radical:
  formation of, 57t
  iron in production of, 22
  lipid peroxidation and, 22, 24f
  production of, 20–21, 21f
Hydrozoa, 449
Hymenoptera, 448–449
Hyperaldosteronism, secondary, 1150
Hyperbilirubinemia, 727, 728, 729f
  neonatal, 732
  primary shunt, 728
Hypercalcemia:
  in cancer, 185, 1149, 1149t
  causes of, 1149, 1149t
Hypercalciuria, idiopathic, 886
Hypercholesterolemia, familial, 224
Hyperemia, 254–256, 255f
  active, 254
  conjunctival, 1508
  liver in, 254, 255f
  lung in, 254
  passive (congestion), 254
  spleen in, 255–256
Hypereosinophilic syndrome, 1408
Hyperglucagonemia, familial, 823
Hyperhemolytic crisis, 1044
Hyperkeratosis:
  epidermolytic, 1206–1207, 1206t, 1207f, 1208f
  follicular, in vitamin A deficiency, 318, 318f
Hyperparathyroid crisis, 1116
Hyperparathyroidism, 1146–1149
  adenoma in, 1146–1147
  bone in, 1346–1348, 1347f
  clinical features of, 1146, 1146f
  hyperplasia in, 1147–1148
  pathogenic pathways of, 1147–1148, 1148f
  secondary, 1348
Hyperpepsinogenemia I, 650
Hyperplasia, 10–11, 12f
  epidermal, 11, 12f
  physiologic, 10
Hyperprolactinemia, 1130
Hypersensitivity reactions, **105–116**
  classification of, 105t
  delayed type, 113–116, 114f–115f
  to environmental chemicals, 294
  type I (immediate or anaphylaxis), 105–106, 107f
  type II (cytotoxic), 106–109, 108f–110f
    antibody-dependent, cell mediated cytotoxicity in, 107–109
    in autoimmune disease, 130–131, 131t
    complement in, 106–107, 108f
  type III (immune complex), 109–113, 111f–112f
    in autoimmune disease, 130–131, 131t
  type IV (cell-mediated), 113–116, 114f–115f

Hypersplenism, 255, 1047, 1064
  in portal hypertension, 780
Hypertension, **477–481**
  atherosclerosis in, 481
  due to autoregulation, 478–480, 480f
  diagnosis of, 478
  effects on kidney, 878–879, 879f
  essential, 478
  etiology of, 478–480, 479f
  ischemic heart disease and, 526
  malignant, 878
  pathology of, 480–481, 480f–481f
  portal, **776–782.** See also Portal hyper-
    tension
  prevalence of, 532
  pulmonary, 254, 621–624. See also Pul-
    monary hypertension
  renin-angiotensin system in, 478
  renovascular, 837, 882–883, 883f
  smoking and, 277
Hypertensive heart disease, 532–533, 533f
Hypertensive hemorrhage, of brain, 1436–
    1438, 1438f–1440f
Hypertensive retinopathy, 1514, 1518f–
    1519f
Hyperthecosis, of ovary, 974, 974f
Hyperthermia, 303–304
  malignant, 303
Hyperthyroidism, **1134–1137**
  apathetic, 1135
  in cancer, 186
  heart in, 537
  ischemic heart disease and, 518
  ocular manifestations of, 1523–1524
  primary, 1134–1137, 1135f–1137f
  secondary, 1137
Hypertrophy, 9, 9f–11f
  myocardial, 9, 11f
  physiologic, 9
Hypervitaminosis D, 324
Hypoalbuminemia:
  in cancer, 187
  in hepatorenal syndrome, 738
Hypocalcemia, in cancer, 186
Hypochlorous acid:
  actions of, 56
  formation of, 57t
Hypogammaglobulinemia:
  Bruton's X-linked infantile, 122–123,
    124f
  malabsorption in, 679
  transient, of infancy, 123
Hypoglycemia, in cancer, 186
Hypokalemic nephropathy, 876, 876f
Hypoparathyroidism, 1145
Hypophosphatasia, 1385
Hypophosphatemic osteomalacia, in can-
    cer, 186
Hypopituitarism, 1125
Hypoplasia, in morphogenesis, 201
Hypoplastic left heart syndrome, 513
Hypospadias, 909
Hypothalamic corticotropin, 1131
Hypothalamic-pituitary axis, 1124
Hypothalamic-pituitary syndromes, 1124–
    1125
Hypothalamus, 1128–1132
  anatomy and physiology of, 1128–1129
  in gonadal dysfunction, 1129–1130
  hamartoma of, 1132
    lesions of, 1132t

Hypothalamus:
  in obesity, 315
  syndromes associated with, 1129
  in thermal regulation, 301
Hypothermia, 301–303
Hypothyroidism, 1139–1140, 1139f
  heart in, 537
  neonatal, 1134
Hypoventilation, idiopathic, pulmonary
    hypertension due to, 622
Hypovolemic shock, 269
Hypoxemia, pulmonary hypertension due
    to, 622
H-zone, of muscle, 1396

Ichthyoses, **1205–1209**
  definition and clinical features of, 1205
  lamellar, 1206t, 1207
  major types of, 1206t
  pathogenesis of, 1207
  pathology of, 1204–1207
  X-linked (sex-linked), 1206t, 1207
Ichthyosis vulgaris, 1206–1207, 1206t,
    1207f–1208f
Icterus, 727, 728, 729f
Icterus gravis, 245
Icterus neonatorum, 239
Ig, quantitation of, 119
IgA, in small intestine, 664
IgA deficiency, 123
IgA heavy chain disease, 1100
IgA nephropathy, 862, 863f–864f, 863t
IgE antibody, in immediate hypersensitiv-
    ity reaction, 105–106
IgG heavy chain disease, 1100
Ileitis, backwash, 686, 697
Ileocecal valve, 686
Ileum:
  anatomy of, 663
  ancylostomiasis of, 436, 437f
  blood and lymphatic supply of, 663
Ileus:
  adynamic, 671
  gallstone, 804
Immersion foot, 302
Immune complexes:
  in glomerulonephritis, 851–852
  in systemic lupus erythematosus, 132–
    133
  tissue injury by, 109–113, 111f–112f
  in tumor cell killing, 184
  in vasculitis, 482
Immune response:
  in alcoholism, 286
  B cells in, 100–101
  in celiac disease, 676–677
  cellular components of, **98–104**
  deficient, conditions promoting, 328
  lymphocytes in, 98–101, 99f
  macrophages in, 101–102, 102t
  in malignant tumors, 181–184, 183f–184f
  mononuclear phagocyte in, 101–102
  NK cells in, 101
  T cells in, 98–99, 100f, 100t
  in transplantation, 116–119, 118f
  in vasculitis, 482
Immune status, assessment of, 119–122,
    120f–122f

Immune surveillance, in tumor cell kill-
    ing, 184
Immune tolerance, 129
Immunoblast, 1023
Immunodeficiency, 122–129
  acquired. See also AIDS
  aspergillosis in, 574
  B cell, 122–123
  combined B cell and T cell, 123–124
  common variable, 123
  cryptococcosis in, 426
  flow cytometric profiles in, 124f–125f
  T cell, 123
  toxoplasmosis in, 413, 413f
Immunologically mediated disorders, **104–
    116**
  type I hypersensitivity in, 105–106, 107f
  type II hypersensitivity in, 106–109,
    108f–110f
  type III hypersensitivity in, 109–113,
    111f–112f
  type IV hypersensitivity in, 113–116,
    114f–115f
Immunologic theory of aging, 32
Impetigo:
  staphylococcal, 382
  streptococcal, 386
Incision, 307
Incisional hernia, 88
Inclusion blennorrhea, 1503
Inclusion conjunctivitis, 347, 1503
Indian childhood cirrhosis, 776
Infant. See Neonate
Infantile hemangioendothelioma, of liver,
    794
Infarct:
  bile, 734, 735f
  of brain, 257, 259f, 1427–1431, 1429f–
    1431f
  common sites of, 258t
  of intestine, 257–258
  of kidney, 258, 883
  lacunar, 257, 1432
  of liver, 787
  of lung, 257, 618–619
  morphology of, 256–257, 257f, 257t
  myocardial. See Myocardial infarct
  of placenta, 983
  of prostate, 930
  size of, determinants of, 256
  of small intestine, 669–671, 671f
  of spleen, 1065
  watershed, 1433–1434, 1434f
  Zahn, 787
Infectious mononucleosis, 338–340, 339f
  gingiva in, 1272
  lymphadenitis in, 1061
  spleen in, 1064
Infertility, 963, 964f
Inflammation, **34–64**
  acute, 35f, 36, 39f
  cellular recruitment in, 48–49, 50f
  chronic, 35f, 36, 39f, 58–59, 58f–61f
  granulomatous, 59–62, 62f–63f
  inflammatory cell activation in, 49–50,
    51f
  macrophages in, 101
  mediators of, 39f
  modulation of inflammatory cell func-
    tion in, 52–54, 52f–53f
  phagocytic cell adherence in, 57–58

Inflammation:
    possible outcomes of, 36
    systemic manifestations of, 62–63
    vascular permeability in, 36–37, 40f
    vasoactive mediators of, **38–48**. *See also*
        under Vasoactive mediators
Influenza virus, respiratory, 343–344
Infraglottic carcinoma, 548
Infraglottis, 545
Inguinal lymph nodes, hyperplasia of,
    1059
Inheritance:
    autosomal dominant, 220, 220f
    autosomal recessive, 224, 224f
    multifactorial, 234–235, 235t
Injury, physical, 306–307
Insect bites, 448–449
Insecticides, 296
Insertional mutagenesis, 173, 174f
Insulin:
    physiologic actions of, 825t
    synthesis and secretion of, 822f, 823,
        824f
Insulinoma, 826f–827f, 827
γ-Interferon, 100t
Interleukin–1:
    actions of, 62–63
    in atherosclerosis, 466
    function of, 101
Interleukin–2, 100t, 101
Interleukin–3, 100t
Intermittent claudication, 471
Interstitial space, 252
Intestinal angina, 672
Intestinal metaplasia, 11, 644–645, 646f,
    647
Intestine:
    large. *See* Colon
    small. *See* Small intestine
Intracellular storage, 13–14
Intramembranous ossification, 1306
Intranuclear inclusion:
    Cowdry type A, 334
    cytomegalic, 338
Intraocular pressure, elevated, 1528
Intraparotid lymph nodes, inflammation
    of, 1282
Intrauterine growth retardation, 238
Intravascular coagulation, disseminated,
    187, 487–488, 737, 1028–1029,
    1028f
Intravascular space, 252
Intravenous leiomyomatosis, 969
Intraventricular hemorrhage, 1438
Intrinsic mutagenesis theory of aging, 32
Invertebrates, marine, 449–450
Involucrum, 1333
Involution failures, 201
Iridopathy, diabetic, 1521–1522
Iris:
    neovascularization of, 1521
    in systemic disease, 1510t
Iron:
    absorption in hemochromatosis, 767–
        768
    cellular metabolism of, 22, 22f, 768
    gastrointestinal absorption of, 768
    in hydroxyl radical production, 22
    intracellular storage of, 14
    total body, increase of, 14
Iron deficiency, anemia in, 1040

Iron poisoning, 299–300
Ischemia:
    atrophy in, 8
    cell injury due to, 17–20
    cytoskeletal alterations due to, 19
    intracellular calcium homeostasis in, 19–
        20
    liver, irreversible cell injury in, 19, 20f
    myocardial. *See* Ischemic heart disease
    oxygen radicals in, 18–19
    phospholipid metabolism in, altered,
        19, 20f
    reperfusion injury in, 18–19
    reversible vs irreversible injury due to,
        17–18
Ischemic colitis, 700–701
Ischemic heart disease, **515–527**. *See also*
        Myocardial infarct; Myocardial
        infarction
    definition of, 515
    etiology of, 516–519, 516t, 517f
    irreversible cell injury in, 19, 20f
    manifestations of, 515
    metabolic and biochemical effects of,
        524
    mortality as function of age in, 465f
Islet cell tumors, **825–830**
    alpha cell, 825, 826
    beta cell, 826f–827f, 827
    D1, 828
    delta cell, 827–828
    enterochromaffin cell, 828
    polypeptide-secreting, 828
    ulcerogenic, 828–830
Islets of Langerhans, 822–823, 822f
    alpha cells of, 822–823, 822f
    beta cells of, 822f, 823
    cellular composition of, 822–823
    delta cells of, 822f, 823
    polypeptide-producing cells of, 823
    secretory products and physiologic ac-
        tions of, 825t
Isochromosome, 212
Isosporiasis, 418–419

Jamaican vomiting illness, 784
James fibers, 500
Japanese B encephalitis, 332
Jaundice, 727, 728
    in drug reactions, 289
    in erythroblastosis fetalis, 245
    in hepatic failure, 735
    hepatocellular mechanisms of, 729f
    idiopathic dyserythropoietic, 728
    neonatal, 732
    in neonate, 239
Jaw:
    ameloblastoma of, 1274, 1276f
    osteomyelitis of, 1272
JC virus, 171, 1455
Jejunitis, ulcerative, 677
Jejunum:
    anatomy of, 663
    blood and lymphatic supply of, 663
    strongyloidiasis of, 437, 437f
Jellyfish, 450
Joints, **1365–1392**
    biaxial, 1365
    cavitation of, 1367, 1368f

Joints:
    diarthrodial, development of, 1367–
        1368, 1368f
    embryologic development of, 1367
    function of, 1367
    polyaxial, 1365
    synovial:
        classification of, 1365–1367
        structures of, 1368–1371
        tumor and tumor-like lesions of, 1386–
            1387
        types of, 1365
        uniaxial, 1365
    vascular and nerve supply of, 1367
Junctional nevus, 1243
Juvenile angiofibroma, of nasopharynx,
    1292–1293, 1293
Juvenile colonic polyps, 708, 708f
Juvenile hemangioma, 493
Juvenile pilocytic astrocytoma, 1469
Juxtacortical osteosarcoma, 1359, 1361f

Kala-azar, 407–408, 408f, 789
Kaposi's sarcoma, 494–495, 1257, 1257f–
    1258f, 1392
    of lymph nodes, 1116
    of oral cavity, 1268, 1269f
Kappa light-chain glomerulosclerosis, 868
Kartagener's syndrome, 592
Karyolysis, 15
Karyorrhexis, 15
Kawasaki's disease, 484
Kayser-Fleischer ring, in Wilson's disease,
    773
K cells, 545
Keloid, 89, 90f, 1296
Keratinocytes, 1197, 1197f
Keratinocytic neoplasia, 1254–1256
Keratinosome, 1197, 1198f
Keratitis, interstitial, 321, 321f
Keratohyaline granule, 1197
Keratolysis, pitted, 394
Keratomalacia, 318, 318f
Keratopathy, band, 1525
Keratosis:
    actinic, 1255, 1255f
    retention, 1207
    seborrheic, 1254–1255
Keratosis follicularis, 1209, 1209f
Kerley B lines, 624
Kernicterus, 245, 728
Kerosene, 295
Kidney, **832–889**
    agenesis of, 837
    amyloid deposits in, 1189, 1190f
    anatomy of, 834–836, 834f–837f
    angiomyolipoma of, 887–888
    Ash-Upmark, 837
    clinical disease syndromes of, 836–837
    congenital abnormalities of, 837–841
    cortical necrosis of, bilateral, 883–884,
        884f
    cystic disease of, 838
    dysplasia of, cystic, 838, 838f
    ectopic, 837
    failure. *See* Renal failure
    glomerular diseases of, 841–869. *See also*
        Glomerulonephritis; Nephrotic
        syndrome

Kidney:
  in gout, 1382–1383
  hepatorenal syndrome of, 737–738
  horseshoe, 837
  in hydronephrosis, 885–886
  hypertension effects on, 878–879, 879f
  hypoplasia of, 837
  infarct of, 258, 883
  lead poisoning in, 298
  medullary cystic disease complex of, 840
  medullary sponge, 840
  in microangiopathic hemolytic anemia, 880
  in multiple myeloma, 1106
  necrotizing papillitis of, 1176
  nephroblastoma of, 887, 887f
  polyarteritis nodosa of, 879–880, 880f
  polycystic disease of, 838, 839f
    adult, 838–839, 839f
    infantile, 839–840, 840f
  renal cell carcinoma of, 888–889, 888f–889f
  in scleroderma, 882
  in shock, 271
  in sickle cell disease, 884
  simple cysts of, 840–841
  stones of, 652, 886, 886f
  in thrombotic thrombocytopenic purpura, 881
  transitional cell carcinoma of, 889
  tubulointerstitial diseases of, 869–877.
    See also Pyelonephritis
  vascular diseases of, 878–884
  vasculature of, 832f
  vasculitis of, 879–880, 880f
  Wegener's granulomatosis of, 880
  Wilms' tumor of, 887, 887f
  wound healing in, 92–93
  in yellow fever, 330
Kidney transplantation, 116–119, 118f, 652
  acute rejection in, 116–117, 118f
  chronic rejection in, 117–118, 118f
  hyperacute rejection in, 116, 118f
Kikuchi's disease, 1061
Kimmelstiel-Wilson disease, 487, 847, 1174–1175, 1175f
Kininase I, 43
Kininase II, 43
Kinins, vasoactive, 42–43, 44f
Klebsiella pneumoniae pneumonia, 378–379, 568
Klebsiella rhinoscleromatis, 1286
Klinefelter's syndrome, 217, 217f, 915–916, 915f
Knee, chondromalacia of, 1371
Köhler's disease, 1326
Koplik's spots, 340
Korean hemorrhagic fever, 331
Korsakoff's psychosis, 1479
Korsakoff's syndrome, 319
Krabbe's disease, 228f, 1463
Krukenberg tumor, 660, 974, 981, 981f
Kugelberg-Welander disease, 1403, 1413
Kupffer cells, of liver, 726
Kuru, 1455–1456
Kwashiorkor, 316–317, 317f
Kyasanur Forest disease, 331

Labyrinthine toxicity, 1301
Labyrinthitis, viral, 1302

Laceration, 307
Lacrimal gland, 1510t
Lactating adenoma, of breast, 1000
Lactation, breast in, 995
Lactiferous sinus, 992
Lactose tolerance test, 675
Lacunar infarct, 257, 1432
Laennec's cirrhosis, 764
LAK cells, tumoricidal, 181
Lamellar ichthyosis, 1206t, 1207
Lamina densa, of basement membrane, 72, 72f
Lamina lucida, of basement membrane, 72, 72f
Lamina rara, of basement membrane, 72, 72f
Laminar necrosis, 1432f–1433f, 1433–1434
Laminin, in basement membrane, 73, 73t
Landry-Guillain-Barré syndrome, 1492
Langerhans cells, 1200f, 1201
Langhans' giant cells, 61, 63f
Large for gestational age infant, 238
Larva currens, 438
Larva migrans:
  cutaneous, 438, 438f
  visceral, 437
Laryngitis, 548
Larynx:
  anatomy and histology of, 544–545, 545f
  carcinoma of, 278
  nodules of, 548
  squamous papilloma of, 548
Lassa fever, 331
Lathyrism, 71
Laurence-Moon-Biedl syndrome, 1124
Lead colic, 297
Lead poisoning, 297–298, 298f
Lecithin:sphingomyelin ratio, 238–239, 239f
Leg, sporotrichosis of, 427, 427f
Legg-Calvé-Perthes disease, 1326
Legionella pneumophilia pneumonia, 569–570
Legionnaires' disease, 365–366, 366f
Legs, varicose veins of, 491
Leiomyoblastomas, of stomach, 655–656
Leiomyoma:
  of cervix, 957
  of stomach, 655–656, 656f
  of uterus, 969, 969f–970f
Leiomyomatosis, intravenous, 969
Leiomyosarcoma:
  of small intestine, 684
  of stomach, 661
  of uterus, 969–970, 971f
Leishmania brasiliensis, 406, 407
Leishmania donovani, 407–408
Leishmania mexicana, 406–407, 407f
Leishmaniasis, 406–408, 407f–408f
  cutaneous, 406–407
  of liver, 789
  mucocutaneous, 406–407
  of nose, 1287
  visceral, 407–408, 408f
Leishmania tropica, 406–407, 407f
Lens:
  common disorders of, 1525–1527
  in diabetes mellitus, 1522–1523
  in systemic disease, 1510t–1511t
Lentigo, 1243
Lentigo maligna melanoma, 1250, 1251f

Leontiasis ossea, 1352
Lepidoptera, 448
Leprosy, 397–401, 398f–400f
  distribution of, 399f
  lepromatous, 398f–400f
  nose in, 1286
  susceptibility to, 400
  tuberculoid, 398f–399f
Leptomeningitis, 1441
Leptospirosis, 351–352, 352f, 790
Lethal midline granuloma, of nose, 1288, 1289f
Letterer-Siwe disease, 1054–1055, 1337
Leukemia, 144
  acute lymphoblastic, 1089–1091, 1090t
    bone marrow in, 1078f, 1090
    FAB morphologic classification in, 1076f, 1090
    immunologic classification in, 1090, 1090t
    lymph nodes in, 1080f, 1090
    meningitis in, 1089
    pathogenesis of, 1089–1090
  acute megakaryoblastic, 1075
  acute monocytic, 1075
  acute nonlymphocytic, 1074–1079
    Auer rods in, 1075, 1075f
    bone marrow in, 1075, 1078f
    clinical manifestations of, 1077–1079
    complications of, 1074
    cytochemical studies in, 1075, 1077f
    dyspoiesis in, 1075
    granulocytic sarcoma in, 1077, 1081f
    hematologic disorders associated with, 1074–1075
    laboratory findings in, 1077
    lymph node in, 1077, 1080f
    morphologic variants in, 1075, 1076f
    risk factors in, 1074, 1074t
  cellular differentiation in, 180
  chicken, 169
  chronic lymphocytic, 1083–1087
    bone marrow in, 1078f, 1083–1086
    geographic and ethnic factors in, 194
    global epidemiology of, 1083, 1084f–1085f
    lymphocytes in, 1086–1087, 1086f
    neoplastic cells in, 1086
    pathophysiology of, 1083
    Rai clinical staging system for, 1087, 1087t
    Richter's syndrome with, 1087
    spleen in, 1083, 1086f
    T-cell, 1087
  chronic myelogenous, 1069–1071
    clinical features of, 1071, 1072t
    hematopathologic features of, 1072t
    laboratory findings in, 1071, 1072t
    leukocyte alkaline phosphatase in, 1071
    Philadelphia chromosome in, 1070
    spleen in, 1070–1071, 1070f
  gingiva in, 1273
  hairy cell, 1088–1089
    bone marrow in, 1078f, 1088
    malignant lymphoma simulating, 1088
    peripheral blood smear in, 1088, 1089f
    spleen in, 1070f, 1088
    TRAP stain in, 1088
  mast cell, 1052

Leukemia:
  myelomonocytic, chronic, 1036t
  prolymphocytic, 1087–1088
Leukemic reticuloendotheliosis, 1088
Leukemoid reaction, 63, 1049
Leukocyte:
  exudation and phagocytosis of, 50f
  flow cytometric analysis of, 122, 122f
  in inflammatory response, 48–50, 50f
  morphology of, abnormal, 1050f
  polymorphonuclear:
    activation of, 49, 51t
    benign disorders of, 1048–1051
    in chronic inflammation, 59
    granules of, 54–55, 56f
    morphology and function of, 56f
    oxygen radical production by, 56–57, 57t
Leukocyte alkaline phosphatase, 1071
Leukocyte function antigen–1 (LFA–1), 58
Leukocyte inhibition factor, 100t
Leukocytosis, in inflammation, 63
Leukodystrophy, metachromatic, 228f, 1463–1464
Leukoencephalopathy, progressive multifocal, 171, 1448, 1451f, 1454–1455, 1454f–1456f
Leukopenia, 63
Leukoplakia, 1267, 1267f
Leukotriene B₄, 106
Leukotriene C₄:
  functions of, 42
  in immediate hypersensitivity reaction, 106
Leukotriene D₄:
  functions of, 42
  in immediate hypersensitivity reaction, 106
Leukotriene E₄:
  functions of, 42
  in immediate hypersensitivity reaction, 106
Leukotrienes, formation of, 47–48, 48f
Leydig cell tumor, of testis, 921, 922f
Libman-Sacks endocarditis, 134, 532
Lice, sucking, 448
Lichen planus, 1226–1229
  definition and clinical features of, 1226–1227
  etiology and pathogenesis of, 1228–1229, 1230f
  pathology of, 1227–1228, 1228f–1229f
Lichen sclerosis, of vulva, 949–950, 950f
Lichen simplex chronicus, 1206
Life span, 29–30, 30f
Ligandin, 727
Lignac-Fanconi syndrome, 1345
Limit dextrinosis, 1410
Lindau's syndrome, 1475
Lindau-von Hippel disease, 493
Lingual thyroid nodule, 1262
Linitis plastica, 658, 659f
Lip, cleft, 235–236, 236f
Lipid metabolism, 466–470, 467t, 468f–469f
  clinical disorders of, 470t
  endogenous pathway of, 467–470, 468f–469f
  exogenous pathway of, 467, 468f–469f
Lipid peroxidation:
  in cellular aging, 32–33

Lipid peroxidation:
  hydroxyl radicals and, 22, 24f
  trichloromethyl radical in, 25–26, 27f
Lipocortin:
  actions of, 48
  in phospholipase A2 regulation, 49
Lipofuscin, 32
Lipogranuloma, sclerosing, of penis, 938
Lipoid nephrosis, 842
Lipoma, 1390
  infiltrating, 1390, 1390f
  intracranial, 1474
  microscopic appearance of, 147, 147f
  of small intestine, 681–682
Lipoprotein:
  classes of, 467
  low-density, in atherosclerosis, 460
Lipoproteinosis, alveolar, 581, 582f
Lipoprotein-X, in primary biliary cirrhosis, 762
Liposarcoma, 1390, 1391f
Lips, diseases of, 1269, 1269f–1270f
Lissencephaly, 1461
Listeriosis, 372
Liver, 722–799
  abscess of:
    amebic, 416
    cholangitic, 788, 788f
  adenoma of, 792–793, 792f
    in oral contraceptive use, 292
  in alcoholism, 284, 284f–285f, 750–760. *See also* Alcoholic liver disease
  amebiasis of, 788–789, 789f
  anatomy of, 723f–726f, 724–726
  angiosarcoma of, 494
  ascariasis of, 789
  bacterial infection of, 787–788, 788f
  bilirubin metabolism in, 727–732
  blood supply of, 724
  carcinogenesis in, chemical, 164–167, 166f
  carcinoma of, 794–796, 796f. *See also* Hepatocellular carcinoma
  cardiac fibrosis of, 787
  cells of, 725–726
  central hyaline sclerosis in, 759, 760f
  cirrhosis of. *See* Cirrhosis
  clonorchiasis of, 441, 443f
  confluent necrosis of, 748–749, 749f
  congestion of:
    chronic passive, 254, 255f, 786–787, 786f
    in heart failure, 502–503, 504f
  in congestive heart failure, 786–787, 786f
  cystic disease of, 794
  echinococcosis in, 446, 790
  failure of, 734–738. *See also* Hepatic failure
  fatty. *See* Fatty liver
  fibrosis of:
    congenital, 794
    onion skin, 767
  flukes of, parasitic, 789–790
  focal nodular hyperplasia of, 793, 793f
  functions of, 726–727
  helminthic infection of, 789–790
  hemangioma of, 794
  hemangiosarcoma of, 786, 797–798
  in hemochromatosis, 769–771, 770f
  hepatitis of, 738–751. *See also* Hepatitis

Liver:
  hepatorenal syndrome of, 737–738
  hydatid cysts of, 446
  infantile hemangioendothelioma of, 794
  infarction of, 787
  ischemia, irreversible cell injury in, 19, 20f
  leishmaniasis in, 789
  in leptospirosis, 790
  lobular architecture of, 724–725, 724f–725f
  in malaria, 789
  metastasis to, 798, 798f
  microscopic structure of, 724–726
  nodular transformation of, 793–794
  nutmeg, 254, 255f, 503, 504f, 786–787, 786f
  pipestem fibrosis of, 441, 443f
  in premature infant, 239
  protozoal infection of, 788–789, 789f
  regeneration of, 83, 86
  schistosomiasis of, 441, 443f
  shock in, 273, 787
  sinusoidal architecture of, 459, 726
  in syphilis, 355, 790
  toxic injury of, 782–786
  toxic necrosis of, 25–27, 27f, 782–786
    due to acetaminophen, 26–27
    due to bromobenzene, 26–27
    due to carbon tetrachloride, 25–26, 27f
    chronic active hepatitis in, 785
    fatty liver due to, 783–784, 783f
    granulomatous hepatitis in, 785
    hyperplastic and neoplastic lesions in, 786
    intrahepatic cholestasis in, 784–785
    mild intralobular hepatitis in, 785
    peliosis hepatis in, 785, 786f
    predictable hepatotoxins in, 782
    vascular lesions in, 785, 786f
    viral hepatitis-like reaction in, 785
    zonal hepatocellular necrosis in, 782f, 783
  transplantation, rejection of, 798–799, 798f–799f
  in tuberculosis, 398f
  veno-occlusive disease of, 779, 785
  in Wilson's disease, 773
  wound healing in, 89, 92, 92f
  in yellow fever, 330, 330f
Loa loa, 432
Lobar sclerosis, 1487, 1489f
Lockjaw, 376
Loiasis, 432
Luetic aneurysm, 489, 489f
Luetic aortitis, 355, 355f, 456, 489, 489f, 518, 540
Luetic vasculitis, 354, 354f
Lung. *See also* Pneumonia; Tuberculosis
  abscess of, 552–553, 552f–553f
  actinomycosis of, 573
  aging, 593
  airspace enlargement in, 593, 593t
  amyloidosis of, 576
  anatomy of, 542f–543f, 545–546
  anthrax in, 358
  ascariasis of, 439
  aspergillosis of, 574, 575f
  atypical mycobacterial infection of, 573
  bacterial infections of, 566–573

Lung:
  black, 13, 595
  blastoma of, 559
  blastomycosis of, 574
  bronchocentric granulomatosis of, 615
  brown induration of, 254, 623
  candidiasis of, 575
  carcinoma of. See Lung cancer
  chronic disease of, peptic ulcer disease and, 653
  chronic obstructive disease of (COPD), 279, 280f
  Churg-Strauss syndrome of, 615
  coccidioidomycosis of, 425–426, 573–574
  coin lesions of, 561–562, 562f
  compensatory overinflation of, 593
  congenital adenomatoid malformation of, 563
  congenital hypoplasia of, 562–563
  congenital intralobar sequestration in, 563
  congenital lobar overinflation of, 593
  congestion of, chronic passive, 254
  cryptococcoma of, 426
  cryptococcosis in, 426, 574
  defense mechanisms of, 547, 547f
  dirofilariasis of, 433, 576
  in Down's syndrome, 593
  edema of, 261–263, 266f, 618–621, 619f. See also Pulmonary edema
  embolism of, 265–267, 266f, **618–621**, 619f. See also Embolism, of lung
  eosinophilic, 432
  eosinophilic granuloma of, 610–612, 611f
  in fetus and neonate, 238–239
  fibrosis of, idiopathic, 609
  in first breath, 240
  fungal infection of, 573–575
  gangrene of, 569
  hamartoma of, 561, 562f
  hemodynamics of, in hepatorenal syndrome, 738
  hemorrhage of, 581–583
  histoplasmosis of, 428, 428f, 573
  honeycomb, 608, 608f
  hypertensive disorders of. See Pulmonary hypertension
  infarction of, 257, 618–619
  interstitium of, 546
  in Legionnaires' disease, 365–366, 366f
  lymphangiomyomatosis of, 612–614
  lymphomatoid granulomatosis of, 615
  lymphoproliferative disorders of, 610
  in melioidosis, 370, 370f
  metastatic calcification of, 577
  in miliary tuberculosis, 397f–398f
  mucormycosis of, 574–575
  nocardiosis of, 393–394, 394f, 573
  oxygen toxicity of, 580
  ozone damage to, 580
  in paracoccidioidomycosis, 424f
  paragonimiasis of, 444
  paraquat poisoning in, 580
  passive congestion of, chronic, 623
  phycomycosis of, 574–575
  in pneumocystosis, 413–414, 414f
  protozoal infection of, 575–576
  pseudolymphoma of, 610
  restrictive, infiltrative, or interstitial disease of, 605–615

Lung:
  in rheumatic heart disease, 531
  right middle lobe syndrome of, 552
  sarcoidal granulomatosis of, necrotizing, 615
  sarcoidosis of, 607–608, 607f
  shock in, 272
  thromboembolism of, 265–267, 266f, 618–619, 619f
  in tularemia, 363, 364f
  vasculature of, disease of, 618–627
  viral infections of, 563–566
  in Wegener's granulomatosis, 484, 485f, 614
  wound healing in, 93–94
  zygomycosis of, 430, 430f
Lung cancer, **553–561**
  adenocarcinoma, 556, 557f
  adenoid cystic carcinoma, 559
  in asbestos workers, 605
  bronchoalveolar, 557–559
  carcinoid tumor, 559, 560f
  carcinosarcoma, 559
  cigarette smoking and, 554
  classification of, 554
  features common to all types of, 554
  large cell undifferentiated, 556
  lymphangitic carcinoma, 560–561
  metastatic, 560–561, 561f
  mucoepidermoid carcinoma, 559
  paraneoplastic syndromes in, 559–560
  primary, 553–560
  small cell carcinoma, 556–557, 558f
  due to smoking, 278–279, 278f–279f
  squamous cell carcinoma, 156f, 554–556, 555f–556f
  in United States, 190, 191f–192f, 192t
Lupus erythematosus:
  cutaneous, **1223–1226**
    acute, 1223
    chronic, 1223
    etiology and pathogenesis of, 1224–1226, 1227f
    pathology of, 1223, 1226f
    subacute, 1223
  discoid, 1223
  systemic, **131–135**, 1222–1223
    complications of, 133f
    as drug reaction, 293
    etiology of, 131–132
    glomerulonephritis in, 133–134, 133f–134f, 864–867, 865f–866f. See also Lupus nephritis
    heart in, 531–532
    immunologic abnormalities in, 132
    lymphadenopathy in, 1062
    pathogenesis of, 132–135
    primary organ systems in, 132t
Lupus nephritis, 133–134, 133f–134f, 864–867, 865f–866f
  classification of, 866
  diffuse proliferative, 133–134, 134f
  focal proliferative, 133, 134f
  hematoxylin bodies in, 865
  interstitial involvement in, 867
  membranous, 134
  mesangeal, 133, 133f
  morphology in, 865–866, 865f–866f
  transformation in, 866
  wire loops in, 865, 866f
Lupus vulgaris, 1285

Luteinizing hormone, 1122
Lutembacher's syndrome, 507
Luteotropic hormone, 1122
Lyme disease, 358
Lymphadenitis, 62
  onchocercal, 433
  suppurative, acute, 1059
  in toxoplasmosis, 412–413
Lymphadenopathy:
  in Burkitt's lymphoma, 339–340
  dermatopathic, 1053
  in sinus histiocytosis, 1053
Lymphangiectasia, 492
  congenital, malabsorption in, 679–680
Lymphangioma:
  capillary, 495
  cavernous, 495
  cystic, 495
  of oral cavity, 1267
Lymphangiomyomatosis, of lung, 612–614
Lymphangitic carcinoma, of lung, 560–561
Lymphangitis, 62, 492
Lymphatic space, 252
Lymphatic system:
  function of, 459
  in inflammation, 62
  of lung, 546
Lymphatic vessels, 492
Lymphedema, 263f
Lymph nodes, 1020, 1020f
  in acute lymphoblastic leukemia, 1080f, 1090
  cervical, hyperplasia of, 1059
  in Gambian trypanosomiasis, 404f, 405
  hyperplasia of, **1057–1063**
    in AIDS, 1061
    angiofollicular lymphoid, 1060–1061
    benign reactive, 1057–1059, 1058f
    extranodal, 1063–1064, 1063t
    follicular, 1059–1061, 1060f–1061f
    giant, 1060–1061
    interfollicular, 1061–1063, 1062f
    in rheumatoid arthritis, 1060
    site of, 1059
    in syphilis, 1060
    in toxoplasmosis, 1060
  inguinal, hyperplasia of, 1059
  intraparotid, 1282
  in leukemia and lymphoma, 1080f
  in lymphogranuloma venereum, 348, 348f
  in metastasis, 153, 153f
  metastatic tumors of, 1116
  mucocutaneous, syndrome of, 484
  in non-Hodgkin's malignant lymphoma, 1080f–1081f, 1094, 1095f
  in onchocerciasis, 433
  reactive hyperplasia of, 153
  in syphilis, 355
  in tuberculosis, 397f
Lymphocyte
  atypical, 1023
  in chronic inflammation, 59
  immune function of, 98–101, 99f
  large granular, 1056
  maturational stages of, 99f
  morphology and function of, 61f
Lymphocytopenia, 1057
Lymphocytosis, 63, 1056–1057, 1057t
Lymphogranuloma venereum, 347–348, 348f
  of female genital tract, 947

Lymphoid cells, benign disorders of, 1054–1064
Lymphoid hyperplasia, benign, of stomach, 656
Lymphoid nodules, 1055–1056
Lymphokines, T cell, 100t
Lymphoma:
  of breast, 1012
  Burkitt's. *See* Burkitt's lymphoma
  cellular differentiation in, 180
  chicken, 169
  of colon, 712
  composite, 1104
  cutaneous T-helper cell, 1257–1258
  diffuse large cleaved cell, 1102–1103
  diffuse large noncleaved cell, 1102–1103, 1102f
  diffuse mixed small and large cell, 1102
  diffuse small cleaved cell, 1101–1102
  follicular large cell, 1101
  follicular small cleaved and large cell, 1101
  follicular small cleaved cell, 1100–1101
  intracranial, 1475
  large cell immunoblastic, 1103
  lymphoblastic, 1103–1104
  Mediterranean:
    abdominal, 1100
    of small bowel, 682–683
  non-Burkitt's, 1104
  non-Hodgkin's malignant, **1091–1108**
    classification of, 1094–1096, 1097t
    cytologic features of, 1098f
    disorders with increased risk of, 1092, 1094t
    etiology of, 1091–1092
    follicular, 1094, 1095f
    general features of, 1093–1094
    global epidemiologic patterns of, 1091, 1094t
    high-grade, 1103–1104
    Hodgkin's disease vs, 1092t
    intermediate grade, 1101–1103
    International Working Formulation for, 1096, 1097t
    light chain restriction in, 1091, 1093f
    low grade, 1096–1101
    Lukes-Collins classification of, 1095–1096, 1097t
    lymph node in, 1080f–1081f, 1094, 1095f
    pediatric vs adult, 1094, 1095t
    Rappaport classification of, 1094–1095, 1097t
    reactive follicular hyperplasia vs, 1094, 1096t
    sites of involvement of, 1099f
  of oral cavity, 1268
  of small bowel, 682–683
  small lymphocytic, 1096–1097, 1100f
  small lymphocytic plasmacytoid, 1097–1100
  small noncleaved cell, 1104
  of stomach, 661
  of thyroid, 1144
  true histiocytic, 1082f, 1083
  of Waldeyer's ring, 1294
  western, of small intestine, 683
Lymphomatoid granulomatosis, of lung, 615

Lymphopoietic system:
  biochemical identification of cell lineage in, 1024t
  cellular differentiation in, 1015t, 1017t
  cellular maturation in, 1015t, 1022–1023, 1023t
  functions of, 1019–1022
  lymph nodes of, 1020, 1020f
  lymphoid tissues of gut and bronchi in, 1020–1021
  morphologic and immunologic evaluation of, 1023–1024, 1023t–1024t
  spleen in, 1021–1022, 1021f
Lymphoproliferative disorders, of lung, 610
Lymphotoxin, 100t
Lysosomal diseases, 226
Lysosomal granule defect, 57t
Lysosomal storage disease, 219
Lysozyme, bactericidal, 54
Lysyl oxidase, in collagen assembly, 71

McArdle's disease, 227f, 1410, 1410f
MacCallum's patch, 529f, 531
McCune-Albright's syndrome, 1124
Macrocytes, oval, 1038
α_2-Macroglobulin, actions of, 55
Macroglobulinemia, Waldenström's, 1097
Macroglossia, 1269–1270
Macrophage:
  alveolar, 547, 547f
  in atherosclerosis, 460, 465–466
  in chronic inflammation, 59, 60f
  enzymes of, 55
  in granuloma formation, 60–61, 62f
  immune function of, 101–102
  in inflammation, 101
  intracellular storage by, 13
  major products of, 102t
  morphology and function of, 59, 59f
  oxygen radical production by, 57
  tingible bodies of, 1020, 1059–1060
  tumoricidal, 183
Macula:
  cherry red, 1529, 1530f
  degeneration of, 1529
Maffucci's syndrome, 1322–1323
Mahaim fibers, 500
Major histocompatibility complex, 99, 102–104, 103f, 104t
  class I antigens in, 102
  class II antigens in, 102, 104
Malabsorption, **672–675**, 674f
  in abetalipoproteinemia, 678–679
  in cancer, 187
  in celiac disease, 675–678, 676f–677f
  clinical features of, 673–675
  in deficiency states, 673
  in diarrhea, 675
  generalized, 673
  in hypogammaglobulinemia, 679
  intestinal phase of, 673, 674f
  laboratory evalation of, 675
  luminal phase of, 672–673, 674f
  in lymphangiectasia, 679–680
  in radiation enteritis, 680
  specific, 673
  in tropical sprue, 680
  in Whipple's disease, 678, 679f

Malacoplakia:
  of prostate, 930
  of testis, 916
  of urinary bladder, 901–903, 902f
Malaria, 408–412, 409f–412f
  geographic distribution of, 408, 409f
  life cycle of, 409, 410f
  liver in, 789
  plasmodial species in, 408
  spleen in, 1064–1065
Malayan filariasis, 431–432
Male infertility, 914f–915f, 915–916
Male urinary tract, **890–941**. *See also individual anatomic parts*
Malformation, 199
Malignant hyperthermia, 303
Malignant melanoma. *See* Melanoma, malignant
Mallory body, 759, 759f
Mallory-Weiss syndrome, 285, 637
Malnutrition, protein-calorie, 316–317
Mammotropic hormone, 1122
Manganese deficiency, 325
Mansonelliasis, 433
Marasmus, 316
Marble bone disease of Albers-Schönberg, 1320
Marburg virus disease, 331
March fracture, 1326
March hemoglobinuria, 1047
Marek's disease virus, 471
Marfan syndrome, 222, 222f
Marine invertebrates, 449–450
Mast cell leukemia, 1052
Mast cells, 1203–1204
  morphology and function of, 40–42, 42f
  proliferative disorders of, 1051–1052, 1052t
  in type I hypersensitivity reaction, 106, 107f
  in urticaria pigmentosa, 1204, 1204f
Mastitis:
  acute bacterial, 997
  granulomatous, 998
  plasma cell, 997
Mastocytoma, solitary, 1052
Mastocytosis, systemic, 1052
Mastoiditis, 1298
May-Hegglin anomaly, 1027
Measles, 340–341, 341f
  bronchiolitis in, 550
  German, 341
  lymphadenitis in, 1061
  pneumonia in, 566
Measles virus pneumonia, 344
Meckel's diverticulum, 665–666, 665f
Meconium ileus, 666
Meconium peritonitis, 225
Mediterranean abdominal lymphoma, 1100
Mediterranean fever, familial, 720, 1183–1184
Mediterranean lymphoma, of small intestine, 682–683
Medulloblastoma, 1472
Megacolon:
  acquired, 688
  congenital, 687–688, 687f–688f
  toxic, in ulcerative colitis, 697
Megakaryoblast, 1022
Megakaryocytes, 1017, 1023

Megakaryocytopenia, 1027
Megaloblastosis, 1037, 1038f
Megaloureter, congenital, 893
Melanocytes, 1199–1200, 1199f
Melanocyte stimulating hormone, 1123
Melanocytic nevi, 1242–1243, 1242f–1243f
    congenital, 1254
Melanofilaments, 1200
Melanoma, malignant:
    acral lentiginous, 1250–1252, 1251f–1253f
    of anal canal, 713
    geographic and ethnic factors in, 193
    intraocular, 1505, 1506f, 1508t
    in vivo-in vitro correlations of, 1249
    lentigo maligna, 1250, 1251f
    level of invasion in, 1252–1253
    lymphocytic response in, 1253, 1254f
    metastatic, 1249
    mucosal lentiginous, 1250
    nodular, 1249–1250, 1249f–1250f
    of oral cavity, 1268
    prognostic indicators in, 1252–1253
    radial growth phase of, 1243–1245,
        1245f
    superficial spreading, 1242–1249
    of vagina, 955
    vertical growth phase of, 1245–1246,
        1246f–1248f
    of vulva, 952
Melanosis coli, 713
Melanosome, 1199–1200, 1199f
Melanotropin, 1123
Melatonin, 1161
Melioidosis, 370–371, 370f
Membrane attack complex, 44, 106
Membranoproliferative glomerulonephri-
        tis, 858–859, 860f–862f
Membranous nephropathy, 845–847, 845f–
        847f
Ménétrier's disease, 647–648, 647f
Meniere's disease, 1301, 1302f
Meningioma, 1472–1474, 1472f–1473f
    of inner ear, 1302
Meningitis, **1441–1446**
    in acute lymphoblastic leukemia, 1089
    bacterial, 1443–1444
    cryptococcal, 426, 1445
    Hemophilus influenzae in, 364, 1444
    listeriosis, 372
    meningococcal, 389, 1444
    organisms in, 1441
    pneumococcal, 388
    purulent, 1441–1443, 1442f
    routes of entry for microorganisms in,
        1443, 1443f
    staphylococcal, 384
    syphilitic, 1445–1446, 1446f–1447f
    tuberculous, 1444–1445, 1444f
Meningocele, 1459
Meningococcal infection, 388–389, 389f
Meningococcal meningitis, 389
Meningococcemia, 389
Meningoencephalitis:
    amebic, 417
    cryptococcal, 426
    hartmannella-acanthameba, 417–418
Meningoencephalomyelitis, 406
Meningomyelocele, 1458f–1459f, 1459
Meningothelial cells, 1472, 1473f
Meningovascular syphilis, 355

Menopause:
    breast in, 995
    hypothalamus in, 1130
Menstrual cycle, 961
    abnormalities of, 962
    effects on breast of, 992–995
    hormonal, ovarian, endometrial
        changes in, 943f
MEN type 1, 1126, 1155f
MEN type 2, 1155f
MEN type 2a, 1143
MEN type 2b, 1143
Mercaptans, in hepatic encephalopathy,
        735
Mercury poisoning, 298–299
Merkel cells, 1201, 1201f
Mesenteric artery, thrombosis of, 671
Mesenteric cyst, 720
Mesenteric vein, thrombosis of, 671
Mesothelioma, 605
    benign (localized), 618
    of heart, 540–541
    malignant, of tunica vaginalis, 924
    peritoneal, 168–169
    pleural, 168–169, 617–618, 617f
Metachromatic leukodystrophy, 228f, 1463
Metal ions, in carcinogenesis, 163
Metals, toxic, 297–300
Metaphysis, 1306, 1307f
    lead lines in, 297
Metaplasia, 11–12, 13f
    intestinal, 11, 644–645, 646f, 647
    squamous, 11, 13f
Metastasis, 151–153
    hematogenous, 152, 152f
    lymphatic, 153, 153f
    skip, 153
Methanol, 295
Methemoglobinemia, hereditary, 1045
Methotrexate, alveolar damage due to,
        581
Miami Beach syndrome, 549
Microabscess, Darier-Pautrier's, 1004
Microaneurysm, retinal capillary, 487
Microcirculation, 38f, 253
Microglandular hyperplasia, of cervix,
        956–957
Microhamartoma, of bile duct, 794
Microorganism:
    body defenses against, 328
    Koch's postulates of, 329
    pathologists criteria of, 329, 329t
Micropinocytosis, 459
Microprolactinoma, 1127
Microsporidiosis, 419–421
Microsporum, 431
Microvasculature, injury to, 36–37, 40f
Microwave radiation, 314
Midline lethal reticulosis of face, 1288,
        1289f
Migration inhibition factor, 100t
Mikulicz cells, 378
Mikulicz's disease, 1277
Milkman-Looser syndrome, 1344
Millipedes, 449
Milroy's disease, 492, 679
Minamata disease, 299
Mites, 448
Mitochondria:
    in irreversible ischemic injury, 17–18
    in reversible cell injury, 5, 7f

Mitochondrial myopathy, 1397, 1400f
Mitral valve:
    in bacterial endocarditis, 534
    in rheumatic heart disease, 528, 528f–
        529f
Mixed connective tissue disease, 138
M-line, of muscle, 1396
MO–1, in phagocytic cell adherence, 58
Moles, 1242–1243, 1242f–1243f
Molluscum infection, of female genital
        tract, 948
Moniliasis. See Candidiasis
Monoblast, 1022
Monoclonal gammopathy, 1065–1066,
        1066f, 1067t
Monocytes:
    enzymes of, 55
    maturation of, 1022–1023
    morphology and function of, 59, 59f
    oxygen radical production by, 57
Monocytosis, 1052–1053, 1053f
Mononuclear phagocyte system, 101–102,
        1018–1019, 1019f
    benign disorders of, 1052–1054, 1054f
    functions of, 1019
    immunologic and functional markers of,
        1023t
    malignant disorders of, 1079–1083
Mononucleosis, infectious, 338–340, 339f
Monosomy, autosomal, 213
Monosomy X, 217–218
Monsters, double, 201
Morphea, 1234
Morphogenesis, errors of, **199–209**
    clinically important, 203–209
    developmental stages and, 200f
    terminology in, 200–203
Morphostasis, 77
Morquio's syndrome, 1315, 1316f
Morton's neuroma, 1495
Mosaicism, 214
Moths, 448
Motilin:
    physiologic actions of, 825t
    synthesis of, 823
Motor unit, 1396
Mountain sickness, 306
Mouse mammary tumor virus, 1005
Mucinous tumor, of ovary, 977
Mucocele:
    of appendix, 715–716, 715f
    of lip, 1270
    in sinusitis, 1284
Mucociliary blanket, respiratory, 547, 547f
Mucocutaneous candidiasis, 123, 424
Mucocutaneous leishmaniasis, 406–407
Mucocutaneous lymph node syndrome,
        484
Mucoepidermoid carcinoma, of lung, 559
Mucopolysaccharides, 74
Mucopolysaccharidoses, 230, 231f
    epiphyseal plate in, 1316f
    heart in, 538, 538f
Mucormycosis:
    of lung, 574–575
    of small intestine, 669
Mucosal lentiginous melanoma, 1250
Mucous glands, tracheobronchial, 545
Mucous neck cells, 641
Mucoviscidosis, 225
Müllerian adenosarcoma, 968

Multifactorial inheritance, 234–235, 235t
Multiple endocrine adenopathy (MEA) syndromes, 830
Multiple endocrine neoplasia (MEN) syndrome, 224, 652
Multiple gestation, 983–985
Multiple sclerosis, 1464–1466
  etiology and pathogenesis of, 1465
  plaque in, 1464–1465, 1464f–1465f
Mumps, 341–342, 1275–1276
Muscle, **1394–1414**
  in alcoholism, 285
  alkaline ATPase reaction for, 1397
  anatomy of, 1395f, 1396–1397
  biopsy of, 1400
  degeneration/regeneration in, 1402f
  denervation of, 1397, 1398f–1400f, 1412–1414
    target fibers in, 1412–1413
    type grouping in, 1413
    type predominance in, 1413
  enzyme histochemical stains for, 1397, 1400f–1401f
  fast twitch, 1396
  inflammatory myopathies of, 1406–1409
  metabolic disease of, 1409–1412
  metabolic profiles of, 1396
  NADH-TR reaction for, 1397, 1400f–1401f
  noninflammatory myopathies of, 1400–1406
  nonspecific esterase reaction for, 1397
  PAS stain for, 1397
  reinnervation of, 1399f
  slow twitch, 1396
  target fiber of, 1397, 1401f
  type I, 1396–1397, 1398f
  type II, 1396–1397, 1398f
  type II atrophy of, 1414, 1414f
Muscle cells, smooth:
  endoreplication of, 455, 457f
  of vasculature, 454–455, 454f
Muscular dystrophy, **1400–1403**
  degeneration/regeneration in, 1400, 1402f
  Duchenne, 234, 234f, 1401–1403, 1404f
  progressive, 1401–1403, 1404f
Mutagenesis, insertional, 173, 174f
Myasthenia gravis, 109, 109f
Mycetoma, 421–422, 421f–422f, 550
Mycobacterial infection, **394–402**
  atypical, 401–402, 401t, 402f, 573
Mycobacterium avium-intracellulare, 451
Mycobacterium chelonei, 402, 402f
Mycobacterium fortuitum, 402
Mycobacterium leprae, 397
Mycobacterium marinum, 401–402
Mycobacterium tuberculosis, 570
Mycobacterium tuberculosis bovis, 394
Mycobacterium tuberculosis hominis, 394
Mycobacterium ulcerans, 401
Mycoplasmal infection:
  of female genital tract, 947
  pneumonia, 566
Mycoplasma pneumoniae, 345–346
Mycoplasmas, 345
Mycosis fungoides, 1104, 1257–1258
Mycotic aneurysm, 490, 1436
Myelinolysis, central pontine, 286, 1466–1467, 1466f–1467f
Myeloblast, 1022

Myelodysplastic syndromes, 1036, 1036t
Myelofibrosis:
  acute, 1075
  with myeloid metaplasia, 1071–1073, 1072t
Myeloma:
  multiple, 1105–1108
    of bone, 1361, 1364f
    bone marrow in, 1078f, 1106
    cause of, 1105
    clinical course and prognosis in, 1108
    clinical symptoms of, 1107
    diagnosis of, 1106, 1107f
    geographic and ethnic factors in, 194
    immunoglobulin abnormalities in, 1106, 1107t
    laboratory findings in, 1107
    nephrosis in, 1106
    paraproteinemia in, 868, 868f
    pathophysiology of, 1105–1106
  solitary, 1105
Myeloma cast nephropathy, 868
Myelomalacia, 1427
Myeloperoxidase:
  cytotoxity of, 55
  deficiency, 57t, 1050
Myeloperoxidase reaction, 57t
Myeloproliferative syndrome, chronic, 1066–1074, 1068f
Myeloproliferative syndromes, acute, 1074–1079
Myiasis, 449
Myoadenylate deaminase deficiency, 1411–1412
Myoblast, 1396
Myocardial hypertrophy, 9, 11f
Myocardial infarct, 257, 515. *See also* Ischemic heart disease
  gross characteristics of, 519–521, 520f
  limitation of size of, 525, 526t
  location of, 519, 519t
    due to coronary artery in, 498, 499f, 519
  microscopic characteristics of, 521–522, 521f–523f
  reperfusion of, 525
  subendocardial, 257, 519, 520t
  transmural, 257, 519, 519t
Myocardial infarction. *See also* Ischemic heart disease
  "at a distance," 518
  clinical diagnosis of, 522–523
  complications of, 523–524
  obesity and, 315
  in oral contraceptive use, 292
  pathology of, 519–522
  personality type and, 519
  smoking and, 277, 277f
  wound healing after, 93f, 94
Myocardial rupture, in myocardial infarction, 523–524
Myocarditis, 535–536, 535t
  in Chagas's disease, 403, 403f
  rheumatic, 527–528, 527f
Myocardium:
  amyloid deposits in, 1192
  degenerative diseases of, 538f
  ischemia of. *See* Ischemic heart disease
  myocyte of, 498–500, 501f, 504, 505f
Myofibrillar degeneration, 522, 524f

Myofibroblasts, morphology and function of, 77, 78f
Myonecrosis, clostridial, 373–374, 374f–375f
Myopathy:
  congenital, 1403–1405, 1407f
  inflammatory, 1406–1409
  lipid, 1411
  mitochondrial, 1397, 1400f
  noninflammatory, 1400–1406
"Myopericarditis," 536
Myophosphorylase deficiency, 1410, 1410f
Myopia, 1531
Myositis ossificans, 1329, 1330f
Myotubular myopathy, 1406, 1407f
Myxedema, 537, 1139
Myxoma, 540, 540f

NADH-TR stain, for muscle, 1397, 1400f–1401f
NADPH oxidase:
  activation of, 55–56
  defect, 57, 57t
Naegleria fowleri, 417
Narcotic lung, 287
Nasofacial zygomycosis, 430
Nasogastric tube, esophagitis due to, 637
Nasopharynx, 1290–1295
  anatomy and function of, 1290–1291
  carcinoma of:
    Epstein-Barr virus in, 171, 339f
    geographic and ethnic factors in, 192
  inflammation of, 1292
  neoplasms of, 1292–1295
    anaplastic carcinoma, 1293–1294, 1294f
    epidermoid carcinoma, 1293
    juvenile angiofibroma, 1292–1293
    rhinosporidiosis of, 430–431, 431f
Necator americanus, 436, 437f
Neck and head, **1260–1303**. *See also individual anatomic parts*
Necrosis:
  caseous, 16, 17t
  coagulative, **15–27**
    calcium deposits in, 16–17, 19f
    ischemia in, 17–20
    morphology of, 14f–18f, 15–16
    pathogenesis of, 16–27
    sequence of events in, 16–17
  fat, 15–16, 16f
  fibrinoid, 16, 18f, 113, 481
  hepatic, confluent, 748–749, 749f
  liquefactive, 15, 16f
  possible outcomes of, 90f–91f
  toxic liver, 25–27, 27f
Necrotizing enterocolitis, 243, 373, 374f–375f
Necrotizing papillitis, of kidney, 1176
Necrotizing venulitis, cutaneous, 1231–1232, 1231f–1233f
Negri body, 1448, 1451, 1451f
Neisseria gonorrhoeae, 390f, 391, 945
Neisseria meningitidis, 388
Nelson's syndrome, 1127
Nemaline myopathy, 1405, 1407f
Nematode disease, **434–440**. *See also individual types*
Nematodes, filarial, 431–433

Neonatal purpura, isoimmune, 1027
Neonate:
    arteriohepatic dysplasia of, 792
    biliary atresia of, 791–792
    birth injury of, 246–247
    botulism in, 376–377
    Chlamydia trachomatis pneumonia in, 566
    congenital anemia of, 245
    effects of maternal smoking on, 280–
        282, 282f
    erythroblastosis fetalis in, 243–246,
        244f–245f
    genetic and developmental disorders of,
        237–247
    hepatitis in, 790–791, 790t, 791f
    hyperbilirubinemia of, 732
    hypothyroidism of, 1134
    jaundice of, 732
    lungs of, 238–239
    respiratory distress syndrome in, 239–
        243, 241f–243f
    sudden infant death syndrome and, 247
    tetanus in, 376
    toxoplasmosis of, 413
    tumors of, 247–248
Neoplasia, **140–195**. *See also individual*
        types; Cancer; Tumor
Neoplasia syndromes, inherited, 189t
Nephritic syndrome, 836
Nephritis:
    glomerulonephritis, 850–864
    Henoch-Schönlein, 862–863
    hereditary, 869
    Heyman, 845
    interstitial, chronic, 836–837, 869
    lupus, 133–134, 133f–134f, 864–867,
        865f–866f. *See also* Lupus nephri-
        tis
    radiation, 310
    tubulointerstitial, drug-induced, 873–874
Nephroblastoma, 248, 887, 887f
Nephrocalcinosis, 875–876, 875t
Nephronophthisis, 840
Nephropathy:
    heroin, 287
    hypokalemic, 876, 876f
    IgA, 862, 863f–864f, 863t
    lead, 298
    membranous, 845–847, 845f–847f
    myeloma cast, 868
    urate, 875, 875f
    vasomotor, 834
Nephrosclerosis, malignant, 879, 879f
Nephrosis:
    biliary, 737
    hemoglobinuric, 409
    lipoid, 842
    myeloma, 1106
Nephrotic syndrome, 836, **841–850**
    amyloidosis in, 848–850, 849f–850f
    in cancer, 188
    diabetic glomerulosclerosis in, 847–848,
        848f–849f
    in drug reaction, 290
    edema in, 261
    epithelial cell disease in, 841–842, 842f–
        843f
    focal segmental glomerulosclerosis in,
        842–845, 844f

Nephrotic syndrome:
    membranous nephropathy in, 845–847,
        845f–847f
Nephrotoxicity, mercurial, 299
Nervous system, **1416–1498**. *See also* Cen-
        tral nervous system; Peripheral
        nervous system
Neural tube defect, 204f
Neurilemoma, 1496–1497, 1496f
Neuroblastoma, 1156–1157, 1157f
    metastasis of, 1157
    olfactory, 1289–1290, 1290f
    rosettes of, 1156, 1157f
Neuroendocrine activity, 1120
Neuroendocrine cells, 1122
Neuroendocrine tumors, of thymus, 1160,
        1161f
Neuroepithelial bodies, 1162
Neurofibrillary tangles, 1486, 1488f
Neurofibroma, 1497–1498, 1497f
Neurofibromatosis, 223–224, 223f, 1498
Neurofibrosarcoma, 1498
Neurofilament protein, 150
Neuroma:
    Morton's, 1495
    plantar, 1495
    traumatic, 94, 94f, 1495
Neuronal heterotopia, 1462
Neuronal metabolic disease, 1478–1479
Neuronal storage disease, 1477–1478
Neuronopathy, 1491
Neuron specific enolase, 149
Neuropathic ulcer, 89
Neuropathy:
    alcoholic, 1493
    amyloid, 1493t, 1494
    cryptogenic, 1494–1495
    in diabetes mellitus, 1492–1493
    dying-back, 1491, 1491f
    hereditary, 1494, 1495t
    hypertrophic, 1492
    inflammatory demyelinating, 1492
    paraneoplastic, 1493t, 1494
    paraproteinemic, 1493t, 1494
    toxic, 1493t, 1494
    uremic, 1493
    vasculitic, 1493
Neurosyphilis, 355–356
Neutropenia, 1049
    cyclic, 1049
Neutrophil:
    activation of, 49, 51f
    qualitative disorders of, 1049–1050
Neutrophilia, 63, 1048–1049, 1049t
Nevus:
    compound, 1242f, 1243
    dermal, 1243, 1243f
    dysplastic, 1243, 1244f
    epithelioid cell, 1254, 1254f
    junctional, 1243
    melanocytic, 1242–1243, 1242f–1243f
        congenital, 1254
    of oral cavity, 1266
Niacin deficiency, 320–321, 320f
Nickel poisoning, 299
Niemann-Pick disease:
    central nervous system in, 1478
    metabolic disturbance in, 228f
Night sweats, 303

Nipple:
    adenoma of, 1004
    inversion of, 996
    morphology of, 996
    Paget's disease of, 1007–1009, 1008f
    supernumerary, 996
Nitrogen dioxide, as respiratory irritant,
        551
Nitrosamines:
    in carcinogenesis, 163
    in esophageal cancer, 639
NK cells, 101
    cytotoxic, 116, 117f
    tumoricidal, 181
Nocardiosis, 393–394, 394f, 573
Nodular fasciitis, 146, 147f, 1389, 1389f
Nodular lymphoid hyperplasia, 708
Noma, 381, 382f, 1264, 1264f
Nondisjunction, chromosomal, 213
Non-Hodgkin's lymphoma. *See* Lym-
        phoma, non-Hodgkin's malig-
        nant
Normoblast, 1022
Norwalk-like viral diarrhea, 342–343
Norwalk virus, in gastroenteritis, 668
Nose, **1282–1290**
    anatomy of, 1282
    cavity, diseases of, 1283–1290
    external and vestibule of, 1282–1283
    fungal infection of, 1286–1287
    Hebra, 378
    in leprosy, 1286
    necrotizing granulomas of, 1287–1288
    neoplasia of, 1288–1290
        carcinoma, 1289, 1290f
        inverted papilloma, 1288, 1289f
        neuroblastoma, 1289–1290, 1290f
        squamous papilloma, 1288, 1289f
    parasitic disease of, 1287
    pathologic processes and adjacent struc-
        tures, 1283t
    pathways for intracranial infection
        from, 1283f
    polyps of, 1284, 1284f–1285f
    as respiratory defense mechanism, 547,
        547f
    saddle, 356
    scleroma of, 1286
    septum of, perforation of, 1284t
    syphilis of, 1284–1285
    tuberculosis of, 1285
Nosebleed, 1282–1283
Nucleolus, in reversible cell injury, 5
Nucleoside phosphorylase deficiency, 124
Nucleus:
    in coagulative necrosis, 14f–15f, 15
    in reversible cell injury, 5
Null cells, 101
Nutmeg liver, 786, 787f
Nutritional disorders, **314–325**. *See also in-*
        dividual types
    mineral deficiency, 325
    obesity, 314–316
    protein-calorie malnutrition, 316–317
    small intestinal absorption in, 628f–629f,
        672. *See also* Malabsorption
    vitamin A deficiency, 318–319
    vitamin B complex deficiency, 319–322
    vitamin C deficiency, 322–323

Nutritional disorders:
vitamin D deficiency, 323–324
vitamin E deficiency, 324
vitamin K deficiency, 324–325

Oat cell carcinoma, of lung, 556–557, 558f
Obesity, **314–316**, 315f
adult onset, 314–315
causes of, 314
complications of, 315, 315f
definition of, 314
hypothalamus in, 315
lifelong, 314–315
pulmonary hypertension due to, 622
treatment of, 316
in type II diabetes mellitus, 1169f, 1170–1171, 1172f
upper body vs lower body, 1171, 1172f
Occupational disease, 276
Ochronosis, 232, 1386
Ocular onchocercal, 433
Odland bodies, 1197, 1197–1199, 1198f
Odontogenic cysts, 1273–1274, 1275f
Odontogenic tumors, 1273–1274, 1275f
Odontoma, 1274
Odynophagia, 632
Olfactory neuroblastoma, 1289–1290, 1290f
Oligodendroglioma, 1470
Oligohydramnios, 202, 202f
Oligomenorrhea, 316, 962
Oliguria, in renal tubular necrosis, 877, 878f
Ollier's disease, 1322–1323, 1322f
Omental cyst, 720
Omentum, greater, 640
Omsk hemorrhagic fever, 331
Onchocerca volvulus, 432–433
Onchocerciasis, 432–433, 1503–1504
Onchocercoma, 432
Oncocytoma, of salivary glands, **1279**
Oncofetal gene expression, 180
Oncogene:
cellular, 158, 159
growth factor interactions with, 175, 176f
retroviral, 173–175, 174t
transfection in, 177–179, 178f
viral, 158
Oncogenic virus, **169–175**
adenovirus as, 173
DNA, 170–173, 172f
Ebstein-Barr virus as, 158, 169–175, 172f, 174f
hepatitis B virus as, 171–173
herpesvirus as, 171
historical overview of, 169–170
papillomavirus as, 170–171
polyomavirus as, 171
poxvirus as, 173
RNA virus (retrovirus) as, 173–175, 174f
Onion-bulb formation, in peripheral nerve, 1491, 1492f
Oophoritis, 973
Ophthalmia neonatorum, 1503
Opsonization:
functions of, 46
in type II hypersensitivity reaction, 107, 108f

Optic atrophy, 1531
Optic disc, edema of, 1531
Optic nerve:
common disorders of, 1531
in systemic disease, 1511t
Oral cavity, **1262–1274**
candidiasis of, 424
carcinoma of, 278
developmental anomalies of, 1262
infections of, 1262–1265
metastases to, 1268
tumors and tumor-like conditions of, 1265–1268
Oral contraceptives:
adenoma of liver due to, 793
drug reactions to, 291–292, 292f
endometrial effects of, 963
Oral thrush, 424
Orbit:
inflammatory pseudotumor of, 1504
in systemic disease, 1511t
Orchitis, 916
Organ primordia, 201
Ornithosis, 346–347, 566
Oroya fever, 379
Orthomyxovirus, respiratory, 343–344
Osmotic pressure gradient, 252
Ossicles, anatomy of, 1261f
Ossification:
endochondral, 1306
heterotopic, 1328
intramembranous, 1306
primary center of, 1311
secondary center of, 1311, 1312f
zone of, 1314
Osteitis, dissecting, 1341f, 1347
Osteitis fibrosa, 1347
Osteitis fibrosa cystica, 1146, 1347–1348
Osteitis fibrosa disseminata, 1362
Osteoarthritis, **1371–1374**
articular cartilage resilience in, 1371
biochemical abnormalities in, 1372–1374
coarse cancellous bone in, 1371
eburnated bone in, 1372, 1374f
etiology of, 1370
histogenesis of, 1372, 1373f
increased unit load in, 1371
pathology in, 1372, 1374f
Osteoblastoma, 1357, 1358f
Osteoblasts, 1308
Osteocalcin, 1308
Osteochondritis dissecans, 1326
Osteochondroma, 1318–1320, 1319f
Osteochondromatosis:
hereditary multiple, 1319
synovial, 1386
Osteoclast, 1309, 1354, 1355f
Osteocytes, 1309, 1309f
Osteodystrophy, renal, 1346
Osteogenesis imperfecta, 223, 1320–1322, 1322f
type I, 1320–1321, 1322f
type II, 1321
type III, 1321
type IV, 1321–1322
Osteoid osteoma, 1357, 1358f
Osteoid seams, 1339
Osteomalacia, 186, 1341f, 1344–1346
Osteomyelitis, **1329–1333**
chronic, 1333

Osteomyelitis:
complications of, 1333
hematogenous, 1329–1332, 1331f
of jaw, 1272
pathogenesis and clinical presentation in, 1329–1333, 1331f–1332f
repair in, 1332–1333
in sinusitis, 1284–1285
staphylococcal, 383
treatment of, 1333
tuberculous, of long bones, 1335
of vertebral bodies, 1332f, 1333
Osteonecrosis, 1326–1328
causes of, 1326
of coarse cancellous bone, 1326
of cortical bone, 1326
corticomedullary, 1349
of femoral head, 1326, 1327f
Osteonectin, 1308
Osteopenia, 1343
Osteopetrosis, 1320, 1321f
Osteophytes, 1371, 1372
Osteoporosis, 1340, 1341f–1343f, 1342–1343, 1342t
classification of, 1342t
diagnosis of, 1343
disuse, 1343f
epidemiology of, 1343
treatment of, 1343
Osteoporosis circumscripta, 1352
Osteoprogenitor cells, 1308
Osteosarcoma, 1357–1359, 1360f
juxtacortical, 1359, 1361f
sunburst pattern in, 1328, 1328f
Ostium primum, 507, 508f
Ostium secundum, 507, 508f
Otitis media, **1297–1299**
acute necrotizing, 1298
acute serous, 1297
acute suppurative, 1298
cholesteatoma in, 1299
cholesterol granuloma in, 1297
chronic serous, 1297
chronic suppurative, 1298–1299, 1298f
complications of, 1299
Otosclerosis, 1300–1301, 1300f–1301f
Oval macrocytes, 1038
Ovary, **972–981**
cysts of, 973–974
functional, 973–974
nonfunctional, 973
endometriosis of, 988f
hyperthecosis of, 974, 974f
inflammation of, 973
radiation injury to, 310
stromal hyperplasia of, 974
torsion of, 973
tumors of, **974–981**
benign, 975
Brenner tumor, 977
choriocarcinoma, 981
classification of, 975f
clear cell adenocarcinoma, 977
clinical staging of, 977t
dysgerminoma, 978–979
embryonal cell carcinoma, 979
endometrioid adenocarcinoma, 977
entodermal sinus, 979
epidemiology of, 974–975
of epithelial origin, 975–977

Ovary:
  germ cell, 978–981
  granulosa-stromal cell, 977–978
  invasive carcinoma, 975–977
  of low malignant potential, 975
  malignant, 975–977
  metastatic, 981
  mucinous adenoma, 977
  serous cystadenoma, 977
  Sertoli-Leydig cell, 978
  sex cord-stromal, 977
  teratoma, 979
  thecoma-fibroma, 978
  yolk sac carcinoma, 979
Overhydration, pathology of, 265
Oxygen:
  alveolar damage due to, 580
  cellular metabolism of, 21f
Oxygen radicals:
  cell injury due to, 20–22, 21f–24f
  in disease, 21, 22f
  iron and, 771
  produced by phagocytic cells, 56, 57t
  production of, 20–21, 21f
  in reperfusion injury, 18–19
Oxyntic cells, 641
Oxytocin, 1123
Ozone, as respiratory irritant, 551, 580

p150,95, in phagocytic cell adherence, 58
Pachygyria, 1461
Pachymeningitis, 1441
Pagetic steal, 1352
Paget's disease, of bone, **1350–1354**
  etiology of, 1351, 1351f
  focal manifestations of, 1352–1354
  fractures in, 1352
  geographic distribution of, 1351
  histologic features of, 1354, 1355f
  radiologic appearance of bone in, 1352,
    1352f
  sarcomatous changes in, 1352–1354
  treatment of, 1354
Paget's disease of epithelium:
  of nipple, 1007–1009, 1008f
  of penis, 939
  of scrotum, 940, 940f
  of vulva, 952, 952f
Palate, cleft, 235–236, 236f, 1367–1368
Pancreas, **808–831**
  aberrant or accessory, 811
  acinar cell of, 808f
  adenocarcinoma of, 279, 279f
  in alcoholism, 284–285
  anatomy of, 810
  annular, 811
  cystadenoma of, 816, 819
  in cystic fibrosis, 225–226, 226f
  cysts of, 811
  developmental defects of, 811
  embryologic development of, 810–811
  endocrine:
    alpha cell tumors of, 825, 826
    beta cell tumors of, 826f–827f, 827
    D1 tumors of, 828
    delta cell tumor of, 827–828
    enterochromaffin cell tumors of, 828
    gastrinoma of, 828–830
    islet cell tumors of, 825–830

Pancreas:
    polypeptide-secreting tumors of, 828
  exocrine:
    benign tumors of, 816, 819
    carcinoma of, 819–821
      complications of, 819, 820f
      Courvoisier's sign in, 819
      desmoplastic reaction in, 820, 821f
      etiology and pathogenesis of, 820–
        821
      gross pathology in, 819, 821f
      locations of, 819
      symptoms of, 819
  islets of, 822–823, 822f
  shock in, 273
Pancreas divisum, 811
Pancreatic cholera, 828
Pancreatic duct obstruction, 813–814
Pancreatic enzymes, in intestinal absorp-
    tion, 672
Pancreatic polypeptide-secreting tumors,
    828
Pancreatic rests, of stomach, 642
Pancreatitis, **811–816**
  acute, 811–816, 812f–813f
    clinical manifestations of, 812–813,
      812f–813f
    fat necrosis in, 15–16, 16f
    hemorrhagic, 812–816, 812f–813f
    pathogenesis of, 813–816, 815f
  chronic, 816, 817f–818f
    calcifying, 284–285, 816, 817f–818f
    complications of, 816, 818f
  edematous, 812
  familial hereditary, 816
  interstitial, 812
  peritonitis in, 720
Panencephalitis, subacute sclerosing,
    1448, 1451f, 1454
Paneth cells, 664
Panniculitis, septal, 1237–1238
Pannus, rheumatoid, 1376
Papillary cystadenoma, of epididymis,
    926, 926f
Papillary fibroelastoma, of heart, 541
Papilledema, 1531
Papillitis, necrotizing, of kidney, 1176
Papilloma, 143
  of gallbladder, 806
  intraductal, of breast, 1004
  inverted:
    of nose, 1288
    of urinary bladder, 904, 904f
  of oral cavity, 1265
  squamous:
    of larynx, 548
    of nose, 1288
  transitional cell, of urinary bladder,
    904–905
Papillomatosis, juvenile, of breast, 999
Papillomavirus, 170–171
  in cervical carcinoma, 957
  Shope, 170
Papulosis, bowenoid, 938–939
Paracoccidioides brasiliensis, 423, 424f
Paracoccidioidomycosis, 423, 424f
Paracrine activity, 1120
Paraffinoma, 553
Paraganglioma, 1157–1158, 1299, 1299f
Paragonimiasis, 441, 444
Paragonimus westermani, 441, 444

Parainfluenza virus, 344
Paralysis, periodic, 1412
Paramyxovirus, 344
Paranasal sinuses, 1282–1290
  anatomy of, 1282
  carcinoma of, 1289, 1290f
  diseases of, 1283–1290
  fungal infections of, 1286–1287
  pathologic processes and adjacent struc-
    tures, 1283t
  pathways for intracranial infection
    from, 1283f
Paraneoplastic neuropathy, 1493t, 1494
Paraneoplastic syndromes, 185, 559–560
Paraphyseal cyst, 1476
Paraproteinemic glomerulonephritis, 867–
    869, 868f
Paraproteinemic neuropathy, 1493t, 1494
Paraquat, alveolar damage due to, 580
Parasitism, 328
  carcinogenesis due to, 169
  of small intestine, 669, 670f
Parathyrinoma, 830
Parathyroid glands, **1145–1146**
  adenoma of, 1146–1147, 1147f
  anatomy, embryology, physiology of,
    1145
  carcinoma of, 1148–1149
  hyperparathyroidism, 1146–1149
  hyperplasia of, 1147–1148
    primary, 1147–1148
    secondary, 1148
    tertiary or autonomous, 1148
  hypoparathyroidism, 1145
  pseudohypoparathyroidism, 1145
  pseudopseudohypoparathyroidism,
    1146
Parathyroid hormone, in calcium homeo-
    stasis, 1338–1339
Parietal cells, 641
Parkinsonism, 1480–1481, 1482f
Parotitis, 1275–1276
  acute suppurative, 1275
  epidemic, 1275–1276
Paroxysmal cold hemoglobinuria, 1046
Paroxysmal nocturnal hemoglobinuria,
    1045
Parrot fever, 346–347
Partial thromboplastin time, 1026t
Patent ductus arteriosus, 243, 507–509
Paterson-Kelly syndrome, 631
Peau d'orange skin, of breast, 1010, 1011
Peliosis hepatis, 785, 786f
Pellagra, 320–321, 320f, 1270
Pelvic inflammatory disease, 946f
Pemphigoid:
  bullous, 1219–1220, 1220f–1221f
  esophagus in, 637
Pemphigus erythematosus, 1216t
Pemphigus foliaceus, 1216f, 1216t
  Brazilian, 1216t
Pemphigus vegetans, 1216t
Pemphigus vulgaris, **1211–1214**
  definition and clinical features of, 1211
  etiology and pathogenesis of, 1213–
    1214, 1214f
  pathology of, 1211–1213, 1213f
Penetrating wound, 307
Penis, **938–940**
  condyloma acuminatum of, 938, 938f
  mesenchymal neoplasms of, 939

Penis:
  metastatic neoplasms of, 940
  Paget's disease of, 939
  sclerosing lipogranuloma of, 938
  sexually transmitted inflammatory lesions of, 938
  squamous cell carcinoma of, 939
    geographic and ethnic factors in, 193
    in situ, 938–939
  verrucous carcinoma of, 939
Peptic ulcer disease, **648–655**
  accelerated gastric emptying in, 651, 652f
  combined gastric and duodenal ulcers in, 655
  complications of, 654–655
  disease associations in, 651–653
  in drug reactions, 289, 649
  duodenal pH in, 651
  epidemiology in, 649
  gastric acid secretion in, 650–651, 652f
  gastric and duodenal factors in, 650–651, 652f
  gastric ulcers in, 651
  genetic factors in, 650
  hemorrhage in, 654
  malignant transformation in, 655
  pathogenesis of, 649–651
  pathology of, 653–654, 654f
  perforation of, 655
  physiologic factors in, 650–651
  psychologic factors in, 650
  pyloric obstruction due to, 655
  risk factors for, 649–650
  due to smoking, 279–280, 649–650
  symptomatology of, 648–649
Perfusion:
  hemodynamic disorders of, **253–258**
  reduced, pathology of, 256–258
  regional, pathologic conditions altering, 256
Perfusion pressure, 252
Periapical abscess, 1271
Periapical granuloma, 1271, 1273f
Periarteritis nodosa, 110
Pericardial tamponade, 264f, 265
Pericarditis, 536, 536f–537f
  constrictive, 536, 537t
  in myocardial infarction, 524
  purulent, 536, 536f
  rheumatic, 528
  in systemic lupus erythematosus, 134
Pericholecystic abscess, 804
Perichondrium, 1311
Pericytes, 459
Periodic paralysis, 1412
Periodontal cyst, apical, 1271
Periodontal tissue, diseases of, 1270–1274
Peripheral blood smear, 1018
Peripheral nervous system, **1490–1498**
  in cancer, 186
  general pathology of, 1490–1492
  nerve trauma in, 1495
  neuropathy of, 1492–1495, 1493t
  structure of, 1490, 1490f
  tumors of, 1495–1498
  wound healing in, 94
Peripheral neuropathy:
  in diabetes mellitus, 1175
  in drug reaction, 289–290
  esophagus in, 633

Peripheral neuropathy:
  motor, in lead poisoning, 297
  thiamine deficiency in, 319–320
Peritoneal dialysis, peritonitis due to, 718–720
Peritoneal effusion, 265
Peritoneum, 717–720
  carcinomatosis of, 151, 152f, 977
  mesenteric and omental cysts of, 720
  mesothelioma of, 168–169, 720–721
  metastatic carcinoma of, 721
Peritonitis:
  bacterial, 717–720
  bile, 720, 804
  chemical, 720
  meconium, 225
  in pancreatitis, 720
  spontaneous bacterial, in portal hypertension, 782
  tuberculous, 720
Peritonsillar abscess, 1292
Peroneal muscular atrophy, 1495t
Peroxisomal proliferation, 9, 10f
Pertussis, 364–365
Petechia, 254
Peutz-Jeghers syndrome, 681, 681f
Peyer's patches, 663, 1020
Peyronie's disease, 938
Phaeomycotic cyst, 429
Phagocytes:
  adherence of, 57–58
  function of, congenital defects in, 57, 57t
  mononuclear, 101–102
Phagocytosis, process of, 54–57, 54f–55f
Phagolysosome, 54, 55f
Phagosome, 54, 54f
Phakomatosis, 188
Pharyngitis, streptococcal, 529–531, 530f
Pharynx, lymphoid tissues of:
  absence or hypoplasia of, 1291
  atrophy of, 1291
  hyperplasia of, 1291
Phenacetin, renal damage due to, 874
Phenomelanin, 1200
Phenylalanine, metabolic pathway of, 230–231
Phenylalanine hydroxylase deficiency, 219
Phenylketonuria, 231, 1478
Pheochromocytoma, 1154–1156
  cytoplasmic granules in, 1156, 1156f
  diagnosis of, 1155
  types of, 1154
Philadelphia chromosome, 175–177, 1070
Phimosis, 938
Phlebitis, 492, 748
Phlebothrombosis, 492
Phocomelia, 205, 205f
Phosphate, metabolism of, 1338–1339
Phosphofructokinase deficiency, 1411
Phospholipase A$_2$:
  activities of, 49, 51f
  bactericidal, 54
Phospholipase C, 49, 51f
Phospholipidosis, fatty liver due to, 784
Phycomycosis, of lung, 574–575
Phyllodes tumor, of breast, 1011–1012, 1012f
Physical injury, 306–307
Phytobezoar, 662
Pick bodies, 1487, 1490f

Pick's disease, 1487, 1489f
Pickwickian syndrome, 622
Picornavirus pneumonia, 345
Pigbel, 373, 374f–375f
Pigmented villonodular synovitis, 1387, 1388f
Pilonidal cyst, 688
Pilosebaceous unit, disorders of, 1238, 1240f–1241f
Pineal gland, 1160–1162
  anatomy, embryology, physiology of, 1160–1161
  neoplasms of, 1161–1162
Pinealoma, 1161–1162, 1475
Pineoblastoma, 1161–1162
Pineocytoma, 1162
Pinguecula, 1525
Pink puffer, 598
Pinta, 357
Pinworm infection, 438–439
Pipestem fibrosis, of liver, 441, 443f
Piroplasmosis, 413
Pitting edema, 261
Pituicytoma, 1125
Pituitary, **1122–1128**
  anterior, syndromes of, 1127–1128
  congenital anomalies of, 1123–1124
  embryology of, 1122
  histology of, 1122, 1123f
  hormone release by, 1119f
  in pregnancy, 1127–1128
  tumors of, 1125–1127
    anterior, 1125–1127
    posterior, 1125
Pituitary adenoma, 1125–1127
  basophilic, 1127
  chromophobe, 1126, 1126f
  oncocytoma, 1127
  somatotropic, 1126–1127
Pituitary cachexia, 1125
Pituitary gonadotropin deficiency, isolated, 1130
Placenta:
  abnormalities of, 982, 982f
  dizygotic, 983
  gross anatomy of, 981–982
  histology of, 982
  hyperplastic abnormalities of, 986f
  infarct of, 983
  infection of, 985–986
  monochorionic-diamniotic, 983–985
  monochorionic-monoamniotic, 985
  monozygotic twin, 983
  in multiple gestation, 983–985
  retroplacental hematoma of, 983
Placenta accreta, 982, 982f
Placenta increta, 982, 982f
Placental site trophoblastic tumor, 987
Placenta percreta, 982, 982f
Placenta previa, 283f, 982, 982f
Plantar neuroma, 1495
Plasma cell mastitis, 997
Plasma cell neoplasia, 1067t
Plasma cell pneumonia, 414
Plasma cells:
  in chronic inflammation, 59
  circulating, 1057
  morphology and function of, 60f
Plasmacytoma:
  extramedullary, 1105, 1106f
  of nasopharynx, 1294

Plasmacytosis:
  of bone marrow, 1056
  peripheral blood, 1057
Plasma fibronectin, 74
Plasma membrane:
  cytoskeletal alterations of, in ischemia,
    19
  fluidization of, 287
  functions of, 4
  in hydropic swelling, 5
  hydroxyl radical damage to, 22
  intracellular calcium homeostasis and,
    19–20
  in irreversible cell injury, 17
  in irreversible ischemic injury, 18
  mechanisms of damage in disease, 28f
  phospholipid metabolism of, in isch-
    emia, 19, 20f
  potentially reversible damage to, 17
  in reversible cell injury, 5
  viral damage to, 24–25, 26f
Plasmin, 42, 55, 474–476
Plasminogen, 474–476, 475f
Plasminogen activator, 55
Plasmodium falciparum, 408–409, 410f
Platelet activating factor:
  functions of, 42
  in immediate hypersensitivity reaction,
    106
Platelet count, 1026
Platelet-derived growth factor, 77
  in atherosclerosis, 460
  cellular ion fluxes due to, 159
  in tumor growth, 158
Platelets:
  aggregation of, 472–474
  aspirin effects on, 1029
  in coronary artery occlusion, 476
  in hemostasis, 1025
  in hemostasis disorders, 1027–1029
  morphology and function of, 38–40, 41f
  pavementing of, 472, 473f
  qualitative or functional disorders of,
    1029
  in thrombosis, 471–472, 472f
Platybasia, 1352
Pleomorphic rhabdomyosarcoma, 1392
Pleomorphism, 147
Pleura, mesothelioma of, 168–169, 617–
  618, 617f
Pleural effusion, 263–265, 605, 616
Pleural plaques, 605, 617
Pleuritis, 568, 616–617
Plicae circularis, 663
Plummer-Vinson syndrome, 631
Pneumatocele, in staphylococcal pneumo-
  nia, 568–569
Pneumatosis cystoides intestinalis, 684–
  686
Pneumococcal meningitis, 388
Pneumococcal pneumonia, 388, 565f, 567–
  568, 567f
Pneumoconiosis, 595, 598–600, 601f
  asbestos, 601f, 604–605, 604f
  coal, 601f, 603–604
Pneumocystis carinii, 413–414, 414f
Pneumocystis carinii pneumonia, 450, 575–
  576, 576f
Pneumocystosis, 413–414, 414f
Pneumonia:
  adenovirus, 344

Pneumonia:
  ascariasis, 439
  atypical, 566
  Chlamydia trachomatis, 566
  community-acquired, 569
  cytomegalovirus, 563
  E. coli, 569
  eosinophilic, 575, 583, 584f
  Friedländer's bacillus, 378–379
  Herpes influenzae, 364
  herpesvirus, 344–345
  interstitial, 608–610
    cellular, 610
    desquamative, 609–610
    giant cell, 610
    lymphoid, 610
    pathogenesis of, 563, 563f–564f
    unusual, 606f, 609
  intra-alveolar (lobar), 563, 563f, 565f
  klebsiella, 568
  Klebsiella pneumoniae, 378–379
  Legionella pneumophilia, 569–570
  Legionnaires', 365–366, 366f
  lipid:
    endogenous (golden), 553
    exogenous, 553
  measles, 344, 566
  Mycoplasma pneumoniae, 345–346, 566
  organizing, 610
  picornavirus, 345
  plasma cell, 414
  pneumococcal, 388, 565f, 567–568, 567f
  pneumocystis, 413–414, 414f
  Pneumocystis carinii, 450, 575–576, 576f
  Pseudomonas aeruginosa, 569
  rubeola, 344
  staphylococcal, 568–569
  streptococcal, 569
  syphilitic, 209, 209f
  varicella, 566
  viral, 343–345
Pneumonia alba, 356
Pneumonitis:
  in drug reaction, 290, 291f
  radiation, 580–581
Pneumoperitoneum, 655
Pneumothorax, 615–616
  spontaneous, 615
  tension, 615
Podagra, 1382
Poisoning, food:
  salmonella, 373, 374f–375f
  staphylococcal, 384
Poison ivy dermatitis, 1232–1233, 1234f–
  1236f
Poliomyelitis, 333, 333f, 1450–1451, 1452f
Polio virus, directly cytopathic, 24, 26f
Pollution, air, 551
Polyarteritis nodosa, 482–483, 483f
  of heart, 532
  of kidney, 879–880, 880f
Polychlorinated biphenyls (PCB), 296
Polychondritis, relapsing, 1296, 1296f
Polycystic ovary syndrome, 973–974, 974f,
  1130
Polycythemia, 1047–1048
  hemodynamics in, 256
  stress, 1048
Polycythemia vera, 1067–1069
  criteria for diagnosis of, 1069t
  hematopathologic features of, 1072t

Polycythemia vera:
  laboratory findings in, 1069, 1072t
  spleen in, 1068, 1070f
Polymenorrhea, 962
Polymicrogyria, 1461–1462, 1461f
Polymorphonuclear leukocyte. See Leukocyte, polymorphonuclear
Polymyositis, 1408–1409, 1408f
  eosinophilic, 1408
  muscle staining in, 1401f
Polymyositis/dermatomyositis, 137–138,
  186
Polyneuropathy, familial amyloidotic,
  1184
Polyomavirus, 170, 171
Polyp:
  adenomatous, 143
  of anal canal, 702
  of cervix, 956
  of colon, 702–709. See also Colon, polyps
    of
    adenomatous, 702f–705f, 703–706
    hyperplastic, 707–708, 707f
    inflammatory, 708
    retention, 708, 708f
  of ear, 1296
  of endometrium, 963, 965f
  juvenile, 708, 708f
  lymphoid, 708
  metaplastic, 707–708, 707f
  of nose, 1284, 1284f
  Peutz-Jeghers, 681, 681f
  of renal pelvis and ureter, 894
  of stomach:
    adenomatous, 656
    hyperplastic, 656
  of urethra, 910, 910f
    adenomatous, 910, 911f
  of vagina, 954
Polypeptide growth factors, 158–159
Polyposis coli, familial, 706, 706f
Polyserositis, familial paroxysmal, 720
Polysplenia, 1064
Pompe's disease, 227f, 1409, 1410f
Pontiac fever, 570
Pontine hemorrhage, 1438, 1439f
Pontine myelinolysis, central, 286, 1466–
  1467, 1466f–1467f
Porcelain gallbladder, 804
Porphyria, hepatic, 290
Portal hypertension, 776–782
  anorectal varices in, 780
  arteriovenous fistula in, 778
  ascites in, 781–782, 781f
  in Budd-Chiari syndrome, 778–779, 779f
  caput Medusae in, 780
  causes of, 777f
  complications of, 779, 780f
  esophageal varices in, 779–780
  in hepatic vein thrombosis, 779, 779f
  idiopathic, 778
  intrahepatic, 777–778
  noncirrhotic, 794
  portal vein thrombosis in, 778
  posthepatic, 778–779, 779f
  prehepatic, 778
  in schistosomiasis, 778
  spleen in, 1065
  splenomegaly in, 778, 780
  spontaneous bacterial peritonitis in, 782
Portal-systemic encephalopathy, 735

Portal triads, 724–725, 724f–725f
Portal vein thrombosis, 778
Postmyocardial infarction syndrome, 524
Post-term infant, 238
Post-transfusion purpura, 1027
Postvaccinial lymphadenitis, 1061
Potter's complex, 202, 202f
Pott's disease, 1332f, 1334–1335, 1334f
Poxvirus, in carcinogenesis, 173
Prealbumin, 1185
   amyloid deposition associated with, 1189
Precocious puberty, 1125, 1129
Preeclampsia, 885, 885f, 983, 984f
Pregnancy:
   acute pyelonephritis in, 870
   breast in, 995
   diabetes mellitus and, 1176
   ectopic, 971–972, 972f
   endometrium in, 961
   fatty liver of, 784
   pituitary in, 1127–1128
   toxemia of, 885, 885f, 983, 984f
Pregnancy tumor, of oral cavity, 1264
Preleukemic disorders, 1053
Premature infant, 237–238. *See also* Neonate
   brain in, 239
   liver in, 239
   respiratory distress syndrome in, 239–243, 241f–243f
Prematurity, retinopathy of, 1523, 1524f
Prenatal diagnosis, 236
Presbyopia, 1527
Prinzmetal's angina, 515, 516
Prions, 1449
Proctitis, ulcerative, 697
Progeria, 32f, 33
Prolactin, 1122
Prolactinoma, 1127
Prolymphocytes, 1086–1087
Pronormoblast, 1022
Proptosis, 1531
Prostacyclin, 47–48, 48f, 473
Prostaglandin E$_2$, 47–48, 48f
Prostaglandin G$_2$, 47–48, 48f
Prostaglandin H$_2$, 47–48, 48f
Prostaglandin I$_2$:
   formation of, 47–48, 48f
   inhibitory effects of, 52–54, 53f
Prostaglandins:
   ductus arteriosus and, 509
   vasodilative, functions of, 43
Prostate, **927–938**
   adenocarcinoma of, 932–937
     ductal, 937
     epidemiology of, 932–934
     etiology and pathogenesis of, 934
     extraprostatic spread of, 934–936
     geographic and ethnic factors in, 193
     histogenesis of, 934
     natural history of, 936–937, 936f
     pathology of, 934, 935f
     staging of, 936–937, 936f
   control of growth of, 928–929
   hyperplasia of, 930–932
     complications of, 931, 933f
     incidence and epidemiology of, 930, 931f
     nodule types in, 931
     pathogenesis of, 930–931

Prostate:
   pathology in, 931–932, 932f–933f
   infarct of, 930
   inflammatory disease of, 929–930
   malacoplakia of, 930
   mesenchymal neoplasms of, 937
   metastatic tumors of, 937–938
   normal structure and embryology of, 927–928
   senescent atrophy of, 928
   squamous cell carcinoma of, 937
   staining techniques for, 928, 929f
   testosterone and estrogen effects on, 928–929
   transitional cell carcinoma of, 937
Prostate-specific antigen, 151
Prostatic acid phosphatase, 151
Prostatitis, 929–930
   chronic, 929
   granulomatous, 930
   nonspecific granulomatous, 930
   nonspecific nongranulomatous, 929–930
Protein:
   AA amyloid, 1185, 1186–1189, 1188f
   adherence, defect in, 57t
   AE amyloid, 1185
   AL amyloid, 1184–1185, 1186, 1187f
   cationic, in leukocytic granules, 54
   cereal, in celiac disease, 675–676, 676f
   glial fibrillary acidic, 150
   glial filament, 150
   neurofilament, 150
   S-100, 150t, 151
   serum, electrophoresis of, 119, 120f
Protein C, 473
Protein-calorie malnutrition, 316–317
Protein kinase C, 159
Protein-losing enteropathy, 187, 679–680
Proteoglycans:
   of cartilage, 1370
   distribution and function of, 74–75
   heparan sulfate, 73, 73t
   in wound healing, 79
Prothrombin time, 1026t
Proto-oncogene, 158, 173
Protozoal disease, **402–421.** *See also individual types*
Protozoal infection, of liver, 788–789, 789t
Pseudoarthrosis, 1325
Pseudocysts, of spleen, 1065
Pseudofracture, in Milkman-Looser syndrome, 1344
Pseudogout, 1385
Pseudohermaphroditism, 915
Pseudohypoparathyroidism, 1145–1146
Pseudolymphoma, 1063
   of lung, 610
   of stomach, 656
Pseudomembranous colitis, 689, 690f
Pseudomembranous enterocolitis, 689
Pseudomonas aeruginosa pneumonia, 569
Pseudomyxoma peritonei, 716, 977
Pseudoneurotrophic joint, 1385
Pseudo-osteoarthritis, 1385
Pseudoparalysis of Parrot, 1335
Pseudopseudohypoparathyroidism, 1146
Pseudopyloric metaplasia, 645
Pseudorheumatoid arthritis, 1385
Pseudoxanthoma elasticum, 1234–1235, 1236f
Psittacosis, 346–347

Psoas abscess, 1334
Psoriasis, 1209–1211, 1210f–1212f
   definition and clinical features of, 1209
   epidermal hyperplasia in, 11, 12f
   etiology and pathogenesis of, 1210–1211, 1212f
   pathology of, 1209–1210, 1210f–1211f
Pterygium, 1525
Puberty:
   breast in, 992
   delayed, hypothalamus in, 1129
   precocious, 1125, 1129
Puerperal sepsis, 386
Pulmonary anthrax, 358
Pulmonary artery:
   anatomy of, 546
   connective tissue tumor of, 626–627
   in hypertension, 621, 621f
   thrombosis of, 621
Pulmonary circulation, fetal, 240
Pulmonary coccidioidomycosis, 425–426
Pulmonary dirofilariasis, 433
Pulmonary edema, 261–263, **624–626,** 625f–626f
   alveolar, 624, 626f
   in heart failure, 502, 503f
   in high-altitude sickness, 306
   hydrostatic, 624
   interstitial, 624
   oncotic, 626
   pathogenesis of, 624, 625f
   permeability, 626
Pulmonary embolism, 265–267, 266f, 618–621, 619f. *See also* Embolism, of lung
Pulmonary emphysema, 279, 280f
Pulmonary eosinophilia, 432
Pulmonary hemorrhage, 581–583
Pulmonary hypertension, 254, **621–624**
   capillary, 623
   cardiac causes of, 623
   emphysema and, 623
   functional flow resistance in, 622
   histopathology of, 621, 621f
   hypoventilation and, 622
   hypoxemia and, 622
   increased blood flow in, 621
   increased resistance to flow in, 622
   large pulmonary artery embolism in, 622
   multiple thromboemboli in, 622
   postcapillary, 623
   precapillary, 622–623
   primary, 622
   venous, 623–624
Pulmonary infarct, 257
Pulmonary paragonimiasis, 444
Pulmonary stenosis, isolated or pure, 512–513
Pulmonary surfactant, fetal, 238–239, 239f
Pulmonary thromboembolism, 265–267, 266f, 618–619, 619f. *See also* Embolism, of lung
Pulmonary vascular system, tumors of, 626–627
Pulmonary vein, anomalous drainage of, 510
Pulmonary veno-occlusive disease, 623–624
Pulpitis, 1271–1272, 1273f
Purine metabolism, 1383

Purpura, 253
  allergic, 1027
  neonatal, isoimmune, 1027
  post-transfusion, 1027
  Schönlein-Henoch, 1027
  senile, 1026
  thrombocytopenic, idiopathic, 1027
  thrombotic thrombocytopenic, 1029
Purulent effusion, 37
Purulent exudate, 37
Pyarthrosis, H. influenzae, 364
Pyelitis cystica, 894
Pyelitis glandularis, 894–895
Pyelonephritis, 869–873
  acute, 869–871
    ascending, 870, 871f
      gross pathology in, 871, 872f
    hematogenous, 870
    mechanism of, 869–870
    in pregnancy, 870
    ureter anatomy in, 870, 871f
  chronic, 871–873, 873f–874f
Pyknosis, 15
Pylephlebitic abscess, 788
Pyle's disease, 1320
Pyloric glands, 641
Pyloric membrane, congenital, 642
Pyloric obstruction, in peptic ulcer dis-
    ease, 655
Pyloric stenosis, congenital, 641–642
Pyocele, in sinusitis, 1284
Pyogenic granuloma:
  of nose, 1282
  of oral cavity, 1263, 1263f
  of vulva, 950
Pyometra, 961
Pyosalpinx, 948
Pyothorax, 568, 616
Pyridoxine deficiency, 321–322
Pyridoxine-dependency syndrome, 322
Pyrimidine dimers, in DNA, due to UV
    radiation, 168
Pyrogen, endogenous, 62–63
Pyrrolizidine alkaloids:
  in carcinogenesis, 163
  in vero-occlusive disease of liver, 779
Pyruvate kinase deficiency, 1043

Q fever, 351, 566
Quinsy, 1292

Rabies, 1451
Racemose cysticercus, 447
Rachischisis, 1459
Rad, 307
Radiation, 307–314
  breast, injury due to, 998
  cancer due to, 310–314
    atom bomb causing, 312
    iatrogenic causes of, 312
    low-level exposure and, 312–314
    occupational exposure causing, 312
  cellular effects of, 22–24, 25f, 307–308
  cystitis in, 903
  enteritis due to, 680
  enterocolitis due to, 702
  esophagitis due to, 637

Radiation:
  gastritis due to, 648
  ionizing, cell injury due to, 22–24, 25f
  microwave, 314
  nephritis due to, 310
  pneumonitis due to, 580–581
  quantitation of, 307
  therapeutic, injury due to, 309–310,
    310f–311f
  ultrasound, 314
  ultraviolet, in carcinogenesis, 167–168
  vasculitis due to, 310, 311f
  whole body, 308–309, 309f
Radiodermatitis, 310, 311f
Ragged red fibers, 1397, 1400f
Rat bite fever, 357–358
Rathke rests, 1122
Reciprocal translocation, chromosomal,
    212
Rectosigmoid ischemic, 701
Rectum:
  adenocarcinoma of, 709–712. See also
    Colorectal cancer
  endometriosis of, 713
Red blood cells:
  drug-mediated immunologic injury of,
    1046–1047
  in malaria, 409, 410f–412f
  normochromic, 1031
  normocytic, 1031
  in type II hypersensitivity reaction, 106–
    107, 108f
Reed-Sternberg cell, 1109–1110, 1110f
Refsum's disease, 1495t
Regeneration, 68, 83, 86
  axial, 68
Reid index, 585, 586f
Relapsing fever, 352–353
Rem, 307
Renal artery, fibromuscular dysplasia of,
    882
Renal cell adenoma, 889
Renal cell carcinoma, 888–889, 888f–889f
Renal failure:
  acute, 271, 836
  chronic, 836
    anemia of, 1037
    peptic ulcer disease and, 652
  in diabetes mellitus, 1174
Renal infarct, 258
Renal osteodystrophy, 1346
Renal pelvis:
  amyloidosis of, 893
  anatomy of, 892
  carcinoma of, 895–896, 896f
  congenital disorders of, 892–893
  diverticulum of, 892
  embryology of, 891f, 892
  fibroepithelial polyps of, 894
  inflammatory disorders of, 893–894
  mesenchymal neoplasms of, 896
  metastatic neoplasms of, 896
Renal stones, 652, 886, 886f
Renal transplantation. See Kidney trans-
    plantation
Renal tubular necrosis:
  acute, 876–877, 877f–878f
    ischemic, 877
    nephrotoxic, 877
    oliguria in, 877, 878f
  in drug reaction, 290

Renal tubules:
  anatomy of, 834
  cortical, wound healing in, 92
  lead nephropathy of, 298
  medullary, wound healing in, 92–93
Renal tubulorrhexis, 92
Renin-angiotensin-aldosterone mecha-
    nism, in shock, 271
Renin-angiotensin system, in hyperten-
    sion, 478
Renovascular hypertension, 837, 882–883,
    883f
Repair, 68–77
  cell proliferation in, 75–77, 76f
  extracellular matrix in, 68–75
Reperfusion injury, 18–19
Resistance vessels, 457
Respiration, first neonatal, 240
Respiratory burst, cellular, 55–56
Respiratory distress syndrome:
  adult, 577–579, 578f–579f, 580t
  neonatal, 239–243, 241f–243f
    causes of, 240
    complications of, 242
    histologic examination in, 242, 242f
    idiopathic, 240–241
    outcome of, 242
    pathogenesis of, 241–242, 241f
    respiratory effort in, 241
Respiratory syncytial virus, 344, 550
Respiratory system:
  anatomy of, 544–546
  embryology of, 546–547
Respiratory tract, staphylococcal infection
    of, 383, 386
Respiratory viruses (pneumonia), 343–345
Reticulocyte, 1022
Reticuloendothelial system, 101
Reticuloendotheliosis, leukemic, 1088
Reticulosis:
  hemophagocytic, 1054
  midline lethal, of face, 1288, 1289f
Retina:
  anatomy of, 1513f
  common disorders of, 1528–1529
  cotton wool spots of, 481, 1509
  detached, 1528–1529, 1528f
  hemorrhage of, 305, 1509
  in systemic disease, 1511t–1512t
Retinal arterioles, in hypertension, 481
Retinal capillaries, in diabetes mellitus,
    487
Retinal capillary basement membrane
    thickening, 1518–1521
Retinal occlusovascular disease, 1509,
    1517t
  central arterial, 1509, 1514f–1515f, 1517t
  central venous, 1509, 1514f, 1516f, 1517t
Retinitis pigmentosa, 1529
Retinoblastoma, 1505–1507, 1506f, 1508t
  gene deletion in, 177
  hereditary, 248
Retinopathy:
  in diabetes mellitus, 1174f, 1175
  diabetic, 1517–1518, 1520f–1522f
  hypertensive, 1514, 1518f–1519f
Retinopathy of prematurity, 1523, 1524f
Retrolental fibroplasia, 1523, 1524f
Retroperitoneal fibrosis, 720
Retroplacental hematoma, 983
Retroviral oncogenes, 173–175, 174f

Reverse transcriptase, 173
Reye's syndrome, 784
Rhabdomyolysis, 1411
   alcoholic, 285
Rhabdomyoma, of heart, 540
Rhabdomyosarcoma, 1391–1392
   alveolar, 1391–1392
   embryonal, 1391
      of nasopharynx, 1295, 1295f
      of vagina, 955–956, 956f
   pleomorphic, 1392
Rh blood group system, 243, 245
Rheumatic fever, 388
Rheumatic heart disease, **527–531**
   anatomic features of, 527–528, 527f–528f
   chronic, 528, 529f
   etiology of, 528–531, 530f
   incidence of, 527
   major and minor clinical manifestations of, 527
   sequelae of, 531
Rheumatoid arthritis, **1374–1381**
   bony ankylosis in, 1379, 1379f
   bronchiolitis and, 591
   cell-mediated immunity in, 1376
   classification and incidence of, 1375
   diagnosis of, 1375
   heart in, 532
   histogenesis of, 1377f
   immune complexes in, 1376
   lymphadenopathy of, 1060
   pathogenesis of, 1375–1376
   pathology of, 1376–1379, 1378f–1379f
   synovial fluid in, 1376, 1379
   treatment of, 1380
   variants of, 1380–1381, 1381f
   viruses in, 1375
Rheumatoid arthritis cells, 1379
Rheumatoid factor, 1375
Rheumatoid nodules, 1379–1380, 1380f
Rhinitis:
   acute, 1283–1284
   allergic, 1284
   chronic, 1283
Rhinocerebral aspergillosis, 1287
Rhinocerebral zygomycosis, 430
Rhinophyma, 1282
Rhinoscleroma, 378, 1286
Rhinosporidiosis, 430–431, 431f, 1287
Rhinosporidium seeberi, 430–431, 431f
Rhinovirus, 345
Riboflavin deficiency, 321, 321f, 1270
Ribosomes, in hydropic swelling, 5, 7f
Rice bodies, 1376
Ricewater stool, 366, 367f
Richter's syndrome, 1087
Rickets, 324, 1344–1346, 1345f
   clinical presentation in, 1344
   epidemiology of, 1344–1345
   epiphyseal plate in, 1344, 1345f
   radiologic and histologic findings in, 1344, 1345f
   vitamin-D resistant, 1345–1346
Rickettsial disease, **349–351**
Rickettsial vasculitis, 486
Riedel's struma, 1138–1139, 1139f
Rift Valley fever, 330
Ring chromosome, 212
Ring of Ranvier, 1314
Risus sardonicus, 376

RNA virus, in carcinogenesis, 173–175, 174f
Robertsonian translocation, chromosomal, 212
Rocky Mountain Spotted fever, 350–351, 486
Rod myopathy, 1405, 1407f
Roentgen, 307
Rokitansky-Aschoff sinuses, 800
Romana's sign, 403
Rosenthal fibers, 1463
Rose spots, 359
Rotavirus:
   in diarrhea, 342
   in gastroenteritis, 668
Rotor's syndrome, 731
Rous sarcoma virus, 169–170
Rubella, 341
   in TORCH complex, 206–208, 206f, 207t
Rubeola, 340–341, 341f
Rubeola pneumonia, 344
Rubeosis iridis, 1521
Russell body, 406, 1056

S–100 protein, 150f, 151
Saber shin, 356
Saccular aneurysm, 1435, 1435f–1436f
Saddle nose, 356
St. Louis encephalitis, 332
Salivary glands:
   adenolymphoma of, 1279, 1280f
   carcinoma of, 1280–1282
      adenoid cystic, 1280–1281, 1281f–1282f
      mucoepidermoid, 1280, 1281f
      pleomorphic adenoma and, 1281
   diseases of, **1274–1282**
   enlargement of, 1274
   hemangioma of, 1281–1282
   inflammation of, 1275–1276
   lymphoepithelial lesions of, 1063–1064
   Mikulicz's disease of, 1277
   monomorphic adenoma of, 1279, 1280f
   oncocytes of, 1279, 1280f
   pleomorphic adenoma (mixed tumor) of, 1278–1279, 1278f–1279f
   Sjögren's syndrome of, 1276–1277, 1277f–1278f
   Warthin's tumor of, 1279, 1280f
Salmonella enteritis, 667
Salmonellosis, 358–362
   bacterial species in, 359
   gastroenteritis in, 359
   nontyphoidal, 667
   septicemia in, 359
   typhoid fever in, 359–362, 361f
Salpingitis:
   chronic, 970–971
   tuberculous, 948, 971
Salpingitis isthmica nodosa, 971
Sandhoff's disease, 228f
Sanfilippo's syndrome, 231f
Saphenous vein bypass graft, autologous, 492
Saprophytism, 328
Sarcocystosis, 419
Sarcoidal granulomatosis, necrotizing, of lung, 615
Sarcoidosis:
   of eye, 1524
   of liver, 778

Sarcoidosis:
   of lung, 607–608, 607f
   of salivary glands, 1277
   of skin, 1235–1237, 1237f
Sarcoma:
   Ewing's, 1360–1361, 1363f
   granulocytic, in leukemia, 1077, 1081f
   Kaposi's, 494–495, 1256, 1257f–1258f, 1392
      of lymph nodes, 1116
      of oral cavity, 1268, 1269f
   of oral cavity, 1268
   osteogenic, 1357–1359, 1360f
   sclerosing endothelial, 627
   synovial, 1392, 1392t
Sarcoma botryoides, of vagina, 955–956, 956f
Sarcoma virus, Rous, 169–170
Sarcomere, 1396
   of heart, 498–500, 501f
Sarcoplasmic reticulum, 1396
Saturnine gout, 1383
Scalded skin syndrome, 384
Scar:
   deficient formation of, 88–89
   hypertrophic, 89
   organization of, 79
Scarlet fever, 386, 1262–1263
Schatzki's mucosal ring, 631–632, 631f, 634f
Scheie's syndrome, 231f
Schilder's disease, 1463
Schiller test, 954, 954f
Schilling test, 675
Schistosoma haematobium, 440–441, 440t, 442f–443f
Schistosoma japonicum, 440–441, 440f, 442f–443f
Schistosoma mansoni, 440–441, 440f, 442f–443f
Schistosomiasis, 440–441, 440t
   embolism in, 620
   portal hypertension due to, 778
Schönlein-Henoch purpura, 1027
Schwannoma, 1474
   acoustic, 1496
   of inner ear, 1302
   malignant, 1498
   of peripheral nervous system, 1496–1497, 1496f
   vestibular, 1302
Sclera, in systemic disease, 1512t
Scleroderma, 136–137, 137f, 1234, 1236f
   esophagus in, 633
   heart in, 532
   kidney in, 882
Scleroma, of nose, 1286
Sclerosing endothelial sarcoma, 627
Sclerosing lipogranuloma, of penis, 938
Sclerosis, progressive systemic, 136–137, 137f, 1234, 1236f. *See also* Scleroderma
Scoliosis, 1318
Scorpions, 447
Scrotum, 940
   Paget's disease of, 940, 940f
   squamous cell carcinoma of, 940
Scrub typhus, vasculitis in, 486
Scurvy, 322–323, 323f
   bleeding in, 1026
   bone formation in, 1316–1317, 1318f
   gingiva in, 1272

Scyphozoa, 450
Seborrheic dermatitis, 321, 321f
Seborrheic keratosis, 1254–1255
Seizure, in intracranial tumor, 1469
Seminal vesicles, 927
Seminoma, of testis, 918–919, 918f
Senile atrophy, 9
Senile cardiac amyloidosis, 539
Senile cataract, 1523
Senile plaque, 1486, 1488f
Senile purpura, 1026
Sentinal node, 660
Septicemia:
    listeriosis, 372
    meningococcal, 389
    S. choleraesuis, 359
    staphylococcal, 383–384
    streptococcal, 388
Septic shock, 269–271
Sequestrum, 1332
Serosanguineous exudate, 37
Serotonin:
    platelet release of, 40
    synthesis of, 823
Serotonin substance P, 825t
Serous adenocarcinoma, of ovary, 977
Serous cystadenoma, of ovary, 977
Serous exudate, 37
Serous inclusion cysts, 973
Sertoli cell tumor, of testis, 921, 923f
Sertoli-Leydig cell tumors, 978
Serum carboxypeptidase N (SCPN), 45–46
Serum protein electrophoresis, 119, 120f
Serum sickness:
    acute, 110, 111f
    in drug reaction, 293
    vasculitis in, 482
Sex chromosome trisomies, 215–217, 216f
Sex cord-stromal tumors, 977–981
Sex-linked disorders, 232–234, 233f
Sexual differentiation, disorders of, 913–915
Sexually transmitted disease, **945–948**
    bacterial, 945–946
    mycoplasmal, 947
    protozoal, 948
    rickettsial, 947
    spirochetal, 946–947
    viral, 947–948
Sézary syndrome, 1105, 1107f, 1260
Sheehan's syndrome, 1125, 1125f
Shiga toxin, 368
Shigellosis, 368, 667
Shin, saber, 209, 356
Shingles, 335
Shock, **268–273**
    adrenals in, 273
    brain in, 273
    cardiogenic, 269, 523
    complications of, 272f
    exocrine pancreas in, 273
    heart in, 271
    host defenses in, 273
    hypovolemic, 269
    intestines in, 272–273
    kidney in, 271
    liver in, 273, 787
    lung in, 272
    mechanisms and types of, 268–271
    pathogenesis of, 269–271, 270f
    pathology of, 271–273

Shock:
    septic, 269–271
    vascular compensatory mechanisms of, 271
Shock lung, 272
Shope papilloma virus, 170
Shunt hyperbilirubinemia, primary, 728
Sialadenitis, 1277f
Sialorrhea, 1274
Sialolithiasis, 1274–1275
Sickle cell crisis, 1044
Sickle cell disease, 1044
    biochemical basis of, 220
    kidney in, 884
Sickle cell trait, 1044
Sideroblast, ringed, 1042
Siderosis:
    Bantu, 769
    definition of, 767
Signet ring carcinoma, of breast, 1009
Signet ring cell, 658, 659f
Silicosis, 600–603, 601f–602f
    acute, 602
    etiology and pathogenesis of, 602–603
    progressive massive fibrosis in, 602, 603f
    simple nodular, 600–602
Silo-filler's disease, 551
Simian B virus encephalitis, 1453
Simian virus, 170
Simmonds disease, 1125
Simon's foci, 395
Sinus histiocytosis, 62, 1053
Sinusitis, acute and chronic, 1284–1285, 1285f
Sinus venosus defect, 507
Siphonaptera, 449
Sipple's syndrome, 830, 1155f
Situs inversus, of stomach, 642
Sjögren's disease, 135–136, 136f
Sjögren's syndrome, 1276–1277, 1277f–1278f
Skeletal muscle, **1394–1414.** *See also* Muscle
Skin, **1194–1259**
    in amebiasis, 417
    anatomy and physiology of, 1197–1205
    appendages of, 1204–1205
    basal cell carcinoma of, 1256, 1256f
    basement membrane of, diseases of, 1215–1229
    candidiasis of, 424
    carcinoma of, geographic and ethnic factors in, 193
    chromomycosis of, 428–429, 429f
    dermal connective tissue diseases of, 1234–1237
    dermis of, 1203
    disease patterns of, 1205
    epidermis of, 1197–1203
        diseases of, 1205–1214
    in hemochromatosis, 771
    larva migrans of, 438, 438f
    layers and vasculature of, 1195f
    leishmaniasis of, 406–407
    mansonelliasis of, 433
    mycetoma of, 421–422, 422f
    necrotizing venulitis of, 1231–1232, 1231f–1233f
    neoplasms of, 1238–1258
        etiology and pathogenesis of, 1238–1239

Skin:
    indirect and direct tumor progression in, 1242–1254
        keratinocytic, 1254–1256
        skin appendage tumors in, 1256
        T-helper cell lymphoma, 1257–1258
        ultraviolet light in, 1239
        vascular, 1257
    in niacin deficiency, 320, 320f
    onchocerciasis, 432–433
    phaeomycotic cyst of, 429
    radiodermatitis of, 310, 311f
    in riboflavin deficiency, 321, 321f
    in sarcoidosis, 1235–1237, 1237f
    sporotrichosis of, 427, 427f
    squamous cell carcinoma of, 1255–1256, 1255f
    staphylococcal infection of, 382–383
    in thermal regulation, 301
    vasculature of, 1204, 1229–1234
    zygomycosis of, 430
Skip metastasis, 153
Sleeping sickness, 404f, 405–406
Slow-reacting substances of anaphylaxis, 41–42
    formation of, 47–48, 48f
    in immediate hypersensitivity reaction, 106
Slow viral infections, of brain, 1455–1456
Small cell carcinoma, of lung, 556–557, 558f
Small for gestational age infant, 238
Small intestine, **662–686**
    adenocarcinoma of, 682
    adenoma of, 681
    in alcoholism, 286
    anatomy of, 662–664
    ancylostomiasis of, 436, 437f
    anisakiasis of, 440
    atresia of, 664–665
    benign tumors of, 681–682
    bleeding in, 716f
    carcinoid tumor of, 683–684, 685f
    celiac disease of, 675–678, 676f–677f
    cell renewal in, 664
    in cholera, 366, 367f
    chronic ischemia of, 672
    congenital disorders of, 664–666
    in Crohn's disease, 694f–695f
    diarrheal diseases of, 666–668. *See also* Diarrhea
    duplications of, 665
    fungal infection of, 669
    immunoproliferative disease of, 682
    infarction of, 257–258, 669–671, 671f
    in isosporiasis, 419
    leiomyosarcoma of, 684
    lipoma of, 681–682
    lymphoma of, 682–683, 683f
    malabsorption in, 672–675, 674f. *See also* Malabsorption
    malignant tumor of, 682–684
    malrotation of, 666
    microscopic anatomy of, 663
    nonocclusive ischemia of, 671
    nutrient absorption in, 628f–629f, 672
    obstruction of, 717f
    parasites of, 669, 670f
    peptic ulcer disease of, **648–655.** *See also* Peptic ulcer disease
    Peutz-Jeghers syndrome in, 681, 681f

Small intestine:
  radiation enteritis of, 680
  resistance to neoplasia of, 680–681
  shock in, 272–273
  stenosis of, congenital, 665
  strongyloidiasis of, 437, 437f
  tuberculosis of, 668–669
  vascular disease of, 669–672
  villi of, 663–664
  Whipple's disease of, 678, 679f
Smallpox, 333 334, 334f
Smoking. *See* Cigarette smoking
Smudge cells, 1087
Snowflake cataract, 1523
Sodium, homeostatic control of, 258–259
Sodium pump, in hydropic swelling, 5
Soft tissue, tumors of, 1387–1392
Solar cheilitis, 1269f
Somatic mutation theory, 31
Somatostatin:
  physiologic actions of, 825t
  synthesis of, 822f, 823
Somatostatinoma, 827–828
Somatotropic hormone, 1122
Sommer's sector, necrosis of, 1433f, 1434
Space of Disse, 726, 726f
Spermatic cord, 926–927
  torsion of, 916
Spermatic cord veins, varicocele of, 924,
    925f
Spermatic granuloma, 926
Spermatocele, 924, 925f
Spherocytosis, hereditary, 1042 1043
Sphincter of Oddi, 724
Sphingolipidoses, 228f, 229–230, 538, 538f
Spiders, 447–448
Spina bifida, 203, 204f, 1458f–1459f, 1459
Spina bifida occulta, 1459
Spinal cord:
  degenerative disorders of, 1484t
  demyelination of, 1039
  injury of, 1427, 1428f–1429f
    hyperextension, 1427, 1428f
    hyperflexion, 1427, 1428f
  radiation injury of, 310
Spinal muscular atrophy, 1403
  infantile, 1413, 1413f
Spine, ankylosing spondylitis of, 1381,
    1381f
Spinocerebellar degeneration, 1482–1487
Spirochetal disease, **351–358**
Spitz tumor, 1254, 1254f
Spleen, 1064–1065
  accessory, 1064
  activated, 1064
  amyloid deposits in, 1189–1190
  anatomy of, 1021–1022, 1021f
  in Burkitt's lymphoma, 340
  in chronic lymphocytic leukemia, 1083,
    1086f
  in chronic myelogenous leukemia,
    1070–1071, 1070f
  congestion of, 255–256, 1065
  cysts of, 1065
  in hairy cell leukemia, 1070f, 1088
  in Hodgkin's disease, 1109, 1109f
  hyperplasia of:
    immunoreactive, 1064
    nonspecific acute reactive, 1064
  infarction of, 1065
  lardaceous, 1190

Spleen:
  in malignant histiocytosis, 1070f, 1082
  in myelofibrosis with myeloid metapla-
    sia, 1070f, 1073
  in polycythemia vera, 1068, 1070f
  red pulp of, 1021–1022, 1021f
  rupture of, 1065
  sago, 1190
  tumors of, 1065
  white pulp of, 1021, 1021f
Splendore-Hoeppli phenomenon, 383,
    393, 427, 427f
Splenic sequestration, 1029
Splenomegaly, 1064, 1064t
  fibrocongestive, 1065
  in portal hypertension, 778, 780
Spondylitis:
  ankylosing, 1381, 1381f
  tuberculous, 1332f, 1334–1335, 1334f
Spongiform degeneration, of brain, 1456,
    1457f
Spongiosum, primary, 1311
Sporothrix schenckii, 427, 427f
Sporotrichosis, 427, 427f
Sprue, celiac (nontropical), 675–678
Sprue, tropical, malabsorption in, 680
Squamous cell carcinoma, 144, 145f
  of cervix, 193, 959, 959t, 960f
  development of, 556
  of larynx, 548, 549f
  of lung, 156f, 554–556, 555f–556f
  microinvasive, in cervix, 959
  of oral cavity, 1267 1268, 1268f
  of penis, 193, 939
  of prostate, 937
  of scrotum, 940
  of skin, 1255–1256, 1255f
  of urinary bladder, 908
  of vagina, 954, 955t
  of vulva, 951–952, 951f, 951t
Squamous metaplasia, 11, 13f
Squamous papilloma:
  of larynx, 548
  of nose, 1288
Staphylococcal infection, **381–385**
  in arthritis, 383
  of bone, 383
  of burns and surgical wounds, 383
  in endocarditis, 384
  in food poisoning, 384, 668
  in meningitis, 384
  in pneumonia, 568–569
  of respiratory tract, 383
  in scalded skin syndrome, 384
  in septicemia, 383 384
  of skin, 382–383
  in toxic shock syndrome, 384
Staphylococcus aureus infection, 382
Staphylococcus epidermidis infection, 385
Staphylococcus saprophyticus infection, 385
Starling's law, 502, 624
Starvation, atrophy in, 8
Status asthmaticus, 589, 590f
Steatorrhea, in cystic fibrosis, 225
Steatosis, of liver, 754–756, 756f
Stein-Leventhal syndrome, 973–974, 974f
Stem cells, 75–76
Stercoral ulcer, 713–714
Steroid myopathy, 1414
Stimulus-response coupling, 49, 51f
Stinging microorganisms, 449–450

Stomach, **640–662**
  adenocarcinoma of, 144
  in alcoholism, 285
  anatomy of, 640–641, 641f
  anthrax of, 358
  antral membrane of, congenital, 642
  antrum of, 640, 641f
  benign lymphoid hyperplasia of, 656
  benign tumors of, 655–656
  bleeding in, 716f
  body (corpus) of, 640, 641f
  carcinoid tumor of, 661
  carcinoma of, **656–661**
    advanced, 657–658, 658f–659f
    clinical features of, 660–661
    colloid or mucinous, 658
    diffuse or infiltrating, 657–658, 659f–
      660f
    early, 658–660, 659f
    geographic and ethnic factors in, 193
    histologic pattern in, 658, 659f
    linitis plastica, 658, 659f
    medullary, 658
    metastasis of, 660
    in migrant populations, 194
    nonerosive gastritis with, 647
    papillary, 658
    pathology of, 657–660, 658f–660f
    polypoid (fungating), 657–658, 660f
    risk factors for, 657
    ulcerating, 657, 658f, 660f
  cardia of, 640, 641f
  congenital disorders of, 641 642
  diverticuli of, 662
  fundus of, 640, 641f
  glands of, 641
  greater curvature of, 640
  histology of, 641
  inflammation of. *See* Gastritis
  leather-bottle, 658, 659f
  leiomyoblastoma of, 655–656
  leiomyoma of, 655–656, 656f
  leiomyosarcoma of, 661
  lesser curvature of, 640
  lymphoma of, 661
  malignant tumors of, 656–661
  metastatic lesions of, 661
  pancreatic rests of, 642
  peptic ulcer disease of, **648–655**. *See also*
    Peptic ulcer disease
  polyps of, hyperplastic or adenoma-
    tous, 656
  pseudolymphoma of, 656
  pylorus of, 640, 641f
  rugae of, 640, 641f
  rupture of, 661
  situs inversus of, 642
  spontaneous perforation of, 661–662
  stress ulcer of, 643
  syphilis of, secondary, 355
  volvulus of, 662
Stomatitis:
  gangrenous, 382f
  herpetic, 1265
Stomatocytosis, hereditary, 1043
Stool:
  occult blood test of, 712
  ricewater, 366, 367f
Storage diseases, 226–230
Strawberry gallbladder, 805
Strawberry hemangioma, 493

Streptococcal infection, **385–391**. *See also individual types*
  antigens and exotoxins in, 385–386
  gonococcal, 389–391, 390f
  groups and subtypes of, 385
  meningococcal, 388–389, 389f
  nonsuppurative complications of, 388
  in pneumonia, 569
  primary, 386
  secondary, 388
  sites and types of, 387f
Streptolysin O, 385–386
Streptolysin S, 385–386
Stress:
  cellular patterns of response to, 4–5
  in peptic ulcer disease, 650
Stress fracture, 1326
Stress polycythemia, 1048
Stress ulcer, 643
Stroke:
  in oral contraceptive use, 291–292
  smoking and, 277
Stromatosis, endometrial, 967
Strongyloides stercoralis, 436–437, 437f
Strongyloidiasis, 436–437, 437f
Struma lymphomatosa, 1138
Struma ovarii, 1137
Sturge-Weber disease, 493
Sturge-Weber syndrome, 1266–1267
Styes, 382, 1504
Subchondral bone cyst, 1372, 1374f
Subchondral bone plate, 1370
Subcutaneous dirofilariasis, 433
Subcutaneous zygomycosis, 429, 429f
Subdural hematoma, 1420–1422, 1421f–1423f
Subsarcolemmic blebs, in ischemia, 19
Sudden death:
  in ischemic heart disease, 515
  in pulmonary embolism, 618
Sudden infant death syndrome, 247
Sulfur dioxide, as respiratory irritant, 551
Sunflower cataract, in Wilson's disease, 773
Superoxide, 20, 21f
Superoxide anion, 57t
Supraglottic carcinoma, 548
Supraglottis, 545
Surgery, obesity and, 316
SV–40 virus, 170, 171
Sweats, night, 303
Swimming pool conjunctivitis, 1503
Swimming pool granuloma, 401–402
Symbiosis, 328
Sympathetic nervous system, in shock, 271
Sympathetic ophthalmia, 1504
Symphyses, 1365
Synaptophysin, 149
Synarthrosis, 1365
Synchondroses, 1365
Syncytiotrophoblast, 981
Syndactyly, 1368
Syndesmoses, 1365
Synostoses, 1365
Synovial chondromatosis, 1386, 1387f
Synovial osteochondromatosis, 1386
Synovial sarcoma, 1392, 1392f
Synovitis:
  localized nodular, 1387
  pigmented villonodular, 1387, 1388f

Synovium:
  anatomy of, 1368–1369
  function of, 1369
Syntropy, 203
Syphilis, 353–356, 946–947
  of bone, 1335–1336, 1335f
  chancre in, 354
  clinical stages of, 353, 353f
  congenital, 208–209, 209f, 356, 1335, 1335f
  heart disease in, 540
  latent, 355
  liver in, 790
  lymphadenitis of, 1060
  meningitis in, 1445–1446, 1446f–1447f
  nose in, 1284–1285
  oral cavity in, 1264
  primary, 354, 354f
  secondary, 354–355
  tertiary, 355–356, 356f
Syphilitic aneurysm, 489, 489f
Syphilitic aortitis, 355, 355f, 456, 489, 489f, 518, 540
Syphilitic vasculitis, 456
Syringoma, 1256, 1256f
  of vulva, 950

Tabes dorsalis, 356, 1445, 1447f
Tabetic crisis, 356
Taboparesis, 356
Taeniae coli, 686
Taenia solium, 446–447, 447f
Talc:
  embolism, 620
  intravenous injection of, 287
Talcosis, 605
Tamponade, pericardial, 264f, 265
Tangier disease, 471
Tarantula, 447
Tardive dyskinesia, 289
Target fiber, 1397, 1401f, 1412–1413
Tarui's disease, 1411
Taussig-Bing malformation, 511–512
Tay-Sachs disease, 229, 229f, 1477
T-cell chronic lymphocytic leukemia, 1087
T-cell leukemia/lymphoma, adult, 1103
T cells, 98–99, 100f, 100t
  in atherosclerosis, 466
  in autoimmune disease, 129–130
  cytotoxic, 113–116, 115f
  in infectious mononucleosis, 338
  lymphokines of, 100t
  mitogenic response assay of, 119, 120f
  ontogeny of, cell markers for, 1024t
  in scleroderma, 136
  in systemic lupus erythematosus, 132
Teeth:
  caries of, 1270–1271, 1272f
  diseases of, 1270–1274
  Hutchinson's, 209, 356
  pulpitis of, 1271–1272, 1273f
Telangiectasia, hereditary hemorrhagic, 1266
Telogen hairs, 1204–1205
Temperature, body, regulation of, 301
Temporal arteritis, 483–484, 484f
Tendon sheath, giant cell tumor of, 1387
Tenosynovitis, localized nodular, 1387

Teratogenesis, timing of exposure in, 199, 200f
Teratogens, 199
Teratology, 199, 200f
Teratoma, 143, 979
  of testis, 919, 920f
Terminal deoxynucleotidyl transferase, 1077t
Testicular adnexa, **922–927**
Testicular feminization, 915
Testicular tunics, 922–924
  adenomatoid tumor of, 924
  fibrous pseudotumor of, 924
  mesothelial cell proliferation in, 924
Testis:
  in alcoholism, 285
  atrophy of, in hemochromatosis, 771
  carcinoma of, geographic and ethnic factors in, 193
  choriocarcinoma of, 918, 919, 921f
  congenital disorders of, 912–915
  embryonal carcinoma of, 919, 919f
  germ cell neoplasms of, 916–919
  gonadal stromal/sex cord tumors of, 921–922
  gonadoblastoma of, 921–922
  gumma of, 356, 356f
  hematopoietic neoplasms of, 922
  inflammatory disorders of, 916
  Leydig cell tumor of, 921, 922f
  malacoplakia of, 916
  metastatic tumors of, 922
  mixed germ cell tumor of, 919
  neoplasms of, histiogenesis of, 917f
  normal structure and embryology of, 911–912
  radiation injury to, 310
  seminoma of, 918–919, 918f
  Sertoli cell tumor of, 921, 923f
  teratoma of, 919, 920f
  torsion of, 916
  yolk sac neoplasm of, 919, 920f
Testosterone, prostate and, 928–929
Tetanospasmin, 374
Tetanus, 374–376, 374f–375f
Tetralogy of Fallot, 510–511, 511f
Thalassemia, 1040–1041
  α-Thalassemia, 1041
  β-Thalassemia, 1040–1041
Thalidomide-induced malformations, 205, 205f
Theca lutein cyst, 973
Thecoma, of ovary, 978
T-helper cell lymphoma, cutaneous, 1257–1258
Thermal-regulatory dysfunction, 301–304
  hyperthermia in, 303–304
  hypothermia in, 301–303
Thiamine deficiency, 319–320, 319f
Thiamine deficiency heart disease, 537
Third ventricle cyst, 1476
Thrombin, generation of, 474
Thrombin time, 1026t
Thromboangiitis obliterans, 485–486, 485f
Thrombocytopenia, 1027
  in alcoholism, 286
  in cancer, 187
  dilutional, 1029
  drug-induced, 1028
  primary hemorrhagic, 1072t, 1073–1074
  in splenic sequestration, 1029

Thrombocytopenic purpura, idiopathic, 1027
Thromboembolism, 472. *See also* Embolism
  of lung, 265–267, 266f, 618–619, 619f
    multiple recurrent, 619
    pulmonary hypertension due to, 622
  in myocardial infarction, 516, 517f, 524
  in oral contraceptive use, 291
  pulmonary, 265–267, 266f
Thrombolysis, 474–476, 475f
Thrombomodulin, 473
Thrombophlebitis:
  in cancer, 187
  of cavernous venous sinus, 1285
  in oral contraceptive use, 291
Thrombosis, 471
  in coronary artery occlusion, 476, 516, 517f
  endothelium in, 472–474, 473f
  of hemorrhoids, 701
  of mesenteric artery, 671
  of mesenteric vein, 671
  platelets in, 471–472, 472f
  of portal vein, 778
  of pulmonary artery, 621
  of venous sinus, 1433
Thrombotic endocarditis, nonbacterial, 187
Thrombotic thrombocytopenic purpura, 881, 1029
Thromboxane A$_2$:
  inhibitory effects of, 53f
  platelet release of, 40
Thrombus:
  canalization of, 477
  dissolution of, 466, 467f
  mural, 267, 269f
    in atherosclerosis, 460
    cocaine use and, 477
    in coronary artery occlusion, 476–477
    in myocardial infarction, 524
    in rheumatic heart disease, 531
  organization of, 466, 466f, 477
Thrush, oral, 424, 1265
Thymolipomas, 1160
Thymoma, 1159–1160, 1160f
  benign, 1159–1160, 1160f
  malignant, 1160
Thymus, 1158–1160
  agenesis and hypoplasia of, 1159
  anatomy, embryology, physiology of, 1158–1159
  hyperplasia of, 1159, 1159f
  neuroendocrine tumors of, 1160, 1161f
  tumors of, 1159–1160
Thyroglobulin, as tumor marker, 151
Thyroglossal duct cyst, 1132, 1262
Thyroid, **1132–1144**
  adenocarcinoma of, papillary, 146, 146f
  adenoma of, 143, 144f, 1140
    atypical, 1140
    follicular, 1140, 1140f
    Hürthle cell, 1140, 1140f
    papillary, 1140
  anatomy, embryology, physiology of, 1132
  carcinoma of, 1141–1144
    adenoma with invasion in, 1141
    follicular, 1141, 1142f–1144f
    medullary, 1141–1143, 1142f, 1144f
    papillary, 1141, 1142f
    undifferentiated, 1144, 1144f

Thyroid:
  disease of, 1523–1524
  histopathology of, 1133f
  hyperthyroidism of, 1134–1137
  hypothyroidism of, 1139–1140, 1139f
  lingual, 1262
  lymphoma of, 1144
  metabolic and inflammatory disease of, 1132–1140
  primary hyperplasia of, 1134–1137
Thyroid cartilage, 544
Thyroiditis, 1137–1139
  autoantibodies in, 109, 109f
  chronic, 1137–1138
  chronic lymphocytic, 1063–1064
  de Quervain's, 1137
  granulomatous, 1137
  nonspecific chronic, 1138
  pseudotuberculous, 1137
  subacute, 1137
Thyroid nodule, lingual, 1132
Thyroid stimulating hormone, 1122–1123
Thyroid storm, 1134
Thyrotoxic heart disease, 537
Thyrotropin, 1122–1123
Thyrotropin releasing factors, 1131
Tick paralysis, 448
Ticks, 448
Tinea barbae, 431
Tinea capitis, 431
Tinea corporis, 431
Tingible body macrophages, 1059–1060
Tissue fibronectin, 74
Tissue typing, 104t
TNM cancer staging system, 157
Tolerance, immune, 129
Tongue:
  diseases of, 1269–1270
  tuberculosis of, 1264, 1265f
Tonofibril, 1197
Tonsillitis, 1292
Tonsils:
  nasopharyngeal, 1291
  palatine, 1291
Tophi, in gout, 1382, 1382f
TORCH complex, 206–208, 206f, 207t, 208f
Toxemia of pregnancy, 885, 885f, 983, 984f
Toxic megacolon, 697
Toxic neuropathy, 1493t, 1494
Toxic shock syndrome, 384, 948
Toxocariasis, 437
Toxoplasma, in TORCH complex, 206–208, 206f, 207t
Toxoplasma gondii, 412
  in encephalitis, 450–451
Toxoplasmosis, 412–413, 412f–413f
  of brain, 1441, 1441f
  lymphadenitis in, 1060, 1061f
Trabeculum, primary, 1311
Trachea:
  anatomy of, 542f–543f, 545
  compression of, 549
  foreign body of, 549
  trauma to, 549
Tracheitis, 548
Tracheobronchial mucous glands, 545
Tracheo-bronchio-pathica-osteoplastica, 548
Tracheo-esophageal fistula, 547 548, 630 631, 630f
Tracheostomy, 549

Trachoma, 347, 1502–1503, 1502f
Transduction, 175
Transfection, 177–179, 178f
Transglottic carcinoma, 548
Transient hypogammaglobulinemia of infancy, 123
Transitional cell carcinoma, 144
Transplantation:
  graft vs host response in, 119
  host vs graft response in, 116–118, 118f
  immune response in, 116 119, 118f
  of kidney, 116–119, 118f
  of liver, rejection of, 798–799, 798f–799f
  rejection of, vascular changes in, 488
Transposition of great arteries, 511–512, 512f
Transtentorial herniation, 1420, 1421f
  in intracranial tumor, 1469
Transthyretin, 1185
Transudate, 616
  definition of, 37
  exudate vs, 503t
Trauma, 306–307
Traumatic neuroma, 1495
Traveler's diarrhea, 369, 667
Trematode disease, **440–444**
Trenchfoot, 302
Treponema pallidum, 353, 353f, 946
Trichinella spiralis, 434, 435f
Trichinosis, 434, 435f
Trichloroethylene, 295
Trichloromethyl radical, 25–26, 27f
Trichobezoar, 662, 662f
Trichomoniasis, 948
Trichophyton, 431
Trichuriasis, 436, 436f
Trichuris trichiura, 436, 436f
Triglyceride, in hepatocyte, 13
Triorthocresyl phosphate (TOCP), 296
Trismus, 376
Trisomy, autosomal, 213–214
Trisomy 13–15, 1462, 1462t
Trisomy 21, 214–215, 215t, 216f
Trophic ulcer, 89
Trophoblast, 981
Tropical eosinophilia, 432, 575, 583
Tropical medicine, 276
Tropical phagedenic ulcer, 381, 381f
Tropical sprue, 680
Trousseau's syndrome, 819
Truncus arteriosus, persistent, 509–510
Trypanosoma brucei gambiense, 404f, 405
Trypanosoma brucei rhodesiense, 404f, 405
Trypanosoma cruzi, 402, 402f
Trypanosomiasis:
  African, 404f, 405–406
  American, 402, 402f
Tsutsugamushi disease, 351
Tuberculoma, 1444–1445, 1444f
Tuberculosis, 394–397, 570–573
  appendicitis in, 715
  arthritis in, 1334–1335, 1334f
  of bone, 1334–1335, 1334f
  caseous necrosis in, 16, 17f
  cavitary, 395, 396f
  clinical and pathologic manifestations of, 570, 570f
  complications of, 571–572
  distribution of, 394
  of endometrium, 962
  of epididymus, 924–926